DISEASES OF POULTRY Ninth Edition

DISEASES OF POULTRY

NINTH EDITION

Edited by **B.W. Calnek**

with

H. John Barnes

C.W. Beard

W.M. Reid

H.W. Yoder, Jr.

Editorial Board for the American Association of Avian Pathologists

Iowa State University Press, Ames, Iowa, USA

Manufactured in the United States of America
♾ This book is printed on acid-free paper.

Ninth edition, 1991

Library of Congress Cataloging-in-Publication Data

Diseases of poultry.–9th ed. / edited by B.W. Calnek . . . [et al.]
p. cm.
Includes bibliographical references.
ISBN 0–8138–0429–9
1. Poultry–Diseases. I. Calnek, B.W.
SF995.D69 1991
636.5′0896–dc20 90–33648

CONTENTS

CONTRIBUTING AUTHORS

D.J. ALEXANDER. Poultry Department, Central Veterinary Laboratory, New Haw, Weybridge, Surrey KT15 3NB, England

JAMES J. ARENDS. Department of Entomology, Agricultural Extension, North Carolina State University, Raleigh, NC 27695–7613

L.H. ARP. Department of Veterinary Pathology, College of Veterinary Medicine, Iowa State University, Ames, IA 50011

R.E. AUSTIC. Department of Poultry and Avian Science, New York State College of Agriculture and Life Sciences, Cornell University, Ithaca, NY 14853

TREVOR J. BAGUST. Commonwealth Scientific and Industrial Research Organization, Division of Animal Health, Private Bag No. 1, Parkville, Victoria 3052, Australia

H. JOHN BARNES. Department of Food Animal and Equine Medicine, College of Veterinary Medicine, North Carolina State University, Raleigh, NC 27606

C.W. BEARD. Southeast Poultry Research Laboratory, Agricultural Research Service, USDA, Athens, GA 30601

H.A. BERKHOFF. Department of Microbiology, Pathology and Parasitology, College of Veterinary Medicine, North Carolina State University, Raleigh, NC 27606

P.M. BIGGS. Willows, London Road, St. Ives, Huntingdon, Cambs PE17 4ES, England

J.M. BRICKER. Intervet America Inc., Millsboro, DE 19966

V. VON BÜLOW. Freie Universitat Berlin, Institut fur Geflugelkrankheiten, D-1000 Berlin 33, Germany

B.W. CALNEK. Department of Avian and Aquatic Animal Medicine, New York State College of Veterinary Medicine, Cornell University, Ithaca, NY 14853

DAVID CAVANAGH. Houghton Laboratory, AFRC Institute for Animal Health, Houghton, Huntingdon, Cambs PE17 2DA, England

H.L. CHUTE. 432 Main Street, Orono, ME 04473

WILLIAM L. CURRENT. Infectious Disease Research (MC7R2), Bldg. B98A/2C, Lilly Corporate Center, Indianapolis, IN 46285

JOHN E. DOHMS. Department of Animal Science and Agricultural Biochemistry, College of Agricultural Sciences, University of Delaware, Newark, DE 19717

C.H. DOMERMUTH. Regional College of Veterinary Medicine, Virginia Polytechnic Institute and State University, Blacksburg, VA 24061

R.T. DUBOSE. Regional College of Veterinary Medicine, Virginia Polytechnic Institute and State University, Blacksburg, VA 24061

J.P. DUCHATEL. Faculty of Veterinary Medicine, University of Liege, Brussels, Belgium

B.C. EASTERDAY. School of Veterinary Medicine, University of Wisconsin-Madison, Madison, WI 53706

J. FABRICANT. Department of Avian and Aquatic Animal Medicine, New York State College of Veterinary Medicine, Cornell University, Ithaca, NY 14853

M.D. FICKEN. Department of Food Animal and Equine Medicine, College of Veterinary Medicine, North Carolina State University, Raleigh, NC 27606

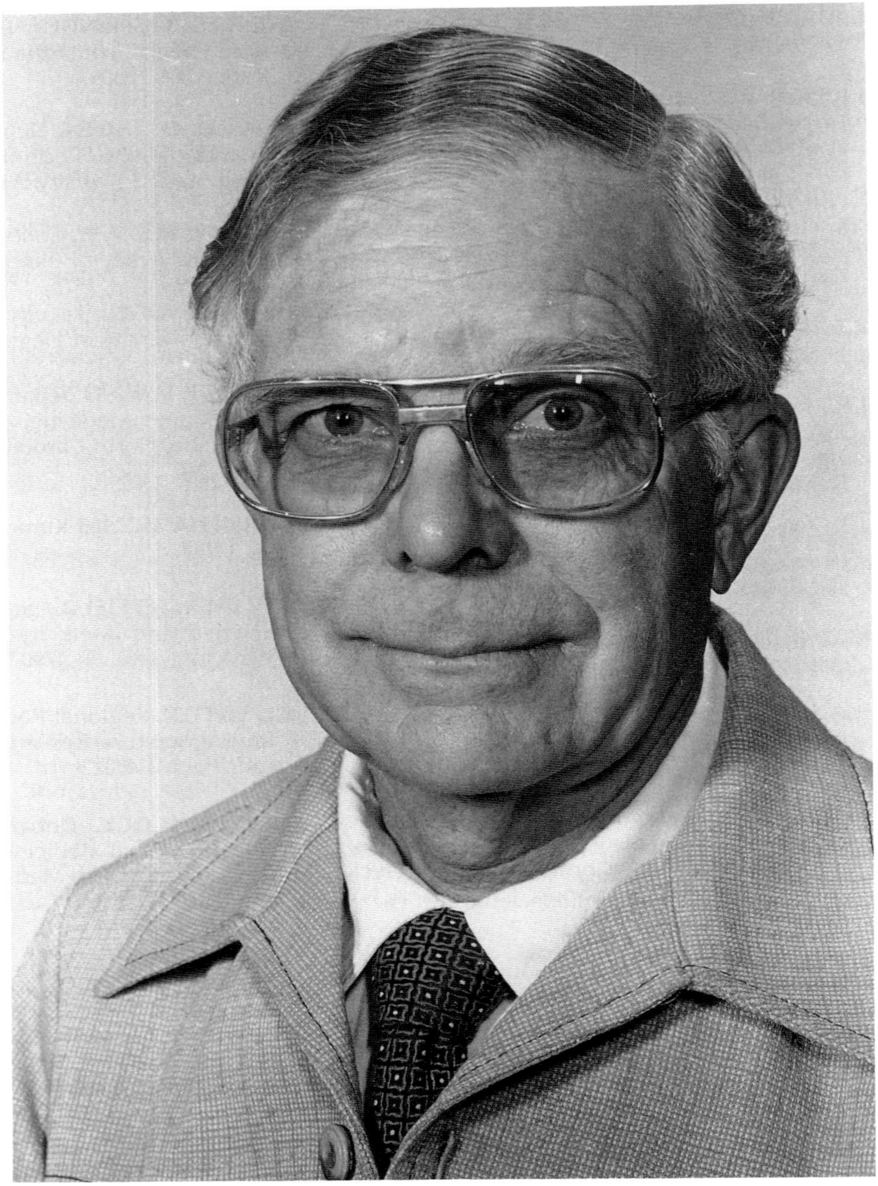

Dedicated to **Melvin S. Hofstad**

FOREWORD

The revised ninth edition of *Diseases of Poultry* is published 6 years after the previous edition and 47 years since the first edition. It is always exciting to turn back the pages of time and reflect on the struggle it was for the first editors, H.E. Biester and Louis Devries, and the 34 contributing authors, to generate the first edition. In the preface, the editors indicated the strategy was to design the first edition using American investigators to emphasize the poultry disease problems and conditions prevailing in the USA. The ninth edition has not only added new contributing authors but has truly expanded its international horizon by adding contributors from Canada, Europe, Asia, and Australia.

The structure of the poultry industry has changed dramatically over the past 50 years not only in the USA, but worldwide. The small family-farm flocks of chickens, turkeys, geese, and ducks have been replaced by large integrated operations with greater emphasis on preventive health and biosecurity programs. However, avian disease problems have no respect for international borders. There is worldwide movement of poultry breeding stock, poultry products, and biologics. Pet birds and free-flying migratory birds and waterfowl may be additional means of introduction of avian disease agents from one country to another. Newcastle disease virus, influenza viruses, and paramyxoviruses are good examples of important pathogens that have been spread in this fashion.

Per capita consumption of poultry products has increased dramatically over the past 50 years, and the industry has become a multibillion dollar enterprise. In USA, for example, the per capita consumption of poultry products now exceeds the consumption of beef and pork. However, the consumer is becoming increasingly sensitive to animal welfare and public health and food safety issues, e.g., *Salmonella enteritidis* infection in humans associated with table eggs. The poultry industry, poultry scientists, and veterinary professionals must make every effort to provide the consumer with safe and wholesome poultry products at a reasonable cost.

The ninth edition has kept up with the explosion of knowledge on the prevention and control of avian diseases, and several newly emerging diseases and infections have been covered. It seems that new emerging problems kept ahead of our ability to control and eliminate existing diseases. Progress has been made through sustained organized industry effort to reduce egg-transmitted and hatchery-disseminated diseases such as pullorum disease, fowl typhoid, mycoplasmosis, and lymphoid leucosis. Preventive use of vaccines has controlled other devastating diseases such as Marek's disease, Newcastle disease, and infectious bronchitis. The poultry industry has relied extensively on the preventive use of vaccines, anticoccidials, and other chemotherapeutic agents and only minimally on biosecurity measures and management practices. The challenge for the 1990's is to utilize our increased knowledge base in an organized industry effort to eliminate some of the existing and emerging disease problems.

Avian diagnosticians, pathologists, industrial veterinarians, regulatory officials, and poultry industry personnel all face many challenges in keeping abreast of the prevention and control of the current and emerging disease problems that are complicated by present-day poultry management practices. The ninth edition serves a highly useful purpose in providing the latest scientific information to the entire spectrum of the poultry industry.

B.S. Pomeroy

PREFACE

The ninth edition of *Diseases of Poultry* follows a long tradition of updating material to keep the text current by incorporating new and pertinent information. The book is intended primarily as a reference that is both comprehensive and practical, covering most of the domestic avian species.

Readers will find a number of format changes in this edition; some simply rearrangements—others entirely new or extensively rewritten material. Previous subchapters accorded chapter status include colibacillosis, reovirus infections, and infectious bursal disease. One new chapter will present clostridial diseases and another will cover viral enteric infections.

Pigeon herpesvirus and goose parvovirus infections are covered for the first time. Also, several newly emerging diseases and infections are described, including the unclassified chicken anemia agent, a picornavirus causing infectious nephritis, a chicken parvovirus thought to be involved in "malabsorption syndrome," a pneumovirus that causes turkey rhinotracheitis and swollen head syndrome in chickens, and an astrovirus involved in enteric infections.

Chapters or subchapters on infectious bronchitis, Newcastle disease, reovirus infection, chicken adenovirus infections, vibrio infections (now campylobacteriosis), bordetellosis, gangrenous dermatitis, necrotic enteritis, botulism, staphylococcosis, streptococcosis, spirochetosis, aspergillosis, poisons, and arbovirus infections have been largely or entirely rewritten by new authors, and new subchapters expanding the coverage of cryptosporidiosis and mycotoxins have been added to reflect the increased knowledge or significance of these conditions. Much of the Vices and Miscellaneous Diseases chapter has also been rewritten and given a new title (Developmental, Metabolic, and Miscellaneous Disorders; Chap. 34) to reflect a change in emphasis.

Many chapters contain increased information on molecular biology of the agent reflecting the quantum leaps being made on that front, and the potential or actual application of this basic information for disease control.

This edition was prepared for the first time using the computer, which will facilitate future revisions. It has also helped accomplish the switch from the author-year to the number style of literature citation in the text. Titles of all references have been included for the first time since the sixth edition in response to strong urging from readers.

Revision is a task requiring efforts of many persons. Of 55 contributors for the eighth edition, 40 were joined by 37 new authors or co-authors in preparing the ninth edition. Authorship, once entirely from the USA, now represents 10 countries. The editorial committee members express their sincere and profound gratitude to all who assisted in the writing and revision of the material found herein.

EDITORIAL COMMITTEE
B.W. Calnek, *Chairman*
H.John Barnes
C.W. Beard
W.M. Reid
H.W. Yoder, Jr.

DISEASES OF POULTRY Ninth Edition

1 PRINCIPLES OF DISEASE PREVENTION: DIAGNOSIS AND CONTROL

D.V. Zander and E.T. Mallinson

INTRODUCTION. This chapter acquaints the reader with basic principles of poultry sanitation and disease prevention and control. It also introduces the student to basic necropsy procedures and provides information on insecticides and disinfectants. For information on specific diagnostic techniques and control measures, the reader is referred to the respective chapters covering specific diseases in this text and to Whiteman and Bickford (46).

This chapter will not cover all the detailed disease-control methods or all types of poultry but will attempt only to outline and illustrate some fundamental concepts. Each poultry enterprise is different; therefore, the basic concepts must be applied according to conditions and facilities existing in individual situations. To keep abreast of the flow of research and information, a constant review of current literature and recommendations applicable to specific diseases, special enterprises, and various geographic areas is necessary. Excellent journal sources of current information are *Avian Diseases, Avian Pathology, Poultry Science,* and *World Poultry Science.* There are many publication and trade journals with special emphasis on particular segments of poultry husbandry, e.g., *Poultry International, International Hatchery Practice, Poultry Digest, Broiler Industry, Egg Industry, Turkey World,* and others including publications in various languages. Standard textbooks on chicken and turkey production, husbandry, and nutrition are other sources of information. A good practical manual on commercial chicken production is North (32).

HOST-PARASITE RELATIONSHIP. Disease results when normal body functions are impaired, and the degree of impairment determines severity of the disease. Disease may occur from deficiency of a vital nutrient or ingestion of a toxic substance. It may result from injury or physical stress with which the bird cannot cope, or it may be the consequence of harmful action of infectious and parasitic agents.

Some nutritional deficiencies are temporary and reversible when the nutrient is supplied in adequate amounts; others are irreversible. Disease resulting from stress is related to its severity and duration. Injuries such as extreme beak trimming tend to persist for a long time and may be permanent. Diseases caused by infectious and parasitic agents are frequently complex and depend upon characteristics of both host and parasite.

Whether disease results from parasitism depends on number, type, and virulence of the parasite; route of entry to the body; and defense status and capabilities of the host. The latter depends partly on the host's prior disease encounters (e.g., infectious bursal disease), nutritional status, genetic ability to organize resistance mechanisms; environmental stresses; and kind and timing of countermeasures employed (drugs, changes of environment).

Some virulent organisms rapidly overcome the resistance of even the healthiest hosts. Less virulent strains or types cause moderate to severe illness, but most birds respond and return to a state of health. Still other strains or types cause no marked reaction, and the host shows little or no obvious signs of ill health. Some infectious agents may not cause dramatic effects themselves but predispose the host to more serious infections by other agents. Some microorganisms are not considered pathogenic because they are usually found in and around individuals considered "normal," but it must be recognized that so-called nonpathogenic and low-pathogenic organisms can also cause serious losses when the right circumstances exist. Severe physical stresses such as chilling, overheating, water deprivation, starvation, and concurrent infection by other disease agents can reduce the host's ability to resist and thus may precipitate a disease condition that can be detected (e.g., clinical mycoplasmosis following infectious bronchitis, or clinical salmonellosis in chilled or water-deprived chicks).

Coccidiosis provides a good example of the relationship between the number of invading organisms and the severity of the resulting infection, since the morbidity and mortality of the host species are usually proportional to the number of coccidial oocysts ingested. A similar situation exists for many other infectious diseases. A mild roundworm infection may not be serious, whereas a severe infection can be very detrimental. The titer of a live virus vaccine may be so low that an immunizing infection does not occur following administration. A good reason for removing moribund and dead birds from a flock is to reduce the number of infectious organisms available to penmates. Thorough washing and disinfecting of a building may not render it sterile, but it can reduce the number of infectious organisms to such a low level that they cannot cause disease.

By following sound disease-preventive practices before and after arrival of new flocks; making sure the flock has adequate, properly placed, good-quality feed and water; applying judicious and timely vaccines and medications; and providing a less stressful environment, the poultry producer can control the probability of a flock becoming infected as well as the severity and outcome of an infection.

Influence of Modern Practices. Avian disease specialists must continually seek new knowledge about the nature and control of specific diseases. Meanwhile, persons responsible for production of poultry meat, table and hatching eggs, chicks and poults, feed ingredients, and mixed feeds should practice the basic techniques and management principles that will prevent occurrence of disease. They should also provide the physical facilities and quarantine capabilities necessary for control and elimination of diseases that occasionally gain entrance so they do not become a continuing problem. Economic losses, sometimes relatively subtle, resulting from disease can mean the difference between success or failure in the poultry business. Those who disregard the basic principles of disease prevention may succeed in times of a favorable market but do not remain competitive when the margin of profit is very small. A new modern enterprise with many good buildings and labor-saving equipment, but constructed and operated without regard to fundamental disease control and eradication principles, may function free of disease for a few years. All too frequently a troublesome disease gains entrance and thereafter becomes a constant, costly burden because of the extreme cost of depopulation required to eradicate it.

When new farms and buildings are designed and constructed, and production is programmed with the objective of excluding diseases or eradicating them when they gain entry, poultry can be maintained free of most harmful diseases in a practical manner with a minimum of effort. The poultry producer who uses fundamental management practices that prevent disease outbreaks has little need for detailed knowledge of the many infectious diseases affecting poultry.

Facilities need not be new to be adequate. Frequently, old farms can be enlarged and production reprogrammed to exclude or eradicate disease. Many old poultry buildings, hatcheries, and feed mills can be redesigned to favor exclusion, eradication, or control of disease. Strict application of disease-preventive management techniques has enabled producers to maintain specific-pathogen-free chickens on farms of standard design and construction (10).

The trend in all agricultural industries continues toward larger units, fewer farmers, and corporate enterprise. The chicken and turkey industries have been leaders in this trend, which has placed emphasis on efficiency of operation and lower costs of production. Survival in the industry has depended upon continual adoption of newer and more efficient practices. It is sometimes forgotten that efficiency in disease prevention is as important as efficiency in cleaning, feeding, bird handling, and egg processing. The resulting evolution of management systems has altered the emphasis in disease control practices and will continue to do so; e.g., the shift in housing of egg-laying flocks from floor pens to cages has altered the approach to control of intestinal diseases and parasites and increased emphasis on control of cannibalism through reduced light intensity and surgical removal of sharp beak tips (beak trimming).

New problems in feed formulation have arisen because certain vitamins and minerals normally found in the litter are not available to caged birds. Windowless, insulated, light- and temperature-controlled poultry houses have reduced environmental stresses from extremes in weather. Chickens in such houses require less feed in cold weather than those without this protection, which necessitates new considerations in feed formulation.

Corporation farming accelerated the move toward integrated control and operation of two or more segments of the industry such as feed manufacturing, breeder-flock management, hatchery operation, pullet rearing, broiler and turkey grow-out phases, laying farm production, egg processing, turkey and broiler slaughter and processing, and even retail distribution. Integration of the industry has concentrated under one decision-making body the disease-control practices for millions of birds as well as several phases in the production chain of eggs and meat. Thus, sound health practices and emergency quarantine measures decided upon by one or a few individuals can be quickly and effectively applied to large numbers of birds. Through integration it has become economically practical to employ veterinarians full time and place responsibility for disease control directly in the hands of specialized avian pathologists. Disease considerations are sometimes reduced to simple cost accounting, whereby the economic loss from a disease and the costs of treating it are weighed against cost of eradication and maintaining the clean status before determining the course of action.

Where established management and industry practices allow or contribute to spread and propagation of some disease agent, attempts are frequently made to deliberately expose flocks to the disease at an opportune time. This practice is successful for many viral diseases and has led to widespread use of specially prepared vaccines. The practice is much less successful for bacterial infections and is more likely to perpetuate the disease. Exposure to culturally altered or selected, naturally occurring attenuated strains of pasteurella, bordetella, and staphylococci have been used with considerable success in turkey flocks (21). Except for prevalent and highly contagious diseases for which effective vaccines are available, it is usually more economical to keep poultry free of disease than to burden them with it deliberately or by accident, provided costs of eradication and maintaining a free status do not exceed costs resulting from outbreaks of the disease. Poultry producers with extremely large, compact, multiple-age, egg-laying enterprises find it more economical to expose pullet flocks to some bacterial agents that are endemic on the layer premises to which they may later be moved (*Hemophilus gallinarum, Mycoplasma gallisepticum*) than to attempt the costly adult depopulation necessary to eradicate infections.

The poultry industry can no longer be considered composed of localized businesses limited to certain states or areas. It is characterized by multistate and even multinational companies moving products daily between locations and to various markets. Because of the high cost of scientific poultry breeding, producers throughout the world depend on a few organizations for their highly efficient breeding and production stocks. In the case of turkeys, most of the world's breeding stock originates in one state of the USA. For such a system to function smoothly and efficiently, widespread and daily shipments of hatching eggs, poults, chicks, started pullets, and adult fowl across state and national boundaries are essential and necessitate reevaluation of old concepts of health regulations. Specialized avian pathologists have evolved to guide the course of health control measures. Diagnostic facilities, both private and government, are available in major poultry-producing areas of the world. Except where importation and use are restricted by government regulation, high-quality vaccines and drugs are available wherever poultry is raised commercially. Breeding of poultry on a scientific basis has created strains of uniform quality with a high degree of resistance against diseases for which satisfactory drugs and vaccines are not available. Good-quality feed is the rule, not the exception.

Yet disease still takes a heavy toll from all types of poultry enterprises. Those who exercise farm management decisions (caretaker, owner, flock supervisor, corporate manager, money lender) have the power to reduce these losses through management for disease control. They must be made aware of the responsibilities and continually encouraged to develop a philosophy of disease prevention through management and concentrate on amortized long-term advantages and not just short-term savings.

Cardinal principles of disease prevention and control are the same for the chicken hobbyist, fancy-bird breeder, and game-bird farmer as for the corporation with several million turkeys, broilers, or laying hens. The backyard flock maintained without regard for disease control can perpetuate a disease that constitutes a threat to a large productive industry. On the other hand, since most such flocks are not vaccinated, they may be susceptible to diseases against which large commercial flocks are protected. The greatest hazard to commercial producers that is created by fancy breeds and backyard flocks is the possible perpetuation of diseases that have been eradicated from the industry. Thus, it is a sound principle of disease prevention that no employee of a commercial unit have any contact with poultry, or pet, or hobby birds at home or elsewhere.

Many producers attempt to save money through substitution of cheaper feed ingredients or unproven equipment and housing or fail to keep equipment operating as the manufacturer recommends. This frequently leads to poor growth or adult performance that is mistakenly attributed to a nonexistent mysterious disease. Considering the capital investment and daily minimum maintenance costs of a flock of chickens, maximum performance (growth, egg production) should be the primary husbandry goal.

With better control over diseases of all kinds, providing optimum bird comfort throughout the house has become a very important management factor in obtaining maximum performance. That is not achieved solely by windowless, insulated, light- and temperature-controlled houses. Such factors as overcrowding, poor beak trimming, uneven temperatures, and uncomfortable air currents on caged birds that cannot move to a more comfortable location also adversely affect performance. Proper orientation of feeders, waterers, and light promote good performance; slight, seemingly insignificant changes from proven systems can have a pronounced adverse effect on performance of both caged and floor-housed flocks of chickens and other commercial fowl. Poor performance of adults is often traceable to detrimental events that occurred during the rearing period.

Meat birds are bred to grow fast and large, but the flocks kept for breeding must have feed intake restricted to prevent obesity and poor adult performance. Feed restriction must be carefully controlled to prevent aggressive birds from getting most of the available feed. Two systems are widely used: daily restriction and skip-a-day feeding. The former requires special feeding equipment or procedures to ensure that feed is presented to the entire flock simultaneously so that all birds begin eating at the same time. In the skip-a-day system, feed is given in larger quantities on alternate days, permitting the recessive birds to obtain their share even if they have to wait their turn to eat. In either system, special provision must be made in formulating feeds to provide adequate coccidiostat and essential nutrients in the reduced amount consumed.

Poultry and game birds are very cannibalistic under any circumstances. Under most modern systems, beak trimming is a virtual necessity, and special machines have been manufactured for this purpose. Beak trimming is performed on birds of various ages, depending on the husbandry system in use. The extremely dim light used in light-tight poultry houses greatly reduces or prevents cannibalism, but chicks reared under natural or bright light frequently have their beaks trimmed lightly at 1 day of age or a few days after delivery to the brooder. This early mild trimming is not severe enough to be permanent; therefore, beaks of such flocks of breeders or commercial layers are frequently trimmed again before maturity. Some methods and ages of early beak trimming can protect chickens from cannibalism throughout life if other management factors (e.g., light intensity) are favorable.

Biosecurity. Biosecurity, safety from transmissible infectious diseases, parasites, and pests, is a term that embodies all of the measures that can or should be taken to prevent viruses, bacteria, fungi, protozoa, parasites, insects, rodents, and wild birds from entering or surviving and infecting or endangering the well being of the poultry flock.

The reader is referred to a series of eight videotapes illustrating biosecurity measures and the many threats to poultry health that biosecurity is designed to prevent. These were produced by the USDA, APHIS, Veterinary Services. Inquire at your state APHIS veterinary office for further information. These professionally filmed tapes are also available from state extension offices and major poultry industry trade associations. They provide graphic biosecurity training for workers, managers, and owners in all types of broiler, layer, turkey, game bird, breeder farm, hatchery, feed mill, transportation, and live-bird market operations.

BIOSECURITY GUIDELINES. Specific disease-prevention guidelines, targeted to different sectors of industry (truckers, service workers, farm owners, catching crews, and others), are often available from university extension specialists. A 14-page booklet, *Biosecurity for Poultry,* published by the Mid-Atlantic States Cooperative Extension Poultry Health and Management Unit and available from the University of Maryland Extension Service, is an informative example of such cooperatively produced guidelines.

SOURCES OF INFECTION AND PROTECTIVE MEASURES AGAINST THEM. Infections gain entrance to a flock from various sources. To understand why various preventive practices are recommended, it is important to review briefly the sources and routes of infection.

Humans. Because of their mobility, duties, curiosity, ignorance, indifference, carelessness, or total concentration on current profit margin, humans constitute one of the greatest potential causes of introduction of disease. Rarely is this because they become infected and shed the disease agent, but rather because they track infectious diseases, use contaminated equipment, or manage their flocks in such a way that spread of disease is inevitable.

Most frequently, footwear is suspected as the means of transport of disease, but hands can become contaminated with exudates when lesions and discharges are examined. Clothing can also become contaminated with dust, feathers, and excrement. At least one avian disease pathogen (Newcastle disease virus) has been found to survive for several days on the mucous membrane of the human respiratory tract and has been isolated from sputum (45).

NEIGHBORS. A frequent source of infection is a disease outbreak at a neighboring farm. Disease inspection visits among producers are a common way of spreading disease. If a neighbor's flock is afflicted with a very interesting new disease, discuss it by telephone. It is best to warn neighbors not to visit when a disease is in progress and by all means do not walk about a neighbor's farm for any purpose.

CONTRACT WORK CREWS. Much of poultry farm procedure requires sporadic use of a crew of several workers, e.g., blood testing, beak trimming, vaccinating, inseminating, sexing, weighing, and moving birds from one location to another. The producer or farm manager frequently has difficulty in assembling a crew who are available and knowledgeable about handling poultry. Therefore, crews who service many poultry enterprises are contracted. Such crews travel about the poultry community, handling many flocks, and must be regarded as a potential source of infection. Thus, they should take stringent precautions to safeguard the health of every flock with which they work.

VISITORS. Disease outbreaks in a community have

been known to follow the path of a careless visitor. If visitors do not enter premises or buildings, they cannot track in diseases.

The source of a new or dreaded disease is often puzzling. World trade and travel are becoming more commonplace. It is not uncommon for a person to leave one farm in the morning and be visiting another farm or place of business in another part of the country or another continent on the same day. Some disease agents can easily survive that time frame. All who travel should be cognizant of this and guard against introduction of disease into their own flocks or onto premises of clients, competitors, friends, or fellow producers when returning from a trip. Protective footwear and clothing are not readily available in all countries and poultry areas. A good preventive measure when returning from a trip is to sanitize shoes and launder all clothing worn on farms.

Recovered Carriers. Carrier birds are those that have apparently recovered from a clinical infection but still retain the infectious organism in some part of the body. While they appear healthy, the infectious agent continues to multiply in the body and to be eliminated into the environment. Like actively infected flocks, they can perpetuate a disease on a farm and constitute a disease threat to other birds. Many commonly occurring diseases are known to be transmitted by carriers. Carrier birds can be a potential source of disease through the various practices noted below.

MULTIPLE AGES. Multiple ages on a premises constitute a serious disease potential from both actively infected fowl and recovered carriers, particularly if birds of differing ages are closely associated through management practices or proximity. Disease agents that result in chronic infections or recovered carriers are passed by various means, including direct contact, to each new susceptible flock brought onto the premises. Serious drops in production may occur in young laying flocks moved onto laying premises where carrier birds from previous disease outbreaks remain.

STARTED PULLETS. Pullets are frequently reared to or near point-of-lay by a specialized pullet rearer or on a separate premises unit belonging to the laying-farm owner. This practice has become established in the industry for many sound reasons. Pullets can, however, be a potential source for introduction of a disease onto a layer farm if they have been exposed on the pullet farm and as a result have become recovered carriers of some disease not existing on the layer farm. Another hazard is assembling mature pullets reared in different geographic areas onto a single layer premises even an all-in, all-out layer premises. Those reared in one area may have been exposed to and recovered from, but are carrying, a disease agent not found in the area where the other pullets were reared.

FORCE-MOLTED HENS. Force-molting of laying hens or breeders is frequently practiced (particularly during times of economic stress) to supply a special market, meet an emergency egg demand, improve declining shell quality, or because it is deemed economical at the time. One advantage of keeping force-molted hens rather than rearing new replacement pullets is that old hens are not apt to suffer a disease that normally occurs during the rearing age. If such flocks are force-molted and held in the same house, there is little danger of disease problems developing. Conversely, a producer who collects spent hens from many poultry farms for molting and mixes them on one premises at one time is running a serious risk, since any of the force-molted groups may be carriers of a disease to which the others are susceptible.

POULTRY SHOW STOCK. Birds exhibited at poultry shows may be exposed to actively infected or symptomless carrier birds of other exhibitors from which they may contract disease. The contact-infected stock may not develop active signs until returned to the owner's farm, where they may then be a source of new infection. Breeders of fancy birds and game birds and youths with poultry projects (4-H, Future Farmers of America) must recognize the extreme hazards of returning birds exhibited in shows and fairs and of introducing partly grown or adult birds for special breeding purposes. A cardinal rule for show stock is that it should never be returned to the owner's farm. If birds must be shown, individuals should be selected that can be sold after the exhibition. If they must be returned, they should be quarantined for several weeks. In some areas, exhibition-type poultry should be vaccinated against some diseases. Check with a local avian pathologist or veterinary diagnostic laboratory.

BREEDING STOCK. Adult stock considered especially desirable for breeding purposes may be symptomless carriers and serve as a source of infection for the breeding farm. It is best to purchase such stock as hatching eggs or day-old chicks and to rear them in an isolated off-farm quarantine area until there is reasonable assurance they are free of infection.

MIXED SPECIES OF POULTRY. One species that is naturally very resistant to a disease may act as a carrier of that disease for another species that is very susceptible. Some death losses and debilitation from enterohepatitis may occur in chickens, but in turkeys the losses can be disastrous. Therefore, even with routine use of drugs to prevent blackhead, the two species should never be run together, and turkeys should not be run on a dirt yard or floor that has recently had chickens on it.

Also, a silent (inapparent) mycoplasma infection in chickens may spread to mycoplasma-free turkeys and erupt into a full-blown case of sinusitis and air sac infection. Other diseases may be rather innocuous in one species of fowl but very serious in another. It is also advisable to keep meat and laying chickens separated, since the same disease may have different economic importance in the two types.

Other Sources

HOSPITAL PEN. Sick birds from several pens collected into one hospital pen or house and later returned to their respective quarters may carry back not only the condition for which they were removed but one or more diseases contracted while in the hospital area. Therefore, hospital pens are not recommended for routine segregation of sick birds except as a way-station enroute to the diagnostic laboratory or crematorium. If and when used for a special purpose (observation, injury, cannibalism), they should be temporary arrangements within the house and should hold birds from only one pen or house.

CULL PEN. Cull pens still exist on some poultry farms. Nonlaying hens are frequently culled from a flock and marketed for meat. Nonproducing hens in good health present no health hazard for humans or poultry. Cull birds in obviously poor health may or may not be afflicted with an infectious disease. The producer should suspect the worst and destroy such birds rather than hold them for slaughter.

BACKYARD AND PET FOWL. Poultry kept as pets or to supply household eggs or meat are just as capable of carrying and transmitting disease as the commercial flock. Pet barnyard fowl of a rare or interesting nature may also carry disease to commercial poultry. The risk to the invested enterprise is too great to permit such a part-time hobby by a resident owner or employee. Cockfighting is banned in many states, but these game fowl seem to be transported around the country, constituting an effective way to carry disease. Some employees may own or handle these fowl and thus could introduce a serious disease to the poultry enterprise where they work. Poultry farm and hatchery owners and workers should be especially cautious about contact with imported ornamental pet birds or migratory waterfowl because they can be symptomless carriers of diseases that are highly virulent for domestic poultry.

LIVE-BIRD MARKETS. These are buildings, usually in the inner cities, in which poultry of all types, ages, and health status are assembled by small buyers to supply a demand for live fowl for those who wish to examine the fowl live prior to slaughter or prefer to kill and dress fowl at home (Fig. 1.1). Such facilities are rarely depopulated, cleaned, and disinfected, and thus are ideal situations for transmission and propagation of poultry diseases. In addition, the hauling equipment and vehicles may not be cleaned and disinfected after each use. Such equipment hauled throughout the poultry industry areas where a few birds of different types or age are bought at various places are excellent means of transmitting diseases. Good managers and owners will keep such buyers and their equipment out of their farms and offices. The live-bird market trade has been strongly associated with the propagation and spread of avian influenza and laryngotracheitis.

Egg-borne Diseases. Egg-borne diseases are transmitted from the infected dam to newly hatched offspring by means of the fertile egg. Some disease agents are carried inside the shell as a result of shedding into the egg prior to addition of the shell and membranes. Others are carried on the shell or penetrate the shell surface through natural pores after the egg is laid.

The agent may gain entrance to the egg as a result of infection of the ovary and ovarian follicles (transovarian transmission), as a result of contamination of the free ovum in the peritoneal cavity, or by contact in the oviduct. Once the shell and membranes are added, the organism enjoys a protected location where it is not easily destroyed. From there it can later invade the developing embryo, and lesions are frequently observed in tissues and organs of offspring at hatching. Transovarian transmission seems to be limited to only a few of the many diseases that affect poultry and most of these have been eradicated from breeding flocks.

When the freshly laid egg cools from body temperature to nest, room, or cool-room temperature, a pressure differential occurs between the inside of the egg and the atmosphere. Any fluid on the shell surface is drawn inward. Motile bacteria are aided by this pressure differential in penetrating the shell. The primary contamination of this nature is from enteric organisms, particularly salmonellae and coliforms, but other types of bacteria and fungi also may be drawn into the egg. For preventive measures, see Breeder Flock Management and Management of Hatching Eggs.

Equipment. Diseases and parasites can be carried on equipment. Cleaning equipment and vehicles usually have accumulations of litter and feces that can be a threat to other farms and houses where they may be transported for succeeding assignments. They should be washed free of litter and droppings before use in another farm area.

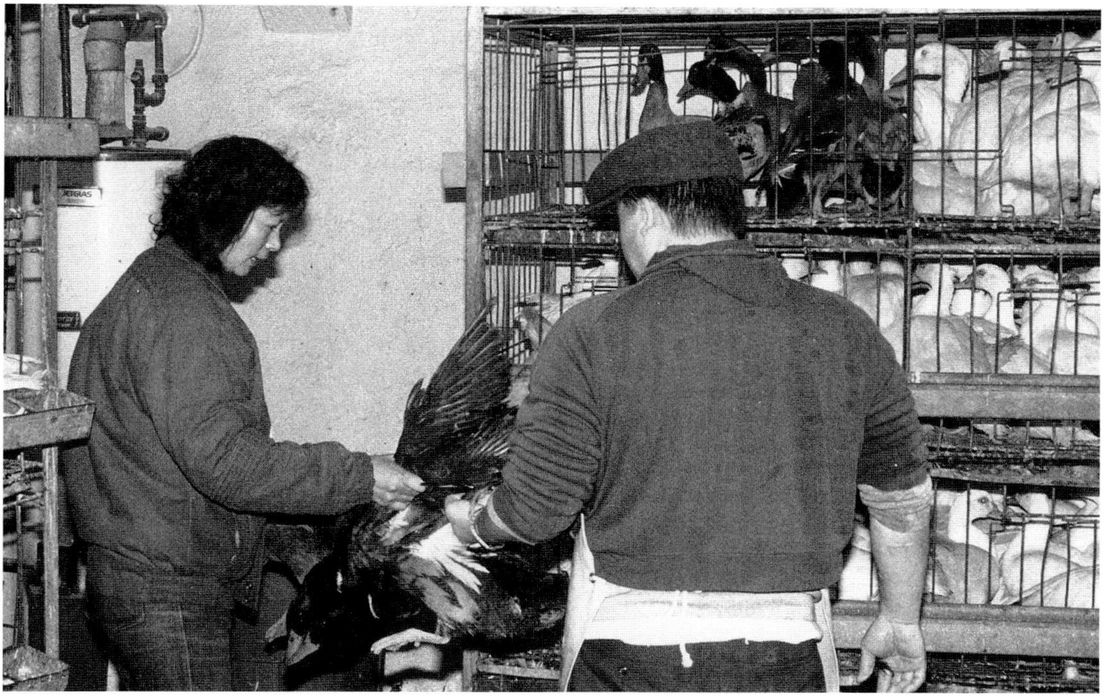

1.1. Urban live-bird market. Live birds are examined, purchased, and either slaughtered and dressed at the market or taken live and slaughtered at home. Such markets are not often depopulated and disinfected, thus can readily propogate and transmit disease. (Univ Maryland)

Mites are frequently found on eggs and can be transported from farm to farm in corrugations of egg cases taken into chicken houses. Wire crates and baskets do not offer these hiding places. Residues of salmonella-contaminated eggs on egg flats may be a potential method of introducing disease. Use of washed and disinfected plastic egg flats and moving of stacked flats of uncased eggs on racks and pallets (see Fig. 1.26) reduce the hazard of transmission of diseases and parasites among farms.

Fowl pox, infectious bursal disease, Marek's disease viruses, coccidia, roundworm eggs, and other infectious material can be carried on crates, footwear, and vehicles, particularly on the floor and foot-control pedals of a vehicle.

Artificial inseminating equipment, particularly reused inseminating tubes, offer an excellent method of transmitting disease.

Poultry-hauling equipment can disseminate infectious material through feathers, feces, blood, exudates, and skin encrustations left in the crates or picked up at the slaughter plant. Hauling equipment should be washed and disinfected after use before being taken to another farm (Fig. 1.2).

Miscellaneous Sources

LABORATORY EXPOSURE. Frequently a producer, particularly a small-flock owner, hobbyist, or gamebird owner, will want to take a bird home after the veterinarian has examined it at the laboratory. While in the receiving area or diagnostic facilities even for a short time, live poultry have a good opportunity to contact some disease agent. Except under special circumstances (exotic birds, valuable pet), no bird should be returned from the laboratory to the farm because it could develop disease and be the source of a new infection on the home premises. The bird should either be sacrificed and necropsied or, if a pet, referred to a private clinician.

A disease may be tracked from laboratory surroundings to a farm by careless laboratory or service workers or the producers. Clean and frequently washed and disinfected laboratory areas are the responsibility of the veterinarian. Precautions against tracking disease from the laboratory to the farm are the responsibility of the producer and service worker.

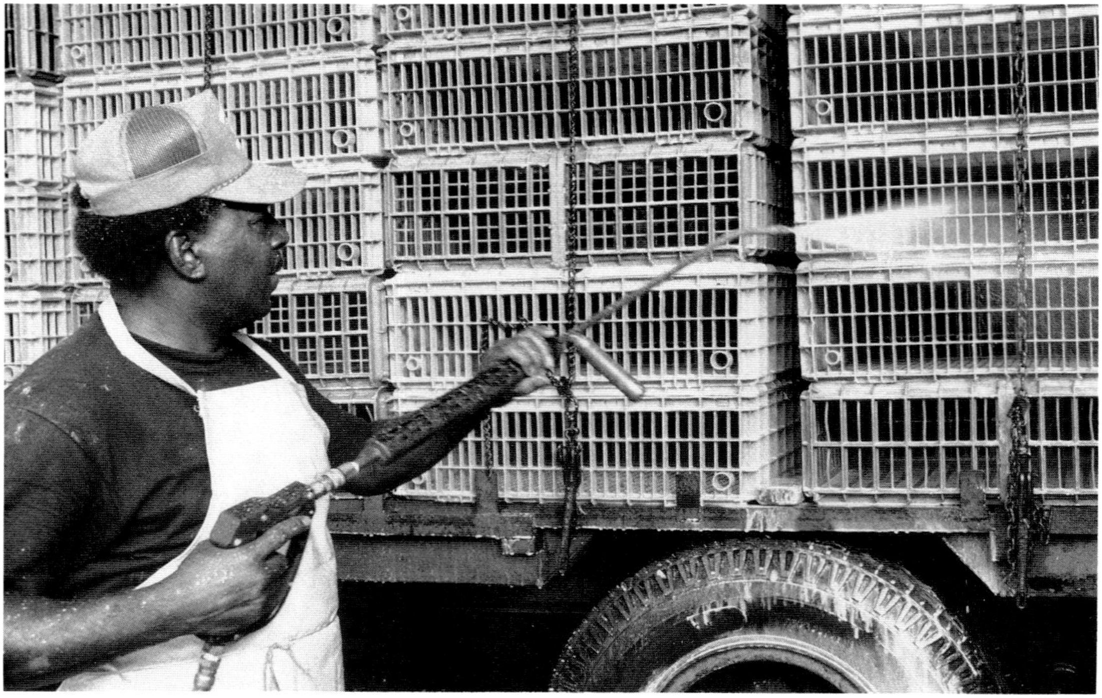

1.2. Soiled vehicles and equipment can carry disease agents. They should be thoroughly washed and disinfected after each live haul. One gram of chicken manure can contain enough viral particles to infect 1 million birds with avian influenza. (USDA)

RODENTS. Rodents contaminate feed and litter with their excrement. They are particularly hazardous to salmonella control, since they are frequently infected with these organisms and can perpetuate the disease on a farm.

HOUSEHOLD PETS. Dogs and cats, like rodents, are capable of harboring enteric organisms that are infectious for poultry. When these pets are not confined to the household area but roam continually among the poultry in the pens and yards, they constitute a serious health hazard. Such pets are just as capable of tracking contaminated material on their feet and in their hair as people.

WILD BIRDS. Wild birds are capable of carrying a variety of diseases and parasites. Some cause illness in the wild birds themselves; for others, the birds act as mechanical carriers. Every effort should be made to prevent their nesting in the poultry area. Imported zoological specimens destined for zoos are not a direct contact threat because the zoos are located in cities, but they should be considered as a potential source of introduction of an exotic disease or parasite. Exotic ornamental pet birds constitute a real hazard because they become widely dispersed and may be purchased by poultry workers. On numerous occasions exotic birds in or destined for pet stores have been found infected with a virulent exotic form of Newcastle disease virus, which in at least one instance was the source of a serious and costly outbreak in poultry. Stringent entry quarantine requirements to apprehend and destroy infected birds provide a good barrier against introduction and dissemination by carrier birds, but failures can occur (illegal smuggling), and producers should be wary of such personal pets. Domestic pigeons can also be a source of dangerous strains of Newcastle disease virus.

INSECTS. Many insects act as transmitters of disease. Some are intermediate hosts for blood or intestinal parasites; others are mechanical carriers of disease through their biting parts. Still others because of their feeding habits and hiding places appear to be reservoirs of disease whereby the infectious agent survives from one flock to the next.

FEED. Some ingredients may contain infectious agents, particularly salmonellae, from contamination at their source or anywhere along the production line or storage areas. Methods are available for sterilizing feed, but they increase cost of the final product. Pelleting, if done properly, is a practical method of greatly reducing contaminants because of the heat generated in the process, but it is not dependable for complete sterilization. Meat meal is the feed ingredient most apt to introduce salmonella species. This hazard can be avoided by using only vegetable protein ingredients supplemented as necessary with synthetic amino acids. Such formulations are recommended for breeder rations if pelleting capabilities are not available.

MANAGEMENT FACTORS IN DISEASE PREVENTION. The more important physical principles of disease prevention include favorable geographic location of the farm in respect to other poultry units, proper location of buildings in relation to each other and to prevailing wind currents, proper design of the building inside and out, and design and positioning of equipment. Long-range planning and programming of the operation, whether large or small, is very important and should consider movement patterns of various vehicles and equipment, work traffic of regular and holiday caretakers and special work crews, feed delivery and storage, and the system for moving eggs and flocks from the farm. An avian pathologist can be helpful in avoiding some common pitfalls, but to avoid high-risk disease situations, consultation should be done when the farm is being designed and the production programmed, rather than after it is developed and serious trouble is evident.

Good disease-prevention practices are perhaps best illustrated as a chain that is only as strong as its weakest link. Many sound principles can be discredited by failure to carry out one or two related ones that are either overlooked or not considered essential. While it may not always be possible to use all the practices, the more that are followed, the greater the chances of avoiding disease outbreaks.

Isolation. Not all producers follow the same disease-control practices. A close neighbor may disregard sound principles and be burdened with diseases until forced out of business by economic pressures. In the meantime, disease agents present on his premises may be blown or carried by various vectors and fomites to adjacent premises; thus a disease may occasionally gain entrance even on well-managed units. Until a disease has been eradicated, it serves as a reservoir and potential source of infection for future flocks on the same premises and those on adjacent premises. The closer the houses of one premises to those of another the more likely is the spread of infection to healthy birds on an adjacent farm.

Some highly concentrated poultry areas have developed because of some favorable condition such as a close market, an available slaughter or processing plant, an accessible feed supply, low-cost land, or favorable climate or zoning. Usually these areas deteriorate into problem zones of disease of one type or another and resemble huge "megafarms" with many managers, each vaccinating, treating, or exposing birds without regard to the programs of others. Since such areas are in competition for markets, several things may happen. Various advantages may offset disease losses, or the additional cost of production resulting from disease prices the product (meat, eggs) out of the market. In extreme cases, products cannot be marketed either because of the disease or the residues from drugs used to control disease. Producers who do not minimize losses go out of business; many abandoned poultry farms are purchased or leased by other poultry producers. Some move their operations to a less concentrated area where they usually escape disease, unless they take their problems with them knowingly or inadvertently through carelessness. Those who remain usually upgrade disease-prevention practices by redesigning houses and reprogramming the production cycle. Frequently, reprogramming proceeds to a system of a single age of fowl, permitting complete depopulation at the end of each rearing or laying cycle.

Another solution to area disease problems where farms are too close even for systematic depopulation to succeed is to develop a coordinated area depopulation and restocking program. All flocks in a reasonably defined geographic area may be marketed at the same time and the houses refilled at the same time. This is more adaptable to broiler production than egg production.

Most serious disease problems could be avoided if a philosophy of premises isolation prevailed from the beginning of an enterprise. No exact minimum distance from other poultry farms can be stated because this is influenced by prevailing winds, climate, type of houses, and other factors. The farther from other poultry farms, the less likelihood of contracting disease from them. Isolation can be effected by taking advantage of segregating space provided by natural or fabricated barriers such as bodies of water, hills, cities or towns, forests, or other interposing agriculture enterprises such as grain, vegetable, or fruit production. The degree of isolation is influenced as much by management philosophy as by economic considerations. This is illustrated by the cluster of farms shown in Fig. 1.3 and the isolated breeding farm shown in Fig. 1.4.

One Age of Fowl per Farm. Removing carriers from a flock and premises is an effective way of preventing a recurrence of some diseases, but it is impossible or impractical for others. The best way to prevent infection from carrier birds is to remove the entire flock from the farm before any

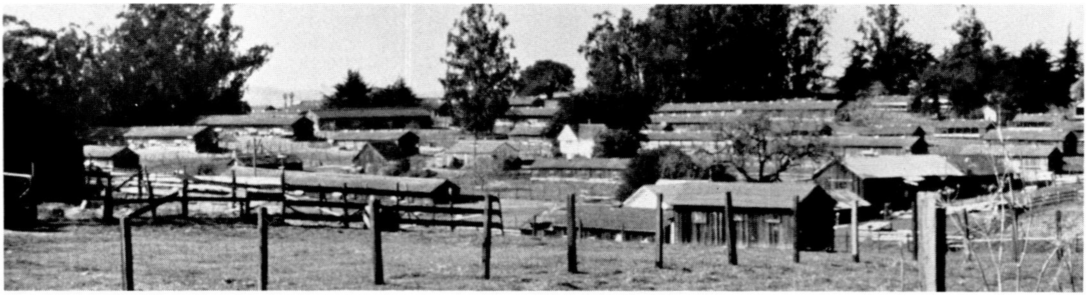

1.3. Farms in this cluster are too close to provide any reasonable degree of isolation. Diseases tend to remain endemic within such a group unless all are depopulated and restocked, but similar clusters of individually owned large farms with more modern physical structures can still be found along with the chronic diseases they perpetuate.

new replacements are added and to rear young stock in complete isolation from older recovered birds on a separated farm segment or preferably on another farm and in an isolated area.

Where birds of different ages exist on a large farm, depopulation seems drastic; but considering mortality, poor performance, and endless drug expense, it could be the most economical solution. Farms and quarantinable farm divisions of up to 100,000 birds of one age prove that size is no deterrent to application of the sound principle of one age of bird per farm or quarantinable segment, with programmed depopulation at the end of the production cycle.

Where only one age of bird is maintained, depopulation occurs each time pullets or poults are moved to the layer or breeder premises, each time the broilers or turkeys are moved to slaughter, and each time the old layers or breeders are sent to market. Should a disease occur, the flock can be quarantined, treated, and handled in the best way possible until its disposal. Depopulated premises are then cleaned out, washed, disinfected, and left idle for as long as possible but at least for 2 wk before new healthy stock is introduced.

Depopulation is most effective in controlling disease agents that do not survive for long outside the bird. This applies to most respiratory infections (mycoplasma infections, infectious coryza, laryngotracheitis). It is least effective in controlling disease agents having a resistant state that survives for long periods in nature (intestinal parasites, clostridia).

Started-pullet and pullet-rearing premises are now an established specialized enterprise in the poultry industry. This system has made layer and breeder farm depopulation more practical and successful. As on multiple-age layer farms, serious disease problems may develop and persist on multiple-age rearing farms until they are reprogrammed for a single age or divided into quarantinable, isolated units.

In addition to sanitary practices, environmental factors (temperature, humidity) play an important part in the time interval necessary to prevent carryover of disease. Disease germs begin to die out slowly after elimination from the body. Some (coryza) die out very quickly; others (parasites, coccidia) survive for months or years, depending on whether they develop a resistant stage and on factors discussed under individual diseases. In general, the longer a premises remains vacant, the lower the number of surviving pathogens.

Functional Units. For certain economic reasons (breeding farm or small specialized market trade), it is not always possible to limit the entire farm to a single age of poultry. In such instances it should be divided into separate quarantinable units or areas for different groups of birds (rearing area, pedigree unit, production groups, experimental birds) (Fig. 1.4). With a suitable arrangement each area is periodically depopulated, cleaned, and sanitized, or can be if necessary. Much stricter security procedures for personnel, bird, and equipment movements are necessary for this type of operation. A very rigid monitoring system is also essential to detect any disease early enough to bring it under control while it is still confined to one quarantinable segment.

There is no reliable formula for minimum distances between houses or units. Windowless and temperature- and ventilation-controlled houses appear to prevent building-to-building and premises-to-premises spread better than open houses. Greater distance can compensate for some inadequacy in building design, human traffic control, and shared equipment. Since each premises and enterprise is different from all others, the poultry

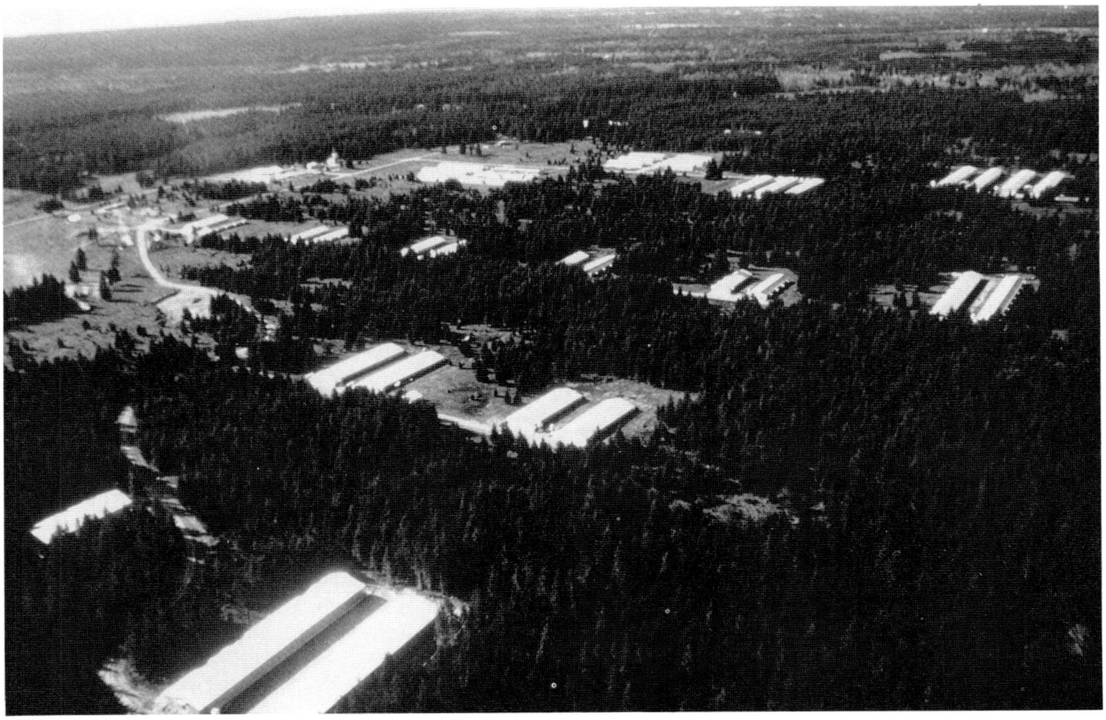

1.4. This isolated breeding farm benefits from several fundamental disease-prevention and control principles. It is isolated from other poultry farms, is surrounded by forestland, and is divided into quarantinable sections separated by woods as well as distance.

producer should seek advice from specialists whose business it is to study diseases and how to prevent and control them.

The most important factor in dividing the farm into segregated units is not so much to facilitate daily separation of farm personnel, equipment, and poultry, but to provide quarantinable units to prevent spread and facilitate elimination of disease, should it occur.

Building Construction

BIRDPROOFING. The first rule in poultry house construction is to exclude free-flying wild birds, since many carry mites and harbor them in their nests. In addition, many species have been found susceptible to some common viral and bacterial diseases of poultry and thus could act as carriers. Turkeys on range are especially vulnerable to infections carried by wild birds. For this reason and for generally improved sanitary practices, the trend is to house turkeys, especially breeder and young growing turkeys, in closed or partially closed birdproof houses. Ducks and other domestic waterfowl are also vulnerable to water-borne diseases and diseases carried by wild birds, especially wild waterfowl and seabirds (gulls, terns, etc.).

Light- and temperature-controlled houses are usually birdproof by reason of their construction (Fig 1.5), but both ventilation and birdproofing are also achievable in open-type houses in hot cli-

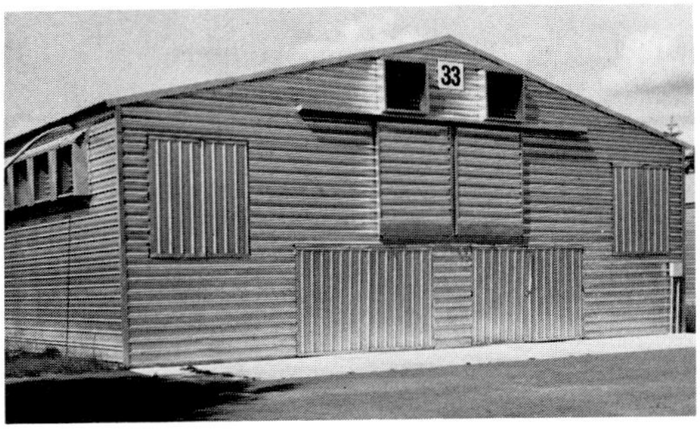

1.5. Light-, temperature-, and ventilation-controlled houses exclude wild birds and most flying insects. Concrete aprons and paved roadways help prevent tracking of soil-borne diseases into the premises.

mates (Fig 1.6). Birdproofing is also an important feature of other buildings on the farm, e.g., clean crate and wood shavings (bedding) storage.

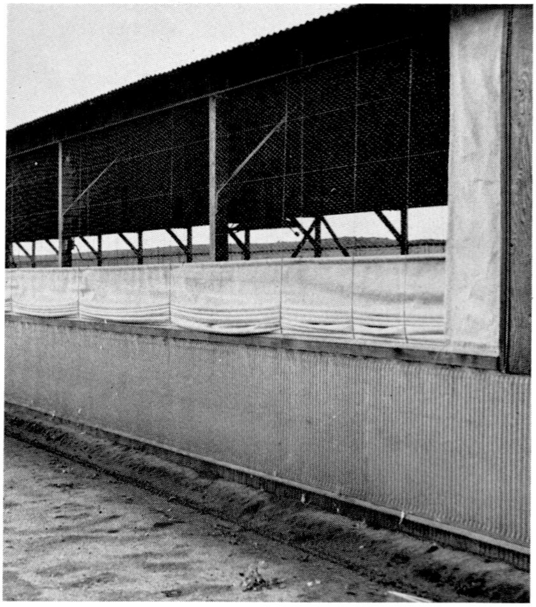

1.6. Wild birds are effectively excluded from this open-type house.

ENTRANCES. An apron of concrete at the entrance to a poultry house helps prevent tracking of disease into the unit (Fig 1.5). Rain and sunshine help keep the apron cleaned and sterilized. A water faucet, boot brush, and covered pan of disinfectant available on the apron for disinfecting footwear are further aids in keeping litter and soil-borne diseases out of the house. The disinfectant is useless, however, unless renewed frequently enough to ensure a potent solution at all times.

VENTILATION. Poultry buildings should be constructed to provide protection against the elements yet not create stress conditions such as excess dust, insufficient ventilation with ammonia buildup, excessive draft, damp litter, and situations leading to injuries by mechanical equipment or sharp objects.

There are many advantages of windowless and temperature-controlled houses, but one serious drawback has been development in some instances of excessively dry and dusty litter. While Anderson et al. (4) could not demonstrate significant deleterious effects of short-term inhalation of dust by test chickens, it has been observed in practice that colibacillosis outbreaks are frequently associated with inhalation of excessive dust, which must be carried from the building with ventilating air. This may require increased air movement, and precautions must be taken to prevent a stream of incoming cold outside air from blowing directly onto chickens that are prevented, by pen (or cage) arrangement, from seeking shelter.

Coccidial oocysts require moisture to develop into the infective stage. Excessively dry litter inhibits their development and may so limit the number of infective oocysts that infection is too light for a good immune reaction. Conversely, improper ventilation can lead to excessively wet litter, which favors the survival and development of coccidia and other parasites.

Ammonia fumes develop in damp litter and droppings. If ventilation is poor and fumes accumulate, they may reach high enough concentration to inhibit growth and performance, cause keratoconjunctivitis, and exacerbate respiratory infections.

Litter will dry better if it can be stirred frequently, but in spite of all efforts, it may remain wet in winter or in humid climates. If wetness and excess ammonia concentration persist, litter should be replaced and ventilation improved.

Proper ventilation is an engineering science; a good policy is to seek professional advice before installing any system. The influence of such environmental conditions as temperature, humidity, radiation, and atmospheric pollutants on virus diseases of poultry has been reviewed by Anderson and Hanson (3).

FLOORS AND CAGES. All surfaces inside the building should be of impervious material (such as concrete) to permit thorough washing and disinfection. It is impossible to sterilize a dirt floor!

Raised slatted floors have been used successfully for years for laying chickens, both for adults and for rearing birds. Such floors have alternating wooden pieces and spaces, each about 3/4 in. wide (Fig 1.7), to permit droppings to fall out of reach of birds and to prevent recycling infection of intestinal parasites and diseases. Since coccidial infection is thus avoided or greatly reduced, poor or no immunity to the parasite develops. This creates no problem for pullets destined for cages or slat-floored laying houses, because immunity to coccidiosis during the laying period in such units would not be an important consideration. However, if such pullets were transferred to litter-floored laying houses, they would very likely become seriously infected with coccidia. Commercial meat birds are inclined to develop leg problems and breast blisters if raised on complete slatted or wire floors. A modification of this system, with part of the floor or yard raised slightly and covered with slats, has been used for broiler breeders. The value of this system is increased further by placing feed and water over the slatted

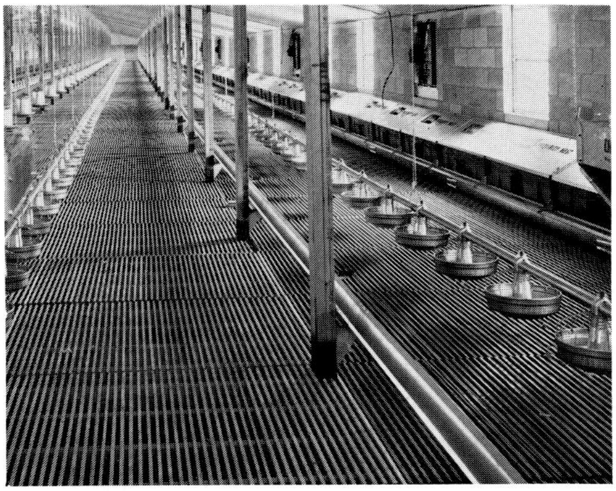

1.7. Slat floors aid in control of intestinal diseases and parasites. Droppings fall through open spaces and out of reach of the flock.

area, which encourages collection of more droppings out of reach of birds.

Keeping laying hens in some type of cage has become an accepted practice in closed houses (Fig. 1.8) and open-type houses found in hot climates (Fig. 1.9). Cages and wire floors are widely used also to rear pullets destined for cages as adults. The system is so successful in preventing intestinal diseases that birds have no opportunity to develop immunity to them. Coccidiosis is almost certain to occur if chickens or other poultry reared in cages are transferred to litter floors. Drugs can be used successfully to control coccidiosis in these birds, but legal restrictions on their use in meat and egg-producing fowl seriously curtail drug choices for this purpose in laying hens. There has been renewed interest in developing suitable cages for breeder turkeys and commercial broilers. Such a development would be a distinct aid in eliminating many disease problems of soil and litter origin.

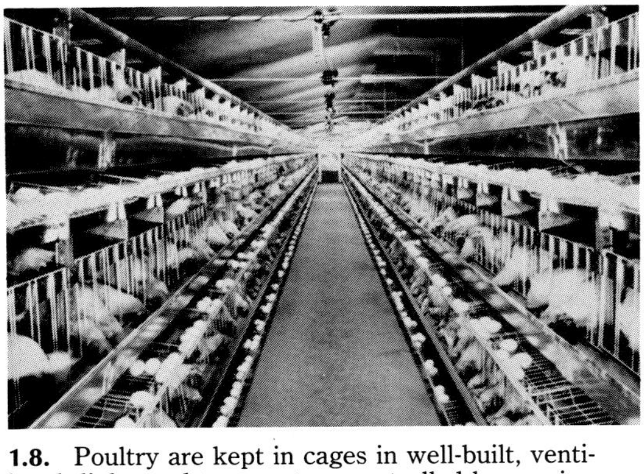

1.8. Poultry are kept in cages in well-built, ventilated, light- and temperature-controlled houses in many countries. Good housing reduces stress associated with variations in weather, and cages reduce intestinal diseases and parasitism.

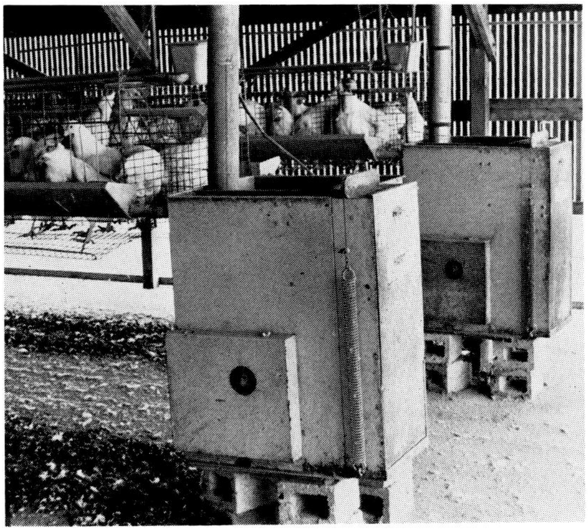

1.9. In hot climates poultry are kept in cages in open-type houses. This practice prevents intestinal diseases and parasitism but subjects birds to temperature extremes. If the house is not birdproof, external parasites can be carried in by wild birds. Medicated feed can be placed in small feed tanks by hand for emergency flock treatment.

FEEDERS AND WATERERS. Rats, mice, and other rodents should be kept out of feed because they may introduce and spread salmonellae or other disease agents that can be the source of an outbreak in the poultry flock.

Litter scratched into feed and water troughs and feed spilled in litter increase intake of litter and litter-borne disease agents; e.g., more coccidial oocysts and less coccidiostat are ingested, and a clinical infection may result. If poultry are permitted to consume litter, considerable mortality and depression can occur from impaction of the gizzard, and litter fragments may cause enteritis by mechanical irritation.

Feed troughs should have some type of guard to keep poultry out (Fig. 1.10) and should not be over-filled so that feed is spilled into litter. Feeders without guards permit defecation into feed, which encourages spread of disease organisms shed in feces. Wet feed in litter or yards attracts wild birds and rodents and provides a good medium for growth of molds, which can cause liver, kidney, immune system, and other damage to the well-being of poultry. Feeders used in turkey yards should be in a covered area designed to protect the feed from rainwater and sunlight to prevent mold growth and vitamin loss. Growing and laying cages for egg production flocks in light- and temperature-controlled houses eliminate most of the problems associated with litter. There are many good automated feeding

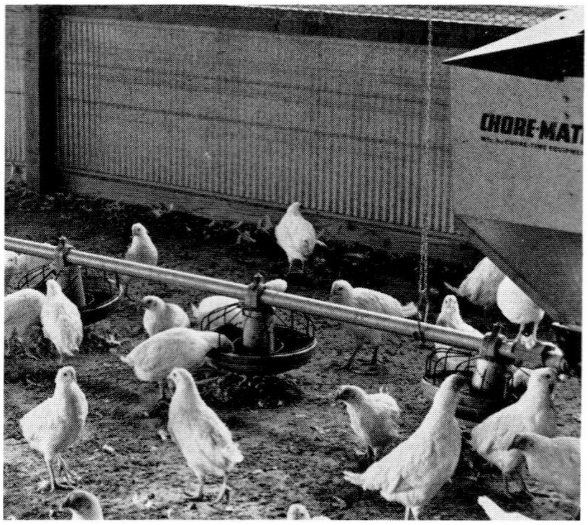

1.10. Small feed tanks between the large bulk tank and the feed trough allow hand dumping of emergency medicated feed. Wire guards keep chickens out of feeders.

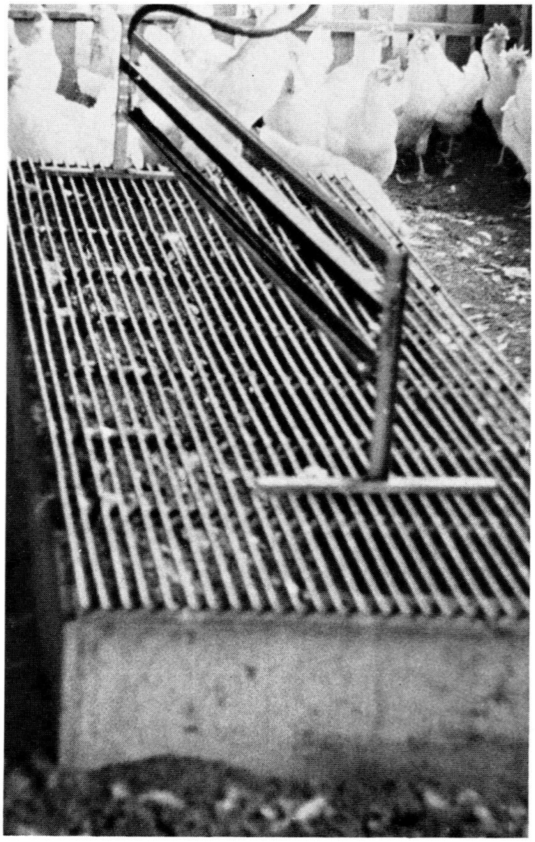

1.11. Raised concrete platform covered with a removable grill on which the waterer is placed. Spilled water collects in the pit and does not wet the litter.

and watering systems available commercially, but sometimes these are not installed or oriented as the manufacturer intended and consequently health problems develop.

Roost areas over screened dropping pits are common in floor-laying and breeder hen houses to keep chickens away from their feces. Screened roost areas are also desirable in rearing houses for layers and breeders to prevent piling by the birds and excessive fouling of litter with feces, which in turn leads to packing and caking. Feeders and waterers over the pits keep the birds on the roost area much of the daytime as well as at night, so most droppings collect out of reach. Spilled water also falls under the roosts, so the litter area stays drier.

Waterers are frequently set or hung over the litter area. In this case, the waterer should be of a type that does not lend itself to spillage (cups, nipples, hanging plastic bells), or a raised slatted frame should be placed under it (Fig. 1.11) with a drain area provided in the floor. Gravel may be added under the frame, or it may be left empty. Here again, the aim is to prevent the litter from becoming wet, which encourages multiplication of coccidia, worms, bacteria, and fungi.

FEED AND WATER MEDICATION. In spite of all precautions, poultry may become sick. This should be recognized from the start, and facilities for quick treatment by medication in water or feed should be provided long before it is needed. When birds are grouped by tens of thousands in one big pen, segregation and treatment of individuals is impractical; mass medication and vaccination are essential if any treatment is to be given.

Feed medication is not the best method of treatment because of the inappetence of sick birds and their inability to compete for feed. Water medication is somewhat better because the sick will frequently drink when they will not eat, but the medicaments that can be administered in water are limited. Mass medication, while not completely successful in curing the sick, may hold the disease in check until the host can respond with a successful immune response. Provision should also be made for mass vaccination through drinking water, as this is an accepted and successful labor-saving practice. If drinking water is chlorinated or otherwise treated, the sanitizing agent may destroy the vaccine, so provision must be made to permit use of untreated or distilled water for mixing and administering water vaccines.

Several methods can be used to reduce, remove, or neutralize chlorine in chlorinated water supplies. The only practical method for dealing with this problem on poultry farms is to add protein to the water when mixing water vaccines. A common practice is to add 1 lb of nonfat dried milk to 50 gal H_2O in tanks or canned liquid nonfat milk mixed with vaccine in a proportioner.

If a building is constructed with a bulk water tank for gravity-flow watering devices, the tank should be of plastic or lined with some nonreactive protective substance and be readily accessible for cleaning and for mixing medicaments. If the watering devices are operated on high pressure, the pipe leading into the pen should have a bypass system with proper valve arrangement so that a medicament proportioner can be installed quickly when needed. A metering device to measure feed and water consumption is useful to keep track of the health of the flock (Fig 1.12). Float-regulated or continuous-flow water troughs can spread disease within a house. Infectious coryza has been observed to spread down cage rows of chickens in the direction of water flow. Use of a watering system with small drinking cups for individual cage units will aid in preventing spread of disease.

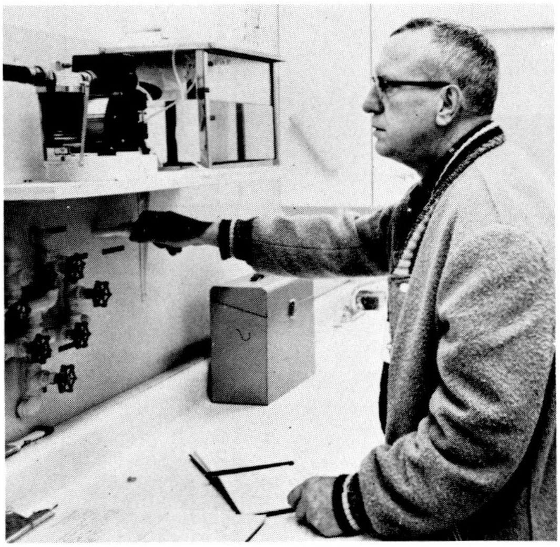

1.12. Control panel and proportioner in a poultry house from which water can be metered or medication introduced into the water.

Bulk feed delivery, metal bulk storage tanks, and automatic feeders are common in modern poultry operations. These eliminate the possibility of rodent contamination since feed is always in closed tanks rather than in bags or open bins, but the system leads to difficulties when short-term emergency medication in feed is desirable and the bulk tank is full. Two alternative systems are useful: an additional smaller bulk tank may be installed just for emergency medicated feed or a small dispensing tank may be interposed between the bulk tank and feed troughs (Figs. 1.9, 1.10) so emergency medicated feed can be put in the smaller tank by hand. Though rarely, if ever, used in commercial poultry operations any longer, disposable paper bags have been developed that eliminate the danger of used feed bags as a mechanical carrier of disease from farm to farm. Users of such pre-bagged rations should be certain that the feed has recently been milled and not old with the risk of lowered vitamin potency.

Personnel Control

COMPANY AND FARM PERSONNEL. Managers, supervisors, and owners are sometimes the worst offenders at breaking sanitation rules. These people frequently visit many different types of poultry enterprises, farms, and farm units, and disease agents do not respect authority or ownership. Such personnel, like veterinarians, should set a good example for the workers. One of the most important aspects of disease control is an awareness on the part of everyone: owner; work force; feed and supply delivery people; egg, bird, and litter haulers; and all who visit or work on poultry farms, that each has an important role in disease prevention. Occasional educational conferences with the assembled work force on health goals and reasons for procedures will foster awareness. This is as important as the preventive measure established, and a good occasion to use the biosecurity action tapes mentioned previously in this chapter.

In designing buildings and farm layout and in programming production and management, it is important to make every disease-preventive practice as easy and efficient as possible. Any procedures that are difficult will probably be done incorrectly.

VISITORS AND CUSTOMERS. For some types of poultry enterprise it is deemed necessary to show the birds, premises, or procedures to visitors. In such cases an observation booth, platform, or fenced area should be provided. Such an area should be sealed off from the poultry pens or hatchery. For maximum security the entry, access road, and observation area should be completely separated from the work area. Such a facility for a hatchery is shown in Fig. 1.13.

Visitors can be a minimum hazard if proper provisions are made to accommodate them and they cooperate fully with strict sanitary rules. When they must enter the poultry quarters, they should wear protective clothing such as clean, laundered, or new disposable coveralls and hat in addition to disinfected rubber overshoes and other footwear, which is most important. Plastic footwear cover has limited use because it is easily punctured by gravel or other sharp objects. The sanitary precautions are most essential when entering floor-brooding and -rearing houses but will also help keep disease out of any house or pen.

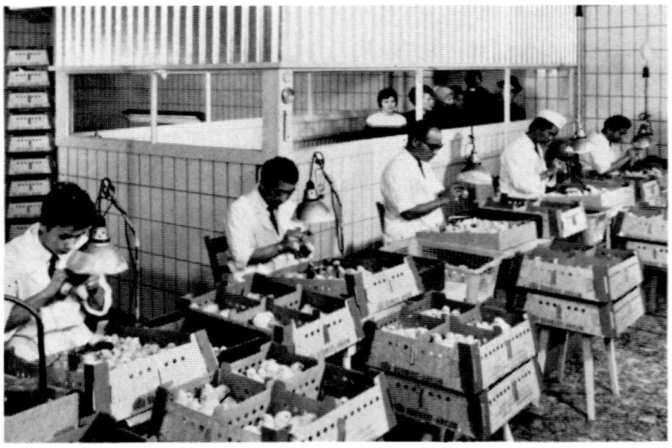

1.13. Sealed observation cubicle permits visitors to observe hatchery operations without tracking disease into the building. The observation booth is reached by a special walkway from a parking lot; the entrance is located far from those used by hatchery personnel.

SANITARY ENVIRONMENTS

Grounds Around Buildings

RODENT CONTROL. Piles of trash and unused equipment are good hiding and breeding places for rats, mice, and ground squirrels, which may serve as reservoirs of disease and contaminate troughs with excrement. Feed spilled or stored in troughs is an attractive food supply; when it is exhausted, rodents will find any available route into the building where they have intimate contact with poultry. Even if buildings are rodentproof, excrement can be tracked in on footwear. It is more difficult to get rid of rodents once the premises are infested than to keep them out initially.

INSECT CONTROL. Many parasites and disease agents are harbored from one generation to another in resident insects (Marek's disease), require an insect for an intermediate stage of development (tapeworms), or are simply carried from bird to bird mechanically or by biting (fowl pox virus). Countermeasures against insects are part of the sanitary environment and cleanup.

Some methods used to keep insects away from buildings are an apron of treated soil to prevent growth of all vegetation, an apron of hard surface material, or a border of well-mowed green grass. Spraying the area around buildings with an insecticide also prevents insect buildup, but the other methods have the additional advantage of reducing fire hazards to the buildings.

A good practice during cleanup is to spray the grounds, litter, and buildings with an insecticide immediately after removing fowl, then allow a few days for effective insect kill before removing litter preparatory to cleaning and disinfection. This is especially important when there is a history of an insect-borne disease in the previous brood. After cleaning, the building should be sprayed again with an insecticide having a residual effect to prevent reinfestation. Professional, integrated rodent- and insect-control services are available in some locations. They may provide cost-effective convenience.

Dead-Bird Disposal

FOCI OF INFECTION. When birds die owing to disease agents, carcasses remain a source of infection for penmates and other poultry on the same or other farms. Also, hopelessly sick birds discharge infectious material into the environment and should be removed from the flock and killed in a manner that will not permit the discharge of blood or exudates (see Diagnostic Procedures). Whether the result of a serious clinical infection or just the usual expected mortality, all carcasses should be disposed of by one of the following methods to prevent dissemination of disease.

COOKING OR RENDERING. Freshly dead poultry, like livestock, can be rendered into fertilizer or other products. The rendering temperature should be sufficient for sterilization and the truck bed used to transport the carcasses washed and disinfected. Cans used to haul the carcasses should be steam cleaned and sterilized. Again, it should be remembered that commercial or contract haulers of dead carcasses may introduce another disease from some other outbreak unless strict precautionary measures are taken.

BURNING. Burning is the most dependable way of destroying infectious material. Many smokeless, odorless incinerators for disposal of animal carcasses are available commercially. These devices are expensive but are handy and suitable for some purposes. Homemade incinerators of various types have also been used successfully, but they may create objectionable odors and air pollution.

BURYING. For losses creating a serious disposal problem and where environmental regulations allow, a deep hole may be dug and the carcasses buried so animals cannot get at them. The best and easiest way is to use a backhoe and dig a deep narrow trench. Each day's collection of dead birds can be deposited and covered until the trench is filled.

PIT OR TANK DISPOSAL. For small losses and normal attrition, a decomposition pit can be used (Fig. 1.14A). A bigger and less elaborate one than that shown can be built, but precautions should be taken to assure that it is not located where it will contaminate drinking water supplies, that the roof or walls will not cave in, that animals will not dig into it, that flies and other insects cannot get into it, and above all that children cannot fall into it. The pit cover should be sealed with tar paper or plastic and be strong enough to hold at least a foot of soil overlay. Where groundwater levels are close to the surface (deltas, lowlands, shorelines), underground pits may be undesirable. An alternative is an aboveground dead bird composting unit.

An electrically heated septic tank for disposal of dead birds and waste products from large poultry farms has been developed by the Agricultural Research Service, USDA, in cooperation with the Maine and Connecticut agricultural experiment stations. The method consists of digesting carcasses and/or waste products in a heated septic tank. Heat is applied at 37.8 C and requires 2–3 kwh/day of electricity to maintain this temperature for the 2 wk needed for destruction of all but the bones of carcasses. The system depends on mesophilic bacteria, which multiply best at 32.2–37.8 C, to accelerate decomposition. Neutralizing the mass at intervals with lime and adding hot water further accelerate the action and speed of decomposition.

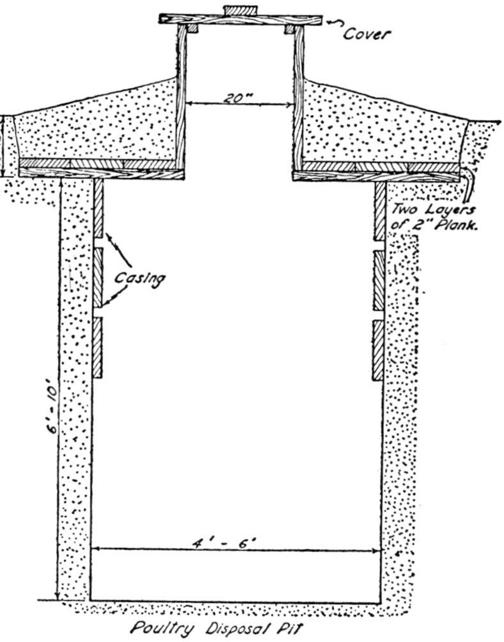

A

B

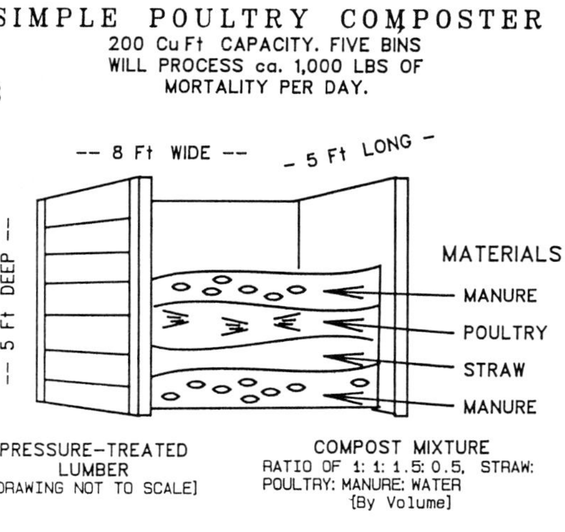

1.14. A. Poultry disposal pit. Such a pit can be made any size that is convenient. B. A simple aboveground poultry carcass composter of 200-ft³ (5.7-m³) capacity. Five such bins will process 1000 lb (455 kg) of carcasses per day. (Courtesy Poultry Sci Dep, Univ Maryland)

COMPOSTING. Aerobic, thermophilic, batch composting of poultry carcasses is a method of disposal developed at the University of Maryland (31). Compost mixtures of straw, whole poultry carcasses, manure, and water in the proportions of 1:1:1.5:0.5, respectively, (1/3 of water added to each layer), decompose rapidly and odorlessly. Composts heat rapidly, attain temperatures of between 145 and 165 F, and reduce soft tissues completely within 14 days. Compost structures and management procedures are simple (Fig. 1.14B). Pathogen survival studies suggest the process is biologically "clean." Attempts to isolate coliform and salmonellalike bacteria and IBD virus have yielded negative results. Composting may be an effective alternative to more traditional dead bird disposal methods, especially where water tables are near the surface.

Buildings and Runs

CLEAN BUILDINGS. A clean sanitized environment is good insurance against disease outbreaks from any cause. Stringent sanitary practices are frequently ineffective because disease is tracked in after the buildings and equipment are cleaned and disinfected or because some step in the total program was omitted and a focus of infection was preserved.

LITTER REMOVAL. When a house is depopulated, the litter or droppings should be removed preparatory to cleaning. With development of huge specialized poultry farms, proper and economical disposal of litter and poultry manure has become a serious problem. There is no clear-cut answer. A general recommendation is to remove it far enough from the buildings so that insects will not crawl or fly back into the houses and to dry it, compost it, or spread it onto fields and work it into the soil. If cleaning is done while chickens are still present (cages), remember that contracted personnel, trucks, and equipment may recently have been on another farm where a disease outbreak occurred.

In some cases the nature of a disease may dictate that some extra precautions (wetting down or soaking with disinfectant, delaying removal, burying, burning) be taken with litter, even though expensive. Any treatment of manure or litter must consider residual effects of the applied compounds on plant life when treated manure is spread on the land. For most disease agents composting of litter or droppings is sufficient. Whatever is done, one must be aware that wherever litter is spilled or piled, it remains as a disease reservoir for varying lengths of time.

OUTSIDE RUNS. In the case of outside runs such as turkey and game-bird ranges, the topsoil should be scraped off and hauled some distance from the poultry. Sunlight and soil activity combine over a long period to destroy most pathogens. Anything that can be done to aid the destruction process is helpful. Removal of organic residues such as leaf beds and manure accumulations helps to reduce the danger for future broods. It is best to rotate the ranges or dirt yards so they stand idle for one complete flock cycle.

WASHING AND DISINFECTING. Once the litter or cage droppings have been removed, cleaning and transfer equipment, feeders, waterers, egg-collecting equipment, walls, floors, roosts or cages, outside concrete or suspended runs, and entries to buildings should be washed thoroughly and disinfected. If the supply of water is limited and washing is not possible, dry cleaning may suffice, if it is thorough and includes scraping and sweeping or vacuuming surfaces, corners, ledges, nests, and feeders. The amount of disinfectant used on dry-cleaned surfaces must be increased over that required for washed surfaces.

If possible to do so efficiently, it is preferable to clean the house without removing equipment. If not, all portable equipment should be removed, soaked with water, then thoroughly washed and dried. A high-pressure water hose is effective. Equipment that cannot be removed should be washed in place and then the entire inside building surface washed clean. If the building has been constructed to facilitate good cleaning, it can be done easily. If not, satisfactory cleaning may not be accomplished at all or only with great effort and expense. A large concrete apron equipped with racks and a high-pressure hose is a good place to clean and stack equipment.

After washing, disinfection is in order (see Disinfectants). There are many good disinfectants sold under trade names; follow the manufacturers' recommendations. The important thing is that the surfaces be clean before application. Disinfectants applied to dirt-encrusted surfaces are ineffective and wasted. Not only are they inactivated by organic material in the dirt, but they never reach the infectious agents beneath it. Thorough washing removes most infectious agents from the house and equipment and leaves a clean surface so the disinfectant can reach those that remain. Two to 4 wk of idleness or "downtime" before a new flock is moved in is additional insurance against carry-over of disease. However, downtime should be considered as an adjunct to, and not a substitute for, thorough cleaning, washing, and disinfection.

BUILT-UP LITTER AND UNCLEANED BUILDINGS. Commercial producers demand chicks and poults that are free of pathogenic microbial agents acquired through egg transmission or from unsanitary hatchery or delivery environments. To maintain this status, it is preferable to place these healthy new flocks in cleaned and disinfected buildings with fresh clean litter. Providing these ideal conditions is expensive because of labor and litter costs. Also, suitable litter materials are becoming less plentiful. In keeping with the constant necessity to reduce production costs and cope with shortages, rearing of several successive flocks on the same (built-up) litter has become an economically acceptable practice with broilers, where the life span is very short and single ages of birds per farm permit complete depopulation at the end of each brood. Commercial producers recognize, however, that cleaning and disinfecting a house or group of houses may become necessary any time excessive economic losses are attributable to a disease that may carry over to the next brood.

The practice of reusing litter is much less attractive for rearing egg-production flocks where the life span usually exceeds 18 mo; it is not acceptable for rearing breeding flocks that produce hatching eggs for new generations. In any case, those who reuse litter should be fully aware of the possible hazards involved and should follow other sound disease control practices to minimize the dangers.

When old litter must be reused, it is good insurance to remove any caked or excessively fouled litter, accumulated feathers, and decomposed carcasses. A layer of fresh clean litter should then be placed under the heating brooders and over the area to which the young will be confined or will spend most of their time the first week or two of life. One disadvantage of multiple brooding on the same litter is the excessive dust that accumulates. Inhalation of the dust provides an avenue of entry to the respiratory tract for bacteria and fungal spores.

HATCHERY MANAGEMENT. The building and equipment in which the fertile egg is converted to a day-old chick, poult, or other fowl and the equipment used to process and deliver it to the farm must be clean and sanitary. An individual hatched from a pathogen-free egg will remain pathogen-free only if it hatches in a clean hatcher, is put in a clean box and held in a clean room where it can breathe clean air, and then is hauled to the farm in a clean delivery van.

Design and Location. A hatchery should be located away from sources of poultry pathogens such as poultry farms, processing plants, necropsy laboratories, rendering plants, and feed mills. It is not good practice to retail poultry equipment and supplies from a hatchery building, since this draws producers and service workers who may introduce contaminating material.

A good hatchery design has a one-way traffic flow from the egg-entry room through egg traying, incubation, hatching, and holding rooms to chick-loading area. The cleanup area and hatch-waste discharge should be off the hatching room, with a separate load-out area. Each hatchery room should be designed for thorough washing and disinfecting. The ventilation system is equally important and must be designed to prevent recirculation of contaminated and dust-laden air. Gentry et al. (15) found that hatcheries with poor floor designs and faulty traffic patterns were highly contaminated compared to those with one-way flow.

Importance of Good Sanitation. Factors that aid in obtaining pathogen-free chicks and poults are hatchery cleanliness and sanitation, well-arranged traffic flow, and well-controlled ventilation. Techniques have been devised for evaluating the sanitary status of commercial hatcheries by culturing fluff samples (49), detecting microbial populations in hatchery air samples (9, 15, 26), and culturing various surfaces in the hatchery (28). By relating results of these techniques to hatchery management, it has been observed by Magwood (27) that bacterial counts of eggshells dropped quickly in clean air and low counts persisted on all surfaces to completion of hatching. Chute and Barden (8) found fungal flora of hatcheries to be related to management and sanitation programs.

To minimize bacterial contamination of eggs and hatching chicks, hatchery premises must be kept free of reservoirs of contamination, which readily become air-borne (27). Trays used for hatching should be thoroughly cleaned with water and then disinfected before eggs are placed in them. This can be done by dipping in a tank of suitable disinfectant (see Disinfectants), washing with hot water or steam followed with disinfectant spray, or fumigating with formaldehyde in the hatcher. Trays and eggs are frequently fumigated together immediately after eggs are transferred to the hatcher. Fumigation is sometimes done during the hatch (at about 10% hatch), but concentrations low enough to avoid harming the hatching chick probably serve only to give the down a pleasing yellow color. Formaldehyde fumigation in one case increased the severity of mold infection rather than overcoming it (50). Wright (47) emphasized the practical meaning of hatchery sanitation and how to attain it. He concluded that no fumigation program should be used to replace cleanliness but rather to supplement it.

As chicks hatch, the exposed embryo fluids collect bacteria from contaminated shells, trays, and ventilating air. The combination of the nutritious fluids and warm temperature forms an excellent environment for bacteria, and they multiply very rapidly (15). The cleaner the air and environment to begin with, the more the bacterial buildup is delayed and, as the hatch progresses, the less likely is the navel to become infected (omphalitis).

BREEDER CODES. The breeder code is a designation used to denote the source of hatching eggs. It usually denotes breeders of the same age on the same or different farms, all breeders on a particular farm, or any other grouping. There is a tendency to keep breeders in larger flocks and to avoid as much as is practical the mixing of hatching eggs from flocks of many different microbial, nutritional, and genetic backgrounds. If breeders are kept free of disease and fed a good ration, hatching eggs are produced clean and properly disinfected, and chicks are hatched and handled in clean surroundings, keeping chicks of different breeder codes separated has little practical meaning other than providing all with more nearly the same level of maternal antibodies against the same diseases. This may permit a more uniform response to vaccines applied to chicks the first 2–3 wk of life when maternal antibodies have a protective effect.

Occasionally a disease is believed to be egg transmitted from a breeder flock to the offspring. When this occurs, the disease nearly always appears in several offspring flocks derived from the same breeder flock(s) and delivered to different farms. On the other hand, a hatch of chicks is frequently divided into deliveries to several farms and a disease occurs in only those delivered to one farm. This indicates that the disease is farm associated and not hatchery or breeder-flock associated.

CHICK SEXERS. Unless the output of one hatchery is so great as to demand their full time, chick sexers may go from one hatchery to another, which introduces the possibility of carrying disease. Most sexers are aware of this hazard and are eager to follow proper procedures. If sexers must also service other hatcheries, facilities should be provided so that their equipment can remain at the hatchery. They should have a clean area in which to change clothes and wash themselves and their equipment and should have clean protective garments to wear. Their habits should be at least as clean as those of the hatchery crew.

FLOCK MANAGEMENT

Handling the Young. Chicks and poults hatch with a reserve food supply in unabsorbed yolk sufficient to sustain them for about 72 hr. Some offspring actually hatch 1 or 2 days before they are taken from the hatcher; therefore, they should receive feed and water as soon as possible, preferably within 24 hr after removal.

BROODER TEMPERATURE. Chilling, overheating, starvation, and dehydration are serious stress producers and can precipitate active disease from latent infections that might otherwise be overcome by the young without detectable symptoms. In a randomly split hatch of chicks from the same group of dams, those delivered to one farm can suffer much greater mortality than those delivered to others. This is associated with differences in environmental stresses and exposure to disease. Young chicks and poults should be kept at a comfortable temperature at all times. The brooder temperature is usually started at 35 C and gradually reduced as the birds mature. While thermometers are helpful, strict adherence to thermometer temperatures without regard to obvious discomfort of chicks or poults is poor practice. An uncomfortable bird lets the caretaker know about it. Its peeping should be heeded and the cause of discomfort corrected regardless of thermometer reading.

COCCIDIOSTATS AND OTHER DRUGS. Floor-reared poultry receive coccidiostatic drugs in feed from the first day to prevent coccidiosis (broilers, turkeys, replacement pullets destined for cage adult housing) or to keep the disease under control until birds develop active immunity (breeder flocks, replacement pullets destined for floor adult housing).

However, immunity depends on a number of factors. The amount of feed and coccidiostat intake may vary among birds, and the number of viable sporulated oocysts will vary with differing humidity, temperature, and litter conditions, even in different areas of large buildings. Depending on the relationship of these variable factors, the coccidial infection may be too mild to elicit good immunity, or it may be so severe that a frank outbreak occurs. There is no special management formula to overcome this dilemma other than a keen awareness of the variable factors and an attempt to maintain the proper physical environment to favor the degree of infection desired (see Chapter 33).

FEED AND WATER CONSUMPTION AND MEDICATION. Scientific feed formulation is the business of highly trained nutrition experts, and quality feeds are the rule, not the exception. However, poultry eat the feed, not the formula, and occasionally problems do arise that are traceable to feed (accidental omission of an ingredient, low-potency vitamin supplement, moldy or toxic contamination of an ingredient).

More important in everyday disease control are variations in feed consumption associated with hot or cold weather; housing changes, breed, type, strain, and age of bird; body weight; rate of lay; energy and fiber content of feed; and particle size of feed ingredients. With a 10–20% lower feed consumption associated with one of these factors, there is also a comparably lower intake of coccidiostat or other medicament in feed. Conversely, an increase in total feed consumption as a result of one of these factors increases total intake of all feed ingredients, including drugs.

Increased water intake during hot weather can spell disaster through overconsumption of water medication, but a given concentration of a drug in water may fail to control a disease under circumstances where consumption is very low, as in very cold weather. Also, if natural sources of water are available, particularly for range turkeys, the intake by some birds from the trough may be light. Many are the tragedies from overdosing due to carelessness; miscalculation; or failure to consider feed and water intake, weather, and other variables. When drugs are used in feed, great care should be exercised in adding the same or other drugs to water.

IMMUNIZATION. Some diseases are so ubiquitous and easily and rapidly spread that it is possible to avoid them only with extreme precautions, and little can be done to alter the course of an outbreak should it occur. Yet prevention through vaccination is relatively harmless and inexpensive. This is particularly true of Marek's disease, infectious bursal disease, Newcastle disease, infectious bronchitis, and avian encephalomyelitis. For these diseases, vaccination at the appropriate time is good common sense and a means of preventing spread of virulent forms.

Encounters with virulent and devastating disease agents have become less frequent. Reliance on emergency drug treatments has declined as a result of increased knowledge of diseases, widespread saturation of the poultry population with mild and attenuated immunizing agents, elimination of egg-borne diseases, improved genetic resistance to disease, and improved health-protecting management practices. As a consequence, minor health improvements have become more significant.

SURGICAL PROCEDURES. Beak trimming is commonly practiced on growing flocks, particularly those destined for cages as adults. When this is done properly there is no serious adverse effect. However, proper beak trimming is more an art than a science, and many birds are permanently handicapped when it is not done properly.

If the operation is done correctly, after the beak tip is removed, the remaining growing tip is cauterized sufficiently with the hot cutter blade to prevent bleeding and regrowth but not so much that the bird develops a sensitive or grotesque beak that interferes with eating and drinking. Proper beak trimming promotes maximum performance. Done improperly, it is probably the greatest single management cause of unsatisfactory performance of laying and breeding stock. Poor performance resulting from improper beak trimming must not be attributed to some mysterious disease. For more detail on cannibalism and beak trimming see Chapter 34. Likewise, other surgical procedures such as removing wattles, combs, or toenails of certain toes must be done by one trained in the procedure if harm to the bird is to be avoided.

Adult Flocks. Modern laying strains are bred for high egg production and broiler stocks for rapid growth and good feed conversion. The most important management factor is maintaining feed, water, and environmental conditions at the optimum condition for hen comfort, which in turn results in maximum efficient production and growth. The same is required of meat birds, turkeys, and other types of breeder hens. The egg production or efficiency of feed use will be a good indicator of the success of the management and the welfare of the flock. Many conditions arise that hamper performance, and it is important not only to keep disease out but to prevent conditions from causing discomfort.

BREEDER-FLOCK MANAGEMENT.

Breeder flocks should be managed so that egg-borne diseases are prevented by whatever techniques are available.

Diet, Health, Parental Immunity. A breeder ration must contain a higher level of many nutrients than does a laying ration. Laying rations sufficient to sustain egg production are not always adequate to sustain good hatchability and health of young offspring. Many times, production is satisfactory in breeder hens, but their embryos or chicks show symptoms and lesions of vitamin deficiency. The breeder ration must be adequate for development of the embryo and the chick as well as performance of the breeder hen.

Breeder hens in poor health for any reason frequently fail to supply the embryo with some vital nutritional factor or perhaps pass some toxic material to the egg; thus, the hatch is poor or chicks are of low quality and must be culled. While this occasionally happens with apparently healthy birds also, a healthy breeder flock is the best insurance of good-quality offspring. Holding hatching eggs too long or under improper storage temperature, humidity, and environment can result in poor-quality chicks.

Baby poultry are delivered into many types of environment. In some areas husbandry methods are such that birds are exposed to disease from the first day of life. In some cases, exposure of very young poultry lacking any maternal antibodies to a disease can lead to significant mortality or economic loss (infectious bronchitis, avian encephalomyelitis, infectious bursal disease, duck virus hepatitis). Where exposure is apt to occur at a very early age, maternal antibody can be a significant aid to prevention of disease. On the other hand, a high level of maternal antibodies can interfere with early immunization. How much maternal immunity is desirable and against how many diseases are debatable subjects and will vary according to the area where poultry are raised and type of rearing facility (cage vs. floor).

Maternal immunity is dissipated gradually and usually does not last more than 2–4 wk after hatch. In modern, well-run layer and breeder replacement-rearing facilities, chicks and poults are well protected, not only against the elements but also against introduction of disease from outside sources, for several weeks or beyond the time that a high initial maternal immunity would be protective. Maternal immunity in chicks is of less concern in such cases. This is not so likely to be true of inadequately sanitized and poorly managed pullet-rearing or broiler grow-out farms where exposure can occur as early as the first day of life to a disease agent carried over from the previous brood in reused built-up litter. In these cases protective maternal antibodies become a very important consideration in preventing disease or reducing losses; vaccinating breeder dams with killed vaccines to give high maternal antibody protection for the offspring has become common practice. Lesions and residues from the carrier for killed vaccines injected into the breast muscle has been cause for carcass condemnation at slaughter.

Interior Egg-borne Diseases. Various techniques are used for preventing disease agents from being transmitted from dam to offspring via the egg. The ideal situation is to have breeders free of all pathogens. For most viral diseases there is still no practical way of obtaining this utopian situation. For others (avian encephalomyelitis) the probability of the infection occurring during the egg-laying period with resultant egg transmission is too great to permit the clean but susceptible status (see Chapter 20).

IMMUNIZATION. In addition to immunization of breeders against several common diseases to prevent adverse effects of inopportune infections on egg production, they are immunized against avian encephalomyelitis during the growing period to ensure that they do not become naturally infected during the period they are producing hatching eggs. While this may not be an absolute guarantee against egg transmission of the virus, it has been a practical means of preventing its serious dissemination through infected offspring. Reluctance to use the vaccine in breeder flocks only encourages this type of dissemination.

TESTING AND REMOVAL OF CARRIERS. Carriers of some transovarially transmitted diseases can be detected by serologic means, and this procedure has been used to eliminate possible egg shedders from breeding flocks. This has proved most successful for pullorum disease and fowl typhoid. The method has been so effective that its application in infected breeder flocks, along with management techniques, has been largely responsible for eradication of these diseases from most commercial poultry enterprises in the USA and many other countries.

TESTING AND SLAUGHTER OF INFECTED FLOCKS. Where infected breeders are detected, the entire flock may be discarded. This method is indicated where testing is not likely to detect all infected birds. It is a costly procedure and not warranted unless there is a definite advantage for the offspring and reasonable assurance that they will not become infected from other sources after delivery to the farm. It has been used successfully for eliminating mycoplasma-infected turkey and chicken breeder flocks.

DESTRUCTION OF AGENT INSIDE THE EGG. A pressure differential between the atmosphere and the inside of the egg has been used to force antibiotics through the shell of incubating eggs to prevent transmission of pathogenic mycoplasmas from dam to offspring. This is done by dipping warm eggs into cold antibiotic solutions or using special vacuum machines (2). Antibiotics have also been injected directly into eggs for this purpose (30).

Elevating the egg temperature has also been used to destroy mycoplasmas inside the egg (51). In this procedure incubator temperature (and internal egg temperature) is gradually raised over a 12- to 14-hr period to the maximum embryo survival temperature, approximately 46.9 C, and then cooled immediately and rapidly to normal incubation temperatures. The procedure usually lowers hatchability.

TREATMENT OF OFFSPRING. Offspring from infected dams may be treated with high levels of antibiotics by injection or feeding or both. This is unreliable but can be a significant adjunct to other methods and can greatly assist in overcoming economic losses from egg-transmitted diseases that are drug sensitive.

Eggshell-borne Diseases. Several procedures are used to overcome shell contamination that arises from intestinal contents and other environmental sources. Control involves preventing shell contamination or destroying organisms before they penetrate the shell.

Egg penetration by bacteria occurs more readily if the shell becomes porous. This occurs in the late life of the breeder hen or when there is a deficiency or imbalance between calcium, phosphorus, and Vitamin D. Respiratory virus infections can also result in porous and poor shells.

MANAGEMENT OF HATCHING EGGS

Clean Hatching Eggs. Very dirty eggs should not be used for hatching. If they must be used, they should be dry-cleaned when gathered. The cleaner the shell surface, the less likelihood there will be for bacterial contamination and shell penetration.

The most important consideration in hatching-egg sanitation is to manage the flock so that eggs are clean when gathered. Many factors enter into accomplishing this goal. Sloping wire-bottom roll-away nests with or without automatic collecting devices generally result in clean eggs and a minimum of bacterial contamination.

Clean eggs can also be produced in conventional box-type nests if nesting material is diligently kept clean by continually replacing soiled material. Egg breakage can be reduced by providing sufficient nests for the peak laying period.

The number of floor and yard eggs can be reduced by proper design and location of nests when maturing pullets need them; location and design will vary with the type of house. Nests should be darkened and ventilated, and hens must be prevented from roosting in them at night because they contaminate the area with fecal deposits.

Keeping the litter dry is an aid in preventing soiled nests and nest material. Proper design and construction of the breeder house to create conditions conducive to keeping litter dry aids disease control at the hatching-egg level. Table-egg breeding stock performs satisfactorily in litterless housing, either all slat or sloping wire-floor houses, and this largely eliminates dirty eggs resulting from tracking litter and feces into the nests. Heavy breeds and turkeys do not perform as well on these floors, so combinations of part slat and part litter are used to aid in litter management.

Measures should be taken to prevent salmonella infections by using salmonella-free feed ingredients particularly meat meal, elimination of these pathogens from mixed feed (pelleting), keeping feed clean by good feeding practices and storage facilities, and keeping natural carriers (rodents, wild birds, pets) out of pens and houses. Preventing salmonellosis and other types of enteric infections also helps prevent wet droppings which contributed to wet litter.

Above all, eggs should be gathered frequently, especially in the early part of the day when most hens visit the nests. They should be gathered in clean, dry equipment and held in a dry, dust-free area.

Fumigation of Eggs. The shell surface of hatching eggs should be disinfected immediately after gathering (on-farm fumigation) (see Fig. 1.26). If fumigation cannot be done on the farm, it should be done as soon as possible thereafter, preferably before eggs enter the hatchery building or at the entrance to the egg-processing area. The more delayed the fumigation, the less effective it is because the bacteria will have had longer to penetrate the shell. Unfumigated eggs raise the possibility of carrying some serious infection into the hatchery when susceptible newly hatched chicks are present (see DISINFECTANTS, FORMALDEHYDE).

Washing and Liquid Sterilization. Washing eggs with warm detergent solution at a temperature (43–51.8 C) always higher than that of the eggs entering the washing machine—at least 16.6 C higher but not to exceed 54 C—followed by sanitizing the shells with a chlorine compound, quarternary ammonia product, or other sanitizing agent is routine for commercial eggs. The procedure has been employed successfully with hatching eggs, but some real disasters have occurred where thousands of eggs were contaminated rather than sanitized when dirty water was used, especially in recirculating washing machines. Even if eggs are washed properly, very dirty eggs should be cleaned first by sanding to prevent excessive pollution of the washing solution and equipment. If the iron content of the wash water exceeds 5 ppm, it favors multiplication of certain types of bacteria and creates a serious egg spoilage problem.

If egg washing is done, it should be only with a type of machine (brush conveyor type using flow-through wash water principle) that will ensure against contamination with dirty wash or rinse water. Very careful supervision is also necessary to see that all equipment is working properly at all times and is cleaned daily. In some types of machines, if the washing system fails, a few eggs can contaminate the water and thus contaminate thousands of others before the problem is detected and corrected. Contaminated eggs in the incubator set off a chain reaction of egg explosions that contaminate surrounding eggs, causing more "exploders" and more contamination. While washing and liquid sterilization of hatching eggs can be done satisfactorily, the procedure is subject to operational difficulties and should not be attempted on a routine basis without full knowledge of the hazards involved.

Whenever cold eggs are moved into a warm, humid atmosphere, moisture condenses on the cold shells (called "sweating"). This moisture provides a medium for growth of bacteria and fungi already present on dirty or unsanitized shells or originates in contaminated warm air around the eggs. Cold eggs should therefore be warmed to room temperature in clean, low-humidity air before placing in an incubator.

STORAGE FACILITIES. After fumigation or other shell sterilization, hatching eggs are frequently stored in a cool room (about 10 C) at the hatchery until set. Cool rooms should be clean and free of mold and bacteria and periodically disinfected to prevent recontamination of shells. Clinical histories indicate that infection in young chicks may sometimes be traceable to fungus-contaminated hatching eggs; infections have been produced experimentally by contaminating shells with fungus spores (50). See Chapter 3 for additional discussion on egg-handling procedures to control salmonellae.

Because of possible health considerations from inhalation of formaldehyde fumes, hatchery workers should be alert for any new and effective shell sterilization compounds and methods which may become available.

HANDLING DISEASE OUTBREAKS

Observe the Normal. Good poultry producers watch feed and water consumption and egg production at all times, but more important, they observe normal sounds and actions of the flock. They sense immediately when any of these conditions are abnormal and interpret them as signs of abnormal health. When this happens, it should be assumed that an infectious disease has gained entry and may be tracked elsewhere during the investigation period. In a modern factory like poultry operation, any disease creates serious disruption in the economical operation of the farm and the plants processing products from it. Serious infectious diseases can create havoc. The following steps should be followed when disease is suspected.

Look for Noninfectious Conditions. Take precautions against tracking an infectious disease that may be present, but investigate management errors immediately. A high percentage of so-called disease problems referred to laboratories for diagnosis are noninfectious conditions related to management: beak trimming errors; consumption of litter and trash; feed and water deprivation; chilling of chicks; injury from rough handling, automatic equipment, or drug injection; electrical failures; cannibalism; smothering; overcrowding; poor arrangement of feeders, waterers, and ventilators; inexpensive low-quality feed ingredients; ingredients causing feed refusal; improper particle size of feed ingredients; and rodent and predator attacks (1, 7). Zander observed a severe drop in egg production in a pathogen-free flock after a 48-hr failure of a mechanical feeder (52). Bell (6) observed marked reduction in lay from water deprivation related to a beak trimming system that resulted in long lower beaks, making it difficult to obtain water when the level was low. These are conditions that do not require services of a diagnostic laboratory. External parasites (mites, lice, ticks) can be determined by producers if they examine affected birds.

Quarantine the Flock. In the event that no management factors can be found, the next step is to set up a quarantine of the pen, building, farm unit area, or entire farm, depending upon its design and programming. If this emergency was anticipated when the farm was laid out and programmed originally, the quarantine will be a minor problem. If the basic principle of "a single age in quarantinable units" was disregarded in original farm planning, a disease outbreak can be an economic disaster. Separate caretakers should be established for affected birds, or at least sick ones should be visited last.

SUBMIT SPECIMENS OR CALL A VETERINARIAN. The owner or caretaker should submit typical specimens to a diagnostic laboratory or call a veterinarian to visit the farm and establish the diagnosis. Owners should seek professional diagnosis rather than trying to hide some disease because of possible public recrimination. Veterinarians and caretakers can and should help dispel this apprehension by maintaining high ethical standards and refraining from discussing one producer's problems with others. Yet there comes a time when all producers must be apprised of a problem. Service workers are frequently requested to examine the flock, select specimens for the laboratory, and initiate first-aid procedures until the veterinarian can be called or visited. If so, they should wear protective footwear and clothing when they enter the house. No other farm should be visited en route to the laboratory.

DIAGNOSIS. It is important to get a diagnosis as soon as possible. The course of action will be determined by the nature of the disease. A producer should not procrastinate for any reason when a disease threatens, or it may get completely out of hand before a diagnosis is made. It is not always possible to treat a disease or check its deleterious effects; but to plan effectively for the future, it is important to identify any and all diseases that occur. A veterinarian should also be aware of the owner's economic plight at such times and render advice and assistance as quickly as information is available or a judgement can be made.

SPECIAL PRECAUTIONS. In addition to causing serious losses in poultry, some diseases (ornithosis, erysipelas, fungal infections) are especially hazardous for humans. When these conditions are suspected or diagnosed, extra precautions must be taken to ensure against human infection. The proper government health authorities should be notified of ornithosis outbreaks, and all handling and processing personnel should be apprised of the disease, hazards, and necessary precautions.

In some states, certain diseases (salmonellosis, ornithosis, laryngotracheitis) must be reported immediately to the state animal disease control authorities so that proper investigation and action can be taken to protect the human population and the poultry industry. Common sense dictates that when a condition suggestive of an exotic disease such as velogenic viscerotropic Newcastle disease, fowl typhoid, or avian influenza is encountered, the proper regulatory authorities should be informed.

Nursing Care. Whether the flock consists of a few hundred individuals or tens of thousands, nursing care plays an important role in the outcome of disease. Additional heat should be supplied to young chicks that begin huddling because of sickness. Clean and fresh (or medicated) water should be available at close range. Temporary, more accessibly located waterers are sometimes necessary during sickness. If water founts are normally located where chickens must jump onto some raised device or turkeys must cross through hot sunlight to reach them, the sick will not have the energy or initiative to seek water. They will soon become dehydrated, an early step on the road to death. Turkey yards should be well drained because birds tend to drink from the closest puddles, which may be thoroughly polluted.

The same principles are true for feed. Sick birds can be encouraged to eat if the caretaker will proceed through the house stirring feed and rattling feed hoppers or adding small quantities of fresh feed. Sometimes a little molasses in feed or water (1 pt/gal) will encourage consumption. Some antibiotics appear to stimulate feed consumption when included in the diet. However, any additive that proves distasteful to the birds should be removed immediately.

Sometimes birds become so depressed and moribund that the caretaker must walk among them frequently to rouse them so they will eat or drink.

Hopelessly sick and crippled birds should be killed in a manner to preclude or control the discharge of blood or exudates (see Diagnostic Procedures). Dead and destroyed birds should be disposed of immediately (see Carcass Disposal).

DRUGS. No drugs should be given until a diagnosis is obtained or a veterinarian consulted. If the wrong drug is given, it can be a useless waste of money, or it may be harmful or even disastrous. If an infectious disease is found and corrective drugs are indicated, they should be used very carefully according to directions.

Strict regulations govern use of drugs in mixed feeds for food-producing animals. For information, write to the U. S. Food and Drug Administration (FDA), 200 C Street SW, Washington DC 20204. A handy reference is the annually updated *Feed Additive Compendium* published by Miller Publishing Co., Minneapolis MN. Feed manufacturers must have FDA clearance to include most drugs in mixed feeds. When treated flocks are to be marketed, a specified period (depending on the drug used) must follow cessation of treatment to allow dissipation of drug residues from tissues before slaughter. If the flock is producing table eggs when treated, the drug must be one permitted for use in laying flocks, or eggs must be discarded during, and for varying lengths of time after, treatment, a costly alternative.

If the flock is producing hatching eggs when it becomes infected and there is danger that egg transmission of the infectious agent from dams to offspring may occur (salmonellosis, mycoplasmosis, avian encephalomyelitis), eggs should not be used for hatching until danger has passed. It should also be kept in mind that in fertile eggs residues of drugs used to treat breeders may occasionally cause abnormalities in some embryos.

DISPOSITION OF THE FLOCK. The flock should not be moved or handled until it has recovered, unless the move is to a more favorable environment as part of the therapy. After treatment, if any, has been completed and the flock appears to be completely healthy, it may be marketed or moved to permanent quarters if such a move is part of the management program. Some healthy carriers may remain. If the flock is moved to another depopulated farm, this will present no problem except that occasionally a disease may flare up from stress of handling and moving. If the recovered flock is moved to a multiple-age farm, carriers can introduce the disease into susceptible flocks already there. If the recovered flock is already in permanent quarters having multiple ages, newly introduced flocks may be exposed and contract the disease, a common occurrence, especially with respiratory and litter-borne diseases.

DIAGNOSTIC PROCEDURES.

There are many satisfactory diagnostic and necropsy methods. The techniques and instruments used by one pathologist may vary considerably from those used by another. Some suggestions are offered here to guide the student and beginner. The goal of the necropsy is to determine the cause of impaired performance, signs, or mortality by examining tissues and organs and to obtain the best specimens possible to carry out microbiologic, serologic, histopathologic, or animal-inoculation tests. It is important that, in the process, infectious materials do not endanger the health of humans, livestock, or other poultry. By proceeding in an orderly fashion, possible clues are less apt to be overlooked, and tissues will not be grossly contaminated prior to examination. Remember that a blood sample or tissue specimen determined later to be superfluous can always be discarded. It's better to save tissues then discard if they are later determined to be unnecessary or unimportant to the diagnosis.

A key to good poultry diagnosis is the art of "seeing the forest as well as the trees." Try to identify the most significant flock problem(s) rather than becoming engrossed in individual bird disorders. Watch for telltale patterns of pathology as presented by the total diagnostic consignment.

The techniques and procedures necessary to make an accurate diagnosis and identify specific disease agents are found in the technical information contained in succeeding chapters of this book and in the following excellent reference manuals: *A Laboratory Manual for Isolation and Identification of Avian Pathogens* (37), *Avian Disease Manual* (46), *Avian Histopathology* (40), and *Diseases of the Domestic Fowl and Turkey, a Colour Atlas* (38). *Atlas of Avian Hematology* (24) should be consulted for detailed information on avian blood elements and methods for preparation and study. New information is continually being presented in the following journals: *Avian Diseases, Avian Pathology, Poultry Science,* the proceedings of several regional poultry disease conferences, and other avian pathology and science journals.

Anamnesis.

The pathologist who has not seen the farm or the flock before attempting to diagnose the problem and recommend corrective measures is at a disadvantage. This can be partially overcome by getting a complete history of the disease and all pertinent events leading to the outbreak. The more information pathologists have about the history and environment, the more directly they can proceed to solution of problems. Unfortunately, the history includes only the situations, events, and signs that the caretaker, owner, service worker, or neighbor has observed and remembered. Knowledge of management factors such as ventilation; feeding and watering systems, accurate records of egg production, feed consumption, feed formulation, and body weight; lighting program; beak trimming practices; brooding and rearing procedures; routine medication and vaccination used; age; previous history of disease; farm location; and unusual weather or farm events may make the difference between diagnosis of the flock problem and the finding of a few miscellaneous conditions in a sample that may or may not be representative. Duration of the signs, the number sick and dead, and when and where they were found dead can be important clues.

Poultry producers have developed a high degree of knowledge about poultry diseases and usually recognize those resulting in dramatic or clear-cut signs and lesions. The veterinarian, therefore, is often confronted with obscure, undramatic, and complicated disease cases requiring extensive investigation. Even if all indications are that reduced performance is most likely due to a management factor, the veterinarian must check all reasonable disease possibilities. This requires a systematic approach to be sure nothing is overlooked.

External Examination. Look for external parasites. Lice and northern fowl mites (*Ornithonyssus silviarum*) can be found on the affected chicken. If red mites (*Dermanyssus gallinae*) or blue bugs (*Argas persicus*) are suspected, examination of roosting areas and cracks and crevices in the houses and around the yards must be made because these species do not stay on birds. See Chapter 30 for diagnosis and identification of external parasites.

The general attitude of live birds and all abnormal conditions should be carefully noted. It is very important to observe evidence of incoordination, tremors, paralytic conditions, abnormal gait and leg weakness, depression, blindness, and respiratory signs before the specimens are killed. It is very helpful to place birds in a cage where they can be observed after they have become accustomed to the surroundings and perform at their best. It is sometimes advisable to save some of the affected birds to observe possible recovery from a transitory condition (transient paralysis), respiratory infection, chemical toxicity, feed or water deprivation on the farm, or overheating during transport to the laboratory.

Examination should be made for tumors, abscesses, skin changes, beak condition, evidence of cannibalism, injuries, diarrhea, nasal and respiratory discharges, conjunctival exudates, feather and comb conditions, dehydration, and the body fleshing condition. These are all useful clues.

Blood Samples. Blood specimens may be taken at this time (or immediately after the bird is killed). Frequently it is desirable to have two (paired) blood samples several days apart to determine a rising or falling titer of antibodies to some disease (Newcastle disease) in the serum. In this case, a blood specimen may be taken from the main (brachial) wing vein or jugular vein or by heart puncture and the bird saved for a second sample.

Venipuncture of the brachial vein is usually the simplest and best method for obtaining blood from turkeys, chickens, and most fowl under field conditions, especially when the bird is to be returned to the flock. Ducks are bled from the saphenous vein near the hock. Expose the vein to view by plucking a few feathers from the ventral surface of the humeral region of the wing. The vein will be seen lying in the depression between the biceps brachialis and triceps humeralis muscles. It is more easily seen if the skin is first dampened with 70% alcohol or other colorless disinfectant. To facilitate venipuncture, extend both wings dorsally by gripping them firmly together in the area of the wing web with the left hand. Insert the needle into the vein of the right wing holding the syringe in the right hand (Fig. 1.15). The needle should be inserted opposite to the direction of blood flow.

Heart puncture can be made anteromedially between the sternum and metasternum (20), laterally through the rib cage, or anteroposteriorly through the thoracic inlet. Only through experience can one learn exactly where and at what angle to insert the needle. It is best to practice these techniques on freshly killed specimens before attempting to bleed live birds. A general rule for the lateral puncture is to form an imaginary

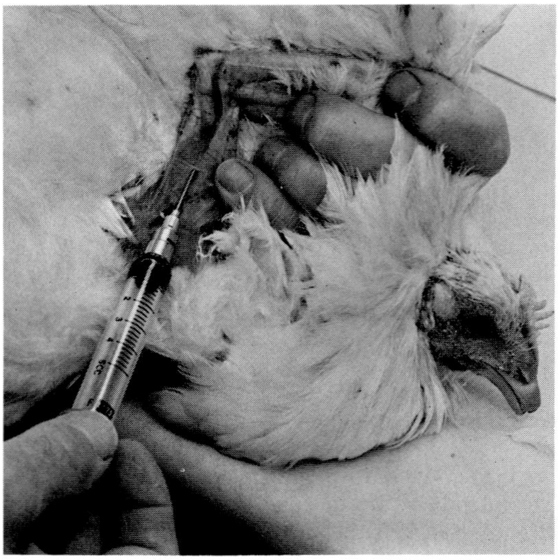

1.15. Obtaining a blood sample from the wing vein.

vertical line at the anterior end, and at a right angle with, the keel, then palpate along that line. The heartbeat can be felt and the needle inserted to the proper depth (Fig. 1.16).

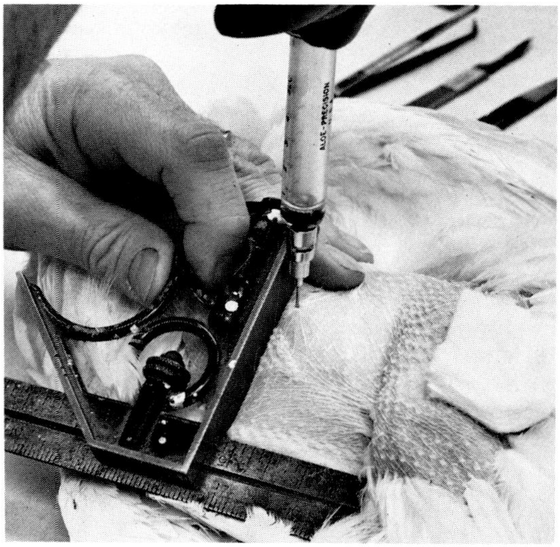

1.16. Approximate location for insertion of the needle for a lateral heart puncture.

For heart puncture through the thoracic inlet, the bird should be held on its back with the keel up. The crop and contents are then pressed out of the way with a finger while the needle is guided along the ventral angle of the inlet. After penetrating the inlet, the needle is directed horizontally and posteriorly along the midline until reaching the heart (Fig. 1.17).

The site for heart puncture between the

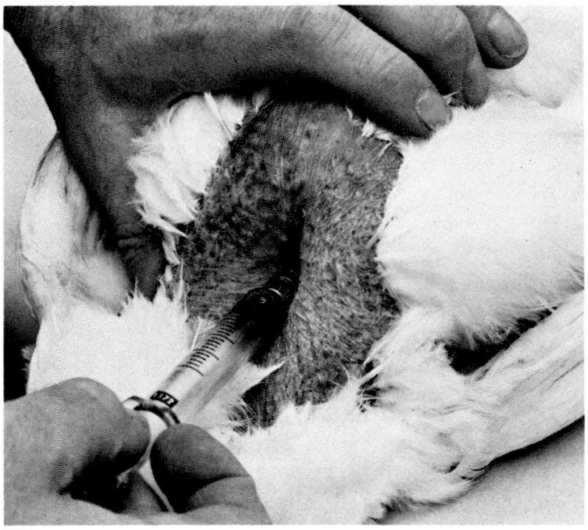

1.17. Heart puncture through the thoracic inlet.

sternum and metasterum is (in a mature chicken) about an inch dorsal and posterior to the anterior point of the keel. The needle is directed at approximately a 45 degree angle in the anteromedial direction toward the opposite shoulder joint. The needle should pass through the angle formed by the sternum and metasternum and directly into the heart (Fig. 1.18). For further details and illustrations, see Hofstad (20).

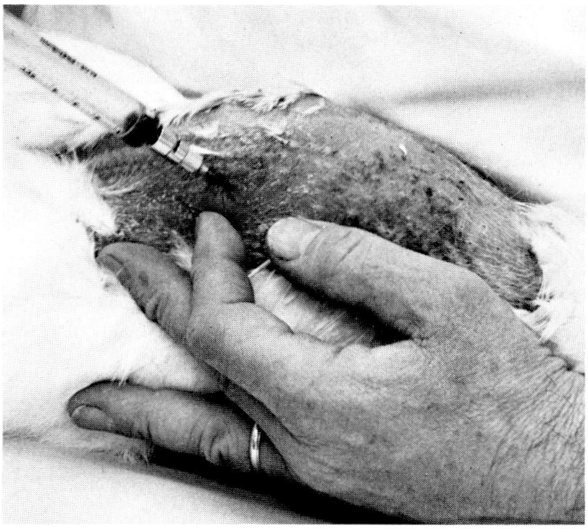

1.18. Heart puncture can be made by inserting the needle between the sternum and metasternum and directing it toward the opposite shoulder joint.

The size and length of the needle required for heart and venipuncture will depend on the size of the bird: for young chicks and poults, a ¾-in. 20-gauge needle; for mature chickens, a 2-in. 20-gauge needle. Mature turkeys may require larger needles. For quick and accurate bleeding, it is essential that the needle be sharp. Very slight vacuum should be developed intermittently to determine when vein or heart puncture has occurred. After vein puncture, steady, slight vacuum should be used to withdraw blood. If vacuum is too great, the vessel wall may be drawn into the needle and plug the beveled opening. It is sometimes necessary to rotate the needle and syringe to be sure the beveled opening is free in the lumen of the vessel.

For most serologic studies, the serum from 2 ml blood is adequate. The blood should be removed aseptically and placed in a clean vial, which is then laid horizontally, or nearly so, until the blood clots. An occasional sample may require a long time to clot. This is especially true of turkey blood. Clotting can be hastened by adding a drop of tissue extract, made by killing and pooling a number of 10- to 12-day-old chicken embryos, grinding in a Waring blender, and freezing for future use. After the clot is firm, the vial may be returned to the vertical position to permit serum to collect in a pool at the bottom. Plastic vials are also available for blood collection. The clot does not adhere to the vial, and special positioning during clotting is unnecessary. Frequently the serum from fat hens will appear milky due to lipids. Placing vials in an incubator will hasten syneresis. A fresh blood sample should never be refrigerated immediately after collection as this will hinder the clotting process. Sera should not be frozen if agglutination tests are to be performed as this frequently causes false-positive reactions.

If an unclotted blood sample is required, it should be drawn into sodium citrate solution at the rate of 1.5 ml 2% solution/10 ml fresh blood or deposited in a vial containing sodium citrate powder at the rate of 3 mg/1 ml whole blood and the mixture quickly shaken. One way to prepare tubes for collecting sterile citrated blood is to add the proper amount of 2% sodium citrate solution to the collecting tubes ahead of time, then sterilize the solution and evaporate the moisture in an oven.

Blood-collecting vials containing the anticoagulant heparin can also be obtained commercially from laboratory supply companies. For certain types of serologic tests, fresh blood can be absorbed on the tips of filter paper strips, dried, and sent to the diagnostic laboratory where antibodies can be recovered for testing by placing pieces of the treated paper into saline solution (Fig. 1.19).

If a blood parasite or blood dyscrasia is suspected, smears of whole blood should be made on clean glass slides previously warmed to promote rapid drying. For staining techniques, see Lucas and Jamroz (24).

A drop of blood for a wet mount or smear may be obtained from very small chicks by pricking the vein on the posteromedial side of the leg or by pricking or cutting the immature comb.

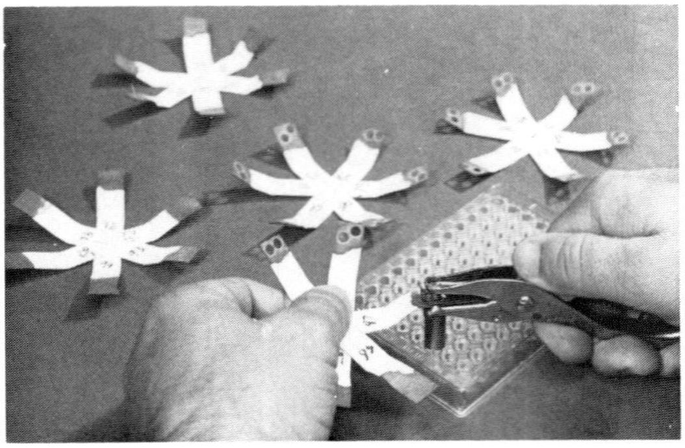

1.19. Blood absorbed on filter paper strips. For antibody testing, serum is recovered by punching out a piece of blood-soaked paper into saline solution. (Beard)

Killing Birds for Necropsy

CERVICAL DISLOCATION. Several methods can be used to kill fowl, and each has certain advantages. The objective is to kill the bird instantaneously so it will not suffer in the process. The quickest way to kill a small bird is to hold both wings over the back with one hand and the head with the other in such a way as to bend the head sharply vertically at the same time it is pulled firmly and quickly forward in a stretching manner (Fig. 1.20). This breaks the neck and spinal cord instantly. Holding both wings prevents agonal flapping and stirring of dust. If the neck is held firmly in the final position until struggling ceases, this prevents agonal regurgitation and aspiration of crop contents into the respiratory passages. Quick cervical luxation, as described, has been considered a humane method of poultry euthanasia by the American Veterinary Medical Association (AVMA) (5).

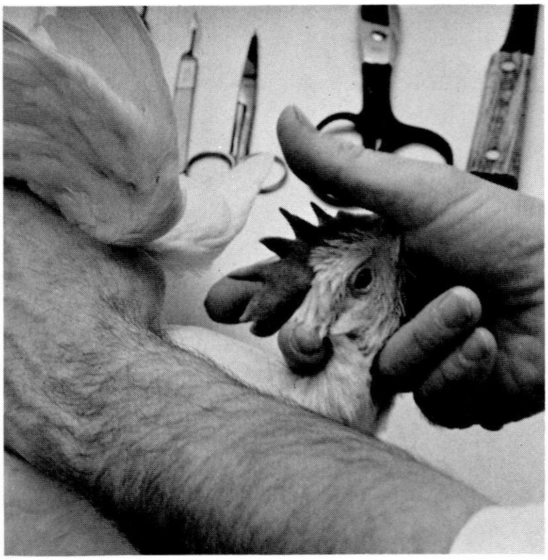

1.20. To kill a small turkey or chicken, grasp wings with one hand and head with the other as shown. Break the neck with one quick pull on the head.

The neck of a young chick can also be broken easily by pressing it firmly against a sharp table edge or by pinching between thumb and index finger or by using the inside, noncutting angles of a surgical scissor as a small burdizzo. Bovine Burdizzo castration forceps can be used for killing large chickens and turkeys. It is difficult for one person to perform this operation and hold the bird at the same time, but it is quite easily done with the aid of an assistant. This technique also prevents agonal regurgitation and aspiration of crop contents into the respiratory passages if the forceps are left clamped until reflex muscle spasms cease.

ELECTROCUTION. Electrocution is a satisfactory method also. Clamps fixed to the end of electrical wires are fastened to the cloaca and mouth (this will assure moist contacts). The wires are then attached by means of a standard plug directly to 110-V alternating house current. A switch is thrown to feed the electric current through the wires. With this system, the bird rarely struggles and thus does not stir up dust or regurgitate crop contents. There is also less danger of agonal hemorrhages occurring or loss of blood when tissue specimens are desired. Obvious hazards to personnel and of short circuits on metal table tops should be recognized.

OTHER. Specimens selected for diagnosis may also be killed by intravenous injection of euthanasic solutions. Another method that would be satisfactory is asphyxiation by placing the specimen in a chamber filled with carbon dioxide (CO_2). Local availability of a CO_2 source may limit utilization of this technique.

Other methods of euthanasia can be found in a report of the AVMA (5). The method selected will depend upon the existing situation: species, size, and number of birds to be necropsied or sacrificed, or tissues, fluids, and cultures to be taken, etc.

Necropsy Precautions. If there is reason to suspect that birds to be necropsied are infected with disease that may be contagious for humans (ornithosis, erysipelas, equine encephalitis), stringent health precautions are essential. The carcass and the necropsy table surface should be wet thoroughly with a disinfectant. Good rubber gloves should be worn, and care should be taken that neither the pathologist nor assistants puncture the skin of their hands or inhale dust or aerosols from tissues or feces. It is advisable to wear a fine-particle respiratory mask to prevent inhalation of contaminated dust. All laboratory personnel who may come in contact with carcasses, tissues, or cultures should be informed of their possible infectious nature and precautions to be taken.

With some notable exceptions (see specific diseases), most commonly encountered poultry disease agents are not considered pathogenic for humans. Nevertheless, it would be wise to wear rubber gloves at all times while performing necropsies, until sufficient experience has been gained to anticipate and recognize possible human health hazards. For a review of poultry diseases in public health, see Galton and Arnstein (14). Examining specimens on metal trays that will fit into an autoclave facilitates quick sterilization of carcasses after necropsy.

Adequate instruments for routine work are necropsy shears to cut bones, enterotome scissors to incise the gut, a necropsy knife to cut skin and muscle, and a scalpel for fine examination of tissues. These should be supplemented with forceps, sterile syringes, needles, vials, and petri dishes for collecting blood samples and tissue specimens as the situation dictates (Fig. 1.21).

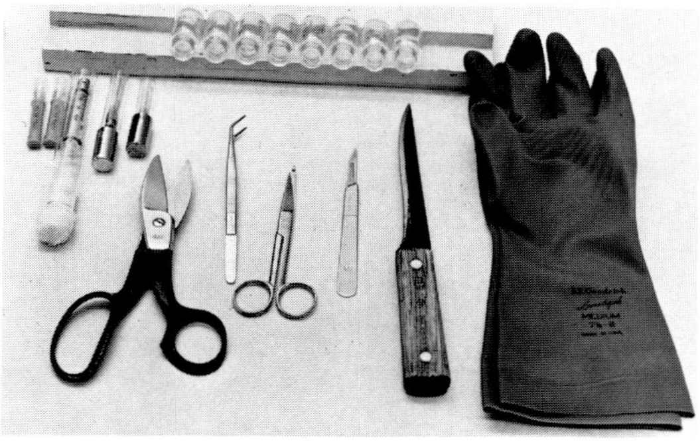

1.21. Instruments and equipment adequate for most necropsies of poultry.

Necropsy Technique. The specimen is laid on its back and each leg in turn is drawn outward away from the body while the skin is incised between the leg and abdomen (Fig. 1.22A). Each leg is then grasped firmly in the area of the femur and bent forward, downward, and outward, until the head of the femur is broken free of the acetabular attachment so that the leg will lie flat on the table.

The skin is cut between the two previous incisions at a point midway between keel and vent. The cut edge is then forcibly reflected forward, cutting as necessary, until the entire ventral aspect of the body, including the neck, is exposed (Fig. 1.22B). Hemorrhages of the musculature, if present, can be detected at this stage.

Either of two procedures is now used to expose the viscera. The necropsy knife is used to cut through the abdominal wall transversely midway between keel and vent and then through breast muscles on each side. Bone shears are used to cut the rib cage and then the coracoid and clavicle on both sides (Fig. 1.22C). With some care, this can be done without severing the large blood vessels. The process may also be done equally well in reverse order, cutting through the clavicle and coracoid and then through the rib cage and abdominal wall on each side. The sternum and attached structures can now be removed from the body and laid aside. The organs are now in full view and may be removed as they are examined (Fig. 1.22D).

If a blood sample has not previously been taken

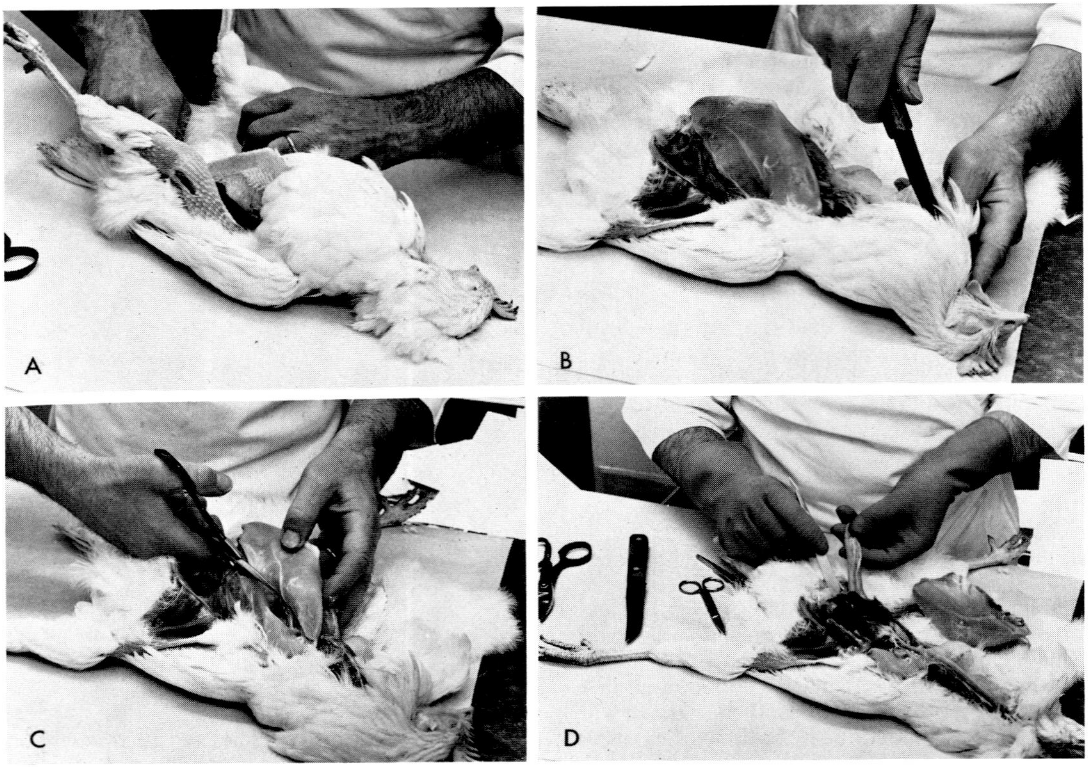

1.22. Pathologists develop their own techniques for necropsy. This technique will aid the beginner. A. Sever skin and fascia between legs and abdomen and break legs out of the acetabular articulation. B. Incise and reflect the skin from vent to beak. C. Remove breast, taking care not to sever large blood vessels. D. Expose viscera for examination.

and the bird was killed just prior to necropsy, a sample can be promptly taken by heart puncture before clotting occurs. Large veins leading into the leg may be incised allowing blood to pool in the region for subsequent collection.

Laboratory Procedures

IMPRESSION SMEARS. If the foregoing procedures have all been done aseptically, the internal organs will not be contaminated; if exudates suggest the need, impression smears with sterile slides can now be taken.

BACTERIAL CULTURES. If gross lesions indicate bacterial cultures are needed, they can be made from unexposed surfaces of the viscera without searing the surface (Fig. 1.23). If contamination has occurred, the surface of the organs should be seared with a hot spatula or other iron designed for that purpose before inserting a sterile culture loop. Care must be taken not to sear and overheat the tissue excessively. It is often desirable to transfer large tissue samples aseptically to a sterile petri dish and take them to the microbiology laboratory for initial culture in cleaner surroundings.

BILE SAMPLES. If infection with a campylobacter is suspected, a bile sample for wet mount examination or bacterial culture can be made at this point.

RESPIRATORY VIRUS ISOLATION. If a respiratory disease is suspected and virus culture or bird passage is desirable, an intact section of lower trachea, the bronchi, and upper portions of the lungs are removed aseptically with sterile scissors and forceps and transferred to a sterile mortar and pestle for grinding or to a sterile petri dish for temporary storage and later grinding. Other tissues (air-sac tissue) can be added aseptically to the sample or transferred to other sterile containers for separate study. The trachea can now be incised; if exudate is present, it can be added to the above collection or saved in separate vials.

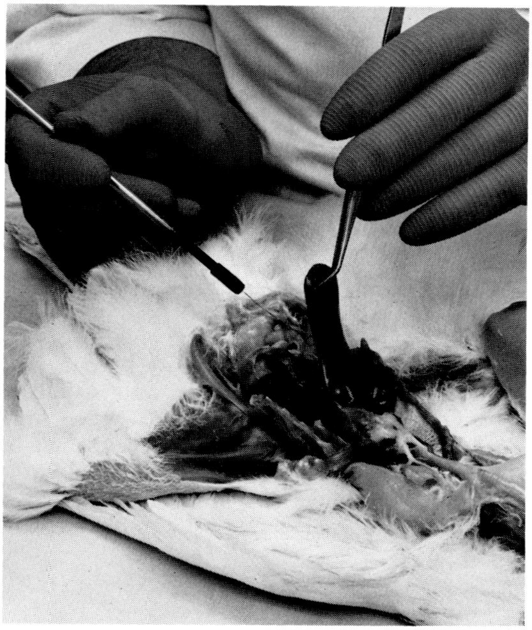

1.23. If the abdominal cavity has been carefully opened, bacterial cultures can be taken from unexposed surfaces of the viscera without fear of extraneous contamination.

Grinding of such specimens is facilitated by adding a portion of sterile sand or, preferably, Alundum (mesh #60) to the mortar contents. Ground tissues are then transferred to sterile covered centrifuge tubes and spun at low speeds to prepare a supernatant fluid free of particulate matter for inoculation into embryos, nutrient media, cell cultures, or experimental birds.

Similar procedures can be followed for initial virus isolation from various parenchymatous organs.

SALMONELLA CULTURES. All other visceral organs should be examined for abnormalities (microabscesses, discoloration, swelling, friability). If abnormalities are observed, inoculum from the affected tissues should be transferred to suitable solid or liquid media for culture before the intestinal tract is opened. Once opened, gross contamination of other organs with gut contents is almost certain to occur. If salmonella infection is suspected, selected sections of the gut are removed with sterile forceps and scissors and placed directly into a sterile mortar and pestle or into a sterile petri dish for later culture. For routine examination, a single section comprising the lower ileum, proximal portions of the ceca and cecal "tonsils," and proximal portion of the large intestine may be used. All are minced and ground aseptically to produce an inoculum. Additional areas of the intestinal tract or tissues of other visceral organs may be added to the gut collection or cultured separately. Alternatively, sterile swabs may be used to obtain samples from the exposed gut lining for salmonella cultures. See Chapter 3 and *A Laboratory Manual for Isolation and Identification of Avian Pathogens* (37) for detailed culture technique.

MISCELLANEOUS. After necessary cultures have been made, the intestine may be laid out on newspaper or tabletop for examination for inflammation, exudates, parasites, foreign bodies, malfunctions, tumors, and abscesses. The various nerves, bone structure, marrow condition, and joints can now be examined. The sciatic nerve can be examined by dissecting away the musculature on the medial side of the thigh. Inside the body cavity, the sciatic plexus is obscured by kidney tissue. These nerves can best be exposed by scraping away the tissue with the blunt end of a scalpel. Nerves of the brachial plexuses are easily found on either side near the thoracic inlet and should be examined for enlargement. Examination of vagus nerves in their entirety should be made, otherwise, short enlargements may be missed.

The ease or difficulty with which bones can be cut with the bone shears is an indication of their condition. The costochondral junctions should be palpated and examined for enlargement ("beading") and the long bones cut longitudinally through the epiphysis to examine for abnormal calcification. Rigidity of the tibiotarsus or metatarsus should be tested by bending and breaking to check for nutritional deficiency. A healthy bone will make an audible snap when it breaks. Bones from a chicken deficient in Vitamin D or minerals may be so lacking in mineral elements that they can be bent at any angle without breaking.

Joint exudate, if present, can be removed after first plucking the feathers and searing the overlying skin with a hot iron. After searing, the skin may be incised with a sterile scalpel and exudate removed with a sterile inoculating loop or swab. Paranasal sinus exudates can be removed and examined in a similar manner.

EXPOSURE AND REMOVAL OF BRAIN. Removing the intact brain is not easy, since meningeal layers are attached firmly to bony structures in some places. The following technique can be performed quickly and is satisfactory for examination and removal of the brain in most instances.

Remove the head at the atlanto-occipital junction and remove the lower mandible. Sear the cut surface and trim away excess loose tissue. Reflect the skin forward over the skull and upper mandible and hold it firmly in that position with one hand. Sterile instruments should be used for the succeeding steps if a portion of the brain is desired for animal inoculation, virus isolation, or fungal or bacterial culture.

With the sterilized tips of heavy-jawed bone shears or strong surgical scissors, nip just through the bone to the cranial cavity on both sides of the head, beginning at the occipital foramen and proceeding forward laterally to the midpoint at the anterior edge of the cranial cavity (Fig. 1.24A). Lift off the cut portion of bone and expose the entire brain (Fig. 1.24B).

If a portion is needed for culture or animal inoculation (e.g., avian encephalomyelitis virus suspect) and also one for histopathologic examination (e.g., vitamin E deficiency), cut the brain medially from anterior to posterior along the midline with a sharp, sterile scalpel and then cut the nerves and attachments carefully from one of the brain halves while the head is tipped upside down, so the loosened portion will fall into a sterile petri dish or mortar and pestle as it is freed (Fig. 1.24C). The second half can now be removed aseptically with sterile, sharp, curved scissors (but without concern for preservation of tissue structure) to a jar of formalin (Fig. 1.24D). Be careful not to contaminate brain tissue intended for virus isolation with instruments that have been in contact with formalin. The separate halves may also be removed in reverse order. If all the brain is required for either purpose, proceed with proper precautions for the purpose intended. If the brain is destined only for sectioning, it may be fixed in situ and then removed. Large brain portions should be incised longitudinally to permit good penetration of fixative.

TISSUES FOR HISTOPATHOLOGIC EXAMINATION. Frequently, stained tissue sections are needed. The quality of the slide is no better than the quality of the specimen and the care taken to preserve it. For good preservation, the tissue pieces should be saved immediately after death from killed birds, especially brain and kidney tissues, which deteriorate rapidly. Specimens should be small to allow

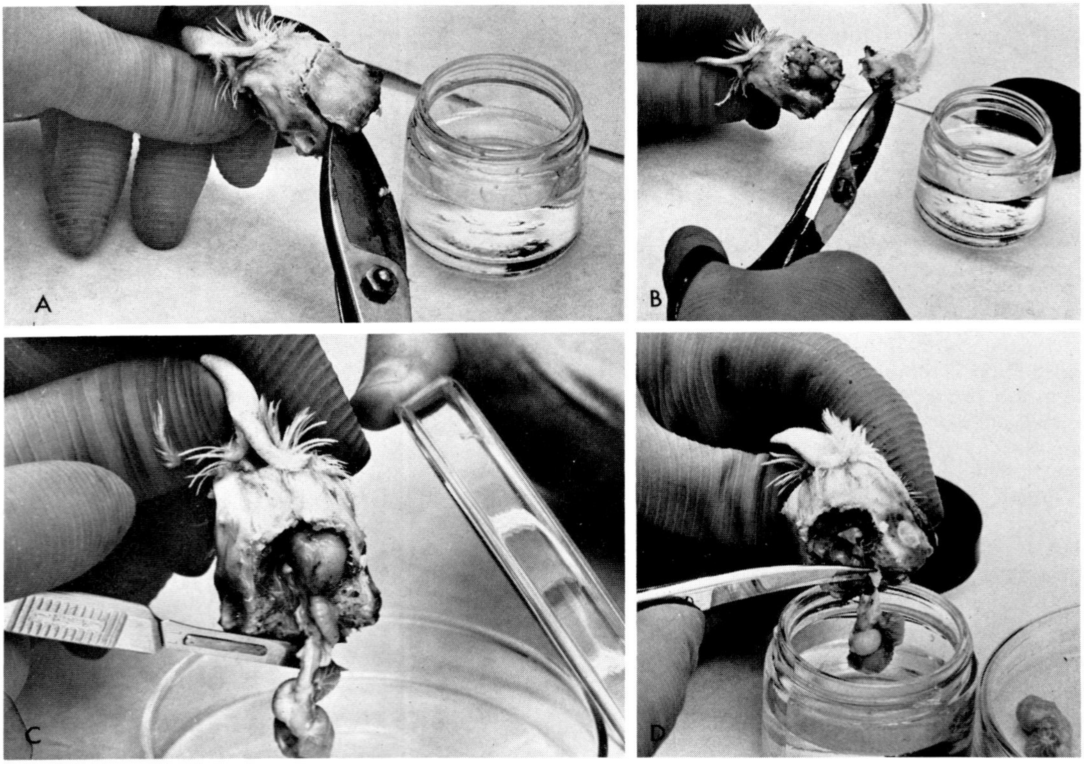

1.24. With a little practice the brain can be removed with a minimum of trauma. A. Incise bone all the way around the periphery of the cranial cavity with heavy bone shears. B. Remove loosened portion of the bony skull. C. Incise brain longitudinally with sterile, sharp scalpel and remove one-half for sterile culture technique. D. Remove second half of brain by dropping it into 10% formalin for histologic techniques.

quick penetration of fixative, gently incised with a sharp scalpel or razor blade to preserve tissue structure, and preserved in 10 times their own volume of 10% formalin or other fixative. Zenker's fixative may be used for all tissues except brain and spinal cord. Bone pieces should be sawed with a sharp bone saw unless thin or soft enough to cut with scissors or scalpel. After proper labeling and dating they should be sent immediately to the processing laboratory.

Lung tissue usually floats on the surface of the fixing solution because of trapped air. Satisfactory fixation can be accomplished by placing absorbent cotton over the tissue, which serves to keep it immersed. Methods to exhaust air from air spaces in lung tissue by creating a vacuum over the fixative can be used but are less satisfactory and may result in artifacts.

After fixing, bone tissue must be decalcified. Nitric acid solution (10 parts nitric acid: 90 parts 70% alcohol) may be used for this purpose; decalcification requires 1 wk or more.

If eye tissue is to be saved for sectioning, a hole should be cut through the scleral wall to allow fixative to quickly penetrate the vitreous body and thus reach the internal eye structures.

Any tissue held too long in formalin fixative becomes excessively hard. If processing is to be delayed, tissues should be transferred to 70% alcohol after 48 hr in fixative. Textbooks on histologic techniques (25, 35, 44) should be consulted for detailed procedures.

PROGRESSIVE EXAMINATION HINTS. The following procedures during the course of necropsy may be helpful to the beginner in checking for some commonly encountered diseases. They are not intended as definitive diagnostic methods. To arrive at a diagnosis, the student and beginning diagnostician must refer to the characteristic signs and lesions, diagnostic procedures, and characteristics of the infectious agent discussed under the specific diseases in succeeding chapters and also to the *Laboratory Manual for Isolation and Identification of Avian Pathogens* (37).

Coccidia. Observe and note the subserosa before incising the intestine. Make wet mount smears of mucosal scrapings from various segments of the intestine and cecal contents and examine directly under the microscope for suspended oocysts and merozoites and stages undergoing development in epithelial cells (tissue stages).

Other Protozoa. Make wet mount smears of affected areas, adding a little warm physiologic saline solution if necessary to provide fluid, and examine under a microscope for hexamita, histomonads, and trichomonads.

Capillarids and Ascarid Larvae. Collect mucous exudate and deep mucosal scrapings and press into a thin layer between two thick pieces of plate glass. Examine before a strong light or under low-power magnification for the presence of parasites. Under magnification, look for double-poled, lemon-shaped eggs in the female capillarids.

Fungi. Make wet mount smears of scrapings of affected areas and add 20% sodium or potassium hydroxide. Digest with frequent warming for 15 min or more and examine under high-power magnification for mold hyphae.

Campylobacters. Examine fresh bile wet mounts under dark-field or phase illumination. Only positive findings may have significance.

Bacteremia and Blood Parasites. Make fresh mounts, preferably with citrated blood, and examine under light- and dark-field illumination for viable organisms. Make fresh blood smears and air dry for staining by Giemsa's, Gram's, Wright's, or other method.

Exudates. If infectious coryza is suspected, make thin smears of clear nasal or sinus exudate for staining by Giemsa's, Gram's, methylene blue, or other method. Inoculate appropriate media or susceptible chickens for isolation of the organism.

Abscesses. Select appropriate culture media suitable for growth of a variety of infectious organisms that may be suspected of causing the abscess. Sear and incise the surface of the abscess and inoculate culture media with the extracted material, using a sterile inoculating loop or swab. Make smears from the abscess on clean glass slides, diluting with a drop of water if the material is too thick. Air dry and flame slides and make Gram's, acid-fast, or any other stain as desired.

Embryo Inoculation for Virus Isolation. For routine virus isolation, centrifuged and/or filtered fine-ground suspensions of suspect tissues (trachea, bronchi, lung, liver, spleen, kidney, brain, bone marrow) or body fluids and exudates may be inoculated into the chorioallantoic cavity and yolk sac and onto the chorioallantoic membrane (CAM) of embryos at various stages of incubation. See specific diseases for virus culture techniques. Also see Cunningham (11) for selection of the proper age of embryo and route of inoculation for various disease agents as well as detailed inoculation procedures. Embryos from specific-pathogen-free dams should be used for culture to be sure any agent recovered originated in the inoculum and not in the dams that produced the eggs. Equally important is assurance that negative cultures are due to absence of infectious agents in inoculum rather than to interference of passive antibodies in eggs. Since the purpose of virus isolation is to determine which may be present, it is advisable to inoculate various ages of embryo by the various routes. Several blind passages may be necessary before the culture attempt can reasonably be considered negative. A simple technique that does not require dropping the CAM has been described (18).

The CAM may be drawn away from the shell (dropped) to facilitate inoculation. First drill or punch a small hole in the shell over the air cell, then slowly drill or punch a second hole through the shell at a point on the side over the embryo. Applying mild suction through a rubber tube over the hole into the air cell causes the CAM to drop away from the inner shell membrane under the second drilled hole. A bright candling light should be used while suction is applied to determine when the CAM has dropped.

For yolk sac inoculation, the needle can be directed through the air cell and directly to the center of the egg. Some yolk can be withdrawn into the syringe to be sure of the location of the needle.

For chorioallantoic cavity inoculation, a hole is drilled over the edge of the air cell at a spot previously marked with the aid of a candling light. The cavity lies adjacent to the shell and can be easily penetrated from that point. All holes should be sealed with suitable sterile material before reincubating.

Cell culture procedures are becoming more common in diagnostic laboratories. Technicians with this capability may inoculate the cell cultures directly with tissue extracts or body fluids, or they may use embryos for primary screening and transfer embryo fluids or extracts to cell culture for further study and identification.

DISPOSING OF THE SPECIMEN. If a disease infectious for humans is suspected, the carcass should be autoclaved, incinerated, or otherwise rendered incapable of causing infection to laboratory or other personnel. Similar precautions should be followed during disposal of carcasses infected with a virulent poultry pathogen that presents a health hazard to the industry. The necropsy area, instruments, and gloves should then be cleaned, washed, and disinfected.

COMMUNICATION. Flock owners are not interested in technical data. They want to know what the problem is and what should be done to correct it and/or how to prevent reoccurrences. Sometimes technical data is necessary to clarify the diagnosis, but the report should be in language and terms that they will understand. A minimum of complicated scientific and medical technology words should be used. When medical terms are apt to be confusing they should always be explained in lay terms.

The report should include the necropsy findings, results of laboratory studies (histopathologic, serologic, cultural), diagnosis (temporary or final), conclusions, and recommendations. The owner is seeking professional advice. The veterinarian should give his/her best conclusions and recommendations based on the facts available. A verbal report or telephone call to the flock owner, manager, or service workers, soon after completion of the necropsy and initial tests is highly advisable. A tentative diagnosis can be offered pending further confirmation.

FLOCK PROFILING. Today's disease problems often represent the sum of various subclinical disorders occurring at different times throughout the life of a flock. Acquisition of the fullest understanding of this sequential collection of serologic and other data concerning multiple pathogens requires disciplined and careful organization. The systematic, graphical presentation of this data is commonly called a "flock profile." The establishment of such profiles is facilitated by enzyme-linked immunosorbent assay (ELISA) technology, because a single basic test system is used to monitor for a broad array of diseases (42).

Snyder et al. (43) demonstrated the value of correlating ELISA profiling data with flock performance. The further evolution and diagnostic advantages of the graphical presentation of ELISA-based flock profiling data in combination with gross and microscopic pathology data was described by Mallinson et al. (29). The method has broad applicability to epizootiologic investigations, field research, and quality control. Baseline profiles can be established both as targets for vaccination goals and as a base from which deviations from the norm may be demonstrated when a field problem is subsequently encountered. Several flock profiling kits and systems are now commercially available. Their value is enhanced when good data retrieval and graphic presentation of data (Fig. 1.25) is combined with the diagnostician's veterinary skills and experience in assimilating medical information and establishing a plausible diagnosis.

DISINFECTANTS.

To disinfect is to free from pathogenic substances or organisms or to render them inert; a disinfectant is an agent or substance that disinfects chiefly by destroying infective agents (pathogenic microorganisms) or rendering them inactive; disinfection is the act or process of destroying pathogenic microorganisms. To sanitize is to reduce microbial populations and keep them from multiplying.

Properties. Among the properties of an ideal disinfectant are low cost per unit of disinfecting value, ready solubility in hard water, relative safety for humans and animals, ready availability, nondestructibility to utensils and fabrics, stability when exposed to air, absence of objectionable or lingering odor, no residual toxicity, effectiveness for a large variety of infectious agents, and no deleterious accumulation of any portion of the disinfectant in meat or eggs. For any disinfectant to be effective in economical quantities it must be applied to surfaces that have first been freed of debris and organic material by thorough scraping, scrubbing, brushing, dusting, and washing with soap or detergent solutions. Many disinfectants are highly efficient but only when these basic cleaning prerequisites have first been met.

Types. Many disinfectants of similar composition are sold under different trade names. Before buying a product with an unfamiliar name, compare types and values with a well-known product. Directions for dilutions given by the manufacturer should be closely followed. Complete discussions of various disinfectants and sterilization methods should be consulted (23, 39). Additional references on disinfectants and their use (17, 34) and textbooks on pharmacology and therapeutics should be consulted.

The virucidal activity of several commercial disinfectants against velogenic viscerotropic Newcastle disease have been determined (48). A list of 48 commercial disinfectants approved for use against avian influenza virus is available from National Emergency Field Operations, Veterinary Services, USDA, 6505 Belcrest Road, Hyattsville MD 20782. The list provides product names, basic formulations, and dilutions along with the names, addresses, and telephone numbers of appropriate distributors or formulators.

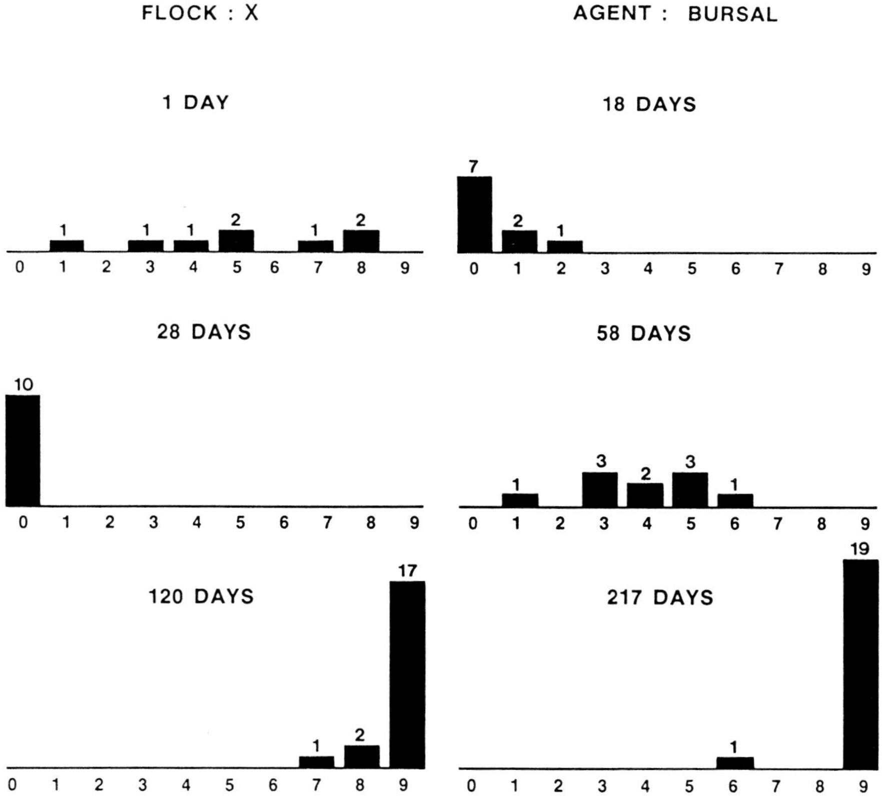

1.25. Temporal graphic distribution of infectious bursal disease ELISA group titer levels at 1, 18, 28, 58, 120, and 217 days of age for a poultry flock. Numbers on the abscissa represent the relative group titer levels obtained by ELISA. Reciprocal endpoint titers of 0–50 are group 0, 51–150 are group 1, 151–300 are group 2, etc., with a titer of >19,200 comprising group 9. Numbers above each bar represent the number of samples reacting at each level on the indicated day of age. (Snyder)

PHENOL (CARBOLIC ACID). Phenol is a chemical substance obtained from coal tar. In its pure form it occurs as colorless needles having a characteristic and familiar odor (Lysol soap). It is usually sold in water solutions and is too expensive for general poultry house use. It is, however, the chemical used as a basis for determining the phenol coefficients of various disinfectants (relative ability to kill specific test organisms when compared to that of phenol). Prindle and Wright (36) present a complete discussion of the phenolic compounds. Commercial disinfectants containing phenolic compounds have been developed and marketed at cost values, which permits wider use in poultry operations. Some have residual activity persisting after they have dried, giving the advantage of continued suppression of bacterial and viral populations on sprayed surfaces.

CRESOLS. Cresol extracts of coal tar products are compounds closely related chemically to phenol and have similar bactericidal properties. They are thick yellow or brown liquids, miscible with water, but only slightly soluble. They form the basis for a large number of commercial brands made by combining cresol with soap.

A list of cresylic disinfectants permitted for use for official disinfection is published periodically by the USDA, Agricultural Research Service, Animal Health Division. This list (41) serves as a guide for use of specific products.

BISPHENOLS. Bisphenols are compounds composed of two phenol molecules modified and joined by various chemical linkages. Halogens, particularly chlorine, have been combined with bisphenols to increase their effectiveness; some of the chlorophenols have high antifungal activity. Bisphenols are frequently combined with other phenolic compounds in disinfectants. Additional information on these compounds is available (19).

PINE OIL. Pine oil has proved satisfactory as a disinfectant and has the advantage of being less injurious to the skin than cresol compounds. The odor is also less objectionable and in fact is rather pleasant, which enhances its desirability for use in offices and lavatory areas. Since it is insoluble in water, it is used in the emulsion form with soap or other emulsifying agent.

HYPOCHLORITES AND CHLORINATED LIME. Chlorine is the basis of disinfectants known as hypochlorites, which contain about 70% available chlorine. Hypochlorites (12) are available as powders containing calcium hypochlorite (CaOCl) and sodium hypochlorite (NaOCl) combined with hydrated trisodium phosphate and as liquids containing NaOCl. Chlorinated lime (bleaching powder), prepared by saturating slaked lime with chlorine gas, was one of the earliest recognized disinfectants. It has been largely supplanted by the more readily available hypochlorites.

Products containing NaOCl are essentially liquids ranging in concentrations from 1 to 15%. The 15% solutions are used to prepare 5% solutions with water for bleaches and sanitizing agents. Germicidal potency of hypochlorites is dependent upon concentration of available chlorine and the pH (acidity) of the solution or upon the amount of hypochlorous acid formed, which, in turn, is dependent upon both factors. The influence of pH, especially in dilute solutions, is even greater than the percentage of available chlorine. Increasing the pH decreases the biocidal activity of chlorine, and decreasing the pH increases the activity. Germicidal activity is speeded up by raising the temperature.

If used according to directions, hypochlorites are highly efficient. Their principal use in the poultry industry is for egg washing and sanitizing and for disinfecting limited areas such as incubators, incubator and hatcher trays and other areas around the hatchery, egg-breaking areas, small brooders, and water and feed containers. They can also be used on cement surfaces. All surfaces to be disinfected with hypochlorite solutions must first be thoroughly cleaned to ensure the greatest efficiency. Stock supplies should be kept in dark, cool places, and containers should be tightly sealed when not in use. Fresh solutions must be prepared daily and periodically tested to assure that proper levels of available chlorine remain. A simple swimming pool test kit may prove helpful for such monitoring. Recently purchased or stored hypochlorites have been found to have wide ranges of concentration values.

All products containing chlorine must be handled with care because free chlorine is destructive to fabrics, leather, and metal.

ORGANIC IODINE COMBINATIONS. Iodine has long been recognized as an effective disinfectant. Many of the disadvantages of earlier products have been overcome by combining iodine in organic complexes, sometimes called "tamed iodine." The term "iodophor" refers to a combination of iodine with a solubilizing agent that slowly liberates free iodine when diluted with water. The term most frequently refers to formulas consisting of iodine complexed with certain types of surfactants that have detergent properties. These complexes are said to enhance the bactericidal activity of iodine and render it nontoxic, nonirritating, and nonstaining if used as directed. The detergent also makes the products water soluble and stable under usual conditions of storage. There is no offensive odor, and the detergent properties impart cleansing activity. See Gershenfeld (16) for additional information on iodine compounds.

A group of commercial iodophors have been developed and marketed for a wide variety of disinfectant uses. Some of these products have a built-in indicator of germicidal activity; as the solution is used up, the normal amber color fades. When the solution is colorless, it is no longer effective. The products can be mixed in cold and hard water. Organic iodine products have a wide variety of uses in the industry. They can be applied without hazard to nearly all surfaces and are useful for disinfecting hatchery and incubator surfaces, incubator and hatcher trays, egg-breaking areas, feeders and fountains, footwear, and poultry buildings. Like other disinfectants, these compounds are most effective on clean surfaces.

QUICKLIME (UNSLAKED LIME, CALCIUM OXIDE). The action of quicklime depends on liberation of heat and oxygen when the chemical comes in contact with water. On the poultry farm, its use is limited to small yard areas that are damp and cannot be exposed to the sun, disinfection of drains and fecal matter, and whitewashes. As quicklime has a caustic action, birds should be kept away from it until it has become thoroughly dry.

FORMALDEHYDE. Formaldehyde (CH_2O) is a gas. It is sold commercially in a 40% solution (37% by weight) with water under the name of formalin. It may also be purchased in the form of a powder known as paraformaldehyde (Paraform, Triformal, Formaldegen). When heated, this powder liberates CH_2O. A suitable heating device is a thermostatically controlled electric pan with a timer that can be controlled from outside the fumigation chamber. Manufacturer's directions on amounts to use for each type of equipment and the means of liberating the gas must be carefully observed.

Formaldehyde is often generated by adding formalin to potassium permanganate ($KMnO_4$) in an earthenware crock or metal container. Because of the heat generated by the chemical reaction, glass containers should not be used. The container should be deep and have a volume several times that of the combined chemicals, because considerable bubbling and splattering takes place. The ratio in liquid measure of formalin is approximately twice the dry measure of $KMnO_4$ (1 g $KMnO_4$/2 ml formalin). If too much formalin is used, the excess will remain in the vessel. If too much $KMnO_4$ is used, the excess remains unchanged and is wasted. Potassium permanganate is poisonous. Both these compounds must be kept in accident-proof containers in a safe place away from work traffic.

A suitable fumigation cabinet must have a source of heat, a fan to circulate the warm humid air and fumigant, a source of humidifying moisture, and a method of generating formaldehyde gas. The box should be air-tight, and have an exhausting device from the fumigation box to the outside of the building. It is much safer to locate fumigation chambers outside of any building and away from human traffic.

Though it is a powerful disinfectant, CH_2O has many disadvantages, especially its volatility, pungent odor, caustic action, and tendency to harden the skin—properties that make it disagreeable to apply. It is extremely irritating to the conjunctiva and mucous membranes, and some people are very sensitive to it. Because of this and other toxic properties, precautions must be taken to prevent its escape into areas where people work. Its chief advantages are that it can be used as a gas or vapor for fumigation of hatching eggs. It is a good disinfectant in the presence of some organic matter, and it does not injure equipment with which it comes in contact. The maximum atmospheric concentration permitted in work areas by some Occupational Safety and Health Administration regulations is 2 ppm. Suitable gas masks should be readily available near fumigation boxes. Formaldehyde can be neutralized with ammonium hydroxide by using a solution of approximately 30% and a quantity not to exceed one-half the quantity of formalin used in the fumigation. Ammonia may be released by sprinkling or spraying in the intake air during evacuation of the fumigation box after the surfaces have dried completely.

Formaldehyde gas is widely used in poultry enterprises for fumigation of hatching eggs to destroy potential pathogenic shell contaminants. See Chapter 3 for detailed information on fumigation to control salmonellae. It is also used at the end of cleanup to fumigate the inside of incubators and hatchers and their contents.

Fumigation of incubators and eggs has been an established practice in the industry and has varied little over the years. Various recommendations have been made for quantities, humidity, temperature, and time for adequate sterilization of shells of hatching eggs. Frequent recommendations specify the following: 60 g $KMnO_4$:120 ml formalin/100 ft^3 (2.8 M^3) cabinet space, 21.1 C, 70% humidity, and 20 min fumigation time. The higher the humidity and temperature, the more effective the fumigation. When fumigation is completed, exhaust ducts are opened and the gas thoroughly exhausted before anyone opens the door to the cabinet.

In modern enterprises, hatching eggs are frequently handled only once and are placed directly into plastic holders (flats), which then travel in stacks through the fumigation, transportation, and storage route and eventually into the incubators. Entire racks, dollies, or pallets of closely stacked flats of eggs are thus fumigated in large boxes (Fig. 1.26). In order to generate adequate concentration of CH_2O and have it penetrate and disinfect the egg shells in the centers of these stacks, there should be increased quantity of

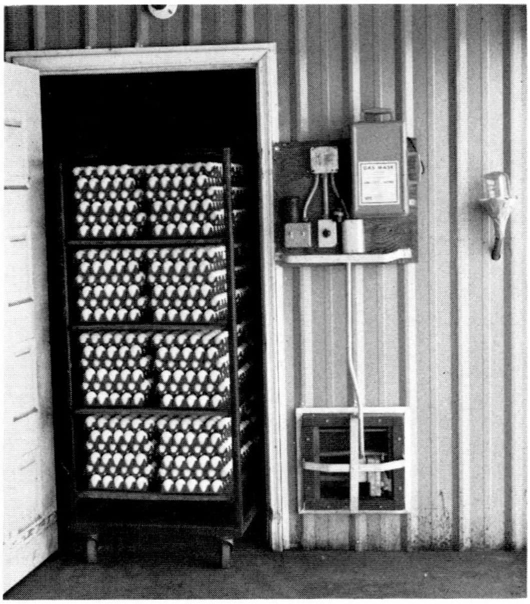

1.26. Hatching eggs are moved in stacked plastic flats on special dollies directly from the poultry house service area into a special room for fumigation prior to transport to the hatchery. Controls for heater, circulating fan, and ventilators; signal lights; formaldehyde dispenser; and gas mask for protection of the worker are placed on the outside near the door.

chemicals (75 g $KMnO_4$:150 ml formalin/100 ft^3), higher humidity (up to 90%), higher temperature (up to 32.2 C), longer time (up to 30 min), and vigorous agitation of the gas during fumigation so it will penetrate the spaces and effectively sanitize surfaces of eggs in the centers of such large stacks. Pressed-paper egg flats tend to trap CH_2O and continue to release the gas during storage and processing. Therefore, CH_2O fumigation should be confined to eggs in plastic flats or wire containers.

CH_2O fumigation is sometimes used to disinfect the inside and contents (including eggs at 18 days of incubation) of hatching machines. Since these machines are inside of the building, this should not be done unless provision is made for adequate ventilation of the gas to the outside of the building when fumigation is completed.

Certain precautions are necessary after fumigation of hatching eggs. The incoming air for exhaustion must be clean, otherwise the humid surface of the egg can become recontaminated. During extremely cold weather, outside air must be warmed before entering the fumigation chamber to avoid overchilling eggs. While humidity is essential for disinfective activity of the CH_2O, the surface of eggs should not become visibly wet during fumigation and should be dry when the eggs leave the fumigator.

Fumigation should not be done in incubators because of the danger of injuring embryos (see Chapter 3). Also, it should not be done at such high concentration after the hatch begins because of the danger of injuring chicks or poults. Formaldehyde may be generated in hatchers by using approximately 20 ml formalin/100 ft^3. The formalin is soaked into enough cheesecloth so it does not drip and hung in the circulating currents in the box. Effectiveness of this method is limited because of the low concentration.

COPPER SULFATE (BLUESTONE). Although copper sulfate ($CuSO_4$) and other salts of copper have a marked toxic effect upon some of the lower forms of life, they are not considered good general disinfectants. Copper sulfate is toxic to algae and fungi and has been used in attempts to stop or prevent outbreaks of fungal diseases. It has been used in the feed at 0.5 lb/ton and sometimes 1 lb/ton for short periods without noticeable toxicity to chickens. Poultry will usually drink water containing $CuSO_4$ at no greater concentration than 1:2000, but a concentration greater than 1:500 may be toxic when given in the only source of water. Turkeys do not like water containing $CuSO_4$ and will seek other supplies if available. A 0.5% solution may be of value for disinfecting feed hoppers, water fountains, and surrounding areas associated with outbreaks of fungal disease.

QUATERNARY AMMONIUM SURFACTANTS. Quaternary ammonium products (quats) are considered to be good disinfectants if used according to directions. They are noncorrosive, water clear, odorless, cationic (+ charged ions), nonirritating to the skin, good deodorants, and have a marked detergent action. They contain no phenols, halogens, or heavy metals and are highly stable and relatively nontoxic. Most quats cannot be used in soapy solutions. All surfaces to be disinfected must be thoroughly rinsed with water to remove any residue of soap or anionic (− charged ions) detergent before using quats for sterilizing purposes. Some hard-water minerals may interfere with their action. See Lawrence (22) for more information on these compounds.

Quats are used for washing eggs and disinfecting hatchery surfaces, incubator and hatcher trays, egg-breaking equipment and areas, feeders and waterers, and footwear, among other uses.

SUNLIGHT AND ULTRAVIOLET RADIATION. Solar radiation has disinfecting properties. However, since the material to be treated must be in thin layers and exposed to direct rays, this method is limited to impervious surfaced yards, concrete and blacktop aprons, and equipment that can be thoroughly cleaned before being exposed. The construction of most poultry houses prevents efficient disinfection by the sun. A cement platform fully exposed to the sun makes a convenient place for treating movable equipment. If properly constructed with a drain, such a platform can be used as a washing and disinfection rack. A concrete apron before the poultry house entry will be washed by rains or can be washed by hose to take advantage of the disinfecting power of the sun's rays on the clean surface (see Fig. 1.5).

There are many types of germicidal (ultraviolet) lamps but not enough scientific evidence is available to warrant a recommendation for their general use in hatcheries or on poultry farms. A complete review of the use of UV radiation in microbiologic laboratories is available (33).

HOT WATER. Hot water adds to the efficiency of most disinfectants and, if applied in the form of boiling water or live steam, is effective without addition of any chemical. Detergents added to systems for generating and disseminating hot water and steam will increase cleaning and decontaminating efficiency. Live steam must be applied directly and at close range to the part to be disinfected.

DRY HEAT. Dry heat in the form of a flame is effective if the flame comes in contact with the pathogen to be killed. All methods involving direct flame are fire hazards and not recommended except possibly on cement surfaces. In tightly controlled circumstances, flames might be used to eliminate hard-to-remove feathers and fluff accumulations.

Other commercial disinfectants, mostly organic compounds, are available under trade names. Many are combinations of several individual disinfectants with complementary properties. Some also have long residual activity. To choose disinfectants wisely, one must continually keep abreast of new product development through current scientific and lay publications.

Residues of disinfectants used to sanitize drinking fountains should be rinsed off with fresh water before water vaccines are given, since they can inactivate the vaccine virus.

DISINFESTANTS (PARASITICIDES, INSECTICIDES, PESTICIDES)

Properties. Disinfestants destroy animal parasites such as lice, mites, ticks, and fleas. They also destroy other undesirable insects (flies, beetles, ants, sow bugs). Some pesticides are highly toxic to humans and livestock. Their use (preferably by a licensed expert as part of a professional, integrated, insect and rodent control service) is recommended only as an adjunct to a properly conducted total sanitary control program. Many disinfectants are also destructive to lice, mites, and other similar parasites, but must come in contact with them. Many pesticides, however, are useless as disinfectants.

Suitable insecticides are those that can be used on or around poultry without causing toxic effects to humans or birds from contact or ingestion and that do not accumulate to harmful levels in edible tissues or eggs as a result of ingestion or absorption.

The list of available and permissible commercial insecticides has declined greatly and changes frequently. Many widely used in the past have been prohibited for use around food animals because of the deposition of insecticides in fatty tissues and eggs. Others have been abandoned because populations of insects become resistant to them. Therefore, it is necessary to keep informed on available effective insecticides through current government, university, and industry literature. In some situations it may be cost effective to contract this complex, changing activity through an agency providing professional insect and pest control services. Biosecurity measures for their employees and equipment must be considered when contemplating such contract services.

The limited number of available commercial parasiticides, their active chemical properties, limitations, tolerances, and various applications, are discussed in detail in Chapter 30. See also Chapter 35 for toxic effects of some insecticides.

Unlike flies, which travel to insecticide baits or over insecticide-treated surfaces, bird ectoparasites are best controlled by bringing the insecticide into contact with the parasite. A wide assortment of housing types and production systems are in use. One application method or system is seldom suitable for all types of housing. The type and form of parasiticide best suited for a particular type of housing and management system should be determined and then used according to directions on the label. Fogging and misting can be effective only if the insecticide can be confined in the building and/or applied (blown) into cracks and crevices and on feathers where parasites are congregated. Otherwise, the effort and expense are largely wasted. Pyrethrum preparations containing synergists can be used in light- and temperature-controlled houses, but the automatic ventilation system must be bypassed and hand controlled during treatment. In high-rise houses, one must be sure to compensate for the large volume of space under the floors by using additional insecticide in a space-calculated application.

A common error is to assume that one application of insecticide will accomplish the objective. Parasite eggs are seldom destroyed; they remain to generate a new population, which must be attacked with a second application 2–3 weeks after the first. In addition, no system, application, or insecticide will result in a 100% parasite kill. Once the parasite gains a foothold, it must be attacked repeatedly. Frequently, alternating insecticides and methods is necessary to effect control. Do not be misled by statements that the birds learn to live with their parasites. Such thinking encourages continuous poor bird performance and a host of problems.

Handling Precautions. Possible hazards to humans and animals from many of the modern pesticides must always be remembered when considering their use. It is best to wear a suitable mask, rubber gloves, and protective clothing when applying insecticides. The most important precaution in handling chemical insecticides is to read the directions, hazards, and antidotes on labels of containers before any use.

A basic rule in handling insecticides is to keep them properly labeled and stored in a locked building reserved for that purpose. Disposal of empty containers and discarded leftover insecticides is becoming more of a hazard and responsibility. Large drums should be returned to the supplier or heated to red hot for 5–10 min. Paper and plastic containers should be burned. Small glass and metal containers should be broken or punctured so no one will use them for any purpose. In addition to the human hazard, discarded insecticides must not pollute lakes or streams nor become a hazard for honeybees. A safe policy is to check with the local environmental protection agency (EPA) for recommendations.

Types

CRUDE OIL, DISTILLATES, SIMILAR COMPOUNDS. Petroleum oils applied to clean buildings and equipment prior to introducing a new flock have been widely used to control lice, mites, and ticks. Oily residues get on the parasites and cause suffocation. They have been effective in getting at parasites in cracks and crevices of the building, but they cannot be applied to parasites on birds. Carbolinium, a wood preservative, also repels mites and other insects for long periods after it is applied. These products are quite messy and smelly and not as effective as many newer products.

NICOTINE SULFATE. A 40% solution of nicotine sulfate (Black Leaf 40) has been widely used to control lice and mites. It is sprayed or painted on perches or floors of cages shortly before the flock settles for the night. In heavily infested birds, it is daubed on the fluff feathers. A 2% nicotine sulfate dust is also available for mite control. It can be dusted into the fluff feathers with a garden duster. The insect-killing properties depend on a substance that volatilizes at body temperature and penetrates the feathers to attack the parasites. In very cold weather volatilization may not occur unless the treated surface is close enough to the bird to be warmed by the body heat. This product is not well adapted for control of turkey parasites where roosting areas are not enclosed.

Though it has been largely replaced by newer products, it remains a very effective parasiticide for lice and mites and is often used when others fail. Whenever nicotine products, particularly the concentrated ones, are applied, workers should be well protected with coveralls, hats, respirators, goggles, and rubber gloves. If the concentrate is spilled, any contaminated clothing should be removed immediately and thoroughly washed and any contaminated skin area washed immediately with soap and water.

SPACE DIFFUSION INSECTICIDES. Pyrethrum products are released as a fog or mist, and the volatile compound permeates the room. Pyrethrum, an extract from plants, has low toxicity for higher forms of life but high toxicity for insects. It is relatively costly and may fail to penetrate adequately through feathers of birds and into insect hiding places. Synthetic forms of pyrethrum are now available commercially.

Vapona or DDVP, a preparation of dichlorvos, is sometimes impregnated into special materials from which it slowly vaporizes and diffuses through the air. This has greatest application in storage and other rooms that are closed and unventilated for long periods (overnight).

SYSTEMIC INHIBITORS. Sulfaquinoxaline, used so extensively in feed and water for control of coccidiosis and many bacterial infections, was found to rid birds of northern fowl mites (13). The product or its metabolites apparently create body conditions objectionable to the parasites (possibly odors), which drive them off the birds. The drug has since been banned from feed for hens laying eggs for human consumption, but other products have been reported to exert similar effects, and some may exert an unsuspected mite-repelling action. Drugs providing this type of mite control seem most effective when incorporated in feed prior to infestation and least effective as a treatment after infestation has become established.

DUSTS AND SPRAYS. Nearly all insecticides adaptable to control of parasites on fowl can be obtained as ready-to-use dusts or in the form of wettable powders, emulsifiable concentrates, or liquid suspensions, all of which can be prepared as sprays. Each has advantages, and suggested uses are supplied with the insecticide.

Chickens dust themselves instinctively. In litter-floor houses insecticide dusts can be added to litter to control mites, according to specifications of the manufacturer. Special dust boxes with added insecticide can be placed in large cages and wire- or slat-floored houses to accomplish the same objective. Dusts can also be applied to birds in cages by using a dust applicator. The dust must be blown into the feathers to get at the parasites.

Although laborious, dusting individual birds can be effective.

The most common method of applying insecticides is by spray. The mixture must be agitated during application to maintain a constant concentration and prevent separation. Sprays are mostly applied to floors and walls, but some can be sprayed on the birds.

None is perfect, and resistance is already known to have developed against some. New products are constantly being developed and tested for effectiveness. Poultry producers should be alert for products, preparations, and local vendors of professional pest-control services most suitable for their type of management system.

The best parasite control is to prevent the initial infestation through wise management practices. Once again, parasite infestations, like bacterial and viral diseases, can be most successfully controlled and eradicated from single-age farms or quarantinable units as part of a total, integrated system of "disease-prevention management" (biosecurity).

REFERENCES

1. Adams, A.W. 1973. Consequences of depriving laying hens of water a short time. Poult Sci 52:1221–1223.
2. Alls, A.A., W.J. Benton, W.C. Krauss, and M.S. Cover. 1963. The mechanics of treating hatching eggs for disease prevention. Avian Dis 7:89–97.
3. Anderson, D.P., and R.P. Hanson. 1965. Influence of environment on virus diseases of poultry. Avian Dis 9:171–182.
4. Anderson, D.P., C.W. Beard, and R.P. Hanson. 1966. Influence of poultry house dust, ammonia, and carbon dioxide on resistance of chickens to Newcastle disease virus. Avian Dis 10:117–188.
5. AVMA. 1986. American Veterinary Medical Association Panel on Euthanasia. J Am Vet Med Assoc 188:252–268.
6. Bell, D. 1966. Water shortages can cut egg production. Poult Trib 72:30.
7. Bierer, B.W., T.H. Eleazer, and D.E. Roebuck. 1965. Effect of feed and water deprivation on chickens, turkeys, and laboratory mammals. Poult Sci 44:768–773.
8. Chute, H.L., and E. Barden. 1964. The fungus flora of chick hatcheries. Avian Dis 8:13–19.
9. Chute, H.L., and M. Gershman. 1961. A new approach to hatchery sanitation. Poult Sci 60:568–571.
10. Chute, H.L., D.R. Stauffer, and D.C. O'Meara. 1964. The production of specific pathogen-free (SPF) broilers in Maine. Maine Agric Exp Sta Bull 633.
11. Cunningham, C.H. 1966. A Laboratory Guide in Virology, 6th Ed. Burgess Publ. Co., Minneapolis.
12. Dychdala, G.R., 1968. Chlorine and chlorine compounds. In C.A. Lawrence, and S.S. Block (eds.), Disinfection, Sterilization, and Preservation, pp. 278–304. Lea & Febiger, Philadelphia.
13. Furman, D.P., and V.S. Stratton. 1963. Control of northern fowl mites, Ornithonyssus sylviarum, with sulphaquinoxaline. J Econ Entomol 56:904–905.
14. Galton, M.M., and P. Arnstein. 1960. Poultry diseases in public health. US Public Health Serv Publ 767.
15. Gentry, R.F., M. Mitrovic, and G.R. Bubash. 1962. Application of Andersen sampler in hatchery sanitation. Poult Sci 61:794–804.
16. Gershenfeld, L. 1968. Iodine. In C.A. Lawrence and S.S. Block (eds.), Disinfection, Sterilization, and Preservation, pp. 329–347. Lea & Febiger, Philadelphia.
17. Glick, C.A., G.G. Gremillion, and G.A. Bodmer. 1961. Practical methods and problems of steam and chemical sterilization. Proc Anim Care Panel 11:37.
18. Gorham, J.R. 1957. A simple technique for the inoculation of the chorioallantoic membrane of chicken embryos. Am J Vet Res 18:691–692.
19. Gump, W.S., and G.R. Walter. 1968. The bisphenols. In C.A. Lawrence and S.S. Block (eds.), Disinfection, Sterilization, and Preservation, pp. 257–277. Lea & Febiger, Philadelphia.
20. Hofstad, M.S. 1950. A method of bleeding chickens from the heart. J Am Vet Med Assoc 116:353–354.
21. Jensen, M.M. 1988. Update on usage and effectiveness of coryza, cholera, and staphylococcal vaccines. Proc 37th West Poult Dis Conf, pp. 54–56, Veterinary Extension, Univ California, Davis.
22. Lawrence, C.A. 1968. Quaternary ammonium surface-active disinfectants. In C.A. Lawrence and S.S. Block (eds.), Disinfection, Sterilization, and Preservation, pp. 430–452. Lea & Febiger, Philadelphia.
23. Lawrence, C.A., and S.S. Block. 1968. Disinfection, Sterilization, and Preservation. Lea & Febiger, Philadelphia.
24. Lucas, A.M., and C. Jamroz. 1961. Atlas of Avian Hematology. USDA Agr Monogr 25.
25. Luna, L.G. 1968. Manual of Histological Staining Methods of the Armed Forces Institute of Pathology, 3rd Ed. Blakiston Div., McGraw-Hill, New York.
26. Magwood, S.E. 1964. Studies in hatchery sanitation. 1. Fluctuations in microbial counts of air in poultry hatcheries. Poult Sci 63:441–449.
27. Magwood, S.E. 1964. Studies in hatchery sanitation. 3. The effect of air-borne bacterial populations on contamination of egg and embryo surfaces. Poult Sci 43:1567–1572.
28. Magwood, S.E., and H. Marr. 1964. Studies in hatchery sanitation. 2. A simplified method for assessing bacterial populations on surfaces within hatcheries. Poult Sci 63:1558–1566.
29. Mallinson, E.T., D.B. Snyder, W.W. Marquardt, and S.L. Gorham. 1988. In B.A. Morris, M.N. Clifford, and R. Jackman (eds.), Immunoassays for Veterinary and Food Analysis-1, pp. 109–117. Elsevier, London and New York.
30. McCapes, R.H., R. Yamamoto, G. Ghazikhanian, W.M. Dungan, and H.B. Ortmayer. 1977. Antibiotic egg injection to eliminate disease. I. Effect of injection methods on turkey hatchability and Mycoplasma meleagridis infection. Avian Dis 21:57–68.
31. Murphy, D.W. 1988. Composting as a dead bird disposal method. Poult Sci 67, Suppl 1:124.
32. North, Mack O. 1984. Commercial chicken production manual, 3rd Ed. AVI Publishing Co., Inc., Westport, CN.
33. Phillips, G.B., and E. Hanel. 1960. Use of ultraviolet radiation in microbiological laboratories. US Govt Res Rep 34:122. (Abstr).
34. Phillips, C.R., and B. Warshowsky. 1958. Chemical disinfectants. Annu Rev Microbiol 12:525.
35. Preece, A. 1965. A Manual for Histological Techniques, 2nd Ed. Little, Brown & Co., Boston.
36. Prindle, R.F., and E.S. Wright. 1968. Phenolic compounds. In C.A. Lawrence and S.S. Block (eds.), Disinfection, Sterilization, and Preservation, pp. 401–429. Lea & Febiger, Philadelphia.
37. Purchase, H.G., L.H. Arp, C.H. Domermuth, and J.E. Pearson. 1989. A Laboratory Manual for Isolation and Identification of Avian Pathogens, 3rd Ed. Am As-

soc Avian Pathol, Kennett Square, PA. (In press).
38. Randall, C.J., 1985. Diseases of the Domestic Fowl and Turkey, a Colour Atlas. Wolfe Medical Publications Ltd., Wolfe House, London.
39. Reddish, G.F. 1957. Antiseptics, Disinfectants, Fungicides and Sterilization, 2nd Ed. Lea & Febiger, Philadelphia.
40. Riddell, C. 1987. Avian Histopathology. Am Assoc Avian Pathol, Kennett Square, PA
41. Saulmon, E.E. 1968. Cresylic disinfectants permitted for use in official disinfection. USDA, ARS, Anim Health Div Memo 586.
42. Snyder, D.B., 1986. Latest developments in the enzyme linked immunosorbent assay (ELISA). Avian Dis 30:19–23.
43. Snyder, D.B., W.W. Marquardt, E.T. Mallinson, E. Russek-Cohen, P.K. Savage, and D.C. Allen. 1986. Rapid serological profiling by enzyme-linked immunosorbent assay. IV. Association of infectious bursal disease serology with broiler flock performance. Avian Dis 30:139–148.
44. Thompson, S.W. 1966. Selected Histochemical and Histopathological Methods. Charles C. Thomas, Springfield, IL.
45. Utterback, W.W., and J.H. Schwartz. 1973. Epizootiology of velogenic viserotropic Newcastle disease in Southern California, 1971–1973. J Am Vet Med Assoc 163:1080–1088.
46. Whiteman, C.E., and A.A. Bickford. 1979. Avian Dis Man Am Assoc Avian Pathol, Kennett Square, PA.
47. Wright, M.L. 1958. Hatchery sanitation. Can J Comp Med Vet Sci 22:62–66.
48. Wright, H.S. 1974. Virucidal activity of commercial disinfectants against velogenic viscerotropic Newcastle disease virus. Avian Dis 18:526–530.
49. Wright, M.L., G.W. Anderson, and N.A. Epps. 1959. Hatchery sanitation. Can J Comp Med Vet Sci 23:288–290.
50. Wright, M.L., G.W. Anderson, and J.D. McConachie. 1961. Transmission of aspergillosis during incubation. Poult Sci 60:727–731.
51. Yoder, H.W., Jr. 1970. Preincubation heat treatment of chicken hatching eggs to inactivate Mycoplasma. Avian Dis 14:75 86.
52. Zander, D.V. 1977. Unpublished observations.

2 NUTRITIONAL DISEASES

R.E. Austic and M.L. Scott

An adequate supply of nutritious food and water is essential for normal growth and development, reproduction, and livability of domestic fowl. More than 36 nutrients are absolutely essential and must be in the diet in appropriate concentrations and balance in order to maximize the ability of poultry to express their genetic potential to grow and reproduce. Often it is the task of the veterinarian to determine whether an ailment is nutritional in its origin or whether nutrition is a contributing factor to a specific clinical problem. Whenever a serious deficiency of one of the essential nutrients occurs, characteristic signs often develop. These are frequently preceded or accompanied by nonspecific signs such as retarded uneven growth, rough-feather development, decreased egg production, and lowered hatchability. When a deficiency is partial, these may be the only signs observed. This makes it difficult to recognize a partial nutritional deficiency, since nonspecific signs may be brought about by a number of causes, including infectious diseases and toxicants.

The quantitative nutrient requirements of the young growing chick and turkey and for light breeds of laying hens are quite well established (5, 97): however the requirements of growing chicks and poults after the first few weeks of age, and the requirements of male and female broiler and turkey breeding fowls for many nutrients have not been determined experimentally.

Food substances of importance in nutrition of poultry are proteins and amino acids, carbohydrates, fats, vitamins, essential inorganic elements, and water.

PROTEINS AND AMINO ACIDS. Proteins are composed of approximately 20 nutritionally important amino acids. The protein requirement represents the collective need for 10 absolutely essential amino acids (arginine, histidine, isoleucine, leucine, lysine, methionine, phenylalanine, threonine, tryptophan, valine), 2 amino acids (cysteine and tyrosine) that can be synthesized from essential amino acids, 2 amino acids essential for the young chick (glycine or serine, proline), plus additional amino acids to satisfy the nitrogen requirement for synthesis of nonessential amino acids, purines, pyrimidines, and other nitrogenous compounds.

Practical ingredients are usually limiting in one or more amino acids. In rations composed of corn and soybean meals as sources of protein, methionine supplementation is usually necessary. Lysine may be slightly deficient in such diets for starting broilers or turkeys unless alternate lysine-rich protein sources or feed-grade lysine are included. Diets based on cereal grains and other protein concentrates such as cottonseed meal, safflower meal, or peanut meal may require both lysine and methionine supplementation. Other amino acids such as threonine, tryptophan, arginine, and isoleucine can become limiting when unusual protein sources are used or when the dietary protein level is reduced. Some of these amino acids are now available from commercial suppliers for supplementation in poultry feeds.

In contrast to the specific signs that may occur as a result of vitamin or mineral deficiencies, the effects of essential amino acid deficiencies are nonspecific – reduced growth, reduced feed consumption, decreased egg production and egg size, and loss of body weight in adults. Marginal amino acid deficiencies often result in increased food intake, or maintenance of food intake with concomitant reduction of body weight gain and lean tissue growth resulting in markedly increased body fat. Severe deficiencies also result in altered body composition. Some amino acids have additional effects. Methionine deficiency may exacerbate choline or vitamin B_{12} deficiencies owing to its role in methyl group metabolism. Lysine deficiency causes impaired pigmentation of Bronze turkey poults (Fig. 2.1), the biochemical basis of which is unknown (49). Arginine deficiency tends to cause the wing feathers to curl upward, giving the chick a distinct ruffled appearance. Several other amino acids have been reported to affect feather growth and structure (116).

When animals are provided with dietary protein in excess of their requirements, the surplus protein is catabolized and the nitrogen released is converted to uric acid. A large excess of protein may cause hyperuricemia and articular gout, particularly in birds that are genetically susceptible (12, 110, 132).

CARBOHYDRATES. This food component is the primary source of metabolizable energy in practical poultry diets. Starch and sucrose are

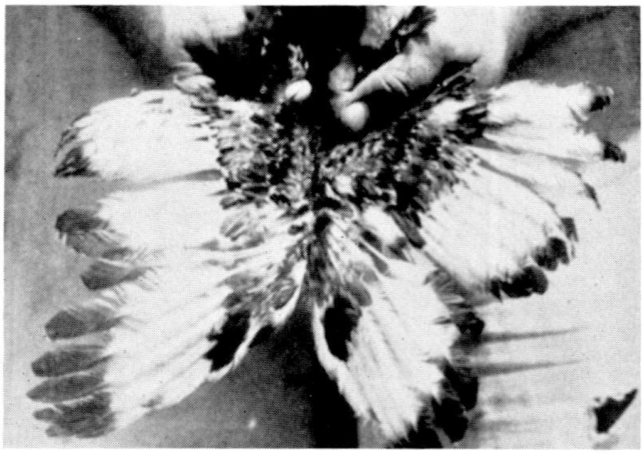

2.1. Lack of normal feather pigmentation in Bronze poult caused by deficiency of lysine.

readily used by the chick. Intestinal lactase activity is low in chickens; this limits the amount of milk sugar (lactose) that can be tolerated. Milk by-products such as whey are excellent sources of B vitamins and although beneficial at low levels, excessive levels in the diet cause growth depression and severe diarrhea. The latter condition, characteristic of lactose intolerance in many species, is caused by influx of water into the lower digestive tract and by microbial fermentation of undigested lactose.

FATS. Fats are important in the diet of poultry as concentrated sources of energy and sources of the essential nutrients, linoleic acid, and arachidonic acid. Linoleic acid cannot be synthesized, but can be converted to arachidonic acid, by poultry or other monogastric animals. Both fatty acids are important constituents of cell organelles, membranes, and adipose tissue and have additional physiologic roles as precursors of prostaglandins. Lack of these fatty acids in the diet of young chicks results in suboptimal growth and enlarged fatty livers (64). Essential fatty acid deficiency in laying hens results in lowered egg production, egg size, and hatchability (93). Reduced concentrations of arachidonic acid and increased concentrations of eicosatrienoic acid in tissue and egg lipids is a characteristic sign of essential fatty deficiency.

Unsaturated fatty acids may undergo oxidative rancidity, with multiple effects: essential fatty acids are destroyed; aldehydes that are formed may react with free amino groups in proteins, reducing amino acid availability; and the active peroxides generated during rancidification may destroy activities of vitamins A, D, and E and water-soluble vitamins such as biotin. Producers of vitamin A supplements have enhanced the stability of this vitamin by mechanical means, wherein minute droplets of vitamin A are enveloped in a stable fat, gelatin, or wax, forming a small bead that prevents most of the vitamin from coming into contact with oxygen until it is digested in the intestinal tract. The addition of synthetic antioxidants to poultry feeds provides further protection of vitamin A and other essential nutrients.

VITAMINS. The term "vitamin" refers to a heterogeneous group of fat-soluble and water-soluble chemical compounds essential in nutrition that bear no structural or necessary functional relationship to each other. All recognized vitamins with the exception of vitamin C are dietary essentials for poultry. Although amounts of various vitamins needed in poultry diets range from parts per million to parts per billion, each is required for normal metabolism and health.

A marked deficiency of a single vitamin in the diet of a chick or poult results in breakdown of the metabolic process in which that particular vitamin is concerned. This causes a vitamin deficiency disease, which in some instances exhibits characteristic macro- or microscopic changes. In several instances a single disease may result from a deficiency of any one of several nutrients. Perosis, for example, occurs in young chicks or poults when the diet is deficient in manganese or any one of the following vitamins: choline, nicotinic acid, pyridoxine, biotin, or folic acid. In young chickens, turkeys, pheasants, and other birds perosis is an anatomic deformity of leg bones that is characterized by enlargement of the tibiometatarsal joint, twisting or bending of the distal end of the tibia and proximal end of the metatarsus, and finally slipping of the gastrocnemius tendon from its condyles. This last lesion causes complete crippling in the affected leg; if both legs are affected, death usually results, since the chick or poult cannot secure food and water. Analysis of the diet may be the only way to determine whether a specific nutritional deficiency is responsible for the condition.

Vitamins A and D and riboflavin are most likely to be deficient if special attention is not given to provide them when feed is formulated. However, because of continued extraction and purification of many common ingredients and the tendency to omit animal proteins and high-fiber ingredients such as alfalfa meal and wheat mill by-products from diets, amounts of several other vitamins have decreased to sometimes deficient levels. These are vitamins E, B_{12}, and K; pantothenic acid, nicotinic acid, biotin, and choline. Poultry rations are usually formulated to contain more than adequate amounts of all vitamins, providing margins of safety to compensate for possible losses during feed processing, transportation, storage, and variations in feed composition and environmental conditions.

VITAMIN A. Vitamin A is essential in poultry

diets for growth, optimal vision, and integrity of mucous membranes. Since epithelial linings of alimentary, urinary, genital, and respiratory systems are composed of mucous membranes, these are the tissues in which lesions of vitamin A deficiency are most readily observed.

Vitamin A aldehyde, or retinal, is a component of visual pigments in sensory cells of the retina within which cis-trans isomerization of the isoprenoid side chain plays an essential role in the detection of light. Evidence suggests that a phosphorylated form of vitamin A serves in the biochemical transfer of mannose and galactose residues to glycoproteins in the synthesis of mucopolysaccarides. The latter may be a key feature of the involvement of vitamin A in the structural integrity of epithelial membranes.

Signs of Deficiency. When adult chickens or turkeys are fed a diet severely deficient in vitamin A, signs and lesions usually develop within 2–5 mo, depending on the amount stored in liver and other tissues of the body. As deficiency progresses, chickens become emaciated and weak and their feathers are ruffled. Egg production decreases sharply, length of time between clutches increases, and hatchability is decreased. A watery discharge from nostrils and eyes is noted, and eyelids are often stuck together. As the deficiency continues, milky white, caseous material accumulates in the eyes. At this stage of the disease, eyes fill with this white exudate to such an extent that it is impossible for the chicken to see unless the mass is removed; in many cases the eye is destroyed. Most signs in adult turkeys are similar to those in chickens (62).

The incidence and severity of blood spots in eggs of chickens is increased in vitamin A deficiency (20). The amount of vitamin A required to minimize blood spot incidence may be slightly higher than the requirement for good production and health of the laying hens (61, 112).

Vitamin A–deficiency signs in chicks and poults are characterized by cessation of growth, drowsiness, weakness, incoordination, emaciation, and ruffled plumage. If deficiency is severe, they may show ataxia not unlike that of vitamin E deficiency (61), although the two conditions can be differentiated by histological examination of the brain (3). In acute vitamin A deficiency, lacrimation usually occurs, and a caseous material may be seen under the eyelids. Xerophthalmia is a definite lesion of vitamin A deficiency; not all chicks and poults exhibit this, because in acute deficiency they often die of other causes before eyes become affected. Increased testes weight, spermatogenesis, and comb development may occur in young cockerels marginally deficient in vitamin A (100). Vitamin A–deficient cocks have decreased sperm counts, reduced sperm motility, and high incidence of abnormal sperm (106).

Pathology. Vitamin A–deficiency lesions first appear in the pharynx and are largely confined to mucous glands and their ducts. The original epithelium is replaced by a keratinizing epithelium that blocks ducts of the mucous glands, causing them to become distended with secretions and necrotic materials. Small white pustules are found in nasal passages, mouth, esophagus, and pharynx and may extend into the crop. Pustules range in size from microscopic lesions to 2 mm in diameter (Fig. 2.2). As the deficiency progresses, lesions enlarge, are raised above the surface of the mucous membrane, and have a depression in the center. Small ulcers surrounded by inflammatory products may appear at the site of these lesions. This condition resembles certain stages of fowl pox, and the two conditions can be differentiated only by microscopic examination. Bacterial and viral infections often occur because of breakdown of the mucous membrane.

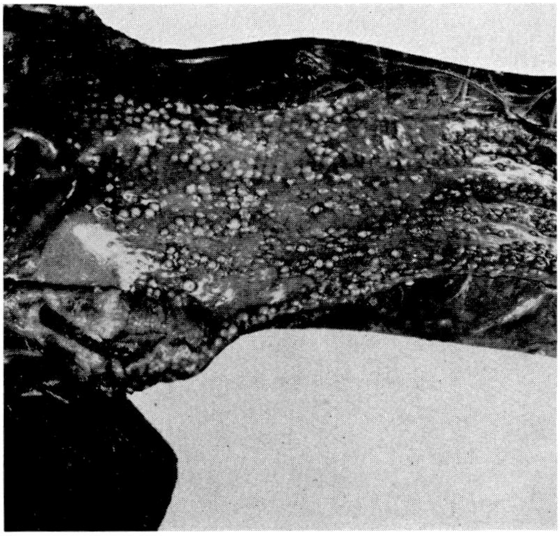

2.2. Pustulelike lesions in pharynx and esophagus due to vitamin A deficiency. (Biester and Schwarte, North Am Vet)

Clinical signs and lesions of vitamin A deficiency of the respiratory tract are variable; it is difficult to differentiate this condition from infectious coryza, fowl pox, and infectious bronchitis. In vitamin A deficiency, thin membranes and nasal plugs are usually limited to the cleft palate and its adjacent epithelium. They may be removed easily without bleeding. Atrophy and degeneration of the respiratory mucous membrane and its glands occur. Later, the original epithelium is replaced by a stratified squamous keratinizing epithelium. In early stages of vitamin A deficiency in chickens, turbinates are filled with seromucoid water-clear masses that may be forced out of the nodules and cleft palate by application of slight pressure. The vestibule becomes plugged and overflows into paranasal sinuses. Exudate may also fill sinuses and other nasal cavities, causing swelling of one or both sides of the face (Fig. 2.3). Mucous membranes, cleared of inflammatory products, appear thin, rough, and dry.

Similar lesions may frequently be found in trachea and bronchi. In early stages these may be difficult to see. As the condition progresses the mucous membrane is covered with a dry, dull, fine film that is slightly uneven, whereas normal membrane is even and moist. In some cases small nodulelike particles may be found in or beneath the mucous membrane in the upper part of the trachea.

Chronic vitamin A deficiency causes damage to the kidney tubules which leads to azotemia and visceral gout in severe cases (132).

Histopathology. The first histologic lesion of vitamin A deficiency is atrophy and deciliation of columnar ciliated epithelium of the respiratory tract (129). Nuclei often present marked karyorrhexis. A pseudomembrane formed by the atrophying and degenerating ciliated cells may hang as tufts on the basement membrane; later these are sloughed. During this process new cylindric or polygonal cells may be formed singly or in pairs and appear as islands beneath the epithelium. These new cells proliferate and their nuclei enlarge, containing less chromatin as they develop. Cell boundaries are less clearly defined; finally the columnar ciliated epithelial lining of nasal cavities and communicating sinuses, trachea, bronchi, and submucous glands are transformed into a stratified squamous keratinizing epithelium. Lesions in glands of tongue (Fig. 2.4), palate, and esophagus are similar to those of the respiratory tract (130).

Histopathologic examination of tissues from nasal passages of chicks serves as a sensitive indicator of borderline deficiencies of vitamin A (72). Chicks receiving suboptimal levels show lesions that resemble in basic character but not in severity those described by Seifried (129) for complete deficiency of vitamin A.

According to Wolbach and Hegsted (158, 159), vitamin A deficiency in young chicks and ducks causes marked retardation and suppression of endochondral bone growth. The proliferating zone is reduced. Hypertrophied cells accumulate, surrounded by uncalcified matrix. Vascular invasion of the epiphyseal cartilage is reduced and exhibits irregular patterns such as branching. The number of endosteal and periosteal osteoblasts is decreased, leading to impaired bone growth and thinning of bone cortex. Bone remodeling is inhibited. Disproportionate growth of brain and spinal cord relative to that of the axial skeleton appears to cause compression of brain tissue. Increased

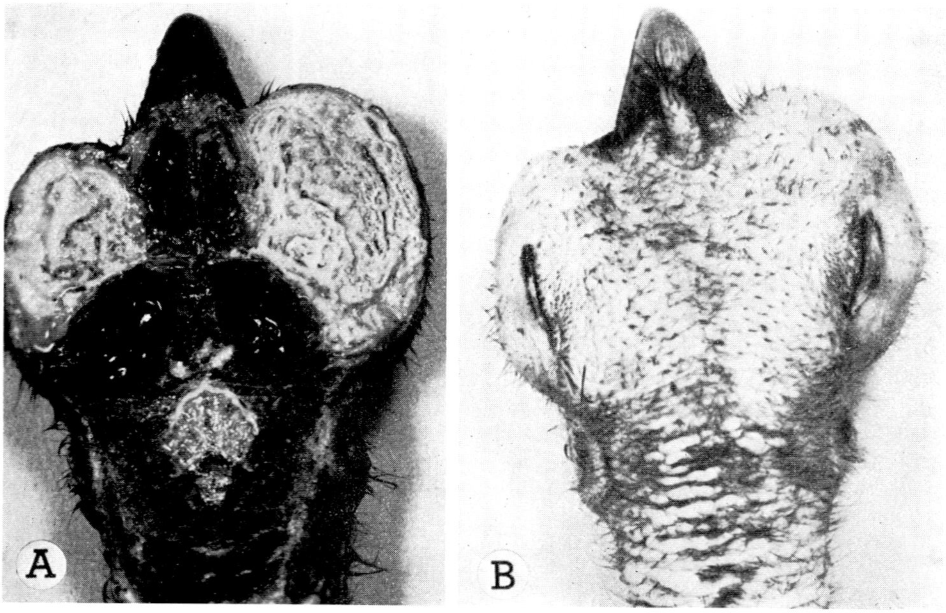

2.3. Extreme case of sinusitis in turkey hen suffering from vitamin A deficiency after being fed 8 mo on a ration containing a low level of vitamin A. A. Saggital section. B. Note massive accumulation of whitish yellow caseous exudate. (Hinshaw)

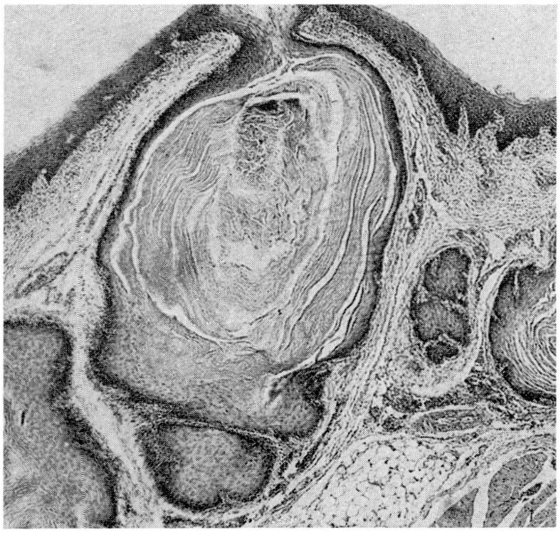

2.4. Cross section through base of tongue showing final stage of process with dilation of glands filled with stratified, more or less keratinized, homogeneous masses. ×50. (130)

cerebrospinal fluid pressure is one of the earliest signs of vitamin A deficiency (162).

Vitamin A deficiency has been reported to decrease hatchability of chicken and turkey eggs and increase mortality of chicks and poults that do hatch (9, 61). Thompson et al. (147) produced a severe vitamin A deficiency in developing embryos by supplementing breeder diets with retinoic acid. This form of vitamin A permits egg production but does not support embryonic development. Embryos die–always in the same stage of development. The complete trunk and head are formed, and the head is rotated slightly to one side. No differentiation of major blood vessels occurs, and an expanded area of vasculosa is seen forming a "blood ring" at the sinus terminalis.

Hypervitaminosis A. Baker et al. (16) reported that the administration of 200 mg retinyl acetate per kg of body weight per day to growing chickens adversely affects skeletal development. Chicks have lighter and shortened tibiae exhibiting widened epiphyseal growth plates with irregular tunneling by blood vessels. Widening results from increased numbers of hyperplastic chondrocytes. Bones exhibit reduced osteoblastic activity and increased bone and blood alkaline phosphatase activity. Ventricular dilation and brain swelling are also observed.

Tang et al. (144) administered 330 or 660 IU vitamin A per kg body weight per day to commercial broilers. Chicks had an unsteady gait and were reluctant to walk within a few days of treatment with excess vitamin A. They became anorexic by 9 days and developed conjunctivitis, adhesions of the eyelids, and encrustations around the mouth. Tibiae had widened epiphyseal growth plates due primarily to accumulation of hypertrophic chondrocytes. These investigators reported other abnormalities of the tibia including hyperosteoidosis and metaphyseal sclerosis. Frontal bones of the skull were thinner and more porous and exhibited thickened osteoid seams.

Signs of hypervitaminosis A in leghorn chicks differed from those of broiler chicks administered similar levels of vitamin A (144). The epiphyseal growth plates in tibiae from leghorn chicks were normal in width, but contained a narrower proliferative/maturation zone and a wider hypertrophic zone. Osteoid seams were normal. Leghorns had normal parathyroid morphology whereas parathyroid hyperplasia was observed in broiler chicks.

It must be noted that the reported histopathology of hypervitaminosis A is not entirely consistent among laboratories. The nature of the cell population contributing to widening of the epiphyseal growth plate differed in the preceding studies (16, 144). Wolbach and Hegstead (160, 161), moreover, reported that vitamin A excess caused narrowing of the growth plate in their early studies involving young chicks and ducks.

Treatment of Deficiency. Poultry found to be severely deficient in vitamin A should be given a stabilized vitamin A preparation at a level of approximately 10,000 IU vitamin A/kg of ration. Absorption of vitamin A is rapid; therefore, chickens or turkeys not in advanced stages of deficiency should respond promptly, except for blindness, which may be permanent.

VITAMIN D. Vitamin D is required by poultry for proper metabolism of calcium and phosphorus in formation of normal skeleton, hard beaks and claws, and strong eggshells.

One of the primary actions of vitamin D is concerned with stimulating gastrointestinal absorption of calcium. The metabolically active form of vitamin D is formed by two enzymatic hydroxylations of cholecalciferol (vitamin D_3), the first yielding 25-hydroxycholecalciferol in liver and the second yielding 1,25-dihydroxycholecalciferol in kidney (40). The latter appears to be a regulatory step, influenced by calcium status and activated by low blood phosphate or parathyroid hormone. Its product is much more potent in promoting calcium absorption and bone mobilization than its precursors, vitamin D_3 and 25-hydroxycholecalciferol. Many other hydroxylation products of 25-hydroxycholecalciferol have been identified. Their biological roles are unknown (7).

Signs of Deficiency. In confined laying hens, signs of deficiency begin to occur about 2–3 mo after they are deprived of vitamin D. The first sign is marked increase in number of thin-shelled and soft-shelled eggs, followed soon after by marked decrease in egg production. Egg production and eggshell strength may vary in a cyclic manner. Several cycles of decreased egg production and shell strength may each be followed by periods of relatively normal production and shell strength.

Individual hens may show temporary loss of use of the legs, with recovery after laying an egg that is usually shell-less. During periods of extreme leg weakness, hens show a characteristic posture that has been described as a "penguin-type squat." Later, beak, claws, and keel become very soft and pliable. The sternum usually is bent and ribs lose their normal rigidity and turn inward at the junction of the sternal and vertebral portions, producing a characteristic inward curve of the ribs along the sides of the thorax.

Vitamin D metabolism has been implicated in problems of eggshell quality. Soares et al. (134) recently reported that two strains of chickens that had been selected for divergence in eggshell strength and thickness differed in their blood concentrations of 1,25-dihydroxycholecalciferol: the strain having higher eggshell quality also had significantly higher concentrations of the vitamin D metabolite. When hens of a commercial strain of leghorns received 30 μg of vitamin D_3 or 5 μg of 1α-hydroxycholecalciferol, the latter resulted in greater tibial calcium and phosphorus content, tibial breaking strength, and eggshell mineralization. Bar et al. (18) reported that the inclusion of 2 or 5 μg/kg of 1,25-dihydroxycholecalciferol in the diet of aging hens increased shell weight and density in the first egg of the clutch and decreased the rate of decline of both measures in subsequent eggs of the clutch. Similar dietary levels of 1α-hydroxycholecalciferol increased shell density and reduced the proportion of cracked eggs in aging hens. The highest level of 1α-hydroxycholecalciferol, however, significantly increased the amount of mortality and culling. Both levels of 1α-hydroxycholecalciferol increased the concentrations of 1,25-dihydroxycholecalciferol in blood and calcium-binding protein (calbindin) in duodenal mucosa.

Hatchability is markedly reduced by vitamin D deficiency. Chicks and poults that do not hatch have a high incidence of chondrodystrophy in which the upper or lower mandible is shortened to the extent that occlusion of the mandibles is abnormal (136, 142). The synthetic vitamin D analogs 25-hydroxycholecalciferol, 1α-hydroxycholecalciferol, and 1,25-dihydroxycholecalciferol support adequate egg production and eggshell strength but only 25-hydroxycholecalciferol is effective in supporting hatchability (1, 7). Evidence strongly suggests that the other two analogs are poorly transported into the egg (8, 133). Manley and coworkers (87) reported that the addition of 1100 ICU of 25-hydroxycholecalciferol to diets of turkey hens that already contained 2200 ICU of vitamin D_3 improved the hatchability of fertile eggs. This interesting observation appears at odds with other evidence that 900 IU of vitamin D_3 per kilogram of diet is adequate for hatchability of turkey eggs (136).

In addition to retarded growth, the first sign of vitamin D deficiency in chicks or poults is rickets, characterized by a severe bone weakness. Between 2 and 3 wk of age beaks and claws become soft and pliable, and birds walk with obvious effort and take a few unsteady steps before squatting on their hocks, which they rest upon while swaying slightly from side to side. Feathering is poor. A marked increase in serum phosphatase is perhaps the first indicator of a borderline rachitic condition.

Pathology. In laying and breeding chicken and turkey hens receiving deficient vitamin D, characteristic changes observed on necropsy are confined to bones and parathyroid glands. The latter become enlarged from hypertrophy and hyperplasia. Bones are soft and break easily. Well-defined knobs are present on the inner surface of the ribs at the costochondral junction (rachitic rosary). Many ribs show evidence of pathologic fracture in this region. In chronic vitamin D deficiency, marked skeletal distortions become apparent. The spinal column may bend downward in the sacral and coccygeal region; the sternum usually shows a lateral bend and an acute dent near the middle of the breast. These changes reduce the size of the thorax with consequent crowding of vital organs.

The most characteristic internal signs of vitamin D deficiency in chicks and poults are a beading of the ribs at their juncture with the spinal column and a bending of the ribs downward and posteriorly (Fig. 2.5). Poor calcification can be observed at the epiphysis of the tibia or femur (Fig. 2.6). Bones of vitamin D–deficient chicks have a reduced calcium content with an increased proportion of osteoid, and a greater proportion of bone mineral is present as a low-density amorphous form of calcium phosphate (42). The ratio of dihydroxylysinonorleucine to hydroxylysinonorleucine in bone collagen is increased (92).

Vitamin D deficiency results in widening of the epiphyseal plate, hypertrophy, and softening of bone. Enlargement of the epiphyseal plate is due initially to widening of the proliferating and hypertrophic zones; as the deficiency progresses, it may be primarily the former (66, 81). Long and coworkers (81) noted that the hypertrophic zone exhibits irregular contours: wider in some areas and narrower in others, among and within affected birds. The widening of the proliferating zone appears to be the result of delayed chondrocyte hypertrophy rather than increased chondrocyte replication (76). As the deficiency pro-

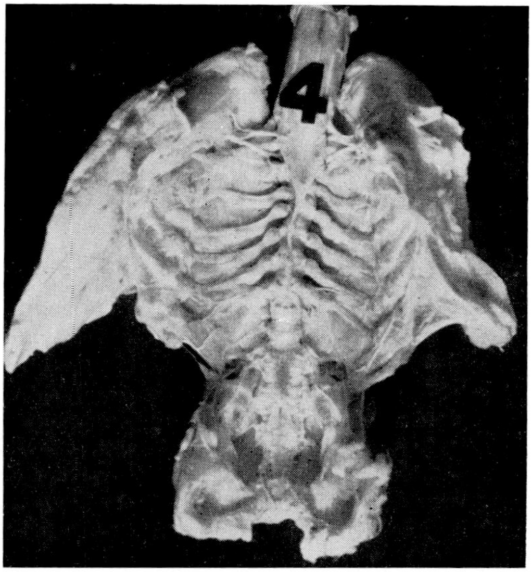

2.5. Rickets in a chicken showing severe beading and curvature of ribs and spinal column.

gresses, the columns of chondrocytes in the degenerating hypertrophic zone of the epiphyseal plate become shortened and thickened and exhibit an irregular pattern of invasion by metaphyseal blood vessels. Irregular patterns of cartilage and bone development occur in the primary and secondary spongiosa (66, 81). Porosity of cortical bone increases due to resorption of bone in haversion canals.

The histopathology of rickets differs significantly depending on the cause of the disease (76, 81–83). Refer to the section on calcium and phosphorus for further information on this topic.

Hypervitaminosis D. Very high levels of vitamin D_3–4 million IU or more/kg diet–causes renal damage from dystrophic calcification of kidney tubules. Calcification may be less often observed in the aorta and other arteries. A moderate excess of vitamin D has been reported to increase the incidence of eggshell pimpling (53). The latter appears to be due to excessive localized calcareous deposits on and within the eggshell that, when scraped off the shell, often expose the underlying eggshell membranes.

Treatment of Deficiency. Hooper et al. (63) found that feeding a single massive dose of 15,000 IU vitamin D_3 cured rachitic chicks more promptly than when generous levels of the vitamin were added to feed. This single oral dose protected cockerels against rickets for 8 wk and pullet chicks for 5 wk. In giving massive doses to rachitic chicks it should be remembered that excess vitamin D can be harmful. The dose should be scaled to the degree of deficiency, and excessive amounts of vitamin D should not be added to feed.

VITAMIN E. Vitamin E deficiency produces encephalomalacia, exudative diathesis, and muscular dystrophy in chicks; enlarged hocks and dystrophy of the gizzard musculature in turkeys; and muscular dystrophy in ducks. Vitamin E also is required for normal embryonic development in chickens, turkeys, and probably ducks.

In its alcoholic form vitamin E is a very effective antioxidant. It is an important protector in feeds of the essential fatty acids and other highly unsaturated fatty acids as well as vitamins A and D_3, carotenes, and xanthophylls. Selenium (Se) at dietary concentrations of 0.04–0.1 parts per million (ppm) has been shown to prevent or cure ex-

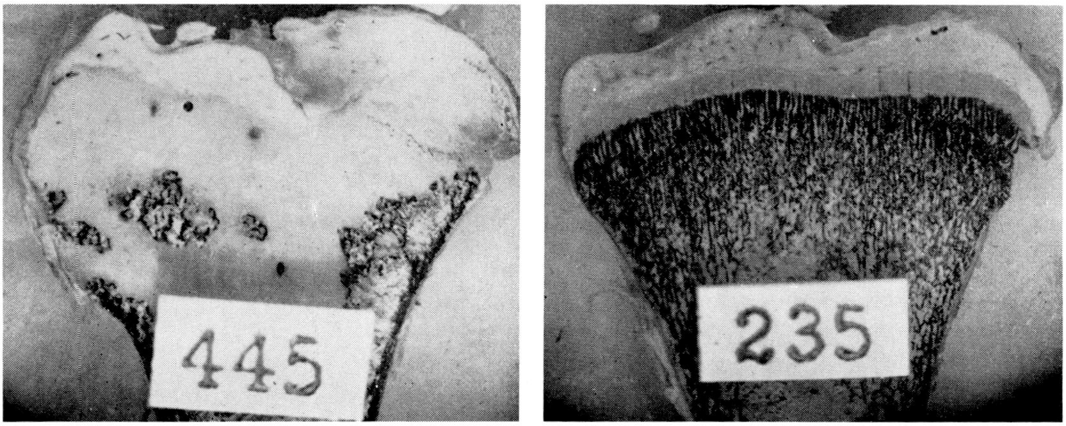

2.6. Tibiae of severely vitamin D-deficient rachitic (445) and normal (235) chick, after staining with silver nitrate and exposure to light.

udative diathesis in vitamin E–deficient chicks (123, 124). Selenium at 0.1–0.2 ppm effectively prevents myopathies of gizzard and heart in young poults (128).

Vitamin E plays a multiple role in poultry nutrition. It is required not only for normal reproduction but also as nature's most effective antioxidant for prevention of encephalomalacia, in a specific role interrelated with action of Se for prevention of exudative diathesis and turkey myopathies, and in another role interrelated with Se and cystine for prevention of nutritional muscular dystrophy.

Signs and Pathology of Deficiency. No outward signs occur in mature chickens or turkeys receiving very low levels of vitamin E over prolonged periods. However, hatchability of eggs from vitamin E–deficient chickens or turkeys is reduced markedly (67). Embryos from hens fed rations low in vitamin E may die as early as the 4th day of incubation or considerably later, depending on severity of the deficiency. Turkey embryos may have bilateral cataracts that can cause blindness (46). Testicular degeneration occurs in males deprived of vitamin E for prolonged periods (4).

ENCEPHALOMALACIA IN CHICKS. Encephalomalacia is a nervous derangement characterized by ataxia, backward or downward retractions of the head (sometimes with lateral twisting), forced movements, increasing incoordination, rapid contraction and relaxation of the legs, and finally complete prostration and death. Even under these conditions, complete paralysis of wings or legs is not observed. The deficiency usually manifests itself between the 15th and 30th days of the chick's life, although it has been known to occur as early as the 7th and as late as the 56th day.

The cerebellum, striatal hemispheres, medulla oblongata, and mesencephalon are affected most commonly in the order named (105). In chicks killed soon after appearance of signs of encephalomalacia, the cerebellum is softened and swollen and the meninges are edematous. Minute hemorrhages are often visible on the surface of the cerebellum. The convolutions are flattened. As much as four-fifths of the cerebellum may be affected, or lesions may be so small they cannot be recognized grossly. A day or two after signs of encephalomalacia appear, necrotic areas present a green-yellow opaque appearance.

In the corpus striatum necrotic tissue is frequently pale, swollen, and wet and in early stages becomes sharply delineated from remaining normal tissue. The greater portion of both hemispheres may be destroyed. In other cases lesions are apparent only on microscopic examination. Medullary lesions are not so readily noted in a macroscopic examination.

Histologically, lesions include circulatory disturbances (ischemic necrosis), demyelination, and neuronal degeneration. Meningeal, cerebellar, and cerebral vessels are markedly hyperemic, and a severe edema usually develops. Capillary thrombosis often results in necrosis of varying extent. In the normal chick cerebellum, myelinated tracts exhibit a strongly positive reaction with Luxol fast blue, whereas in affected chicks the staining reaction is markedly diminished, diffusely or locally accentuated (Fig. 2.7). Degenerative neuronal changes occur everywhere but are most prominent in Purkinje cells and in large motor nuclei. Ischemic cell change is most frequently encountered. Cells are shrunken and intensely hyperchromatic, and the nucleus is typically triangular. Peripheral chromatolysis with the Nissl substance packed along the periphery of the cell nucleus is also common.

Signs of encephalomalacia in turkey poults are similar to those observed in chicks (68).

EXUDATIVE DIATHESIS IN CHICKS. Exudative diathesis is an edema of subcutaneous tissues (Fig. 2.8) associated with abnormal permeability of capillary walls. In severe cases chicks stand with their legs far apart as a result of accumulation of fluid under the ventral skin. This green-blue viscous fluid is easily seen through the skin since it usually contains some blood components from slight hemorrhages that appear throughout the breast and leg musculature and in the intestinal walls. Distention of the pericardium and sudden deaths have been noted. Chicks suffering from exudative diathesis show a low ratio of albumin to globulins in blood (52).

Onset of exudative diathesis coincides with appearance of peroxides in tissues. Noguchi et al. (101) proposed that vitamin E in the capillary membranes and the Se-containing enzyme glutathione peroxidase of plasma protect the capillary membrane against oxidative damage. This may explain the dual role of vitamin E and Se in prevention of exudative diathesis and other vitamin E/Se-responsive diseases (126, 139).

MUSCULAR DYSTROPHY IN CHICKENS, DUCKS, AND TURKEYS. When vitamin E deficiency is accompanied by a sulfur amino acid deficiency, chicks show signs of muscular dystrophy, particularly of the breast muscle, at about 4 wk of age. The condition is characterized by light-colored streaks of easily distinguished affected bundles of muscle fibers in the breast (Fig. 2.9). A similar dystrophy occurs throughout all skeletal muscles of the body in vitamin E–deficient ducks.

The initial histologic change is hyaline degeneration. Mitochondria undergo swelling, coalesce, and form intracytoplasmic globules. Later, muscle fibers are disrupted transversely (Fig. 2.10, lower part). Extravasation separates groups

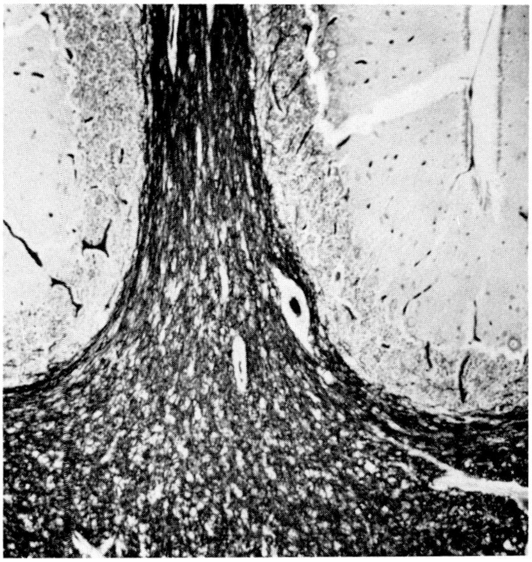

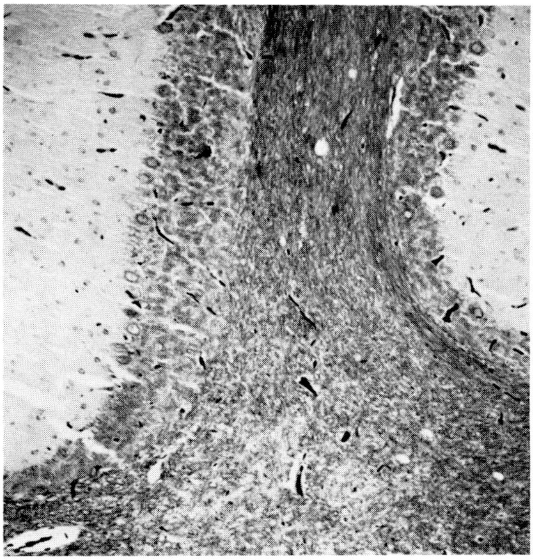

2.7. Cerebellum of normal chick (*left*) and chick with encephalomalacia (*right*). Note poor staining reaction of the myelinated tract in the affected cerebellum. Luxol Fast Blue, ×120.

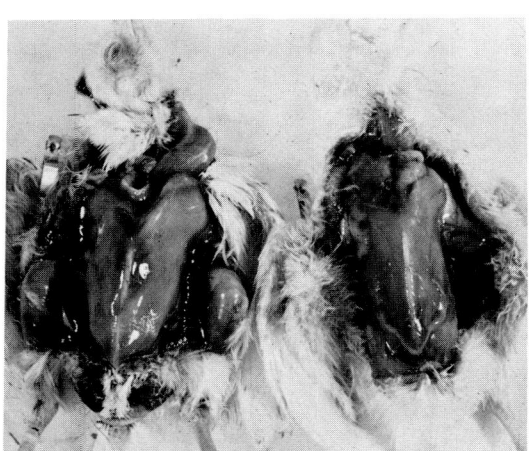

2.8. Exudative diathesis in chicks.

of muscle fibers and individual fibers. The transuded plasma usually contains erythrocytes and heterophilic leukocytes. In more chronic conditions, reparative processes dominate the picture. There is a pronounced proliferation of cell nuclei and also fibroplasia (Fig. 2.10, upper part), leaving a scar in the degenerate muscle.

Vitamin E and Se deficiency in chickens and especially in turkeys may result in an extreme myopathy of the gizzard (Fig. 2.11) and heart muscles (128).

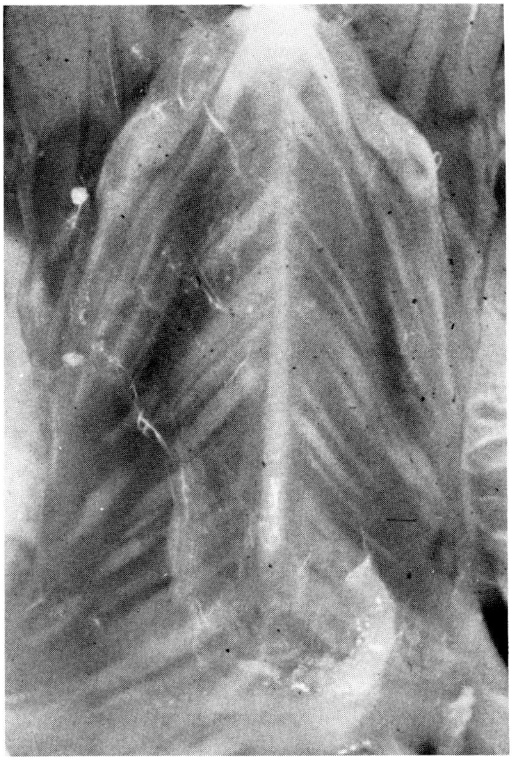

2.9. Muscular dystrophy in chicks.

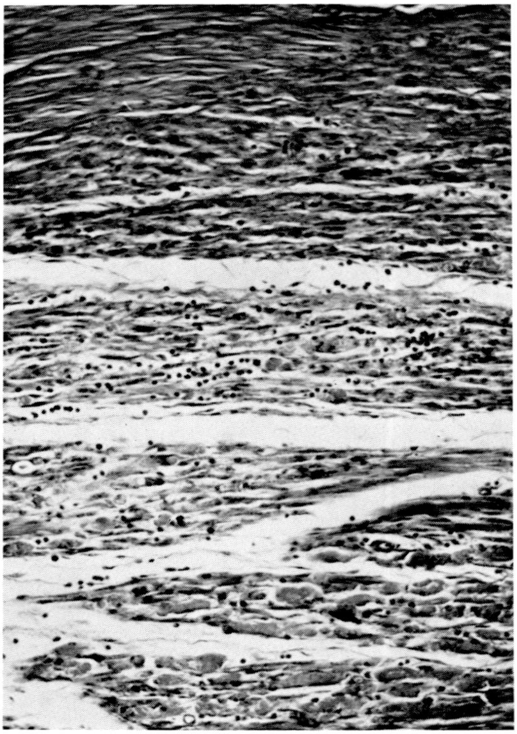

2.10. Pectoral muscle of chick with muscular dystrophy. Upper part shows proliferation of muscle nuclei and fibroblasts; lower part shows disruption of muscle fibers and separation of fibers and bundle fibers by edema. Dark spots in edema are heterophilic leukocytes. H & E, ×180.

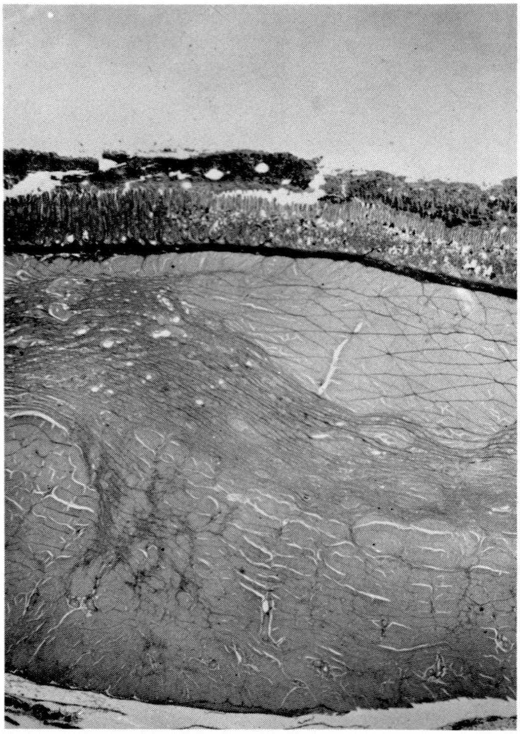

2.11. Gizzard. Chronic vitamin E deficiency in turkey showing extensive scar formation. Van Gieson, ×10.

ENLARGED HOCK DISORDER IN TURKEYS. Turkeys receiving diets low in vitamin E and also containing readily oxidizable fats or oils may develop characteristic hock enlargements and bowed legs at approximately 2–3 wk of age (122). If poults are allowed to continue on these diets, hock enlargements usually disappear by the time the poults are 6 wk of age, only to reappear in more severe form when they reach 14–16 wk, especially in toms raised on wire or slat floors. Creatine excretion is increased and muscle creatine levels are reduced. The need for vitamin E may be related to a protection of biotin that otherwise might be destroyed in presence of rancidifying fats or oils (125).

Treatment of Deficiency. If not too far advanced, exudative diathesis and muscular dystrophy in chicks are readily reversed by administration of proper levels of vitamin E and Se by injection, by oral dosing, or in feed. Encephalomalacia may or may not respond to treatment with vitamin E, depending on extent of damage to the cerebellum. Gizzard myopathy in turkeys is prevented by supplementing deficient diets with vitamin E or Se. It is not affected by the dietary level of sulfur amino acids.

VITAMIN K. Vitamin K is required for synthesis of prothrombin. It is a cofactor in the post-translational carboxylation of glutamic acid in prothrombin and a protein in bone, osteocalcin. The product, gamma-carboxyglutamic acid, is anionic at physiologic pH and functions in the binding of Ca^{++} to protein during blood-clotting. In the absence of vitamin K, an abnormal prothrombin, lacking gamma-carboxyglutamic acid, is secreted into the body by the liver (50). Since prothrombin is an important part of the blood-clotting mechanism, deficiency of vitamin K results in markedly prolonged blood-clotting time; an affected chick or poult may bleed to death from a slight bruise or other injury.

Signs and Pathology of Deficiency. Signs of vitamin K deficiency occur most frequently 2–3 wk after chicks are placed on a vitamin K-deficient diet. Presence of sulfaquinoxaline in feed or drinking water may increase incidence and severity of the condition. Large hemorrhages appear on the breast, legs, wings, and/or in the abdominal cavity. Chicks show an anemia that may result partly from loss of blood but also from development of a hypoplastic bone marrow. Although blood-clotting time is a fairly good measure of vitamin K deficiency, a more accurate one is obtained by determining prothrombin time. Inadequate vitamin K in breeder diets causes increased embryo mortality late in incubation. Dead embryos appear hemorrhagic.

Treatment of Deficiency. Within 4–6 hr after vitamin K is administered to deficient chicks, blood clots normally, but recovery from anemia or disappearance of hemorrhages cannot be expected to take place promptly.

THIAMIN (VITAMIN B_1). Thiamin is converted in the body to an active form, thiamin pyrophosphate, which is an important cofactor in oxidative decarboxylation reactions and aldehyde exchanges in carbohydrate metabolism. Deficiency of thiamin leads to extreme anorexia, polyneuritis, and death.

Signs and Pathology of Deficiency. Polyneuritis is observed in mature chickens approximately 3 wk after they are placed on a thiamin-deficient diet. In young chicks it may appear before 2 wk of age. Onset is sudden in young chicks but more gradual in mature birds. Anorexia is followed by loss of weight, ruffled feathers, leg weakness, and an unsteady gait. Adult chickens often show a blue comb. As the deficiency progresses, apparent paralysis of muscles occurs, beginning with the flexors of the toes and progressing upward, affecting the extensor muscles of legs, wings, and neck. The chicken characteristically sits on its flexed legs and draws back the head in a "stargazing" position (Fig. 2.12). Retraction of the head is due to paralysis of the anterior muscles of the neck. The chicken soon loses ability to stand or sit upright and topples to the floor where it may lie with the head still retracted.

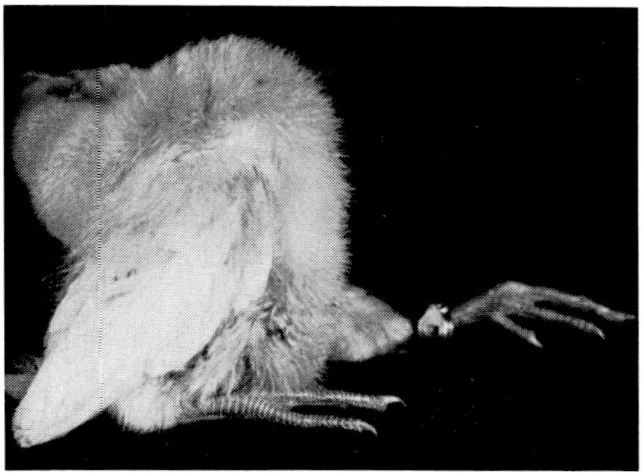

2.12. Typical stargazing pose displayed by chick suffering from thiamin deficiency.

The body temperature may drop to as low as 35.6 C. A progressive decrease in respiration rate occurs. Adrenal glands hypertrophy more markedly in females than males. The cortex is affected to a greater extent than the medulla. Apparently the degree of hypertrophy determines the degree of edema, which occurs chiefly in the skin. The epinephrine content of the adrenal gland increases as the organ hypertrophies. Atrophy of genital organs is more pronounced in males than females. The heart shows a slight degree of atrophy; the right side may be dilated, the auricle being more frequently affected than the ventricle. Atrophy of the stomach and intestinal walls may be sufficiently severe to be easily noted.

Crypts of Lieberkühn in the duodenum of deficient chicks become dilated (54). Mitosis of epithelial cells in the crypts decreases markedly; in advanced stages of deficiency the mucosal lining disappears, leaving a connective tissue framework. Necrotic cells and cell debris accumulate in the enlarged crypts (Fig. 2.13). Exocrine cells of the pancreas show cytoplasmic vacuolation with formation of hyaline bodies.

Treatment of Deficiency. Chickens suffering from thiamin deficiency respond in a matter of a few hours to oral administration of the vitamin. Since thiamin deficiency causes extreme anorexia, supplementing feed with the vitamin is not a reliable treatment until after chickens have recovered from acute deficiency.

RIBOFLAVIN (VITAMIN B_2). Riboflavin is a cofactor in many enzyme systems in the body. Examples of riboflavin-containing enzymes are: NAD- and NADP-cytochrome reductases, succinic dehydrogenase, acyl dehydrogenase, diaphorase, xanthine oxidase, L- and D-amino acid oxidases, L-hydroxy acid oxidases, and histaminase, some of which are vitally associated with oxidation-reduction reactions involved in cell respiration.

Signs and Pathology of Deficiency. When chicks are fed a diet deficient in riboflavin, they grow very slowly and become weak and emaciated; their appetite is fairly good; diarrhea develops between the 1st and 2nd wk. Chicks do not walk except when forced to, and then frequently walk on their hocks with the aid of their wings. Toes are curled inward when both walking and resting (Fig. 2.14). Chicks are usually found in a resting position. The wings often droop as though it were impossible to hold them in the normal position. Leg muscles are atrophied and flabby, and the skin is dry and harsh. Young chicks in ad-

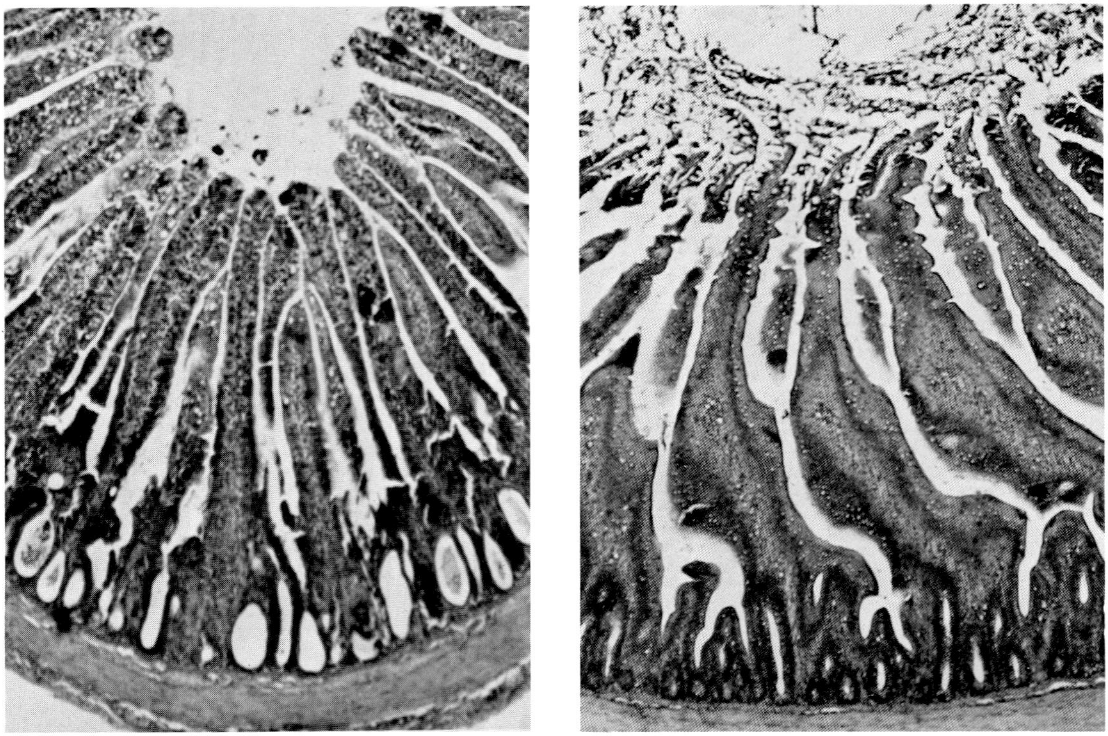

2.13. Duodenum from thiamin-deficient chick, with severe dilation of crypts of Lieberkühn (*left*). Control (*right*). ×30.

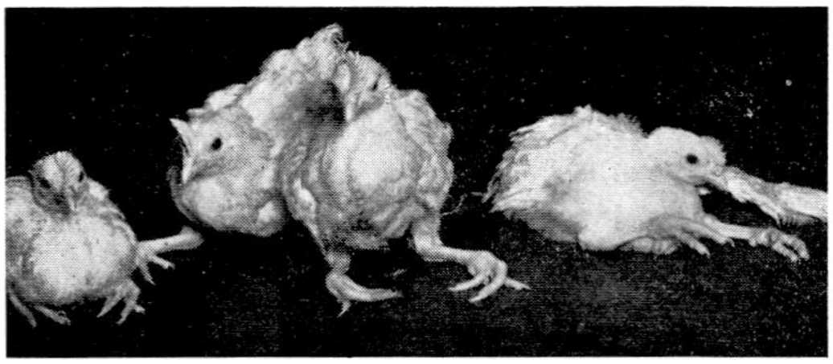

2.14. Riboflavin deficiency (curly toe).

vanced stages of deficiency do not move around but lie with their legs sprawled out.

A deficiency of riboflavin in the diet of hens results in decreased egg production, increased embryonic mortality, and an increase in size and fat content of the liver. Hatchability of eggs decreases within 2 wk after hens are fed a riboflavin-deficient diet but improves to near normal levels within 7 days after adequate amounts of riboflavin are added to the diet. Embryos that fail to hatch from eggs of hens fed diets low in this vitamin are dwarfed and show a high incidence of edema, degeneration of Wolffian bodies, and defective down. The down is referred to as "clubbed" and results from failure of the down feathers to rupture the sheaths, causing feathers to coil in a characteristic way.

Riboflavin deficiency in young turkeys is characterized by poor growth and incrustations in the corners of the mouth and on the eyelids. Severe dermatitis of the feet and shanks—marked by edematous swelling, desquamation, and deep fissures—appears in some deficient poults (90).

In severe cases of riboflavin deficiency chicks show marked swelling and softening of sciatic and brachial nerves. Sciatic nerves usually undergo the most pronounced changes, sometimes reaching a diameter four to five times normal size. Histologic examination of affected nerves shows degenerative changes in myelin sheaths of the main peripheral nerve trunks. This may be accompanied by axis-cylinder swelling and fragmentation. Schwann cell proliferation, myelin changes, gliosis, and chromatolysis occur in the spinal cord. In cases of curled-toe paralysis, degeneration of the neuromuscular end plate and muscle tissues is often found. Riboflavin is probably also essential for myelin metabolism of the main peripheral nerve trunks. No gross dystrophy develops, although muscle fibers are in some cases completely degenerated. The sciatic nerve exhibits myelin degeneration in one or more branches. Similar changes are apparent in the brachial nerve trunks.

The nervous system of embryos that fail to hatch from eggs laid by hens fed riboflavin-deficient diets has degenerative changes very much like those described in riboflavin-deficient chicks (45).

Chicks fed riboflavin-deficient diets develop pancreatic and duodenal lesions as described for thiamin deficiency in addition to the more classic nervous signs (54).

Treatment of Deficiency. Fig. 2.15 shows a 35-day-old poult prostrate from riboflavin deficiency, with curled-toe paralysis. This same poult was standing with toes extended normally 5 days later after having been given two 100-μg doses of riboflavin. This amount should be sufficient for treatment of riboflavin-deficient chicks or poults, followed by incorporation of an adequate level in the ration. However, when the curled-toe deformity is of long standing, irreparable damage has occurred and administration of riboflavin no longer cures the condition.

PANTOTHENIC ACID. Pantothenic acid is a component of coenzyme A, which is involved in formation of citric acid, synthesis and oxidation of fatty acids, oxidation of keto acids resulting from deamination of amino acids, acetylation of choline, and many other reactions.

Signs and Pathology of Deficiency. Signs of pantothenic acid deficiency in chicks are difficult to differentiate from those of biotin deficiency; deficiencies of either result in dermatitis, broken feathers, perosis, poor growth, and mortality. Pantothenic acid–deficient chicks are characterized by retarded and rough feather growth. Chicks are emaciated, and definite crusty scablike lesions appear in corners of the mouth. Eyelid margins are granular, and small scabs develop on them. Eyelids frequently are stuck together by a viscous exudate; they are contracted, and vision is restricted (Fig. 2.16). There is slow sloughing of the keratinizing epithelium of the skin. Outer layers of skin between the toes and on bottoms of the feet sometimes peel off; small cracks and fissures appear at these points. These cracks and fissures enlarge and deepen so that chicks move

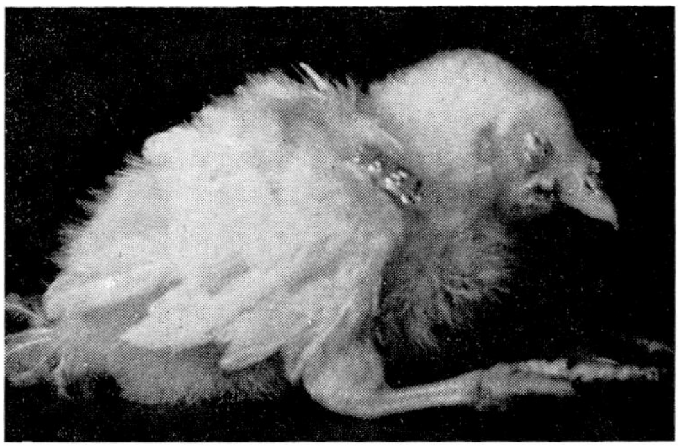

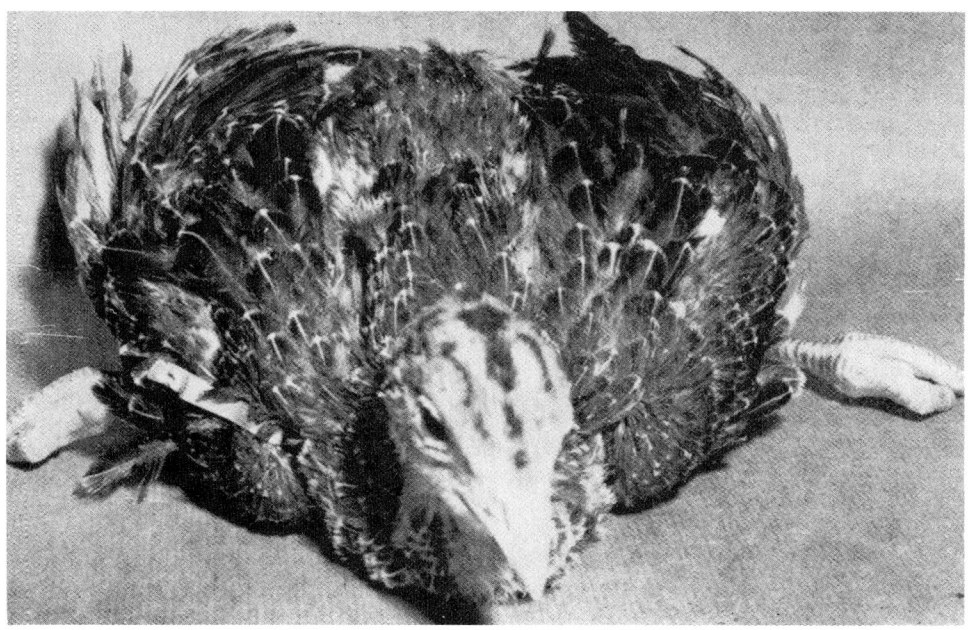

2.16. Dermatosis of pantothenic acid deficiency in the chick.

2.15. A 35-day-old poult showing riboflavin deficiency with curled-toe paralysis. This poult completely recovered 5 days after receiving two 100-μg doses of riboflavin. (Richardson)

about very little. In some cases skin layers of the feet of deficient chicks cornify, and wartlike protuberances develop on the balls of the feet.

Necropsy shows the presence of a puslike substance in the mouth and an opaque gray-white exudate in the proventriculus (114). The liver is hypertrophied and may vary in color from a faint to dirty yellow. The spleen is slightly atrophied. Kidneys are somewhat enlarged. Nerves and myelinated fibers of the spinal cord show myelin degeneration (111). These degenerating fibers occur in all segments of the cord down to the lumbar region.

Pantothenic acid is required in the diet of breeding hens for normal hatchability of eggs (51). Beer et al. (21) observed that the peak day of embryonic mortality depends on the degree of pantothenic acid deficiency and that borderline deficiencies produce extremely weak chicks that fail to survive unless injected immediately with pantothenic acid (200 μg intraperitoneally). Subcutaneous hemorrhage and severe edema are signs of pantothenic acid deficiency in the developing chicken embryo (21).

Pantothenic acid deficiency in chicks produces duodenal and pancreatic lesions as described under thiamin deficiency (but of lesser extent), dermatosis, and severe ataxia progressing to inability to stand. In addition there is pronounced lymphocytic necrosis and lymphoid depletion in the bursa of Fabricius, thymus, and spleen (54).

Treatment of Deficiency. Pantothenic acid deficiency appears to be completely reversible, if not too far advanced, by oral treatment or injection with the vitamin followed by restoration of an adequate level in the diet.

NICOTINIC ACID (NIACIN). Nicotinic acid is the vitamin component in two important coenzymes, nicotinamide adenine dinucleotide (NAD) and nicotinamide adenine dinucleotide phosphate (NADP), which are extensively involved in carbohydrate, fat, and protein metabolism. They are especially important in metabolic reactions that furnish energy. One or both coenzymes take part in the anaerobic and aerobic oxidation of glucose, glycerol synthesis and catabolism, fatty acid synthesis and oxidation, and oxidation of acetyl coenzyme A via the Krebs cycle.

Niacin-Tryptophan-Pyridoxine Interrelationships. Tryptophan pyrrolase catalyzes the initial reaction in the major metabolic pathway of tryptophan catabolism. Picolinic carboxylase regulates an important branchpoint in the pathway at which an intermediate either enters a sequence of reactions resulting in its degradation to carbon dioxide, water, and ammonia or enters a biosynthetic pathway leading to NAD synthesis. Picolinic carboxylase catalyzes the first reaction in the degradative pathway, whereas the first reaction in the NAD pathway occurs nonenzymatically. High picolinic carboxylase activity limits the synthesis of NAD from tryptophan.

Key enzymes in the metabolism of tryptophan require vitamin B_6 as a cofactor, and limit the overall pathway in vitamin B_6 deficiency. Briggs et al. (27) first showed that niacin requirements of chicks and hens depend on the level of tryptophan in the diet. When tryptophan is marginally adequate, chickens are able to synthesize approximately 1 mg of niacin from 45 mg of dietary tryptophan (17, 32, 43). Ducks in contrast are much less efficient: approximately 1 mg niacin can be synthesized from 175 mg of dietary tryptophan (32). This difference in efficiency of conversion of tryptophan to niacin is reflected in a markedly higher niacin requirement for ducks than chicks. It has been attributed to relatively high picolinic carboxylase activity in ducks (32, 43).

Signs and Pathology of Deficiency. The main sign of nicotinic acid deficiency in young chicks, turkeys, and ducks is an enlargement of the hock joint and bowing of the legs similar to perosis (127). The main difference between this condition and the perosis of manganese or choline deficiency is that in nicotinic acid deficiency the Achilles tendon rarely slips from its condyles. Scott (122) showed that both nicotinic acid and vitamin E are required for prevention of the disorder in turkeys. Briggs (26) described further signs of nicotinic acid deficiency as inflammation of the mouth, diarrhea, and poor feathering. Hock disorders and lesions of the mouth were prominent in ducks and chicks respectively in recent studies of Chen (32). Niacin/tryptophan deficiency in chicks produces duodenal and pancreatic lesions comparable to those of thiamin deficiency (54).

Ringrose et al. (115) observed reduced feed consumption and body weight, decreased rate of egg production, and reduced hatchability of eggs when hens were fed a semipurified diet based on casein and gelatin as the sources of protein and lacking in supplemental niacin. No signs of pathology were observed. Based on their data, the authors suggested that 0.8 mg and 1.0 mg niacin/hen/day were required in order to maintain egg production and hatchability, respectively. However, no evidence has been obtained of any need to supplement practical diets of mature poultry with nicotinic acid (2).

Treatment of Deficiency. Supplementing a deficient ration with required amounts of nicotinic acid supplementation has little or no effect on cases that have progressed to the extent that the tendon has slipped from its condyles (perosis) or on advanced cases of enlarged hock disorder in adult tom turkeys.

PYRIDOXINE (VITAMIN B_6). Pyridoxine is required in several enzymes, particularly those concerned in transamination and decarboxylation of amino acids. The coenzymes are pyridoxal phosphate and pyridoxamine phosphate.

Signs and Pathology of Deficiency. Pyridoxine-deficient chicks show depressed appetite, poor growth, perosis, and characteristic nervous signs. Chicks show jerky, nervous movements of the legs when walking and often undergo extreme spasmodic convulsions that usually terminate in death. During these convulsions chicks may run aimlessly about, flapping their wings and falling to their sides or rolling completely over on their backs, where they perform rapid jerking motions with their feet and heads. These signs may be distinguished from those of encephalomalacia (vitamin E deficiency) by the relatively greater intensity of activity of the chicks during a seizure, which results in complete exhaustion and often death.

Gries and Scott (55) observed that chicks fed very low levels of pyridoxine (up to 2.2 mg B_6/kg diet) combined with a high protein level (31%) have classic nervous signs. Intermediate levels (2.5–2.8 mg B_6/kg diet) combined with 31% protein cause severe perosis but no nervous signs. The consequence is bone curvature. If the diet contains 22% protein, even the lowest levels of pyridoxine (1.9 mg/kg diet) fail to induce nervous signs, perosis, or even lowered growth rate. The function of pyridoxine in amino acid metabolism is reflected in an increased requirement when high levels of protein are fed.

In adult birds pyridoxine deficiency causes marked reduction of egg production and hatchability as well as decreased feed consumption, loss of weight, and death.

BIOTIN. Biotin is a cofactor in carboxylation and decarboxylation reactions involving fixation of carbon dioxide. These reactions have important roles in anabolic processes and in nitrogen metabolism.

Signs and Pathology of Deficiency. In biotin deficiency the dermatitis of the feet and skin around the beak and eyes is similar to that of pantothenic acid deficiency (Fig. 2.17). Thus in making a differential diagnosis, it is usually necessary to examine composition of the diet.

Perosis is a sign of biotin avitaminosis in growing chickens and turkeys. Biotin-deficiency signs in chicks include various other abnormalities of the tibia. Bain et al. (15) reported that chicks fed a purified diet devoid of biotin had shortened tibiae, higher bone density and bone ash, and an abnormal pattern of bone modelling: the median side of the mid-diaphyseal cortex was thicker than the lateral side in chicks fed the biotin-free diet, whereas the opposite pattern existed for chicks fed the same diet supplemented with adequate biotin. This raises the possibility that biotin may have a role in varus deformities of the limb (15).

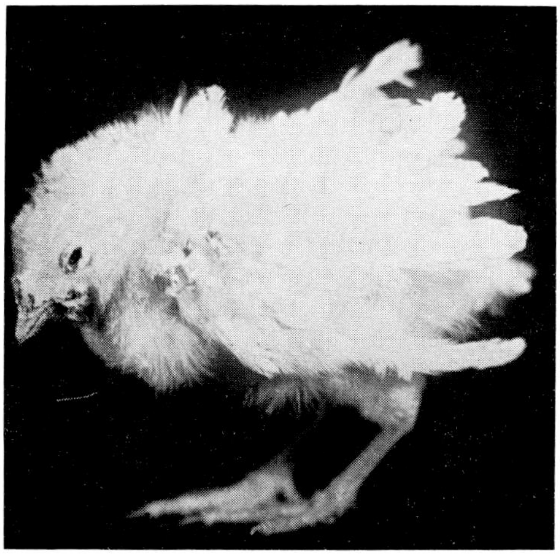

2.17. Biotin-deficient chick.

Biotin is essential for embryonic development (35, 36). Embryos from hens fed biotin-deficient diets developed syndactylia, an extensive webbing between the third and fourth toes. Many embryos that fail to hatch are chondrodystrophic—characterized by reduced size, a parrot beak, severely crooked tibia, shortened or twisted tarsometatarsus, shortened bones of the wing and skull, and shortening and bending of the scapula. Two peaks of embryonic mortality may occur: one during the 1st wk and a second during the last 3 days of incubation.

Robel and Christensen (117) recently reported that the injection of 87 μg of D-biotin into eggs of large white turkey hens that had been held under commercial conditions resulted in approximately 4–5% higher hatchability of their eggs. The reason for the improvement is not known; however, the authors suggest that biotin levels or biotin availability in the egg may have been low.

Fatty liver and kidney syndrome (FLKS) is a biotin-responsive condition that has been observed in broiler chicks. Chicks exhibit depressed growth; fatty infiltrations of liver, kidney, and heart; decreased plasma glucose; increased plasma-free fatty acids; and increased ratio of C16:1 to C18:0 fatty acids in liver and adipose tissue (108, 149). High dietary protein or fat reduces or eliminates mortality, whereas high protein or fat increases the signs of biotin deficiency. Fasting exacerbates FLKS and its associated mortality (149). Fasting decreases blood glucose concentrations and increases plasma-free fatty acids. Pyruvic carboxylase, a biotin-containing enzyme, is decreased in activity in FLKS biotin deficiency

(108). It has been suggested that biotin deficiency impairs gluconeogenesis as a result of low activity of this enzyme, leading to increased conversion of pyruvate to fatty acids. Chicks having FLKS frequently do not have the characteristic signs of biotin deficiency. It is quite possible that this condition is not a simple biotin deficiency but involves other unrecognized nutritional or environmental factors.

Recently, biotin has been suspected of having a role in "acute death syndrome" (or "sudden death syndrome") in broiler chickens. Biotin deficiency alters the unsaturated fatty acid profile in tissue lipids in such a manner as to suggest that it impairs the conversion of linoleic acid to arachidonic acid (148). The latter is a precursor of the prostaglandins, prostocyclin I_2 and thromboxane A_2, which have marked effects on the vascular system. The concentration of biotin in liver was reported to be depressed in chicks that exhibited acute death syndrome (75). Hulan et al. (65) had previously reported that dietary biotin reduced the incidence of acute death syndrome in broiler chicks. However, this effect was not observed in other treatments in the same experiment in which combinations of biotin, pyridoxine, and thiamine providing similar, or two- and four-fold higher, concentrations of biotin were included in the diet. The role of biotin in acute death syndrome remains obscure.

Biotin bioavailability for chickens and turkeys varies greatly among practical feed ingredients (48, 94, 150). Biotin is no more than 10% available in some grains but almost completely available in others. This is an important consideration in formulating diets to satisfy the biotin requirements of poultry.

Treatment of Deficiency. Patrick et al. (107) and Jukes and Bird (69) reported that injection or oral administration of a few micrograms of biotin was sufficient to prevent biotin-deficiency signs in chicks and turkey poults.

FOLIC ACID (FOLACIN). Folic acid is a part of the enzyme system concerned in single-carbon metabolism. It is involved in synthesis of purines and the methyl groups of such important metabolites as choline, methionine, and thymine. Folic acid, therefore, is required for normal nucleic acid metabolism and formation of the nucleoproteins required for cell multiplication.

Signs and Pathology of Deficiency. Folic acid deficiency in chicks is characterized by poor growth, very poor feathering, anemia, and perosis. Folic acid is required for pigmentation in feathers of Rhode Island Red and black leghorn chicks. Thus folic acid, lysine, copper, and iron appear to be required for prevention of achroma of feathers in colored poultry.

A deficiency in the breeding diet of chickens or turkeys causes a marked increase in embryonic mortality. Embryos die soon after pipping the air cell. According to Sunde et al. (140, 141), a deformed upper mandible and bending of the tibiotarsus are lesions of embryonic deficiency. Poults show a characteristic cervical paralysis and die within 2 days after the onset of these signs unless folic acid is administered immediately. Poults show only a slight anemia.

Folic acid deficiency in chicks causes megaloblastic arrest of erythrocyte formation in bone marrow, which results in a severe macrocytic anemia as one of the first signs in chicks. White cell formation also is reduced, causing a marked agranulocytosis.

Folic Acid–Choline Interrelationship. Folic acid has a central role in methyl group metabolism. Young et al. (163) observed that when a diet for chicks is deficient in folic acid, an increase in the dietary level of choline reduces, but does not completely prevent, the incidence and severity of perosis.

Treatment of Deficiency. A single intramuscular (IM) injection of 50–100 μg pure pteroylglutamic (folic) acid causes a peak reticulocyte response within 4 days in severely anemic folic acid–deficient chicks (118). Hemoglobin values and growth rates return to normal within 1 wk. Addition of 500 μg folic acid/100 g feed caused recovery comparable to that obtained with injection of the vitamin.

VITAMIN B_{12} (COBALAMIN). Vitamin B_{12} is concerned in nucleic acid and methyl synthesis and carbohydrate and fat metabolism. One of its main enzyme functions involves isomerization of methylmalonyl coenzyme A to form succinyl CoA.

Signs and Pathology of Deficiency. Signs of vitamin B_{12} deficiency are slow growth, decreased efficiency of feed utilization, mortality, and reduced egg size and hatchability. Specific signs for vitamin B_{12} deficiency have not been demonstrated in growing or mature poultry. Vitamin B_{12} deficiency has been reported to cause myelin degeneration in chicks. Some investigators have detected increased total phospholipids and decreased levels of galactolipids from deficient chicks, suggesting impaired myelin maturation (73). Perosis may occur in vitamin B_{12}-deficient chicks or poults when their diets lack choline, methionine, or betaine as sources of methyl groups. Addition of vitamin B_{12} may prevent perosis under these conditions because of its effect on the synthesis of methyl groups.

Vitamin B_{12}-deficient embryos have a peak in mortality at the 17th day of incubation, reduced size, myoatrophy of the legs, diffuse hemorrhages, perosis, edema, and fatty liver (99, 103).

Treatment of Deficiency. Peeler et al. (109) showed that intramuscular injection of 2 μg vitamin B_{12}/hen increased hatchability of eggs from vitamin B_{12}–deficient hens from approximately 15% to 80% within 1 wk. Addition of 4 mg vitamin B_{12}/ton breeding ration is sufficient to maintain maximum hatchability and to produce chicks having sufficient stores of the vitamin to prevent any deficiency during the first few weeks of life. Similar injections of young chicks followed by supplementation of the chick ration also will correct the deficiency.

CHOLINE. Choline is present in acetylcholine in body phospholipids and acts as a methyl source in synthesis of methyl-containing compounds such as methionine, creatine, and N-methylnicotinamide. Choline per se does not act as a methyl donor but first must be oxidized to the compound betaine, which can then donate one of its three methyl groups to a methyl acceptor such as homocysteine or glycocyamine for formation of methionine or creatine, respectively.

Signs and Pathology of Deficiency. In addition to poor growth, the outstanding sign of choline deficiency in chicks and poults is perosis. Young turkeys have a high requirement for choline and therefore will show a high incidence of severe perosis unless special care is taken to supplement the diet with choline. Perosis is first characterized by pinpoint hemorrhages and a slight puffiness about the hock joint, followed by an apparent flattening of the tibiometatarsal joint caused by rotation of the metatarsus. The metatarsus continues to twist and may become bent or bowed so that it is out of alignment with the tibia. When this condition exists, the leg cannot adequately support the bird. The articular cartilage is deformed and the Achilles tendon slips from its condyles.

When laying pullets that have received high-choline rearing diets are fed severely deficient diets, percentage of fat in the liver increases. In livers of choline-deficient chickens, fat content is higher in females than males. However, choline deficiency is rare in adult chickens and turkeys fed practical rations. Nesheim et al. (98) showed that pullets fed high choline levels during the 8- to 20-wk growing period are more likely to show fatty livers when placed on purified low-choline laying diets than pullets fed minimum levels during the same growth period. These results indicate that maturing chickens can synthesize choline but will not fully develop this ability if given diets containing ample amounts.

Treatment of Deficiency. If choline deficiency is noted in chicks or poults before severe signs of perosis have developed, the deficiency can be cured by supplementing the ration with sufficient choline to meet the requirements. Once the tendon has slipped in chicks or poults suffering from choline deficiency, the damage is irreparable.

ESSENTIAL INORGANIC ELEMENTS. Essential mineral elements are as important as amino acids and vitamins in maintenance of life, well-being, and production in poultry. They enter into composition of bones and give the skeleton the rigidity and strength needed to support the soft tissues. Minerals combine with protein, lipids, and other substances that make up the soft tissues. They take part in maintenance of osmotic pressure and acid-base balance and exert specific effects on the ability of muscles and nerves to respond to stimuli. Minerals also are necessary for activation of many enzymes of the body.

The inorganic elements essential for maintenance of well-being are calcium; phosphorus; magnesium; potassium; sodium; chlorine; and the trace elements manganese, iron, copper, zinc, iodine, molybdenum, and selenium. Fluorine in small amounts is a constant constituent of several tissues, particularly bones. Traces of this element may be essential or at least beneficial for some species, but no direct evidence has been obtained with poultry. Analyses of individual mineral constituents in the body of chickens show that major portions of calcium, phosphorus, magnesium, and zinc are present in bones. Other essential elements are distributed largely in muscles, other soft tissues, and body fluids.

CALCIUM AND PHOSPHORUS. Calcium (Ca) and phosphorus (P) are closely associated in metabolism, particularly in bone formation. The major portion of dietary Ca is used for bone formation in growing chicks or poults and for eggshell formation in mature hens. Ca also is essential for clotting of blood, and is required along with sodium and potassium for normal beating of the heart. Ca is an important factor in the regulation of cellular metabolism and processes.

In addition to its role in bone formation, P is an essential component of purine nucleotides and other phosphorylated compounds involved in the transfer or conservation of free energy in biochemical reactions. It exercises important functions in metabolism of carbohydrates and fats, and enters into composition of important constituents of all living cells. Salts formed from it play an important part in maintenance of the acid-base balance.

The utilization of Ca and P depends on presence of an adequate amount of vitamin D in the diet. In vitamin D deficiency, the deposition of these minerals in bones of growing chicks and poults is reduced, and the quantity of Ca in eggshells is decreased.

According to Long and associates (81, 82, 83), deficiencies of Ca and P in the diet of growing broiler chicks cause rickets, which differs in histopathology and differs also from the rickets of vitamin D deficiency. Tibiae from chicks that had been fed a diet containing 0.3% Ca from the time of hatching showed, by 2 wk, a widening of the proliferating prehypertrophic zone of epiphyseal cartilage and irregular contours in the boundary between the zones of proliferating and hypertrophic cartilage (82). Irregular cartilage columns and elongated epiphyseal vessels were present. By 4 wk, the epiphyseal growth plate had widened and in some cases extended as a cartilaginous plug into the metaphysis. Histologically, the proliferating and hypertrophic zones were irregular and often contained areas of nonviable cells. The hypertrophied zone was markedly widened in some chicks by 4 wk. Metaphyseal blood vessels invaded along the lateral, but not the apical, region of the cartilagenous plug; cartilage columns of the metaphysis were thickened and irregular. The investigators note that the pathology is similar to that of tibial dyschondroplasia.

According to Long et al. (83), P deficiency (0.2% available dietary P) and Ca excess (2.24% Ca and 0.45% available P) resulted in similar abnormalities of the tibiae. Several histological abnormalities were observed, but most conspicuous was a marked lengthening of the cartilage columns of the degenerating hypertrophied epiphyseal cartilage and metaphyseal primary spongiosa. Some chicks were unable to stand at 4 wk, displaying a spraddle-legged posture. Folding fractures and bowing or rotation of the tibiotarsus were frequently observed.

Julian et al. (71) observed that P-deficient chicks had increased respiratory rates and were polycythemic. Blood CO_2 and O_2 were decreased, presumably due to poor rib strength and infolding, which interfered with respiratory movements of the rib cage. Birds died of right ventricular failure, often accompanied by ascites.

In laying hens Ca deficiency results in reduced egg production and thin-shelled eggs as well as a tendency to deplete Ca content of the bones, first by complete removal of the medullary bone followed by a gradual removal of the cortical bone. Finally, bones become so thin that spontaneous fractures may occur, especially in vertebrae, tibiae, and femurs. This condition may be associated with a syndrome commonly termed "cage layer fatigue" (113). While a marginal Ca deficiency has often been found to be a triggering agent in cage layer fatigue, the syndrome apparently is not due to a simple deficiency of Ca but also involves other etiological factors not yet identified.

Excess Calcium. Shane et al. (131) fed leghorn pullets diets containing 3.0% Ca and 0.4% P from 8 to 20 wk of age. Nephrosis and visceral gout were observed in the high Ca treatment by 16 wk of age. Wideman et al. 1985 (151) provided replacement pullets diets containing excess (3.25%) or adequate (1.0%) levels of Ca in combinations with moderate (0.6%) or low (0.4%) available P from 7 wk until 18 wk of age. All birds received a commercial layer diet during the laying period. Pullets fed on the 3.25% Ca diets developed a high incidence of urolithiasis by 18 wk, which persisted or increased in the laying period through 51 wk of age. Low levels of dietary P during the rearing period exacerbated the effect of excess Ca.

MAGNESIUM. Magnesium (Mg) is essential for carbohydrate metabolism and for activation of many enzymes, especially those involved in phosphorylation reactions. It is essential for bone formation, about two-thirds being present in bone chiefly as a carbonate. Eggshells contain about 0.4% Mg.

Almquist (6) observed that chicks fed a Mg-deficient diet grew slowly for approximately 1 wk and then ceased growing and became lethargic. When disturbed, these chicks frequently passed into a brief convulsion accompanied by gasping and finally into a comatose state, sometimes ending in death. Mg-deficiency signs of poults are similar to those of chicks (138).

Excess Magnesium. Ordinary feeds supply enough Mg in practical poultry diets to meet requirements. It is possible, however, that under certain conditions rations may contain excess Mg, producing detrimental effects including reduced growth rate and bone ash in chicks and decreased egg size, eggshell thinning, and diarrhea in hens (33, 91, 137).

SODIUM AND CHLORINE (SALT). Sodium (Na) as chloride (Cl), carbonate, and phosphate is found chiefly in blood and body fluids. Na is connected intimately with maintenance of membrane potentials, cellular transport processes, and the regulation of the hydrogen ion concentration of blood. Chloride, the major mineral anion in extracellular fluid, plays a role in fluid and ionic balance.

Signs of Deficiency. Animals receiving diets deficient in Na not only fail to grow but also develop softening of bones, corneal keratinization, gonadal inactivity, adrenal hypertrophy, changes in cellular function, impairment of food utilization, and decrease in both plasma and special fluid volumes. Cardiac output drops; mean arterial pressure falls; the hematocrit increases; elasticity of subcutaneous tissue decreases; adrenal function is impaired; and a state of shock results, which if uncorrected terminates in death.

Chicks fed a diet containing no added salt show retarded growth with decreased efficiency of food utilization. Lack of salt in the diet of laying hens results in an abrupt decrease of egg production and reduced egg size, loss of weight, and cannibalism. Salt deprivation in turkeys impairs egg production and hatchability (58). Leach and Nesheim (78) observed that chicks fed a purified diet containing 0.24% Na and 0.4% potassium required 0.12% chlorine. They produced Cl deficiency by feeding young chicks a purified diet containing 190 mg Cl/kg diet. Chicks exhibited extremely poor growth rate, high mortality, hemoconcentration, dehydration, and reduced blood Cl. In addition, deficient chicks showed nervous signs characteristic of Cl deficiency. When startled they fell forward with their legs outstretched behind them and lay paralyzed for several minutes, then appeared quite normal until frightened again (Fig. 2.18).

Excess Salt. Large amounts of salt in the ration are toxic to chickens. The lethal dose is approximately 4 g/kg body weight. Young chicks appear to be more susceptible to toxic effects of salt than older chickens. Signs of salt intoxication include inability to stand, intense thirst, pronounced muscular weakness, and convulsive movements preceding death. There are lesions in many organs, particularly hemorrhages and severe congestion in gastrointestinal tract, muscles, liver, and lungs. Excess Na resulted in ascites, right ventricular hypertrophy, and right ventricular failure in broiler chickens (70). Matterson et al. (88) fed day-old poults graded quantities of salt for 23 days and observed 25% edema and 25% mortality at 4.0% salt but none at 2.0%. Swayne et al. (143), however, described a case of accidental salt poisoning in 5- to 11-day-old poults in which a diet contained 1.85% salt. Signs included respiratory distress, ascites, hydropericardium, hydrothorax, and sudden death.

POTASSIUM. Potassium (K) is found primarily in the cellular compartment of the body; soft tissues of the chicken contain more than three times as much K as Na. As a major cation in intracellular fluid, K has an essential role in the maintenance of membrane potential and cellular fluid balance and participates directly in numerous biochemical reactions. K is necessary for normal heart activity, reducing contractility of the heart muscle and favoring relaxation.

Signs of Deficiency. The main effect of K deficiency is overall muscle weakness characterized by weak extremities, poor intestinal tone with distention, cardiac weakness, and weakness of the respiratory muscles and their ultimate failure. Severely affected individuals may exhibit tetanic seizures followed by death. Low levels of K in laying diets cause decreased egg production and eggshell thinning (77). A low K level in the vital organs of animals may occur during severe stress. Plasma K is elevated, causing the kidney (acting under influence of the adrenocortical hormone) to discharge K into the urine. During adaptation to stress, the muscle will begin to retrieve its lost K. As liver glycogen is restored, K returns to the liver. This may result in temporary prolongation of the general K deficiency throughout the body. High temperature results in increased loss of K in the urine (39).

DIETARY BALANCE OF MACROMINERALS. Studies in many laboratories during the past two decades have determined that the balance among dietary minerals has a profound effect on acid-base balance and certain developmental, metabolic, and physiological functions in poultry (95). Balance has been expressed in several ways. One expression is dietary undetermined anion (dUA), sometimes referred to as mineral cation-anion balance (14). It is defined as follows: dUA = (Na + K + Ca + Mg) − (Cl + P + S), in which all values are expressed in milliequivalents per kg of

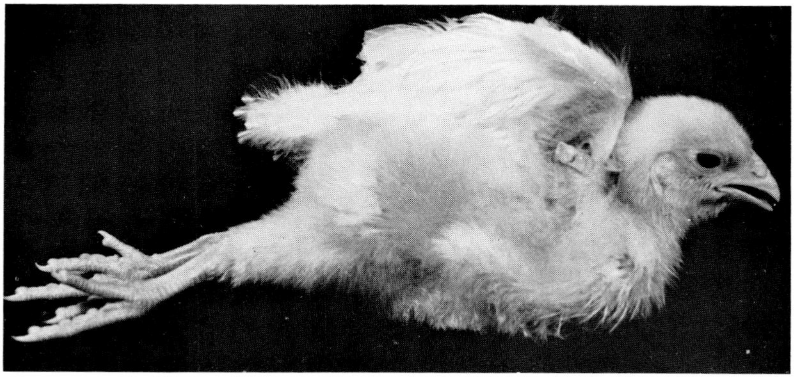

2.18. Characteristic sign of chloride deficiency.

diet and valences are assumed to be +1 for Na and K, +2 for Ca and Mg, −1 for Cl, −1.75 for P, and −2 for S. P and S are assumed to be inorganic. Trace minerals are excluded because of their insignificant contributions to the overall mineral balance. Another term, dietary electrolyte balance, emphasizes the balance among the strong electrolytes (Na + K − Cl).

A positive value of dUA represents the net dietary concentration of organic anions. If the value is negative, a very unusual condition, it is a measure of the net hydrogen ion content of the diet. Minerals differ in their chemical properties and metabolism. Therefore, while dUA provides an indication of the qualitative effect, it is not an accurate predictor of the quantitative effect of the diet on acid-base balance.

Diets rich in mineral anions, particularly Cl, tend to cause metabolic acidosis and result in disturbances of Ca metabolism, increased incidence and severity of tibial dyschondroplasia in immature fowls, and reduced eggshell calcification in laying hens. Effects on tibial development (44, 57, 79, 121) and eggshells (13) are exacerbated when Ca is limiting.

A dietary combination of excessive Ca and low P results in the excretion of an alkaline urine (151) as would be predicted from dUA. The urolithiasis observed in replacement pullets by Wideman et al. (151) under these conditions may be due in part to the increased pH of urine. Alkaline conditions favor the precipitation of divalent mineral salts. Increasing the dietary acid load has been used to reduce uroliths in some mammals. The potentially adverse effects of low dUA on bone development and eggshell quality should be considered before such treatment is attempted in poultry.

Manganese. Manganese (Mn) is an activator of several enzymes and is required for normal growth and reproduction, and prevention of perosis.

In addition to its perosis-preventing properties, Mn is necessary for formation of normal bones. Wilgus et al. (155, 156) observed that leg bones of chicks fed perosis-producing diets frequently were thickened and shortened. Mn also has been reported to be necessary for maximum eggshell quality.

Lyons and Insko (86) found that Mn deficiency resulted in very low hatchability of fertile eggs and chondrodystrophy in embryos. The peak of mortality for such embryos occurred on the 20th and 21st days of incubation. Chondrodystrophic embryos were characterized by very short, thickened legs, short wings, parrot beak, globular contour of head, protruding abdomen, and retarded down and body growth. Marked edema was noted in about 75% of these embryos. The Mn content of eggs producing chondrodystrophic embryos was less than that of normal eggs.

Chicks hatched from eggs produced by hens fed a diet deficient in Mn sometimes exhibit ataxia, particularly when excited (31). The head may be drawn forward and bent underneath the body or retracted over the back. Ataxic chicks grow normally and reach maturity but fail to recover completely. They also retain the short bones characteristic of embryos and newly hatched chicks from Mn-deficient dams (30).

Iodine. Traces of iodine (I) are required for normal functioning of the thyroid gland in poultry as in other animals. Thyroxine contains approximately 65% I and acts as an important regulating agent in body metabolism. When the intake of I is suboptimal, the thyroid tissue enlarges and goiter results.

Wilgus et al. (157) reported that I deficiency results in enlarged thyroid and in some cases lower body weight in growing chicks. They observed congenital goiter in baby chicks hatched from hens receiving 0.025 ppm I in the ration. Rogler et al. (119) observed mortality late in incubation. Hatching time was delayed. Embryo size was reduced and yolk-sac resorption was retarded. Use of 0.25% iodized salt in chicken and turkey rations should prevent development of I deficiency. This would supply 0.175 ppm in addition to that contained in the diet. Christensen and Ort (34) recently reported that dietary supplements of iodine increased the permeability of eggshells and hatchability of turkey eggs.

Iodine deficiency in poultry has been largely offset by widespread use of I either in iodized salt or as part of the trace mineral premix.

Copper. Copper (Cu) is essential for formation of hemoglobin. In absence of Cu, dietary iron is absorbed and deposited in the liver and elsewhere, but hemoglobin synthesis does not occur. Cu deficiency in chicks results in anemia, characterized by reduced numbers of circulating erythrocytes and impaired feather pigmentation in colored breeds of fowl (38).

Copper is a component of several enzymes that participate in redox reactions. Lysyl oxidase is a Cu-containing enzyme that catalyses oxidation of lysine residues in formation of the cross-linking structure desmosine in elastin. Cu deficiency decreases the cross-linking. This weakens the structure of elastin, leading to aortic rupture in poultry. Thinning of the tertiary bronchial mantle in lungs may also result from decreased cross-linking of elastin (28); however, observations on birds fed high levels of cadmium appear inconsistent with this view (80). Cu deficiency has been reported to decrease cross-linking in bone collagen and to increase bone fragility (104, 120). Cu is a component of superoxide dismutase and cytochrome oxidase, both of which have decreased activities in

Cu-deficient chicks (22).

A deficiency of Cu in laying hens causes reduced egg production, increased egg size, and abnormal eggshell calcification. Eggshell abnormalities include shell-less eggs, misshapen eggs, wrinkled eggshells, and reduced eggshell thickness. The palisade layer of the eggshell appears normal; however, the mammillary layer has enlarged mammillary knobs and increased spacing between knobs. This may be related to abnormal structure of eggshell membranes caused by a decrease in lysine cross-linking (19).

Excess Copper. Excessive dietary levels of Cu have been reported to cause abnormalities of the gizzard. Fisher et al. (47) reported that dietary Cu levels ranging from 205 ppm to 605 ppm resulted in a rough, thickened gizzard lining in broiler chicks, the severity of the lesion increasing as the Cu level of the diet increased. The highest Cu level caused markedly thickened and folded linings having a warty appearance. Histological examination revealed thickening of the koilin layer, sloughing of epithelial cells into the area under the koilin layer, and the inclusion of clusters of sloughed cells within the koilin layer. Wight et al. (154) observed similar lesions in chicks receiving 2000 and 4000 ppm Cu. They noted gizzard erosions and fissures in the gizzard lining, hemorrhages under the koilin layer, and a mucoid material adhering to the mucosa of the proventriculus.

IRON. Iron (Fe) is an essential component of heme, the porphyrin nucleus of hemoglobin and the cytochromes, and is a component of several enzymes including catalase, peroxidase, phenylalanine hydroxylase, tyrosinase, and proline hydroxylase.

Iron deficiency results in a hypochromic, microcytic anemia and reduced concentration of nonheme Fe in plasma and prevents normal feather pigmentation in breeds having colored plumage (38, 60). A deficiency in laying hens also causes anemia in the developing chick embryo and reduced hatchability (96). Chicks that survive incubation are weak and listless; however, they recover when given supplemental Fe.

The hemoglobin level of hens falls with the beginning of egg production, but this apparently is not related to the Fe or Cu content of the diet. Since the hemoglobin level rises rapidly with onset of broodiness, it is more probable that low levels prevailing in egg production are caused by changes in hormone activity rather than Fe or Cu deficiencies.

ZINC. Traces of zinc (Zn) appear to be necessary for life in all animals. It is a constituent of the enzyme carbonic anhydrase and is necessary for activation of several other enzymes.

Deficiency signs include retarded growth; poor feathering; enlarged hocks (Fig. 2.19); short, thickened long bones; scaling of the skin and dermatitis, particularly on the feet; and an awkward arthritic gait (102, 164). Zn-deficient chicks exhibit increased hematocrit, which is due to redistribution of body water rather than altered water intake (25).

Histologic lesions include hyperkeratinization of skin of the shank and feet and parakeratosis of the esophagus. Nucleoli of the crop epithelium are enlarged and contain increased amounts of RNA. Alkaline phosphatase and alcohol dehydrogenase, two Zn-containing enzymes, exhibit reduced activities in the crop and esophagus (153). Reduced alkaline phosphatase activity is also observed in epiphyseal cartilage. Starcher et al. (135) found that activity of the Zn-dependent enzyme collagenase is reduced in the tibia during Zn deficiency. They suggest that effects of Zn on bone may be the result of decreased bone collagen turnover. Bettger et al. (23, 24) reported evidence of an interrelationship between vitamin E and Zn. Arthritic gait and epidermal lesions were reduced by vitamin E and exacerbated by polyunsaturated fatty acids.

Ducks exhibit poor growth and epidermal lesions of the feet, particularly interdigital webs (152). Pathology of the epidermis is evident in the interdigital web, mucous membrane of the tongue, and epithelium in other parts of the gastrointestinal tract. Hyperkeratosis and acanthosis characterize the tongue and interdigital web lesions. Intercellular spacing between prickle cells and basal cells is increased and number of desmo-

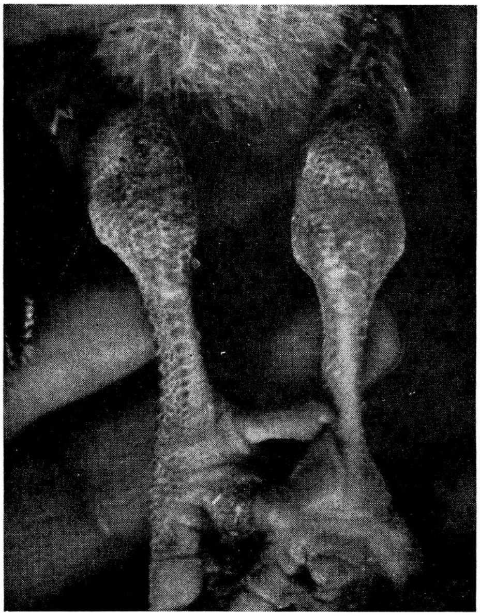

2.19. Enlarged hocks in poult caused by zinc deficiency.

somes is diminished. Prickle cells have an abnormal structure, enlarged nuclei and nucleoli, and decreased content of free ribosomes, tonofilaments, and other structures.

The Zn requirement of poults is higher than for chicks. Thus poults are more likely to show enlarged hocks and poor feathering of Zn deficiency unless special supplements are added to the diet. The most dramatic embryonic abnormalities resulting from nutritional deficiency appear when the breeding diet contains excess Ca and P, is high in phytic acid, and is deficient in Zn. Zn-deficient embryos may have only a head and complete viscera but no spinal column beyond a few vertebrae and no wings, body wall, or legs (74).

Chickens maintained on a Zn-deficient diet are unable to produce antibodies against T-cell-dependent antigens even though lymphocytes are capable of immunoglobulin production (29).

Excess Zinc. Excessive dietary levels of Zn (e.g. 20,000 ppm as zinc oxide) induce molt in laying hens (37). Zn results in abrupt decline in egg production and onset of molt followed by rapid resumption of egg laying after dietary Zn concentrations are returned to normal. Excess Zn results in inanition, which is presumably responsible for initiating the molt (89). High levels of Zn result in accumulation of Zn in tissues and pathological changes in the gizzard and pancreas. Chicks exhibit a rough, pale-colored gizzard lining, which may show evidence of fissures and, less frequently, ulceration (41, 154). Histological examination reveals epithelial desquamation and infiltration of inflammatory cells. Pancreases exhibit dilated acinar lumina and degenerative changes in acinar cells. The latter include loss of zymogen granules, vacuolization of the cytoplasm, and the presence of hyaline bodies and other electron-dense debris (154).

Large excesses of dietary Zn such as those used to induce a molt result in reduced activity of the selenium-dependent enzyme, plasma glutathione peroxidase. Selenium administration restores glutathione peroxidase activity but fails to prevent pathological changes in the gizzard and pancreas (154). Lesser excesses of Zn (i.e., up to 2000 ppm) did not affect plasma or hepatic glutathione peroxidase activity, but interfered with exocrine function of the pancreas and plasma and tissue concentrations of alpha-tocopherol in chicks fed a purified diet but not in chicks fed a practical diet (84, 85).

Selenium. Selenium (Se) has been shown to be an essential mineral for both chicks and poults. Se prevents development of exudative diathesis in young chickens and myopathy of gizzard and heart in young turkeys (123, 124, 128). Vitamin E and Se have a mutual sparing effect in prevention of these diseases (see Vitamin E).

Chicks severely deficient in Se exhibit poor growth and feathering, impaired fat digestion, and pancreatic atrophy and fibrosis (145, 146). Gries and Scott (56) performed a time-sequence study of pancreatic lesions, which began at 6 days of age with vacuolation and hyaline body formation in the exocrine pancreas. As the deficiency progressed, cytoplasm degenerated until acini were represented by rings of cells with a central lumen embedded in fibrous tissue (Fig. 2.20). Addition of 0.1 ppm Se as Na_2SeO_3 to the diet caused

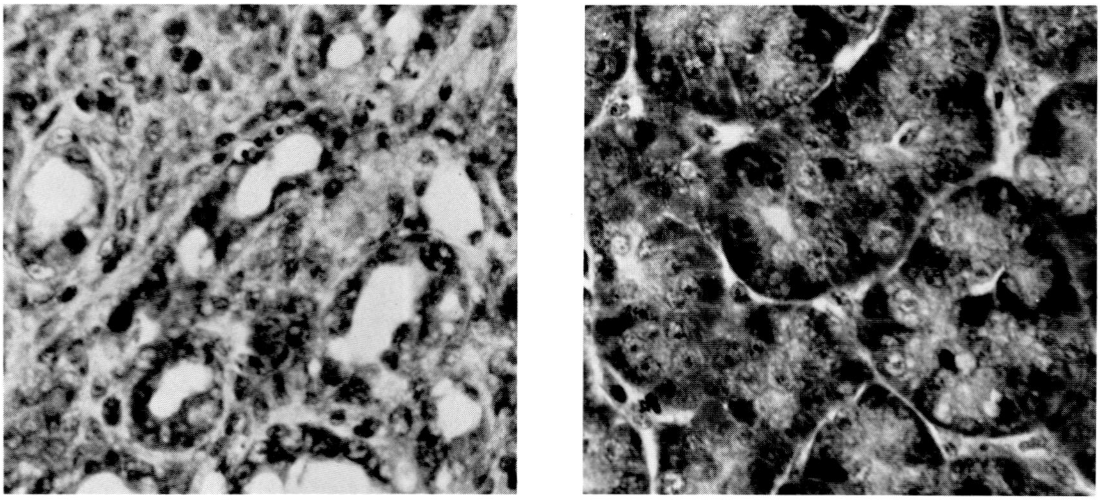

2.20. Pancreas from selenium-deficient chick. Acini consist of degenerating cells forming central lumen with extensive interstitial fibrosis (*left*). Control (*right*). ×250.

complete pancreatic acinar regeneration within 2 wk and a marked clinical recovery.

High plasma tocopherol levels were maintained by feeding 100 IU vitamin E/kg and bile salts to enhance its absorption. This greatly reduced incidence of exudative diathesis, which did not appear until the pancreas in chicks had degenerated severely.

WATER. Water (H_2O) holds a unique position in nutrition mainly due to its physical properties. Because of its solvent and polar properties it acts as a transport medium for other nutrients and products of metabolism and enhances cell reactions. Because of its high specific heat it can absorb the heat of reactions produced in oxidation of carbohydrates and fats with little rise in temperature. H_2O evaporates readily, removing many calories from the body as latent heat of vaporization. These and many other functions explain why the animal is able to exist much longer without food than without H_2O.

Unlike larger farm animals, chickens and turkeys must have access to a continuous H_2O supply since they drink only small amounts at a time. An insufficient amount results in decreased growth and egg production.

The quantity of water drunk by chicks is correlated directly with salt content of the diet (59). Austic (11) reported that equimolar additions to the diet of Na and K in the form of bicarbonate salts resulted in similar increases in water intake of broiler chicks. When added to the diet as Ca chloride in substitution for Ca carbonate, Cl increased water intake, but only about one-half as much as equivalent amounts of Na and K. Excess dietary protein and deficiencies of amino acids result in increased water intake (10). The effect of protein is presumably due to increased excretion of nitrogen and minerals such as P and sulfur that are constituents of protein.

REFERENCES

1. Abdulrahim, S.M., M.B. Patel, and J. McGinnis. 1979. Effects of vitamin D_3 and D_3 metabolites in production parameters and hatchability of eggs. Poult Sci 58:858–863.
2. Adams, R.L., and C.W. Carrick. 1967. A study of the niacin requirement of the laying hen. Poult Sci 46:712–718.
3. Adamstone, F.B. 1947. Histologic comparisons of the brains of vitamin A-deficient and vitamin E-deficient chicks. Arch Pathol 43:301–312.
4. Adamstone, F.B., and L.E. Card. 1934. The effects of vitamin E deficiency on the testis of the male fowl (Gallus domesticus). J Morphol 56:339–359.
5. Agricultural Research Council. 1975. Nutrient requirement of farm livestock. No. 1. Poultry. Agricultural Research Council (London).
6. Almquist, H.J. 1942. Magnesium requirement of the chick. Proc Soc Exp Biol Med 49:544–545.
7. Ameenuddin, S., M.L. Sunde, and M.E. Cook. 1985. Essentiality of vitamin D_3 and its metabolites in poultry nutrition: A review. World Poult Sci J 41:52–63.
8. Ameenuddin, S., M.L. Sunde, and H.F. DeLuca. 1987. Lack of response of bone mineralization of chicks fed egg yolks from hens on dietary 1,25-dihydroxycholecalciferol. Poult Sci 66:1829–1834.
9. Asmundson, V.S., and F.H. Kratzer. 1952. Observations of vitamin A deficiency in turkey breeding stock. Poult Sci 31:71–73.
10. Austic, R.E. 1979. Nutritional influences on water intake in poultry. Proc Cornell Nutr Conf, pp. 37–41. Syracuse, NY.
11. Austic, R.E. 1981. Sodium, potassium, and chlorine ratios in broiler nutrition. Proc Carolina Poult Nutr Conf, pp. 1–5. Charlotte, NC.
12. Austic, R.E., and R.K. Cole. 1972. Impaired renal clearance of uric acid in chickens having hyperuricemia and articular gout. Am J Physiol 223:525–530.
13. Austic, R.E., and K. Keshavarz. 1988. Interaction of dietary calcium and chloride and the influence of monovalent minerals on eggshell quality. Poult Sci 67:750–759.
14. Austic, R.E., and J.F. Patience. 1988. Undetermined anion in poultry diets: Influence on acid-base balance, metabolism and physiological performance. CRC Crit Rev Poult Biol 1:315–345.
15. Bain, S.D., J.W. Newbrey, and B.A. Watkins. 1988. Biotin deficiency may alter tibiotarsal bone growth and modeling in broiler chicks. Poult Sci 67:590–595.
16. Baker, J.R., J.M. Howell, and J.N. Thompson. 1967. Hypervitaminosis A in the chick. Br J Exp Pathol 48:507–512.
17. Baker, D.H., N.K. Allen, and A.J. Kleiss. 1973. Efficiency of tryptophan as a niacin precursor in the young chick. J Anim Sci 36:299–302.
18. Bar, A., S. Striem, J. Rosenberg, and S. Hurwitz. 1988. Egg shell quality and cholecalciferol metabolism in aged laying hens. J Nutr 118:1018–1023.
19. Baumgartner, S., D.J. Brown, E. Salevsky, Jr., and R.M. Leach, Jr. 1978. Copper deficiency in the laying hen. J Nutr 108:804–811.
20. Bearse, G.F., C.F. McClary, and H.C. Saxena. 1953. Blood spot incidence and the vitamin A level of the diet. Poult Sci 32:888.
21. Beer, A.E., M.L. Scott, and M.C. Nesheim. 1963. The effects of graded levels of pantothenic acid on the breeding performance of White Leghorn pullets. Br Poult Sci 4:243–253.
22. Bettger, W.J., J.E. Savage, and B.L. O'Dell. 1979. Effects of dietary copper and zinc on erythrocyte superoxide dismutase activity in the chick. Nutr Rep Int 19:893–900.
23. Bettger, W.J., P.G. Reeves, J.E. Savage, and B.L. O'Dell. 1980. Interaction of zinc and vitamin E in the chick. Proc Soc Exp Biol Med 163:432–436.
24. Bettger, W.J., P.G. Reeves, E.A. Moscatelli, J.E. Savage, and B.L. O'Dell. 1980. Interaction of zinc and polyunsaturated fatty acids in the chick. J Nutr 110:50–58.
25. Bettger, W.J., J.E. Savage, and B.L. O'Dell. 1981. Extracellular zinc concentration and water metabolism in chicks. J Nutr 111:1013–1019.
26. Briggs, G.M. 1946. Nicotinic acid deficiency in turkey poults and the occurrence of perosis. J Nutr 31:79–84.
27. Briggs, G.M., A.C. Groschke, and R.J. Lillie. 1946. Effect of proteins low in tryptophane on growth of chickens and on laying hens receiving nicotinic acid-low rations. J Nutr 32:659–675.
28. Buckingham, K., C.S. Heng-Khoo, M. Dubick, M. Lefevre, C. Cross, L. Julian, and R. Rucker. 1981. Copper deficiency and elastin metabolism in avian lung. Proc Soc Exp Biol Med 166:310–319.

29. Burns, R.B. 1983. Antibody production suppressed in the domestic fowl (Gallus domesticus) by zinc deficiency. Avian Pathol 12:141-146.

30. Caskey, C.D., and L.C. Norris. 1940. Micromelia in adult fowl caused by manganese deficiency during embryonic development. Proc Soc Exp Biol Med 44:332-335.

31. Caskey, C.D., L.C. Norris, and G.F. Heuser. 1944. A chronic congenital ataxia in chicks due to manganese deficiency in the maternal diet. Poult Sci 23:516-520.

32. Chen, B.-J. 1989. Studies on the conversion of tryptophan to niacin in chickens and ducks. Ph.D. Thesis, Cornell Univ, Ithaca, NY.

33. Chicco, C.F., C.B. Ammerman, P.A. van Walleghem, P.W. Waldroup, and R.H. Harms. 1967. Effects of varying dietary ratios of magnesium, calcium, and phosphorus in growing chicks. Poult Sci 46:368-373.

34. Christensen, V.L., and J.F. Ort. 1988. Effect of dietary iodine on the permeability and hatchability of large white turkey eggs. Poult Sci 67:67. (Suppl) (Abstr).

35. Couch, J.R., W.W. Cravens, C.A. Elvehjem, and J.G. Halpin. 1948. Relation of biotin to congenital deformities in the chick. Anat Rec 100:29-48.

36. Cravens, W.W., W.H. McGibbon, and E.E. Sebesta. 1944. Effect of biotin deficiency on embryonic development in the domestic fowl. Anat Rec 90:55-64.

37. Creger, C.R., and J.T. Scott. 1980. Using zinc oxide to rest laying hens. Poult Dig 39:230-232.

38. Davis, P.N., L.C. Norris, and F.H. Kratzer. 1962. Iron deficiency studies in chicks using treated isolated soybean protein diets. J Nutr 78:445-453.

39. Deetz, L.E., and R.C. Ringrose. 1976. Effect of heat stress on the potassium requirement of the hen. Poult Sci 55:1765-1770.

40. DeLuca, H.F. 1971. Vitamin D: A new look at an old vitamin. Nutr Rev 29:179-181.

41. Dewar, W.A., P.A.L. Wight, R.A. Pearson, and M.J. Gentle. 1983. Toxic effects of high concentrations of zinc oxide in the diet of the chick and laying hen. Br Poult Sci 24:397-404.

42. Dickson, I.R., and E. Kodicek. 1979. Effect of vitamin D deficiency on bone formation in the chick. Biochem J 182:429-435.

43. DiLorenzo, R.N. 1972. Studies of the genetic variation in tryptophan-nicotinic acid conversion in chicks. Ph.D. Thesis, Cornell Univ, Ithaca, NY.

44. Edwards, H.M., Jr. 1984. Studies on the etiology of tibial dyschondroplasia in chickens. J Nutr 114:1001-1013.

45. Engel, R.W., P.H. Phillips, and J.G. Halpin. 1940. The effect of a riboflavin deficiency in the hen upon embryonic development of the chick. Poult Sci 19:135-142.

46. Ferguson, T.M., R.H. Rigdon, and J.R. Couch. 1956. Cataracts in vitamin E deficiency: An experimental study in the turkey embryo. Am Med Assoc Arch Ophthalmol (NY) 55:346-355.

47. Fisher, C., A.P. Laursen-Jones, K.J. Hill, and W.S. Hardy. 1973. The effect of copper sulphate on performance and the structure of the gizzard in broilers. Br Poult Sci 14:55-68.

48. Frigg, M. 1984. Available biotin content of various feed ingredients. Poult Sci 63:750-753.

49. Fritz, J.C., J.H. Hooper, J.L. Halpin, and H.P. Moore. 1946. Failure of feather pigmentation in bronze poults due to lysine deficiency. J Nutr 31:387-396.

50. Garvey, W.T., and R.E. Olson. 1978. In vitro vitamin K-dependent conversion of precursor to prothrombin in chick liver. J Nutr 108:1078-1086.

51. Gillis, M.B., G.F. Heuser, and L.C. Norris. 1948. Pantothenic acid in the nutrition of the hen. J Nutr 35:351-363.

52. Goldstein, J., and M.L. Scott. 1956. An electrophoretic study of exudative diathesis in chicks. J Nutr 60:349-359.

53. Goodson-Williams, R., D.A. Roland, Sr., and J.A. McGuire. 1986. Effects of feeding graded levels of vitamin D_3 on egg shell pimpling in aged hens. Poult Sci 65:1556-1560.

54. Gries, C.L., and M.L. Scott. 1972. The pathology of thiamin, riboflavin, pantothenic acid, and niacin deficiencies in the chick. J Nutr 102:1269-1285.

55. Gries, C.L., and M. L. Scott. 1972. The pathology of pyridoxine deficiency in chicks. J Nutr 102:1259-1267.

56. Gries, C.L., and M.L. Scott. 1972. Pathology of selenium deficiency in the chick. J Nutr 102:1287-1296.

57. Halley, J.T., T.S. Nelson, L.K. Kirby, and Z.B. Johnson. 1987. Effect of altering dietary mineral balance on growth, leg abnormalities, and blood base excess in broiler chicks. Poult Sci 66:1684-1692.

58. Harms, R.H., R.E. Buresh, and H.R. Wilson. 1985. Sodium requirement of the turkey hen. Br Poult Sci 26:217-220.

59. Heuser, G.F. 1952. Salt additions to chick rations. Poult Sci 31:85-88.

60. Hill, C.H., and G. Matrone. 1961. Studies on copper and iron deficiencies in growing chickens. J Nutr 73:425-431.

61. Hill, F.W., M.L. Scott, L.C. Norris, and G.F. Heuser. 1961. Reinvestigation of the vitamin A requirements of laying and breeding hens and their progeny. Poult Sci 40:1245-1254.

62. Hinshaw, W.R., and W.E. Lloyd. 1934. Vitamin-A deficiency in turkeys. Hilgardia 8:281-304.

63. Hooper, J.H., J.L. Halpin, and J.C. Fritz. 1942. The feeding of single massive doses of vitamin D to birds. Poult Sci 21:472. (Abstr).

64. Hopkins, D.T., and M.C. Nesheim. 1967. The linoleic acid requirement of chicks. Poult Sci 46:872-881.

65. Hulan, H.W., F.G. Proudfoot, and K.B. McRae. 1980. Effect of vitamins on the incidence of mortality and acute death syndrome ("flip-over") in broiler chickens. Poult Sci 59:927-931.

66. Itakura, C., K. Yamasaki, and M. Goto. 1978. Pathology of experimental vitamin D deficiency rickets in growing chickens. 1. Bone. Avian Pathol 7:491-513.

67. Jensen, L.S., M.L. Scott, G.F. Heuser, L.C. Norris, and T.S. Nelson. 1956. Studies on the nutrition of breeding turkeys. I. Evidence indicating a need to supplement practical turkey rations with vitamin E. Poult Sci 35:810-816.

68. Jortner, B.S., J.B. Meldrum, C.H. Domermuth, and L.M. Potter. 1985. Encephalomalacia associated with hypovitaminosis E in turkey poults. Avian Dis 29:488-498.

69. Jukes, T.H., and F.H. Bird. 1942. Prevention of perosis by biotin. Proc Soc Exp Biol Med 49:231-232.

70. Julian, R.J. 1987. The effect of increased sodium in the drinking water on right ventricular hypertrophy, right ventricular failure, and ascites in broiler chickens. Avian Pathol 16:61-71.

71. Julian, R.J., J. Summers, and J.B. Wilson. 1986. Right ventricular failure and ascites in broiler chicks caused by phosphorus-deficient diets. Avian Dis 30:453-459.

72. Jungherr, E. 1943. Nasal histopathology and liver storage in subtotal vitamin A deficiency of chickens. Conn Agric Exp Stn Bull 250, pp. 1-36.

73. Kalemegham, R., and K. Krishnaswamy. 1975. Myelin lipids in vitamin B_{12} deficiency in chicks. Life Sci 16:1441-1445.

74. Kienholz, E.W., D.E. Turk, M.L. Sunde, and W.G.

Hoekstra. 1961. Effects of zinc deficiency in the diets of hens. J Nutr 75:211–221.
75. Kratzer, F.H., J.L. Buenrostro, and B.A. Watkins, 1985. Biotin related abnormal fat metabolism in chickens and its consequences. Ann NY Acad Sci 447:401–402.
76. Lacy, D.L., and W.E. Huffer. 1982. Studies on the pathogenesis of avian rickets. I. Changes in epiphyseal and metaphyseal vessels in hypocalcemic and hypophosphatemic rickets. Am J Pathol 109:288–301.
77. Leach, R.M., Jr. 1974. Studies on the potassium requirement of the laying hen. J Nutr 104:684–686.
78. Leach, R.M., Jr., and M.C. Nesheim. 1963. Studies on chloride deficiency in chicks. J Nutr 81:193–199.
79. Leach, R.M., Jr., and M.C. Nesheim. 1972. Further studies on tibial dyschondroplasia (cartilage abnormality) in young chicks. J Nutr 102:1673–1680.
80. Lefevre, M., H. Heng, and R.B. Rucker. 1982. Dietary cadmium, zinc, and copper: Effects on chick lung morphology and elastin cross-linking. J Nutr 112:1344–1352.
81. Long, P.H., S.R. Lee, G.N. Rowland, and W.M. Britton. 1984. Experimental rickets in broilers: Gross, microscopic, and radiographic lesions. III. Vitamin D deficiency. Avian Dis 28:933–943.
82. Long, P.H., S.R. Lee, G.N. Rowland, and W.M. Britton. 1984. Experimental rickets in broilers: Gross, microscopic, and radiographic lesions. II. Calcium deficiency. Avian Dis 28:921–932.
83. Long, P.H., S.R. Lee, G.N. Rowland, and W.M. Britton. 1984. Experimental rickets in broilers: Gross, microscopic, and radiographic lesions. I. Phosphorus deficiency and calcium excess. Avian Dis 28:460–474.
84. Lü, J., and G.F. Combs, Jr. 1988. Effect of excess dietary zinc on pancreatic exocrine function in the chick. J Nutr 118:681–689.
85. Lü, J., and G.F. Combs, Jr. 1988. Excess dietary zinc decreases tissue α-tocopherol in chicks. J Nutr 118:1349–1359.
86. Lyons, M., and W.M. Insko, Jr. 1937. Chondrodystrophy in the chick embryo produced by manganese deficiency in the diet of the hen. Ky Agric Exp Stn Bull 371. pp. 61–75.
87. Manley, J.M., R.A. Voitle, and R.H. Harms. 1978. The influence of hatchability of turkey eggs from the addition of 2,4-hydroxycholecalciferol to the diet. Poult Sci 57:290–292.
88. Matterson, L.D., H.M. Scott, and E. Jungherr. 1946. Salt tolerance of turkeys. Poult Sci 25:539–541.
89. McCormick, C.C., and D.L. Cunningham. 1984. High dietary zinc and fasting as methods of forced resting: A performance comparison. Poult Sci 63:1201–1206.
90. McGinnis, J., and J.S. Carver. 1947. The effect of riboflavin and biotin in the prevention of dermatitis and perosis in turkey poults. Poult Sci 26:364–371.
91. McWard, G.W. 1967. Magnesium tolerance of the growing and laying chicken. Br Poult Sci 8:91–99.
92. Mechanic, G.L. 1977. The qualitative and quantitative crosslink chemistry of collagen matrices. Adv Exp Med Biol 86B:699–708.
93. Menge, H.C., C. Calvert and C.A. Denton. 1965. Further studies of the effect of linoleic acid on reproduction in the hen. J Nutr 86:115–119.
94. Misir, R., and R. Blair. 1988. Biotin bioavailability of protein supplements and cereal grains for starting turkey poults. Poult Sci 67:1274–1280.
95. Mongin, P. 1981. Recent advances in dietary anion-cation balance: Applications in poultry. Proc Nutr Soc 40:285–294.
96. Morck, T.A., and R.E. Austic. 1981. Iron requirements of white leghorn hens. Poult Sci 60:1497–1503.
97. National Research Council. 1984. Nutrient requirements of poultry. National Academy of Sciences. Washington, DC.
98. Nesheim, M.C., R.M. Leach, Jr., and M.J. Norvell. 1967. The effect of rearing diet on choline deficiency in hens. Proc 1967 Cornell Nutr Conf, pp. 57–60. Buffalo, NY.
99. Noble, R.C., and J.H. Moore. 1966. Some aspects of the lipid metabolism of the chick embryo. In C. Horton-Smith and E.C. Amoroso (eds.), Physiology of the Domestic Fowl, pp. 87–102. Oliver and Boyd, London.
100. Nockels, C.F., and E.W. Kienholz. 1967. Influence of vitamin A deficiency on testes, bursa fabricius, adrenal and hematocrit in cockerels. J Nutr 92:384–388.
101. Noguchi, T., A.H. Cantor, and M.L. Scott. 1973. Mode of action of selenium and vitamin E in prevention of exudative diathesis in chicks. J Nutr 103:1502–1511.
102. O'Dell, B.L., P.M. Newberne, and J.E. Savage. 1958. Significance of dietary zinc for the growing chicken. J Nutr 65:503–518.
103. Olcese, O., J.R. Couch, J.H. Quisenberry, and P.B. Pearson. 1950. Congenital anomalies in the chick due to vitamin B_{12} deficiency. J Nutr 41:423–431.
104. Opsahl, W., H. Zeronian, M. Ellison, D. Lewis, R.B. Rucker, and R.S. Riggins. 1982. Role of copper in collagen cross-linking and its influence on selected mechanical properties of chick bone and tendon. J Nutr 112:708–716.
105. Pappenheimer, A.M., M. Goettsch, and E. Jungherr. 1939. Nutritional encephalomalacia in chicks and certain related disorders of domestic birds. Conn Agric Exp Stn Bull 229.
106. Paredes, J.R., and T.P. Garcia. 1959. Vitamin A as a factor affecting fertility in cockerels. Poult Sci 38:3–7.
107. Patrick, H., R.V. Boucher, R.A. Dutcher, and H.C. Knandel. 1941. Biotin and prevention of dermatitis in turkey poults. Proc Soc Exp Biol Med 48:456–458.
108. Pearce, J., and D. Balnave. 1978. A review of biotin deficiency and the fatty liver and kidney syndrome in poultry. Br Vet J 134:598–609.
109. Peeler, H.T., R.F. Miller, C.W. Carlson, L.C. Norris, and G.F. Heuser. 1951. Studies of the effect of vitamin B_{12} on hatchability. Poult Sci 30:11–17.
110. Peterson, D.W., W.H. Hamilton, and A.L. Lilyblade. 1971. Hereditary succeptibility to dietary induction of gout in selected lines of chickens. J Nutr 101:347–354.
111. Phillips, P.H., and R.W. Engel. 1939. Some histopathological observations on chicks deficient in the chick antidermatitis factor in pantothenic acid. J Nutr 18:227–232.
112. Reid, B.L., B.W. Heywang, A.A. Kurnick, M.G. Vavich, and B.J. Hulett. 1965. Effect of vitamin A and ambient temperature on reproductive performance of white leghorn pullets. Poult Sci 44:446–452.
113. Riddell, C., C.F. Helmboldt, E.P. Singsen, and L.D. Matterson. 1968. Bone pathology of birds affected with cage layer fatigue. Avian Dis 12:285–297.
114. Ringrose, A.T., L.C. Norris, and G.F. Heuser. 1931. The occurrence of a pellagra-like syndrome in chicks. Poult Sci 10:166–177.
115. Ringrose, R.C., A.G. Manoukas, R. Hinkson, and A.E. Teeri. 1965. The niacin requirement of the hen. Poult Sci 44:1053–1065.
116. Robel, E.J. 1977. A feather abnormality in chicks fed diets deficient in certain amino acids. Poult Sci 56:1968–1971.
117. Robel, E.J., and V.L. Christensen. 1987. Increasing hatchability of turkey eggs with biotin egg injections. Poult Sci 66:1429–1430.

118. Robertson, E.I., G.F. Fiala, M.L. Scott, L.C. Norris, and G.F. Heuser. 1947. Response of anemic chicks to pteroylglutamic acid. Proc Soc Exp Biol Med 64:441-443.
119. Rogler, J.C., H.E. Parker, F.N. Andrews, and C.W. Carrick. 1959. The effects of an iodine deficiency on embryo development and hatchability. Poult Sci 38:398-405.
120. Rucker, R.B., R.S. Riggins, R. Laughlin, M.M. Chan, M. Chen, and K. Tom. 1975. Effects of nutritional copper deficiency on the biomechanical properties of bone and arterial elastin metabolism in the chick. J Nutr 105:1062-1070.
121. Sauveur, B., and P. Mongin. 1978. Tibial dyschondroplasia, a cartilage abnormality in poultry. Ann Biol Anim Biochem Biophys 18:87-98.
122. Scott, M.L. 1953. Prevention of the enlarged hock disorder in turkeys with niacin and vitamin E. Poult Sci 32:670-677.
123. Scott, M.L. 1962. Anti-oxidants, selenium, and sulfur amino acids in the vitamin E nutrition of chicks. Nutr Abstr Rev 32:1-8.
124. Scott, M.L. 1962. Vitamin E in health and disease of poultry. Vitam Horm 20:621-632.
125. Scott, M.L. 1968. Rediscovery of biotin as a factor for prevention of leg weakness in turkeys. Feedstuffs 40:24-26.
126. Scott, M.L. 1980. Advances in our understanding of vitamin E. Fed Proc 39:2736-2739.
127. Scott, M.L., and G.F. Heuser. 1954. Studies on leg weakness in turkeys, ducks, and geese. Proc 10th Wld Poult Congr, pp. 255-258. Edinburgh, Scot.
128. Scott, M.L., G. Olson, L. Krook, and W.R. Brown. 1967. Selenium-responsive myopathies of myocardium and of smooth muscle in the young poult. J Nutr 91:573-583.
129. Seifried, O. 1930. Studies on A-avitaminosis in chickens. I. Lesions of the respiratory tract and their relation to some infectious diseases. J Exp Med 52:519-531.
130. Seifried, O. 1930. Studies on A-avitaminosis in chickens. II. Lesions of the upper alimentary tract and their relation to some infectious diseases. J Exp Med 52:533-538.
131. Shane, S.M., R.J. Young, and L. Krook. 1969. Renal and parathyroid changes produced by high calcium intake in growing pullets. Avian Dis 13:558-567.
132. Siller, W.G. 1981. Renal pathology of the fowl – A review. Avian Pathol 10:187-262.
133. Soares, J.H., Jr., M.R. Swerdel, and M.A. Ottinger. 1979. The effectiveness of vitamin D analog 1 $-OH-D_3$ in promoting fertility and hatchability in the laying hen. Poult Sci 58:1004-1006.
134. Soares, J.H., Jr., M.A. Ottinger, and E.G. Buss. 1988. Potential role of 1,25 dihydroxycholecalciferol in egg shell calcification. Poult Sci 67:1322-1328.
135. Starcher, B.C., C.H. Hill, and J.G. Madaras. 1980. Effect of zinc deficiency on bone collagenase and collagen turnover. J Nutr 110:2095-2102.
136. Stevens, V.I., R. Blair, R.E. Salmon, and J.P. Stevens. 1984. Effect of varying levels of dietary vitamin D_3 on turkey hen egg production, fertility and hatchability, embryo mortality, and incidence of embryo beak malformations. Poult Sci 63:760-764.
137. Stillmak, S.J., and M.L. Sunde. 1971. The use of high magnesium limestone in the diet of the laying hen. I. Egg production. Poult Sci 50:553-564.
138. Sullivan, T.W., 1964. Studies on the dietary requirement and interaction of magnesium with antibiotics in turkeys to 4 weeks of age. Poult Sci 43:401-405.
139. Sunde, R.A., and W.G. Hoekstra. 1980. Structure, synthesis, and function of glutathione peroxidase. Nutr Rev 38:265-273.
140. Sunde, M.L., W.W. Cravens, H.W. Bruins, C.A. Elvehjem, and J.G. Halpin. 1950. The pteroylglutamic acid requirement of laying and breeding hens. Poult Sci 29:220-226.
141. Sunde, M.L., W.W. Cravens, C.A. Elvehjem, and J.G. Halpin. 1950. The effect of folic acid on embryonic development of the domestic fowl. Poult Sci 29:696-702.
142. Sunde, M.L., C.M. Turk, and H.F. DeLuca. 1978. The essentiality of vitamin D metabolites for embryonic chick development. Science 200:1067-1069.
143. Swayne, D.E., A. Shlosberg, and R.B. Davis. 1986. Salt poisoning in turkey poults. Avian Dis 30:847-852.
144. Tang, K.-N., G.N. Rowland, and J.R. Veltmann, Jr. 1985. Vitamin A toxicity: Comparative changes in bone of the broiler and leghorn chicks. Avian Dis 29:416-429.
145. Thompson, J.N., and M.L. Scott. 1969. Role of selenium in the nutrition of the chick. J Nutr 97:335-342.
146. Thompson, J.N., and M.L. Scott. 1970. Impaired lipid and vitamin E absorption related to atrophy of the pancreas in selenium-deficient chicks. J Nutr 100:797-809.
147. Thompson, J.N., J.M. Howell, G.A.J. Pitt, and C.I. Houghton. 1965. Biological activity of retinoic acid ester in the domestic fowl: Production of vitamin A deficiency in the early chick embryo. Nature (London) 205:1006-1007.
148. Watkins, B.A., and F.H. Kratzer. 1987. Dietary biotin effects on polyunsaturated fatty acids in chick tissue lipids and prostaglandin E_2 levels in freeze-clamped hearts. Poult Sci 66:1818-1828.
149. Whitehead, C.C., D.W. Bannister, A.J. Evans, W.G. Siller, and P.A.L. Wight. 1976. Biotin deficiency and fatty liver and kidney syndrome in chicks given purified diets containing different fat and protein levels. Br J Nutr 35:115-125.
150. Whitehead, C.C., J.A. Armstrong, and D. Waddington. 1982. The determination of the availability to chicks of biotin in feed ingredients by a bioassay based on the response of blood pyruvate carboxylase (EC 6.4.1.1) activity. Br J Nutr 48:81-88.
151. Wideman, R.F., Jr., J.A. Closser, W.B. Roush, and B.S. Cowen. 1985. Urolithiasis in pullets and laying hens: Role of dietary calcium and phosphorus. Poult Sci 64:2300-2307.
152. Wight, P.A.L., and W.A. Dewar. 1976. The histopathology of zinc deficiency in ducks. J Pathol 120:183-191.
153. Wight, P.A.L. and W.A. Dewar. 1979. Some histochemical observations on zinc deficiency in chickens. Avian Pathol 8:437-451.
154. Wight, P.A.L., W.A. Dewar, and C.L. Saunderson. 1986. Zinc toxicity in the fowl: Ultrastructural pathology and relationship to selenium, lead, and copper. Avian Pathol 15:23-38.
155. Wilgus, H.S., Jr., L.C. Norris, and G.F. Heuser. 1937. The role of manganese and certain other trace elements in the prevention of perosis. J Nutr 14:155-167.
156. Wilgus, H.S., Jr., L.C. Norris, and G.F. Heuser. 1937. The effect of various calcium and phosphorus salts on the severity of perosis. Poult Sci 16:232-237.
157. Wilgus, H.S., Jr., G.S. Harshfield, A.R. Patton, L.P. Ferris, and F.X. Gassner. 1941. The iodine requirements of growing chickens. Poult Sci 20:477. (Abstr).

158. Wolbach, S.B., and D.M. Hegsted. 1952. Vitamin A deficiency in the chick. Skeletal growth and the central nervous system. Arch Pathol 54:13–29.

159. Wolbach, S.B., and D.M. Hegsted. 1952. Vitamin A deficiency in the duck. Skeletal growth and the central nervous system. Arch Pathol 54:548–563.

160. Wolbach, S.B., and D.M. Hegsted. 1952. Hypervitaminosis A and the skeleton of growing chicks. Arch Pathol 54:30–38.

161. Wolbach, S.B., and D.M. Hegsted. 1953. Hypervitaminosis A in young ducks. The epiphyseal cartilages. Arch Pathol 55:47–54.

162. Woolam, D.H.M., and J.W. Millen. 1955. Effect of vitamin A deficiency on the cerebro-spinal fluid pressure of the chick. Nature (London) 175:41–42.

163. Young, R.J., L.C. Norris, and G.F. Heuser. 1955. The chicks requirement for folic acid in the utilization of choline and its precursors betaine and methylaminoethanol. J Nutr 55:353–362.

164. Young, R.J., H.M. Edwards, Jr., and M.B. Gillis. 1958. Studies on zinc in poultry nutrition. II. Zinc requirement and deficiency symptoms of chicks. Poult Sci 37:1100–1107.

3 SALMONELLOSIS

INTRODUCTION

G.H. Snoeyenbos and J.E. Williams

Avian salmonellosis is an inclusive term designating a large group of acute or chronic diseases of fowl caused by any one or more members of the bacterial genus *Salmonella,* which is a member of the large family Enterobacteriaceae.

The genus *Salmonella,* named for the late eminent USDA veterinarian, Daniel E. Salmon, is composed of over 2100 serotypes, which include the group previously classified as *Arizona hinshawii.* Except for the arizona group, until 1966 most motile salmonella were designated with a serotype (serovar) name corresponding to the geographic site of initial isolation. Serotypes identified after that date have been designated by antigenic formulae.

Kauffmann (2) proposed that the genus *Salmonella* be divided into four subgenera based on biochemical reactions. This division was adopted by the 8th edition of *Bergey's Manual* (1), which included the *Salmonella arizonae* as the type species of subgenus III. In the most recent 9th edition of *Bergey's Manual* (3), a new subgenus V was added. In this chapter, various serotypes are designated in the traditional manner, and the genus *Salmonella* is discussed as a single group of organisms without division into subgenera of subspecies serotypes.

Domestic poultry constitutes the largest single reservoir of salmonella organisms existing in nature. Among all animal species the salmonellae are most frequently reported from poultry and poultry products, partly because of the large population at risk and the active nationwide programs for their isolation and identification.

The two relatively host-specific and nonmotile members of the genus, *S. pullorum* and *S. gallinarum,* causative organisms of pullorum disease and fowl typhoid respectively, are discussed in separate sections as the diseases are distinctly different from each other in important respects, and they are both different from the diseases resulting from the motile salmonellae.

The motile salmonellae are divided for clarity of discussion into sections on the *Arizona salmonella* and *Paratyphoid salmonella.* The latter groups frequently infect or gut-colonize a very broad range of warm- and cold-blooded animal species including humans. Infections in poultry flocks are very common but seldom result in acute systemic form except in young birds under stressful conditions including other infectious diseases, inadequate diet or feed, or water deprivation. Unusually pathogenic strains occur occasionally. Phage type 4 of *Salmonella enteritidis* has been a major problem in parts of central and western Europe for a number of years and has recently become extensively distributed in England. Some strains produce as high as 20% mortality in chicks. Major egg-borne infections in humans have been attributed to transovarian transmission. Similar egg-borne public health problems in the USA, particularly in the northeast, have occurred with increasing frequency for the past 10 yr. These outbreaks have been caused by several other phage types that have not usually been related to unusual virulence in chickens. Most food-borne salmonella infections in humans have been preceded by improper food handling, which allows extensive growth of the bacterium prior to consumption.

With the great expansion of the poultry industry, the widespread occurrence of avian salmonellosis has ranked it as one of the most important egg-borne bacterial diseases of poultry. As these infections recognize no international boundaries and few host barriers, nationwide programs to control them have been beset with numerous obstacles (4). Avian salmonellosis is a problem of economic concern to all phases of the poultry industry from production to marketing. Pet store owners, zoological park administrators, pigeon and fancy-bird raisers, and those interested in wild game are also concerned with these diseases. As they occur in poultry and poultry products, the normally motile salmonellae are also of major interest to those in the public health field.

REFERENCES

1. Buchanan, R.E., and N.E. Gibbons. 1974. Bergey's Manual of Determinative Bacteriology, 8th Ed. Williams and Wilkins, Baltimore.

2. Kauffmann, F. 1966. The Bacteriology of Enterobacteriaceae, Williams and Wilkins, Baltimore.
3. Krieg, N.R., and J.G. Holt. 1984. Bergey's Manual of Systematic Bacteriology, 9th Ed. Vol. 1, Williams and Wilkins, Baltimore/London.
4. Snoeyenbos, G.H. 1985. Proc Int Symp on Salmonella. Am Assoc Avian Pathol, Kennett Square, PA.

PULLORUM DISEASE

G.H. Snoeyenbos

INTRODUCTION. The term pullorum disease (PD) is used to designate infections of avian species by *Salmonella pullorum.* The disease is most commonly spread by true egg transmission. It usually occurs in an acute systemic form in chicks and poults but in adults is most often localized and chronic.

"Bacillary white diarrhea" was used to designate the disease until the term "pullorum disease" was proposed in 1929; the latter term has since gained almost universal acceptance. In some areas of the world, including parts of Europe, *S. pullorum* and *S. gallinarum* are considered to be the same species. Reports of PD from these areas sometimes indicate either PD or fowl typhoid. The disease was once enzootic in many areas of the world but has been reduced in incidence to the point where it is rare in most advanced poultry-producing areas. Virtual if not total eradication of PD has been secured in some areas.

The major economic loss from PD in the USA is indirect and due to the necessity of testing substantially all breeding flocks of chickens and turkeys to ensure freedom from infection. Occasional infections in humans have been produced by massive exposure following ingestion of contaminated foods and are characterized by rapid onset of severe signs of acute enteric infection followed by prompt recovery without treatment.

HISTORY. The etiologic agent of PD was discovered by Rettger in 1899 and described by him as a "fatal septicemia of young chicks" (44). In a later report he designated it as "white diarrhea" (45) and shortly thereafter expanded the term to "bacillary white diarrhea" to distinguish it from other diseases of chicks. Reports in the lay press at the turn of the century, cited by Rettger and Plastridge (46), indicated that PD was widespread in the USA and many foreign countries and caused mortality in chick flocks ranging upward to 100%. Losses were so high that intensive husbandry of chickens was seriously threatened. During 1900–1910, investigators proved that PD was an egg-borne infection. The cycle involved an infected hen laying infected eggs, from which infected chicks would hatch; they could remain infected throughout life.

In 1913 Jones (36) announced the practical application of a macroscopic tube agglutination test for detection of carriers of the organism. Extensive evaluation and development of this test for control and eradication of PD were carried out in several eastern states, allowing inauguration of official state testing programs toward the close of the decade.

PD was first recognized in turkeys in 1928 by Hewitt (31) and within several years was identified in this species in several states and foreign countries. According to Hinshaw and McNeil (34), it was introduced into turkeys from chickens principally by contact with infected chickens in commercial hatcheries or by brooding chicks and poults together. By 1940 PD was widespread in turkeys and responsible for severe economic losses.

Early epidemiologic investigations demonstrated the possibility of transmission of infection in incubators and hatchers. The progressive development, starting in the late 1890s, of large hatcheries that used eggs from many flocks contributed a major means of disseminating PD.

The major economic loss from PD and the promise of securing control through use of the agglutination test stimulated organization of the Conference of Investigators and Workers in Bacillary White Diarrhea Control in 1928 (32), composed first of representatives from the New England states and later (3) enlarged to include other eastern states and provinces in Canada. This conference made a major contribution through concerted efforts to bring about standardization and uniformity of methods to stimulate an interest in practical eradication from breeding flocks.

The Conference of Research Workers in Animal Diseases of North America (4) formulated "Standard Methods of Diagnosis of Pullorum Disease in Barnyard Fowl," which were adopted by the US Livestock Association in 1932 and have served as valuable guides in combating PD.

In 1931 Schaffer et al. (54) announced development of a modified whole-blood test method in which stained antigen is employed. In view of its apparent simplicity, it has been widely used.

A voluntary National Poultry Improvement

Plan administered by state agencies cooperating with the USDA, designed in part to secure control of PD in chickens, became operative in 1935. A National Turkey Improvement Plan organized along the same general lines became operative in 1943. Although these plans were recognized as being inadequate in many respects when formulated, they represented highly significant steps toward reducing the incidence of PD. The glaring scientific shortcomings of the initial plans, which tolerated a low level of infection in officially tested flocks, reflected interests of the industry that had helped formulate them. Industry cooperation was clearly essential for success of a control program of this scope. The plans allowed states to exceed minimum national requirements, with the result that the state industries with the most stringent requirements generally made the most rapid progress in gaining control of PD. A series of modifications of these plans in succeeding years has removed a number of the initial inadequacies. Total eradication on a national basis appears technically feasible but awaits commitment of the industry to this ultimate goal.

INCIDENCE AND DISTRIBUTION

Chickens. PD is worldwide in distribution and has been found in substantially all poultry-producing areas of the world. It is not clear whether it originated in the USA or in some other country. The geographic incidence is closely related to organized control efforts; such efforts have yielded variable results but in some areas have resulted in virtual if not complete eradication.

Turkeys. PD was first reported in poults in Minnesota by Hewitt (31) and soon became widespread. Essentially all characteristics were found to be similar in chickens and turkeys. Extension of infection to turkeys was largely a result of contact with infected chickens in mixed hatching or growing operations. By 1939 PD had become sufficiently established in California breeding stock to stimulate development of a state control program. Many other turkey-producing areas were encountering similar problems.

ETIOLOGY

Classification. *S. pullorum* is a member of the family Enterobacteriaceae, is highly host-adapted, and is one of the few members of the genus that is nonmotile. It is in serogroup D according to the Kauffmann-White schema. Beginning with the 7th edition of *Bergey's Manual,* the designation *S. gallinarum* has been used for both *S. pullorum* and *S. gallinarum,* which has resulted in confusion by combining two pathogens with significantly different biochemical and epizootiologic characteristics.

Morphology and Staining. The organism is a long slender rod (0.3–0.5 × 1–2.5 μm) with slightly rounded ends. It readily stains with ordinary basic aniline dyes and is gram-negative. The cells occur singly, with chains of more than two bacilli rarely found. An occasional filament and large cell may be found in smear preparations. It is nonmotile, nonliquefying, nonchromogenic, nonsporogenic, and facultatively anaerobic.

Growth Requirements. *S. pullorum* grows readily on beef agar or broth and on other media of comparable nutritive value. Selective media should be avoided for isolation because some strains are particularly sensitive. Yoshida and Sato (89) isolated a desoxycholate-sensitive strain and Carlson and Snoeyenbos (16) found a strain that failed to grow on either brilliant green or salmonella-shigella agar but grew satisfactorily on bismuth-sulfite and MacConkey agars.

Stokes and Bayne (61) showed that *S. gallinarum* was of intermediate growth rate between the slow growth of *S. pullorum* and the rapid rate of most salmonellae. They later demonstrated that *S. pullorum* is apparently unique among microorganisms in lacking ability to oxidatively assimilate a variety of amino acids and that this characteristic may explain the slow growth rate (62).

Colonial Morphology. On meat extract agar (pH 7.0–7.2) heavily seeded with inoculum, the colonies appear discrete, smooth, glistening, homogeneous, entire, dome-shaped, transparent, and varying in form from round to angular. On liver infusion agar the growth is even more luxuriant and markedly translucent. Crowded colonies remain small (1 mm or less), but isolated colonies may attain a diameter of 3–4 mm or more. Surface markings may appear as the colony increases in size and age, but as a rule the young colony on a heavily seeded plate changes little with age. Occasionally, abnormal morphologic strains are encountered.

Resistance to Chemical and Physical Agents. *S. pullorum* may survive for years in a favorable environment. It is less resistant to heat, and probably to chemicals and adverse environmental factors, than most paratyphoid salmonellae.

Biochemical Properties. The following substances are fermented with acid, with or without gas production: arabinose, dextrose, galactose, levulose, mannitol, mannose, rhammose, and zylose. Substances not fermented include adonite, dextrin, dulcitol, erythrol, glycerol, inositol, inulin, lactose, raffinose, sucrose, salicin, sorbite, and starch. Maltose is fermented very infrequently. Variation in behavior of some strains may be observed occasionally, especially in regard to gas production. Litmus milk remains practically unchanged. Indole and acetylmethylcarbinol are not formed. Ornithine is rapidly decarboxylated. Hydrogen sulfide (H_2S) is produced more slowly than by most salmonellae, and nitrates are reduced.

Workers in the USA have regarded *S. pullorum* and *S. gallinarum* as distinct species since their initial isolation. Trabulsi and Edwards (68) reviewed the evidence, based primarily on occasional fermentation of maltose by *S. pullorum* isolates and occasional fermentation of dulcitol upon prolonged incubation by isolates of *S. gallinarum*, which led some workers to conclude that the organisms belonged to a single species. Detailed biochemical studies of approximately 100 cultures of both *S. pullorum* and *S. gallinarum* demonstrated that only the ornithine decarboxylase test gave an absolute separation of the two. All the *S. pullorum* cultures produced rapid decarboxylation of ornithine, whereas none of the *S. gallinarum* cultures gave positive reactions within a 7-day observation period. They concluded that *S. pullorum* and *S. gallinarum* constitute two distinct biochemical types.

Antigenic Structure and Toxins. The first evidence of antigenic form variation of *S. pullorum* was provided by Younie in 1941 (90), who found infection in the progeny of a flock negative to a standard agglutination test. Serum from infected chicks agglutinated homologous strain antigens but not standard antigens. Edwards and Bruner (18) explored the nature of the antigenic characteristics of *S. pullorum* and later extended these observations (19). The antigenic composition was shown to be 9, 12_1, 12_2, 12_3; presence of an O-1 antigen has been recognized in publications of the Kauffmann-White schema. Form variation involves antigens 12_2 and 12_3, with standard strains containing a large amount of 12_3 and a very small amount of 12_2, whereas in variant strains the content of the two antigens is reversed. Edwards and Bruner (18) recognized that standard strains of *S. pullorum* contained a small percentage of cells with strong 12_2 antigen and considered this to be the normal form of the organism. Later reports by Gwatkin and Bond (27), Williams et al. (84), and Snoeyenbos et al. (59), among others, showed that initial field isolates are usually rather unstable unless they are in the variant form. Extensive examination of individual colonies, sometimes through successive transfers, is necessary to accurately determine the antigenic form of a culture. Most isolates tend to stabilize during passage on artificial media. Standard form cultures usually contain a small percentage of 12_2 predominant colonies even after long artificial cultivation. Variant form cultures are often pure or nearly pure for 12_2 and 12_3 factors. Colonies of intermediate strains are usually mixtures of 12_2 and 12_3 predominant colonies, or rarely are uniform and contain appreciable amounts of both factors in individual colonies. Strains may also vary in content of the O-1 antigen. There is no evidence to indicate antigenic variation of *S. gallinarum.*

Williams (78, 79) reported that standard, intermediate, and variant types could be differentiated with an ammonium sulfate sedimentation test. An ammonium sulfate concentration of 310 g/L completely cleared the supernatant fluid of standard type suspensions but had little or no effect on suspensions of the variant type and only partially cleared suspensions of intermediate types. A concentration of 470 g/L was required to clear suspensions of variant and intermediate types.

Early reports of incidence of the variant antigenic type of *S. pullorum* in the USA indicated that as high as one-third of the isolates from some areas of the country were of the variant type; by 1950 only 13% of total isolates were of that type (80), a reduction believed to be a result of extensive use of polyvalent testing antigens.

Tsubokura (69, 70) reported a series of experiments to elucidate the relationship between *S. pullorum* and the bacteriophages found to be associated with them. He indicated that phage typing could be of value for type identification, epidemiologic investigations, and genetic studies of *S. pullorum.*

Blaxland et al. (12) reviewed publications to that date bearing on the relationship between *S. pullorum* and *S. gallinarum* and reported studies on 1007 cultures of *S. pullorum* and 608 of *S. gallinarum.* They concluded that antigenic differences between the two organisms, represented by absence of antigenic variation in cultures of *S. gallinarum* and established biochemical and epidemiologic differences, provided evidence that the two are separate and distinct species.

S. pullorum contains a thermostable toxin to which several rodents are susceptible. Since the chick is resistant to the toxin, it probably plays no role in the disease process in this species.

PATHOGENESIS AND EPIZOOTIOLOGY

Natural Hosts. Although the chicken appears to be the natural host of *S. pullorum,* the turkey has also proved to be an important host. The high degree of adaptation of *S. pullorum* for the chicken, and to a lesser degree for the turkey, appears to have severely restricted pathogenicity for other hosts. In these hosts, infection is usually lifelong. Infections in other species have usually been minor and of little long-term significance.

Significant differences in susceptibility have been found among breeds of chickens. The lighter breeds, particularly leghorns, have had fewer reactors within infected flocks than found in heavy breeds. Hutt and Crawford (35) reviewed previous work explaining the mechanism of genetic resistance and reported success in developing resistant and susceptible lines of Rhode Island Reds, New Hampshires, and crosses between the two. Differentiation was based on selection for high and low body temperatures during the first 6 days of life. Lines with high body temperature, indicating a superior thermoregulatory mechanism, were significantly more resistant to mortality following challenge than lines with low body temperature. This work has considerable academic significance because of the unique example of developing genetically resistant lines without using infection as a means of separation. Also, the composition of the B blood group, the major histocompatibility locus of the chicken, influences antibody response and probably mortality reported by Pevzner et al. (41, 42).

Test results over a period of years show a greater percentage of reactors among females than males. The reason for this difference has not been determined but may be related to the sequestered nature of local infection of ovarian follicles.

AGE OF HOST COMMONLY INFECTED. Mortality from PD is usually confined to the first 2–3 wk of age. Severens et al. (56) concluded that resistance increases rapidly during the first 5–10 days in chicks coincident with increases in blood lymphocytes and body temperature. Acute infections in adult chickens, particularly among brown egg-producing strains, has occasionally been reported from a variety of areas. Mortality in semimature and mature turkeys has also been observed.

A substantial percentage of chickens and turkeys that survive retain the infection with or without the presence of lesions.

Unusual Hosts. Naturally occurring infections in animals other than the chicken or turkey have usually been a result of direct or indirect exposure to infected chickens. Naturally infected birds include ducks, guinea fowl, pheasants, quail, sparrows, canaries, European bullfinches, hawk-headed parrots, and urus. Several other avian species have been experimentally infected. Naturally or experimentally infected mammals include chimpanzees, rabbits, guinea pigs, chinchillas, pigs, kittens, foxes, dogs, swine, mink, calves, and wild rats (*Rattus norvegicus*). Recognition of this potentially wide range of hosts caused many people to suspect that infection was so prevalent that efforts to eliminate it in poultry would be fruitless. The striking progress achieved in eliminating *S. pullorum* from most domestic poultry has demonstrated that other birds and mammals are of little importance in epidemiology of the disease.

Human salmonellosis caused by *S. pullorum* has occasionally been reported. Mitchell et al. (39) reviewed earlier reports and recorded what appeared to be the first extensive food-borne outbreak. McCullough and Eisele (38) produced salmonellosis with four strains of *S. pullorum* by feeding 1.3–4 billion organisms. The pathogen was recovered from stools on the 1st or 2nd day of illness only and was not recovered when fed at levels lower than those producing illness. Explosive onset of illness, high fever, prostration, and prompt recovery were noteworthy.

Transmission. The primary role of infected hatching eggs in transmitting infection was recognized early in the course of investigations. As many as a third of the eggs laid by infected hens contain *S. pullorum,* chiefly as a result of contamination of the ovum following ovulation. Although *S. pullorum* may penetrate the shell following lay, this route of infection is probably of minor importance (85).

Watanabe et al. (76) found that eggs from some infected hens carried levels of agglutinins in the yolk comparable to those circulating in the serum of the hen. When *S. pullorum* was inoculated into the yolk of such eggs, they survived much longer than control embryos and sometimes hatched as infected chicks that died later. Such antibody protection is probably critical to prevent embryonic mortality in infected eggs and to allow successful egg transmission.

Transmission of infection during hatching from infected to uninfected chicks can result in extensive dissemination that is only partially prevented by fumigation of the hatcher. Transmission may also occur within a flock as a result of cannibalism of infected birds, egg eating, and entry of *S. pullorum* through wounds. Infection from eating contaminated feed has been demonstrated experimentally. Since *S. pullorum* has rarely been demonstrated in feed, in contrast to frequent contamination by the paratyphoid salmonellae, this avenue of infection is probably of little significance.

Botts et al. (14) reported that *S. pullorum* disappeared more rapidly from built-up litter than from new corncob litter. Tucker (71) made similar observations and found that survival time varied in built-up litter from 11 wk in new litter to 3 wk in old litter. A correlation was found between survival time and moisture level of litter, which favored survival in dry litter. Turnbull and Snoeyenbos (72) reported that ammonia elaborated by microflora of moist, long-used litter sharply increased the pH of available water to the point that litter was actively salmonellacidal.

Signs. PD was first recognized among young chicks, and the malady may be considered as principally a chick or poult disease. Characteristics in both the chick and poult are so nearly identical that they may be considered as one. PD occasionally is subclinical even when originating from egg transmission.

CHICKS AND POULTS. If birds are hatched from infected eggs, moribund and dead birds may be observed in the incubator or within a short time after hatching. They manifest somnolence, weakness, and loss of appetite; death may follow suddenly. In some instances evidence of PD is not observed until 5–10 days after hatching, but it gains momentum during the following 7–10 days. The peak of mortality usually occurs during the 2nd or 3rd wk of life. In some instances the birds exhibit lassitude, an inclination to huddle together under the hover, inappetence, drooping of wings, somnolence, and distorted body appearance. Affected birds frequently exhibit a shrill cry when voiding excreta and commonly develop an accumulation of chalk-white excreta, sometimes stained greenish brown, in and around the vent.

Labored breathing or gasping may be observed as a result of extensive pathology of the lungs. Anderson et al. (1) found that lesions in lungs of chicks that died from PD occurred as frequently in those infected orally as in those infected by an aerosol. Survivors may be greatly retarded in their growth and appear underdeveloped and poorly feathered. Van Roekel (74) reported in 1931 that among 29 chicks that were 6 wk old and exposed to infection when 72 hr old, the range in weight varied from 90 to 558 g. In most instances it is advisable to destroy survivors, clean and disinfect quarters, and replace with clean stock. Chicks retarded in growth do not mature into vigorous, well-developed laying or breeding birds. However, some survivors may not reveal any great setback in growth but develop to maturity even though harboring the infection. Flocks that have passed through a serious outbreak usually have a high percentage of carriers at maturity.

Evans et al. (20) reported blindness associated with salmonellosis in chicks. In one case *S. pullorum* was isolated from the anterior chamber of the eye and from the tibiotarsal joint. Fluctuating swelling of the tibiotarsal and the humeroradial and ulnar articulations have been ascribed to *S. pullorum* infection in chicks. Ferguson et al. (21) and others observed a relatively high incidence of localization of infection, which produced lameness and obvious swelling in joints and adjacent synovial sheaths of chicks. Similar lesions in turkey poults have been reported. These observations suggest that some strains of the organism may have a predilection for these tissues.

ADULTS. PD in a maturing or adult flock does not manifest characteristics of an acute infection as a rule. Infection may spread within a flock for a long time without producing distinct signs. Infected birds may exhibit few or no signs and usually cannot be detected by their physical appearance.

Variable degrees of reduction in egg production, fertility, and hatchability, largely dependent upon the incidence of infection within a flock, is usually observed.

Occasionally, acute infections occur in semimature and mature flocks. Depression, anorexia, diarrhea, and dehydration are prominent signs.

Morbidity and Mortality. Both morbidity and mortality are highly variable in chickens and turkeys and are influenced by age, strain susceptibility, nutrition, flock management, and characteristics of exposure. Mortality may vary from no losses to 100% in serious outbreaks. The greatest losses usually occur during the 2nd wk after hatching, with a rapid decline during the 3rd and 4th wk of age. Morbidity is often much higher than mortality, with some of the affected birds recovering spontaneously. Birds hatched from an infected flock and raised on the same premises will usually exhibit less mortality than those subjected to the stress of shipping.

Gross Lesions

CHICKS AND POULTS. In birds that die suddenly in the early stages of brooding, lesions are limited. The liver is enlarged and congested, and the normal yellow color may be streaked with hemorrhages. In the septicemic form an active hyperemia may be found in other organs. The yolk sac and its contents reveal slight or no alteration. In more protracted cases interference with yolk absorption may occur, and yolk sac contents may be yellowish and of creamy or caseous consistency. Necrotic foci or nodules may be present in cardiac muscle, liver, lungs (Fig. 3.1), ceca, large intestine (Fig. 3.2D), and gizzard muscle. Pericarditis may be observed in some instances. The liver may reveal punctiform hemorrhages and focal necrosis (Fig. 3.2A,B). The spleen may be enlarged and kidneys congested or anemic, with ureters prominently distended with urates. The ceca may contain a caseous core, sometimes tinted with blood. The wall of the intestine may be thickened. Frequently, peritonitis is manifested. Doyle and Mathews (17) report that the liver is the most consistent seat of gross lesions and is followed in order of frequency by lungs, heart, gizzard, and ceca. Among chicks only a few days old, lung lesions may consist of only a hemorrhagic pneumonia, whereas in older chicks yellowish gray hepatization may be found. Nodules in the myocardium may attain sufficient size to cause a marked distortion in the shape of the heart (Fig. 3.2C).

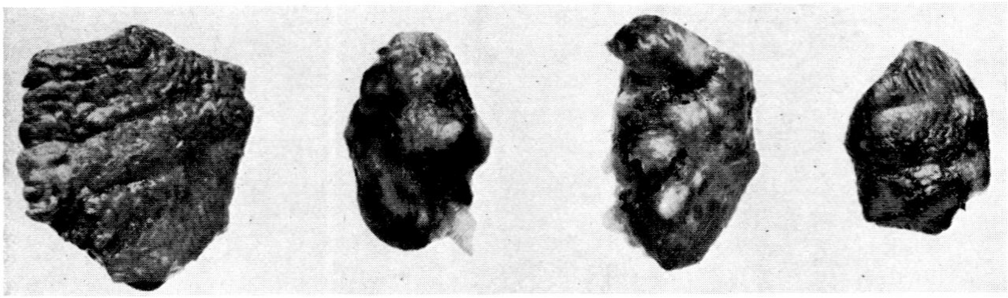

3.1. Normal lung (17-day-old chick) (*no. 1 from left*). Pullorum-infected lungs exhibiting pneumonia and multiple abscesses (16-day-old chick) (*nos. 2, 3, 4)*.

ADULTS. Lesions found most frequently in the chronic carrier hen are misshapen, discolored, cystic ova (Fig. 3.2E), peritonitis, and frequently an acute or chronic pericarditis. The involved ova usually contain oily and caseous material enclosed in a thickened capsule. These degenerated ovarian follicles may be closely attached to the ovary, but frequently they are pedunculated and may become detached from the ovarian mass. In such cases they may become embedded in the adipose tissue of the abdominal cavity. Ovarian and oviduct dysfunction may lead to abdominal ovulation or oviduct impaction, which in turn may bring about extensive peritonitis and adhesions of the abdominal viscera. Ascites may also develop, particularly in the turkey. Advanced lesions of this type seldom fail to yield *S. pullorum* on culture.

Lesions less extensive in nature may involve the heart. Quite frequently, pericarditis is observed in both females and males. Changes in the pericardium, epicardium, and pericardial fluid appear to depend on the duration of the disease process. In some cases the pericardium exhibits only a slight translucency and the pericardial fluid may be increased and turbid. In the more advanced stages the pericardial sac is thickened and opaque and the pericardial fluid is greatly increased in amount, containing considerable exudative material. This may be followed by permanent thickening of the pericardium and epicardium and partial obliteration of the pericardial cavity by the adhesions. Occasionally, small cysts containing amber-colored, caseous material may be found embedded in the abdominal fat or attached to the gizzard or intestines.

The pancreas is frequently infected, with or without gross focal lesions. The organism can usually be recovered from such processes. In the male the infection is frequently found in reproductive organs. In adults acute infections that produce lesions indistinguishable from acute *S. gallinarum* infections may also occur.

Histopathology. Doyle and Mathews (17) state that in young chicks the livers show hyperemia, hemorrhages, focal degeneration, and necrosis (Fig. 3.3) and that accumulation of endothelial leukocytes that replace the degenerated or necrotic liver cells is a characteristic cell reaction of the liver to *S. pullorum* infection.

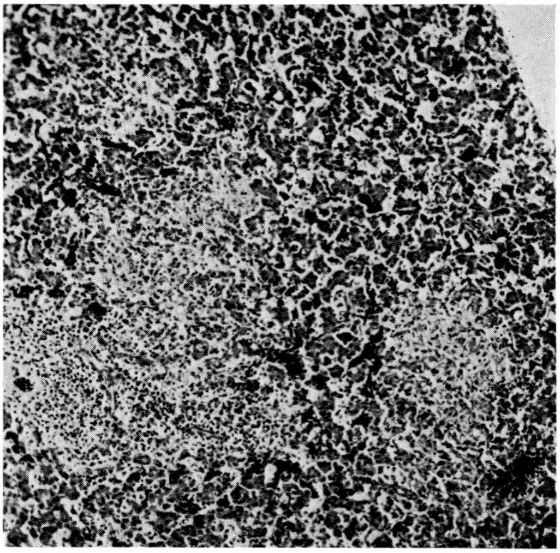

3.3. Liver revealing focal degeneration and necrosis. ×100.

Lesions are often extensive but not specific. Suganuma (64) studied 459 field cases of PD that included chicks and adult hens and roosters. The main pathologic changes observed were endothelial cell proliferative foci of the liver; focal necrosis of the myocardium; catarrhal bronchitis; catarrhal enteritis in chicks; and interstitial inflammation of liver, lungs, and kidneys. Serositis, particularly in the pericardium, pleuroperitoneum, and serosa of the intestinal tract and mesentery, was found in a high percentage of cases and regarded as the most characteristic lesion of the disease. This inflammatory change

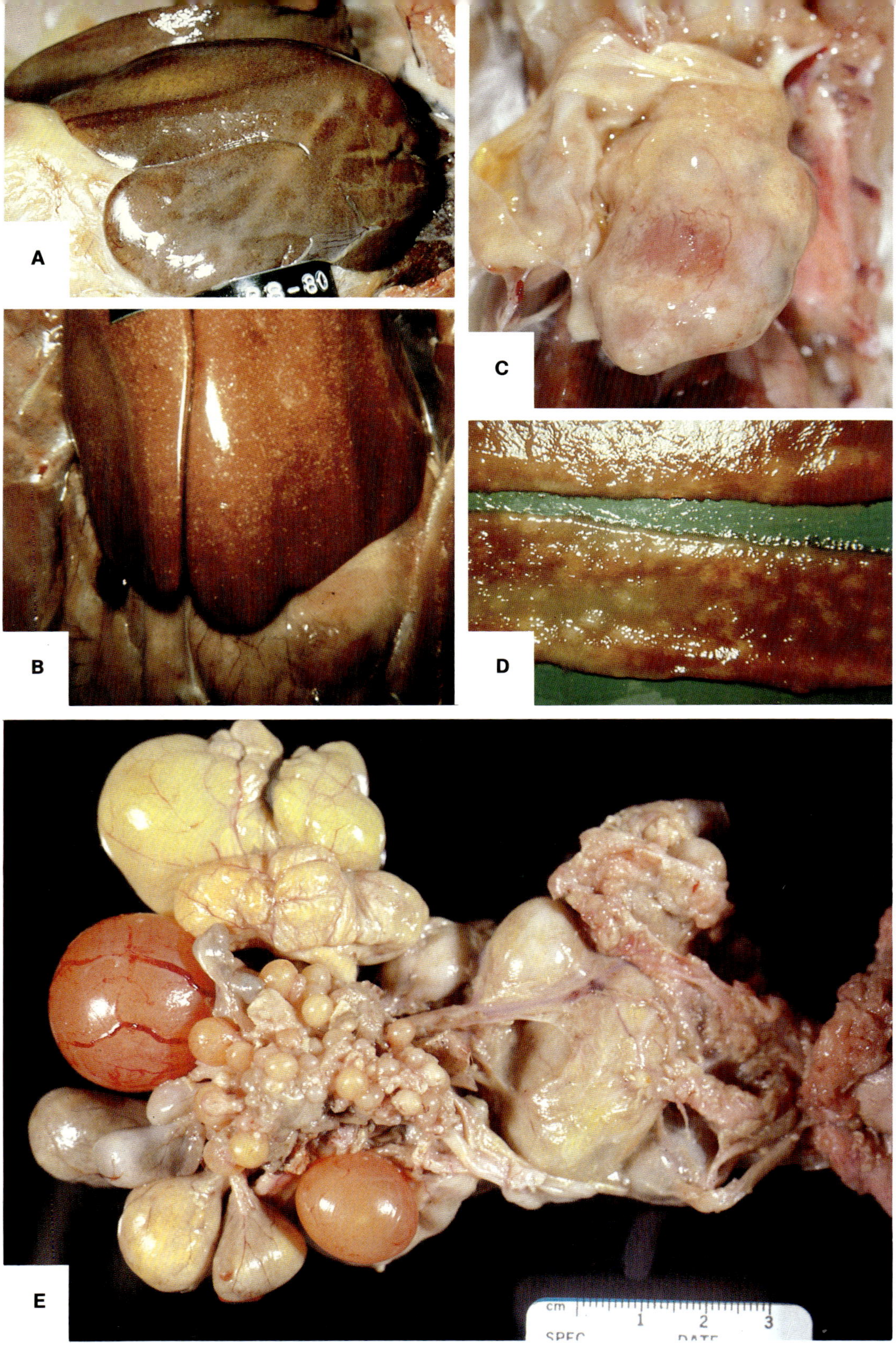

3.2. Gross lesions associated with *S. pullorum* infection in chickens. A, B. Enlarged livers showing discoloration and hemorrhagic areas (A) or congestion and small necrotic foci (B). (Glass). C. Nodular lesions in the heart; note the thickened yellowish pericardium (reflected). (Shivaprasad). D. Necrotic foci in the intestine. (Glass). E. Ovarian lesions and salpingitis. (Shivaprasad)

consisted of infiltration of lymphocytes, lymphocytic cells, plasma cells, and heterophils and proliferation of fibroblastic and histiocytic cells without accompanying exudative changes. Pericarditis was rarely observed.

Histopathologic lesions in turkeys apparently have not been studied and reported. They could be expected to be substantially identical to those found in the chicken.

Immunity. Buxton (15) found that chicks orally infected at 4 days did not produce detectable agglutinating antibodies until 20–40 days of age and did not achieve maximum antibody production until approximately 100 days. Intravenous injection of 15-day-old chicken embryos with killed *S. pullorum* resulted in a marked reduction in ability of the hatched chick to produce agglutinins following challenge with live *S. pullorum* later in life.

Birds infected at maturity usually produce agglutinating antibodies within 3–10 days following infection, which persist at varying levels for the duration of infection. Although such antibody production represents an immune response, the possible role of agglutinating antibodies in modifying the course of infection in the host is little understood. The general success in eradication of infection by elimination of carriers has not encouraged comprehensive investigation of the immune mechanism. High-titered serum from infected birds supports multiplication of *S. pullorum* in vitro; agglutinating antibodies in vivo probably serve a function in localizing infection. Gupta and Mallick (26) reported that the 9R vaccine strain of *S. gallinarum* administered to baby chicks provided significant protection against challenge with *S. pullorum* 14 days later.

DIAGNOSIS.

A definitive diagnosis of PD requires isolation and identification of *S. pullorum*. Flock history and signs are of limited value in arriving at a diagnosis because of the similarity to a number of other diseases. Lesions, particularly in severely affected chicks and poults, may be highly suggestive and used as a basis for a tentative diagnosis. Positive serologic findings are of major value in detecting infection in a control program but should not be considered adequate for a definitive diagnosis. Delay of 3–10 or more days in appearance of agglutinating antibodies following infection often results in mortality before antibody development.

Isolation of *S. pullorum*. Acute PD is characterized by a systemic infection that allows ready isolation from most body tissues. In such infections the liver is usually prominently involved and is a preferred organ to culture. Lesions that may occur in the spleen, myocardium or pericardium, lungs, gizzard, pancreas, or yolk sac are also dependable for isolation. A bacteriologic inoculating loop is satisfactory for transferring adherent tissues to culture media from chicks and poults; a cotton swab is preferable for making cultures from older birds since a larger amount of tissue is transferred.

Beef infusion agar in petri dishes is satisfactory for isolation by direct inoculation. Any other media of comparable nutritive value may also be used. Media containing inhibitory substances such as brilliant green and desoxycholate are occasionally also inhibitory for salmonellae and should be used only if required because of decomposition of the specimens.

CHRONIC INFECTIONS. Cultural examination to identify localized chronic infections, represented by the carrier detected by serologic tests, must be detailed if reasonable accuracy is to be secured. A detailed outline for examination of such specimens is given in the National Poultry Improvement Plan and Auxiliary Provisions (NPIP) (5). This procedure may be summarized briefly as follows.

Grossly normal or diseased internal organs should be cultured directly on veal infusion (VI) and brilliant green (BG) agar plates and incubated 48 hr at 37 C. In addition, portions of the internal organs should be pooled, ground, or blended in 10 times their volume of VI broth; 10-ml aliquots of the suspension are transferrable to 100 ml of both VI and tetrathionate BG (TBG) broth and incubated 24 hr at 37 C. The broths are then plated on VI and BG agar and incubated and examined after 24 and 48 hr. If contamination with proteus or pseudomonas is a problem, platings can be done on BG sulfapyridine (BGS) agar.

The digestive tract should be cultured using individual cotton swabs for the upper, middle, and lower intestinal tract including both the ceca and rectum-cloaca area. The swabs should be deposited in 10 ml TBG broth, incubated, and plated as previously described for the internal organs. In addition, portions of the gut should be pooled, ground, or blended in 10 times their volume of TBG broth. Ten ml of the suspension from the digestive tract are transferred to 100 ml TBG broth and incubated at 42 or 37 C for 24 hr. The higher incubation temperatures for TBG broth reduce populations of competitive contaminants common in gut tissue.

Suspect colonies are transferred to triple-sugar-iron (TSI) agar and lysine-iron (LI) agar and incubated at 37 C for 24 hr. Cultures revealing typical reactions of salmonellae or arizonae on TSI or LI agar slants should be identified by appropriate biochemical and other tests. All salmonella cultures should be serologically typed.

Use of nonselective media demands careful aseptic techniques but has the advantage of more dependably securing isolation of *S. pullorum*. Also, other bacteria capable of producing cross-reactions with pullorum antigen may be more dependably demonstrated.

Identification of Cultures. Most isolates of *S. pullorum* produce typical reactions and can be identified promptly without resorting to a large bank of differential media. Familiarity with the characteristic small, smooth, translucent colony on nutrient media after 24 hr of incubation often allows tentative identification. Careful initial culture of tissues on nonselective media should usually result in pure cultures. If pure cultures are not secured or if an enrichment medium has been used, it is often advantageous to transfer individual colonies to TSI agar slants for preliminary differentiation. *S. pullorum* on such slants produces a red slant with a yellow butt that shows delayed blackening from H_2S production.

The following reactions, which can be determined within 24 hr and provide identification of a number of other common pathogens, allow identification of most isolates:

Dextrose	fermented with gas
Lactose	not fermented
Sucrose	not fermented
Mannitol	fermented with gas
Maltose	usually not fermented
Dulcitol	not fermented
Indole	not produced
Urea	not hydrolyzed
Motility	nonmotile
Agglutination	positive with group D antiserum

Additional differential tests described under Etiology are necessary to identify isolates that produce nontypical reactions (chiefly fermentation of maltose or no gas production). Decarboxylation of ornithine by *S. pullorum* is the single most dependable test for differentiating maltose-fermenting *S. pullorum* strains from *S. gallinarum*.

Differential Diagnosis. Signs and lesions produced by PD are not pathognomonic. Even the broadest spectrum of lesions that may develop in the chick, poult, or adult bird may be duplicated by infections with *S. gallinarum*. Other salmonella infections produce lesions of liver, spleen, and intestines that cannot be distinguished grossly or microscopically from those produced by PD. Aspergillus or other molds may produce similar lesions in lungs. Occasionally, *S. pullorum* localizes in major joints and tendon sheaths of considerable numbers of chicks and produces signs and lesions like those of *Mycoplasma synoviae* and other infectious agents that localize at these sites.

Local infections of *S. pullorum* in the adult carrier, particularly of the pericardium and ovary, may appear identical to those produced by other bacterial infections such as coliforms, staphylococci, micrococci, and other salmonellae. Birds of any age may be infected with *S. pullorum* and fail to show grossly discernible lesions.

A definitive diagnosis of PD can be made only following isolation and identification of *S. pullorum*.

TREATMENT. Reasonably effective prophylactic and therapeutic drugs were first discovered among the sulfonamides. Since that time other compounds including nitrofurans and several antibiotics have been found to be effective in reducing mortality from PD. No drug or combination of drugs has been found that is capable of eliminating infection from a treated flock. Sulfonamides in particular frequently suppress growth and may interfere with feed and water intake and egg production. Therapy, therefore, may have short-range economic merit but is no substitute for a sound eradication program.

Sulfonamides. Severans et al. (57) appear to have been the first to report on the efficacy of sulfonamide medication for control of mortality from PD. They found that among seven sulfonamides tested, sulfadiazine and sulfamerazine were the most effective in reducing chick mortality. Sulfathiazole and sulfaguanadine were intermediate in effectiveness; sulfasuxidine, phthalylsulfathiazone and sulfanilamide were least effective. Mullen (40), in an extensive field trial in poults, found that a 0.5% level of sulfamerazine in mash for the first 5 days apparently reduced mortality in progeny of infected breeders from approximately 17 to 4%. A litter-eating problem developed if the medication period was extended beyond 5 days. Bottorff and Kiser (13) found sulfadiazine, sulfamethazine, and sulfamerazine to be equally effective in preventing chick mortality, which was reduced in the medicated groups from a minimum of 30% to a maximum of 56% compared to untreated controls. A maximum drug level of 0.75% in starter mash was used for either 5 or 10 days starting at 1 day of age. Mortality recurred in all groups beginning 5 days after drug withdrawal. They made the significant observation, not found by Severens (56), that 90% of all survivors reacted to the whole-blood test for PD when tested at 12 wk of age.

Pomeroy et al. (43) tested the efficacy of nine sulfonamides against PD in chicks. Sulfadiazine, sulfamerazine, sulfapyrazine, sulfaquinoxaline, and sulfamethazine were the most effective of the drugs tested. Sulfadiazine, sulfapyrazine, and sulfamethazine were not effective in reducing mortality in poults experimentally infected with *S. pullorum*. The authors concluded that results obtained from chicks treated with sulfonamides should not be considered applicable to turkeys. They found, as had Bottorff and Kiser (13), that appreciable numbers of infected birds remained among medicated survivors.

Nitrofurans. Smith (58) appears to have been the first to report tests of nitrofurazone for treatment of PD. In trials reported, a concentration of 0.04% furazolidone in feed for a 10- to 14-day period beginning shortly after exposure was highly effective in preventing mortality and carriers among chicks. Under conditions of the trial, furazolidone was superior to either chloramphenicol or sulfamerazine. Gordon and Tucker (24) and Wilson (86, 87) used furazolidone in mash at a 0.04% concentration and in some instances appeared to have eliminated *S. pullorum* from carrier birds. Henderson et al. (29) fed chickens 0.011% furazolidone in feed for 5 wk starting at time of artificial exposure at 9–14 wk of age. Infection developed in some birds during treatment without concurrent antibody development. They concluded that furazolidone interferes with antibody production and should not be used for a least 6 wk before testing for PD. Richey and Morgan (48) found infection in survivors of chickens treated at levels as high as 0.066% furazolidone from the 85th to the 20th day postexposure. Francis (22) found that 0.011% furazolidone in feed significantly reduced mortality from PD but that *S. pullorum* was still being excreted after the 4-wk treatment period.

Bierer (10) found furaltadone-water medication effective in reducing mortality in chicks infected with *S. pullorum.*

Antibiotics. Limited trials with chloramphenicol were reported by Smith (58). A 0.5% concentration in feed for 10 days following experimentally induced infection sharply reduced mortality but left many infected chicks. Chlortetracycline at a 200-mg/kg level in the ration was found by Grausgruber and Kissling (25) to suppress mortality in orally infected day-old chicks. The authors did not find interference with isolation of *S. pullorum* from infected chicks or adverse effect on agglutinin development, even if the drug was administered for prolonged periods.

Colinstin was found by Biondi and Schiavo (11) and Schiavo and Biondi (55) to increase survival of infected chicken embryos and to markedly increase survival of infected chicks. *S. pullorum* was isolated from treated survivors.

Stuart and Keenum (63) were unable to recover *S. pullorum* from infected eggs treated by spraying the shells with neomycin sulfate prior to incubation.

Tacconi et al. (65) found a 5-day treatment of either 150 or 225 mg/L in drinking water of the aminoglycoside apromycin to be highly effective in preventing morbidity in chicks exposed at 3 days with medication starting 24 hr later. The treatment did not eliminate infection.

Drug Resistance. Karyagin (37) found that the minimum inhibitory concentration of chlortetracycline for 24 isolates of *S. pullorum* varied between 1.25 and 12.5 μg/ml. Resistance was increased as much as 32 times after passages in increasing amounts of antibiotics. These strains lost pathogenicity for chicks, and their biochemical properties changed. Relatively resistant strains with unchanged biochemical properties were obtained from infected birds treated with chlortetracycline. Similar changes in the 24 isolates in susceptibility, biochemical properties, and virulence occurred following passage in media containing increasing amounts of nitrofurazone. Increased resistance without decrease in virulence was found in isolates from birds treated with nitrofurazone. Sarkisov and Trishkina (53) were unable to demonstrate increased resistance to chlortetracycline following a 30-day medication period.

PREVENTION AND CONTROL. It has long been established that chicken and turkey flocks can be developed and maintained free of PD by adhering to well-defined procedures. In the simplest sense it may be stated that the only requirement is to establish breeding flocks free of *S. pullorum* and to hatch and rear their progeny under circumstances that preclude direct or indirect contact with infected chickens or turkeys.

Management Procedures. Commonly accepted methods of management to prevent introduction of infectious agents are generally applicable to prevent introduction of *S. pullorum.* The fact that egg transmission plays a dominant role in spread of infection makes it mandatory that only eggs from flocks known to be free of PD be introduced into hatcheries. Hinshaw et al. (33) demonstrated that *S. pullorum* could be spread through the air of forced-draft incubators. Fumigation of incubators and hatchers with formaldehyde was originally developed to decrease spread of PD and to destroy residual infection during cleaning between hatches. Fumigation may have been of some benefit in the past when the disease was rampant, but it no longer has more than historic significance as an aid in control of PD. The reader interested in fumigation methods is referred to discussion of this subject under Paratyphoid Infections.

There should be no mixing of pullorum-free stock at any time with other poultry or confined birds not known to be free of the disease. This principle applies on a farm basis; infected stock on a farm, even if in separate pens or buildings, compromises the status all other birds on the farm.

Elimination of Carriers. Investigations already reviewed, which established that PD was transmitted through the egg, suggested a method of attack to secure control. The foundation of the control program was established in 1913 by Jones (36), who reported use of a macroscopic tube agglutination test (TA) for detecting infected chickens. The test was promptly applied in state programs to eliminate the disease from flocks by detection and removal of reactors.

Early field testing results indicated that removal of reactors following a single test usually was not sufficient for complete elimination of infected birds from a flock. Such results may be expected because of three possible intercurrent characteristics: 1) serum agglutinin titers of infected birds tend to fluctuate and may for brief periods fail to produce significant agglutination at the usual dilution of 1:25 or 1:50; 2) there is a delay of at least several days between infection and development of agglutinins; 3) environmental contamination may exist following removal of reactors, which may serve as a source of infection at a later date.

SEROLOGIC TESTS. As the obvious value of a serologic testing program as a tool to gain control of PD became apparent, many investigators worked diligently to evaluate, refine, and modify the system. In addition to the macroscopic test, a rapid serum (RS) test was introduced by Runnels et al. (51), and a stained antigen whole-blood (WB) test was developed by Schaffer et al. (54). Gwatkin et al. (28) concluded that the WB and TA tests were equally satisfactory for testing chickens. Winter et al. (88) found, as had with others, that the WB test was not satisfactory for testing turkeys. Williams and Whittemore (81) developed a microagglutination (MA) test system using tetrazolium-stained antigen, which is as dependable as the TA test and offers important advantages in economy.

The NPIP (5), which details testing methods, accepts four for testing chickens: standard TA test, WB test, RS test, and MA test. Of the four, only the WB test is not accepted for testing turkeys. Testing for accreditation is allowed after chickens and turkeys reach approximate immunologic maturity at 16 wk of age.

In contrast to US requirements for producing antigen from cells grown on the surface of appropriate agar, Tanaka (66) developed a WB test antigen, now officially used in Japan, that is grown in a continuous-flow broth culture system. As marked differences in antigenicity occur with duration of continuous culture, with agglutinability increasing over time, it is necessary to blend sublots to secure desired agglutinability. Prior to blending of sublots the production protocol includes collecting cells by centrifugation, washing twice in physiologic saline, heating at 80 C for 30 min to reduce sensitivity, adding phenol to a final concentration of 0.5%, adjusting concentration to McFarland scale 1, and staining with malachite green to a concentration of 0.1%.

Serologic evidence of infection should be confirmed by bacteriologic examination of one or more reactors. If only suspicious reactions are observed in a flock, the birds reacting most strongly should be submitted to a laboratory for retesting and a careful bacteriologic examination. In routine testing, flocks should not be condemned as infected on the basis of doubtful or atypical reactions, because such reactions may be from infections other than *S. pullorum.*

NONPULLORUM REACTORS. Nonpullorum reactions occasionally cause problems of interpretation. A variety of bacteria possessing antigens in common with or closely related to those of *S. pullorum* may infect birds and produce an agglutinin response. Garrard et al. (23) reported that nonpullorum reactions occurred more frequently with variant than with standard form antigens. Infections with coliforms, micrococci, and streptococci—particularly those belonging to Lancefield group D—were found to be responsible for a large percentage of nonpullorum reactions in chickens. Absorption tests indicated that the 12_2 factor was most frequently responsible for the cross-reactions. Other salmonellae with antigens common to *S. pullorum* may also produce cross-reactions. Among many workers who found avian serums reactive with pullorum antigens from infection with other bacteria were Bergqvist et al. (9). They reported that *Staphylococcus epidermidis, Micrococcus* sp., *Aerobacter aerogenes, Proteus* sp., *Escherichia coli,* and species of *Arizona, Providence,* and *Citrobacter,* often infecting gonads, were responsible for many nonpullorum reactions. Infections with *Salmonella gallinarum* produce antibodies indistinguishable from *S. pullorum;* and the paratyphoids, particularly those in group D, may also produce cross-reactions. Isolates from viscera of nonpullorum reactors, which are agglutinated by that individual's serum as well as by pullorum-positive serum, may be presumed to be the cause of reaction.

Nonpullorum reactors may range from one to a few birds in a flock to as high as 30–40%. The character of the agglutination may range from typical to atypical and the titer of the serums from low to high. In some flocks in which a very high percentage of birds reacted strongly to the WB test, serum titers were no greater than 1:40 or 1:80 by the TA test. Titration of serum from 20 to 30 birds in such flocks allows determination of the flock status, since an *S. pullorum* infection would result in a substantial percentage of samples with much higher titer. A similar approach is useful in flocks recently vaccinated with attenuated (9R) *S. gallinarum,* which may cause a transient, low-titer serologic response. If there are only a few reactors, serum titration is not dependable, as infected birds sometimes have low titers.

Detailed bacteriologic examination of representative reactors is often the only dependable method of determining the pullorum status of a flock. It is usually the only method of distinguishing between infections by *S. pullorum* and *S. gallinarum*, which is of major epizootiologic importance. The serum of birds infected with bacteria antigenically related to *S. pullorum* often produces a low titer with an atypical type of agglutination; at times both the titer and character of agglutination are indistinguishable from those produced by PD. If no conclusive evidence of pullorum infection can be found, the flock should be regarded as negative. Occasionally, it is advisable to retest groups of birds to clarify their status.

MISCELLANEOUS TESTS. A number of additional tests have been employed as a means of detecting infected birds. An intradermal test applied to the wattle was described by Ward and Gallagher (75). Rettger and Plastridge (46) summarized the work of several investigators with intradermal tests and concluded that the agglutination tests were more dependable.

Stephanov et al. (60) reported that an allergin prepared from a live culture of 9R *S. gallinarum* detected more reactors from pullorum-typhoid than a serum drop agglutination test.

Williams (77) described a "spot test" for detection of infected chickens, which may serve as a useful adjunct to the agglutination test, especially in flocks in which suspicious reactors are detected.

A flocculation test was described by Roznowski and Foltz (50). The antigen, which produced promising results from the limited work reported, was prepared by coating cholesterol crystals with an ectoantigen extract of *S. pullorum.*

Rice and Gwatkin (47) compared an indirect complement-fixation test to the agglutination test. The test was too involved and expensive for routine work but offered promise for differentiating nonpullorum reactors from true reactors. Aoki et al. (7) used an agar gel precipitin test to detect infected birds. The test was consistently negative with serums that produced nonspecific reactions with an agglutination test.

A rapid hemagglutination (HA) test with chloroform or ethyl alcohol–washed antigens was reported by Ungureanu and Grecianu (73) to be specific and to produce a higher titer than produced by the TA test. Sapre and Mehta (52) described an indirect HA test for *S. pullorum* that detected antibodies earlier and in dilutions four times greater than by a bacterial agglutination test.

Andrews (2) saturated serodisks with serum and with whole blood of infected pheasants. TA tests of whole-blood eluates from PD were unreadable, and the plate agglutination test of eluates was only about one-half as accurate as the serum TA test. Heutgens (30) found that juices of either fresh or frozen muscle of affected chickens produced positive reactions with the whole-blood test when TA titers of the donor birds were 640 or higher.

Williams and Whittemore (81, 82, 83) developed a microantiglobulin test (MAG) for paratyphoid infections of poultry that is fully capable of detecting agglutinating antibodies against *S. pullorum* with the use of group D antigen. Enhancement of agglutinin activity by antiglobulin results in greatly increased titers compared to most test systems. Thain and Blanford (67) found the MAG test comparable in sensitivity to conventional agglutination tests. The MAG test was superior to the others in detecting birds with low titers. It would be expected that the later test, developed to detect agglutinins for group D salmonella, would sometimes yield false-positive results from infection by other members of this group.

Beaudette (8) reported that infected hens with high serum titers laid eggs with high albumen titers. Thain and Blanford (67) made similar observations.

Rozanska and Kirzajew (49) used a phenol extract of *S. pullorum* for a gel precipitation test that compared favorably to standard agglutination tests.

NATIONAL CONTROL PROGRAM. The NPIP (5) details specific criteria for establishing and maintaining official US pullorum/typhoid–clean flocks and hatcheries. These criteria are based on farm and hatchery management to prevent direct or indirect contact with infected stock and annual testing of all (or a representative portion) flocks.

If an attempt is made to free a flock of infection, retesting of the infected flock should be done at 2- to 4-wk intervals until two consecutive negative tests of the entire flock are secured at not less than a 21-day interval. In the majority of cases, infection can be eliminated from the flock through short-interval testing. Two or three retests are often sufficient to detect all infected birds (Table 3.1) Occasionally, infection continues to spread within a flock and the disease cannot be eliminated by repeated testing.

AREA ERADICATION. Early efforts to control PD were of necessity based on the objective of eliminating infection from individual flocks and from flocks of individual hatchery and breeding organizations. In some states initial testing in the 1920s indicated an infection rate of 20% of chickens tested. Efforts to eliminate infection resulted in a progressive decline in incidence of infections in both chickens and turkeys (Tables 3.2, 3.3). Since at least the early 1970s, all major commercial poultry breeding flocks in the USA have been free of PD. A reservoir of infection exists in small

Table 3.1. Retesting data of 10 infected flocks

Flock Number	Test	First Test	Second Test	Third Test	Fourth Test	Fifth Test	Subsequent Season
1	No. of birds tested	189	152	48	...	...	467
	Percentage reactors	1.59	0	0	...	...	0
2	No. of birds tested	369	256	218	...	...	232
	Percentage reactors	0.54	0.39	0	...	...	0
3	No. of birds tested	125	98	91	...	...	201
	Percentage reactors	20.00	4.08	0	...	...	0
4	No. of birds tested	243	262	223	179	...	199
	Percentage reactors	11.11	1.15	0	0	...	0
5	No. of birds tested	464	444	433	397	...	1087
	Percentage reactors	2.37	0.45	0	0	...	0
6	No. of birds tested	1765	1559	1508	1108	767	1796
	Percentage reactors	3.17	0.13	0	0	0	0
7	No. of birds tested	2079	1929	1811	1648	1337	2132
	Percentage reactors	3.17	1.09	0	0	0	0
8	No. of birds tested	704	691	610	422	...	693
	Percentage reactors	8.24	8.83	0.16	0	...	0
9	No. of birds tested	2722	2413	2284	1929	...	3707
	Percentage reactors	1.80	0.54	0.48	0	...	0
10	No. of birds tested	640	440	399	352	339	747
	Percentage reactors	27.34	4.32	1.00	0	0	0

Table 3.2. Pullorum disease testing summary of US chickens in commercial flocks during 51-yr period

Item	1935–36	1949–50	1962–63	1974–75	1986–87
No. of flocks	9191	111,422	21,272	4139	3716
No. of birds	4,329,364	37,237,674	35,236,200	24,904,143	36,769,824
Percentage of positive tests	3.66	0.72	0.005	0.000006	0.000005
Birds in pullorum-clean flocks	257,577	13,302,642	33,517,824	24,902,812	36,767,855

Source: (6).

Table 3.3. Pullorum disease testing summary of US turkeys during 43-yr period

Item	1943–44	1949–50	1962–63	1974–75	1986–87
No. of flocks	2489	4717	2297	817	660
No. of birds	982,904	2,340,574	3,879,861	2,882,958	3,917,589
Percentage of positive tests	2.00	0.39	0.003	0	0
Birds in pullorum-clean flocks	...	...	...	2,882,958	3,917,589

Source: (6).

flocks. In 1987 the NPIP reported infection in 18 such flocks. This reservoir of infection may be larger than indicated, since not all states have a program to test noncommercial and exhibition poultry. Experience indicates that the usual separation of commercial and noncommercial poultry is quite effective in preventing transmission of *S. pullorum* between these populations. Nevertheless, infected backyard flocks pose some danger to commercial flocks. It is necessary to continue to test commercial breeding flocks to allow early identification of accidental infections from noncommercial poultry.

The American Association of Avian Pathologists in 1965 voted to go on record endorsing as a philosophy an effort to eradicate PD. It was significant that this body, composed of people with broad experience with the disease from all standpoints, considered eradication both possible and practical. It appears that a program to eradicate PD should be based on regulatory action that includes as a minimum: mandatory reporting of all diagnoses; epidemiologic investigations and quarantine of all infected and suspicious flocks; and limiting public exhibition and interstate movement of all chickens, turkeys, and hatching eggs unless accompanied by a history indicating freedom from PD.

REFERENCES

1. Anderson, G.W., J.B. Cooper, J. C. Jones, and C.L. Morgan. 1948. Sulfonamides in the control of pullorum disease. Poult Sci 27:172–175.

2. Andrews, R.D. 1963. Evaluation of tests for pullorum and Newcastle disease with whole-blood samples collected on serodiscs. Avian Dis 7:193–196.

3. Anonymous. 1930. Eastern states conference on laboratory workers in pullorum disease control. J Am Vet Med Assoc 77:259–263.

4. Anonymous. 1933. Report of the conference of official research workers in animal diseases of North America on standard methods of pullorum disease in barnyard fowl. J Am Vet Med Assoc 82:487–491.

5. Anonymous. 1984. The National Poultry Improvement Plan and Auxiliary Provisions. USDA, APHIS, Hyattsville, MD.
6. Anonymous. 1988. The National Poultry Improvement Plan. USDA, APHIS #91-43. Hyattsville, MD.
7. Aoki, S., M. Kashiwazaki, S. Sato, H. Watase, and C. Sakamato. 1963. Application of agar-jell precipitin test to the diagnosis of pullorum disease. Nat Inst Anim Health Q 3:175-184.
8. Beaudette, F.R. 1923. Agglutinins for Bacterium pullorum in hens' eggs. J Immunol 8:493-499.
9. Bergqvist, E., S. Rosende, and R. Bauer. 1973. Factors which can disturb the hemagglutination test in the diagnosis of pullorum disease: Isolation and identification of microorganisms which react nonspecifically with pullorum antigen. Agric Tec (Santiago) 33:204-208.
10. Bierer, B.W. 1961. Furaltadone water medication against naturally induced Salmonella pullorum infection in stressed floor broilers. Avian Dis 5:333-336.
11. Biondi, E., and A. Schiavo. 1966. Action of colimycin (colistin) on Salmonella pullorum. III. Studies in chicks. Zooprofilassi. 21:637-658.
12. Blaxland, J.D., W.J. Sojka, and A.M. Smither. 1956. A study of Salmonella pullorum and Salmonella gallinarum strains isolated from field outbreaks of disease. J Comp Pathol Ther 66:270-277.
13. Bottorff, C.A., and J.S. Kiser. 1947. The use of sulfonamides in the control of pullorum disease. Poult Sci 26:335-339.
14. Botts, C.W., L. C. Ferguson, J.M. Birkeland, and A.R. Winter. 1952. The influence of litter on the control of salmonella infections in chicks. Am J Vet Res 13:562-565.
15. Buxton, A. 1954. Antibody production in avian embryos and young chicks. J Gen Microbiol 10:398-410.
16. Carlson, V.L., and G.H. Snoeyenbos. 1974. Comparative efficacies of selenite and tetrathionate broths for the isolation of salmonella serotypes. Am J Vet Res 35:711-718.
17. Doyle, L.P., and F.P. Mathews. 1928. The pathology of bacillary white diarrhea in chicks. Purdue Univ Agric Exp Stn Res Bull 323.
18. Edwards, P.R., and D.W. Bruner. 1946. Form variation in Salmonella pullorum and its relation to X strains. Cornell Vet 36:318-324.
19. Edwards, P.R., D.W. Bruner, E.R. Doll, and G.S. Hermann. 1948. Further notes on variation in Salmonella pullorum. Cornell Vet 38:257-262.
20. Evans, W.M., D.W. Bruner, and M. C. Peckham. 1955. Blindness in chicks associated with salmonellosis. Cornell Vet 45:239-247.
21. Ferguson, A.E., M.C. Connell, and R.B. Truscott. 1961. Isolation of Salmonella pullorum from the joints of broiler chicks. Can Vet J 2:143-145.
22. Francis, D.W. 1960. Treatment of natural infection of Salmonella pullorum in day-old chicks with furazolidone. Avian Dis 4:63-73.
23. Garrard, E.H., W.H. Burton, and J.A. Carpenter. 1948. Non-pullorum agglutination reactions. Proc 8th World's Poult Congr, pp. 626-631.
24. Gordon, R.F. and J. Tucker. 1955. The treatment of chronic carriers of Salmonella pullorum with furazolidone. Vet Rec 67:116-118.
25. Grausgruber, W., and R. Kissling. 1964. Influence of antibiotic food supplements on bacteriological and serological diagnosis of pullorum disease. Wien Tieraerztl Monatsschr 51:814-822.
26. Gupta, B.R., and B.B. Mallick. 1977. Use of 9R strain of S. gallinarum as vaccine against S. pullorum infection in chicks. India Vet J 54:331-333.
27. Gwatkin, R., and E.W. Bond. 1947. Studies in pullorum disease. XIX. Examination of colonies from regular and variant form cultures of Salmonella pullorum. Can J Comp Med Vet Sci 11:282-289.
28. Gwatkin, R., I. Moynihan, C.W. Traves, and W. Roach. 1941. Comparison of the whole blood and tube agglutination test for pullorum disease. Sci Agric 21:335-349.
29. Henderson, W., G.L. Morehouse, and R. F. Cross. 1960. The effect of furazolidone on Salmonella pullorum and agglutination titers in chickens. Avian Dis 4:223-230.
30. Heutgens, H.W. 1964. A rapid method for determination of S. gallinarum-pullorum antibodies in poultry meat by the muscle juice press method and antibody reaction. Inaug Diss Tieraerztl, Hochschule, Hannover.
31. Hewitt, E.A. 1928. Bacillary white diarrhea in baby turkeys. Cornell Vet 18:272-276.
32. Hinshaw, W.R. 1928. New England Conference of Laboratory Workers in Bacillary White Diarrhea Control. J Am Vet Med Assoc 73:263-264.
33. Hinshaw, W.R., C.W. Upp, and J.M. Moore. 1926. Studies on transmission of bacillary white diarrhea in incubators. J Am Vet Assoc 68:631-641.
34. Hinshaw, W.R., and E. McNeil. 1940. Eradication of pullorum disease from turkey flocks. Proc 44th Annu Meet US Livestock Sanit Assoc, pp. 178-194.
35. Hutt, F.B., and R.D. Crawford. 1960. On breeding chicks resistant to pullorum disease without exposure thereto. Can J Genet Cytol 2:357-370.
36. Jones, F.S. 1913. The value of the macroscopic agglutination test in detecting fowls that are harboring Bacterium pullorum. J Med Res 27:481-495.
37. Karyagin, V.W. 1964. Development of resistance of Salmonella pullorum. I. To biomycin. II. To Furazolidone. Nauchn Tr, pp. 31-49.
38. McCullough, N.B., and C.W. Eisele. 1951. Experimental human salmonellosis. IV. Pathogenicity of strains of Salmonella pullorum obtained from spray-dried whole egg. J Infect Dis 89:259-265.
39. Mitchell, R.B., F.C. Garlock, and R.H. Broh-Kahn. 1946. An outbreak of gastro-enteritis presumably caused by Salmonella pullorum. J Infect Dis 79:57-62.
40. Mullen, F.E. 1946. Sulfamerazine as a prophylactic in pullorum disease in poults. J Am Vet Med Assoc 108:163-164.
41. Pevzner, I., A.W. Nordskog, and M.L. Kaeberle. 1975. Immune response and the B blood group locus in chickens. Genetics 80:753-759.
42. Pevzner, I.Y., H.A. Stone, and A.W. Nordskog. 1981. Immune response and disease resistance in chickens. I. Selection for high and low titer to Salmonella pullorum antigen. Poult Sci 60:920-926.
43. Pomeroy, B.S., R. Fenstermacher, and M.H. Roepke. 1948. Sulfonamides in the control of salmonellosis of chicks and poults. J Am Vet Med Assoc 112:296-303.
44. Rettger, L.F. 1900. Septicemia among young chickens. NY Med J 71:803-805.
45. Rettger, L.F. 1909. Further studies on fatal septicemia in young chickens or "white diarrhea." J Med Res 21:115-123.
46. Rettger, L.F., and W.N. Plastridge. 1932. Pullorum disease of domestic fowl. Monogr Storrs Agric Exp Stn Bull 178.
47. Rice, C.E., and R. Gwatkin. 1949. Studies in pullorum disease. XXVI. A comparison of the titers obtained by indirect complement-fixation and agglutination methods for turkey sera. Cornell Vet 39:183-194.
48. Richey, D.J., and C.L. Morgan. 1960. The effects of furazolidone on chicken Salmonella pullorum carriers. Avian Dis 4:48-63.
49. Rozanska, M., and F. Kirzajew. 1977. Value of the

agar gel-precipitin test to discover fowls infected with Salmonella pullorum. Med Weter 33:615–619.

50. Roznowski, E.P., and V.D. Foltz. 1958. Flocculation tests for pullorum disease. Am J Vet Res 19:478–482.

51. Runnels, R.A., C.J. Coon, H. Farley, and F. Thorp. 1927. An application of the rapid-method agglutination test to the diagnosis of bacillary white diarrhea infection. J Am Vet Med Assoc 70:660–662.

52. Sapre, V.A., and M.L. Mehta. 1967. Indirect hemagglutination test for the diagnosis of salmonellosis in poultry. Indian Vet J 44:647–652.

53. Sarkisov, A.Kh., and E.T. Trishkina. 1966. Antibiotic sensitivity of Salmonella pullorum isolated from chicks on farms where antibiotics have been used over a long period. Tr Vses Inst Eksp Vet 32:224–230.

54. Schaffer, J.M., A.D. MacDonald, W.J. Hall, and H. Bunyea. 1931. A stained antigen for the rapid whole blood test for pullorum disease. J Am Vet Med Assoc 79:236–240.

55. Schiavo, A., and E. Biondi. 1966. Action of colimycin (colistin) on Salmonella pullorum. II. Studies on chick embryos. Zooprofilassi 21:69–79.

56. Severens, J.M., E. Roberts, and L.E. Card. 1944. A study of the defense mechanism involved in hereditary resistance to pullorum disease of the domestic fowl. J Infect Dis 75:33–46.

57. Severens, J.M., E. Roberts, and L.E. Card. 1945. The effect of sulfonamides in reducing mortality from pullorum disease in the domestic fowl. Poult Sci 24:155–158.

58. Smith, H.W. 1954. The treatment of Salmonella pullorum infection in chicks with furazolidone, sulphamerazine, and chloramphenicol. Vet Rec 493–496.

59. Snoeyenbos, G.H., A.M. Crotty, and H. Van Roekel. 1950. Some antigenic characteristics of Salmonella pullorum. Am J Vet Res 11:221–225.

60. Stephanov, V., P. Ivanov, and I. Sizov. 1974. On the diagnosis of typhos-pulorosis during life in poultry. Vet Sci (Sofia) 11:72–77.

61. Stokes, J.L., and H.G. Bayne. 1957. Growth rates of salmonella colonies. J Bacteriol 74:200–206.

62. Stokes, J.L., and H.G. Bayne. 1961. Oxidative assimilation of amino acids by salmonellae in relation to growth rates. J Bacteriol 81:118–125.

63. Stuart, E.E., and R.D. Keenum. 1970. Preincubation treatment of chicken hatching eggs infected with Salmonella pullorum. Avian Dis 14:87–95.

64. Suganuma, Y. 1960. Histopathological studies of serositis of pullorum disease. Jpn J Vet Sci 22:175–182.

65. Tacconi, G., G. Astrybal, and G. Bertorotta. 1987. Evaluation of the efficacy of apromycin against Salmonella pullorum infection in chickens. Avian Pathol 16:319–326.

66. Tanaka, S. 1975. Production of pullorum antigen by continuous submerged culture. Jpn Agric Res Q 9:60–65.

67. Thain, J.A., and T.B. Blandford. 1981. A long-term serological study of a flock of chickens naturally infected with Salmonella pullorum. Vet Rec 109:136–138.

68. Trabulsi, L.R., and P.R. Edwards. 1962. The differentiation of Salmonella pullorum and Salmonella gallinarum by biochemical methods. Cornell Vet 52:563–569.

69. Tsubokura, M. 1965. Studies of Salmonella pullorum phage. I. Isolation of phages and their properties. Jpn J Vet Sci 27:179–188.

70. Tsubokura, M. 1966. Studies on Salmonella pullorum phage. V. Conversion of subtypes of S. pullorum by phage. Jpn J Vet Sci 28:35–40.

71. Tucker, J. F. 1967. Survival of salmonella in built-up litter for housing of rearing and laying fowl. Br Vet J 123:92–103.

72. Turnbull, P.C.B., and G.H. Snoeyenbos. 1973. The role of ammonia, water activity, and pH in the salmonellacidal effect of long-used poultry litter. Avian Dis 17:72–86.

73. Ungureanu, C., and A. Grecianu. 1963. Improvement of antigen for the rapid haemagglutination test for pullorum disease. Lucrarile Inst Patol Igiena Anima Buchuresti 12:315–322.

74. Van Roekel, H. 1931. Eleventh annual report on eradication of pullorum disease in Massachusetts. Mass Agric Exp Stn Control Ser Bull 58.

75. Ward, A.R., and B.A. Gallagher. 1917. An intradermal test for Bacterium pullorum infection in fowls. USDA Bull 517.

76. Watanabe, S., T. Nagai, K. Hashimoto, T. Kume, and R. Sakazaki. 1960. Studies on salmonella infection in hens' eggs during incubation. VII. Transmission to eggs of agglutinins and immunity from hens infected with S. pullorum. Bull Nat Inst Anim Health (Tokyo) 39:37–41.

77. Williams, J.E. 1951. Use of the spot test in the diagnosis of pullorum disease. Poult Sci 30:125–131.

78. Williams, J.E. 1953. Antigenic studies using ammonium sulfate. I. The relative sedimentation effect of ammonium sulfate on the various antigenic types of Salmonella pullorum. Am J Vet Res 14:458–462.

79. Williams, J.E. 1953. Antigenic studies using ammonium sulfate. II. The macroscopic ammonium sulfate sedimentation test for distinguishing the antigenic forms of Salmonella pullorum. Am J Vet Res 14:465–470.

80. Williams, J.E., and A.D. MacDonald. 1955. The past, present, and future of salmonella antigens for poultry. Proc Annu Meet Am Vet Med Assoc, pp. 333–339.

81. Williams, J.E., and A.D. Whittemore. 1971. Serological diagnosis of pullorum disease with the microagglutination system. Appl Microbiol 21:394–399.

82. Williams, J.E., and A.D. Whittemore. 1972. Microantiglobulin test for detecting Salmonella typhimurium agglutinins. Appl Microbiol 23:931–937.

83. Williams, J.E., and A.D. Whittemore. 1973. Microtesting for avian salmonellosis. Proc 77th Annu Meet US Anim Hlth Assoc, pp. 607–613.

84. Williams, J.E., B.S. Pomeroy, R. Fenstermacher, and A. Holland. 1949. The incidence of variant pullorum in Minnesota. Cornell Vet 39:129–135.

85. Williams, J.E., L.H. Dillard, and G.O. Hall. 1968. The penetration patterns of Salmonella typhimurium through the outer structures of chicken eggs. Avian Dis 12:445–466.

86. Wilson, J.E. 1955. The use of furazolidone in the treatment of infections of day-old chicks with S. pullorum, S. gallinarum, S. typhimurium, and S. thompson. Vet Rec 67:849–853.

87. Wilson, J.E. 1956. The treatment of carriers of Salmonella pullorum and Salmonella gallinarum with furazolidone. Vet Rec 68:748–751.

88. Winter, A.R., B. Burkhart, and H. Widley. 1952. Further studies on the whole blood and tube methods of testing turkeys for Salmonella pullorum infection. Poult Sci 31:399–404.

89. Yoshida, I., and S. Sato. 1960. The isolation of desoxycholate-sensitive strains of Salmonella pullorum from chickens in a naturally infected flock. Avian Dis 8:394–402.

90. Younie, A.R. 1941. Fowl infection like pullorum disease. Can J Comp Med Vet Sci. 5:164–167.

FOWL TYPHOID

B.S. Pomeroy and K.V. Nagaraja

INTRODUCTION. Fowl typhoid (FT) is a septicemic disease of domesticated birds. The course may be acute or chronic. The mortality may be moderate or very high, depending largely on the virulence of the inciting organism *Salmonella gallinarum*. It appears to be primarily a disease of chickens and turkeys; in exceptional cases ducks, pheasants, peacocks, guinea fowl, and a few other birds are attacked.

There have been no reported outbreaks of FT in commercial poultry in the USA since 1980 (4). However, two cases of FT in backyard flocks were reported in 1988. The elimination of FT in the USA is related to the pullorum-typhoid control program of the National Poultry Improvement Plan (NPIP) (3). When the control of FT was included in the NPIP in 1954, it resulted in the treatment of FT in the same category as pullorum disease. Cost of the pullorum-typhoid control program has been reduced in states classified as U.S. pullorum-typhoid clean, which permits testing of a sample of primary breeding flocks and elimination of testing of parent flocks.

S. gallinarum is rarely isolated from humans and has little public health significance (25, 64, 82). The 1987 annual report of U.S. Center for Disease Control reported seven isolations of *S. gallinarum* from humans in 1975–87 (84).

HISTORY. In 1888 a chicken breeder in England lost 400 chickens as a result of an infectious disease at first considered to be fowl cholera; 200 of these birds died in the first 2 mo of the outbreak. Specimens were sent to Klein (55) for necropsy and diagnosis. He reported it chiefly as an infectious enteritis. The intestinal mucosa and serosa were inflamed, and feces appeared thin and greenish yellow. The spleen was enlarged two to three times; the liver was also somewhat enlarged, soft, flabby, and moist. The cause was an organism he named *Bacillus gallinarum*. The same year he reported the disease among grouse, and in 1893 a similar disease among pheasants. The disease was investigated by Smith in Rhode Island in 1894 and more fully by Moore in Virginia and Maryland in 1895. Moore (71) described the disease as "infectious leukemia" and named the organism *B. sanguinarium*.

Klein (55) observed small numbers of bacilli in the blood. They were nonmotile, gram-negative, and easily cultivated. Chickens inoculated subcutaneously became sick in 5–6 days and died 2–3 days later. A similar disease was described by Lucet (67) in France. Lignieres and Zabala (66) described a disease that was probably identical to Klein's disease. The catarrhal enteritis and swollen spleen attracted attention; gram-negative bacilli were observed in the blood. They were different from those described by Klein (55) in that they first coagulated and later peptonized milk with an alkaline reaction.

Curtice (26) studied the disease in Rhode Island and named it "fowl typhoid." In Germany it was observed by Pfeiler and Rehse (79). Van Straaten and Te Hennepe (105) in Holland described the disease very fully.

On the basis of necropsy observation, Klein (55) believed it was not cholera but a special disease. His suspicion was soon confirmed; he ascertained that the newly discovered organism was different morphologically and biologically from that of fowl cholera.

INCIDENCE AND DISTRIBUTION. FT is worldwide in distribution. Canada, the USA, and several European countries report low incidence or complete absence of FT, but Mexico and countries in Central and South America and Africa have reported a dramatic increase of the disease in poultry flocks (5, 19, 20, 68, 85).

ETIOLOGY

Classification. The causative agent of FT belongs to the genus *Salmonella* within the family Enterobacteriaceae. It has received the following names: *Bacillus gallinarum, B. sanguinarium, B. typhi gallinarum alacalifaciens, B. paradysenteriae gallinarum, Eberthella sanguinaria, Shigella gallinarum, Salmonella gallinarum,* and *S. enteritidis* serotype *gallinarum*.

Morphology and Staining. The organism is a relatively short plump rod about 1.0–2.0 μm long and 1.5 μm in diameter. The bacilli mostly occur singly but are occasionally united in pairs. They have a tendency to stain a little more heavily at the poles than in the center. They are gram-negative, form no spores, have no capsules, and are nonmotile.

Growth Requirements. *S. gallinarum* grows readily on beef extract or infusion agar or in tryptose broth and other nutrient media adjusted to pH 7.2. It is aerobic, facultatively anaerobic, and grows best at 37 C. The organism will grow in selective enrichment media such as selenite F and tetrathionate broths and on differential plating media such as MacConkey's, bismuth sulfite, salmonella-shigella, deoxycholate, deoxycholate citrate lactose sucrose, and brilliant green agars.

Colony Morphology. On meat extract or infusion agar (pH 7.0–7.2) colonies are small, blue-gray, moist, circular, and entire. Gelatin colonies are small, grayish white, and entire. Gelatin stab growth has a slight grayish white surface with filiform growth in the stab and no liquefaction. Growth in broth is turbid with heavy flocculent sediment.

Biochemical Properties. Over the years numerous studies have been made comparing fermentation reactions of isolates of *S. pullorum* and *S. gallinarum* (see PULLORUM DISEASE). The following substances are usually metabolized with acid and without gas production: arabinose, dextrose, galactose, mannitol, mannose, rhamnose, xylose, fructose, maltose, dulcitol, and isodulcitol. Substances not fermented are lactose, sucrose, glycerol, salicin, and sorbitol. Ornithine is not decarboxylated, and D-tartrate is used. Cysteine hydrochloride gelatin supports growth of *S. gallinarum.* These media are helpful in differentiating *S. pullorum* and *S. gallinarum.* Indole is not formed and nitrates are reduced to nitrites.

Resistance to Chemical and Physical Agents. In general, resistance of this organism is about the same as that of other members of the typhoid and paratyphoid groups. The FT organism is killed within 10 min at 60 C. It remains viable in the dark for 20 days in ordinary and distilled water but dies in 24 hr when exposed to sunlight. When dried on glass plates and kept in the dark, the organism retains its viability for 89 hr; under action of direct sunlight it is killed in a few minutes. The organism is killed by phenol in a 1:1000 dilution, by bichloride of mercury in a 1:20,000 dilution, by 1% potassium permanganate in 3 min, and by 2% formalin in 1 min. Agar cultures rapidly lose their pathogenic character, although they retain their antigenic properties for some time. *S. gallinarum* in the virulent state can be demonstrated in the bone marrow of carcasses 3 mo after chickens have died of FT. No doubt under certain conditions it lives for much longer periods. Kaupp and Dearstyne (52) reported that although direct sunlight destroyed the organism in a short time, it remained viable for 20 days when stored in water in the dark.

In Moore's (73) national survey of FT, 75% of the states reporting were uncertain as to persistence of the organism in soil, and 25% claimed it persisted from year to year.

In experiments of Hall et al. (44) there was little danger of starting an outbreak in susceptible birds when they were put into a FT-contaminated pen 1 wk or more after removal of all sick birds. It was evident that the causative organism did not survive long after leaving the bird's body.

Orr and Moore (76) tested *S. gallinarum* for longevity under various conditions. In cloth in the dark at room temperature, organisms remained alive for 228 days; on plastic cover slips some were viable up to 93 days. Organisms in distilled water in diffused light at room temperature were viable up to the time the water evaporated (88 days). *S. gallinarum* retained viability up to 43 days when subjected to daily freezing and thawing. A liver naturally infected with *S. gallinarum* was divided, one-half being kept at 7 C and the other half at −20 C. Organisms in the liver kept at 7 C survived 2 wk, while those kept at −20 C were still alive at 148 days, even though they were accidentally thawed twice.

Smith (88) found that the average survival time of *S. gallinarum* in feces from infected chickens was 10.9 days when kept in a range house and 2 days less in the open. Survival time was longer in naturally dried specimens than in those kept moist.

Tucker (102) found that *S. gallinarum* persisted from 3 wk in old built-up litter to 11 wk in new litter. When the infected pens were left unoccupied, survival time in both types was increased to more than 30 wk.

Antigenic Structure and Toxins. *S. gallinarum* possesses the O antigens 1, 9, 12. There does not appear to be form variation involving 12 antigens as in *S. pullorum* (10, 16, 29, 62, 106) (see PULLORUM DISEASE).

Smith and Ten Broeck (90) found a toxin in filtrates of broth cultures of *S. gallinarum.* It appeared in the culture at the end of 2 days at 37 C and caused prompt death of a rabbit by the intravenous (IV) route. Death resulted within 2 hr and in many respects was like anaphylactic shock. It was probably an endotoxin, stable at 60 C for 1 hr. Boiling for 15 min reduced its activity.

Smith et al. (92) studied effects of IV injections of *S. gallinarum* endotoxin resulting in clinical illness within a few hours; with significant falls in body temperature, bursa weight, main hematologic parameters, serum iron (SI), and transferrin saturation; and an increase in unsaturated iron-binding capacity. Most responses returned to normal within 24–48 hr following a single injection except bursa weight, SI values, and total and differential blood cell white counts.

Pathogenicity. Pathogenicity of FT cultures has proved decidedly variable in the hands of different investigators, probably because they used cultures varying widely in virulence. Like most pathogenic microorganisms, *S. gallinarum* loses virulence rapidly on artificial media; hence, cultures should be passaged serially in their natural host, the chicken, before testing pathogenicity of the organism. Pathogenicity of such cultures is best maintained in the lyophilized or frozen state. With a uniformly pathogenic culture, most commonly used routes of exposure of chickens prove fatal.

Hall et al. (43) found that feeding mash moistened with a broth culture of a stable virulent strain of *S. gallinarum* was an effective way of testing susceptibility to FT. Of 20 groups of birds totaling 382 that were challenged by adding a broth culture of virulent strains of *S. gallinarum* to their mash, 367 (96%) died of FT.

Sorrells et al. (94) found that freezing (−75 C) and storage (−20 C) resulted in a heterogeneous population of dead, metabolically injured, and unharmed cells. Pathogenicity was evaluated by observing percentage of mortality after injecting injured or uninjured cells into separate sets of chicks. The mortality difference attributed to wholly uninjured versus predominantly injured populations was small but consistent ($p < 0.05$).

Barrow et al. (9) studied four strains of *S. gallinarum* that possessed both an 85-kilobase and a 2.5-kilobase plasmid. Each plasmid was eliminated in turn from one of the strains by transposon labeling and curing at 42 C. Elimination of the small plasmid had no effect on the high virulence of the strain for newly hatched and 2-wk-old chickens orally exposed whereas no mortality occurred in birds inoculated with bacteria from which the large plasmid had been eliminated. Reintroduction of the large plasmid completely restored virulence and demonstrated that the large plasmid contributed toward virulence in FT in chickens.

PATHOGENESIS AND EPIZOOTIOLOGY

Natural and Experimental Hosts. The disease was originally encountered in chickens and reported among grouse and pheasants (55). Natural outbreaks occur in chickens; turkeys; guinea fowl; peafowl; ducklings; and game birds such as quail, grouse, and pheasants. Lucet (67) described what was probably an outbreak of the disease in turkeys but claimed that ducks, geese, and pigeons were not susceptible. Donatien et al. (27) consider palmipeds to be refractory but found the turkey, guinea fowl, and peafowl among the susceptible species; ducks and geese were resistant. Pfeiler and Roepke (80) mentioned pheasants, turkeys, and guinea fowl as susceptible in natural outbreaks but that ducks, geese, and pigeons are not, although a duck inoculated with a culture died a few days later. Kaupp and Dearstyne (53), Te Hennepe (98), and Beck and Eber (15) observed the disease in ducks. Kaupp and Dearstyne (54) stated that turkeys are less susceptible than chickens and that guineas, though slightly susceptible, yield to artificial inoculation. Fox (32) isolated *B. sanguinarium* from an outbreak of disease among parrots in the Philadelphia Zoological Garden. Beck and Eber (15) reported on loss from *B. gallinarum* infection in ducklings 1–14 days old. Truche (101) found that pheasants, swans, grouse, sparrows, ring doves, and ostriches commonly became infected but that ducks, geese, and turkeys were more resistant. Johnson and Anderson (48) reported outbreaks of the disease in ducklings, turkeys, and guinea fowl. The infection has been observed in wild birds, quail, grouse, and pheasants. These birds are susceptible by feeding or injection of cultures. Te Hennepe (99) stated that FT had decreased in the Netherlands between 1929 and 1939 from a point at which it caused 8% of the total deaths in adult birds to 0.7%. This was considered to be due to greater interest in poultry diseases and improved care of poultry. El-Dine (30) in Egypt stated that FT was often mistaken for fowl cholera. He reported the disease mainly in chickens and turkeys and stated that it had been reported in peacocks but had never been seen in pigeons, geese, or ducks. A vaccine was used to confer immunity.

Reports on susceptibility of pigeons have been variable. Klein (55) reported no success following subcutaneous (SC) injection of cultures. Lucet (67) was unable to infect pigeons with 1 ml SC doses; Moore (71) killed pigeons within 8 days with 2 ml of a broth culture. Pfeiler and Roepke (80) killed pigeons by injecting 1 ml of a 24-hr broth culture, but the heart blood of these birds would not cause infection in a second pigeon. Kaupp and Dearstyne (53) caused the pigeon to become sick on the 3rd or 4th day with recovery on the 15th day. Kraus (63) produced death in a pigeon within 4 days by using 1 ml of a 24-hr broth culture of the FT organism. Te Hennepe and Van Straaten (100) claimed that pigeons were not always susceptible to inoculation with these organisms. At the Animal Disease Station in 1946, four pigeons were killed in an average period of 4.5 days by intraperitoneal or intramuscular inoculation with 1 ml of a 5-hr broth culture of *S. gallinarum.*

Assoku and Penhale (7) assessed various factors in studying pathogenesis of FT. In acute FT there is severe hemolytic anemia, with loss of more than 70% of the original total circulating erythrocytes. The authors suggested that the modification of the erythrocytes in vivo by endotoxin leads to their clearance by the reticuloendothelial system (RES) with subsequent development of hemolytic anemia. A functional impairment of the erythrophagocytic and endotoxin-detoxifying function of the RES develops, resulting in increased susceptibility to endotoxin and leading rapidly to death.

Although FT frequently has been spoken of as a disease of adult birds, Beaudette (12), Beach and Davis (11), Martinaglia (69), and Komarov (58) reported the disease in young chicks. Moore

(73), in a nationwide survey of FT, reported that workers in 11 states found the disease to be commoner in birds under 6 mo, those in 16 states believed the disease to be more prevalent in older fowl, and workers in 10 states found little difference in age susceptibility. Hall et al. (44) reported that in 25 hatches from typhoid reactors in their 2nd yr of lay, about every 4th hatch experienced a FT outbreak; losses up to 6 mo of age amounted to 33.4% of the chicks hatched. Monthly distribution of mortality was: 25.6%, 13.5%, 24.9%, 19.2%, 13.8%, and 2.7% for months 1-6, respectively.

As in pullorum disease, FT losses often begin at hatching time; conversely, FT losses continue to laying age.

Epizootiologically, there are a few peculiarities in regard to FT. Van Heelsbergen (104) found it very difficult, in some cases at least, to infect chickens from a region in which FT is indigenous. If chickens are imported from a part of the country where the disease is not known, infection was rather easy. It was suggested that the bacteriophage or acquired immunity is probably partly responsible.

St. John-Brooks and Rhodes (95) found that strains of *S. gallinarum* produced lesions in young chicks indistinguishable from those associated with pullorum disease.

Transmission, Carriers, Vectors. Like most other bacterial diseases, FT is spread in several ways. The infected bird (reactor and carrier) is by far the most important means of perpetuation and spread. Such birds may infect not only their own but succeeding generations through egg transmission. Evidence of egg transmission of *S. gallinarum* was reported by Beaudette (12, 13) and Beach and Davis (11).

Nobrega and Bueno (75) cultured 1465 fresh infertile eggs from 52 hens shown to be chronic carriers of FT. These were reactors from three different flocks where severe outbreaks of FT among chicks had been experienced. Incidence of *S. gallinarum* in eggs from the three lots of fowl was 2.8%, 0%, and 1.73%, respectively.

Moore (72) recovered *S. gallinarum* from 8.9% of 395 eggs cultured from a pen of 21 FT reactors, some naturally and some artificially infected. He also conducted FT transmission experiments. No evidence was produced to indicate transmission of disease by flies, mating, or air currents; rats and turkey buzzards were found capable of transmitting FT. Boney (17) isolated *S. gallinarum* from 1 turkey egg of 374 cultured from a flock of pullorum reactors.

Gordeuk et al. (38) found that FT is transmitted from artificially infected birds to normal ones by cohabitation. The mortality among contact birds was 60.9% in four experiments with duplicate groups.

After culturing over 10, 000 eggs from two flocks, one naturally and one artificially infected, Hall et al. (44) found that 50% of typhoid reactors laid infected eggs, and an average of 6% of all unhatched eggs were infected with *S. gallinarum*. That these infected eggs laid by typhoid carriers are highly virulent and may be the means of starting new outbreaks of FT in laying flocks is indicated by six feeding trials in which 27 birds ranging in age from 8 wk to 1 yr were fed one or more infected eggs mixed in their mash; death resulted in 21 of the birds in an average period of 10 days. These investigators also reported that of 906 chicks hatched from these reactors, 296 (32.6%) died of the disease during the first 6 mo; the heaviest loss was in the 1st mo.

Rao et al. (83) recovered *S. gallinarum* from 13 of 36 (36%) eggs from a reactor flock.

Jordan (50) recovered, by a single swab, *S. gallinarum* from fresh feces of 4 of 13 birds acutely ill of FT. Single cloacal swabs were positive in 15 of 47 (31.9%). A total of 377 cloacal swabs were taken at intervals from 36 reactors that had recovered from FT 3-18 mo previously, but only 1 bird was positive for *S. gallinarum*.

Jordan (51) reported isolation of *S. gallinarum* from eggs laid by reactors to the rapid whole blood test: from 3 of 23 eggs (13%) from 4 recovered birds, from 13 of 274 eggs (4.75%) from 10 naturally recovered birds, from none of 217 eggs from 4 recovered birds treated with chloramphenicol, and from 25 of 226 eggs (11%) from 2 recovered birds that received nitrofurazone. Both *S. pullorum* and *S. gallinarum* were isolated from different eggs from 1 bird.

Attendants, feed dealers, chicken buyers, and visitors who travel from house to house and from farm to farm may carry infection unless precautions are taken to disinfect footwear, hands, and clothing. Trucks, crates, and feed sacks may also be contaminated. Wild birds, animals, and flies may be important mechanical spreaders, especially if they have been feeding on carcasses of dead birds or offal from packing plants or hatcheries.

Incubation Period. Rao et al. (83) reported *S. gallinarum* to be equally pathogenic to susceptible chicks and adults under natural conditions. The incubation period is 4-5 days, although this varies with virulence of the organism. The course of FT is about 5 days. In a flock the losses may extend over 2-3 wk, with a tendency for recurrence.

Signs. Although FT is encountered more frequently in growing and adult chickens and turkeys, it may be encountered in young chicks and poults infected by egg transmission. Signs noted in young chicks and poults are quite similar to pullorum disease but not specific for either disease.

CHICKS AND POULTS. If birds are hatched from infected eggs, moribund and dead chicks may be seen on the hatching trays when the hatch is removed from the incubator. Others show somnolence, poor growth, weakness, inappetence, and adherence of whitish material to the vent. Labored breathing or gasping may be noted as a result of lung involvement.

GROWING AND MATURE FOWL. An acute outbreak in chickens may begin by a sudden drop in feed consumption, with birds being droopy and ruffled and having pale heads and shrunken combs. Body temperature may increase 1–3 C within 2–3 days after exposure and remain high until a few hours before death. Death may occur within 4 days after exposure but usually in 5–10 days.

In turkeys there may be increased thirst, inappetence, listlessness, tendency to separate from healthy birds, and green to greenish-yellow diarrhea. Body temperature increases several degrees to as high as 44–45 C; before death it may drop to below normal. Losses may occur with no apparent previous clinical signs. The initial outbreak usually causes the heaviest mortality, followed by intermittent recurrence with less severe loss (46).

Morbidity and Mortality. Both morbidity and mortality may vary in chicken and turkey flocks. Following extensive investigations of FT in chickens, Hall et al. (44) reported that mortality varied from 10 to 50% or more; the loss in two lots of chicks hatched from FT reactors was 92.8% within 16 days in one lot and 93.5% within 11 days in the other. Seasonal influence of FT is coincidental with the period of most active egg production.

In turkeys losses may be as severe as in chickens. Hinshaw (46) reported average mortality in 4 outbreaks studied was 26.5%.

Gross Lesions

CHICKENS. In peracute cases few or no gross tissue changes are observed. In prolonged cases marked changes begin to appear, the commonest of which are swelling and redness of liver, spleen, and kidneys. These lesions are frequently seen in young birds. In subacute and chronic stages, greenish brown or bronze and swollen livers are commonly seen (see Fig. 3.2A). Other changes include grayish white foci of the miliary type in the liver and myocardium; pericarditis; peritonitis from ruptured ova; hemorrhagic, misshapen, and discolored ova; and catarrhal inflammation of intestines. In young chicks grayish white foci may sometimes be observed in lungs, heart, and gizzard, as in pullorum disease.

Gauger (34) isolated the FT organism from focal lesions in testicles of a rooster. The culture was pathogenic for other roosters by inoculation and feeding. Although various focal lesions had been described, this was the first reported case in testicles.

Rao et al. (83) reported presence of a hemorrhagic band in the proventricular submucosa and cyanotic instead of anemic comb and wattles in the adult.

Smith (89) produced FT in chickens by oral administration of *S. gallinarum.* Infection took place in the intestinal tract, with localization in the intestinal wall, liver, and spleen. This was followed by bacteremia and death or chronic disease with proliferative lesions in intestinal and heart walls. Of 300 nine-wk-old cockerels, 45% died of the acute disease and 15% in the chronic stage. *S. gallinarum* was shed in feces up to 2–3 mo post infection. This was associated with focal infection in the intestinal wall.

TURKEYS. Lesions resemble those observed in chickens. Because of the short duration of FT, birds nearly always die while in good flesh. Muscles of the breast have a tendency to be congested and often appear as if partially cooked. The heart is usually swollen and contains small grayish necrotic areas or petechiae; in a few cases both have been observed. The liver is friable and consistently enlarged two to three times its normal size; it is bronze- to mahogany-colored or covered with a mixture of bronze- and mahogany-colored streaks. Pinpoint areas of necrosis have been noted. On cutting the organ, the blood flows readily. The spleen is always enlarged two to three times its normal size, is friable, and appears mottled. In most birds the lungs present a parboiled appearance and often are firmer than normal because of minute caseated abscesses. Kidneys are usually enlarged and may show some petechiae.

The crop usually contains food, which suggests paralysis of the digestive tract, since birds seldom eat after clinical signs appear. The mucous membrane of the proventriculus sloughs readily. The gizzard contains food, and the lining is easily removed. With a few exceptions the intestine appears anemic when viewed from the exterior and ulcerations of the mucous membrane may be visible through the serosa. Ulceration is most severe in the duodenum; a few ulcers 1–4 mm in diameter have been observed throughout the intestine, extending to the ceca.

The enlarged mahogany- or bronze-streaked liver, enlarged spleen, areas of necrosis in the heart, and grayish lungs are pathognomonic. Hemorrhagic enteritis (especially of the duodenum) and marked ulceration of the intestine, although uncommon in chickens, are more or less consistent lesions in turkeys. *S. gallinarum* can readily be isolated from all organs. In birds that have been dead for some time, pure cultures are more easily isolated from bone marrow than from liver, spleen, or heart blood.

Johnson and Pollard (49) described the following necropsy findings in young poults: increased percentage of large retained yolks; slightly enlarged somewhat friable, creamy white liver, the surface of which was mottled with slight hemorrhagic areas; and slight congestion in the anterior duodenum. Crops, gizzards, and intestines were always devoid of food, indicating inappetence for several hours before death. In adult carriers there is (as in pullorum disease) a predilection for the reproductive organs.

DUCKS. Beck and Eber (15) recognized great losses from *S. gallinarum* infection among ducklings 1–14 days old. The disease picture was similar to that observed in pullorum infection in chicks. Ducklings were sick only a short time. Anatomic changes were hemorrhage in the pericardium, slight swelling of spleen, and catarrhal inflammation of lungs and intestines. Small necrotic foci in lungs, as frequently observed in chicks with pullorum disease, did not occur. In adult ducks, changes of the ovary and yolk were frequently the same as those found in adult hens. FT organisms were isolated from the misshapen yolks.

GUINEA FOWL. Beaudette (14) stated that FT in guinea fowl was interesting because affected birds showed respiratory symptoms characterized by severe congestion, with collection of mucus in the nasal cleft and trachea. Lungs were congested, and the organism could be isolated from nasal exudate.

Histopathology. Dyakov (28) reported finding a diffuse parenchymatous hepatitis and severe fatty dystrophy in acute FT, with occasional small necrotic foci in the parenchyma that was sometimes infiltrated with lymphocytes. The myocardium showed infarcts and large areas of fibrinoid necrosis and sclerosis. Changes in the kidney, pancreas, intestine, and brain were similar to those in fowl cholera. There was severe hyperplasia of the reticuloendothelial system, particularly in the sinuses.

Garren and Barber (33) studied the effect of FT on weight and histologic changes in the pituitary, thyroid, and adrenal glands and bursae of Fabricius in young New Hampshire (NH), Rhode Island Red (RIR), and white leghorn (WL) chickens. There were no statistically significant differences between the thyroid weights of the control and experimental groups. However, in the thyroid glands of chickens dying of FT, the flat epithelial lining of the follicles showed decreased activity compared to cuboidal epithelium possessing the rounded nuclei characteristic of an active gland. Thyroid appearance similar to that of chickens infected with typhoid was induced in the control group by restricting feed and water intake. In the infected chickens there was marked hypertrophy of interrenal tissue, individual cells of interrenal tissue were larger, and cytoplasm was less dense. Only a small amount of medullary tissue remained. There was hypertrophy of the pituitary without consistent histologic changes. Lymphatic follicles of the bursa of Fabricius were found in various stages of involution, suggesting a loss of cells from the follicles accompanied by a metaplasia of the cuboidal cells separating the medulla and cortex. Areas of cystlike formation were more numerous in infected birds than in controls. The WL chickens survived the test period, whereas mortality of NH chickens was 85% and of RIR chickens 100%. The only pronounced changes in tissues of the WL chickens were decreases in bursa weight and size of the follicles, but no alterations.

Kokosharov et al (57) found necrobiotic and degenerative lesions in the epithelial cells of seminiferous tubules as well as disturbances in the process of spermatogenesis in experimentally induced infection in adult male chickens.

Hematology. Birds inoculated with FT organisms experienced changes in the packed cell volume (PCV) and buffy coat value. As the disease progressed in the acute stage and anemia developed, the PCV dropped, accompanied by hemolysis visible in the plasma. The lowest PCV recorded was 16.1%, compared to normal levels of 28.4–32.9% (average 30.7%). The average buffy coat value before inoculation was 1.08%; after inoculation it showed a steady increase until death, 2.6–5.6%, with an average value of 3.7%.

In the subacute disease severe anemia was not found, and erythrocyte fragility was not in evidence. There was a slight reduction in PCV, but normal values returned after recovery. Buffy coat values increased and reached a peak between days 10 and 16. When birds recovered, buffy coat values also returned to normal.

In the acute infection, total white blood cell (WBC) count increased steadily to two to three times original value (Table 3.4). The heterophil count increased, but lymphocytes and other cells remained in normal range (1, 8).

Kokosharov and Todorova (56) studied changes in the iron content, erythrocytes, and hemoglobulin in the blood of mature heavy-breed chickens with experimentally induced acute FT. It was found that blood serum iron dropped abruptly as early as the second day whereas the level of iron in the liver rose. The erythrocyte count dropped as early as the second day following infection, hematocrit value of the blood dropped considerably on the third day, with gradually lowering values up to the 7th day. All of these changes were found to precede the onset of the first clinical signs of the disease. The values of the hematolog-

Table 3.4. Total and differential WBC counts for chickens infected orally with virulent strain of *S. gallinarum*

	Total WBC $\times 10^3/mm^3$	Throm.	Lymph.	Het.	Mon.	Bas.	Eos.
				(%)			
Before inoculation	66.2	55	26	11	4	1	3
After inoculation							
Day 1	69.7	50	26	12	7	1	4
2	87.7	48	26	18	6	1	1
3	94.4	41	29	22	8	...	...
4	133.1	34	22	31	6	2	5
5	150.7	31	27	27	8	3	4
6	136.3	31	24	29	9	2	5
7	136.7	23	28	30	7	4	8
8	159.4	36	24	24	6	2	8

Source: (1).
Note: Of the four chickens in this group, one died on day 6, two on day 7, and one on day 9.

ic indices with birds that survived came back to normal after the 14th day of infection. The authors' hypothesis regarding the pathogenesis of acute typhoid was that the lowered amount of serum iron disturbed the synthesis of hemoglobin and hence the maturity of erythrocytes, substantiating their lower count.

Immunity. Buxton and Allan (22) conducted a series of experiments indicating that during early stages of FT, circulating leukocytes develop a marked susceptibility to cytophilic antibodies in serum and later to bacterial polysaccharide. It was also shown that humoral antibodies, demonstrable by the antiglobulin hemagglutination (HA) test, have cytophilic properties. The results suggest that during acute infection cellular antigen-antibody reactions occur, which may result in development of a hypersensitive reaction.

Buxton and Davies (23) used bacterial agglutination, and antiglobulin HA tests to detect antibody production during development of *S. gallinarum* infection in chickens. The antiglobulin HA test detected serum antibodies as early as 1 day after oral infection, and antibodies were detected in all birds at the time of death. Accumulation of bacterial polysaccharide in tissues of infected birds was detected by a HA test. High but variable concentrations occurred in different organs of chickens that died from the disease. In birds that had recovered from an acute infection, the concentration was low or undetectable. The authors postulated that an antigen-antibody reaction, developing as an anaphylactic type of hypersensitivity, may be closely associated with the production of signs and death of chickens infected with *S. gallinarum*.

Allan et al. (2) found that following oral infection with live *S. gallinarum* organisms, serum collected on the 9th day and tested for presence of hemagglutinating antibody (using erythrocytes modified with a Westphal lipopolysaccharide extract of *S. gallinarum*) had a high titer; on Sephadex fractionation and ultracentrifugation it showed a marked immunoglobulin M (IgM) response.

Allan and Duffus (1) studied immune responses in chickens developing acute and subacute clinical signs. In the former an unusually high concentration of incomplete IgG antibodies was produced. Neither complete nor incomplete IgM specific antibodies were found to correlate with clinical signs. Studies on the immunologic response to heat-killed *S. gallinarum* and to the purified somatic antigen confirmed it was only when chickens were inoculated with the live organism and became clinically ill that this high titer of incomplete IgG was found.

Horsfall et al. (47), using a bactericidal assay for presence of antibody, found that 1-day-old chicks had little natural antibody against *S. gallinarum*. Adult hens had relatively higher levels.

Cameron et al. (24) studied chicks given cyclophosphamide during the first 3–5 days of life. There was a marked depression in their humoral antibody response to sheep red blood cells and brucella antigen but no effect on their ability to develop tuberculin sensitivity or on their immune response to live *S. gallinarum* vaccine. Administration of methylprednisolone acetate, hydrocortisone acetate, azathioprim, and 6-mercaptopurine to 6-, 10-, or 12-wk-old chickens neither selectively depressed the humoral or cellular response nor affected the immune response to live *S. gallinarum* vaccine. Similarly, the immune response could not be depressed by thymectomy or antilymphocyte globulin. Immunity to *S. gallinarum* after administration of a live avirulent vaccine thus did not appear to be dependent on a humoral immune mechanism but probably on cellular immunity, although this could not be proved.

DIAGNOSIS. A definitive diagnosis of FT requires isolation and identification of *S. gallinarum*. Flock history, signs, and lesions may be highly suggestive of FT. In growing and mature birds serologic findings may be helpful in making a tentative diagnosis.

Isolation of *S. gallinarum*. Acute FT is characterized by a systemic infection. *S. gallinarum* may be isolated from most of the visceral organs. The liver and spleen are usually involved and are preferred organs to culture. Lesions may occur in lungs, heart, and gizzard; these organs are dependable sites to culture. In the young chick and poult the yolk sac may be cultured. A bacteriologic inoculating loop or cotton swab is satisfactory to transfer material to culture media.

Beef extract or infusion or tryptose agar in tubes or petri dishes is satisfactory for primary isolation. Enrichment broths or selective media may also be used if tissues are decomposed.

Chronic FT is characterized by localized infection; infected organs may not show gross lesions. If a bird is submitted to the laboratory as a carrier detected by serologic tests, detailed culturing of internal organs is necessary. An outline for this examination is given under Pullorum Disease.

Identification of Cultures. *S. gallinarum* may be identified by bacteriologic and serologic methods. If pure cultures are obtained on primary isolation from tissues, special media may be inoculated. If cultures are mixed, single colony isolations may be made on triple-sugar iron agar slants. *S. gallinarum* produces a red slant with a yellow butt with gas production and delayed blackening from hydrogen sulfide production (31, 107).

The following reactions occurring within 24 hr allow identification:

Dextrose	fermented with no gas
Lactose	not fermented
Sucrose	not fermented
Mannitol	fermented with no gas
Maltose	fermented with no gas
Dulcitol	fermented with no gas
Ornithine	not fermented
Indole	not produced
Urea	not hydrolyzed
Motility	nonmotile
Agglutination	positive with group D antiserum

Additional differential tests are described under Etiology.

Serology. Several serologic tests for FT have been used under experimental and laboratory conditions: bacterial agglutination, HA, antiglobulin HA, and indirect HA. The standard procedure in the USA for detection of breeding flocks chronically infected with *S. gallinarum* is to use the standard strains of *S. pullorum* (1, 9, 12_3) for tube and serum plate antigens and both standard (1, 9, 12_3), and variant (1, 9, 12_2) strains of *S. pullorum* for the polyvalent, rapid, whole-blood plate antigens. These antigens will detect flocks infected with either *S. pullorum* or *S. gallinarum*.

Numerous investigators involved in development of control programs for FT compared antigens prepared from various isolates of *S. gallinarum* with *S. pullorum* antigens with variable results (36, 41, 45, 59, 60–62, 65, 70, 74).

Techniques and procedures for official testing of chicken and turkey breeding flocks and interpretations of tests are described in detail in the latest revision of the NPIP (3).

Giurov and Kostov (37) have suggested the use of a stable erythrocyte antigen for rapid diagnosis of FT and pullorum disease (PD).

TREATMENT. Effective prophylactic and therapeutic drugs have been developed against FT and have a role in salvaging infected flocks. In Canada and the USA every effort is being made to eradicate the disease. In the USA the Food and Drug Administration has approved use of sulfaquinoxaline and nitrofurans (furazolidone) (6).

Various sulfonamides have been used in treatment of FT: sulfathiazole, sulfamerazine, sulfadiazine, sulfamethazine, and sulfaquinoxaline. In the feed 0.1% sulfaquinoxaline is used for 2–3 days and 0.05% for 2 additional days if necessary. The water-soluble form may be used at the level of 0.04% for 2–3 days and repeated if necessary. The withdrawal period is a minimum of 10 days before slaughtering for food (81).

Numerous reports have indicated effectiveness of the nitrofurans in treatment of FT. Furazolidone is used at 0.011% level in the feed for 2 wk, followed by 0.0055% continuously until the flock is marketed. The withdrawal period is a minimum of 5 days before slaughtering for food (81).

Smith et al. (93) studied 22 strains isolated from five countries experiencing outbreaks of FT and found 20 were more resistant to furazolidone in vitro than 6 strains isolated in the UK in the 1950s. Furazolidone given continuously in feed did not control experimental infections in chickens exposed to most of the resistant strains. Earlier studies (42, 96, 97) with isolates in the USA identified a similar problem.

Numerous antibiotics have been tried in treatment of FT: streptomycin, chloromycetin, and chlortetracycline; none is approved for use in poultry raised for food in the USA (81).

In one natural and two experimental outbreaks of FT, Hall et al. (45) saw no benefit from administration of bacteriophage either in drinking water in the experimental outbreak or by SC injection in the natural outbreak.

PREVENTION AND CONTROL. FT is a good example of a disease that has decreased in incidence in the USA by application of basic procedures involving control programs aimed at breeding flocks, judicious use of effective drugs in control and treatment of outbreaks, and recognition of the importance of environment as a source of reinfection.

Flocks can be developed and maintained free of FT by following well-defined management programs. Inclusion of FT in the NPIP programs in 1954 recognized the importance of egg transmission in the cycle of this infection. Under the NPIP (3) chicken and turkey breeding flocks and their progeny are recognized as free of PD and FT. As with PD, chickens and turkeys are primary hosts of *S. gallinarum;* free-flying birds and other fowl are not major reservoirs of the infection. Thus eradication of these diseases from chicken and turkey breeding flocks will go a long way toward their total elimination from commercial poultry flocks. In some areas contaminated poultry ranges and pond water provide excellent means of perpetuation of FT.

Silva et al. (87) found that native intestinal microflora of chickens protective against paratyphoid salmonellae appeared to be partially protective against *S. gallinarum* and abbreviated its excretion time in WL chicks. Both treated and untreated groups of meat-type chicks were infected more frequently than comparable groups of WL chicks. The authors concluded that the low level of protection provided by competitive exclusion would not prove useful in practical control of FT.

Management Procedures. Management practices should be broadly applied to prevent introduction of FT as well as other infectious diseases into a poultry population:

1. Chicks and poults should be obtained from sources free of PD and FT.
2. Chicks and poults should be placed in an environment that can be cleaned and sanitized to eliminate any residential salmonellae from previous flocks (see Resistance to Chemical and Physical Agents).
3. Chicks and poults should receive pelletized, crumbled feed to minimize the introduction of *S. gallinarum* and other salmonellae through contaminated feed ingredients. Use of feed ingredients free of salmonellae is highly desirable.
4. Introduction of salmonellae from outside sources must be minimized.
    a. Free-flying birds are commonly found to be carriers of salmonellae, but *S. gallinarum* is rarely encountered. Poultry houses should be birdproof.
    b. Rats, mice, rabbits, and other pests may be carriers of salmonellae but are rarely found infected with *S. gallinarum*. Nevertheless, poultry houses should be rodentproof.
    c. Insect control is important, particularly against flies, poultry mites, and the lesser mealworm. These pests may provide a means of survival of salmonellae and other avian pathogens in the environment.
    d. Other animals such as dogs and cats may be carriers of salmonellae but rarely *S. gallinarum.* These animals should be kept from the poultry house.
    e. Potable drinking water must be used, or chlorinated water should be provided. In some areas surface water is collected in open ponds for use as drinking water for livestock and poultry.
    f. Humans may be mechanical carriers of the organism on footwear and clothing as well as poultry equipment, processing trucks, and poultry crates. Every precaution should be made to prevent introduction of *S. gallinarum* by fomites.
    g. Proper disposal of dead birds is essential. *S. gallinarum* will survive in poultry carcasses for weeks, depending on ambient temperatures (18, 44, 102, 103).

Eradication Program. Principles established for identification and elimination of PD-infected flocks under the NPIP are applicable to FT.

The essentials of an eradication program for an area are:

1. PD and FT must be mandatory reportable diseases.
2. Outbreaks are placed under quarantine, and infected flocks are marketed under supervision.
3. All reports of PD and FT are investigated by an authorized state or federal official.
4. Importation regulations shall require shipments of poultry and hatching eggs to be from sources considered free of PD and FT.
5. Regulations shall require poultry going to public exhibition to be from flocks free from PD and FT.
6. Total participation of poultry breeding flocks and hatcheries shall be required in a pullorum-typhoid control program such as NPIP programs or equivalent.

Thirty-four states in the USA had qualified under the above program as pullorum-typhoid-clean states by 1988.

Immunization. In the USA, federally licensed *S. gallinarum*-killed bacterins are no longer produced. Live modified vaccines as used in other countries are not permitted in the USA.

Various investigators have evaluated killed and modified live vaccines. Pomeroy (81) reviewed some of the early research work on use of immunizing agents to prevent and control FT. With the upsurge of FT in many countries, studies on use of 9R strain as an oral vaccine or as an injectable vaccine with oil adjuvants have been reported. Gupta and Mallick (39) observed that 9R strain administered orally gave significant protection against challenge with the virulent strain if chicks were pretreated with sodium bicarbonate or magnesium carbonate 10 min before vaccination. The same authors (40) reported that incorporation of Freund's complete adjuvant into 9R live vaccine given subcutaneously resulted in protection up to 32 wk. The 9R strain was not recovered from eggs laid by immunized pullets. Padmanaban et al. (77) studied live and killed vaccines with and without Freund's complete adjuvant using 9R and other strains of *S. gallinarum.* Live vaccines with adjuvant gave the best protection, followed by live vaccines without adjuvants. Comparison of response to various serologic tests and survival after challenge indicated that a humoral immune response was not essential for protection.

Silva et al. (86) concluded from extensive studies on use of 9R strains in WL and meat-type and brown egg-producing strains of chickens that protection against mortality in highly susceptible stock exposed to virulent strains may be severely limited. Vaccinated birds appear capable of transmitting 9R and pathogenic strains through the egg, and some vaccinated birds develop antibodies that produce reactions in serologic tests for pullorum-typhoid.

Bouzoubaa et al. (21) found that outer membrane proteins from *S. gallinarum* gave better protection than formalin-killed, whole-cell bacterin. Addition of an oil adjuvant to the protein appeared to increase the efficiency of the vaccine. When protein was given to chickens at 400 μg/100g of live weight, it produced 100% protection against oral challenge with *S. gallinarum.*

Bouzoubaa (19) found that outer membrane proteins from *S. gallinarum* gave better protection than 9R live vaccine in terms of clearance of the pathogenic strain from internal organs. Potential egg transmission of 9R and pathogenic strains following challenge of birds vaccinated with 9R either orally or subcutaneously was indicated by ovarian infection. In another experiment the oil-adjuvanted outer membrane protein vaccine reduced egg-transmission in an experimentally infected group of layers to zero by the 3rd wk post-vaccination whereas it remained stable (25–36%) in unvaccinated controls. Also, studies (19) were directed at delayed-type hypersensitivity reaction (DTH) as a measure of cell-mediated immunity in birds vaccinated with protein extracts and whole cell bacterin. The results indicated the presence of DTH in most birds given protein vaccine and no DTH in birds receiving whole cell bacterin.

Host Resistance. Breeding and selection for strains of chickens resistant to FT have not been applied from a practical standpoint but may have to be explored along with other approaches to control serious losses occurring in some areas of the world. In the USA, Canada, and some European countries, emphasis has been placed on a control and eradication program by testing and selecting clean breeding flocks.

Pomeroy (81) reviewed some of the early research on selection for resistant strains, and Gavora and Spencer (35) reviewed the area of breeding for genetic resistance and the need to develop adequate methods for measurements of general disease resistance and its incorporation into breeding plans. Pevzner et al. (78) used *S. pullorum* to study mortality differences within B blood group genotypes in chickens and were able to show a difference based on mortality between selected groups.

Research reports have suggested that nutrition may have an influence on resistance to *S. gallinarum* infection in chickens (81). In countries where FT is a serious problem, nutrition may affect FT mortality in commercial flocks used for meat and egg production. However, there has been no practical use of nutrition to complement a control and eradication program in countries having a severe problem with FT.

Aflatoxicosis had no added effect on body weight and mortality in *S. gallinarum*-infected chickens (91).

REFERENCES

1. Allan, D., and W.P. Duffus. 1971. The immunopathology in fowls (Gallus domesticus) of acute and subacute Salmonella gallinarum infection. Res Vet Sci 12:140–151.

2. Allan, D., W.P.H. Duffus, and D.A. Higgins. 1968. Measurement of antigen-antibody complexes in Salmonella gallinarum infection. Immunol 14:575–581.

3. Anonymous. 1985. The National Poultry Improvement Plan and Auxiliary Provisions. USDA, APHIS, Beltsville, MD.

4. Anonymous. 1987. 1986 Summary of commercial poultry disease reports. Avian Dis 31:926–978.

5. Anonymous. 1987. Animal Health Yearbook. FAO, Rome.

6. Anonymous. 1988. Feed Additive Compendium–a guide to the use of drugs in medicated animal feed, pp. 1–358. Miller Publishing Co., Minneapolis, MN.

7. Assoku, R.K.G., and W.J. Penhale. 1974. The pathogenesis of fowl typhoid: The influence of anaemia and erythrocyte clearance on the susceptibility of the fowl to bacterial endotoxin. J Comp Pathol 84:443–453

8. Assoku, R.K.G., W.J. Penhale, and A. Buxton. 1970. Hematological changes in acute experimental Salmonella gallinarum infections in chickens. J Comp Pathol 80:473–485.

9. Barrow, P.A., J.M. Simpson, M.A. Lovell, and M.M. Binns. 1987. Contribution of Salmonella gallinarum large plasmid toward virulence in fowl typhoid. Infect Immun 55:388–392.

10. Bassiouni, A., M. Rifai, and K. Abbasi. 1966. The influence of the somatic factor 0–1 on the agglutination reactions for detecting Salmonella gallinarum-pullorum infections. Vet Med J Giza 12:369–376.

11. Beach, J.R., and D.E. Davis. 1927. Acute infection in chicks and chronic infection of the ovaries of hens caused by the fowl typhoid organisms. Hilgardia 2:411–424.

12. Beaudette, F.R. 1925. The possible transmission

of fowl typhoid through the egg. J Am Vet Med Assoc 67:741-745.
13. Beaudette, F.R. 1930. Fowl typhoid and bacillary white diarrhea. Proc 11th Int Vet Congr 3:705-723.
14. Beaudette, F.R. 1938. An outbreak of fowl typhoid in guineas. J Am Vet Med Assoc 92:695-698.
15. Beck, A., and R. Eber. 1929. Die wichtigsten bakteriellen Kükenerkrankungen. Ihre Diagnose, Differentialdiagnose und Bekämpfung. Z Infekt Haustiere 35:76-95.
16. Blaxland, J.D., W.J. Sojka, and A.M. Smither. 1956. A study of Salmonella pullorum and Salmonella gallinarum strains isolated from field outbreaks of disease. J Comp Pathol Ther 66:270-277.
17. Boney, W.A., Jr. 1947. Isolation of Shigella gallinarum from turkey eggs. Am J Vet Res 8:133-135.
18. Botts, C.W., L.C. Ferguson, J.M. Birkeland, and A.R. Winter. 1952. The influence of litter on the control of salmonella infections in chicks. Am J Vet Res 13:562-565.
19. Bouzoubaa, K. 1988. Membrane proteins from Salmonella gallinarum for protection against fowl typhoid. PhD Thesis. Institute of Agronomy and Veterinary Medicine, Hassan II, Rabat, Morocco.
20. Bouzoubaa, K. and K.V. Nagaraja. 1984. Epidemiological studies on the incidence of salmonellosis in chicken breeder/hatchery operations in Morocco. In G.H. Snoeyenbos (ed.), Proc Int Symp Salmonella, New Orleans, p. 337. Am Assoc Avian Pathol, Kennett Square, PA.
21. Bouzoubaa, K., K.V. Nagaraja, J.A. Newman and B.S. Pomeroy. 1987. Use of membrane proteins from Salmonella gallinarum for prevention of fowl typhoid infection in chickens. Avian Dis 31:699-704.
22. Buxton, A., and D. Allan. 1963. Studies on immunity and pathogenesis of salmonellosis. I. Antigen-antibody reactions on circulating leucocytes of chickens infected with Salmonella gallinarum. Immunology 6:520-529.
23. Buxton, A., and J.M. Davies. 1963. Studies on immunity and pathogenesis of salmonellosis. II. Antibody production and accumulation of bacterial polysaccharide in the tissues of chickens infected with Salmonella gallinarum. Immunology 6:530-538.
24. Cameron, C.M., O.L. Brett, and W.J.P. Fuls. 1974. The effect of immunosuppression on the development of immunity to fowl typhoid. Onderstepoort J Vet Res 41:15-21.
25. Cloud, O.E. 1943. Perforation with peritonitis from Shigella gallinarum (Var Duisburg). Med Bull Veterans' Adm 19:335-336.
26. Curtice, C. 1902. Fowl typhoid. RI Agric Exp Stn Bull 87.
27. Donatien, A., E. Plantureaux, and F. Lestoquard. 1923. La typhose aviaire en Algerie. Annu Inst Pasteur d'Algerie 1:585.
28. Dyakov, L. 1966. Pathology of acute fowl typhoid with reference to differential diagnosis. Nauchni Tr Visshiya Vet Med Inst Sofia 16:13-22.
29. Edwards, P.R., D.W. Bruner, E.R. Doll, and G.S. Hermann. 1948. Salmonella infections of fowls. Cornell Vet 38:257-262.
30. El-Dine, H.S. 1939. Important diseases of poultry in Egypt and their control. Proc 7th World's Poult Congr, pp. 229-231.
31. Ellis, E.M., J.E. Williams, E.T. Mallinson, G.H. Snoeyenbos, and W.J. Martin. 1976. Culture Methods for the Detection of Animal Salmonellosis and Arizonosis, pp. 9-87. Iowa State Univ Press, Ames.
32. Fox, H. 1923. Diseases of Captive Wild Animals and Birds, 1st Ed. Lippincott, Philadelphia.
33. Garren, H.W., and C.W. Barber. 1955. Endocrine and lymphatic gland changes occurring in young chickens with fowl typhoid. Poult Sci 34:1250-1258.
34. Gauger, H.C. 1934. A chronic carrier of fowl typhoid with testicular focalization. J Am Vet Med Assoc 84:248-251.
35. Gavora, J.S., and J.L. Spencer. 1978. Breeding for genetic resistance to disease: specific or general. World's Poult Sci J 34:137-148.
36. Geissler, H. 1958. Comparison of agglutination of different antigens in infection with Salmonella gallinarum-pullorum. Berl Muench Tieraerztl Wochenschr 71:328-330.
37. Giurov, B. and G. Kostov. 1983. Erythrocyte antigen for the rapid intravital diagnosis of fowl typhoid and pullorum disease. Vet Med Nauki 20(9):18-24.
38. Gordeuk, S., Jr., P.J. Glantz, E.W. Callenbach, and W.T.S. Thorp. 1949. Transmission of fowl typhoid. Poult Sci 28:385-391.
39. Gupta, B.R., and B.B. Mallick. 1976. Immunization against fowl typhoid. 1. Live oral vaccine. Indian J Anim Sci 46:502-505.
40. Gupta, B.R., and B.B. Mallick. 1976. Immunization against fowl typhoid. 2. Live adjuvant vaccine. Indian J Anim Sci 46:546-551.
41. Gwatkin, R., and L. Dzenis. 1951. Fowl Typhoid. 1. Comparison of antigenicity of sixteen gallinarum antigens. Can J Comp Med Vet Sci 15:15-20.
42. Hall, C.F., and H.T. Cartrite. 1961. Observations on strains of Salmonella gallinarum apparently resistant to furazolidone. Avian Dis 5:382-392.
43. Hall, W.J., D.H. Legenhausen, and A.D. Macdonald. 1948. A summary of results of fowl typhoid investigations. Proc 20th Annu Meet Northeast Conf Lab Workers in Pullorum Dis Control, p. 55.
44. Hall, W.J., D.H. Legenhausen, and A.D. Macdonald. 1949. Studies on fowl typhoid. 1. Nature and dissemination. Poult Sci 28:344-362.
45. Hall, W.J., D.H. Legenhausen, and A.D. Macdonald. 1949. Studies on fowl typhoid II. Control of the disease. Poult Sci 28:344-362.
46. Hinshaw, W.R. 1930. Fowl typhoid of turkeys. Vet Med 25:514-517.
47. Horsfall, D.J., Rowley, and C.R. Jenkins. 1970. The titre of bactericidal antibody against Salmonella gallinarum in chicks. Immunol 18:595-598.
48. Johnson, E.P., and G.W. Anderson. 1933. An outbreak of fowl typhoid in guinea fowls (Numida meleagris). J Am Vet Med Assoc 82:258-259.
49. Johnson, E.P. and M. Pollard. 1940. Fowl typhoid in turkey poults. J Am Vet Med Assoc 6:243-244.
50. Jordan, F.T.W. 1956. The occurrence of Salmonella gallinarum in the feces in fowl typhoid. Poult Sci 35:1026-1029.
51. Jordan, F.T.W. 1956. The transmission of Salmonella gallinarum through the egg. Poult Sci 35:1019-1025.
52. Kaupp, B.F., and R.S. Dearstyne. 1924. Chronic carriers in fowl typhoid. J Am Vet Med Assoc 64:329-333.
53. Kaupp, B.F., and R.S. Dearstyne. 1924. Fowl typhoid: A comparison of various European strains with those of North America. Poult Sci 3:119-127.
54. Kaupp, B.F., and R.S. Dearstyne. 1925. The differential diagnosis of fowl cholera and fowl typhoid. J Am Vet Med Assoc 67:249-259.
55. Klein, E. 1889. Über eine epidemische Krankheit der Hühner, verursacht durch einer Bacillus-Bacillus gallinarum. Zentralbl Bakteriol Parasitenkd Abt I Orig 5:689-93.
56. Kokosharov, T, and T. Todorova. 1987. Changes in the iron content, erythrocytes and hemoglobin in the blood of poultry with acute experimental fowl typhoid.

Vet Med Nauki 24(5):44-51
57. Kokosharov, T., I. Petkov, and I. Dzhurova. 1984. Cocks with experimentally induced acute typhoid. Vet Med Nauki 21:18-26.
58. Komarov, A. 1932. Fowl typhoid in baby chicks. Vet Rec 12:1455-1457.
59. Kösters, J. 1965. Antigenic structure and serological behaviour. I. Distribution of individual antigens in various strains. Berl Muench Tieraerztl Wochenschr 78:211-213.
60. Kösters, J. 1965. Antigenic structure and serological behaviour of Salmonella gallinarum. II. Antibody formation against various S.gallinarum strains. Berl Muench Tieraerztl Wochenschr 78:290-291.
61. Kösters, J. 1965. Antigenic structure and serological behaviour of Salmonella gallinarum. III. Differentiation of nonspecific agglutination reactions. Berl Muench Tieraerztl Wochenschr 78:314-315.
62. Kösters, J., and H. Geissler. 1966. The selection of Salmonella gallinarum-pullorum strains for production of a standardized agglutination antigen. Berl Muench Tieraerztl Wochenschr 79:276-278.
63. Kraus, E.J. 1918. Zur Kenntnis des Hühnertyphus. Zentralbl f. Bakteriol Parasitenkd Abt I Orig 82:282-303.
64. Lerche, Von M. 1939. Salmonellainfektionen beim Geflügel und ihre Bedeutung fur die Epidemiologie der Salmonellabakterien. Proc 7th World's Poult Congr, pp. 274-278.
65. Lerche, Von M., and E. Roots. 1958. Preparation of S.gallinarum-pullorum antigens for agglutination reaction. Berl Muench Tieraerztl Wochenschr 71:431-432.
66. Lignieres, J., and Zabala. 1905. Sur une nouvelle maladie des poules. Bull Soc Cent Med Vet 59:453-456.
67. Lucet, A. 1891. Dysenterie epizootique des poules et des dindes. Ann Inst Pasteur 5:312-331.
68. Lucio, B., M. Padron, and A. Mosqueda. 1984. Fowl typhoid in Mexico. In G.H. Snoeyenbos (ed.), Proc Int Symp Salmonella, pp. 382-383. Am Assoc Avian Pathol, Kennett Square, PA.
69. Martinaglia, G. 1929. A note on Salmonella gallinarum infection of ten-day-old chicks and adult turkeys. J S Afr Vet Med Assoc 1:35-36.
70. Molnar, I., and G. Nagy, 1959. Production of fowl typhoid antigens by fermentation. Magy Allatorv Lapja 14:386-387.
71. Moore, V.A. 1895. Infectious leukemia in fowls – a bacterial disease frequently mistaken for fowl cholera. USDA BAI 12th, 13th Annu Rep, pp.185-205.
72. Moore, E.N. 1946. Fowl typhoid transmission. Del Agric Exp Stn Bull 262:21.
73. Moore, E.N. 1946. The occurrence of fowl typhoid. Del Agric Exp Stn Bull Cir. 19:20.
74. Moore, E.N. 1947. The agglutination test as a means of detecting fowl typhoid infections. Cornell Vet 37:21-28.
75. Nobrega, P., and R.C. Bueno. 1942. Sobre a presenca da Salmonella gallinarum nos ovos de galinhas portadoras de tifo aviario. Arq Inst Biol (Sao Paulo) 13:17-20.
76. Orr, B.B., and E.N. Moore. 1953. Longevity of Salmonella gallinarum. Poult Sci 32:800-805.
77. Padmanaban, V.D., K.R. Mittal, and B.R. Gupta. 1981. Cross protection against fowl typhoid: Immunization trials and humoral immune response. Dev Comp Immun 5:301-312.
78. Pevzner, I.Y., C.L. Trowbridge, A.W. Nordskog, and L.B. Crittenden. 1978. Mortality differences associated with divergent selection for immune response to Salmonella pullorum within B Blood Group genotypes in chickens. Poult Sci 57:1180.
79. Pfeiler, W., and A. Rehse. 1913. Bacillus typhi gallinarum alcalifaciens und die durch ihn verursachte Hühnerseuche. Mitt Kaiser Wilhelm Inst Landwirtsch Bromberg 5:306-321.
80. Pfeiler, W., and E. Roepke. 1917. Zweite Mitteilung uber das Auftreten des Huhnertyphus und die Eigenschaften seines Erregers. Zentralbl Bakteriol Parasitenkd Abt I Orig 79:125-139.
81. Pomeroy, B.S. 1984. Fowl Typhoid. In M.S. Hofstad, H.J. Barnes, B.W. Calnek, W.M. Reid, and H.W. Yoder, Jr. (eds.), Diseases of Poultry, 8th Ed., pp. 79-91. Iowa State Univ Press, Ames.
82. Popp, L. 1947. Fowl typhoid organisms as the cause of gastroenteritis in man. J Am Vet Med Assoc 111:314. (Abstr)
83. Rao, S.B.V., S. Narayanan, D.R. Ramnani, and J. Das. 1952. Avian salmonellosis: Studies on Salmonella gallinarum. Indian J Vet Sci 22:199-208.
84. Salmonella Surveillance. 1987. Annu Summ Centers for Disease Control, Atlanta, GA.
85. Silva, E.N. 1984. The Salmonella gallinarum problem in Central and South America. In G.H. Snoeyenbos (ed.), Proc Int Symp Salmonella, pp. 150-156. Am Assoc Avian Pathol, Kennett Square, PA.
86. Silva, E.N., G.H. Snoeyenbos, O.M. Weinack, and C.F. Smyser. 1981. Studies on the use of 9R strain of Salmonella gallinarum as a vacccine in chickens. Avian Dis 25:38-52.
87. Silva, E.N., G.H. Snoeyenbos, O.M. Weinack, and C.F. Smyser. 1981. The influence of native gut microflora on the colonization and infection of Salmonella gallinarum in chickens. Avian Dis 25:68-73.
88. Smith, H.W. 1955. The longevity of Salmonella gallinarum in the faeces of infected chickens. J Comp Pathol Ther 65:267-270.
89. Smith, H.W. 1955. Observations on experimental fowl typhoid. J Comp Pathol 65:37-54.
90. Smith, T.H., and C. Ten Broeck. 1915. Agglutination affinities of a pathogenic bacillus from fowls (fowl typhoid) (Bacterium Sanguinarium Moore) with the typhoid bacillus of man. J Med Res 31:503-521.
91. Smith, J.W., W.R. Prince, and P.B. Hamilton. 1969. Relationship of aflatoxicosis to Salmonella gallinarum infections of chickens. Appl Microbiol 18:946-947.
92. Smith, I.M., S.T. Licence, and R. Hill. 1978. Haematological, serological and pathological effects in chicks of one or more intravenous injections of Salmonella gallinarum endotoxin. Res Vet Sci 24:154-160.
93. Smith, H.W., J.F.Tucker, and M. Lovell. 1981. Furazolidone resistance in Salmonella gallinarum: The relationship between in vitro and in vivo determinations of resistance. J Hyg (Camb) 87:71-81.
94. Sorrells, K.M., M.L. Speck, and J.A. Warren. 1970. Pathogenicity of Salmonella gallinarum after metabolic injury by freezing. Appl Microbiol 19:39-43.
95. St. John-Brooks, R., and M. Rhodes. 1923. The organisms of the fowl typhoid group. J Pathol Bacteriol 26:433-39.
96. Stuart, E.E., R.D. Keenum, and H.W. Bruins. 1962. Experimental studies on an isolate of Salmonella gallinarum apparently resistant to furazolidone. Avian Dis 7:294-303.
97. Stuart, E.E., R.D. Keenum, and H.W. Bruins. 1967. The emergence of a furazolidone-resistant strain of Salmonella gallinarum. Avian Dis 11:139-45.
98. Te Hennepe, B.J.C. 1924. Combating poultry diseases by the state serum institute at Rotterdam. Proc 2nd World's Poult Congr, pp. 219-228.

99. Te Hennepe, B.J.C. 1939. Combating poultry diseases in the Netherlands. Proc 7th World's Poult Congr, pp. 224–227.

100. Te Hennepe, B.J.C., and Van Straaten, H. 1921. Fowl septicemia. Trans 1st World's Poult Congr 1:259.

101. Truche, C. 1923. De la typhose aviaire. Ann Inst Pasteur 37:478–497.

102. Tucker, J.F. 1967. Survival of salmonellae in built-up litter for housing of rearing and laying fowls. Br Vet J 123:92–103.

103. Van Es, L., and J.F. Olney. 1940. An inquiry into the influence of environment on the incidence of poultry diseases; fowl typhus. Nebr Agric Exp Stn Res Bull 118.

104. Van Heelsbergen, T. 1929. Handbuch der Geflugelkrankheiten und Geflugelzucht. Ferdinand Enke, Stuttgart. p. 135.

105. Van Straaten, H., and B.J.C. Te Hennepe. 1919. Die kleinsche Hühnerseuche. Folia Microbiol 5:103–125.

106. Williams, J.E. and M.E. Harris. 1956. Antigenic studies using ammonium sulfate. IV. The sedimentation effect of ammonium sulfate on Salmonella gallinarum. Am J Vet Res 17:535–537.

107. Williams, J.E., E.T. Mallinson, and G.H. Snoeyenbos. 1980. Salmonellosis and Arizonosis. In S.B. Hitchner, C.H. Domermuth, H.G. Purchase, and J.E. Williams (eds.), Isolation and Identification of Avian Pathogens, 2nd Ed., pp. 1–8. Am Assoc Avian Pathol, Kennett Square, PA.

PARATYPHOID INFECTIONS

K.V. Nagaraja, B.S. Pomeroy, and J.E. Williams

INTRODUCTION. Moore (201) recorded the first authentic case of paratyphoid (PT) infection in domestic poultry when he described an outbreak of infectious enteritis in pigeons. Early historic reports on PT infections in all avian species were reviewed by Henning (145) and Williams (345).

National interest in avian salmonellosis has been stimulated by public concern for foods of highest quality, which has in turn required the poultry industry to take measures to eliminate salmonellae from its operations in an attempt to offer products free of the organisms.

The Salmonella Committee of the US Animal Health Association has published an annual report in its yearly proceedings, providing a review of regulatory considerations in control programs for salmonella infections in poultry. These reports cover current problems relating to salmonellae in food-producing animals. Published in the proceedings are the annual reports of the salmonella serotyping data accumulated at National Veterinary Services Laboratories (NVSL), Animal Plant Health Inspection Service (APHIS), USDA.

Workshops or symposia on avian salmonellosis were held in 1970 (9), 1976 (11) and 1984 (14). Snoeyenbos (291) stated that the limited available evidence suggests that perhaps 75% of chicken and turkey populations in the USA have been infected with one or more salmonella serotypes at some stage of their life. In 1978, the US Advisory Committee on Salmonella issued its recommendations for reduction and control of salmonellosis (12); only a few have actually been implemented. Rigby et al. (252) found *Salmonella typhimurium* to be the most common salmonella isolated from quarantined imported birds in Canada, and discussed the possible public health significance of exotic salmonella serotypes or those resistant to several antimicrobials introduced by exotic birds. Bullis (62) traced the history of avian salmonelloses in the USA. In the last few years there has been a dramatic increase of human cases of *S. enteritidis* in the USA, Canada, and Europe. In the USA, epidemiologic observations suggest that grade A eggs or egg-containing dishes were associated with many of the human outbreaks (307).

INCIDENCE, DISTRIBUTION, ECONOMIC IMPORTANCE. PT infections of poultry exist in all parts of the world. However, it has often been found that particular serotypes that previously were rare may become increasingly common in one region or country. The more commonly isolated salmonella serotypes in poultry in any country are usually characteristic of that locale and not subject to extreme fluctuation of isolation frequency over short periods, although their rank in frequency of isolation may change. The majority of new serotypes being added constantly to the genus *Salmonella* are usually not commonly found in nature; approximately 70% of salmonella disease outbreaks at any one time in both animals and humans are due to no more than 10 or 12 serotypes.

Serologic Surveys of Avian Cultures. Moran (203) noted that *S. typhimurium* was encountered four times as often in turkeys as chickens in the USA in 1957. *S. heidelberg* and *S. infantis,* which had not been reported in fowl in the USA in earlier reports, composed 8 and 6.7%, respectively, of cultures from chickens. Sanders et al. (259) reported that in 1963 about 61% of all nonhuman isolates were obtained from chickens, turkeys, other wild and domestic fowl, and eggs and egg products.

Martin and Ewing (191) found that 33 salmonella serotypes accounted for almost 80% of isolates from animal sources, including poultry. Bruner (58) encountered 43 serotypes of salmonellae among 482 cultures from turkeys; 40 among 1694 cultures from chickens; 17 among 874 cultures from ducks; and 24 among 79 cultures from animal feeds during a survey extending over a 22-yr period in New York. Ferris and Frerichs (106) reported the results of serotyping of 1284 cultures from turkeys, 918 from chickens and 366 from feed; 58 different serotypes were reported from turkeys, 57 from chickens and 56 from feed. *S. heidelberg* was the most common serotype isolated from turkeys and chickens.

Serotypes from Chickens and Turkeys in the USA. A total of 203 PT serotypes isolated from chickens and/or turkeys in the USA are listed in Table 3.5. Five new types not previously seen from poultry have been reported since the 8th edition of this book. Information included in the table has been developed from published reports and data supplied by diagnostic laboratories, regulatory agencies, typing centers, and research workers in various areas. Original references to the description of most of the salmonella types included in the table are listed by Kauffmann (158) or Kelterborn (161).

Some of the types listed have not been associated with disease outbreaks but were recovered from intestines of birds that were apparently normal carriers, in some cases only on a single occasion. However, most of the cultures were derived from acute, fatal infections in young chicks or poults and were isolated from internal organs or intestinal contents. Isolations from unabsorbed yolks, ovarian cysts, and oviducts represent only a small percentage of the culture types listed.

Worldwide Avian Salmonellosis. Buxton (65) noted that worldwide 90 types of PT organisms have been reported from 12 species of fowl. Many serotypes were reported to have caused only a few minor epizootics and some to have been isolated only from apparently healthy birds. The reader seeking reference material on host species, origin, and distribution of salmonella types occurring in poultry around the world is referred to Buxton's excellent review.

Economic Importance. From an economic viewpoint PT infections are among the bacterial diseases most important to the hatching industry. They result in high death losses among all types of young poultry. One estimate cited economic loss to the US poultry industry from PT infections at approximately $77 million annually (189). Jackson et al. (152) described a severe outbreak of *S. typhimurium* infection costing many hundred thousands of dollars in an integrated poultry organization in Australia.

Purchase (239) called attention to the fact that an eradication program for salmonella infections would likely cost the consumer far more than could be justified by benefits derived from such eradication. Nevertheless, practical control of salmonella contamination can be achieved through progressive application of new technology developed through research. Finn and Mehr (107) calculated that it would require $12.68 of expenditure on eradication of salmonellae from poultry to generate $1.00 of benefit from the program.

Because of its chronic nature and the difficulty of eradication, PT is capable of terminating breeding operations in which large amounts of money may have been invested. The infection has a definite stunting effect on surviving birds and a debilitating influence on poultry of all ages, increasing their susceptibility to many other diseases.

Roberts (253) estimated that medical costs and lost productivity from food-borne salmonellosis in the USA totaled $553–988 million annually. Adverse publicity from salmonella outbreaks such as *S. enteritidis* or salmonella contamination of poultry meat has had severe economic impact on the industry.

ETIOLOGY

Morphology and Staining. Organisms of the PT group are defined as serologically related, gram-negative, and nonsporogenic bacilli. They usually measure 0.4–0.6 × 1–3 μm, but occasionally they form short filaments (Fig. 3.4). They are normally motile by means of peritrichous flagella, but nonmotile variants with or without flagella may be encountered under natural conditions.

Growth Requirements. PT is a facultative anaerobe readily cultivated on initial isolation (from sources other than feces) on simple beef extract and beef infusion agars and broths. Optimum growth temperature is 37 C. Stock cultures can be maintained viable in paraffin-corked plain agar stabs for many years without transplanting. Kokolios et al. (170) demonstrated that salmonellae can remain viable for as long as 40 yr in such simple media as soft agar sealed in glass ampules at room temperature.

Colony Morphology. Typical colonies of PT on agar culture are round, slightly raised, and glistening with smooth edges. Colonies are generally 1–2 mm in diameter depending on degree of

Table 3.5. Paratyphoids isolated from chickens and/or turkeys in the USA

S. aberdeen (F)	*S. daytona* (C_1)	*S. kiambu* (B)	*S. reading* (B)
S. adelaide (O)	*S. decatur* (C_1)	*S. kralingen* (C_3)	*S. richmond* (C_1)
S. agama (B)	*S. denver* (C_1)	*S. kingston* (B)	*S. rubislaw* (F)
S. agona (B)	*S. derby* (B)	*S. kottbus* (C_2)	*S. rutgers* (E_1)
S. akanji (C_2)	*S. drypool* (E_2)	*S. lexington* (E_1)	*S. saint-paul* (B)
S. alabama (D_1)	*S. dublin* (D_1)	*S. lille* (C_1)	*S. san-diego* (B)
S. alachua (O)	*S. duesseldorf* (C_2)	*S. lindenburg* (C_2)	*S. san-juan* (C_1)
S. albany (C_3)	*S. eastbourne* (D_1)	*S. litchfield* (C_2)	*S. saphra* (I)
S. amager (E_1)	*S. edinburg* (C_1)	*S. livingstone* (C_1)	*S. schwarzengrund* (B)
S. amersfoort (C_1)	*S. eimsbuettel* (C_1)	*S. loma-linda* (D_1)	*S. seegefeld* (E_1)
S. amherstiana (C_3)	*S. enteritidis* (D_1))	*S. lomita* (C_1)	*S. senftenberg* (E_4)
S. amsterdam (E_1)	*S. epicrates* (E_1)	*S. london* (E_1)	*S. shomron* (K)
S. anatum (E_1)	*S. essen* (B)	*S. madelia* (H)	*S. shubra* (B)
S. aqua (N)	*S. fayed* (C_2)	*S. mampong* (G_1)	*S. siegburg* (K)
S. arechavaleta (B)	*S. florida* (H)	*S. manchester* (C_2)	*S. simsbury* (E_4)
S. arkansas (E_3)	*S. fresno* (D_2)	*S. manhattan* (C_2)	*S. sinstorf* (E_1)
S. atlania (G_2)	*S. gaminara* (I)	*S. manila* (E_2)	*S. stanley* (B)
S. babelsberg (M)	*S. gege* (N)	*S. mbandaka* (C_1)	*S. stellenbosch* (D_1)
S. bardo (C_3)	*S. georgia* (C_1)	*S. meleagridis* (E_1)	*S. sundsvall* (H)
S. bareilly (C_1)	*S. gera* (T)	*S. memphis* (K)	*S. takoradi* (C_2)
S. bere (X)	*S. give* (E_1)	*S. menston* (C_1)	*S. taksony* (E_4)
S. berkeley (U)	*S. good* (L)	*S. menhaden* (E_3)	*S. tallahassee* (C_2)
S. berlin (J)	*S. gojenberg* (G_2)	*S. mgulani* (P)	*S. tel-aviv* (M)
S. berta (D_1)	*S. grumpensis* (G_2)	*S. miami* (D_1)	*S. tennessee* (C_1)
S. bietri (N)	*S. haardt* (C_3)	*S. mikawasima* (C_1)	*S. thomasville* (E_3)
S. binza (E_2)	*S. hadar* (C_2)	*S. minneapolis* (E_3)	*S. thompson* (C_1)
S. blegdam (D_1)	*S. halmstad* (E_2)	*S. minnesota* (L)	*S. treforest* (Gr. 51)
S. blockley (C_2)	*S. hamburg* (D_1)	*S. mission* (C_1)	*S. tuebingen* (E_2)
S. bornum (C_1)	*S. hamilton* (*goerlitz*) (E_2)	*S. molade* (C_3)	*S. tulear II* (C_2)
S. bovis morbificans (C_2)	*S. harrisonburg* (E_2)	*S. montevideo* (C_1)	*S. typhi* (D_1)
S. bradford (B)	*S. hartford* (C_1)	*S. muenchen* (*oregon*) (C_2)	*S. typhimurium* (B)
S. braenderup (C_1)	*S. hato* (B)	*S. muenster* (E_1)	*S. typhimurium* var.
S. brandenberg (B)	*S. hauten* (U)	*S. newbrunswick* (E_2)	*copenhagen* (B)
S. bredeney (B)	*S. havana* (G_2)	*S. new-haw* (E_2)	*S. typhi-suis* (C_1)
S. broughton (E_4)	*S. heidelberg* (B)	*S. newington* (E_2)	*S. uganda* (E_1)
S. budapest (B)	*S. hidalgo* (C_2)	*S. newport* (*pueris*) (C_2)	*S. uno* (C_2)
S. california (B)	*S. hillbrow* (J)	*S. nienstedten* (C_1)	*S. urbana* (N)
S. cambridge (E_2)	*S. hvittingfoss* (I)	*S. norwich* (C_1)	*S. vejle* (E_1)
S. canoga (E_3)	*S. illinois* (E_3)	*S. ohio* (C_1)	*S. virchow* (C_1)
S. caracas (H)	*S. indiana* (B)	*S. onarimon* (D_1)	*S. virginia* (C_3)
S. carrau (H))	*S. infantis* (C_1)	*S. onderstepoort* (H)	*S. weltevreden* (E_1)
S. cerro (K)	*S. iverness* (P)	*S. oranienberg* (C_1)	*S. westerstede* (E_4)
S. champaign (Q)	*S. irumu* (C_1)	*S. ordonez* (G_2)	*S. westhampton* (E_1)
S. chester (B)	*S. israel* (D_1)	*S. orion* (E_1)	*S. wichita* (G_1)
S. choleraesuis (C_1)	*S. istanbul* C_3)	*S. oslo* (C_1)	*S. worcester* (G_1)
S. cholerae-suis var.	*S. java* (B)	*S. panama* (*italiana*) (D_1)	*S. worthington* (G_1)
kunzendorf (C_1)	*S. javiana* (D_1)	*S. paratyphi A* (A)	*S. yovokome* (C_2)
S. clackamas (B)	*S. jerusalem* (C_1)	*S. paratyphi B* (B)	*S. zanzibar* (E_1)
S. colorado (C_1)	*S. johannesburg* (R)	*S. pensacola* (D_1)	*S. zehlendorf* (N)
S. concord (C_1)	*S. kaapstad* (B)	*S. pomona* (M)	
S. corvallis (C_3)	*S. kentucky* (C_3)	*S. poona* (G_1)	
S. cubana (G_2)	*S. kentucky* var. *jerusalem* (C_3)	*S. putten* (G_2)	

Note: Letter in parentheses indicates antigenic group in the Kauffmann-White scheme to which each serotype belongs. Five new paratyphoids were isolated from chickens and/or turkeys in the USA since the 8th edition of this book.

dispersion on the plates. Rough colonies may be encountered among recently isolated strains and those maintained in the laboratory on artificial media. Smooth broth cultures show a thick homogeneous turbidity with no pellicle and very little sediment after incubation for 24 hr. Rough cultures in broth have a heavy granular sediment and an almost clear supernatant fluid.

Biochemical Properties. The following biochemical reactions, as described by Edwards and Ewing (90), are typical of practically all members of the PT group:

Dextrose	fermented with gas
Lactose	not fermented
Sucrose	not fermented
Mannitol	fermented with gas
Maltose	fermented with gas
Dulcitol	usually fermented with gas
Salicin	not fermented

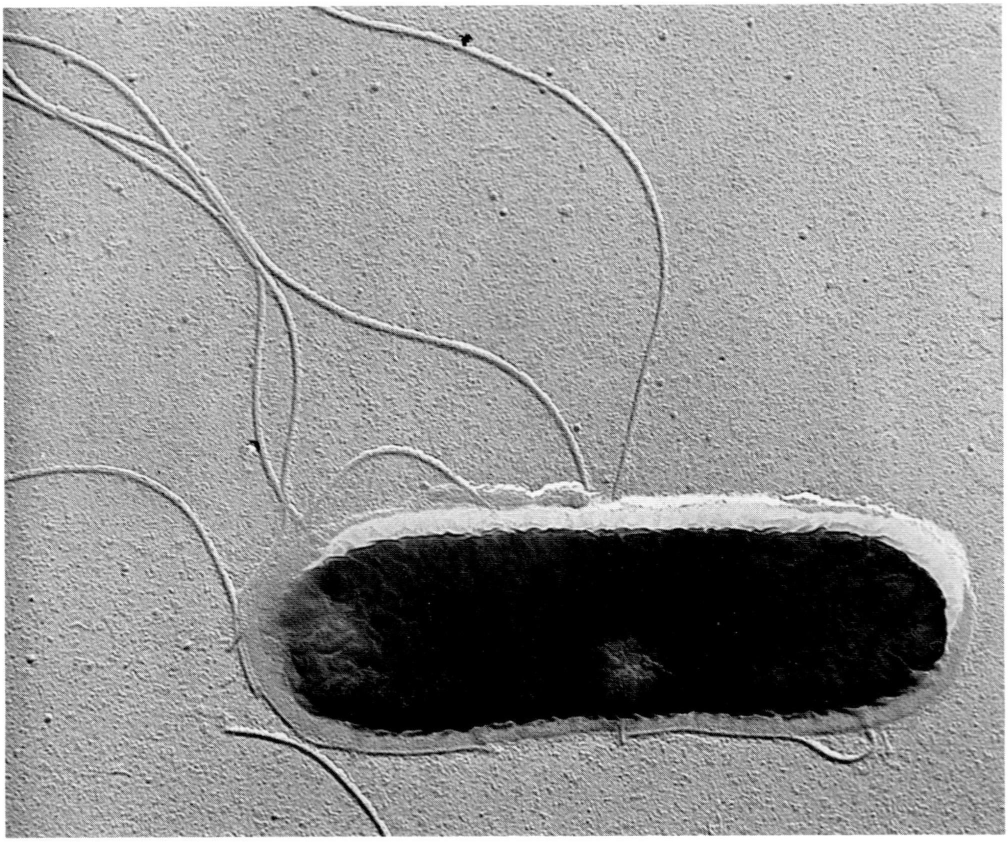

3.4. Electron micrograph of single flagellated cell of *S. typhimurium*. Chromium shadowed, ×14,000.

Sorbitol	fermented with gas
Adonitol	not fermented
Inositol	fermented or not fermented
Indole	not produced
Methyl red	positive
Voges-Proskauer	negative
Simmons' citrate	usually utilized
Hydrogen sulfide	usually positive
Urea	not hydrolyzed
Gelatin	rarely liquefied
Potassium cyanide	negative
Nitrates	reduced
Motility	positive
Decarboxylases	positive
Lysine	
Arginine	positive, usually delayed
Ornithine	positive
Malonate	negative
Phenylalanine deaminase	negative

Cultures that do not possess the above characteristics may be excluded from the PT group unless it can be established that they possess antigens of known salmonella types. *S. typhimurium* var. *copenhagen,* a frequent cause of paratyphoid infection of pigeons, usually forms no acid in maltose broth when isolated from this species. Consequently, this organism is sometimes confused with *S. pullorum* on initial examination. For a comprehensive review of the biochemical reactions of PT organisms, see Ewing and Ball (99), Kauffmann (159), Edwards and Ewing (90) and Ewing (98).

Resistance to Chemical and Physical Agents

HEAT, COLD, DISINFECTANTS. The fact that salmonellae are able to survive and multiply readily in the environment is an important factor in transmission and spread of the disease. PT organisms have simple growth requirements and multiply in a wide variety of media, provided the other parameters such as pH, temperature, and salt are not in the prohibitive range. Organisms are quite susceptible to heat and most common disinfectants. Bayne et al. (33) found it took only 5 min exposure to heat at 60 C to destroy 3×10^8 *S. typhimurium* cells/g ground chicken meat. Henning (145), working with *S. dublin* in South Africa, found that organisms survived at least 1069 days in infected manure that had been dried in the incubator for 48 hr and then bottled and kept in the laboratory.

Browne (54) reported that salmonellae lived 13 mo on poultry carcasses quick-frozen at −37 C and stored at −21 C. Cresylic acid, lye, and phenolic compounds are frequently employed in disinfection of poultry premises. Formaldehyde is also widely used as a disinfectant, particularly as a fumigant for eggs, incubators, hatchery rooms, and buildings. Formaldehyde and formaldehyde-containing compounds have been shown to be very effective in eliminating salmonellae from the soil and turkey facilities (235).

LITTER, FEEDSTUFFS, DUST. Brownell et al. (56) were unable to isolate salmonellae from litter taken 39 or 51 days after experimentally infected birds were removed. Several workers (104, 293, 322) reported that salmonellae do not persist as long in built-up litter as in fresh litter. Turnbull and Snoeyenbos (326) reported that the salmonellacidal activity of chicken litter was the result of two principal factors: a water activity unfavorable to salmonella cell viability and high pH from ammonia dissolved in available moisture of the litter. Morgan-Jones (205) noted that mature broiler litter is a hostile environment for salmonellae and it becomes more inhibitory as it matures. There is less agreement on the role of the indigenous microflora.

Smyser et al. (288) found that *S. typhimurium* had a short survival period in feed contaminated with fewer than 10 organisms/g and held at room temperature. Survival in feed was longer at 4 C than at room temperature.

Smyser et al. (289) recovered *S. heidelberg* from contaminated litter, grit, feed, and dust held for extended periods at room temperature. Litter was positive at 7 mo, when last tested. Williams and Benson (355) found that *S. typhimurium* survived at least 18 mo at 11 C in both feed and litter; 16 mo in feed and 18 mo in litter at 25 C; and about 40 days in feed and only 13 days in litter at 38 C. Salmonellae have been found to survive for months in sludge and on pastures, which is of great importance to maintenance of environmental contamination cycles.

Simmons (280) reported a lethal action of dazomet on salmonellae in naturally contaminated litter.

FECES AND HATCHERY FLUFF. Morse and Duncan (207) indicated that salmonellae will live for 28 mo in naturally infected avian feces; however, Berkowitz et al. (38) found that salmonellae inoculated into samples of poultry feces declined to very low numbers or disappeared within 1 mo. Salmonellae survived in hatchery fluff samples stored at room temperature for as long as 5 yr (200).

SOIL, WATER, VEGETATION. Mair and Ross (187) reported that *S. typhimurium* survived in urban garden soil for at least 280 days, and salmonellae were isolated from soil taken from turkey pens or ranges that had not been in use for 6–7 mo (6, 262). The organisms survived best in soil when organic material was present (312).

ANTIGENIC FORMULAS AND TYPE DISTRIBUTION IN POULTRY. There is marked variation in somatic and flagellar antigenic structure of salmonella types infecting poultry. Organisms representative of most of the major antigenic groups in the Kauffmann-White scheme have been isolated from chickens and turkeys.

In 1986, the 10 most frequently identified serotypes isolated from chickens were in serogroups B, C, D, and E, and those from turkeys in serogoups B, C, E, G, and *S. arizonae* (18:Z4, Z32). However, in 1987 and 1988, isolates of *S. enteritidis* dramatically increased (106).

Toxins. The pathogenic properties of salmonellae are due to endotoxins closely associated with the somatic portion of the organism. Vestal and Stephens (331) suggested that differences in pathogenicity of salmonella serotypes for chicks may be because the cells of some types are rapidly lysed following injection, with release of a large quantity of endotoxin causing early mortality. Other serotypes, it was believed, must build up to a large number of cells over several days before sufficient endotoxin is released to cause mortality. *S. enteritidis* has the capability to produce hazardous levels of enterotoxins under appropriate conditions (28, 301). Koo et al. (171) found that salmonella cytotoxin present in cell lysates inhibited protein synthesis, thus providing a molecular explanation for the cellular damage in intestinal cells caused by the cytotoxin during experimental salmonellosis.

Pathogenicity. Mortality from PT infections is encountered most frequently during the first 2 wk after hatching, with the highest losses occurring between the 6th and 10th days. The infection seldom causes mortality in birds more than 1 mo old. Pigeons, parakeets, and canaries may be cited as exceptions; the disease occurs more often in the acute form in adults of these species. Williams (348) described an outbreak of *S. thompson* infection with 30% mortality in older chicks.

Fagerberg et al. (102) demonstrated that as chicks reach about 1 wk of age, experimental salmonella infections are no longer lethal. Gordon

(123) noted that salmonella infection rarely causes clinical disease in chicks over 3 wk of age, and even then mortality may be high only when other adverse conditions are present. Unfortunately, however, a high proportion of survivors are likely to remain carriers and become symptomless excreters. If these birds are used as breeders, they will continue the cycle of infection; if they are broilers, they will serve to infect the packing station environment at slaughter. O'Brien (221), in England, reported increased mortality in broiler chickens caused by *S. enteritidis* phage type 4. Benson and Eckroade (36) reported differences among isolates of *S. enteritidis* from chickens in the USA; some may be more invasive and more virulent than others. Restriction endonuclease fingerprints of the plasmid and genomic DNA of these isolates indicated distinct differences between the various isolates. *S. enteritidis* was isolated from egg yolk, from dead-in-shell eggs from breeder hens, and from ovaries from layers. A phage typing scheme for *S. enteritidis* has been developed (334) in Great Britain and has been used as an epidemiological marker. Phage typing schemes have been used in several countries including the USA. Nagaraja et al. (216), using restriction endonuclease analysis on several isolates of *S. enteritidis* from animal and human origin, were able to detect differences in their genomic DNA. Among the isolates from animal origin, three distinct types were recognized. Plasmid groups may contribute to the pathogenic potential of salmonella serotypes including *S. enteritidis, S. typhimurium,* and *S. heidelberg* (234).

YOUNG BIRDS. Mortality rates among broods of young birds under natural conditions vary from negligible to 10–20%; however, mortality rates of 80% or higher are encountered in severe outbreaks.

Bierer (40) found poults extremely susceptible to *S. typhimurium* infection during the first 48 hr after hatching. Mitrovic (199) reported that day-old poults were very susceptible to experimental infection with *S. reading,* with a mortality of 40%, whereas 2-wk-old poults were highly resistant.

In contrast to poults, chicks usually do not exhibit high mortalities when infected experimentally, although Sieburth and Johnson (276) reported 50% mortality in day-old chicks given $10^{3.5}$ viable organisms of orally administered *S. typhimurium* organisms. Thaxton et al. (315) and Soerjadi et al. (302) found that lowering the brooding temperature (18–24 C) considerably increased the level of mortality caused by *S. worthington* or *S. typhimurium* infection in newly hatched chicks. It was concluded that a normal body temperature is essential for neonatal chickens to resist PT infections.

Snoeyenbos et al. (295) demonstrated that 10 salmonella serotypes spread rapidly from infected day-old chicks to penmates reared on litter, but mortality was confined chiefly to the infected principals and was low. Clinical signs were minimal or undetected.

Experimental efforts to produce chronic PT infection in chicks and poults by oral inoculation often result in a transitory disease. Organisms can be isolated from tissues and intestines for a few weeks following the acute phase of infection but not after 1–2 mo. In field cases, the course of the disease may be longer than that seen under controlled experimental conditions.

Sadler et al. (256) found that the older the chickens, the greater the number of *S. typhimurium* organisms required to infect them. Excretion rates in feces on the 38th, 73rd, and 94th day postinfection were only 8, 1, and 0.5%, respectively.

Mortality under natural conditions varies depending on environment, strain of infecting organism, and presence of concurrent infections. Sieburth and Johnson (276) found that the bluecomb agent (turkey coronavirus), when administered to susceptible chicks in conjunction with *S. typhimurium,* increased mortality from 29 to 67%.

Boonchuvit and Hamilton (49) reported significant interaction resulting in increasing mortality in chickens fed aflatoxins and infected with PT organisms. Enlarged livers developed from which salmonellae could be isolated with increased frequency, and antisalmonella agglutinins increased dramatically in infected birds. In further studies, Boonchuvit et al. (50) found that T-2 toxin increased mortality from PT infections in chickens, but agglutinin titers were unaltered. Wyatt and Hamilton (376) demonstrated that broiler chicks with a natural congenital infection of *S. worthington* required a lower concentration of dietary aflatoxin (0.625 μg/g) to depress growth than was required in uninfected chicks (2.50 μg/g).

Leaney et al. (178) used cloacal inoculation to establish a quantitatively reproducible intestinal and systemic salmonella infection in hatchlings, and considered it a possibly important infection route in natural circumstances. Arakawa et al. (18) exposed chickens to salmonellae for 5 consecutive days and infected them with coccidia. There was a significant increase in number of salmonellae in coccidia-infected ceca and livers when compared with those of birds given salmonella alone. There have been several similar reports showing the increased ability of salmonellae organisms to invade the cecal and intestinal mucosa when birds are infected with various species of coccidia (19, 20, 109, 110, 163, 206, 310).

ADULT BIRDS. Adult birds infected with PT organisms generally show no outward signs; however, they may serve as intestinal carriers of the infection over long periods (223). PT infections exhibit no selectivity in their pathogenicity for specific strains or breeds of birds. Savov et al. (265) produced ascending genital tract infection in 49 hens by instilling *S. typhimurium* labeled with ^{32}P into the cloaca. The organism was present on the shell of 30 of 95 eggs and in the yolk of 1 egg. It was recovered from the cloaca, oviduct, and ovarian follicles but not viscera. Cox et al. (75) found approximately 25% of laying hens to pass salmonellae in their feces following experimental oral infection. Less than 10% of egg samples from the same birds were salmonella-positive; only 1 egg yielded the organisms from its contents, and none of the tissues taken from the birds at the end of the experiment carried salmonellae.

Lee et al. (179) found that intravenous (IV) inoculation of 1×10^6 *S. typhimurium* organisms into adult chickens established infection in the liver, spleen, and intestinal tract of all birds. The organism persisted in these sites until day 9, after which it was cleared rapidly from all sites. Detectable levels of agglutinating and hemagglutinating antibodies were still found in serum and bile at 6 wk postinfection. Cell-mediated immunity was detected at day 14.

PATHOGENESIS AND EPIZOOTIOLOGY

Natural and Experimental Hosts. PT infections occur in most species of warm- and cold-blooded animals. Many of the salmonella serotypes, particularly members of Kauffmann's subgenus II, have appeared only in cold-blooded animals. Among domestic poultry, PT infections are most frequently encountered in turkeys and chickens. Smith (282) reviewed the epizootiology of salmonella infections in poultry with a complete discussion of all natural sources.

TURKEYS. PT infections are more prevalent in turkeys than in any other domestic avian species. Pfaff (225, 226) was the first to report on occurrence of PT in turkeys. Pomeroy and Fenstermacher (229) first observed this infection in turkeys in 1932. Hinshaw and McNeil (148) found that *S. typhimurium* accounted for approximately 50% of the PT outbreaks in turkeys investigated by them. McBride et al. (193) investigated the incidence of salmonellae in 25 turkey flocks entering a processing plant. Considerable flock-to-flock variability was found (0–72%), with one-third of the flocks having greater than 10% infection. Certain growers were found to ship salmonella-infected flocks repeatedly. There was no difference in infection levels between hens, toms, and broilers, and the seasonal effect was not significant. This study has shown that it is possible to pinpoint specific salmonella-infected flocks that may be contributing to dissemination of salmonellae in the plant. Pomeroy et al. (232) reported that approximately 50% of turkey candidate flocks tested from 1980–84 were infected with one or more serotypes of salmonellae.

Bagley and Ramsay (21) isolated 46 serotypes during an 11-yr monitoring program in an integrated turkey operation. Serogroups B, C, and E represented 82.6% of all isolates. Feed and ingredients were the major source (71%) of new serotypes entering the operation.

CHICKENS. In 1899, Mazza (192) was one of the first to describe a PT epizootic among chickens in various parts of northern Italy. Since that time, various workers have reported many outbreaks of salmonellosis in chickens due to a variety of species including *S. thompson, S. typhimurium, S. anatum, S. bareilly, S. california, S. london, S. montevideo,* and *S. newington* (124, 278, 311, 373). Losses ranged from 20 to 100%. Little correlation was found between salmonella serotypes in feed ingredients and those identified from the flocks.

Generally, mortality was a problem only in young birds. Resistance of chickens to salmonella infection increased rapidly with age with infection levels dropping significantly by the 3rd to 5th week (86, 210). Therefore, special attention should be given to prevention of infection of chicks during the brooding period.

Rigby and Pettit (248) found that infection spread rapidly through chicks on new litter contaminated by infected seeders. As the flock matured, fewer of the birds examined were infected, and the number of organisms in their ceca and feces decreased. Subjecting chickens to transport stress did not increase shedding or detectable infection. McGarr et al. (196) found that one of five infected breeder flocks was transmitting salmonellae vertically to progeny. Infected broiler flocks introduced salmonellae to the processing plants and many of the salmonellae serotypes found on carcasses at consumer outlets were similar to those found on broiler-flock farms. A total of 228 salmonella isolates were recovered from 7875 samples examined. Rigby et al. (251) were unable to isolate salmonellae from a 4160-bird broiler flock even though nest litter samples from four of the eight parent flocks were positive. Processed carcasses yielded salmonellae, and the most likely source was plastic transport crates. The crate washer did not reduce incidence of contaminated crates.

Kapoor et al. (156) studied the epidemiology of salmonellosis in poultry on an organized poultry farm; two outbreaks of *S. bareilly,* one in chickens and one in quail, were traced back to a breeding hen. *S. richmond* and *S. stanley* were isolated from other chickens and fish meal as well as from rats on the farm. Native breeds of poultry were free from salmonellae.

Van Roekel (329) reviewed salmonellae in poultry and eggs.

GEESE AND DUCKS. Young geese and ducks are quite susceptible to PT infection, and outbreaks often become epizootic. Vuillaume and Labatut (332) discussed salmonella carriers among geese.

Rettger and Scoville (246) described *S. anatum* as the cause of a disease in ducks known as "keel" (from "keel over," i.e., die suddenly). This term has come to be accepted as a synonym for PT infection as it occurs in ducks, but may be a misnomer since there are often protracted signs (237). Truscott (318) reported a severe outbreak of *S. moscow* infection in ducklings. This salmonella type had not previously been identified from fowl in North America.

Dougherty (84) noted that PT infection is enzootic in ducks on Long Island; according to Price et al. (237) 93% of positive cultures during 1950–60 were *S. typhimurium* and only 1% were *S. anatum*. Bisgaard (42) reported a high incidence of *S. typhimurium* in the intestinal tract of ducks maintained on free range or in open houses. Proper egg washing and confinement of duck breeders will minimize the problem of salmonellosis in ducklings (24).

PIGEONS. The pigeon fancier usually refers to PT infection as "megrims." Gauger et al. (116) published a comprehensive study of pigeon infection with *S. typhimurium* var. *copenhagen*. These authors listed 26 references to PT epizootics in pigeons. Over 97% of all cultures of *S. typhimurium* isolated from pigeons were *S. typhimurium* var. *copenhagen* (92, 208, 375). This organism, unlike typical *S. typhimurium* strains, lacks the somatic antigen 5 and does not ferment maltose (286). It is a unique example of a PT type exhibiting host specificity and has resulted in most investigators suspecting direct or indirect association with pigeons as the source of infection when this type is encountered in other species of animals, although Wuthe (375) noted that it does not seem to spread to other animals.

Pigeons surviving PT outbreaks often become chronic carriers, excreting the organisms intermittently in feces. Epizootics may occur among adult flocks, especially if resistance is lowered by other conditions. Van Ulsen (330) found feces from 1 of 25 carrier pigeons positive, and Müller (208) suggested that pigeons should test salmonella-negative before exhibitions or flying contests.

OTHER BIRDS. Goodchild and Tucker (122) presented an excellent review of the literature on salmonella infections in wild birds. The most common serotypes involved were *S. typhimurium* and *S. typhimurium* var. *copenhagen*. Graham (130) studied an outbreak of PT among quail in which *S. oranienburg* was found to be the causative organism.

Parrots, canaries, and budgerigars all have been found infected with *S. typhimurium* or *S. heidelberg*, with mortality sometimes reaching 50% (35, 64, 65, 139, 160). Several serotypes have been isolated from seagulls and mallard ducks (65, 258, 360), and Oelke and Steiniger (222) reported isolation of salmonellae from penguins and skuas in Antarctica. The organisms were more frequently isolated from chicks than adult birds.

The frequency of isolations of salmonellae and the extremely wide range of wild-bird species found infected by many workers in widely separated areas of the world (354) suggest that paratyphoid infections are nondiscriminatory and only require access to the organisms. Sometimes, infections can be linked to obvious sources, e.g., sewage outfalls or treatment plants, animal clinics, quarantine stations, etc. The possibility that infections in wild birds could result in spread to humans and domestic animals has been noted (150, 317). Readers interested in salmonellosis as a disease of wild birds should refer to Davis et al. (79).

OTHER ANIMALS. PTs are common pathogens of all species of domestic and wild mammals. Cattle, swine, sheep, goats, dogs, cats, horses, mink, foxes, and reptiles are among the many animal species that may be chronically infected, healthy carriers and shed the organisms in large numbers in feces. In these animals, PT usually occurs as an acute disease only in the very young or in old debilitated animals under extreme stress conditions. For a review of salmonella infections of animals other than poultry, see Buxton (65).

Rats and mice are frequently intestinal carriers of PT organisms, particularly *S. typhimurium* and *S. enteritidis*. When *S. enteritidis* is encountered in poultry, it is logical to suspect these rodents as a possible source of the infection. Sato et al. (263) found wild rats to spread salmonella infections to poultry flocks. Goyal and Singh (129) studied sources of salmonellae on a poultry farm and found that rodents, free-flying birds, and lizards were the most important.

Krabisch and Dorn (172) isolated salmonellae from 20.9% of 349 carrier vectors living in direct contact with broiler flocks. Contaminated vectors included mice, beetles, flies, and cats. No salmonellae were isolated from 13 rats.

INSECTS AND PARASITES. Salmonellae have also been isolated from various insects including flies, fleas, beetles, and cockroaches. It is known that *S. enteritidis* can be transmitted through the complete life cycle of flies and that the infection may continue as long as 4 wk within flies (131).

PT isolations have been made from a variety of insects including bluebottle (*Calliphora* sp.) flies, houseflies, ticks, lice, fleas, cockroaches, and lessor mealworms and from freshly collected *Ascaridia galli* (63, 136, 160, 309). Geissler and Kösters

(117) fed an *S. thompson* culture to adult beetles and larvae about to pupate. Infection was demonstrated in adults for up to 15 days and in newly emerged beetles infected as larvae. It is considered that the presence of the insects in chicken houses could cause salmonella infections in successive batches of birds.

HUMANS. In the U.S. approximately 40,000 salmonellosis cases are reported annually to Centers for Disease Control (CDC), Atlanta, Georgia, and it is estimated that 2 million cases actually occur with 2,000 deaths (253). Statistics compiled by CD C from 1973 to 1984 showed that chicken was implicated in only 5% of salmonellosis outbreaks for which the vehicle was known.

Beef or veal accounted for 19%, pork for 7%, dairy products for 6% and turkeys for 9%. Microbiological examination of broilers at the processing level revealed the rate of salmonella contamination was 36.9% in a 1979 survey and 35.2% in a 1982–84 survey (87). In Canada, the number of laboratory-confirmed cases of human salmonellosis was approximately 10,000 annually (153). The prevalence of salmonella in chicken carcasses in 1983 was 50.6%, turkeys 68.8%, geese 60%, pork 11.6% and beef 1.5% (37). There are several reviews of human salmonellosis and the importance of animals (including poultry) as a source of infection (7, 59–61, 277, 324). Recent reports of human cases caused by *S. enteritidis* have implicated grade A eggs and egg products as a vehicle for the salmonella (307).

Cohen and Blake (71) reported poultry to be the most important source of salmonella infections for humans. Rowe et al. (254) reported that *S. hadar* is now the second commonest salmonella serotype isolated from cases of food poisoning in England and Wales. Turkeys are the main reservoir of the organism. The subject of salmonella organisms on processed poultry intended for market sale has been discussed by Dougherty (85), Watson and Brown (335), Cox et al. (76), Campbell et al. (67), and Williams (349).

Borland (51) noted that poultry may acquire a wide range of salmonella serotypes from various sources, including feeds, breeding flocks, rodents, wild birds, and other vectors. Clinical disease is uncommon, but all infections are important as potential sources of food poisoning in humans. McGarr et al. (195) called attention to the high incidence of salmonella contamination of consumer poultry products and discussed the problem of elimination of these organisms at the various stages of poultry production and carcass processing. A rise in multiple resistance of the strains has made large-scale antibiotic therapy ineffective.

Since pasteurization became mandatory for raw, frozen, and dried chicken egg products in interstate shipment in 1966, salmonella outbreaks in humans from this source have ceased. Fresh shell eggs have never posed a salmonella problem for humans until recently (307). For a review of the past history of eggs and egg products as a source of human salmonellosis, see Cunningham (77), Williams and Hobbs (362), or Williams (349).

Transmission, Carriers, Vectors. Wide distribution of organisms contributes to their rapid spread. Bowmer (53) noted that most poultry flocks are exposed to salmonellae at some stage of their lives. Frequent isolation of organisms from eggs has resulted in reference to the disease as an egg-borne infection. However, it is important to distinguish between direct ovarian transmission and transmission through shell penetration.

DIRECT OVARIAN TRANSMISSION. PT infections of turkeys may occasionally be directly transmitted through the ovaries; the rate of egg infection is low. Yamamoto et al. (377) isolated *S. typhimurium* from ovaries of an experimentally infected adult turkey.

Direct ovarian transmission is apparently uncommon in chickens. Mundt and Tugwell (209) were unable to recover salmonellae from contents of eggs laid by white leghorn pullets experimentally infected orally and intravenously with various types of PT organisms. However, the organisms were recovered from shells of eggs laid 24 days postinfection and from feces after 35 days. Forsythe et al. (108) were unable to establish a localized infection of the reproductive tracts of hens by direct ovarian inoculation of *S. anatum;* none of the eggs produced by such hens was contaminated.

Snoeyenbos et al. (294) isolated motile salmonellae from the ovary, peritoneal cavity, or both sites from a total of 63 semimature or mature chickens of 1050 submitted for bacteriologic examination as serologic reactors to pullorum-typhoid antigen. In a few cases, pathologic ovarian follicles were found, and the pathogen was isolated on direct plate cultures. It was suggested that at least some non-host-adapted salmonellae produce local infections of the ovary and peritoneum of laying chickens, allowing contamination of egg contents prior to shell formation. Although the incidence of such infection is probably low, these studies suggest that true egg transmission may sometimes occur. *S. enteritidis* is occasionally egg transmitted (36). Apparently there are strain differences since Morales-Diaz (202) found that the Benson strain of *S. enteritidis* infected the magma of the egg directly, whereas the Rochester strain failed to infect eggs even when the hens were shedding organisms in the feces.

EGGSHELL CONTAMINATION AND PENETRATION

Fecal Carrier. Fecal contamination of eggshells during laying or from contaminated nests, floor, or incubators after laying is of foremost importance in spread of the disease. Intestinal carriers of the organisms are common. Buxton and Gordon (66) reported an instance in which *S. thompson* infected the gallbladder of a chicken and the organisms were excreted in feces for at least 18 mo. Board et al. (48) reported isolation of only one salmonella strain, *S. senftenberg,* from the shell of a lightly soiled egg during an extensive survey of microbial contamination of eggshells and egg-packing materials. The main source of salmonella contamination of contents of chicken eggs appears to be shell contamination resulting from fecal contact (108, 198). Smyser et al. (289) isolated *S. heidelberg* from contents of only a small percentage of eggs laid by hens known to be intestinal carriers of the organisms. Most isolations from shell surfaces resulted from eggs being contaminated in the nests.

Shell Penetration. Schalm (266) demonstrated that *S. typhimurium* in fecal material smeared on the surface of chicken eggs was capable of penetrating the shell and multiplying within the egg. Several workers have since concluded that eggshell contamination with subsequent penetration can be involved in transmission of salmonellae (26, 114, 155, 169, 279), although rates of contamination from infected birds may be low (26) or absent (25). Thus, PT organisms might be introduced into the incubator by contaminated eggs, with subsequent spread to hatched chicks or poults. Organisms that have gained entrance into the egg are able to multiply rapidly in the yolk and subsequently infect the developing embryo, which may die or hatch to serve as a source of infection for other young birds. Egg albumen has very little inhibitory effect on salmonellae that penetrate the shell (1). A historic review, dating to 1895, of experimental studies of salmonella penetration of chicken eggshells was presented by Williams et al. (372).

Gordon and Tucker (125) found *S. menston* on the shell and in membranes, albumen, and yolks of eggs from chickens fed the organisms. Williams et al. (372) found that *S. typhimurium* penetrated all outer structures of chicken eggs after as few as 6 min incubation at 37.2 C. Defects in shell structure, including cracks, rather than shell thickness determined the degree to which salmonellae could penetrate into eggs. Moisture aided penetration. Chicken eggs were more resistant to shell penetration by *S. typhimurium* as embryonic development took place (357).

Gauger and Greaves (114) recovered *S. typhimurium* from both shells and contents of eggs from experimentally infected turkeys. Penetration of turkey eggshells may occur within a few hours and continue for many days (308). Williams and Dillard (358) demonstrated that turkey eggshells without pigmentation have more gross openings and were thinner than speckled eggshells, and were much more likely to be penetrated by *S. typhimurium.*

Simmons et al. (281) reported that salmonellae survived better on the surface of eggs at lower temperatures, but that shell penetration was less. A higher relative humidity contributed to growth of organisms on the shell. Sauter and Peterson (264) reported progressive decrease of penetration of chicken eggshells by salmonellae as eggshell quality increased.

With *S. enteritidis,* there were strain differences in egg penetration, survival in the albumin, and migration from albumin to yolk (greater with the Rochester than the Benson strain) (202).

INCUBATOR, HATCHERY, BROODER, ENVIRONMENT. Contaminated eggshells, down, dust, and other debris of the hatch may also serve as a source of infection in the incubator. From the incubator, organisms may be distributed by air currents throughout the hatchery. Samples of air taken within the hatchery may remain positive for several weeks or months, and the infection may spread to subsequent hatches through this means. Gauger and Greaves (115) demonstrated that contaminated drinking water could serve as a source of the disease in an infected environment, and Adler et al. (2) recovered *S. typhimurium* from dust, litter, and feathers for 71, 44, and 37 days, respectively, following experimental oral infection of poults.

PT infection, when established in the brooder, is rapidly transmitted by inhalation, fecal contamination of feed and water, or direct consumption of fecal matter by young birds. Repeated passage of the organism results in an infection of increased severity.

The disease may be transmitted directly to young birds from older fowl that are asymptomatic chronic intestinal carriers and also by fomites such as footwear, feed bags, shipping crates, or brooding equipment. Rigby and Pettit (249) found that carriage of *S. typhimurium* was significantly higher among birds placed in shipping crates than among uncrated controls, mainly as a result of an increase in cecal carriers (from 23.5 to 61.5%). Twenty-four chickens placed in crates contaminated with *S. alachua* all became carriers. These results indicate that chickens exposed to salmonellae in shipping crates under transport conditions may readily become infected and begin to shed organisms within 24 hr.

POULTRY FEEDS. Williams (353, 354) comprehensively reviewed salmonellae in poultry feeds, covering all important references pertaining to incidence, distribution, and sources of salmonellae in poultry feeds; methods of isolation and identification of the organisms; and methods of control and elimination. The role of poultry feeds and feed ingredients in the epidemiology of salmonellosis in poultry and humans also has been reviewed (91, 111, 231). With widespread distribution of salmonellae in poultry feeds, it is difficult to try to control the disease.

Poultry feeds may be a common and very important source of PT organisms. The level of contamination is normally low; however, infection can result from 1 organism/1–15 g feed (125, 140).

The National Marine Fisheries Service of the US Department of Commerce offers an effective national voluntary cooperative program (112) that provides guidelines and analyzes and surveys plants three times a year to ascertain the status of salmonella contamination in fish meal. Walker (333) reviewed the experience of the USDA in cooperation with the states in evaluating both the presence of salmonellae in feed and feed ingredients during the 1960s and a subsequent program aimed at eliminating salmonellae from animal and fish proteins used in animal feeds. Also a brief review was made of the 5-yr study in California aimed at establishing salmonella-free turkey flocks.

Hacking (134) found a direct correlation between salmonella serotypes isolated from poultry feed and those from the litter of flocks receiving the feed. MacKenzie and Bains (184) similarly observed a significant correlation between salmonella serotypes isolated from raw feed ingredients and those from finished carcasses. It appeared that a significant reduction in carcass contamination could be achieved by minimizing salmonellae in meat and grain constituents of poultry feed. Egger (93) reported that in 1975–77, 908 salmonellae of 60 different serotypes were identified from 6019 samples of poultry feeds of animal origin from 23 countries submitted to the Swiss Veterinary Directorate's Meat Bacteriology Section. Bhatia and McNabb (39) traced dissemination of salmonella infection from fluff and meconium collected at the hatchery to feed and litter at the farm and ultimately to carcasses rinsed at the processing plant. The same serotypes were involved, and properly pelleted feed did not seem to be an important source of infection.

Using salmonella-free feed is not a panacea that will stop all animal infections, but it is an important step in reducing them; it is necessary that this measure be instituted first so that other parts of the animal cycle can be assessed with regard to their true role in perpetuation of infections (362). Active programs aimed at eliminating the organisms need to be undertaken immediately. Recommended sanitation guidelines for salmonella control in the processing of poultry feeds and animal by-products and industrial fishery products are available (16).

OTHER ANIMAL SOURCES AND HUMANS. Rats and mice are frequent carriers of the organisms, and their droppings may contaminate feed. Pigeons, sparrows, and various other species of wild birds may also serve as a source of infection for domestic poultry flocks. Attention has already been drawn to dogs, cats, swine, cattle, sheep, and goats as sources of PT infections for poultry. Human contact must also be recognized as a possible source; this may involve not only caretakers but also human waste products. Hinshaw et al. (149) record instances of humans transmitting the infection to poults. Poultry may serve as a source of salmonellosis for other animal species on the farm.

DIRECT SPREAD AMONG ADULT AND YOUNG CHICKENS. In transmission among adult poultry, feces of infected carriers are probably the most common source of the organisms. The bacterial population and nature of the environment are among many factors that determine the extent of such transmission. Snoeyenbos et al. (293) did not find direct transmission of established salmonella flock infections between houses, even though there was ample opportunity for transfer of large numbers of salmonellae from pen to pen. Litter from pens containing chicks known to be infected with *S. montevideo* yielded a high percentage of positive samples (87.5%) during the first 16 wk but a very low percentage thereafter. On the other hand, Snoeyenbos et al. (296) reported that salmonella transmission from pens contaminated by the previous generation appeared to be a major means of perpetuating infection between generations.

Signs. Signs of PT infections closely resemble those observed in pullorum disease, fowl typhoid, avian arizonosis, and several other diseases. Young birds with generalized salmonella infections may show signs and lesions identical to any acute septicemia caused by a wide variety of bacteria including *Escherichia coli.* Joint involvement caused by PT organisms in all avian species may be mistaken for synovitis or bursitis caused by other infectious agents.

YOUNG BIRDS. Basically, PT infection is a disease of young fowl, with environmental conditions, degree of exposure, and presence of concurrent infections having an important influence on severity of an outbreak. In acute outbreaks, with deaths occurring in the incubator or during the first few days after hatching, no signs may be noted. In such instances infection is acquired by egg transmission or early incubator exposure. A high proportion of pipped and unpipped eggs containing dead embryos may be observed.

Signs of PT infections in all species of young fowl are very similar and include a progressive state of somnolence evidenced by a tendency to stand in one position with head lowered, eyes closed, wings drooping, and feathers ruffled; marked anorexia and increased water consumption; profuse, watery diarrhea with pasting of the vent; and a tendency of the birds to huddle together near the source of heat. Respiratory signs are not commonly observed.

In poults infected orally with broth cultures of *S. typhimurium,* losses started 2–3 days and stopped 2 wk postexposure (228). When signs are observed in young birds 1 wk of age or older, contact exposure or an outside source of the disease should be considered.

Blindness and conjunctivitis in chicks are frequently associated with salmonellosis (97, 176). Laursen-Jones (177) reported unilateral blindness in 12-day-old broiler chicks from *S. typhimurium.* At 28 days the main feature was a circular caseous plaque that seemed to fill the eyeball, which was shrunken. Dwivedi and Malhotra (89) dosed chicks with *S. typhimurium, S. saint-paul,* and *S. kentucky;* blindness developed in 40–50% of the chicks infected with *S. typhimurium* or *S. saint-paul* due to opacity of the cornea membrane.

Dougherty (83) and Price et al. (237) found that ducklings infected with PT usually die slowly, tremble and gasp for air, and very often have pasted vents. Eyelids frequently become swollen and edematous. Rasmussen (242) described the frequency with which *S. typhimurium* is associated with arthritis in ducks.

Das et al. (78) reported that pigeons with salmonellosis demonstrated anorexia, greenish diarrhea, droopiness, and death within 2–3 days. Infected squabs are often retarded in growth, underweight, and exhibit a general depression and listlessness accompanied by a partial or complete inappetence (100).

ADULT BIRDS. Mature fowl generally exhibit no outward signs of the infection. Acute outbreaks in semimature and adult birds under natural conditions are rare.

Experimental PT infection of adult chickens and turkeys by the parenteral or oral route of administration results in an acute disease of short duration. Signs during the acute stage include inappetence, increased water consumption, diarrhea, dehydration, and general listlessness. Recovery is rapid in most cases, and death losses do not usually exceed 10%. Kashiwazaki et al. (157) described the signs and pathologic findings during a field outbreak of *S. typhimurium* infection in adult chickens. Watery diarrhea, general depression and listlessness, droopy wings, and ruffled feathers were listed.

Gross Lesions and Histopathology

YOUNG BIRDS. Lesions may be entirely absent in extremely severe outbreaks. In outbreaks permitting development of advanced cases, lesions most commonly observed are emaciation, dehydration, coagulated yolks, congested liver and spleen with hemorrhagic streaks or pinpoint necrotic foci, congested kidneys, and pericarditis with adhesions. However, heart and lung lesions are not as frequently observed as in pullorum disease. Hemorrhagic enteritis involving the duodenum is a common occurrence in poults. Cecal cores are occasionally observed. Ballantyne (27) reported that caseous ceca were found in 33% of poults infected with *S. oranienburg,* in 46% infected with *S. typhimurium,* and in 20% infected with *S. newport.* Caseous ceca also occurred in 33% of chicks with *S. typhimurium* infection.

Lukas and Bradford (183) classified necropsy findings of PT outbreaks in poults during a survey in California: 1) systemic involvement with lesions such as pericarditis, necrotic foci in the liver and heart, air sac involvement, central nervous system disturbance, and severe catarrhal enteritis with cecal cores (20.8% of specimens); 2) uncomplicated catarrhal enteritis (33.2% of specimens); 3) enteritis complicated with coccidiosis, hexamitiasis, or sinusitis and air sac infection (28.4% of specimens); 4) other findings such as water starvation, ascites, mycosis (15% of specimens); and 5) no gross lesions (2.5% of specimens). *S. typhimurium* was most frequently involved in systemic cases; other types such as *S. anatum* and *S. manhattan* were commoner in cases with uncomplicated diarrhea.

Anderson and Stephens (4) found that infection of chicks with either *S. anatum* or *S. heidelberg* resulted in development of severe heterophilic leukopenia and significant increase in percentage of both juveniles and lymphocytes by 48 hr postinoculation. Sidoli (271) observed purulent panophthalmia with corneal hyperplasia in 18 of 60 chicks that died during an outbreak of salmonellosis. Cantini and Rossi (68) reported that about 5% of 4000 female chicks infected with *S. typhimurium* exhibited a lesion in one eye only. The conjunctiva, cornea, and pupil were affected, and a grayish yellow spherical mass about 4 mm in diameter appeared in the anterior chamber. Williams (348) described an outbreak of *S. thompson* infection in chicks with severe fibropurulent perihepatitis and pericarditis identical to that observed in air sac disease.

Kodama et al. (168) demonstrated that bactericidal activity of splenic phagocytes from 0-day-old chicks was higher against *S. senftenberg* than *S. pullorum* and similar to that of the phagocytes from 2-mo-old chickens, indicating that the splenic phagocytes had acquired the activity before hatching.

Bayer et al. (32) infected 1-day-old chicks with *S. typhimurium.* The impact on the intestinal mucosa was observed by scanning and transmission electron microscopy (EM). Salmonella-infected birds had areas of intestinal mucosa devoid of microvilli; probably this interfered with nutrient absorption. Using both light microscopy and EM, Turnbull and Richmond (325) studied penetration patterns of *S. enteritidis* in chick intestines. In epithelial cells, bacteria were enclosed within membrane-bound vacuoles and appeared undamaged by intracellular passage.

Price et al. (237), in necropsy studies of ducklings infected with salmonellae, found necrotic foci in the liver, cheesy plugs in the ceca, impaction of the rectum, and blanching of the kidneys. Rasmussen (242) described the pathology of arthritis in slaughter ducks, predominantly from *S. typhimurium* infection. Among 827 arthritic ducks, *S. typhimurium* was isolated from 12% of inflamed hock joints, 75% of knee joints, and 52% of hip joints. Sokkar and Bassiouni (306) found that White Pekin ducks experimentally infected with *S. typhimurium* developed prominent splenic lesions, which consisted of fibrinoid deposits that replaced the lymphoid follicles after lymphocytic necrosis.

Arthritis is commonly observed in paratyphoid infection of pigeons. It most frequently involves the wing joints and is evident as soft subcutaneous swellings. Swelling of the eyelids is also common in pigeons. Das et al. (78) described yellow-green fibrinous deposits in the oral cavity, at the base of the tongue, and on the upper palate of pigeons infected with *S. typhimurium.*

ADULT BIRDS. Acutely infected adult fowl may reveal congested and swollen liver, spleen, and kidneys and hemorrhagic or necrotic enteritis, pericarditis, and peritonitis. Khera et al. (162) described an outbreak of avian salmonellosis in maturing pullets and hens caused by *S. stanley.* The disease was characterized by necrotic and hyperplastic lesions in the oviduct and suppurative and necrotic lesions in the ovaries, simulating *S. pullorum* infection. Lesions often progressed to generalized peritonitis.

Sapre and Mehta (261) artificially infected chickens with salmonellae and found significant hematologic changes that could be correlated with specific antibody titer increases. There was a decrease in packed-cell volume, hemoglobin, and total erythrocyte count but an increase in erythrocyte sedimentation rate, buffy coat, and total leukocyte count.

Leg weakness in mature birds is not uncommon. Higgins et al. (146) encountered a flock of 24-wk-old turkeys infected with PT in which 10% of the birds were so severely affected with an arthritic condition they were unsuitable for marketing. Chaplin and Hamilton (70) reported synovitis in turkeys, similar to that ascribed to staphylococcal infection, following intravenous inoculation of broth cultures of *S. thompson.*

Adult chronic carriers of PT infections are often submitted for necropsy as reactors to serologic tests for pullorum disease or *S. typhimurium* infection. Emaciation; necrotic ulcers in the intestines; enlarged liver, spleen, or kidneys; nodules on the heart; and distorted ovules may occasionally be noted. Pathologic changes in ovarian tissues as a result of PT infection are not so distinctive or common as those observed in chronic carriers of pullorum disease. Chronically infected adults frequently exhibit no lesions. This is particularly true of intestinal carriers.

DIAGNOSIS. Clinical observations and necropsy findings may be suggestive of PT infection when a supportive history is available and may permit one to reach a tentative diagnosis as a basis for early treatment or control recommendations. However, the final diagnosis depends on isolation and identification of causative organisms; these procedures require approximately 48–72 hr.

Faddoul and Fellows (101) found that in 78% of the positive consignments from chickens and 70% of those from turkeys, salmonellae were isolated only from the intestinal tract, where they have a predilection to establish a chronic infection in the ceca. Turnbull and Snoeyenbos (327, 328) found a preference of salmonellae for caudal regions. The crop appeared to be a potential reservoir of persisting infection at all ages, and major sites of movement of bacteria to internal tissues were the crop and the ceca.

Brownell et al. (56) found that sampling of both cecal contents and cecal tonsils of chickens was superior for salmonella isolation to sampling of either alone or any other area of the intestinal tract. Gerlach (119) reported that in chickens infected orally with salmonellae, the organisms persisted in the ceca, whereas in birds exposed by egg infection the organisms were found almost exclusively in the jejunum.

Snoeyenbos et al. (293) suggested that detection of PT-infected flocks on a practical basis remains one of the most serious unsolved problems in controlling salmonellosis of poultry, and that litter samples can be used to detect salmonella-infected chicken flocks.

The reliability of cloacal swab cultures as a diagnostic procedure for PT infection seems to be limited, since fecal excretion of the organisms may be intermittent (186, 369). Thus, failure to isolate the organisms did not prove absence of infection in flocks. Recovery of salmonellae from cloacas or from dead-in-shell embryos indicated the likelihood of clinical disease in the progeny. Brown et al. (57) orally infected cockerals with *S. typhimurium* and observed cloacal shedding only shortly after infection.

Culture of floor litter was more effective than serologic tests or cloacal swab culture for detecting experimental *S. typhimurium* infection (223), and nest litter gave the highest frequency of isolations in comparisons of various environmental sampling to detect organisms (293).

According to Higgins et al. (147), dust may be contaminated even after houses are disinfected, and fresh feces were a more reliable source than litter for detecting salmonellae.

Fluff samples collected in hatcheries have proved to be a very effective method of detecting PT infections early. Miura et al. (200) sampled 300 hatchery fluff samples from commercial hatcheries in Japan and found 52.7% infected with salmonellae. Bacteriologic examination of yolk material from embryos dying between days 19 and 21 proved a practical method of detecting carrier flocks in Great Britain (34).

Weinack et al. (337) found that chicks infected at 1 day of age yielded the highest level of positive cloacal swab cultures, whereas exposure of older birds gave maximal serologic titers, which persisted after salmonellae could no longer be isolated from cloacal swabs or environmental samples.

Culture of the shell and shell membranes is an effective procedure for detecting contaminated eggs (132). Harvey and Price (143) recommended that in culturing animal feeds, four 25-g samples be examined from each consignment, and provided specific procedures for enrichment and plating of cultures.

Isolation and Identification of Causative Agent. Harvey and Price (143), Ellis et al. (96), and Williams et al. (373) presented detailed outlines of standard laboratory procedures for effective isolation of PT organisms from poultry tissues, eggs, embryos, feed, and vaccines as well as various environmental sources, including litter. Recently, the American Feed Industries Association (16) published a booklet entitled Recommended Salmonella Control Guidelines for Processors of Livestock and Poultry Feeds, outlining sampling and analysis procedures for feed and feed ingredients. For further information on liquid and solid media discussed in this section, see Ewing (98).

CULTURE. For direct culture of fresh organs of diseased birds, tissues are seared and transfers streaked with a loop or swab on the surface of slants or plates of a nutrient medium such as veal infusion agar. Cultures are read after incubation for 24 and 48 hr at 37 C. Tissues can also be triturated and enriched in a selective broth for 24 and 48 hr at 37 C prior to plating on a selective agar as discussed below. All fecal samples as well as specimens in a state of decomposition are enriched in a selective broth for 24–48 hr, preferably incubated at 42–43 C, prior to plating on selective agar.

Fresh hatching eggs can best be cultured by triturating both the shell and membranes without contents and incubating in selective broth for 24 and 48 hr at 37 C before plating on selective agar. It is difficult to isolate salmonellae from contents of fresh eggs; this is more readily accomplished with contents of incubated eggs enriched in nutrient and selective broths. The yolk sac and its contents provide the best source for recovery of salmonellae from the embryos. For cloacal swab cultures from living birds, a moistened cotton swab is inserted into the cloaca and then withdrawn. The swab is incubated for 24 and 48 hr at 37 or 42 C in selective enrichment broth and plated on selective agar.

Air in a hatchery can be examined for salmonellae by exposing open plates of selective agar at various points during a hatch. Fluff samples can also be collected, cultured in enrichment broth, and then plated on selective agar. Litter from floors or nests can be cultured in enrichment broth at 42 C prior to plating at 24 and 48 hr.

Standard requirements for testing vaccines for salmonella contaminants have been issued by Veterinary Services of the USDA (10). Vaccine samples should be collected from the bulk suspension; 5 ml of the liquid vaccine suspension should be used to inoculate each 100 ml of nutrient and 100 ml of selective enrichment broth incubated at 37 C and plated on selective agar after 24 and 48 hr.

Rapid confirmation procedures for suspect salmonella colonies include using a Minitek system in conjunction with serologic tests (73) and noncommercial microtests in conjunction with API 20E for rapid identification of Enterobacteriaceae (118).

MEDIA. The most popular selective enrichment broths for PT isolation include tetrathionate broth base with 1:100,000 brilliant green (BG), selenite BG sulfa, and selenite F. These media are available commercially dehydrated and may be tubed in 10-ml amounts or dispensed in wide-mouthed flasks in 100-ml quantities for triturated tissues. A 10% inoculum of the specimen is made into these broths.

Solid selective plating media for isolation of PTs include BG, BG sulfa, salmonella-shigella, MacConkey's, and Hektoen agars. BG is probably the most widely used and preferred solid medium for isolation of PTs.

Smyser and Snoeyenbos (285) found that tetrathionate BG broth incubated at 42 C yielded a maximum number of salmonella isolations from rendered animal by-products and was superior to the enrichment/serology method. Harrington et al. (138) found that by compositing samples of animal by-products they were able to get culture results very similar to those obtained using standard methods.

Kumar et al. (174) observed that selenite BG with sulfapyridine and tetrathionate BG broths were equally effective in isolating salmonellae. Smyser and Snoeyenbos (284) found selenite BG sulfa broth incubated for 48 hr at 43 C to be the preferred enrichment medium for isolation of salmonellae from poultry litter and animal feed. Pourciau and Springer (236) reported that secondary enrichment of cultures in tetrathionate BG broth substantially increased salmonella recovery over that achieved with primary tetrathionate BG broth or primary selenite crystal broth.

Preenrichment in lactose broth prior to transfer to a selective broth has been recommended for any specimen in which salmonellae have been stressed in some way. This is particularly important in culturing materials such as poultry feeds. Although enrichment broths for isolation of salmonellae have conventionally been incubated at 37 C, a temperature of 42–43 C is particularly favorable for recovering salmonellae from feces-contaminated specimens.

Selective agar plates should be examined for colony types with a Quebec counter after both 24 and 48 hr of incubation at 37 C. On BG agar, salmonella colonies are usually transparent pink to deep fuchsia, surrounded by the reddened medium.

Usually two or three colonies are selected from plates with many typical colonies; if colonies are doubtful, more should be selected for transfer. The procedure is as follows: first stab the needle to the bottom of the butt of a tube of triple-sugar iron (TSI) agar and then streak the slant surface. With the same unheated needle inoculate a tube of lysine iron (LI) agar directly by stabbing the butt of the medium twice and streaking the slant. The TSI and LI agar tubes are incubated at 37 C for approximately 24 hr.

In TSI agar salmonellae will reveal an alkaline slant and acid (yellow) butt, with gas bubbles in the agar and a blackening due to hydrogen sulfide (H_2S) production that often obscures the acid reaction in the butt, of the tube. In LI agar slants salmonellae will show lysine decarboxylation with a purple (alkaline) slant and alkaline or neutral butt with slight blackening owing to H_2S production.

Cultures revealing typical reactions of salmonellae on TSI and LI agar slants are transferred to biochemical broths and other media for final identification. These media and the reactions of PT, arizona, and citrobacter organisms on them are listed in Table 3.6. Some members of the *Citrobacter* genus, a group of nonpathogenic enteric organisms, can be confused with PTs; therefore, typical reactions of this group are included.

Table 3.6. Typical reactions of paratyphoid, arizona, and citrobacter cultures on diagnostic media

Media	Paratyphoid	Arizona	Citrobacter
Dextrose	+	+	+
Lactose	–	(–)	d
Sucrose	–	–	d
Mannitol	+	+	+
Maltose	+	+	+
Dulcitol	+	–	d
Malonate	–	+	d
Urease	–	–	d
Potassium cyanide	–	–	+
Gelatin	–	(–)	–
Lysine decarboxylase	+	+	–
Beta-galactosidase	–	+	+ or –
Jordan's tartrate	+	–	+
Motility	+	+	+

Note: Abbreviations: + = positive with gas formation within 1–2 days incubation; (+) = positive reaction after 3 or more days; – = no reaction; (–) = most arizonae from avian sources ferment lactose only after 7–10 days; + or – = majority of strains positive, occasional cultures negative; d = different reactions, (+) or –.

Blackburn and Ellis (44) noted that 15.6% of salmonellae isolated from dried milk products and milk-drying plants fermented lactose. While these types of cultures are apparently rarely encountered among those from poultry, it is essential that bismuth sulfite agar be used for their detection in cases where they are suspected. Cox and Williams (74) reported use of six fermentation broths (dextrose, lactose, sucrose, mannitol, maltose, dulcitol) along with TSI and LI agars for salmonella identification and adapted readings to a miniaturized system.

Williams and Benson (356) studied the in vitro inhibitory effect of sodium nalidixate for 206 avian salmonella cultures of varying serotypes in liquid and on solid media. Salmonella cultures were much more resistant to lethal effects of sodium nalidixate in veal infusion broth than on a solid medium. The use of xylose lysine agar and BG agar containing Novobiocin increased the isolation of salmonellae (188).

IMMUNOFLUORESCENCE. Thomason (316) reviewed the current status of immunofluorescent methodology for identification of salmonellae. Fluorescent antibody (FA) procedures for detection of salmonellae in animal by-products and poultry feeds have been reported (95, 105, 137). However, these techniques have had only limited application to date for detecting salmonellae in avian tissues and fecal material. Information on their use and usefulness is available from several sources (22, 30, 31, 96, 245, 316). Smyser and Snoeyenbos (287) found that FA examination of litter samples can be expedited by using sample pools, but there was a high percentage of false-positive reactions.

Serology

SEROLOGIC TYPING. All salmonellae isolated in pure culture and identified biochemically should be submitted for serologic typing. They can be sent to the Salmonella Serotyping Laboratory, National Veterinary Services Laboratories, P.O. Box 844, Ames, Iowa 50010.

SEROLOGIC TESTING PROCEDURES. Procedures for serologic detection of adult carriers or PT infections have not been accepted or applied on the scale of those employed for detection of pullorum disease and fowl typhoid. Specific methodology for conducting the serologic tests discussed here will be referenced under each test and has been described elsewhere (8).

Macroscopic Tube Agglutination Test. The tube agglutination (TA) test for *S. typhimurium* has been most widely applied in testing turkey breeding flocks, but also in most other species of fowl, for PT. In 1983, approximately nine states in the USA were using the macroscopic TA test on a large scale to detect *S. typhimurium* in turkey breeding flocks; Minnesota and Texas have official blood-testing programs.

Intestinal carriers may reveal no serologic response by the TA test, and titers of birds that do react may fluctuate widely (66, 230, 289).

Specific antigens must be prepared for each salmonella type and laboratory personnel must be thoroughly familiar with salmonella serology and variations that may arise during testing procedures. Representative reactors to the TA test should be submitted for complete bacteriologic examination and laboratory confirmation of presence of the infection.

DeLay et al. (80) tested 593,341 turkeys with *S. typhimurium* antigens by the TA method; 4486 of the 7578 positive birds were from flocks subsequently found to have *S. typhimurium* carriers. The O antigen was found to be most useful in detecting carriers; birds positive to both O and H antigens were most likely to yield *S. typhimurium* on culture. They emphasized that a testing program for *S. typhimurium* is most effective when it is possible to practice complete replacement of all flocks shown to harbor carriers.

Studies by several workers (see 354) suggested that the TA test is useful in identifying infected flocks but that efficiency is sometimes low and correlation between serologic response and isolation of salmonellae is variable and often poor.

Rapid Serum Plate Test. Very limited application has been made of the rapid serum plate (SP) test for avian PT infections. Bierer and Vickers (41) found that the test, using stained antigen for *S. typhimurium,* was superior to the TA or the rapid whole-blood (WB) test in detecting turkeys demonstrated bacteriologically to be carriers of the organism. However, serologic tests were not entirely effective in detecting the infection. Kumar et al. (173) reported development of a new SP test for detection of *S. typhimurium* infection in turkey flocks. This test was more sensitive than the microagglutination test or the TA test for detecting reactors.

Rapid Whole-Blood Test. Blaxland et al. (47) described the preparation and use of a stained whole-blood *S. typhimurium* antigen for testing chickens, turkeys, and ducks by the rapid macroscopic plate method. Although they showed close agreement between TA and WB tests, and Smith et al. (283) found it to be of some value early after experimental infection, others considered it to be unreliable (263) and insensitive (369).

Indirect Hemagglutination Test. An indirect hemagglutination (HA) test (260, 272–276) may be of value in screening for detection of salmonella infections of poultry. Chicken erythrocytes sensitized with antigen liberated from boiled bacterial cells are used in the test. Polyvalent antigen was capable of detecting several antigenic types of the infection. It was stated that the indirect HA test, unlike the agglutination test, detected antibodies in chickens receiving furazolidone treatment. Hemagglutinins appeared earlier than conventional agglutinins, were 10–15 times higher, and persisted longer. Smith et al. (283) reported that the indirect HA test was most useful in detecting specific salmonella antibody in chickens.

Microagglutination and Microantiglobulin Tests. Williams and Whittemore (364), reported a microagglutination (MA) test and a sensitive and specific microantiglobulin (MAG) test for detection of agglutinins to *S. typhimurium* in poultry flocks. The MAG test enhanced titers as much as 16 times, and these persisted at a significant level for as long as 4 mo. Methodology in application of the MA and MAG tests in poultry flocks for detection of salmonella serogroups B, C, and D has been reviewed (15, 350, 365). Williams and Whittemore (367) used the MA and MAG tests to determine the antibody response of chickens ranging in age from 1 day to 126 days. In all groups 6 wk old or older, a high and continuing level of group B antibody was demonstrated by the MAG test but not by the MA test, which agreed very closely with the TA test. Serologic response was maximal at about 15 wk or later. Kumar et al. (173) found that the MAG test was superior to all other tests in detecting PT-infected birds.

The MAG test was found to be more sensitive and reliable than the TA, MA, rapid WB, and rapid SP tests in determining prior exposure of chickens to *S. typhimurium* infection (369). Also, when used with bird and litter culture, it proved to be the most reliable means of detecting naturally occurring salmonella infections (368). Several studies have confirmed the superiority of the MAG test over other serological tests and cultural methods for detecting infection with *S. typhimurium* (314), *S. thompson* and *S. pullorum* (370), *S. infantis* (217), and others (313).

Lee et al. (179) prepared a tetrazolium-stained *S. typhimurium* antigen for use in the MA test.

Other Tests. Rice et al. (247) applied the modified direct complement-fixation test for detection of salmonella antibodies in heat-inactivated turkey serum. Reactions recorded with partially purified somatic antigens were group-specific. Magwood and Annau (185) adsorbed crude and partially purified extracts containing salmonella somatic antigens on polystyrene latex particles, which were used in agglutination tests to detect salmonella agglutinins in turkey serum. The antigen revealed serologic specificity and was agglutinated by antibodies for the homologous salmonella groups.

PT Antigens. Various procedures have been recommended for preparation of antigens for use in conducting serologic tests for PT of poultry (8, 363). Presently, all testing being applied nationally for *S. typhimurium* infection is conducted using an antigen of the somatic (O) type. No official tests are being carried out for the detection of flagellar (H) agglutinins. The techniques usually employed in the USA for the preparation of TA antigen closely follow recommended methods (8).

A single strain of *S. typhimurium,* designated P-10, is used for preparation of TA antigen in the USA (346). This strain possesses only O antigens, since it is naturally nonmotile, unlike most group B organisms in the Kauffmann-White scheme. Strain P-10, which has antigens 4, 5, and 12, grows very well on common laboratory media. It yields an antigen of high stability and excellent sensitivity. The culture is best maintained by transferring every 3 mo to new nutrient agar stabs that are maintained in the dark at room temperature. With only a few exceptions, the recommendations for pullorum-typhoid TA antigen and its standardization can be applied to the TA antigen for *S. typhimurium* and most other salmonella serotypes. Several antigen strains may need to be examined before a satisfactory one is found; hypersensitivity is the main problem.

Kumar et al. (173) developed a rose bengal-stained rapid SP antigen having a low cell density and a pH of 6.0. Williams and Whittemore (369) used a tetrazolium-stained MA test antigen (no pH adjustment) for conducting rapid SP tests.

Most rapid WB antigens for PT infections are prepared the same as rapid WB pullorum-typhoid antigens (8). Gwatkin and Dzenis (133) prepared *S. typhimurium* rapid WB antigens for testing chickens using K medium and beef infusion agar. Kashiwazaki et al. (157) described a malachite green-stained rapid WB antigen that was used with some success for detection of *S. typhimurium* infection in chickens.

Williams and Whittemore (366) described procedures for preparing tetrazolium-stained *S. pullorum* (group D) and *S. typhimurium* (group B) microtest antigens on solid media. The same procedure can also be used to prepare salmonella group C microtest antigen using a naturally nonmotile variant of group C. Microtest antigens are available commercially.

Enzyme-linked Immunosorbent Assay (ELISA). Nagaraja et al. (212, 214) developed a sensitive and specific ELISA for use in the detection of *S. arizonae* infection in turkey breeder flocks. Outer membrane protein antigens extracted from *S. arizonae* were used as antigens.

TREATMENT

Chemotherapy. There are numerous publications on the use of sulfonamides, antibiotics, nitrofurans in the treatment of PT infections in chickens and turkeys (354). In the USA, furazolidone and injectable gentamicin and spectinomycin are approved for use (17). Williams and Whittemore (371) administered five antimicrobial agents in drinking water of chicks. If they were administered before infection, the drugs reduced the number of positive isolations of *S. typhimurium* from cloacal swabs. Sodium nalidixate was the most effective agent, followed in effectiveness by gentamicin, sulfathiazole, sulfamethazine, and chloramphenicol. Birds removed from treatment were found to be active carriers of *S. typhimurium.* There is experimental evidence to indicate some drugs actually increased the amount of salmonella excreted (29).

Competitive Exclusion. Royal and Mutimer (255) found that anaerobic cultures of poultry cecal contents grown in nutrient broth bufferred at pH 5.5 inhibited growth of *S. typhimurium.* Further, it was reported that when 1- to 2-day-old chicks were given normal intestinal contents or alimentary tract flora of adult birds prior to oral infection with *S. infantis,* colonization of their ceca was prevented and they were free of infection 1–2 wk later whereas controls were still infected (218, 241). Feed ingesta, cultured cecal microflora, and feces from adult chickens had the same protective property when fed to young birds, apparently due to anaerobes (220, 269, 297), and the method was found suitable for mass application. Lloyd et al. (181) reported similar resistance induction against *S. typhimurium* and suggested the term "competitive exclusion" to describe this phenomenon. They thought protection resulted from rapid establishment of a conventional indigenous microflora that inhibits establishment and growth by the invading enteric pathogen. Snoeyenbos et al. (299) reported that chicks monocolonized by salmonellae had persistent and undiminished colonization of all levels of the GI tract whereas those treated with a native protective microflora were infrequently colonized. Reciprocal protection was provided by native chicken and turkey intestinal microflora in chicks and poults; chicken and turkey microflora appeared to be equally effective in protecting the two species (339).

Nurmi and Rantala (219) found that zinc bacitracin administered to birds or mixed with in vitro cultures of intestinal flora did not influence the protective effect against salmonella colonization of intestinal cultures from adult birds, but normal intestinal flora did lose its preventive effect when cultured with furazolidone.

Snoeyenbos et al. (297) reported that protection by these methods was substantial for 63 days, the longest period tested, although it could be overcome by severe exposure; protection was poor, however, when the culture was given simultaneously with the challenge and was absent when given after challenge (269). Soerjadi et al. (303), on the other hand, found protection as early as 2 hr posttreatment with optimal protection by 32 hr. Good protection can be obtained with as little as 10^{-4} g of feces or 10^{-2} ml of a fourth serial fecal subculture (45).

Snoeyenbos et al. (298) found that protective intestinal microflora of chickens was readily transferred to penmates and apparently to birds in adjacent pens. The microflora not only minimized infection resulting from exposure following colonization of the gut with microflora but significantly abbreviated the period of infection when introduced after a salmonella infection was established in chicks. A hypothesis involving specificity of attachment between the glycocalyces of the protective microflora and of the intestinal mucosa was offered as the likely mechanism of protection. Soerjadi et al. (305) demonstrated adherence of salmonellae to cecal mucosa using scanning EM. In chicks treated with selected fecal microflora there was early colonization by adherent bacteria interconnected with fibers forming a matt of microflora that may be responsible for preventing colonization of salmonellae in the ceca.

Weinack et al. (338) evaluated salmonella protection based on culture of cloacal and fecal samples by enrichment methods plus enumeration of salmonellae in fresh droppings collected from test groups. Fresh fecal suspensions were somewhat more dependable than anaerobic cultures in providing a high level of protection against subsequent salmonella infection.

In three separate trials, Rigby and Pettit (250) treated groups of broiler chicks with a lyophilized extract of breeder-flock litter, an anaerobic culture of this extract, and an anaerobic culture of adult chicken feces, respectively. At 3 days of age they were exposed to *S. typhimurium* infection and reared to market age when the incidence of infection was found to be significantly lower in treated chickens than in untreated controls.

Soerjadi et al. (304) investigated competitive exclusion of salmonellae using various avian lactobacilli, which reduced the number of salmonellae adhering to the crop mucosa by 1–2 $\log_{10}$. Treatment with lactobacilli did not lower either the number of chickens shedding salmonellae or the number of salmonellae adhering to the mucosa of the cecum. Lactobacilli as a single bacterial treatment played a minor role in protecting the crop, but no protection of the cecum was demonstrated.

Pivnick et al. (227) treated chicks orally with 24–hr anaerobic cultures of feces from mature chickens 1 day after hatching, and challenged with *S. typhimurium* in the drinking water 2 days later. The lower third of the intestinal tract was examined for salmonellae on day 11 or 12. Treated chicks were about 1000-fold more resistant to infection by salmonellae than untreated chicks. Cultures were protective after inoculation directly into the crop or added to the drinking water, and could be held at −70 C for 21 days, serially subcultured daily up to four times, or diluted to 1:80 in drinking water containing 4% skim milk powder without losing their protective effect.

There have been several reports on the principal of competitive exclusion (5, 23, 127, 128, 151, 175, 197, 243, 244, 270, 300, 340–342). A comprehensive review of the efficacy and mechanism of competitive exclusion was published by Schleifer (268). Until a defined beneficial microflora is commercially available, the wide use of crude intestinal material should be viewed cautiously to prevent the transmission of unknown viral and bacterial agents. In addition, the widespread use of antisalmonella drugs in starter feeds and drinking water and by injection in baby chicks and poults may have detrimental effects on beneficial intestinal microflora.

PREVENTION AND CONTROL. A number of control programs have been initiated by various groups in Europe (135, 165, 344), with some success attributable to aspects such as control of imports, central control of hatching eggs and breeding units, issuance of guidelines to combat poultry salmonellosis, establishment of breeding centers, monitoring programs using serologic tests, and strict control of salmonella infections of animals.

The NPIP has no specific disease control program for PT except the newly developed U.S. Sanitation Monitored Program – Turkeys and Egg

Type Chickens. Minnesota has a specific regulatory program for *S. typhimurium* in turkeys in which any candidate turkey breeding flock found infected with *S. typhimurium* has to be marketed (232). The Minnesota breeder hen industry has also targeted its unofficial program at the top ten human salmonellae (215).

The major production factors contributing to infection and contamination of chickens and turkeys are 1) breeder-hatchery, 2) environment of poultry farm, and 3) feed. Recommendations have been outlined for control of salmonellosis in chickens and turkeys (15).

Breeder-Hatchery. The primary breeder, commercial breeder, and hatchery play a key role in the control and reduction of salmonellosis in egg- and meat-type chickens, turkeys, and other fowl.

Flocks that are known to have carried the infection at any age should not be used as sources of hatching eggs, even if they have been on antibiotic therapy, since carriers can still result (113). Early disposal of such flocks is usually the most desirable program to follow. All replacement stock and hatching eggs should be obtained from a source that is known to be PT-free. Birds should be maintained at all times in an environment where exposure is kept at a minimum. Morgan-Jones (204) found salmonellae were not isolated from empty, cleaned, and fumigated poultry houses, and only rarely from feed but were isolated from the environment of the chicks. Water in the troughs rather than feed appeared to be the major source of infection or reinfection during rearing.

Many reports have concluded that preventive measures such as PT-free breeders, feed sanitation, hatching-egg sanitation, segregation of eggs from known clean flocks from those of known infected flocks, and general hygiene at the breeder-flock and hatchery levels are fundamental to salmonella control (3, 82, 88, 164, 190, 290, 349).

Marthedal (190) noted that there is no doubt that introduction of a number of preventive measures in Denmark has contributed to reduction of frequency of salmonellosis in Danish poultry and consequently in humans. Fairbrother (103) concluded that eradication of salmonellae from the poultry industry is not possible with current scientific knowledge and technology, but control is both feasible and essential. A detailed program for prevention of avian salmonella infections in breeding flocks and hatcheries has been outlined and general management procedures and methods given for disinfection of salmonella-infected buildings (13).

In breeder flocks, systematic bacteriologic monitoring of the grandparent flocks and their progeny, plus the highest standards of hygiene, can help to produce parent stocks that are free of salmonellae.

Rodents and other pests around poultry yards serve as an important source of salmonellae for semimature and adult flocks, contaminating feed supplies and water as well as litter and poultry yards. An active rodent eradication campaign is an essential part of the general salmonella control program. Dogs, cats, sheep, cattle, horses, swine, and wild birds should never have access to poultry operations.

Goetz (121) reported an incident in which it was necessary to abandon turkey-raising operations because *S. typhimurium* was indigenous in the wildlife of the area. The organism was isolated from gopher snakes, ground squirrels, and owls shot on the premises.

Housing should be designed to be both rodentproof and birdproof to aid in control of avian PT infections (144, 154).

Litter-sample culturing can be used as a reasonably accurate and practical method for detecting salmonella-infected breeder flocks (296). Weston (343) found that on primary breeding farms and multiplying farms most salmonella contamination was from "resident" serotypes on particular farms and in certain buildings. In some buildings the same serotype has been isolated each year for up to 10 yr.

Lindgren (180) outlined the Swedish program to eliminate salmonellae from poultry breeder flocks based on hygienic housing and management and monitoring for salmonellae. Positive broiler flocks were destroyed and the premises cleaned and disinfected before restocking.

Williams (352) destroyed salmonellae by spraying litter with 4 or 6% formalin solutions with intermittent litter turnover. Extreme caution in using formalin is required for personnel safety (see Chapter 1).

In Great Britain methyl bromide has been examined as a sanitizing agent (140). Unlike formaldehyde, methyl bromide was found to have considerable penetrating power, but it may not completely kill all salmonellae present, and it is adversely affected by low temperature and high moisture (141, 142, 323).

A 5-yr study by Pomeroy et al. (233) indicated that turkey breeder flocks can be maintained free of salmonella and arizona organisms. Turkeys received pelletized feed with no animal by-products, but with fish solubles. Samples cultured during a 4-yr period of intensive monitoring did not reveal the presence of salmonella and arizona organisms, and there was no seroconversion.

During a period of 16 mo, Dorn et al. (82) reared a broiler parent flock of 230 birds and kept them salmonella-free as a result of hygiene. Propionic acid was added to feed of parent stock and broiler chickens. Although they did not succeed in production of completely salmonella-free broilers, these investigations showed some possibilities and methods to reduce salmonella contamination in broiler production.

When encountered in valuable breeding stock, PT infections constitute a particular problem. Special measures are necessary in such cases, and eradication efforts often extend over a period of several years and involve considerable financial loss.

HATCHERY AND EGG SANITATION

Egg Production, Collection, Handling, Storing. Use of only clean eggs for hatching purposes will lessen chances of introducing the infection into the incubator through fecal contamination. Adequate numbers of clean nests should be provided. There is a growing interest in use of wire floors and rollaway nests for hatching-egg flocks (Fig. 3.5).

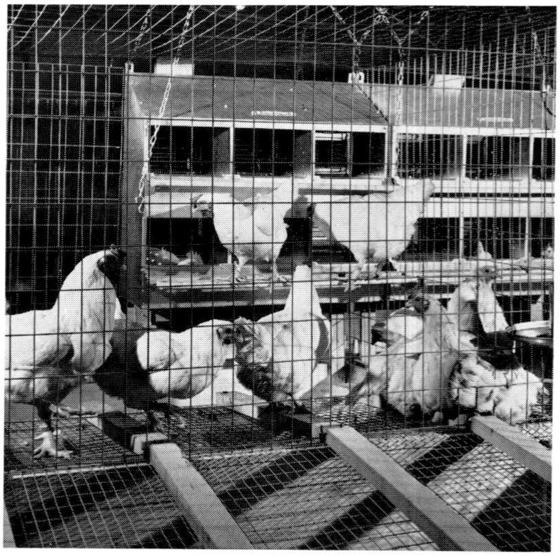

3.5. Wire-floored houses with rollaway nests for production of hatching eggs with a minimum of fecal contamination. (Indian River Poultry Farms, Lancaster, PA)

Perhaps one of the most promising methods for prevention of salmonellosis in poultry flocks will be production of hatching eggs on wire floors equipped with rapid, mechanized means of removal, followed by immediate egg fumigation. Fertility levels of 95–97% have been obtained with white leghorn breeders housed at $\frac{2}{3}$ ft^2 space/bird on sloping wire floors, with a ratio of males to females of 1:12. Quarles et al. (240) and Carter et al. (69) demonstrated that much less bacterial shell contamination occurred when eggs were collected from wire-floored houses with sloping floors than from houses with conventional nests and litter floors, and several workers have noted that infected birds placed on wire in clean facilities rapidly lose their infected status (55, 69, 240, 289).

Eggs should be collected at frequent intervals, fumigated, and stored in a cool place for as short a period as possible before setting. Cleaned and disinfected containers should be used in collecting eggs, and the collector should be certain not to serve as a source of contamination from organisms that may be present on clothing or hands. Dirty eggs should not be used for hatching purposes and should be collected in a separate container from hatching eggs. Cleaning eggs with cold water or wiping with a damp cloth hastens bacterial penetration and facilitates transfer of infection from egg to egg (126). It is best to remove dirt and dried feces from eggs by dry sanding (Fig. 3.6).

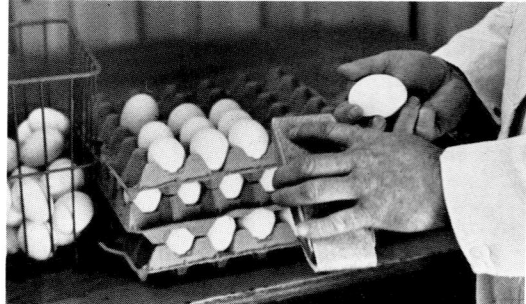

3.6. Dry-sanding soiled eggs immediately after collection. Abrasive must be changed frequently to prevent spread of contamination.

Chlorine and quaternary ammonium compounds are the most effective and practical disinfectants for sanitizing hatching eggs (336). Ghazikhanian et al. (120) recommended that they be dipped in antibiotic and disinfectant solution, and injected with antibiotics. Newly hatched poultry should be injected with antibiotics, feeds should be pelletized, and a clean and sanitary environment should be provided. These procedures have been used to reduce and eliminate salmonella infections at the primary breeder level.

Racks or crates used for storing eggs should be new or properly cleaned and disinfected. Contact with eggs should be kept at a minimum during storage, since one egg may serve as a source of contamination for many others. If it is necessary to transport eggs before setting, new crates are essential; dirty crates should never be used. Attention to sanitation on the farm at the supply-flock level to obtain salmonella-free hatching eggs is an essential part of a PT control program.

Egg Treatment. Egg-dipping and -spraying procedures are used to destroy salmonellae on the surface of hatching eggs prior to penetration of the organisms through the shell and shell membranes. To be effective, such procedures must be properly applied immediately after egg collection. Disinfectants used to wash eggs after exposure to salmonella organisms for ½ hr did not alter penetration patterns, since organisms had already penetrated the shells and were not reached (359).

Wash solutions can become excessively contaminated with organic matter and bacteria to the extent that dipping practices can do more harm than good. For this reason they are not universally recommended or applied for prevention of egg-borne salmonellosis.

Quaternary ammonium compounds, formalin, sodium hydroxide, and sodium orthophenylphenate have been studied for many years for dipping and washing hatching eggs. Gordon et al. (126) studied germicidal effects of nine chemical dipping solutions for destruction of *S. typhimurium* and *S. thompson* experimentally deposited on shells of chicken eggs. Most of the compounds effectively sanitized the shell surfaces and did not affect flavor of the egg contents or hatchability of dipped eggs.

Lucas et al. (182) dipped preinfected turkey hatching eggs in kanamycin, neomycin, and spectinomycin. The first two were effective in reducing *S. saint paul* infection of eggs; low levels of infection of turkey eggs with *S. typhimurium* were not significantly reduced by either. Several workers have used gentamicin as an external treatment for surface contamination and found it to be effective (94, 257, 292), but not after organisms had reached the thick albumin.

Preincubation Fumigation. Early fumigation of hatching eggs with formaldehyde gas on the farm has been found to be very effective in prevention of egg-borne PT infections. Williams (347) found that up to 99.8% of aerobic bacteria on the surface of brown-shell eggs could be destroyed by fumigation of 20 min.

Early fumigation (preferably within 2 hr after laying) is essential; in the event PT organisms are on the shells at setting time, penetration is likely to have already occurred in the incubator, and fumigation will be of no benefit. Furthermore, developing embryos may be killed if the fumigation period is too long or the formaldehyde level is too high when fumigation is performed later. With early fumigation, formaldehyde levels up to five times those used for routine preincubation fumigation of hatching eggs did not adversely affect egg hatchability (361).

When an air-borne infection of salmonellae has become established, it may be necessary to fumigate the entire hatchery. Fumigation procedures are covered in detail in Chapter 1.

Cleaning Incubators and Hatching Rooms. After each hatch, incubators should be thoroughly cleaned of debris, washed with detergent and hot water, disinfected, and fumigated with a high level of formaldehyde gas. At least 1.2 ml formalin (40%) and 0.6 $KMnO_4/ft^3$ incubator space should be used, with an exposure period of 1 hr. General disinfection procedures for incubators and hatching rooms and additional recommendations on formaldehyde fumigation of incubators are discussed in Chapter 1.

Hatchery Sanitation. Restrictions should be placed on hatchery personnel to ensure that they do not introduce infections into the hatchery from older fowl or from other animals with which they come in contact in their daily operations. It should be determined that no human carriers exist among the personnel. Visitors to the hatching area should be restricted. Boxes used to ship birds should be new and trucks employed for transporting operations should be kept clean and be frequently disinfected. There should be a constant campaign to eliminate rats, mice, and flies in the vicinity of the hatchery.

Environment of Poultry Farm. For prevention of PT infections during brooding it is important that young birds be constantly isolated from sources of infection. Olesiuk et al. (224) reported that transmission of *S. typhimurium* among chicks occurred rapidly on new litter, but slowly on used litter; used litter might contribute to a control program but it must be free of salmonellae.

Personnel in contact with older birds and other animals should take precautions not to introduce the infection through droppings that may adhere to shoes, clothing, or hands. It is a good practice under these conditions to wear rubber boots that can be disinfected and coveralls that can be changed frequently. All other animals should be restricted from the brooding area.

Gordon and Tucker (125) found that when salmonella-contaminated feed is given to poultry, water containers may become infected either by fecal contamination or by birds carrying infected food on their beaks. Multiplication of the organisms under these conditions is rapid. Feed and water containers should be situated where they cannot be contaminated by droppings and should be frequently cleaned and disinfected. Live steam is very effective.

A detailed sanitation program was outlined for the turkey breeder industry and is applicable for chicken industry (235).

Feed. Several recent reports indicate that salmonella contamination of feed ingredients has not materially changed over the past 20 years (46, 72, 353). The American Protein Producers Industry initiated a salmonella-reduction program of animal proteins in 1984. A benchmark program was established to determine the current status of salmonella contamination of animal proteins. Samples were tested from a large number of plants in 1985 and 1986; 2906 of 6009 (48.3%) were salmonella-positive. The Minnesota Turkey Breeder Hen Committee recommended that breeder-flock owners use pelletized feed for breeder candidates that is free of animal by-products, or prepared with known salmonella-free by-products. Since 1981, the number of the breeder flocks fed animal by-products in mash rations has gone from 16 to 0%.

Immunization. Bacterins and attenuated live cultures for use as vaccines in prevention of avian PT infections have been studied experimentally but have never had wide application under field conditions in the USA, until recently.

INACTIVATED ANTIGENS. Khera et al. (162) reported use of a formalized broth culture vaccine prepared from a strain of *S. stanley* during an outbreak caused by this serotype in a chicken flock. After vaccination, mortality from this infection ceased.

McCapes et al. (194) used four isolates of *S. typhimurium* to prepare a whole-broth, aluminum hydroxide-adsorbed bacterin for vaccination of turkey hens. Poults from vaccinated dams exhibited measurable resistance to yolk sac challenge with both *S. typhimurium* and *S. schwarzengrund* but not with *S. anatum*.

Immunity to challenge was evident after oral inoculation of chicks with a heat-inactivated *S. typhimurium* vaccine (43, 81); the antigen reached the circulation from the intestine and stimulated antibodies, and challenge caused a booster effect.

Autogenous bacterins in an oil-emulsion preparation were very effective in breaking the salmonella cycle in a turkey breeder-hatchery operation (211), and *S. arizonae* bacterins reduced egg transmission of *S. arizonae* in infected breeder flocks (213).

Truscott (319) added multivalent antigen preparations of sonicated lyophilized cells derived from up to six different salmonella serotypes in decreasing levels to broiler feed throughout the life of the birds. Several preliminary experiments challenging chicks with some of the homologous serotypes via contaminated feed showed that salmonellae were cleared more rapidly from treated chicks than from untreated controls and that fewer isolations of salmonellae were made from their ceca.

Vaccination with *S. typhimurium* endotoxin also induced protective antibodies in chickens and turkeys (320, 321).

LIVE VACCINES. Botes (52) tested live attenuated cultures and found their immunogenicity to be proportional to their virulence. Attenuation, to the point of complete avirulency, sacrificed a considerable part of immunizing potency.

Knivett and Stevens (166) orally vaccinated 1-day-old chicks with a live attenuated strain of *S. dublin* and subsequently challenged them with *S. typhimurium;* growth of the challenge organism in the liver was considerably reduced or prevented. Neither vaccination with live salmonella cultures administered in water nor furazolidone therapy is adequately effective once a salmonella pathogen is established in intestines of a chicken (167). Schimmel et al. (267) found that a streptomycin-dependent mutant strain of *S. typhimurium* was well tolerated when given orally to chicks and laying hens and shortened excretion of field strains of salmonellae.

Pritchard et al. (238) found that 1-day-old chicks vaccinated orally with live *S. typhimurium* galactose epimerase mutant (G30D) and challenged orally after 14 days with a field strain of *S. typhimurium* had statistically significant reductions in fecal shedding, salmonella-carrier status at slaughter, salmonellae in the broiler house environment, and serologic response in the 4th wk after challenge.

REFERENCES

1. Adler, H.E. 1965. Salmonella in eggs–an appraisal. Food Technol 19:191–192.

2. Adler, H.E., M.A. Nilson, and W.J. Stadelman. 1953. A study of turkeys artificially infected with Salmonella typhimurium. Am J Vet Res 14:246–248.

3. Almlof, J. 1977. National approach to salmonella control. In D.A. Barnum (ed.), Proc Int Symp on Salmonella and Prospects for Control, pp. 239–252. Univ Guelph, Ontario, Canada.

4. Anderson, E.L., and J.F. Stephens. 1970. Changes in the differential leukocyte count of chicks inoculated with salmonella. Appl Microbiol 19:726–730.

5. Anderson, W.R., W.R. Mitchell, D.A. Barnum, and R.J. Julian. 1984. Practical aspects of competitive exclusion for the control of salmonella in turkeys. Avian Dis 28:1071–1078.

6. Anonymous. 1967. Annual Report (1966)–Food Protection and Toxicology Center, Univ Calif, Davis.

7. Anonymous. 1969. An evaluation of the salmonella problem. Nat Acad Sci, Washington, DC, Publ 1683, pp. 67–95.

8. Anonymous. 1971. Methods for Examining Poultry Biologies and for Identifying and Quantifying Avian Pathogens. Nat Acad Sci, Washington, DC, pp. 190–214.

9. Anonymous. 1971. American Association of Avian Pathologists Salmonellosis Workshop, 1970. USDA, APHIS, Hyattsville, MD.

10. Anonymous. 1973. Animals and animal products.

Code of Federal Regulations, pt. 113.30. USDA, Washington, DC.
11. Anonymous. 1976. Proc Salmonella Symp. Am Assoc Avian Pathol, College Station, Tex.
12. Anonymous. 1978. Recommendations for Reduction and Control of Salmonellosis. Rep US Advis Comm on Salmonella. Food Safety Qual Serv, USDA, Washington, DC.
13. Anonymous. 1979. Salmonella Infection in Poultry. Dep Agric Fish Scotland, Welsh Off, Leafl 298.
14. Anonymous. 1984. Proc Int Symposium on Salmonella, pp. 1–384. Am Assoc Avian Pathol, Kennett Square, PA.
15. Anonymous. 1985. The National Poultry Improvement Plan and Auxiliary Provisions. USDA, APHIS-VS, Hyattsville, MD.
16. Anonymous. 1988. Recommended salmonella control guidelines for processors of livestock and poultry feeds. American Feed Industries, Inc, Arlington, VA.
17. Anonymous. 1988. Feed Additive Compendium–a guide to the use of drugs in medicated animal feed, pp. 1–358. Miller Publishing Co, Minneapolis, MN.
18. Arakawa, A., E. Baba, and T. Fukata. 1981. Eimeria tenella infection enhances Salmonella typhimurium infection in chickens. Poult Sci 60:2203–2209.
19. Baba, E., T. Fukata, and A. Arakawa. 1985. Factors influencing Salmonella typhimurium infection in Eimeria tenella-infected chickens. Am J Vet Res 46:1593–1596.
20. Baba, E., M. Yaono, T. Fukata and A. Arakawa. 1985. Infection by Salmonella typhimurium, S. agona, S. enteritidis, or S. infantis of chicks with caecal coccidiosis. Br Poult Sci 26:505–511.
21. Bagley, R.A., and M.J. Ramsay. 1980. An eleven year study of salmonella serotypes in an integrated turkey operation. Proc 29th West Poult Dis Conf, pp. 218–221. Acapulco, Mexico.
22. Bahl, A.K., M.C. Kumar, M.D. York, and B.S. Pomeroy. 1975. Direct immunofluorescent technique in diagnosis of experimental salmonellosis of turkeys. Avian Dis 19:59–66.
23. Bailey, J.S., L.C. Blankenship, N.J. Stern, N.A. Cox, and F. McHan. 1988. Effect of anticoccidial and antimicrobial feed additives on prevention of Salmonella colonization of chicks treated with anaerobic cultures of chicken feces. Avian Dis 32:324–329.
24. Baker, R.C., and R.A. Qureshi. 1985. The frequency of salmonellae on duck eggs. Poult Sci 64:646–652.
25. Baker, R.C., J.P. Goff, and E.J. Mulnix. 1980. Salmonella recovery following oral and intravenous inoculation of laying hens. Poult Sci 59:1067–1072.
26. Baker, R.C., J.P. Goff, and J.F. Timoney. 1980. Prevalence of salmonellae on eggs from poultry farms in New York state. Poult Sci 59:289–292.
27. Ballantyne, E.E. 1953. Salmonella infections of poultry in Alberta. Proc 90th Annu Meet Am Vet Med Assoc, pp. 355–358.
28. Baloda, S.B., A. Faris, K. Krovacek, and T. Wadstrom. 1983. Cytotoxic enterotoxins and cytotoxic factors produced by Salmonella enteritidis and Salmonella typhimurium. Toxicology 21:785–796.
29. Barrow, P.A., H.S. Williams, and J.F. Tucker. 1984. The effect of feeding diets containing avoparcin on the excretion of salmonellas by chickens experimentally infected with natural sources of salmonella organisms. J Hyg 93:439–444.
30. Bassiouni, A., and E. Palliola. 1970. Immunofluorescent technique in the diagnosis of experimental salmonellosis of fowls. 1. Use of somatic antigens and antiserum. Vet Ital 21:20–32.
31. Bassiouni, A., and E. Palliola. 1970. Immunofluorescent technique in the diagnosis of experimental salmonellosis in poultry. II. Influence of enrichment technique and of various antisera. Vet Ital 21:642–647.
32. Bayer, R.C., M. Gershman, T.A. Bryan, and J.H. Rittenburg. 1977. Degeneration of the mucosal surface of the small intestine of the chicken in salmonella infection. Poult Sci 56:1041–1042.
33. Bayne, H.G., J.A. Garibaldi, and H. Lineweaver. 1965. Heat resistance of Salmonella typhimurium and Salmonella senftenberg 775 W in chicken meat. Poult Sci 44:1281–1284.
34. Beattie, W.E. 1960. Avian infection with Salmonella thompson–observations. Poult Sci 39:1233.
35. Beaudette, F.R., and P.R. Edwards. 1926. The etiology of a canary bird epizootic. J Bacteriol 12:51–55.
36. Benson, C.E., and R.J. Eckroade. 1988. Salmonella enteritidis isolated from poultry-related sources–recommendations for isolation and characterization. J Am Vet Med Assoc 192:1784.
37. Bentley, A.H. 1984. The salmonella situation in Canada. In G.H. Snoeyenbos (ed.), Proc Int Symposium on Salmonella, pp. 54–63. Am Assoc Avian Pathol, Kennett Square, PA.
38. Berkowitz, J.H., D.J. Kraft, and M.S. Finstein. 1974. Persistence of salmonellae in poultry excreta. J Environ Qual 3:158–161.
39. Bhatia, T.R.S., and G.D. McNabb. 1980. Dissemination of Salmonella in broiler chicken operations. Avian Dis 24:616–624.
40. Bierer, B.W. 1960. Effect of age factor on mortality in Salmonella typhimurium infection in turkey poults. J Am Vet Med Assoc 137:657–658.
41. Bierer, B.W., and C.L. Vickers. 1960. Nitrofuran medication for experimental Salmonella typhimurium infection in poults. Avian Dis 4:22–37.
42. Bisgaard, M. 1981. Arthritis in ducks. 1. Aetiology and public health aspects. Avian Pathol 10:11–21.
43. Bisping, W., I. Dimitriadis, and M. Seippel. 1971. Versuche zür oralen Immunisierung von Hühnern mit hitzinaktivierter Salmonella-vakzine. 1. Impf-und Infektionsversuche an Hühnerküken. Zentralbl Veterinaermed [B] 18:306–311.
44. Blackburn, B.O., and E.M. Ellis. 1973. Lactose-fermenting salmonella from dried milk and milk-drying plants. Appl Microbiol 26:672–674.
45. Blanchfield, B., M.A. Gardiner, and H. Pivnick. 1982. Nurmi concept for preventing infection of chicks by Salmonella: Comparison of fecal suspensions and fecal cultures administered into the crop and in drinking water. J Food Prot 45:345–347.
46. Blankenship, L.C., D.A. Shackelford, N.A. Cox, D. Burdick, J.S. Bailey, and J.E. Thomson. 1984. Survival of salmonellae as a function of poultry feed processing conditions. In G.H. Snoyenbos (ed.), Proc Int Symp Salmonella, pp.211–220. Am Assoc Avian Pathol, Kennett Square, PA.
47. Blaxland, J.D., W.J. Sojka, and A.M. Smither. 1958. Avian Salmonellosis in England and Wales 1948–56, with comment on its prevention and control. Vet Rec 70:374–382.
48. Board, R.G., J.C. Ayres, A.A. Kraft, and R.H. Forsythe. 1964. The microbiological contamination of egg shells and egg packing materials. Poult Sci 43:584–595.
49. Boonchuvit, B., and P.B. Hamilton. 1975. Interaction of aflatoxin and paratyphoid infections in broiler chickens. Poult Sci 54:1567–1573.
50. Boonchuvit, B., P.B. Hamilton, and H.R. Burmeister. 1975. Interaction of T-2 toxin with salmonella infections of chickens. Poult Sci 54:1693–1696.

51. Borland, E.D. 1975. Salmonella infection in poultry. Vet Rec 97:406–408.
52. Botes, H.J.W. 1965. Live vaccines in the control of salmonellosis. J S Afr Vet Med Assoc 36:461–474.
53. Bowmer, E.J. 1964. The challenge of salmonellosis: Major public health problem. Am J Med Sci 247:467–501.
54. Browne, A.S. 1949. The public health significance of salmonella on poultry and poultry products. Ph.D. diss., Univ California, Berkeley.
55. Brownell, J.R., and W.W. Sadler. 1967. Salmonella carriers. Proc West Poult Dis Conf, pp. 14–16.
56. Brownell, J.R., W.W. Sadler, and M.J. Fanelli. 1969. Factors influencing the intestinal infections of chickens with Salmonella typhimurium. Avian Dis 13:804–816.
57. Brown, D.D., J.G. Ross, and A.F.G. Smith. 1975. Experimental infection of cockerels with Salmonella typhimurium. Res Vet Sci 18:165–170.
58. Bruner, D.W. 1973. Salmonella cultures typed during the years 1950–1971 for the service laboratories of the New York State Veterinary College at Cornell University. Cornell Vet 63:138–143.
59. Bryan, F.L. 1972. Emerging foodborne diseases. 1. Their surveillance and epidemiology. J Milk Food Technol 35:618–625.
60. Bryan, F. 1980. Foodborne diseases in the United States associated with meat and poultry. J Food Prot 43:140–155.
61. Bryan, F. 1981. Current trends in foodborne salmonellosis in the United States and Canada. J Food Prot 44:394–401.
62. Bullis, K.L. 1977. The history of avian medicine in the U.S. III. Salmonellosis. Avian Dis 21:430–435.
63. Buriro, S.N. 1980. Occurrence and isolation of microorganisms from Argus (persicargas) persicus oken. Z Angew Entomol 89:22–25.
64. Burkhart, D.M., R.W. Wolfgang, and P.D. Harwood. 1962. Salmonellosis in parakeets and canaries treated with nitrofurans in the drinking water. Avian Dis 6:275–283.
65. Buxton, A. 1957. Salmonellosis in Animals. A review. Commonw Agric Bur, Farnham Royal, Bucks, England.
66. Buxton, A., and R.F. Gordon. 1947. The epidemiology and control of Salmonella thompson infection of fowls. J Hyg 45:265–281.
67. Campbell, D.F., S.S. Green, C.S. Custer, and R.W. Johnston. 1982. Incidence of salmonella in fresh dressed turkeys raised under Salmonella-controlled and uncontrolled environments. Poult Sci 61:1962–1967.
68. Cantini, G., and C. Rossi. 1972. Salmonellosis affecting the eyes of chicks. Atti Conv Patol Aviare 10:73–75.
69. Carter, T.A., R.F. Gentry, and G.O. Bressler. 1973. Bacterial contamination of hatching eggs and chicks produced by broiler breeders housed in litter-slat and sloping floor management systems. Poult Sci 52:2226–2236.
70. Chaplin, W.C., and C.M. Hamilton. 1957. A synovitis in turkeys produced by Salmonella thompson. Poult Sci 36:1380–1381.
71. Cohen, M.L., and P.A. Blake. 1977. Trends in foodborne salmonellosis outbreaks: 1963–1975. J Food Prot 40:798–800.
72. Cover, M.S., J.T. Gary, and S.F. Binder. 1984. Reduction of standard plate counts, total coliform counts, and salmonella by pelletizing animal feeds. In G.H. Snoeyenbos (ed.), Proc Int Symp on Salmonella, pp. 221–231. Am Assoc Avian Pathol, Kennett Square, PA.
73. Cox, N.A., and A.J. Mercuri. 1976. Rapid confirmation of suspect salmonella colonies by use of Minitek system in conjuction with serological tests. J Appl Bacteriol 41:389–394.
74. Cox, N.A., and J.E. Williams. 1976. A simplified biochemical system to screen salmonella isolated from poultry for serotyping. Poult Sci 55:1968–1971.
75. Cox, N.A., B.H. Davis, A.B. Watts, and A.R. Colmer. 1973. Salmonella in the laying hen. 1. Salmonella recovery from viscera, feces, and eggs following oral inoculation. Poult Sci 52:661–666.
76. Cox, N.A., A.J. Mercuri, D.A. Tanner, M.O. Carson, J.E. Thomson, and J.S. Bailey. 1978. Effectiveness of sampling methods for salmonella detection on processed broilers. J Food Prot 41:341–343.
77. Cunningham, F.E. 1986. Egg-product pasteurization. In W.J. Stadelman and O.J. Cotterill (eds.), Egg Science and Technology, pp. 243–268. Avi, Westport, CN.
78. Das, M.S., M.B. Chakravorty, and G.K. Ghosh. 1959. Occurrence of avian salmonellosis in West Bengal. Indian Vet J 36:403–408.
79. Davis, J.W., R.C. Anderson, L. Karstad, and D.O. Trainer. 1971. Infectious and Parasitic Diseases of Wild Birds. Iowa State Univ Press, Ames.
80. DeLay, P.D., T.W. Jackson, E.E. Jones, and D.E. Stover. 1954. A testing service for the control of Salmonella typhimurium infection in turkeys. Am J Vet Res 15:122–129.
81. Dimitriadis, I., and W. Bisping. 1971. Studies on oral immunization of fowls with heat inactivated salmonella vaccine. 2. Serological studies on the occurrence of antibodies and a "booster effect." Zentralbl Veterinaermed [B] 18:337–346.
82. Dorn, P., P. Krabisch, F.W. Klein, R. Pakosta, and W. Rapp. 1980. Research on salmonella-free production of broilers. Dtsch Tieraerztl Wochenschr 87:10–17.
83. Dougherty, E. 1953. Disease problems confronting the duck industry. Proc 90th Annu Meet Am Vet Med Assoc, pp. 359–365.
84. Dougherty, E. 1961. The pathology of paratyphoid infection in the White Pekin duck, particularly the lesions in the central nervous system. Avian Dis 5:415–430.
85. Dougherty, T.J. 1974. Salmonella contamination in a commercial poultry (broiler) processing operation. Poult Sci 53:814–821.
86. Dougherty, T. 1976. A study of salmonella contamination in broiler flocks. Poult Sci 55:1811–1815.
87. Dubert, W.H. 1988. Assessment of salmonella contamination in poultry—past, present, and future. Poult Sci 67:944–949.
88. Dungan, W.M. 1976. Rationale for the control of salmonellae: Turkey breeder and multiplier flocks, Proc Salmonella Symp, pp. 21–26. Am Assoc Avian Pathol. Kennett Square, PA.
89. Dwivedi, P., and F.C. Malhotra. 1973. Relative pathogenicity and pathogenesis of some salmonella serotypes in young chicks. I. Clinical signs and growth response. Indian J Poult Sci 8:241–46.
90. Edwards, P.R., and W.H. Ewing. 1972. Identification of Enterobacteriaceae. Burgess Publishing Co., Minneapolis.
91. Edwards, P.R., and M.M. Galton. 1967. Salmonellosis. In C.A. Brandly and C. Cornelius (eds.), Advances in Veterinary Science, pp. 1–63. Academic Press, New York.
92. Edwards, P.R., D.W. Bruner, and A.B. Moran. 1948. Salmonella infections in fowls. Cornell Vet 38:247–256.
93. Egger, L. 1978. Die Bedeutung von Salmonellen in Futtermitteln tierischer Herkunft für die Verseuch-

ung von Schlachtgeflügel und die Ansteckung von Menschen. Inaug. diss., Veterinar-Medizenische Fakultat., Zurich.
94. El-Attar, A.F. 1973. Procedures for the elimination of Salmonella typhimurium from chicken hatching eggs by dipping. M.S. thesis, Cornell Univ, Ithaca, NY.
95. Ellis, E.M., and R. Harrington, Jr. 1969. A direct fluorescent antibody test for salmonella. Arch Environ Health 19:876–881.
96. Ellis, E.M., J.E. Williams, E.T. Mallinson, G.H. Snoeyenbos, and W.J. Martin. 1976. Culture Methods for the Detection of Animal Salmonellosis and Arizonosis, pp. 9–87. Iowa State Univ Press, Ames.
97. Evans, W.M., D.W. Bruner, and M.C. Peckham. 1955. Blindness in chicks associated with Salmonellosis. Cornell Vet 45:239–247.
98. Ewing, W.H. 1986. Edwards and Ewing's Identification of Enterobacteriaceae. Elsevier, New York.
99. Ewing, W.H., and M.M. Ball. 1966. The Biochemical Reactions of Members of the Genus Salmonella. US Dep HEW, NCDC, Atlanta, GA.
100. Faddoul, G.P., and G.W. Fellows. 1965. Clinical manifestations of paratyphoid infection in pigeons. Avian Dis 9:377–381.
101. Faddoul, G.P., and G.W. Fellows. 1966. A five-year survey of the incidence of salmonellae in avian species. Avian Dis 10:296–304.
102. Fagerberg, D.J., C.L. Quarles, J.A. Ranson, R.D. Williams, L.P. Williams, Jr., C.B. Hancock, and S.L. Seaman. 1976. Experimental procedure for testing the effects of low level antibiotic feeding and therapeutic treatment on Salmonella typhimurium var. copenhagen infection in broiler chicks. Poult Sci 55:1848–1857.
103. Fairbrother, J.G. 1978. Salmonella problems in poultry and poultry products. Proc 16th World Poult Congr, pp. 90–114.
104. Fanelli, M.J., W.W. Sadler, and J.R. Brownell. 1970. Preliminary studies of persistence of salmonella in poultry litter. Avian Dis 14:131–141.
105. Fantasia, L.D. 1969. Accelerated immunofluorescence procedure for the detection of salmonella in foods and animal by-products. Appl Microbiol 18:708–713.
106. Ferris, K., and W.M. Frerichs. 1988. Salmonella serotypes from animals and related sources reported during the fiscal year 1988. Proc 92nd Annu Meet US Anim Health Assoc 92:349–378.
107. Finn, P.J., and B. Mehr. 1977. A benefit-cost analysis of eradicating salmonella infection in chicken meat produced in Canada. In D.A. Barnum (ed.), Proc Int Symp Salmonella and Prospects for Control, pp. 203–238. Guelph, Ontario, Canada.
108. Forsythe, R.H., W.J. Ross, and J.C. Ayres. 1967. Salmonella recovery following gastro intestinal and ovarian inoculation in the domestic fowl. Poult Sci 46:849–855.
109. Fukata, T., E. Baba, and A. Arakawa. 1984. Growth of Salmonella typhimurium in the caecum of gnotobiotic chickens with Eimeria tenella. Res Vet Sci 37:230–233.
110. Fukata, T., E. Baba, and A. Arakawa. 1987. Invasion of Salmonella typhimurium into the cecal wall of gnotobiotic chickens with Eimeria tenella. Poult Sci 66:760–761.
111. Galton, M.M., J.H. Steele, and K.W. Newell. 1964. In E. Van Oye (ed.), The World Problem of Salmonellosis, pp.421–444. Junk, The Hague, Netherlands.
112. Garrett, E.S., and R. Hamilton. 1971. Sanitation guidelines for control of salmonella in the production of fish meal. Nat Marine Fish Serv Circ 354. US Dept Commerce, Washington, DC.
113. Garside, J.S., R.F. Gordon, and J.F. Tucker. 1960. The emergence of resistant strains of Salmonella typhimurium in the tissues and alimentary tracts of chickens following the feeding of an antibiotic. Res Vet Sci 1:184–199.
114. Gauger, H.C., and R.E. Greaves. 1946. Bacteriological examination of shells and contents of eggs laid by turkeys naturally or artificially infected with Salmonella typhimurium. Poult Sci 25:119–123.
115. Gauger, H.C., and R.E. Greaves. 1946. Isolations of Salmonella typhimurium from drinking water in an infected environment. Poult Sci 25:476–478.
116. Gauger, H.C., R.E. Greaves, and F.W. Cook. 1940. Paratyphoid of pigeons. NC State Coll Agric Exp Stn Bull 62, pp.3–71.
117. Geissler, H., and J. Kösters. 1972. Die hygienische Bedeutung des Getreideschimmelkäfers (Alphitobius diaperinus panz.) in der Geflügelmast. Dtsch Tieraerztl Wochenschr 79:178–180.
118. George, S., and G.H.G. Davis. 1979. Rapid identification of Enterobacteriaceae by using noncommercial micro-tests in conjunction with API 20E profile data. J Clin Microbiol 10:399–403.
119. Gerlach, H. 1971. Verlauf von Salmonelleninfektionen bei Hühnerküken. Arch Gefluegelkd 35:102–104.
120. Ghazikhanian, G.Y., R. Yamamoto, R.H. McCapes., W.M. Dungan, and H.B. Ortmayer. 1980. Combination dip and injection of turkey eggs with antibiotics to eliminate Mycoplasma meleagridis infection from a primary breeding stock. Avian Dis 24:57–70.
121. Goetz, M.E. 1962. The control of paracolon and paratyphoid infections in turkey poults. Avian Dis 6:93–99.
122. Goodchild, W.M., and J.F. Tucker. 1968. Salmonellae in British wild birds and their transfer to domestic fowl. Br Vet J 124:95–101.
123. Gordon R.F. 1977. Avian salmonellosis. In Poultry Diseases, pp. 24–33. Baillière Tindall, London.
124. Gordon, R.F., and A. Buxton. 1946. A survey of avian salmonellosis in Great Britain. Br Vet J 102:187–206.
125. Gordon, R.F., and J.F. Tucker. 1965. The epizootiology of Salmonella menston infection of fowls and the effect of feeding poultry food artificially infected with salmonella. Br Poult Sci 6:251–264.
126. Gordon, R.F., E.G. Harry, and J.F. Tucker. 1956. The use of germicidal dips in the control of bacterial contamination of the shells of hatching eggs. Vet Rec 68:33–38.
127. Goren, E., W.A. de Jong, P. Doornebal, J.P. Koopman, and H.M Kennis. 1984. Protection of chicks against Salmonella infantis infection induced by strict anaerobically cultured intestinal microflora. Vet Q 6:22–26.
128. Goren, E., W.A. de Jong, P. Doornebal, J.P. Koopman, and H.M Kennis. 1984. Protection of chicks against salmonella infection induced by spray application of intestinal microflora in the hatchery. Vet Q 6:73–79.
129. Goyal, S.M., and I.P. Singh. 1970. Probable sources of salmonellae on a poultry farm. Br Vet J 126:180–184.
130. Graham, R. 1936. Salmonella isolated from baby quail. J Am Vet Med Assoc 88:763–764.
131. Greenberg, B. 1959. Persistence of bacteria in the developmental stages of the house fly. 1. Survival of enteric pathogens in the normal and aseptically reared host. Am J Trop Med Hyg 8:405–411.
132. Greenfield, J., C.H. Bigland, and H.D. McCausland. 1971. Detection of salmonella contaminated

eggs. Poult Sci 50:652–653.
133. Gwatkin, R., and L. Dzenis. 1954. Salmonellosis. I. Agglutination tests in experimental infection in chickens. Can J Comp Med Vet Sci 18:155–167.
134. Hacking, W.C. 1977. Salmonella in feed and environment. In D.A. Barnum (ed.), Proc Int Symp Salmonella and Prospect for Control, pp. 58–70. Univ Guelph, Ontario, Canada.
135. Hansen, H.C., and H.E. Marthedal. 1974. Avian Salmonellosis in chickens in Denmark with special reference to Salmonella typhimurium. Proc 15th World Poult Congr and Exposition, pp. 575–577. New Orleans, LA.
136. Harein, P.K., E. De las Casas, B.S. Pomeroy, and M.D. York. 1970. Salmonella spp. and serotypes of Escherichia coli isolated from lesser meal worm collected from poultry brooder houses. J Econ Entomol 63:80–82.
137. Harrington, R., Jr., E.M. Ellis, E.T. Mallinson, M. Ranck, and E. Solee. 1970. An evaluation of a fluorescent antibody technique for the detection of salmonellae in animal by-products, feeds, and tissues. J Am Vet Med Assoc 157:1898–1900.
138. Harrington, R., Jr., B.O. Blackburn, and C.D. Murphy. 1972. The efficiency of dry composting for detecting salmonella in animal by-products. Proc 76th Annu Meet US Anim Health Assoc, pp. 565–567.
139. Harrington, R., Jr., B.O. Blackburn, and D.R. Cassidy. 1975. Salmonellosis in canaries. Avian Dis 19:827–829.
140. Harry, E.G., and W.B. Brown. 1974. Fumigation with methyl bromide—applications in the poultry industry—a review. World's Poult Sci J 30:193–216.
141. Harry, E.G., W.B. Brown, and G. Goodship. 1972. The disinfecting activity of methyl bromide on various microbes and injected materials under controlled conditions. J Appl Bacteriol 35:485–491.
142. Harry, E.G., W.B. Brown, and G. Goodship. 1973. The influence of temperature and moisture on the disinfecting activity of methyl bromide on infected poultry litter. J Appl Bacteriol 36:343–350.
143. Harvey, R.W.S., and T.H. Price. 1974. Isolation of salmonellas. Monogr Ser 8. Her Majesty's Stationery Office, London.
144. Heard, T.W. 1969. Housing and salmonella infections. Vet Rec 85:482–484.
145. Henning, M.W. 1939. The antigenic structure of salmonellas obtained from domestic animals and birds in South Africa. Onderstepoort J Vet Sci Anim Ind 13:79–189.
146. Higgins, W.A., J.B. Christiansen, and C.H. Schroeder. 1944. A Salmonella enteritidis infection associated with leg deformity in turkeys. Poult Sci 23:340–341.
147. Higgins, R., R. Malo, E. Rene-Roberge, and R. Gauthier. 1982. Studies on the dissemination of salmonella in nine broiler-chicken flocks. Avian Dis 26:26–33.
148. Hinshaw, W.R., and E. McNeil. 1943. The use of the agglutination test detecting Salmonella typhimurium carriers in turkey flocks. Proc 47th Annu Meet US Livest Sanit Assoc, pp. 106–121.
149. Hinshaw, W.R., E. McNeil, and T.J. Taylor. 1944. Avian salmonellosis: Types of salmonella isolated and their relation to public health. Am J Hyg 40:264–278.
150. Hudson, C.B., and D.C. Tudor. 1957. Salmonella typhimurium infection in feral birds. Cornell Vet 47:394–395.
151. Impey, C.S., G.C. Mead, and M. Hinton. 1987. Influence of continuous challenge via the feed on competitive exclusion of salmonella from broiler chicks. J Appl Bacteriol 63:139–146.
152. Jackson, C.A.W., M.J. Lindsay, and F. Shiel. 1971. A study of the epizootiology and control of Salmonella typhimurium infection in a commercial poultry organization. Aust Vet J 47:485–491.
153. Jamieson, B.R. 1987. Salmonella control program in Canada. Proc 91st Annu Meet US Anim Health Assoc, pp.451–455.
154. Junnila, W.A., K.A. Jordan, M.C. Kumar, and B.S. Pomeroy. 1972. House design can aid disease control. Poult Dig 31:277–279.
155. Kapoor, K.N., H.V.S. Chauhan, and B.R. Gupta. 1980. Epidemiological and pathological studies in outbreaks of Salmonella bareilly infection in chickens and quails. Indian Vet J 57:536–538.
156. Kapoor, K.N., H.V.S. Chauhan, and B.R. Gupta. 1981. Studies on the epidemiological and other aspects of salmonellosis on an organized poultry farm. Indian Vet J 58:261–265.
157. Kashiwazaki, M., S. Aoki, T. Horiuchi, S. Shoya, and S. Namioka. 1966. An outbreak of paratyphoid infection due to Salmonella typhimurium in adult chickens. Nat Inst Anim Health Q (Tokyo) 6:144–151.
158. Kauffmann, F. 1966. The Bacteriology of Enterobacteriaceae. Williams & Wilkins Co., Baltimore.
159. Kauffmann, F. 1972. Serological Diagnosis of Salmonella Species. Williams & Wilkins, Baltimore.
160. Kaye, D., H.R. Shinefield, and E.W. Hook. 1961. The parakeet as a source of salmonellosis in man. Report of a case. N Engl J Med 264:868–869.
161. Kelterborn, E. 1967. Salmonella species. First isolations, names, and occurrence. Junk, The Hague, Netherlands.
162. Khera, S.S., S.B.V. Rao, and K.K. Agarwal. 1965. Avian salmonellosis—an outbreak of egg peritonitis simulating Salmonella pullorum infection caused by Salmonella stanley. Indian J Vet Sci 35:126–130.
163. Kim, S., T. Fukato, E. Baba, and A. Arakawa. 1985. Effects of infection with Eimeria tenella upon Salmonella typhimurium infection in the gnotobiotic chicks. Scanning electron microscopic study. Zentralbl Bakteriol Mikrobiol Hyg (A) 260:238–246.
164. Kingston, D.J., and R. Shapcott. 1980. Reduction of Salmonella spp in and the elimination of S. typhimurium from a commercial broiler breeding and growout operation. Proc 117th Annu Meet Am Vet Med Assoc, pp. 94.
165. Klingler, K. 1972. Control of salmonellosis in the Swiss poultry industry. Schweiz Arch Tierheilkd 114:519–528.
166. Knivett, V.A., and W.K. Stevens. 1971. The evaluation of a live salmonella vaccine in mice and chickens. J Hyg 69:233–245.
167. Knivett, V.A., and J.F. Tucker. 1972. Comparison of oral vaccination or Furazolidone prophylaxis for Salmonella typhimurium infection in chicks. Br Vet J 128:24–34.
168. Kodama, H., G. Sato, and T. Mikami. 1976. Age-dependent resistance of chickens to salmonella in vitro:phagocytic and bactericidal activities of splenic phagocytes. Am J Vet Res 37:1091–1094.
169. Köhler, B., K. Vogel, H. Kühn, W. Rabsch, H.G. Rummler, L. Schulze, and W. Schöll. 1979. Epizootiologie der Salmonella-typhimurium Infektion beim Huhn. Arch Exp Veterinaermed 33:281–298.
170. Kokolios, H., C. Paizis, F. Bredakis, and A.P. Georgopoulos. 1970. Survival of salmonella in soft agar. Public Health Rep 85:841–842.
171. Koo, F.C., J.W. Peterson, C.W. Houston, and N.C. Molina. 1984. Pathogenesis of experimental

salmonellosis: Inhibition of protein synthesis by cytotoxin. Infect Immun 43:93–100.
172. Krabisch, P., and P. Dorn. 1980. Zur epidemiologischen Bedeutung von Lebendvektoren bei der Verbreitung von Salmonellen in der Geflügelmast. Berl Muench Tieraerztl Wochenschr 93:232–235.
173. Kumar, M.C., M.D. York, J.E. Williams, A.D. Whittemore, B.S. Pomeroy, and L.T. Ausherman. 1974. Development of a serum-plate antigen for detection of Salmonella infections in turkeys. Proc 17th Annu Meet Am Assoc Vet Lab Diag, pp. 19–32.
174. Kumar, M.C., M.D. York, and B.S. Pomeroy. 1976. Comparison of tetrathionate and selenite enrichment broths for isolations of Arizona Hinshawii 7:1,7,8 and various serotypes of salmonella. Proc 19th Annu Meet Am Assoc Vet Lab Diag, pp. 179–188.
175. Lafont, J.P., A. Bree, M. Naciri, P. Yvore, J.F. Guillot, and E. Chaslus-Dancla. 1983. Experimental study of some factors limiting competitive exclusion of salmonella in chickens. Res Vet Sci 34:16–20.
176. Lannek, N., N.O. Lindgren, and T. Nilsson. 1962. Therapeutical experiments with a new nitrofuran compound. Avian Dis 6:228–238.
177. Laursen-Jones, A.P. 1968. Blindness in chicks associated with Salmonella typhimurium infection. Vet Rec 83:205.
178. Leaney, N., G.N. Cooper, and G.D.F. Jackson. 1978. Percloacal infection of chickens with Salmonella typhimurium. Vet Microbiol 3:155–165.
179. Lee, G.M., G.D.F. Jackson, and G.N. Cooper. 1981. The role of serum and biliary antibodies and cell-mediated immunity in the clearance of S. typhimurium from chickens. Vet Immunol Immunopathol 2:233–252.
180. Lindgren, N.O. 1973. Avian salmonellosis: A programme for its control in Sweden. Proc 5th Congr World Vet Poult Assoc, pp. 691–724. Munich, Germany.
181. Lloyd, A.B., R.B. Cumming, and R.D. Kent. 1977. Prevention of Salmonella typhimurium infection in poultry by pretreatment of chickens and poults with intestinal extracts. Aust Vet J 53:82–87.
182. Lucas, T.E., M.C. Kumar, S.H. Kleven, and B.S. Pomeroy. 1970. Antibiotic treatment of turkey hatching eggs preinfected with salmonella. Avian Dis 14:455–462.
183. Lukas, G.N., and D.R. Bradford. 1954. Salmonellosis in turkey poults as observed in routine necropsy of 1148 cases. J Am Vet Med Assoc 125:215–218.
184. MacKenzie, M.M., and B.S. Bains. 1976. Dissemination of salmonella serotypes from raw feed ingredients to chicken carcasses. Poult Sci 55:957–960.
185. Magwood, S.E., and E. Annau. 1961. The adsorption of somatic antigens of salmonella by polystyrene latex particles. Can J Comp Med Vet Sci 25:69–73.
186. Magwood, S.E., and C.H. Bigland. 1962. Salmonellosis in turkeys: Evaluation of bacteriological and serological evidence in infection. Can J Comp Med Vet Sci 26:151–159.
187. Mair, N.S., and A.I. Ross. 1960. Survival of S. typhimurium in the soil. Mon Bull Minist Health, Public Health Lab Serv 19:39–41.
188. Mallinson, E.T., C.R. Tate, R.G. Miller, and E. Russek-Cohen. 1988. Practical salmonella sampling and testing techniques for poultry farms. Report of the Committee on Salmonella. Proc 92nd Annu Meet US Anim Health Assoc 92:384–385.
189. Marsh, G.A. 1976. The salmonella problem. Poult Dig 35:417–418.
190. Marthedal, H.E. 1977. The occurrence of salmonellosis in poultry in Denmark 1935–75 and the controlling program established. In D.A. Barnum (ed.), Proc Int Symp on Salmonella and Prospects for Control, pp. 78–94. Univ Guelph, Ontario, Canada.
191. Martin, W.J., and W.H. Ewing. 1969. Prevalence of serotypes of salmonella. Appl Microbiol 17:111–117.
192. Mazza, C. 1899. Bakteriologische Unterseuchungen uber einer neuerdings aufgetretene Hühnerepizootie. Zentralbl Bakteriol Parasitenkd Abt I Orig 26:181–185.
193. McBride, G.B., B. Brown, and B.J. Skura. 1978. Effect of bird type, growers and season on the incidence of salmonellae in turkeys. J Food Sci 43:323–326.
194. McCapes, R.H., R.T. Coffland, and L.E. Christie. 1967. Challenge of turkey poults originating from hens vaccinated with Salmonella typhimurium bacteria. Avian Dis 11:15–24.
195. McGarr, C., W.R. Mitchell, H.C. Carlson, and D.A. Barnum. 1976. The transfer of Salmonella from poultry and calves through the food chain. Proc 20th Congr World Vet Poult Assoc, pp. 799–804. Thessaloniki, Greece.
196. McGarr, C., W.R. Mitchell, H.C. Carlson, and N.A. Fish. 1980. An epidemiological study of salmonellae in broiler chicken production. Can J Public Health 71:47–57.
197. McHan, F., N.A. Cox, J.S. Bailey, L.C. Blankenship, and N.J. Stern. 1988. The influence of physical and environmental variables on the in vitro attachment of Salmonella typhimurium to the ceca of chickens. Avian Dis 32:215–219.
198. Mellor, D.B., and G.J. Banwart. 1965. Salmonella derby contamination of eggs from inoculated hens. J Food Sci 30:333–336.
199. Mitrovic, M. 1956. First report of paratyphoid infection in turkey poults due to Salmonella reading. Poult Sci 35:171–174.
200. Miura, S., G. Sato, and T. Miyamae. 1964. Occurrence and survival of salmonella organisms in hatcher chick fluff from commercial hatcheries. Avian Dis 8:546–554.
201. Moore, V.A. 1895. On a pathogenic bacillus of the hog-cholera group associated with a fatal disease in pigeons. USDA BAI Bull 8, pp. 71–76.
202. Morales-Diaz, H.S. 1989. The influence of Salmonella enteritidis in the egg industry. Ph.D. diss., Cornell Univ, Ithaca, NY.
203. Moran, A.B. 1959. Salmonella in animals: A report for 1957. Avian Dis 3:85–88.
204. Morgan-Jones, S.C. 1980. The occurrence of salmonellae during the rearing of broiler birds. Br Poult Sci 21:463–470.
205. Morgan-Jones, S.C. 1981. The interaction of Salmonella typhimurium and the indigenous bacteria in poultry litter. Soc Gen Microbiol Q 8:269.
206. Morishima, H., E. Baba, T. Fukata, and A. Arakawa. 1984. Effect of Eimeria tenella infection in chickens fed the feed artificially contaminated with Salmonella typhimurium. Poult Sci 63:1732–1737.
207. Morse, E.V., and M.A. Duncan. 1974. Salmonellosis – an enviromental health problem. J Am Vet Med Assoc 165:1015–1019.
208. Müller, H. 1972. Salmonellae found in poultry with particular reference to pigeons. Monatsh Veterinaermed 27:575–578.
209. Mundt, J.O., and R.L. Tugwell. 1958. The relationship of the chicken egg to selected paratyphoids. Poult Sci 37:415–420.
210. Murphy, C.D. 1969. Detection of low level salmonella contamination of feed and potential infectivity for poultry. M.S. thesis, Texas A&M Univ, College Station.
211. Nagaraja, K.V., J.A. Newman, and B.S. Pome-

roy. 1984. Use of adjuvant vaccine for the control of salmonella infections in turkeys. In G.H. Snoeyenbos (ed.), Proc Int Symp on Salmonella, pp. 374–375. Am Assoc Avian Path, Kennett Square, PA.

212. Nagaraja, K.V., D.A. Emery, L.F. Sherlock, J.A. Newman, and B.S. Pomeroy. 1984. Detection of Salmonella arizonae in turkey flocks by ELISA. Proc 27th Annu Meet Am Assoc Vet Lab Diag, pp.185–204.

213. Nagaraja, K.V., M.C. Kumar, J.A. Newman, and B.S. Pomeroy. 1985. Control of Salmonella arizonae infection in turkey breeder flocks by immunization. J Am Vet Med Assoc 187:309.

214. Nagaraja, K.V., L.T. Ausherman, D.A. Emery, and B.S. Pomeroy. 1986. Update on enzyme linked immunosorbent assay for its field application in the detection of Salmonella arizonae infection in breeder flocks of turkeys. Proc 29th Annu Meet Am Assoc Vet Lab Diag, pp. 347–356.

215. Nagaraja, K.V., B.S. Pomeroy, L.T. Ausherman, and K.A. Friendshuh. 1987. Salmonella control programs in Minnesota turkey industry. Proc 23rd World Vet Congress, p. 317. Montreal, Canada.

216. Nagaraja, K.V., C.J. Kim, and B.S. Pomeroy. 1988. DNA fingerprinting of S. enteritidis from humans and animals. Report of the Committee on Salmonella. Proc 92nd Annu Meet US Anim Health Assoc 92:347–348.

217. Nazari, A.A. 1977. The use of microantiglobulin test in detection of salmonella carriers in chicken flocks. J Vet Fac Univ Tehran 33:68–74.

218. Nurmi, E., and M. Rantala. 1973. New aspects of salmonella infection in broiler production. Nature 241:210–211.

219. Nurmi, E., and M. Rantala. 1974. The influence of zinc bacitracin on the colonization of Salmonella infantis in the intestine of broiler chickens. Res Vet Sci 17:24–27.

220. Nurmi, E., E. Seuna, and M. Raevuori. 1977. Prevention of salmonellosis in broiler chickens. In D.A. Barnum (ed.), Proc Int Symp on Salmonella and Prospects for Control, pp. 71–77. Univ Guelph, Ontario, Canada.

221. O'Brien, J.D.P. 1988. Salmonella enteritidis infection in broiler chickens. Vet Rec 259:2103–2107.

222. Oelke, H., and F. Steiniger. 1973. Salmonella in adelie penguins (Pygoscelis adeliae) and South polar skuas (Catharacta maccormicki) on Ross island, Antarctica. Avian Dis 17:568–573.

223. Olesiuk, O.M., V.L. Carlson, G.H. Snoeyenbos, and C.F. Smyser. 1969. Experimental Salmonella typhimurium infection in two chicken flocks. Avian Dis 13:500–508.

224. Olesiuk, O.M., G.H. Snoeyenbos, and C.F. Smyser. 1971. Inhibitory effect of used litter on Salmonella typhimurium transmission in the chicken. Avian Dis 15:118–124.

225. Pfaff, Fr. 1921. Eine Truthuhnerseuche mit Paratyphus-Befund. Z Infekt Haustiere 22:285–292.

226. Pfaff, Fr. 1921. Schweinerotlaufbakterien als Erreger einer chronischen Hühnerseuche. Z Infekt Haustiere 22:293–298.

227. Pivnick, H., B. Blanchfield, and J.-Y. D'Aoust. 1981. Prevention of salmonella infection in chicks by treatment with fecal cultures from mature chickens (Nurmi culture). J Food Prot 44:909–916.

228. Pomeroy, B.S. 1944. Salmonellosis of turkeys. Ph.D. diss., Univ Minnesota.

229. Pomeroy, B.S., and R. Fenstermacher. 1939. Paratyphoid infections in turkeys. J Am Vet Med Assoc 94:90–97.

230. Pomeroy, B.S., and R. Fenstermacher. 1943. Salmonella infections in breeding turkeys. Am J Vet Res 4:199–208.

231. Pomeroy, B.S., Y. Siddiqui, and M.K. Grady. 1965. Salmonella in animal feeds and feed ingredients. Proc Nat Conf on Salmonellosis, pp. 74–77. US Dept HEW, NCDC, Atlanta, GA.

232. Pomeroy, B.S., K.V. Nagaraja, H. Olson, L.T. Ausherman, S.C. Nivas, and M.C. Kumar. 1984. Control of Salmonella infections in turkeys in Minnesota. In G.H. Snoeyenbos (ed.), Proc Int Symp on Salmonella, pp. 115–125. Am Assoc Avian Pathol, Kennett Square, PA.

233. Pomeroy, B.S., K.V. Nagaraja, L.T. Ausherman, I.L. Peterson, and K.A. Friendshuh. 1989. Studies of feasibility of producing salmonella-free turkeys. Avian Dis 33:1–7.

234. Poppe, C., and C.L. Gyles. 1987. Relation of plasmids to virulence and other properties of salmonella from avian sources. Avian Dis 31:844–854.

235. Poss, P.E. 1984. Cleaning and disinfection programs in the turkey breeder industry. In G.H. Snoeyenbos (ed.), Proc Int Symp on Salmonella, pp. 131–141. Am Assoc Avian Pathol, Kennett Square, PA.

236. Pourciau, S.S., and W.T. Springer. 1978. Evaluation of secondary enrichment for detecting salmonella in bobwhite quail. Avian Dis 22:42–45.

237. Price, J.I., E. Dougherty, and D.W. Bruner. 1962. Salmonella infection in White Pekin ducks. A short summary of the years 1950–60. Avian Dis 6:145–147.

238. Pritchard, D.G., S.C. Nivas, M.D. York, and B.S. Pomeroy. 1978. Effects of Gal-E mutant of Salmonella typhimurium of experimental salmonellosis in chickens. Avian Dis 22:562–575.

239. Purchase, H.G. 1979. Are we ready for a national Salmonella control program? Rev Infect Dis 1:600–606.

240. Quarles, C.L., R.F. Gentry, and G.O. Bressler. 1970. Bacterial contamination in poultry houses and its relationship to egg hatchability. Poult Sci 49:60–66.

241. Rantala, M., and E. Nurmi. 1973. Prevention of the growth of Salmonella infantis in chicks by the flora of the alimentary tract of chickens. Br Poult Sci 14:627–630.

242. Rasmussen, P.G. 1962. Salmonella typhimurium – ledbetaendelser hos slagteaender: Ledbetaendelsernes aetiologi og fjerkraekontrolmaessige bedommelse. Nord Vet Med 14:39–52.

243. Reid, C.R., and D.A. Barnum. 1983. Evaluation of turkey cecal microflora in protecting day-old poults from Salmonella typhimurium challenge. Avian Dis 27:632–643.

244. Reid, C.R., and D.A. Barnum. 1985. The effects of treatments of cecal contents on their protective properties against salmonella in poults. Avian Dis 29:1–11.

245. Renault, L., J.P. Labadie, N. Miramont, J. Vaissaire, and C. Maire. 1975. Importance of immunofluorescence in the rapid diagnosis of avian salmonellas. Bull Acad Vet Fr 48:52–59.

246. Rettger, L.F., and M. Scoville. 1920. Bacterium anatum, N.S. The etiologic factor in a widespread disease of young ducklings known in some places as "Keel." J Infect Dis 26:217–229.

247. Rice, C.E., S.E. Magwood, and E. Annau. 1960. A modified direct complement-fixation test for the detection of antibodies for salmonella antigens in turkey sera. Can Vet J 1:132–137.

248. Rigby, C.E., and J.R. Pettit. 1979. Some factors affecting Salmonella typhimurium infection and shedding in chickens raised on litter. Avian Dis 23:442–455.

249. Rigby, C.E., and J.R. Pettit. 1980. Changes in the salmonella status of broiler chickens subjected to simulated shipping conditions. Can J Comp Med 44:374–381.

250. Rigby, C.E., and J.R. Pettit. 1980. Observations on competitive exclusion for preventing Salmonella typhimurium infection of broiler chickens. Avian Dis 24:604-615.

251. Rigby, C.E., J.R. Pettit, M.F. Baker, A.H. Bentley, M.O. Solomons, and H. Lior. 1980. Sources of salmonellae in an uninfected commercially-processed broiler flock. Can J Comp Med 44:267-274.

252. Rigby, C.E., J.R. Pettit, G. Papp-Vid, J.L. Spencer, and N.G. Willis. 1981. The isolation of salmonellae, Newcastle disease virus and other infectious agents from quarantined imported birds in Canada. Can J Comp Med 45:366-370.

253. Roberts, T. 1986. The economic losses due to selected foodborne diseases. Proc 90th Annu Meet US Animal Health Assoc, pp. 336-353.

254. Rowe, B., M.L.M. Hall, L.R. Ward, and J.D.H. de Sa. 1980. Epidemic spread of Salmonella hadar in England and Wales. Br Med J 280:1065-1066.

255. Royal, W.A., and M.D. Mutimer. 1972. Inhibition of Salmonella typhimurium by fowl caecal cultures. Res Vet Sci 13:184-185.

256. Sadler, W.W., J.R. Brownell, and M.J. Fanelli. 1969. Influence of age and inoculum level on shed pattern of Salmonella typhimurium in chickens. Avian Dis 13:793-803.

257. Saif, Y.M., and S.M. Shelly. 1973. Effect of gentamicin sulfate dip on salmonella organisms in experimentally infected turkey eggs. Avian Dis 17:574-581.

258. Salisbury, R.M. 1958. Salmonella infections in animals and birds in New Zealand. NZ Vet J 6:76-86.

259. Sanders, E., P.S. Brachman, E.A. Friedman, J. Goldsby, and C.E. McCall. 1965. Salmonellosis in the United States. Results of nationwide surveillance. Am J Epidemiol 81:370-384.

260. Sapre, V.A., and M.L. Mehta. 1969. Diagnostic potentialities of indirect hemagglutination test in chicken artificially infected with salmonella. Indian Vet J 46:183-190.

261. Sapre, V.A., and M.L. Mehta. 1970. Hematological changes in salmonella infections in poultry. Indian J Anim Sci 40:456-463.

262. Sato, G. 1967. Detection of salmonella and arizona organisms from soil of empty turkey yards. Jpn J Vet Res 15:53-55.

263. Sato, G., T. Miyamae, and S. Miura. 1970. A long-term epizootiological study of chicken salmonellosis on a farm with reference to elimination of paratyphoid infection by cloacal swab culture test. Jpn J Vet Res 18:47-62.

264. Sauter, E.A., and C.F. Peterson. 1974. The effect of eggshell quality on penetration by various salmonellae. Poult Sci 53:2159-2163.

265. Savov, D., A. Vrigazov, N. Dimitrov, and N. Gromkov. 1974. Salmonelite i salmonelozite v Bulgariya, pp. 265-271. Acad Sci, Sofia, Bulgaria.

266. Schalm, O.W. 1937. Study of a partyphoid infection in chicks. J Infect Dis 61:208-216.

267. Schimmel, D., K. Linde, G. Marx, and K. Ziedler. 1974. Use of a SMD mutant of Salmonella typhimurium in chicks. Arch Exp Veterinaermed 28:551-558.

268. Schleifer, J.H. 1985. A review of the efficacy and mechanism of competitive exclusion for the control of Salmonella in poultry. World's Poult Sci J 41:72-82.

269. Seuna, E. 1979. Sensitivity of young chickens to Salmonella typhimurium var. copenhagen and S. infantis infection and the preventive effect of cultured intestinal microflora. Avian Dis 23:392-400.

270. Seuna, E., K.V. Nagaraja, and B.S. Pomeroy. 1985. Gentamicin and bacterial culture (Nurmi culture) treatments either alone or in combination against experimental Salmonella hadar infection in turkey poults. Avian Dis 29:617-629.

271. Sidoli, L. 1971. Clinical and postmortem observations on cases of localization of Salmonella typhimurium in the eyes of fowls. Vet Ital 22:335-341.

272. Sieburth, J.M. 1957. The effect of furazolidone on the cultural and serological response of Salmonella typhimurium infected chickens. Avian Dis 1:180-194.

273. Sieburth, J.M. 1957. Indirect hemagglutination studies on salmonellosis of chickens. J Immunol 78:380-386.

274. Sieburth, J.M. 1958. The indirect hemagglutination test in the avian salmonella problem. Am J Vet Res 19:729-735.

275. Sieburth, J.M. 1960. Stable, standardized, sensitized chicken erythrocytes for the polyvalent salmonella indirect hemagglutination test. Am J Vet Res 21:1084-1089.

276. Sieburth, J.M., and E.P. Johnson. 1957. Observations on stress factors and serological response in Salmonella typhimurium infection in chicks. Avian Dis 1:122. (Abstr).

277. Silliker, J.H. 1982. The Salmonella problem—current status and future detection. J Food Prot 45:661-666.

278. Silva, E.N., and O. Hipólito. 1978. Occurrence of salmonella serotypes in chickens (Brazil). Proc 16th World Poult Congr, pp. 388-394.

279. Silva, E.N., and O. Hipólito. 1978. Salmonella strains isolated from the digestive tract of breeding chickens and apparently normal turkeys and in chick embryos. Proc 16th World Poult Congr, pp. 701-706.

280. Simmons, G.C. 1973. Use of Dozomet as a poultry litter fumigant for salmonellas. Aust Vet J 49:268.

281. Simmons, E.R., J.C. Ayres, and A.A. Kraft. 1970. Effect of moisture and temperature on ability of salmonella to infect shell eggs. Poult Sci 49:761-768.

282. Smith, H.W. 1971. The epizootiology of salmonella infection in poultry. In R.F. Gordon and B.M. Freeman (eds.), Poultry Disease and World Economy, pp. 37-46. British Poultry Science, Edinburgh, Scotland.

283. Smith, P.J., M. Larkin, and N.H. Brooksbank. 1972. Bacteriological and serological diagnosis of salmonellas of fowls. Res Vet Sci 13:460-67.

284. Smyser, C.F., and G.H. Snoeyenbos. 1969. Evaluation of several methods of isolating salmonellae from poultry litter and animal feedstuffs. Avian Dis 13:134-141.

285. Smyser, C.F., and G.H. Snoeyenbos. 1971. Enrichment serology compared with a direct-culture procedure for isolating salmonellae from rendered animal by-products. Avian Dis 15:581-587.

286. Smyser, C.F., and G.H. Snoeyenbos. 1972. A pigeon host-adapted type of Salmonella typhimurium var. copenhagen. Avian Dis 16:270-277.

287. Smyser, C.F., and G.H. Snoeyenbos. 1976. Examination of poultry litter for Salmonellae by direct culture and fluorescent antibody technique. Avian Dis 20:545-551.

288. Smyser, C.F., J. Bacharz, and H. Van Roekel. 1963. Detection of Salmonella typhimurium from artificially contaminated poultry feed and animal by-products. Avian Dis 7:423-434.

289. Smyser, C.F., N. Adinarayanan, H. Van Roekel, and G.H. Snoeyenbos. 1966. Field and laboratory observations on Salmonella heidelberg infections in three chicken breeding flocks. Avian Dis 10:314-329.

290. Snoeyenbos, G.H. 1976. Symposium synopsis.

Proc Salmonella Symp, pp. 79-80. Am Assoc Avian Pathol, Kennett Square, PA.

291. Snoeyenbos, G.H. 1977. Salmonella infection at the farm level. In D.A. Barnum (ed.), Proc Int Symp on Salmonella and Prospects for Control, pp. 41-47. Univ Guelph, Ontario, Canada.

292. Snoeyenbos, G.H., and V.L. Carlson. 1973. Gentamicin efficacy against Salmonella and Arizonae in eggs as influenced by administration route and test organism. Avian Dis 17:673-682.

293. Snoeyenbos, G.H., V.L. Carlson, B.A. McKie, and C.F. Smyser. 1967. An epidemiological study of salmonellosis of chickens. Avian Dis 11:653-667.

294. Snoeyenbos, G.H., C.F. Smyser, and H. Van Roekel. 1969. Salmonella infections of the ovary and peritoneum of chickens. Avian Dis 13:668-670.

295. Snoeyenbos, G.H., V.L. Carlson, C.F. Smyser, and O.M. Olesiuk. 1969. Dynamics of salmonella infection in chicks reared on litter. Avian Dis 13:72-83.

296. Snoeyenbos, G.H., B.A. McKie, C.F. Smyser, and C.R. Weston. 1970. Progress in identifying and maintaining Salmonella-free commercial chicken breeding flocks. Avian Dis 14:683-696.

297. Snoeyenbos, G.H., O.M. Weinack, and C.F. Smyser. 1978. Protecting chicks and poults from salmonellae by oral administration of "normal" gut microflora. Avian Dis 22:273-287.

298. Snoeyenbos, G.H., O.M. Weinack, and C.F. Smyser. 1979. Further studies on competitive exclusion for controlling salmonellae in chickens. Avian Dis 23:904-914.

299. Snoeyenbos, G.H., A.S. Soerjadi, and O.M. Weinack. 1982. Gastrointestinal colonization by Salmonellae and pathogenic Escherichia coli in monoxenic and holoxenic chicks and poults. Avian Dis 26:566-575.

300. Snoeyenbos, G.H., O.M. Weinack, A.S. Soerjadi, B.M. Miller, D.E. Woodward, and C.R. Weston. 1985. Large-scale trials to study competitive exclusion of salmonella in chickens. Avian Dis 29:1004-1011.

301. Sobeh, F.Y., and D.V. Vadehra. 1984. Comparison of enterotoxin production by Salmonella enteritidis in laboratory media, milk and meat. Indian J Med Res 79:28-34.

302. Soerjadi, A.S., J.H. Druitt, A.B. Lloyd, and R.B. Cumming. 1979. Effect of environmental temperature on susceptibility of young chickens to Salmonella typhimurium. Aust Vet J 55:413-417.

303. Soerjadi, A.S., S.M. Stehman, G.H. Snoeyenbos, O.M. Weinack, and C.F. Smyser. 1981. Some measurements of protection against paratyphoid Salmonella and Escherichia coli by competitive exclusion in chickens. Avian Dis 25:706-712.

304. Soerjadi, A.S., S.M. Stehman, G.H. Snoeyenbos, O.M. Weinack, and C.F. Smyser. 1981. The influence of lactobacilli on the competitive exclusion of paratyphoid salmonellae in chickens. Avian Dis 25:1027-1033.

305. Soerjadi, A.S., R. Rufner, G.H. Snoeyenbos, and O.M. Weinack. 1982. Adherence of salmonella and native gut microflora to the gastrointestinal mucosa of chicks. Avian Dis 26:576-584.

306. Sokkar, S.M., and A.A. Bassiouni. 1974. Fibrinoid change in the spleen of ducks experimentally infected with Salmonella typhimurium. Zentralbl Veterinaermed Reihe [B] 21:632-637.

307. St. Louis, M.E., D.L. Morse, M.E. Potter, T.M. DeMelfi, J.J. Guzewich, R.V. Tauxe, and P.A. Blake. 1988. The emergence of grade A eggs as a major source of Salmonella enteritidis infections. J Am Med Assoc 259:2103-2107.

308. Stover, D.E. 1964. Hatching egg sanitation and fumigation for disease control. Bull Calif Dep Agric 53:147-150.

309. Tacal, J.V., Jr., and C.F. Meñez. 1967. Salmonella studies in the Philippines. VII. The isolation of Salmonella derby from abattoir flies and chicken ascarids. Phillipp J Vet Med 6:106-111.

310. Takimoto, H., E. Baba, T. Fukata, and A. Arakawa. 1984. Effects of infection of Eimeria tenella, E. acervulina, and E. maxima upon Salmonella typhimurium infection in chickens. Poult Sci 63:478-484.

311. Talbot, N.T., and A.M. Rampling. 1966. Chicken mortality due to Salmonella newington in Port Moresby. Aust Vet J 42:308.

312. Tannock, G.W., and J.M.B. Smith. 1972. Studies on the survival of Salmonella typhimurium and Salmonella bovis-morbificans on soil and sheep faeces. Res Vet Sci 13:150-153.

313. Thain, J.A. 1980. An evaluation of the microantiglobulin test in monitoring experimental salmonella group C infections in chickens. Res Vet Sci 28:212-216.

314. Thain, J.A., and G.A. Cullen. 1978. Detection of Salmonella typhimurium of chickens. Vet Rec 102:143-145.

315. Thaxton, P., R.D. Wyatt, and P.B. Hamilton. 1974. The effect of environmental temperature on paratyphoid infection in neonatal chicken. Poult Sci 53:88-94.

316. Thomason, B.M. 1981. Current status of immunofluorescent methodology for salmonellae. J Food Prot 44:381-384.

317. Tizard, I.R., N.A. Fish, and J. Harmeson. 1979. Free flying sparrows as carriers of salmonellosis. Can Vet J 20:143-144.

318. Truscott, R.B. 1956. Salmonella moscow isolated from ducks in Ontario. Can J Comp Med Vet Sci 20:345-346.

319. Truscott, R.B. 1981. Oral Salmonella antigens for the control of salmonella in chicks. Avian Dis 25:810-820.

320. Truscott, R.B., and G.W. Friars. 1972. The transfer of endotoxin induced immunity from hens to poults. Can J Comp Med Vet Sci 36:64-68.

321. Truscott, R.B., and A.N. Sajnani. 1972. Studies on the serological and immunological response of chickens to endotoxin and endotoxoid. Can J Comp Med Vet Sci 36:170-177.

322. Tucker, J.F. 1967. Survival of salmonella in built-up litter for housing of rearing and laying fowls. Br Vet J 123:92-103.

323. Tucker, J.F., W.B. Brown, and G. Goodship. 1974. Fumigation with methyl bromide of poultry foods artificially contaminated with salmonella. Br Poult Sci 15:587-595.

324. Turnbull, P.C.B. 1979. Food poisoning with special reference to salmonella—its epidemiology, pathogenesis and control. Clin Gastroenterol 8:663-714.

325. Turnbull, P.C.B., and J.E. Richmond. 1978. A model of salmonella enteritis: The behaviour of Salmonella enteritidis in chick intestine studies by light and electron microscopy. Br J Exp Pathol 59:64-75.

326. Turnbull, P.C.B., and G.H. Snoeyenbos. 1973. The roles of ammonia water activity and pH in the salmonellacidal effect of long-used poultry litter. Avian Dis 17:72-86.

327. Turnbull, P.C.B., and G.H. Snoeyenbos. 1974. Experimental salmonellosis in the chicken. I. Fate and host response in alimentary canal, liver, and spleen. Avian Dis 18:153-177.

328. Turnbull, P.C.B., and G.H. Snoeyenbos. 1974. Experimental salmonellosis in the chicken. 2. Fate of a temperature sensitive filamentous mutant. Avian Dis 18:178-185.

329. Van Roekel, H. 1965. Salmonella in poultry and eggs. Proc Nat Conf Salmonellosis, pp. 78-83. Atlanta, GA.

330. Van Ulsen, F.W. 1977. Darminfecties bij postduiven, Tijdschr Diergeneeskd 102:696-697.
331. Vestal, O.H., and J.F. Stephens. 1966. The relative pathogenicity of selected paratyphoids for chicks. Avian Dis 10:502-507.
332. Vuillaume, A., and R. Labatut. 1977. Incidence of Salmonella typhimurium and S. enteritidis infections in the Landes Department in a flock of breeding geese. Rev Med Vet 128:661-666.
333. Walker, J.W. 1977. Salmonella in feed. In D.A. Barnum (ed.), Proc Int Symp on Salmonella and Prospects for Control, pp. 48-57. Univ Guelph, Ontario, Canada.
334. Ward, L.R., J.D. de Sa, and B. Rowe. 1987. A phage typing scheme for S. enteritidis. Epidemiol Infect 99: 291-294.
335. Watson, W.A., and J.M. Brown. 1975. Salmonella infection and meat hygiene: Poultry meat. Vet Rec 96:351-353.
336. Weand, D.C., and A.G. Horsting. 1978. Sanitation of hatching eggs. Proc 16th World Poult Congr, pp. 797-808.
337. Weinack, O.M., C.F. Smyser, and G.H. Snoeyenbos. 1979. Evaluation of several methods of detecting salmonella in groups of chickens. Avian Dis 23:179-193.
338. Weinack, O.M., G.H. Snoeyenbos, and C.F. Smyser. 1979. A supplemental test system to measure competitive exclusion of salmonella by native microflora in the chicken gut. Avian Dis 23:1019-1030.
339. Weinack, O.M., G.H. Snoeyenbos, C.F. Smyser, and A.S. Soerjadi. 1982. Reciprocal competitive exclusion of Salmonella and Escherichia coli by native intestinal microflora of the chicken and turkey. Avian Dis 26:585-595.
340. Weinack, O.M., G.H. Snoeyenbos, A.S. Soerjadi, and C.F. Smyser. 1985. Influence of temperature, social, and dietary stress on development and stability of protective microflora in chickens against S. typhimurium. Avian Dis 29:1177-1183.
341. Weinack, O.M., G.H. Snoeyenbos, A.S. Soerjadi, and C.F. Smyser. 1985. Therapeutic trials with native intestinal microflora for Salmonella typhimurium infections in chickens. Avian Dis 29:1230-1234.
342. Weinack, O.M., G.H. Snoeyenbos, and A.S. Soerjadi. 1985. Further studies on competitive exclusion of Salmonella typhimurium by lactobacilli in chickens. Avian Dis 29:1273-1276.
343. Weston, C.R. 1976. Epidemiology of salmonella in commercial primary breeding and multiplier flocks. Proc Salmonella Symp, pp. 18-20. Am Assoc Avian Pathol, Kennett Square, PA.
344. Wierup, M., and B. Nordblom 1984. The salmonella control program in Sweden with special reference to poultry. In G.H. Snoeyenbos (ed.), Proc Int Symposium on Salmonella, pp. 94-101. Am Assoc Avian Pathol, Kennett Square, PA.
345. Williams, J.E. 1965. Paratyphoid and Arizona infections. In H.E. Biester and L.H. Schwarte (eds.), Diseases of Poultry, 5th Ed., pp. 260-328. Iowa State Univ Press, Ames.
346. Williams, J.E. 1968. History, morphology, and biochemical and antigenic properties of Salmonella typhimurium strain P-10. Avian Dis 12:512-517.
347. Williams, J.E. 1970. Effect of high-level formaldehyde fumigation on bacterial populations on the surface of chicken hatching eggs. Avian Dis 14:386-392.
348. Williams, J.E. 1972. Observations on Salmonella thompson as a poultry pathogen. Avian Pathol 1:69-73.
349. Williams, J.E. 1972. Paratyphoid infections. In M.S. Hofstad, B.W. Calnek, C.F. Helmboldt, W.M Reid, and H.W. Yoder, Jr. (eds.), Diseases of Poultry, 6th Ed., pp. 135-202. Iowa State Univ Press, Ames.
350. Williams, J.E. 1976. Rationale for the control of salmonellae: Eggs and hatchery. Proc Salmonella Symposium, pp. 27-29. Am Assoc Avian Pathol, Kennett Square, PA.
351. Williams, J.E. 1978. Microtest methodology for the detection of avian salmonella infections. Proc 16th World Poult Congr, pp. 1412-1416.
352. Williams, J.E. 1980. Formalin destruction of salmonellae in poultry litter. Poult Sci 59:2717-2724.
353. Williams, J.E. 1981. Salmonellas in poultry feeds – a worldwide review. III. Methods in control and elimination. World's Poult Sci J 37:6-25. 97-105.
354. Williams, J.E. 1984. Paratyphoid infections. In M.S. Hofstad., H.J. Barnes, B.W. Calnek, W.M. Reid, and H.W. Yoder, Jr. (eds.), Diseases of Poultry, 8th Ed., pp. 91-129. Iowa State Univ Press, Ames.
355. Williams, J.E., and S.T. Benson. 1978. Survival of Salmonella typhimurium in poultry feed and litter at three temperatures. Avian Dis 22:742-747.
356. Williams, J.E., and S.T. Benson. 1978. Antibacterial properties of sodium nalidixate against avian salmonellae in liquid and on solid media. Poult Sci 57:1546-1549.
357. Williams, J.E., and L.H. Dillard. 1968. Salmonella penetration of fertile and infertile chicken eggs at progressive stages. Avian Dis 12:629-635.
358. Williams, J.E., and L.H. Dillard. 1969. Salmonella penetration of the outer structures of white and speckled shell turkey eggs. Avian Dis 13:203-210.
359. Williams, J.E., and L.H. Dillard. 1973. The effect of external shell treatments on salmonella penetration of chicken eggs. Poult Sci 52:1084-1089.
360. Williams, R.B., and M.W. Dodson. 1960. Salmonella in Alaska. Public Health Rep 75:913-916.
361. Williams, J.E., and C.D. Gordon. 1970. The hatchability of chicken eggs fumigated with increasing levels of formaldehyde gas before incubation. Poult Sci 49:560-564.
362. Williams, L.P., and B.C. Hobbs. 1975. Enterobacteriaceae infections. In W.T. Hubbert, W.F. McCulloch, and P.R. Schnurrenberger (eds.), Diseases Transmitted from Animals to Man, pp. 33-109. Charles C. Thomas, Springfield, IL.
363. Williams, J.E., and A.D. MacDonald. 1955. The past, present, and future of salmonella antigens for poultry. Proc 92nd Annu Meet Am Vet Med Assoc, pp. 333-339.
364. Williams, J.E., and A.D. Whittemore. 1972. Microantiglobulin test for detecting Salmonella typhimurium agglutinins. Appl Microbiol 23:931-937.
365. Williams, J.E., and A.D. Whittemore. 1973. Microtesting for avian salmonellosis. Proc 77th Annu Meet US Anim Health Assoc, pp. 607-613.
366. Williams, J.E., and A.D. Whittemore. 1973. Avian salmonella-stained microtest antigens produced on solid media. Appl Microbiol 26:1-3.
367. Williams, J.E., and A.D. Whittemore. 1975. Influence of age on the serological response of chickens to Salmonella typhimurium infection. Avian Dis 19:745-760.
368. Williams, J.E., and A.D. Whittemore. 1976. Field applications of MA and MAG tests for detection of avian salmonellosis. Proc 80th Annu Meet US Anim Health Assoc, pp. 297-303.
369. Williams, J.E., and A.D. Whittemore. 1976. Comparison of six methods of detecting Salmonella typhimurium infection of chickens. Avian Dis 20:728-734.
370. Williams, J.E., and A.D. Whittemore. 1979. Serological response of chickens to Salmonella thompson and Salmonella pullorum infections. J Clin Microbiol 9:108-114.
371. Williams, J.E., and A.D. Whittemore. 1980. Bac-

teriostatic effect of five antimicrobial agents on salmonellae in the intestinal tract of chickens. Poult Sci 59:44–53.

372. Williams, J.E., L.H. Dillard, and G.O. Hall. 1968. The penetration patterns of Salmonella typhimurium through the outer structures of chicken eggs. Avian Dis 12:445–466.

373. Williams, J.E., E.T. Mallinson, and G.H. Snoeyenbos. 1980. Salmonellosis and Arizonosis. In S.B. Hitchner, C.H. Domermuth, H.G. Purchase, and J.E. Williams (eds.), Isolation and Identification of Avian Pathogens, pp. 1–8. Am Assoc Avian Pathol, Kennett Square, PA.

374. Wilson, J.E. 1944. Observations on paralysis and some current conditions in poultry problems. Vet Rec 56:521–524.

375. Wuthe, H.H. 1971. Untersuchungen uber Typen der Salmonella typhimurium bei Haustauben in Schleswig-Holstein und ihre mögliche epizootologische Bedeutung. Berl Muench Tieraerztl Wochenschr 84:290–292.

376. Wyatt, R.D., and P.B. Hamilton. 1975. Interaction between Aflatoxicosis and a natural infection of chickens with salmonella. Appl Microbiol 30:870–872.

377. Yamamoto, R., H.E. Adler, W.W. Sadler, and G.F. Stewart. 1961. A study of Salmonella typhimurium infection in market-age turkeys. Am J Vet Res 22:382–387.

ARIZONOSIS

K.V. Nagaraja, B.S. Pomeroy, and J.E. Williams

INTRODUCTION. *Salmonella arizonae* is a subspecies of the genus *Salmonella* based on relatedness of the deoxyribonucleic acids of all the various kinds of salmonellae (24). Since 1984, arizona isolates have been identified with salmonella terminology. Members of the arizona group originally were recovered from cold-blooded animals (8), but since have been isolated from a wide variety of animals including poultry. In turkeys, it is one of the most frequently identified serotypes (28) in the USA and it is related to serious mortality and morbidity losses.

The disease caused by *S. arizonae* serotypes in poultry is indistinguishable clinically from salmonellosis and is referred to as arizona infection or avian arizonosis (AA). *S. arizonae* isolates may be distinguished from other salmonellae based on biochemical characteristics.

AA poses a problem of considerable economic importance to the turkey industry through reduced production and hatchability (16, 17, 35, 47, 57, 83, 87). There are several reviews available (3, 4, 42).

HISTORY. The first-described culture was isolated from fatally infected reptiles (8), although Lewis and Hitchner (62) had previously reported recovery of slow lactose-fermenting bacteria from a disease of chicks resembling salmonellosis. This infection was probably due to a member of the arizona group and may represent the first report of AA. AA was first reported in poultry in Great Britain in 1968 (53).

INCIDENCE AND DISTRIBUTION. AA occurs worldwide wherever poultry is raised. *S. arizonae* 18:Z4, Z32 is widely distributed in turkey-raising areas of the USA; very high rates of isolation were reported in California in 1968 and 1969, descending to a low point in 1972 (65). AA may have been eliminated from the turkey industry in Great Britain (88); no outbreaks were reported during 1976–86 (5).

ETIOLOGY

Classification. Since 1939 repeated attempts have been made to find a generally acceptable taxonomic position for this group of bacteria; several classification systems have been used and a wide variety of names and designations has been applied to the organisms.

Edwards and associates (cited in 64), established the biochemical and antigenic similarity of the arizonae and salmonellae. Enough differences were found between the groups, however, to justify classification of the arizonae in a separated genus. Kauffmann and Edwards (55) first employed the name *Arizona arizonae,* which was also used by Ewing (21) for members of the genus *Arizona* (genus II of the tribe Salmonellae). A new type species name *Arizona hinshawii* had been proposed by Ewing (23) to pay honor to the pioneering work of W.R. Hinshaw on AA in turkeys, reptiles, and other animals. Kauffmann (54) subsequently included the arizonae in his subgenus III of the genus *Salmonella,* designating them *S. arizonae* and listing their antigenic formulas only in the simplified Kauffmann-White scheme. The arizonae have been classified in the *Salmonella* genus in the 8th edition of Bergy's Manual (7) and all organisms in the group are designated *Salmonella arizonae.*

Ewing and his colleagues (22, 25–27, 64) have further clarified the definition by which the biochemical and antigenic characteristics of members of the genus *Arizona* may be readily differentiated from other Enterobacteriaceae. The terminology used by Centers for Disease Control will be will be followed in this subchapter, e.g., *S. arizonae,* 18:Z4, Z32.

Morphology and Staining. The *S. arizonae* resemble other enteric organisms. They are gram-negative nonsporogenic bacilli that are motile by peritrichous flagella.

Growth Requirements. Members can be readily cultivated on ordinary liquid and solid laboratory media, revealing an abundant growth similar to that of the salmonellae. Most cultures grow very well on salmonella-shigella and brilliant-green agars as well as other solid media recommended for isolation of salmonellae. On initial isolation, colonies usually resemble those of salmonellae but may develop an indicator change typical of lactose fermenters after incubation for several days or weeks. Rapid lactose-fermenting strains, rare in poultry, cannot be distinguished from normal coliforms, which are usually inhibited by these media. Routine use of bismuth sulfite plating medium was recommended (19, 42, 64) to aid in preliminary recognition of lactose-fermenting arizona strains before they are possibly discarded as coliforms.

Biochemical Properties. Cultures possessing the following biochemical characteristics are almost invariably classifiable serologically as members of *S. arizonae* (12, 24, 26).

Dextrose	fermented with gas
Lactose	fermented, as a rule, slowly or promptly
Sucrose	not fermented, as a rule
Mannitol	fermented with gas
Maltose	fermented with gas
Dulcitol	not fermented
Inositol	not fermented
Indole	not produced, as a rule
Methyl red	positive
Voges-Proskauer	negative
Jordan's tartrate	no reaction
Hydrogen sulfide	positive
Urea	not hydrolyzed
Gelatin	liquified slowly
Potassium cyanide	negative, as a rule
Nitrates	reduced
Motility	positive
Beta-galactosidase	positive
Decarboxylases	
Lysine	positive
Arginine	positive, usually delayed
Ornithine	positive
Malonate	positive
Phenylalanine deaminase	negative

Most isolates from poultry, unlike salmonellae, ferment lactose usually within 7–10 days incubation. Failure of cultures to ferment dulcitol and inositol or to use D-tartrate, their slow liquefaction of gelatin, and their positive reactions in sodium malonate and beta-galactosidase are most useful in distinguishing them from other members of the salmonella group.

A summary tabulation of biochemical and other differential tests for identification of paratyphoid, arizona, and citrobacter strains is presented in Table 3.6 (see also Table 11.1 in 24).

CITROBACTERS. For purposes of classification and identification, the *S. arizonae* must be differentiated not only from other salmonellae but also from the antigenically related genus *Citrobacter* of the tribe Salmonellae (see Table 3.6). Members of this genus are not known to be pathogenic for poultry, but from a diagnostic standpoint they may be confused with salmonella cultures on initial isolation from fecal specimens. The former Bethesda-Ballerup "paracolons" (*P. intermedium*) are included in the genus *Citrobacter* along with cultures previously classified as *Escherichia freundii.*

Resistance to Chemical and Physical Agents. Arizonae are readily destroyed by heat and common disinfectants but have survived in contaminated water for 5 mo, in contaminated feed for 17 mo, in soil on turkey ranges for 6–7 mo, and on materials and utensils in poultry houses for 5 to 25 or more wk (2, 31, 56, 57, 76, 80). Resistance properties are very similar to those of salmonellae.

Antigenic Structure. *S. arizonae* strains are related serologically to the salmonellae and other Enterobacteriaceae, and procedures for study and identification of their antigenic structure are identical to those for paratyphoid organisms. Both somatic (O) and flagellar (H) components are demonstrable.

The serotype nomenclature system used in designating members of the genus *Salmonella* has been applied to *S. arizonae.* In writing antigenic formulas, commas are used to separate O antigen factors, a colon to distinguish the O and H antigens, commas to separate H antigenic factors within a single phase, and a hyphen or dash to separate the first phase from the second and the second from the third, etc. Thus the monophasic type species would be designated *S. arizonae* 18:Z4,Z32.

Pathogenicity. *S. arizonae* can invade the bloodstream, especially of young fowl; high mortality has been reported (16). Lewis and Hitchner (62) recorded mortality of 32–50% in chicks from the infection. Others have observed mortality generally between 10 and 50%, with chicks or poults especially susceptible within the first few days after hatching and with mortality continuing for up to 3–4 wk (1, 15, 44, 57, 75, 87). Geissler and Youssef (30) inoculated or dipped chicken eggs with *S. arizonae;* 100% and 40–79% of embryos in the respective groups died during the incubation period. Hatchability for the latter group varied from 0 to 21–70%, with evidence that the organisms penetrated to the inner structures of the eggs.

Worcester (98) noted that *S. arizonae* can penetrate the wall of the intestinal tract and stay there indefinitely.

PATHOGENESIS AND EPIZOOTIOLOGY

Natural and Experimental Hosts. *S. arizonae* recognize no host barriers and are widely distributed in nature in a variety of avian, mammalian, and reptilian species (9, 15–17, 64, 78, 84, 96, 97).

Among poultry, AA is most frequently encountered in turkeys. Greenfield (39) noted that AA in chickens does not appear to be economically important, although chickens are affected by AA both naturally and experimentally (15, 62, 86).

Dougherty (10) isolated *S. arizonae* from duck livers, revealing lesions very similar to those produced by paratyphoid infections.

For a review of AA as a human disease causing gastroenteritis and frequently more serious enteric fever and focal infections, see Guckian et al. (45), Martin et al. (64), Williams and Hobbs (94), Johnson et al. (52), and Weiss et al. (90).

Transmission, Carriers, Vectors. The transmission cycle of AA in poultry is identical with that established for motile salmonellae (see Paratyphoid Infections). Infected adult birds are frequently intestinal carriers and spreaders of *S. arizonae* for long periods (14). Wild birds (67), rats and mice (35), and reptiles (46, 48) have been cited as common sources of the organisms for poultry flocks.

Intestinal infections have been reported (47, 82), and Adler and Rosenwald (1) reported that AA in adult turkeys is confined primarily to the intestinal tract.

Transmission of AA through eggs has been reported by many workers (6, 14–17, 37, 47), and recovery of *S. arizonae* from ovaries of adult turkeys (29, 47, 83) suggests that transovarian transmission can occur. Direct contamination of the ovary by systemic infection can follow ingestion of the organisms (58, 83, 85). Perek et al. (74) isolated *S. arizonae* from semen of cockerels.

S. arizonae from fecal contamination have a penetration pattern through the shell and shell membranes of chicken eggs very similar to that of *S. typhimurium* when incubated at 37.2 C, resulting in frequent presence of the organisms in chicken and turkey eggs (14, 37, 83, 93). Fecal contamination may spread the infection from other animal species to poultry. Goetz (35) found an AA rate of 90% in rats and 50% in mice on the premises of a turkey farm where the infection was a problem in poults. Various types of wild birds, reptiles, and many common animal species can also infect poultry flocks.

AA is transmitted in the incubator and brooder by direct contact and through contaminated feed and water (20, 57).

Signs. While signs of AA in poultry are not specific, infected poults and chicks may appear listless and develop diarrhea, leg paralysis, twisted necks, and pasting of the down around the vent. There may be blindness caused by caseous material covering the retina (57, 86). Infected birds tend to sit on their hocks and huddle together. Nervous signs, including convulsions, may follow brain infection in poults (51, 73).

Sato and Adler (83) noted that clinical signs of AA are rarely seen in adult turkeys and they seldom die from this infection.

Gross Lesions and Histopathology. West and Mohanty (91) presented a very comprehensive review of pathologic changes noted in AA of poults. Lesions in poults naturally infected with *S. arizonae* were found to be comparable to lesions induced by paratyphoid organisms. Most organs had inflammatory, degenerative, and/or necrotic changes. Changes were acute in central nervous system and ocular tissues and subacute in tissues of other organs.

Lesions described by Lewis and Hitchner (62) in experimentally infected chicks were typical of a generalized septicemia and included peritonitis; retained yolk sacs; enlarged yellowish, mottled, or inflamed livers; and discolored hearts.

Marked congestion of the duodenum and ocher or mottled livers are common in AA (47). Goetz and Quortrup (36) found caseous plugs similar to those seen in pullorum disease in arizonae-infected poults, and Hinshaw and McNeil (47) noted that *S. arizonae*-infected adult turkeys had small caseous mesenteric lesions and cystic ovules. Yellowish, caseous exudates in air sacs and abdominal cavities may also be seen, and there may be retained yolks (57, 82).

Sari et al. (79) reported striking lesions in the brain and Silva et al. (86) found caseous material in the cortical region.

DIAGNOSIS.

Signs and lesions are of little value in differentiating AA from other salmonella infections. Findings on necropsy must be substantiated by recovery and identification of the causative bacteria. In AA the organisms can usually be recovered from liver, spleen, heart blood, lungs, kidneys, unabsorbed yolk, and intestines.

Birds with generalized AA infection may show signs and lesions typical of any acute septicemia caused by a wide variety of bacteria. The heavy, yellowish white, cheesy exudate covering the retinas of poults with AA infection can be confused with lesions of aspergillosis. Nervous signs associated with AA infection may resemble those of Newcastle disease or other diseases affecting the nervous system.

Isolation and Identification of Causative Agent. Cultural procedures identical to those outlined and discussed under Paratyphoid Infections are employed for isolation and identification of arizonae. Standard methods for isolation and biochemical or serological identification of *S. arizonae* from poultry tissues, eggs and embryos, and environmental samples have been described (19, 24, 88, 95). Bismuth sulfite medium can be used for plating enrichment broths in addition to brilliant green (BG) sulfa if desired. The two serotypes of *S. arizonae* common in turkeys are slow lactose fermenters and therefore identical to paratyphoids on initial isolation on BG agar.

Selenite cystine broth may be used in enrichment of fecal and organic tissue cultures (57, 82, 83). Selenite broth incubated at 43 C yielded fewer isolations of arizonae than did tetrathionate or selenite F broth at 35 C (40).

Forty-nine strains of *S. arizonae* isolated from turkeys all had similar cultural and biochemical characteristics, varying only in use of citrate and melibiose (89). Most *S. arizonae* strains were sensitive only to chloramphenicol and nalidixic acid among the antibiotics tested. Kumar et al. (59) found that selenite BG with sulfapyridine (SBGS) and tetrathionate BG broths gave comparable results with *S. arizonae,* but at 48 hr there was considerable reduction in recovery of arizonae from SBGS in tubes initially inoculated with high numbers of organisms. Littell (63) described a differential plating medium for isolation of *S. arizonae* that produces a uniform reaction of both lactose-negative and lactose-positive *S. arizonae* and differentiates them from other salmonellae.

Snoeyenbos and Smyser (87) believed that litter culturing may aid epidemiologic studies and identify infected turkey flocks as part of a control program. Greenfield and Bigland (41) noted that culture of turkey litter might be a useful means of detecting insidious AA.

Culture of turkey shell membranes and shells is recommended over yolk material for rapid detection of arizonae-contaminated eggs (11, 43, 77).

Serology. Serologic analysis of cultures is essential in epizootiologic studies of AA of fowl; cultures can be submitted to the Salmonella Serotyping Laboratory, National Veterinary Services Laboratories P.O. Box 844, Ames, IA 50010, for biochemical characterization and antigenic typing.

Edwards and Galton (13) noted that it is essential to use a polyvalent *S. arizonae* antiserum in preliminary examination of cultures, since arizona types may not be agglutinated by salmonella polyvalent antiserum. Kowalski and Stephens (57) employed formolized broth cultures and *S. arizonae* polymonophasic antiserum in serologic identification of arizonae cultures. Snoeyenbos and Smyser (87) used *S. arizonae* flagellar polyvalent, salmonella flagellar Z32, and salmonella somatic 18 antisera in screening cultures suspected to be *S. arizonae.*

TREATMENT. Chemotherapy may reduce losses in acute outbreaks of AA and may be recommended to prevent spread of the disease in market flocks. Williams (92) reviewed various treatments for AA. In the USA the only drugs approved by the Food and Drug Administration for treatment of AA are furazolidone and antibiotic injectables, gentamicin and spectinomycin. These injectables, given at the hatchery, have dramatically controlled the acute losses and morbidity that may occur during the first 3 wk of age. Isolates of *S. arizonae* resistant to gentamicin have been reported (18, 49).

Ghazikhanian et al. (34) reviewed the program of a primary breeder to reduce and eliminate *S. arizonae* from a basic breeding operation. A combination antibiotic hatching-egg treatment (dipped and injected) was successful in producing *S. arizonae*-free pedigree stock (33, 66). In addition to the egg treatment program, an autogenous oil-emulsion *S. arizonae* bacterin was used on infected flocks to reduce transmission. Because of contamination of ranges, a new capital building program was initiated (total confinement, paved floors, birdproof). A cleaning and disinfecting program was initiated after each depopulation and the facilities were monitored to determine the effectiveness of the program. Finally, special emphasis was placed on frequent egg collection practices. Only pelleted feed containing no animal or poultry by-products was used. The program has been highly successful.

PREVENTION AND CONTROL. Because *S. arizonae* is egg transmitted, primary breeding stock must be developed free of *S. arizonae.* The control program at the multiplier/breeder level is dependent on having available *S. arizonae*-free stock. Management procedures outlined under Paratyphoid Infections are applicable for the control and reduction of AA. The program outlined by Ghazikhanian et al. (34) for the primary breeder level is applicable to the multiplier level except for the treatment of hatching eggs with antibiotics. Total confinement, birdproof and rodentproof buildings that can be cleaned and disinfected, quality feed and feed ingredients, and microbiological monitoring at the hatchery and breeder farm levels are essential.

Serologic Testing. Serologic tests have not been entirely effective in detecting or controlling AA in turkeys (1, 76, 98).

Methods for preparing and using *S. arizonae* antigens for serologic testing of chickens and turkeys have been outlined (4).

Timms (88) found that the most reliable and satisfactory methods for detecting *S. arizonae* at various stages of infection in adult turkeys were the rapid serum plate (SP) test and the somatic tube agglutination (TA) test. The rapid whole-blood (WB) test was found to be a useful tool in testing large numbers of birds in the field, but it required confirmation by the TA test. Uses of the agar gel diffusion, indirect hemagglutination, immunofluorescent, and H agglutination tests in providing supporting evidence of infection were discussed. Lamont and Timms (61) reported use of O and H TA tests, the rapid WB test, and agar gel precipitin tests for detection of AA in turkeys. They also found the rapid WB test particularly useful for flock screening.

Sato and Adler (82, 83) used a formalin-treated broth culture of actively motile arizona strains in preparing H antigen, and ethanol-treated cell suspension from beef heart infusion agar for O antigen. They found that naturally infected turkeys had positive O agglutination reactions at some time during the period they were observed; however, some of the same birds were negative when tested with H antigen. The H agglutinins disappeared earlier then O agglutinins. Not all infected birds revealed positive O agglutinin tests at time of necropsy. There was little correlation between serologic results and persistence of infection.

Kumar et al. (60) developed a tetrazolium-stained microagglutination (MA) test antigen for detection of *S. arizonae* infections in turkeys. The MA test was demonstrated to be far more sensitive and superior to the TA and SP tests in detecting turkeys infected *S. arizonae*. Attempts to detect infection with the microantiglobulin test were unsuccessful.

Adult carriers may lack detectable antibodies 12–14 wk after exposure and infected turkey hens go through an antibody-negative phase at 16–20 wk of age when most breeder flocks are tested (60, 88). When the ovary becomes activated following a lighting regime at 28–32 wk of age, antibodies may be detectable. At that stage in the breeding cycle it is too late to eliminate the flocks. Greenfield (38) noted that antibody titers do not persist for lengthy periods and may not be detectable in birds with subclinical infections.

Nagaraja et al. (69, 71) found an ELISA using outer-membrane proteins extracted from *S. arizonae* as antigens to be sensitive and specific for the detection of *S. arizonae* infection in breeder flocks of turkeys. It was considered to be a valuable tool to determine which breeder flock is infected, allowing the hatchery program to be adjusted to reduce *S. arizonae* dissemination at the time of hatching.

Immunization. Several types of bacterins have been applied to turkey breeding stock. Holte (50) found that vaccinated breeders exposed to *S. arizonae* 18:Z4,Z32 had reduced shedding and were protected from systemic infection, thus preventing egg-transmission of arizonae. Parental immunity was found to be transmitted to poults of vaccinated hens.

Sato and Adler (81) found varying degrees of protection afforded by arizona bacterins in both mice and turkeys. A formalin-treated whole culture in aluminum hydroxide gel provided the best protection, based on the number of organisms that migrated to the spleen following intramuscular challenge. In turkeys a chrome-alum-treated arizona bacterin provided protection against both oral and intraperitoneal challenge (68). Fecal shedding for the first 3 wk after challenge may be reduced by immunization with bacterins (1).

Gerlach et al. (32) found serum from unimmunized turkey hens had both bacteriostatic and bactericidal effects on cultures of *S. arizonae* 18:Z4,Z32, but there was no inhibitory activity in the serum of birds vaccinated with arizona bacterin or in serum from naturally infected breeders. Inhibition of growth was not associated with presence of agglutinating antibodies; in fact, the opposite appeared to be true. In contrast, a bactericidal substance in the albumen of eggs from vaccinated turkeys was reported (1).

Ghazikhanian et al. (34) reported encouraging results using oil-emulsion bacterins; egg transmission following challenge was reduced from 12% in nonvaccinated controls to 2% in vaccinated turkeys. Vaccination against *S. arizonae* infection with a mineral oil–adjuvanted vaccine was evaluated in turkey breeder flocks under laboratory and field situations by Nagaraja et al. (70, 72). The results were encouraging; it was possible to obtain *S. arizonae*–free progeny from vaccinated breeder flocks held in infected environments.

REFERENCES

1. Adler, H.E., and A.S. Rosenwald. 1968. Paracolon control–what we know and need to know. Turkey World 43:18.

2. Anonymous. 1967. Salmonella and Arizona group of infections of avian origin. Annu Rep 1966, pp. 24–29. Food Prot Toxicol Cent, Univ Calif, Davis.

3. Anonymous. 1976. Proc Salmonella Symp. Am Assoc Avian Pathol, Kennett Square, PA.

4. Anonymous. 1984. Proc Int Symp on Salmonella. G.H. Snoyenbos (ed.). Am Assoc Avian Pathol, Kennett Square, PA.

5. Anonymous. 1986. Animal salmonellosis. Annual summaries, survey of drug resistance in Salmonellae. Ministry of Agriculture Fisheries and Food. Welsh Office Agriculture Department. Department of Agriculture and Fisheries for Scotland.
6. Bruner, D.W., and M.C. Peckham. 1952. An outbreak of paracolon infection in turkey poults. Cornell Vet 42:22-24.
7. Buchanan, R.E., and N.E. Gibbons. 1974. Bergey's Manual of Determinative Bacteriology, 8th Ed., pp. 290-340. Williams & Wilkins, Baltimore, MD.
8. Caldwell, M.E., and D.L. Ryerson. 1939. Salmonellosis in certain reptiles. J Infect Dis 65:242-245.
9. Cambre, R.C., D.E. Green, E.E. Smith, R.J. Montali, and M. Bush. 1980. Salmonellosis and arizonosis in the reptile collection at the National Zoological Park. J Am Vet Med Assoc 177:800-803.
10. Dougherty, E. 1953. Disease problems confronting the duck industry. Proc 90th Annu Meet Am Vet Med Assoc, pp. 359-365.
11. Dovadola, E., and F. Carlotto. 1969. Bacteriological survey for arizona infection in turkey eggs. Results and discussion. Vet Ital 20:304-311.
12. Edwards, P.R., and W.H. Ewing. 1972. Identification of Enterobacteriaceae. Burgess Publishing Co., Minneapolis, MN.
13. Edwards, P.R., and M.M. Galton. 1967. Salmonellosis. In C.A. Brandly and C. Cornelius (eds.), Adv Vet Sci 11:1-63. Academic Press, New York.
14. Edwards, P.R., W.B. Cherry, and D.W. Bruner. 1943. Further studies on coliform bacteria serologically related to the genus Salmonella. J Infect Dis 73:229-238.
15. Edwards, P.R., M.G. West, and D.W. Bruner. 1947. Arizona group of paracolon bacteria. Kentucky Agric Exp Stn Bull 499. Lexington.
16. Edwards P.R., A.C. McWhorter, and M.A. Fife. 1956. The Arizona group of Enterobacteriaceae in animals and man. Bull WHO 14: 511-528
17. Edwards, P.R., M.A. Fife, and C.H. Ramsey. 1959. Studies on the arizona group of Enterobacteriaceae. Bacteriol Rev 23:155-174.
18. Ekperigin, H.E., S. Jang, and R.H. McCapes. 1983. Effective control of a gentamicin-resistant Salmonella arizonae infection in turkey poults. Avian Dis 27:822-829.
19. Ellis, E.M., J.E. Williams, E.T. Mallinson, G.H. Snoeyenbos, and W.J. Martin. 1976. Culture Methods for the Detection of Animal Salmonellosis and Arizonosis, pp. 9-87. Iowa State Univ Press, Ames.
20. Erwin, L.E. 1955. Examination of prepared poultry feeds for the presence of salmonella and other enteric organisms. Poult Sci 34:215-216.
21. Ewing, W.H. 1963. An outline of nomenclature for the family Enterobacteriaceae. Int Bull Bacteriol Nomencl Taxon 13:95-110.
22. Ewing, W.H. 1967. Revised Definitions for the Family Enterobacteriaceae, Its Tribes and Genera. US Dep HEW, NCDC, Atlanta, GA.
23. Ewing, W.H. 1969. Arizona hinshawii. Int J Syst Bacteriol 19:1.
24. Ewing, W.H. 1986. Edwards and Ewing's Identification of Enterobacteriaceae. Elsevier Science Publication Co. Inc., New York.
25. Ewing, W.H., and M.M. Ball. 1966. The Biochemical Reactions of Members of the Genus Salmonella. US Dep HEW, NCDC, Atlanta, GA.
26. Ewing, W.H., and M.A. Fife. 1966. A summary of the biochemical reactions of Arizona arizonae. Int J Syst Bacteriol 16:427-433.
27. Ewing, W.H., M.A. Fife, and B.R. Davis. 1965. The Biochemical Reactions of Arizona arizonae. US Dep HEW, NCDC, Atlanta, GA.
28. Ferris, K., and W.M. Frerichs. 1987. Salmonella serotypes from animals and related sources reported during the fiscal year 1987. Proc 92nd Annu Meet US Anim Health Assoc, pp. 349-362. US Anim Health Assoc, Richmond, VA.
29. Gauger, H.C. 1946. Isolation of a type 10 paracolon bacillus from an adult turkey. Poult Sci 25:299-300.
30. Geissler, H., and Y.I. Youssef. 1979. The effect of infection with Arizona hinshawii on chicken embryos. Avian Pathol 8:157-161.
31. Geissler, H., and Y.I. Youssef. 1981. Persistence of Arizona hinshawii in or on materials used in poultry houses. Avian Pathol 10:359-363.
32. Gerlach, H., H.E. Adler, and A.S. Rosenwald. 1968. Research Note: Observations on immune factors associated with arizona group infection in turkeys. Avian Dis 12:681-686.
33. Ghazikhanian, G.Y., R. Yamamoto, R.H. McCapes, W.M. Dungan, and H.B. Ortmayer. 1980. Combination dip and injection of turkey eggs with antibiotics to eliminate Mycoplasma meleagridis infection from a primary breeding stock. Avian Dis 24:57-70.
34. Ghazikhanian, G.Y., B.J. Kelly, and W.M Dungan. 1984. Salmonella arizonae control program. In G.H. Snoeyenbos (ed.), Proc Int Symp on Salmonella, pp. 142-149. Am Assoc Avian Pathol, Kennett Square, PA.
35. Goetz, M.E. 1962. The control of paracolon and paratyphoid infections in turkey poults. Avian Dis 6:93-99.
36. Goetz, M.E., and E.R. Quortrup. 1953. Some observations of the problem of arizona paracolon infections in poults. Vet Med 48:58-60.
37. Goetz, M.E., E.R. Quortrup, and J.E. Dunsing. 1954. Investigations of arizona paracolon infections in poults. J Am Vet Med Assoc 124:120-121.
38. Greenfield, J. 1972. Studies on Arizona in turkeys: Isolation and antibiotic control. Diss Abstr Int B, pp. 489-490.
39. Greenfield, J. 1976. Proc Salmonella Symposium, pp. 70-78. Am Assoc Avian Pathol, Kennett Square, PA.
40. Greenfield, J., and J.C. Bankier. 1969. Isolation of salmonella and arizona using enrichment media incubated at 35 and 43 C. Avian Dis 13:864-871.
41. Greenfield, J., and C.H. Bigland. 1971. Isolation of arizona from specimens grossly contaminated with competitive bacteria. Avian Dis 15:604-608.
42. Greenfield, J., C.H. Bigland, and T.W. Dukes. 1971. The genus Arizona with special reference to arizona disease in turkeys. Vet Bull 41:605-612.
43. Greenfield, J., C.H. Bigland, and H.D. McCausland. 1971. Culture of shell and shell membranes for efficient isolation of arizona from turkey hatching eggs. Avian Dis 15:82-88.
44. Greenfield, J., C.H. Bigland, H.D. McCausland, and C.W. Wood. 1972. Control of arizona disease in turkeys by poult injection. Poult Sci 51:523-526.
45. Guckian, J.E., E.H. Byers, and J.E. Perry. 1967. Arizona infection of man. Arch Int Med 119:170-175.
46. Hinshaw, W.R., and E. McNeil. 1944. Gopher snakes as carriers of salmonellosis and paracolon infections. Cornell Vet 34:248-254.
47. Hinshaw, W.R., and E. McNeil. 1946. The occurrence of type 10 paracolon in turkeys. J Bacteriol 51:281-280.
48. Hinshaw, W.R., and E. McNeil. 1947. Lizards as carriers of salmonella and paracolon bacteria. J Bacteriol 53:715-718.
49. Hirsh, D.C., J.S. Ikeda, L.D. Martin, B.J. Kelly, and G.Y. Ghazikhanian. 1983. R plasmid-mediated gentamicin resistance in salmonella isolated from turkeys

and their environment. Avian Dis 27:766–772.
50. Holte, R.J.A. 1965. Paracolon arizona immunization trials in turkeys. Proc 69th Annu Meet US Livest Sanit Assoc, pp. 539–542.
51. Jamison, S.L. 1956. Paracolon infections. Pac Poult 62:40–42.
52. Johnson, R.H., L.I. Lutwick, G.A. Huntley, and K.L. Vosti. 1976. Arizona hinshawii infections. New cases, antimicrobial sensitivities and literature review. Ann Intern Med 85:587–592.
53. Jordan, F.T.W., P.H. Lamont, L. Timms, and D.A.P. Grattan, 1976. The eradication of Arizona 7:1,7,8 from a turkey breeding flock. Vet Rec 99:413–415.
54. Kauffmann, F. 1966. The Bacteriology of Enterobacteriaceae. Williams & Wilkins, Baltimore, MD.
55. Kauffmann, F., and P.R. Edwards. 1952. Classification and Nomenclature of Enterobacteriaceae. Int Bull Bacteriol Nomencl Taxon 2:2–8.
56. Kowalski, L.M., and J.F. Stephens. 1967. Persistence of Arizona paracolon 7:1,7,8 in feed and water. Poult Sci 46:1586–1587.
57. Kowalski, L.M., and J.F. Stephens. 1968. Arizona 7:1,7,8 infection in young turkeys. Avian Dis 12:317–326.
58. Kumar, M.C., S.C. Nivas, A.K. Bahl, M.D. York, and B.S. Pomeroy. 1974. Studies on natural infection and egg transmission of Arizona hinshawii 7:1,7,8 in turkeys. Avian Dis 18:416–426.
59. Kumar, M.C., M.D. York, and B.S. Pomeroy. 1976. Comparison of tetrathionate and selenite enrichment broth for isolations of Arizona hinshawii 7:1,7,8 and various serotypes of salmonella. Proc 19th Annu Meet Am Assoc Vet Lab Diagn, pp. 179–188.
60. Kumar, M.C., M.D. York, and B.S. Pomeroy. 1977. Development of microagglutination test for detecting Arizona hinshawii 7:1,7,8 infection in turkeys. Am J Vet Res 38:255–257.
61. Lamont, P.H., and L. Timms. 1972. Experimental infection of turkey poults with Arizona serotype 7:1,7,8. Br Vet J 128:129–137.
62. Lewis, K.H., and E.R. Hitchner. 1936. Slow lactose fermenting bacteria pathogenic for baby chicks. J Infect Dis 59:225–235.
63. Littell, A.M. 1977. Plating medium for differentiation of Salmonella arizonae from other salmonellae. Appl Environ Microbiol 33:485–487.
64. Martin, W.J., M.A. Fife, and W.H. Ewing. 1967. The Occurrence and Distribution of the Serotypes of Arizona. US Dep HEW, NCDC, Atlanta, GA.
65. Mayeda, B., R.H. McCapes, and W.F. Scott. 1978. Protection of day-old poults against Arizona hinshawii challenge by preincubation streptomycin egg treatment. Avian Dis 22:61–70.
66. McCapes, R.H., R. Yamamoto, H.B. Ortmayer, and W.F. Scott. 1975. Injecting antibiotics into turkey hatching eggs to eliminate Mycoplasma meleagridis infection. Avian Dis 19:506–514.
67. McClure, H.E., W.C. Eveland, and A. Kase. 1957. The occurrence of certain Enterobacteriaceae in birds. Am J Vet Res 18:207–209.
68. Miyamae, T., and H.E. Adler. 1967. Comparative studies on immunogenicity of Arizona (7:1,7,8) adjuvant bacterins in mice and turkeys. Avian Dis 11:380–392.
69. Nagaraja, K.V., D.A. Emery, L.F. Sherlock, J.A. Newman, and B.S. Pomeroy. 1984. Detection of Salmonella arizonae in turkey flocks by ELISA. Proc Am Assoc Vet Lab, pp. 185–203.
70. Nagaraja, K.V., M.C. Kumar, J.A. Newman, and B.S. Pomeroy. 1985. Control of Salmonella arizonae infection in turkey breeder flocks by immunization. J Am Vet Med Assoc 187:309.
71. Nagaraja, K.V., L.T. Ausherman, D.A. Emery, and B.S. Pomeroy. 1986. Update on enzyme-linked immunosorbent assay for its field application in the detection of Salmonella arizonae infection in breeder flocks of turkeys. Proc Am Assoc Vet Diag, pp. 347–356.
72. Nagaraja, K.V., C.J. Kim, and B.S. Pomeroy. 1988. Prophylactic vaccines for the control and reduction of salmonella in turkeys. Proc. 92nd Annu Meet US Anim Health Assoc, pp. 347–348. US Anim Health Assoc, Richmond, VA.
73. Perek, M. 1957. Isolation of a paracolobactrum organism pathogenic to chickens. J Infect Dis 101:8–10.
74. Perek, M., M. Elian, and E.D. Heller. 1969. Bacterial flora of semen and contamination of the reproductive organs of the hen following artificial insemination. Res Vet Sci 10:127–132.
75. Renault, L., J. Vaissaire, C. Maire, and P. Motte. 1972. Identification of Arizona arizonae from turkeys in France. Bull Acad Vet Fr 45:53–55.
76. Rosenwald, A.S. 1965. New facts on paracolon control. Poult Meat 2:25.
77. Saif, Y.M., L.C. Ferguson, and K.E. Nestor. 1971. Treatment of turkey hatching eggs for control of Arizona infection. Avian Dis 15:448–461.
78. Sambyal, D.S., and V.K. Sharma. 1972. Screening of free-living animals and birds for Listeria, Brucella, and Salmonella infections. Br Vet J 128:50–55.
79. Sari, I., M. Lakatos, S. Toth, Z. Nemes, and G. Szeifert. 1979. Arizona salmonellosis of turkeys in Hungary. II. Aetiology and histopathology. Magy Allatorv Lapja 34:610–615.
80. Sato, G. 1967. Detection of salmonella and arizona organisms from soil of empty turkey yards. Jpn J Vet Res 15:53–55.
81. Sato, G., and H.E. Adler. 1966. A study on the efficacy of arizona bacterin in turkeys. Avian Dis 10:239–246.
82. Sato, G., and H.E. Adler. 1966. Bacteriological and serological observations on turkeys naturally infected with Arizona 7:1,7,8. Avian Dis 10:291–295.
83. Sato, G., and H.E. Adler. 1966. Experimental infection of adult turkeys with arizona group organisms. Avian Dis 10:329–336.
84. Sharma, V.K., Y.K. Kaura, and I.P. Singh. 1970. Arizona infection in snakes, rats, and man. Indian J Med Res 58:409–412.
85. Silva, E.N., and O. Hipólito. 1978. Salmonella strains isolated from the digestive tract of breeding chickens and apparently normal turkeys and in chick embryos. Proc 16th World's Poult Congr, pp. 701–706.
86. Silva, E.N., O. Hipólito, and R. Grecchi. 1980. Natural and experimental Salmonella arizonae 18:Z4, Z32 (Ar. 7:1,7,8) infection in broilers. Bacteriological and histological survey of eye and brain lesions. Avian Dis 24:631–636.
87. Snoeyenbos, G.H., and C.F. Smyser. 1969. Research Note–isolation of Arizona 7:1,7,8 from litter of pens housing infected turkeys. Avian Dis 13:223–224.
88. Timms, L. 1971. Arizona infection in turkeys in Great Britain. J Med Lab Technol [Br] 28:150–156.
89. Valeri, A., C. Marenzi, F. Enice, and T. Rampin. 1976. Study of biochemical characteristics of Salmonella arizonae isolates from turkeys. Clin Vet 99:422–429.
90. Weiss, S.H., M.J. Blaser, F.P. Paleologo, R.E. Black, A.C. McWhorter, M.A. Asbury, G.P. Carter, R.A. Feldman, and D.J. Brenner. 1986. Occurrence and distribution of serotypes of the Arizona subgroup of Salmonella strains in the United States from 1967 to 1976. J Clin Microbiol 23:1056–1064.
91. West, J.L., and G.C. Mohanty. 1973. Arizona hinshawii infection in turkey poults: Pathologic changes. Avian Dis 17:314–324.
92. Williams, J.E. 1984. Avian arizonosis. In M.S.

Hofstad, H.J. Barnes, B.W. Calnek, W.M. Reid, and H.W. Yoder, Jr. (eds.), Diseases of Poultry, 8th Ed., pp. 130–140. Iowa State Univ Press, Ames.

93. Williams, J.E., and L.H. Dillard. 1968. Penetration of chicken egg shells by members of the Arizona group. Avian Dis 12:645–649.

94. Williams, L.P., and B.C. Hobbs. 1975. Enterobacteriaceae infections. In W.T. Hubbert, W.F. McCulloch, and P.R. Schnurrenberger (eds.), Diseases Transmitted from Animals to Man, pp. 33–109. Charles C. Thomas, Springfield, IL.

95. Williams, J.E., E.T. Mallinson, and G.H. Snoeyenbos. 1980. Salmonellosis and Arizonosis. In S.B. Hitchner, C.H. Domermuth, H.G. Purchase, and J.E. Williams (eds.), Isolation and Identification of Avian Pathogens, pp. 1–8. Am Assoc Avian Pathol, Kennett Square, PA.

96. Windingstad, R.W., D.O. Trainer, and R. Duncan. 1977. Salmonella enteritidis and Arizona hinshawii isolated from wild sandhill cranes. Avian Dis 21:704–707.

97. Winsor, D.K., A.P. Bloebaum, and J.J. Mathewson. 1981. Gram-negative aerobic, enteric pathogens among intestinal microflora of wild turkey vultures (Cathartes aura) in west central Texas. Appl Environ Microbiol 42:1123–1124.

98. Worcester, W.W. 1965. Californian report results of test on paracolon control. Feedstuffs 37:6.

4 COLIBACILLOSIS

W. B. Gross

INTRODUCTION. *Escherichia coli* infections include colibacillosis, colisepticemia, Hjarre's disease, coligranuloma, peritonitis, salpingitis, synovitis, omphalitis, air sac disease, and all other disease conditions caused entirely or partly by *E. coli*. Collectively, these diseases are responsible for significant economic losses to the poultry industry. The various serotypes are intestinal inhabitants of all animals; therefore, their distribution is widespread. Avian strains of *E. coli* are not recognized as important causes of infections in other animals, including man. Most serotypes isolated from poultry are pathogenic only for birds.

INCIDENCE AND DISTRIBUTION. Various strains of *E. coli* probably infect most mammals and birds. Clinical disease is reported most often in chickens, turkeys, and ducks.

E. coli is a common inhabitant in the intestinal tracts of animals at a concentration of 10^6/g or less. Its presence in drinking water is considered indicative of fecal contamination. Among normal chickens, 10–15% of intestinal coliforms belong to potentially pathogenic serotypes (19). Intestinal strains are not necessarily the same serotype as those from the pericardial sac of the same bird. Egg transmission of pathogenic *E. coli* is common and can be responsible for high chick mortality. Pathogenic coliforms are more frequent in the gut of newly hatched chicks than in eggs from which they hatched (20), which suggests rapid spread after hatching. The most important source of egg infection seems to be fecal contamination of the surface with subsequent penetration of the shell and membranes. Coliform bacteria can be found in litter and fecal matter. Dust in poultry houses may contain 10^5–10^6 *E. coli*/g. These bacteria persist for long periods, particularly when dry (18). There was a reduction of 84–97% in 7 days following wetting of dust with water. Feed is often contaminated with pathogenic coliforms that can be destroyed by hot pelleting. Rodent droppings often contain pathogenic coliforms. Pathogenic serotypes can also be introduced into poultry flocks through contaminated well water (26).

ETIOLOGY. *E. coli* is a gram-negative, nonacid-fast, uniform-staining, nonspore-forming bacillus, usually 2–3 × 0.6 μm. The organism may be variable in size and shape. Many strains are motile and have peritrichous flagella.

Growth Requirements. *E. coli* grows on ordinary nutrient media at temperatures of 18–44 C or lower. On agar plates incubated for 24 hr at 37 C, colonies are low, convex, smooth, and colorless. They are usually 1–3 mm in diameter with granular structure and an entire margin. *E. coli* grows well in broth, producing turbid growth.

Biochemical Properties. Acid and gas are produced in glucose, maltose, mannitol, xylose, glycerol, rhamnose, sorbitol, and arabinose but not in dextrin, starch, or inositol. A few strains require up to 1 wk to ferment lactose. Fermentation of adonitol, sucrose, salicin, raffinose, and dulcitol is variable. *E. coli* produces positive methyl red and negative Voges-Proskauer reactions; hydrogen sulfide is not produced on Kligler's medium. It does not grow in the presence of potassium cyanide, attack urea, liquefy gelatin, or grow in citrate medium. *E. coli* isolates from poultry have similar biochemical properties to those from other sources.

Antigenic Structures. Various serotypes of *E. coli* are classified according to the Ewing scheme (10). Knowledge about the antigenic structure of *E. coli* and its antigenic relationship to other species has been reviewed by Sojka (33). The current classification lists over 154 O antigen, 89 K antigen, and 49 H antigen serotypes.

O ANTIGEN. The O (somatic) antigen is the endotoxin liberated on autolysis of smooth cells. It is composed of a polysaccharide-phospholipid complex with a protein fraction resistant to boiling. Ewing et al. (10) and Sojka (33) discussed methods of preparing O antisera, which agglutinate antigen at high titers (usually over 1:2560) when the antigen-antibody mixture is incubated at 50 C for 24 hr.

K ANTIGEN. K (capsular) antigens are polymeric acids containing 2% reducing sugars. They are associated with virulence, are on the surface of the cell, interfere with O agglutination, and can be removed by heating to 100 C for 1 hr; however, some strains require heating for 2½ hr at 121 C. On the basis of heat stability, K antigens are subdivided into L, A, and B forms. Antisera are prepared in rabbits by inoculating live organisms intravenously. Tube agglutination titers are determined by incubating antigen-antibody mixtures at 37 C for 2 hr and overnight at 4 C. Titers are low (1:100–1:400). Most of these antigens can be identified by the slide agglutination test (serum diluted 1:2–1:10).

H ANTIGEN. H (flagellar) antigens are not often used in antigenic identification of *E. coli* isolates and are not correlated with pathogenicity. They are proteins that are destroyed by heating to 100 C. Tube agglutination tests are read after incubation at 37 C for 2 hr. Siccardi (31) found 57% of the 607 isolates he studied to be motile.

Surveys have been made in many parts of the world to determine serotypes most frequently associated with poultry disease. Over many years the most common serotypes have been 01, 02, 035, and 078. Many other serotypes have been found less frequently while some pathogenic isolates do not belong to known serotypes or are untypable.

PATHOGENESIS AND EPIZOOTIOLOGY.

Siccardi (31) tested all known *E. coli* serotypes for their ability to kill 13-day-old embryos following allantoic inoculation and to cause pericarditis and mortality in 3-wk-old chicks following air sac inoculation. Seventy-four of 154 (48%) serotypes were pathogenic for chicks, embryos, or both. Other serotypes might have been found pathogenic if other routes of inoculation had been used.

Neither endotoxins nor hemolysins are associated with disease-producing ability of *E. coli* in birds. Pathogenic and nonpathogenic isolates of *E. coli* are similar in biochemical characteristics and drug sensitivities (6, 29). Pathogenic isolates are reported to differ from nonpathogenic isolates by their ability to bind congo red dye (2), grow in the presence of low concentrations of iron, and adhere to epithelial surfaces by means of pili (filamentous hairlike proteinaceous surface appendages) (9, 27). Exogenous iron increases pathogenicity (3).

E. coli–related airsacculitis and pericarditis, may follow infection with group I and II adenoviruses, reoviruses, coronaviruses, and infectious bursal disease viruses (8, 22, 23, 28, 29).

Embryo and Early Chick Mortality.

Between 0.5 and 6% of eggs from normal hens contain *E. coli*. Experimentally inoculated hens may shed *E. coli* in up to 26% of their eggs. Pathogenic strains accounted for 43 of 245 isolates from dead embryos (18). Normal yolk sac contents change from viscid, yellow-green to watery, yellow-brown or caseous material when contaminated with *E. coli*. The bacterium can occasionally be isolated from normal-appearing yolk. *E. coli* was present in yolk sacs of about 70% of chicks with "mushy chick disease," which was characterized by edema and infected yolk (17). Other commonly isolated bacteria were *Proteus* spp., *Bacillus* spp., and enterococci.

Fecal contamination of eggs is considered to be the most important source of infection. Other sources may be ovarian infection or salpingitis. The incidence of infection increases shortly after hatching and is reduced after about 6 days.

Yolk sac of embryos is the focus of infection (Fig. 4.1). Many embryos die before hatching, particularly late in incubation. Some die at or shortly after hatching, with losses continuing up to 3 wk. Siccardi (31) found as few as 10 organisms of serotype 01a:K1:H7 would cause 100% mortality in day-old chicks when injected into the yolk sac. Chicks with yolk sac infection also often have inflammation of the navel (omphalitis). Chicks or poults living more than 4 days may have pericarditis as well as infected yolks indicating systemic spread of the organism from the yolk sac. There may be no embryo or chick mortality, the only manifestation of infected yolk sacs being retained infected yolk and reduced weight gain.

The microscopic reaction in the wall of infected yolk sacs appears to be mild. The wall is edematous. There is an outer connective tissue zone followed by a layer of inflammatory cells containing heterophils and macrophages, a layer of giant cells, a zone of necrotic heterophils and masses of bacteria, and then the inner infected yolk contents (Fig. 4.2). In some yolk sacs there are a few plasma cells.

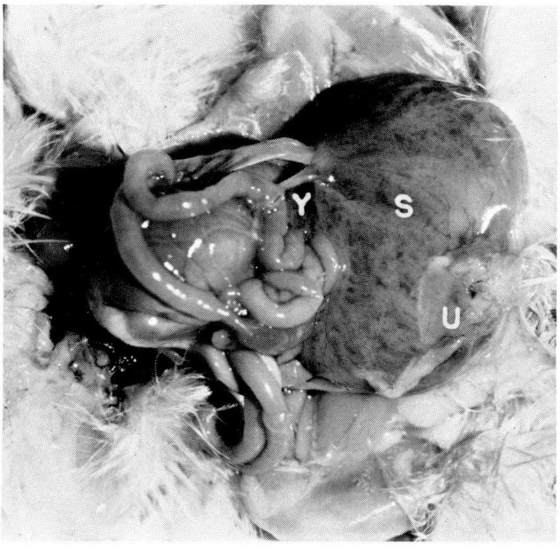

4.1. Coliform-infected yolk sac of 6-day-old chick showing yolk stalk (*Y*), yolk sac (*S*), and umbilicus (*U*).

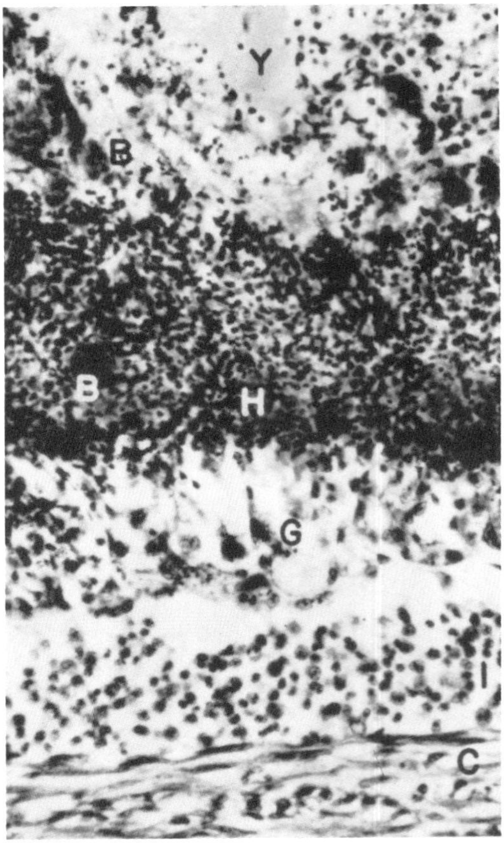

4.2. Wall of coliform-infected yolk sac, showing outer connective tissue layer of yolk sac wall (*C*), layer of inflammatory cells containing heterophils and macrophages (*I*), layer of giant cells (*G*), zone of necrotic heterophils (*H*) containing masses of bacteria (*B*), and yolk (*Y*). H & E, ×220.

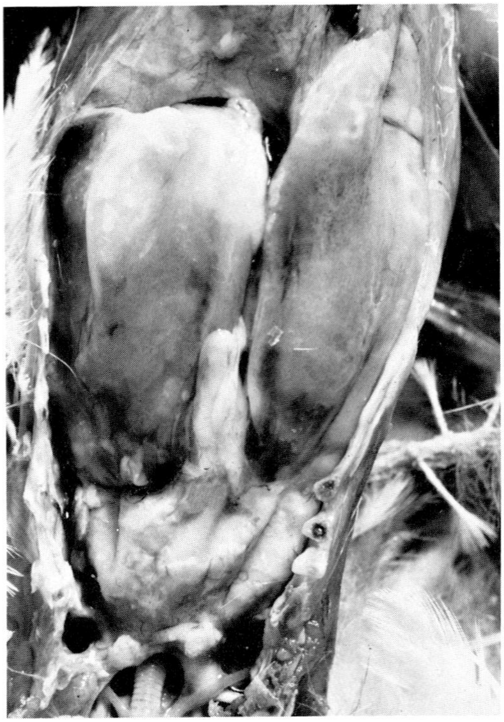

4.3. Coliform pericarditis and perihepatitis.

Omphalitis and yolk sac infection have been experimentally reproduced in ducks by exposing eggs to *E. coli* broth cultures (30). Dipping eggs at 18 days of incubation resulted in a higher incidence of infection than dipping at 1 day. Low brooding temperature or fasting increases incidence of infection and mortality.

Respiratory Tract Infection. *E. coli* often infects respiratory tracts of birds concurrently infected with various combinations of infectious bronchitis viruses (IBV); Newcastle disease viruses (NDV), including vaccine strains; and mycoplasmas. Apparently the damaged respiratory tract becomes extremely susceptible to invasion by *E. coli* entering via a respiratory route (13). The resulting disease is commonly called air sac disease or chronic respiratory disease (CRD). Pericarditis and perihepatitis are also often present (Fig. 4.3). Less commonly, panophthalmitis, salpingitis, and infections in bones and synovial structures may occur following sepsis. Air sac disease occurs chiefly in 5- to 12-wk-old chickens with a maximum incidence at 6–9 wk. Important economic losses result from morbidity, mortality, and condemnation of birds at time of slaughter.

Lesions of uncomplicated coliform infection can easily be reproduced by inoculating pathogenic *E. coli* into the air sac. Airsacculitis occurs within 1 hr. Bacteremia and pericarditis may develop in 6 hr. In birds that survive, lesions are well developed 48 hr postinoculation. Most mortality occurs during the first 5 days. Recovery is usually rapid if birds survive initial infection, although a few with persistent anorexia become emaciated and die.

Mycoplasmal infection results in increased susceptibility to *E. coli* about 12–16 days after inoculation, and susceptibility persists for at least 30 days. Respiratory tracts infected with IBV or NDV in addition to mycoplasma become more susceptible to *E. coli;* the susceptible period begins earlier and persists longer. Infection with IBV or NDV alone results in a lower level of susceptibility to *E. coli* aerosols than mixed infection.

Five days after administration of a vaccine strain of NDV there was reduced clearance of aerosol-administered *E. coli.* Microscopically, the pseudostratified, columnar epithelium of the trachea was replaced by 3–8 layers of immature nonciliated cells (12). Mixed IBV-*E. coli* infections were more severe than those caused by single-agent infections (21, 32). Although uninfected chicken respiratory tracts are relatively resistant to inhaled *E. coli,* losses have been reported without signs of respiratory disease (4). Socialization, environmental stresses, strain of chicken, and their interactions influence susceptibility to air-sac injection and aerosol exposure to *E. coli.*

Inhaled coliform-contaminated dust has been considered one of the most important sources for infecting susceptible air sacs. Exposure to chicken house dust and ammonia results in deciliation of the upper respiratory tract of birds (24, 28), which allows inhaled *E. coli* to infect air sacs.

Pathology. Infected air sacs are thickened and often have caseous exudate on the respiratory surface. Microscopically, the earliest changes consist of edema and heterophil infiltration. Mononuclear phagocytes are frequently seen 12 hr after inoculation. Later, mononuclear phagocytes are very common, with giant cells along margins of necrotic areas. There is fibroblast proliferation and accumulation of vast numbers of necrotic heterophils in caseous exudate. Lesions of predisposing respiratory disease are usually present and consist of lymphoid follicles, epithelial hyperplasia, and epithelium-lined air passages that may contain heterophils (Fig. 4.4).

PERICARDITIS. Most *E. coli* serotypes cause pericarditis after they become septicemic. Pericarditis is usually associated with myocarditis and results in marked changes in the electrocardiogram (14), often before macroscopic lesions appear. The pericardial sac becomes cloudy and epicardium becomes edematous and covered with a light-colored exudate. The pericardial sac often fills with a light yellow, fibrinous exudate. Microscopically, at first there are many heterophils in the epicardium. In less than 24 hr, macrophages become more numerous. Within the myocardium, particularly close to the epicardium, there are accumulations of lymphoid cells, and by 7–10 days there are many plasma cells (Fig. 4.5). Pericarditis-myocarditis results in reduction of carotid artery blood pressure from a norm of about 150 to 40 mm mercury just before death.

SALPINGITIS. When the left greater abdominal air sac is infected by *E. coli,* many females develop chronic salpingitis characterized by a large caseous mass in a dilated thin-walled oviduct. The caseous mass contains numerous necrotic heterophils and bacteria that persist for months. Size of the caseous mass may increase with time. Affected birds frequently die during the first 6 mo

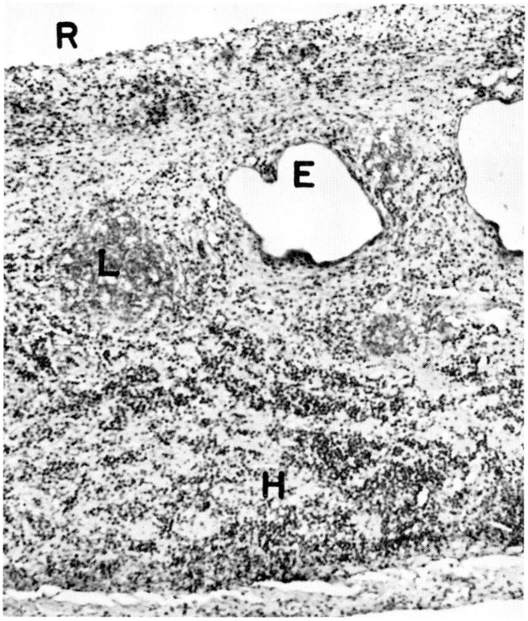

4.4. Air sac infected with *M. gallisepticum* followed by *E. coli* aerosol exposure. Section shows respiratory surface (*R*), epithelium-lined air passages (*E*), lymphoid follicles (*L*), and area containing many heterophils (*H*). H & E, ×110.

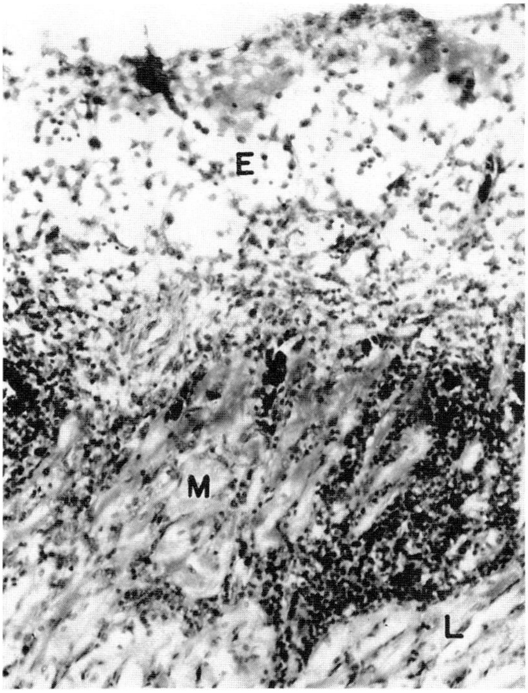

4.5. Coliform-infected heart wall showing epicardium (*E*) that is edematous and contains mononuclear inflammatory cells and myocardium (*M*) that contains large infiltrations of lymphoid cells (*L*). H & E, ×100.

postinfection; those surviving rarely lay eggs. Salpingitis may also occur following entry of coliform bacteria from the cloaca in laying hens.

Tissue reaction in the oviduct is surprisingly mild, consisting largely of heterophil accumulation just under the epithelium. High estrogenic activity seems to be associated with coliform growth in the oviduct. Infection can be reproduced by injecting large (10^9) doses of bacteria into the uterus or oviduct. Stilbestrol implants increase susceptibility and result in increased numbers of coliforms in the oviduct.

PERITONITIS. Coliform infection of the peritoneal cavity occurs in laying hens and is characterized by acute mortality, fibrin, and free yolk. Infection occurs when bacteria ascending through the oviduct grow rapidly in yolk material that has been deposited in the peritoneal cavity (15).

ACUTE SEPTICEMIA. An acute infectious disease resembling fowl typhoid and fowl cholera from which *E. coli* can be isolated is sometimes seen in mature and growing chickens and turkeys. Affected birds are in good flesh and have full crops, which indicates the acute nature of the infection. The most characteristic lesions are green liver and congested pectoral muscles. In some cases, small, white, foci in the liver have been described. As in less acute coliform septicemia, there is a tendency toward pericarditis and peritonitis. There are no reports of experimental reproduction of the condition.

SYNOVITIS. Isolates of *E. coli* have been recovered from joint infections of chickens. Lesions can be reproduced following intravenous inoculation of a broth culture of certain isolates. Synovitis is frequently a sequel to septicemia. Many birds recover in about 1 wk, while others remain chronically infected and may become emaciated.

PANOPHTHALMITIS. Panophthalmitis is an uncommon manifestation of *E. coli* septicemia. There is hypopyon, usually of one eye, which is blind (Fig. 4.6). Most birds die shortly after onset of lesions, although some recover. Microscopically, there are infiltrations of heterophils and mononuclear phagocytes throughout the eye, and giant cells form around necrotic areas. The choroid becomes hyperemic, and there is complete destruction of the retina.

COLIGRANULOMA. Coligranuloma (Hjarre's disease) of chickens and turkeys is characterized by granulomas in liver, ceca, duodenum, and mesentery, but not spleen (Fig. 4.7). It is a relatively uncommon coliform disease; however, individual flocks may have mortality as high as 75%. Serosal lesions resembling leukotic neoplasms are sometimes caused by *E. coli*. There is confluent coagulation necrosis involving as much as half the liver.

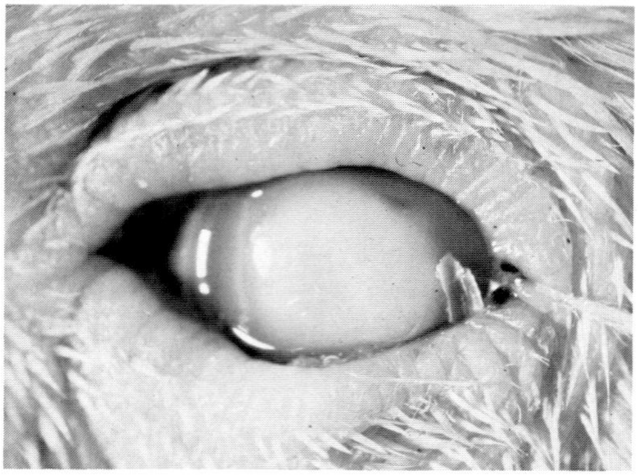

4.6. Coliform panophthalmitis of left eye of chicken.

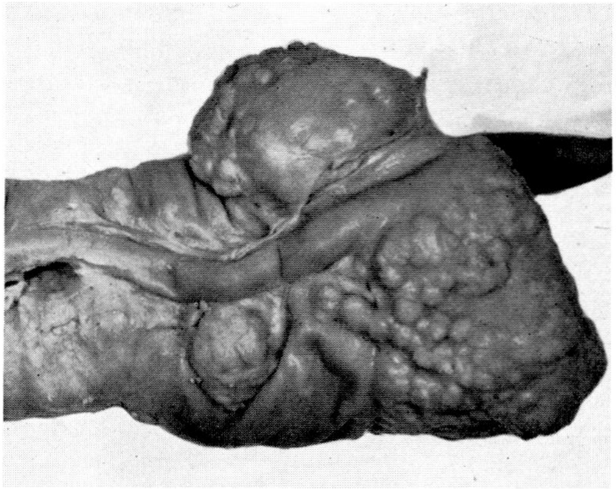

4.7. Cecum containing granulomas. (Hjarre)

Only scattered heterophils are seen, and at the edge of the necrotic areas there are a few giant cells. This lesion is possibly the precursor to Hjarre's disease.

SWOLLEN HEAD SYNDROME. *E. coli* can be isolated from an edematous swelling of the head of broilers due to damage to capillaries following repeated intraperitoneal injections of *E. coli* or by combined coronavirus–*E. coli* challenge (11, 22).

COLIFORM SEPTICEMIA OF DUCKS. The commonest causes of pericarditis, perihepatitis, and airsacculitis in ducklings are *E. coli, Pasteurella anatipestifer,* and salmonellae, although other agents may produce similar necropsy findings. Coliform septicemia of ducks is characterized by moist, granular to curdlike exudate on abdominal and thoracic viscera and surfaces of air sacs. Exudate varies in thickness. A characteristic odor is often noted when affected birds are necropsied. The liver is frequently swollen, dark, and bile stained. The spleen is swollen and dark. The organism (often 078) can usually be recovered from any internal organ.

Coliform septicemia occurs throughout the growing season but becomes more frequent in late fall and winter. All ages of ducklings are susceptible. Distribution of losses suggests individual farms, rather than hatcheries, are the source of infection.

Differential diagnosis involves distinguishing coliform infection from other bacterial infections. *P. anatipestifer* infection is characterized by more limited involvement of the respiratory tract and a dry, thin, transparent covering over visceral organs. When exudate is thick, it is yellow and firm. Casts of such thick exudates may be found in nasal sinuses, respiratory tract, and oviducts. *P. anatipestifer* is more difficult to recover by cultural means. It is most frequently isolated from respiratory tract, heart blood, and brain of affected birds, and less frequently from other internal organs. Dual infections of ducklings with *E. coli* and *P. anatipestifer* are seldom encountered.

ENTERITIS. While there are a few reports of enteritis in poultry in which *E. coli* has been suggested as playing a part, there has not been enough conclusive research to indicate it as the etiology. Feeding *E. coli* to chickens with mild *E. brunetti* infection results in severe hemorrhagic typhlitis (25).

DIAGNOSIS

Isolation and Identification of Causative Agent. Material should be streaked on eosin methylene blue (EMB), MacConkey's, or tergitol 7 agar, as well as noninhibitory media. Care must be taken to avoid fecal contamination of samples to be cultured. A presumptive diagnosis of *E. coli* infection can be made if most of the colonies are characteristically dark with a metallic sheen on EMB agar, bright pink with precipitate in medium on MacConkey's agar, and yellow on tergitol 7 agar. Strains of *E. coli* rarely can be slow lactose fermenters and appear as nonlactose-fermenting colonies. A definite diagnosis of *E. coli* can be made based on the organism's characteristics (see Etiology). Antigenic identification of the isolate might be helpful, particularly when done as part of epidemiologic investigation.

Differential Diagnosis. Lesions similar to those described as being caused by *E. coli* can be caused by many other organisms.

Synovitis-arthritis can also be caused by viruses, mycoplasmas, staphylococci, salmonellae, *Streptobacillus moniliformis,* and other organisms. A great variety of organisms such as *Aerobacter* spp., *Klebsiella* spp., *Proteus* spp., salmonellae, *Bacillus* spp., staphylococci, enterococci, or clostridia are frequently isolated (often as mixed cultures) from yolk sacs of embryos and chicks (17). Pericarditis can also be caused by chlamydia. Peritonitis is sometimes caused by pasteurellae or streptococci. Airsacculitis can be caused by other bacteria, mycoplasmas, and chlamydia. Acute septicemic diseases are caused by pasteurellae, salmonellae, streptococci, and other organisms. Liver granulomas have many causes, including anaerobic bacteria belonging to the genera *Eubacterium* and *Bacteroides.*

TREATMENT. *E. coli* may be sensitive to many drugs such as ampicillin, chloramphenicol, chlortetracycline, neomycin, nitrofurans, gentamicin, ormethiprim-sulfadimethoxine, nalidixic acid, oxytetracycline, polymyxin B, spectinomycin, streptomycin, and sulfa drugs. Isolates of *E. coli* from poultry are frequently resistant to one or more drugs. It is imperative to determine the drug sensitivity of *E. coli* strains involved in a disease outbreak so ineffective drugs can be avoided. Even a highly effective drug may not result in improvement of the flock if too little is used or it is incapable of reaching the site of infection.

PREVENTION AND CONTROL. Effective inactivated vaccines against serotypes 02:K1 and 078:K80 have been produced (1, 5, 7). An inactivated 078 vaccine protected ducks (30).

Multivalent vaccines made from pili, containing low levels (180 μg) of protein per dose, reduced the severity of challenge infection (16). Absorbed sera indicate pili of serotypes 01, 02, and 078 are antigenically different (34). Passive immunization results in increased clearance of bacteria from blood and increased resistance to aerosol challenge (23).

E. coli infection of the respiratory tract of birds can be reduced by raising mycoplasma-free birds and reducing exposure of birds to viruses causing respiratory diseases. Proper ventilation will reduce respiratory tract damage and exposure.

There are no known methods for reducing the level of pathogenic *E. coli* in the intestinal tract and feces, although consideration that 1) pelleted feed has fewer *E. coli* than mash, 2) rodent droppings are a source of pathogenic *E. coli,* and 3) contaminated water can contain high numbers of the organism, should not be overlooked. Pathogenic strains of *E. coli* can be competitively excluded from intestines of chicks by seeding them with native microflora from resistant chickens (35). Infection with *Mycoplasma gallisepticum* and/or infectious bronchitis virus induces protected chickens to shed *E. coli* (36).

The most important source for transmission of pathogenic *E. coli* between flocks is fecal contamination of hatching eggs. Transmission can be reduced by fumigating or disinfecting eggs within 2 hr after they are laid and discarding cracked eggs or those with obvious fecal contamination. If infected eggs are broken during incubation, the contents are a serious source of infection to others, especially when personnel and egg-handling equipment are contaminated. Eggs are particularly susceptible just before hatching. Methods for preventing incubator and hatcher dissemination are unknown. However, venting incubators and hatchers to the outside and having as few breeder flocks as possible represented in each unit will help reduce losses. Contaminated chicks survive better if kept warm and not starved. High protein diets and increased vitamin E levels apparently favor survival.

REFERENCES

1. Arp, L.H. 1982. Effect of passive immunization on phagocytosis of blood-borne Escherichia coli in spleen and liver of turkeys. Am J Vet Res 43:1034–1040.

2. Berkhoff, H.A., and A.C. Vinal. 1986. Congo red medium to distinguish between invasive and non-invasive Escherichia coli pathogenic for poultry. Avian Dis 30:117–121.

3. Bolin, C.A. 1986. Effects of exogenous iron on Escherichia coli septicemia of turkeys. Am J Vet Res 47:1813–1816.

4. Carlson, H.C., and G.R. Whenham. 1968. Coliform bacteria in chicken broiler house dust and their possible relationship to coli-septicemia. Avian Dis 12:297–302.

5. Cessi, D. 1979. Prophylaxis of Escherichia coli infection in fowls with emulsified vaccines. Clinica Vet 102:270–278.

6. Cloud, S.S., J.K. Rosenberger, P.A. Fries, R.A. Wilson, and E.M. Odor. 1985. In vitro and in vivo characterization of avian Escherichia coli. I. Serotypes, metabolic activity, and antibiotic sensitivity. Avian Dis 29:1084–1093.

7. Deb, J.R., and E.G. Harry. 1978. Laboratory trials with inactivated vaccines against Escherichia coli 02:K1 infection in fowls. Res Vet Sci 24:308–313.

8. Dhillon, A.S. 1986. Pathology of avian adenovirus serotypes in the presence of Escherichia coli in infectious-bursal-disease-virus infected specific-pathogen-free chickens. Avian Dis 30:81–86.

9. Dho, M., and J.P. Lafont. 1984. Adhesive properties and iron uptake ability in Escherichia coli lethal and nonlethal for chicks. Avian Dis 29:1016–1025.

10. Ewing, W.H., H.W. Tatum, B.R. Davis, and R.W. Reavis. 1956. Studies on the serology of the Escherichia coli group. US Dept Health, Educ, and Welfare, Publ Health Serv, p. 42. Atlanta, GA.

11. Fernandez, A., A. Gazquez, A. Mendez, E. Mozos, and A. Jover. 1986. Morphopathology of the adenohypophysis of chickens in shock induced by Escherichia coli. Avian Dis 30:247–254.

12. Ficken, M.D., J.F. Edwards, J.C. Lay, and D.E. Tveter. 1987. Tracheal mucus transport rate and bacterial clearance in turkeys exposed by aerosol to La Sota strain of Newcastle disease virus. Avian Dis 31:241–248.

13. Gross, W.B. 1961. The development of "air sac disease." Avian Dis 5:431–439.

14. Gross, W.B. 1966. Electrocardiographic changes of Escherichia coli infected birds. Am J Vet Res 27:1427–1436.

15. Gross, W.B., and P.B. Siegel. 1959. Coliform peritonitis of chickens. Avian Dis 3:370–373.

16. Gyimah, J.E., B. Panigrahy, and J.D. Williams. 1986. Immunogenicity of an Escherichia coli multivalent pilus vaccine in chickens. Avian Dis 30:687–689.

17. Harry, E.G. 1957. The effect on embryonic and chick mortality of yolk contamination with bacteria from the hen. Vet Rec 69:1433–1440.

18. Harry, E.G. 1964. The survival of E. coli in the dust of poultry houses. Vet Rec 76:466–470.

19. Harry, E.G., and L.A. Hemsley. 1965. The association between the presence of septicaemic strains of Escherichia coli in the respiratory and intestinal tracts of chickens and the occurrence of coli septicaemia. Vet Rec 77:35–40.

20. Harry, E.G., and L.A. Hemsley. 1965. The relationship between environmental contamination with septicaemia strains of Escherichia coli and their incidence in chickens. Vet Rec 77:241–245.

21. Ibragimov, A.A., V.S. Oskolpov, and Y.R. Golod. 1983. Pathogenesis and diagnosis of mixed respiratory infections in fowls. Veterinarya (Moscow) 12:33–36.

22. Morley, A.J., and D.K. Thomson. 1984. Swollen-head syndrome in broiler chickens. Avian Dis 28:238–243.

23. Myers, R.K., and L.H. Arp. 1987. Pulmonary clearance and lesions of lung and air sac in passively immunized and unimmunized turkeys following exposure to aerosolized Escherichia coli. Avian Dis 31:622–628.

24. Nagaraja, K.V., D.A. Emery, K.A. Jordan, V. Sivanandan, J.A. Newman, and B.S. Pomeroy. 1984. Effect of ammonia on the quantitative clearance of Escherichia coli from lungs, air sacs, and livers of turkeys aerosol vaccinated against Escherichia coli. Am J Vet Res 45:392–95.

25. Nagi, M.S., and W.J. Mathey. 1972. Interaction of Escherichia coli and Eimeria brunetti in chickens. Avian Dis 16:864–873.

26. Nagi, M.S., and L.G. Raggi. 1972. Importance to "airsac" disease of water supplies contaminated with pathogenic Escherichia coli. Avian Dis 16:718–723.

27. Naveh, M.W., T. Zusman, E. Skutelsky, and E.Z. Ron. 1984. Adherence pili in avian strains of Escherichia coli: Effect on pathogenicity. Avian Dis 28:651–661.

28. Oyetunde, O.O.F., R.G. Thomson, and H.C. Carlson. 1978. Aerosol exposure of ammonia, dust, and Escherichia coli in broiler chickens. Can Vet J 19:187–193.

29. Rosenberger, J.K., P.A. Fries, S.S. Cloud, and R.A. Wilson. 1985. In vitro and in vivo characterization of avian Escherichia coli. II. Factors associated with pathogenicity. Avian Dis 29:1094–1107.

30. Sandhu, T.S., and H.W. Layton. 1985. Laboratory and field trials with formalin-inactivated Escherichia coli (078)–Pasteurella anatipestifer bacterin in White Pekin ducks. Avian Dis 29:128–135.

31. Siccardi, F.J. 1966. Identification and disease producing ability of Escherichia coli associated with E. coli infection of chickens and turkeys. MS thesis, Univ Minnesota.

32. Smith, H.W., J.K.A. Cook, and Z.E. Parsell. 1985. The experimental infection of chickens with mixtures of infectious bronchitis virus and Escherichia coli. J Gen Virol 66:777–786.

33. Sojka, W.J. 1965. Escherichia coli in domestic animals and poultry. Commonwealth Agric Bur, Farnham Royal, England, pp. 231.

34. Suwanichkul, A., B. Panigrahy, and R.M. Wagner. 1987. Antigenic relatedness and partial amino acid sequences of pili of Escherichia coli serotypes O1, O2, and O78 pathogenic for poultry. Avian Dis 31:809–813.

35. Weinack, O.M., G.H. Snoeyenbos, C.F. Smyser, and A.S. Soerjadi. 1981. Competitive exclusion of intestinal colonization of Escherichia coli in chicks. Avian Dis 25:696–705.

36. Weinack, O.M., G.H. Snoeyenbos, C.F. Smyser, and A.S. Soerjadi-Liem. 1984. Influence of Mycoplasma gallisepticum, infectious bronchitis, and cyclophosphamide on chickens protected by native intestinal microflora against Salmonella typhimurium or Escherichia coli. Avian Dis 28:416–425.

5 PASTEURELLOSIS

INTRODUCTION

K.R. Rhoades and R.B. Rimler

Pasteurellosis is a general term used to designate a group of diseases caused by pasteurellae and by pasteurellaelike bacteria such as *Yersinia pseudotuberculosis*. In poultry these diseases are fowl cholera; pseudotuberculosis; goose influenza; and *Pasteurella anatipestifer, P. haemolytica,* and *P. gallinarum* infections. Goose influenza is similar to *P. anatipestifer* infection, and there is reason to believe that the causative bacterium *P. septicaemiae* is identical to *P. anatipestifer*. Therefore, goose influenza will not be included as a separate disease but will be discussed under *P. anatipestifer* infection. *P. haemolytica* and *P. gallinarum* are discussed under differential diagnosis of fowl cholera.

FOWL CHOLERA

K.R. Rhoades and R.B. Rimler

INTRODUCTION. Fowl cholera (FC) (avian cholera, avian pasteurellosis, avian hemorrhagic septicemia) is a contagious disease affecting domesticated and wild birds. It usually appears as a septicemic disease associated with high morbidity and mortality, but chronic or benign conditions often occur. This disease is of historical importance because of its role in early development of bacteriology and because it was one of four diseases for which the Veterinary Division of the USDA was created to investigate.

HISTORY. Several epornitics among fowl occurred in Europe during the latter half of the 18th century. The disease was studied in France by Chabert in 1782 and in 1836 by Mailet, who first used the term "fowl cholera." Huppe in 1886 referred to "hemorrhagic septicemia," and Lignieres in 1900 used the term "avian pasteurellosis." Benjamin in 1851 gave a good description of the disease and demonstrated that it could be spread by cohabitation. With this knowledge of the disease he formulated procedures for its prevention. At about the same time Renault, Reynal, and Delafond demonstrated its transmissibility to various species by inoculation. In 1877 and 1878 Perroncito of Italy and Semmer of Russia observed in tissues of affected birds a bacterium that had a rounded form and occurred singly or in pairs. In 1879 Toussaint isolated the bacterium and proved it was the sole cause of the disease (43).

Pasteur (105) isolated the organism and grew pure cultures in chicken broth. In further studies Pasteur (106, 107) used the FC organism to perform his classic experiments in attenuation of bacteria for use in producing immunity. Salmon (132) appears to have been the first to study the disease in the USA. However, a good description of disease signs was reported as early as 1867 in Iowa where losses of chickens, turkeys, and geese had occurred (7).

INCIDENCE AND DISTRIBUTION. FC occurs sporadically or enzootically in most countries. Sometimes it causes high mortality; at others, losses are nominal. Alberts and Graham (2) reported a loss of 68% within 6 days in a flock of 5½-mo-old turkeys. Vaught et al. (140) reported that over 1000 wild geese died of FC in one night. In studying the chronic respiratory form in chickens, Hall et al. (46) observed that mortality was low but infection persisted for at least 4 yr.

FC is more prevalent in late summer, fall, and winter. This seasonal occurrence is one of circumstance rather than lowered resistance, except that chickens become more susceptible as they reach maturity.

ETIOLOGY

Classification. *Pasteurella multocida* is the causative agent of FC. When pronouncing *multocida* the accent should be on the *ci* (15) rather than on the *to* as given in the 7th and 8th editions of *Bergey's Manual.* In the past the bacterium has been given many names, including *Micrococcus gallicidus,* 1883; *M. cholerae gallinarum,* 1885; *Oc-*

topsis cholerae gallinarum, 1885; *Bacterium cholerae gallinarum,* 1886; *Bacillus cholerae gallinarum,* 1886; *P. cholerae-gallinarum,* 1887; *Coccobacillus avicidus,* 1888; *P. avicida,* 1889; *Bacterium multicidum,* 1899; *P. avium,* 1903; *Bacillus avisepticus,* 1903; *Bacterium avisepticum,* 1903; *Bacterium avisepticus,* 1912; and *P. aviseptica,* 1920 (15, 18).

For a while each isolate of *P. multocida* was named according to the animal from which it was isolated, such as *P. avicida* or *P. aviseptica, P. muricida* or *P. muriseptica.* In 1929 it was suggested that all isolates be referred to as *P. septica* (145). This name was used mainly in the UK and can be found in recent literature. *Pasteurella multocida,* proposed by Rosenbusch and Merchant (130), is now accepted as the official name in *Bergey's Manual* and is used exclusively throughout the world.

Morphology and Staining. *P. multocida* is a gram-negative, nonmotile, non-spore-forming rod occurring singly, in pairs, and occasionally as chains or filaments. It measures 0.2–0.4 × 0.6–2.5 μm but tends toward pleomorphicity after repeated subculture. A capsule can be demonstrated in recently isolated cultures, using indirect methods of staining (Fig. 5.1). In tissues, blood, and recently isolated cultures the organism stains bipolar (Fig. 5.2). Pili have been reported (41, 115).

Growth Requirements. *P. multocida* grows aerobically or anaerobically. The optimal growth temperature is 37 C. The optimal pH range is 7.2–7.8, but growth can occur in the range 6.2–9.0, depending upon composition of the medium. In liquid media, maximum growth is obtained in 16–24 hr. The broth becomes cloudy, and in a few days a sticky sediment collects. With some isolates a flocculent precipitate occurs.

The bacterium will grow on meat infusion media; growth is enhanced when the medium is enriched with peptone, casein hydrolysate, or avian serum. Blood or serum from some animals inhibits growth of *P. multocida.* Inhibition is greatest from blood of horses, cattle, sheep, and goats; blood of chickens, ducks, swine, and water buffalo has little or no inhibitory action (131). Several selective media for isolation have been described (22, 23, 38, 82, 94, 137). Chemically defined media have been described by Jordan (76), Watko (142), Wessman and Wessman (144), and Flossmann et al. (36). Berkman (11) found that pantothenic acid and nicotinamide are essential for growth. Dextrose starch agar with 5% avian serum is an excellent medium for isolating and growing *P. multocida.*

Colonial Morphology and Related Properties. Colonial morphology observed with obliquely transmitted light is one of the most useful characteristics in the study of *P. multocida.* On primary isolation from birds with FC, colonies may be iridescent, sectored with various intensities of iridescence, or blue with little or no iridescence (Fig. 5.3). Iridescence is related to the presence of a capsule. The term "fluorescent" used to describe colonies in older literature should be considered synonymous with iridescent; the latter is the appropriate term.

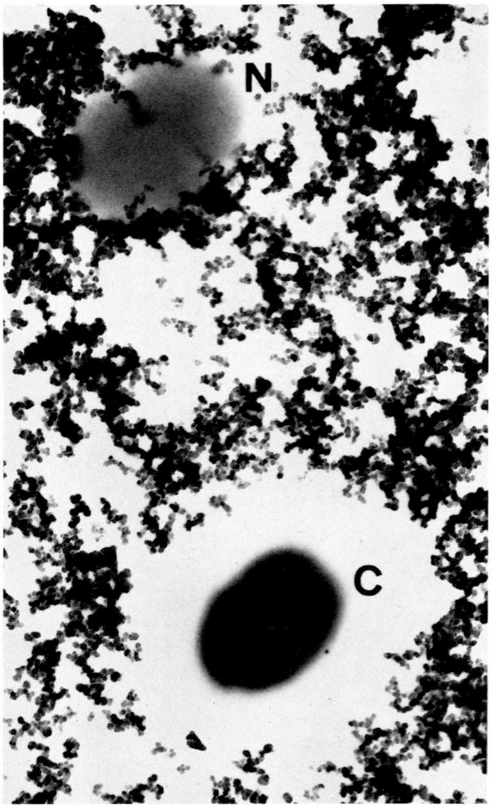

5.1. Electron micrograph of *P. multocida*-encapsulated cell (*C*) and nonencapsulated cell (*N*) suspended in India ink. ×19,000.

The composition of the medium determines to a certain extent the degree and type of iridescence. Occasionally an isolate produces blue colonies; when serum is added to the medium, sectored or iridescent colonies are sometimes produced. Examination of 18- to 24-hr colonies with a stereomicroscope using obliquely transmitted light (Fig. 5.4) is helpful when observing colonial morphology (64). Iridescent colonies on primary isolation from acute cases of FC are circular (2–3 mm), smooth, convex, translucent, glistening, and butyrous and show a tendency to coalesce. As the colony ages, it usually loses these distinguishing properties, becomes larger and viscous, and may adhere to the medium when

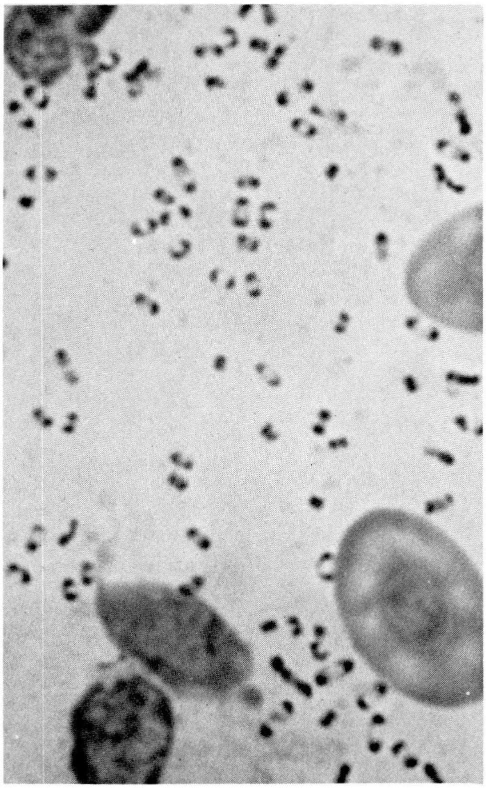

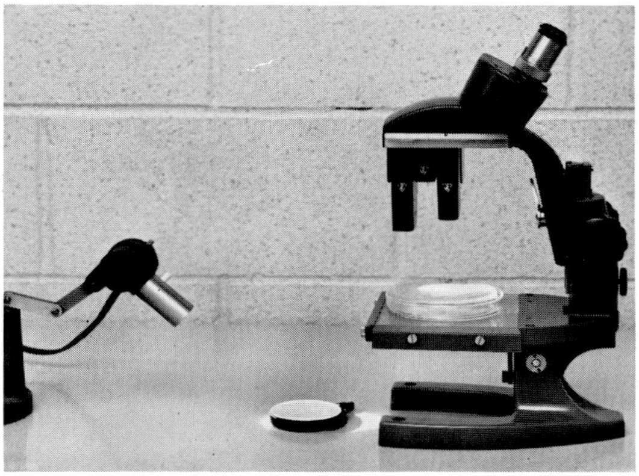

5.4. Arrangement of stereomicroscope with obliquely transmitted light for evaluation of colonial morphology.

5.2. *Pasteurella multocida* in liver imprint from chicken with acute FC (note bipolarity). Wright's stain, ×2500.

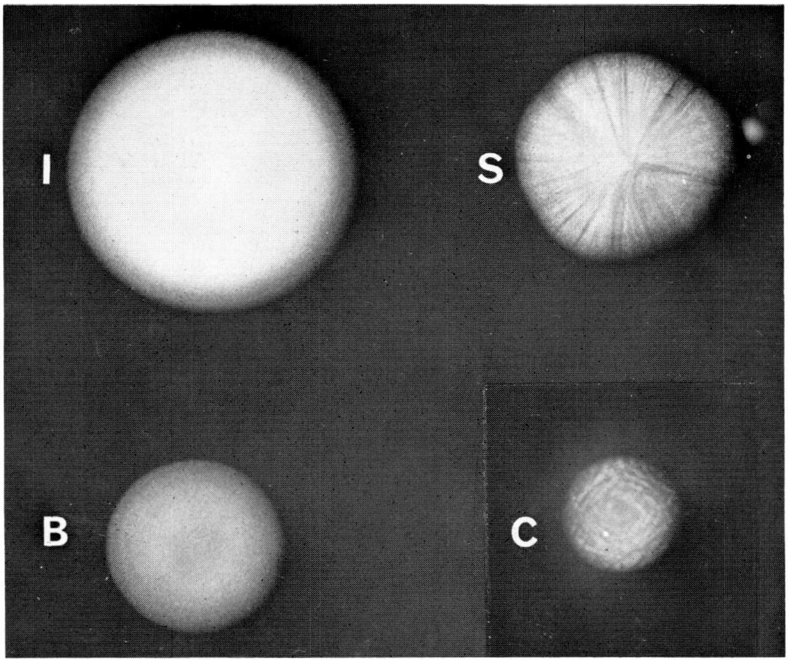

5.3. *Pasteurella multocida* 20-hr colonies on dextrose starch agar viewed with obliquely transmitted lighting (see Fig. 5.4); (*I*) iridescent, (*S*) sectored, (*B*) blue, and (*C*) rough. ×20.

picked with an inoculating needle. Blue colonies often isolated from birds with the chronic type of cholera or derived by dissociation of iridescent colonies are circular (1–2 mm), smooth, slightly convex or flat, translucent, butyrous, and discrete. The watery mucoid colonies produced by encapsulated strains from the respiratory tract of cattle, swine, sheep, rabbits, and humans are not iridescent but gray (58).

Anderson et al. (5) observed that a highly virulent isolate, which produced smooth colonies, later dissociated on subculture and produced rough colonies. Organisms from the smooth colonies were approximately 3–4 million times more virulent for pigeons than those from rough colonies. Hughes (66) studied the colonial morphology of 210 cultures from cases of FC and distinguished three types. The iridescent type was associated with outbreaks of acute FC and was highly virulent. The blue type was of low virulence and occurred in flocks in which cholera was enzootic. The third type was intermediate in its properties of iridescence and virulence.

Heddleston et al. (59) reported that a virulent isolate of *P. multocida* of avian origin produced iridescent colonies that dissociated in vitro and produced blue colonies. Organisms from blue colonies also mutated and produced gray colonies, which have not been reported in primary cultures from birds. Cells from iridescent colonies occurred singly or in pairs, did not agglutinate in immune serum, were encapsulated, and were virulent for chickens, turkeys, rabbits, and mice when administered on mucous membranes of the upper air passages. Cells from blue colonies occurred singly or in pairs, were agglutinated by immune serum, were unencapsulated, and were avirulent when applied to mucous membranes of chickens and mice but were virulent for rabbits and slightly virulent for turkeys. Cells from gray colonies occurred only as chains (Fig. 5.5) and were unencapsulated and avirulent. Killed organisms from all three colonial forms induced immunity in chickens. Antigens extracted with hot saline from highly virulent encapsulated cells of iridescent colonies by Yaw and Kakavas (146) actively immunized chickens and mice, whereas less virulent unencapsulated cells from blue colonies immunized chickens more effectively than mice.

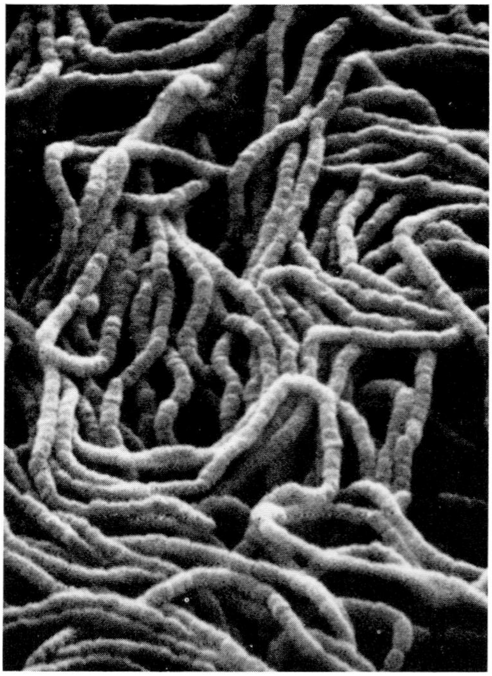

5.5. Scanning electron micrograph showing chain formation of *P. multocida* from gray colony (laboratory mutant). ×8000.

Physiologic Properties. The physiologic properties of *P. multocida* are used for identification. *P. multocida* does not produce gas but produces oxidase, catalase, peroxidase, and a characteristic odor. Unlike most gram-negative bacteria, it is sensitive to penicillin. The results of 29 other physiologic tests with 948 cultures of avian origin are shown in Table 5.1.

Significant differential characteristics are listed in Table 5.2.

Table 5.1. Physiologic properties of 948 *P. multocida* cultures of avian origin

Test	% Positive
Arabinose	7.4
Dextrin	0.6
Dulcitol	2.6
Fructose	100.0
Galactose	99.8
Gelatin	0.0
Glucose	100.0
Glycerol	93.3
Hemolysis	0.0
Hydrogen sulfide	97.5
Indol	99.6
Inositol	0.0
Inulin	0.0
Lactose	1.6
Litmus milk	0.7
MacConkey's agar	0.1
Maltose	0.0
Mannitol	99.5
Mannose	99.6
Motility	0.0
Nitrate reduction	100.0
Raffinose	2.7
Rhamnose	0.0
Salicin	0.0
Sorbitol	97.6
Sucrose	100.0
Trehalose	4.1
Urease	0.0
Xylose	77.4

Source: From (54).

Table 5.2. Differential tests for *P. multocida, P. anatipestifer, P. haemolytica, P. gallinarum,* and *Y. pseudotuberculosis*

	Pasteurella				*Yersinia*
Test	*multocida*	*anatipestifer*	*haemolytica*	*gallinarum*	*pseudotuberculosis*
Hemolysis	−	−	+	−	−
MacConkey's agar	−	−	+U	−	+U
Indol	+	−	−	−	−
Motility	−	−	−	−	+
Gelatin	−	+U	−	−	−
Catalase	+	+	+U	−	+
Oxidase	+	+	+	+	−
Urease	−	V	−	−	+
Glucose	+	−	+	+	+
Lactose	−U	−	+U	−	−
Sucrose	+	−	+	+	−
Maltose	−U	−	−U	+	+

Note: U = usually; V = variable.

Resistance to Chemical and Physical Agents. *P. multocida* is easily destroyed by ordinary disinfectants, sunlight, drying, or heat, being killed within 15 min at 56 C and 10 min at 60 C. A 1% solution of formaldehyde, phenol, sodium hydroxide, betapropiolactone, or glutaraldehyde and a 0.1% solution of benzalkonium chloride killed within 5 min 4.4×10^8 organisms of *P. multocida*/ml suspended in 0.85% saline solution at 24 C.

Das (22) observed that cotton swabs saturated with blood from infected mice contained viable organisms after 118 hr but not after 166 hr (at which time the swabs were completely dry); films of blood on glass contained viable organisms after 24 hr but not after 30 hr. Das also reported that infected blood sealed in glass tubes and held in a cold room contained viable organisms after 221 days. Skidmore (136) observed that the organism survived in dried turkey blood on glass for 8 days but not for 30 days at room temperature. In studies of the influence of environment on the incidence of FC, Van Es and Olney (139) found the infection hazard had apparently disappeared from a poultry yard 2 wk after occurrence of the last death and removal of birds.

Influence of temperature on viability and virulence of *P. multocida* was studied by Nobrega and Bueno (100), who observed that broth cultures stored in sealed tubes at an average room temperature of 17.6 C were still virulent after 2 yr; at 2–4 C they were nonviable after 1 yr. With controlled experiments Dimov (28) observed that *P. multocida* died rapidly in soils with moisture content of less than 40%. At a moisture content of 50% and temperature of 20 C, it survived for 5–6 days at pH 5.0, 15–100 days at pH 7.0, and 24–85 days at pH 8.0. A culture survived without loss of virulence for 113 days in soil with 50% moisture at 3 C and pH 7.15.

Cultures may be maintained without dissociation or loss of virulence in the lyophilized state or sealed in glass tubes and stored at 4 C or colder (143). Lyophilized cultures tested after 26 yr were still virulent for chickens, and a culture sealed in a rubber-stoppered bottle containing beef infusion broth with 50% horse serum and held at room temperature was virulent after 26 yr (51).

Serotyping and Other Methods of Grouping Strains. Serologic typing is based on methods that detect specific capsule and somatic antigens. Specific capsule serogroup antigens are recognized using passive hemagglutination tests (19). Five serogroups (A, B, D, E, F) are currently recognized (126). Carter (19) studied numerous isolates from various animals and found serogroups A and D were isolated from fowl and other animals. In a study of isolates representing a variety of avian hosts, Rhoades and Rimler (118) found organisms belonging to serogroups A, B, D, and F.

Somatic serotyping has been done by tube agglutination test (96) and gel diffusion precipitin test methods (61). Comparison studies by Brogden and Packer (16) indicated that a serotype determined by one method did not correlate with a serotype determined by the other method. Often, cultures that represented a single somatic serotype in a particular test represented more than one serotype in the other test. Because of its simplicity, the gel diffusion precipitin test is used routinely in the USA, and its popularity is increasing throughout the world. The test uses antisera prepared in chickens and heat-stable antigens extracted from formalinized saline suspensions of the bacteria. The heat-stable antigens form lines of identity with lipopolysaccharide-protein complexes from culture supernatants (61). Somatic serotype specificity seems to be determined by the lipopolysaccharide component of a complex (123). Heddleston et al. (61) found there was good correlation, though not absolute, between the gel diffusion precipitin test and the immune response in chickens and turkeys. Rimler and Phillips (125) found that lipopolysaccharide combined with carrier protein protected chickens against FC. To date, 16 somatic serotypes have been described (17), all of which have been isolated from avian hosts. Rosenbusch and Merchant (130) placed isolates of *P. multocida* into three groups on the basis of fermentation of xylose, arabinose, and dulcitol. Group I fermented arabinose and dulcitol but not xylose; group II fermented xylose but not arabinose or dulcitol; group III was variable but more nearly like group I. Dorsey (31) studied fermentation reactions of 409 isolates of fowl origin and found 81.42% were of group I, 16.87% of group II, and 1.71% of group III; 23 isolates could not be grouped on the basis of these reactions. Donahue and Olson (29) studied 214 isolates from turkeys: 0.47% were in group I; 83.64% in group II; 1.4% in group III; and 14% did not correlate with any of the groups.

Phage sensitivity as a basis for grouping *P. multocida* has been investigated. Rifkind and Pickett (122) found 84 of 118 isolates from various hosts were sensitive to one or more of 16 bacteriophages. Kirchner and Eisenstark (80) examined 25 cultures of avian origin and found that 11 were lysogenic. They divided the 11 bacteriophages into five groups as to their host range and into three groups on plaque morphology. Karaivanov and Mraz (79) identified 87% of 77 cultures of *P. multocida* using one strain of bacteriophage. Saxena and Hoerlein (133) demonstrated lysogeny in 63 of 112 cultures from various hosts. One phage caused lysis of 8 different cultures; many were lysogenic for only 1 or 2 cultures. Gadberry and Miller (37) showed that 32 of 61 isolates were sensitive to 1 or more of 3 phages. Isolates of *P. haemolytica, P. gallinarum, P. ureae, P. pneumotropica,* and 3 species of the genus *Yersinia* were resistant to lysis. Results of these investigations demonstrated the possibility of a phage grouping system for *P. multocida.*

Pathogenicity. Pathogenicity or virulence of *P. multocida* in relation to FC is complex and variable, depending on the strain, host species, and variations within the strain or host and conditions of contact between the two. The ability of *P. multocida* to invade and reproduce in the host is enhanced by the presence of a capsule (see Fig. 5.1) that surrounds the organism (86). Loss of ability of a virulent strain to produce the capsule results in loss of virulence (59). Many isolates from cases of fowl cholera have large capsules but are of low virulence. Therefore, virulence is apparently related to some chemical substance associated with the capsule rather than with its physical presence.

P. multocida usually enters tissues of birds through mucous membranes of the pharnyx or upper air passages, but it may also enter through the conjunctiva or cutaneous wounds. Hughes and Pritchett (67) were unable to infect chickens by placing a culture in a gelatin capsule and inserting it into the esophagus, but chickens were infected when culture was dropped on the roof of the nasal cleft. Arsov (8) infected birds by mouth, using ^{32}P-labeled culture, and observed that the portal of infection was the mucous membrane of the mouth and pharnyx but not the esophagus, crop, or proventriculus. The eustachian tube was suggested by Olson and McCune (102) as the most likely route of infection, since it localizes in air spaces of the cranial bone, middle ear, and meninges.

Turkeys are much more susceptible than chickens to infection with *P. multocida,* and mature chickens are more susceptible than young ones (50). Hungerford (68) observed heavy losses in mature chickens but no losses in birds up to 16 wk of age in a case involving 90,000 birds. When testing infectivity of an isolate or susceptibility of a host, cohabitation is the most natural method of exposure. However, unless the host is highly susceptible and the isolate highly invasive, results may be slow. Therefore, it is often advantageous to swab the nasal cleft with cotton saturated with the culture; if a more severe exposure is required, culture can be injected parenterally.

Toxicity. A dried culture filtrate of *P. multocida* was first demonstrated to produce signs of toxicity in chickens by Pasteur (105). Salmon (132) repeated this work and described signs resulting from toxicity similar to those observed in cases of acute FC. Kyaw (83), using the developing chick embryo in the study of pathogenesis, suggested that a toxin was produced in vivo by *P. multocida.* Rhoades (117) observed acute general passive hyperemia in chickens that died from acute FC. This lesion was considered to be indicative of shock and was attributed to action of endotoxin.

Endotoxins. Endotoxins are produced by all *P. multocida,* both virulent and nonvirulent. They may contribute to virulence, however, invasion and multiplication of a strain are necessary for production of sufficient quantities of endotoxin in vivo to contribute to pathologic processes.

Pirosky (111) obtained an endotoxin from *P. multocida* of avian origin by the trichloroacetic acid extraction procedure of Boivin. Heddleston and Rebers (55) demonstrated that a loosely bound endotoxin could be washed from *P. multocida* with cold formalinized saline solution. This endotoxin was a nitrogen-containing phosphorylated lipopolysaccharide, readily inactivated under mild acid conditions. Signs of acute FC were induced in chickens by injection of fractional amounts of endotoxin. The LD_{50} for chicken embryos was 5.2 μg via the chorioallantoic membrane; the LD_{50} for mice was 194 μg via the peritoneal cavity. One dose of 1.9 mg injected intravenously killed five of six 19-day-old turkeys; the median death time was only 3 hr. The endotoxin was present in the vascular system of turkeys with FC and could be detected with the Limulus lysate test and antiserum in the gel diffusion precipitin test. The serologic specificity of the endotoxin was associated with the lipopolysaccharide. Free endotoxin induced active immunity.

Purified lipopolysaccharides of each of the Heddleston serotypes were prepared by Rimler et al. (127). The lipopolysaccharides were similar to those of other gram-negative bacteria. Week-old poults were relatively resistant to the lethal effects of purified lipopolysaccharides from two highly pathogenic FC strains of *P. multocida* (119). In poults, the lipopolysaccharides did not provoke a dermal Shwartzman reaction and lethality was not enhanced by a liver-damaging substance, a histamine-releasing substance, or surgical bursectomy.

Protein Toxins. Heat-labile protein toxins have been found in serogroup A and D strains isolated from different animal species. Nielsen et al. (99) found 6 of 10 turkey strains produced heat-labile protein toxins; the strains were not serotyped. Four serogroup D strains isolated from turkeys were found to contain a heat-labile toxin (120). Sonicated suspensions of these strains produced dermonecrotic lesions in turkey skin and were lethal to poults. Antiserum prepared against the heat-labile toxin from a swine strain neutralized the ability of the avian strain sonicates to produce dermonecrosis (121). Baba and Bito (9) chemically purified a protein toxin from an avian stain.

PATHOGENESIS AND EPIZOOTIOLOGY

Natural and Experimental Hosts. Most reported outbreaks of FC affected chickens, turkeys, ducks, or geese. However, this disease also affects other types of poultry, game birds raised in captivity, companion birds, birds in zoos, and wild birds. The wide range of avian hosts in which FC has been reported suggests that all types of birds are susceptible.

Among types of poultry, turkeys are most affected. Most or all in an infected flock may die within a few days. The disease usually occurs in young mature turkeys, but all ages are highly susceptible. Under experimental conditions 90–100% of mature turkeys may die within 48 hr when exposed to a highly virulent strain of *P. multocida* by swabbing the palatine cleft or by contact with infected birds.

The disease in turkeys was first reported in detail by DeVolt and Davis (27), who described an outbreak in a flock of 175 turkeys in Maryland, where the mortality was 17%. Alberts and Graham (2) described outbreaks in four flocks of turkeys in which mortality was 17–68%. They emphasized that environmental stressors such as changes in climate, nutrition, injury, and excitement may have influenced the incidence and course of the disease.

Death losses from FC in chickens usually occur in laying flocks, because this age bird is more susceptible than younger chickens. Chickens less than 16 wk of age are generally quite resistant. FC that occurs in young chickens is often in conjunction with some other malady and usually is caused by infection with serotype 1. However, recent outbreaks of FC in six flocks of 20- to 46-day-old broilers resulted from infections with serotypes 3; 1,3; and 3,4. Experimental challenge of 5-wk-old broilers with two representative strains (serotypes 3 and 1,3) resulted in mortality and lameness. In naturally infected chickens, mortality usually ranges from 0–20%, but greater losses have been reported. Reduced egg production and persistent localized infection often occur. Chickens are more susceptible to FC after withdrawal of feed and water or after abrupt change of diet (14). Heat or rough treatment on a shaking machine increased the incidence in chickens exposed experimentally (77, 78).

Under experimental conditions 90–100% of mature chickens exposed by swabbing the palatine cleft may die within 24–48 hr, depending on the strain of *P. multocida* used, but only 10–20% usually die within a 2-wk period when exposed by contact with infected birds. Pritchett et al. (113) observed mortality of 35–45% in three houses of pullets. In one house 45% of the birds died within 4 wk. In a flock of 45 birds that had survived an acute outbreak the previous year, no losses were observed, but the number of birds with localized lesions increased during winter. In South Carolina and adjoining areas, FC exists mainly as a persistent, subacute, chronic disease that clinically resembles avian monocytosis (12).

Domestic geese and ducks are also highly susceptible to FC. Curtice (21) reported the disease in geese in Rhode Island, where about 3200 of a flock of 4000 died in a short period. Van Es and Olney (139) recognized the marked susceptibility of geese to FC in using them to test for persistence of viable organisms in lots after removal of infected chickens. FC in ducks is a serious problem on Long Island, where it was diagnosed on 32 of 68 commercial duck farms. Losses usually occur in ducks over 4 wk of age, and mortality may reach 50% (33).

Birds of prey, waterfowl, and other birds kept in zoological gardens occasionally succumb to infection. *P. multocida* has been isolated from over 50 species of feral birds. During a 2½-year survey Faddoul et al. (34) isolated *P. multocida* from 13 (seven species) of 248 feral birds submitted to the diagnostic laboratory. Jaksic et al. (74) described an acute epornitic among pheasants in which 1700 died. An outbreak in the San Francisco Bay area was reported to have been responsible for an estimated loss of 40,000 waterfowl (129). Gershman et al. (39) observed a serious outbreak among eider ducks (*Somateria mollissima*) in their nesting area 6 mi off the coast of Maine, where over 200 birds died and more than 100 nests were lost. Over 60,000 waterfowl died of FC during the winter of 1956–57 at the Muleshoe National Wildlife Refuge in Texas (75). Rosen (128) reported there are two areas in the USA where fowl cholera is enzootic in waterfowl–the Muleshoe National Wildlife Refuge and the north central area of California. Both locations have had periodic outbreaks since 1944.

P. multocida from birds with FC will usually kill rabbits and mice, but other mammals are resistant to infection. According to Heddleston and Watko (57), rabbits, mice, pigeons, and sparrows died of acute septicemia when exposed intranasally to an isolate of *P. multocida* from an acute case of FC; rats, ferrets, guinea pigs, a sheep, a pig, and a calf did not show any clinical response to the same organism. One of 5 rats, 1 of 2 mink, and 11 of 19 mice fed viscera of infected chickens developed nasal infection, pneumonia, and fatal septicemia respectively. A calf died of acute septicemia less than 18 hr after intramuscular (IM) exposure. Guinea pigs exposed by IM inoculation developed necrosis at the inoculation site; those exposed intraperitoneally usually died.

Horses, cattle, sheep, pigs, dogs, and cats are refractory to oral inoculation, and subcutaneous (SC) inoculation results in localized abscesses. However, all these animals may succumb to intravenous inoculation.

Transmission, Carriers and Vectors. How FC is introduced into a flock is often impossible to determine. Chronically infected birds are considered to be a major source of infection. The only limit to the duration of the chronic carrier state is the life span of the infected bird. Free-flying birds having contact with poultry may be a source of FC organisms. Transmission of the organism through the egg seldom if ever occurs. A study of more than 2000 fresh and embryonated eggs from chickens infected with chronic FC yielded no evidence that *P. multocida* was transmitted through the egg (135).

Pritchett et al. (113, 114) and Pritchett and Hughes (112) examined three infected commercial flocks of white leghorns for *P. multocida* and found that many birds harbored the organism in nasal clefts. Presence of the bacterium was related to severity of upper respiratory infection in the flocks. They concluded that the enzootic focus of infection was healthy nasal carriers. These studies as well as those of Van Es and Olney (139) and Hall et al. (46) proved that survivors of an epornitic of FC may be reservoirs of infection. Dorsey and Harshfield (32) reported a higher incidence of FC during late summer and fall in South Dakota. Carrier birds among the older flock, held over for a second year, provided a reservoir of infection for young susceptible pullets housed with them.

Most species of farm animals may be carriers of *P. multocida*. Generally, these organisms, except for those from swine and possibly those from cats, are avirulent for fowl. Iliev et al. (70) isolated *P. multocida* from tonsils of 34 of 75 slaughtered cattle, 14 or 27 sheep, and 102 of 162 pigs. Isolates from cattle and sheep were not pathogenic for fowl, but all 18 isolates from pigs in areas where FC was common were highly pathogenic for fowl. Only 2 of 47 isolates from pigs in areas having low incidence of FC were pathogenic. Iliev et al. (71) also reported that healthy pigs that were carriers of *P. multocida* transmitted infection to fowl in the same enclosure. Two isolates, serotypes 1:A and 5:A, from lungs of pigs with pneumonia, were studied by Murata et al. (95). Serotype 5:A was highly virulent for chickens, and serotype 1:A was avirulent. They found no cross-immunity in chickens between the 2 serotypes.

Gregg et al. (44) isolated two cultures from raccoons, which were pathogenic for turkeys. They suggested that racoons are a reservoir of *P. multocida* and the organisms may be transmitted to turkeys via the raccoon bite.

Contaminated crates, feed bags, or any equipment used previously for poultry may serve in introducing FC into a flock. Organisms are disseminated throughout the carcasses of birds that die of acute FC, and may serve as an infection source, especially since fowl tend to consume such carcasses. Hendrickson and Hilbert (63) were able to isolate *P. multocida* from the blood of a naturally infected chicken for 49 days preceding death. They noticed rapid increase in the number of organisms immediately preceding and following death, and the organisms remained viable 2 mo at 5–10 C. Serdyuk and Tsimokh (134) demonstrated experimentally that sparrows, pigeons, and rats could become infected with *P. multocida* when exposed to chickens with FC and that they in turn could infect susceptible chickens. Sparrows and pigeons carried organisms without showing clinical signs, but 10% of infected rats developed acute pasteurellosis.

The possibility that insects may serve as vectors of FC has been investigated. Skidmore (136) experimentally transmitted FC to turkeys by feeding them flies that had previously fed on infected blood. He pointed out that under natural conditions, ingestion of flies might be a means of introducing the disease into a flock. Transmission by flies, however, is probably not common, as indicated by studies of Van Es and Olney (139). Although FC was maintained in two lots of chickens during the height of the fly season, there was no spread of the disease to adjoining lots separated only by poultry netting. Iovcev (73) observed that larvae, nymphs, and adult ticks (*Argas persicus*) contained *P. multocida* after feeding on infected hens. Petrov (109) demonstrated that the red mite (*Dermanyssus gallinae*) became infected with *P. multocida* after feeding on infected birds, but the mite did not transmit the organism.

Heddleston and Wessman (58) showed that 27 cultures of *P. multocida* from the upper respiratory tract of humans were not pathogenic for turkeys. However, humans can become infected and may infect poultry via excretion from the nose or mouth.

Dissemination of *P. multocida* within a flock is primarily by excretions from the mouth (Fig. 5.6), nose, and conjunctiva of diseased birds that contaminate their environment, particularly feed and water. Feces very seldom contain viable *P. multocida;* however, Reis (116) found the organism in feces from one of nine birds just before death. In the remaining eight birds the organisms were isolated only in feces collected from the cloacae of dead birds. Iliev et al. (72) demonstrated that *P. multocida* labeled with ^{32}P was inactivated in the proventriculus, and feces contained no viable *P. multocida.* Turkeys drinking from the same water trough with those experimentally infected with *P. multocida* developed FC (103).

Signs

ACUTE. Signs of infection in acute FC are often present for only a few hours before death. Unless infected birds are observed during this period, death may be the first indication of disease. Signs that often occur are fever, anorexia, ruffled feathers, mucous discharge from the mouth, diarrhea, and increased respiratory rate. Cyanosis often occurs immediately prior to death and is most evident in unfeathered areas of the head, such as comb and wattles. Fecal material associated with the diarrhea is initially watery and whitish in color but later becomes greenish and contains mucus. Birds that survive the initial acute septicemic stage may later succumb to debilitating effects of emaciation and dehydration, may become chronically infected, or may recover.

CHRONIC. Chronic FC may follow an acute stage of the disease or result from infection with organisms of low virulence. Signs are generally related to localized infections. Wattles (Fig. 5.7), sinuses, leg or wing joints, foot pads, and sternal bursae often become swollen. Exudative conjunctival (Fig. 5.8) and pharyngeal lesions may be observed, and torticollis (Fig. 5.9) sometimes occurs. Tracheal rales and dyspnea may result from respiratory tract infections. In the past the term

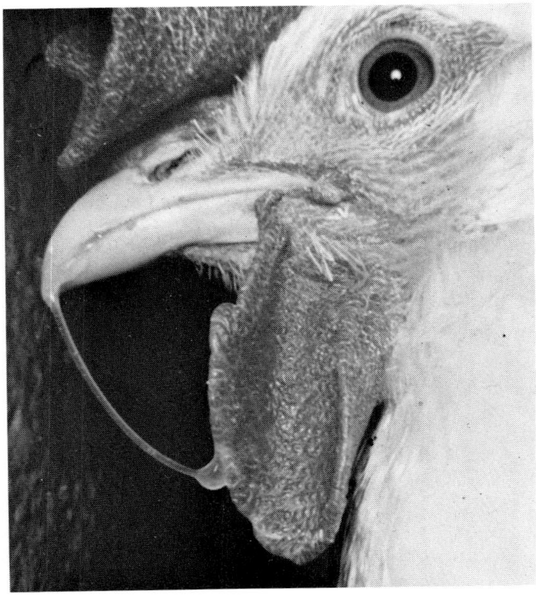

5.6. Acute FC; mucous excretion from the mouth contains large numbers of *P. multocida* that can contaminate feed and water.

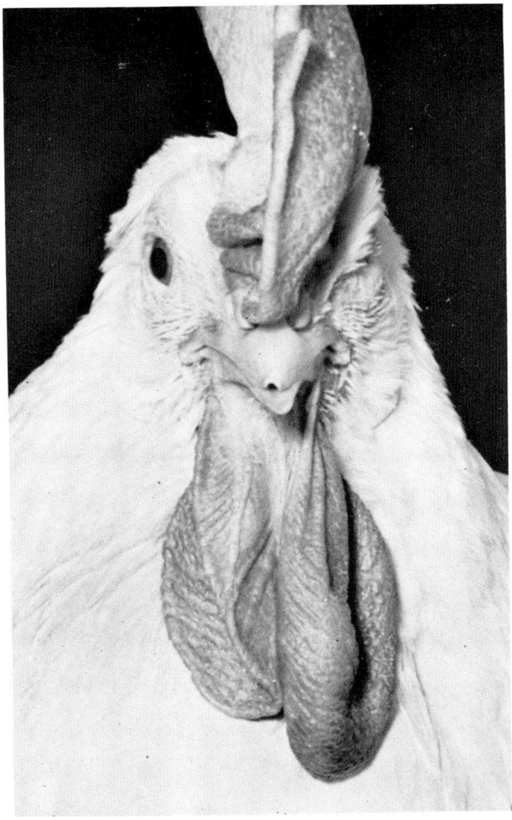

5.7. Chronic FC; swollen wattle resulting from localized infection.

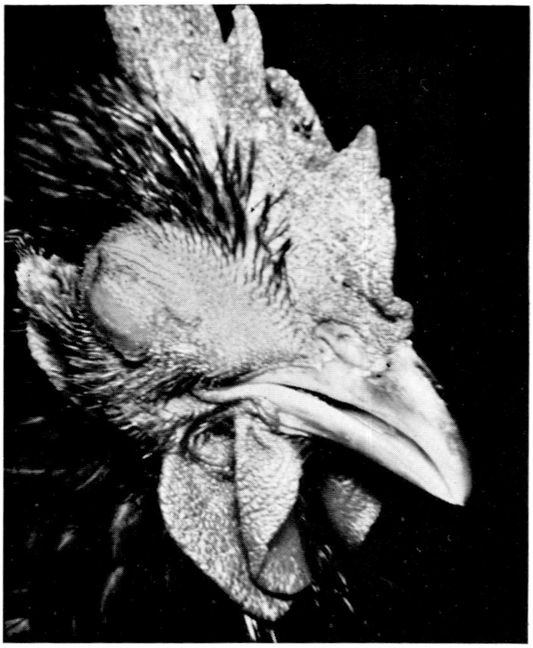

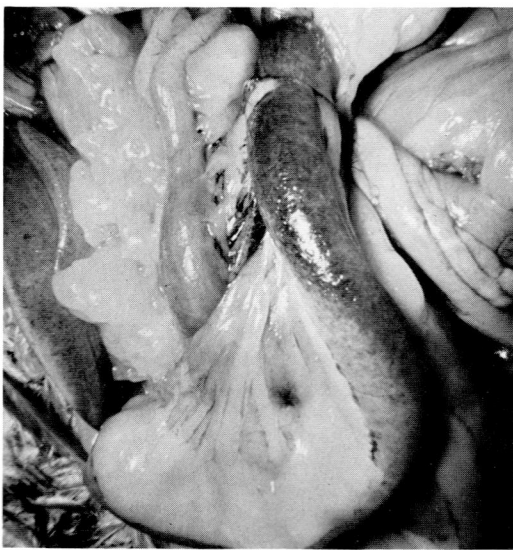

5.8. Chronic FC; serous inflammation of conjunctiva.

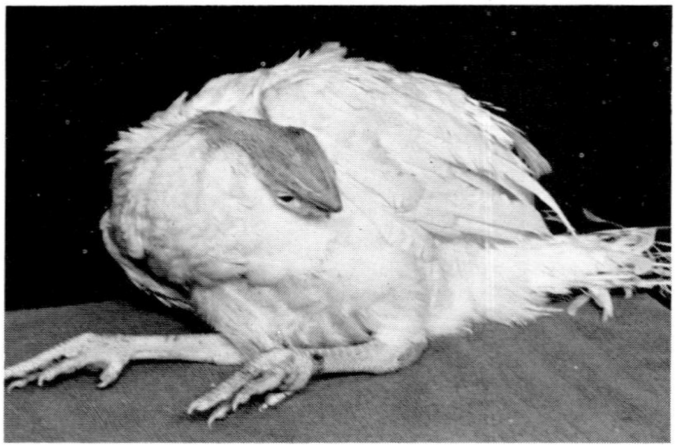

5.9. Chronic FC; torticollis resulting from meningeal infection.

"roup" was used to indicate a condition in which signs were associated with chronic infections of cephalic mucous membranes. The term was not limited to FC but included other diseases as well. Chronically infected birds may succumb, remain infected for long periods, or recover.

Gross and Microscopic Lesions. Lesions of FC are not constant but vary in type and severity. The greatest variation is related to the course of the disease, whether acute or chronic. Although it is convenient for descriptive purposes to refer to either acute or chronic FC, it is sometimes difficult to categorize the disease in this manner. Signs of infection and lesions that occur may be intermediate to those described for acute and chronic forms.

ACUTE. When the course of the disease is acute, most of the postmortem lesions are associated with vascular disturbances. General hyperemia usually occurs, is most evident in veins of the abdominal viscera, and may be quite pronounced in small vessels of the duodenal mucosa (Figs. 5.10, 5.11). Large numbers of bacteria can usually be observed microscopically in the hyperemic vessels. Petechial and ecchymotic hemorrhages are frequently found and may be widely distributed. Subepicardial (Fig. 5.12A) and subserosal hemorrhages are common, as are hemorrhages in the lung, abdominal fat, and intestinal mucosa. Increased amounts of pericardial and peritoneal fluid frequently occur. Disseminated intravascular clotting or fibrinous thrombosis has been observed in chickens and ducks that died from acute experimentally induced FC (69, 104).

Livers of acutely affected birds may be swollen and usually contain multiple small focal areas of coagulative necrosis (Fig. 5.12B) and heterophilic infiltration (Fig. 5.13). Some of the less virulent *P. multocida* do not produce necrotic foci in the liver. Heterophilic infiltration also occurs in lungs and certain other parenchymatous organs (117). Lungs of turkeys are affected more severely than those of chickens, with pneumonia being a common sequela. Large amounts of viscid mucus may be observed in the digestive tract, particularly in the pharynx, crop, and intestine.

5.10. Acute FC; hyperemia of chicken duodenum.

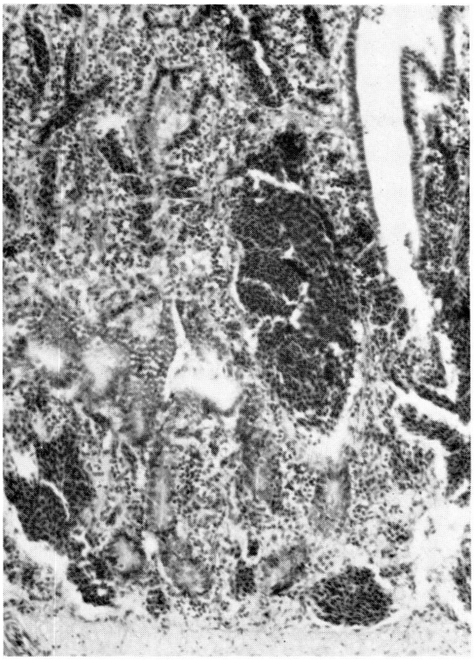

5.11. Acute FC; marked hyperemia of chicken duodenum. H & E, ×150.

Ovaries of laying hens are commonly affected. Mature follicles often appear flaccid; thecal blood vessels, which are normally easily observed, are less evident (Fig. 5.12C). Yolk material from ruptured follicles may be found in the peritoneal cavity. Immature follicles and ovarian stroma are often hyperemic.

CHRONIC. Chronic FC is usually characterized by localized infections, in contrast to the septicemic nature of the acute disease. These generally become suppurative and may be widely distributed anatomically. They often occur in the respiratory tract and may involve any part, including sinuses and pneumatic bones (Fig. 5.14). Pneumonia (Fig. 5.15) is an especially common lesion in turkeys. Infections of the conjunctiva and adjacent tissues occur (see Fig. 5.8), and facial edema may be observed. Localized infections may also involve the hock joints (Fig. 5.12D), foot pads, peritoneal cavity, and oviduct.

Chronic localized infections can involve the middle ear and cranial bones and have been reported to result in torticollis. In turkeys torticollis and eventual death can be associated with infections of the cranial bones, middle ear, and meninges. In a study of naturally infected turkeys exhibiting torticollis, Olson (101) described lesions at these sites. The outstanding gross lesion was yellowish caseous exudate in air spaces of the calvarial bones. Heterophilic infiltration and fi-

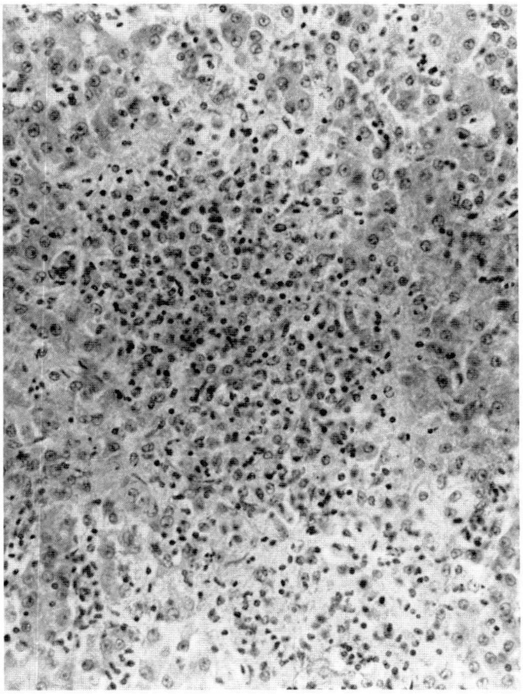

5.13. Acute FC; coagulative necrosis and heterophilic infiltration in turkey liver. H & E, ×375.

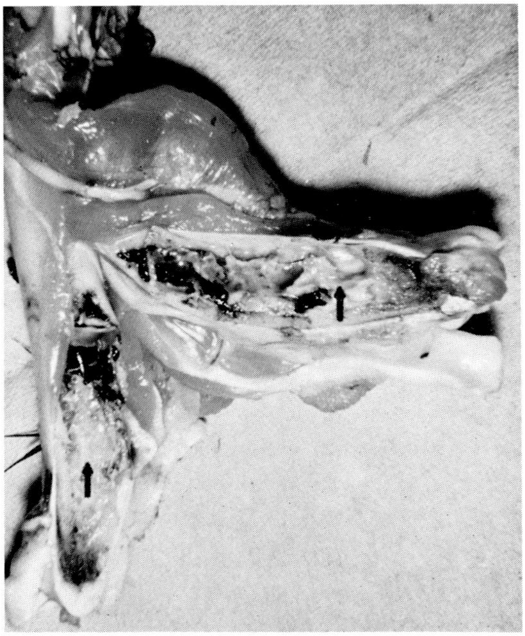

5.14. Chronic FC; caseous exudate (*arrows*) in turkey humerus.

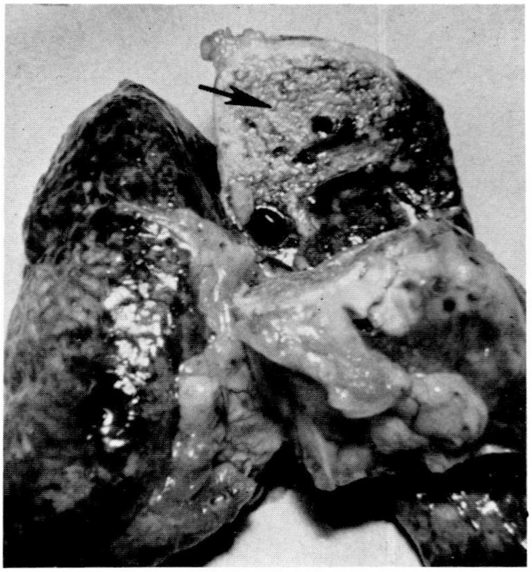

5.15. Chronic FC; pneumonic area (*arrow*) in turkey lung.

brin were consistently observed in the air spaces, middle ear, and meninges. Multinuclear giant cells were often associated with necrotic masses of heterophils in air spaces. Similar lesions were found in experimentally exposed turkeys (102). Localized meningeal infections (Fig. 5.16) without involvement of cranial bones or the middle ear have been observed in turkeys exhibiting torticollis, as have cerebellar infections (35).

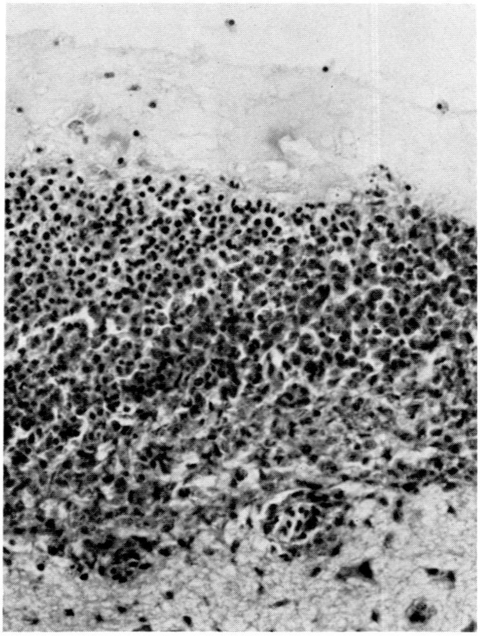

5.16. Chronic FC; fibrinosuppurative meningitis in turkey. H & E, ×400.

Immunity. Pasteur (107) used an avirulent culture attenuated by prolonged growth on artificial medium and produced immunity that protected fowl against subsequent exposure. In field use his method did not prove practical because uniform attenuation could not be obtained and heavy losses sometimes occurred in vaccinated flocks.

Since Pasteur's classic work there have been numerous attempts to produce efficient vaccines against FC, but results have not been consistent. However, there can be little doubt that a substantial but not absolute immunity can be induced in fowl by using killed *P. multocida* vaccines under controlled conditions (10, 52). Killed *P. multocida* vaccines are usually prepared by growing selected immunogenic strains on a suitable medium and suspending in formolized saline solution. The killed organisms are usually incorporated with an adjuvant and injected subcutaneously.

Under field conditions, losses from FC sometimes occur in vaccinated flocks. This failure may be due to improperly prepared or administered vaccine or immune impaired birds. Heddleston and Reisinger (56) demonstrated that stress caused by changing the social or peck order of vaccinated males as well as fowl pox infection in chickens at time of vaccination and exposure significantly reduced the efficacy of vaccination. In experimental studies (110) the manifestation of acquired resistance was impaired in turkeys vaccinated against *P. multocida* while receiving aflatoxin in their feed. It was also observed that an isolate of *P. multocida* recovered from a FC outbreak in previously vaccinated turkeys differed serologically from the culture used in preparing vaccine (60).

In experimental studies Heddleston and Rebers (54) showed that bacterins prepared with tissues from infected turkeys or live *P. multocida* administered in drinking water will induce immunity in turkeys against a different immunogenic type. A bacterin prepared with bacteria grown on conventional agar media did not induce cross-immunity. These studies indicate that *P. multocida* produces a wider spectrum of immunogens in vivo than in vitro. Rimler (124) showed that turkeys vaccinated with in vivo–grown *P. multocida* and challenged with the homologous strain produced serum that passively immunized poults against five different serotypes. Bierer and others at Clemson University stimulated renewed interest in live FC vaccine administered in drinking water. Bierer and Derieux (13) demonstrated good immunity in 14-wk-old turkeys that were given a live culture of *P. multocida* (CU strain, previously CS-148) in drinking water 2 wk before challenge exposure. However, the vaccine killed 4.2% of 120 turkeys. Best results were obtained by inocu-

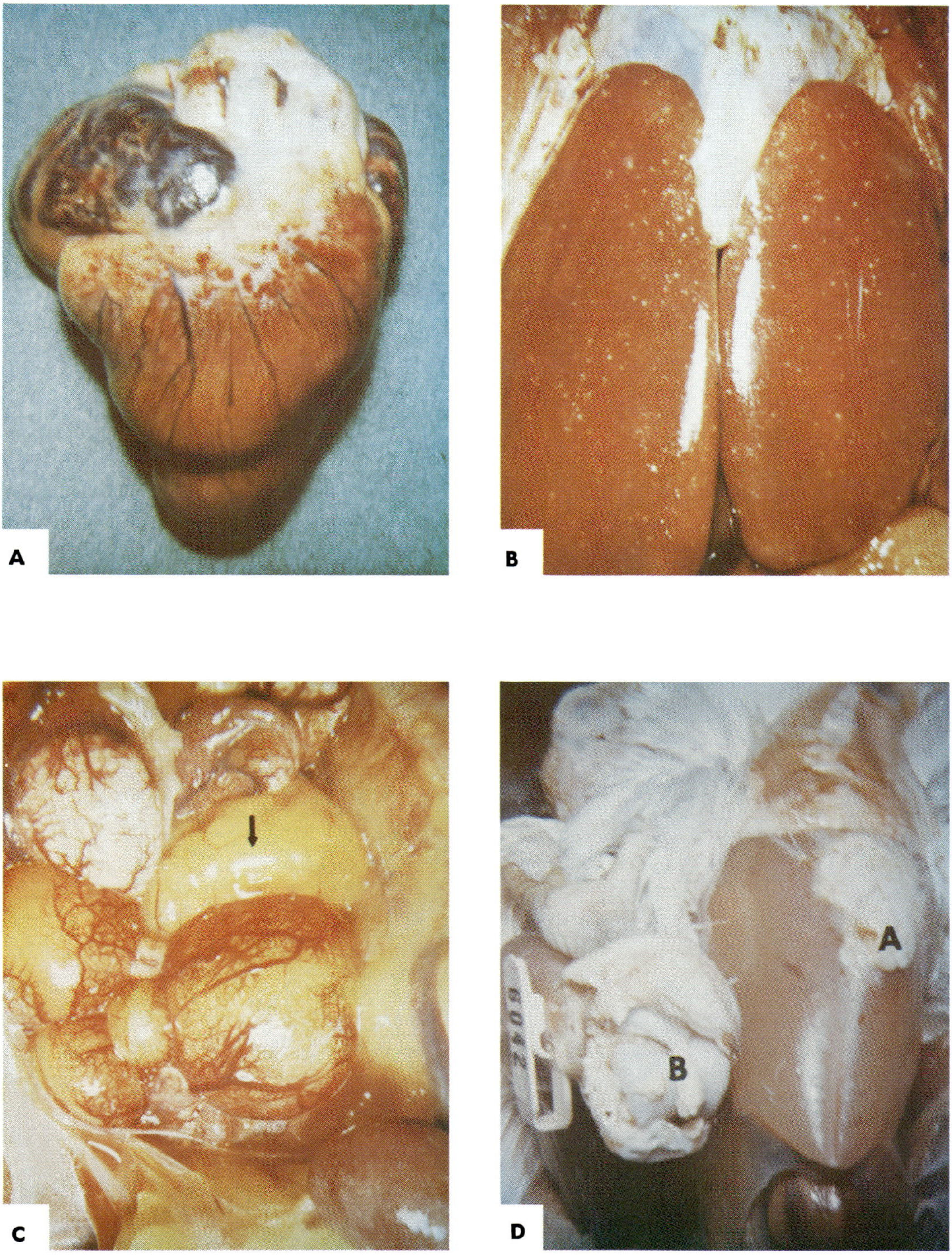

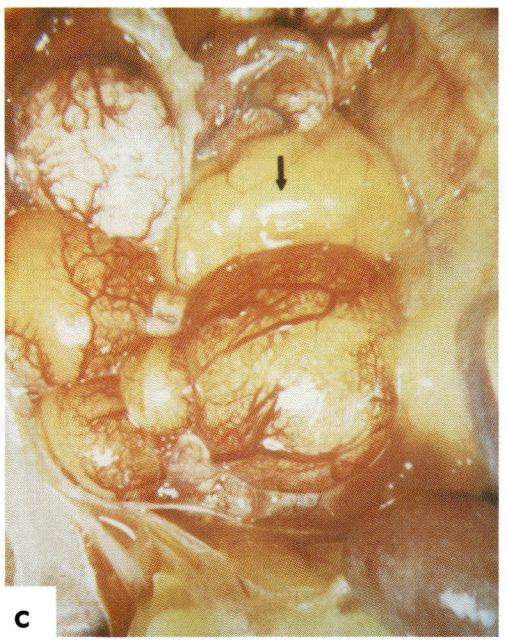

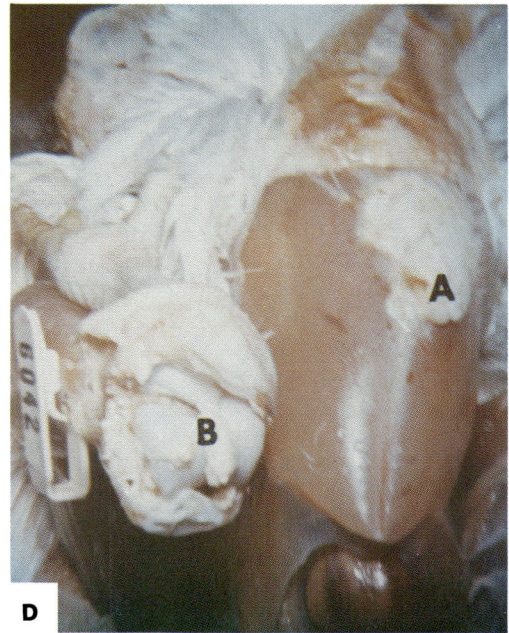

5.12. A. Acute FC; subepicardial hemorrhages in a chicken. B. Acute FC; multiple necrotic foci in chicken liver. C. Acute FC; flaccid ovarian follicle (*arrow*) with thecal blood vessels less evident than normal. D. Chronic FC; caseous exudate in sternal bursa (*A*) and hock joint (*B*) of turkey.

lating 8-wk-old turkeys with a killed bacterin and then administering the live vaccine 2 wk later; the live vaccine killed only 2.5% of 120 turkeys. Derieux and Bierer (26) stated that good immunity may be obtained in 6-wk-old turkeys by administering 2 doses of vaccine in drinking water on the same day and repeating the vaccination 4 wk later. However, no data were given as to duration of immunity or number of turkeys killed by vaccination. The CU strain administered in drinking water was immunologically less effective in chickens than in turkeys. It was more effective in chickens when administered by wing-web or SC inoculation than in drinking water (25). Live vaccines are commercially available for oral administration to turkeys and parenteral administration to chickens.

Maheswaran et al. (85) also induced immunity in turkeys with live vaccines via drinking water; they suggested that the vaccine induced localized but not systemic protection. In other studies Heddleston et al. (62) showed that serum from birds vaccinated via drinking water would induce passive immunity in chicks and turkeys.

Passive immunity for prevention of FC was studied in 1892 by Kitt, who used immune horse serum. This method was employed frequently, but because of the short duration of passive immunity it is presently used little if at all. Bolin and Eveleth (14) reported that *P. multocida* antiserum prepared in chickens gave maximum protection 16–24 hr after injection; protection began to decline after 48 hr and had disappeared after 192 hr.

DIAGNOSIS. A presumptive diagnosis of FC may be made from clinical observations, necropsy findings, or isolation of *P. multocida;* a conclusive diagnosis should be based on all three. Signs and lesions of the disease were described previously.

Isolation and Identification of Causative Agent. *P. multocida* can be isolated readily from viscera of birds that die of acute FC and usually from lesions of chronic cases; it is less likely to be isolated from dehydrated, emaciated survivors of an acute outbreak. A tentative diagnosis of acute FC can be made by demonstrating bipolar organisms in liver imprints (see Fig. 5.2) using Wright's stain. Immunofluorescent microscopy can be used to identify *P. multocida* in tissue or exudate (87).

Bone marrow, heart blood, liver, meninges, or localized lesions are preferred for culturing. To isolate *P. multocida,* sear the tissue or exudate with a spatula and obtain a specimen by inserting a sterile cotton swab or wire loop through the seared surface. If birds are living, squeeze mucus from the nostril or insert a cotton swab into the nasal cleft. Transfer the specimen to peptone broth and streak on dextrose starch agar containing 5% chicken serum or other suitable media. Specimens may also be streaked on MacConkey's and blood agar media to aid in identification.

Colonies characteristic of *P. multocida* (described under Etiology) are transferred to dextrose starch agar slants incubated 18–24 hr. Tubes of phenol red broth base containing 1% glucose, lactose, sucrose, mannitol, and maltose respectively are then inoculated with growth from the slant. Fermentation of glucose, sucrose, and mannitol without gas is characteristic of *P. multocida.* Lactose is usually not fermented, but some avian isolates will ferment it. Inoculate 2% tryptose in 0.85% saline solution, incubate 24 hrs at 37 C and test for indole (Kovac's test). Indole is almost always produced by *P. multocida.* There should be no hemolysis of blood and no growth on MacConkey's agar (Table 5.2).

Inoculation of animals may be used as an aid in isolating *P. multocida* from contaminated materials. Rabbits, hamsters, or mice are inoculated subcutaneously or intraperitoneally with 0.2 ml exudate or minced tissue. If *P. multocida* is present, the animal usually dies within 24–48 hr and the organism can be isolated in pure culture from heart, blood, or liver.

Serologic diagnosis of FC by rapid whole-blood agglutination, serum plate agglutination, or agar diffusion tests has limited value in chronic cholera and no value with the acute form of the disease.

Differential Diagnosis. *P. gallinarum* and *P. haemolytica* are two closely related bacteria that may be isolated from diseased poultry and incorrectly identified as *P. multocida* (53). *P. gallinarum* was first described by Hall et al. (46), who isolated it along with *P. multocida* from chickens with other maladies characterized by inflammation of the upper respiratory tract. The gel diffusion precipitin test shows a common antigen between *P. gallinarum* and *P. multocida.* Clark and Godfrey (20) found *P. gallinarum* associated with a respiratory disease complex of chickens in southern California. Gilchrist (40), in a survey of avian respiratory diseases in New South Wales, reported finding *P. gallinarum, P. haemolytica,* and *P. multocida.* Harbourne (48) isolated *P. haemolytica* on four occasions from livers of young chickens and turkeys. *P. haemolytica* was isolated from young chickens with salpingitis, which was often accompanied by nasal catarrh, helminth infection, or leukosis; the organism was also isolated from lungs of fowl with chronic respiratory disease and infectious bronchitis (98). Matthes et al. (88) isolated *P. haemolytica* from chickens with a septicemia. Chloramphenicol was effective in treatment. Hacking and Pettit (45) reported on eight cases of *P. haemolytica* in pullets and laying hens: five cases involved egg production, with some birds showing peritonitis or salpingitis; three cases involved mortality; some birds had enteritis, enteritis and hepatitis, or respiratory infection. In most cases *P. haemolytica* was thought to be a secondary pathogen.

Differential characteristics of various species of pasteurella that may be isolated from poultry are listed in Table 5.2.

TREATMENT. Antibacterial chemotherapy has been used extensively with varying success in treatment of FC, depending to a large extent on the promptness of treatment and drug used. Sensitivity testing is often advantageous, since strains of *P. multocida* vary in susceptibility to chemotherapeutic agents (30, 141) and resistance to treatment may develop, especially during prolonged use of these agents.

Sulfonamides. Several of the sulfonamides have been employed both experimentally and in natural outbreaks. The main disadvantages of the sulfonamides are their bacteriostatic instead of bactericidal action, inability to cure localized abscesses, and toxic effect on birds. Kiser et al. (81) reported 63–85% reduction in mortality from experimentally produced FC compared to untreated controls when using sulfamethazine and sodium sulfamethazine. In natural outbreaks mortality was reduced 45–75%. Favorable results were obtained with 0.5–1% of the drug in food or 0.1% in drinking water.

Alberts and Graham (3) employed 0.5% sulfamerazine in mash feed for 5 days in a field outbreak of FC in turkeys. Mortality was 1.9% in the treated group compared with 50% in untreated birds. FC recurred four times after cessation of treatment, and each time losses were arrested after turkeys were again given the sulfamerazine-mash mixture. In experimental infection in turkeys, sodium sulfamerazine at oral dosage rates of 143 and 107.25 mg/kg body weight effectively reduced mortality. In chickens 0.2% sodium sulfamerazine in drinking water or 0.4% sulfamerazine in mash checked mortality in an established outbreak 2 days after treatment was started (1). Sulfaquinoxaline in amounts of 0.01–0.05% in drinking water was completely prophylactic in experimental FC when treatment was started 24 hr before birds were inoculated. Peterson (108) treated two natural outbreaks in turkey flocks successfully with 1:2000–1:4000 dilution of the drug in drinking water. He found sulfamethazine and sodium sulfamerazine also were markedly effective in reducing experimental FC; sulfadiazine, sulfathiazole, and sulfanilamide were much less so. Sulfaquinoxaline was used by Delaplane (24) at the rate of 0.1% or 0.05% in mash in prophylaxis of FC in chickens. Nelson (97) reported favorable results in controlling mortality in turkeys with a concentration of 0.025% sulfaquinoxaline in drinking water for 5–7 days; he stated also that its administration 1 day out of 4 usually controls later mortality and permits the grower to finish birds for market. Dorsey and Harshfield (32) confirmed the usefulness of several sulfonamide drugs in checking losses from FC if treatment is carried out in early stages of an outbreak. They also noted frequent recurrence of mortality after treatment was discontinued and unsatisfactory results of treatment after the disease had become chronic.

Sulfaethoxypyridazine was reported by Stuart et al. (138) to be effective in controlling FC in chickens and turkeys. Effectiveness of the drug was dependent in part on size of dose and duration and promptness of treatment. Sulfadimethoxine, used alone or potentiated with ormetoprim, was found to be safe, palatable, and effective against experimentally induced FC in chickens and turkeys (90–93). Anderson et al. (6) reported that sulfachloropyrazine administered in drinking water was effective in preventing mortality in experimentally exposed chickens.

Antibiotics. Streptomycin given intramuscularly (IM) in a dose of 150,000 μg prevented deaths in adult turkeys when administered before or at the time of inoculation of *P. multocida.* When treatment was delayed for 6–24 hr or dosage was reduced, chronic infection resulted (89). Penicillin, streptomycin, penicillin and streptomycin together, and oxytetracycline (administered IM at the time of experimental exposure of chickens) all possessed activity as therapeutic agents (12). Chlortetracycline reduced losses in chicks about 80% when given at the rate of 40 mg/kg body weight IM 30 min after parenteral inoculation of the organism (84). Chicks that received mash containing 1 mg/g had 50% fewer losses than untreated controls. In an outbreak of FC in pheasants, however, Alberts and Graham (4) did not observe any beneficial results when 1 mg/g mash was fed. When chlortetracycline was given IM, a slight reduction in mortality was recorded. Novobiocin administered in feed or water reduced death losses in experimentally exposed turkeys (47). Chloramphenicol (20 mg/kg body weight) in a single IM injection was effective in treating FC, but in flocks where FC and fowl typhoid or fowl pox were concurrently present, chloramphenicol treatment was not successful (65). A chloramphenicol-dexamethasone-pyribenzamine combination was used successfully with vaccination in treatment of FC in breeding turkeys. Respiratory problems, which occurred 1 wk after the initial outbreak, responded readily to IM administration of this drug combination (42). Water-soluble erythromycin at the rate of 1 lb/50 gal drinking water halted mortality in two flocks of Muscovy ducklings infected with *P. multocida* (49).

Antibiotics used in rations at very low levels for promotion of growth, according to the experiments of Dorsey and Harshfield (32), did not significantly influence the course of FC infection in inoculated birds. At therapeutic levels, birds that received penicillin and streptomycin in feed died at about the same rate as controls. No deaths occurred in groups that received sulfaquinoxaline or sulfamerazine. These workers found oxytetracycline and chlortetracycline effective also in preventing mortality in experimental FC in a small flock of laying birds; mortality was 80% in an untreated group compared to 12% in a group receiving mash containing oxytetracycline at the level of 500 g/ton. In six natural outbreaks, oxytetracycline at this level in feed checked mortality, but losses returned in three flocks after withdrawal of the antibiotic.

PREVENTION AND CONTROL

Management Procedures. Prevention of FC can be effected by eliminating reservoirs of *P. multocida* or by preventing their access to poultry flocks. Good management practices, with emphasis on sanitation (see Chapter 1), are the best means of preventing FC. Unlike many bacterial diseases, FC is not a disease of the hatchery. Infection therefore occurs after birds are in the hands of the producer, and consideration must be given to the many ways that infection might be introduced into a flock.

The primary source of infection is usually sick birds or those that have recovered and still carry the causative organism. Only young birds should be introduced as new stock; they should be raised in a clean environment completely isolated from other birds. Isolation should be extended to housing. Unless separate houses can be provided for first- and second-year layer flocks, the older flock should be marketed in its entirety. Different species of birds should not be raised on the same premises. The danger of mixing birds from different flocks cannot be overemphasized. Farm animals (particularly pigs, dogs, and cats) should not have access to the poultry area. Water fountains should be self-cleaning and feeders covered to prevent contamination as much as possible.

The fact that *P. multocida* has been recovered from many species of free-flying birds warrants consideration of this source of infection to poultry, with measures taken to prevent their association with the flock. Raising turkeys in areas where FC is a serious problem may warrant their confinement in houses where free-flying birds, rodents, and other animals can be excluded. If an outbreak of FC occurs, the flock should be quarantined and disposed of as soon as economically feasible. All housing and equipment should be cleaned and disinfected before repopulation.

Immunization. Vaccination should be considered in areas where FC is prevalent, but it should not be substituted for good sanitary practice. Commercially produced bacterins and live vaccines are available.

REFERENCES

1. Alberts, J.O. 1950. The prophylactic and therapeutic properties of sulfamerazine in fowl cholera. Am J Vet Res 11:414–420.
2. Alberts, J.O., and R. Graham. 1948. Fowl cholera in turkeys. North Am Vet 29:24–26.
3. Alberts, J.O., and R. Graham. 1948. Sulfamerazine in the treatment of fowl cholera in turkeys. Am J Vet Res 9:310–313.
4. Alberts, J.O., and R. Graham. 1951. An observation on aureomycin therapy of fowl cholera in pheasants. Vet Med 46:505–506.
5. Anderson, L.A.P., M.G. Coombes, and S.M.K. Mallick. 1929. On the dissociation of Bacillus avisepticus. Indian J Med Res 29:611–622.
6. Anderson, N.G., W.C. Alpaugh, and C.O. Baughn. 1974. Effect of sulfachloropyrazine in the drinking water of chickens infected experimentally with fowl cholera. Avian Dis 18:410–415.
7. Anonymous. 1867. Poultry Diseases, USDA Monthly Rep, pp. 216–217.
8. Arsov, R. 1965. The portal of infection in fowl cholera. Nauchni Tr Vissh Vet Med Inst 14:13–17.
9. Baba, T., and Y. Bito. 1966. Studies on the toxin of Pasteurella multocida. Jpn J Bacteriol 21:711–714.
10. Bairey, M.H. 1975. Immune response to fowl cholera antigens. Am J Vet Res 36:575–578.
11. Berkman, S. 1942. Accessory growth factor requirements of the members of the genus Pasteurella. J Infect Dis 71:201–211.
12. Bierer, B.W. 1962. Treatment of avian pasteurellosis with injectable antibiotics. J Am Vet Med Assoc 141:1344–1346.
13. Bierer, B.W., and W.T. Derieux. 1972. Immunologic response of turkeys to an avirulent Pasteurella multocida vaccine in the drinking water. Poult Sci 51:408–416.
14. Bolin, F.M., and D.F. Eveleth. 1951. The use of biological products in experimental fowl cholera. Proc 88th Annu Meet Am Vet Med Assoc, pp. 110–112.
15. Breed, R.S., E.G.D. Murray, and N.R. Smith. 1957. Bergey's Manual of Determinative Bacteriology, 7th Ed. Williams & Wilkins, Baltimore, MD.
16. Brogden, K.A., and R.A. Packer. 1979. Comparison of Pasteurella multocida serotyping systems. Am J Vet Res 40:1332–1335.
17. Brogden, K.A., K.R. Rhoades, and K.L. Heddleston. 1978. A new serotype of Pasteurella multocida associated with fowl cholera. Avian Dis 22:185–190.
18. Buchanan, R.E., J.G. Holt, and E.F. Lessel. 1966. Index Bergeyana. Williams & Wilkins, Baltimore, MD.
19. Carter, G.R. 1955. Studies on Pasteurella multocida. I. A hemagglutination test for the identification of serological types. Am J Vet Res 16:481–484.
20. Clark, D.S., and J.F. Godfrey. 1960. Atypical Pasteurella infections in chickens. Avian Dis 4:280–290.
21. Curtice, C. 1902. Goose septicemia. Univ Rhode Island Agric Exp Stn Bull 86:191–203.
22. Das, M.S. 1958. Studies on Pasteurella septica (Pasteurella multocida). Observations on some biophysical characteristics. J Comp Pathol Ther 68:288–294.
23. de Jong, M.F., and G.H.A. Borst. 1985. Selective media for the isolation of P. multocida and B. bronchiseptica. Vet Rec 116:167.

24. Delaplane, J.P. 1945. Sulfaquinoxaline in preventing upper respiratory infection of chickens inoculated with infective field material containing Pasteurella avicida. Am J Vet Res 6:207-208.
25. Derieux, W.T. 1978. Responses of young chickens and turkeys to virulent and avirulent Pasteurella multocida administered by various routes. Avian Dis 22:131-139.
26. Derieux, W.T., and B.W. Bierer. 1975. The CU strain of Pasteurella multocida. Proc 24th West Poult Dis Conf, pp. 64-66.
27. DeVolt, H.M., and C.R. Davis. 1932. A cholera-like disease in turkeys. Cornell Vet 22:78-80.
28. Dimov, I. 1964. Survival of avian Pasteurella multocida in soils at different acidity, humidity, and temperature. Nauchni Tr Vissh Vet Med Inst Sofia 12:339-345.
29. Donahue, J.M., and L.O. Olson. 1972. Biochemic study of Pasteurella multocida from turkeys. Avian Dis 16:501-505.
30. Donahue, J.M., and L.O. Olson. 1972. The in vitro sensitivity of Pasteurella multocida of turkey origin to various chemotherapeutic agents. Avian Dis 16:506-511.
31. Dorsey, T.A. 1963. Studies on fowl cholera. I. A biochemic study of avian Pasteurella multocida strains. Avian Dis 7:386-392.
32. Dorsey, T.A., and G.S. Harshfield. 1959. Studies on control of fowl cholera. South Dakota State Univ Agric Exp Stn Bull 23:1-18.
33. Dougherty, E. 1953. Disease problems confronting the duck industry. Proc 90th Annu Meet Am Vet Med Assoc, pp 359-365.
34. Faddoul, G.P., G.W. Fellows, and J. Baird. 1967. Pasteurellosis in wild birds in Massachusetts. Avian Dis 11:413-418.
35. Fenstermacher, R., and B.S. Pomeroy. 1941. Encephalitislike symptoms in turkeys associated with a Pasteurella sp. Cornell Vet 31:295-301.
36. Flossmann, K.D., H. Feist, M. Hofer, and W. Erler. 1974. Untersuchungen uber chemisch definierte nahrmedien fur Pasteurella multocida und P. haemolytica. Z Allg Mikrobiol 14:29-38.
37. Gadberry, J.L., and N.G. Miller. 1977. Use of bacteriophages as an adjunct in the identification of Pasteurella multocida. Am J Vet Res 38:129-130.
38. Garlinghouse, L.E., R.F. DiGiacomo, G.L. Van Hoosier, and J. Condon. 1971. Selective media for Pasteurella multocida and Bordetella bronchiseptica. J Lab Anim Sci 31:39-42.
39. Gershman, M., J.F. Witter, H.E. Spencer, and A. Kalvaitis. 1964. Epizootic of fowl cholera in the common eider duck. J Wildl Manage 28:587-589.
40. Gilchrist, P. 1963. A survey of avian respiratory disease. Aust Vet J 39:140-144.
41. Glorioso, J.C., G.W. Jones, H.G. Rush, L.J. Pentler, C.A. Darif, and J.E. Coward. 1982. Adhesion of type A Pasteurella multocida to rabbit pharyngeal cells and its possible role in rabbit respiratory tract infection. Infect Immun 35:1103-1109.
42. Grant, G., A.M. Russell, and D.McK. Fraser. 1968. Treatment of fowl cholera. Vet Rec 83:419.
43. Gray, H. 1913. Some diseases of birds. In E.W. Hoare (ed.), A System of Veterinary Medicine, Vol. 1, pp. 420-432. Alexander Eger, Chicago.
44. Gregg, D.A., L.O. Olson, and E.L. McCune. 1974. Experimental transmission of Pasteurella multocida from raccoons to turkeys via bite wounds. Avian Dis 18:559-564.
45. Hacking, W.C., and J.R. Pettit. 1974. Pasteurella hemolytica in pullets and laying hens. Avian Dis 18:483-486.
46. Hall, W.J., K.L. Heddleston, D.H. Legenhausen, and R.W. Hughes. 1955. Studies on pasteurellosis. I. A new species of Pasteurella encountered in chronic fowl cholera. Am J Vet Res 16:598-604.
47. Hamdy, A.H., and C.J. Blanchard. 1970. Effect of novobiocin on fowl cholera in turkeys. Avian Dis 14:770-778.
48. Harbourne, J.F. 1962. A hemolytic coccobacillus recovered from poultry. Vet Rec 74:566-567.
49. Hart, L. 1963. Treatment of duck cholera with erythromycin. Aust Vet J 39:92-93.
50. Heddleston, K.L. 1962. Studies on pasteurellosis. V. Two immunogenic types of Pasteurella multocida associated with fowl cholera. Avian Dis 6:315-321.
51. Heddleston, K.L. 1970. Personal communication.
52. Heddleston, K.L. 1972. Avian Pasteurellosis. In M.S. Hofstad, B.W. Calnek, C.F. Helmboldt, W.M. Reid, and H.W. Yoder, Jr. (eds.), Diseases of Poultry, 6th Ed., pp. 219-241. Iowa State Univ Press, Ames.
53. Heddleston, K.L. 1975. Pasteurellosis. In S.B. Hitchner, C.H. Domermuth, H.G. Purchase, and J.E. Williams (eds.), Isolation and Identification of Avian Pathogens, pp. 38-51. Am Assoc Avian Pathol, Kennett Square, PA.
54. Heddleston, K.L., and P.A. Rebers. 1972. Fowl cholera: Cross-immunity induced in turkeys with formalin-killed in-vivo-propagated Pasteurella multocida. Avian Dis 16:578-586.
55. Heddleston, K.L., and P.A. Rebers. 1975. Properties of free endotoxin from Pasteurella multocida. Am J Vet Res 36:573-574.
56. Heddleston, K.L., and R.C. Reisinger. 1960. Studies on pasteurellosis. IV. Killed fowl cholera vaccine adsorbed on aluminum hydroxide. Avian Dis 4:429-435.
57. Heddleston, K.L., and L.P. Watko. 1963. Fowl cholera: Susceptibility of various animals and their potential as disseminators of disease. Proc 67th Annu Meet US Livest Sanit Assoc, pp. 247-251.
58. Heddleston, K.L., and G. Wessman. 1975. Characteristics of Pasteurella multocida of human origin. J Clin Microbiol 1:377-383.
59. Heddleston, K.L., L.P. Watko, and P.A. Rebers. 1964. Dissociation of a fowl cholera strain of Pasteurella multocida. Avian Dis 8:649-657.
60. Heddleston, K.L., J.E. Gallagher, and P.A. Rebers. 1970. Fowl cholera: Immune responses in turkeys. Avian Dis 14:626-635.
61. Heddleston, K.L., J.E. Gallagher, and P.A. Rebers. 1972. Fowl cholera: Gel diffusion precipitin test for serotyping Pasteurella multocida from avian species. Avian Dis 16:925-936.
62. Heddleston, K.L., P.A. Rebers, and G. Wessman. 1975. Fowl cholera: Immunologic and serologic response in turkeys to live Pasteurella multocida vaccine administered in the drinking water. Poult Sci 54:217-221.
63. Hendrickson, J.M., and K.F. Hilbert. 1932. The persistence of P. avium in the blood and organs of fowls with spontaneous fowl cholera. J Infect Dis 50:89-97.
64. Henry, B.S. 1933. Dissociation in the genus Brucella. J Infect Dis 52:374-402.
65. Horvath, Z., M. Padanyi, and Z. Palatka. 1962. Chloramphenicol in the treatment of fowl cholera. Magy Allatory Lapja 17:332-336.
66. Hughes, T.P. 1930. The epidemiology of fowl cholera. II. Biological properties of P. avicida. J Exp Med 51:225-238.
67. Hughes, T.P., and I.W. Pritchett. 1930. The epidemiology of fowl cholera. III. Portal of entry of P. avicida; reaction of the host. J Exp Med 51:239-248.
68. Hungerford, T.G. 1968. A clinical note on avian cholera. The effect of age on the susceptibility of fowls.

Aust Vet J 44:31-32.

69. Hunter, B., and G. Wobeser. 1980. Pathology of experimental avian cholera in mallard ducks. Avian Dis 24:403-414.

70. Iliev, T., R. Arsov, I. Dimov, G. Girginov, and E. Iovcev. 1963. Swine, cattle, and sheep as carriers and latent sources of pasteurella infection for fowl. Nauchni Tr Vissh Vet Med Inst Sofia 11:281-288.

71. Iliev, T., R. Arsov, E. Iovcev, and G. Girginov. 1963. Role of swine in the epidemiology of fowl cholera. Nauchni Tr Vissh Vet Med Inst Sofia 11:289-293.

72. Iliev, T., R. Arsov, and V. Lazarov. 1965. Can fowls, carriers of Pasteurella, excrete the organism in faeces? Nauchni Tr Vissh Vet Med Inst 14:7-12.

73. Iovcev, E. 1967. The role of Argas persicus in the epidemiology of fowl cholera. Angew Parasitol 8:114-117.

74. Jaksic, B.L., M. Dordevic, and B. Markovic. 1964. Fowl cholera in wild birds. Vet Glasnik 18:725-730.

75. Jensen, W.I., and C.S. Williams. 1964. Botulism and fowl cholera. In J. P. Linduska (ed.), Waterfowl Tomorrow, pp. 333-341. US Government Printing Office, Washington, D.C.

76. Jordan, R.M.M. 1952. The nutrition of Pasteurella septica. II. The formation of hydrogen peroxide in a chemically-defined medium. Br J Exp Pathol 33:36-45.

77. Juszkiewicz, T. 1966. Hyperthermia and prednisolone acetate as provocative factors of Pasteurella multocida infection in chickens. Pol Arch Weter 10:141-151.

78. Juszkiewicz, T. 1966. Effects of shaking and premedication with methylprednisolone on some biochemical indices associated with Pasteurella multocida infection of cockerels. Pol Arch Weter 10:129-140.

79. Karaivanov, L., and O. Mraz. 1973. Use of phagodiagnostics in Pasteurella multocida. Acta Vet (Brno) 42:195-200.

80. Kirchner, C., and A. Eisenstark. 1956. Lysogeny in Pasteurella multocida. Am J Vet Res 17:547-548.

81. Kiser, J.S., J. Prier, C.A. Bottorff, and L.M. Greene. 1948. Treatment of experimental and naturally occurring fowl cholera with sulfamethazine. Poult Sci 27:257-262.

82. Knight, D.P., J.E. Paine, and D.C.E. Speller. 1983. A selective medium for Pasteurella multocida and its use with animal and human species. J Clin Pathol 36:591-594.

83. Kyaw, M.H. 1944. Pathogenesis of Pasteurella septica infection in developing chick embryo. J Comp Pathol 54:200-206.

84. Little, P.A. 1948. Use of Aureomycin in some experimental infections in animals. Ann NY Acad Sci 51:246-253.

85. Maheswaran, S.K., J.R. McDowell, and B.S. Pomeroy. 1973. Studies on Pasteurella multocida. I. Efficacy of an avirulent mutant as a live vaccine in turkeys. Avian Dis 17:396-405.

86. Manninger, R. 1919. Concerning a mutation of the fowl cholera bacillus. Zentralbl Bakteriol Abt I Orig 83:520-528.

87. Marshall, J.D. 1963. The use of immunofluorescence for the identification of members of the genus Pasteurella in chemically fixed tissues. PhD diss, Univ Maryland.

88. Matthes, S., H. Loliger, and H.J. Schubert. 1969. Enzootisches Auftreten der Pasteurella hemolytica beim Huhn. Dtsch Tieraerztl Wochenschr 76:94-95.

89. McNeil, E., and W.R. Hinshaw. 1948. The effect of streptomycin on Pasteurella multocida in vitro, and on fowl cholera in turkeys. Cornell Vet 38:239-246.

90. Mitrovic, M. 1967. Chemotherapeutic efficacy of sulfadimethoxine against fowl cholera and infectious coryza. Poult Sci 46:1153-1158.

91. Mitrovic, M., and J.C. Bauernfeind. 1971. Efficacy of sulfadimethoxine in turkey diseases. Avian Dis 15:884-893.

92. Mitrovic, M., G. Fusiek, and E.G. Schildknecht. 1969. Antibacterial activity of sulfadimethoxine potentiated mixture (Ro 5-0013) in chickens. Poult Sci 48:1151-1155.

93. Mitrovic, M., G. Fusiek, and E.G. Schildknecht. 1971. Antibacterial activity of sulfadimethoxine potentiated mixture (Rolfenaid) in turkeys. Poult Sci 50:525-529.

94. Morris, E.J. 1958. Selective media for some Pasteurella species. J Gen Microbiol 19:305-311.

95. Murata, M., T. Horiuchi, and S. Namioka. 1964. Studies on the pathogenicity of Pasteurella multocida for mice and chickens on the basis of O-groups. Cornell Vet 54:293-307.

96. Namioka, S., and M. Murata. 1961. Serological studies on Pasteurella multocida. II. Characteristics of somatic (O) antigen of the organism. Cornell Vet 51:507-521.

97. Nelson, C.L. 1955. The veterinarian in poultry practice. Proc 92nd Annu Meet Am Vet Med Assoc, pp. 306-310.

98. Nicolet, J., and H. Fey. 1965. Role of Pasteurella haemolytica in salpingitis of fowls. Schweiz Arch Tierheilkd 107:329-334.

99. Nielsen, J.P., Bisgaard, M., and K.B. Pedersen. 1986. Production of toxin in strains previously classified as Pasteurella multocida. Acta Path Microbiol Immunol Scand [Sect B] 94:203-204.

100. Nobrega, R., and R.C. Bueno. 1950. The influence of the temperature on the viability and virulence of Pasteurella avicida. Bol Soc Paulista Med Vet 8:189-194.

101. Olson, L.D. 1966. Gross and histopathological description of the cranial form of chronic fowl cholera in turkeys. Avian Dis 10:518-529.

102. Olson, L.D., and E.L. McCune. 1968. Experimental production of the cranial form of fowl cholera in turkeys. Am J Vet Res 29:1665-1673.

103. Pabs-Garnon, L.F., and M.A. Soltys. 1971. Methods of transmission of fowl cholera in turkeys. Am J Vet Res 32:1119-1120.

104. Park, P.Y. 1982. Disseminated intravascular coagulation in experimental fowl cholera of chickens. Korean J Vet Res 22:211-219.

105. Pasteur, L. 1880. Sur les maladies virulents et en particulier sur la maladie appelee vulgairement cholera des poules. CR Acad Sci 90:239-248, 1030-1033.

106. Pasteur, L. 1880. De l'attenuation du virus du cholera des poules. CR Acad Sci 91:673-680.

107. Pasteur, L. 1881. Sur les virus-vaccins du cholera des poules et du charbon. CR Travaux Congr Int Dir Stn Agron Sess Versailles, pp. 151-162.

108. Peterson, E.H. 1948. Sulfonamides in the prophylaxis of experimental fowl cholera. J Am Vet Med Assoc 113:263-266.

109. Petrov, D. 1975. Studies on the gamasid red mite of poultry, Dermanyssus gallinae, as a carrier of Pasteurella multocida. Vet Med Nauk (Bulg) 12:32-36.

110. Pier, A.C., K.L. Heddleston, S.J. Cysewski, and J.M. Patterson. 1972. Effect of aflatoxin on immunity in turkeys. II. Reversal of impaired resistance to bacterial infection by passive transfer of plasma. Avian Dis 16:381-87.

111. Pirosky, I. 1938. Sur l'antigen glucidolipidique des Pasteurella. CR Soc Biol 127:98-100.

112. Pritchett, I.W., and T.P. Hughes. 1932. The epidemiology of fowl cholera. VI. The spread of epidemic and endemic strains of Pasteurella avicida in laboratory

populations of normal fowl. J Exp Med 55:71–78.

113. Pritchett, I.W., F.R. Beaudette, and T.P. Hughes. 1930. The epidemiology of fowl cholera. IV. Field observations of the "spontaneous" disease. J Exp Med 51:249–258.

114. Pritchett, I.W., F.R. Beaudette, and T.P. Hughes. 1930. The epidemiology of fowl cholera. V. Further field observations of the spontaneous disease. J Exp Med 51:259–274.

115. Rebers, P.A., A.E. Jensen, and G.A. Laird. 1988. Expression of pili and capsule by the avian strain P-1059 of Pasteurella multocida. Avian Dis 32:313–318.

116. Reis, J. 1941. On the presence of Pasteurella avicida in feces of infected birds. Arq Inst Biol (Sao Paulo) 12:307–309.

117. Rhoades, K.R. 1964. The microscopic lesions of acute fowl cholera in mature chickens. Avian Dis 8:658–665.

118. Rhoades, K.R., and R.B. Rimler. 1987. Capsular groups of Pasteurella multocida isolated from avian hosts. Avian Dis 31:895–898.

119. Rhoades, K.R., and R.B. Rimler. 1987. Effects of Pasteurella multocida endotoxins on turkey poults. Avian Dis 31:523–526.

120. Rhoades, K.R., and R.B. Rimler. 1988. Toxicity and virulence of capsular serogroup D Pasteurella multocida strains isolated from turkeys. J Am Med Assoc 192:1790.

121. Rhoades, K.R., and R.B. Rimler. 1988. Unpublished data.

122. Rifkind, D., and M.J. Pickett. 1954. Bacteriophage studies on the hemorrhagic septicemia Pasteurellae. J Bacteriol 67:243–246.

123. Rimler, R.B. 1984. Comparisons of serologic responses of white leghorn and New Hampshire red chickens to purified lipopolysaccharides of Pasteurella multocida. Avian Dis 28:984–989.

124. Rimler, R.B. 1987. Cross-protection factor(s) of Pasteurella multocida: Passive immunization of turkeys against fowl cholera caused by different serotypes. Avian Dis 31:884–887.

125. Rimler, R.B., and M. Phillips. 1986. Fowl cholera: Protection against Pasteurella multocida by ribosome-lipopolysaccharide vaccine. Avian Dis 30:409–415.

126. Rimler, R.B., and K.R. Rhoades. 1987. Serogroup F, a new capsule serogroup of Pasteurella multocida. J Clin Microbiol 25:615–618.

127. Rimler, R.B., P.A. Rebers, and M. Phillips. 1984. Lipopolysaccharides of the Heddleston serotypes of Pasteurella multocida. Am J Vet Res 45:759–763.

128. Rosen, M. 1971. Avian Cholera. In J.W. Davis, L.H. Karstad, D.O. Trainer, and R.C. Anderson (eds.), Infectious and Parasitic Diseases of Wild Birds, pp. 59–74. Iowa State Univ Press, Ames.

129. Rosen, M.N., and A.I. Bischoff. 1949. The 1948–49 outbreak of fowl cholera in birds in the San Francisco Bay area and surrounding counties. Calif Fish Game 35:185–192.

130. Rosenbusch, C., and I.A. Merchant. 1939. A study of the hemorrhagic septicemia Pasteurellae. J Bacteriol 37:69–89.

131. Ryu, E. 1961. Studies on Pasteurella multocida. VI. The relationship between inhibitory action of blood and susceptibility of animals to Past. multocida. Jpn J Vet Sci 23:357–361.

132. Salmon, D.E. 1880. Investigations of fowl cholera. Rep US Comm Agric, pp. 401–445.

133. Saxena, S.P., and A.B. Hoerlein. 1959. Lysogeny in Pasteurella. I. Isolation of bacteriophages from Pasteurella strains isolated from shipping fever and those from other infectious processes. J Vet Anim Husb 3:53–66.

134. Serdyuk, H.G., and P.F. Tsimokh. 1970. Role of free-living birds and rodents in the distribution of pasteurellosis. Veterinariia 6:53–54.

135. Simms, B.T. 1951. Rep Chief Bur Anim Indust, USDA, p. 44–45.

136. Skidmore, L.V. 1932. The transmission of fowl cholera to turkeys by the common house fly (Musca domestics Linn) with brief notes on the viability of fowl cholera microorganisms. Cornell Vet 22:281–285.

137. Smith, I.M., and A.J. Baskerville. 1983. A selective medium for isolation of P. multocida in nasal specimens from pigs. Br Vet J 139:476–486.

138. Stuart, E.E., R.D. Keenum, and H.W. Bruins. 1966. Efficacy of sulfaethoxypyridazine against fowl cholera in artificially infected chickens and turkeys, and its safety in laying chickens and broilers. Avian Dis 10:135–145.

139. Van Es, L., and J.F. Olney. 1940. An inquiry into the influence of environment on the incidence of poultry diseases. Univ Nebraska Agric Exp Stn Res Bull 118, pp. 17–21.

140. Vaught, R.W., H.C. McDougle, and H.H. Burgess. 1967. Fowl cholera in waterfowl at Squaw Creek National Wildlife Refuge, Missouri. J Wildl Manage 31:248–253.

141. Walser, M.M., and R.B. Davis. 1975. In vitro characterization of field isolates of Pasteurella multocida from Georgia turkeys. Avian Dis 19:525–532.

142. Watko, L.P. 1966. A chemically defined medium for growth of Pasteurella multocida. Can J Microbiol 12:933–937.

143. Watko, L.P., and K.L. Heddleston. 1966. Survival of shell-frozen, freeze-dried, and agar slant cultures of Pasteurella multocida. Cryobiology 3:53–55.

144. Wessman, G.E., and G. Wessman. 1970. Chemically defined media for Pasteurella multocida and Pasteurella ureae, and a comparison of their thiamine requirements with those of Pasteurella haemolytica. Can J Microbiol 16:751–757.

145. Wilson, G.S., and A.A. Miles. 1964. Topley and Wilson's Principles of Bacteriology and Immunity. Williams & Wilkins, Baltimore, MD.

146. Yaw, K.E., and J.C. Kakavas. 1957. A comparison of the protection-inducing factors in chickens and mice of a type 1 strain of Pasteurella multocida. Am J Vet Res 18:661–664.

PSEUDOTUBERCULOSIS

K.R. Rhoades and R.B. Rimler

INTRODUCTION. Avian pseudotuberculosis (AP) is a contagious disease of domesticated and wild birds. It is characterized by an acute septicemia of short duration, followed by chronic focal infections that result in caseous nodules resembling the tubercules of tuberculosis. Research on this disease has been limited, and most publications on this disease are case reports.

HISTORY AND DISTRIBUTION. The causative agent, *Yersinia (Pasteurella) pseudotuberculosis,* was first isolated from a guinea pig inoculated with material from a subcutaneous tubercular lesion on the forearm of a child (13). Since then the organism has been isolated from many species of mammals and birds. In describing a case of AP in a blackbird, Beaudette (2) gave an extensive review of the disease in birds. He credited Riech in 1889 and Kinyoun in 1906 with making the first isolation from birds in Europe and the USA respectively.

AP has been reported in many countries and probably occurs throughout the world. It occurs sporadically in domestic poultry and occasionally causes severe losses in turkeys. However, because of minor economic importance, it has received little research attention.

ETIOLOGY

Classification. The bacterium, *Y. pseudotuberculosis,* has been given many names (3, 16): *Bacillus pseudotuberculosis,* 1889; *Bacterium pseudotuberculosis,* 1900; *Streptobacillus pseudotuberculosis-rodentium,* 1894; *Bacterium pseudotuberculosis-rodentium,* 1896; *Corynebacterium pseudotuberculosis,* 1925; *Pasteurella pseudotuberculosis,* 1929; *C. rodentium,* 1932; *C. pseudotuberculosis-rodentium,* 1933; *Malleomyces pseudotuberculosis-rodentium,* 1933; *Shigella pseudotuberculosis,* 1935; *Y. rodentium,* 1944; *P. rodentium,* 1944; *P. pseudotuberculosis-rodentium,* 1947; *Cillopasteurella pseudotuberculosis-rodentium,* 1953; and *Y. pseudotuberculosis,* 1974.

Morphology and Staining. *Y. pseudotuberculosis* is a gram-negative rod, 0.5 × 0.8–5.0 μm. Coccoid and long filamentous forms also occur. The coccoid forms usually show some bipolar staining. According to Cook (7) it is slightly acid-fast, which can be demonstrated in imprint smears using a modified Ziehl-Nielsen staining method. Neither spores nor visible capsules are formed, although at 22 C an envelope may be seen in India ink preparations. Single rods occasionally show peritrichous flagellae, which develop at temperatures between 20 and 30 C.

Growth Requirements and Colonial Morphology. *Y. pseudotuberculosis* grows in the presence or absence of oxygen; optimal temperature is 30 C. Burrows and Gillett (4) studied seven strains of various serotypes and observed that some grown at 28 C required thiamine or pantothenate. At 37 C most strains could grow with the addition of any three of four factors–glutamic acid, thiamine, cystine, and pantothenate; other strains required all four factors and nicotinamide.

Good growth occurs in peptone broth. Growth at 22 C is diffuse, with some clumped masses and occasionally ring and pellicle formation. Cultivation at 37 C, especially in acid media, accelerates dissociation. On peptone or infusion agar media it forms colonies that are smooth to slimy, granular, translucent, grayish yellow, butyrous, and 0.5–1 mm in diameter. On agar medium containing blood, colonies grow to 2–3 mm in diameter by the 2nd day. At 37 C colonies are thin, dry, and irregular, with rough edges. Growth occurs on MacConkey's agar. *Y. pseudotuberculosis* is motile at 25 C but not at 37 C. Motility is best demonstrated in semisolid medium.

Physiologic Properties. *Y. pseudotuberculosis* metabolizes many compounds without producing gas. The following properties are characteristic of *Y. pseudotuberculosis:*

Arabinose	fermented
Dextrin	fermented
Fructose	fermented
Glucose	fermented
Glycerol	fermented
Maltose	fermented
Mannitol	fermented
Mannose	fermented
Melibiose	fermented
Rhamnose	fermented
Trehalose	fermented
Xylose	usually fermented
Salicin	usually fermented
Sucrose	not fermented
Dulcitol	not fermented
Inositol	not fermented
Lactose	not fermented
Raffinose	not fermented
Sorbitol	not fermented
Urease	produced
Catalase	produced
Ammonia	produced
Hydrogen sulfide	usually not produced
Nitrates	reduced
Methylene blue	reduced
Blood	not hemolyzed
Indole	not produced

Gelatin	not liquified
MacConkey's agar	usually growth

Differential characteristics are presented in Table 5.3.

Resistance to Chemical and Physical Agents. *Y. pseudotuberculosis* is easily destroyed by sunlight, drying, heat, or ordinary disinfectants. It remains viable for years on sealed agar slants or when lyophilized.

Antigenic Structure. Somatic and flagellar antigens are used to characterize strains of *Y. pseudotuberculosis.* Fifteen somatic antigens are demonstrable by agglutination and agglutination-adsorption serologic tests. These heat-stable somatic antigens are used to differentiate 6 serotypes; 4 of which have 2 subtypes each (16). Five heat-labile flagellar antigens are recognized, but are infrequently used for antigenic characterization. Antigens and serotypes are indicated in Table 5.4.

Additional serotypes VII and VIII, and an additional subtype, IIC, have been proposed (21). Among strains isolated from birds, serotype I is most common, followed by II and IV. Serotype III is rare and V and VI have not been reported from birds (19).

Thal (20) studied 186 strains of *Y. pseudotuberculosis;* of these, 33 were isolated from eight species of birds. All were biochemically identical; there were five serologically distinct groups. Most strains in group III produced thermolabile exotoxins that were convertible to toxoids. Experimentally, antiinfection immunity was produced with live avirulent strains, thus protecting against infection with atoxic strains and subtoxic culture doses of toxic strains. Antitoxic immunity protected against toxin and to a degree against infection with toxic strains, but not against infection with atoxic strains.

Mair (12) studied the type distribution of *Y. pseudotuberculosis* in Great Britain during 1961–64; 177 strains were isolated from 39 different species of mammals and birds. Sixty-five isolates were from 26 species of birds; 39 of these were type IA, 16 type IB, 6 type IIA, 2 type IIB, and 2 type IV. Of 17 isolates from turkeys, 9 were type IA and 8 were type IB. In studies of 22 strains isolated from birds in New Zealand, 7 were serotype I and 15 were serotype II (9).

Table 5.4. Serotypes and antigens of *Y. pseudotuberculosis*

Serotype	Subtype	O antigens	H antigens
I	A	1, 2, 3	a, c
	B	1, 2, 4	a, c
II	A	1, 5, 6	a, d
	B	1, 5, 7	a, d
III	-	1, 8	a
IV	A	1, 9, 11	a, b; b
	B	1, 9, 12	a, b, d
V	A	1, 10, 14	a; a, b, e
	B	1, 10, 15	a
VI	-	1, 13	a

PATHOGENESIS AND EPIZOOTIOLOGY

Natural and Experimental Hosts. AP has been reported in turkeys, ducks, geese, chickens, guinea fowl, companion birds, and wild birds. It has also been reported in many species of mammals. Of the laboratory animals, guinea pigs, rabbits, mice, monkeys, and baboons are quite susceptible; white rats and hamsters are refractory. Ground squirrels can become infected and may play a role in transmission to turkeys (22).

AP occurs occasionally in turkeys; losses have been as high as 80% (1, 10,15, 18, 22, 23).

AP among stock doves in Hampshire, England, was observed by Clapham (5). In a search for the source of infection, *Y. pseudotuberculosis* was isolated from a lark, wood pigeon, jackdaw, rook, and hare. This author also isolated the organism from gray partridge, pheasants, and bobwhite quail. Outbreaks in Denmark affected pigeons, canaries, snow buntings, waxwings, and a turkey (14). An epornitic of AP in common grackles (*Quiscalus quiscula*) occurred at a major winter roost in Maryland (6). Mortality and morbidity were extensive and continued for several weeks until spring roost breakup. Occurrence of extensive infection in a large migratory bird population has major epizootiologic significance.

Transmission, Pathogenesis, Incubation Period. Body excretions of diseased birds or mammals may contaminate soil, food, or water and are important factors in dissemination of AP. Predisposing causes are apparently important; as a rule, the only birds affected are those whose resistance has been lowered by inadequate feeding, exposure to cold, or worm infection. Very young birds are particularly susceptible. During cold and wet

Table 5.3. Differential characteristics of *Y. pseudotuberculosis, Y. pestis,* and *Y. enterocolitica*

	Yersinia		
Test	*pseudotuberculosis*	*pestis*	*enterocolitica*
Urease	+	–	+
Ornithine decarboxylase	–	–	+
Adonitol	+	–	–
Cellobiose	–	–	+
Motility at 22 C	+	–	+

weather in the fall, considerable losses may occur among young turkeys. In susceptible birds the organism gains entrance to the bloodstream through breaks in the skin or through the mucous membranes, perhaps mostly in the digestive tract. Thus a bacteremia is established. Usually the bacteremic condition is of short duration, but the bacteria are not all destroyed. Some establish foci of infection in one or more organs such as liver, spleen, lungs, or intestines, giving rise to tubercularlike lesions. Such lesions have also been found in the mesentery and breast muscles.

The incubation period of artificial infection varies considerably and depends on the virulence of the organism, amount of inoculum, avenue of introduction, and host species. Sparrows and canaries were very susceptible and may die in 1–3 days from small doses of organisms injected subcutaneously, intramuscularly, or intraperitoneally. Feeding of cultures is usually ineffective unless some intestinal inflammation is present to act as a predisposing influence. Canaries fed mustard seed to cause intestinal irritation sickened 5 days after being given cultures by mouth; death resulted 2 days later. Judging from various reports, the incubation period may vary from 3 to 6 days in acute attacks and 2 wk or more in chronic cases.

Signs. Signs vary considerably. In very acute cases birds may die suddenly without warning or may live a few hours or days after showing the first signs. Such cases are usually marked by sudden appearance of diarrhea and manifestations of acute septicemia. More often, however, the course of this disease extends over 2 or more wk, in which case the signs appear 2–4 days before death. In such cases birds will show weakness, dull and ruffled feathers, and difficult breathing. Diarrhea is also a common sign. Occasionally, the disease will run a more protracted course, and emaciation and extreme weakness or paralysis may be evident. Such manifestations as stiffness, difficulty in walking, droopiness, somnolence, constipation, and discoloration of the skin have also been observed. In early stages of the chronic form of the disease, birds may eat normally, but the appetite is usually completely lost 1 or 2 days before death.

Lesions. When deaths occur early in the septicemic stage of the disease, enteritis and enlarged livers and spleens may be the only lesions. Later, miliary necrotic foci become evident in visceral organs, particularly livers and spleens, and in muscle. Enteritis, varying in severity from catarrhal to hemorrhagic, is common. Serous cavities sometimes contain an increased amount of fluid. Osteomyelitis sometimes occurs in affected turkey flocks (22, 23), causing caseous necrotic foci near the growth plates of long bones in some cases (22). Degenerative myopathy has also been observed in affected turkey flocks with locomotor difficulties (8).

DIAGNOSIS.

A definitive diagnosis can be established only by isolation and identification of the organism, since the signs and lesions are very similar to those of several other diseases such as fowl cholera, fowl typhoid, paratyphoid, spirochetosis, tuberculosis, and certain neoplastic diseases.

Isolation and Identification. Primary isolation is made by streaking specimens from affected tissues on blood or trypticase soy agar or by inoculating trypticase soy broth, followed by streaking onto agar after 3–5 hr incubation at 37 C. The medium of Patterson and Cook (17) is recommended for isolation of *Y. pseudotuberculosis* from feces. The surface of the agar is inoculated by streaking a suspension of 10% feces in phosphate buffer (pH 7.6) and incubating at 37 C for 24–48 hr. Identification is based primarily on physiologic characteristics as described in the section on physiologic properties.

Differential Diagnosis. The bacterium *Y. pseudotuberculosis* is quite similar in many respects to *Y. pestis* and *Y. enterocolitica.* Although these two organisms are not likely to be encountered in poultry, they may be carried by rodents having access to the poultry area. A summary of differential tests of *Y. pseudotuberculosis, Y. pestis,* and *Y. enterocolitica* is listed in Table 5.3.

An unusual strain of *Y. pseudotuberculosis* with similarities to *Salmonella pullorum* was isolated from turkey hens by Kiliam et al. (11). It resembled *S. pullorum* on brilliant green agar; was agglutinated by *S. pullorum* antiserum; produced acid but not gas from glucose and mannitol; and did not ferment lactose, sucrose, maltose, dulcitol, or salicin. Antiserum from sensitized guinea pigs, chickens, and turkeys, which agglutinated homologous antigen, failed to agglutinate either *S. pullorum* or *S. typhimurium.*

TREATMENT AND PREVENTION.

Little current information is available on the use of chemotherapeutic agents for treatment of pseudotuberculosis in birds. In one case, treatment of affected turkeys with chloramphenicol and streptomycin sulphate (0.6 g and 0.5 g/l respectively) in drinking water for 2 days, followed by tetracycline (0.5 g/l) for 4 days resulted in decreased death losses; no relapse occurred (8). In another case, treatment with high levels of tetracycline in the feed seemed to arrest the disease, but surviving turkeys were later condemned at processing because of septicemic lesions (22). Vaccines are not available for use in preventing avian pseudotuberculosis; therefore, prevention is limited to use of good management procedures (see Chapter 1).

REFERENCES

1. Adamec, Z., and K. Matousek. 1965. Pseudotuberculosis in turkeys. Veterinarstvi 15:158–160.
2. Beaudette, F.R. 1940. A case of pseudotuberculosis in a blackbird. J Am Vet Med Assoc 97:151–157.
3. Buchanan, R.E., J.G. Holt, and E.F. Lessel. 1966. Index Bergeyana. Williams & Wilkins, Baltimore, MD.
4. Burrows, T.W., and W.A. Gillett. 1966. The nutritional requirements of some Pasteurella species. J Gen Microbiol 45:333–345.
5. Clapham, P.A. 1953. Pseudotuberculosis among stock-doves in Hampshire. Nature 172:353.
6. Clark, M.C., and L.N. Locke. 1962. Case report: Observations on pseudotuberculosis in common grackles. Avian Dis 6:506–510.
7. Cook, R. 1952. A method of demonstrating Pasteurella pseudotuberculosis in smears from animal lesions. J Pathol Bacteriol 64:228–229.
8. Hinz, K.H., E.F. Kaleta, B. Stiburek, G. Glunder, and K. Tessler. 1981. Eine durch Yersinia pseudotuberculosis bei Mastputen verursachte Myopathie. Dtsch Tieraerztl Wochenschr 88:352–354.
9. Hodges, R.T., M.G. Carman, and W.J. Mortimer. 1984. Serotypes of Yersinia pseudotuberculosis recovered from domestic livestock. N Z Vet J 32:11–13.
10. Karlsson, K.F. 1945. Pseudotuberkulos hos honsfaglar. Scand Vet Tidskr 35:673–687.
11. Kiliam, J.G., R. Yamamoto, W.E. Babcock, and E.M. Dickenson. 1962. An unusual aspect of Pasteurella pseudotuberculosis in turkeys. Avian Dis 6:403–405.
12. Mair, N.S. 1965. Sources and serological classification of 177 strains of Pasteurella psuedotuberculosis isolated in Great Britain. J Pathol Bacteriol 90:275–278.
13. Malassez, L., and W. Vignal. 1883. Tuberculose zoologique (forme on espice de tuberculose sans bacillis). Arch Physiol Norm Pathol Ser 3, 2:369–412.
14. Marthedal, H.E., and G. Velling. 1954. Pasteurellosis and pseudotuberculosis among fowls in Denmark. Nord Vet Med 6:651–665.
15. Mathey, W.J., Fr., and P.J. Siddle. 1954. Isolation of Pasteurella pseudotuberculosis from a California turkey. J Am Vet Med Assoc 125:482–483.
16. Mollaret, H.H., and E. Thal. 1974. Yersinia. In R.E. Buchanan and N.E. Gibbons (eds.), Bergey's Manual of Determinative Bacteriology, pp. 330–332. Williams & Wilkins, Baltimore, MD.
17. Paterson, J.S., and R. Cook. 1963. A method for the recovery of Pasteurella pseudotuberculosis from faeces. J Pathol Bacteriol 85:241–242.
18. Rosenwald, A.S., and F.M. Dickinson. 1944. A report on Pasteurella pseudotuberculosis infection in turkeys. Am J Vet Res 5:246–249.
19. Stovell, P.L. 1980. Pseudotubercular yersiniosis. In J. H. Steele, H. Stoenner, W. Kaplan, and M. Torten (eds.), CRC Handbook Series in Zoonoses, Sect A, Vol II, pp. 209–256. CRC Press, Inc., Boca Raton, FL.
20. Thal, E. 1954. Untersuchungen ueber Pasteurella pseudotuberculosis unter besonder Beruecksichtigun ihres immunologisches Verhaltens. Thesis, Berlingska Boktryckeriet, Lund, Sweden.
21. Tsubokura, M., K. Otsuki, Y. Kawasoka, H. Fukushima, K. Ikemure, and K. Kanazawa. 1984. Addition of new serogroups and improvement of the antigenic designs of Yersinia pseudotuberculosis. Curr Microbiol 11:89–92.
22. Wallner-Pendleton, E., and G. Cooper. 1983. Several outbreaks of Yersinia pseudotuberculosis in California turkey flocks. Avian Dis 27:524–526.
23. Wise, D.R., and P.K. Uppal. 1972. Osteomyelitis in turkeys caused by Yersinia pseudotuberculosis. J Med Microbiol 5:128–130.

PASTEURELLA ANATIPESTIFER INFECTION

T.S. Sandhu, K.R. Rhoades, and R.B. Rimler

INTRODUCTION. *Pasteurella anatipestifer* (PA) infection is a contagious disease of domestic ducks, turkeys, and various other birds. It is also known as new duck disease, duck septicemia, anatipestifer syndrome, anatipestifer septicemia, and infectious serositis. It occurs as an acute or chronic septicemia characterized by fibrinous pericarditis, perihepatitis, airsacculitis, caseous salpingitis, and meningitis. The respiratory tract may also be infected without showing clinical signs. PA infection accounts for major economic losses to the duck industry due to high mortality, weight loss, and condemnations.

Signs and lesions of PA infection in ducks and those reported in geese affected with "goose influenza" (31) are similar; the causal agents *P. anatipestifer* and *P. septicaemiae* cannot be differentiated on the basis of reported characteristics. Therefore, goose influenza will not be described as a separate disease.

HISTORY AND DISTRIBUTION. PA infection was first described in 1932 in White Pekin ducks from three farms on Long Island, N.Y. (25). The report referred to a new disease, which became known in the area as "new duck disease." The disease started in 7- to 10-wk-old ducks with about 10% mortality, and later spread to younger ducklings of about 3 wk of age. Six years later the disease was observed in ducks from a commercial farm in Illinois and was reported as "duck septicemia" (16). The designation "infectious serositis" was given by Dougherty et al. (13) after a comprehensive pathologic study. The term PA infection was recommended by Leibovitz (30) to identify the disease specifically caused by *P. anatipestifer* and to differentiate it from other infections with similar pathology.

The disease occurs worldwide and has been recognized in countries that have intensive duck production (43).

ETIOLOGY

Classification. The causative bacterium was isolated and characterized by Hendrickson and Hilbert (25), who called it *Pfeifferella anatipestifer.* Bruner and Fabricant (10) studied and compared its characteristics with those of *Brucella, Pasteurella, Moraxella, Actinobacillus,* and *Haemophilus.* They concluded that the organism had more in common with *Moraxella* spp. and suggested the name *Moraxella anatipestifer.* However, it was listed in the seventh edition of Bergey's Manual of Determinative Bacteriology as *Pasteurella anatipestifer* (8). A valid taxonomic placement of PA is uncertain; it is currently placed as species *incertae sedis* in the ninth edition of *Bergey's Manual of Systematic Bacteriology* (32). Comparison of DNA base composition, DNA-DNA homology, and cellular fatty-acid profile has indicated its exclusion from the genus *Moraxella* as well as *Pasteurella* (5, 32). Piechulla et al. (38) have suggested the transfer of PA to the *Flavobacterium/Cytophaga* group (family Cytophagaceae) on the basis of low but significant DNA binding and production of menaquinones and branched-chain fatty acids.

To date 12 serotypes exist, including 8 identified by agar-gel precipitin reaction (7, 46). Numerical designation of PA serotypes has been suggested to eliminate confusion and to standardize serotype nomenclature for recognition of new types (7). Harry (18) reported 8 serotypes (A through H) on the basis of agglutination reaction; later 8 more (I through P) were identified (7). Four of these (E, F, J, K) were lost in storage, while serotypes N and O were found to be identical. Seven serotypes (1 through 7) have been differentiated by agar-gel precipitin reaction (9). One more, serotype 8, was reported by Sandhu and Harry (46). Two new serotypes have been isolated in Denmark (7).

Morphology and Staining. PA is a gram-negative, nonmotile, non-spore-forming rod occurring singly, in pairs, and occasionally as filaments. The cells vary from 0.2–0.4 μm in width and 1–5 μm in length. Many cells stain bipolar with Wright's stain, and a capsule can be demonstrated in preparations with India ink.

Growth Requirements and Colonial Morphology. The organism grows well on chocolate agar, blood agar, or trypticase soy agar. Growth on trypticase soy agar can be enhanced by the addition of 0.05% yeast extract. Growth is more abundant with increased carbon dioxide (16). Hendrickson and Hilbert (25) described the organism as a strict aerobe on the basis of results obtained with the pyrogallic acid and sodium hydroxide procedure for removing oxygen. However, since carbon dioxide would also be depleted by reacting with the sodium hydroxide, neither oxygen nor carbon dioxide was available to the organism. Although some strains of PA grew at an incubation temperature of 45 C, no growth was observed at 4 C or 55 C (4); maximum growth usually occurs in 48–72 hr when incubated at 37 C in a candle jar.

Colonies on blood agar, when grown 24 hr at 37 C in a candle jar, are 1–2 mm in diameter, convex, entire, transparent, glistening, and butyrous. Some strains produce slimy growth. Colonies on clear media are iridescent when observed with obliquely transmitted light. Incubation in the candle jar is recommended for good growth as it increases carbon dioxide and moisture, both of which are favorable for growth.

Biochemical Characteristics. Carbohydrates are not fermented, although some researchers have reported acid production in glucose, maltose, inositol, and fructose by some strains (2, 4). Gelatin is usually liquefied and litmus milk may slowly turn alkaline. Indole and hydrogen sulfide are not produced. Nitrate is not reduced to nitrite, and starch is not hydrolyzed. There is no growth on MacConkey agar and no hemolysis of blood agar. PA is oxidase- and catalase-positive; phosphatase is produced (19). Some strains produce urease. Arginine and hippurate are hydrolyzed (17). Differential characteristics are listed in Table 5.2 (see Fowl Cholera).

Resistance to Chemical and Physical Agents. Most PA strains do not survive on solid media for more than 3–4 days at 37 C or room temperature; cultures in broth may be viable for 2–3 wk when stored at 4 C. Incubation at 55 C for 12–16 hr resulted in nonviability of the organism (4). PA has been reported to survive in tap water and turkey litter for 13 and 27 days, respectively (6). PA is sensitive to penicillin, novobiocin, chloramphenicol, lincomycin, streptomycin, gentamicin, erythromycin, ampicillin, bacitracin, neomycin, and tetracycline but resistant to kanamycin and polymyxin B (4).

PATHOGENESIS AND EPIZOOTIOLOGY

Natural and Experimental Hosts. PA infection is primarily a disease of domestic ducks. Ducklings of 1–8 wk of age are highly susceptible. Ducklings under 5 wk of age usually die 1–2 days after signs appear; older birds may survive longer. The disease is rare in breeder ducks. Natural outbreaks of PA have been reported in turkeys (24, 50). Recent outbreaks in turkeys in

California and Minnesota have shown that PA is a potential pathogen of domestic turkeys (36, 48). PA has also been isolated from pheasants (11), chickens (41), and waterfowl (14, 28, 35, 39, 49).

Adverse environmental conditions or concomitant disease often predispose the birds to outbreaks of PA infection. Mortality may vary from 5 to 75%.

The disease can be produced in healthy ducks by exposure to PA. There is wide variation, however, in severity of the disease depending on the strain of the organism and the route of exposure. Mortality can be produced most consistently by injection of the organism intravenously, subcutaneously, into the foot pad, or into the infraorbital sinus. The disease can also be reproduced by intraperitoneal, intramuscular, or intratracheal routes of exposure. Attempts to produce the disease by oral inoculation of PA have been unsuccessful (3, 21).

Chickens, geese, pigeons, rabbits, and mice were reported to be refractory to infection with PA; guinea pigs succumbed to inoculation of large doses intraperitoneally (16, 25). However, Heddleston (23) observed that 8×10^6 organisms inoculated into the foot pad killed 5 of 7 day-old chicks; 4×10^6 organisms produced the same signs and lesions in 2-wk-old White Chinese goslings as were produced in White Pekin ducklings. Infection takes place via the respiratory tract (30) or through wounds of the skin, particularly of the feet (3).

Signs. Signs most often observed are listlessness, ocular and nasal discharge, mild coughing and sneezing, greenish diarrhea, ataxia (Fig. 5.17), tremor of head and neck, and coma. Affected ducklings show inability to move with the brood. Surviving ducks may be stunted (37).

Lesions. The most obvious gross lesion in ducks is fibrinous exudate, which involves serosal surfaces in general but is most evident in the pericardial cavity and over the surface of the liver (Figs. 5.18, 5.19, 5.20); similar lesions have been reported in turkeys and other birds. In addition to fibrin, the exudate contains a few inflammatory cells, primarily mononuclear cells and heterophils.

Fibrinous airsacculitis is common. Mononuclear cells are the predominant cell type in the exudate. Multinuclear giant cells and fibroblasts may be observed in chronic cases (13). Lungs of infected ducks may be unaffected; there may be interstitial cellular infiltration and proliferation of lymphoid nodules adjacent to parabronchi (37); or there may be an acute fibrinopurulent pneumonia (16).

Liver lesions observed in the acute stage of the disease are mild periportal mononuclear leukocytic infiltration and cloudy swelling and hydropic degeneration of parenchymal cells. In less acute cases, moderate periportal lymphocytic infiltration may be observed (37).

Infections of the central nervous system can produce a fibrinous meningitis. Spleens may be enlarged and mottled. Mucopurulent exudate in nasal sinuses and caseous exudate in oviducts have been observed in PA infection (13). Jortner et al. (27) studied lesions in the central nervous system of naturally infected ducklings and described diffuse fibrinous meningitis with leukocytic infiltration in and around the walls of menin-

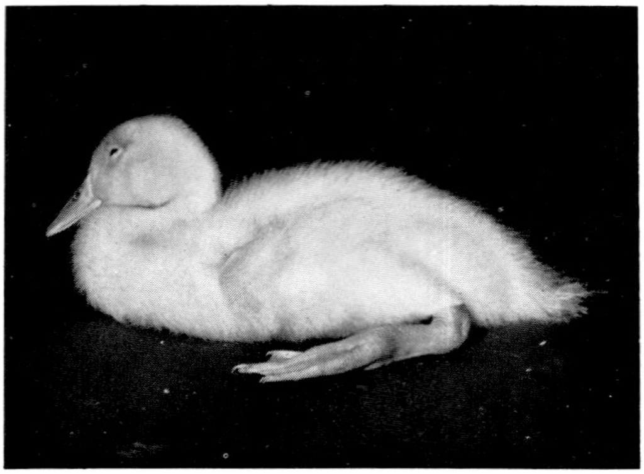

5.17. *Pasteurella anatipestifer* infection. Duckling is incoordinated and droopy.

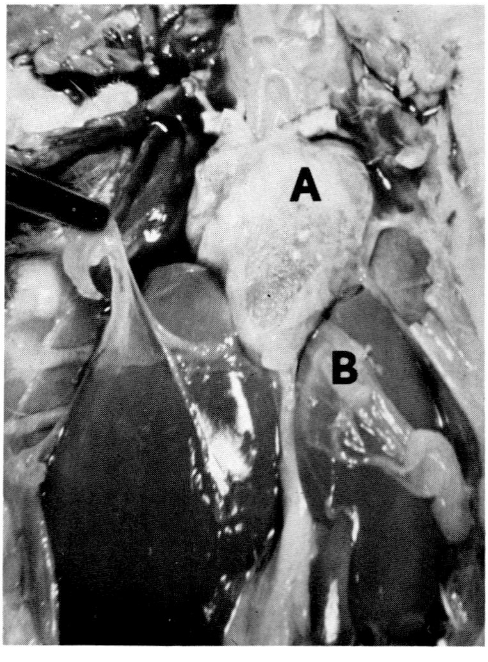

5.18. *Pasteurella anatipestifer* infection; fibrinous epicarditis (*A*), pericarditis, and perihepatitis (*B*). Forceps hold exudate from surface of liver.

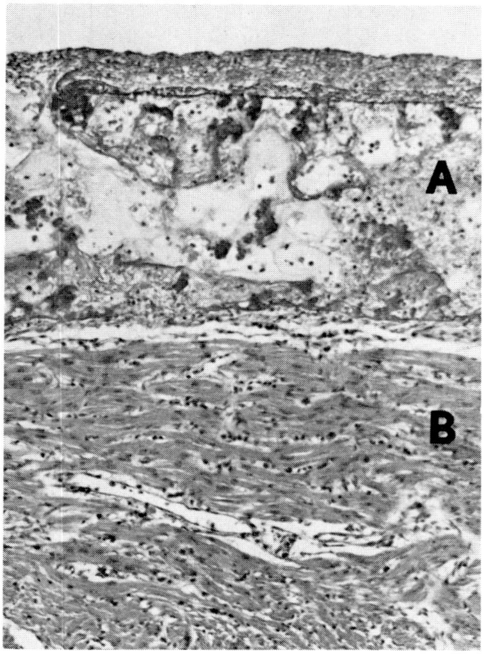

5.19. *Pasteurella anatipestifer* infection; fibrinous exudate (*A*) over surface of heart (*B*). H & E, ×150.

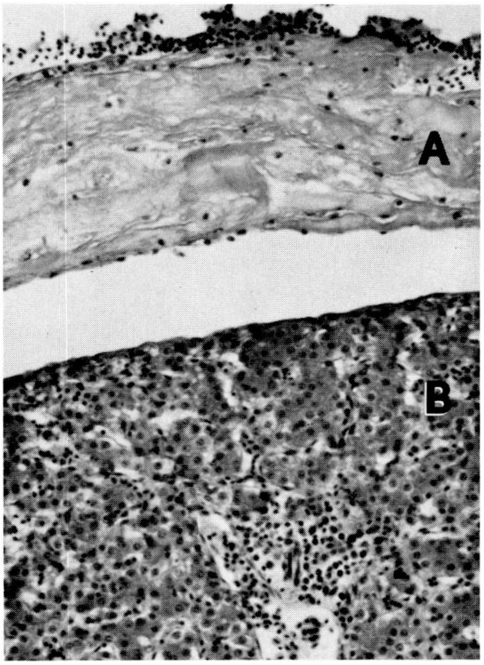

5.20. *Pasteurella anatipestifer* infection; fibrinous exudate (*A*) over surface of liver (*B*). H & E, ×300.

geal blood vessels. Extensive exudate was observed in the ventricular system. Slight to moderate leukocytic and microglial infiltrates were observed in subpial and periventricular brain tissue.

Chronic localized infections usually occur in skin and occasionally in joints. Skin lesions are in the form of necrotic dermatitis on the lower back or around the vent. Yellowish exudate is observed between skin and fat layers.

Immunity. Ducklings that recover from the disease are resistant to subsequent infection (2, 16, 25). Inactivated bacterins have been used in ducks to prevent PA infection. Ducks vaccinated with formalin-inactivated bacterins and subsequently challenged with strains representing serotypes 1, 2, and 5 developed homologous but not heterologous protection. A trivalent bacterin containing these strains provided protection against challenge with each, but the protection lasted only a short time (42). Harry and Deb (20) evaluated effectiveness of several types of bacterins and conducted a field trial with a formalin-inactivated bacterin. A single dose of oil-emulsion bacterin provided longer lasting immunity in ducklings (15, 42). Passive protection of progeny may be obtained by immunization of the female breeder ducks; this protection may last for about 2 wk.

DIAGNOSIS.

Although a presumptive diagnosis may be made from clinical signs and necropsy findings, a definite diagnosis should be based on isolation and identification of PA.

Isolation and Identification. The bacterium can be isolated most readily when birds are in the acute stage of the disease. Suitable tissues for culturing the organism are heart blood, brain, air sacs, bone marrow, lung, liver, and exudates from the lesions. Specimens should be taken aseptically, streaked over blood agar or trypticase soy agar, and incubated in a "candle jar" at 37 C for 24–72 hr. Isolated colonies should be selected for inoculation of the differentiating media and identified on the basis of characteristics listed in Table 5.2 (see FOWL CHOLERA). Serotype identification can be established by the rapid slide agglutination test with specific antisera.

Immunofluorescent procedures can be used to identify PA in tissue or exudate from infected birds (33). Hatfield et al. (22) described an enzyme-linked immunosorbent assay (ELISA) that was more sensitive than the agglutination test to detect serum antibodies in ducks.

Differential Diagnosis. PA infection should be differentiated from other septicemic diseases caused by *P. multocida, E. coli, Streptococcus faecium,* and salmonellae. Since these diseases produce gross lesions indistinguishable from those caused by PA, diagnosis must include isolation and identification of the causal organism. Differential diagnosis of PA should also include chlamydiosis, especially in turkeys and in areas where the latter is a serious problem.

Goose influenza (31) and PA infection are probably the same disease except that one has been described as a disease of geese and the other as a disease of ducks. Information in the literature about the characteristics of the respective causative agents leads one to believe they are the same organism (26, 47). Riemer (40), who was one of the first to study the disease in geese, used the term *septicaemia anserum exsudativa*. He found that the causative bacterium was more pathogenic for geese than ducks, but the lesions were the same in both species when they were exposed artificially.

TREATMENT. Antibiotics and sulfa drugs have been tried for treatment of PA with varying degrees of success. Sulfamethazine, 0.2–0.25%, in drinking water or feed was reported to prevent the onset of clinical signs in ducks exposed experimentally to PA (2). Sulfaquinoxaline at levels of 0.025 or 0.05% in feed was effective in reducing mortality in field and experimental infections (12, 45). Medicated feeds containing novobiocin (0.0303–0.0368%) or lincomycin (0.011–0.022%) were reported to be highly effective in reducing mortality when started 3 days prior to experimental infection. A combination of sulfadimethoxine and ormetoprim, when administered at 0.02–0.12% levels in feed, prevented or reduced mortality and gross lesions in experimentally exposed ducks (34, 45). Tetracyclines were of little value for treatment of PA infection (1, 45). Subcutaneous injection of lincomycin-spectinomycin, penicillin, or a combination of penicillin and dihydrostreptomycin were reported to be effective in reducing mortality in artificially infected ducklings (45).

PREVENTION AND CONTROL. Inactivated bacterins have been reported to prevent or reduce mortality due to PA (20, 29,42). Since immunity induced by bacterins is serotype-specific, an ideal bacterin should contain cells of predominant serotypes to provide an effective protection. A bacterin containing serotypes 1, 2, and 5 has been used in the USA. Ducklings are vaccinated at 2 and 3 wk of age to provide adequate protection up to market age (29). A single inoculation of oil-emulsified bacterin has been reported to produce better and longer lasting protection, but it may cause unfavorable lesions at the site of inoculation (15, 42).

A live PA vaccine, developed against serotypes 1, 2, and 5, has been reported to provide significant protection against experimental or field infections with virulent organisms when administered to day-old ducklings by aerosol or in drinking water (44). The vaccine strains grew in the upper respiratory tract and produced a humoral antibody response. The vaccine was reported to be avirulent to day-old ducklings when administered by aerosol or injection into the infraorbital sinus, and was safe in ducks up to 10 back-passages using the contact-exposure method.

REFERENCES

1. Ash, W.J. 1967. Antibiotics and infectious serositis in White Pekin ducklings. Avian Dis 11:38–41.
2. Asplin, F.D. 1955. A septicaemic disease of ducklings. Vet Rec 67:854–858.
3. Asplin, F.D. 1956. Experiments on the transmission of a septicaemic disease of ducklings. Vet Rec 68:588–590.
4. Bangun, A., D.N. Tripathy, and L.E. Hanson. 1981. Studies of Pasteurella anatipestifer: An approach to its classification. Avian Dis 25:326–337.
5. Bangun A., J.L. Johnson, and D.N. Tripathy. 1987. Taxonomy of Pasteurella anatipestifer. 1. DNA base composition and DNA-DNA hybridization analysis. Avian Dis 31:43–45.
6. Bendheim U., and A. Even-Shoshan. 1975. Survival of Pasteurella multocida and Pasteurella anatipestifer in various natural media. Refu Vet 32:40–46.
7. Bisgaard, M. 1982. Antigenic studies on Pasteurella anatipestifer, species incertae sedis, using slide and tube agglutination. Avian Pathol 11:341–350.
8. Breed, R.S., E.F. Lessel, Jr., and E. Heist Clise. 1957. Genus I. Pasteurella Trevisan, 1887. In R.S. Breed, E.G.D. Murray, and N.R. Smith (eds.), Bergey's Manual of Determinative Bacteriology, 7th Ed., pp.395–402. Williams & Wilkins, Baltimore, MD.
9. Brogden, K.A., K.R. Rhoades, and R.B. Rimler. 1982. Serologic types and physiologic characteristics of 46 avian Pasteurella anatipestifer cultures. Avian Dis 26:891–896.
10. Bruner, D.W., and J. Fabricant. 1954. A strain of Moraxella anatipestifer (Pfeifferella anatipestifer) isolated from ducks. Cornell Vet 44:461–464.
11. Bruner, D.W., C.I. Angstrom, and J.I. Price. 1970. Pasteurella anatipestifer infection in pheasants. A case report. Cornell Vet 60:491–494.
12. Dean, W.F., J.I. Price, and L. Leibovitz. 1973. Effect of feed medicaments on bacterial infections in ducklings. Poult Sci 52:549–558.
13. Dougherty, E., L.Z. Saunders, and E.H. Parsons. 1955. The pathology of infectious serositis of ducks. Am J Pathol 31:475–487.
14. Eleazer, T.H., H.G. Blalock, J.S. Harrell, and W.T. Derieux. 1973. Pasteurella anatipestifer as a cause of mortality in semiwild pen-raised mallard ducks in South Carolina. Avian Dis 17:855–857.
15. Floren, U., P.K. Storm, and E.F. Kaleta. 1988. Pasteurella anatipestifer sp.i.c. bei Pekingenten:Pathogenitätsprüfungen und Immunisierung mit einer inaktivierten, homologen, monovalenten (serotyp 6/B) Lemulsionsvakzine. Dtsch Tierärztl. Wochenschr 95:210–214.
16. Graham, R., C.A. Brandly, and G.L. Dunlap. 1938. Studies on duck septicemia. Cornell Vet 28:1–8.
17. Grimes, T.M., and L.E. Rosenfeld. 1972. Pasteurella anatipestifer infection in ducks in Australia. Aust Vet J 48:367–368.
18. Harry, E.G. 1969. Pasteurella (Pfeifferella) anatipestifer serotypes isolated from cases of anatipestifer

septicaemia in ducks. Vet Rec 84:673.
19. Harry, E.G. 1981. Personal communication.
20. Harry, E.G., and J.R. Deb. 1979. Laboratory and field trials on a formalin inactivated vaccine for the control of Pasteurella anatipestifer septicaemia in ducks. Res Vet Sci 27:329-333.
21. Hatfield, R.M., and B.A. Morris. 1988. Influence of the route of infection of Pasteurella anatipestifer on the clinical and immune responses of White Pekin ducks. Res Vet Sci 44:208- 214.
22. Hatfield, R.M., B.A. Morris, and R.R. Henry. 1987. Development of an enzyme-linked immunosorbent assay for the detection of humoral antibody to Pasteurella anatipestifer. Avian Pathol 16:123-140.
23. Heddleston, K.L. 1972. Infectious serositis. In M.S. Hofstad, B.W. Calnek, C.F. Helmboldt, W.M. Reid, H.W. Yoder, Jr. (eds.). Diseases of Poultry, 6th Ed., pp.246-251. Iowa State Univ Press, Ames.
24. Helfer, D.H., and C.F. Helmboldt. 1977. Pasteurella anatipestifer infection in turkeys. Avian Dis 21:712-715.
25. Hendrickson, J.M., and K.F. Hilbert. 1932. A new and serious septicemic disease of young ducks with a description of the causative organism, Pfeifferella anatipestifer, N.S. Cornell Vet 22:239-252.
26. Hinz, K.-H., H. Grebe, and M. Knapp. 1976. Moraxella septicaemiae-Infektion bei Gnsen. Zentralbl Veterinaermed [B] 23:341-345.
27. Jortner, B.S., R. Porro, and L. Leibovitz. 1969. Central-nervous-system lesions of spontaneous Pasteurella anatipestifer infection in ducklings. Avian Dis 13:27-35.
28. Karstad, L., P. Lusis, and J.R. Long. 1970. Pasteurella anatipestifer as a cause of mortality in captive wild waterfowl. J Wildl Dis 6:408-413.
29. Layton, H.W., and T.S. Sandhu. 1984. Protection of ducklings with a broth-grown Pasteurella anatipestifer bacterin. Avian Dis 28:718-726.
30. Leibovitz, L. 1972. A survey of the so-called “anatipestifer syndrome “. Avian Dis 16:836-851.
31. Levine, N.D. 1965. Goose influenza (septicaemia anserum exsudativa). In H.E. Biester, and L.H. Schwarte (eds.), Diseases of Poultry, 5th Ed., pp.469-471. Iowa State Univ Press, Ames.
32. Mannheim, W. 1984. Family III. Pasteurellaceae Pohl 1981a, 382. In N.R. Krieg and J.G. Holt (eds.), Bergey's Manual of Systematic Bacteriology, 9th Ed., Vol. 1, pp. 550-557. Williams & Wilkins, Baltimore, MD.
33. Marshall, J.D., Jr., P.A. Hansen, and W.C. Eveland. 1961. Histobacteriology of the genus Pasteurella. 1. Pasteurella anatipestifer. Cornell Vet 51:24-34.
34. Mitrovic, M., E.G. Schildknecht, G. Maestrone, and H.G. Luther. 1980. Rofenaid in the control of Pasteurella anatipestifer and Escherichia coli infections in ducklings. Avian Dis 24:302-308.
35. Munday, B.L., A. Corbould, K.L. Heddleston, and E.G. Harry. 1970. Isolation of Pasteurella anatipestifer from black swan (Cygnus atratus). Aust Vet J 46:322-325.
36. Nagaraja, K.V. 1988. Personal communication.
37. Pickrell, J.A. 1966. Pathologic changes associated with experimental Pasteurella anatipestifer infection in ducklings. Avian Dis 10:281-288.
38. Piechulla, K., S. Pohl, and W. Mannheim. 1986. Phenotypic and genetic relationships of so-called Moraxella (Pasteurella) anatipestifer to the Flavobacterium/Cytophaga group. Vet Microbiol 11:261-270.
39. Pierce, R.L., and M.W. Vorhies. 1973. Pasteurella anatipestifer infection in geese. Avian Dis 17:868-870.
40. Riemer. 1904. Kurze Mitteilung ber eine bei Gnsen beobachtete exsudative Septikmie und deren Erreger. Zentralbl Bakteriol I Abt Orig 37:641-648.
41. Rosenfeld, L.E. 1973. Pasteurella anatipestifer infection in fowls in Australia. Aust Vet J 49:55-56.
42. Sandhu, T. 1979. Immunization of White Pekin ducklings against Pasteurella anatipestifer infection. Avian Dis 23:662-669.
43. Sandhu, T.S. 1986. Important diseases of ducks. In D.J. Farrell and P. Stapleton (eds.), Duck Production Science and World Practice, pp.111-134. Univ of New England, Australia.
44. Sandhu, T.S. 1987. Pasteurella anatipestifer live vaccine: Laboratory and field trials in White Pekin ducklings. Proc 23rd World Vet Congr, p. 325. Montreal, Canada.
45. Sandhu, T.S., and W.F. Dean. 1980. Effect of chemotherapeutic agents on Pasteurella anatipestifer infection in White Pekin ducklings. Poult Sci 59:1027-1030.
46. Sandhu, T., and E.G. Harry. 1981. Serotypes of Pasteurella anatipestifer isolated from commercial White Pekin ducks in the United States. Avian Dis 25:497-502.
47. Smith, J.E. 1974. Genus Pasteurella Trevisan 1887. In R.E. Buchanan and N.E. Gibbons (eds.), Bergey's Manual of Determinative Bacteriology, 8th Ed., pp. 370-373. Williams & Wilkins, Baltimore, MD.
48. Smith, J.M., D.D. Frame, G. Cooper, A.A. Bickford, G.Y. Ghazikhanian, and B.J. Kelly. 1987. Pasteurella anatipestifer infection in commercial meat-type turkeys in California. Avian Dis 31:913-917.
49. Wobeser, G., and G.E. Ward. 1974. Pasteurella anatipestifer infection in migrating whistling swans. J Wildl Dis 10:466-470.
50. Zehr, W.J., and J. Ostendorf, Jr. 1970. Pasteurella anatipestifer in turkeys. Avian Dis 14:557-560.

6 TUBERCULOSIS

Charles O. Thoen and Alfred G. Karlson

INTRODUCTION. Tuberculosis of poultry is a contagious disease caused by *Mycobacterium avium.* It is characterized by its chronicity; persistence in a flock when once established; and tendency to induce unthriftiness, decreased egg production, and finally death. Although the incidence of tuberculosis in chickens has been reduced to a low level, tuberculosis remains an important problem in captive exotic birds. The importance of tuberculosis in birds in zoo aviaries is emphasized by lack of efficacious vaccines or suitable drug-treatment regimens.

The literature contains a number of instances in which it was claimed that *M. avium* was responsible for a tuberculous infection in humans. In the USA, the first case of avian tuberculosis (AT) in humans (with adequate proof) was published in 1947 (15).

With decline in incidence of tuberculosis in humans, increasing interest is directed toward mycobacteria other than *M. tuberculosis,* so that more isolations of *M. avium* are being recognized (13, 74). Recent information indicates *M. avium*–complex infection is common in patients with acquired immune deficiency syndrome (AIDS) (21, 33, 72). *M. avium* serotype 1, the organism most commonly isolated from birds, has been isolated from patients with AIDS (5, 20, 25). However, serotypes of *M. avium* isolated from humans are usually different from those commonly isolated from chickens.

HISTORY. AT in chickens was first recognized as a related but separate entity by Cornil and Mégnin (11). Koch (35) maintained for many years that tubercle bacilli were always the same regardless of the species in which they might occur. However, Rivolta and later Maffucci (39) showed that the microorganism of AT in chickens is dissimilar to that of bovine tuberculosis. Koch (36) finally abandoned his previous position and declared that tuberculosis of poultry is unlike tuberculosis of humans and that the disease in humans is dissimilar to that of cattle.

Although AT in chickens has long been recognized as a contagious disease, it has continued to spread throughout most of the world. With available information on the nature of AT, its eradication is entirely feasible. The more important reasons for its elimination are: 1) affected birds are unthrifty, 2) tuberculous chickens are undesirable for human food, 3) diseased birds produce fewer eggs, 4) tuberculous chickens are the source of tuberculosis of sheep and especially of swine, 5) avian tubercle bacilli are capable of sensitizing cattle to mammalian tuberculin, and 6) avian tubercle bacilli have been isolated from lesions in humans. Unfortunately, in the USA presence of AT in chickens continues to be accepted with a certain complacency, and we have failed to formulate a program that can be expected to eradicate the disease. The noteworthy results obtained in eradication of bovine tuberculosis should stimulate the attack on the disease in chickens.

The occurrence of AT in birds in zoo aviaries has become of additional importance, since the disease causes increased economic losses. Certain species of exotic birds have increased in value as they near extinction, thereby increasing the significance of mortalities from AT. Management problems concerning control of the disease are magnified, since exotic species are often maintained for years. A major obstacle in elimination of AT in zoological gardens is related to the ability of the organism to survive in the soil and lack of adequate procedures for cleaning and disinfecting contaminated premises.

INCIDENCE AND DISTRIBUTION. AT in chickens is worldwide in distribution but occurs most frequently in the North Temperate Zone. The highest incidence of infection in the USA occurs in flocks of the north central states–North Dakota, South Dakota, Kansas, Nebraska, Minnesota, Iowa, Missouri, Wisconsin, Illinois, Michigan, Indiana, and Ohio. Available data indicate that in some areas more than 50% of the flocks may be infected (67). Incidence of the disease in western and southern states is low. The explanation for this is not entirely obvious, although there are several possible contributing factors such as climate, flock management, and duration of infection. The necessity of keeping birds closely confined during winter provides favorable conditions for spread of the disease.

The difficulty of tuberculin-testing all chickens in the USA, or even a majority of the flocks, makes it impossible to obtain exact data on incidence of tuberculous infection of chickens. In 1972 AT was the cause for condemning 0.04% of 186.9 million mature chickens slaughtered under federal inspection (67). However, this figure may be deceiving because the chickens may not be representative of the average farm flock. Furthermore, visual inspection may not disclose all infected birds.

There has been significant reduction in the prevalence of AT, owing in considerable part to the changing concept of poultry husbandry. Increasing emphasis has been placed on the desirability of maintaining all-pullet flocks rather than older hens.

In Canada the incidence of AT in chickens varies greatly in different areas–from 1 to 26%. It occurs in some Latin American countries, but the incidence is variable–low in Brazil, common in Uruguay, widespread in Venezuela as of 1946, and reported in Argentina. Isolated cases of avian tubercle bacillus infections in humans have been found in various Latin American countries (44).

Considerable information exists on occurrence of AT in certain European countries. It is said to be rare in Finland (53, 71) but not uncommon in Norway (17) and Denmark (2). AT occurs in Germany (22) and Great Britain (38). In Australia AT is unknown in Queensland and West Australia but occurs in other states. In South Africa the incidence in poultry is low (34). It is rare also in Kenya and Rhodesia (44). Infections probably occur in domestic and wild fowl in other countries, but the incidence and distribution cannot be determined because bacteriologic studies are not universally done. AT has been reported in lesser flamingoes in Kenya (10). Disease in swine from *M. avium* has been reported in countries other than the foregoing (59) and in humans (37). Further discussion on prevalence of tuberculosis in animals may be found in Myers and Steele (44).

Age in Relation to Incidence. AT appears to be less prevalent in young fowl, not because the younger birds are more resistant to infection but because in older birds the disease has had a greater opportunity to become established through a longer period of exposure. Although tuberculous lesions are usually less severe in young chickens than adult birds, extensive or generalized AT in young chickens has been observed. Such birds are an important source of dissemination of virulent tubercle bacilli and must be considered a menace to other fowl and susceptible mammals.

Schack-Steffenhagen and Seeger (46) found *M. avium* in livers of 3.38% of mature chickens imported into Germany from Holland and the USA but could not demonstrate the microorganisms in broilers. They concluded that tuberculosis is commoner in older birds.

Tuberculosis causes important death losses in exotic birds of zoo aviaries (43). The significance of these findings is emphasized by reports of disease in valuable endangered species. Numerous reports are also available on tuberculosis in pet birds.

ETIOLOGY.

The most common cause of AT in chickens in the USA is *M. avium* serotypes 1 and 2 (60). In Europe *M. avium* serotype 3 has been isolated from birds; however, this organism has not been isolated from domestic birds in the USA (48). Serotype 3 was cultured from a tree duck being held for importation into the USA (63). Some other serotypes of *M. avium* (previously called *M. intracellulare*) isolated from humans have not been found to cause progressive disease in chickens.

The most characteristic feature of *M. avium* is its acid-fastness. The organisms are bacillary in character; clublike, curved, and crooked forms are also seen in some preparations. Cords are not formed. Branching infrequently occurs. Most of the bacteria have rounded ends and vary in length from 1 to 3 μm. Spores are not produced, and the organism is nonmotile. Reproduction of the avian tubercle bacillus is by simple fission. Spherical or conical granules occur in the endoplasm anywhere along the length of the bacterium.

Cultural Distinctions. The avian tubercle bacillus is not as exacting in its temperature requirements as the human and bovine forms. The avian form will grow at temperatures ranging from 25 to 45 C, although the most favorable temperature range is 39–45 C. *M. avium* is aerobic. On original isolation, growth is enhanced by an atmosphere of 5–10% carbon dioxide (52).

For original isolation from naturally infected material, one of the special media designed for culturing tubercle bacilli is desirable. Both glycerinated and nonglycerinated media are satisfactory, but colonies are larger if the medium contains glycerin (Fig. 6.1). Some strains of *M. avium* require mycobactin as a growth factor for initial and subsequent growth (40). On media containing whole egg or egg yolk and incubated at 37.5–40 C, the bacteria usually become evident in 10 days to 3 wk as small, slightly raised, discrete, grayish white colonies. If the inoculum is rich in bacteria, colonies will be numerous and may tend to coalesce into granulated masses. Colonies are hemispheric and do not penetrate the medium. They gradually change from grayish white to light ocher and become darker as age of the culture increases. Karlson et al. (31) described a culture of *M. avium* that was bright yellow but typical in all other respects.

Subcultures on solid media show evidence of growth within a few days and reach maximal development in 3–4 wk. Such cultures usually appear moist and unctuous, the surface eventually

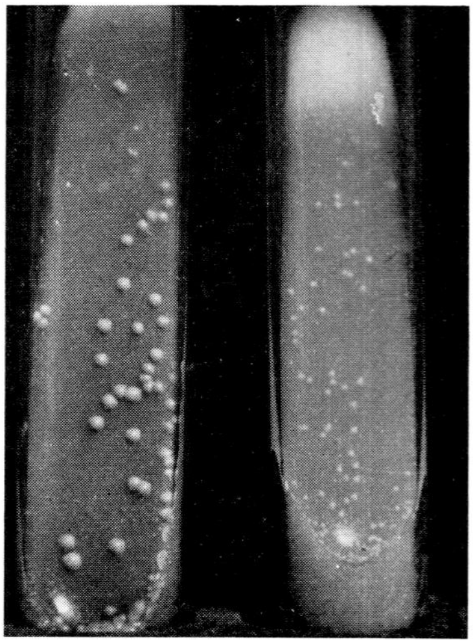

6.1. *Mycobacterium avium;* primary isolation on egg yolk agar showing enhancement of growth in presence of glycerin (*left*) compared with growth on nonglycerinated medium (*right*).

becoming roughened. The growth is creamy or sticky and is readily removable from the underlying medium. In liquid media growth occurs at the bottom as well as at the surface. Growth usually may be dispersed readily by shaking to form a turbid suspension, which is in contrast to the flocculent or granular growth of mammalian tubercle bacilli.

A definite relationship appears to exist between type of colony and virulence. Studies comparing cultures isolated from tuberculous chickens and certain similar nonchromogenic mycobacteria from humans showed that pure cultures with smooth transparent colonies were virulent for chickens; in contrast, variants with smooth-domed or rough colonies were avirulent for chickens regardless of source. The loss of virulence in *M. avium* has been associated with change from transparent to domed colonies on culture media (56).

Biochemical Properties. Cultures of *M. avium* and certain nonchromogenic strains from humans and swine have been studied with an attempt to delineate differences. There appear to be no significant biochemical distinctions between *M. avium* serotypes 1, 2, and 3 (avian tubercle bacilli)–known to be virulent for chickens–and serotypes 4–20–previously called "Battey" bacilli or *M. intracellulare* and having less virulence for chickens (42, 66). However, *M. avium* has features that separate it from other species or groups of mycobacteria (12).

M. avium does not produce niacin, does not hydrolyze Tween-80, is peroxidase-negative, produces catalase, does not have urease or arylsulfatase, and does not reduce nitrate; there are variations in these features, particularly in results of tests for arylsulfatase. Mycobacteria possess amidases that appear to be specific for certain species or closely related groups; e.g., avian tubercle bacilli are singularly lacking in certain amidases except for pyrazinamidase and nicotinamidase (8).

Detailed discussions of the biochemical features of *M. avium* and related microorganisms may be found in Karlson and Thoen (29).

Sensitivity to Antituberculosis Drugs. Generally, *M. avium* is resistant to the commonly used antituberculosis drugs compared to *M. tuberculosis* and *M. bovis.* On approximately 50 strains of *M. avium* from chickens and swine and 11 from humans, the authors found that in egg yolk agar most strains will grow in 10 μg but not in 50 μg of streptomycin/ml, in more than 10 μg of p-aminosalicylic acid/ml, and in more than 40 μg isoniazid/ml medium. On the same kind of medium a relative resistance was shown to ethambutol, ethionamide, viomycin, and pyrazinamide. The inhibitory concentration is variable, depending on the medium and procedure. Other reports are in agreement that *M. avium* has a high degree of resistance to antituberculosis agents (12). However, synergistic effects of antimycobacterial drug combinations (i.e., ethambutol and rifampicin) on *M. avium* complex have been reported (24).

Serotypes. The notable contributions of Schaefer (47) have demonstrated a number of serotypes of *M. avium* that appear to be stable even during years of artificial culture. These studies indicate that strains of *M. avium* can be identified by serologic procedures, including those that have lost their virulence for fowl. A numbering scheme has been developed for reporting *M. avium* serotypes (76). Serotypes 1, 2, and 3 occur mainly in animals, whereas 4–20 are commonly found in humans (60). Some serotypes of *M. avium* found in animals have also been isolated from humans (75). Ability to identify stable serotypes of *M. avium* provides a means for studying origin and distribution of specific strains.

A micromethod has been developed for identifying serotypes of *M. avium,* allowing for savings in time and materials compared to the tube agglutination test (61). The method is simple and can be conducted in microtiter plates in most diagnostic laboratories.

PATHOGENESIS AND EPIZOOTIOLOGY

Natural and Experimental Hosts

FOWL. All species of birds can be infected with *M. avium.* Generally speaking, domesticated fowl or captive exotic birds are affected more frequently than those living in a wild state. AT may occur in ducks, geese, swans, peacocks, pigeons, turkeys, and captive and wild birds. Parrots and canaries may also be infected. Reports of AT in domestic fowl other than chickens have been made by Scrivner and Elder (51), Feldman (14), and Francis (18).

AT is uncommon among wildfowl. However, in wild birds that frequent farm premises where AT is prevalent in chickens, the disease may be expected to develop. Pheasants seem to be unusually susceptible to infection by the avian tubercle bacillus; the disease has also been observed in sparrows, crows, barn owls, cowbirds, blackbirds, eastern sparrow hawks, starlings, wood pigeons, and whooping cranes.

TURKEYS. Turkeys are not commonly affected with AT. The disease in most instances is contracted from infected chickens and is chronic in character. Information regarding AT in turkeys has been contributed by Hinshaw et al. (23), who examined a total of 88 birds at necropsy; AT was found in 45 (51.15%). The disease was found in only 1 of 11 birds less than 1 yr of age, whereas 28 of 43 (65.12%) over 2 yr of age were tuberculous. Additional information on the disease in turkeys may be found in Feldman (14) and Francis (18).

WILD BIRDS. Accounts of AT in wild birds and reviews of the literature may be found in Feldman (14), McDiarmid (41), Francis (18), Hoybraten (26), Bickford et al. (6), Schaefer et al. (48), and Karlson (28).

AT is common among birds in many zoological gardens. In the unnatural environment of captivity the incidence frequently equals or even exceeds that for domestic fowl (43). The infectious agent in nearly all instances is the avian tubercle bacillus (57). Tuberculosis in parrots may also be due to either the human or bovine type of bacillus (1).

MAMMALS. The avian tubercle bacillus has a definite pathogenicity for some important species of domesticated mammals and at least a slight pathogenicity for others (14, 18). This should be recognized if the problem of eliminating tuberculosis is to be attacked and eventually solved.

Under conditions of natural exposure it is very exceptional for extensive tuberculosis caused by *M. avium* to develop in mammals other than rabbits and swine. Infection may occur, but the disease in most mammals remains localized. However, microorganisms may multiply in tissues for a considerable period and induce sensitivity to tuberculin. Although spontaneous infection of mammals may not be of comparable severity to that which develops in fowl, it is possible to produce extensive changes in many species of mammals by introducing the infective agent artificially. The relative pathogenicity of *M. avium* for many of the domesticated mammals is summarized in Table 6.1.

Table 6.1. Comparative pathogenicity of *M. avium* for certain mammals

Animal	Susceptibility
Cat	Highly resistant
Cattle	Infection occurs; usually localized
Deer	Infection reported
Dog	Highly resistant
Goat	Assumed to be relatively resistant
Guinea pig	Relatively resistant
Hamster	Susceptible (intratesticularly)
Horse	Assumed to be highly resistant
Human	Highly resistant
Marsupial	Infection reported
Mink	Readily infected
Monkey	Highly resistant
Mouse	Relatively resistant
Rabbit	Readily infected
Rat	Relatively resistant
Sheep	Moderately susceptible
Swine	Readily infected

In the USA and Europe *M. avium* serotype 2 is the commonest cause of tuberculous lesions in swine (27, 62, 73). Tuberculosis will remain an unnecessary economic burden on the swine industry until it is eliminated from chickens and other barnyard fowl. There has been a gradual but definite decrease of tuberculosis in swine in the USA (67–69). One reason for the decrease may be the lower incidence in poultry as a result of the increasing practice of maintaining all-pullet flocks (59).

Transmission. The tremendous number of tubercle bacilli exuded from ulcerated tuberculous lesions of the intestine in poultry creates a constant source of virulent bacteria. Although other sources of infection exist, none equals infective fecal material in dissemination of AT. Fecal discharges may contain tubercle bacilli from lesions of the liver and mucosa of the gallbladder expelled through the common duct. The respiratory tract is also a potential source of infection, especially if lesions occur in tracheal mucosa.

The contaminated environment containing bacilli-laden soil and litter is the factor of greatest importance in transmission of the disease to uninfected animals. The longer the premises have been occupied by infected birds and the more concentrated the poultry population, the more prevalent the infection is likely to be.

Avian tubercle bacilli may persist in soil for a long time. Schalk et al. (49) found a contaminated barnyard to have viable and virulent *M. avium* in litter and soil after 4 yr. These workers also demonstrated that bacteria remained viable in carcasses buried 3 ft deep for 27 mo. Virulent strains of *M. avium* have been found to survive in sawdust for 168 days at 20 C and 244 days at 37 C (50). This ability to survive outside the host presents a serious hazard to domestic and wild fowl and swine.

ROLE OF EGGS. The possibility that AT might be transmitted through eggs from tuberculous hens has long been pertinent. It has been demonstrated many times that some artificially inoculated eggs will hatch, and that chicks hatched from such eggs will be infected with tubercle bacilli. Such observations are of doubtful importance to the fundamental question: Are eggs from naturally infected chickens likely to produce tuberculous chicks? The most convincing evidence to the contrary is furnished by Fitch and Lubbenhusen (16) and Schalk et al. (49), who raised many hundreds of chicks hatched from eggs of naturally infected hens without AT being observed in a single instance. Similar conclusions have been reached by others (14, 18). However, *M. avium* has been isolated by culture of eggs from naturally infected chickens. In Germany, Fritzsche and Allam (19) found that avian tubercle bacilli were demonstrable in 3.55% of 899 eggs from 58 flocks in which AT existed. In contrast, of 650 eggs from seven commercial poultry farms only 0.31% had *M. avium;* these came from a single large farm where a few tuberculin-positive chickens were found. Also, these workers found that avian tubercle bacilli would not survive in eggs after 6 min of boiling; in preparation of scrambled eggs 2 min of frying was sufficient to kill the bacteria. Studies in Poland by Bojarski (7) revealed that *M. avium* could be cultured from 8% of 175 eggs from naturally infected hens. However, avian tubercle bacilli were recovered by culture from 8 (33.3%) of 24 eggs from artificially infected hens.

OTHER SOURCES. Other sources of dissemination of avian tubercle bacilli are carcasses of tuberculous fowl that die of the disease and offal from chickens dressed for food. It is also conceivable that cannibalism might play a part in transmission.

Avian tubercle bacilli may be carried by persons whose shoes have become soiled with fecal matter. Equipment used in care and maintenance of infected poultry (crates and feed sacks) also might be responsible for transfer of infective bacteria from diseased to healthy flocks.

Wild birds and pigeons may be infected with avian tubercle bacilli and are therefore capable of spreading *M. avium* to poultry flocks. Swine may have ulcerative intestinal lesions from avian tubercle bacilli and thus constitute a source of infection for other animals and birds. Birds such as sparrows, starlings, and pigeons that feed in farmyards are also potential sources.

Signs. Few signs of the disease in chickens are pathognomonic. However, if the disease is prevalent in a flock, several or most of the signs may be evident in different birds.

Ordinarily, if the infection has progressed sufficiently to affect physical condition, the bird will be less lively than its penmates. The affected fowl fatigues easily and appears depressed. Although appetite usually remains good, progressive and striking loss of weight commonly occurs, especially noticeable in the breast muscles (Fig. 6.2). The pectoral muscles are often atrophied, and the breastbone becomes very prominent and may be deformed. In extreme instances most of the body fat eventually disappears, and the face of the affected bird appears smaller than normal.

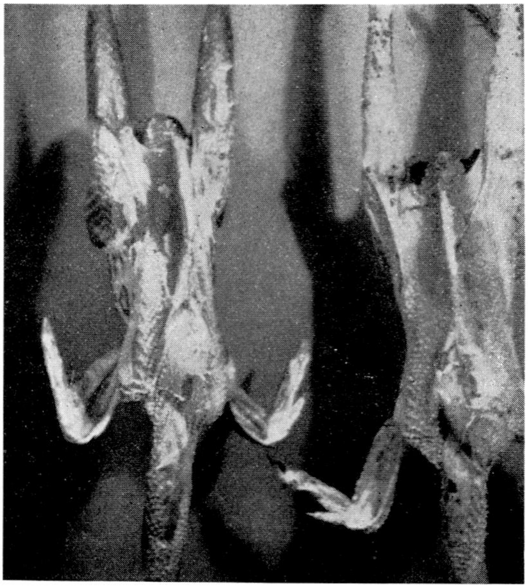

6.2. Carcasses of tuberculous chickens from flock in which disease was rampant. Note extreme atrophy of pectoral muscles.

Feathers assume a dull and ruffled appearance. Comb, wattles, and earlobes often become anemic and thinner than normal, and the uncovered epidermis has a peculiar dryness. Occasionally, however, the comb and wattles have a bluish discoloration. Icterus, indicative of hepatic changes, may be noted.

Even though the disease is severe, the temperature of the affected bird remains within the normal range. In many instances the bird reveals a unilateral lameness and walks with a peculiar jerky hopping gait, probably the result of tuberculous involvement of bone marrow of the leg. Infrequently, a wing may droop, owing to tuberculous involvement of the humeral scapulocoracoid articulation, which may rupture and discharge fluid or caseous material. Paralysis from tuberculous arthritis sometimes occurs.

If the affected chicken is greatly emaciated, one may detect nodular masses along the intestine by palpation of the abdomen. However, the great hypertrophy of the liver of many tuberculous birds may make this procedure difficult or impossible. Most tuberculous chickens have lesions along the intestinal tract; if these are ulcerative, severe diarrhea results. The enteric disturbance induces extreme weakness, and the affected bird assumes a sitting position as a result of exhaustion.

Affected birds may die within a few months or live for many, depending on severity or extent of the disease. A bird may die suddenly as a consequence of hemorrhage from rupture of the affected liver or spleen.

Gross Lesions. Lesions are seen most frequently in liver, spleen, intestines, and bone marrow. The bacillemia, which probably occurs intermittently and perhaps early in most instances, provides for a generalized distribution of lesions. None of the tissues, with the possible exception of the central nervous system, appears to be immune from infection. Some of the organs, such as heart, ovaries, testes, and skin, are affected infrequently and cannot be considered organs of predilection. Francis (18) reviewed the available literature and found that for turkeys, ducks, and pigeons, lesions predominate in liver and spleen but occur also in many other organs.

AT in fowl is characterized by occurrence of irregular grayish yellow or grayish white nodules of varying sizes in organs of predilection such as liver, spleen and intestine (Figs. 6.3, 6.4, 6.5). Involvement of liver and spleen results in hypertrophy, which is often significant; fatal hemorrhage from rupture may result. The tuberculous nodule varies in size from a barely discernible structure to a huge mass that may measure several centimeters in diameter. Large nodules frequently have an irregular knobby contour, with smaller granulations or nodules often present over the surface. Lesions near the surface in such organs as liver and spleen are enucleated easily from adjacent tissues. Nodules are firm but can be incised easily, since mineral salts are not present. On cross section a fibrous nodule containing a variable number of small yellowish foci or a single soft yellowish central region, which is frequently caseous, may be observed. The latter is surrounded by a fibrous capsule, the continuity of which often is interrupted by small circumscribed necrotic foci. The fibrous capsule varies in thickness and consistency, depending on size and duration of lesions. It is barely discernible or apparently absent in small lesions and measures 0.1–0.2 cm in thickness in larger nodules.

Number of lesions is also variable, ranging from a few to innumerable. It is rather common to

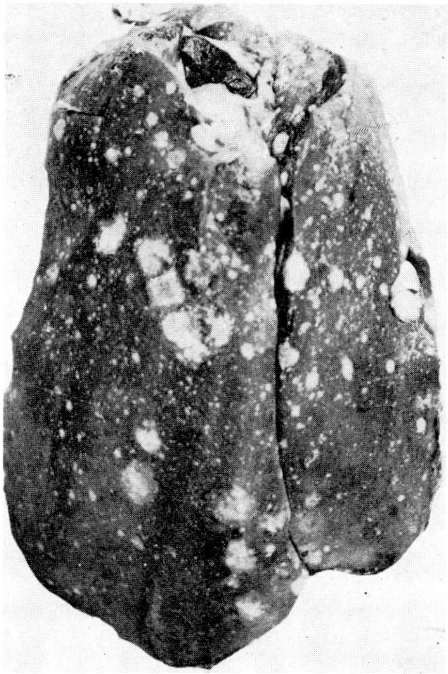

6.3. Tuberculous lesions in liver of naturally infected chicken.

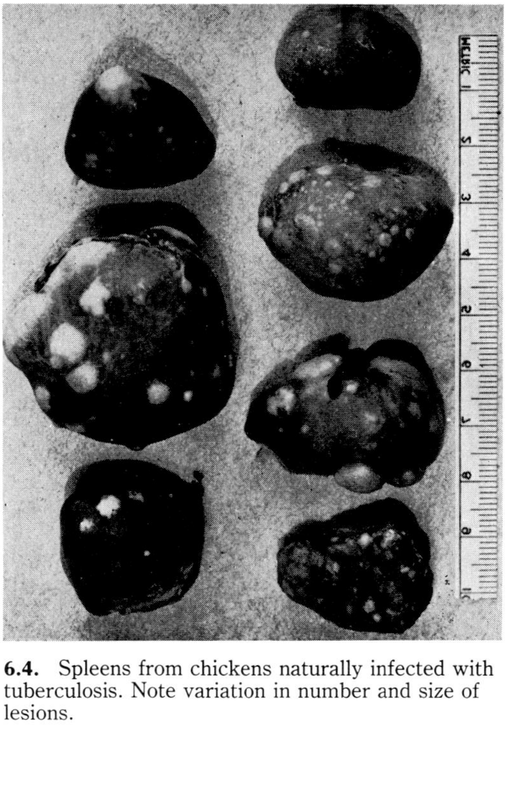

6.4. Spleens from chickens naturally infected with tuberculosis. Note variation in number and size of lesions.

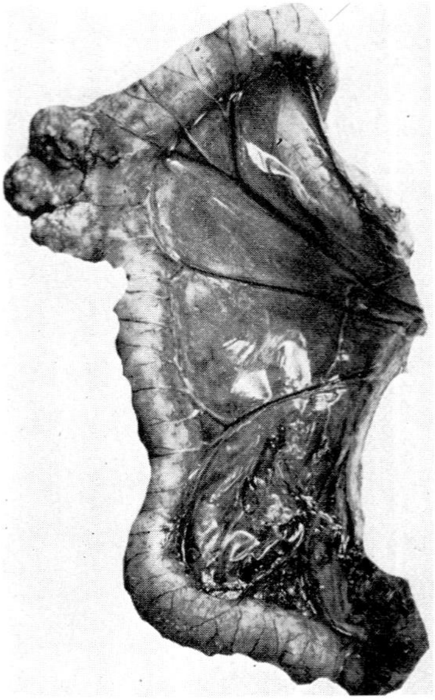

6.5. Large, nodulated tuberculous lesions in wall of small intestine of chickens.

observe a few nodular lesions in organs such as liver and spleen associated with an enormous number of lesions of minute to moderate size. Variation in size is a consequence of successive episodes or reinfection from previously established lesions, usually of the same organ. Involvement of lungs is usually less severe than that of liver or spleen (Fig. 6.6).

The marked tendency of the disease to disseminate to several organs indicates that tuberculous bacillemia is common. This tendency of the bacilli to circulate within the bloodstream provides the explanation for frequent involvement of bone marrow (Figs. 6.7, 6.8). Infection of bone marrow probably occurs very early in the course of the disease and is characterized by hypertrophy of myeloid tissues; by disappearance of most of the bony spicules; and finally by formation of tuberculous nodules, which may be numerous and visible to the unaided eye or few and microscopic.

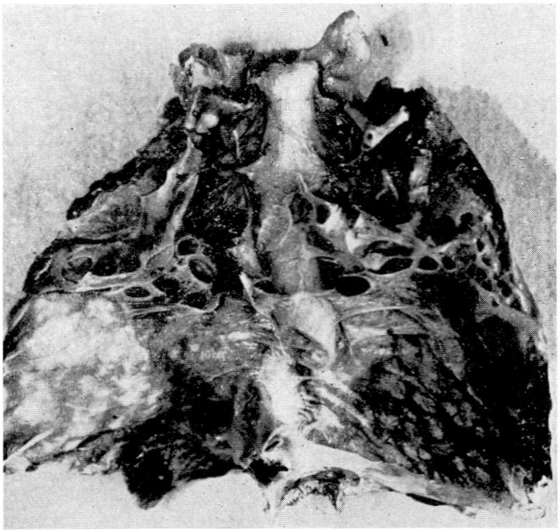

6.6. Unusually massive tuberculous involvement of lung of naturally infected chicken.

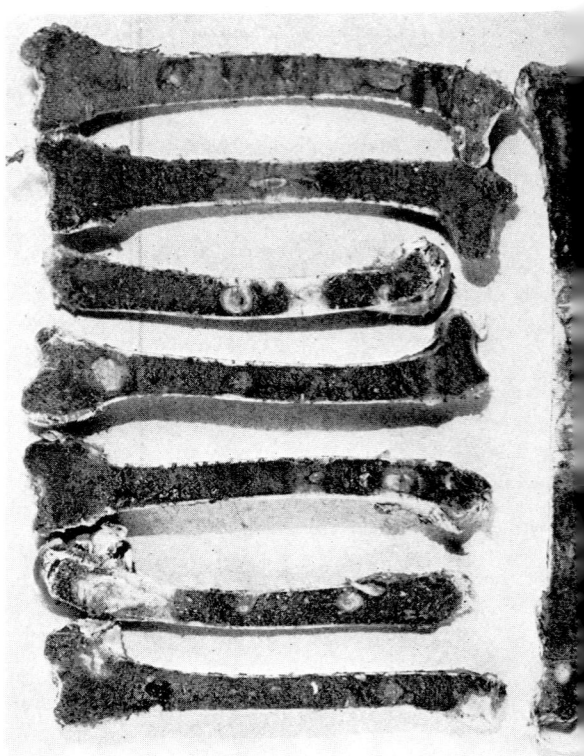

6.7. Several femurs and one tibia from chickens naturally infected with tuberculosis, showing lesions in myeloid tissue and some well-marked osteoplastic changes caused by the infection.

Histopathology. In chickens the tubercle may be observed experimentally 10–14 days postinfection as a closely packed collection of pale-staining cells with vesiculated nuclei. These epithelioid cells are derived from fixed tissue elements known as histiocytes. The latter cells phagocytose tubercle bacilli early in the reactive process.

The cellular mass or primary tubercle gradually expands as histiocytes proliferate at the periphery; within 3–4 wk signs or retrogression can be detected in epithelioid cells in the central zone. This retrogression is due partly to the avascularity of the structure and partly to the toxic substances of the tubercle bacilli. As the cellular mass becomes larger, epithelioid cells have a

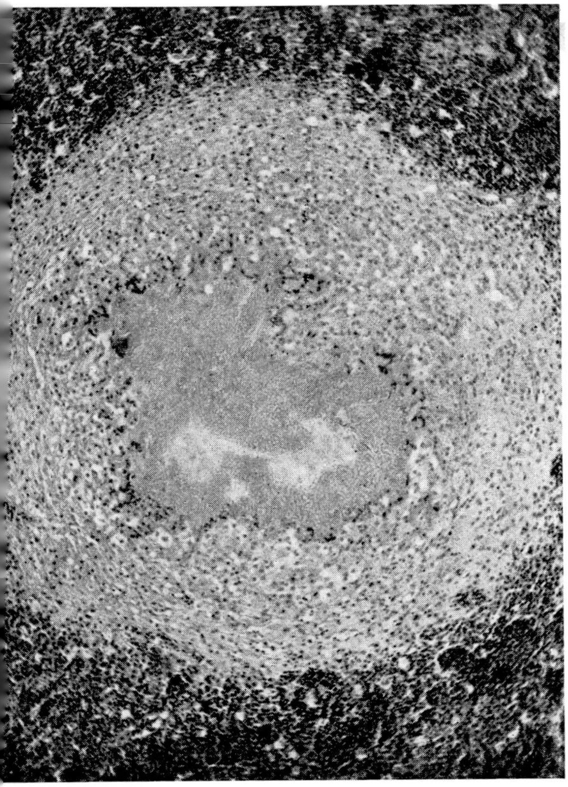

6.8. Small tuberculous nodule in bone marrow of naturally infected chicken. Central necrotic region is surrounded by zone of dense connective tissue. ×100.

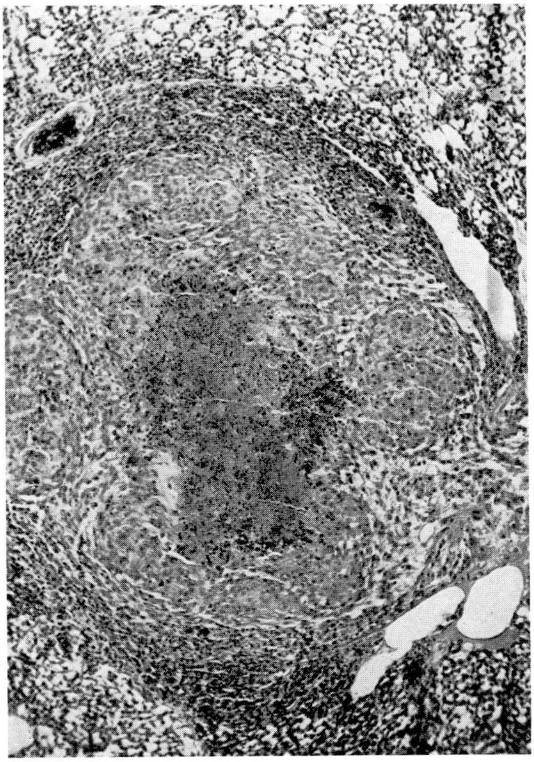

6.9. Developing tubercle in lung of chicken. ×100.

tendency to fuse and form syncytia. Outlines of the individual cells become less distinct or disappear. Vacuoles appear, and the staining reaction is more acidophilic. This is followed within a week or so by a necrobiotic change resembling coagulation necrosis. Nuclei or epithelioid cells become pyknotic and may disappear; the cellular mass, except the peripheral portion, becomes fused and stains deeply with eosin. The tubercle bacilli have multiplied and appear singly or in clumps throughout the necrotic tissue.

While the epithelioid cells in the central zone undergo necrobiotic changes, there persists an outer zone of epithelioid syncytia appearing as a mantle around the entire periphery. From these, giant cells are developed, the nuclei of which are situated distally to the central zone of necrosis; the cells are arranged rather frequently in palisade formation. Large vacuoles often occur in cytoplasm of giant cells. Immediately peripheral to the zone of giant cells there is a more or less diffuse collection of epithelioid cells and their progenitors, histiocytes (Fig. 6.9). Fibrocytes and minute blood vascular channels also occur near the outer portion of the peripheral area. Although bacilli are more numerous in the central or necrotic zone of the tubercle, they are also found in large numbers in the epithelioid zone adjacent and distal to giant cells.

The final phase in formation of a tubercle is development of a zone of encapsulation consisting of fibrous connective tissue, histiocytes, some lymphocytes, and an occasional eosinophilic granulocyte. New tubercles develop in the epithelioid zone immediately peripheral to giant cells. Consequently, a tubercle, as recognized grossly, consists of the original or parent tubercle and several smaller or adjacent ones.

The nature of the degenerative process in the central zone of the tubercle is somewhat unusual in that the integrity of the cells is maintained for a considerable period before disintegration. Caseous necrosis eventually occurs and may affect all or part of the central zone.

Calcification of the tubercle rarely occurs in fowl. Amyloidlike degeneration of portions or the surrounding parenchymal element sometimes is observed in liver, spleen, and kidney.

Acid-fast bacilli occur in great numbers in smears of lesions and appropriately stained sections (Fig. 6.10).

Microscopically, lesions of AT in turkeys vary

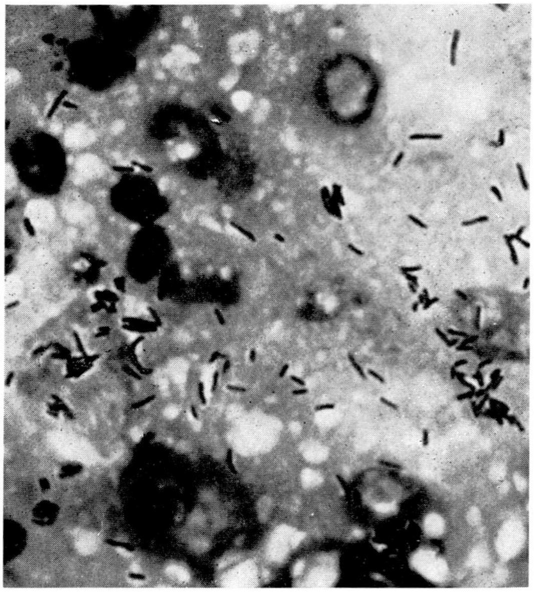

6.10. Numerous acid-fast tubercle bacilli in smear preparation from small lesion of lung of naturally infected chicken. Ziehl-Neelsen, ×1600.

considerably. In some, tubercles like those seen in AT of chickens are present. In other instances lesions are diffuse, with extensive destruction of surrounding parenchyma. Cytoplasmic masses or large giant cells may be numerous, and large numbers of eosinophilic granulocytes are commonly present. Some lesions become circumscribed by a broad, dense zone of fibrous connective tissue.

Detailed descriptions of gross and microscopic lesions of AT in the different organs of birds will be found in Feldman (14), Francis (18), and Thoen et al. (65).

Immunity. The capacity of *M. avium* complex to produce progressive disease may be related to certain complex lipids present in the cell wall, such as cord factor, sulfur-containing glycolipids (sulfatides), or strongly acidic lipids (58). However, it appears that the effect of these components alone or together on phagosome-lysosome fusion cannot account for virulence. Delayed-type hypersensitivity (DTH) develops following exposure to mycobacteria; once activated, macrophages demonstrate an increased capacity to kill intracellular *M. avium* (54). The DTH responses are mediated by lymphocytes, which release lymphokines that act to attract, immobilize, and activate blood-borne mononuclear cells at the site where virulent bacilli or their products exist. Recently, it has been reported that tumor necrosis factor, alone or in combination with interleukin-2, but not gamma interferon, is associated with macrophage killing of *M. avium* serotype 1 (4). The DTH that develops contributes to accelerated tubercle formation and is in part, responsible for cell-mediated immunity in tuberculosis. Activated macrophages that lack sufficient subcellular microbicidal components to kill virulent tubercle bacilli are destroyed by the intracellular growth of the organism, and a lesion develops. Available information indicates a combination of toxic lipids and factors released by virulent *M. avium* may 1) cause disruption of the phagosome, 2) inhibit phagolysosome formation, 3) interfere with release of hydrolytic enzymes from the attached lysosomes, and/or 4) inactivate lysosomal enzymes released into the cytoplasmic vacuole. The role of cyclic guanine monophospate (GMP) or the ratio of cyclic GMP to cyclic adenosine monophosphate (AMP) in altering mononuclear cell functions in naturally occurring *M. avium* infections needs investigation. Available information suggests that toxic oxygen metabolites are not responsible for killing in activated macrophages (54). However, the significance of hydrogen peroxide or of activated oxygen radical(s), such as superoxide anions and singlet oxygen, in resistant macrophages of birds exposed to virulent *M. avium* remains to be elucidated.

DIAGNOSIS.

A presumptive diagnosis of AT in fowl can usually be made on the basis of gross lesions. However, finding acid-fast organisms in smears of infected liver, spleen, or other organs stained with a stain such as Ziehl-Neelsen is very helpful in diagnosis. Inoculation of suitable media to isolate and identify the causative agent is necessary for definite diagnosis of AT (29).

Tuberculin Test. When administered properly, the tuberculin test provides a satisfactory procedure for determining presence of AT in a flock.

TECHNIQUE. Equipment consists of a sterile tuberculin syringe (1-ml capacity) and a supply of sterile 25–26 gauge hypodermic needles 0.5 in. (1.3 cm) in length. Absorbent cotton and 70% alcohol should also be available. Tuberculin should be that prepared for intradermic use from avian tubercle bacilli. That prepared from mammalian strains of tubercle bacilli may elicit positive reactions in tuberculous chickens, but results are generally unsatisfactory. The reactions to avian tuberculin are usually more pronounced.

The bird should be restrained so that the head is entirely immobile. The surface of the wattle should be cleaned with alcohol; other attempts to clean or disinfect the skin are unnecessary. The needle is inserted carefully into the lateral aspect of the dermis, and 0.03–0.05 ml tuberculin is injected into the tissue. The purified protein derivative tuberculin presently supplied by the USDA is prepared from synthetic liquid culture medium on which *M. avium* strain D-4 has grown for 8 wk (3).

The tuberculoproteins are precipitated using ammonium sulfate. The protein concentration is adjusted to 1 mg phosphorus/ml with phosphate-buffered saline. A small bleb or diffuse blanched area will appear where tuberculin was deposited. Although fairly satisfactory results may follow if tuberculin is injected into subcutaneous tissue, it is a better practice to inject it intradermally.

REACTION. After 48 hr the chickens are examined. The opposite uninjected wattle is used for comparison. A positive reaction is indicated by soft swelling in tissues of the injected wattle (Fig. 6.11). Some reactions are small; others result in pronounced swelling that increases the thickness of the wattle one to five times. The swelling is due largely to edema that occurs in the zone of connective tissue lying between layers of the dermis. To a lesser extent, swelling is due to increased width of the corium, which is filled with closely packed mononuclear histiocytic cells, a few eosinophilic granulocytes, and a variable number of lymphoid cells and lymphocytes. After 48 hr the swelling gradually subsides and usually disappears within 5 days.

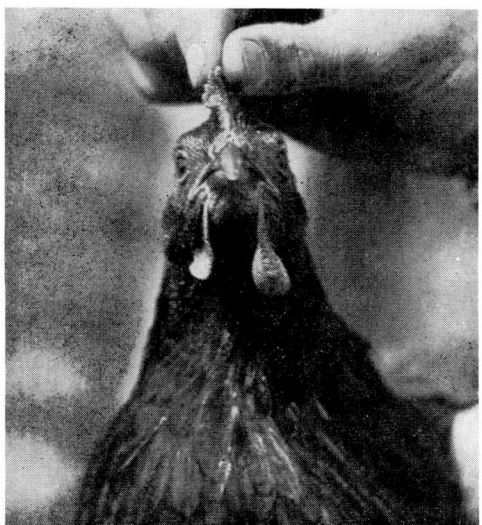

6.11. Positive reaction in left wattle of tuberculous chicken 48 hr after intradermal injection of avian tuberculin.

Sometimes a negative reaction will appear in a bird that is definitely tuberculous; conversely, a positive result is sometimes obtained in chickens in which signs of AT cannot be demonstrated. In the latter instance, failure to find lesions does not imply that tubercle bacilli are not present in tissues of the chicken. If the disease is in an early stage, lesions are likely to be too small to be noted grossly or too few to be found by ordinary methods of examination. A definitely positive tuberculin test indicates that the bird has been exposed to avian tubercle bacilli.

Tuberculin is a bacteria-free concentrated filtrate prepared from a liquid culture of tubercle bacilli and, as used for diagnosis of AT in chickens, may be considered harmless to normal birds. If retests are done after an interval of 1 mo, false-positive reactions will not occur. In chickens the usual diagnostic dose of tuberculin does not sensitize the nontuberculous bird to subsequent injections of the same product.

The tuberculin test has been used to a limited extent in diagnosing AT of turkeys. However, for the most part results have been less satisfactory than for chickens. Certain difficulties are encountered also in tuberculin testing of pigeons and ducks. For pigeons Svrcek et al. (55) applied the test in the submandibular area. For Japanese quail tuberculin may be injected intradermally in the area around the vent (32). The test is of limited value in diagnosing AT in these birds.

Usefulness of the tuberculin test in diagnosis of AT in turkeys has not been adequately established. Hinshaw et al. (23), using avian tuberculin, injected the snood, mucosa of the cloaca, wattle, skin of the edge of the wing web, and skin at the center of the wing web. Test results indicated that reactions in the wattle agreed with the findings at necropsy in only 11.1% of the birds, and that there was agreement between the tuberculin reaction in the wing web and findings at necropsy in 75.68% of the birds. From the meager information available, one must conclude that the intradermic tuberculin test has been less reliable for detecting AT in turkeys than in chickens. It would seem desirable to investigate reliability of the rapid agglutination test as a means of detecting AT in live turkeys.

Serology

RAPID AGGLUTINATION TEST. A whole-blood agglutination test of possible diagnostic value for AT in fowl was described by Karlson et al. (30). The antigen is a 10% suspension of avian tubercle bacilli in 0.85% sodium chloride solution containing 0.5% phenol. Blood is obtained by pricking the comb with a sharp instrument such as an 18-gauge needle. A drop of fresh blood is mixed with a drop of antigen on a warm plate. Appearance of agglutination in 1 min is considered a positive test, as shown in Fig 6.12.

In chickens the whole-blood agglutination test may have a reliability comparable to that of the tuberculin test. Hiller et al. (22) compared the agglutination test and the tuberculin test in flocks where, on the same farm, so-called nonspecific tuberculin reactions were found in cattle. In 290 flocks, 38.3% of the birds reacted to the serologic test compared to 18.4% to the tuberculin test;

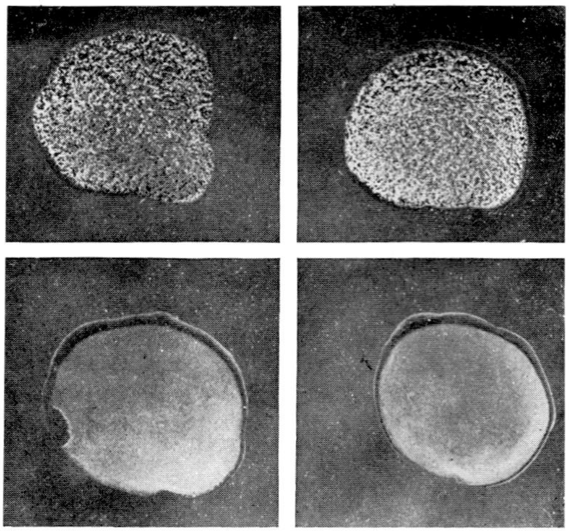

6.12. Results of four tests from four different chickens, two of which were tuberculous and two not. Upper row shows characteristic agglutination. Blood was obtained from tuberculin-positive chickens, and lesions were found at necropsy. Lower row shows failure to agglutinate. Negative reactions agreed with results of tuberculin tests; lesions not found at necropsy. (from 30).

77.2% had postmortem or bacteriologic evidence of AT. It was concluded that the agglutination test was more useful than the tuberculin test for detecting infected birds in a diseased flock; however, occurrence of false-positive agglutination reactions in healthy birds is a drawback.

ENZYME-LINKED IMMUNOSORBENT ASSAY (ELISA). ELISA has been described for use in detecting mycobacterial antibodies in serums of chickens experimentally inoculated with *M. avium* serotype 2 (64). Positive ELISA reactions were observed in serums of chickens 2, 4, 6, and 8 wk after intramuscular (IM) inoculation; no reactions were observed in uninfected controls. Tuberculin skin tests did not induce positive reactions in uninfected chickens. ELISA has also been used for detecting antibodies in serums of tuberculous birds maintained in captivity (9). Since only a small amount of serum is required, the test may be of practical value for use in diagnosis of AT in small species as well as exotic birds without wattles. ELISA reagents can be readily standardized. Moreover, the test is a rapid, simple procedure that can be readily automated to allow for screening large numbers of birds.

Serologic procedures offer certain practical advantages. Birds need to be handled only once, and samples of blood submitted for agglutination tests for pullorum disease may be examined for presence of specific mycobacterial antibodies. Reliability of serologic tests for use in detection of AT in captive exotic and wild fowl should be explored.

Differential Diagnosis. The most expedient way to diagnose the disease is by necropsy. Lesions are rather characteristic, but other conditions must be differentiated. These include neoplasia, enterohepatitis, and possibly fowl cholera and fowl typhoid. Presence of numerous acid-fast bacilli in lesions is especially significant because they do not occur in any other known disease of chickens. Proof of diagnosis depends on laboratory studies to establish the microorganism as *M. avium*.

TREATMENT.

Antituberculosis drugs are not often used to treat domestic fowl. However, combinations of these drugs have been utilized in treatment of certain exotic birds maintained in captivity (70). Clinical remission was observed in three birds that received a combination of isoniazid (30 mg/kg), ethambutol (30 mg/kg), and rifampicin (45 mg/kg). The recommended duration of therapy was 18 mo provided there are no adverse side effects. Additional investigations are needed to develop suitable regimens for treatment of tuberculosis in various exotic herds.

PREVENTION AND CONTROL.

Widespread distribution of the disease, its high incidence in some areas, and importance of the poultry and swine industries make it imperative that measures be devised for control and eradication.

The tuberculin test is of considerable practical value. Removal of chickens that react eliminates many foci of infection. The test enables detection of many infected fowl before the disease reaches a severe or chronic state; if repeated tests are made and reactors removed, dissemination of the bacteria to the environment may be reduced. The whole-blood agglutination test also may serve to detect infected birds. Hiller et al. (22) concluded that this rapid serologic test was more useful than the tuberculin test for detecting tuberculous chickens in a diseased flock.

If the residual flock is permitted to occupy the same contaminated premises, a continuing source of infection remains. This provides opportunity for new infections to occur indefinitely, since avian tubercle bacilli may remain viable and virulent in the soil for years. Neither the tuberculin nor agglutination test can be depended on for detection of every tuberculous fowl. As long as one infected bird remains in a flock, dissemination of the disease to healthy fowl is possible. Consequently, means other than the tuberculin test must be used if a more satisfactory control of AT is to be expected.

It has been stated frequently that AT can be controlled if all birds in the flock are disposed of after the first laying season. The practice is commendable, especially since it is economically sound from the point of view of egg production. Older birds usually produce fewer eggs; furthermore, mortality from nonbacterial disease such as neoplasia is greater among older hens than pullets. Another factor in favor of disposal of old stock is that AT is usually more severe in older birds, which as a consequence are more likely to become depots of dissemination.

Use of vaccines containing inactivated and/or live mycobacteria for protecting chickens against tuberculosis has been evaluated (45). The best results were obtained in chickens vaccinated with live *M. intracellulare* serotype 6 (*M. avium* serotype 6) given orally. These fowl showed 70% protection after IM challenge with *M. avium.* Encouraging results were also reported in chickens after combined IM vaccination with inactivated plus live *M. intracellulare* serotype 7 and serotype Darden (*M. avium* serotypes 7 and 19). Additional investigations are needed to confirm the efficacy of various vaccines in exotic birds.

Procedures for establishing and maintaining AT-free flocks should include the following: 1) Abandon old equipment and establish other facilities on new soil. Ordinarily it is impractical to render an infected environment satisfactorily safe by disinfection. 2) Provide proper fencing or other measures to prevent unrestricted movement of chickens, thus preventing exposure from previously infected premises. 3) Eliminate the old flock, burning carcasses of birds that show lesions of tuberculosis. 4) Establish a new flock in the new environment from AT-free stock. 5) Eliminate from swine herds all reactors to avian and mammalian tuberculin. If chickens in a clean flock are prevented from access to an infected environment and are protected against accidental exposure to tubercle bacilli, it is reasonable to believe they will remain free from AT.

The measures just mentioned are not complicated. Additional profits that will accrue from an AT-free flock maintained in a hygienic environment will compensate for the initial expense and work. The general health of birds will be better, and disease other than AT will be controlled more satisfactorily. Benefits will also be reflected in a decrease in tuberculosis in swine. The importance of AT in infection of swine is such that if chickens were maintained entirely separate and apart, the incidence of tuberculosis of swine from *M. avium* would be reduced.

Recommendations for control of AT in exotic birds include the following: 1) Prevent contact with tuberculous birds; premises and housing previously used by them are to be avoided. 2) Quarantine additions to the aviary for 60 days and retest with avian tuberculin. Studies should be made to confirm the validity of vaccination trials made in chickens for protection of various exotic species against the disease.

REFERENCES

1. Ackerman, L.J., S.C. Benbrook, and B.C. Walton. 1974. Mycobacterium tuberculosis infection in a parrot (Amazona farinosa). Annu Rev Respir Dis 109:388–390.
2. Andersen, S. 1965. The distribution of avian tuberculosis in Denmark. Medlemsbl Dan Dyrlaegeforen 2:54–59.
3. Angus, R.D. 1978. Production of reference PPD tuberculins for veterinary use in the United States. J Biol Stand 6:221–228.
4. Bermudez, L., and L. Young. 1988. Tumor necrosis factor, alone or in combination with IL-2, but not IFN-γ, is associated with macrophage killing of Mycobacterium avium complex. J Immunol 140:3006–3013.
5. Bertram, M. Inderlied, C. Yadegar, S. Kolanoski, P. Yamada, and Young, L. 1986. Confirmation of the beige mouse model for study of disseminated infection with Mycobacterium avium complex. J Infect Dis 154:194–195.
6. Bickford, A.A., G.H. Ellis, and H.E. Moses. 1966. Epizootiology of tuberculosis in starlings. J Am Vet Med Assoc 149:312–318.
7. Bojarski, J. 1968. Occurrence of Mycobacterium in eggs of tuberculin-positive hens. Med Weter 24:21–23.
8. Bonicke, R. 1962. Identification of mycobacteria by biochemical methods. Bull Int Union against Tuberc 32:13–68.
9. Bush, M.A., R.J. Montali, C.O. Thoen, E.E. Smith, W. Peritino, and D.W. Johnson. 1978. Avian tuberculosis: status of antemortem diagnostic procedures. Proc 1st Int Birds in Captivity Symp, pp. 185–195.
10. Cooper, J.E., L. Karstad, and E. Boughton. 1975. Tuberculosis in lesser flamingos in Kenya. J Wildl Dis 11:32–36.
11. Cornil, V., and P. Mégnin. 1884. Tuberculose et diphtherie des gallinaces. CR Soc Biol 36:617–621.
12. Engbaek, H.C., E.H. Runyon, and A.G. Karlson. 1971. Mycobacterium avium Chester: Designation of neotype strain. Int J System Bacteriol 21:192–196.
13. Falk, G.A., S.J. Hadley, F.E. Sharkey, M. Liss, and C. Muschenheim. 1973. Mycobacterium avium infections in man. Am J Med 54:801–810.
14. Feldman, W.H. 1938. Avian Tuberculosis Infections. Williams & Williams, Baltimore, MD.
15. Feldman, W.H. 1947. Animal tuberculosis and its relationship to the disease in man. Ann NY Acad Sci 48:469–505.
16. Fitch, C.P., and R.E. Lubbenhusen. 1928. Completed experiments to determine whether avian tuberculosis can be transmitted through eggs of tuberculous fowls. J Am Vet Med Assoc 72:636–649.
17. Fodstad, F.H. 1967. A survey of mycobacterial infections detected in animals in Norway in 1966. Medlemsbl Nor Veterinaerforen 19:314–327.
18. Francis, J. 1958. Tuberculosis in Animals and Man: A Study in Comparative Pathology. Cassell, London.
19. Fritzsche, K., and M.S.A.M. Allam. 1965. The contamination of hen eggs with mycobacteria. Arch Lebensmittelhyg 16:248–250.
20. Good, R.C. 1985. Opportunistic pathogens in the genus Mycobacterium. Annu Rev Microbiol 39:347–369.
21. Greene, J., G. Sidhu, S. Lewin, J. Levine, H. Masur, M. Simberkoff, P. Nicholas, R. Good, S. Zolla-Pazner, A. Pollock, R. Tapper, and M. Holzman. 1982. Mycobacterium avium-intracellulare: A cause of disseminated life-threatening infection in homosexuals and drug abusers. Ann Int Med 97:539–546.
22. Hiller, K., T. Schliesser, G. Fink, and P. Dorn. 1967. Zur serologischen Diagnose der Huhnertuberku-

lose. Berl Muench Tieraerztl Wochenschr 80:212–216.

23. Hinshaw, W.R., K.W. Niemann, and W.H. Busic. 1932. Studies of tuberculosis of turkeys. J Am Vet Med Assoc 80:765–777.

24. Hoffner, S.E., S.B. Svenson, and G. Kallenius. 1987. Synergistic effects of antimycobacterial drug combinations on Mycobacterium avium complex determined radiometrically in liquid medium. Eur J Clin Microbiol 6:530–535.

25. Horsburgh, C.R., Jr., U.G. Mason, D.C. Farhi, and M.D. Iseman. 1985. Disseminated infection with Mycobacterium avium-intracellulare. Medicine 64:36–48.

26. Hoybraten, P. 1959. Tuberkulose tiefeller nos fuglen. Nord Vet Med 11:780–786.

27. Jorgensen, J.B. 1978. Serological investigations of strains of Mycobacterium avium and Mycobacterium intracellulare isolated from animals and nonanimal sources. Nord Vet Med 30:155–162.

28. Karlson, A.G. 1978. Avian Tuberculosis. In R.J. Montali (ed.), Mycobacterial Infections of Zoo Animals, pp. 21–24. Smithsonian Institution Press, Washington.

29. Karlson, A.G., and C.O. Thoen. 1980. Tuberculosis. In S.B. Hitchner, C.H. Domermuth, H.G. Purchase, and J.E. Williams (eds.), Isolation and Identification of Avian Pathogens, 2nd Ed., pp 36–39. Am Assoc Avian Pathol, Kennett Square, PA.

30. Karlson, A.G., M.R. Zinober, and W.H. Feldman. 1950. A whole blood rapid agglutination test for avian tuberculosis. Am J Vet Res 11:137–141.

31. Karlson, A.G., C.L. Davis, and M.L. Cohn. 1962. Skotochromogenic Mycobacterium avium from a trumpeter swan. Am J Vet Res 23:575–579.

32. Karlson, A.G., C.O. Thoen, and R. Harrington. 1970. Japanese quail: Susceptibility to avian tuberculosis. Avian Dis 14:39–44.

33. Kiehn, T., F. Edwards, P. Brannon, A. Tsang, M. Maio, J. Gold, E. Whimbey, B. Wong, K. McClatchy, and D. Armstrong. 1985. Infections caused by Mycobacterium avium complex in immunocompromised patients: Diagnosis by blood culture and fecal examination, antimicrobial susceptibility tests, and morphological and seroagglutination characteristics. J Clin Microbiol 21:168–173.

34. Kleeberg, H.H. 1975. Tuberculosis and other Mycobacterioses. In W.T. Hubbert, W.F. McCulloch, and P.R. Schnurrenberger (eds.), Diseases Transmitted from Animals to Man, 6th Ed., pp.303–360. Charles C. Thomas, Springfield, IL.

35. Koch, R. 1890. Ueber bakteriologische Forschung. Wien Med Bl 13:531–535.

36. Koch, R. 1902. Address before the second general meeting. Trans Br Congr Tuberc 1:23–35.

37. Kubin, M., and E. Matuskova. 1968. Serological typing of mycobacteria for tracing possible sources of avian mycobacterial infections in man. Bull WHO 39:657–662.

38. Lesslie, I.W., and K.J. Birn. 1967. Tuberculosis in cattle caused by the avian type tubercle bacillus. Vet Rec 80:559–564.

39. Maffucci, A. 1890. Beitrag zur Aetiologie der Tuberkulose (Huhnertuberculose). Zentralbl Allg Pathol Pathol Anat 1:409–416.

40. Matthews, P.R.J., J.A. McDiarmid, P. Collins, and A. Brown. 1977. The dependence of some strains of Mycobacterium avium on mycobactin for initial and subsequent growth. J Med Microbiol 2:53–57.

41. McDiarmid, A. 1948. The occurence of tuberculosis in the wild wood-pigeon. J Comp Pathol Ther 58:128–133.

42. Meissner, G., K.H. Schroder, G.E. Amadio, W. Anz, S. Chaparas, H.W.B. Engel, P.A. Jenkins, W. Kappler, H.H. Kleeberg, E. Kubala, M. Kubin, D. Lauterbach, A. Lind, M. Magnusson, Z.D. Mikova, S.R. Pattyn, W.B. Schaefer, J.L. Stanford, M. Tsukamura, L.G. Wayne, I. Willers, and E. Wolinsky. 1974. A cooperative numerical analysis of nonscoto- and nonphoto-chromogenic slowly growing mycobacteria. J Gen Microbiol 83:207–235.

43. Montali, R.J., M. Bush, C.O. Thoen, and E. Smith. 1976. Tuberculosis in captive exotic birds. J Am Vet Med Assoc 169:920–927.

44. Myers, J.A., and J.H. Steele, 1969. Bovine Tuberculosis: Control in Man and Animals. Warren H. Green, St. Louis.

45. Rossi, L. 1974. Immunizing potency of inactivated and living Mycobacterium avium and Mycobacterium intracellulare vaccines against tuberculosis of domestic fowls. Acta Vet Brno 43:133–138.

46. Schack-Steffenhagen, G., and J. Seeger. 1967. Untersuchungen uber das Vorkommen von Geflugeltuberkelbakterien beiauslandischen Schlachthuhnern. Zentralbl Bakteriol Parasitenkd Abt I [orig] 202:204–211.

47. Schaefer, W.B. 1965. Serologic identification and classification of the atypical mycobacteria by their agglutination. Am Rev Respir Dis 92:85–93.

48. Schaefer, W.B., J.V. Beer, N.A. Wood, E. Boughton, P.A. Jenkins, and J. Marks. 1973. A bacteriological study of endemic tuberculosis in birds. J Hyg (Camb) 71:549–557.

49. Schalk, A.F., L.M. Roderick, H.L. Foust, and G.S. Harshfield. 1935. Avian Tuberculosis: Collected Studies. North Dakota Agric Exp Stn Tech Bull 279.

50. Schliesser, T., and A. Weber. 1973. Untersuchungen uber die Tenazitat von Mykobakterien der Gruppe III nach runyon in Sagemehleinstreu. Zentralbl Veterinaermed [B] 20:710–714.

51. Scrivner, L.H., and C. Elder. 1931. Cutaneous and subcutaneous tuberculosis in turkeys. J Am Vet Med Assoc 79:244–247.

52. Stafseth, H.J., R.J. Biggar, W.W. Thompson, and L. Neu. 1934. The cultivation and egg-transmission of the avian tubercle bacillus. J Am Vet Med Assoc 85:342–359.

53. Stenberg, H., and A. Turunen. 1968. Differentiation of mycobacteria isolated from domestic animals. Zentralbl Veterinaermed [B] 15:494–503.

54. Stokes, R., I. Orme, and F. Collins. 1986. Role of mononuclear phagocytes in expression of resistance and susceptibility to Mycobacterium avium infections in mice. Infect Immun 54:811–819.

55. Svrcek, S., O.J. Vrtiak, B. Kapitancik, T. Pauer, and Z. Koppel. 1966. Wild birds and domestic pigeons as sources of avian tuberculosis. Rozhl Tuberk 26:659–67.

56. Thoen, C.O. 1979. Factors associated with pathogenicity of mycobacteria. In R. Schlessinger (ed.), Microbiology – 1979, pp. 162–167. Am Soc Microbiol, Washington, DC.

57. Thoen, C.O., and Himes, E.M. 1981. Tuberculosis. In J.W. Davis, L.H. Karstad, and D.O. Trainer (eds.), Infectious Diseases of Wild Mammals, 2nd Ed., pp. 263–274. Iowa State Univ Press, Ames.

58. Thoen, C.O., and Himes, E. M. 1986. Mycobacterium. In L. L. Gyles and C.O. Thoen (eds.), Pathogenesis of Bacterial Infections in Animals, pp. 26–37. Iowa State Univ Press, Ames.

59. Thoen, C.O., and A.G. Karlson. 1981. Tuberculosis. In A.D. Leman, R.D. Glock, W.L. Mengeling, R.H.C. Penny, E. Scholl, and B. Straw (eds.), Diseases of Swine, 5th Ed., pp.508–516. Iowa State Univ Press, Ames.

60. Thoen, C.O., A.G. Karlson, and A.F. Ranney. 1972. Epidemiology of infections with serotypes of Mycobacterium avium complex in swine and other species. Proc 76th Annu Meet US Anim Health Assoc, pp.423–426.

61. Thoen, C.O., J.L. Jarnagin, and M.L. Champion. 1975. Micromethod for serotyping strains of Mycobacterium avium. J Clin Microbiol 1:469–471.

62. Thoen, C.O., J.L. Jarnagin, and W.D. Richards. 1975. Isolation and identification of mycobacteria from porcine tissues: a three year summary. Am J Vet Res 36:1383–1386.

63. Thoen, C.O., E.M. Himes, and J.H. Campbell. 1976. Isolation of Mycobacterium avium serotype 3 from a white-headed tree duck. Avian Dis 20:587–592.

64. Thoen, C.O., W.G. Eacret, and E.M. Himes. 1978. An enzyme-labeled antibody test for detecting antibodies in chickens infected with Mycobacterium avium serotype 2. Avian Dis 22:162–168.

65. Thoen, C.O., A.G. Karlson, and E.M. Himes. 1981. Mycobacterial infections in animals. Rev Infect Dis 3:960–972.

66. Thoen, C.O., E.M. Himes, and A.G. Karlson. 1984. Mycobacterium avium complex. In G.P. Kubica and L.G. Wayne (eds.), The Mycobacteria: A sourcebook, pp. 1251–1275. Marcel Dekker, New York.

67. USDA. 1973. Statistical Summary. Federal Meat and Poultry Inspection for Calendar Year 1972. MPI-I.

68. USDA. 1979. Statistical Summary. Federal Meat and Poultry Inspection for Calendar Year 1978. MPI-I.

69. USDA. 1985. Statistical Summary. Federal Meat and Poultry Inspection for Calendar Year 1984. MPI-I.

70. Vanderheyden, N. 1986. Avian tuberculosis: Diagnosis and attempted treatment. In Proc 1986 Annu Meet Assoc Avian Vet, pp. 203–211.

71. Vasenius, H. 1965. Tuberculosislike lesions in slaughter swine in Finland. Nord Vet Med 17:17–21.

72. Wallace, J.M., and J.B. Hannah. 1988. Mycobacterium avium complex infection in patients with the acquired immunodeficiency syndrome. Chest 93:926–932.

73. Weber, A., T. Schliesser, J.M. Schultze, and U. Bertelsmann. 1976. Serologische Typendifferenzierung aviarer Mykobacterienstamme isoliert von Schlachtrindern. Zentralbl Bakterial [orig A] 235:202–206.

74. Wiesenthal, A.M., K.E. Powell, J. Kopp, and J.W. Spindler. 1982. Increase in Mycobacterium avium complex isolation among patients admitted to a general hospital. Public Health Rep 97:61–65.

75. Wolinsky, E. 1979. Nontuberculous mycobacteria and associated diseases. Am Rev Respir Dis 119:107–159.

76. Wolinsky, E., and W.B. Schaefer. 1973. Proposed numbering scheme for mycobacterial serotypes by agglutination. Int J System Bacteriol 23:182–183.

7 INFECTIOUS CORYZA

R. Yamamoto

INTRODUCTION. Infectious coryza (IC) is an acute respiratory disease of chickens caused by *Haemophilus paragallinarum.* The clinical syndrome has been described in the early literature as roup, contagious or infectious catarrh, cold, and uncomplicated coryza (98). Since the disease proved to be infectious and primarily affected nasal passages, the name "infectious coryza" was adopted (3). IC may occur in growing chickens and layers; the greatest economic losses result from an increased number of culls and marked reduction (10–40%) in egg production. The disease is limited primarily to chickens and has no public health significance.

HISTORY. As early as 1920 Beach (2) believed that IC was a distinct clinical entity. The etiologic agent eluded detection for a number of years since the disease was often masked in mixed infections and with fowl pox in particular. In 1931 De Blieck (17) isolated the causative agent and named it *Bacillus hemoglobinophilus coryzae gallinarum.*

INCIDENCE AND DISTRIBUTION. IC is a disease of economic significance in many parts of the world. In the USA the disease is most prevalent in California and the southeastern states.

ETIOLOGY

Classification. Early workers classified the causative agent of IC as *H. gallinarum* because of its requirement for both *X*-(hemin) and *V*-(nicotinamide adenine dinucleotide, NAD) factors for growth (21, 87). This designation went unchallenged until Page in 1962 (62) found that all of his isolates required only the *V*-factor for growth. Since then isolates recovered from various parts of the world have been shown to require only the *V*-factor (9, 26, 58, 68). This has led to the proposal and general acceptance of a new species, *H. paragallinarum* (104), for organisms requiring only the *V*-factor. *H. gallinarum* and *H. paragallinarum* are identical in all other growth characteristics and disease producing potential (68). These observations in addition to the apparent abrupt change in the *X*-factor requirement of all isolates recovered worldwide since 1962 have led some workers to question the validity of tests used by earlier workers in classifying their isolates as *H. gallinarum* (68). Indeed, a recent study suggests that the early descriptions of the causative agent of IC as an *X*- and *V*-factor-dependent organism were incorrect (11).

Morphology and Staining. *H. paragallinarum* is a gram-negative, polar-staining, nonmotile bacterium. In 24-hr cultures it appears as short rods or coccobacilli 1–3 μm in length and 0.4–0.8 μm in width, with a tendency for filament formation. A capsule may be demonstrated in virulent strains (23, 80). The organism undergoes degeneration within 48–60 hr, showing fragments and indefinite forms. Subcultures to fresh medium at this stage will again yield the typical rod-shaped morphology. Bacilli may occur singly, in pairs, or as short chains (87). The organism detected in the sinus exudate of infected chickens has bipolar staining characteristics (Fig. 7.1).

Growth Requirements. The reduced form of NAD (NADH) (1.56–25 μg/ml medium) (62, 71) or its oxidized form (20–100 μg/ml) (76) and sodium chloride (NaCl) (1.0–1.5%) (71) are essential for

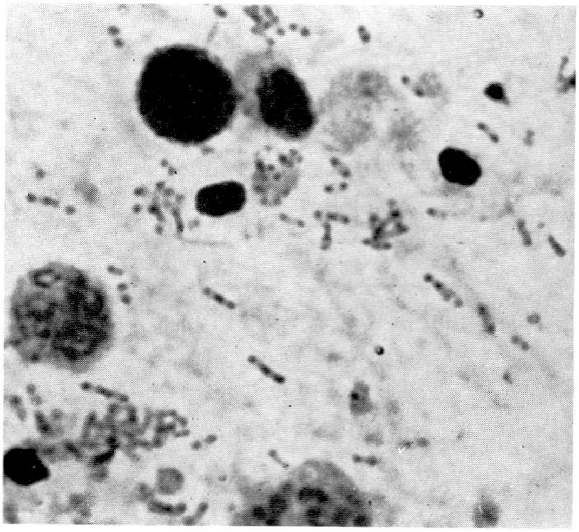

7.1. *Hemophilus paragallinarum* in film of nasal exudate. ×810.

growth. Chicken serum (1%) is required by some strains (23), whereas others merely show improved growth with this supplement (9). Brain-heart infusion (BHI), tryptose agar, and chicken meat infusion are some basal media to which supplements are added (23, 49, 76). More complex media are used to obtain dense growth of organisms for characterization studies (4, 67, 68). The pH of various media varies from 6.9 to 7.6. A number of bacterial species excrete *V*-factor that will support growth of *H. paragallinarum* (62).

The organism is commonly grown in an atmosphere of 5% carbon dioxide; however, CO_2 is not an essential requirement since the organism is able to grow under reduced oxygen tension or anaerobically (21, 62).

The minimal and maximal temperatures of growth are 25 and 45 C, respectively, the optimal range being 34–42 C. The organism is commonly grown at 37–38 C.

Colony Morphology. Tiny dewdrop colonies up to 0.3 mm in diameter develop on suitable media. In obliquely transmitted light, mucoid (smooth) iridescent and rough noniridescent and other intermediate colony forms have been observed (25, 68, 77, 79).

Biochemical Properties. Variations in fermentation patterns observed in a number of early studies do not reflect differences in biotypes (62) but rather may be due to differences in media and methods used (23). Using phenol red broth enriched with NaCl (1%), NADH (25 μg/ml), chicken serum (1%), and carbohydrates (1%) in a standard test procedure, a large number of strains from various parts of the world were tested. All isolates produced acid in fructose, glucose, and mannose; none fermented trehalose or galactose. Acid production in other sugars was variable or did not occur (4, 28, 58, 68). A heavy inoculum was essential to obtain reproducible results (4). *H. paragallinarum* is the only avian hemophilus that does not ferment trehalose or galactose (4), and it is catalase-negative. It shares with other avian hemophili common characteristics of reducing nitrate and fermenting glucose, having oxidase and alkaline phosphatase activities, and failing to produce indole or hydrolyse urea or gelatin (7).

The requirement for *X*-factor may be determined by the porphyrin test and for *V*-factor by growing the organism on a semisynthetic medium with and without NADH (68). Commercial *X*- or *V*-factor-containing discs are not reliable (7). Additional tests are described by Rimler (68) and Blackall (7).

Resistance to Chemical and Physical Agents. *H. paragallinarum* is a delicate organism that is inactivated rather rapidly outside the host. Infectious exudate suspended in tap water is inactivated in 4 hr at ambient temperature; when suspended in saline the exudate is infectious for at least 24 hr at 22 C. Exudate or tissue remains infectious when held at 37 C for 24 hr and, on occasion, up to 48 hr; at 4 C exudate remains infectious for several days. At temperatures of 45–55 C, hemophilus cultures are killed within 2–10 min. Infectious embryonic fluids treated with 0.25% formalin are inactivated within 24 hr at 6 C, but the organism survived for several days under similar conditions when treated with thimerosal, 1:10,000 (99).

The organism may be maintained on blood agar plates by weekly passages. Young cultures maintained in a "candle jar" will remain viable for 2 wk at 4 C. Chicken embryos 6–7 days old may be inoculated with single colonies or broth cultures via the yolk sac; yolk from embryos dead in 24–48 hr will contain a large number of organisms that may be frozen at −20 to −70 C or lyophilized. Titers in frozen yolk material may drop 100-fold; consequently, serial embryo passages should be made at monthly intervals to maintain cultures by this method. The organism has survived for at least 10 yr in the lyophilized state (98).

Antigenic Structure. Page (62) classified his organisms of *H. paragallinarum* with the plate agglutination test into serovars A, B, and C. While Page's serovar A strain 0083 and B strain 0222 are available today, all the serovar C strains were lost during the mid-1960s. Matsumoto and Yamamoto (56) isolated strain Modesto (M), which was later classified as a serovar C strain by Rimler et al. (70), based on tests with a rabbit anti-C serum.

Based on Page's agglutination typing scheme, isolates from Germany were classified as serovars A and B (24), from Spain as A, B, and C (63) and from Australia and South Africa as A and C (8). In independent studies from Japan, Kato and Tsubahara (42) described three serovars, I, II, and III, but later studies indicated that II and III were variants of I (36, 78). Sawata et al. (78) extended Kato and Tsubahara's study and identified two serovars, 1 and 2. Serovar I, represented by strain 221, was designated 1 and a new serovar represented by strain H-18 was designated 2. Later, serovars 1 and 2 were found to correspond to Page's serovars A and C (49, 80).

Hinz (24) was the first investigator to describe a heat-labile type-specific antigen and a heat-stable common antigen for strains of serovar A and B. Subsequently, a detailed antigenic analysis was performed by Sawata et al. (79) using encapsulated strains forming iridescent colonies of serovar 1 (A) and 2 (C). The study based on the agglutination test with immune rabbit serum revealed serovar-specific, heat-labile, trypsin-sensitive antigens designated L1 and L2. Three common antigens between the two serovars were identified. One was heat-labile and trypsin-sensitive (designated L3), another was heat-labile and trypsin-resistant (designated HL), and the third was heat-stable and trypsin-resistant (designated HS). Several studies showed correlation between agglutination serovar specificity and immunotype specificity (10, 48, 70). Chickens vaccinated with bacterin prepared from one serovar were protected only against homologous challenge. The protection was correlated with serovar-specific L1 and L2 antigens (48). These antigens may be polysaccharide (35), protein (50), or glycoprotein (34) in nature.

Nonencapsulated variants forming low or no iridescent colonies possessed only the common antigens and failed to induce protective immunity (48). Page's serovar B strains (Spross, 0222) were in this category and therefore considered to be variants of serovar A or C that had lost their type-specific antigen (49, 80).

Strains of both serovars A and C possess antigenic determinants capable of hemagglutinating erythrocytes. They differ, however, in that untreated cell suspensions of serovar A will hemagglutinate fresh erythrocytes of various animals (36, 47, 81), whereas both antigen and erythrocytes must be chemically treated before hemagglutination will occur with organism of serovar C (81). Two hemagglutinins (HA) were identified in cell suspensions of serovar A strain 221 (94, 95). Type 1 HA had biologic and immunologic properties similar to agglutination serovar-specific L1 antigen. Type 2 HA had similar characteristics as the agglutination serovar-common HL antigen.

When used in the hemagglutination-inhibition (HI) test against antisera from chickens immunized with strains of serovars A, B, or C, type 1 HA was found to be serovar A–specific (36). Two strains of serovar B, (Spross, 2403-Hinz) were also classified into serovar A, confirming an earlier observation (49) that some strains of serovar B may be variants of A or C. Type 2 HA reacted with serums of all strains, confirming that it represents a common antigen shared by all three serovars.

In a separate study Sawata et al. (82) described three types of HA located in the outer membrane of organisms of serovar A. They were named HA-L1, HA-HL, and HA-HS because their biologic and immunologic properties were similar to the agglutination antigens L1, HL, and HS. Antigens HA-L1 and HA-HL were found to be similar to type 1 and 2 HA discovered by Yamaguchi and Iritani (94). Similar to the agglutination L1 antigen, the HA-L1 antigen induced serovar-specific protective immunity in chickens (46, 50, 83).

Iritani et al. (35) extracted a heat-labile polysaccharide antigen from cells of a serovar 2 (C) strain that had properties similar to serovar C–specific L2 antigen. In contrast to type 1 HA of serovar A, this antigen failed to agglutinate chicken erythrocytes.

Serovar 2 (C) strains were rendered hemagglutinable by sonication of potassium thiocyanate–treated cells and reacting them with glutaraldehyde-fixed chicken erythrocytes. This HA antigen had biologic and immunologic properties similar to those of the agglutination serovar C–specific L2 antigen, and was designated HA-L2. Similar to serovar A type 1 HA (HA-L1) antigen, the HI antibody response detected by the HA-L2 antigen following vaccination correlated with protective immunity (81).

Based on heat-stable determinants, Hinz (27) used the agar-gel precipitin (AGP) test to classify *H. paragallinarum* into six serovars. The value of such a system is questionable because it does not allow for ready identification of different immunotypes.

Kume et al. (51) proposed a classification based on the HI test using potassium thiocyanate–treated and –sonicated cells, rabbit-immune serums, and glutaraldehyde-fixed chicken erythrocytes. This system was based on serovar-specific and -common hemagglutinins (HA-L antigens). In essence, Page's serovars A, C, and B were elevated to serogroups I, II, and III and seven serovars (HA-1 to HA-7) were recognized among the three serogroups: three each for I and II and one for III. While strains Spross and 0222 of Page's serovar B were not included in the study, some of the strains that Hinz (24) had classified into serovar B were typed by the new system into serogroup I, while those remaining were identified as members of group III. Of interest was the finding that the serovar-specific antigens seemed to be unique to the geographic origin of the strains. Furthermore, the common HA-L antigens shared by serovars within serogroups seemed to be important in inducing serogroup-specific immunity.

Many isolates that were nontypeable in Page's agglutination scheme were easily typed using Kume's HI procedure (20). Recently an eighth serovar was recognized in Australia (20).

A serum bactericidal test has been described that is capable of classifying isolates of *H. paragallinarum* to the same subdivision as in the HI scheme (84).

Soluble whole-cell proteins of strains of serovars A, B, and C showed two major banding patterns by sodium dodecyl sulfate polyacrylamide gel electrophoresis. There was no apparent correlation between the profiles and the serotyping scheme (12).

During the past 10 yr much has been learned about the antigenic structure, function, and relationships of *H. paragallinarum.* It is evident, however, that the status of Page's serovar B needs further clarification.

Pathogenicity. At least three virulence-associated antigens have been described in *H. paragallinarum,* none of which induce protective immunity. One is lipopolysaccharide isolated from culture supernatant fluids of strains of serovars A and C (33). This antigen may be similar to the agglutination common HS antigen, and it causes toxic signs in chickens following bacterin administration. Another is a polysaccharide isolated from strains of serovars A and C. This antigen, which causes hydropericardium in chickens, may be similar to the agglutination common L3 antigen or it may originate from the capsule (34). The third antigen is the hyaluronic acid–containing capsule that appears to be responsible for eliciting signs of coryza (77). In another study it was suggested that a toxin released from capsular organisms during in vivo multiplication was responsible for the clinical disease (52).

Pathogenic strains of *H. paragallinarum* adhere firmly to cultured chicken embryo fibroblasts in vitro and to tracheal mucosal epithelium in vivo (92). Both the serovar-specific L and HA-L antigens (77) and capsular material (45, 86) seem to be responsible for adherence and colonization of the respiratory mucosa. The capsule seems to protect the organism against the bactericidal action of normal serum (85).

In vivo dissociation of encapsulated pathogenic organisms to nonencapsulated nonpathogenic forms and dissociation in the reverse direction were described by Kato (39) and Hinz (25).

PATHOGENESIS AND EPIZOOTIOLOGY

Natural and Experimental Hosts. The chicken is the natural host for *H. paragallinarum;* all ages are susceptible. Chicks 3–5 days of age were somewhat resistant, but coryza was routinely produced in 7-day-old chicks by intranasal inoculation (21). Beach and Schalm (3) found that chickens 4 wk to 3 yr of age were susceptible but observed considerable individual variation in resistance. Kato and Tsubahara (43) reproduced typical signs of coryza in 90% of chickens 4–8 wk of age and 100% of chickens 13 wk of age and older. The incubation period was shortened and the course of the disease tended to be longer in older birds.

IC has been diagnosed infrequently in pheasants (18), and single cases were reported in guinea fowl (98) and companion birds (19). A severe outbreak involving a flock of 10, 000 Japanese quail (*Coturnix coturnix*) was traced to infected pullets raised on the same premise (66). The following species are refractory to experimental infection: turkey, pigeon, sparrow, duck, crow, rabbit, guinea pig, and mouse (98, 99).

Transmission, Carriers, Vectors. Chronic or healthy carrier birds serve as the main reservoir of infection. IC seems to occur most frequently in fall and winter, although such seasonal patterns may be coincidental to management practices (e.g., introduction of susceptible replacement pullets onto farms where IC is present). On farms where multiple-age groups are brooded and raised, spread of the disease to successive age groups can almost be predicted; infection occurs in a matter of 1–6 wk after such birds are moved from the brooder house to growing cages near older groups of infected birds (14).

Sparrows could not be implicated as vectors; however, epidemiologic studies suggest air-borne transmission as a possible means of introduction of IC on to isolated ranches (100).

Incubation Period. The characteristic feature of the disease is a coryza of short incubation that develops within 24–48 hr after intranasal or intrasinus inoculation with either culture or exudate. The intrasinus method will more consistently induce disease (68). Susceptible birds exposed by contact to infected cases usually have signs of the disease in 1–3 days.

Duration of the disease varies with the inoculum and virulence of the organism (77). The coryza produced by culture was of much shorter duration (6–14 days) than that produced by infectious sinus exudate (50 days or more) (59, 87). The organism rapidly lost virulence following artificial cultivation, which accounted for the shorter duration of the culture-induced disease; 30–40 transfers on artificial media rendered the organism completely avirulent in most cases (59). However, since these studies were conducted at a time when *Mycoplasma gallisepticum* was still an unknown entity, the prolonged course of the exudate-induced disease could very well have been from an infection complicated with this and possibly other agents. A coryza of short incubation and long duration has since been convincingly demonstrated in mixed infections of *H. paragallinarum* and *M. gallisepticum* (1, 60). Conversely, Schalm and Beach (87) showed that virulence of attenuated laboratory cultures could be increased to simulate the exudate-induced disease by rapid serial passages through chickens.

Signs. The most prominent features are involvement of nasal passages and sinuses with a serous to mucoid nasal discharge, facial edema, and conjunctivitis. Figure 7.2 illustrates the typical facial edema. Swollen wattles may be evident, particularly in males. Infections of the lower respiratory tract may occur, causing rales (3).

Birds may have diarrhea, and feed and water consumption usually is decreased; in growing birds this means an increased number of culls,

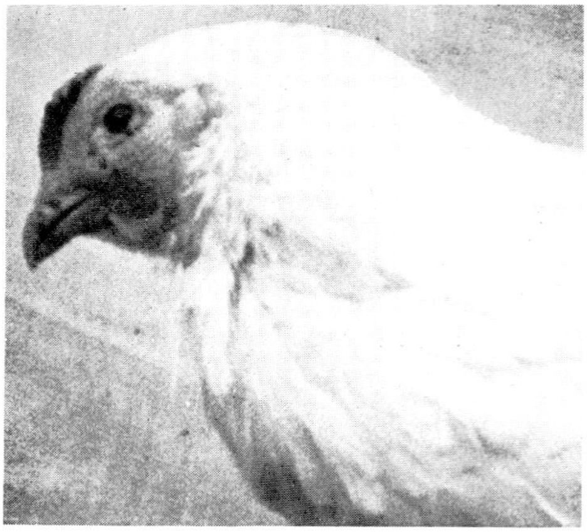

7.2. Artificial infection with IC showing facial edema.

and in laying flocks a reduction in egg production. A foul odor may be detected in flocks where the disease has become chronic and complicated with other bacteria.

Morbidity and Mortality. Virulence of the organism may alter the course of the disease. While highly toxigenic strains such as those described by Delaplane et al. (18) may cause high mortality, IC is usually characterized by low mortality and high morbidity. Variations in breed resistance may also influence the clinical picture (5). Complicating factors such as poor housing, parasitism, and inadequate nutrition may add to severity and duration.

IC is usually more severe and prolonged, with resulting increased mortality, when complicated with other agents such as fowl pox, *M. gallisepticum,* infectious bronchitis, pasteurella, and infectious laryngotracheitis (98).

Gross Lesions. *H. paragallinarum* produces an acute catarrhal inflammation of mucous membranes of nasal passages and sinuses. There is frequently a catarrhal conjunctivitis and subcutaneous edema of face and wattles. Pneumonia and airsacculitis is rarely present.

Histopathology. Fujiwara and Konno (22) studied the histopathologic response of chickens from 12 hr to 3 mo after intranasal inoculation. Changes in the nasal cavity, infraorbital sinuses, and trachea consisted of sloughing, disintegration, and hyperplasia of mucosal and glandular epithelia, and edema and hyperemia with heterophil infiltration in the tunica propria of the mucous membranes. Pathologic changes first observed at 20 hr reached maximum severity by 7–10 days, with subsequent repair occurring within 14–21 days. In birds with involvement of the lower respiratory tract, acute catarrhal bronchopneumonia was observed, with heterophils and cell debris filling the lumen of secondary and tertiary bronchi; epithelial cells of air capillaries were swollen and showed hyperplasia. Catarrhal inflammation of airsacs was characterized by swelling and hyperplasia of the cells, with abundant heterophil infiltration. In addition, a pronounced infiltration of mast cells was observed in the lamina propia of the mucous membrane of the nasal cavity (86). The products of mast cells, heterophils, and macrophages may be responsible for the severe vascular changes and cell damage leading to coryza.

Immunity. Chickens that have recovered from active infection possess varying degrees of immunity to reexposure. Pullets that have experienced IC during their growing period are generally protected against a later drop in egg production. Resistance to reexposure among individual birds may develop as early as 2 wk after initial exposure by the intrasinus route (75). Antigens of *H. paragallinarum* associated with virulence and protection have been described (see Antigenic Structure; Pathogenicity). Information is not available on passive immunity to *H. paragallinarum* infection.

DIAGNOSIS

Isolation and Identification of Causative Agent. Many different media have been developed to support growth of *H. paragallinarum* (49, 61, 68). While *H. paragallinarum* is considered to be a fastidious organism, it is not difficult to isolate, requiring simple media and procedures. Specimens should be taken from two or three chickens in the acute stage of the disease (1–7 days postinfection). Skin under the eyes is seared with a hot iron spatula and an incision made into the sinus cavity with sterile scissors. A sterile cotton swab is inserted deep into the sinus cavity where the organism is most often found in pure form. Tracheal and air sac exudates also may be taken on sterile swabs. The swab is streaked on a blood agar plate, which is then cross-streaked with a staphylococcus and incubated at 37 C in a large screw-cap jar in which a candle is allowed to burn out. *Staphylococcus epidermidis* (62) or *S. hyicus* (9), which are commonly used as "feeders," should be pretested because not all strains actively produce the V-factor.

Diagnosis of IC may be based on a history of a rapidly spreading disease in which coryza is the main manifestation, with isolation of a catalase-negative, gram-negative bacterium showing satellitic growth. The organism may be characterized more fully by biochemical and serologic tests (7).

Another efficient diagnostic procedure is to inoculate the sinus exudate or culture into two or three normal chickens by the intrasinus route.

The production of a coryza in 24–48 hr is diagnostic; however, the incubation period may be delayed up to 1 wk if only a few organisms are present in the inoculum, such as in long-standing cases.

Nonpathogenic hemophili have been described that are strongly catalase-positive, grow aerobically, require *V*-factor for growth, and ferment trehalose or galactose; most strains produce a yellow pigment. These organisms, named *H. avium* (26, 28), should not be confused with *H. paragallinarum.* The reader is referred to the review of Blackall (7) for this and other *V*-factor-requiring organisms that have been isolated from the avian species.

Serology. Commonly used serologic tests include plate or tube agglutination (31, 49, 101), AGP (31, 75), and HI (31, 52).

Since common antigens (L3, HL, HS) are shared by the three serovars, an agglutination antigen prepared from one serovar may be used to detect antibodies to all three serovars. *H. paragallinarum* agglutinins are detected 7–14 days postinfection and may persist up to 1 yr or longer. The test may be used to check flocks for evidence of past infection prior to their movement if one is concerned about introducing infection through carrier birds. The test has been used to follow the immune response in bacterin efficacy studies and for antigenic analysis of serovars.

Autoagglutination and nonagglutination observed with some antigen preparations may be obviated in some cases by treating the cells with trypsin (32) and hyaluronidase (70), respectively. Others have found that trypsin destroys functional determinant groups (77).

A serovar-specific agglutination test was developed by adsorbing polysaccharide antigens (L1 and L2) onto latex particles (96); it seems to be effective in detecting recent (3-wk) infections.

The AGP test will detect antibodies 2 wk postinfection or postvaccination and for at least 11 wk (31, 75). The test also has been used in antigenic analysis of strains (27, 36).

An HI test for serovar A uses whole bacterial cells and fresh chicken erythrocytes. Kato's strain 221 has been used most commonly as the antigen although other strains of serovar A will hemagglutinate chicken erythrocytes (49, 68). Many factors such as type of basal media, chicken serum concentration, and length of incubation of cultures will influence the yield and quality of the HA antigen (30, 88). The chicken erythrocyte phenotype can influence reactivity of the HA antigen (36). Treatment of the erythrocytes with trypsin or formalin will increase the sensitivity of the test (37). Glutaraldehyde-fixed erythrocytes also have been used (83). Trypsin and hyaluronidase treatment of cells of strain 221 will enhance its HA activity (29, 30, 77, 82); hyaluronidase treatment, which removes the hyaluronic acid capsule, will also enable some nonhemagglutinating strains to hemagglutinate (68). The HI test does not detect antibody as early as agglutination or AGP tests in infected or immunized birds (31, 41). The test detects antibodies to the serovar-specific HA-L1 antigen that is closely correlated with protective immunity (41, 46, 52, 61, 81).

The finding that serovar 2 (C) strains can be made to hemagglutinate by the use of potassium thiocyanate–treated and sonicated cells and glutaraldehyde-fixed chicken erythrocytes has yielded a useful HI test to evaluate protective potency of serovar C vaccines (81, 97). The test detects antibodies to the serovar-specific HA-L2 antigen, which correlate with protective immunity. Others have reported that this test was not satisfactory for evaluating protective potency of serovar C vaccines (90). The test has not been used extensively as a method for detecting antibodies in infected chickens (97). For both HI tests it may be necessary to pretreat the sera with erythrocytes to eliminate nonspecific hemagglutinins.

Other serologic tests include the direct complement fixation, indirect HA, and direct fluorescent antibody tests (99).

Differential Diagnosis. *H. paragallinarum* infection must be differentiated from other diseases, such as chronic respiratory disease, chronic fowl cholera, fowl pox, and A-avitaminosis, which produce similar clinical signs. Since *H. paragallinarum* infections often occur in mixed infections, one should consider the possibility of other bacteria or viruses as complicating IC, particularly if mortality is high and the disease takes a prolonged course (see Pathogenicity; Morbidity and Mortality).

TREATMENT. Various sulfonamides and antibiotics are useful in alleviating the severity and course of IC; however, none of the therapeutic agents has been found to be bactericidal and drug resistance does develop (6, 65). Relapse often occurs after treatment is discontinued, and the carrier state is not eliminated (99). Erythromycin and oxytetracycline are two commonly used antibiotics.

Drugs in combination found effective in treatment of IC include sulfachloropyrazine-sulfadimidine (13), chlortetracycline-sulfadimethoxine (44), sulfachloropyridazine-trimethoprim (53, 64, 89), sulfadimethoxine-trimethoprim (74), and sulfamonomethoxine-ormetoprim (54, 91). A new macrolide antibiotic, miporamicin (102), and a new quinolone derivative, esafloxacin (73), show promise against *H. paragallinarum* infections. Dihydrostreptomycin and some sulfa drugs act synergistically (13, 40). Strains of *H. paragallinarum* resistant to various antibiotics did not carry plasmids (6).

PREVENTION AND CONTROL

Management Procedures. Since recovered carrier birds are the main source of infection, practices such as buying breeding males or started chicks should be discouraged. Only day-old chicks should be secured for replacement purposes unless the source is known to be free of IC. Isolation rearing and housing away from old stock are desirable practices. To eliminate the agent from a farm it is necessary to depopulate the infected or recovered flock(s) because birds in such flocks remain reservoirs of infection. After cleaning and disinfection of equipment and houses the premises should be allowed to remain vacant for 2–3 wk before restocking with clean birds.

Immunization. Commercial bacterins prepared from chicken embryos (14), broth (15), or cell culture (93) may be autogenous or may contain strains of two to three serovars. The products, inactivated with formalin or thimerosal, must contain at least 10^8 colony-forming units (CFU)/ml to be effective. They may contain adjuvants, stabilizers, or saline diluents. Bacterins that are generally injected subcutaneously or intramuscularly in birds between 10 and 20 wk of age yield optimal results when injected 3–4 wk prior to an expected natural outbreak. Two injections given approximately 4 wk apart before 20 wk of age seem to result in better performance of layers than a single injection. When administered to growing birds the bacterin reduces losses from complicated respiratory disease. Chickens vaccinated with the chicken embryo product at 16 wk of age maintained a significant degree of immunity to challenge up to 27 wk (99).

Broth bacterins are more effective than egg-propagated products (16, 55). The organism has been propagated in chicken meat infusion, BHI, modified Casman broth, and other complex media to titers of 10^8 or greater CFU/ml in 24–36 hr (10, 99). Bacterins inactivated with thimerosal and adsorbed with aluminium hydroxide were more effective than those inactivated with formalin and emulsified in mineral oil (10). However, in another study a significant protection was induced by bacterins prepared with mineral oil (15). The bacterin was ineffective when administered intranasally (10) and induced better protection when injected into the leg versus breast muscle (38). Broth bacterins confer significant immunity for about 9 mo (10, 47, 55, 56).

As mentioned earlier, immunity induced by bacterins is serovar-specific and is closely correlated with serovar-specific L and HA-L antigens; antibodies detected by the serovar-specific HI tests correlate with protective immunity (see Serology). The finding of Rimler and Davis (69) that live organisms induce a broader-based cross-protection between serovars suggests that a common antigen may be important in conferring immunity. The discrepancy in these two observations might be due to differences in quality of the immunogen (bacterin vs. live organism), inoculation methods, challenge strain, dose, etc. (47). Irrespective of this question, one cannot disregard the importance of immunotype specificity in bacterin preparation. Since dissociation of *H. paragallinarum* is a common phenomenon (79), care should be taken in selecting the proper colonies, media, and incubation period to obtain the most immunogenic product. On the other hand, strains of serovar 2 (C) seem to be inherently less immunogenic than those of serovar 1 (A) (47).

Mixed bacterins containing inactivated infectious bronchitis, Newcastle disease, and *H. paragallinarum* have been described (61, 103). A combined *H. paragallinarum–M. gallisepticum* bacterin was reported to provide protection against transient and chronic coryza (72). However, antibody response to *H. paragallinarum* was suppressed in chickens inoculated with a similar product (57).

Another approach to prevention of IC in endemic areas has been the practice of controlled exposure. The usual procedure is to vaccinate birds between 15 and 18 wk of age and expose them to the live organism at 20 wk. Autogenous organisms or isolates of known characteristics should be used since different serovars may vary in their cross-protection. Vaccination with live viruses should be avoided during hemophilus exposure. Individual birds showing severe signs may be treated with antibiotics. Controlled exposure should be performed under careful veterinary supervision.

REFERENCES

1. Adler, H.E., and R. Yamamoto. 1956. Studies on chronic coryza (Nelson) in the domestic fowl. Cornell Vet 46:337–343.
2. Beach, J.R. 1920. The diagnosis, therapeutic, and prophylaxis of chicken-pox (contagious epithelioma) of fowls. J Am Vet Med Assoc 58:301–312.
3. Beach, J.R., and O.W. Schalm. 1936. Studies of the clinical manifestions and transmissibility of infectious coryza of chickens. Poult Sci 15:466–472.
4. Blackall, P.J. 1983. An evaluation of methods for the detection of carbohydrate fermentation in avian Haemophilus species. J Microbiol Methods 1:275–281.
5. Blackall, P.J. 1983. Development of a vaccine against infectious coryza. In Disease Prevention and Control in Poultry Production. Proc #66 Post-graduate Comm Vet Sci, Univ of Sydney, pp. 99–104.
6. Blackall, P.J. 1988. Antimicrobial drug resistance and the occurrence of plasmids in Haemophilus paragallinarum. Avian Dis 32:742–747.
7. Blackall, P.J. 1989. The avian haemophili. A review. Clin Microbiol Rev 2:270–277.
8. Blackall, P.J., and L.E. Eaves. 1988. Serological classification of Australian and South African isolates of

Haemophilus paragallinarum. Aust Vet J 63:362-363.
9. Blackall, P.J., and G.G. Reid. 1982. Further characterization of Haemophilus paragallinarum and Haemophilus avium. Vet Microbiol 7:359-367.
10. Blackall, P.J., and G.G. Reid. 1987. Further efficacy studies on inactivated, aluminum-hydroxide-adsorbed vaccines against infectious coryza. Avian Dis 31:527-532.
11. Blackall, P.J., and R. Yamamoto. 1989. "Haemophilus gallinarum"—a re-examination. J Gen Microbiol 135:469-474.
12. Blackall, P.J., and R. Yamamoto. 1989. Whole-cell protein profiles of Haemophilus paragallinarum as detected by polyacrylamide gel electrophoresis. Avian Dis 33:168-173.
13. Buys, S.B. 1972. Hemophilus coryza: Therapy with selected drugs. J S Afr Vet Assoc 43:383-389.
14. Clark, D.S., and J.F. Godfrey. 1961. Studies of an inactivated Hemophilus gallinarum vaccine for immunization of chickens against infectious coryza. Avian Dis 5:37-47.
15. Coetzee, L., E.J. Rogers, and L. Velthuysen. 1983. The production and evaluation of a Haemophilus paragallinarum (infectious coryza) oil emulsion vaccine in laying birds. In Disease Prevention and Control in Poultry Production. Proc #66 Post-graduate Comm Vet Sci, Univ of Sydney, pp. 277-283.
16. Davis, R.B., R.B. Rimler, and E.B. Shotts, Jr. 1976. Efficacy studies on Haemophilus gallinarum bacterin preparations. Am J Vet Res 37:219-222.
17. De Blieck, L. 1932. A haemoglobinophilic bacterium as the cause of contagious catarrh of the fowl (coryza infectiosa gallinarum). Vet J 88:9-13.
18. Delaplane, J.P., L.E. Erwin, and H.O. Stuart. 1934. A hemophilic bacillus as the cause of an infectious rhinitis (coryza) of fowls. R I Agric Exp Stn Bull 244.
19. Dolphin, R.E., and D.E. Olsen. 1978. Bacteriology of companion birds. Vet Med Small Anim Clin 73:359-361.
20. Eaves, L.E., D.G. Rogers, and P.J. Blackall. 1989. Comparison of hemagglutinin and agglutinin schemes for the serological classification of Haemophilus paragallinarum and proposal of a new hemagglutinin serovar. J Clin Microbiol 27:1510-1513.
21. Eliot, C.P., and M.R. Lewis. 1934. A hemophilic bacterium as a cause of infectious coryza in the fowl. J Am Vet Med Assoc 84:878-888.
22. Fujiwara, H., and S. Konno. 1965. Histopathological studies on infectious coryza of chickens. I. Findings in naturally infected cases. Nat Inst Anim Health Q (Tokyo) 5:86-96.
23. Hinz, K.H. 1973. Beitrag zur Differenzierung von Haemophilus Stämmen aus Hühnern. I. Mitteilung: Kulturelle und biochemische Untersuchungen. Avian Pathol 2:211-229.
24. Hinz, K.H. 1973. Beitrag zur Differenzierung von Haemophilus Stämmen aus Hühnern. II. Mitteilung: Serologische Untersuchungen im Objekttrger-Agglutinations-Test. Avian Pathol 2:269-278.
25. Hinz, K.H. 1976. Beitrag zur Differenzierung von Haemophilus Stämmen aus Hühnern. IV. Mitteilung: Untersuchungen Über die Dissoziation von Haemophilus paragallinarum. Avian Pathol 5:51-66.
26. Hinz, K.H. 1980. Differentiation of Haemophilus paragallinarum and Haemophilus avium by phenotypical characteristics. Proc 2nd Int Symp Vet Lab Diag 3:347-350.
27. Hinz, K.H. 1981. Serological differentiation of Haemophilus paragallinarum strains by their heat stable antigens. In M. Kilian, W. Frederiksen, and E.L. Biberstein (eds.), Haemophilus, Pasteurella, and Actinobacillus, pp. 111-120. Academic Press, New York.
28. Hinz, K.H., and C. Kunjara. 1977. Haemophilus avium a new species from chickens. Int J Syst Bacteriol 27:324-329.
29. Iritani, Y., and S. Hidaka. 1976. Enhancement of hemagglutinating activity of Haemophilus gallinarum by trypsin. Avian Dis 20:614-616.
30. Iritani, Y., S. Hidaka, and K. Katagiri. 1977. Production and properties of Haemophilus gallinarum. Avian Dis 21:39-49.
31. Iritani, Y., G. Sugimori, and K. Katagiri. 1977. Serologic response to Haemophilus gallinarum in artificially infected and vaccinated chickens. Avian Dis 21:1-8.
32. Iritani, Y., K. Katagiri, and K. Tsuji. 1978. Slide-agglutination test of Haemophilus gallinarum antigen treated by trypsin to inhibit spontaneous agglutination. Avian Dis 22:793-797.
33. Iritani, Y., S. Iwaki, and T. Yamaguchi. 1980. Properties of heat-stable antigen in the culture supernate of Haemophilus paragallinarum. Jpn J Vet Sci 42:635-641.
34. Iritani, Y., K. Katagiri, and H. Arita. 1980. Purification and properties of Haemophilus paragallinarum hemagglutinin. Am J Vet Res 41:2114-2118.
35. Iritani, Y., S. Iwaki, and T. Yamaguchi. 1981. Biological activities of crude polysaccharide extracted from two different immunotype strains of Haemophilus gallinarum in chickens. Avian Dis 25:29-37.
36. Iritani, Y., S. Iwaki, T. Yamaguchi, and T. Sueishi. 1981. Determination of types 1 and 2 hemagglutinins in serotypes of Haemophilus paragallinarum. Avian Dis 25:479-483.
37. Iritani, Y., T. Yamaguchi, K. Katagiri, and H. Arita. 1981. Hemagglutination inhibition of Haemophilus paragallinarum type 1 hemagglutinin by lipopolysaccharide. Am J Vet Res 42:689-690.
38. Iritani, Y., K. Kunihiro, T. Yamaguchi, T. Tomii, and Y. Hayashi. 1984. Difference of immune efficacy of infectious coryza vaccine by different site of injection in chickens. J Jpn Soc Poult Dis 20:182-185.
39. Kato, K. 1967. Personal communication.
40. Kato, K. 1968. Infectious coryza of chickens. VII. Effectiveness of sulfamonomethoxine in the treatment of experimental Haemophilus infections. J Jpn Vet Med Assoc 21:349-358.
41. Kato, K. 1970. Nature of hemagglutination inhibition antibody response and its relationship to protection in infectious coryza. Jpn J Vet Sci 32:263 (Suppl).
42. Kato, K., and H. Tsubahara. 1962. Infectious coryza of chickens. II. Identification of isolates. Bull Nat Inst Anim Health 45:21-26 [Engl summ Nat Inst Anim Health Q (Tokyo) 2:239].
43. Kato, K., and H. Tsubahara. 1962. Infectious coryza of chickens. III. Susceptibility of chickens of different ages. Bull Nat Inst Anim Health 45:27-32 [Engl summ Nat Inst Anim Health Q (Tokyo) 2:239-240].
44. Kato, K., H. Tsubahara, and O. Taniguchi. 1967. Infectious coryza of chickens. VI. Therapeutic effect of chlortetracycline-sulfadimethoxine tablets (CTC-SD) on chickens experimentally infected with Hemophilus gallinarum and on chickens involved in mixed infections with Hemophilus gallinarum and Mycoplasma gallisepticum. Bull Natl Inst Anim Health 55:35-39 [Engl summ Nat Inst Anim Health Q (Tokyo) 7:233].
45. Kotani, T., Y. Odagiri, and T. Horiuchi. 1988. Light and electron microscopic observation of chicken nasal mucosa infected with Haemophilus paragallinarum. Proc 18th World's Poult Congr, pp. 1311-1313.
46. Kume, K., and A. Sawata. 1984. Immunologic properties of variants dissociated from serotype 1 Haemophilus paragallinarum strains. Jpn J Vet Sci 46:49-56.

47. Kume, K., A. Sawata, and Y. Nakase. 1980. Haemophilus infections in chickens. 3. Immunogenicity of serotypes 1 and 2 strains of Haemophilus paragallinarum. Jpn J Vet Sci 42: 673-680.

48. Kume, K., A. Sawata, and Y. Nakase. 1980. Relationship between protective activity and antigen structure of Haemophilus paragallinarum serotypes 1 and 2. Am J Vet Res 41:97-100.

49. Kume, K., A. Sawata, and Y. Nakase. 1980. Immunologic relationship between Page's and Sawata's serotype strains of Haemophilus paragallinarum. Am J Vet Res 41:757-760.

50. Kume, K., A. Sawata, and T. Nakai. 1983. Serologic and immunologic studies on three types of hemagglutinin of Haemophilus paragallinarum serotype 1 organisms. Jpn J Vet Sci 45:783-792.

51. Kume, K., A. Sawata, T. Nakai, and M. Matsumoto. 1983. Serological classification of Haemophilus paragallinarum with a hemagglutinin system. J Clin Microbiol 17:958-964.

52. Kume, K., A. Sawata, and T. Nakai. 1984. Clearance of the challenge organisms from the upper respiratory tract of chickens injected with an inactivated Haemophilus paragallinarum vaccine. Jpn J Vet Sci 46:843-850.

53. Linster, N., and K.-H. Hinz. 1983. In-vivo efficacy of sulfachlorpyridazine and the combination sulfachlorpyridazine-trimethoprim against Haemophilus paragallinarum. Dtsch Tieraerztl Wochenschr 90:170-173.

54. Lu, Y. S., D.F. Lin, H.J. Tsai, K.S. Tsai, Y.L. Lee, and T. Lee. 1983. Drug sensitivity test of Haemophilus paragallinarum isolated in Taiwan. Taiwan J Vet Med Anim Husb 41:73-76.

55. Matsumoto, M., and R. Yamamoto. 1971. A broth bacterin against infectious coryza: Immunogenicity of various preparations. Avian Dis 15:109-117.

56. Matsumoto, M., and R. Yamamoto. 1975. Protective quality of an aluminum hydroxide absorbed broth bacterin against infectious coryza. Am J Vet Res 36:579-582.

57. Matsuo, K., C. Kuniyasu, S. Yamada, and S. Susumi. 1978. Suppression of immunoresponses to Haemophilus gallinarum with nonviable Mycoplasma gallisepticum in chickens. Avian Dis 22: 552-561.

58. Narita, N., O. Hipólito, and J.A. Bottino. 1978. Studies on infectious coryza of chickens. I. The biochemical and serological characteristics of 17 Haemophilus strains isolated in Brazil. Proc 16th World's Poult Congr 5:685-692.

59. Nelson, J.B. 1933. Studies on an uncomplicated coryza of the domestic fowl. I. The isolation of a bacillus which produces a nasal discharge. J Exp Med 58:289-295.

60. Nelson, J.B. 1938. Studies on an uncomplicated coryza in the domestic fowl. IX. The cooperative action of Haemophilus gallinarum and the coccobacilliform bodies in the coryza of rapid onset and long duration. J Exp Med 67:847-855.

61. Otsuki, K., and Y. Iritani. 1974. Preparation and immunological response to a new mixed vaccine composed of inactivated Newcastle disease virus, inactivated infectious bronchitis virus, and inactivated Haemophilus gallinarum. Avian Dis 18:297-304.

62. Page, L.A. 1962. Hemophilus infections in chickens. I. Characteristics of 12 Hemophilus isolates recovered from diseased chickens. Am J Vet Res 23:85-95.

63. Pages Mante, A., and L. Costa Quintana. 1986. Efficacy of polyvalent inactivated oil vaccine against avian coryza. Med Vet 3:27-36.

64. Poernomo, P., and P. Ronohardjo. 1987. Efficacy of cosumix plus in broilers with coryza (Haemophilus paragallinarum infection). Penyakit Hewan 19:6-10.

65. Reece, R.L., and P.J. Coloe. 1985. The resistance to antimicrobial agents of bacteria isolated from pathological conditions of birds in Victoria, 1978 to 1983. Aust Vet J 62:379-381.

66. Reece, R.L., D.A. Barr, and A.C. Owen. 1981. The isolation of Haemophilus paragallinarum from Japanese quail (correspondence). Austr Vet J 57:350-351.

67. Reid, G.G., and P.J. Blackall. 1987. Comparison of adjuvants for an inactivated infectious coryza vaccine. Avian Dis 31:59-63.

68. Rimler, R.B. 1979. Studies of the pathogenic avian haemophili. Avian Dis 23:1006-1018.

69. Rimler, R.B., and R.B. Davis. 1977. Infectious coryza: In vivo growth of Haemophilus gallinarum as a determinant for cross protection. Am J Vet Res 38:1591-1593.

70. Rimler, R.B., R.B. Davis, and P.K. Page. 1977. Infectious coryza: Cross-protection studies, using seven strains of Haemophilus gallinarum. Am J Vet Res 38:1587-1589.

71. Rimler, R.B., E.B. Shotts, Jr., J. Brown, and R.B. Davis. 1977. The effect of sodium chloride and NADH on the growth of six strains of Haemophilus species pathogenic to chickens. J Gen Microbiol 98:349-354.

72. Rimler, R.B., R.B. Davis, R.K. Page, and S.H. Kleven. 1978. Infectious coryza: Preventing complicated coryza with Haemophilus gallinarum and Mycoplasma gallisepticum bacterins. Avian Dis 22:140-150.

73. Sakaguchi, Y., K. Kouno, T. Kojima, H. Yoshida, M. Nakai, S. Matsumoto, H. Katae, and S. Nakamura. 1988. Esafloxacin, a new quinolone derivative: Its in vitro antibacterial activity against chicken pathogens. Proc 18th World's Poult Congr, pp. 1265-1266.

74. Sakai, T., and S. Nagao. 1987. Experimental infection of chickens with Haemophilus paragallinarum and therapeutic efficacy of TA-068W. Bull Coll Ag Vet Med Nihon Univ 40:228-235.

75. Sato, S., and M. Shifrine. 1964. Serologic response of chickens to experimental infection with Hemophilus gallinarum, and their immunity to challenge. Poult Sci 43:1199-1204.

76. Sato, S., and M. Shifrine. 1965. Application of the agar gel precipitation test to serologic studies of chickens inoculated with Haemophilus gallinarum. Avian Dis 9:591-598.

77. Sawata, A., and K. Kume. 1983. Relationships between virulence and morphological or serological properties of variants dissociated from serotype 1 Haemophilus paragallinarum strains. J Clin Microbiol 18:49-55.

78. Sawata, A., K. Kume, and Y. Nakase. 1978. Haemophilus infections in chickens. 2. Types of Haemophilus paragallinarum isolates from chickens with infectious coryza, in relation to Haemophilus gallinarum strain No.221. Jpn J Vet Sci 40:645-652.

79. Sawata, A., K. Kume, and Y. Nakase. 1979. Antigenic structure and relationship between serotypes 1 and 2 of Haemophilus paragallinarum. Am J Vet Res 40:1450-1453.

80. Sawata, A., K. Kume, and Y. Nakase. 1980. Biologic and serologic relationships between Page's and Sawata's serotypes of Haemophilus paragallinarum. Am J Vet Res 41:1901-1904.

81. Sawata, A., K. Kume, and Y. Nakase. 1982. Hemagglutinin of Haemophilus paragallinarum serotype 2 organisms: Occurrence and immunologic properties of hemagglutinin. Am J Vet Res 43:1311-1314.

82. Sawata, A., K. Kume, and T. Nakai. 1984. Hemagglutinin of Haemophilus paragallinarum serotype 1 organisms. Jpn J Vet Sci 46:21-29.

83. Sawata, A., K. Kume, and T. Nakai. 1984. Relationship between anticapsular antibody and protective

activity of a capsular antigen of Haemophilus paragallinarum. Jpn J Vet Sci 46:475-486.

84. Sawata, A., K. Kume, and T. Nakai. 1984. Serologic typing of Haemophilus paragallinarum based on serum bactericidal reactions. Jpn J Vet Sci 46:909-912.

85. Sawata, A., K. Kume, and T. Nakai. 1984. Susceptibility of Haemophilus paragallinarum to bactericidal activity of normal and immune chicken sera. Jpn J Vet Sci 46:805-813.

86. Sawata, A., T. Nakai, K. Kume, H. Yoshikawa, and T. Yoshikawa. 1985. Intranasal inoculation of chickens with encapsulated or nonencapsulated variants of Haemophilus paragallinarum: Electron microscopic evaluation of the nasal mucosa. Am J Vet Res 46:2346-2353.

87. Schalm, O.W., and J.R. Beach. 1936. Studies of infectious coryza of chickens with special reference to its etiology. Poult Sci 15:473-482.

88. Sueishi, T., Y. Hayashi, and Y. Iritani. 1982. Use of gonococcal agar medium for preparation of antigen of Haemophilus paragallinarum hemagglutinin. Avian Dis 26:186-190.

89. Sumano Lopez, H., and L. Ocampo Camberos. 1987. Comparative pharmacokinetics of three sulfonamide-trimethoprim combinations in healthy White Leghorn pullets and pullets with infectious coryza (Haemophilus gallinarum). Vet Mexico 18:21-26.

90. Takagi, M., S. Ohta, and K. Kato. 1986. Haemagglutination inhibition antibody response in chickens to inactivated infectious coryza serotype C vaccine. Bull Nat Inst Anim Health 89:11-17.

91. Takahata, T., M. Takei, and M. Kato. 1988. Efficacy of the combination of sulfamonomethoxine and ormetoprim against experimentally induced infectious coryza in chickens. Proc 18th World's Poult Congr, pp. 1282-1283.

92. Ueda, S., Y. Nagasawa, T. Suzuki, and M. Tajima. 1982. Adhesion of Haemophilus paragallinarum to cultured chicken cells. Microbiol Immunol 26:1007-1016.

93. Wichmann, R.W., and A.C. Wichmann. 1983. The cultivation of Haemophilus gallinarum (Haemophilus paragallinarum) in tissue culture and the use of these cultures in the preparation of a bacterin for the prevention of infectious coryza. Proc 32nd West Poult Dis Conf, pp. 7-10.

94. Yamaguchi, T., and Y. Iritani. 1980. Occurrence of two hemagglutinins on Haemophilus paragallinarum strain 221 and comparison of their properties. Jpn J Vet Sci 42:709-711.

95. Yamaguchi, T., S. Iwaki, and Y. Iritani. 1980. Serological and immunological differences between two hemagglutinins of Haemophilus paragallinarum strain 221. Jpn J Vet Sci 42:713-715.

96. Yamaguchi, T., S. Iwaki, and Y. Iritani. 1981. Latex agglutination test for measurement of type-specific antibody to Haemophilus paragallinarum in chickens. Avian Dis 25: 988-995.

97. Yamaguchi, T., Y. Iritani, and Y. Hayashi. 1988. Serological response of chickens either vaccinated or artificially infected with Haemophilus paragallinarum. Avian Dis 32:308-312.

98. Yamamoto, R. 1972. Infectious coryza. In M.S. Hofstad, B.W. Calnek, C.F. Helmboldt, W.M. Reid, and H.W. Yoder, Jr. (eds.), Diseases of Poultry, 6th Ed., pp. 272-281. Iowa State Univ Press, Ames.

99. Yamamoto, R. 1978. Infectious coryza. In M.S. Hofstad, B.W. Calnek, C.F. Helmboldt, W.M. Reid, and H.W. Yoder, Jr. (eds.), Diseases of Poultry, 7th Ed., pp. 225-232. Iowa State Univ Press, Ames.

100. Yamamoto, R., and G.T. Clark. 1966. Intra and interflock transmission of Haemophilus gallinarum. Am J Vet Res 27:1419-1425.

101. Yamamoto, R., and D.T. Somersett. 1964. Antibody response in chickens to infection with Haemophilus gallinarum. Avian Dis 8:441-453.

102. Yamamoto, K., S. Tateyama, T. Sakai, N. Watanabe, N. Watanabe, Y. Hattori, M. Suzuki, and M. Kozasa. 1988. Myplabin (miporamicin), a new macrolide antibiotic. II. Clinical effects of Myplabin premix against respiratory mycoplasmosis and infectious coryza in chickens. Proc 18th World's Poult Congr, pp. 1256-1258.

103. Yoshimura, M., S. Tsubaki, T. Yamagami, R. Sugimoto, S. Ide, Y. Nakase, and S. Masu. 1972. The effectiveness of immunization to Newcastle disease, avian infectious bronchitis, and avian infectious coryza with inactivated combined vaccines. Kitasato Arch Exp Med 45:165-179.

104. Zinnemann, K., and E.L. Biberstein. 1974. Haemophilus. In R.E. Buchanan, and N.E. Gibbons (eds.), Bergey's Manual of Determinative Bacteriology, 8th Ed., pp. 364-370. Williams & Wilkins, Baltimore, MD.

8 MYCOPLASMOSIS

INTRODUCTION

Harry W. Yoder, Jr.

The number of species designations for mycoplasma of avian origin has increased rapidly during recent years. Thus, it has become necessary to briefly introduce the numerous species in this preliminary section followed by more complete discussions of the most significant members: *M. gallisepticum, M. meleagridis,* and *M. synoviae.* Then a final section will present brief discussions on several species which are becoming of greater concern.

HISTORY. *Mycoplasma* spp. were probably first encountered in chickens during the 1930s by Nelson (18, 19), and the condition designated "chronic respiratory disease" was described in 1943 by Delaplane and Stuart (6). The infection in turkeys was described by Dodd (9) in 1905 and was named "infectious sinusitis" in 1938 by Dickinson and Hinshaw (7). Markham and Wong (17) and Van Roekel and Olesiuk (24) reported almost simultaneously in the early 1950s on the successful cultivation of the organisms from chickens and turkeys and noted their similarity. Other early reports (11, 13) described some of the cultural and biochemical characteristics of mycoplasma (probably *M. gallisepticum*) from chickens and turkeys. Comparative studies indicated that their isolates were all antigenically similar.

Characterization. Mycoplasma species from avian sources generally require a protein-rich medium containing 10–15% added animal serum. Swine serum is more often used that horse serum. Further supplementation with some yeast-derived component is often beneficial. Growth of *M. synoviae* requires the addition of nicotinamide adenine dinucleotide (NAD).

Mycoplasma organisms tend to grow rather slowly, usually prefer 37–38 C, and are rather resistant to thallium acetate and penicillin, which are frequently employed in media to retard growth of contaminant bacteria and fungi. Colonies form on agar media incubated in an especially moist area for 3–10 days at 37 C. Typical colonies are very small (0.1–1.0 mm), smooth, circular, and somewhat flat with a more dense central elevation (see Fig. 8.4). Variations in colony morphology have been described, but cannot be relied upon to differentiate the various serotypes or species. Individual cells vary from 0.2 to 0.5 μm and are basically coccoid to coccobacilliform, but slender rods, filaments, and ring forms have been described employing Giemsa-stained films.

Fermentation of carbohydrates is variable, but all species may be divided into those that ferment glucose with acid production and those that do not. Glucose is frequently added to broth media to enhance growth of the carbohydrate-fermenting species and to provide an indication of growth when glucose fermentation produces acid in media containing added phenol red, which then becomes yellow.

Other characteristics that aid in the differentiation of species are reduction of 2,3,5-triphenyl tetrazolium (which becomes red) or reduction of neotetrazolium (which becomes blue). The presence of phosphatase activity is often evaluated, as is the presence of arginine decarboxylase. Most species that do not ferment dextrose use the amino acid arginine as their major source of energy. However, isolates of *M. iowae* ferment dextrose and hydrolyze arginine.

One very useful characteristic of at least *M. gallisepticum* (MG), *M. meleagridis* (MM), and *M. synoviae* (MS) is that selected strains cause hemagglutination of erythrocytes from chickens or turkeys. Special hemagglutinating antigens have been developed for application in the very important hemagglutination-inhibition serological tests for these three very important species.

Serotyping. Mycoplasma species representing different serotypes became apparent during early studies by Adler et al. (1). Yamamoto and Adler (25, 26) characterized 5 serotypes; Kleckner (14) described 8, designated A–H, including the previous 5. Twelve serotypes (A–L) were characterized by Yoder and Hofstad (27), and 19 (A–S) by Dierks et al. (8). Numerous characteristics were described, but the final serotyping procedure was based primarily on agglutination titrations. Several of those 19 serotype designations were either deleted or combined as further research employing additional serological procedures was evaluated. Direct staining of mycoplasma colonies on agar surfaces with specific fluorescent antibody as reported by Talkington and Kleven (23) has frequently been employed to type cultures of MG, MS, MM and others during recent years. Similarly, culture identification has been conducted by agar-gel diffusion procedures described by Aycardi et al. (2) and by Nonomura and Yoder (20). More recent studies employing monoclonal antibody, restriction endonucleases, and nucleic acid hybridizations will be discussed in the sections of this chapter.

Pathogenicity. Studies to determine the relative pathogenicity of mycoplasma inoculated into embryonating eggs, chickens, turkeys, and other avian species will be discussed in subsequent sections of this chapter.

Classification. Considerable progress has been made to avoid further confusion caused by the early serotype designations of various avian mycoplasmas. Following rather detailed studies the early species designations of *M. gallisepticum, M. gallinarum, M. iners, M. meleagridis,* and *M. synoviae* have become commonly employed in the literature; a continuing list of new species designations have been published. *M. gallopavonis, M. iowae, M. pullorum, M. gallinaceum,* and *M. columbinasale* were named in 1982 (12) for some of the previously characterized serotypes. *M. columbinum* was named for an isolate from the trachea of pigeons and *M. columborale* from the oropharynx of pigeons (21). *M. lipofaciens* was named for an isolate from the sinus of a chicken (4). *M. glycophilum* was named for an isolate obtained from the oviduct of a chicken (10), *M. cloacale* was described as an isolate from the cloaca of turkeys (3), and *M. anseris* was reported from geese (5). *Ureaplasma gallorale* was named for an isolate from the oropharynx of a chicken (15), and other reports have mentioned *Ureaplasma* spp. from turkey cloacal areas. Studies on a *Ureaplasma* isolated from the semen of turkeys was reported to be somewhat pathogenic (22).

Almost all of the species of mycoplasma isolated from avian sources are included in the ninth edition of *Bergey's Manual* (16). A summary of the characteristics of mycoplasma species isolated from avian sources is presented in Table 8.1.

REFERENCES

1. Adler, H.E., R. Yamamoto, and J. Berg. 1957. Strain differences of pleuropneumonia-like organisms of avian origin. Avian Dis 1:19–27.

2. Aycardi, E.R, D.P. Anderson, and R.P. Hanson. 1971. Classification of avian mycoplasmas by gel diffusion and growth inhibition tests. Avian Dis 15:434–447.

3. Bradbury, J., and M. Forrest. 1984. Mycoplasma cloacale, a new species isolated from a turkey. Int J Syst Bact 34:389–392.

4. Bradbury, J., M. Forrest, and A. Williams. 1983. Mycoplasma lipofaciens, a new species of avian origin. Int J Syst Bact 33:329–335.

5. Bradbury, J.M., F.T.W. Jordan, T. Shimizu, L. Stipkovits, and Z. Varga. 1988. Mycoplasma anseris sp. nov. found in geese. Int J Syst Bact 38:74–76.

6. Delaplane, J.P., and H.O. Stuart. 1943. The propagation of a virus in embryonated chicken eggs causing a chronic respiratory disease of chickens. Am J Vet Res 4:325–332.

7. Dickinson, E.M., and W.R. Hinshaw. 1938. Treat-

Table 8.1. Characteristics of avian mycoplasma

Mycoplasma Species	Usual Host	Glucose Fermentation	Arginine Hydrolysis	Phosphatase Activity
M. gallisepticum	Chicken, turkey	+	–	–
M. synoviae	Chicken, turkey	+	–	–
M. meleagridis	Turkey	–	+	+
M. iowae	Turkey, chicken	+	+	–
M. gallopavonis	Turkey	+	–	–
M. cloacale	Turkey	–	+	–
M. gallinarum	Chicken	–	+	–
M. gallinaceum	Chicken	+	–	–
M. pullorum	Chicken	+	–	–
M. iners	Chicken	–	+	–
M. lipofaciens	Chicken	+	+	–
M. glycophilum	Chicken	+	–	+ or –
M. columbinasale	Pigeon	–	+	+
M. columbinum	Pigeon	–	+	–
M. columborale	Pigeon	+	–	–
M. anatis	Duck	+	–	+
M. anseris	Goose	–	+	–
Acholeplasma[a] *laidlawii*	Various	+	–	+ or –
Ureaplasma[b] *gallorale*	Chicken	–	–	
Ureaplasma spp.	Turkey	–	–	

[a]*Acholeplasma,* a sister genus in the family Mycoplasmataceae, consists of mycoplasmalike organisms that do not require a source of sterol for growth and are saprophytic. They sometimes grow at room temperature.

[b]*Ureaplasma,* another sister genus, consists of mycoplasmalike organisms that do not utilize glucose or arginine, but hydrolyze urea. Some species of *Ureaplasma* are possibly of pathogenic significance in avian species.

ment of infectious sinusitis of turkeys with argyrol and silver nitrate. J Am Vet Med Assoc 93:151–156.
8. Dierks, R.E., J.A. Newman, and B.S. Pomeroy. 1967. Characterization of avian Mycoplasma. Ann NY Acad Sci 143:170–189.
9. Dodd, S. 1905. Epizootic pneumo-enteritis of the turkey. J Comp Pathol Ther 18:239–245.
10. Forrest, M., and J. Bradbury. 1984. Mycoplasma glycophilum, a new species of avian origin. J Gen Microbiol 130:597–603.
11. Grumbles, L.C., E. Phillips, W.A. Boney, Jr., and J.P. Delaplane. 1953. Cultural and biochemical characteristics of the agent causing infectious sinusitis of turkeys and chronic respiratory disease of chickens. Southwest Vet 6:166–168.
12. Jordan, F.T.W., H. Erno, G.S. Cottew, K.H. Hinz, and L. Stipkovits. 1982. Characterization and taxonomic description of five Mycoplasma serovars (serotypes) of avian origin and their elevation to species rank and further evaluation of the taxonomic status of Mycoplasma synoviae. Int J Syst Bact 32:108–115.
13. Jungherr, E.L., R.E. Luginbuhl, M. Tourtellotte, and W.E. Burr. 1955. Significance of serological testing for chronic respiratory disease. Proc 92nd Annu Meet Am Vet Med Assoc, pp. 315–321.
14. Kleckner, A.L. 1960. Serotypes of avian pleuropneumonia-like organisms. Am J Vet Res 21:274–280.
15. Koshimizu, K., R. Harasawa, I.J. Pan, H. Kotani, M. Ogata, E.B. Stephens, and M.F. Barile. 1987. Ureaplasma gallorale sp. nov. from the oropharynx of chickens. Int J Syst Bact 37:333–338.
16. Kreig, N.R., and J.G. Holt. 1984. Bergey's Manual of Systematic Bacteriology, 9th Ed., Vol. 1, pp. 740–793. Williams & Wilkins, Baltimore/London.
17. Markham, F.S., and S.C. Wong. 1952. Pleuropneumonia-like organisms in the etiology of turkey sinusitis and chronic respiratory disease of chickens. Poult Sci 31:902–904.
18. Nelson, J.B. 1933. Studies on an uncomplicated coryza of the domestic fowl. II. The relation of the "Bacillary" coryza to that produced by exudate. J Exp Med 58:297–304.
19. Nelson, J.B. 1939. Growth of the fowl coryza bodies in tissue culture and in blood agar. J Exp Med 69:199–209.
20. Nonomura, I., and H.W. Yoder, Jr. 1977. Identification of avian Mycoplasma isolates by the agar gel precipitin test. Avian Dis 21:370–381.
21. Shimizu, T., H. Erno, and H. Nagatomo. 1978. Isolation and characterization of Mycoplasma columbinum and Mycoplasma columborale, two new species from pigeons. Int J Syst Bact 28:538–546.
22. Stipkovits, L., A. Rashwan, and M.Z. Sabry. 1978. Studies on pathogenicity of turkey Ureaplasma. Avian Pathol 7:577–582.
23. Talkington, F.D., and S.H. Kleven. 1983. A classification of laboratory strains of avian Mycoplasma serotypes by direct immunofluorescence. Avian Dis 27:422–429.
24. Van Roekel, H., and Olga M. Olesiuk. 1953. The etiology of chronic respiratory disease. Proc 90th Annu Meet Am Vet Med Assoc, pp. 289–303.
25. Yamamoto, R., and H.E. Adler. 1958. Characterization of pleuropneumonia-like organisms of avian origin. I. Antigenic analysis of seven strains and their comparative pathogenicity for birds. J Infect Dis 102:143–152.
26. Yamamoto, R., and H.E. Adler. 1958. Characteristics of pleuropneumonia-like organisms of avian origin. II. Cultural, biochemical, morphological and further serological studies. J Infect Dis 102:243–250.
27. Yoder, H.W., Jr., and M.S. Hofstad. 1964. Characterization of avian Mycoplasma. Avian Dis 8:481–512.

MYCOPLASMA GALLISEPTICUM INFECTION

Harry W. Yoder, Jr.

INTRODUCTION. *Mycoplasma gallisepticum* (MG) infection is commonly designated as chronic respiratory disease (CRD) of chickens and infectious sinusitis of turkeys. It is characterized by respiratory rales, coughing, nasal discharge, and frequently sinusitis in turkeys. Clinical manifestations are usually slow to develop and the disease has a long course. Air sac disease designates a severe airsacculitis that is the result of *M. gallisepticum* infection complicated by some respiratory virus infection and usually *Escherichia coli* (see also section on *M. synoviae*).

Economic and Public Health Significance. Airsacculitis in chickens and airsacculitis and sinusitis in turkeys can cause significant condemnations at slaughter. Most of this loss is related directly or indirectly to *M. gallisepticum* infection, with or without complicating factors. Economic losses from down-grading of carcasses, reduced feed and egg-production efficiency, and increased medication costs are additional factors that make this one of the costliest disease problems confronting the industry. Conducting adequate prevention and control programs is also expensive. The disease is of little or no public health significance.

HISTORY. The first accurate description of the disease in turkeys was probably made in 1905 by Dodd (28) in England under the name "epizootic pneumoenteritis." Dickinson and Hinshaw (26) named the disease "infectious sinusitis" of turkeys in 1938.

Nelson (78) described coccobacilliform bodies associated with an infectious coryza in chickens in 1935. Later he associated them with the coryza of slow onset and long duration and eventually was able to grow the coccobacilliform bodies in embryonating eggs, tissue culture, and cell-free medium.

In 1943 Delaplane and Stuart (25) isolated and cultivated an agent in embryos isolated from chickens with CRD and later from turkeys with sinusitis. In the early 1950's Markham and Wong (72) and Van Roekel and Olesiuk (106) reported on successful cultivation of the organisms from chickens and turkeys, noting their similarity, and suggested they were members of the pleuropneumonia group (*Mycoplasma* spp.)

INCIDENCE AND DISTRIBUTION. The disease has become an important flock problem in chickens and turkeys in all areas of the USA. It appears to be worldwide in distribution.

The incidence has decreased considerably during the past 20 yr of extensive control programs within the poultry industry. However, the continuation of MG infection in many large multiple-age commercial egg production units is a major problem, and will be discussed further in the control and prevention sections.

ETIOLOGY

Classification. *M. gallisepticum* is a pathogenic species within the genus *Mycoplasma* of the family Mycoplasmataceae as recently discussed in the ninth edition of *Bergey's Manual* (61).

Morphology and Staining. The organism stains well with Giemsa stain but is weakly gram-negative. It is generally coccoid, approximately 0.25–0.5 μm (Fig. 8.1). Some variation in morphology has been found by electron microscopy (EM). Shifrine et al. (92) studied the edge of growing colonies and concluded that elementary cells were hexagonal and originated from within larger cells or by fragmentation of peripheral filaments. Use of thin-section techniques with negative staining has made it possible to study their ultrastructure and modes of multiplication. Domermuth et al. (29) noted internal cellular dense bodies that appeared to be developing elementary bodies. Similar dense bodies were observed in protrusions (buds) extending from the cell surface (Fig. 8.2). Ribosomes were present in some of their preparations (Fig. 8.3). Dutta et al. (31) noted similar internal dense areas within mother cells, in cell protrusions, and in daughter cells. Part of the growth cycle resembled budding. It is probable that more than one mode of cell replication can occur, depending on various cell and environmental conditions. Tajima et al. (96) described capsular material associated with MG cells in contact with chicken tracheal epithelium based on EM studies. Further reports on the interaction of MG cells with tracheal epithelium are discussed in the section on histopathology.

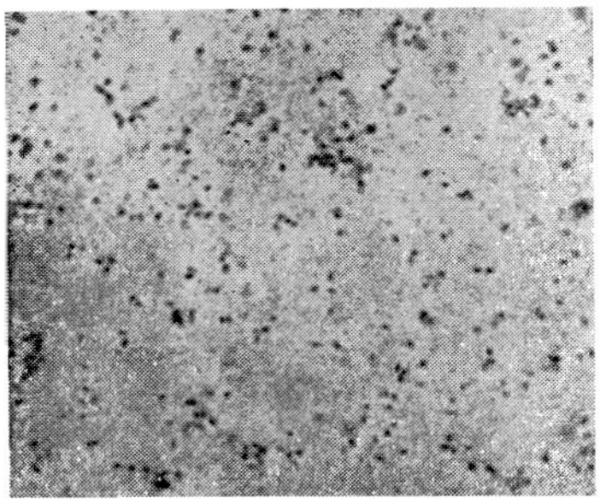

8.1. Smear of sedimented broth culture of *M. gallisepticum.* Giemsa, ×885. (47)

Growth Requirements. *M. gallisepticum* requires a rather complex medium enriched with 10–15% heat-inactivated swine, avian, or horse serum. Several types of liquid or agar media will support growth of mycoplasmas of avian origin, with certain purposes altering the final choice. Liquid medium is desirable for antigen production, but use of a broth overlay on an agar slant apparently is of some added value for making original isolations and maintaining cultures. Media and techniques for antigen production have been described (40, 108). Growth generally is optimal in medium at approximately pH 7.8 incubated at 37–38 C. Colonies form on agar medium containing the usual mycoplasma ingredients but require prolonged incubation (2–5 days) in a very moist atmosphere.

Frey et al. (36) developed a medium (see *M. synoviae* section) that incorporated all essential ingredients including yeast autolysate and dextrose. When prepared with 10–15% swine serum it is a convenient and very efficient medium for cultivation of most mycoplasmas. Inclusion of phenol red and dextrose makes it possible to detect growth in tubes employed in mass culturings, as does addition of 0.0025% 2,3,5-triphenyl tetrazolium chloride as an indicator (118).

MG may also be propagated in embryonated chicken eggs (see Pathogenicity; Isolation and Identification of Causative Agent).

Colony Morphology. *M. gallisepticum* can be grown on serum-enriched agar medium inoculated with broth or agar culture material. It often is very difficult to obtain colony growth directly from original exudates. Inoculated agar plates must be incubated at 37 C in a very moist atmosphere for 3–5 days. Evidence of colony growth is best studied with the aid of a dissecting microscope with indirect lighting. Characteristic colonies appear as tiny, smooth, circular, translucent masses with a dense, raised central area (Fig. 8.4). They rarely are more than 0.2–0.3 mm in diameter and frequently occur in ridges along the

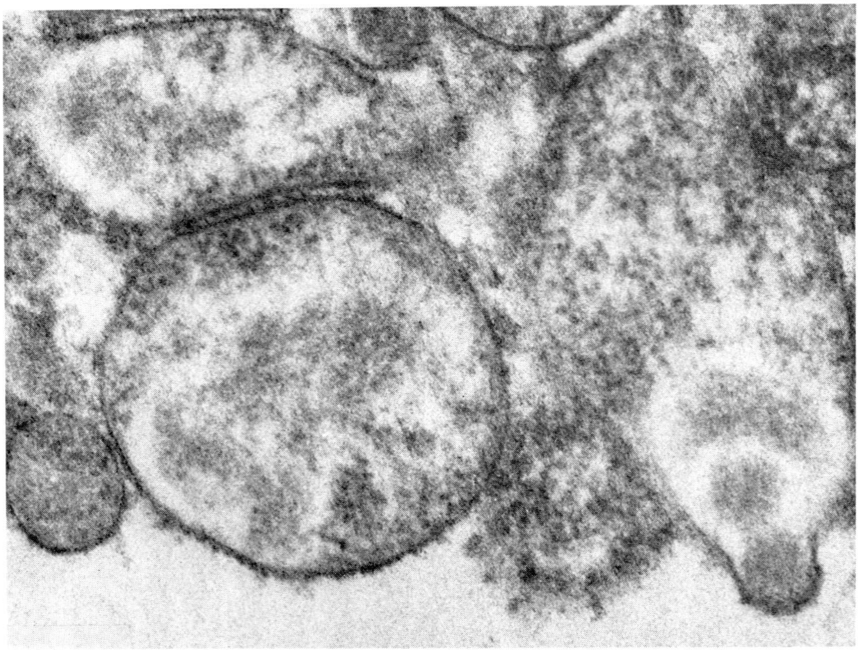

8.2. Electron micrograph of thin section of *M. gallisepticum* strain W, 96-hr culture. Small elementary body (*lower left*) contains cytoplasm of marked electron density. One semilunar and two spherical condensations are located with a protrusion of the cell membrane (*lower right*). ×94,000. (29)

streak line, since closely adjacent colonies readily coalesce. Variations in colonies of isolates representing numerous species of avian mycoplasma have been noted (27, 118), but the species designation of an organism cannot be determined by its colony characteristics.

Biochemical Properties. Biochemical and related biologic properties of MG have been reported by numerous workers. It ferments glucose and maltose, with production of acid but not gas. It does not ferment lactose, dulcitol, or salicin. Sucrose is rarely fermented; results with galactose, fructose, trehalose, and mannitol are variable. It does not hydrolyze arginine and is phosphatase-negative. It reduces 2,3,5-triphenyl tetrazolium (becomes red) and neotetrazolium (becomes blue). MG causes complete hemolysis of horse erythrocytes incorporated into agar medium, and agglutinates turkey and chicken erythrocytes. See further discussion of the hemagglutination-inhibition (HI) test under Serology.

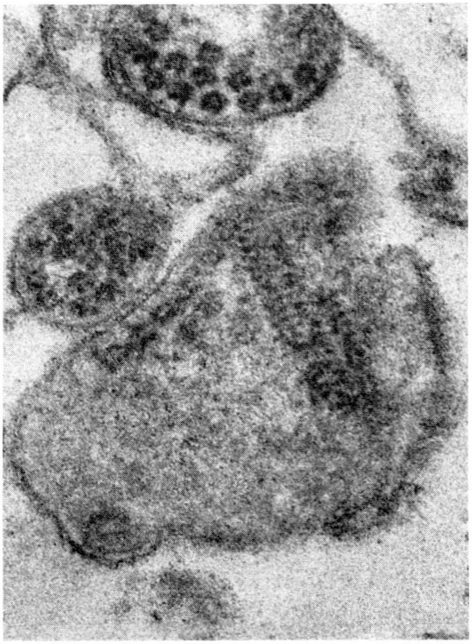

8.3. Electron micrograph of thin section of *M. gallisepticum* strain JA, 96-hr culture. Cells with ribosomes arranged in corncoblike pattern in longitudinal section; others seen on cross section. ×94,000. (29)

Resistance to Chemical and Physical Agents. It is assumed that most of the commonly employ-

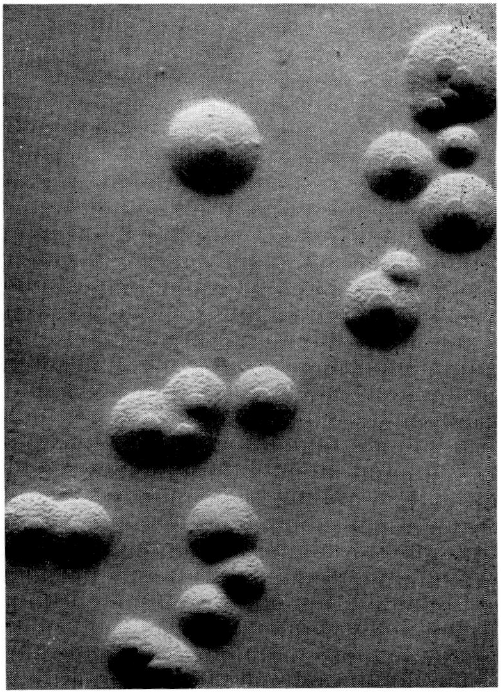

8.4. Colonies of *M. gallisepticum* on 20% chicken serum agar plates. ×40. (47)

ed chemical disinfectants are effective against MG. Inactivation has been produced by phenol, formalin, beta propiolactone, and merthiolate. Its resistance to penicillin and low concentration (1:4000) of thallous acetate make these valuable additives to mycoplasma culture media as inhibitors of bacterial and fungal contamination.

The organism remained viable in chicken feces 1–3 days at 20 C, on muslin cloth 3 days at 20 C or 1 day at 37 C, and in egg yolk 18 wk at 37 C or 6 wk at 20 C (21). Broth suspensions of infective chorioallantoic membrane (CAM) lost their infectivity after 1 hr of exposure at 46 C, after 20 min at 50 C, or by the 3rd wk at 5 C (47). However, other workers (80) found allantoic fluid remained infective 4 days in the incubator, 6 days at room temperature, and 32–60 days in the refrigerator. Yoder (112) found that MG was inactivated in infected chicken hatching eggs that just reached 45.6 C during a 12- to 14-hr heating procedure. Yoder and Hofstad (118) found that broth cultures remained viable 2–4 yr when stored at −30 C. They also recovered viable MG from lyophilized broth culture stored at 4 C at least 7 yr and from lyophilized infective chicken turbinates stored at 4 C for 13–14 yr. Yoder (116) recently found that numerous broth cultures of MG and various other serotypes that had been frozen at −60 C since 1965 were viable upon subculturing more than 20 yr later. *M. synoviae* (MS) and *M. meleagridis* (MM) were not included. Sets of broth cultures including MG, MS, and MM were viable when subcultured after 10 yr at −60 C. One ampule of MG culture lyophilized in 1959 and stored at 4 C was viable when subcultured at 23 yr. Numerous other lyophilized broth cultures including MG, MS, and MM were routinely found to be viable when subcultured at 10–15 yr. Kleven (58) studied the stability of F strain MG in powdered skim milk, phosphate-buffered saline (PBS), tryptose phosphate broth, and distilled water stored at 4, 22, and 37 C. It was stable in all diluents for 24 hr when stored at 4 or 22 C. When stored at 37 C it was stable in PBS for up to 24 hr.

Strain Classification. Various strains within MG should not be confused with the numerous serotypes that have been characterized from avian sources within the entire genus *Mycoplasma.* Certain isolates of *M. gallisepticum* have come to be known more commonly by their isolate designations, which sometimes are called strains. The S6 strain of Zander (3, 33, 123) was an early pathogenic isolate from the brain of a turkey with infectious sinusitis. The A5969 strain was given that designation by Jungherr et al. (51) for a pathogenic culture supplied by Van Roekel. The A5969 strain has become a standard strain for various antigen productions. The F strain of MG, which is so commonly used in current live culture vaccination programs (20, 37, 87), is a relatively mild strain that apparently originated from studies by van der Heide (105) employing the Connecticut F strain. However, the original F isolate was described by Yamamoto and Adler (111) as a typical pathogenic strain. That strain was used by Luginbuhl et al. (68) in Connecticut for live culture vaccination of young broiler breeder replacement flocks to reduce possible egg-transmission of MG in the subsequent breeder flocks. The R strain of MG was isolated by Dale Richey at the Univ. of Georgia Poultry Disease Research Center in 1963 from a chicken with airsacculitis. Yoder (113) employed the pathogenic R strain for inactivated MG bacterin studies. The R strain has been widely used for bacterin production and as a pathogenic strain for MG challenge studies (37, 85, 120).

Pathogenicity

INOCULUM. Isolates of MG vary widely in their relative pathogenicity, depending on the nature of the isolate, its method of propagation, and the number of passages through which it has been maintained. Infective yolk from inoculated embryonated chicken eggs was often considered to be more infective than broth-passaged mycoplasma.

CHICKENS AND TURKEYS. Pathogenicity for chickens and turkeys was studied by numerous researchers in early studies often employing cultures that represented serotypes other than the typical pathogenic MG. However, there is ample evidence to conclude that turkeys are more susceptible than chickens; inoculated turkeys develop more severe sinusitis, airsacculitis, and tendovaginitis. Lin and Kleven (65) determined that the live F strain of MG was relatively more pathogenic for turkeys than usually noted in chickens. Inoculation by the intraocular, intranasal, or intratracheal routes often results in fewer and milder lesions than intrasinus or intra-air sac inoculation. Turkeys sometimes do not develop sinusitis unless cultures are injected directly into the sinus. Inoculation of the tendovaginal cavity in the region of the hock and foot pad of chickens usually results in the production of antibodies and sometimes severe to moderate tendovaginitis, while inoculated air sacs in the same chicken may show little or no gross response. MG infection is frequently associated with a complexity of environmental and disease agents involved, as discussed further under Morbidity and Mortality.

EMBRYONATED CHICKEN EGGS. Inoculation of broth cultures or exudates containing MG into 7-day-old embryonated chicken eggs via the yolk sac route usually results in embryo deaths within 5–7 days. One or more yolk passages may be necessary before typical deaths and lesions are produced. Dwarfing, generalized edema, liver necrosis, and enlarged spleens are most typical. The organism reaches its highest concentration in the yolk sac, yolk, and CAM just prior to embryo death. Recent studies (64) showed that MG strains varied in their in ovo pathogenicity and their chicken pathogenicity. Embryo mortality due to virulent MG was blocked in eggs containing maternal MG antibodies.

Inoculation of embryonated chicken eggs is rarely employed for the isolation of avian mycoplasma now that adequate media are available.

PATHOGENESIS AND EPIZOOTIOLOGY

Natural and Experimental Hosts. *M. gallisepticum* infection occurs naturally in chickens and turkeys. However, it has also been isolated from natural infections in pheasants (*Phasianus colchicus*), chukar partridge (*Alectoris graeca*), peafowl (*Pavo cristatus*), bobwhite quail (*Colinus virginianus*), and Japanese quail (*Coturnix coturnix japonica*). MG was isolated from a golden pheasant (*Chrysolophus pictus*) in Australia by Reece et al. (84) and from a yellow-naped Amazon parrot (*Amazona ochrocephala auropalliata*) by Bozeman et al. (14). The isolation of MG from ducks has been reported from England (49) and from Yugoslavia (11). Reports on the isolation of MG from geese have come from France (19) and from Yugoslavia (12). The report by Davidson et al. (24) concerning MG isolated from wild turkeys (*Meleagris gallopavo*) notes that involved turkeys were in confinement, not free-living in their natural habitat.

The author is aware of publications concerning mycoplasma isolations from various other free-flying birds, but the significance of occasionally reported MG has not been clearly established. Similarly, attempts to determine its pathogenicity for various free-flying birds have not been very conclusive.

Transmission. Direct contact of susceptible birds with infected carrier chickens or turkeys causes outbreaks of the disease; it is also spread by air-borne dust or droplets. Spread by contact with contaminated equipment is commonly assumed, but has not been well documented. The infection is often transmitted through the egg in chickens and turkeys. MG was isolated from the oviduct of infected chickens and semen of infected roosters (118). Egg transmission has been successfully produced following experimental infection of susceptible chickens by a number of researchers (13, 35, 37, 119, 120). A recent report (91) noted that culturing the vitelline membrane of fresh eggs provided more isolations of MG than did culturing 18-day-old embryos.

Incubation Period. Early investigators found the incubation period to vary from 6–21 days in experimental transmission. Sinusitis often develops in experimentally inoculated turkeys within 6–10 days. Under natural conditions it is very difficult to determine the exact date of exposure; so many variables seem to influence the onset and extent of clinical infection that meaningful incubation periods cannot be stated. Numerous chicken and turkey flocks develop clinical infection near the onset of egg production, suggesting a low level of inherent infection (probably due to egg transmission) that precipitates from a series of stressing events. This apparent long extension of the incubation period is especially common in offspring of infected chickens or turkeys hatched from eggs dipped in antibiotic solutions for control of MG infection. The possible role of contamination from other sources of infection is not always clear and can rarely be proved beyond reasonable doubt. Many isolates of MG obtained by Truscott et al. (104), Mallinson and Rosenstein (70) and Yoder (115) seem to represent this newer kind of infection with delayed onset in which serologic evidence first appears between the 26th and 38th wk of age, usually without clinical signs.

Signs

CHICKENS. The most characteristic signs of the natural disease in adult flocks are tracheal rales, nasal discharge, and coughing. Feed consumption is reduced and birds lose weight. In laying flocks, egg production declines but is usually maintained at a lowered level. However, flocks may have serologic evidence of infection with no obvious clinical signs, especially if they encountered the infection at a younger age and have partially recovered. Male birds frequently have the most pronounced signs, and the disease is often more severe during winter. In broiler flocks most outbreaks occur between 4 and 8 wk of age. Signs are frequently more marked than those observed in mature flocks. Severe outbreaks observed in broilers are frequently due to complications (see Morbidity and Mortality).

TURKEYS. A nasal discharge with foaming of eye secretions frequently precedes the more typical swelling of the paranasal sinuses from sinusitis. Sometimes partial to complete closing of the eyes results from severe sinus swelling (Fig. 8.5). Appetite remains near normal as long as the bird can see to eat. As the disease progresses the affected birds become thin. Tracheal rales, coughing, and labored breathing may become evident if tracheitis or airsacculitis is present. In breeding flocks there may be a drop in egg production or at least a lowered production efficiency.

Morbidity and Mortality

CHICKENS. The infection usually affects nearly all chickens in a flock but is variable in severity and duration. It tends to be more severe and of longer duration in the cold months and affects younger birds more severely than mature birds, although there may be a considerable loss from lowered egg production.

While MG is considered the primary cause of chronic respiratory disease, other organisms frequently cause complications. Severe air sac infection, frequently designated as complicated CRD or air sac disease, is undoubtedly the condition more commonly encountered in the field. Newcastle disease (ND) or infectious bronchitis (IB) may precipitate outbreaks of MG infection. *E. coli* has been found to be a frequent complicating organism. The effect of MG, *E. coli,* and IB virus (IBV) infections alone or together in chickens was studied by Gross (39) and Fabricant and Levine (34). They reproduced a severe air sac infection when all three agents were combined. They further noted that *E. coli* could not readily infect the air sac unless they were previously invaded by MG alone or in combination with either IBV or ND virus (NDV). Several investigators have noted increased severity and duration of the disease when both MG and IBV were present.

Mortality is usually negligible in adult flocks, but there can be a reduction in the number of birds in production (16). In broilers the mortality may be low in uncomplicated disease to as much as 30% in complicated outbreaks, especially during the colder months. Retarded growth, down-grading of carcasses, and condemnations constitute further losses.

TURKEYS. The disease affects most turkeys in a flock, although some may not exhibit sinusitis, and the lower respiratory form of the infection

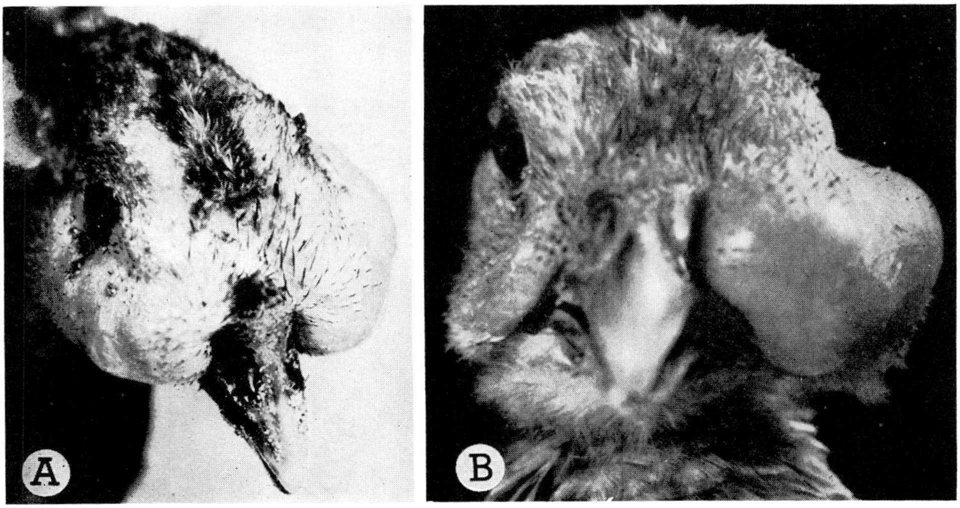

8.5. A. Advanced case of infectious sinusitis involving both sides of face. B. Similar case after exudate in one sinus was removed. (Hinshaw)

may be most prominent. The infection will last for weeks and months in untreated flocks. Condemnations primarily result from airsacculitis and related systemic effects rather than from sinusitis as such.

Gross Lesions. Gross lesions consist primarily of catarrhal exudate in nasal and paranasal passages, trachea, bronchi, and air sacs. Sinusitis is usually most prominent in turkeys but is also observed in chickens and other affected avian hosts. Air sacs frequently contain caseous exudate, although they may only present a "beaded" or lymphofollicular appearance. Some degree of pneumonia may be observed. In severe cases of typical air sac disease in chickens, there is fibrinous or fibrinopurulent perihepatitis and pericarditis along with massive airsacculitis. *M. gallisepticum*-induced salpingitis of chickens and turkeys was reported by Domermuth et al. (30).

Histopathology. The microscopic pathology in chickens and turkeys was studied by Van Roekel et al. (107) and in turkeys by Hitchner (45). They found marked thickening of the mucous membrane of the affected tissues from infiltration with mononuclear cells and hyperplasia of the mucous glands (Fig. 8.6). Focal areas of lymphoid hyperplasia were commonly found in the submucosa (Figs. 8.7, 8.8, 8.9). In the lungs, in addition to pneumonic areas and lymphofollicular changes, granulomatous lesions were also found. Detailed examination of MG-infected chicken air sacs via light microscopy, scanning EM, and histomorphic evaluation was reported by Trampel and Fletcher (102). Ultrastructural details of the interaction of MG with the tracheal epithelium of chickens was studied by Tajima et al. (95). Similar studies with infected tracheal ring explants were reported by Abu-Zahr and Butler (1) and Takagi and Arakawa (97). Dykstra et al. (32) employed EM, including scanning studies, to show the cytopathological changes induced in chicken tracheal epithelium and in tracheal ring cultures inoculated with pathogenic MG. They especially showed exfoliation of ciliated epithelial cells prior to those cells evidencing loss of cilia.

Immunity. Birds that have recovered from clinical signs of the disease have some degree of immunity. Such flocks, however, carry the organism and can transmit the disease to susceptible

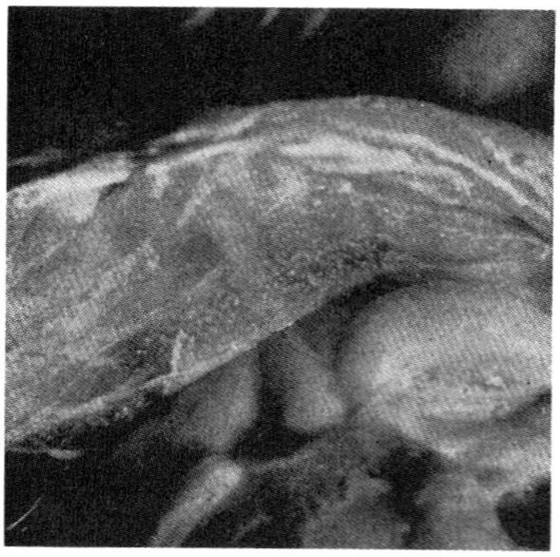

8.7. Lymphofollicular or "beading" reaction in air sac of experimentally inoculated turkey. (107)

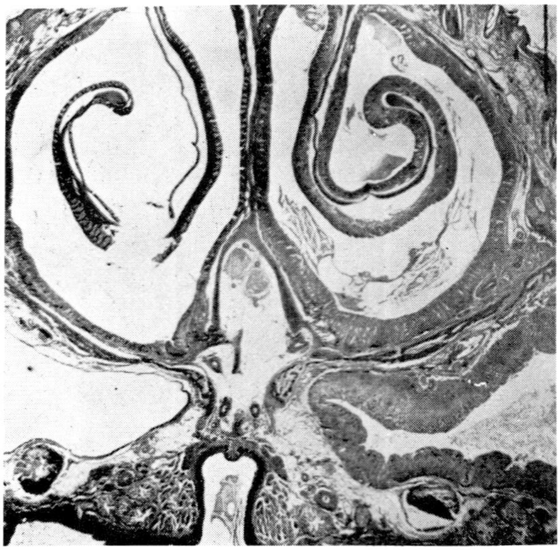

8.6. Section through nasal passages and sinuses of experimental chicken. Unilateral mucosal thickening of sinus and nasal passage. ×6. (107)

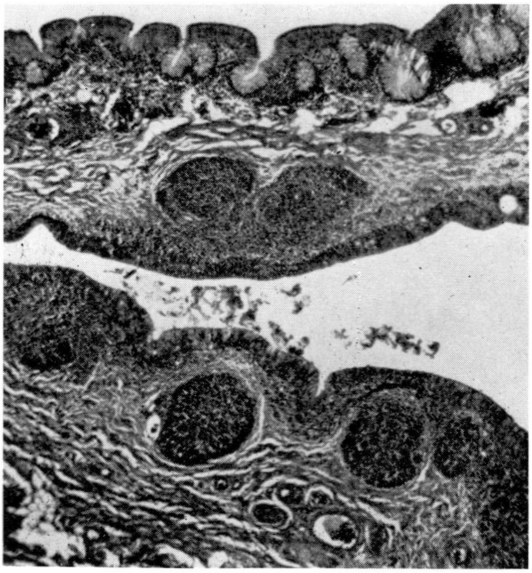

8.8. Section of sinus in chicken. Subepithelial infiltration of mononuclear cells and lymphofollicular reaction. ×36. (107)

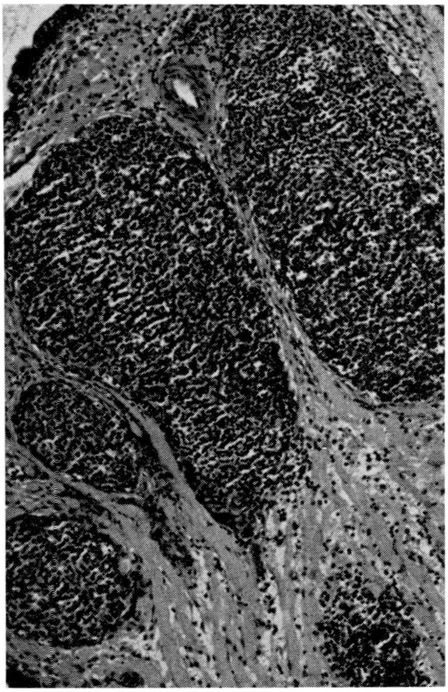

8.9. Air sac of 7-wk-old experimental chicken. Lymphofollicular reaction. ×100. (107)

stock by contact or by egg transmission to their progeny. A review of the literature concerning the immune response to MG is included in the report by Luginbuhl et al. (68). Adler et al. (4) determined the importance of the bursa of Fabricius in development of resistance and serologic response to the organism. A more comprehensive discussion is presented in the section on Immunization.

DIAGNOSIS

Isolation and Identification of Causative Agent. Suspensions of tracheal or air sac exudates, turbinates, lungs, or fluid sinus exudate may be cultured directly in suitable broth or agar overlay medium. Culturing swabs taken from the choanal cleft (palatine fissure) proved to be adequate for isolating MG (17). In Frey's medium (36) supplemented with 10–15% horse or swine serum, extraneous bacterial contamination is usually controlled by inclusion of thallous acetate (1:4000) and penicillin (up to 2000 IU/ml). MG has been isolated from rooster semen (118), and from oviducts (30, 118). Although *M. meleagridis* is frequently isolated from turkey cloacal swabs, MG has been similarly isolated from the cloacal areas of turkeys (109) and chickens (6, 69).

Cultures should be incubated at least 5–7 days at 37 C. Growth may not be evident, but 2 or 3 serial passages at 3- to 5-day intervals may increase the number of isolations. Inclusion of 2,3,5-triphenyl tetrazolium or phenol red with sufficient dextrose provides a growth indicator system. *M. gallisepticum* reduces triphenyl tetrazolium to produce a red color in the medium, or it ferments dextrose to change phenol red to a yellow color as the medium becomes acid.

Cultures can be further identified by preparing Giemsa-stained films that should reveal small coccoid organisms, often in clumps, when examined through the oil immersion lens of a microscope (see Fig. 8.1). Enriched agar medium may be inoculated from the broth cultures to study colonial morphology. The inoculated plates must be incubated at 37 C in a very moist atmosphere 3–5 days before being examined for typical mycoplasma colonies. The hemagglutinating ability of cultures may also be determined. Sinuses, air sacs, or tendon sheaths of young chickens or turkeys may be inoculated to determine pathogenicity of the culture. Sections prepared for histopathology may also be of aid in making a diagnosis.

The inoculation of 7-day-old embryonated chicken eggs via the yolk sac with original exudates may be employed as a further means of isolating MG, but the inoculum must be relatively free from bacterial contamination. Death of embryos should occur within 5–8 days, but one serial passage or more of harvested yolk material might be required before embryo deaths and typical lesions are noted.

However, proof that isolates truly are MG must be determined by serologic procedures. Antigens can be prepared and then tested with known MG antiserum. Although such testing of recently isolated cultures is rarely very satisfactory. Another method is to test the serum from experimentally inoculated chickens or turkeys with known MG antigen.

Identification of mycoplasma cultures is generally conducted in various research laboratories employing one or more of the following procedures. The use of direct immunofluorescence employing colonies on the surface of agar plates was reported to be very effective for culture identification by Talkington and Kleven (98, 99). Somewhat varied applications of the direct immunofluorescence procedure have been reported to be effective for the identification of MG and MS cultures (73, 77).

The agar-gel precipitin test has also been used to identify cultures by Aycardi et al. (9) and by Nonomura and Yoder (79). The direct immunoperoxidase test system was reported to be effective for the identification of MG and MS cultures (48), but that procedure is more commonly employed in an enzyme-linked immunosorbent assay (ELISA) procedure for detecting antibodies in serum.

Distinct differences in the protein banding patterns of various MG strains by the polyacrylamide gel electrophoresis procedure were reported to distinguish vaccine F strain from the usual standard MG cultures S6 and A5969 (56). Kleven et al. (59) compared various strains of MG by restriction endonuclease analysis and HI procedures. They found that hemagglutination antigen prepared from the standard MG strain A5969 was relatively insensitive for detecting HI antibodies to many of the strains of MG studied. Several distinct groupings of strains, not closely related to standard MG strains, were readily detected by restriction endonuclease analysis. Similarly, Kleven et al. (60) employed the restriction endonuclease DNA analysis and DNA-DNA hybridization procedures to distinguish between the F vaccine strain and standard MG strains S6 and A5969. Similar methods and results were also reported by Khan et al. (55). A further procedure that could also distinguish the F vaccine strain from the standard MG strains employed the use of ribosomal RNA gene probes (122).

Serology. Serologic procedures are available to aid in diagnosis of MG infection. A positive serologic test, together with history and signs typical of the disease, would allow a presumptive diagnosis pending isolation and identification of the organisms. The rapid serum plate (SP) test is performed by mixing a drop of serum with a drop of commercially available stained antigen on a white porcelain or glass plate and mixing. After mixing to make a spot about 2 cm in diameter, the plate is rotated gently and the test is read within 2 min. Clumping of the stained antigen with clearing of the suspension constitutes a positive reaction.

The tube agglutination test was a common procedure, especially within the MG control program in turkeys during the 1960s and 1970s, but is rarely used anymore.

The HI test is used almost routinely to confirm reactors detected by the SP procedure or the more recent ELISA test. The detailed procedure for HI tests is presented by Hitchner et al. (46), including the very frequently employed microtiter HI system described by Ryan (88).

Piela et al. (83) reported on the use of a saline and chloroform extract of yolk from fresh eggs as a substitute for serum for the detection of antibodies by the ELISA and HI tests for MG; the former was confirmed by Mohammed et al. (75). Coleman et al. (22) employed one part of fluid yolk with two parts of saline without the hazards of added solvents. Yoder and Hopkins (120) confirmed that the yolk-saline suspension compared favorably with the serum from the same hen in the HI procedure.

The ELISA procedure has been used by several groups of researchers in an attempt to devise a test that would be more sensitive and more specific than either the SP or HI test for MG antibodies. Talkington et al. (101) reported their ELISA test to be less sensitive, but more specific than the SP test, and more sensitive than the HI test for MG. Workers in Japan (110) detected MG antibodies in sera and in tracheal washings by ELISA. Australian studies (43) used the ELISA procedure to differentiate MG and MS antibodies in sera, but there were some nonspecific reactions that were not reduced by heat inactivation, mercaptoethanol or neuraminidase treatment. While studying two commercial ELISA assay kits for MG, Avakian et al. (8) showed high rates of nonspecific positive reactions when testing serum from birds given various inactivated poultry disease vaccines, although HI tests were negative. Opitz and Cyr (81) employed Triton X-100-solubilized MG and MS antigens in the ELISA and found them to be more specific and sensitive than other antigens tested.

During the 1970s atypical MG serological test results were encountered in some chicken breeding flocks with histories of being free of MG. The usually normal appearing flocks started to have a small percent of MG SP test reactors at 28–36 wk of age. Mallinson and Rosenstein (70) and Yoder (115) noted that HI titers were rarely over 1:80, and the percent of SP reactors often did not exceed 20–40% of the flock during several months of study. The atypical reactor problems seemed to be associated with “variant” MG strains. Isolation of MG often required repeated attempts. Truscott et al. (104) considered the infection to be caused by MG of low virulence which seemed to be egg transmitted. Yoder (115) agreed that the strains involved appeared to be of low virulence and spread slowly within the flocks, and that egg transmission appeared to be the most likely means of transmission.

Many isolates readily produced airsacculitis when broilers were given cultures by aerosol. The challenged broilers became positive on the MG SP test and developed moderate to high HI titers. However, other reports (71, 89) have shown some variant strains of MG that do not readily react with standard MG antigens in HI tests. Kleven et al. (59) reported that some of the HI-variant strains differed from standard MG strains in restriction endonuclease studies.

Nonspecific (false-positive) reactions to mycoplasma plate test antigens have followed the use of some inactivated, oil-emulsion poultry vaccines (15, 23, 86). More recently Glisson et al. (38) and Yoder (117) studied several MG and MS plate agglutination antigens employed with positive- and negative-control sera and sera from chickens inoculated with various inactivated (mostly oil-emulsion) commercial poultry disease vaccines. Numerous serum plate reactions appeared within 2–3 wk postvaccination and generally persisted for several weeks. The plate test reactions were noted with both MG and MS antigens, although the degree and duration of the reactions varied with the vaccine and the source of the testing antigen. Reactions seemed to be strongest from birds given vaccines of tissue culture origin, but one bacterin containing aluminum hydroxide gel also caused nonspecific reactions. The nonspecific plate reactor sera gave negative HI results. Yoder (117) was unable to prevent the nonspecific reactions by heat inactivation or by addition of mercaptoethanol, dithiothreitol, or 3 M sodium chloride solution.

Differential Diagnosis

CHICKENS. Care must be taken to differentiate *M. gallisepticum* infection from other common respiratory diseases of chickens. ND and IB or their antibodies may be present as separate entities or as part of the complicated CRD problem. Infectious coryza and fowl cholera (FC) usually can be identified by cultural studies. MS infection may be present alone or in addition to MG. Application of both serologic and cultural test procedures may be necessary in some cases.

TURKEYS. Presence of a respiratory disease including sinusitis in a turkey flock may at times be due to such things as FC, ornithosis, MS infection, or vitamin A deficiency as well as the more usual MG. Specific cultural and serologic procedures are needed to differentiate them. Avian influenza A infection might also be considered.

TREATMENT. MG is susceptible to certain antibiotics: streptomycin, oxytetracycline, chlortetracycline, erythromycin, magnamycin, spiramycin, tylosin, lincomycin and spectinomycin. However, some strains of MG have been reported to be rather resistant to streptomycin, erythromycin, spiramycin, and tylosin.

Various antibiotics and chemicals were injected or administered in the feed or water during the 1960s for the treatment of CRD. Results of treatment studies have been variable, probably reflecting the different complicating infections present in a wide spectrum of age groups under diverse conditions. In many cases it is doubtful if the small increase in weight gains or egg production and moderate reduction of carcass condemnations are sufficient to cover cost of treatment. However, some more commonly employed treatments that tend to provide favorable results include use of oxytetracycline or chlortetracycline at 200 g/ton feed for at least several days. Such broad-spectrum antibiotics have been potentiated with approximately 0.5% terephthalic acid and sometimes a reduced calcium ration. However, terephthalic acid is not cleared by the US Food and Drug Administration for use in poultry rations. Tylosin has been injected subcutaneously at 3–5 mg/lb body weight or administered at 2–3 g/gal drinking water for 3–5 days. Administration of very low levels of tylosin in feed to MG-exposed layers in multiple-age complexes was found to lessen egg production losses (82). Tiamulin was reported to be effective against development of airsacculitis in chickens and turkeys (10).

Hamdy (42) reported that a combination of lincomycin and spectinomycin was effective in controlling experimental complicated airsacculitis in young chickens. The minimum inhibitory concentrations of kitasamycin, tiamulin, and tylosin for MG were reported by Jordan and Knight (50).

Medication of Breeders. Attempts to eliminate egg transmission of MG by medication of breeder flocks or their progeny with streptomycin, dihydrostreptomycin, oxytetracycline, chlortetracycline, erythromycin, or tylosin have generally been able to produce considerable reduction in rate of MG infection but generally were not adequate to obtain entirely infection-free flocks.

Egg Dipping. Fabricant and Levine (34) and others (41, 94) used egg dipping as a means of getting antibiotics into hatching eggs to eliminate egg-transmitted MG. Eggs warmed to 37.8 C were immersed in cold (1.7–4.4 C) antibiotic solutions (especially tylosin or erythromycin at 40–1000 ppm) for 15–20 min. Because of the temperature differential the cooling of the egg contents caused antibiotic to be pulled in through the eggshell. This procedure was later replaced by a pressure differential (vacuum) system as reported by Alls et al. (5). In general, these methods greatly reduced, but sometimes did not completely eliminate, the possibility of egg transmission. The influence on hatchability was not consistently favorable, and bacterial contamination was troublesome at times. However, in the judgment of the author, egg dipping in antibiotic solutions has made it possible to obtain sufficient MG-free flocks to provide the poultry industry with a nucleus for producing clean progeny for large flocks, resulting in MG-free chicken and turkey breeder flocks in the USA. Serologic testing and selection of negative flocks for breeders are practical only when clean breeder flocks are established and reproduced.

Egg Inoculation. Injection of lincomycin-spectinomycin into the air cell of hatching eggs was reasonably effective in controlling MG infection in experimentally inoculated eggs (103). Further studies were conducted, including work within the poultry industry, but reports from such are not readily available. Antibiotic injection studies employing turkey hatching eggs are discussed in the section on *M. meleagridis* infection.

Egg Heating. Still another approach to breaking the egg transmission cycle was reported by Yoder (112). Room temperature (25.6 C) eggs were heated in a forced-air incubator during a 12-

to 14-hr period to reach an internal temperature of 46.1 C. Hatchability was sometimes reduced 8–12%, but MG and MS appeared to be inactivated. Similar success was reported by Meroz et al. (74) in Israel. Field studies have been extensive, with adequate success apparent in many cases and only 2–3% reduction of hatchability (114).

PREVENTION AND CONTROL

Management Procedures. Maintaining chicken and turkey flocks free of MG infection is only possible by obtaining replacement flocks that are known to be free of the infection, and rearing them in strict isolation to avoid introduction of the disease. Establishing and maintaining the MG-clean status of breeder flocks can be accomplished by participation in control programs.

Control Programs. Both turkey and chicken breeders have generally adopted the various state-supported MG-control programs within the National Poultry Improvement Plan (NPIP) as prescribed in their Plans and Auxiliary Provisions (7). In general, flocks that are progeny of normal MG-clean flocks must undergo blood testing of at least 10% of the flock (not less than 300 birds) when more than 4 mo of age and be found MG-negative serologically to be declared MG-clean. Chicken flocks also must have subsequent negative tests on at least 150 birds at intervals not more than 90 days. Proved reactor flocks must not be used as breeders. Special provisions for testing multiplier flocks include the use of smaller numbers of blood samples, and permits the use of yolk-saline suspensions from eggs to be tested by HI or ELISA procedures.

Immunization

INACTIVATED MG BACTERINS. In the late 1970s it became apparent that MG was becoming a lingering problem in some large multiple-age, egg-laying complexes. Most of the replacement pullets were obtained from MG-clean sources, but often became infected by the time they were in production. Yoder (113) studied an MG bacterin employing an improved oil-emulsion adjuvant system reported by Stone et al. (93), even though MG bacterins generally had not seemed to be very effective, as reviewed by Adler (2). However, MG bacterin with oil-emulsion adjuvant protected young chickens against intrasinus challenge with virulent MG and commercial egg layers against MG-induced drops in egg production (44). Some workers confirmed that such bacterins could protect broilers against airsacculitis (53, 121) or against reductions in egg production in layers (120), while others (54) did not detect much effect of bacterin in commercial egg layers with endemic MG infection. Yet another report (90) concluded that the application of an inactivated oil-emulsion MG bacterin in an endemically MG-infected flock for two consecutive generations had resulted in MG-clean third generation chickens. Talkington and Kleven (100) noted that there was only limited protection against MG colonization of the trachea of chickens challenged after vaccination with inactivated oil-emulsion MG bacterin. Other reports (120, 121) also noted tracheal infection following challenge after use of MG bacterin.

Live Culture Vaccination. Early studies on the use of live cultures of MG in young replacement pullets prior to being housed in large multiple-age egg-laying complexes was reported in 1977 by van der Heide (105). He employed the rather mild Connecticut F strain of MG as did Carpenter et al. (20) in Pennsylvania. Numerous other studies concerning live F strain MG vaccination have been published.

Glisson and Kleven (37) studied the relative efficacy of live F strain and MG bacterin in protecting against MG-challenged hens against production losses or egg transmission of MG. All vaccinated groups had better egg production and less egg transmission than controls. Hens vaccinated with two doses of MG bacterin had the longest lag before egg transmission. In a large-scale field study Branton and Deaton (16) evaluated the use of live F strain MG in three strains of commercial egg layers in an endemic MG complex. Egg weight and eggshell strength were similar for all three strains of chickens with no differences from the unvaccinated controls. Less mortality in F strain–vaccinated hens of some strains gives the appearance of better egg production, based on production per hen housed. Further studies (18) showed that vaccination with live F strain at 45 wk of age (postproduction peak) had no effect on oviduct function as judged by eggshell strength and thickness, and egg quality. Egg transmission of live F strain MG did not occur in hens vaccinated by ocular exposure, but did occur in hens given F strain by aerosol. However, egg transmission was considerably greater when live R strain was administered by either route (66). Other reports (67, 87) showed protection against airsacculitis in broilers aerosol-challenged with virulent R strain following ocular vaccination with live F strain. Levisohn and Dykstra (63) also found that F strain could protect against airsacculitis induced by MG challenge, but F strain colonization on the tracheal epithelium did not block infection by the pathogenic MG strain. Kleven (57) reported that pullets given live F strain by ocular inoculation did not readily transmit the infection to broilers in pens in the same house when separated by an isle or empty pen.

Carpenter et al. (20) reported on the relative performance of MG-clean and F strain–vaccinated laying hens on farms in Pennsylvania with endemic MG infection. They concluded that, on the average, layers maintained free of MG infection laid 15.7 more eggs, and F strain–vaccinated layers 7.0 more eggs, per hen housed, than did the MG infected layers. Similarly, Mohammed et al. (76) determined the economic impact of MG and MS infection in commercial layers in California. They concluded that MG-infected flocks produced 5–12 fewer eggs per hen and F strain–vaccinated flocks 6 eggs less per hen, compared to uninfected flocks. They estimated that the total loss due to MG infection in commercial layers in California for 1984 was approximately seven million dollars.

Young chicks immunized with selected temperature-sensitive mutants of the S6 strain of MG by intranasal inoculation and then challenged via the air sac with virulent S6 were noted to have less airsacculitis than controls (52, 62).

REFERENCES

1. Abu-Zahr, M.N., and M. Butler. 1978. Ultrastructural features of Mycoplasma gallisepticum in tracheal explants under transmission and stereoscan electron microscopy. Res Vet Sci 24:248–253.

2. Adler, H.E. 1976. Immunological response to Mycoplasma gallisepticum. Theriogenology 6:87–91.

3. Adler, H.E., R. Yamamoto, and J. Berg. 1957. Strain differences of pleuropneumonialike organisms of avian origin. Avian Dis 1:19–27.

4. Adler, H.E., B.J. Bryant, D.R. Cordy, M. Shifrine, and A.J. DaMassa. 1973. Immunity and mortality in chickens infected with Mycoplasma gallisepticum: Influence of the bursa of Fabricius. J Infect Dis 127:61–68. (Suppl).

5. Alls, A.A., W.J. Benton, W.C. Krauss, and M.S. Cover. 1963. The mechanics of treating hatching eggs for disease prevention. Avian Dis 7:89–97.

6. Amin, M.M., and F.T.W. Jordan. 1979. Infection of the chicken with a virulent or avirulent strain of Mycoplasma gallisepticum alone and together with Newcastle disease virus or E. coli or both. Vet Microbiol 4:35–45.

7. Anonymous. 1985. The National Poultry Improvement Plan and Auxiliary Provisions. USDA, APHIS. Beltsville, MD.

8. Avakian, A.P., S.H. Kleven, and J.R. Glisson. 1988. Evaluation of the specificity and sensitivity of two commercial enzyme-linked immunosorbent assay kits, the SP agglutination test, and the hemagglutination-inhibition test for antibodies formed in response to Mycoplasma gallisepticum. Avian Dis 32:262–272.

9. Aycardi, E.R., D.P. Anderson, and R.P. Hanson. 1971. Classification of avian mycoplasmas by gel diffusion and growth inhibition tests. Avian Dis 15:434–447.

10. Baughn, C.O., W.C. Alpaugh, W.H. Linkenheimer, and D.C. Maplesden. 1978. Effect of tiamulin in chickens and turkeys infected experimentally with avian Mycoplasma. Avian Dis 22:620–626.

11. Bencina, D., T. Tadina, and D. Dorrer. 1988. Natural infection of ducks with Mycoplasma synoviae and Mycoplasma gallisepticum and mycoplasma egg transmission. Avian Pathol 17:441–449.

12. Bencina, D., T. Tadina, and D. Dorrer. 1988. Natural infection of geese with Mycoplasma gallisepticum and Mycoplasma synoviae and egg transmission of the mycoplasmas. Avian Pathol 17:925–928.

13. Benton, W.J., M.S. Cover, and F.W. Melchior. 1967. Mycoplasma gallisepticum in a commercial laryngotracheitis vaccine. Avian Dis 11:426–429.

14. Bozeman, L.H., S.H. Kleven, and R.B. Davis. 1984. Mycoplasma challenge studies in budgerigars (Melopsittacus undulatus) and chickens. Avian Dis 28:426–434.

15. Bradbury, J.M., and F.T.W. Jordan. 1972. Studies on the absorption of certain medium proteins to Mycoplasma gallisepticum and their influence on agglutination and haemagglutination reactions. Camb J Hyg 70:267–278.

16. Branton, S.L., and J.W. Deaton. 1985. Egg production, egg weight, eggshell strength, and mortality in three strains of commercial layers vaccinated with F strain Mycoplasma gallisepticum. Avian Dis 29:832–837.

17. Branton, S.L., H. Gerlach, and S.H. Kleven. 1984. Mycoplasma gallisepticum isolation in layers. Poult Sci 63:1917–1919.

18. Branton, S.L., B.D. Lott, J.W. Deaton, J.M. Hardin, and W.R. Maslin. 1988. F strain Mycoplasma gallisepticum vaccination of postproduction-peak commercial leghorns and its effect on egg and eggshell quality. Avian Dis 32:304–307.

19. Buntz, B., J.M. Bradbury, A. Vuillaume, and D. Rousselot-Paillet. 1986. Isolation of Mycoplasma gallisepticum from geese. Avian Pathol 15:615–617.

20. Carpenter, T.E., E.T. Mallinson, K.F. Miller, R.F. Gentry, and L.D. Schwartz. 1981. Vaccination with F-strain Mycoplasma gallisepticum to reduce production losses in layer chickens. Avian Dis 25:404–409.

21. Chandiramani, N.K., H. Van Roekel, and O.M. Olesiuk. 1966. Viability studies with Mycoplasma gallisepticum under different environmental conditions. Poult Sci 45:1029–1044.

22. Coleman, M.A., M. Young, J.P. Donahoe, R. Mohan, and R. Fertel. 1982. Using egg yolk washing to monitor MS/MG and Newcastle antibody titers in egg and meat type breeders. Proc 3rd Annu Meet Southern Poult Sci Soc, p. 7. Atlanta, GA.

23. Cullen, G.A., and L.M. Timms. 1972. Diagnosis of Mycoplasma infection in poultry previously vaccinated with killed adjuvant vaccines. Br Vet J 128:94–100.

24. Davidson, W.R., V.F. Nettles, C.E. Couvillion, and H.W. Yoder. 1982. Infectious sinusitis in wild turkeys. Avian Dis 26:402–405.

25. Delaplane, J.P., and H.O. Stuart. 1943. The propagation of a virus in embryonated chicken eggs causing a chronic respiratory disease of chickens. Am J Vet Res 4:325–332.

26. Dickinson, E.M., and W.R. Hinshaw. 1938. Treatment of infectious sinusitis of turkeys with argyrol and silver nitrate. J Am Vet Med Assoc 93:151–156.

27. Dierks, R.E., J.A. Newman, and B.S. Pomeroy. 1967. Characterization of avian Mycoplasma. Ann NY Acad Sci 143:170–189.

28. Dodd, S. 1905. Epizootic pneumo-enteritis of the turkey. J Comp Pathol Ther 18:239–245.

29. Domermuth, C.H., M. Nielsen, E.A. Freundt, and A. Birch-Andersen. 1964. Ultrastructure of Mycoplasma species. J Bacteriol 88:727–744.

30. Domermuth, C.H., W.B. Gross, and R.T. Dubose. 1967. Mycoplasmal salpingitis of chickens and turkeys. Avian Dis 11:393–398.

31. Dutta, S.K., R.E. Dierks, and B.S. Pomeroy. 1965. Electron microscopic studies of the morphology and the stages of development of Mycoplasma gallisepticum. Avian Dis 9:241–251.

32. Dykstra, M.J., S. Levisohn, O.J. Fletcher, and S.H. Kleven. 1985. Evaluation of cytopathologic

changes induced in chicken tracheal epithelium by Mycoplasma gallisepticum in vivo and in vitro. Am J Vet Res 46:116–122.

33. Fabricant, J. 1958. A re-evaluation of the use of media for the isolation of pleuropneumonialike organisms of avian origin. Avian Dis 2:409–417.

34. Fabricant, J., and P.P. Levine. 1962. Experimental production of complicated chronic respiratory disease infection ("air sac" disease). Avian Dis 6:13–23.

35. Fabricant, J., and P.P. Levine. 1963. Infection in young chickens for the prevention of egg transmission of Mycoplasma gallisepticum in breeders. Proc 17th World Vet Congr, pp. 1469–1474.

36. Frey, M.L., R.P. Hanson, and D.P. Anderson. 1968. A medium for the isolation of avian mycoplasmas. Am J Vet Res 29:2163–2171.

37. Glisson, J.R., and S.H. Kleven. 1984. Mycoplasma gallisepticum vaccination: Effects on egg transmission and egg production. Avian Dis 28:406–415.

38. Glisson, J.R., J.F. Dawe, and S.H. Kleven. 1984. The effect of oil-emulsion vaccines on the occurrence of nonspecific plate agglutination reactions for Mycoplasma gallisepticum and M. synoviae. Avian Dis 28:397–405.

39. Gross, W.B. 1961. The development of "air sac disease." Avian Dis 5:431–439.

40. Hall, C.F. 1962. Mycoplasma gallisepticum antigen production. Avian Dis 6:359–362.

41. Hall, C.F., A.I. Flowers, and L.C. Grumbles. 1963. Dipping of hatching eggs for control of Mycoplasma gallisepticum. Avian Dis 7:178–183.

42. Hamdy, A.H. 1970. Therapeutic effect of Lincospectin on airsacculitis in chickens. Avian Dis 14:706–714.

43. Higgins, P.A., and K.G. Whithear. 1986. Detection and differentiation of Mycoplasma gallisepticum and M. synoviae antibodies in chicken serum using enzyme-linked immunosorbent assay. Avian Dis 30:160–168.

44. Hildebrand, D.G., D.E. Page, and J.R. Berg. 1983. Mycoplasma gallisepticum–laboratory and field studies evaluating the safety and efficacy of an inactivated MG bacterin. Avian Dis 27:792–802.

45. Hitchner, S.B. 1949. The pathology of infectious sinusitis of turkeys. Poult Sci 28:106–118.

46. Hitchner, S.B., C.H. Domermuth, G. Purchase, and J.E. Williams (eds.). 1980. Isolation and Identification of Avian Pathogens, 2nd Ed. Am Assoc Avian Pathol, Kennett Square, PA.

47. Hofstad, M.S. 1959. Chronic respiratory disease. In H.E. Biester and L.H. Schwarte (eds.), Diseases of Poultry, 4th Ed., pp. 320–330. Iowa State Univ Press, Ames.

48. Imada, Y., I. Nonomura, S. Hayashi, and S. Tsurubuchi. 1979. Immunoperoxidase technique for identification of Mycoplasma gallisepticum and M. synoviae. Nat Inst Anim Health Q (Tokyo) 19:40–46.

49. Jordan, F.T.W., and M.M. Amin. 1980. A survey of mycoplasma infections in poultry. Res Vet Sci 28:96–100.

50. Jordan, F.T.W., and D. Knight. 1984. The minimum inhibitory concentration of kitasamycin, tylosin, and tiamulin for Mycoplasma gallisepticum and their protective effect on infected chicks. Avian Pathol 13:151–162.

51. Jungherr, E.L., R.E. Luginbuhl, M. Tourtellotte, and W.E. Burr. 1955. Significance of serological testing for chronic respiratory disease. Proc 92nd Annu Meet Am Vet Med Assoc, pp. 315–321.

52. Karaca, K., and K.M. Lam. 1986. Effect of temperature-sensitive Mycoplasma gallisepticum vaccine preparations and routes of inoculation on resistance of white leghorns to challenge. Avian Dis 30:772–775.

53. Karaca, K., and K.M. Lam. 1987. Efficacy of commercial Mycoplasma gallisepticum bacterin (MG-Bac) in preventing air-sac lesions in chickens. Avian Dis 31:202–203.

54. Khan, M.I., D.A. McMartin, Y. Yamamoto, and H.B. Ortmayer. 1986. Observations on commercial layers vaccinated with Mycoplasma gallisepticum (MG) bacterin on a multiple-age site endemically infected with MG. Avian Dis 30:309–312.

55. Khan, M.I., B.C. Kirkpatrick, and R. Yamamoto. 1987. A Mycoplasma gallisepticum strain-specific DNA probe. Avian Dis 31:907–909.

56. Khan, M.I., K.M. Lam, and R. Yamamoto. 1987. Mycoplasma gallisepticum strain variations detected by sodium dodecyl sulfate-polyacrylamide gel electrophoresis. Avian Dis 31:315–320.

57. Kleven, S.H. 1981. Transmissibility of the F strain of Mycoplasma gallisepticum in leghorn chickens. Avian Dis 25:1005–1018.

58. Kleven, S.H. 1985. Stability of the F strain of Mycoplasma gallisepticum in various diluents at 4, 22, and 37 C. Avian Dis 29:1266–1268.

59. Kleven, S.H., C.J. Morrow, and K.G. Whithear. 1988. Comparison of Mycoplasma gallisepticum strains by hemagglutination-inhibition and restriction endonuclease analysis. Avian Dis 32:731–741.

60. Kleven, S.H., G.F. Browning, D.M. Bulach, E. Ghiocas, C.J. Morrow, and K.G. Whithear. 1988. Examination of Mycoplasma gallisepticum strains using restriction endonuclease DNA analysis and DNA-DNA hybridisation. Avian Pathol 17:559–570.

61. Kreig, N.R., and J.G. Holt. 1984. Bergey's Manual of Systematic Bacteriology, 9th Ed. Vol. 1, pp. 740–793. Williams & Wilkins, Baltimore/London.

62. Lam, K.M., K. Karaca, and A.A. Bickford. 1986. Response of chickens to inoculation with a temperature-sensitive mutant of Mycoplasma gallisepticum. Avian Dis 30:382–388.

63. Levisohn, S., and M.J. Dykstra. 1987. A quantitative study of single and mixed infection of the chicken trachea by Mycoplasma gallisepticum. Avian Dis 31:1–12.

64. Levisohn, S., J.R. Glisson, and S.H. Kleven. 1985. In ovo pathogenicity of Mycoplasma gallisepticum strains in the presence and absence of maternal antibody. Avian Dis 29:188–197.

65. Lin, M.Y., and S.H. Kleven. 1982. Pathogenicity of two strains of Mycoplasma gallisepticum in turkeys. Avian Dis 26:360–364.

66. Lin, M.Y., and S.H. Kleven. 1982. Egg transmission of two strains of Mycoplasma gallisepticum in chickens. Avian Dis 26:487–495.

67. Lin, M.Y., and S.H. Kleven. 1982. Cross-immunity and antigenic relationships among five strains of Mycoplasma gallisepticum in young leghorn chickens. Avian Dis 26:496–507.

68. Luginbuhl, R.E., M.E. Tourtellotte, and M.N. Frazier. 1967. Mycoplasma gallisepticum control by immunization. Ann NY Acad Sci 143:234–238.

69. MacOwan, K.J., C.J. Randall, and T.F. Brand. 1983. Cloacal infection with Mycoplasma gallisepticum and the effect of inoculation with H120 infectious bronchitis vaccine virus. Avian Pathol 12:497–503.

70. Mallinson, E.T., and M. Rosenstein. 1976. Clinical, cultural, and serologic observations of avian mycoplasmosis in two chicken breeder flocks. Avian Dis 20:211–215.

71. Mallinson, E.T., R.J. Eckroade, and S.H. Kleven. 1981. In vivo bioassay and supplemental serologic techniques for the detection of Mycoplasma in suspect

breeding chickens. Avian Dis 25:1077–1082.

72. Markham, F.S, and S.C. Wong. 1952. Pleuropneumonialike organisms in the etiology of turkey sinusitis and chronic respiratory disease of chickens. Poult Sci 31:902–904.

73. May, J.D., S.L. Branton, and M.A. Cuchens. 1988. Identification of Mycoplasma gallisepticum and M. synoviae by flow cytometry. Avian Dis 32:513–516.

74. Meroz, M., D. Hadash, and Y. Samberg. 1973. Elimination of avian Mycoplasma organisms by heat treatment of eggs prior to incubation–some technical aspects. Refu Vet 30:101–109.

75. Mohammed, H.O., R. Yamamoto, T.E. Carpenter, and H.B. Ortmayer. 1986. Comparison of egg yolk and serum for the detection of Mycoplasma gallisepticum and M. synoviae antibodies by enzyme-linked immunosorbent assay. Avian Dis 30:398–408.

76. Mohammed, H.O., T.E. Carpenter, and R. Yamamoto. 1987. Economic impact of Mycoplasma gallisepticum and M. synoviae in commercial layer flocks. Avian Dis 31:477–482.

77. Morse, J.W., J.T. Boothby, and R. Yamamoto. 1986. Detection of Mycoplasma gallisepticum by direct immunofluorescence using a species-specific monoclonal antibody. Avian Dis 30:204–206.

78. Nelson, J.B. 1935. Cocco-bacilliform bodies associated with an infectious fowl coryza. Science 82:43–44.

79. Nonomura, I., and H.W. Yoder, Jr. 1977. Identification of avian Mycoplasma isolates by the agar gel precipitin test. Avian Dis 21:370–381.

80. Olesiuk, O.M., and H. Van Roekel. 1952. Cultural attributes of the chronic respiratory disease agent. Proc 24th Annu Conf Northeast Lab Workers in Pullorum Disease Control. (Abstr).

81. Opitz, H.M., and M.J. Cyr. 1986. Triton X-100-solubilized Mycoplasma gallisepticum and M. synoviae ELISA antigens. Avian Dis 30:213–215.

82. Ose, E.E., R.H. Wellenreiter, and L.V. Tonkinson. 1979. Effects of feeding tylosin to layers exposed to Mycoplasma gallisepticum. Poult Sci 58:42–49.

83. Piela, T.H., C.M. Gulka, V.J. Yates, and P.W. Chang. 1984. Use of egg yolk in serological tests (ELISA and HI) to detect antibody to Newcastle disease, infectious bronchitis, and Mycoplasma gallisepticum. Avian Dis 28:877–883.

84. Reece, R.L., L. Ireland, and D.A. Barr. 1986. Infectious sinusitis associated with Mycoplasma gallisepticum in game-birds. Aust Vet J 63:167–168.

85. Rimler, R.B., R.B. Davis, R.K. Page, and S.H. Kleven. 1978. Infectious coryza: Preventing complicated coryza with Haemophilus gallinarum and M. gallisepticum bacterins. Avian Dis 22:140–150.

86. Roberts, D.H. 1970. Nonspecific agglutination reactions with Mycoplasma gallisepticum antigens. Vet Rec 87:125–126.

87. Rodriguez, R., and S.H. Kleven. 1980. Evaluation of a vaccine against Mycoplasma gallisepticum in commercial broilers. Avian Dis 24:879–889.

88. Ryan, T.B. 1973. The use of microtiter hemagglutination-inhibition in Mycoplasma gallisepticum testing program. Proc US Anim Health Assoc 77:593–595.

89. Sahu, S.P., and N.O. Olson. 1981. Characterization of an isolate of Mycoplasma WVU 907 which possesses common antigens to Mycoplasma gallisepticum. Avian Dis 25:943–953.

90. Sasipreeyajan, J., D.A. Halvorson, and J.A. Newman. 1985. Bacterin to control the vertical transmission of Mycoplasma gallisepticum in chickens. Avian Dis 29:1256–1259.

91. Sasipreeyajan, J., D.A. Halvorson, and J.A. Newman. 1987. Comparison of culturing Mycoplasma gallisepticum from fresh eggs and 18-day-old embryos. Avian Dis 31:556–559.

92. Shifrine, M., J. Pangborn, and H.E. Adler. 1962. Colonial growth of Mycoplasma gallisepticum observed with the electron microscope. J Bacteriol 83:187–192.

93. Stone, H.D., M. Brugh, S.R. Hopkins, H.W. Yoder, and C.W. Beard. 1978. Preparation of inactivated oil-emulsion vaccines with avian viral or Mycoplasma antigens. Avian Dis 22:666–674.

94. Stuart, E.E., and H.W. Bruins. 1963. Preincubation immersion of eggs in erythromycin to control chronic respiratory disease. Avian Dis 7:287–293.

95. Tajima, M., T. Nunoya, and T. Yagihashi. 1979. An ultrastructural study on the interaction of Mycoplasma gallisepticum with the chicken tracheal epithelium. Am J Vet Res 40:1009–1014.

96. Tajima, M., T. Yagihashi, and T. Nunoya. 1985. Ultrastructure of mycoplasmal capsules as revealed by stabilization with antiserum and staining with ruthenium red. Jpn J Vet Sci 47:217–223.

97. Takagi, H., and A. Arakawa. 1980. The growth and cilia-stopping effect of Mycoplasma gallisepticum 1RF in chicken tracheal organ cultures. Res Vet Sci 28:80–86.

98. Talkington, F.D., and S.H. Kleven. 1983. A classification of laboratory strains of avian Mycoplasma serotypes by direct immunofluorescence. Avian Dis 27:422–429.

99. Talkington, F.D., and S.H. Kleven. 1984. Research note: Additional information on the classification of avian Mycoplasma serotypes. Avian Dis 28:278–280.

100. Talkington, F.D., and S.H. Kleven. 1985. Evaluation of protection against colonization of the trachea following administration of Mycoplasma gallisepticum bacterin. Avian Dis 29:998–1003.

101. Talkington, F.D., and S.H. Kleven, and J. Brown. 1985. An enzyme-linked immunosorbent assay for the detection of antibodies to Mycoplasma gallisepticum in experimentally infected chickens. Avian Dis 29:53–70.

102. Trampel, D.W., and O.J. Fletcher. 1981. Light microscopic, scanning electron microscopic, and histomorphometric evaluation of Mycoplasma gallisepticum induced airsacculitis in chickens. Am J Vet Res 42:1281–1289.

103. Truscott, R.B., and A.E. Ferguson. 1975. Studies on the control of Mycoplasma gallisepticum in hatching eggs. Can J Comp Med 39:235–239.

104. Truscott, R.B., A.E. Ferguson, H.L. Ruhnke, J.R. Pettit, A. Robertson, and G. Speckmann. 1974. An infection in chickens with a strain of Mycoplasma gallisepticum of low virulence. Can J Comp Med 38:341–343.

105. van der Heide, L. 1977. Vaccination can control costly chronic respiratory disease in poultry. Res Rep, Connecticut Storrs Agr Expt Stn 47:26.

106. Van Roekel, H., and O.M. Olesiuk. 1953. The etiology of chronic respiratory disease. Proc 90th Annu Meet Am Vet Med Assoc, pp. 289–303.

107. Van Roekel, H., J.E. Gray, N.L. Shipkowitz, M.K. Clarke, and R.M. Luchini. 1957. Etiology and pathology of the chronic respiratory disease complex in chickens. Univ Mass Agr Expt Stn Bull 486.

108. Vardaman, T.H. 1967. A culture medium for the production of Mycoplasma gallisepticum antigen. Avian Dis 11:123–129.

109. Varley, J., and F.T.W. Jordan. 1978. The response of turkey poults to experimental infection with strains of M. gallisepticum of different virulence and with M. gallinarum. Avian Pathol 7:383–395.

110. Yagihashi, T., and M. Tajima. 1986. Antibody responses in sera and respiratory secretions from chick-

ens infected with Mycoplasma gallisepticum. Avian Dis 30:543–550.
111. Yamamoto, R., and H.E. Adler. 1956. The effect of certain antibiotics and chemical agents on pleuropneumonialike agents of avian origin. Am J Vet Res 17:538–542.
112. Yoder, H.W., Jr. 1970. Preincubation heat treatment of chicken hatching eggs to inactivate Mycoplasma. Avian Dis 14:75–86.
113. Yoder, H.W., Jr. 1979. Serologic response of chickens vaccinated with inactivated preparations of Mycoplasma gallisepticum. Avian Dis 23:493–506.
114. Yoder, H.W., Jr. 1985. Unpublished data.
115. Yoder, H.W., Jr. 1986. A historical account of the diagnosis and characterization of strains of Mycoplasma gallisepticum of low virulence. Avian Dis 30:510–518.
116. Yoder, H.W., Jr. 1988. Unpublished data.
117. Yoder, H.W., Jr. 1989. Nonspecific reactions to Mycoplasma serum plate antigens induced by inactivated poultry disease vaccines. Avian Dis 33:60–68.
118. Yoder, H.W., Jr., and M.S. Hofstad. 1964. Characterization of avian Mycoplasma. Avian Dis 8:481–512.
119. Yoder, H.W., Jr., and M.S. Hofstad. 1965. Evaluation of tylosin in preventing egg transmission of Mycoplasma gallisepticum in chickens. Avian Dis 9:291–301.
120. Yoder, H.W., Jr., and S.R. Hopkins. 1985. Efficacy of experimental inactivated Mycoplasma gallisepticum oil-emulsion bacterin in egg layer chickens. Avian Dis 29:322–334.
121. Yoder, H.W., Jr., S.R. Hopkins, and B.W. Mitchell. 1984. Evaluation of inactivated Mycoplasma gallisepticum oil-emulsion bacterins for protection against airsacculitis in broilers. Avian Dis 28:224–234.
122. Yogev, D., S. Levisohn, S.H. Kleven, D. Halachmi, and S. Razin. 1988. Ribosomal RNA gene probes to detect intraspecies heterogeneity in Mycoplasma gallisepticum and M. synoviae. Avian Dis 32:220–231.
123. Zander, D.V. 1961. Origin of S6 strain Mycoplasma. Avian Dis 5:154–156.

MYCOPLASMA MELEAGRIDIS INFECTION

R. Yamamoto

INTRODUCTION. *Mycoplasma meleagridis* (MM) (N strain PPLO, H serotype) is the cause of an egg-transmitted disease of turkeys in which the primary lesion is an airsacculitis in the progeny. Other manifestations include decreased hatchability, skeletal abnormalities, and poor growth performance. The organism is a specific pathogen of turkeys and has no public health significance.

The economic loss to the US turkey industry resulting from MM-related hatchability losses and cost of egg treatment to control egg-borne infection has been estimated at $9.4 million/yr (24).

HISTORY. Adler et al. (3) were the first to show that airsacculitis in day-old poults could be associated with a mycoplasma other than *M. gallisepticum* (MG). The clinical syndrome of airsacculitis and/or associated skeletal abnormalities has been called day-old type airsacculitis (70), airsacculitis deficiency syndrome (92), and turkey syndrome-65 (TS-65) (119).

INCIDENCE AND DISTRIBUTION. MM is distributed worldwide, and the incidence of MM-associated airsacculitis is very high (20–65%) in naturally infected cull poults. While incidence of air sac lesions is greater in cull vs. first-run poults (42), such surveys reflect the ubiquitous nature of the organism in the turkey population. MM-free turkeys have become available on a commercial scale (51).

ETIOLOGY

Classification. *M. meleagridis* (137) was designated as the N strain by Adler et al. (3) and placed in the H serotype by Kleckner (64), Yoder and Hofstad (146), and Dierks et al. (33).

Morphology and Staining. Giemsa-stained smears of broth cultures of MM show coccoid bodies approximately 0.4 μm in diameter, similar to those of MG (137, 146). They appear singly, in pairs, or in small clusters.

Ultrastructure studies (115) showed that MM did not possess bleb structures typical of MG but had thicker fibrils in the central nuclear area. In both species, ribosomes were distributed in uniform rinds around the cell peripheries. Similar studies by others (52) revealed that the predominant morphotype of MM was a spherical form ranging from 200 to 700 nm in diameter. Other forms (chains of streptococcuslike cells) suggested replication by binary fission. Similar forms, including short filaments, have been observed by scanning electron microscopy (59). An acidic mucopolysaccharide capsule was demonstrated. The DNA of strain 17529 was found to have a guanine and cytosine (GC) base composition of 27.0 to 28.1% and a genome size of $4.2 \pm 0.5 \times 10^8$ daltons, both figures being at the lower range exhibited by mycoplasma (4).

Growth Requirements. *M. meleagridis* is a facultative anaerobe. Growth is optimal at 37–38 C and slight at 40–42 C. Most isolates do not adapt readily to broth media (40, 123). Serum and yeast extract (autolysate) are essential ingredients for optimal growth. Swine and horse serums are satisfactory, but chicken and turkey serums are not (123).

A number of media have been described for cultivation of MM (123). A satisfactory broth consists of PPLO broth powder (Difco) (2.1%), yeast autolysate (Sigma) (1%), and heat-inactivated (56 C for 30 min) horse serum (15%) (79, 97, 137). For solid medium, Bacto agar (1.2%) is added to the formulation. The pH of the final medium is 7.5–7.8. Fresh yeast extract (56) may be substituted for the dehydrated product. If the yeast product is obtained from a new source, it should be pretested for its growth-promoting activity. Another commonly used medium is Frey's FM (43) described under *MYCOPLASMA SYNOVIAE* INFECTION. A broth medium, designated SP-4, containing cell culture medium components supports excellent growth of MM (40).

The fastidious and delicate nature of this organism is exemplified in the observation that from time to time certain batches of media do not support growth of the organism. In such cases the source of the problem often can be traced to one of the ingredients such as the serum, yeast supplement, basal medium, or agar.

Colony Morphology. Colonies on agar medium after 2–3 days incubation appear small and flat (0.04–0.2 mm in diameter), with rough-appearing centers of ill-defined nipples. Nippling of the colonies is more prominent in laboratory-adapted strains than in fresh isolates (137).

Biochemical Properties. The organism does not ferment dextrose or other carbohydrates or reduce tetrazolium salts (137, 146) but uses arginine (58) and has phosphatase activity (60). Horse erythrocytes when incorporated at the 2% level into turkey meat infusion agar are hemolyzed by *M. meleagridis* (146).

Resistance to Chemical and Physical Agents. Very little is known about resistance of MM to chemical and physical agents. However, it is assumed that most chemical disinfectants would be effective against it (21).

In broth at pH 8.4–8.7, MM may survive up to 25–30 days at high titers, 10^7 colony-forming units (CFU)/ml (32). Freshly seeded cultures on agar will survive for at least 6 days at room temperature (137). The organism survives for at least 6 hr in the air (8). In vitro inactivation of four strains of MM at 45 C varied from 6 to 24 hr, while at 47 C inactivation of two strains occurred between 40 and 120 min (74).

Isolates of MM may be maintained for at least 2 mo by mincing colonies on agar in 3% sucrose and freezing at −20 to −70 C. Yoder and Hofstad (146) found broth-overlaid agar slant cultures to be viable after at least 2 yr storage at −30 C. Lyophilized cultures remain viable for at least 5 yr (137). The organism does not decline substantially in turkey semen during cryopreservation and subsequent thawing (41).

Antigenic Structure. *M. meleagridis* is antigenically unrelated to all other avian mycoplasmas. The agglutination (3, 146), fluorescent antibody (FA) (30), antiglobulin (2), growth and metabolic inhibition (33, 40,87), and complement-fixation (44, 85) tests have been used to identify MM.

A few isolates possess hemagglutination activity (96, 114,137). When hemagglutinating and nonhemagglutinating strains of MM were compared by polyacrylamide gel electrophoresis and simple and two-dimensional immunoelectrophoresis, minor antigenic differences were observed in the latter test only (40). Rhoades (102) showed that the determinant group(s) responsible for hemagglutination differed from that of agglutination.

The organism possesses a heat-stable lipid or polysaccharide toxin that causes an increase in ceruloplasmin activity when injected intravenously into chickens (31). The relationship of this toxin to the capsular material described by Green and Hanson (52) and to hemagglutinating activity is not known. However, hemagglutinating activity is not an essential component for virulence since strains lacking this activity may be highly pathogenic (137, 143).

Pathogenicity. Pathogenic and nonpathogenic strains of *M. meleagridis* were described by Ghazikhanian and Yamamoto (48, 49). Of three strains studied, one failed to multiply in vivo, another multiplied but failed to produce lesions, while the third multiplied and produced airsacculitis. Zhao et al. (147) showed by sodium dodecyl sulphate-polyacrylamide electrophoresis that these strains differed in their cell protein profiles. Strain variations may account for the variability in clinical manifestations attributed to this organism (38).

PATHOGENESIS AND EPIZOOTIOLOGY

Natural and Experimental Hosts. *M. meleagridis* is a specific pathogen of turkeys transmitted both vertically and horizontally. When injected into turkey embryos by the yolk sac route, the organism is capable of producing a high incidence of airsacculitis but causes minimal mortality (127). High infectivity and low mortality caused by MM in turkey embryos under experimental and natural conditions indicates it has attained an ideal host-parasite relationship.

When inoculated into the yolk sac of chicken embryos, MM will grow to high titers without causing high mortality (130, 146). Turkeys of all ages are susceptible to air sac infection with MM when inoculated via the air sac or trachea (69, 80,126). Chickens are refractory to infection with MM .(1, 125). Reports concerning presence of MM in Japanese quail, peacocks, and pigeons (123) have not been confirmed.

Transmission

VERTICAL TRANSMISSION. The organism is perpetuated primarily through egg transmission. Infection of the female reproductive tract occurs primarily by insemination with mycoplasma-contaminated semen (69, 79, 81, 121, 139). By this route of infection, average airsacculitis rates of 10–25% in first-run poults over a season's lay have been reported under commercial and experimental conditions (69, 79, 139). Egg-transmission rate among individual hens may vary from 10 to 60% (139). However, there is apparently no regular pattern as to sequence of infected eggs laid (79). Transmission starts out at a low rate during the first 2–3 wk of lay, reaches a maximum at midseason, and gradually declines toward the end of the laying season (16, 69). There seems to be some intracyclic fluctuation in the transmission pattern during the laying season (69, 139), but it has not been possible to relate such changes to the insemination schedule.

Egg transmission does not occur in hens in which the organism is found only in the upper respiratory tract (sinus) (69, 79, 121) and is minimal in hens infected via air sac and subsequently inseminated with clean semen (69).

A comparative study of persistence of *M. meleagridis, M. synoviae,* and *M. gallisepticum* in the genitalia of adult turkeys indicated that MM favored this environment more than the others (133).

Although the exact site in the reproductive system where the organism penetrates the developing egg is not known, it appears not to be in the gonads; numerous isolation attempts from ovules of hens known to be transmitting the organism have generally failed to yield it (79, 121, 139). Furthermore, egg transmission occurs at a high rate in absence of active airsacculitis.

The organism has been recovered frequently from various sites of the oviduct, with greatest frequency in the vagina and uterus (81, 139). In hens inseminated with contaminated semen the organism was found as high as the magnum (69). Joshi and Yamamoto (63) indicated that high levels of infection in the uterovaginal region were not sustained in hens repeatedly inseminated with contaminated semen, although they did transmit the organism through their eggs.

The organism has been isolated from the shell membrane and vitelline membrane–yolk of preincubated eggs from naturally infected turkeys, but at higher rates from the latter (10–12%) than former (2–4%) sites (51). Mycoplasma counts of 10^3–10^5 CFU/vitelline membrane have been obtained (128). Thus, while the organism has the potential to infect the developing egg at various sites in the oviduct, the critical site appears to be in the area of the fimbria or magnum.

While gross lesions (if any) in poults at time of hatch from infected dams are limited to air sacs, the organism may be widely distributed in various tissues including feathers, skin, sinus, trachea, lungs, air sac, bursa of Fabricius, intestine and cloaca (11, 93, 99), and hock joint (122). Cloacal infection detected at hatching can persist through maturity; semen taken from such males will contain mycoplasma (121, 141). The organism remains localized in the region of the cloaca and phallus and does not ascend the vas deferens or testes (97, 121). Histologic study of the phallus and accessory organs suggests that a possible site of localization is the region of the submucosal gland (45). Mycoplasma isolation rates from the phallus or semen of turkeys from naturally infected flocks may range from 13 to 32%.

M. meleagridis may infect the oviduct of virgin hens by way of an endogenous infection early in life (76) or an ascending infection from foci in the cloaca or bursa of Fabricius after the occluding plate is perforated at sexual maturity (75). Infection rates of 19–57% have been found in flocks in which cultures were taken from the vagina of virgin females. While such hens probably contribute to the overall egg-transmission rate, particularly when the incidence is high, venereal infection (from artificial insemination) plays a major role in initiating and sustaining the egg-transmission rate during the laying season (66, 69, 135).

HORIZONTAL TRANSMISSION. Direct and indirect transmission of *M. meleagridis* may occur at any stage of the bird's life. Direct transmission by the air-borne route may occur within a hatchery (69) or flock (132), or on occasion between flocks separated by 1/4 mile (51). Air-borne transmission usually results in a high infection rate (up to 100%), which remains localized in the sinus and trachea (69, 79); in young birds (brooding and growing periods), however, the organism may localize in the genitalia of approximately 5% of the birds when infected by the respiratory route (132).

Indirect transmission results from management practices including sexing, palpation of hens, artificial insemination, and vaccination whereby mycoplasmas are manually carried from infected to noninfected turkeys via contaminated hands, clothing, and equipment (51).

Lateral transmission apparently is of little significance once a bird has reached sexual maturity. Thus, infected adult females have been placed in cages adjacent to noninfected females with no evidence of egg transmission occurring in the latter. Similarly, clean males held in the same room with phallus-infected males were found to produce noninfected semen throughout the production period (121, 134).

Signs. Despite a high incidence of airsacculitis that may occur in poults from infected dams, respiratory signs are rarely observed.

While not a consistent feature of the disease, a skeletal abnormality called TS-65 or airsacculitis deficiency syndrome may be associated with *M. meleagridis* infection (95). The syndrome, which includes signs of bowing, twisting, and shortening of the tarsometatarsal bone, hock joint swelling, and deformation of cervical vertebrae, has been reproduced experimentally in MM-free poults (13, 84, 117, 120, 142). Stunting and abnormal feathering are additional features of the disease (13). While the problem develops during the first 12 wk of life, the greatest incidence occurs between 1 and 6 wk (119). The serum protein pattern of affected poults reveals reduced albumen-to-globulin ratios mainly from elevated gammaglobulins and reduced albumen and is suggestive of chronic infection (22). However, Wise and Fuller (117) were unable to demonstrate a drastic decrease in serum albumen concentration in 7- to 21-day-old poults with MM-induced TS-65 syndrome.

M. meleagridis acts synergistically in producing severe airsacculitis with *M. iowae* (105) and sinusitis with *M. synoviae* (101). In a flock naturally infected with MM and *M. synoviae,* sinusitis was estimated to be 2.1% in males and 0.13% in females (101). While it is generally believed that neither agent alone is capable of producing sinusitis, field cases have been encountered recently in which only MM has been isolated from sinus exudate (29).

Morbidity and Mortality. Two points should be clarified regarding MM-associated diseases. First, various clinical manifestations mentioned in the previous section are primarily associated with embryonic infection via egg transmission. Lateral transmission that may occur after hatching may lead to a high infection rate but usually not to clinical disease. Thus, transmission of MM after hatching is important only if concern is for eradication. Second, infection, even via egg transmission, does not invariably lead to a disease process. What determines whether an infected bird or hatch will or will not develop disease is not clear, but such factors as MM strains of varying virulence, environmental stresses, and secondary infections may influence the picture. It has been suggested that the prerequisite for development of skeletal problems is a generalized infection as it occurs in natural egg-borne infection (120). It has also been hypothesized, based on in vivo and in vitro data, that the organism may deprive the embryo of biotin, resulting in abnormal development (13, 15). Yamamoto et al. (142) postulated that the organism may compete for arginine, an essential amino acid for proper bone development. However, other studies indicate that MM strains of different virulence do not vary in their arginine metabolism; also, significant differences in plasma arginine between infected (with leg abnormalities) and noninfected poults were not observed (58).

In affected flocks, skeletal abnormalities may be observed in 5–10% of the birds but on occasion may reach higher levels. Not all cases progress to an irreversible state (119). Peterson (91) found a positive correlation of skeletal lesions, airsacculitis, and high agglutination titers to MM in poults with TS-65 syndrome. Incidence of the disease seems to increase with progression of the laying season. Mortality is due primarily to cannibalism of affected birds. The problem is not associated with a particular strain of bird, but the male seems to be more susceptible.

A number of other conditions (reduced hatchability, poor growth performance, condemnation at processing due to airsacculitis) have been suggested as being directly or indirectly related to infection with MM.

REPRODUCTIVE PERFORMANCE. *M. meleagridis* does not adversely affect egg production or fertility and does not cause early incubation mortality (28, 131). It causes late incubation (25–28 days) mortality in artificially (24, 131) and naturally (34) infected turkey embryos. It has been estimated that industry losses from MM in untreated eggs are approximately 5–6% of fertile eggs (36). Edson (34), using risk analysis, determined the mortality rates of embryos naturally infected with MM and/or an unidentified mycoplasma. The analysis showed that embryos infected with MM, unidentified mycoplasma, and both agents were 5, 7, and 25 times more likely to die than the mycoplasma-free embryos. The unidentified mycoplasma was later identified as *M. iowae* (124), a common parasite of turkeys known to reduce hatchability (104).

GROWTH PERFORMANCE. A significant advantage in weight gain was observed with *M. meleagridis*-free vs. infected poults (12, 86, 119). Nelson et al. (84) distributed MM-free and infected eggs in large numbers to 11 cooperators in eight states to study the leg weakness syndrome under commercial conditions. Results indicated that the total daily mortality, number of cull poults, and skeletal deformity were much lower in the clean poults.

Conversely, others (23, 26, 27) in large field trials were unable to demonstrate any advantage of MM-free over infected turkeys of both sexes concerning mortality, weight gain, and feed conversion from hatch to 23 wk of age. Possible reasons for the divergent results of different investigators have been enumerated under Morbidity and Mortality.

AIR SAC LESIONS AND CONDEMNATIONS. Airsacculitis has been reported to be one of the major causes of condemnation of fryer-roaster turkeys, particularly in the central USA (5, 71). *M. meleagridis* has been implicated as the underlying cause of such condemnations in view of its widespread distribution and high prevalence within individual turkey flocks. Since air sac lesions caused by uncomplicated MM infection regress in a matter of 15–16 wk (9, 141), it would appear that other agents or factors may be involved in the overall picture. Anderson et al. (5) observed a twofold or greater increase in incidence of air sac lesions caused by MM in turkeys raised to 12 wk of age in a high-dust environment.

Brown and Nestor (20) suggested that turkeys selected for low plasma ACTH following cold stress were more resistant to MM infection than those selected for high ACTH levels. Saif et al. (107) reproduced complicated airsacculitis with MM and *Escherichia coli* in poults and suggested that environmental factors were important in aggravating MM-induced air sac lesions. Mixed infections of MM and *M. iowae* also accentuate the severity of air sac lesions (105). A number of interacting factors thus may contribute to complicated air sac lesions in young turkeys.

Gross Lesions. Air sac lesions seen in day-old poults are generally confined to thoracic air sacs. These lesions are characterized by thickening of the walls with adherence of a yellow exudate to the tissue and occasionally presence of various sized flecks of caseous material free in the lumen (3). Extension of such lesions to the abdominal air sacs is a common occurrence by 3–4 wk of age.

It is also possible for the organism to be present in air sacs of day-old poults exhibiting no lesions; in such cases air sac lesions may develop in 3–5 wk (9). Lesions produced by *M. meleagridis* when not mixed with *M. iowae* are not as extensive or fulminating as those described for *M. gallisepticum* (33, 70).

Skeletal lesions when present are usually associated with severe airsacculitis (91). Sternal bursitis (126), synovitis (107), and ascites (117) are additional lesions observed in experimental infections. The sinusitis produced by MM and *M. synoviae* in mixed infections contains clear mucus to caseous exudate (101).

Histopathology. In embryonic infection with *M. meleagridis*, exudative airsacculitis and pneumonia were the only inflammatory lesions seen. Lesions that developed at 25–28 days of age were related to maturation of inflammatory cells. Air sac lesions consisted predominantly of heterophils with some mononuclear cells, including lymphocytes and varying amounts of fibrin and cellular debris. Epithelial necrosis was seen in severely affected air sacs. Mononuclear cells and fibrin were the prominent features of lung lesions (49, 99). Significant or marked microscopic changes in other organs in embryos or poults were not observed despite invasion of the organism into many of these sites (49).

In 7-wk-old poults infected with MM by the air sac route, lymphocytic perivascular infiltration and fibrinocellular exudate were observed in 2 days. Some areas of the air sac epithelium became hyperplastic and others underwent necrosis at about 4–8 days. Lymphoid follicles were observed in 16 days. When examined by electron microscopy, the follicles were found to be surrounded by collagen bundles (encapsulated), composed of hemocytoblasts of bursal origin, and presumed to be involved in antibody formation (100). Essentially similar sequential changes have been observed by others in poults infected as embryos or at 1–3 days of age (6, 49, 82).

Wise et al. (119) indicated that gross and microscopic long-bone lesions of TS-65 were similar to those observed in perosis of dietetic origin. The main lesions were seen in proximal ends of the long bones. Cartilage farthest from blood vessels descending into the proliferative zone from the cartilaginous epiphysis lacked cell density and contained abnormal-appearing chondrocytes. In long-standing cases of 6–8 wk or longer, growth plates often were normal, suggestive of repair, even though the bones were grossly deformed. These cellular changes in the proliferative zone of the growth plates were seen in all long bones examined, suggestive of a generalized response. It was postulated that the mycoplasma causes a secondary block of nutrients to the growth plates.

A secondary lesion in the medial side of the proximal end of the tarsometatarsal bone of chronic cases with varus deformity was described as a dyschondroplasia or chondrodystrophy and was believed to be the consequence of partial failure of the metaphyseal blood supply at the growth plates (119).

Mild mononuclear cell infiltration was observed in the periarticular region of the hock joint in 2-wk-old poults inoculated with MM intravenously (94).

The most prominent lesion in hens infected by the vaginal route was focal encapsulated accumulation of lymphocytes present most frequently in the fimbria, uterus, and vagina. Plasma cells and heterophils were also present in significant numbers in the lamina propria of the reproductive tract. The encapsulated follicles were believed to be active in antibody formation (98). Similar lesions in the reproductive tract of turkeys infected with MM were described by Ball et al. (7).

Gerlach et al. (45) examined histologically the phallus and accessory structures of males experimentally infected with MM. The only significant change was an extensive lymphofollicular formation in the region of the mucous-type glands in the submucosa of the lymphfold.

Immunity

ACTIVE. Turkeys inoculated intravenously or by the respiratory route with *M. meleagridis* were resistant to reinfection when challenged by the same route 21 wk later. However, there was no correlation between antibody titer and resistance (80). Repeated injections of 20-wk-old hens with live MM failed to induce protective immunity or reduce egg transmission (116).

When hens that had been vaginally infected artificially with MM culture or with contaminated semen were subsequently inseminated with clean semen, the organism was eliminated from the vagina within 4–14 wk, while hens continuously inseminated with contaminated semen maintained a high incidence of infection (66, 69). On the other hand, insemination with clean semen of virgin hens known to be vaginal carriers of MM resulted in high egg-transmission rate and persistence of oviduct infection (34, 135). In the first-mentioned studies, it appears that an active immune mechanism was functioning to eliminate the organism after removal of the source of infection, i.e., contaminated semen. Persistence of infection in the latter study may be an expression of immune tolerance in hens infected by egg transmission.

Yamamoto et al. (140) found that hens infected with MM via the oviduct during one breeding season were free from such infection at the start of the second laying season; among five adult males infected via the phallus, the organism persisted for 55–344 days. These findings are consistent with the observation that declines in the egg-transmission rate during the latter part of the laying season may be related to an active immune and/or physiologic mechanism. A study by Ortiz et al. (88) suggests that embryonic infection of the bursa of Fabricius by MM results in impairment of the secondary antibody response to innate or inactivated antigens such as dinitrophenyl bovine globulin, *Salmonella pullorum,* or Newcastle disease virus.

PASSIVE. Maternal antibodies (agglutinins) may be detected in a high percentage of poults from infected dams and persist for approximately 2 wk post-hatching. Such antibodies appear not to protect against development of air sac lesions in infected embryos (80, 139). Conversely, purified IgM and IgG antibodies when injected into the yolk sac of infected embryos significantly reduced embryo mortality and the incidence of leg deformities in hatched poults, but it did not reduce air sac lesions or isolation rates when compared to controls (17).

DIAGNOSIS

Isolation and Identification of Causative Agent. *M. meleagridis* may be readily isolated on several commercially available and laboratory-prepared media (see Growth Requirements).

Ortmayer et al. (90) developed a mass screening cultural technique for isolation of MM from the genital tract of turkeys. The procedure, which is modified after Adler et al. (3), uses Difco PPLO base and a broth-overlay enrichment technique.

For large sampling studies in the field (e.g., cultures from the vagina or phallus), specimens taken on swabs and placed into overlay broth facilitates transport to the laboratory as well as serving as an initial enrichment. Thallium acetate (1:4000) and penicillin (1000 units/ml) are inhibitors added to agar plates, slants, and broth. Polymyxin B (100 units/ml) may be added to the broth portion of the overlay to facilitate isolation of MM from highly contaminated sources such as the cloaca and phallus. Mycostatin (50 units/ml) may be added to the agar and broth to inhibit fungi (81).

Once growth is apparent in original isolation medium, usually after 4–6 days of incubation, agar plates are streaked and placed in a sealed container with added moisture. Plates are incubated at 37 C for 5–7 days before being examined for colonies under the dissecting microscope and are incubated at least 10 days before being discarded as negative.

M. meleagridis may be selectively isolated from specimens containing mixed cultures by adding to the medium immune serum against the undesired mycoplasma (18). MM may be differentiated from other chicken and turkey mycoplasmas by its inability to utilize glucose and its ability to metabolize arginine and phosphate (phosphatase activity) (58, 60, 111, 146). Isolates of MM are distinct in colony morphology from other species found in the reproductive tract on primary isolation (125), but definitive identification must be made by serology. While a number of procedures have been described (see Antigenic Structure), the direct (30) and indirect (18) fluorescent antibody (FA) tests and growth-inhibition (33) are particularly useful. Immune inactivation may occur by either a complement-dependent or independent pathway (74). For the FA test, colony imprints on coverslips may be prepared and examined immediately or stored at −20 or −70 C for several mo. Nonviable organisms may be recognized by immunofluorescence (62).

Serology. Rapid plate (RP) and tube agglutination (TA) tests are effective in detecting *M. meleagridis* infections. Antibodies are detected in poults hatched from infected eggs in 3 wk and in turkeys infected by contact in 4–5 wk. Birds with active air sac lesions may have high agglutinin titers, while those with localized infections in the sinus or phallus may be negative or show low titers (1, 80, 141). The RP test may be quantified by performing it on serially diluted serums. A reaction at a dilution of 1:5 is significant (141, 143), but for flock diagnosis some samples should react at 1:10 or higher. Each lot of antigen should be pretested with a standard positive serum for its reactive quality at higher serum dilutions.

Kleven and Pomeroy (65) found that the RP test detected IgM, the TA test detected both IgM and IgG, and the hemagglutination-inhibition (HI) test detected IgG most efficiently. However, the early HI antibody response of turkeys to high doses of MM given intravenously was of the IgM class (103).

While nonhemagglutinating laboratory strains of MM do not elicit high HI antibody responses in turkeys, the HI test is very effective in detecting such antibodies in naturally infected birds (102). It seems that field infections with MM occur with strains possessing hemagglutinating activity, but this characteristic is quickly lost for most strains when they are cultivated on laboratory media (102). Furthermore, since the antigenic determinant(s) responsible for hemagglutination differs from that of agglutination (102), it is possible to find individual turkeys in an infected flock whose serum will be positive in the HI and negative in the TA test; the reverse situation may also occur (143).

The HI test developed by Rhoades (96) has been recommended as a primary test in eradication programs because of its greater specificity over the TA test (114). However, its greatest use will probably be as a confirmatory test. Yamamoto et al. (143) adapted the HI test to the microtest system. Using four units of antigen, titers of 1:40 were considered suspects and 1:80 or greater as reactors. When used as a confirmatory test to the RP in field testing, a positive HI signifies infection, while a negative HI requires a more conservative interpretation and may involve use of other confirmatory tests or follow-up testing for final diagnosis (144). The micro-HI test has been used to identify false-positive RP reactions (136) in flocks recently vaccinated with *Erysipelothrix* vaccine (14).

A microagglutination test has been developed that may have practical application in large-scale testing programs (129), while the enzyme-linked immunosorbent assay may serve as another confirmatory test (89).

Differential Diagnosis. Air sac lesions caused by *M. meleagridis* must be differentiated from those caused by *M. gallisepticum,* other *Mycoplasma* serotypes, and possibly other agents. However, based on high lesion rates in poults from dams free from *M. gallisepticum,* a tentative diagnosis of MM infection could be made, since other agents produce such lesions only sporadically if at all. *M. synoviae* and *M. iowae* must be considered as possible synergists with MM when embryo mortality, sinusitis, or airsacculitis is observed.

TREATMENT. Antibiotics having in vitro activity against *M. meleagridis* include gentamicin (109), tylosin, chloramphenicol, tetracycline (138), spectinomycin-lincomycin (54), tiamulin, spectinomycin, and spiramycin (73). In turkey embryo trials with two isolates, it was found that tylosin was the most active; tetracycline, chlortetracycline, and streptomycin were variable; and erythromycin showed no activity. Different isolates varied in their sensitivity to certain antibiotics, which points out the importance of prior sensitivity testing of several isolates before mass medication programs are contemplated (138).

A combination of lincomycin and spectinomycin administered at 2 g/gal of water for 5 days (55), or tiamulin at a concentration of 0.025% in the drinking water for 3 days (113), were found to have therapeutic activity against MM infections. Eprofloxacin, a quinolone derivative, also has been shown to have promise for the treatment of MM mixed infections (19). Parenteral injections or water medication with tylosin of turkeys in production have not been successful in reducing the egg-transmitted disease (16, 71). However, dipping of hatching eggs in antibiotic solutions significantly reduces incidence of air sac infection (10, 71, 91, 108) concomitant with improved hatchability (71, 108), improved performance (10, 83), reduced incidence of skeletal deformities (83, 91), and reduced condemnation at processing (71, 83).

Tylosin (1000–3000 ppm) or gentamicin (400–1000 ppm) along with a disinfectant such as quaternary ammonium compound (250 ppm) are commonly used in dip solutions. More recently, josamycin was reported to be more effective than doxycycline or tylosin in eliminating mycoplasma from dipped turkey eggs (112). The compatibility of any new antibiotic or disinfectant should be determined before its use in the system (21). For the temperature differential method, eggs previously warmed to 35–37 C are dipped in antibiotic solution (maintained at 2–8 C) for 5–20 min. For the pressure differential method, a vacuum of 25 cm mercury is drawn on a sealed tank containing eggs immersed in antibiotic solution. The vacuum is released after 5–10 min and the eggs are removed after another 5–10 min.

Hofstad (57) injected tylosin tartrate (0.5–1.0 mg/dose) via the air cell of turkey eggs prior to incubation and was successful in producing MM-free poults in 6 of 12 trials.

McCapes et al. (77, 78) injected antibiotics into the small end of fresh eggs, which gave greater assurance than dipping that every egg received a proper dose of antibiotic(s). Elmahi and Hofstad (39) also demonstrated potential usefulness of this technique of egg injection for eliminating MM. Heat treatment of eggs (145) was not effective in eliminating MM from turkey eggs (53, 61, 119).

Treatment of turkey semen with tylosin (67) or gentamicin (106) to eliminate MM was not successful.

PREVENTION AND CONTROL

Management Procedures. In an eradication program, management should provide an educational program for its staff on the idiosyncracies of *M. meleagridis* infection, its transmission and nature of the disease. It is essential that all personnel are committed to maintaining a high level of sanitation and security of the farm.

Since MM is essentially a venereal infection, strict sanitary procedures must be practiced during collection of semen and insemination of hens to minimize cross-contamination. Manual transmission of MM from infected to noninfected oviducts may be prevented if the inseminator avoids touching the vaginal mucosa (35). Such procedures as determining presence of an egg in the uterus by vaginal palpation may lead to increased incidence of vaginal carriers (79). Since the organism may be present in the cloaca of day-old poults, strict sanitary procedures to reduce cross-contamination during sexing should be considered. Hatchery-borne infections and lateral transmissions during production brooding and growing periods are possibilities that must be considered.

Immunization. Vaccines are not available for prevention of MM infection in turkeys.

Eradication. Basic principles and procedures for production of MM-free breeders include: 1) Reduction of infection to minimal levels by serology and culture. Egg-transmission rate can be reduced significantly by using males that are not genital carriers and by practicing the hygienic method of insemination (35). A male that yields three consecutive negative cultures from the phallus (or semen) may be considered free of infection. The infection rate can be reduced even further by eliminating vaginal carriers. Even a single sampling will identify most carriers. Cultures from males are taken a few weeks before their use as breeders, while those from females may be taken before (cloaca) or during (vagina) egg production. 2) Treatment of eggs with an effective antibiotic(s) by dipping and/or injection. 3) Hatching of eggs in MM-free hatchers and isolation rearing of the turkeys. 4) Serologic and cultural monitoring of the treated flock.

Using the general principles outlined above, MM-free turkeys have been produced experimentally (123) and commercially (50, 51, 72, 86, 118). A treatment regimen that was used to eradicate MM from a primary breeder consisted of dipping eggs in a solution of gentamicin sulfate (750–900 ppm) followed by injection with a solution containing 0.6 mg gentamicin and 2.4 mg tylosin/dose into the small end of the egg (51). Depending on the strain of turkeys from which the eggs originated, this procedure depressed hatchability by 10% or greater. Therefore, pretrials should be conducted before embarking on a large program. The possibility of developing resistant strains of *Mycoplasma* should be kept in mind, particularly at the primary breeder level where treated birds must necessarily be recycled in the operation (47, 77, 120).

Serologic and cultural monitoring of flocks on an eradication program is conducted at 16 wk of age and periodic intervals thereafter.

Edson et al. (37) developed an equation based on the Poisson distribution to predict the chance of success of eradicating *M. meleagridis*: $p(0) = e^{-na\beta h}$, where the probability of success $p(0)$ was described by n, the number of eggs treated; a, the pretreatment infection rate of the eggs; β, the treatment failure rate; and h, the hatchability of treated eggs. Decreasing the size of any or all of the four parameters increases likelihood of eradication. This predictive equation is a useful quantitative decision-making tool for management.

An economic decision analysis technique was described by Carpenter et al. (25) to assist commercial multiplier breeders in determining the economic advantage of eradicating MM. With the availability of MM-free stocks from primary breeders (46), the possibility exists for multiplier breeders and commercial producers to raise turkeys free of this agent (46, 68). A program for certifying freedom from MM infection of turkey breeding stocks under the National Poultry Improvement Plan became effective on January 1, 1983 (110).

REFERENCES

1. Adler, H.E. 1958. A PPLO slide agglutination test for the detection of infectious sinusitis of turkeys. Poult Sci 37:1116–1123.

2. Adler, H.E., and A.J. DaMassa. 1964. Enhancement of Mycoplasma agglutination titers by use of antiglobulin. Proc Soc Exp Biol Med 116:608–610.

3. Adler, H.E., J. Fabricant, R. Yamamoto, and J. Berg. 1958. Symposium on chronic respiratory diseases of poultry. I. Isolation and identification of pleuropneumonia-like organisms of avian origin. Am J Vet Res 19:440–447.

4. Allen, T.C. 1971. Base composition and genome size of Mycoplasma meleagridis deoxyribonucleic acid. J Gen Microbiol 69:285–286.

5. Anderson, D.P., R.R. Wolfe, F.L. Cherms, and W.E. Roper. 1968. Influence of dust and ammonia on the de-

velopment of air sac lesions in turkeys. Am J Vet Res 29:1049–1058.

6. Arya, P.L., J.H. Sautter, and B.S. Pomeroy. 1971. Pathogenesis and histopathology of airsacculitis in turkeys produced by experimental inoculation of day-old poults with Mycoplasma meleagridis. Avian Dis 15:163–176.

7. Ball, R.A., V.B. Singh, and B.S. Pomeroy. 1969. The morphologic response of the turkey oviduct to certain pathogenic agents. Avian Dis 13:119–133.

8. Beard, C.W., and D.P. Anderson. 1967. Aerosol studies with avian Mycoplasma. I. Survival in the air. Avian Dis 11:54–59.

9. Bigland, C.H. 1969. Natural resolution of air sac lesions caused by Mycoplasma meleagridis in turkeys. Can J Comp Med 33:169–172.

10. Bigland, C.H. 1970. Experimental control of Mycoplasma meleagridis in turkeys by the dipping of eggs in tylosin and spiramycin. Can J Comp Med 34:26–30.

11. Bigland, C.H. 1972. The tissue localization of Mycoplasma meleagridis in turkey embryos. Can J Comp Med 36:99–102.

12. Bigland, C.H., and M.L. Benson. 1968. Mycoplasma meleagridis ("N" -Strain Mycoplasma-PPLO): Relationship of airsac lesions and isolations in day-old turkeys (Meleagridis gallopavo). Can Vet J 9:138–141.

13. Bigland, C.H., and F.T.W. Jordan. 1974. Experimental relationship of biotin and Mycoplasma meleagridis in the etiology of turkey syndrome 1965. Proc 23rd West Poult Dis Conf and 8th Poult Health Symp, pp. 55–61. Davis, CA.

14. Bigland, C.H., and J.J. Matsumoto. 1975. Nonspecific reaction to Mycoplasma antigens caused in turkey sera by Erysipelothrix insidiosa bacterins. Avian Dis 19:617–621.

15. Bigland, C.H., and M.W. Warenycia. 1978. Effects of biotin, folic acid, and pantothenic acid on the growth of Mycoplasma meleagridis, a turkey pathogen. Poult Sci 57:611–618.

16. Bigland, C.H., W. Dungan, R. Yamamoto, and J. C. Voris. 1964. Airsacculitis in poults from different strains of turkeys. Avian Dis 8:85–92.

17. Bigland, C.H., M.W. Warenycia, and M. Denson. 1979. Specific immune gammaglobulin in the control of Mycoplasma meleagridis. Poult Sci 58:319–328.

18. Bradbury, J.M., and M. McClenaghan. 1982. Detection of mixed Mycoplasma species. J Clin Micro 16:314–318.

19. Braunius, W.W. 1987. Effect of Baytril (Bay Vp 2674) on young turkeys with respiratory infection. Tijdschr Diergeneeskd 112:531–533.

20. Brown, K.I., and K.E. Nestor. 1974. Interrelationships of cellular physiology and endocrinology with genetics. 2. Implications of selection for high and low adrenal response to stress. Poult Sci 53:1297–1306.

21. Brunner, H., and G. Laber. 1985. Chemotherapy of Mycoplasma infections. In S. Razin and M.F. Barile (eds.), The Mycoplasma IV Mycoplasma Pathogenicity, pp. 403–450. Academic Press, Orlando, FL.

22. Butler, E.J., A.W. Pearson, and C.C. Wannop. 1970. Biochemical abnormalities associated with turkey syndrome '65. Vet Rec 86:617–620.

23. Carpenter, T.E. 1983. A microeconomic evaluation of the impact of Mycoplasma meleagridis infection in turkey production. Prev Vet Med 1:289–301.

24. Carpenter, T.E., R.K. Edson, and R. Yamamoto. 1981. Decreased hatchability of turkey eggs caused by experimental infection with Mycoplasma meleagridis. Avian Dis 25:151–156.

25. Carpenter, T.E., R. Howitt, R. McCapes, R. Yamamoto, and H.P. Riemann. 1981. Formulating a control program against Mycoplasma meleagridis using economic decision analysis. Avian Dis 25:260–271.

26. Carpenter, T.E., H.P. Riemann, and C.E. Franti. 1982. The effect of Mycoplasma meleagridis infection and egg dipping on the weight-gain performance of turkey poults. Avian Dis 26:272–278.

27. Carpenter, T.E., H.P. Riemann, and R.H. McCapes. 1982. The effect of experimental turkey embryo infection with Mycoplasma meleagridis on weight, weight gain, feed consumption, and conversion. Avian Dis 26:689–695.

28. Cherms, F.L., and M.L. Frey. 1967. Mycoplasma meleagridis and fertility in turkey breeder hens. Avian Dis 11:268–274.

29. Chin, R.P. 1988. Personal communication.

30. Corstvet, R.E., and W.W. Sadler. 1964. The diagnosis of certain avian diseases with the fluorescent antibody technique. Poult Sci 43:1280–1288.

31. Curtis, M.J., and G.A. Thornton. 1973. The effect of heat killed Mycoplasma gallisepticum and M. meleagridis on plasma caeruloplasmin activity in the fowl. Res Vet Sci 15:399–401.

32. DaMassa, A.J., and H.E. Adler. 1969. Effect of pH on growth and survival of three avian and one saprophytic Mycoplasma species. Appl Microbiol 17:310–316.

33. Dierks, R.E., J.A. Newman, and B.S. Pomeroy. 1967. Characterization of Avian Mycoplasma. Ann NY Acad Sci 143:170–189.

34. Edson, R.K. 1980. Mycoplasma meleagridis infection of turkeys: Motivation, methods, and predictive tools for eradication. PhD diss., Univ California, Davis.

35. Edson, R.K., D. Massey, R. Yamamoto, and H.B. Ortmayer. 1978. Factors affecting the spread of Mycoplasma meleagridis during artificial insemination. Proc 18th Annu Turkey Meet, Univ Calif, Fresno.

36. Edson, R.K., R. Yamamoto, H.B. Ortmayer, and D.E. Massey. 1979. The effect of Mycoplasma meleagridis on hatchability of turkey eggs. Proc 28th West Poult Dis Conf and 13th Poult Health Symp, pp. 24–29. Davis, CA.

37. Edson, R.K., R. Yamamoto, and T.B. Farver. 1987. Mycoplasma meleagridis of turkeys: Probability of eliminating egg-borne infection. Avian Dis 31:264–271.

38. El-Ebeedy, A.A., M.E.S. Easa, M.Z. Sabey, M.A. Hafez, A.M. Ammar, and A. Rashwan. 1982. Pathological changes in air sacs and lungs of turkey poults after experimental inoculation with different isolates of Mycoplasma meleagridis. J Egypt Vet Med Assoc 42:91–100.

39. Elmahi, M.M., and M.S. Hofstad. 1979. Prevention of egg transmission of Mycoplasma meleagridis by antibiotic treatment of naturally and experimentally infected turkey eggs. Avian Dis 23:88–94.

40. Elmahi, M.M., R.F. Ross, and M.S. Hofstad. 1982. Comparison of seven isolates of Mycoplasma meleagridis. Vet Microbiol 7:61–76.

41. Ferrier, W.T., H.B. Ortmayer, F.X. Ogasawara, and R. Yamamoto. 1982. The survivability of Mycoplasma meleagridis in frozen-thawed turkey semen. Poult Sci 61:379–381.

42. Fox, M.L., and C.H. Bigland. 1970. Differences between cull and normal turkeys in natural infection with Mycoplasma meleagridis at one day of age. Can J Comp Med 34:285–288.

43. Frey, M.L., R.P. Hanson, and D.P. Anderson. 1968. A medium for the isolation of avian mycoplasmas. Am J Vet Res 29:2163–2171.

44. Frey, M.L., S.T. Hawk, and P.A. Hale. 1972. A division by micro-complement fixation tests of previously reported avian mycoplasma serotypes into iden-

tification groups. Avian Dis 16:780–792.
45. Gerlach, H., R. Yamamoto, and H.B. Ortmayer. 1968. Zur Pathologie der Phallus-Infektion der Puten mit Mycoplasma meleagridis. Arch Gefluegelkd 32:396–399.
46. Ghazikhanian, G.Y. 1983. Progress in maintaining Mycoplasma meleagridis–negative turkey breeding flocks. Avian Dis 27:326–329. (Abstr).
47. Ghazikhanian, G., and R. Yamamoto. 1969. Tylosin resistant strains of Mycoplasma meleagridis. Proc 18th West Poult Dis Conf, pp. 36–37. Davis, CA.
48. Ghazikhanian, G., and R. Yamamoto. 1974. Characterization of pathogenic and nonpathogenic strains of Mycoplasma meleagridis: In ovo and in vitro studies. Am J Vet Res 35:425–430.
49. Ghazikhanian, G., and R. Yamamoto. 1974. Characterization of pathogenic and nonpathogenic strains of Mycoplasma meleagridis: Manifestations of disease in turkey embryos and poults. Am J Vet Res 35:417–424.
50. Ghazikhanian, G., R. Yamamoto, R.H. McCapes, W.M. Dungan, C.T. Larsen, and H.B. Ortmayer. 1980. Antibiotic egg injection to eliminate disease. II. Elimination of Mycoplasma meleagridis from a strain of turkeys. Avian Dis 48–56.
51. Ghazikhanian, G., R. Yamamoto, R.H. McCapes, W.M. Dungan, and H.B. Ortmayer. 1980. Combination dip and injection of turkey eggs with antibiotics to eliminate Mycoplasma meleagridis infection from a primary breeding stock. Avian Dis 24:57–70.
52. Green, F., III, and R.P. Hanson. 1973. Ultrastructure and capsule of Mycoplasma meleagridis. J Bacteriol 116:1011–1018.
53. Grimes, T.M. 1972. Means of obtaining Mycoplasma-free turkeys in Australia. Aust Vet J 48:124.
54. Hamdy, A.H., C.J. Farho, C.J. Blanchard, and M.W. Glenn. 1969. Effect of lincomycin and spectinomycin on airsacculitis of turkey poults. Avian Dis 13:721–728.
55. Hamdy, A.H., Y.M. Saif, and C.W. Kasson. 1982. Efficacy of lincomycin-spectinomycin water medication on Mycoplasma meleagridis airsacculitis in commercially reared turkey poults. Avian Dis 26:227–233.
56. Hayflick, L. 1965. Tissue cultures and mycoplasmas. Tex Rep Biol Med 23:285–303.
57. Hofstad, M.S. 1974. The injection of turkey hatching eggs with tylosin to eliminate Mycoplasma meleagridis infection. Avian Dis 18:134–138.
58. Ibrahim, A.A., and R. Yamamoto. 1977. Arginine catabolism by Mycoplasma meleagridis and its role in pathogenesis. Infect Immun 18:226–229.
59. Ibrahim, A.A., and R. Yamamoto. 1977. Morphology and growth cycle of Mycoplasma meleagridis viewed by scanning-electron microscopy. Avian Dis 21:415–421.
60. Jordan, F.T.W. 1983. Recovery and identification of avian mycoplasmas. In J.G. Tully and S. Razin (eds.), Methods in Mycoplasmology, Vol 2, Diagnostic Mycoplasmology, pp. 69–79. Academic Press, New York.
61. Jordan, F.T.W., and M.M. Amin. 1978. The influence of preincubation heating of turkey eggs on Mycoplasma infection. Avian Pathol 7:349–355.
62. Jordan, F.T.W., B.L. Nutor, and S. Bozkur. 1982. The survival and recognition of Mycoplasma meleagridis grown at 37 C and then maintained at room temperature. Avian Pathol 11:123–129.
63. Joshi, C.S., and R. Yamamoto. 1968. Unpublished data.
64. Kleckner, A.L. 1960. Serotypes of avian pleuropneumonia-like organisms. Am J Vet Res 21:274–280.
65. Kleven, S.H., and B.S. Pomeroy. 1971. Characterization of the antibody response of turkeys to Mycoplasma meleagridis. Avian Dis 15:291–298.
66. Kleven, S.H., and B.S. Pomeroy. 1971. Role of the female in egg transmission of Mycoplasma meleagridis in turkeys. Avian Dis 15:299–304.
67. Kleven, S.H., B.S. Pomeroy, and R.C. Nelson. 1971. Ineffectiveness of antibiotic treatment of semen in the prevention of egg transmission of Mycoplasma meleagridis in turkeys. Poult Sci 50:1522–1526.
68. Kolb, G.E. 1983. Mycoplasma meleagridis eradication status in commercial turkeys. Avian Dis 27:329. (Abstr).
69. Kumar, M.C., and B.S. Pomeroy. 1969. Transmission of Mycoplasma meleagridis in turkeys. Am J Vet Res 30:1423–1436.
70. Kumar, S., R.E. Dierks, J.A. Newman, C.I. Pfow, and B.S. Pomeroy. 1963. Airsacculitis in turkeys. I. A study of airsacculitis in day-old poults. Avian Dis 7:376–385.
71. Kumar, M.C., S. Kumar, R.E. Dierks, J.A. Newman, and B.S. Pomeroy. 1966. Airsacculitis in turkeys. II. Use of tylosin in the control of the egg transmission of Mycoplasma spp. other than Mycoplasma gallisepticum in turkeys. Avian Dis 10:194–198.
72. Kumar, M.C., B.S. Pomeroy, W.M. Dungan, and C.T. Larsen. 1974. Development of Mycoplasma gallisepticum, M. synoviae, and M. meleagridis–free primary turkey breeding flocks. Proc 15th World's Poult Congr, pp. 353–355.
73. Levisohn, S. 1981. Antibiotic sensitivity patterns in field isolates of Mycoplasma gallisepticum as a guide to chemotherapy. Isr J Med Sci 17:661–666.
74. Matsumoto, M., and R. Yamamoto. 1971. Inactivation of Mycoplasma meleagridis by immune serum or heat treatment. Proc 20th West Poult Dis Conf and 5th Poult Health Symp, pp. 70–74.
75. Matzer, N., and R. Yamamoto. 1970. Genital pathogenesis of Mycoplasma meleagridis in virgin turkey hens. Avian Dis 14:321–329.
76. Matzer, N., and R. Yamamoto. 1974. Further studies on the genital pathogenesis of Mycoplasma meleagridis. J Comp Pathol 84:271–278.
77. McCapes, R.H., R. Yamamoto, H.B. Ortmayer, and W.F. Scott. 1975. Injecting antibiotics into turkey hatching eggs to eliminate Mycoplasma meleagridis infection. Avian Dis 19:506–514.
78. McCapes, R.H., R. Yamamoto, G. Ghazikhanian, W. M. Dungan, and H. B. Ortmayer. 1977. Antibiotic egg injection to eliminate disease. I. Effect of injection methods on turkey hatchability and Mycoplasma meleagridis infection. Avian Dis 21:57–68.
79. Mohamed, Y.S., and E.H. Bohl. 1967. Studies on the transmission of Mycoplasma meleagridis. Avian Dis 11:634–641.
80. Mohamed, Y.S., and E.H. Bohl. 1968. Serologic studies on Mycoplasma meleagridis in turkeys. Avian Dis 12:554–566.
81. Mohamed, Y.S., S. Chema, and E.H. Bohl. 1966. Studies on Mycoplasma of the "H" serotype (Mycoplasma meleagridis) in the reproductive and respiratory tracts of turkeys. Avian Dis 10:347–352.
82. Moorhead, P.D., and Y.M. Saif. 1970. Mycoplasma meleagridis and Escherichia coli infections in germfree and specific pathogen free turkey poults: Pathologic manifestations. Am J Vet Res 31:1645–1653.
83. Nelson, R.C. 1968. Personal communication.
84. Nelson, R.C., W.M. Dungan, and C.T. Larsen. 1974. Comparison of the performance of Mycoplasma meleagridis-free and infected poults. Proc 23rd West Poult Dis Conf and 8th Poult Health Symp, pp. 66–69. Davis, CA.

85. Newman, J.A. 1967. The detection and control of Mycoplasma meleagridis. PhD diss., Univ Minnesota.
86. O'Brien, J.D.P. 1979. Effect of Mycoplasma meleagridis on hatchability. Proc 28th West Poult Dis Conf and 13th Poult Health Symp, pp. 29–31.
87. Ogra, M.S., and E.H. Bohl. 1970. Growth-inhibition test for identifying Mycoplasma meleagridis and its antibody. Avian Dis 14:364–373.
88. Ortiz, A.M., R. Yamamoto, A.A. Benedict, and A.P. Mateos. 1981. The immunosuppressive effect of Mycoplasma meleagridis on nonreplicating antigens. Avian Dis 25:954–963.
89. Ortmayer, H.B., and R. Yamamoto. 1981. Mycoplasma meleagridis antibody detection by enzyme-linked immunosorbent assay (ELISA). Proc 30th West Poult Dis Conf and 15th Poult Health Symp, pp. 63–66.
90. Ortmayer, H.B., R. Yamamoto, and E.E. Grass. 1975. Mass screening for Mycoplasma in the genitalia of turkeys by cultural method. Poult Sci 54:1802.
91. Peterson, I.L. 1968. Field significance of Mycoplasma meleagridis infection. Poult Sci 47:1708–1709. (Abstr).
92. Pohl, R. 1969. Airsacculitis and pantothenic acid biotin deficiency in turkeys in New Zealand. NZ Vet J 7:183.
93. Reis, R., and R. Yamamoto. 1971. Pathogenesis of single and mixed infections caused by Mycoplasma meleagridis and Mycoplasma gallisepticum in turkey embryos. Am J Vet Res 32:63–74.
94. Reis, R., J.M.L. DaSilva, and R. Yamamoto. 1970. Pathologic changes in the joint and other organs of turkey poults after intravenous inoculation of Mycoplasma meleagridis. Avian Dis 14:117–125.
95. Report of Working Party. (R.F. Gordon, chairman). 1965. A new syndrome in turkey poults. Vet Rec 77:1292.
96. Rhoades, K.R. 1969. A hemagglutination-inhibition test for Mycoplasma meleagridis antibodies. Avian Dis 13:22–26.
97. Rhoades, K.R. 1969. Experimentally induced Mycoplasma meleagridis infection of turkey reproductive tracts. Avian Dis 13:508–519.
98. Rhoades, K.R. 1971. Mycoplasma meleagridis infection: Reproductive tract lesions in mature turkeys. Avian Dis 15:722–729.
99. Rhoades, K.R. 1971. Mycoplasma meleagridis infection: Development of lesions and distribution of infection in turkey embryos. Avian Dis 15:762–774.
100. Rhoades, K.R. 1971. Mycoplasma meleagridis infection: Development of air sac lesions in turkey poults. Avian Dis 15:910–922.
101. Rhoades, K.R. 1977. Turkey sinusitis: Synergism between Mycoplasma synoviae and Mycoplasma meleagridis. Avian Dis 21:670–674.
102. Rhoades, K.R. 1978. Comparison of Mycoplasma meleagridis antibodies demonstrated by tube agglutination and hemagglutination-inhibition test. Avian Dis 22:633–638.
103. Rhoades, K.R. 1978. Inhibition of avian mycoplasmal hemagglutination by IgM type antibody. Poult Sci 57:608–610.
104. Rhoades, K.R. 1981. Pathogencity of strains of the IJKNQR group of avian mycoplasmas for turkey embryos and poults. Avian Dis 25:104–111.
105. Rhoades, K.R. 1981. Turkey airsacculitis: Effect of mixed mycoplasmal infections. Avian Dis 25:131–135.
106. Saif, Y.M., and K.I. Brown. 1972. Treatment of turkey semen to eliminate Mycoplasma meleagridis. Turkey Res, Ohio Agric Res Cent, Wooster, OH, pp. 49–50.
107. Saif, Y.M., P.D. Moorhead, and E.H. Bohl. 1970. Mycoplasma meleagridis and Escherichia coli infections in germfree and specific pathogen free turkey poults: Production of complicated airsacculitis. Am J Vet Res 31:1637–1643.
108. Saif, Y.M., K.E. Nestor, and K.E. McCracken. 1970. Tylosin tartrate absorption of turkey and chicken eggs dipped using pressure and temperature differentials. Poult Sci 49:1641–1649.
109. Saif, Y.M., L.C. Ferguson, and K.E. Nestor. 1971. Treatment of turkey hatching eggs for control of Arizona infection. Avian Dis 15:448–461.
110. Schar, R.D., and I.L. Peterson. 1982. The national poultry improvement plan – an update (with reference to the control of salmonellosis and mycoplasmosis). Proc US Anim Health Assoc 86:445–453.
111. Shimizu, T., and T. Yagihashi. 1980. Isolation of Mycoplasma meleagridis from turkeys in Japan. Jpn J Vet Sci 42:41–47.
112. Sokkar, I.M., A.M. Soliman, S. Mousa, and M.Z. El-Demerdash. 1986. In-vitro sensitivity of mycoplasma and associated bacteria isolated from chickens and turkeys and ducks at the area of Upper Egypt. Assiut Vet Med J 15:243–250.
113. Stipkovits, L., G. Laber, and E. Schultze. 1977. Prophylactical and therapeutical efficacy of tiamuline in mycoplasmosis of chickens and turkeys. Poult Sci 56:1209–1215.
114. Thornton, G.A., D.R. Wise, and M.K. Fuller. 1975. A Mycoplasma meleagridis haemagglutination-inhibition test. Vet Rec 96:113–114.
115. Uppal, P.K., D.R. Wise, and M.K. Boldero. 1972. Ultrastructural characteristics of Mycoplasma gallisepticum, M. gallinarum, and M. meleagridis. Res Vet Sci 13:200–201.
116. Vlaovic, M.S., and C.H. Bigland. 1971. The attempted immunization of turkey hens with viable Mycoplasma meleagridis. Can J Comp Med 35:338–341.
117. Wise, D.R., and M.K. Fuller. 1975. Experimental reproduction of turkey syndrome 65 with Mycoplasma meleagridis and Mycoplasma gallisepticum and associated changes in serum protein characteristics. Res Vet Sci 19:201–203.
118. Wise, D.R., and M.K. Fuller. 1975. Eradication of Mycoplasma meleagridis from a primary turkey breeder enterprise. Vet Rec 96:133–134.
119. Wise, D.R., M.K. Boldero, and G.A. Thornton. 1973. The pathology and aetiology of turkey syndrome '65 (T.S.65). Res Vet Sci 14:194–200.
120. Wise, D.R., M.K. Fuller, and G.A. Thornton. 1974. Experimental reproduction of turkey syndrome '65 with Mycoplasma meleagridis. Res Vet Sci 17:236–241.
121. Yamamoto, R. 1967. Localization and egg transmission of Mycoplasma meleagridis in turkeys exposed by various routes. Ann NY Acad Sci 143:225–233.
122. Yamamoto, R. 1971. Unpublished data.
123. Yamamoto, R. 1978. Mycoplasma meleagridis infection. In M.S. Hofstad, B.W. Calnek, C.F. Helmboldt, W.M. Reid, and H.W. Yoder, Jr. (eds.), Diseases of Poultry, 7th Ed., pp. 250–260. Iowa State Univ Press, Ames.
124. Yamamoto, R. 1988. Unpublished data.
125. Yamamoto, R., and C.H. Bigland. 1964. Pathogenicity to chicks of Mycoplasma associated with turkey airsacculitis. Avian Dis 8:523–531.
126. Yamamoto, R., and C.H. Bigland. 1965. Experimental production of airsacculitis in turkey poults by inoculation with "N"-type Mycoplasma. Avian Dis 9:108–118.
127. Yamamoto, R., and C.H. Bigland. 1966. Infectiv-

ity of Mycoplasma meleagridis for turkey embryos. Am J Vet Res 27:326–330.
128. Yamamoto, R., and M. Matsumoto. 1970. Unpublished data.
129. Yamamoto, R., and A. Ortiz. 1974. Microtiter agglutination test for Mycoplasma meleagridis. Proc 15th World Poult Congr, pp. 171–172.
130. Yamamoto, R., and H.B. Ortmayer. 1966. Pathogenicity of Mycoplasma meleagridis for turkey and chicken embryos. Avian Dis 10:268–272.
131. Yamamoto, R., and H.B. Ortmayer. 1967. Effect of Mycoplasma meleagridis on reproductive performance. Poult Sci 46:1340. (Abstr).
132. Yamamoto, R., and H.B. Ortmayer. 1967. Hatcher and intraflock transmission of Mycoplasma meleagridis. Avian Dis 11:288–295.
133. Yamamoto, R., and H.B. Ortmayer. 1967. Localization and persistence of avian mycoplasma in the genital system of the mature turkey. J Am Vet Med Assoc 150:1371. (Abstr).
134. Yamamoto, R., and H.B. Ortmayer. 1968. Unpublished data.
135. Yamamoto, R., and H.B. Ortmayer. 1969. Egg transmission of Mycoplasma meleagridis in naturally infected turkeys under different mating systems. Poult Sci 48:1893. (Abstr).
136. Yamamoto, R., and H.B. Ortmayer. 1970. Unpublished data.
137. Yamamoto, R., C.H. Bigland, and H.B. Ortmayer. 1965. Characteristics of Mycoplasma meleagridis sp.n., isolated from turkeys. J Bacteriol 90:47–49.
138. Yamamoto, R., C.H. Bigland, and H.B. Ortmayer. 1966. Sensitivity of Mycoplasma meleagridis to various antibiotics. Poult Sci 45:1139. (Abstr).
139. Yamamoto, R., C.H. Bigland, and I.L. Peterson. 1966. Egg transmission of Mycoplasma meleagridis. Poult Sci 45:1245–1257.
140. Yamamoto, R., H.B. Ortmayer, and C.S. Joshi. 1968. Persistance of Mycoplasma meleagridis in the genitalia of experimentally infected turkeys. Poult Sci 47:1734. (Abstr).
141. Yamamoto, R., H.B. Ortmayer, and M. Matsumoto. 1970. Standardization and application of Mycoplasma meleagridis agglutination test. Proc 14th World Poult Congr Sci Comm 3:139–148.
142. Yamamoto, R., F.H. Kratzer, and H.B. Ortmayer. 1974. Recent research on Mycoplasma meleagridis. Proc 23rd West Poult Dis Conf and 8th Poult Health Symp, pp. 53–54.
143. Yamamoto, R., H.B. Ortmayer, and R.K. Edson. 1978. Micro-hemagglutination-inhibition test for Mycoplasma meleagridis. Proc 16th World's Poult Congr 9:1417–1427.
144. Yamamoto, R., H.B. Ortmayer, and R.K. Edson. 1979. Serology of Mycoplasma meleagridis. Proc 28th West Poult Dis Conf and 13th Poult Health Symp, p. 23.
145. Yoder, H.W., Jr. 1970. Preincubation heat treatment of chicken hatching eggs to inactivate mycoplasma. Avian Dis 14:75–86.
146. Yoder, H.W., Jr., and M.S. Hofstad. 1964. Characterization of avian mycoplasma. Avian Dis 8:481–512.
147. Zhao, S., R. Yamamoto, G.Y. Ghazikhanian, and M.I. Khan. 1988. Antigenic analysis of three strains of Mycoplasma meleagridis of varying pathogenicity. Vet Microbiol 18:373–377.

MYCOPLASMA SYNOVIAE INFECTION

S.H. Kleven, G.N. Rowland, and N.O. Olson

INTRODUCTION. *Mycoplasma synoviae* (MS) infection most frequently occurs as a subclinical upper respiratory infection. It may cause air sac infection when combined with Newcastle disease (ND), infectious bronchitis (IB), or both. At other times MS becomes systemic and results in infectious synovitis, an acute to chronic infectious disease of chickens and turkeys, involving primarily the synovial membranes of joints and tendon sheaths producing an exudative synovitis, tenovaginitis, or bursitis.

HISTORY. Infectious synovitis was first described and associated with a mycoplasma by Olson et al. (48, 49). A respiratory form of *M. synoviae* infection occurs (51) and air sac infection results with some isolates of *M. synoviae* when combined with ND and IB vaccination (36). See Jordan (27, 28) and Timms (70) for reviews of the MS literature.

INCIDENCE AND DISTRIBUTION. Infectious synovitis was observed primarily in growing birds 4–12 wk of age in broiler-growing regions of the USA during the 1950s and 1960s. During the 1970s and 1980s the synovitis form was rarely observed in chickens, but the respiratory form was seen more frequently. Infection without apparent clinical signs is not unusual. MS infection occurs frequently in multi age commercial layers (43, 54). Infectious synovitis usually appears in turkeys when they are 10–20 wk old. Breeding stock from all major commercial breeds of chickens and turkeys is largely free of infection. MS is worldwide in distribution.

ETIOLOGY

Classification. Lecce (40) noted mycoplasmas as satellites adjacent to *Micrococcus* colonies. This was confirmed by Chalquest and Fabricant (13), who incorporated nicotinamide adenine dinucleotide (NAD) in their medium. It was designated as serotype S by Dierks et al. (16). Olson et al. (52) studied several isolates and proposed the name *M. synoviae,* which was subsequently confirmed as a separate species (29).

Identification is based on typical colony and cell morphology, biochemical characteristics, special requirements for growth, and serologic reactions. Immunofluorescence of mycoplasma colonies is the most rapid and reliable method for identification of field isolates.

Morphology and Staining. In Giemsa-stained preparations *M. synoviae* cells appear as pleomorphic coccoid bodies approximately 0.2 μm in diameter. Ultrastructural studies of avian synovium reveal MS in endocytotic vesicles. The mycoplasma cells are round or pear-shaped with granular ribosomes. They are 300–500 nm in diameter, lack a cell wall, and are bounded by a triple-layered unit membrane (75). An extracellular surface layer has been demonstrated by electron microscopy with ruthenium red and negative-staining (1).

Growth Requirements. Nicotinamide adenine dinucleotide is required for growth (13); however, it may be possible to substitute nicotinamide for the more expensive NAD for production of antigens (15). Serum is essential for growth, and swine serum is preferred (12). Growth on agar is accomplished by incubation of plates in a closed container to prevent dehydration of the agar. The optimum temperature is 37 C.

On primary isolation, tissue antigens, toxins, and antibodies may be present; therefore, a small inoculum transfer within 24 hr or making dilutions of the inoculum in broth is recommended. All transfers are made with a pipette using a 10% inoculum. Inoculation of broth medium with a cotton swab from the trachea, choanal cleft, or synovial or air sac lesion is satisfactory. Direct plating onto agar plates may result in colonies at 4–5 days of incubation, but isolation in broth is more sensitive. Broth cultures should be incubated until a color change of the phenol red indicator from red to orange or yellow is noted (usually after 3–7 days); the culture should then be transferred to an agar plate and subcultured into another broth culture. MS is sensitive to low pH; therefore, cultures incubated for more than a few hours after the phenol red indicator has changed to yellow (<pH 6.8) may no longer be viable. Plates are observed for the presence of mycoplasma colonies after 4–7 days using a microscope with indirect or low-intensity lighting at a magnification of approximately ×30.

Excellent growth is obtained using a modification of Frey's medium (18) as outlined below; adjust pH to 7.8 with 20% NaOH and filter-sterilize.

Mycoplasma broth base (BBL)	22.5 g
Dextrose	3.0 g
Swine serum	120.0 ml
Nicotinamide adenine dinucleotide (NAD)	0.1 g
Cysteine hydrochloride	0.1 g
Phenol red (1%)	2.5 ml
Thallium acetate (10%)*	5.0 ml
Potassium penicillin G*	1,000,000 units
Distilled H_2O	1000.0 ml

*For potentially contaminated specimens, an extra 20 ml of 1% thallium acetate and 2,000,000 units of penicillin per liter may be added. Ampicillin (200–1000 mg/l) may be substituted for penicillin.

For agar plates use 1% of a purified agar such as ionagar #2, Noble agar, or Difco purified agar. All components except cysteine, NAD, serum, and penicillin are sterilized by autoclaving at 121 C for 15 min. Cool to 50 C and aseptically add the above components, which have been sterilized by filtration and warmed to 50 C. Pour plates to a depth of approximately 5 mm. Phenol red may be eliminated from agar plates.

Colony Morphology. Colonies on solid media are best observed with a dissecting microscope at ×30 using indirect lighting; they appear as raised, round, slightly latticed colonies with or without centers. Colonies are from less than 1 up to 3 mm in diameter, depending on number of colonies present, suitability of medium, and age of culture. Growth is seen on solid medium in 3–7 days.

Biochemical Properties. Biochemical characteristics of *M. synoviae* have been described (13, 16, 79). MS ferments glucose and maltose with production of acid but not gas in suitably enriched media. It does not ferment lactose, dulcitol, salicin, or trehalose. MS is phosphatase-negative (29). Some isolates are capable of hemagglutinating chicken and turkey erythrocytes. Its ability to reduce tetrazolium salts appears to be very limited.

Resistance to Chemical and Physical Agents. Resistance to disinfectants has not been determined but is probably similar to other mycoplasmas. Day-old chicks placed in contaminated chicken houses that had been cleaned and disinfected and maintained empty for 1 wk did not become infected (19). *M. synoviae* is not stable at pH 6.8 or lower. It is sensitive to temperatures above 39 C. It will withstand freezing; however, the titer is reduced. Endpoints have not been reached, but in yolk material MS is viable at least 7 yr at −63 C and after 2 yr at −20 C. Broth cultures maintained frozen at −70 C or lyophilized cultures maintained at 4 C are viable for several years.

Antigenic Structure. Serum plate agglutination (SPA) (50), tube agglutination (TA) (73), hemagglutination (72), agar-gel precipitin (AGP) (67), and enzyme-linked immunosorbent assay (ELISA) (25, 55, 58) antigens have been studied.

Available information indicates a single serotype of *M. synoviae* (16, 52), and DNA-DNA hybridization techniques show little heterogeneity among MS strains (82, 83). However, as with *M. gallisepticum* (38), MS strains can be differentiated using restriction endonuclease analysis of DNA.

Serum from chickens infected with MS occasionally agglutinates *M. gallisepticum* plate antigen (52, 53). The reverse occurs less frequently. Roberts and Olesuik (66) suggested that the cross-reactions were related to presence of the rheumatoid factor and could be stimulated by tissue reactions. There are also epitopes shared by *M. gallisepticum* and MS (2, 10, 83). Species-specific monoclonal antibodies against MS have been produced (56). Cross-reactions are minimal when the hemagglutination inhibition (HI) or TA test is used.

Pathogenicity. There is considerable variation among isolates in their ability to produce disease; many isolates cause little or no clinical disease. Passage in embryos, tissue culture, or broth reduces its ability to produce typical infection. Embryo passage appears to have less effect on pathogenicity than broth passage. *M. synoviae* isolated from air sac lesions are more apt to cause airsacculitis while those isolated from synovia are more apt to produce synovitis (37). Airsacculitis is exacerbated by vaccination against Newcastle disease or infectious bronchitis (36, 69), or any respiratory infection. The severity of the airsacculitis depends on the virulence of the infectious bronchitis virus used in conjunction with MS (26). Air sac lesions are greatly enhanced by cold environmental temperatures (81). Infectious bursal disease causes immunosuppression in chickens, and dual infection with MS results in more severe air sac lesions (21). A rheumatoid factor associated with the euglobulin fraction is present in serum of affected chickens (59).

PATHOGENESIS AND EPIZOOTIOLOGY

Natural and Experimental Hosts. Chickens, turkeys, and guinea fowl (57) are the natural hosts of *M. synoviae.* Ducks (6), geese (7), pigeons (5, 61), Japanese quail (5), and red-legged partridge (60) have been found to be naturally infected. Pheasants and geese (68), ducks (78), and budgerigars (8) are susceptible by artificial inoculation. House sparrows (35) could be artificially infected, but are quite resistant. Rabbits, rats, guinea pigs, mice, pigs, and lambs are not susceptible to experimental inoculation (49).

Natural infection in chickens has been observed as early as 1 wk but acute infection is generally seen when chickens are 4–16 wk old and turkeys are 10–24 wk old. Acute infection occasionally occurs in adult chickens. Chronic infection follows the acute phase and may persist for the life of the flock. The chronic stage may be seen at any age and in some flocks may not be preceded by an acute infection.

Airsacculitis occurs in day-old and older turkeys in MS-infected flocks. Air sac inoculation of mycoplasma-free turkeys results in airsacculitis (20, 64). Inoculation of 18-day-old chicken embryos via the yolk sac resulted in synovitis and airsacculitis in the chicks (9). MS may be isolated from lesions during the acute phase of the disease, but infection of the upper respiratory tract is permanent (36).

Transmission. Lateral transmission occurs readily by direct contact. *M. synoviae* has been demonstrated in the respiratory tract of contact control chickens 1–4 wk following infection of the principals (51). Spread between batteries in the same room occurs. In many respects the spread appears to be similar to that of *M. gallisepticum* (46) except that it is more rapid. However, slow-spreading infections have been reported (76). Transmission occurs via the respiratory tract, and usually 100% of the birds become infected, although none or only a few develop joint lesions.

Vertical transmission occurs in naturally and artificially infected chickens (11). Using the agglutination test, it is possible to demonstrate infection in dams and offspring even though no clinical signs have been seen in either. However, many flocks hatched from infected dams remain free of infection. Vertical transmission plays a major role in spread of MS in chickens and turkeys. Thus all eggs used for live virus vaccine production should be obtained from MS-free flocks. Experimental infection of broiler breeders resulted in MS in the trachea of day-old progeny, infertile eggs, and dead-in-shell embryos 6–31 days postinoculation (71). When commercial breeder flocks become infected during egg production, egg-transmission rate is highest during the first 4–6 wk after infection; transmission thereafter may cease, but infected flocks may shed at any time.

Incubation Period. Infectious synovitis has been seen in 6-day-old chicks, suggesting that the incubation period can be relatively short in birds infected by egg transmission. The incubation period following contact exposure is generally 11–21 days. Antibodies may be detected before clinical disease becomes evident. In birds experimentally infected by inoculation at 3–6 wk of age with joint exudate from infected birds or yolk from infected embryos, the order of susceptibility and incubation period is as follows: footpad, 2–10 days; intravenous, 7–10 days; intracranial, 7–10 days; intraperitoneal, 7–14 days; intrasinus, 14–20 days; conjunctival instillation, 20 days. Birds are also susceptible to intramuscular inoculation. Intratracheal inoculation results in infection of the trachea and sinus as early as 4 days and readily spreads to contact birds. Air sac lesions are at a maximum 17–21 days after aerosol challenge (36). The incubation period varies with titer and pathogenicity of the inoculum.

Signs

CHICKENS. The first observable signs in a flock affected with infectious synovitis are pale comb, lameness, and retarded growth. As the disease progresses, feathers become ruffled and the comb shrinks. In some cases the comb is bluish red. Swellings usually occur around joints, and breast blisters are common. Hock joints and foot pads are principally involved, but in some birds most joints are affected. However, birds are occasionally found with a generalized infection but not with apparent swelling of the joints. Birds become listless, dehydrated, and emaciated. Although birds are severely affected, many continue to eat and drink if placed near feed and water. A greenish discoloration of droppings, which contain large amounts of uric acid or urates, is frequently seen. Acute signs described above are followed by slow recovery; however, synovitis may persist for the life of the flock. In other instances the acute phase is absent or not noticed and only a few chronically infected birds are seen in a flock. Chickens infected via the respiratory tract may show slight rales in 4–6 days or may be asymptomatic.

Air sac infection may occur at any age but is most often observed as a cause of condemnation in broilers (33). Under field conditions most air sac lesions resulting from *M. synoviae* infection occur in winter. Progeny of MS-infected breeders may have increased air sac condemnations, reduced weight gains, and reduced feed efficiency.

Experimental aerosol inoculation of hens with MS resulted in a detectable drop in egg production 1 wk postchallenge; by 2 wk production dropped 18%, and by 4 wk production returned to normal (41). However, with natural infection of adults there is little or no effect on egg production or egg quality (44, 54).

TURKEYS. *M. synoviae* generally causes the same type of signs in turkeys as in chickens. Lameness is the most prominent sign. Warm fluctuating swellings of one or more joints of lame birds are usually found. Occasionally there is enlargement of the sternal bursa. Severely affected birds lose weight, but many that are less severely affected make satisfactory weight gains when separated from the flock. In experimentally infected turkeys (49) the first noticeable sign is failure to grow (Fig. 8.10).

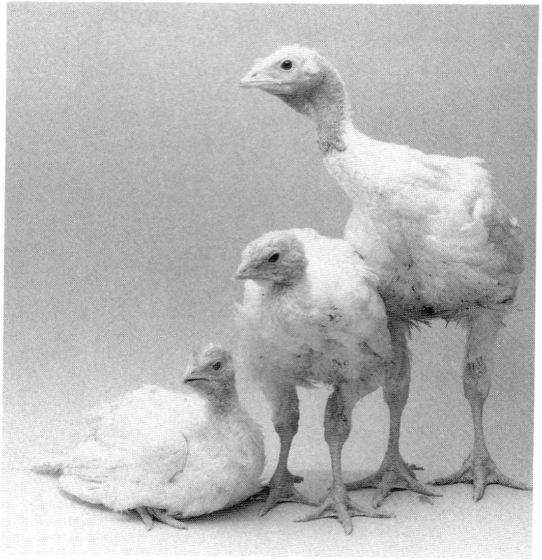

8.10. Two experimental turkeys with infectious synovitis (*left*) and control turkey (*right*) of the same age.

Respiratory signs are not usually observed in turkeys, but MS has been isolated from sinus exudates obtained from turkey flocks exhibiting a very low incidence of sinusitis. Rhoades (63) described a synergistic effect of MS and *M. meleagridis* in producing sinusitis in turkeys. Foot pad inoculation of turkeys results in total cessation of egg production.

Morbidity and Mortality

CHICKENS. Morbidity in flocks with clinical synovitis varies from 2 to 75%, with 5–15% being most usual. Respiratory involvement is generally asymptomatic, but 90–100% of the birds may actually be infected. Mortality is usually less than 1%, ranging up to 10%. In experimentally infected chickens mortality may vary from 0 to 100%, depending on route of inoculation and dose of inoculum.

TURKEYS. Morbidity in infected flocks is usually low (1–20%), but mortality from trampling and cannibalism may be significant.

Gross Lesions

CHICKENS. In early stages of the infectious synovitis form of the disease, chickens frequently have a viscous creamy to gray exudate involving synovial membranes of the tendon sheaths (Fig. 8.11), joints, and keel bursa, and hepatosplenomegaly. Kidneys are usually swollen, mottled, and pale. As the disease progresses caseous exudate may be found involving tendon sheaths, joints, and extending into muscle and air sacs. Articular surfaces, particularly of the hock and shoulder joints, become variably thinned to pitted over time (Fig. 8.12). Generally no gross lesions are seen in the upper respiratory tract. In the respiratory form of the disease, airsacculitis may be present.

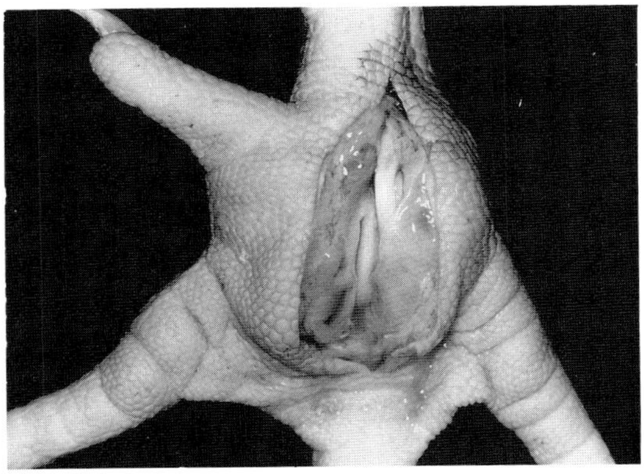

8.11. Incised swollen foot pad of 8-wk-old turkey with granulation tissue and purulent exudate surrounding digital flexors. Similar lesions can be seen in chickens.

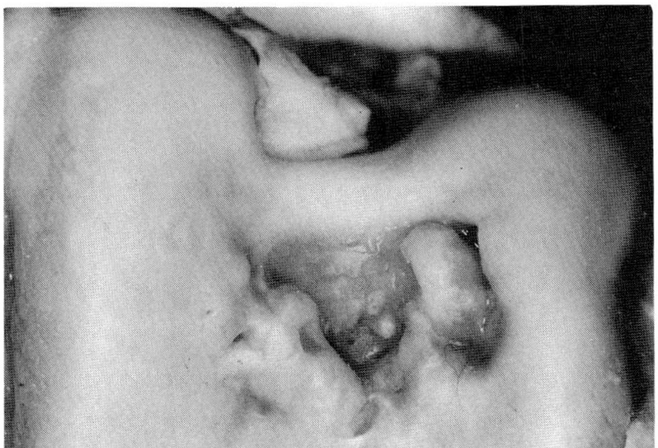

8.12. Ulceration of articular surface of distal tibiotarsus from a chicken with infectious synovitis.

TURKEYS. Swellings of the joints may not be as prominent as in chickens, but fibrinopurulent exudate is frequently present when the joints are opened. Lesions in the respiratory tract are variable.

Histopathology. The histopathology of infectious synovitis (30, 32, 68) in chickens and respiratory disease caused by *M. synoviae* in chickens (17) and turkeys (20, 65) has been described.

The joints, particularly of the foot and hock, have an infiltrate of heterophils and fibrin into joint spaces and along tendon sheaths. The synovial membranes are hyperplastic with villous formation and a diffuse to nodular subsynovial infiltrate of lymphocytes and macrophages (Fig. 8.13). Cartilage surfaces, over time, become discolored, thinned, or pitted. Air sacs may have a mild lesion consisting of edema, capillary proliferation, and the accumulation of heterophils and necrotic debris on the surface, to more severe lesions with hyperplasia of epithelial cells, a diffuse infiltrate of mononuclear cells, and caseous necrosis. Other lesions reported to be associated with infectious synovitis are hyperplasia of the macrophage-monocyte system associated with the sheathed arteries of the spleen, lymphoid infiltrates in the heart, liver, and gizzard, and thymic and bursal atrophy. Cardiac pathology has been described in detail (31).

Immunity. Chickens exposed intranasally to *M. synoviae* were resistant to subsequent foot pad challenge (51). Chickens immunized intranasally with a temperature-sensitive mutant of MS were protected against airsacculitis for at least 21 wk (45). Parenteral inoculation of MS frequently overwhelms the bird before adequate resistance can develop. Resistance to lesions induced by MS is bursa-dependent (39, 74), while thymus-dependent lymphocytes may be needed for the development of macroscopic synovial lesions (39).

DIAGNOSIS

Isolation and Identification. Positive diagnosis may be made by isolation and identification of *M. synoviae.* Isolation from lesions in acutely infected birds is not difficult, but in the chronic stages of infection viable organisms may be no longer present in lesions. Isolation from the upper respiratory tract is more reliable in chronically infected birds (for medium and isolation methods, see Growth Requirements). The fluorescent antibody technique using colony imprints (14) or intact colonies (3) may be used for identification.

Serology. Antigen is available commercially for the SPA test. Adequate directions for use are given with each package. Generally 0.02 ml serum is mixed with an equal amount of antigen on a glass plate, which is gently rotated and observed for agglutination. Nonspecific reactors occur in some flocks when using the SPA test (22), especially in flocks that have been vaccinated with oil-emulsion vaccines against various agents. *M. gallisepticum* antigen may be agglutinated on

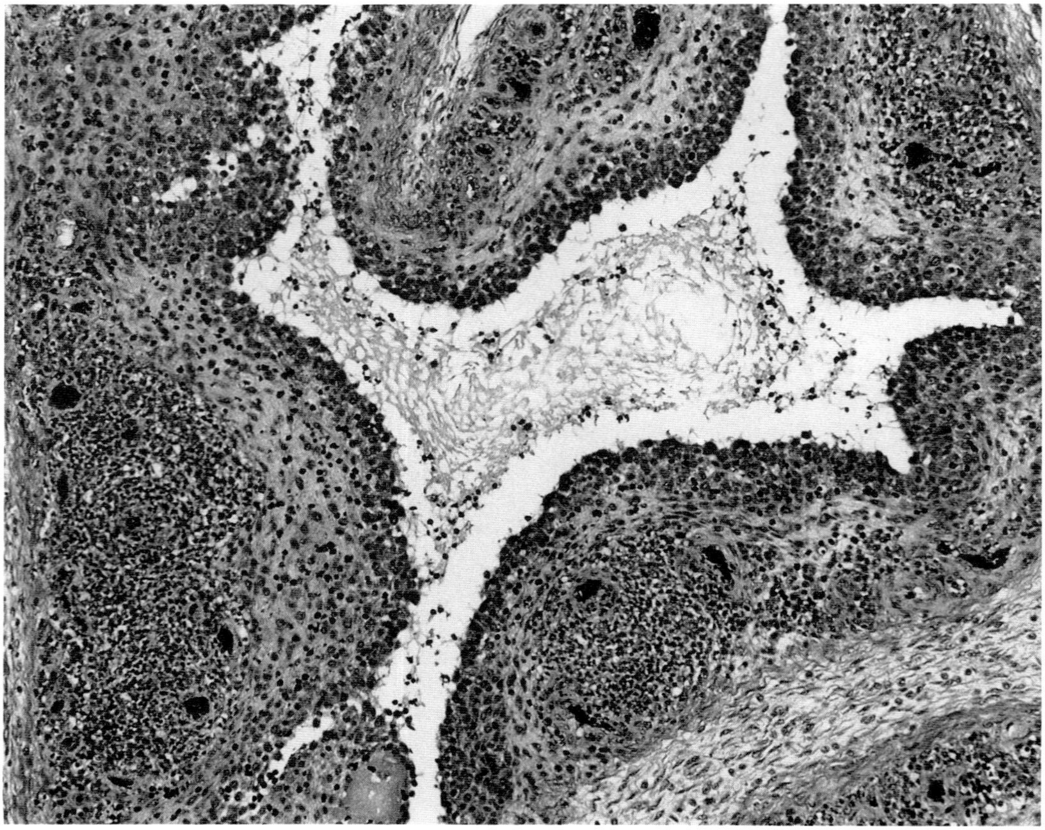

8.13. Hyperplastic synovial membrane with multiple subsynovial lymphoid aggregates from a 7-wk-old turkey with infectious synovitis.

occasion, but the reaction is somewhat delayed and usually lower in titer (53). To confirm specificity of the reaction, the HI test is used (72). Further confirmation may be made by isolation and identification of *M. synoviae* from the upper respiratory tract (67).

Antigen should be tested with known positive and negative serums each day. It requires 2–4 wk for antibodies to develop in infected birds (50). See Jordan (27) and Timms (70) for further information.

Turkeys produce a low level of antibody following respiratory infection; therefore, agglutination may not be effective in determining the MS status of a flock. Significant antibodies develop following foot pad inoculation only (20, 62). Various commercial antigens vary in their ability to detect agglutinins in turkeys. Culture and HI testing may be required in some cases to detect infection.

Differential Diagnosis. A presumptive diagnosis may be made on the basis of pale comb, droopiness, emaciation, leg weakness, breast blisters, enlarged foot pads or hock joints, splenomegaly, and enlarged liver or kidneys. Bacteria that cause synovitis or arthritis must be eliminated by bacteriologic procedures. *Staphylococcus aureus, E. coli,* pasteurellae, and salmonellae may also be present as primary causes of synovitis. *M. gallisepticum* may also be a cause of breast blisters and joint lesions (49, 52).

Fibrosis of metatarsal extensor or digital flexor tendons and lymphocytic infiltration of the myocardium associated with the viral arthritis agent help to differentiate it from *M. synoviae* (42). Serum from viral tenosynovitis-infected chickens does not agglutinate MS antigen, but one must bear in mind that MS agglutinins may be present without obvious joint involvement. See Chapter 27 for procedures for the diagnosis of viral tenosynovitis.

In cases with respiratory involvement, *M. gallisepticum* and other causes of respiratory disease should be eliminated.

TREATMENT. *M. synoviae* is susceptible in vitro to several antibiotics, including tylosin, chlortetracycline, lincomycin, oxytetracycline, spectinomycin, spiromycin, tetracycline, and tiamulin (34, 77). In contrast to *M. gallisepticum,* MS isolates appear to be resistant to erythromycin (77). Acquired antibiotic resistance has not been reported for MS, although earlier isolates seem to respond more poorly to chlortetracycline than later isolates (47). Generally, suitable medication is of value in preventing airsacculitis or synovitis, but treatment of existing lesions is less effective. Antibiotic medication will not eliminate MS infection from the flock.

A summary of data obtained from field and experimental studies indicates that chlortetracycline (50–100 g/ton of feed) given continuously will provide satisfactory control of infectious synovitis in chickens. Higher concentrations (approximately 200 g/ton) are required to control synovitis after infection has occurred. In turkeys, prophylactic levels of 200 g/ton are required. Effectiveness of chlortetracycline may be related to the MS isolate involved (47).

Soluble lincomycin-spectinomycin (2 g/gal of drinking water) is of value in preventing airsacculitis in broilers (23) and turkey poults (24). Tiamulin in the drinking water (0.006–0.025%) has been shown to be effective in preventing airsacculitis and synovitis in chickens (4). Other products have been used, but their value in treatment of MS has not been adequately studied.

PREVENTION AND CONTROL. *M. synoviae* is egg transmitted, and the only effective method of control is to select chickens or turkeys from MS-free flocks. Most primary breeding stocks are free of infection, and MS-free sources of replacement breeding stocks should be available. Effective biosecurity measures should be used to prevent introduction of the infection.

Outbreaks of MS infection in broilers can often be traced to a specific breeder flock. Usually by the time the infected breeder flock is found, egg transmission is low or no longer of clinical significance. Antibiotic treatment of breeders is not effective in eliminating MS; thus the decision to slaughter infected parent breeder flocks is usually made on an economic basis. If such flocks are kept for egg production, progeny should be hatched separately and isolated from MS-free flocks.

Treatment of eggs with antibiotics such as tylosin by egg dipping or egg inoculation or heat treatment (80) of hatching eggs has been used in basic broiler breeders to prevent egg transmission of MS (see chapter on *M. gallisepticum*). Exposure of breeders before the onset of egg production with virulent MS will reduce egg transmission and should only be used in flocks in which infection will almost certainly occur. An inactivated, oil-emulsion bacterin is commercially available, but its role in the control of MS has not been adequately studied.

REFERENCES

1. Ajufo, J.C., and K.G. Whithear. 1980. The surface layer of Mycoplasma synoviae as demonstrated by the negative staining technique. Res Vet Sci 29:268–270.
2. Avakian, A.P., and S.H. Kleven. 1989. The humoral immune response of chickens to Mycoplasma gallisepticum and potential causes of false positive reactions in avian Mycoplasma serology. 1989. Zent Bakteriol Mikrobiol Hyg. (In press).
3. Baas, E.J., and D.E. Jasper. 1972. Agar block technique for identification of mycoplasmas by use of fluorescent antibody. Appl Microbiol 23:1097–1100.
4. Baughn, C.O., W.C. Alpaugh, W.H. Linkenheimer, and D.C. Maplesden. 1978. Effect of tiamulin in chickens and turkeys infected experimentally with avian mycoplasma. Avian Dis 22:620–626.
5. Bencina, D., T. Tadina, and D. Dorrer. 1987. Mycoplasma species isolated from six avian species. Avian Pathol 16:653–664.
6. Bencina, D., T. Tadina, and D. Dorrer. 1988. Natural infection of ducks with Mycoplasma synoviae and Mycoplasma gallisepticum and Mycoplasma egg transmission. Avian Pathol 17:441–449.
7. Bencina, D., T. Tadina, and D. Dorrer. 1988. Natural infection of geese with Mycoplasma gallisepticum and Mycoplasma synoviae and egg transmission of the mycoplasmas. Avian Pathol 17:925–928.
8. Bozeman, L.H., S.H. Kleven, and R.B. Davis. 1984. Mycoplasma challenge studies in budgerigars (Melopsittacus undulatus) and chickens. Avian Dis 28:426–434.
9. Bradbury, J.M., and L.J. Howell. 1975. The response of chickens to experimental infection "in ovo" with Mycoplasma synoviae. Avian Pathol 4:277–286.
10. Bradley, L.D., D.B. Snyder, and R.A. Van Deusen. 1988. Identification of species-specific and interspecies-specific polypeptides of Mycoplasma gallisepticum and Mycoplasma synoviae. Am J Vet Res 49:511–515.
11. Carnaghan, R.B.A. 1961. Egg transmission of infectious synovitis. J Comp Pathol 71:279–285.
12. Chalquest, R.R. 1962. Cultivation of the infectious-synovitis-type pleuropneumonia-like organisms. Avian Dis 6:36–43.
13. Chalquest, R.R., and J. Fabricant. 1960. Pleuropneumonia-like organisms associated with synovitis in fowls. Avian Dis 4:515–539.
14. Corstvet, R.E., and W.W. Sadler. 1964. The diagnosis of certain avian diseases with the fluorescent antibody technique. Poult Sci 43:1280–1288.
15. DaMassa, A.J., and H.E. Adler. 1975. Growth of Mycoplasma synoviae in a medium supplemented with nicotinamide instead of B-nicotinamide adenine dinucleotide. Avian Dis 19:544–555.
16. Dierks, R.E., J.A. Newman, and B.S. Pomeroy. 1967. Characterization of avian mycoplasma. Ann NY Acad Sci 143:170–189.
17. Fletcher, O.J., D.P. Anderson, and S.H. Kleven. 1976. Histology of air sac lesions induced in chickens by contact exposure to Mycoplasma synoviae. Vet Pathol 13:303–314.
18. Frey, M.L., R.P. Hanson, and D.P. Anderson. 1968. A medium for the isolation of avian mycoplasmas. Am J Vet Res 29:2163–2171.
19. Furuta, K., Y. Makino, K. Komi, Y. Nakamura, and S. Oda. 1985. Sanitization of a chicken house contaminated with mycoplasmas. Jpn Poult Sci 22:126–133.
20. Ghazikhanian, G., R. Yamamoto, and D.R. Cordy. 1973. Response of turkeys to experimental infection with Mycoplasma synoviae. Avian Dis 17:122–136.
21. Giambrone, J.J., C.S. Eidson, and S.H. Kleven.

1977. Effect of infectious bursal disease on the response of chickens to Mycoplasma synoviae, Newcastle disease virus, and infectious bronchitis virus. Am J Vet Res 38:251–253.

22. Glisson, J.R., J.F. Dawe, and S.H. Kleven. 1984. The effect of oil-emulsion vaccines on the occurrence of nonspecific plate agglutination reactions for Mycoplasma gallisepticum and M. synoviae. Avian Dis 28:397–405.

23. Hamdy, A.H., S.H. Kleven, E.L. McCune, B.S. Pomeroy, and A.C. Peterson. 1976. Efficacy of Linco-spectin water medication on Mycoplasma synoviae airsacculitis in broilers. Avian Dis 20:118–125.

24. Hamdy, A.H., Y.M. Saif, and C.W. Kasson. 1982. Efficacy of lincomycin-spectinomycin water medication on Mycoplasma meleagridis airsacculitis in commercially reared turkey poults. Avian Dis 26:227–233.

25. Higgins, P.A., and K.G. Whithear. 1986. Detection and differentiation of Mycoplasma gallisepticum and Mycoplasma synoviae antibodies in chicken serum using enzyme-linked immunosorbent assay. Avian Dis 30:160–168.

26. Hopkins, S.R., and H.W. Yoder, Jr. 1982. Influence of infectious bronchitis strains and vaccines on the incidence of Mycoplasma synoviae airsacculitis. Avian Dis 26:741–752.

27. Jordan, F.T.W. 1975. Avian mycoplasma and pathogenicity—a review. Avian Pathol 4:165–174.

28. Jordan, F.T.W. 1981. Mycoplasma-induced arthritis in poultry. Isr J Med Sci 17:622–625.

29. Jordan, F.T.W., H. Erno, G.S. Cottew, K.H. Hinz, and L. Stipkovits. 1982. Characterization and taxonomic description of five mycoplasma serovars (serotypes) of avian origin and their elevation to species rank and further evaluation of the taxonomic status of Mycoplasma synoviae. Int J Syst Bacteriol 32:108–115.

30. Kawakubo, Y., K. Kume, and M. Yoshioka. 1980. Histo- and immuno-pathological studies on experimental Mycoplasma synoviae infection of the chicken. J Comp Pathol 90:457–467.

31. Kerr, K.M., and N.O. Olson. 1967. Cardiac pathology associated with viral and mycoplasmal arthritis in chickens. Ann NY Acad Sci 143:204–217.

32. Kerr, K.M., and N.O. Olson. 1970. Pathology of chickens inoculated experimentally or contact-infected with Mycoplasma synoviae. Avian Dis 14:291–320.

33. King, D.D., S.H. Kleven, D.M. Wenger, and D.P. Anderson. 1973. Field studies with Mycoplasma synoviae. Avian Dis 17:722–726.

34. Kleven, S.H., and D.P. Anderson. 1971. In vitro activity of various antibiotics against Mycoplasma synoviae. Avian Dis 15:551–557.

35. Kleven, S.H., and W.O. Fletcher. 1983. Laboratory infection of house sparrows (Passer domesticus) with Mycoplasma gallisepticum and Mycoplasma synoviae. Avian Dis 27:308–311.

36. Kleven, S.H., D.D. King, and D.P. Anderson. 1972. Airsacculitis in broilers from Mycoplasma synoviae: Effect on air-sac lesions of vaccinating with infectious bronchitis and Newcastle virus. Avian Dis 16:915–924.

37. Kleven, S.H., O.J. Fletcher, and R.B. Davis. 1975. Influence of strain of Mycoplasma synoviae and route of infection on development of synovitis or airsacculitis in broilers. Avian Dis 19:126–135.

38. Kleven, S.H., G.F. Browning, D.M. Bulach, E. Ghiocas, C.J. Morrow, and K.G. Whithear. 1988. Examination of Mycoplasma gallisepticum strains using restriction endonuclease DNA analysis and DNA-DNA hybridisation. Avian Pathol 17:559–570.

39. Kume, K., Y. Kawakubo, C. Morita, E. Hayatsu, and M. Yoshioka. 1977. Experimentally induced synovitis of chickens with Mycoplasma synoviae: Effects of bursectomy and thymectomy on course of the infection for the first four weeks. Am J Vet Res 38:1595–1600.

40. Lecce, J.G. 1960. Porcine polyserositis with arthritis: Isolation of a fastidious pleuropneumonia-like organism and Hemophilus influenzae suis. Ann NY Acad Sci 79:670–676.

41. Lott, B.D., J.H. Drott, T.H. Vardaman, and F.N. Reece. 1978. Effect of Mycoplasma synoviae on egg quality and egg production of broiler breeders. Poult Sci 57:309–311.

42. MacDonald, J.W., C.J. Randall, M.D. Dagless, and D.A. McMartin. 1978. Observations on viral tenosynovitis (viral arthritis) in Scotland. Avian Pathol 7:471–482.

43. Mohammed, H.O., T.E. Carpenter, R. Yamamoto, and D.A. McMartin. 1986. Prevalence of Mycoplasma gallisepticum and M. synoviae in commercial layers in southern and central California. Avian Dis 30:519–526.

44. Mohammed, H.O., T.E. Carpenter, and R. Yamamoto. 1987. Economic impact of Mycoplasma gallisepticum and M. synoviae in commercial layer flocks. Avian Dis 31:477–482.

45. Nonomura, I., and Y. Imada. 1982. Temperature-sensitive mutant of Mycoplasma synoviae. I. Production and selection of a nonpathogenic but immunogenic clone. Avian Dis 26:763–775.

46. Olson, N.O., and K.M. Kerr. 1967. The duration and distribution of synovitis-producing agents in chickens. Avian Dis 11:578–585.

47. Olson, N.O., and S.P. Sahu. 1976. Efficacy of chlortetracycline against Mycoplasma synoviae isolated in two periods. Avian Dis 20:221–229.

48. Olson, N.O., J.K. Bletner, D.C. Shelton, D.A. Munro, and G.C. Anderson. 1954. Enlarged joint condition in poultry caused by an infectious agent. Poult Sci 33:1075. (Abstr).

49. Olson, N.O., D.C. Shelton, J.K. Bletner, D.A. Munro, and G.C. Anderson. 1956. Studies of infectious synovitis in chickens. Am J Vet Res 17:747–754.

50. Olson, N.O., K.M. Kerr, and A. Campbell. 1963. Control of infectious synovitis. 12. Preparation of an agglutination test antigen. Avian Dis 7:310–317.

51. Olson, N.O., H.E. Adler, A.J. DaMassa, and R.E. Corstvet. 1964. The effect of intranasal exposure to Mycoplasma synoviae and infectious bronchitis on development of lesions and agglutinins. Avian Dis 8:623–631.

52. Olson, N.O., K.M. Kerr, and A. Campbell. 1964. Control of infectious synovitis. 13. The antigen study of three strains. Avian Dis 8:209–214.

53. Olson, N.O., R. Yamamoto, and H. Ortmayer. 1965. Antigenic relationship between Mycoplasma synoviae and Mycoplasma gallisepticum. Am J Vet Res 26:195–198.

54. Opitz, H.M. 1983. Mycoplasma synoviae infection in Maine's egg farms. Avian Dis 27:324–326.

55. Opitz, H.M., J.B. Duplessis, and M.J. Cyr. 1983. Indirect micro-enzyme-linked immunosorbent assay ELISA for the detection of antibodies to Mycoplasma synoviae and Mycoplasma gallisepticum. Avian Dis 27:773–786.

56. Panangala, V.S., M.Y. Hwang, L.H.Lauerman, S.H. Kleven, J.J. Giambrone, M. Gresham, and A. Mitra. 1989. Immunoenzymatic test with monoclonal antibodies for detection of avian Mycoplasma gallisepticum and M. synoviae antibodies. Zent Bakteriol Mikrobiol Hyg. (In press).

57. Pascucci, S., N. Maestrini, S. Govoni, and A. Prati. 1976. Mycoplasma synoviae in the guinea-fowl. Avian Pathol 5:291–297.

58. Patten, B.E., P.A. Higgins, and K.G. Whithear. 1984. A urease-ELISA for the detection of mycoplasma

infections in poultry. Aust Vet J 61:151–155.
59. Porter, P., and K.R. Gooderham. 1966. Changes in serum proteins and identification of a rheumatoid factor in a field outbreak of avian infectious synovitis. Res Vet Sci 7:25–34.
60. Poveda, J.B., A. Fernandez, J. Carranza, M. Hermoso, and J.A. Perea. 1986. Isolation of Mycoplasma synoviae from the red-legged partridge (Alectoris rufa). Avian Pathol 15:797–802.
61. Reece, R.L., L. Ireland, and P.C. Scott. 1986. Mycoplasmosis in racing pigeons. Aust Vet J 63:166–167.
62. Rhoades, K.R. 1975. Antibody responses of turkeys experimentally exposed to Mycoplasma synoviae. Avian Dis 19:437–442.
63. Rhoades, K.R. 1977. Turkey sinusitis: Synergism between Mycoplasma synoviae and Mycoplasma meleagridis. Avian Dis 21:670–674.
64. Rhoades, K.R. 1981. Turkey airsacculitis: Effect of mixed mycoplasmal infections. Avian Dis 25:131–135.
65. Rhoades, K.R. 1987. Airsacculitis in turkeys exposed to Mycoplasma synoviae membranes. Avian Dis 31:855–860.
66. Roberts, D.H., and O.M. Olesuik. 1967. Serological studies with Mycoplasma synoviae. Avian Dis 11:104–119.
67. Sahu, S.P., and N.O. Olson. 1976. Evaluation of broiler breeder flocks for nonspecific Mycoplasma synoviae reaction. Avian Dis 20:49–64.
68. Sevoian, M., G.H. Snoeyenbos, H.I. Basch, and I.M. Reynolds. 1958. Infectious synovitis. I. Clinical and pathological manifestations. Avian Dis 2:499–513.
69. Springer, W.T., C. Luskus, and S.S. Pourciau. 1974. Infectious bronchitis and mixed infections of Mycoplasma synoviae and Escherichia coli in gnotobiotic chickens. I. Synergistic role in the airsacculitis syndrome. Infect Immun 10:578–589.
70. Timms, L.M. 1978. Mycoplasma synoviae: A review. Vet Bull 48:187–198.
71. Vardaman, T.H. 1976. The resistance and carrier status of meat-type hens exposed to Mycoplasma synoviae. Poult Sci 55:268–273.
72. Vardaman, T.H., and H.W. Yoder, Jr. 1969. Preparation of Mycoplasma synoviae hemagglutinating antigen and its use in the hemagglutination-inhibition test. Avian Dis 13:654–661.
73. Vardaman, T.H., and H.W. Yoder. 1971. Preparation of Mycoplasma synoviae antigen for the tube agglutination test. Avian Dis 15:462–466.
74. Vardaman, T.H., K. Landaeth, S. Whatley, L.J. Dreesen, and B. Glick. 1973. Resistance to Mycoplasma synoviae is bursal dependent. Infect Immun 8:674–676.
75. Walker, E.R., M.H. Friedman, N.O. Olson, S.P. Sahu, and H.F. Mengoli. 1978. An ultrastructural study of avian synovium infected with an arthrotropic Mycoplasma, Mycoplasma synoviae. Vet Pathol 15:407–416.
76. Weinack, O.M., G.H. Snoeyenbos, and S.H. Kleven. 1983. Strain of Mycoplasma synoviae of low transmissibility. Avian Dis 27:1151–1156.
77. Whithear, K.G., D.D. Bowtell, E. Ghiocas, and K.L. Hughes. 1983. Evaluation and use of a micro-broth dilution procedure for testing sensitivity of fermentative avian mycoplasmas to antibiotics. Avian Dis 27:937–949.
78. Yamada, S., and K. Matsuo. 1983. Experimental infection of ducks with Mycoplasma synoviae. Avian Dis 27:762–765.
79. Yamamoto, R., C.H. Bigland, and H.B. Ortmayer. 1965. Characteristics of Mycoplasma meleagridis, sp.n., isolated from turkeys. J Bacteriol 90:47–49.
80. Yoder, H.W., Jr. 1970. Preincubation heat treatment of hatching eggs to inactivate mycoplasma. Avian Dis 14:75–86.
81. Yoder, H.W., Jr., L.N. Drury, and S.R. Hopkins. 1977. Influence of environment on airsacculitis: Effects of relative humidity and air temperature on broilers infected with Mycoplasma synoviae and infectious bronchitis. Avian Dis 21:195–208.
82. Yogev, D., S. Levisohn, S.H. Kleven, D. Halachmi, and S. Razin. 1988. Ribosomal RNA gene probes to detect intraspecies heterogeneity in Mycoplasma gallisepticum and M. synoviae. Avian Dis 32:220–231.
83. Yogev, D., S. Levisohn, and S. Razin. 1989. Genetic and antigenic relatedness between Mycoplasma gallisepticum and Mycoplasma synoviae. Vet Microbiol 19:75–84.

OTHER MYCOPLASMAL INFECTIONS

S.H. Kleven

MYCOPLASMA IOWAE INFECTION

INTRODUCTION. *Mycoplasma iowae* is generally associated with reduced hatchability and embryo mortality in turkeys. It has been shown experimentally to induce mortality in turkey and chicken embryos and mild to moderate airsacculitis and leg abnormalities in chickens and turkeys.

HISTORY. The Iowa 695 strain of avian mycoplasma was isolated and characterized by Yoder and Hofstad (43) and was subsequently designated avian serotype I (44). Avian mycoplasma serotypes I, J, K, N, Q, and R were classified into separate groups by Dierks et al. (17), and they were later characterized as a single, related group (2, 4, 20). The organism was later named *Mycoplasma iowae* (23).

INCIDENCE AND DISTRIBUTION. In addition to North America, *M. iowae* has been reported in western Europe (22), eastern Europe (5), and India (30). It is presumed to be worldwide in distribution.

ETIOLOGY

Classification. *M. iowae* identification is based on colony and cell morphology typical of mycoplasmas, special requirements for growth, and serologic reactions. Immunofluorescence of mycoplasma colonies (3) is the most rapid and reliable method for identification of field isolates.

Morphology and Staining. As with other mycoplasmas, *M. iowae* stains gram-negative, and with Giemsa staining or dark-field examination the organisms appear coccobacillary in form and show some pleomorphism. By electron microscopy, pleomorphism is evident and cells are bounded by a triple-layered cell membrane and lack a cell wall (23).

Growth Requirements. Like other mycoplasmas, *M. iowae* has complex growth requirements, one of which is cholesterol. Incubation is at 37 C, and growth occurs either aerobically or with added CO_2 (23). Recovery of *M. iowae* from tissues appears to be more successful by direct plating on agar than by inoculation of broth (1). Although several formulations of mycoplasma medium have been used successfully, the formulation described by Bradbury (8) works well.

Colony Morphology. Colonies are characteristic of mycoplasmas and show typical fried egg morphology on solid media and are 0.1–0.3 mm in diameter (43).

Biochemical Properties. *M. iowae* ferments glucose aerobically and anaerobically, utilizes arginine, does not utilize urea, is phosphatase negative, does not produce film and spots, and does not reduce tetrazolium chloride (23). It has the ability to grow in the presence of 0.5–1.0% bile salts (35).

Resistance to Chemical and Physical Agents. Resistance to *M. iowae* to disinfectants has not been determined, but it is probably similar to other mycoplasmas, which are inactivated by proper cleaning and disinfection.

Antigenic Structure. The antigenic structure of *M. iowae* has not been well studied. Agglutination (43) and enzyme-linked immunosorbent assay (ELISA) (24) have been studied, but the antibody response is not strong (14, 15); nonspecific reactions have been a problem with ELISA (24). There appears to be significant antigenic diversity among strains of *M. iowae* (9).

Pathogenicity. There is variability in the pathogenicity and virulence of *M. iowae* strains (32, 43). Experimental infection with *M. iowae* causes mortality in chicken and turkey embryos (13, 29, 32, 43). It induces mild to moderate airsacculitis in turkeys (17, 32, 43) as well as leg lesions in both chickens and turkeys (11, 12, 15, 43). However, there are no clinical reports describing airsacculitis or leg problems in chickens or turkeys, or embryo mortality in chickens, under field circumstances. Under field conditions it is felt to be responsible for embryo mortality and reduced hatchability in turkeys (9).

PATHOGENESIS AND EPIZOOTIOLOGY

Natural and Experimental Hosts. The natural host for *M. iowae* is the turkey, but isolation from chickens is not uncommon (5, 43). *M. iowae* has also been isolated from yellow-naped Amazon parrots (7).

Transmission, Carriers, Vectors. Only avian species are known to be infected with *M. iowae*. Egg transmission occurs in turkeys (29, 43). Infection may be spread venereally, and under modern methods of insemination infected semen may play a role in dissemination (34).

Signs. No clinical signs are observed. Eggs from infected turkey breeders may have reduced hatchability (usually 2–5%) because of embryos that die during the later stages of incubation. In many affected flocks hatchability returns to normal in 1–2 mo (25).

Gross Lesions. Lesions in affected embryos consist primarily of stunting and congestion with various degrees of hepatitis, edema, and splenomegaly (29, 43). Airsacculitis in inoculated chickens and turkeys is ordinarily mild to moderate and similar to lesions caused by other mycoplasmas (17, 32, 43). Inoculation of day-old poults results in stunting, poor feathering, tenosynovitis, and leg abnormalities including chondrodystrophy, rotated tibia, toe deviations, and sometimes erosion of the articular cartilage of the hock joint and rupture of the digital flexor tendon (15, 43). Similar leg lesions may be observed in experimental chicks, including rupture of the digital flexor tendon, but lesions ordinarily are less severe than in turkeys (14). Inoculation of turkey poults with *M. iowae* may result in bursal atrophy (10). Lesions have not been reported under field conditions, perhaps because infected embryos do not hatch.

Histopathology. After inoculation of day-old poults, lesions of the spleen consist of reticular cells with macrophages, plasma cells, and heterophils in the parenchyma. The bursa of Fabricius has localized congestion with infiltration of plasma cells, heterophils, and reticular cells. Macrophages, lymphocytes, heterophils, and plasma cells are seen in the lamina propria of the duodenum, ileum, and cecal tonsils. There is little obvious change observed in cartilage and tendon except for edema in the tendon sheaths (15). After air sac inoculation of turkey poults, lesions consist of thickened air sacs that contain large numbers of inflammatory cells, primarily lymphocytes. In some areas lymphoid follicles are observed. Exudate on the mucosal surface contains fibrin and inflammatory cells (32).

Immunity. Very little information is available on immunity to *M. iowae,* although antibody responses have been observed (24, 43). Older birds are more resistant than newly hatched poults or chicks. The disappearance of embryo mortality in progeny of infected turkey breeders after 1–2 mo suggests that immunity develops.

DIAGNOSIS

Isolation and Identification. *M. iowae* is present in high numbers in dead embryos (13, 29). After inoculation of turkey poults, *M. iowae* can be isolated from a variety of tissues, especially from the gastrointestinal tract or from cloacal swabs, but isolations become less frequent with age; organisms could not be recovered after 12 wk (15, 36). Isolation of *M. iowae* from oviduct, semen, and phallus of adult chickens and turkeys has been reported (30, 34,43). Cotton swabs from the appropriate tissue are streaked on agar plates and incubated 4–5 days or longer at 37 C. Typical mycoplasma colonies can be readily identified by immunofluorescence (3).

Serology. Although agglutination and ELISA tests have been used for experimental infections (24, 43), there is no reliable serological test available for widespread clinical use.

Differential Diagnosis. *M. iowae* infection should be considered in cases of low hatchability in turkeys, especially when there is evidence of late embryo mortality. Although it is not recognized as a significant cause of clinical tenosynovitis, *M. iowae* should be considered as a possibility in cases where there is no apparent explanation for leg problems, including tenosynovitis, especially in young turkeys.

TREATMENT. There is no recognized treatment for *M. iowae* infection. It is presumed that *M. iowae* has antibiotic susceptibility patterns similar to other mycoplasmas. Dipping hatching eggs in solutions containing a new quinolone carboxylic acid derivative (enrofloxacin) has been shown to significantly reduce losses in hatchability under field conditions (25), and, although not proven, other antibiotics may also be useful in egg-dipping programs.

PREVENTION AND CONTROL. The best method of control is to maintain flocks free of *M. iowae;* however, because of unreliability of serological tests and difficulties involved in isolating *M. iowae* from older birds, this may be difficult.

MYCOPLASMA GALLINARUM INFECTION

M. gallinarum has not been considered to be one of the pathogenic avian mycoplasma species. However, there is one report of consistent isolation from air sacs and tracheas from a series of broiler flocks that were having higher than normal condemnations due to airsacculitis. One of those isolates had the ability to induce airsacculitis when given in conjunction with Newcastle disease/infectious bronchitis vaccine (26).

It was originally classified as avian serotype B (17, 44) and was named *Mycoplasma gallinarum* (18). It appears to grow well on all commonly used avian mycoplasma media, and has characteristics common to all mycoplasmas, including cell and colony morphology, absence of a cell wall, and a requirement for cholesterol. It does not ferment glucose but reduces tetrazolium, is positive for arginine decarboxylase, and exhibits the film and spots phenomena (4).

M. gallinarum is isolated primarily from chickens, but it may also been found in turkeys (6, 22). It has been isolated from jungle fowl (33), ducks (19), and pigeons (31) and is considered to be worldwide in distribution. *M. gallinarum* is commonly isolated as a contaminant during attempts to isolate *M. gallisepticum* or *M. synoviae,* especially from adult chickens. Isolation of *M. gallinarum* from chicken embryos (6) suggests the possibility of egg transmission. It is readily identified by immunofluorescence of colonies on agar (3). No serological test is available.

AVIAN UREAPLASMAS

Ureaplasmas differ from mycoplasmas primarily in their ability to hydrolyze urea (28). There are several reports of isolation of avian ureaplasmas (21, 27). These organisms subsequently received the name *Ureaplasma gallorale* (28). There are no reports of avian ureaplasma isolation in North America.

Very little is known about the pathogenicity. Artificial challenge of chickens produced no clinical signs or macroscopic lesions (27). Turkeys and chickens challenged with a turkey ureaplasma isolated in Hungary developed fibrinous airsacculitis and serological responses (37). Ureaplasmas were also isolated in Eastern Europe from turkeys that were experiencing problems with reduced fertility (38).

MYCOPLASMA INFECTIONS OF GEESE

Three serologically and biochemically distinct mycoplasma species were isolated from geese in Europe (40). One of these was further characterized and named *Mycoplasma anseris* (16), another was subsequently identified as *Mycoplasma cloacale* (41), and the third was designated strain 1220. Clinically, they have been associated with reductions in egg production, egg transmission, infertility, inflammation of the cloaca and phallus, and lack of weight gain in hatched goslings (39, 41, 42), but proof of etiology is unclear because mixed mycoplasma species were isolated. Strain 1220, on experimental inoculation of goose embryos and day-old goslings, resulted in embryo mortality and reduced growth of young goslings (42). More work needs to be done to clarify the role of these mycoplasmas in the field syndromes described.

REFERENCES

1. Amin, M.M., and F.T.W. Jordan. 1978. A comparative study of some cultural methods in the isolation of avian mycoplasma from field material. Avian Pathol 7:455-470.

2. Aycardi, E.R., D.P. Anderson, and R.P. Hanson. 1971. Classification of avian mycoplasmas by gel diffusion and growth inhibition tests. Avian Dis 15:434-447.

3. Baas, E.J., and D.E. Jasper. 1972. Agar block technique for identification of mycoplasmas by use of fluorescent antibody. Appl Microbiol 23:1097-1100.

4. Barber, T.L., and J. Fabricant. 1971. A suggested reclassification of avian mycoplasma serotypes. Avian Dis 15:125-138.

5. Bencina, D., I. Mrzel, T. Tadina, and D. Dorrer. 1987. Mycoplasma spp. in chicken flocks with different management systems. Avian Pathol 16:599-608.

6. Bencina, D., D. Dorrer, and T. Tadina. 1987. Mycoplasma species isolated from six avian species. Avian Pathol 16:653-664.

7. Bozeman, L.H., S.H. Kleven, and R.B. Davis. 1984. Mycoplasma challenge studies in budgerigars (Melopsittacus undulatus) and chickens. Avian Dis 28:426-434.

8. Bradbury, J.M. 1977. Rapid biochemical tests for characterization of the Mycoplasmatales. J Clin Microbiol 5:531-534.

9. Bradbury, J.M. 1983. Mycoplasma iowae – an avian Mycoplasma with unusual properties. Yale J Biol Med 56:912.

10. Bradbury, J.M. 1984. Effect of Mycoplasma iowae infection on the immune system of the young turkey. Isr J Med Sci 20:985-988.

11. Bradbury, J.M., and A. Ideris. 1982. Abnormalities in turkey poults following infection with Mycoplasma iowae. Vet Rec 110:559-560.

12. Bradbury, J.M., and J. McCarthy. 1981. Rupture of the digital flexor tendons of chickens after infection with Mycoplasma iowae. Vet Rec 109:428-429.

13. Bradbury, J.M., and J.D. McCarthy. 1983. Pathogenicity of Mycoplasma iowae for chick embryos. Avian Pathol 12:483-496.

14. Bradbury, J.M., and J.D. McCarthy. 1984. Mycoplasma iowae infection in chicks. Avian Pathol 13:529-543.

15. Bradbury, J.M., A. Ideris, and T.T. Oo. 1988. Mycoplasma iowae infection in young turkeys. Avian Pathol 17:149-171.

16. Bradbury, J.M., F.T.W. Jordan, T. Shimizu, L. Stipkovits, and Z. Varga. 1988. Mycoplasma anseris sp. nov. found in geese. Int J Syst Bacteriol 38:74-76.

17. Dierks, R.E., J.A. Newman, and B.S. Pomeroy. 1967. Characterization of avian mycoplasma. Ann NY Acad Sci 143:170-189.

18. Edward, D.G., and E.A. Freundt. 1956. The classification and nomenclature of organisms of the pleuropneumonia group. J Gen Microbiol 14:197-207.

19. El-Ebeedy, A.A., I. Sokkar, A. Soliman, A. Rashwan, and A. Ammar. 1987. Mycoplasma infection of ducks. I. Incidence of mycoplasmas, acholeplasmas and associated E. coli and fungi at Upper Egypt. Isr J Med Sci 23:529.

20. Frey, M.L., S.T. Hawk, and P.A. Hale. 1972. A division by micro-complement fixation tests of previously reported avian Mycoplasma serotypes into identification groups. Avian Dis 16:780-792.

21. Harasawa, R., K. Koshimizu, I.-J. Pan, and M.F. Barile. 1985. Genomic and phenotypic analyses of avian ureaplasma strains. Jpn J Vet Sci 47:901-909.

22. Jordan, F.T.W., and M.M. Amin. 1980. A survey of mycoplasma infections in domestic poultry. Res Vet Sci 28:96-100.

23. Jordan, F.T.W., H. Erno, G.S. Cottew, K.H. Hinz, and L. Stipkovits. 1982. Characterization and taxonomic description of five mycoplasma serovars (serotypes) of avian origin and their elevation to species rank and further evaluation of the taxonomic status of Mycoplasma synoviae. Int J Syst Bacteriol 32:108-115.

24. Jordan, F.T.W., C. Yavari, and D.L. Knight. 1987. Some observations on the indirect ELISA for antibodies to Mycoplasma iowae serotype I in sera from turkeys considered to be free from Mycoplasma infections. Avian Pathol 16:307-318.

25. Kleven, S.H. 1988. Unpublished data.

26. Kleven, S.H., C.S. Eidson, and O.J. Fletcher. 1978. Airsacculitis induced in broilers with a combination of Mycoplasma gallinarum and respiratory viruses. Avian Dis 22:707-716.

27. Koshimizu, K., H. Kotani, T. Magaribuchi, T. Yagihashi, K. Shibata, and M. Ogata. 1982. Isolation of ureaplasmas from poultry and experimental infection in

chickens. Vet Rec 110:426–429.
28. Koshimizu, K., R. Harasawa, I.-J. Pan, H. Kotani, M. Ogata, E.B. Stephens, and M.F. Barile. 1987. Ureaplasma gallorale sp. nov. from the oropharynx of chickens. Int J Syst Bacteriol 37:333–338.
29. McClenaghan, M., J.M. Bradbury, and J.N. Howse. 1981. Embryo mortality associated with avian Mycoplasma serotype I. Vet Rec 108:459–460.
30. Rathore, B.S., G.C. Mohanty, and B.S. Rajya. 1979. Isolation of mycoplasma from oviducts of chickens and their pathogenicity. Ind J Microbiol 19:192–197.
31. Reece, R.L., L. Ireland, and P.C. Scott. 1986. Mycoplasmosis in racing pigeons. Aust Vet J 63:166–167.
32. Rhoades, K.R. 1981. Turkey airsacculitis: Effect of mixed mycoplasmal infections. Avian Dis 25:131–135.
33. Shah-Majid, M. 1987. A case-control study of Mycoplasma gallinarum in the male and female reproductive tract of indigenous fowl. Isr J Med Sci 23:530.
34. Shah-Majid, M., and S. Rosendal. 1986. Mycoplasma iowae from turkey phallus and semen. Vet Rec 118:435.
35. Shah-Majid, M., and S. Rosendal. 1987. Evaluation of growth of avian mycoplasmas on bile salt agar and in bile broth. Res Vet Sci 43:188–190.
36. Shah-Majid, M., and S. Rosendal. 1987. Oral challenge of turkey poults with Mycoplasma iowae. Avian Dis 31:365–369.
37. Stipkovits, L., A. Rashwan, and M.Z. Sabry. 1978. Studies on pathogenicity of turkey ureaplasma. Avian Pathol 7:577–582.
38. Stipkovits, L., P.A. Brown, R. Glavits, and R.J. Julian. 1983. The possible role of ureaplasma in a continuous infertility problem in turkeys. Avian Dis 27:513–523.
39. Stipkovits, L., J.M. Bove, M. Rousselot, P. Larrue, M. Labat, and A. Vuillaume. 1984. Studies on mycoplasma infection of laying geese. Avian Pathol 14:57–68.
40. Stipkovits, L., Z. Varga, M. Dobos-Kovacs, and M. Santha. 1984. Biochemical and serological examination of some Mycoplasma strains of goose origin. Acta Vet Hung 32:117–125.
41. Stipkovits, L., Z. Varga, G. Czifra, and M. Dobos-Kovacs. 1986. Occurrence of Mycoplasmas in geese affected with inflammation of the cloaca and phallus. Avian Pathol 15:289–299.
42. Stipkovits, L., Z. Varga, R. Glavits, F. Ratz, and E. Molnar. 1987. Pathological and immunological studies on goose embryos and one-day-old goslings experimentally infected with a Mycoplasma strain of goose origin. Avian Pathol 16:453–468.
43. Yoder, H.W., Jr., and M.S. Hofstad. 1962. A previously unreported serotype of avian mycoplasma. Avian Dis 6:147–160.
44. Yoder, H.W., Jr., and M.S. Hofstad. 1964. Characterization of avian mycoplasma. Avian Dis 8:481–512.

9 CAMPYLOBACTERIOSIS

Simon M. Shane

INTRODUCTION. Campylobacteriosis has emerged as a significant zoonotic condition affecting a wide range of food and companion animals, in addition to exotic and free-living avian and mammalian species (11). The occurrence of a disease termed "avian vibrionic hepatitis" was extensively documented during the decade commencing in 1965 (40). This condition was retrospectively attributed to *Campylobacter jejuni* infection (89), although contemporary epidemiological evidence fails to support any association between *C. jejuni* and the classic syndrome characterized by hepatopathy (115).

Since various species of domestic poultry serve as reservoir hosts of *C. jejuni* (60, 83), infection is significant primarily in relation to food-borne enterocolitis (34) in consumers of broilers (46), turkeys (2), and possibly eggs (105).

AVIAN VIBRIONIC HEPATITIS

This syndrome was originally described in New Jersey as a chronic hepatodegeneration characterized by low morbidity and variable mortality in mature egg-production flocks by Tudor (124). Subsequent studies in Texas by Delaplane et al. (23) yielded an agent from field cases that could be propagated in 7-day chicken embryos inoculated via the yolk sac. An apparently similar syndrome, "avian infectious hepatitis" (AIH), was first reported by Winterfield and Sevoian (133) from five flocks in Massachusetts with 35% depression in egg production, morbidity of 10%, and cumulative flock mortality of 15%. Gross lesions comprised focal to diffuse hepatic necrosis and subcapsular hemorrhage. Histological examination revealed lymphocytic and granulocytic foci and bile duct proliferation. It was possible to reproduce hepatopathy in young chicks and mature hens using yolk fluid from embryonated eggs inoculated with liver homogenate from field cases (102). Subsequent work showed the agent to be between 0.3μ and 0.5μ long and sensitive to oxytetracycline and furazolidone (134). Studies on the isolation of the AIH agent confirmed the suitability of the embryonic yolk sac for propagation (101). Investigations performed by Hofstad et al. (49) on isolates derived from field cases of AIH in Iowa yielded a curved, vibriolike microorganism that was embryolethal. This agent was also sensitive to tetracyclines and furazolidone.

During 1955–58 similar vibriolike organisms (VLOs) were isolated by Peckham (88) from 29 field cases of hepatitis syndrome, which was diagnosed on the basis of flock history, clinical signs, and gross lesions. These VLOs were isolated either by inoculating embryonated eggs with a suspension of liver from affected birds, or by culturing bile on blood agar medium. It is considered significant that liver necrosis could be induced in susceptible chicks after four passages of the agent on blood agar incubated at 37 C under microaerobic conditions. Based on the characterization of the microorganism and its resemblance to isolates obtained from field cases by other workers, the syndrome was termed "avian vibrionic hepatitis" (AVH).

The isolation of a group of thermophilic VLOs from cases of human enterocolitis (61) stimulated comparisons between these organisms and avian isolates derived from cases of AIH/AVH (29). Both groups of microaerophilic curved rods produced catalase and were less tolerant to sodium chloride than VLOs of human origin.

A relationship between the VLOs and the hepatitis syndrome was indicated by the results of studies conducted in New York State (45). Vibriolike organisms were recovered from 47% of bile samples obtained from 30 field cases classified as presumptive AIH/AVH on the basis of history, clinical observations, and gross lesions. In contrast, VLOs were cultured from only 2% of 173 submissions not corresponding to the profile for AIH/AVH. Both brilliant green agar and blood agar were demonstrated to be suitable for culture of VLOs from bile, and yielded a 32% recovery rate compared to 35% using embryos.

Studies on field isolates derived from laying flocks in Ontario showed that VLOs isolated from either bile or cecal contents of specific birds showed identical biochemical and serological criteria. It was also noted that VLOs derived from various submissions showed differences in pathogenicity and ability to colonize the cecum (123).

In assessing the literature relating to the AIH/AVH complex, it is evident that a field syndrome in commercial laying hens occurred prior to and during the mid-1960s. The syndrome was characterized by low morbidity and mortality with degeneration of the liver as the principal diagnostic feature. The current enigma facing pathologists and epidemiologists is the complete disappearance of the condition as a clinical entity from the United States and western Europe.

Studies conducted during the past few years have failed to reproduce hepatopathy using strains of *C. jejuni* derived either from humans or avian species (97, 98). It is noted that only enteritis, characterized by diarrhea, can be induced by infecting newly hatched chicks (131), as well as mammalian food animals (27), exotics (70), and companion species (28).

There are two speculative explanations for the disappearance of the AIH/AVH complex. The original condition may have been caused by a pathogen other than the VLO that was isolated; however, the experimental reproduction of the condition with an agent cultured on artificial media tends to disprove this hypothesis (88). It is more probable that the VLO interacted synergistically as an opportunist with some other pathogen (132), analogous to the association between *C. jejuni* and parvovirus in dogs (31) or with immunosuppressive or debilitating agents in humans (72). The primary pathogen or cofactor may have subsequently been eliminated by comprehensive immunization programs introduced during the mid-1960s. There is no conclusive experimental evidence to indicate the VLOs isolated from cases of AIH/AVH complex were in fact campylobacters. Attempts in 1985 to propagate and characterize the agent recovered from frozen lyophilized yolk material stored since 1960 were unsuccessful (19).

CAMPYLOBACTERIOSIS

ETIOLOGY. Campylobacteriosis is attributed to infection by thermophilic members of the genus *Campylobacter* (100). The three species of clinical significance, *C. jejuni, C. coli,* and *C. laridis,* are microaerophilic, gram-negative, spiral, uniflagellate organisms that demonstrate characteristic darting motility when examined under dark-field illumination (109).

Classification. The nomenclature of the genus *Campylobacter* has been subject to frequent changes in response to emerging biochemical and taxonomic criteria. Various classification schemes for the genus have been described (37, 57), which clearly designate *C. jejuni,* the predominant organism isolated from avian hosts, as a separate and valid species (112), not a subspecies of *C. fetus* as in early literature. The phylogeny of the campylobacters has been evaluated on the basis of 16S ribosomal ribonucleic acid sequencing, with *C. jejuni, C. coli,* and *C. laridis* included in homology group I (122). *C. jejuni* is the most frequently occurring member of the thermophilic triad, but *C. coli* may occasionally be isolated from the intestinal tract of poultry and derived meat products (79, 96). *C. laridis,* previously referred to as NARTC (nalidixic acid–resistant thermophilic campylobacters) (6), is the remaining species in the related thermophilic group and is isolated mainly from free-living marine birds such as gulls (*Larus* spp.) (55).

Morphology and Staining. Campylobacters are spirally curved rods that appear S-shaped or in "gull-wing" forms, and range in size from 0.2μ to 0.8μ in diameter and 0.5μ to 6.0μ in length. All species are motile and possess a single polar flagellum, although bipolar cells are occasionally observed (111). Campylobacters are gram-negative, but require a fuchsin-based counterstain because of their relative inability to take up saffranin (99).

Growth Requirements. The campylobacters of clinical significance show optimal growth on artificial media at 43 C (109), although minimal growth occurs at 37 C.

Campylobacters are microaerophilic, and satisfactory propagation requires an atmosphere comprising 5% oxygen, 10% carbon dioxide, and 85% nitrogen (93). Purchase of a commercial gas mixture is recommended for laboratories conducting routine isolation of campylobacters. An analysis of alternative methods of achieving a microaerobic environment, including commercial gas packs, torbal and candle jars, or application of Fortner's principle, has demonstrated various disadvantages relating to decreased growth, extended incubation periods, or high cost (41).

Appropriate methods of transport and storage of campylobacters are necessary because these organisms are sensitive to desiccation. An enriched semisolid brucella medium incorporating 10% ovine blood can be used to maintain viability of cultures for transport at 25 C for up to 3 wk (129). Six alternative transport media were compared in a structured study of *C. jejuni* survival. Cary-Blair medium with decreased agar content was superior to Stuart's medium for storage periods exceeding 7 days at 25 C (71). Both Stuart's fluid medium and Cary-Blair semisolid transport medium are commercially available in plastic tubes with accompanying rayon-tipped swabs to facilitate sampling of biological material for subsequent submission to a diagnostic laboratory.

In the late 1970s selective media containing antimicrobial compounds were introduced, simplifying the isolation and propagation of campylobacters (86). Commercial media contain brucella agar; blood agar base; ovine, bovine, or equine blood; and various antibiotic additives, including bacitracin, novobiocin, trimethoprim, actidone, cycloheximide, cephalothin, and colistin. Differences in source of blood and antibiotic content of media have been evaluated under field and laboratory conditions. Medium BU-40 was shown to be superior to both Skirrow's and Butzler's media in terms of efficiency of isolation of *C. jejuni* (77). Preston medium, a selective agar incorporating lysed horse blood and antibiotics, yielded higher isolation rates of *C. jejuni* than Skirrow's, Butzler's, Blaser's, or Campy-BAP media. Recovery can be enhanced by preincubation in Preston enrichment broth (14). A semisolid medium has been developed for transport and enrichment of fecal specimens, which enhances the rate of recovery of *C. jejuni* from patients receiving antibiotic therapy and from their contacts (17). A blood-free selective medium containing charcoal has been shown to be as effective in isolating *C. jejuni* as conventional Skirrow's medium (59). Campy-Choc Agar, a charcoal- and blood-free medium, compared favorably with three conventional media that yielded a 0.3% *C. jejuni* isolation rate in a survey of 2890 human fecal specimens (127).

The current status of isolating enteric pathogens, including campylobacters, has been extensively reviewed with specific reference to selection and preparation of samples, preenrichment, and selective plating. Despite the introduction of immunoassays and gene probes, conventional media provide acceptable selectivity and inhibition for diagnostic and survey purposes (35).

Colonial Morphology. The incubation period for detecting colonial growth generally exceeds 24 hr. With a low concentration of organisms in the inoculum, or when an inhibitory medium is used, incubation for up to 72 hr may be required to observe colony formation (77). On primary isolation, colonies may be either flat, translucent, and gray with a tendency to coalesce, or be raised, opaque, and brown-gray with discrete margins (111). The presence of swarming colonies is attributed to higher moisture content of freshly prepared media in contrast to the discrete colonies formed on media that has aged for a few days prior to inoculation (15). Colonies are nonhemolytic on blood agar (112).

Biochemical Properties. As campylobacters are unable to ferment carbohydrates, energy is derived from the degradation of amino acids. The three thermophilic species of clinical significance all reduce selenite, are oxidase and catalase positive, and are indole negative (109). Differentiation between *C. jejuni, C. coli,* and *C. laridis* is based on nalidixic acid sensitivity and hippurate hydrolysis (Table 9.1).

Table 9.1. Differentiation among catalase-positive *Campylobacter* species according to biochemical characteristics

Species	Growth at 25 C	Growth at 42 C	Nalidixic Acid Sensitivity[a]	Hippurate Hydrolysis
C. fetus	+	–	R	–
C. coli	+	+	S	–
C. jejuni	–	+	S	+
C. laridis	–	+	R	–

Source: (110).
[a]R = resistant; S = sensitive.

An evaluation of various biochemical characteristics of 264 cultures permitted differentiation between eight species or subspecies of *Campylobacter* (48). The additional properties of DNA hydrolysis and rapid production of hydrogen sulfide were incorporated into an extended biotyping scheme for the three species (Table 9.2) (66).

Other sources have defined up to eight biotypes of *C. jejuni* based on hydrolysis of DNA and hippurate and growth on charcoal-yeast extract agar (48). Details concerning biochemical reactions of the thermophilic campylobacters have been comprehensively reviewed with specific reference to differential characteristics to distinguish between field isolates (109, 37, 112).

Table 9.2. Biotyping scheme for *C. jejuni, C. coli,* and *C. laridis*

Test	*C. jejuni*				*C. coli*		*C. laridis*	
	I[a]	II	III	IV	I	II	I	II
Hippurate hydrolysis	+	+	+	+	–	–	–	–
Rapid H_2S test	–	–	+	+	–	–	+	+
DNA hydrolysis	–	+	–	+	–	+	–	+

Source: (66).
[a]Biotype.

Resistance to Physical and Chemical Agents and Antibiotics

PHYSICAL AGENTS. Campylobacters are extremely sensitive to desiccation. A suspension of *C. jejuni* impregnated onto a filter paper strip will not survive beyond 2 hr at 20 C (71). Infectivity is retained for up to 4 wk in water at 4 C (8), but *C. jejuni* can remain viable in milk for 3 wk at 4 C and for 24 hr at 25 C (94).

A comprehensive study on the survival of *C. jejuni* in biological systems showed the organism could multiply in bile stored for 2 mo at 37 C, but was rapidly destroyed in human urine at the same temperature. At 4 C, *C. jejuni* retained viability for 3 wk in feces and 5 wk in urine (9). *C. jejuni* persisted for a 10-day period on chicken portions stored at either −9 C or −12 C, and contamination could be detected after 182 days storage at −20 C (135).

Lyophilized cultures of *C. jejuni* in brucella broth containing 0.16% agar and blood retain viability for many years. When cryoprotective agents such as dimethyl sulfoxide or glycerol are added to heavy suspensions of the organism in brucella broth, survival exceeds 3 yr at −80 C (112).

Irradiation pasteurization at a dose of 1.0 kGy from a cobalt-60 source effectively eliminated *C. jejuni* surface contamination at a level of 10^3 colony-forming units (CFU)/cm^2 (136).

CHEMICAL RESISTANCE. The in vitro sensitivity of *C. jejuni* to various disinfectants was assessed using three strains of the organism isolated from diarrheic human patients. A 1:200,000 solution of 5% sodium hypochlorite and a 2.5% solution of 10% formaldehyde both destroyed *C. jejuni* within 15 min. Contact with 0.15% organic phenol, a 1:50, 000 quaternary-ammonium compound, or 0.125% glutaraldehyde killed a 10^7 CFU suspension of *C. jejuni* within 1 min (130). Resistance to chemical agents is increased by the protective action of biological material. In a comparative study of the efficacy of chemical disinfectants used in the food industry, it was shown that 3% succinic acid, 0.5% glutaraldehyde, and 25 ppm poly-(hexamethylenebiguanide hydrochloride) were all able to significantly reduce the level of *C. jejuni* contamination on the surface of chicken drumsticks. Chlorine levels below 120 ppm were ineffective under conditions simulating immersion in poultry processing plant tanks (136).

ANTIBIOTIC SENSITIVITY. The antibiotic sensitivity of the three thermophilic campylobacters has been extensively documented (58, 112). A study conducted in Sweden showed close similarity in antibiotic sensitivity between approximately 75 isolates derived from diarrheic human patients and from processed broilers. The majority of isolates were sensitive to erythromycin and doxycycline, although a high proportion of strains were resistant to the tetracyclines, and an acceptable response to gentamicin, chloramphenicol, and carbenicillin was obtained (119). Similar results were achieved in an investigation involving 403 human fecal isolates from patients admitted to a hospital in Brussels, and 276 food animal isolates, including 107 derived from chickens. Furazolidone was shown to be the most effective compound, with most human and animal isolates also sensitive to erythromycin and gentamicin. Approximately 26% of the chicken strains were resistant to tetracycline (126). In evaluating the efficacy of 16 antimicrobial compounds against 103 clinical isolates of *C. jejuni,* kanamycin and gentamicin were shown to be completely effective, in contrast to tetracycline, penicillin G, and erythromycin. Approximately 38%, 36%, and 13% of the isolates were resistant to these three compounds, respectively (74). The biochemical mechanisms and genetic aspects of antibiotic resistance in campylobacters have been comprehensively reviewed in relation to quinolones, tetracyclines, aminoglycosides, and macrolides (121).

Serotyping.

A significant advance in serotyping *C. jejuni* was achieved with the introduction of the Penner scheme based on soluble, heat-stable O antigens derived from surface lipopolysaccharides (90). Antisera produced in rabbits can be applied to a passive hemagglutination technique to identify 60 serotypes of *C. jejuni.* Subsequent studies showed that *C. jejuni* and *C. coli* have individual antigens, with minimal commonality between species (91). The alternative Lior serotyping scheme is based on heat-labile H antigens (67). This system is read using slide agglutination and requires multiple absorption of heterogenous antisera. In a comparison between the two schemes, the Penner technique was found to be marginally more specific than the Lior system, and although requiring more equipment, was faster under practical conditions in a diagnostic laboratory (87).

Bacterial restriction endonuclease DNA analysis (BRENDA), a relatively new technique, has been used to differentiate campylobacters. An epidemiologic study has demonstrated that 50% of a sample of 316 isolates of *C. jejuni,* representing 11 of 60 BRENDA types, were common to both humans and poultry (54).

PATHOGENESIS AND EPIZOOTIOLOGY

Natural Hosts.

Poultry serve as primary reservoir hosts of thermophilic campylobacters (38). Up to 90% of broilers may be infected (7), while 100% of turkeys (65, 69, 71), and 88% of domestic ducks (92) may harbor the organisms.

Various species of *Campylobacter* have been isolated from free-ranging pigeons in the USA (70) and Japan (62). Infection has been recorded among game birds, including partridges, pheasants (128), and quail (75). Campylobacters have been isolated from marine birds such as puffins (56) and gulls (55), from waders (36), and from migratory Anseriformes (84). Approximately 8% of samples taken from 8 species (Columbiformes and Passeriformes) in a Japanese investigation yielded *C. jejuni*. It was noted that numerically higher recovery rates were obtained from scavengers and omnivores than from granivores (51). The prevalence of *C. jejuni* in avian species is a function of the intensity of surveillance, since diligent collection and culturing will generally reveal intestinal infection in many orders of birds within a specific area.

Experimental Hosts. The wide range of laboratory animal species susceptible to *C. jejuni* includes rabbits, mice, rats, hamsters, and primates (30). Animal models for campylobacter enterocolitis in humans include mice (12), hamsters (32), and ferrets (33).

Campylobacters can be propagated in vitro in tissue culture systems, including Chinese hamster ovary cells (42), HeLa cells (25), and human epithelial cell lines (16). Fertile chicken eggs serve as a convenient system for isolation and propagation of campylobacters. Both *C. jejuni* and *C. coli* infection of embryos can be achieved by either the chorioallantoic route or by direct intravenous injection on the 11th day of incubation (26). The embryo system can be used as a model to differentiate between the relative virulence of various strains of *C. jejuni* and *C. coli* derived from cases of human and animal enterocolitis.

Transmission. Despite the fact that *C. jejuni* is prevalent as an intestinal commensal in floor-housed turkeys, broiler breeders, and layer-type breeder chickens, there is no evidence to show that campylobacters can be transmitted vertically by either transovarian infection or by penetration of the eggshell after oviposition. An extensive survey failed to demonstrate *C. jejuni* in fertile turkey eggs and poults derived from a flock known to carry the organism (1). Another study showed that *C. jejuni* did not penetrate the shells of eggs produced by cage-housed hens, despite recovery of the organism from the intestinal tract and feces (24). Infrequent isolation of *C. jejuni* from the inner and outer membranes of refrigerated eggs is attributable to shell damage. Failure to demonstrate *C. jejuni* within or on the surface of table eggs was confirmed in field studies conducted on 3 farms in Louisiana (105) and on 23 units in New York (5). It is possible to induce egg penetration by immersion in a suspension of *C. jejuni* (81), or by using either temperature or pressure differential techniques (20). It is concluded that under practical commercial conditions desiccation will destroy organisms on the surface of clean eggs within a short period following oviposition. Artificial contamination of eggs with a fecal suspension of *C. jejuni* showed that viability did not exceed 16 hr, and that 50% of the artificially contaminated eggshells were free of viable campylobacters within 10 hr (105). Rejection of grossly soiled eggs, physical removal of small quantities of fecal material adherent to the shell surface, and fumigation or chemical disinfection within 2 hr of collection will all reduce the possibility of egg-borne transmission of campylobacters (106).

Experiments have conclusively demonstrated that contamination of feed and water by chronic intestinal carriers transmits *C. jejuni* to susceptible contacts (76). This study also showed that intestinal infection persisted for at least 63 days in broilers housed on wire-mesh floors, which prevented coprophagy.

Houseflies (*Musca domestica*), which can acquire *C. jejuni* from contaminated litter, are capable of transmitting infection to susceptible chicks under controlled experimental conditions (104). A field investigation that revealed 50% of houseflies in the vicinity of a poultry farm were infected with *C. jejuni* (95) and the recovery of the organism from cockroaches (125) imply that insects may play a role in transmission of campylobacteriosis. The presence of *C. jejuni* in the feces of domestic sparrows captured in a turkey house suggests the role of free-living birds in introducing infection into commercial poultry flocks (1, 113).

Surveys on broilers (80) and turkey flocks (1) showed that chicks and poults remain uninfected for up to 3 wk when placed into thoroughly disinfected houses containing new litter. Both *C. jejuni* and *C. coli* can be introduced into houses by nonconfined companion animals, vermin, and footwear contaminated with feces and litter (3). Campylobacters are spread rapidly within flocks by horizontal, fecal-oral infection. Consumption of fecally contaminated feed and litter, and nonchlorinated water dispensed from trough-type drinkers contribute to dissemination of the organism (38). Poultry strains of *C. jejuni* have a marked capacity to spread horizontally among chicks in hatchers during the last 24 hr of incubation, and with subsequent post-hatch processing. Artificial infection of one chick in a hatcher resulted in recovery of *C. jejuni* from the intestines of 70% of the contact chicks after 24 hr (21).

Incubation Period. *C. jejuni* colonized the intestinal tracts of 62% of a batch of susceptible day-old broiler chicks within 24 hr of administration of either 10^2 CFU by the intracloacal route, or 10^4 CFU instilled into the crop. The proportion of chicks yielding *C. jejuni* on cloacal swabs increased to 88% and 97%, respectively, on the third and fourth days postinfection (107). In Japanese quail *C. jejuni* could be recovered from feces (4 CFU/g) 1 day after receiving an oral dose of 10^8 CFU (73).

Signs. The severity of clinically detectable changes, usually confined to depression and diarrhea, is dependent on infective dose, strain of *C. jejuni* or *C. coli,* and age of the host. Concurrent environmental stress factors or intercurrent disease and immunosuppression may exacerbate the pathogenicity of *C. jejuni.*

A pathogenic, invasive strain of *C. jejuni* isolated from diarrheic human patients in Mexico produced diarrhea in 88% of a batch of day-old chicks that received 10^8 organisms orally. Within 24–72 hr, affected chicks showed depression, fecal saturation of the vent plumage, and watery droppings, which persisted for 8 days. Mortality of 32% was recorded in infected chicks from which *C. jejuni* could be isolated from the heart blood and intestinal tract (97). Infection of holoxenic (conventionally reared) chicks with *C. jejuni* in a trial designed to investigate competitive exclusion resulted in transient diarrhea (114). Similar observations were made in broiler chicks that were inoculated with 10^3–10^6 CFU of *C. jejuni* derived from diarrheic patients in Bangladesh (98).

In contrast, experimental infections have not produced any clinical abnormalities in broiler chicks aged either 2–3 days or 3 wk, although intestinal colonization was achieved by inoculation via both the oral and cloacal routes (107). In a comparison of age susceptibility, diarrhea was induced in chicks within 12 hr of hatch compared to birds 3 days of age, which were unaffected by an oral dose of 10^9 CFU. Signs of *C. jejuni* infection included diarrhea, characterized by the presence of mucus and blood, commencing 6 hr after inoculation and extending for 10 days. Recurrence of diarrhea was noted in the subjects housed on raised wire-mesh floors, which inhibited coprophagy (131).

Gross Lesions. The principal change associated with *C. jejuni* infection in chicks is the distention of the intestinal tract extending from the distal duodenal loop to the bifurcation of the ceca. Accumulation of mucus and watery fluid occurs (98), and depending on the cytotoxic properties of the *Campylobacter* involved, hemorrhages may be present (131), consistent with observations in human campylobacteriosis (63).

The presence of red or yellow mottling of the liver parenchyma was noted in newly hatched chicks subjected to contact infection by toxigenic and invasive strains of *C. jejuni* during the last 24 hr of incubation (21). This observation may relate to an experiment in which focal hepatic necrosis was induced in 60% of a batch of experimentally infected chicks that received the immunosuppressive agent cyclophosphamide. Untreated control chicks infected with *C. jejuni* failed to show liver lesions (115). It is likely that an intact and functional immune system is required to prevent dissemination of the organism from the intestinal tract (13).

Histological Lesions. Histological changes attributed to *C. jejuni* infection include congestion and mononuclear cell infiltration of the lamina propria and destruction of mucosal cells in the entire intestinal tract. Edema of the mucosa was noted in the ileum and ceca, with accumulation of mucus, erythrocytes, mononuclear cells, and a few polymorphonuclear cells in the lumen. Within 48 hr of infection, hyperplasia and villous atrophy were evident in the distal jejunum. Electron microscopy revealed the presence of campylobacters within and between cells of the epithelium and lamina propria (131).

In mild cases characterized by distention of the jejunum, microscopic changes were confined to submucosal edema with gram-negative curved rods adherent to the brush border and within enterocytes (98).

DIAGNOSIS. Thermophilic campylobacters can be isolated from feces and cecal and jejunal contents. With systemic infection the organism can also be recovered from liver tissue, bile, and blood. Because of the sensitivity of campylobacters to desiccation, special precautions are required when submitting fecal or other biological material to a diagnostic laboratory. It is advisable to sample using a commercially available transport system such as a rayon-tipped swab, which is inserted into a tube containing Cary-Blair medium. Bile samples can be obtained by direct aspiration from the gall bladder using a sterile tuberculin syringe.

Isolation of thermophilic campylobacters requires incubation of cultures for 48–72 hr at 43 C in a microaerobic atmosphere. Selective media are required to suppress the growth of contaminants in fecal and other biological samples (86). Differentiation between *C. jejuni, C. coli,* and *C. laridis,* and their biotypes, can be achieved by applying the criteria of incubation temperature, nalidixic acid sensitivity, hippurate hydrolysis, and hydrogen sulfide production (66, 110). A serotyping scheme, such as the Penner system, can be used to identify specific organisms for epidemiologic investigations (91).

PUBLIC HEALTH SIGNIFICANCE. Human campylobacteriosis is a food-borne condition of emerging significance (10, 22,103). During 1984 the *Campylobacter* isolation rate in the USA attained 4.9/100,000 population, with *C. jejuni* representing 99% of the species cultured (120). This estimate grossly understates the actual prevalence of campylobacteriosis, which may be responsible for 2.1 million cases annually in the USA (78). Projections of cost associated with diagnosis and treatment of human campylobacteriosis, including lost productivity and deaths, range from $700 million to $1400 million per annum.

Early studies on the epidemiology of intestinal campylobacteriosis in human populations demonstrated that consumption of chicken meat was a significant risk factor (11, 82, 108). The high carriage rate of campylobacters in the intestinal tract of broilers (44) and turkeys (68) contributes to contamination during processing (39). This is reflected in high levels of *C. jejuni* on poultry meat (85). Recovery of campylobacters from chicken carcasses is approximately six times higher than from pork or beef, and ranges from 30 to 100% of specimens surveyed (116).

The association of campylobacters with poultry meat represents a significant potential for human food-borne infection under conditions of defective handling, inadequate refrigeration, and improper preparation (50). The correlation between specific *C. jejuni* and *C. coli* serotypes in poultry and in diarrheic humans has been documented, with Penner groups 2, 5, 7, 9, and 22 predominating (4). The staff of poultry processing plants are exposed to campylobacteriosis by handling contaminated material, and the condition may be regarded as an occupational disease (43, 53). An outbreak of *Campylobacter* enteritis in Sweden involved 71% of a group of 24 temporary workers who became ill within 2 wk of commencing employment in a poultry plant. In contrast, only 30% of the long-term employees were infected (18). The dynamics of *Campylobacter* contamination of poultry meat and its relationship to human intestinal infection have been extensively documented following completion of a comprehensive epidemiologic study conducted in King County, Washington (46, 47).

Based on field surveys showing a low prevalence of eggshell contamination with *C. jejuni,* and the sensitivity of the organism to desiccation and approved industrial egg-washing compounds, it is unlikely that campylobacteriosis is attributable to consumption of commercially produced table eggs (52).

PREVENTION AND CONTROL. It is impractical to apply preventive action to reduce campylobacter infection in broiler flocks reared on litter. Although extreme biosecurity measures may limit the introduction of campylobacters into breeding farms, current practices in the US broiler industry contribute to infection before depletion. Under commercial conditions, unrestricted movement of personnel, recycling of litter, and the use of earth-floor convection-ventilated housing subject to ingress by flies, vermin, and possibly wild birds, all contribute to colonization of the intestinal tract with *C. jejuni* and *C. coli* (103). Since coprophagy ensures rapid horizontal spread within a flock (76), the expedient of multitier mesh-floor growing would be required to reduce or obviate transmission. Thorough decontamination, including removal of litter and disinfection of equipment and buildings, followed by a rest period of at least 7 days, will effectively eliminate residual campylobacters in poultry housing (34).

Despite early studies showing the benefits of competitive exclusion of campylobacters by natural intestinal flora (115), recent trials have failed to show any significant benefit in reducing *Campylobacter* infection in vivo (107). This finding is attributed to the association of *C. jejuni* with the intraluminal mucin layer, and the failure of the organism to adhere to enterocytes (118).

Although it is unrealistic to attempt elimination of *Campylobacter* infection during the growing period, it is possible to ameliorate processing-plant contamination by disinfecting transport coops and by withholding feed for at least 8 hr prior to flock depletion. Postprocessing decontamination of carcasses and portions with chemical solutions will reduce the level of *C. jejuni.* A 0.5% acetic or lactic acid rinse effectively limits levels of viable organisms under controlled laboratory conditions (117). Subsequent studies have shown that 120 ppm chlorine, warm succinic acid, and 0.5% glutaraldehyde all reduced *C. jejuni* contamination of drumsticks (136). Gamma radiation of poultry meat at subradicidation (pasteurization) levels of 1–5 kGy using a cobalt-60 source will eliminate campylobacters without inducing any undesirable organoleptic or biochemical changes in the product (64).

REFERENCES

1. Acuff, G.R., C. Vanderzant, F.A. Gardner, and F.A. Golan. 1982. Examination of turkey eggs, poults, and brooder house facilities for Campylobacter jejuni. J Food Prot 45:1279–1281.
2. Acuff, G.R., C. Vanderzant, M.O. Hanna, J.G. Ehlers, F.A. Golan, and F.A. Gardner. 1986. Prevalence of Campylobacter jejuni in turkey carcass processing and further processing of turkey products. J Food Prot 49:712–717.
3. Annan-Prah, A., and M. Janc. 1988. The mode of spread of Campylobacter jejuni/coli to broiler flocks. Zentralbl Veterinaermed [B] 35:11–18.
4. Annan-Prah, A., and M. Janc. 1988. Chicken-to-human infection with Campylobacter jejuni and Campylobacter coli: Biotype and serotype correlation. J Food Prot 51:562–564.
5. Baker, R.C., M.D.C. Paredes, and R.A. Qureshi. 1987. Prevalence of Campylobacter jejuni in eggs and poultry meat in New York State. Poult Sci 66:1766–1770.

6. Benjamin, J., S. Leaper, R.J. Owen, and M.B. Skirrow. 1983. Description of Campylobacter laridis, a new species comprising the nalidixic acid-resistant thermophilic Campylobacter (NARTC) group. Curr Microbiol 8:231-238.

7. Blaser, M.J. 1982. Campylobacter jejuni and food. Food Technol 36:89-92.

8. Blaser, M.J., F.M. LaForce, N.A. Wilson, and W.L.L. Wang. 1980. Reservoirs for human campylobacteriosis. J Infect Dis 141:665-669.

9. Blaser, M.J., H.L. Hardesty, B. Powers, and W.-L.L. Wang. 1980. Survival of Campylobacter fetus subsp. jejuni in biological milieus. J Clin Microbiol 11:309-313.

10. Blaser, M.J., P. Checko, C. Bopp, A. Bruce, and J.M. Hughes. 1982. Campylobacter enteritis associated with foodborne transmission. Am J Epidemiol 116:886-894.

11. Blaser, M.J., D.N. Taylor, and R.A. Feldman. 1983. Epidemiology of Campylobacter jejuni infections. Epidemiol Rev 5:157-176.

12. Blaser, M.J., D.J. Duncan, G.H. Warren, and W-L.L. Wang. 1983. Experimental Campylobacter jejuni infection of adult mice. Infect Immun 39:908-916.

13. Blaser, M.J., P.F. Smith, J.E. Repine, and K.A. Joiner. 1988. Pathogenesis of Campylobacter fetus infections. J Clin Invest 81:1434-1444.

14. Bolton, F.J., D. Coates, P.M. Hinchliffe, and L. Robertson. 1983. Comparison of selective media for isolation of Campylobacter jejuni/coli. J Clin Pathol 36:78-83.

15. Buck, G.E., and M.T. Kelly. 1981. Effect of moisture content of the medium on colony morphology of Campylobacter fetus subsp. jejuni. J Clin Microbiol 14:585-586.

16. Bukholm, G., and G. Kapperud. 1987. Expression of Campylobacter jejuni invasiveness in cell cultures coinfected with other bacteria. Infect Immun 55:2816-2821.

17. Chan, F.T.H., and A.M.R. Mackenzie. 1986. Evaluation of primary selective media and enrichment methods for Campylobacter species isolation. Eur J Clin Microbiol 5:162-164.

18. Christenson, B., Å. Ringer, C. Blücher, H. Billaudelle, K.N. Gundtoft, G. Eriksson, and M. Böttiger. 1983. An outbreak of Campylobacter enteritis among the staff of a poultry abbatoir in Sweden. Scand J Infect Dis 15:167-172.

19. Clark, A.G. 1986. The effect of toxigenic and invasive human strains of Campylobacter jejuni on broiler hatchability and health. Proc 35th West Poult Dis Conf, pp. 25-27.

20. Clark, A.G., and D.H. Bueschkens. 1985. Laboratory infection of chicken eggs with Campylobacter jejuni by using temperature or pressure differentials. Appl Environ Microbiol 49:1467-1471.

21. Clark, A.G., and D.H. Bueschkens. 1988. Horizontal spread of human and poultry-derived strains of Campylobacter jejuni among broiler chicks held in incubators and shipping boxes. J Food Prot 51:438-441.

22. Cruickshank, J.G. 1986. Salmonella and Campylobacter infections, an update. J Small Anim Pract 27:673-681.

23. Delaplane, J.P., H.A. Smith, and R.W. Moore. 1955. An unidentified agent causing a hepatitis in chickens. Southwest Vet 8:356-361.

24. Doyle, M.P. 1984. Association of Campylobacter jejuni with laying hens and eggs. Appl Environ Microbiol 47:533-536.

25. Fauchere, J.L., A. Rosenau, M. Veron, E.N. Moyen, S. Richard, and A. Pfister. 1986. Association with HeLa cells of Campylobacter jejuni and Campylobacter coli isolated from human feces. Infect Immun 54:283-287.

26. Field, L.H., V.L. Headley, J.L. Underwood, S.M. Payne, and L.J. Berry. 1986. The chicken embryo as a model for Campylobacter invasion: Comparative virulence of human isolates of Campylobacter jejuni and Campylobacter coli. Infect Immun 54:118-125.

27. Firehammer, B.D., and L.L. Myers. 1981. Campylobacter fetus subsp. jejuni: Its possible significance in enteric disease of calves and lambs. Am J Vet Res 42:918-922.

28. Fleming, M.P. 1983. Association of Campylobacter jejuni with enteritis in dogs and cats. Vet Rec 113:372-374.

29. Fletcher, R.D., and W.N. Plastridge. 1964. Difference in physiology of Vibrio spp. from chickens and man. Avian Dis 8:72-75.

30. Fox, J.G. 1982. Campylobacteriosis – a "new" disease in laboratory animals. Lab Anim Sci 32:625-637.

31. Fox, J.G., R. Moore, and J.I. Ackerman. 1983. Campylobacter jejuni-associated diarrhea in dogs. J Am Vet Med Assoc 183:1430-1433.

32. Fox, J.G., S. Zanotti, H.V. Jordan, and J.C. Murphy. 1986. Colonization of Syrian hamsters with streptomycin resistant Campylobacter jejuni. Lab Anim Sci 36:28-31.

33. Fox, J.G., J.I. Ackerman, N. Taylor, M. Claps, and J.C. Murphy. 1987. Campylobacter jejuni infection in the ferret: An animal model of human campylobacteriosis. Am J Vet Res 48:85-90.

34. Franco, D.A. 1988. Campylobacter species: Considerations for controlling a foodborne pathogen. J Food Prot 51:145-153.

35. Fricker, C.R. 1987. The isolation of salmonellas and campylobacters. J Appl Bacteriol 63:99-116.

36. Fricker, C.R., and N. Metcalfe. 1984. Campylobacters in wading birds (Charadrii): Incidence, biotypes, and isolation techniques. Zentralbl Bakteriol Mikrobiol Hyg [B] 179:469-475.

37. Garcia, M.M., M.D. Eaglesome, and C. Rigby. 1983. Campylobacters important in veterinary medicine. Vet Bull 53:793-818.

38. Genigeorgis, C. 1986. Significance of campylobacter in poultry. Proc 35th West Poult Dis Conf pp. 54-59.

39. Genigeorgis, C., M. Hassuneh, and P. Collins. 1986. Campylobacter jejuni infection on poultry farms and its effect on poultry meat contamination during slaughtering. J Food Prot 49:895-903.

40. Gerlach, H., and I. Gylstorff. 1967. Untersuchungen über biochemische Eigenschaften, Pathogenität und Resistenzspektrum gegen Antibiotika bei Vibrio metschnikovi. Berl Müench Tierärztl Wochenschr 80:153-155, 161-164.

41. Goossens, H., M. De Boeck, H. Van Landuyt, and J.-P. Butzler. 1984. Isolation of Campylobacter jejuni from human feces. In J.-P. Butzler (ed.), Campylobacter Infection in Man and Animals, pp. 39-50. CRC Press, Inc, FL.

42. Goossens, H., E. Rummens, S. Cadranel, J.-P. Butzler, and Y. Takeda. 1985. Cytotoxic activity on Chinese hamster ovary cells in culture filtrates of Campylobacter jejuni/coli. Lancet ii:511.

43. Grados, O., N. Bravo, J.-P. Butzler, and G. Ventura. 1983. Campylobacter infection: An occupational disease risk in chicken handlers. Campylobacter II, Proc Int Workshop on Campylobacter Infect, p. 162.

44. Grant, I.H., N.J. Richardson, and V.D. Bokkenheuser. 1980. Broiler chickens as potential source of Campylobacter infections in humans. J Clin Microbiol 11:508-510.

45. Hagan, J.R. 1964. Diagnostic techniques in avian vibrionic hepatitis. Avian Dis 8:428-437.

46. Harris, N.V., D. Thompson, D.C. Martin, and C.M. Nolan. 1986. A survey of Campylobacter and other bacterial contaminants of pre-market chicken and retail poultry and meats, King County, Washington. Am J Public Health 76:401-406.

47. Harris, N.V., N.S. Weiss, and C.M. Nolan. 1986. The role of poultry and meats in the etiology of Campylobacter jejuni/coli enteritis. Am J Public Health 76:407-411.

48. Hébert, G.A., D.G. Hollis, R.E. Weaver, M.A. Lambert, M.J. Blaser, and C.W. Moss. 1982. 30 years of campylobacters: Biochemical characteristics and a biotyping proposal for Campylobacter jejuni. J Clin Microbiol 15:1065-1073.

49. Hofstad, M.S., E.H. McGehee, and P.C. Bennett. 1958. Avian infectious hepatitis. Avian Dis 2:358-364.

50. Istre, G.R., M.J. Blaser, P. Shillam, and R.S. Hopkins. 1984. Campylobacter enteritis associated with undercooked barbecued chicken. Am J Public Health 74:1265-1267.

51. Ito, K., Y. Kubokura, K. Kaneko, Y. Totake, and M. Ogawa. 1988. Occurrence of Campylobacter jejuni in free-living wild birds from Japan. J Wildl Dis 24:467-470.

52. Izat, A.L., and F.A. Gardner. 1988. Incidence of Campylobacter jejuni in processed egg products. Poult Sci 67:1431-1435.

53. Jones, D.M., and D.A. Robinson. 1981. Occupational exposure to Campylobacter jejuni infection. Lancet i:440-441.

54. Kakoyiannis, C.K., P.J. Winter, and R.B. Marshall. 1988. The relationship between intestinal Campylobacter species isolated from animals and humans as determined by BRENDA. Epidemiol Infect 100:379-387.

55. Kaneuchi, C., T. Imaizumi, Y. Sugiyama, Y. Kosako, M. Seki, T. Itoh, and M. Ogata. 1987. Thermophilic campylobacters in seagulls and DNA-DNA hybridization test of isolates. Jpn J Vet Sci 49:787-794.

56. Kapperud, G., O. Rosef, O.W. Røstad, and G. Lid. 1983. Isolation of Campylobacter fetus subsp. jejuni from the common puffin (Fratercula arctica) in Norway. J Wildl Dis 19:64-65.

57. Karmali, M.A., and M.B. Skirrow. 1984. Taxonomy of the genus Campylobacter. In J.-P. Butzler (ed.), Campylobacter Infection in Man and Animals, pp. 1-20. CRC Press, Inc, Boca Raton, FL.

58. Karmali, M.A., S. De Grandis, and P.C. Fleming. 1981. Antimicrobial susceptibility of Campylobacter jejuni with special reference to resistance patterns of Canadian isolates. Antimicrob Agents Chemother 19:593-597.

59. Karmali, M.A., A.E. Simor, M. Roscoe, P.C. Fleming, S.S. Smith, and J. Lane. 1986. Evaluation of a blood-free, charcoal-based, selective medium for the isolation of Campylobacter organisms from feces. J Clin Microbiol 23:456-459.

60. Kasrazadeh, M., and C. Genigeorgis. 1987. Origin and prevalence of Campylobacter jejuni in ducks and duck meat at the farm and processing plant level. J Food Prot 50:321-326.

61. King, E.O. 1957. Human infections with Vibrio fetus and a closely related vibrio. J Infect Dis 101:119-128.

62. Kinjo, T., M. Morishige, N. Minamoto, and H. Fukushi. 1983. Prevalence of Campylobacter jejuni in feral pigeons. Jpn J Vet Sci 45:833-835.

63. Klipstein, F.A., R.F. Engert, H. Short, and E.A. Schenk. 1985. Pathogenic properties of Campylobacter jejuni: Assay and correlation with clinical manifestations. Infect Immun 50:43-49.

64. Lambert, J.D., and R.B. Maxcy. 1984. Effect of gamma radiation of Campylobacter jejuni. J Food Sci 49:665-667.

65. Lammerding, A.M., M.M. Garcia, E.D. Mann, Y. Robinson, W.J. Dorward, R.B. Truscott, and F. Tittiger. 1988. Prevalence of Salmonella and thermophilic Campylobacter in fresh pork, beef, veal, and poultry in Canada. J Food Prot 51:47-52.

66. Lior, H. 1984. New, extended biotyping scheme for Campylobacter jejuni, Campylobacter coli, and "Campylobacter laridis." J Clin Microbiol 20:636-640.

67. Lior, H., D.L. Woodward, J.A. Edgar, L.J. Laroche, and P. Gill. 1982. Serotyping of Campylobacter jejuni by slide agglutination based on heat-labile antigenic factors. J Clin Microbiol 15:761-768.

68. Luechtefeld, N.W., and W.-L.L. Wang. 1981. Campylobacter fetus subsp. jejuni in a turkey processing plant. J Clin Microbiol 13:266-268.

69. Luechtefeld, N.W., and W.-L.L. Wang. 1982. Animal reservoirs of Campylobacter jejuni. In D.G. Newell (ed.), Campylobacter. Epidemiology, Pathogenesis, and Biochemistry, pp. 249-252. MTP Press, Lancaster, England.

70. Luechtefeld, N.W., R.C. Cambre, and W.-L.L. Wang. 1981. Isolation of Campylobacter jejuni from zoo animals. J Am Vet Med Assoc 179:1119-1122.

71. Luechtefeld, N.W., W.-L.L. Wang, M.J. Blaser, and L.B. Reller. 1981. Evaluation of transport and storage techniques for isolation of Campylobacter fetus subsp. jejuni from turkey cecal specimens. J Clin Microbiol 13:438-443.

72. Mandal, B.K., P. De Mol, and J.-P. Butzler. 1984. Clinical aspects of Campylobacter infections in humans. In J.-P. Butzler (ed.), Campylobacter Infection in Man and Animals, pp. 21-31. CRC Press, Inc, Boca Raton, FL.

73. Maruyama, S., and Y. Katsube. 1988. Intestinal colonization of Campylobacter jejuni in young Japanese quails (Coturnix coturnix japonica). Jpn J Vet Sci 50:569-572.

74. Michel, J., M. Rogol, and D. Dickman. 1983. Susceptibility of clinical isolates of Campylobacter jejuni to sixteen antimicrobial agents. Antimicrob Agents Chemother 23:796-797.

75. Minakshi, S.C.D., and A. Ayyagari. 1988. Isolation of Campylobacter jejuni from quails: An initial report. Br Vet J 144:411-412.

76. Montrose, M.S., S.M. Shane, and K.S. Harrington. 1985. Role of litter in the transmission of Campylobacter jejuni. Avian Dis 29:392-399.

77. Morris, G.K., C.A. Bopp, C.M. Patton, and J.G. Wells. 1982. Media for isolating Campylobacter. Arch Lebensmittelhyg 33:151-153.

78. Morrison, R.M., and T. Roberts. 1985. Potential public health benefits of irradiating fresh chicken, pork, and beef. In Food irradiation: New perspectives on a controversial technology. US Government Printing Office, Serial 99-14, pp. 1038-1064.

79. Munroe, D.L., J.F. Prescott, and J.L. Penner. 1983. Campylobacter jejuni and Campylobacter coli serotypes isolated from chickens, cattle, and pigs. J Clin Microbiol 18:877-881.

80. Neill, S.D., J.N. Campbell, and J.A. Greene. 1984. Campylobacter species in broiler chickens. Avian Pathol 13:777- 785.

81. Neill, S.D., J.N. Campbell, and J.J. O'Brien. 1985. Egg penetration by Campylobacter jejuni. Avian Pathol 14:313-320.

82. Norkrans, G., and Å. Svedhem. 1982. Epidemiological aspects of Campylobacter jejuni enteritis. J Hyg 89:163-170.

83. Oosterom, J., S. Notermans, H. Karman, and G.B. Engels. 1983. Origin and prevalence of Campylobacter

jejuni in poultry processing. J Food Prot 46:339–344.
84. Pacha, R.E., G.W. Clark, E.A. Williams, and A.M. Carter. 1988. Migratory birds of central Washington as reservoirs of Campylobacter jejuni. Can J Microbiol 34:80–82.
85. Park, C.E., Z.K. Stankiewicz, J. Lovett, and J. Hunt. 1981. Incidence of Campylobacter jejuni in fresh eviscerated whole market chickens. Can J Microbiol 27:841–842.
86. Patton, C.M., S.W. Mitchell, M.E. Potter, and A.F. Kaufmann. 1981. Comparison of selective media for primary isolation of Campylobacter fetus subsp. jejuni. J Clin Microbiol 13:326–330.
87. Patton, C.M., T.J. Barrett, and G.K. Morris. 1985. Comparison of the Penner and Lior methods for serotyping Campylobacter spp. J Clin Microbiol 22:558–565.
88. Peckham, M.C. 1958. Avian vibrionic hepatitis. Avian Dis 2:348–358.
89. Peckham, M.C. 1984. Avian vibrio infections. In M.S. Hofstad, H.J. Barnes, B.W. Calnek, W.M. Reid, and H.W. Yoder, Jr (eds.), Diseases of Poultry, 8th Ed, pp 221–231. Iowa State Univ Press, Ames.
90. Penner, J.L., and J.N. Hennessy. 1980. Passive hemagglutination technique for serotyping Campylobacter fetus subsp. jejuni on the basis of soluble heat-stable antigens. J Clin Microbiol 12:732–737.
91. Penner, J.L., J.N. Hennessy, and R.V. Congi. 1983. Serotyping of Campylobacter jejuni and Campylobacter coli on the basis of thermostable antigens. Eur J Clin Microbiol 2:378–383.
92. Prescott, J.F., and C.W. Bruin-Mosch. 1981. Carriage of Campylobacter jejuni in healthy and diarrheic animals. Am J Vet Res 42:164–165.
93. Prescott, J.F., and D.L. Munroe. 1982. Campylobacter jejuni enteritis in man and domestic animals. J Am Vet Med Assoc 181:1524–1530.
94. Robinson, D.A., and D.M. Jones. 1981. Milk-borne campylobacter infection. Br Med J 282:1374–1376.
95. Rosef, O., and G. Kapperud. 1983. House flies (Musca domestica) as possible vectors of Campylobacter fetus subsp jejuni. Appl Environ Microbiol 45:381–383.
96. Rosef, O., B. Gondrosen, and G. Kapperud. 1984. Campylobacter jejuni and Campylobacter coli as surface contaminants of fresh and frozen poultry carcasses. Int J Food Microbiol 1:205–215.
97. Ruiz-Palacios, G.M., E. Escamilla, and N. Torres. 1981. Experimental Campylobacter diarrhea in chickens. Infect Immun 34:250–255.
98. Sanyal, S.C., K.M.N. Islam, P.K.B. Neogy, M. Islam, P. Speelman, and M.I. Huq. 1984. Campylobacter jejuni diarrhea model in infant chickens. Infect Immun 43:931–936.
99. Schwartz, R.H., C. Bryan, W.J. Rodriguez, C. Park, and P. McCoy. 1983. Experience with the microbiologic diagnosis of Campylobacter enteritis in an office laboratory. Pediatr Infect Dis 2:298–301.
100. Sebald, M., and M. Véron. 1963. Teneur en bases de l'ADN et classification des vibrions. Ann Inst Pasteur (Paris) 105:897–910.
101. Sevoian, M., and B.W. Calnek. 1959. Avian infectious hepatitis. III. Treatment of chickens in egg production. Avian Dis 3:302–311.
102. Sevoian, M., R.W. Winterfield, and C.L. Goldman. 1958. Avian infectious hepatitis. I. Clinical and pathological manifestations. Avian Dis 2:3–18.
103. Shane, S.M., and M.S. Montrose. 1985. The occurrence and significance of Campylobacter jejuni in man and animals. Vet Res Commun 9:167–198.
104. Shane, S.M., M.S. Montrose, and K.S. Harrington. 1985. Transmission of Campylobacter jejuni by the housefly (Musca domestica). Avian Dis 29:384–391.
105. Shane, S.M., D.H. Gifford, and K. Yogasundram. 1986. Campylobacter jejuni contamination of eggs. Vet Res Commun 10:487–492.
106. Shanker, S., A. Lee, and T.C. Sorrell. 1986. Campylobacter jejuni in broilers: The role of vertical transmission. J Hyg 96:153–159.
107. Shanker, S., A. Lee, and T.C. Sorrell. 1988. Experimental colonization of broiler chicks with Campylobacter jejuni. Epidemiol Infect 100:27–34.
108. Skirrow, M.B. 1982. Campylobacter enteritis the first five years. J Hyg 89:175–184.
109. Skirrow, M.B., and J. Benjamin. 1980. '1001' Campylobacters: Cultural characteristics of intestinal campylobacters from man and animals. J Hyg 85:427–442.
110. Skirrow, M.B., and J. Benjamin. 1980. Differentiation of enteropathogenic campylobacter. J Clin Pathol 33:1122.
111. Smibert, R.M. 1978. The genus Campylobacter. Ann Rev Microbiol 32:673–709.
112. Smibert, R.M. 1984. Genus Campylobacter Sebald and Veron 1963, 907[AL]. In N.R. Krieg and J.G. Holt (eds.), Bergey's Manual of Systematic Bacteriology, Vol 1. pp 111–118. Williams & Wilkins, Baltimore, MD.
113. Smitherman, R.E., C.A. Genigeorgis, and T.B. Farver. 1984. Preliminary observations on the occurrence of Campylobacter jejuni at four California chicken ranches. J Food Prot 47:293– 298.
114. Soerjadi, A.S., G.H. Snoeyenbos, and O.M. Weinack. 1982. Intestinal colonization and competitive exclusion of Campylobacter fetus subsp. jejuni in young chicks. Avian Dis 26:520–524.
115. Soerjadi-Liem, A.S., G.H. Snoeyenbos, and O.M. Weinack. 1984. Comparative studies on competitive exclusion of three isolates of Campylobacter fetus subsp. jejuni in chickens by native gut microflora. Avian Dis 28:139–146.
116. Stern, N.J., M.P. Hernandez, L. Blankenship, K.E. Deibel, S. Doores, M.P. Doyle, H. Ng, M.D. Pierson, J.N. Sofos, W.H. Sveum, and D.C. Westhoff. 1985. Prevalence and distribution of Campylobacter jejuni and Campylobacter coli in retail meats. J Food Prot 48:595–599.
117. Stern, N.J., P.J. Rothenberg, and J.M. Stone. 1985. Enumeration and reduction of Campylobacter jejuni in poultry and red meats. J Food Prot 48:606–610.
118. Stern, N.S., J.S. Bailey, L.C. Blankenship, N.A. Cox, and F. McHan. 1988. Colonization characteristics of Campylobacter jejuni in chick ceca. Avian Dis 32:330–334.
119. Svedhem, Å, B. Kaijser, and E. Sjögren. 1981. Antimicrobial susceptibility of Campylobacter jejuni isolated from humans with diarrhoea and from healthy chickens. J Antimicrob Chemother 7:301–305.
120. Tauxe, R.V., D.A. Pegues, and N. Hargrett-Bean. 1987. Campylobacter infections: The emerging national pattern. Am J Public Health 77:1219–1221.
121. Taylor, D.E., and P. Courvalin. 1988. Mechanisms of antibiotic resistance in Campylobacter species. Antimicrob Agents Chemother 32:1107–1112.
122. Thompson, L.M., III, R.M. Smibert, J.L. Johnson, and N.R. Krieg. 1988. Phylogenetic study of the genus Campylobacter. Int J Syst Bacteriol 38:190–200.
123. Truscott, R.B., and P.H.G. Stockdale. 1966. Correlation of the identity of bile and cecal vibrios from the same field cases of avian vibrionic hepatitis. Avian Dis 10:67– 73.
124. Tudor, D.C. 1954. A liver degeneration of unknown origin in chickens. J Am Vet Med Assoc 125:219–220.
125. Umunnabuike, A.C., and E.A. Irokanulo. 1986. Isolation of Campylobacter subsp. jejuni from Oriental

and American cockroaches caught in kitchens and poultry houses in Vom, Nigeria. Int J Zoon 13:180–186.

126. Vanhoof, R., H. Goossens, H. Coignau, G. Stas, and J.-P. Butzler. 1982. Susceptibility patterns of Campylobacter jejuni from human and animal origins to different antimicrobial agents. Antimicrob Agents Chemother 21:990–992.

127. Van Landuyt, H.W., J.-M. Fossépré, and B. Gordts. 1987. A blood-free medium for isolation of thermophilic Campylobacter species. Eur J Clin Microbiol 6:201–203.

128. Volkheimer, A., and H.-H. Wuthe. 1986. Campylobacter jejuni/coli bei Rebhühnern (Perdix perdix L.) und Fasanen (Phasianus colchicus L.). Berl Müench Tierärztl Woschenschr 99:374.

129. Wang, W.-L.L., N.W. Luechtefeld, L.B. Reller, and M.J. Blaser. 1980. Enriched brucella medium for storage and transport of cultures of Campylobacter fetus subsp. jejuni. J Clin Microbiol 12:479–480.

130. Wang, W.-L.L., B.W. Powers, N.W. Luechtefeld, and M.J. Blaser. 1983. Effects of disinfectants on Campylobacter jejuni. Appl Environ Microbiol 45:1202–1205.

131. Welkos, S.L. 1984. Experimental gastroenteritis in newly-hatched chicks infected with Campylobacter jejuni. J Med Microbiol 18:233–248.

132. Winkenwerder, W., and T. Maciak. 1964. Vibrionenfunde bei Hühnern aus erkrankten Beständen und bei Schlachthühnern. Dtsch Tierärztl Wochenschr 71:625–627.

133. Winterfield, R.W., and M. Sevoian. 1957. Isolation of a causal agent of an avian hepatitis. Vet Med 52:273–274.

134. Winterfield, R.W., M. Sevoian, and C.L. Goldman. 1958. Avian infectious hepatitis. II. Some characteristics of the etiologic agent. Effect of various drugs on the course of the disease. Avian Dis 2:19–39.

135. Yogasundram, K., and S.M. Shane. 1986. The viability of Campylobacter jejuni on refrigerated chicken drumsticks. Vet Res Commun 10:479–486.

136. Yogasundram, K., S.M. Shane, R.M. Grodner, E.N. Lambremont, and R.E. Smith. 1987. Decontamination of Campylobacter jejuni on chicken drumsticks using chemicals and radiation. Vet Res Commun 11:31–40.

10 ERYSIPELAS

J.M. Bricker and Y.M. Saif

INTRODUCTION. Erysipelas in birds is generally an acute, fulminating infection of individuals within a flock. The infection and disease have been reported from many different vertebrate species, either as a contaminant (fish) or an infection. It is caused by *Erysipelothrix rhusiopathiae,* which also causes swine erysipelas in pigs and erysipeloid in humans.

Outbreaks of economic significance are uncommon in avian species other than turkeys. Occasional death of individual birds within a flock have been reported, and a few economically significant outbreaks in chickens and ducklings have occurred (41). *E. rhusiopathiae* has caused outbreaks of erysipelas in pheasants, ducks, geese, guinea fowl, coturnix quail, and chukars (13, 21, 28, 32, 33, 52, 53, 64).

Erysipelas not only causes death but frequently affects male fertility and contributes to processing losses because of condemnation, or downgrading, resulting from postmortem evidence of septicemia. Egg production is often depressed in affected chicken flocks.

Erysipeloid in humans may be a local or septicemic, occasionally fatal, infection. It is most common in fish handlers, butchers, kitchen workers, veterinarians, and turkey growers. Silberstein (60) reported endocarditis and encephalitis in humans treated with penicillin. Presumptive diagnoses of the infection have been made in turkey flocks as a result of infection of a turkey handler or insemination crew member. In most cases the disease is preceded by an injury such as a cut.

HISTORY. Sporadic cases were reported in various avian species prior to 1936. Beaudette and Hudson (4) first described the economic significance of the disease in North American turkeys; other outbreaks were reported shortly thereafter. Use of widespread artificial insemination of turkeys made prevention of erysipelas a major problem facing producers of turkey hatching eggs. With confinement-growing of turkeys, the disease has decreased in importance, except in endemic areas.

Following introduction of bacterins in the early 1950s and availability of penicillin for treatment, various preventive programs based on vaccination and/or treatment have been developed. Despite this, cases of postinsemination erysipelas still occur in turkey hens as do sporadic outbreaks in commercial flocks.

INCIDENCE AND DISTRIBUTION. *E. rhusiopathiae* is worldwide in distribution. The adaptiveness of the organism is indicated by its ability to infect a wide variety of vertebrate species. It has been isolated from tissues of birds, mammals, reptiles, and amphibians, as well as surface slime of fish.

Outbreaks of erysipelas in poultry occur sporadically, though locations exist in the world where the disease is endemic. Though the disease in turkeys has been reported more frequently among males than females, there is no evidence of differing susceptibility between sexes. Field observations suggest the portal of entry (skin) is breached more frequently in males, but the incidence in hens has increased due to artificial insemination and more frequent handling.

ETIOLOGY

Classification. *E. rhusiopathiae* (formerly *E. insidiosa*) belongs to the family Lactobacillaceae (12). The organism is a gram-positive bacillus, which tends to decolorize easily, especially in older cultures, and form long filaments. It does not form spores, is not acid-fast, and is nonmotile. Barber (3) and Nelson and Shelton (48) reported that it resembles *Listeria* sp.; however, they demonstrated marked cultural differences between them. It resembles mycobacteria since it has a high lipid content in its cell wall (almost 30%). Similar to some gram-negative bacteria, it has a rather low hexosamine content, but differs from them in having a limited complement of amino acids (37).

Morphology and Staining. The cellular morphology of *E. rhusiopathiae* is variable. Cells isolated from smooth colonies or tissues of acutely infected birds are straight, slender, or slightly curved rods measuring 0.2–0.4 by 0.8–2.5 μm,

The authors gratefully acknowledge the groundwork laid by the previous authors, Drs. A.S. Rosenwald and R.E. Corstvet.

and may occur singly or in short chains. Organisms from older cultures or rough colonies are filamentous rods and may form masses that resemble mycelia. These filamentous rods usually appear somewhat thickened and may appear beaded following staining. The filamentous form begins to appear after several passages on artificial media. Both short rods and short filaments may be observed from a single colony (intermediate colony type).

Growth Requirements. *E. rhusiopathiae* is facultatively anaerobic and grows readily though sparsely on ordinary culture media and moderately well in thioglycollate broth and various other broths containing serum or serum components. It grows especially well in deep stabs of semisolid medium prepared by adding 0.5% agar to tryptose phosphate broth. Reduced oxygen or increased carbon dioxide (5–10%) enhances growth, but neither is necessary to support growth. Smith (61) described the appearance of growth in a meat infusion broth culture at 24 hr as, "a faint opalescence . . ., which on shaking was resolved for the moment into delicate rolling clouds." The addition of serum to broth media supports heavier growth with a powdery sediment forming after 24 hr. Protein hydrolysates, glucose, and certain detergents such as Tween 80 also enhance growth. *E. rhusiopathiae* grows in a temperature range from 4 C (slow growth) to 42 C with an optimal range of 35–37 C. The optimal pH for growth is mildly alkaline, pH 7.4–7.8. Oleic acid and riboflavin have been reported to be essential for growth. The organism does not form a pellicle.

Colony Morphology. Three different colony types have been described for *E. rhusiopathiae.* Smooth colonies are dewy, colorless to bluish gray, and of pinpoint size (0.5–0.8 mm) with smooth edges. Most strains of *E. rhusiopathiae* and organisms isolated directly from infected tissues form this colony type. Some strains, however, form rough colonies, which are opaque, flat, dry, and of pinhead size (1–2 mm) with irregular or lobed edges. Dissociation from smooth to rough colony type results in intermediate colonies. Most strains produce a narrow zone of alpha hemolysis in a medium containing 5–10% horse or bovine blood after 2–3 days incubation at 37 C in an atmosphere of 5–10% carbon dioxide.

Biochemical Properties. *E. rhusiopathiae* ferments glucose, galactose, dextrose, fructose, maltose, lactose, and levulose without gas production. Lead acetate agar or triple-sugar iron (TSI) agar is usually blackened indicating hydrogen sulfide (H_2S) production, and xylose is occasionally fermented. Strains that do not produce H_2S have been isolated (6). Litmus milk is occasionally acidified slightly without coagulation. A test-tube brush type of growth (lateral radiating projections) occurs 48 hr postinoculation in gelatin stab culture incubated at 21 C. The organism is catalase-negative, does not produce indole, does not reduce nitrites, is Voges-Proskauer and methyl red–negative, does not hydrolyze esculin, and does not reduce 0.1% methylene blue. White and Shuman (69) found the fermentation pattern varied with the medium, indicator, and method of measuring acid production; the most dependable medium was Andrade's base plus serum. Of three methods used to measure acid production (chemical indicator, change in pH, production of titratable acidity), they found the chemical indicator gave the most valid, reproducible results.

Resistance to Chemical and Physical Agents. *E. rhusiopathiae* is fairly resistant to various environmental and chemical factors. It is very resistant to desiccation, may survive smoking and pickling processes used for processing meat, and may remain viable in frozen or chilled meat, dried blood, decaying carcasses or fish meal. Apart from tissues, it is killed at 70 C in 5–10 min. Vallee (65) suggested the organism remained viable in soil and multiplied in alkaline soils during warm weather. However, Wood (72), reported that under experimental conditions, *E. rhusiopathiae* was inactivated in soil at different rates when parameters of temperature, pH, and organic matter content were tested. Temperature exerted the greatest effect on viability. Populations of the pathogen survived 35 days at 3 C and 2 days at 30 C. Organisms did not survive longer than 11–18 days under various conditions of organic matter content and pH. *E. rhusiopathiae* is destroyed in a short time by a 1:1000 concentration of bichloride of mercury, 0.5% sodium hydroxide solution, 3.5% liquid cresol, or a 5% solution of phenol. The organism is resistant to 0.001% crystal violet, 0.5% potassium tellurite, and can grow in the presence of 0.1% sodium azide.

Antigenic Structure and Toxins. Cross-immunity and cross-agglutination studies have demonstrated that essentially all strains of *E. rhusiopathiae* possess at least one or more common antigens. These antigens are heat-labile and consist of protein or a complex of protein, carbohydrate, and lipid. Flagellar and capsular antigens are not present, because *E. rhusiopathiae* possesses neither a capsule nor flagella.

A heat-stable antigen (cell wall peptidoglycan) is used to differentiate *E. rhusiopathiae* into serotypes. These antigens are easily extracted from the organism using acid or by autoclaving a washed, whole-cell, inactivated culture for 1 hr at 121 C. Determination of serotype is accomplished with a double-diffusion gel system using specific hyperimmune rabbit sera. The preferred system for serotyping *E. rhusiopathiae* isolates is a numerical system described by Kuscera (40). Using the numerical system, strains previously designated as types A or B now become types 1 and 2 respectively. Currently, 24 serotypes have been described (designated 1–24), in addition to strains not possessing a type-specific antigen, which are designated type N. Subtypes of some serotypes exist and are designated by a number followed by a lowercase letter. The majority of *E. rhusiopathiae* strains isolated from poultry fall into three major serotypes: types 1 (with subtypes 1a and 1b), 2, and 5 (20, 64, 75). The immunizing antigen (protective antigen) is discussed under the section entitled Prevention and Control. *E. rhusiopathiae* does not produce any known toxins.

Strain Classification. Strain classification is primarily based on serologic, not biologic or biochemical activity. White and Shuman (69) noted the fermentation pattern of a particular strain did not vary to any great extent. There is no reported correlation between serologic group or biochemical pattern of strains of *E. rhusiopathiae* isolated from birds, and production of septicemic, urticarial, or endocardial forms of erysipelas, or of the carrier state (7, 68).

Pathogenicity. *E. rhusiopathiae* is pathogenic for turkeys at any age or sex following exposure by a variety of parenteral routes. Infection and disease are also produced in turkeys inoculated orally with chicken embryo yolk-propagated organisms (15) or when allowed to feed on viscera of turkeys that died from erysipelas. However, several workers have reported difficulty in reproducing consistent mortality with *E. rhusiopathiae* isolates of avian origin experimentally (2, 22). Reducing the number of passages on artificial media to an absolute minimum appears essential to maintaining virulence of the organism. Boyer and Brown (9) maintained virulence of an *E. rhusiopathiae* strain by storing infected liver at 4 C, which served as a source of the organism for further bird passage.

In addition to turkeys, other avian species are susceptible to infection with *E. rhusiopathiae,* both experimentally and under field conditions; serious losses have been reported in chickens, ducks, and geese following natural outbreaks of the disease. Experimentally, Malik (43) demonstrated that virulent cultures of *E. rhusiopathiae* administered parenterally produced septicemia in chickens less than 14 days old. However, in older chickens, septicemia could be produced only by intrapalpebral or subconjunctival installation of the pathogen along with injury to that tissue. Administration of hydrocortisone not only increased susceptibility to *E. rhusiopathiae* but shortened the course of infection and increased mortality, thus appearing to increase virulence.

Parenteral injection of most avian strains of the organism regularly kills mice (*Mus musculus*), pigeons, and turkeys, but guinea pigs and chickens usually survive. Iliadis et al. (34) reported pigeons were more susceptible to intravenous than oral inoculation.

The mechanisms by which the organism causes disease are still not well understood. The enzyme hyaluronidase was initially thought to be involved in the virulence of *E. rhusiopathiae,* but later studies revealed no association with hyaluronidase production and pathogenicity of a particular strain (49). The enzyme neuraminidase appears to correlate better with virulence of *E. rhusiopathiae* isolates. This enzyme is produced during logarithmic growth and the amount of enzyme activity was reported by Müller (45) to be lower in strains of lower virulence or avirulent strains compared to highly virulent isolates. However, no apparent relationship exists between the amount of neuraminidase activity and serotype. In a review of erysipelas, Wood (73) noted that specific antibody to this enzyme from *E. rhusiopathiae* was identified in a commercial erysipelas antiserum produced in horses and serum of rabbits hyperimmunized with *E. rhusiopathiae* neuraminidase. The rabbit preparation was shown to induce some protection in mice following challenge with the organism. *E. rhusiopathiae* neuraminidase has not been shown to have toxic activity and must be produced in large amounts to be active in pathogenesis, a condition that probably exists in the septicemic form of the disease.

The reason why different isolates of *E. rhusiopathiae* vary dramatically in pathogenicity is not known. Attempts to establish relationships between chemical structure, antigenic structure, or morphology with virulence have failed. Though neuraminidase is implicated to play a role in the pathogenesis of *E. rhusiopathiae* infection, there are probably other factors as yet undetermined that contribute to virulence of the organism.

PATHOGENESIS AND EPIZOOTIOLOGY.

Van Es and McGrath (66) cited Nocard and Leclainche as noting in 1903 that "at the present state of our knowledge it is impossible to explain the mysterious behavior of the contagion." Basically this is still true. Corstvet (15) reported fecal shedding of the organism in a few birds up to 41 days postinoculation. In other experiments the organism was found to persist in blood for several weeks postinoculation (19). The organism can survive in soil (8, 74), which probably serves as a source of the organism. Though soil is known to harbor the organism for long periods under certain conditions, and swine and sheep as well as various species of wildlife can harbor the organism, no clear-cut relationship has been established between presence of infection in prior years among the same species (e.g., turkeys) and subsequent outbreaks among flocks (55).

Natural and Experimental Hosts. The organism has been isolated from turkeys, chickens, ducks, geese, mud hens, eared grebes, parrots, sparrows, canaries, finches, thrushes, blackbirds, doves, quail, wild mallards, white storks, herring gulls, golden eagles, pheasant, starlings, peacocks, parakeets, swine, sheep, cattle, marine and freshwater fish, various captive wild birds and mammals, chipmunks, meadow and house mice, dolphins, and crocodiles (6, 8, 74, 23, 27, 35, 36, 38, 41). From the reports it appears the susceptibilities of various avian populations differ. Genetic resistance may play a role in susceptibility to disease based on a report of an outbreak in turkeys with different genetic background (58).

Experimental hosts include the pigeon, turkey, chicken, budgerigar, mouse, and rat (8, 25, 26).

Transmission, Carriers, Vectors. The actual portal of entry and pathogenesis of *E. rhusiopathiae* infection in birds (and in animals other than humans) has not been definitely established. Contaminated material as the source of infection and entry through breaks in the mucous membranes or skin have been suggested.

Cannibalism and fighting among birds apparently result in increased losses. Permitting carcasses of infected dead birds to remain on the premises to be picked at or eaten by penmates also increases the spread and increases losses at unpredictable rates.

Experimentally, Corstvet (15) obtained up to 50% mortality in turkeys by oral inoculation of freshly isolated virulent organisms grown in chicken embryo yolk sac. Broth culture instilled orally, intranasally, or into the conjunctival sac (without damaging the membrane) was not infectious (29). Corstvet (15) and Bricker and Saif (11) found subcutaneous (SC) inoculation of virulent cultures resulted in local multiplication followed by septicemia, with 80–100% mortality in susceptible turkeys.

Sadler and Corstvet (57) and Corstvet et al. (19) showed that a few turkeys infected subcutaneously remained carriers for variable periods. Asymptomatic carriers of *E. rhusiopathiae* could not be detected before or after necropsy. The number of organisms used to challenge turkeys, route of inoculation (oral or parenteral), administration of antibiotics, time after vaccination and challenge, and age of the turkey apparently did not influence this carrier state, which is produced in very few birds. Isolations of *E. rhusiopathiae* from carriers are most frequent from cecal tonsils, liver, large intestine, heart, and blood (17, 19, 57). Xu et al. (75) reported a total of 95 isolates obtained from the pharynx of healthy chickens, ducks, and geese.

The role of vectors in transmission is not known. Wellmann (67) found that this pathogen could be transmitted mechanically from sick mice to pigeons by the stable fly, horse fly, mosquito, and other biting flies.

An outbreak of erysipelas in chickens in England was reported by Hall (30). Some pullets escaped from their pen, gained access to an area contaminated 8 yr previously with feces from pigs with erysipelas, and were returned to the same pens. Only chickens in these pens were affected; confined pullets not so exposed remained healthy.

Madsen (42) suggested that rain washing contaminated feces from a sheep corral initiated an outbreak in turkeys on range. Polner et al. (53) reported an outbreak in geese that had access to several hundred acres of pasture, which was the initial site of a demolished pig farm and had been used for 5 yr for fattening sheep prior to the outbreak. Fish meal and fish in general have been cited as probable sources of infection for avian species (8, 29, 47).

Incubation Period. In natural outbreaks the incubation period cannot be readily ascertained. Experimental SC inoculation of turkeys with 10^4–10^6 organisms usually kills most of them in 44–70 hr; a few may die after 96–120 hr. With oral exposure, signs of disease generally occur 2–3 days later than with SC inoculation and with a lower death rate. Occasionally a turkey dies 2–3 wk after oral exposure. A SC inoculum of 10^2 instead of 10^4 or 10^6 organisms delays clinical signs by about 24 hr. Incubation period does not seem to vary among turkeys 7, 12, 16, and 20 wk of age or between sexes.

Signs

TURKEYS. Outbreaks usually start suddenly, with losses of one to several birds; owners may suspect that deaths are from poisoning, stampede injuries, or predators. A few droopy birds (especially toms) may be noticed, but these individuals are usually easily aroused. Just prior to death some birds may be very droopy, with unsteady gait. Some may have cutaneous lesions; affected males may have swollen, discolored turgid snoods (fleshy tubular appendage on dorsal surface of head) and dewlaps (Fig. 10.1). Some turkeys are now "desnooded" shortly after hatching; as a result snood lesions are less frequently seen. Gradual emaciation, weakness, and signs of anemia occur in some cases where endocarditis is the cause of death; other turkeys with vegetations (especially vaccinated birds) may die suddenly without signs, probably as a result of emboli. Sudden losses of hens 4–5 days after artificial insemina-

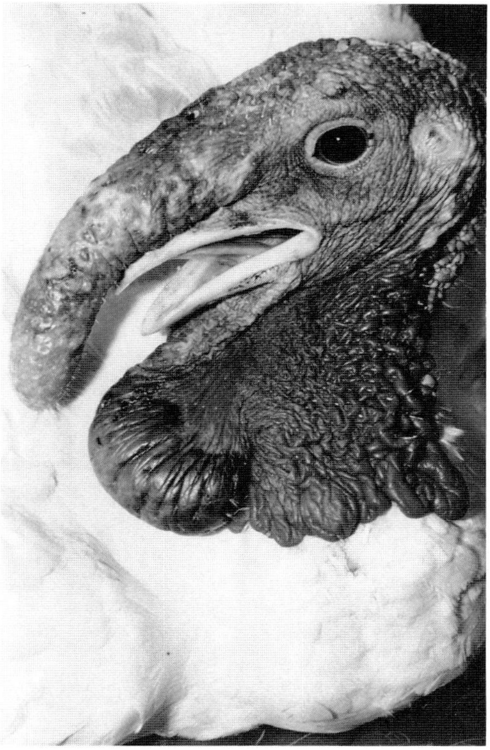

10.1. Turkey with erysipelas. Snood and dewlap are swollen; there is an infarct along dewlap margin, sharply demarcated firm adjacent, viable tissue. (Barnes)

tion with peritonitis, perineal congestion, and skin discoloration have been reported.

OTHER BIRDS. Main clinical signs in chickens are general weakness, depression, diarrhea, and sudden death. In laying chickens, egg production may be decreased. However, Kilian et al. (38) reported no immediate drop in egg production in laying pullets, although signs were evident; later there was about a 50–70% drop. Affected ducks, geese, pheasant, and quail generally are depressed, have diarrhea, and die suddenly.

Morbidity and Mortality. Morbidity and mortality are frequently about the same in unvaccinated turkeys. In other species of poultry, morbidity and mortality rates are also approximately equal since most sick birds die. However, in immunized flocks, some birds may be depressed and recover. Both morbidity and mortality vary from sickness or death of occasional birds in good condition to sudden loss of several within 24–48 hr. Mortality ranges from much less than 1% to as high as 25–50% of a given group, though adjacent groups may not be affected. Mortality ranges could vary due to prior immunization or early treatment. Mortality rates vary among different avian species.

Gross Lesions. In natural outbreaks, lesions are suggestive of generalized septicemia. The following lesions have been observed in different outbreaks in turkeys: generalized congestion; degeneration of fat on the anterior edge of the thigh; degeneration and hemorrhage in pericardial fat; petechial hemorrhage in abdominal fat; hemorrhage in heart muscle; and a friable, enlarged, and possibly mottled liver, spleen, and usually kidney. Other gross lesions may be fibrinopurulent exudate in joints and pericardial sac, fibrin plaques on heart muscle, thickening of the proventriculus and gizzard wall with ulceration, small yellow nodules in ceca, catarrhal or sanguinocatarrhal enteritis, vegetative endocarditis, dark crusty skin lesions, a turgid irregular reddish-purple snood in toms, hydropericardium, and distended visceral blood vessels (55). Other lesions noted with varying frequency in field outbreaks were diffuse skin reddening and a dirty brick red muscle color. Some birds, which died, had no lesions other than slight catarrhal enteritis and petechiae in heart fat.

In experimental infections, lesions observed in natural outbreaks are seen except endocarditis, which is rare in experimentally infected birds unless previously vaccinated. In some field cases and in birds vaccinated twice or more with bacterin and intravenously challenged, congestive heart failure with vegetations of the atrioventricular valves (sometimes extending as much as 7 cm into the aorta) have been found. Asymptomatic carrier turkeys are usually free of gross lesions.

In at least two field outbreaks in laying hens, lesions in endocardium, joints, and skin were not observed (6). In ducks, geese, and pheasants, lesions are similar to those of other avian species, with addition of dark congested areas in foot webs of ducks.

Histopathology. Generally, histopathologic features of acute erysipelas in turkeys reflect gross findings, and specific cellular alterations are those expected in septicemic infections (5). Vascular changes dominate with generalized engorgement of blood vessels and sinusoidal channels in virtually all organs. While there may be a strong central (cardiac or vasomotor) basis for vascular congestion, there is also evidence of direct vascular damage. Intravascular aggregations of bacteria, accompanied by fibrin thrombi, are frequent in capillaries, sinusoids, and venules. Overt hyalinization of walls of affected vessels is common. Edema and hemorrhage, especially prominent in lung and heart (Fig. 10.2), provide additional evidence of severe vascular damage. In

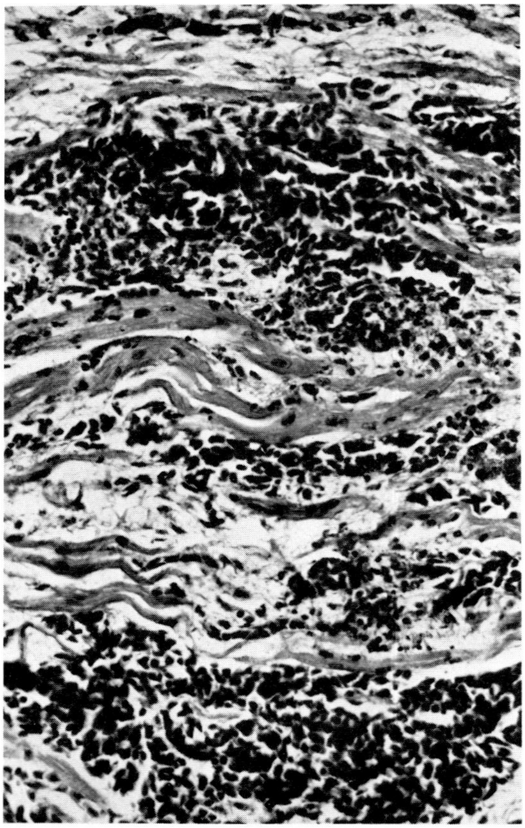

10.2. Acute erysipelas, turkey heart. Interstitial hemorrhages and separation of myocardial fibers (edema). H & E, ×100.

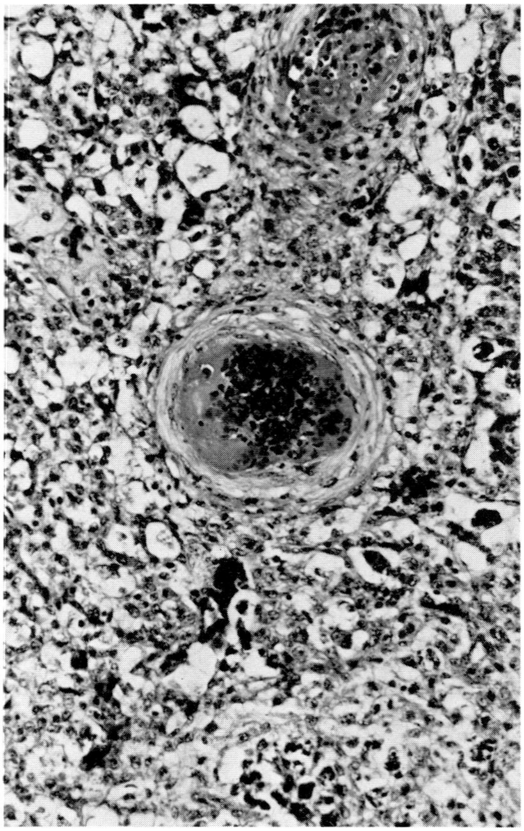

10.3. Acute erysipelas, turkey liver. Fibrin thrombus containing bacterial aggregates in the central portal blood vessel. Severe vacuolar degeneration of surrounding hepatocytes and several large basophilic sinusoidal, reticuloendothelial (Kupffer) cells are evident. H & E, ×100.

addition, rounding up of vascular endothelial cells and reticuloendothelial (RE) cells of sinusoids is a consistent histologic finding. Engulfed bacteria are readily demonstrated in RE cells in liver and spleen.

Damage to parenchymal cells is generalized in acute erysipelas, especially in liver, spleen, and kidney. Changes in hepatic cells range from cloudy swelling with cellular dissociation to overt coagulative necrosis. Focal or massive necrosis, apparently related to thrombosis of major portal vessels, is seen occasionally, but diffuse degenerative changes are more common (Fig. 10.3). In spleen, the earliest change is necrosis and lysis of lymphoid elements, which progresses to nearly total loss of lymphocytes, with hyalinization of sheathed arteries of white pulp and necrosis of surrounding reticular elements (Fig. 10.4). Epithelium of proximal renal tubules undergoes early degenerative change in affected turkeys characterized by swelling, dissociation, and separation from the basement membrane; overt coagulative necrosis is rare (5, 63). It is not unusual to find degenerative changes or necrosis in other organs (lung, heart, pancreas, gastrointestinal tract, skeletal muscle, and skin), however, these are less remarkable or frequent as changes in liver, spleen, and kidney. Regardless of site of involvement, hemorrhage and fibrin deposition frequently accompany parenchymal necrosis.

The cellular inflammatory component of peracute or acute erysipelas lesions is minimal. In scarified skin of turkeys infected by this route there may be extensive heterophil infiltration, congestion, edema, and necrosis. Cellular inflammatory response as judged from examination of field cases is more prominent in turkeys with subacute or chronic disease. Heterophil and mononuclear leukocytic infiltration, as well as proliferation of RE cells, can be found around necrotic lesions in liver, spleen, heart valves, and synovial membranes of joints. The pathology of experimentally induced subacute or chronic erysipelas in turkeys has not been reported.

In acute erysipelas in chickens, histopathologic

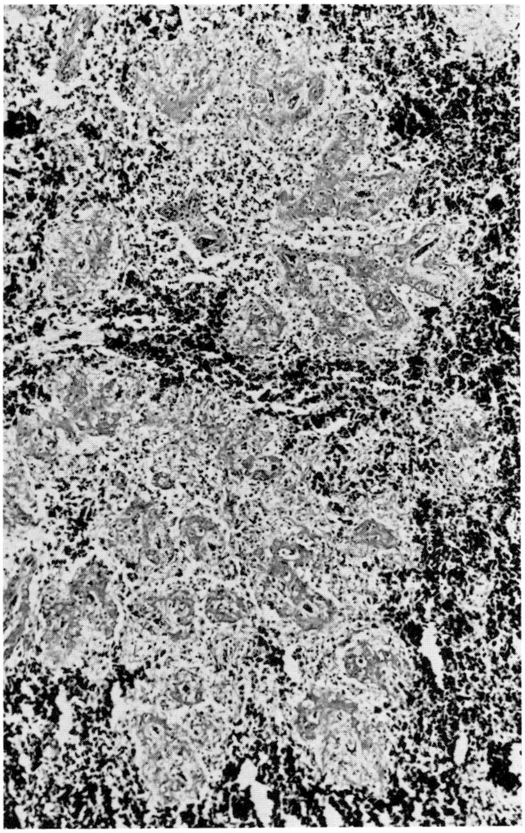

10.4. Acute erysipelas, turkey spleen. Hyalinized sheathed arteries within two malpighian corpuscles and nearly total depletion of lymphocytes are evident. Surrounding sinusoids are engorged with erythrocytes. H & E, ×100.

alterations were similar to those described for turkeys (6).

Immunity

ACTIVE. Birds recovered from acute infections have a high degree of resistance to reinfection and death. Killed bacterins, the current commercially available immunoprophylactic agent for immunization of turkeys against erysipelas, will prevent disease under both experimental and field conditions. Bacterin, in conjunction with penicillin at the beginning of an outbreak, will usually control losses. Long-lasting immunity is not achieved by single bacterin injection in turkeys. The immune response is improved when two or more doses are given at intervals of at least 2–4 wk. Experiments with 4- to 7-wk-old turkeys have shown a decline in protective immunity 4–5 wk postvaccination.

Krasnodebska-Depta and Janowska (39) reported that 28- and 30-wk-old turkeys vaccinated with a bacterin made for swine were resistant to challenge 2 mo postvaccination. Aerosol immunization of ducks with an erysipelas vaccine has been reported to be highly effective in eliminating the disease (46).

Osebold (50) reported limited protection with a live vaccine strain when administered subcutaneously to turkeys followed by subsequent challenge with a virulent strain. Bricker and Saif (11) reported on an effective level of protection in turkeys vaccinated through the drinking water with a live serotype 1a strain of *E. rhusiopathiae* followed by challenge with the homologous serotype. Two vaccine doses, administered 2–3 wk apart, were necessary to induce a sufficient protective response that lasted at least 3 wk following administration of the second vaccine dose. Administration of this live vaccine directly into the esophagus of turkeys did not induce a protective immune response. It is speculated that lymphoid tissue in the pharyngeal region plays a role in induction of an immune response to organisms introduced by the drinking water route.

PASSIVE. Treatment with swine erysipelas antiserum (horse origin) alone is said to be of some value if administered early, but it is not practical because of expense and lack of uniform efficacy. Antiserum and penicillin have been successfully used in ducks (54).

DIAGNOSIS

Isolation and Identification of Causative Agent. Sudden losses of adolescent turkeys in good flesh but with septicemic lesions, intramuscular and subpleural ecchymotic and suffusion hemorrhages, and erysipeloid swelling of the snood are indicative of erysipelas. Also significant is a marked hemorrhagic condition of skin and facial and muscular tissues of the breast. In many cases, predominant losses will be in males, but in breeding flocks, sudden losses in hens with peritonitis and subcutaneous and cutaneous discoloration following insemination suggest *E. rhusiopathiae* infection. Diagnosis is further validated by procedures described below and by Corstvet (16).

Confirmation of erysipelas depends on demonstration and identification of *E. rhusiopathiae.* A rapid presumptive diagnosis can be made by the presence of clumps and segregated gram-positive, beaded, slender, pleomorphic rods in liver, spleen, or heart blood or bone marrow smears. Particularly helpful with decomposed specimens are bone marrow cultures and smears.

Isolation of *E. rhusiopathiae* from sick birds that are killed and then cultured is neither as easy nor as frequently positive as culturing liver, spleen, or bone marrow from dead birds. Isolation from endocardial tissues is facilitated by finely mincing lesions before inoculating enrichment broth. Detecting the organism from a carrier requires multiple samples from various tissues.

Useful inhibitory media include sodium azide–crystal violet medium (51) and tryptose phosphate broth medium with 5% horse serum plus kanamycin, neomycin, vancomycin, and novobiocin (71). These media, while satisfactory, do not completely prevent growth of other organisms (particularly samples of intestinal contents) and may inhibit growth of some strains of *E. rhusiopathiae* (10). For primary isolation, recovery is facilitated by inoculating biplates containing 5% blood agar and sodium azide–crystal violet medium, followed by incubation in an atmosphere of 5–10% CO_2 or reduced oxygen. Ordinary atmosphere is suitable after a few passages on artificial media. Typical colonies composed of gram-positive rods should be selected and placed in triple-sugar iron (TSI) agar or Kligler's lead acetate medium and incubated for 24 hr at 37 C. An excellent presumptive test for *E. rhusiopathiae* is a blackening (due to H_2S production) before there is a noticeable change in the medium color.

The mouse, pigeon, or budgerigar may be used for a confirmatory protection test using erysipelas antiserum (the *E. rhusiopathiae* isolate, however, must be pathogenic for the test species chosen). One group of experimental animals is inoculated parenterally with a 24-hr culture of the isolate; another is inoculated with *E. rhusiopathiae* antiserum and immediately thereafter with the isolate. The unprotected group should die within 4 days, whereas animals receiving antiserum will live. *E. rhusiopathiae* may be detected in tissues using the fluorescent antibody technique (44, 48), which may also be used as a confirmatory test in diagnosis (16).

Serology. Information regarding the nature of immunity induced in turkeys following natural exposure to *E. rhusiopathiae* or to erysipelas vaccines is scarce. Infected birds that recover appear to be solidly immune. Plate, tube, and microagglutination tests, in addition to passive hemagglutination, hemagglutination-inhibition, complement-fixation, growth agglutination, and growth inhibition tests have been used in swine erysipelas research, but their usefulness for avian erysipelas has not been fully studied. Agglutination titers have been reported to be usually 160 or higher in antibiotic-treated recovered turkeys and turkeys that are carriers for the organism. Sikes and Tumlin (59), however, suggested that titers of 40 or greater are indicative of *E. rhusiopathiae* infection in turkeys. Currently, it is not known whether one particular serotype or strain of the organism is effective in detecting antibodies to other serologic types or strains of *E. rhusiopathiae*. At the present time, these tests are mainly useful for research studies only.

Differential Diagnosis. Fowl cholera, *E. coli* infections, salmonellosis, and peracute Newcastle disease might be confused with the acute septicemic form of the disease (16). The less common forms of the disease (urticaria and endocarditis) may be caused by other miscellaneous bacterial agents or possibly fungal pathogens. All the above mentioned agents are easily differentiated from *E. rhusiopathiae* by gram staining or biochemical activity. *Lactobacillus* sp., which may occasionally be isolated from intestinal tracts or livers of poultry and is biochemically similar to *Erysipelothrix,* may be differentiated using the highly selective Packer's medium containing sodium azide and crystal violet. Gram staining, growth on Packer's medium, and the typical reaction pattern in TSI medium or Kligler's lead acetate medium are excellent presumptive tests. Confirmatory diagnosis is by fluorescent antibody test or animal pathogenicity tests.

TREATMENT. The antibiotic of choice for an outbreak in market or breeder turkeys is a rapid-acting form of penicillin. Any antibiotic should be used under veterinary supervision according to current treatment procedure. Label directions should be followed carefully. As soon as diagnosis is definitely established, potassium or sodium penicillin should be administered intramuscularly at the rate of about 10^4 units/lb body weight simultaneously with a full dose of erysipelas bacterin. Control has usually been attained by giving penicillin (10^6 units/gal) in drinking water for 4 or 5 days to all birds in the flock when a presumptive diagnosis is made. All birds in the affected flock should be treated. Some recommendations suggest use of procaine penicillin or other longer-acting derivatives; under certain circumstances these may be used successfully, but in outbreaks, rapid-acting formulations are almost mandatory. A combination of longer-acting and rapid-acting antibiotic formulations may provide best control if individual SC or intramuscular (IM) injection is feasible and cost effective. However, especially in meat-bird flocks, catching and handling each bird may be impractical or even harmful. Sterile abscesses and downgrading may follow IM injections.

Care should be taken to observe required withdrawal periods for the antibiotic used. Turkeys, and possibly other birds with advanced signs of the disease at treatment, often will not recover.

Experimental use of certain antibiotics, including penicillin, will control the infection but not eliminate carriers. Antibiotics other than penicillin may increase carriers in a flock of turkeys (18).

Comparative studies are lacking on efficacy of various antibiotics for controlling *E. rhusiopathiae* infection in avian populations. Erythromycin and broad-spectrum antibiotics have been found effective. In vitro studies have shown the organism to be resistant to neomycin (24). Sulfonamides and oral oxytetracycline are not effective treatments.

Beneficial management practices in handling an outbreak of erysipelas in turkeys include thorough decontamination of equipment, prompt removal of dead birds and other carrion from premises, encouraging adequate feed and water intake, and handling birds as little and as gently as possible or practical. If unlimited range is available, it might be desirable to move the flock to clean ground, but such a practice may contaminate the new range.

PREVENTION AND CONTROL

Management Procedures. It has been suggested, though not established, that various environmental factors may make avian species more susceptible to *E. rhusiopathiae* infection. Field observations suggest that the beginning of rainy, cold weather, which frequently coincides with sexual maturity, is related to outbreaks of erysipelas in turkeys; this may also apply to flocks of other avian species. Source of the organism may be contaminated feed, soil, or decaying matter; infected carrier birds in the flock; or infected rodents. Apparently, the relationship between environmental factors and disease does not apply to cases involving individually confined birds, as in a zoo.

It is impossible to make clear-cut and specific recommendations for preventive or control management. A general suggestion is to use clean, disinfected equipment and rotate turkey ranges away from previously contaminated areas. Certain disinfectants, notably 1–2% sodium hydroxide (lye) solutions, are effective against *E. rhusiopathiae;* phenols, cresols and related disinfectants, iodine, and certain household soaps are moderately effective (31).

With no specific and effective recommendations for management control of this disease in turkeys, it is recommended that birds be properly immunized in areas where erysipelas is known to occur.

Immunization. The current immunoprophylactic agent for immunization of turkeys against erysipelas is the formalin-inactivated, aluminum hydroxide–adsorbed, whole-cell *E. rhusiopathiae* bacterin. These bacterins were initially developed for use in swine but were also shown to be effective in preventing erysipelas in turkeys (1, 2, 14). Only certain strains of *E. rhusiopathiae* belonging to serotype 2, however, have been effective for use in bacterins. These strains are highly immunogenic because they produce a "soluble immunizing substance" that is released when the organism is grown in a complex medium containing serum (62). This soluble immunizing substance is adsorbed and precipitated by aluminum hydroxide, which also adsorbs whole cells. Presence of this soluble substance is considered necessary for production of an effective bacterin. For more details on the protective antigen, see White and Verwey (70) and Rothe (56).

A regimen of immunization can be suggested for meat turkeys and breeder hens. In areas of high risk, a single dose of bacterin given subcutaneously at the dorsal surface of the neck behind the atlas should be given to meat turkeys. The original investigation and demonstration of efficacy were based on intramuscular injection of bacterin; however, because of the possibility of sterile abscesses (with downgrading at slaughter), SC inoculation is now used. For turkey breeders, at least two doses of bacterin given 4 wk apart, should be administered prior to onset of egg production. The first dose may be given at 16–20 wk of age (at selection time) and an additional dose (2 ml/hen, 4 ml/tom) just prior to beginning of lay.

Since the disease is sporadic in other avian species, immunization is not generally recommended for them. Effective immunization of mice or swine is not an adequate demonstration of the ability of a bacterin to protect turkeys. Cultures avirulent for turkeys and without immunogenicity for them may kill mice or provide protection. Immunizing capacity for turkeys can be properly assessed only with challenge of vaccinated turkeys.

Though live erysipelas vaccines for swine have been around for over 30 yr, little information is available on their usefulness in turkeys. Osebold et al. (50) reported limited success after administration of a live culture vaccine subcutaneously to 9-mo-old turkeys followed by challenge with a virulent *E. rhusiopathiae* isolate 3 mo later. Experimentally, Bricker and Saif (11) demonstrated protection in turkeys vaccinated via the drinking water with a live type 1a erysipelas vaccine licensed for use in swine. At least two vaccine treatments consisting of two doses each (4×10^9 organisms/dose) administered 2–3 wk apart induced significant protection in vaccinates following challenge with the homologous serotype. An oral vaccine for erysipelas in turkeys would be advantageous because of its ease of administration and elimination of the need to handle individual birds, which may induce stress.

Improved vaccines, properly used, adequate testing of the biologicals, planned immunization programs based on flock and premise history, and proper diagnosis of disease outbreaks as a basis for prompt treatment must be combined for effective prevention of erysipelas.

REFERENCES

1. Adler, H.E., and M.A. Nilson. 1952. Immunization of turkeys against swine erysipelas with several types of bacterins. Can J Comp Med Vet Sci 16:390–393.

2. Adler, H.E., and G.R. Spencer. 1952. Immunization

of turkeys and pigs with an erysipelas bacterin. Cornell Vet 42:238–246.

3. Barber, M. 1939. A comparative study of Listerella and Erysipelothrix. J Pathol Bacteriol 48:11–23.

4. Beaudette, F.R., and C.B. Hudson. 1936. An outbreak of acute swine erysipelas infection in turkeys. J Am Vet Med Assoc 88:475–488.

5. Bickford, A.A., R.E. Corstvet, and A.S. Rosenwald. 1978. Pathology of experimental erysipelas in turkeys. Avian Dis 22:503–518.

6. Bisgaard, M., and P. Olsen. 1975. Erysipelas in egg-laying chickens: Clinical, pathological, and bacteriological investigations. Avian Pathol 4:59–71.

7. Bisgaard, M., V. Nørrung, and N. Tornme. 1980. Erysipelas in poultry. Prevalence of serotypes and epidemiological investigations. Avian Pathol 9:355–362.

8. Blackmore, D.K., and G.L. Gallagher. 1964. An outbreak of erysipelas in captive wild birds and mammals. Vet Rec 76:1161–1164.

9. Boyer, C.I., Jr., and J.A. Brown. 1957. Studies on erysipelas in turkeys. Avian Dis 1:42–52.

10. Bratberg, A.M. 1981. Observations on the utilization of a selective medium for the isolation of Erysipelothrix rhusiopathiae. Acta Vet Scand 22:55–59.

11. Bricker, J.M., and Y.M. Saif. 1988. Use of a live oral vaccine to immunize turkeys against erysipelas. Avian Dis 32:668–673.

12. Buchanan, R.E., and N.E. Gibbons. 1974. Bergey's Manual of Determinative Bacteriology, 8th Ed., p. 597. Williams & Wilkins, Baltimore, MD.

13. Butcher, G., and B. Panigrahy. 1985. An outbreak of erysipelas in chukars. Avian Dis 29:843–845.

14. Cooper, M.S., G.R. Personeus, and B.R. Choman. 1954. Laboratory studies on the vaccination of mice and turkeys with an Erysipelothrix rhusiopathiae vaccine. Can J Comp Med Vet Sci 18:83–92.

15. Corstvet, R.E. 1967. Pathogenesis of Erysipelothrix insidiosa in the turkey. Poultry Sci 46:1247. (Abstr).

16. Corstvet, R.E. 1980. Erysipelas. In S.B. Hitchner, C.H. Domermuth, H.G. Purchase, and J.E. Williams (eds.), Isolation and Identification of Avian Pathogens, pp. 23–26. Am Assoc Avian Pathol, Kennett Square, PA.

17. Corstvet, R.E., and C.H. Holmberg. 1968. The carrier state of Erysipelothrix insidiosa in turkeys. Poultry Sci 47:1662.

18. Corstvet, R.E., and C. Howard. 1974. Evaluation of certain antibiotics in relation to the carrier state of Erysipelothrix rhusiopathiae (insidiosa) in turkeys. J Am Vet Med 165:744.

19. Corstvet, R.E., C.A. Holmberg, and J.K. Riley. 1970. 14th Congr Mund Avic Commun Sci 3:149–158.

20. Cross, G.M.J., and P.D. Claxton. 1979. Serological classification of Australian strains of Erysipelothrix rhusiopathiae isolated from pigs, sheep, turkeys, and man. Aust Vet J 55:77–81.

21. Dhillon, A.S., R.W. Winterfield, H.L. Thacker, and J.A. Richardson. 1980. Erysipelas in domestic White Pekin ducks. Avian Dis 24:784–787.

22. Dickinson, E.M., A.C. Jerstad, H.E. Adler, M. Cooper, W.E. Babcock, E.E. Johns, and C.A. Bottorff. 1953. The use of an Erysipelothrix rhusiopathiae bacterin for the control of erysipelas in turkeys. Proc 90th Annu Meet Am Vet Med Assoc, pp. 370–375.

23. Faddoul, G.P., G.W. Fellows, and J. Baird. 1968. Erysipelothrix infection in starlings. Avian Dis 12:61–66.

24. Fuzi, M. 1963. A neomycin sensitivity test for the rapid differentiation of Listeria monocytogenes and Erysipelothrix rhusiopathiae. J Pathol Bacteriol 85:524–525.

25. Geissinger, H.D. 1968. Acute and chronic Erysipelothrix rhusiopathiae infection in rats. Zentralbl Veterinaermed [B] 15:392–405.

26. Geissinger, H.D. 1968. Acute and chronic Erysipelothrix rhusiopathiae infection in white mice. J Comp Pathol Ther 78:79–88.

27. Geraci, J.R., R.M. Sauer, and W. Medway. 1966. Erysipelas in dolphins. Am J Vet Res 27:597–606.

28. Graham, R., N.D. Levine, and H.R. Hester. 1939. Erysipelothrix rhusiopathiae associated with a fatal disease in ducks. J Am Vet Med Assoc 95:211–216.

29. Grenci, C.M. 1943. The isolation of Erysipelothrix rhusiopathiae and experimental infection of turkeys. Cornell Vet 33:56–60.

30. Hall, S.A. 1963. A disease in pullets due to Erysipelothrix rhusiopathiae. Vet Rec 75:333–334.

31. Hinshaw, W.R. 1965. Erysipelas. In H.E. Biester and L.H. Schwarte (eds.), Diseases of Poultry, 5th Ed., pp. 1271–1276. Iowa State Univ Press, Ames.

32. Hudson, C.B. 1949. Erysipelothrix rhusiopathiae infection in fowl. J Am Vet Med Assoc 115:36–39.

33. Hudson, C.B., J.J. Black, J.A. Bivins, and D.C. Tudor. 1952. Outbreaks of Erysipelothrix rhusiopathiae infection in fowl. J Am Vet Med Assoc 121:278–284.

34. Iliadis, N., T. Tsangaris, H. Kaldrymidou, and S. Lekas. 1983. Experimentelle infektion mit Erysipelothrix insidiosa bei puten und tauben. Wien Tierärztl Monatsschr 70:282–285.

35. Jasmin, A.M., and J. Baucom. 1967. Erysipelothrix insidiosa infections in the caiman (Caiman crocodilus) and the American crocodile (Crocodilus acutus). Am J Vet Clin Pathol 1:173–177.

36. Jensen, W.I., and S.E. Cotter. 1976. An outbreak of erysipelas in eared grebes (Podiceps nigricollis). J Wildl Dis 12:583–86.

37. Kalf, G.F., and T.G. White. 1963. The antigenic components of Erysipelothrix rhusiopathiae. II. Purification and chemical characterization of a type-specific antigen. Arch Biochem 102:39–47.

38. Kilian, J.G., W.E. Babcock, and E.M. Dickinson. 1958. Two cases of Erysipelothrix rhusiopathiae infection in chickens. J Am Vet Med Assoc 133:560–562.

39. Krasnodebska-Depta, A., and I. Janowska. 1980. Wlasciwosci immunogenne niektorych szczepow wloskowca rozycy dla indikow. Med Weter 36:331–33. (Abstr Vet Bull 51:81).

40. Kuscera, G. 1973. Proposal for standardization of the designations used for serotypes of Erysipelothrix rhusiopathiae (Migula) Buchanan. Int J Syst Bacteriol 23:184–188.

41. Levine, N.D. 1965. Erysipelas. In H.E. Biester and L.H. Schwarte (eds.), Diseases of Poultry, 5th Ed., pp. 461–469. Iowa State Univ Press, Ames.

42. Madsen, D.E. 1937. An erysipelas outbreak in turkeys. J Am Vet Med Assoc 91:206–208.

43. Malik, Z. 1962. Pokusy s experimentalnou vnimavostou kurciat voci mikrobe Erysipelothrix rhusiopathiae. Vet Cas 11:89–94.

44. Marshall, J.D., W.C. Eveland, and C.W. Smith. 1959. The identification of viable and nonviable Erysipelothrix insidiosa with fluorescent antibody. Am J Vet Res 20:1077–1080.

45. Müller, H.E. 1981. Neuraminidase and other enzymes of Erysipelothrix rhusiopathiae as possible pathogenic factors. In H. Deicher (ed.), Arthritis: Models and Mechanisms, pp. 58–67. Springer-Verlag, Berlin.

46. Müller, H.E., and G. Reetz. 1980. Die aerosolimmunislerung von enten mit spirovak-rotlauf-impfstoff "Dessau." Arch Exp Veterinaermed 34:55–57.

47. Murase N., K. Suzuki, and T. Nakahara. 1959. Studies on the typing of Erysipelothrix rhusiopathiae. II. Serological behaviours of the strains isolated from

fowls including those from cattle and humans. Jpn J Vet Sci 21:177-181.
48. Nelson, J.D., and S. Shelton. 1963. Immunofluorescent studies of Listeria monocytogenes and Erysipelothrix insidiosa. Application to clinical diagnosis. J Lab Clin Med 62:935-942.
49. Nørrung, V. 1970. Studies on Erysipelothrix insidiosa s. rhusiopathiae. I. Morphology, cultural features, biochemical reactions, and virulence. Acta Vet Scand 11:577-585.
50. Osebold, J.W., E.M. Dickinson, and W.E. Babcock. 1950. Immunization of turkeys against Erysipelothrix rhusiopathiae with avirulent live culture. Cornell Vet 40:387-391.
51. Packer, R.A. 1943. The use of sodium azide (NaN_3) and crystal violet in a selective medium for streptococci and Erysipelothrix rhusiopathiae. J Bacteriol 46:343-349.
52. Panigrahy, B., and C.F. Hall. 1977. An outbreak of erysipelas in coturnix quails. Avian Dis 21:708-710.
53. Polner, T., G. Cajdacs, F. Kemenes, G. Kucsera, and J. Durst. 1984. Stress effect of plucking as modulation of hosts' defence in birds. Ann Immunol Hung 23:211-224.
54. Reetz, G., and L. Schulze. 1978. Rotlaufinfektion bei mastenten. Monatsh Veterinaermed 33:170-173.
55. Rosenwald, A.S., and E.M. Dickinson. 1941. Swine erysipelas in turkeys. Am J Vet Res 2:202-213.
56. Rothe, F. 1982. Das protektive antigen des rotlaufbakteriums (Erysipelothrix rhusiopathiae). II. Mitteilung: die weitere charakterisierung des protektiven antigens. Arch Exp Vet Med 36:255-267.
57. Sadler, W.W., and R.E. Corstvet. 1965. The effect of Erysipelothrix insidiosa infection on wholesomeness of market turkeys. Am J Vet Res 26:1429-1436.
58. Saif, Y.M., K.E. Nestor, R.N. Dearth, and P.A. Renner. 1984. Possible genetic variation in resistance of turkeys to erysipelas and fowl cholera. Avian Dis 28:770-773.
59. Sikes, D., and T.J. Tumlin. 1967. Further studies on the Erysipelothrix insidiosa tube agglutination test. Am J Vet Res 28:1177-1181.
60. Silberstein, E.P. 1965. Erysipelothrix endocarditis. Report of a case with cerebral manifestations. J Am Med Assoc 191:862-864.
61. Smith, T. 1885. Second Annual Report of the Bureau of Animal Industry, p. 187. USDA, Washington, DC.
62. Traub, E. 1947. Immunisierung gegen schweinerotlauf mit konzentrierten adsorbatimpfstoffen. Monatch veterinaermed 2:165-172.
63. Tsangaris, T., N. Iliadis, E. Kaldrymidou, T. Lekkas, E. Tsiroyannis, and E. Artopios. 1980. Experimenteller rotlauf der tuten nach sintravenöser infection mit Erysipelothrix insidiosa I elektronen-mikroskopische befunde inden nieren. Zentralbl Veterinaermed [B] 27:705-13.
64. Vaissaire, J., P. Desmettre, G. Paille, G. Mirial, and M. Laroche. 1985. Erysipelothrix rhusiopathiae: agent du rouget dans les differentes especes animales. Donn-es actuelles. Bull Acad Vet Fr 58:259-265.
65. Vallee, M. 1930. Sur l'etiologie du rouget. Rev Pathol Comp 30:857-858. (Abstr).
66. Van Es, L., and C.B. McGrath. 1936. Swine erysipelas. Nebraska Agric Exp Stn Res Bull 84:1-47.
67. Wellmann, G.G. 1950. The transmission of swine erysipelas by a variety of blood-sucking insects to pigeons. Zentralbl Bakteriol Parasitenkd Abt I Orig 155:109-115.
68. White, T.G., and G.F. Kalf. 1961. The antigenic components of Erysipelothrix rhusiopathiae. I. Isolation and serological identification. Arch Biochem 95:458-463.
69. White, T.G., and R.D. Shuman. 1961. Fermentation reactions of Erysipelothrix rhusiopathiae. J Bacteriol 82:595-599.
70. White, R.R., and W.F. Verwey. 1970. Isolation and characterization of a protective antigen-containing particle from culture supernatant fluids of Erysipelothrix rhusiopathiae. Infect Immun 1:380-386.
71. Wood, R.L. 1965. A selective liquid medium utilizing antibiotics for isolation of Erysipelothrix insidiosa. Am J Vet Res 26:1303-1308.
72. Wood, R.L. 1973. Survival of Erysipelothrix rhusiopathiae in soil under various environmental conditions. Cornell Vet 63:390-410.
73. Wood, R.L. 1986. Erysipelas. In A.D. Leman, R. Straw, R.D. Glock, W.L. Mengeling, R.H.C. Penny, and E. Scholl (eds.), Diseases of Swine, 6th Ed., p. 576. Iowa State Univ Press, Ames.
74. Woodbine, M. 1950. Erysipelothrix rhusiopathiae. Bacteriology and chemotherapy. Bacteriol Rev 14:161-178.
75. Xu, K.Q., X.F. Hu, C.H. Gao, Q.Y. Lu, and J.H. Wu. 1984. Studies on the serotypes and pathogenicity of Erysipelothrix rhusiopathiae isolated from swine and poultry. Chin J Vet Med 10:9-11.

11 CLOSTRIDIAL DISEASES

INTRODUCTION

Clostridial infections associated with four disease conditions in poultry or game birds are described in this chapter. *Clostridium colinum* is the cause of ulcerative enteritis, *C. perfringens* and *C. septicum* have been isolated from cases of necrotic enteritis or gangrenous dermatitis, and *C. botulinum* is the etiology of botulism. Toxins produced by the clostridial organisms are responsible for the pathology of some of these conditions; in other cases, the organisms are relatively innocuous unless there are cofactors such as coccidiosis or immunosuppressive infections. Infectious bursal disease and infection with the chicken anemia agent are examples of the latter.

ULCERATIVE ENTERITIS (QUAIL DISEASE)

H.A. Berkhoff

INTRODUCTION. Ulcerative enteritis (UE) is an acute bacterial infection in young chickens, poults, and upland game birds characterized by sudden onset and rapidly increasing mortality. The disease was first seen in enzootic proportions in quail and was therefore named "quail disease." It has since been established that many avian species other than quail are susceptible, and the species designation has been superseded by the term "ulcerative enteritis."

Infection of humans has not been reported.

HISTORY. One of the first to report quail disease in the USA was Morse (31). The next two decades yielded several scattered reports of outbreaks in quail and grouse (1, 17, 26, 27, 37). Infection in wild turkeys was reported by Shillinger and Morley (40), and Bullis and Van Roekel (11) first reported the disease in domestic poults. Other domestic birds found susceptible were pigeons (18, 35) and chickens (40, 45). Pheasants, blue grouse, and California quail were added to the list of susceptible game birds by Buss et al. (12).

Chronologic events leading to isolation and precise identification of the etiologic bacterium are detailed by Bass (2, 4), Peckham (32, 33), and Berkhoff et al. (8).

INCIDENCE AND DISTRIBUTION. Distribution of UE is worldwide; a number of reports have originated from England (19), Germany (39), and India (21, 41, 42).

UE is an important disease problem in some concentrated poultry-raising areas (10) and a threat to gamebirds either in confinement or in the wild.

ETIOLOGY. Morley and Wetmore (29) reported isolation of a bacterium from the liver of a diseased quail, with which they reproduced UE in quail. The organism was described as a gram-positive, pleomorphic, aerobic, nonmotile rod and named *Corynebacterium perdicum*. It did not grow on solid media, and grew poorly in fluid media. Upon subculture the organism quickly lost virulence.

Bass (3) described isolation of a gram-negative, anaerobic bacillus from intestine and liver of infected quail. He was able to reproduce the clinical syndrome by feeding quail thioglycolate broth cultures.

Peckham (32, 33) reported isolation of a gram-positive, anaerobic, spore-forming rod following yolk sac inoculation of chicken embryos. This organism produced UE lesions in inoculated quail. The anaerobe was reisolated from inoculated quail, fulfilling Koch's postulates. Peckham (33) reported isolation of a similar anaerobe from chickens and turkeys affected with UE and established that UE in chickens, turkeys, and quail was caused by the same organism. Berkhoff et al. (9) cultured the etiologic anaerobe on solid media, which allowed study of its biochemical characteristics for the first time.

Classification. The organism is a new species of *Clostridium* named *Clostridium colinum* (6, 9).

The author wishes to acknowledge Dr. M.C. Peckham for his previous contribution to this chapter.

Morphology and Staining. *C. colinum* is a 1 × 3–4 μm rod that occurs singly as a straight or slightly curved rod with rounded ends. Spores are subterminal and oval in shape (Fig. 11.1), but only a few strains readily form spores on usual media.

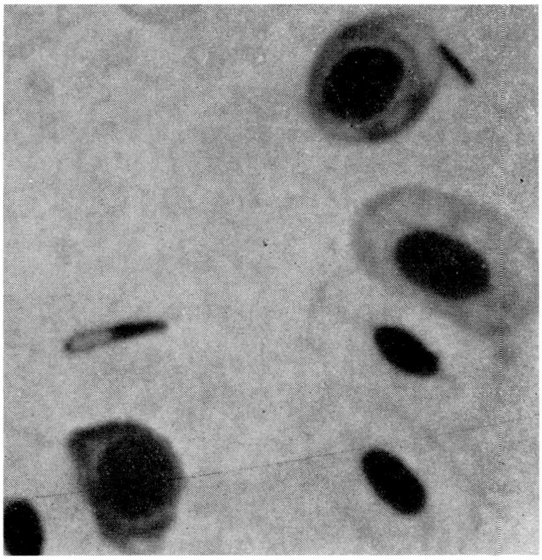

11.1. Blood smear from quail with UE. Note two bacteria, one of which has a subterminal spore. ×2700. (Peckham)

Growth Requirements. The organism is fastidious in its growth requirements, needing an enriched medium and anaerobic conditions. The best medium for isolating *C. colinum* is tryptose-phosphate agar (Difco) to which 0.2% glucose and 0.5% yeast extract are added. The pH is adjusted to 7.2 and the medium is then sterilized by autoclaving. After cooling to 56 C, 8% horse plasma is added, and the medium is poured into Petri dishes. Prereduced plates are inoculated with material from liver lesions and incubated anaerobically for 1–2 days (43). Optimum growth temperature is 35–42 C. Growth in broth media, prepared as above but without agar, can be detected as early as 12–16 hr postinoculation. Actively growing cultures produce gas. Gas production continues for no more than 6–8 hr, after which growth settles to the bottom of the tube (6). Subcultures should be made from actively growing broth cultures still producing gas; later transfers may be unsuccessful.

Biochemical Characteristics. The following carbohydrates are fermented: glucose, mannose, raffinose, sucrose, and trehalose. Fructose and maltose are weakly fermented. Mannitol is fermented only by some strains, one of which is type strain (ATCC 27770). Carbohydrates not fermented are: arabinose, cellobiose, erythritol, glycogen, inositol, lactose, melezitose, melibiose, rhamnose, sorbitol, and xylose. Fermentation products of this organism are acetic and formic acid (6, 9).

Esculin is hydrolyzed. Starch hydrolysis is usually negative; only two strains have been found to cause starch hydrolysis. The type strain does not hydrolyze starch. Nitrite and indole are not produced. Milk is unchanged and casein is not digested. Good growth occurs in Chopped Meat Carbohydrate (CMC) broth. Pyruvate and lactate are not utilized. Gelatin is not liquefied. Catalase, urease, lipase, and lecithinase are not produced.

Resistance to Chemical and Physical Agents. The anaerobe, by virtue of its spore-forming characteristic, is extremely resistant to chemical agents and physical changes. Spores of *C. colinum* are resistant to octanol and chloroform (9). Yolk cultures have remained viable after 16 yr at −20 C and survive heating at 70 C for 3 hr, 80 C for 1 hr, and 100 C for 3 min (33).

Pathogenicity. Berkhoff et al. (8) reported pure cultures of *C. colinum* grown anaerobically were highly pathogenic for quail when administered orally. The experimental disease appeared either in an acute form with birds dying around the 3rd day postinoculation, or in a more chronic form with deaths occurring after 1–2 wk.

PATHOGENESIS AND EPIZOOTIOLOGY

Natural and Experimental Hosts. UE is found in a wide range of avian hosts, but quail are undoubtedly among the most susceptible species. Natural infections have been found in the following: common bobwhite quail (*Colinus virginianus*), California quail (*Lophortyx california*), Gambel quail (*L. gambelii*), mountain quail (*Oreortyx picta*), scaled quail (*Callipepla squamata*), and sharp-tailed grouse (*Pedioecetes phasianellus*) (31); ruffed grouse (*Bonasa umbellus*) (27); domestic turkeys (*Meleagris gallopavo*) and chickens (*Gallus gallus*) (16, 40); European partridge (*Perdix perdix*) and wild turkeys (*M. gallopavo*) (16); chukar partridge (*Alectoris graeca*) (28); pigeons (*Columba livia*) (18); pheasants (*Phasianus colchicus*) and blue grouse (*Dendragapus obscurus*) (12); and crested quail (*L.c. californicus*) (19). Winterfield and Berkhoff (44) reported an outbreak of UE in robins (*Turdus migratorius*) and isolated *C. colinum* from the liver. This was the first evidence of UE in passerine birds.

Although chickens are frequently infected naturally, experimental infections can be readily produced only in quail. UE is more frequently seen in young birds. It occurs in chickens 4–12 wk (33), turkeys 3–8 wk (11), and quail 4–12 wk of age. An outbreak has been reported in adult quail (22).

Outbreaks in chickens often accompany or follow coccidiosis, aplastic anemia, infectious bursal disease, or stress conditions. The observation that coccidiosis and stress play an important role in outbreaks of UE in chickens was demonstrated by Davis (14), who was the first to produce UE in 5-wk-old chicks previously infected with *Eimeria brunetti* or *E. necatrix*. UE developed only in chicks with dual infection.

Transmission. Under natural conditions UE is transmitted through droppings; birds become infected by ingesting contaminated feed, water, or litter. The organism produces spores, resulting in permanent contamination of premises after an outbreak has occurred. Berkhoff et al. (9) showed that at least 10^7 viable cells of *C. colinum* administered orally were required to experimentally reproduce UE in quail.

The carrier status of recovered birds or survivors in a flock has not been critically studied. Morris (30) considered the chronic carrier to be one of the most important factors in perpetuation of UE and used a complement-fixation (CF) test to detect them.

Incubation Period. Following experimental infection in quail, the acute form of UE results in death within 1–3 days. The course of the disease in a flock lasts approximately 3 wk, with peak mortality occurring 5–14 days postinoculation.

Signs. Birds dying from acute disease may exhibit no premonitory signs. They are usually well muscled and fat and have feed in the crop. Quail often exhibit watery white droppings. As UE progresses, infected birds become listless and humped up, with eyes partly closed, and feathers dull and ruffled. Extreme emaciation with atrophy of pectoral muscles is seen in birds affected 1 wk or longer.

Morbidity and Mortality. Mortality in young quail may be as high as 100% in a matter of a few days. Chicken losses typically range from 2 to 10%.

Gross Lesions. Acute lesions in quail are characterized by marked hemorrhagic enteritis in the duodenum. Small punctate hemorrhages may be visible in the intestinal wall.

In birds that have survived infection for several days, inflammatory changes are followed by necrosis and ulceration, which may occur in any portion of the intestine and ceca (Fig. 11.2). Early lesions are characterized by small yellow foci with hemorrhagic borders, which may be seen on serosal and mucosal surfaces (Fig. 11.3C, D). As ulcers increase in size, the hemorrhagic border tends to disappear. Ulcers may be lenticular or roughly circular in outline, sometimes coalescing to form large necrotic diphtheritic patches. The lenticular shape is more common in the upper portion of the intestine. Ulcers may be deep in the mucosa; in older lesions they may be superficial and have raised edges (Fig. 11.4). Ulcers in ceca may have a central depression filled with dark-staining material that cannot be rinsed off. Perforation of ulcers frequently occurs, resulting in peritonitis and intestinal adhesions.

Liver lesions vary from light yellow mottling to large, irregular yellow areas along the edges (Fig. 11.3A). Other liver lesions are disseminated gray foci or small, yellow circumscribed foci, sometimes surrounded by a pale yellow halo. Spleen may be congested, enlarged, and hemorrhagic (Fig. 11.3B). Gross lesions are absent in other or-

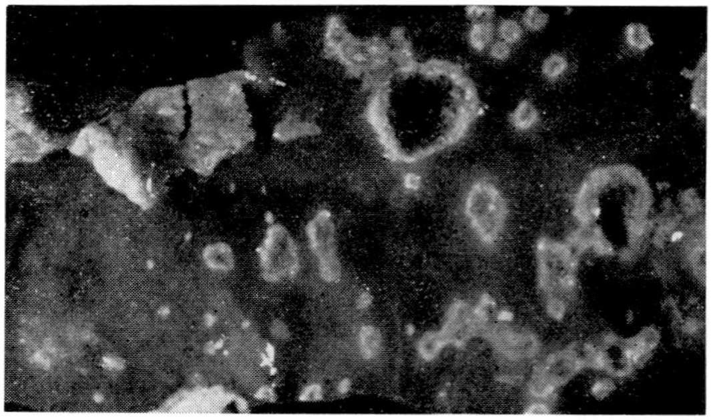

11.4. Craterlike ulcerations in intestines from natural case of UE in poult. (Peckham)

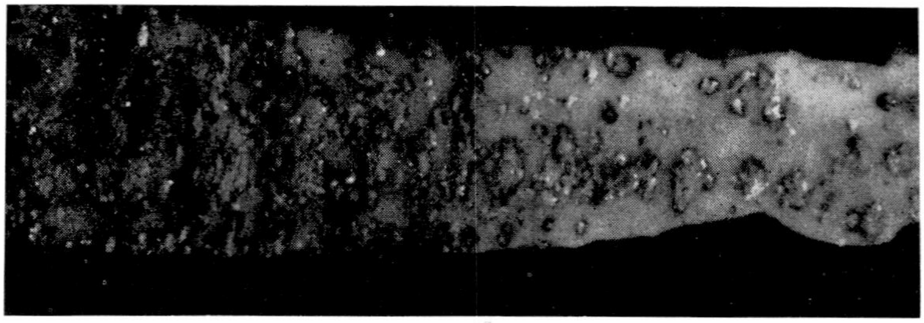

11.2. Ulceration of intestinal mucosa of chicken with UE. (Peckham)

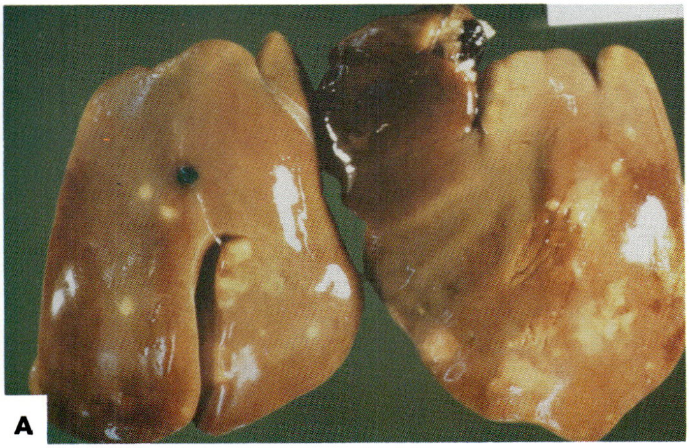

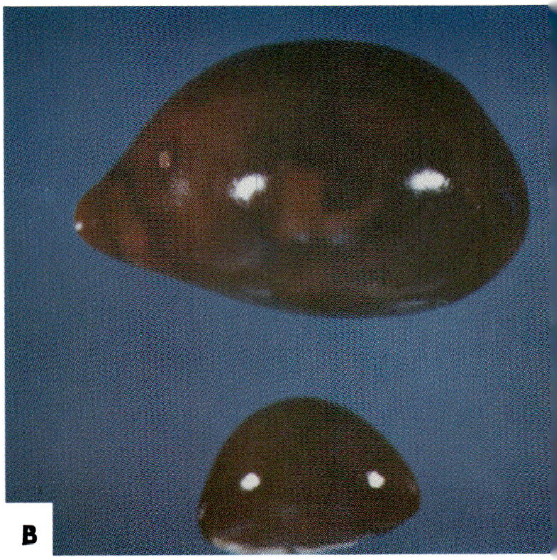

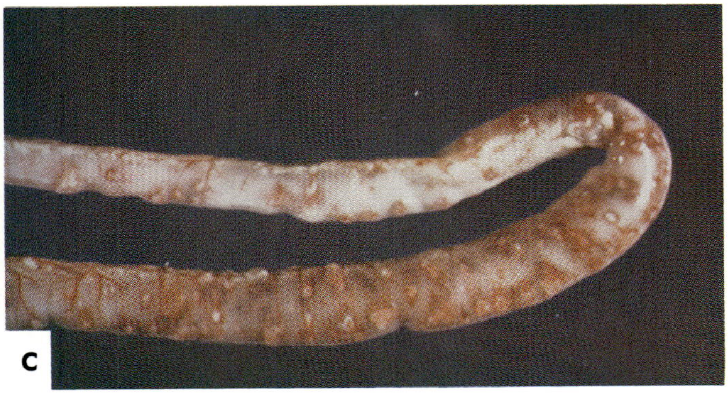

11.3. Lesions of UE. A. Focal areas of necrosis in chicken liver. B. Enlarged hemorrhagic and necrotic spleen compared to normal spleen below. C. Yellowish lenticular ulcers visible through serosal surface of intestine. D. Ulceration of intestinal mucosa of affected bird. (Peckham)

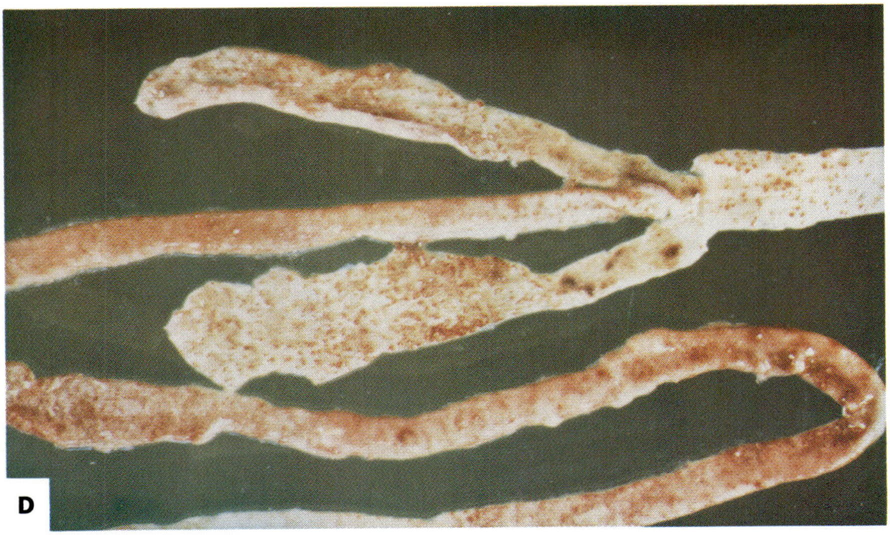

gans. Peckham (33) described an unusual lesion of UE in poults characterized by a necrotic diphtheritic membrane occupying the middle third of the intestine. This combination of necrosis and sloughing of intestinal mucosa appeared similar to lesions produced by *E. brunetti* infection in chickens.

Histopathology. For a description of the histopathology of UE in quail see Durant and Doll (16). Intestinal sections from acute cases reveal desquamation of mucosal epithelium, edema of intestinal wall, vascular engorgement, and lymphocytic infiltration. The lumen of the intestine contains desquamated epithelium, blood cells, and fragments of mucosa. Early ulcers resemble small hemorrhagic necrotizing areas involving villi and extending into the submucosa. Cells adjacent to these areas exhibit coagulation necrosis with karyolysis and karyorrhexis. Lymphocytic and granulocytic infiltration occurs adjacent to necrosis. Small clumps of bacteria are often present in necrotic tissue. Older ulcers appear as thick masses of granular, acidophilic coagulated material mixed with cellular detritus and bacteria (Fig. 11.5). Infiltrations of granulocytes and lymphocytes surround the ulcer (Fig. 11.6). Small blood vessels near ulcers are occasionally occluded by bacteria. Liver lesions are clearly demarcated necrotic foci scattered throughout the parenchyma (19) (Fig. 11.7).

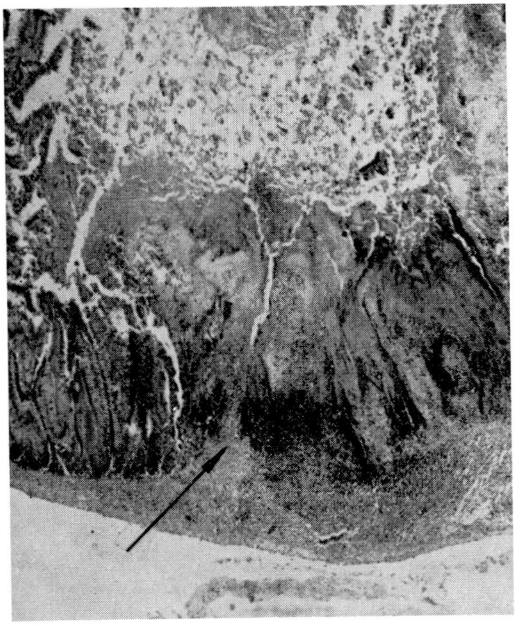

11.5. Transverse section of quail intestine with large ulceration. ×80. (Peckham)

Immunity. In some cases it appears that active immunity develops in survivors of a natural outbreak. Kirkpatrick et al. (23) challenged 22 such survivors without any noticeable effect. By contrast, susceptible controls had 85% mortality. However, it has been observed that survivors in groups treated with antibiotics may remain highly susceptible to infection (25, 34).

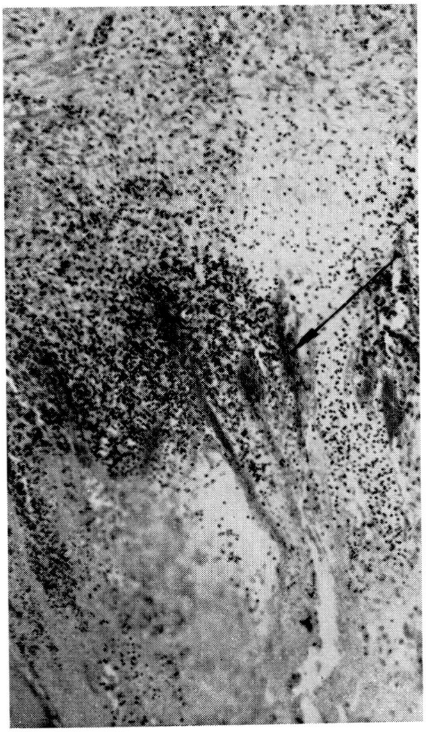

11.6. Higher magnification of area indicated by arrow in Fig. 11.5. Note cellular infiltration and dark linear masses (*arrow*) of bacteria. ×160.

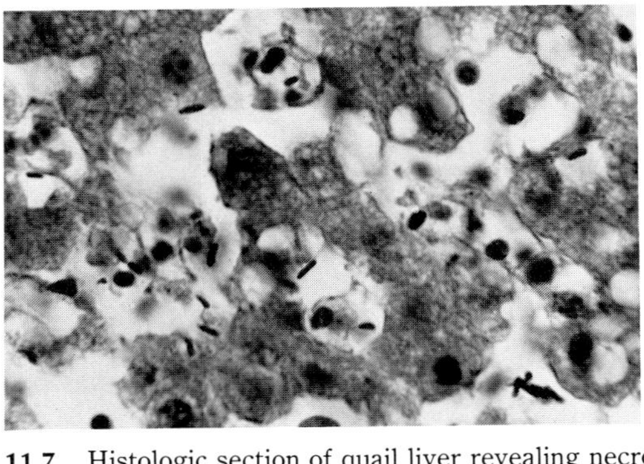

11.7. Histologic section of quail liver revealing necrosis and presence of UE organisms. Gram, ×2700. (Peckham)

DIAGNOSIS. Diagnosis of UE can be made on the basis of gross postmortem lesions. The presence of typical intestinal ulcerations accompanied by necrosis of the liver and an enlarged, hemorrhagic spleen suffices for clinical diagnosis. As an aid in diagnosis, necrotic liver tissue can be crushed between two slides, fixed by heat, and stained by Gram's method. Large gram-positive rods, subterminal spores, and free spores can be seen. If necessary, *C. colinum* can be isolated from liver or spleen (see Isolation and Identification of Causative Agent).

Berkhoff and Kanitz (7) described a fluorescent antibody (FA) test for diagnosis of UE. The FA test proved highly specific, and there was 100% correlation between a presumptive diagnosis based on gross lesions and confirmation with the test.

Berkhoff (5) reported use of the agar-gel immunodiffusion test for diagnosis of UE. Soluble bacterial antigens that reacted with antisera prepared against *C. colinum* were found in high concentrations in intestinal contents. These antigens were identical to bacterial antigens present in culture filtrates of *C. colinum*. However, antigens were not species-specific, as some strains of *C. perfringens* types A and C have cross-reacting antigens. This cross-reactivity among clostridial species makes this test unreliable for diagnostic purposes.

Isolation and Identification of Causative Agent. A clinical diagnosis of UE can be confirmed by isolation and identification of *C. colinum*. Because the organism is often present in the liver in pure culture, isolation from liver rather than from ulcerative, intestinal lesions is recommended. *C. perfringens* may be present as a secondary invader but is easy to recognize (43).

Berkhoff et al. (8) described in detail a technique for isolation of the organism on artificial media under anaerobic conditions (see Growth Requirements).

On anaerobic plates colonies are white, circular, convex, and semitranslucent. Cells are 3–4 μm long. Sporulation is rarely seen in artificial media, but if spores are present, they are oval and subterminal. Sporogenic cells are much longer and thicker than nonsporing cells. *C. colinum* resembles *C. difficile* most closely. These two organisms can be differentiated on cultural characteristics. *C. difficile* hydrolyses gelatin and is unable to ferment raffinose, whereas *C. colinum* is inactive on gelatin and readily ferments raffinose (43).

Differential Diagnosis. Among similar diseases that must be differentiated from UE are coccidiosis, necrotic enteritis, and histomoniasis. Frequently, coccidiosis precedes or accompanies UE (Fig. 11.8). Both diseases may be present in the same or different specimens submitted for diagnosis (32, 45). Bullis and Van Roekel (11) noted that coccidiosis and UE were often associated in poults. Buss et al. (12) found coccidia in pheasants affected with UE. It is imperative that a differential diagnosis between coccidiosis and UE be made because medication for each disease is distinct. Furthermore, both diseases may occur

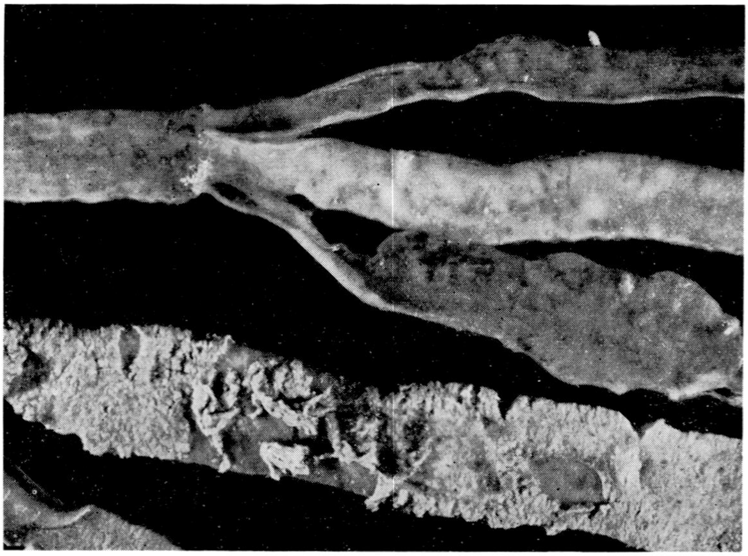

11.8. Combined UE and *E. brunetti* coccidial infection in intestine of chicken. Note small ulcers in ceca and rectum. Diphtheritic membrane is due to coccidial infection. (Peckham).

simultaneously warranting two different medications.

A condition described as necrotic enteritis frequently occurs in broiler-raising areas. Although there was much controversy that UE and necrotic enteritis were the same disease, Davis et al. (15) demonstrated conclusively that they were distinct. Helmboldt and Bryant (20) described gross and histopathologic differentiation of necrotic enteritis and UE.

Histomoniasis produces caseous cores in ceca and necrotic areas of varying size in the liver. This combination of cecal and liver lesions seen in chickens, poults, and other birds makes it imperative that cecal ulcerations and liver necrosis of UE be distinguished from histomoniasis. An enlarged hemorrhagic spleen and intestinal ulcerations are characteristic of UE. Histologic examination of the liver or ceca will reveal histomonads.

TREATMENT. Early reports of unsuccessful sulfonamide chemotherapy were published by Churchill and Coburn (13) and Rosen and Bischoff (38). Kirkpatrick et al. (23–25) and Kirkpatrick and Moses (22) reported that streptomycin administered by injection or in water or feed had a prophylactic and therapeutic value against UE in quail. Streptomycin at a level of 60 g/ton of feed gave complete protection when administered prophylactically. One gram streptomycin/gal drinking water gave complete protection when administered prior to or concomitant with artificial infection. Peckham and Reynolds (36) reported on the efficacy of furazolidone, bacitracin, streptomycin, and chlortetracycline in control of experimental UE in quail. Their results confirmed those of Kirkpatrick et al. (25). In addition they found 100 g bacitracin/ton feed gave complete protection.

PREVENTION AND CONTROL

Management Procedures. Since the infectious organism is in the droppings and remains viable indefinitely in litter, it is recommended on problem farms to remove contaminated litter and use clean litter for each brood. In chickens, avoid stresses caused by overcrowding, keep coccidiosis under control, and use preventive measures against viral diseases, which may act as a stressor and cause immunosuppression.

The most effective drugs are bacitracin or streptomycin. Bacitracin is used in the feed at a concentration of 0.005–0.01%, streptomycin at 0.006%. Either drug can be given in the drinking water prophylactically or therapeutically.

Game farm managers should exercise caution with regard to overgrazing ranges or overcrowding birds. Placing birds on 0.5-in. wire mesh is recommended on farms where the disease is a problem. Survivors of an outbreak may be carriers and should not be mixed with unexposed birds.

REFERENCES

1. Barger, E.H., S.E. Park, and R. Graham. 1934. A note on so-called quail disease. J Am Vet Med Assoc 84:776–783.
2. Bass, C.C. 1939. Observations on the specific cause and the nature of "quail disease" or ulcerative enteritis in quail. Proc Soc Exp Biol Med 42:375–380.
3. Bass, C.C. 1941. Quail disease–some important facts about it. Louisiana Conserv Rev Summer, pp. 11–14.
4. Bass, C.C. 1941. Specific cause and nature of ulcerative enteritis of quail. Proc Soc Exp Biol Med 46:250–52.
5. Berkhoff, G.A. 1975. Ulcerative enteritis–clostridial antigens. Am J Vet Res 36:583–585.
6. Berkhoff, H.A. 1985. Clostridium colinum sp. nov., nom. rev., the causative agent of ulcerative enteritis (quail disease) in quail, chickens, and pheasants. Int J Syst Bacteriol 35:155–159.
7. Berkhoff, G.A., and C.L. Kanitz. 1976. Fluorescent antibody test in diagnosis of ulcerative enteritis. Avian Dis 20:525–533.
8. Berkhoff, G.A., S.G. Campbell, and H.B. Naylor. 1974. Etiology and pathogenesis of ulcerative enteritis ("quail disease"). Isolation of the causative anaerobe. Avian Dis 18:186–194.
9. Berkhoff, G.A., S.G. Campbell, H.B. Naylor, and L.DS. Smith. 1974. Etiology and pathogenesis of ulcerative enteritis ("quail disease"). Characterization of the causative anaerobe. Avian Dis 18:195–204.
10. Bryant, E.S., W. Gerencer, E.T. Mallinson, and G. Stein. 1973. Report of the committee on nomenclature and reporting of disease, Northeastern Conference on Avian Disease. Avian Dis 17:904–911.
11. Bullis, K.L., and H. Van Roekel. 1944. Uncommon pathological conditions in chickens and turkeys. Cornell Vet 34:312–319.
12. Buss, I.O., R.D. Conrad, and J.R. Reilly. 1958. Ulcerative enteritis in the pheasant, blue grouse, and California quail. J Wildl Manage 22:446–449.
13. Churchill, H.M., and D.R. Coburn. 1945. Sulfonamide drugs in the treatment of ulcerative enteritis of quail. Vet Med 40:309–311.
14. Davis, R.B. 1973. Ulcerative enteritis in chickens: Coccidiosis and stress as predisposing factors. Poult Sci 52:1283–1287.
15. Davis, R.B., J. Brown, and D.L. Dawe. 1971. Quail–biological indicators in the differentiation of ulcerative and necrotic enteritis of chickens. Poult Sci 50:737–740.
16. Durant, A.J., and E.R. Doll. 1941. Ulcerative enteritis in quail. Missouri Agr Exp Stn Res Bull 325:3–27.
17. Gallagher, B.A. 1924. Ulcerative enteritis in quail. Am Game Prot Assoc Bull (Apr):14–15.
18. Glover, J.S. 1951. Ulcerative enteritis in pigeons. Can J Comp Med Vet Sci 15:295–297.
19. Harris, A.H. 1961. An outbreak of ulcerative enteritis amongst bobwhite quail (Colinus virginianus). Vet Rec 73:11–13.
20. Helmboldt, C.F. and E.S. Bryant. 1971. The pathology of necrotic enteritis in domestic fowl. Avian Dis 15:775–780.
21. Katiyar, A.K., A.G.R. Pillai, R.P. Awadhiya, and J.L. Vegad. 1986. An outbreak of ulcerative enteritis in chickens. Indian J Anim Sci 56:859–862.

22. Kirkpatrick, C.M., and H.E. Moses. 1953. The effects of streptomycin against spontaneous quail disease in bobwhites. J Wildl Manage 17:24–28.
23. Kirkpatrick, C.M., H.E. Moses, and J.T. Baldini. 1950. Streptomycin studies in ulcerative enteritis in bobwhite quail. I. Results of oral administration of the drug to manually exposed birds in the fall. Poult Sci 29:561–569.
24. Kirkpatrick, C.M., H.E. Moses, and J.T. Baldini. 1952. The effects of several antibiotic products in feed on experimental ulcerative enteritis in quail. Am J Vet Res 13:99–100.
25. Kirkpatrick, C.M., H.E. Moses, and J.T. Baldini. 1952. Streptomycin studies in ulcerative enteritis in bobwhite quail. II. Concentrations of streptomycin in drinking water suppressing the experimental disease. Am J Vet Res 13:102–104.
26. LeDune, E.K. 1935. Ulcerative enteritis in ruffed grouse. Vet Med 30:394–395.
27. Levine, P.P. 1932. A report on an epidemic disease in ruffed grouse. Trans 19th Am Game Conf, pp. 437–41.
28. Levine, P.P., and F.C. Goble. 1947. Diseases of grouse, pp. 401–442. In G. Bump et al. (eds.), The Ruffed Grouse. NY State Conserv Dep, Albany.
29. Morley, L.C., and P.W. Wetmore. 1936. Discovery of the organism of ulcerative enteritis. Proc N Am Wildl Conf, Senate Comm. Print, 74th Congress, pp. 471–473. 2nd session, Washington, DC.
30. Morris, J.A. 1948. The use of the complement fixation test in the detection of ulcerative enteritis in quail. Am J Vet Res 9:102–103.
31. Morse, G.B. 1907. Quail disease in the United States. USDA, BAI Circ 109.
32. Peckham, M.C. 1959. An anaerobe, the cause of ulcerative enteritis ("quail disease"). Avian Dis 3:471–478.
33. Peckham, M.C. 1960. Further studies on the causative organism of ulcerative enteritis. Avian Dis 4:449–456.
34. Peckham, M.C. 1962. Studies on immunization against ulcerative enteritis in quail. Annu Rep NY State Vet Coll, 1961–62, p. 60.
35. Peckham, M.C. 1963. Poultry diagnostic accessions. Annu Rep NY State Vet Coll, 1962–63.
36. Peckham, M.C., and R. Reynolds. 1962. The efficacy of chemotherapeutic drugs in the control of experimental ulcerative enteritis in quail. Avian Dis 6:111–118.
37. Pickens, E.N., H.M. DeVolt, and J.E. Shillinger. 1932. An outbreak of quail disease in bobwhite quail. Maryland Conservationist 9:18–19.
38. Rosen, M.N., and A.I. Bischoff. 1949. Field trials of sulfamethazine and sulfaquinoxaline in the treatment of quail ulcerative enteritis. Cornell Vet 39:195–197.
39. Schneider, J., and K. Haass. 1968. Beobachtungen zur ulceroesen Enteritis (quail disease) bei Huehnerkueken. Berl Muench Tieraerztl Wochenschr 81:466–468.
40. Shillinger, J.E., and L.C. Morley. 1934. Studies on ulcerative enteritis in quail. J Am Vet Med Assoc 84:25–35.
41. Shukla, P.K., and B.S. Rajya. 1968. Affections of the lower alimentary tract of domestic fowl: 1–on the occurrence and morphology of ulcerated enteritis simulating "quail disease." Indian Vet J 45:10–13.
42. Sing, N., M.S. Kwatra, and M.S. Oberoi. 1984. An outbreak of ulcerative enteritis ("quail's disease") in broilers in Punjab. Indian J Poult Sci 19:277–279.
43. Smith, L.DS. 1980. Clostridial infections. In S.B. Hitchner, C.H. Domermuth, H.G. Purchase, and J.E. Williams (eds.), Isolation and Identification of Avian Pathogens, pp. 33–35. Am Assoc Avian Pathol, Kennett Square, PA.
44. Winterfield, R.W., and G.A. Berkhoff. 1977. Ulcerative enteritis in robins. Avian Dis 21:328–330.
45. Witter, J.F. 1952. Observations on apparent complications of coccidiosis in broiler flocks. Proc 24th Annu Conf Lab Workers in Pullorum Dis Control, Univ Maine.

NECROTIC ENTERITIS

M.D. Ficken

HISTORY, INCIDENCE, AND DISTRIBUTION. Necrotic enteritis (NE) in domestic chickens was first described by Parish in 1961 (44–46), who reproduced the disease with a strain of *Clostridium welchii* (*C. perfringens*). It subsequently has been reported from most areas of the world where poultry is produced (6, 12, 18, 19, 32, 34, 36, 40, 42, 60).

ETIOLOGY. The cause of NE is *C. perfringens* types A (4, 8, 13, 33, 38, 43, 59, 62) or C (21, 33, 42, 46, 49). Some isolates of *C. perfringens* from cases of NE do not yield enough toxin in vitro to permit typing (33, 37). Alpha toxin produced by *C. perfringens* types A and C and beta toxin produced by *C. perfringens* type C are those believed responsible for intestinal mucosal necrosis, the characteristic lesion of NE. Both have been detected in feces of chickens with NE (33). Alpha toxin, obtained from broth culture supernatant fluids of *C. perfringens* type A (4, 43), is capable of producing characteristic intestinal lesions in conventional (5) or germ-free chickens (25).

C. perfringens can be readily isolated on blood agar plates incubated anaerobically at 37 C overnight and is indicated by colonies surrounded by an inner zone of complete hemolysis and an outer zone of discoloration and incomplete hemolysis (with rabbit, human, or sheep blood) composed of short to intermediate gram-positive rods without spores. Positive identification of the organism is made by inoculation of differential media (1). Most strains ferment glucose, maltose, lactose, and sucrose; do not ferment mannitol; and variably ferment salicin. Principal products of fermentation are acetic and butyric acid. Gelatin is hydrolyzed, milk is digested, and there is no indole production. Growth on egg yolk agar demonstrates presence of lecithinase and absence of lipase production. Subculturing on egg yolk agar plates, one-half of which have been spread with *C. perfringens* antitoxin, and incubating anaerobically overnight, will produce a zone of precipitation around colonies on control sides of the plate and little or no precipitation on sides spread with antitoxin (1).

PATHOGENESIS AND EPIZOOTIOLOGY.

Natural outbreaks of NE have been reported in chickens from 2 wk to 6 mo of age. A majority of reports of NE have been in 2- to 5-wk-old broiler chickens raised on litter (6, 12, 26, 30 32, 36, 40, 42, 60). However, outbreaks in 3- to 6-mo-old commercial layers raised in floor pens have also been reported (18, 34), and outbreaks of NE and coccidiosis have been reported in 12- to 16- wk-old cage-reared layer replacement pullets (17, 24).

C. perfringens can be found in feces, soil, dust, contaminated feed and litter, or intestinal contents (33, 35). In various outbreaks of NE, contaminated feed (19, 24, 62) and contaminated litter (61) have been incriminated as sources of infection.

Reports vary on the numbers of *C. perfringens* that can be consistently isolated from intestinal tracts of normal chickens. Johansson and Sarles (31) and Shapiro and Sarles (51) reported the principal obligate anaerobic bacterium in the intestinal tract of chickens to be *C. perfringens.* Other investigators have isolated it only sporadically and in low numbers from small intestine of normal chickens ranging in age from recently hatched to 5 mo of age (10, 11, 49, 52, 58). Smith (53), by manipulating the diet, demonstrated an increase in the proportion of *C. perfringens* in the intestinal tract; therefore, it has been postulated that *C. perfringens* numbers within the intestinal tract, and onset of intestinal clostridial disease in chickens, may be precipitated by the nature of the ration (42). High levels of fishmeal (32, 59) or high levels of wheat (16) in the diet can predispose to and/or exacerbate outbreaks of NE.

Damage to the intestinal mucosa is another predisposing factor for NE (2, 59). Factors such as high-fiber litter (59), or various strains of coccidia (3, 7, 8, 9, 30, 49), combined with higher than normal numbers of *C. perfringens,* can result in NE. NE has been experimentally reproduced in chickens (8, 20, 27, 28, 29, 47, 48), turkeys (23), and Japanese quail (21). In conventional chickens, the incidence can be from 1.3–37.3% and as high as 62.0% in specific-pathogen-free chicks (8). NE can be reproduced by rearing chickens on litter in facilities where the disease has previously occurred (28, 29, 39, 61); feeding feed contaminated with *C. perfringens* (38, 59); administering vegetative cultures of *C. perfringens* intravenously (15), orally (15), or into the crop (8); intraduodenal administration of broth cultures of *C. perfringens* (4), bacteria-free crude toxins of *C. perfringens* (5), or a combination of *C. perfringens* and its toxins (2, 9); or by dosing chickens with sporulated oocysts of *Eimeria* spp. and feeding vegetative cultures of *C. perfringens* or *C. perfringens*-contaminated feed (3, 7, 8, 9).

Signs and Lesions.

Clinical signs in natural outbreaks include marked to severe depression, decreased appetite, reluctance to move, diarrhea, and ruffled feathers (6, 14, 30, 36, 42, 44, 60). Clinical illness is very short; often birds are just found acutely dead.

Gross lesions in natural outbreaks are usually confined to the small intestine, primarily jejunum and ileum (6, 14, 30, 42, 60); however, cecal lesions have been described (37). Intestines are often friable and distended with gas. The mucosa is lined by a loosely to tightly adherent pseudomembrane, which is yellow or green in appearance. Flecks of blood have been reported, but hemorrhage is not a prominent feature. Experimentally, gross lesions characterized by a gray, thickened mucosa in the duodenum and jejunum may be observed as early as 3 hr following inoculation of *C. perfringens* (4). By 5 hr, there is necrosis of the intestinal mucosa which progresses, over time, to a severe fibrinonecrotic enteritis with formation of a diphtheritic membrane (8, 49).

Microscopic changes in natural outbreaks are characterized primarily by severe necrosis of the intestinal mucosa with an abundance of fibrin admixed with cellular debris adherent to the necrotic mucosa (14, 30, 37, 42, 60). Initial lesions develop at the apices of villi, and are characterized by sloughing of epithelium and colonization of the exposed lamina propria with bacilli, accompanied by coagulation necrosis. Areas of necrosis are surrounded by heterophils. Progression of lesions usually occurs from villi apices to crypts. Necrosis may extend into the submucosa and muscular layers of the intestine. Numerous large bacilli are often observed attached to cellular debris. In birds that survive, regenerative changes consist of crypt epithelial cell proliferation with a corresponding increase in mitotic figures. Epithelial cells are primarily cuboidal, with a relative decrease in goblet and columnar epithelial cells. Villi are relatively short and flat. In many outbreaks, various sexual and asexual stages of coccidia are found in the intestine (30, 37, 42).

Microscopic changes after experimental inoculation of *C. perfringens* (4) occur as early as 1 hr following challenge, and consist of slight edema and dilation of vessels in the lamina propria, sloughed epithelial cells in the intestinal lumen, and occasional heterophils and mononuclear cells in the lamina propria. By 3 hr, marked edema, resulting in detachment of the epithelial cell layer from the lamina propria, mostly at the apex of villi, has occurred. Mononuclear cell infiltration of the lamina propria is more marked than earlier. At 5 hr, there is marked coagulation necrosis of the epithelial layer and lamina propria at villus tips, resulting in villus shortening. Colonization of organisms may be prominent on necrotic tissues and apices of exposed lamina propria. Blood vessels are very congested and occasionally occluded by hyaline thrombi. By 8–12 hr there is massive necrosis of villi, in some instances reaching to the crypts, characterized by areas of amorphous eosinophilic-staining material and cell nuclei. Fibrin and cellular debris are present in the lumen.

DIAGNOSIS. Diagnosis of NE can be made based on the typical gross and microscopic lesions and isolation of the causative agent. In field cases of NE, *C. perfringens* can be readily isolated from intestinal contents, scrapings of intestinal wall, or hemorrhagic lymphoid nodules by anaerobic incubation overnight at 37 C on blood agar plates (55) and identified as described under ETIOLOGY.

Diseases that must be differentiated from NE are ulcerative enteritis (UE) and *Eimeria brunetti* infection. UE is caused by *C. colinum* (see Ulcerative Enteritis); characteristic gross lesions are multiple areas of necrosis and ulceration in the distal small intestine and ceca and areas of necrosis in the liver. As described previously, lesions of NE are usually confined to jejunum and ileum with little or no involvement of ceca or liver. These distinguishing characteristics should allow differentiation of NE and UE. Isolation and identification of the causative agent will confirm the diagnosis. *E. brunetti* infection (see Coccidiosis) causes gross lesions similar to those produced by *C. perfringens;* however, microscopic examination of fecal smears, impressions, or intestinal sections should demonstrate the presence or absence of coccidia. Finally, NE and coccidiosis often occur simultaneously in a flock and demonstration of one or both agents is warranted.

TREATMENT AND PREVENTION. Experimentally, in vivo, a number of antibiotics placed in the feed reduce the numbers of *C. perfringens* shed in feces (54, 56, 57). These include virginiamycin, nitrovin, tylosin, penicillin, ampicillin, bacitracin, furazolidone, and efrotomycin.

Outbreaks of NE can be effectively treated by administration of lincomycin (28, 29), bacitracin (48), oxytetracycline (6), penicillin (34, 38), or tylosin tartrate (34) in the water. Bacitracin (47, 61), lincomycin (39), virginiamycin (22, 27), penicillin (42), avoparcin (41, 47), and nitrovin (41) have been shown to be effective in preventing and controlling NE when placed in the feed.

REFERENCES

1. Allen, S. D. 1985. Clostridium. In E.H. Lennette, A. Balows, W.J. Hausler, Jr., and H.J. Shadomy (eds.), Manual of Clinical Microbiology, 4th Ed., pp. 434–444. American Society for Microbiology, Washington, DC.
2. Al-Sheikhly, F., and A. Al-Saieg. 1980. Role of coccidia in the occurrence of necrotic enteritis of chickens. Avian Dis 24:324–333.
3. Al-Sheikhly, F., and R.B. Truscott. 1977. The pathology of necrotic enteritis of chickens following infusion of broth cultures of Clostridium perfringens into the duodenum. Avian Dis 21:230–240.
4. Al-Sheikhly, F., and R.B. Truscott. 1977. The pathology of necrotic enteritis of chickens following infusion of crude toxins of Clostridium perfringens into the duodenum. Avian Dis 21:241–255.
5. Al-Sheikhly, F., and R.B. Truscott. 1977. The interaction of Clostridium perfringens and its toxins in the production of necrotic enteritis of chickens. Avian Dis 21:256–263.
6. Bains, B.S. 1968. Necrotic enteritis of chickens. Aust Vet J 44:40.
7. Balauca, N. 1976. Experimentelle reproduktion der nekrotischen enteritis beim huhn. I. Mitteilung. Mono- und polyinfektionen mit Clostridium perfringens und kokzidien unter berucksichtigung der kafighaltung. Arch Exp Veterinaermed 30:903- 912.
8. Balauca, N. 1978. Experimentelle untersuchungen uber die Clostridien infektion und intoxikation bei geflugeln, unter besonderer berucksichtigung der kokzidiose. Arch Vet 13:127–141.
9. Balauca, N., B. Kohler, F. Horsch, R. Jungmann, and E. Prusas. 1976. Experimentelle reproduktion der nekrotischen enteritis des huhnes. II. Mitteilung. Weitere mono- und polyinfektionen mit Cl. perfringens und kokzidien unter besonderer berucksichtigung der bodenhaltung. Arch Exp Veterinaermed 30:913–923.
10. Barnes, E.M., G.C. Mead, D.A. Barnum, and E.G. Harry. 1972. The intestinal flora of the chicken in the period 2 to 6 weeks of age, with particular reference to the anaerobic bacteria. Br Poult Sci 13:311–326.
11. Barnes, E.M., C.S. Impey, and D.M. Cooper. 1980. Manipulation of the crop and intestinal flora of the newly hatched chick. Am J Clin Nutr 33:2426–2433.
12. Bernier, G., and R. Filion. 1971. Necrotic enteritis in broiler chickens. J Am Vet Med Assoc 158:1896–1897.
13. Bernier, G., R. Filion, R. Malo, and J.B. Phaneuf. 1974. Enterite necrotique chez le poulet de gril. II. Caracteres des souches de Clostridium perfringens isolees. Can J Comp Med 38:286–291.
14. Bernier, G., J.B. Phaneuf, and R. Filion. 1974. Enterite necrotique chez le poulet de gril. I. Aspect clinicopathologique. Can J Comp Med 38:280–285.
15. Bernier, G., J.B. Phaneuf, and R. Filion. 1977. Enterite necrotique chez le poulet de gril. III. Etude des facteurs favorisant la multiplication de Clostridium perfringens et la transmission experimentale de la maladie. Can J Comp Med 41:112–116.
16. Branton, S.L., F.N. Reece, and W.M. Hagler, Jr. 1987. Influence of a wheat diet on mortality of broiler chickens associated with necrotic enteritis. Poult Sci 66:1326–1330.
17. Broussard, C.T., C.L. Hofacre, R.K. Page, and O.J. Fletcher. 1986. Necrotic enteritis in cage-reared commercial layer pullets. Avian Dis 30:617–619.
18. Chakraborty, G.C., D. Chakraborty, D. Bhattacharyya, S. Bhattacharyya, U.N. Goswami, and H.M. Bhattacharyya. 1984. Necrotic enteritis in poultry in West Bengal. Indian J Comp Microbiol Immunol Infect Dis 5:54–57.
19. Char, N.L., D.I. Khan, M.R.K. Rao, V. Gopal, and G. Narayana. 1986. A rare occurrence of clostridial infections in poultry. Poult Adviser 19:59–62.
20. Cowen, B.S., L.D. Schwartz, R.A. Wilson, and S.I. Ambrus. 1987. Experimentally induced necrotic enteritis in chickens. Avian Dis 31:904–906.
21. Cygan, Z., and J. Nowak. 1974. Nekrotyczne zapalenie jelit u kurczat. II. Wlasciwosci toksynogenne szczepow Cl. perfringens C i proby zakazenia przepiorek japonskich. Med Weter 30:262–265.
22. Davis, R., R.G. Oakley, M. Free, C. Miller, and R. Rivera. 1980. Profilaxis de la enteritis necrotica con la virginiamicina. Proc 29th West Poult Dis Conf, pp. 117–119.
23. Fagerberg, D.J., B.A. George, W.R. Lance, and

C.R. Miller. 1984. Clostridial enteritis in turkeys. Proc 33rd West Poult Dis Conf, pp. 20–21.

24. Frame, D.D., and A.A. Bickford. 1986. An outbreak of coccidiosis and necrotic enteritis in 16-week-old cage-reared layer replacement pullets. Avian Dis 30:601–602.

25. Fukata, T., Y. Hadate, E. Baba, T. Uemura, and A. Arakawa. 1988. Influence of Clostridium perfringens and its toxin in germ-free chickens. Res Vet Sci 44:68–70.

26. Gardiner, M.R. 1967. Clostridial infections in poultry in western Australia. Aust Vet J 43:359–360.

27. George, B.A., C.L. Quarles, and D.J. Fagerberg. 1982. Virginiamycin effects on controlling necrotic enteritis infection in chickens. Poult Sci 61:447–450.

28. Hamdy, A.H., R.W. Thomas, D.D. Kratzer, and R.B. Davis. 1983. Lincomycin dose response for treatment of necrotic enteritis in broilers. Poult Sci 62:585–588.

29. Hamdy, A.H., R.W. Thomas, R.J. Yancey, and R.B. Davis. 1983. Therapeutic effect of optimal lincomycin concentration in drinking water on necrotic enteritis in broilers. Poult Sci 62:589–591.

30. Helmboldt, C.F., and E.S. Bryant. 1971. The pathology of necrotic enteritis in domestic fowl. Avian Dis 15:775–780.

31. Johansson, K.R., and W.B. Sarles. 1948. Bacterial population changes in the ceca of young chickens infected with Eimeria tenella. J Bacteriol 56:635–647.

32. Johnson, D.C., and C. Pinedo. 1971. Gizzard erosion and ulceration in Peru broilers. Avian Dis 15:835–837.

33. Kohler, B., S. Kolbach, and J. Meine. 1974. Untersuchungen zür nekrotischen Enteritis der Hühner. 2. Mitt.: Microbiologische Aspekte. Monatsh Veterinaermed 29:385–391.

34. Kohler, B., G. Marx, S. Kolbach, and E. Bottcher. 1974. Untersuchungen zür nekrotischen Enteritis der Hühner. 1. Mitt.: Diagnostik und Bekämpfung. Monatsh Veterinaermed 29:380–384.

35. Komnenov, V., M. Velhner, and M. Katrinka. 1981. Importance of feed in the occurrence of clostridial infections in poultry. Vet Glas 35:245–249.

36. Long, J. R. 1973. Necrotic enteritis in broiler chickens. I. A review of the literature and the prevalence of the disease in Ontario. Can J Comp Med 37:302–308.

37. Long, J.R., and R.B. Truscott. 1976. Necrotic enteritis in broiler chickens. III. Reproduction of the disease. Can J Comp Med 40:53–59.

38. Long, J.R., J.R. Pettit, and D.A. Barnum. 1974. Necrotic enteritis in broiler chickens. II. Pathology and proposed pathogenesis. Can J Comp Med 38:467–474.

39. Maxey, B.W., and R.K. Page. 1977. Efficacy of lincomycin feed medication for the control of necrotic enteritis in broiler-type chickens. Poult Sci 56:1909–1913.

40. Morch, J. 1974. Necrotic enteritis in broilers in Denmark. Proc 15th World's Poult Congr Expo, pp. 290–292.

41. Morch, J. 1982. Undersogelser med vaekstfremmende foderadditiver specielt med henblik pa forebyggelse af nekrotiserende enteritis hos kyllinger. Nord Vet Med 34:377–387.

42. Nairn, M.E., and V.W. Bamford. 1967. Necrotic enteritis of broiler chickens in western Australia. Aust Vet J 43:49–54.

43. Niilo, L. 1978. Enterotoxigenic Clostridium perfringens type A isolated from intestinal contents of cattle, sheep, and chickens. Can J Comp Med 42:357–363.

44. Parish, W.E. 1961. Necrotic enteritis in the fowl (Gallus gallus domesticus). I. Histopathology of the disease and isolation of a strain of Clostridium welchii. J Comp Pathol 71:377–393.

45. Parish, W.E. 1961. Necrotic enteritis in the fowl. II. Examination of the causal Clostridium welchii. J Comp Pathol 71:394–404.

46. Parish, W.E. 1961. Necrotic enteritis in the fowl. III. The experimental disease. J Comp Pathol 71:405–413.

47. Prescott, J.F. 1979. The prevention of experimentally induced necrotic enteritis in chickens by avoparcin. Avian Dis 23:1072–1074.

48. Prescott, J.F., R. Sivendra, and D.A. Barnum. 1978. The use of bacitracin in the prevention and treatment of experimentally induced necrotic enteritis in the chicken. Can Vet J 19:181–183.

49. Shane, S.M., D.G. Koetting, and K.S. Harrington. 1984. The occurrence of Clostridium perfringens in the intestine of chicks. Avian Dis 28:1120–1124.

50. Shane, S.M., J.E. Gyimah, K.S. Harrington, and T.G. Snider III. 1985. Etiology and pathogenesis of necrotic enteritis. Vet Res Commun 9:269–287.

51. Shapiro, S.K., and W.B. Sarles. 1949. Microorganisms in the intestinal tract of normal chickens. J Bacteriol 58:531–544.

52. Smith, H.W. 1959. The effect of the continuous administration of diets containing tetracyclines and penicillin on the number of drug-resistant and drug-sensitive Clostridium welchii in the faeces of pigs and chickens. J Pathol Bacteriol 77:79–93.

53. Smith, H.W. 1965. The development of the flora of the alimentary tract in young animals. J Pathol Bacteriol 90:495–513.

54. Smith, H.W. 1972. The antibacterial activity of nitrovin in vitro: The effect of this and other agents against Clostridium welchii in the alimentary tract of chickens. Vet Rec 90:310–312.

55. Smith, L.DS. 1980. Clostridial infections. In S.B. Hitchner, C.H. Domermuth, H.G. Purchase, and J.E. Williams (eds.), Isolation and Identification of Avian Pathogens, pp. 33–35. Creative Printing Co., Inc., Endwell, NY.

56. Stutz, M.W., S.L. Johnson, and F.R. Judith. 1983. Effects of diet and bacitracin on growth, feed efficiency, and populations of Clostridium perfringens in the intestine of broiler chicks. Poult Sci 62:1619–1625.

57. Stutz, M.W., S.L. Johnson, F.R. Judith, and B.M. Miller. 1983. In vitro and in vivo evaluations of the antibiotic efrotomycin. Poult Sci 62:1612–1618.

58. Timms, L. 1968. Observations on the bacterial flora of the alimentary tract in three age groups of normal chickens. Br Vet J 124:470–477.

59. Truscott, R.B., and F. Al-Sheikhly. 1977. Reproduction and treatment of necrotic enteritis in broilers. Am J Vet Res 38:857–861.

60. Tsai, S.S., and M.C. Tung. 1981. An outbreak of necrotic enteritis in broiler chickens. J Chin Soc Vet Sci 7:13–17.

61. Wicker, D.L., W.N. Isgrigg, J.H. Trammell, and R.B. Davis. 1977. The control and prevention of necrotic enteritis in broilers with zinc bacitracin. Poult Sci 56:1229–1231.

62. Wijewanta, E.A., and P. Seneviratna. 1971. Bacteriological studies of fatal Clostridium perfringens type-A infection in chickens. Avian Dis 15:654–661.

GANGRENOUS DERMATITIS

M.D. Ficken

HISTORY, INCIDENCE, DISTRIBUTION. In 1930, Niemann (34) described severe necrosis of muscle and subcutaneous tissue following intramuscular inoculations with *Clostridium welchii* (*C. perfringens*) isolated from heart blood and liver of two chickens. In 1931, Dutch workers (5) isolated *C. perfringens, C. septicum,* and *C. novyi* from chickens dying of wound infections following collection of blood samples for pullorum testing. In 1939, Fenstermacher and Pomeroy (15) described death of turkey breeder hens from wound infections at the time of mating, from which they isolated *C. perfringens, C. septicum,* and *C. sordellii.* Subcutaneous emphysema in chickens, from which *C. perfringens* and cocci were isolated, was described by Israeli workers in 1950 (38). Since 1963, reports of gangrenous dermatitis (GD) have been made from various parts of the world including Argentina (4), Belgium (18), Germany (23, 27), India (9), USA (17, 40), and UK (16). GD also has been given a variety of names including necrotic dermatitis, gangrenous cellulitis, gangrenous dermatomyositis, avian malignant edema, gas edema disease, and wing rot.

ETIOLOGY. Causes of GD are *C. septicum* (16, 17, 22, 23, 41), *C. perfringens* type A (4, 9, 27, 45), and *Staphylococcus aureus* (6, 8, 18, 27), either singly or in combination (17, 24, 27, 40), with combined infections generally more severe.

S. aureus (see STAPHYLOCOCCOSIS) and *C. perfringens* (see Necrotic Enteritis) can be isolated and identified as described elsewhere. Culture for *C. septicum* should be carried out anaerobically on blood agar plates containing 2.5% agar, which will reduce the ability of *C. septicum* to swarm over the plate surface (42). Incubation is for 1–2 days at 37 C. Positive identification of the organism is made by inoculation of differential media (1). *C. septicum* ferments glucose, maltose, lactose, and salicin, but not sucrose or mannitol. Principal products of fermentation are acetic and butyric acid. Gelatin is hydrolyzed. Milk is not digested and indole is not produced. Growth on egg yolk agar demonstrates an absence of lecithinase and lipase production. Spores are oval and subterminal in location.

PATHOGENESIS AND EPIZOOTIOLOGY. Natural outbreaks of GD have been reported in chickens from 17 days to 20 wk of age. A majority of reports of GD have been in 4- to 8-wk-old broiler chickens (6, 8, 16, 17, 22–24, 27, 40). However, outbreaks in 6- to 20-wk-old commercial layers (17, 40), 20-wk-old broiler breeders (18), and chickens following caponization (45) have also been reported. In turkeys, fatalities in breeder hens due to clostridia and gram-positive cocci have been reported (15). Suspected cases of clostridial dermatitis have also been observed in turkeys on range and in breeder toms following semen collection (known locally as "bubbly tail"); however, the causative agent was not positively identified.

Clostridia are distributed in soil, feces, dust, contaminated litter or feed, and intestinal contents (1, 26). Staphylococci are ubiquitous and common inhabitants of skin and mucous membranes of poultry and areas where poultry are hatched, reared, and processed (see STAPHYLOCOCCOSIS).

In many instances, GD is believed to occur as a sequel to disease produced by other infectious agents such as infectious bursal disease (IBD) and avian adenovirus infections, including inclusion body hepatitis (IBH) virus (8, 16, 24, 29, 33, 39). Researchers have demonstrated both GD and IBH occur as sequelae to IBD (14, 39). In addition, some outbreaks of GD have been breeder-flock associated, i.e., progeny from a specific breeder flock consistently develop GD when placed (19), and lack of antibody to IBD virus in broiler breeders correlates with increased susceptibility of their progeny to dermatitis (39). Another condition predisposing chickens to GD is blue wing disease (BWD), which has been reported from Sweden, where it was first described, West Germany, Denmark, Great Britain, Belgium, and Poland (11). Characteristic lesions of this disease are intracutaneous, subcutaneous, and intramuscular hemorrhages and edema (12) with atrophy of thymus, spleen, and bursa of Fabricius (13). GD often occurs secondarily to the skin hemorrhages. Numerous avian reoviruses and chick anemia agent (CAA) have been isolated from chickens affected with BWD (7, 11). Engstrom and associates (13) have postulated BWD is caused by dual infection of CAA and a reovirus. Apparently, a compromised immune system is the underlying predisposing factor allowing GD to occur.

GD has been experimentally reproduced in chickens (17, 22, 23, 27, 40) and turkeys (40). In chickens, fatal disease, with lesions similar to those in natural outbreaks, has been reproduced with intramuscular or subcutaneous inoculations of *C. septicum, C. perfringens* type A, or *S. aureus,* either singly or in combination, with combined infections more severe. In turkeys, intramuscular inoculations with *C. septicum* isolated from chickens caused death in less than 24 hr with circumscribed lesions at the inoculation site.

Signs and Lesions. Clinical signs in natural outbreaks of GD include varying degrees of depression, incoordination, inappetence, leg weakness, and ataxia (16, 17, 22, 23, 40). The period of illness is short, usually less than 24 hr; birds are often just found acutely dead. Mortality ranges from 1 to 60% (16).

Gross lesions consist of dark, moist areas of skin, usually devoid of feathers, overlying wings, breast, abdomen, or legs (9, 16, 17, 22, 23, 40). Extensive blood-tinged edema, with or without gas (emphysema), is present beneath affected skin. Underlying musculature is discolored gray or tan, and may contain edema and gas between muscle bundles. In some cases, emphysema and serosanguineous fluid are present in subcutaneous tissue, but there is no loss of integrity in the overlying skin (24). Most cases report no internal lesions; however, discrete white foci (necrosis) in the liver (8, 40) and small flaccid bursae of Fabricius (8, 24), the latter presumably due to IBD virus infection, have been reported.

Microscopic changes are characterized by edema and emphysema with numerous basophilic large bacilli and/or small cocci within subcutaneous tissues (8, 40). Severe congestion, hemorrhage, and necrosis of underlying skeletal muscle is often present. Livers, if affected, contain small, randomly scattered, discrete areas of coagulation necrosis with intralesion bacteria. Cloacal bursal changes, in cases suspected to have concurrent IBD, are characterized by extensive follicular necrosis and atrophy (8, 24).

DIAGNOSIS.

Diagnosis of GD can be made by the typical gross and microscopic lesions and isolation of the causative agent(s). In field cases of GD, staphylococci and clostridia can be isolated from exudates of skin and subcutaneous tissue or underlying muscle (8, 9, 17, 23, 40). Identification of the causative agent(s) can be done as described under ETIOLOGY.

Since occurrence of GD seems to be preceded by other infectious agents affecting immunologic defensive systems of the bird, diagnosis of the underlying etiology is necessary. Infections with IBD virus, avian adenoviruses, and CAA and reoviruses must be determined, as these can predispose GD.

A variety of skin conditions must be differentiated from GD. Dermatitis caused by mycotic agents, *Rhodotorula mucilaginosa* (3), *R. glutins* (35), *Candida albicans* (28), and *Aspergillus fumigatus* (46), can be differentiated from GD by demonstration of fungal elements in impression smears or tissue sections, and by isolation and identification of the agent. Contact, or ulcerative, dermatitis ("breast burn") of broiler chickens (20, 31) and plantar pododermatitis of turkeys (30) are conditions characterized by erosions and ulcers accompanied by acute inflammatory changes over the breast, hock, and plantar surface of the feet. A strong correlation between wet or poor litter and these conditions is present (30, 32). Scabby hip dermatitis is a syndrome of broilers that, like contact dermatitis, is a nonspecific dermatitis with ulceration and secondary bacterial infection (21). Lesions originate as a scratch around the lumbar and sacral regions, and are strongly correlated with high stocking densities resulting in feather breakage and dermal entrance of bacteria (21, 37). To differentiate GD from these conditions, demonstration of poor environmental conditions and/or overcrowding and lack of a primary infectious etiology is warranted. Vesicular lesions involving the wattles, comb, shanks, and feet have been described in chickens (25, 36, 43), and have been suspected or proven to be due to ingestion of the fungus *Cladosporium herbarum*, producing an ergotlike disease, or *Amni visnaga* seeds, which lead to photosensitization. These invariably occur only on unfeathered areas of the skin and should be easily differentiated. Squamous cell carcinoma of the skin of chickens, the cause of which is undetermined, leads to ulceration of the epidermis which usually is infected with bacteria and may be difficult to differentiate from GD by gross examination (44). Demonstration of cords and nests of neoplastic epithelial cells within the dermis by microscopy is necessary to diagnose this entity. Finally, a number of nutritional deficiencies and genetically slow-feathering male chickens may serve as underlying causes of dermatitis (10).

TREATMENT AND PREVENTION.

Outbreaks of GD have been effectively treated by administration of chlortetracycline (22), oxytetracycline (40), erythromycin (40), penicillin (8, 24), or copper sulfate (2) in the water and chlortetracycline (23, 40) or furoxone (23) in the feed. However, in many instances, antibiotics used for control have had little success (16, 18, 19, 27). Failure of treatment is usually attributed to the underlying etiology, usually viral, which is not controlled. Administration of a mixed clostridial bacterin at 1 day of age has been shown to reduce losses in flocks due to GD (19); however, its use at present is not widespread.

REFERENCES

1. Allen, S.D. 1985. Clostridium. In E.H. Lennette, A. Balows, W.J. Hausler, Jr., and H.J. Shadomy (eds.), Manual of Clinical Microbiology, 4th Ed., pp. 434–444. Am Soc Microbiol, Washington, DC.

2. Awaad, M.H.H. 1986. A research note on the treatment of naturally induced gangrenous dermatitis in chickens by copper sulfate. Vet Med J Giza Egypt 34:121–124.

3. Beemer, A.M., S. Schneerson-Porat, and E.S. Kut-

tin. 1970. Rhodotorula mucilaginosa dermatitis on feathered parts of chickens: An epizootic on a poultry farm. Avian Dis 14:234–239.

4. Bianco, O., J. Quinones, J. Bergesio, M. Demo, and C. Pajaro. 1985. Dermatitis gangrenosa en pollos parrilleros: dos brotes en Rio Cuarto. Vet Arg 19:879–883.

5. Bliek, L. de, and J. Jansen. 1931. Gasoedeem bij kippen na bloedtappen. Tijdschr Diergeneeskd 58:513–518.

6. Bootes, B.W., and G. Slennet. 1964. Staphylococcosis in chickens. Aust Vet J 40:238–239.

7.Bülow, V., R. Rudolph, and B. Fuchs. 1986. Erhohte pathogenitat des erregers der aviaren infektiosen anamie bei huhnerkuken (CAA) bei simultaner infektion mit virus der marekschen krankheit (MDV), bursitisvirus (IBDV) oder reticuloendotheliosevirus (REV). Zentrabl Veterinaermed [B] 33:93–116.

8. Cervantes, H.M., L.L. Munger, D.H. Ley, and M.D. Ficken. 1988. Staphylococcus-induced gangrenous dermatitis in broilers. Avian Dis 32:140–142.

9. Char, N.L., D.I. Khan, M.R.K. Rao, V. Gopal, and G. Narayana. 1986. A rare occurrence of clostridial infection in poultry. Poult Adviser 19:59–62.

10. Clarke, W.E. 1974. Dermatitis in broiler chickens. Pract Nutr 8:5–7.

11. Engström, B.E. 1988. Blue wing disease of chickens: Isolation of avian reovirus and chicken anaemia agent. Avian Pathol 17:23–32.

12. Engström, B.E., and M. Luthman. 1984. Blue wing disease of chickens: Signs, pathology, and natural transmission. Avian Pathol 13:1–12.

13. Engström, B.E., O. Fossum, and M. Luthman. 1988. Blue wing disease of chickens: Experimental infection with a Swedish isolate of chicken anaemia agent and an avian reovirus. Avian Pathol 17:33–50.

14. Fadly, A.M., R.W. Winterfield, and H.J. Olander. 1976. Role of the bursa of Fabricius in the pathogenicity of inclusion body hepatitis and infectious bursal disease viruses. Avian Dis 20:467–477.

15. Fenstermacher, R., and B.S. Pomeroy. 1939. Clostridium infection in turkeys. Cornell Vet 29:25–28.

16. Fowler, N.G., and S.N. Hussaini. 1975. Clostridium septicum infection and antibiotic treatment in broiler chickens. Vet Rec 96:14–15.

17. Frazier, M.N., W.J. Parizek, and E. Garner. 1964. Gangrenous dermatitis of chickens. Avian Dis 8:269–273.

18. Froyman, R., L. Deruyttere, and L.A. Devriese. 1982. The effect of antimicrobial agents on an outbreak of staphylococcal dermatitis in adult broiler breeders. Avian Pathol 11:521–525.

19. Gerdon, D. 1973. Effects of a mixed clostridial bacterin on incidence of gangrenous dermatitis. Avian Dis 17:205–206.

20. Greene, J.A., R.M. McCracken, and R.T. Evans. 1985. A contact dermatitis of broilers – clinical and pathological findings. Avian Pathol 14:23–38.

21. Harris, G.C., Jr., M. Musbah, J.N. Beasley, and G.S. Nelson. 1978. The development of dermatitis (scabby-hip) on the hip and thigh of broiler chickens. Avian Dis 22:122–130.

22. Helfer, D.H., E.M. Dickinson, and D.H. Smith. 1969. Clostridium septicum infection in a broiler flock. Avian Dis 13:231–233.

23. Hinz, K.H., M. Knapp, U. Lohren, and J. Batke. 1975. Gasodemerkrankung bei broilern. Dtsch Tierärztl Wochenschr 82:307–310.

24. Hofacre, C.L., J.D. French, R.K. Page, and O.J. Fletcher. 1986. Subcutaneous clostridial infection in broilers. Avian Dis 30:620–622.

25. Hoffman, H.A. 1939. Vesicular dermatitis in chickens. J Am Vet Med Assoc 95:329–332.

26. Kohler, B., S. Kolbach, and J. Meine. 1974. Untersuchungen zur nekrotischen enteritis der huhner 2. Mitt.: microbiologische aspekte. Monatsh Veterinaermed 29:385–391.

27. Kohler, B., V. Bergmann, W. Witte, R. Heiss, and K. Vogel. 1978. Dermatitis bei broilern durch Staphylococcus aureus. Monatsh Veterinaermed 33:22–28.

28. Kuttin, E.S., A.M. Beemer, and M. Meroz. 1976. Chicken dermatitis and loss of feathers from Candida albicans. Avian Dis 20:216–218.

29. Long, R.V. 1973. Necrotic dermatitis. Poult Dig 32:20–22.

30. Martland, M.F. 1984. Wet litter as a cause of plantar pododermatitis, leading to foot ulceration and lameness in fattening turkeys. Avian Pathol 13:241–252.

31. Martland, M.F. 1985. Ulcerative dermatitis in broiler chickens: The effects of wet litter. Avian Pathol 14:353–364. 1985.

32. McIlroy, S.G., E.A. Goodall, and C.H. McMurray. 1987. A contact dermatitis of broilers – epidemiological findings. Avian Pathol 16:93–105.

33. Monreal, G. 1984. Nachweis von neutralisierenden antikorpern gegen 11 serotypen der aviaren adenoviren. Arch Gefluegelkd 48:245–250.

34. Niemann, K. W. 1930. Clostridium welchii infection in the domesticated fowl. J Am Vet Med Assoc 77:604–606.

35. Page, R.K., O.J. Fletcher, C.S. Eidson, and G.E. Michaels. 1976. Dermatitis produced by Rhodotorula glutins in broiler-age chickens. Avian Dis 20:416–421.

36. Perek, M. 1958. Ergot and ergotlike fungi as the cause of vesicular dermatitis (sod disease) in chickens. J Am Vet Med Assoc 132:529–533.

37. Proudfoot, F.G., and H.W. Hulan. 1985. Effects of stocking density on the incidence of scabby hip syndrome among broiler chickens. Poult Sci 64:2001–2003.

38. Radan, M, and N. Rautenstein-Arasi. 1950. Anaerobic subcutaneous emphysema of poultry. Nature 166:442.

39. Rosenberger, J.K., S. Klopp, R.J. Eckroade, and W.C. Krauss. 1975. The role of the infectious bursal agent and several avian adenoviruses in the hemorrhagic-aplastic-anemia syndrome and gangrenous dermatitis. Avian Dis 19:717–729.

40. Saunders, J.R., and A.A. Bickford. 1965. Clostridial infections of growing chickens. Avian Dis 9:317–326.

41. Shirasaka, S., and Y. Benno. 1982. Isolation of Clostridium septicum from diseased chickens in broiler farms. Jpn J Vet Sci 44:807–809.

42. Smith, L.DS. 1980. Clostridial infections. In S.B. Hitchner, C.H. Domermuth, H.G. Purchase, and J.E. Williams (eds.), Isolation and Identification of Avian Pathogens, pp. 33–35. Creative Printing Co., Inc., Endwell, NY.

43. Trenchi, H. 1960. Ingestion of Ammi visnaga seeds and photosensitization – the cause of vesicular dermatitis in fowls. Avian Dis 4:275–280.

44. Turnquest, R.U. 1979. Dermal squamous cell carcinoma in young chickens. Am J Vet Res 40:1628–1633.

45. Weymouth, D.K., M. Gershman, and H.L. Chute. 1963. Report of Clostridium in capons. Avian Dis 7:342–343.

46. Yamada, S., S. Kamikawa, Y. Uchinuno, Y. Tominaga, K. Matsuo, H. Fujikawa, and K. Takeuchi. 1977. Avian dermatitis caused by Aspergillus fumigatus. J Jpn Vet Med Assoc 30:200–202.

BOTULISM

John E. Dohms

INTRODUCTION. Botulism is an intoxication caused by exotoxin of *Clostridium botulinum*. Synonyms are limberneck and Western duck sickness.

The disease occurs in free-ranging and confinement-reared poultry and feral birds. The majority of avian cases are caused by *C. botulinum* type C, although outbreaks due to other toxin types have been described (10, 33). The public health significance of avian type C botulism outbreaks is considered minimal (3, 25). Four human type C botulism intoxications have been reported, but are not well documented (22, 25). No human cases of type C botulism have been associated with concurrent outbreaks of avian botulism (25, 49). However, nonhuman primates have succumbed to type C botulism after toxin inoculation (52), and captive monkeys died after eating chicken contaminated with type C toxin (47).

HISTORY. Dickson reported the first case of botulism in chickens in 1917 (8). Both chickens and humans developed the disease after ingestion of home-canned vegetables. The cause of Western duck sickness, first recognized in the USA in the early 1900s, was later found to be *C. botulinum* type C toxin (17, 26). Botulism in chickens was reported following ingestion of fly larvae of the genus *Lucilia* in 1923 and the first *C. botulinum* type C strains were isolated from these invertebrates (2). Historical reviews of avian botulism are available (6, 10, 31, 42).

Although many early cases occurred in free-ranging poultry, more recent epornitics have occurred in intensively reared broiler chickens (10, 38, 48).

INCIDENCE AND DISTRIBUTION. The disease has affected poultry and waterfowl worldwide (14). Modern methods of poultry husbandry were thought to have reduced the incidence of botulism by preventing free-ranging poultry from eating toxin-contaminated food sources. However, severe cases have been reported in modern broiler flocks reared in confinement. These cases have been reviewed (10, 48). All types of wild birds and both avian and mammalian predators and scavengers have been affected during type C botulism outbreaks in wild birds (25); ducks are most often affected (42). Botulism has been reported in pheasants reared on game farms (42).

Botulism in ducks, broiler chickens, and pheasants occurs more frequently and with greater severity during warmer months. However, outbreaks in broiler chickens have been reported in winter (11, 39).

ETIOLOGY. *C. botulinum* is a gram-positive, spore-forming bacterium capable of elaborating a potent exotoxin under appropriate environmental conditions (33). The species consists of a diverse group of anaerobic bacteria including four cultural (I-IV) and eight antigenically different toxigenic groupings (A, B, C alpha, C beta, D, E, F, and G). Human disease has been associated mainly with types A, B, E, and F while A, C, and E have caused disease in birds (50). Cases of botulism in chickens, ducks, pheasants, and turkeys in natural or commercial settings have been caused primarily by the type C toxigenic group (10, 42, 48).

Morphology and Staining. The gram-positive cells of *C. botulinum* type C measure 4–6 × 1.0 μm, often occurring singly or in short chains. The vegetative cell is motile. Subterminal or occasional terminal endospores are present in aging cultures (33). A cell wall lysin is responsible for rapid autolysis of the organism and causes gram-variable staining in older cultures. Toxin is released during autolysis (4). Type C spores are more easily heat inactivated than type A and B spores (33), but are more resistant to heat than type E spores (45). The time required to cause a 10-fold reduction in spore viability at 101 C (D value), was 2.44 min for a terrestrial type C strain (45).

Culture group III contains nonproteolytic or weakly proteolytic type C and D toxigenic types. Cultivation and cultural characteristics of this group have been reviewed (23, 50). *C. botulinum* requires an available water content (a_w) of 0.92 for growth and toxin production (40). The type C toxigenic grouping is further subdivided into C alpha and C beta subtypes based on their toxigenic properties (33).

Toxins. Botulism toxins are among the most potent toxins known (30). Type C toxin is produced under anaerobic conditions at temperatures between 10–47 C with optimum toxin production between 35–37 C (33).

Type C alpha cultures produce three toxins; C1, C2, and small amounts of type D toxin (15). C1 and D toxin production is mediated by bacteriophage. Type C strains, cured of their prophage, can be converted to type D organisms by infection with phage purified from type D strains. The reciprocal is also true (15). Type C beta strains, lacking bacteriophage coding for C1 and D toxins, produce only C2 toxin; genes coding for C2 toxin are not phage associated (15). Because of the interconvertibility of C alpha and C beta strains, the relevance of C alpha and C beta toxigenic grouping has been questioned (15).

The C1 and D, together with A, B, E, and F, toxins are synthesized as a single nontoxic polypeptide that is cleaved by proteases to produce a

140,000 to 167,000 dalton dichain neurotoxin (46). A 98,000 dalton heavy chain and a 53,000 dalton light chain, held together by an interchain disulfide bond, are not toxic when dissociated (51).

The site of neurotoxin action is the peripheral cholinergic nerve terminus. Free toxin binds to the cell membrane, translocates, and reacts intracellularly to block release of acetylcholine. When the cholinergic nerve ending is a motor endplate, the muscle is paralyzed (46). Binary C2 toxin, though not neurotoxic, requires trypsin activation and causes increased membrane permeability in a variety of cultured tissues (37, 46). Ducks and geese inoculated intravenously with C2 toxin showed cardiopulmonary symptoms (24, 37). In mice, C2 toxin has enterotoxic properties (37). The role of C2 toxin in natural botulism outbreaks is presently unclear.

Chickens, turkeys, pheasants, and peafowl are susceptible to types A, B, C, and E but not D or F toxin (18). Chickens are most sensitive to types A and E given intravenously but relatively resistant to type C1 intoxication (12, 18, 34, 40, 41). In contrast, ducks and pheasants are more susceptible to C1 toxin (20, 18). Compared to other toxins, C1 and C2 are more readily absorbed by chickens when given orally (18). As broiler chickens age, they become less susceptible to C1 toxin. At hatching, the chicken lethal dose−50% (LD_{50}) was $10^{3.0}$ mouse-LD_{50}/kg body weight compared to $10^{6.3}$ mouse-LD_{50}/kg body weight at 8 wk of age (11).

PATHOGENESIS AND EPIZOOTIOLOGY

Natural And Experimental Hosts. Type C botulism has occurred in many species of birds including chickens, turkeys, ducks, and pheasants. In wildlife outbreaks, 117 avian species in 22 families are believed to have been affected (25). Outbreaks in aviaries have occurred (49). Mammalian species affected by type C toxin include mink, ferrets, cattle, pigs, dogs, horses, and a variety of zoo mammals (33). Fish succumbed to type C botulism during outbreaks on fish farms (49). Type C botulism in ruminants fed poultry manure has caused serious economic loss (16). Laboratory rodents are fully susceptible to type C toxin; mice are useful in the bioassay for toxin detection and typing.

In a study of 27 outbreaks in broiler chickens, ages ranged from 2 to 8 wk of age with a mean of 6.2 ± 1.7 wk (11). Outbreaks in older broiler chickens have been reported (3). Paradoxically, at these ages, broiler chickens are relatively resistant to C1 toxin (11).

Incubation Period. Experimental subcutaneous, intravenous, or oral inoculation of type C toxin in chickens and ducks produced clinical signs identical to those observed in field outbreaks. Morbidity and mortality were dose related. With high levels of toxin, disease appears within hours. With low toxin doses, onset of paralysis occurs within 1–2 days (12, 18, 20).

Transmission. *C. botulinum* type C is distributed worldwide, wherever large populations of wild and domestic birds are found. Type C organisms readily grow in the gastrointestinal tract of birds and are considered obligate parasites (50). Type C spores are commonly found in and around poultry and pheasant farms (11, 29, 48). Presence of organisms in the gastrointestinal tract of wild and domestic birds and the fact that spores are resistant to inactivation favors spread of this organism (25).

Signs. Clinical signs of botulism in chickens, turkeys, pheasants, and ducks are similar (6, 10, 42). In chickens, flaccid paralysis of legs, wings, neck, and eyelids are predominant features of the disease. Paralytic signs progress cranially from the legs to include wings, neck, and eyelids. Initially, affected birds are found sitting and are reluctant to move. If coaxed to walk, they appear lame. Wings droop when paralysed. Limberneck, the original and common name for botulism, precisely describes the paralysis of the neck (Fig. 11.9). Because of eyelid paralysis, birds appear comatose and may seem dead. Gasping has been reported when birds are handled. Death is caused by cardiac and respiratory failure (50).

Affected chickens have ruffled feathers, which may fall out with handling. Quivering of certain feather tracts has been observed. Broiler chickens showing signs of botulism may have diarrhea with excess urates in the loose droppings.

Morbidity And Mortality. Morbidity and mortality are related to the amount of acquired toxin. Low levels of intoxication produce little mortality and morbidity, which can confuse diagnosis. In severe cases, up to 40% mortality has been observed in broiler flocks (10, 39).

Western duck sickness is one of the most devastating diseases of waterfowl. Mortality, although difficult to estimate in wild birds, was reportedly greater than 100,000 birds on separate occasions (6, 25). Such losses have a major impact on wildlife populations (25). In other cases, outbreaks in small lakes have been limited to the relatively few waterfowl in these habitats (1, 48). Epornitics in pheasants reared on game farms have had mortality as high as 40,000 birds (42).

Pathology. Necropsy findings in chickens with type C botulism are unremarkable. Most authors report a lack of gross or microscopic lesions.

Pathogenesis. Type C botulism can be caused

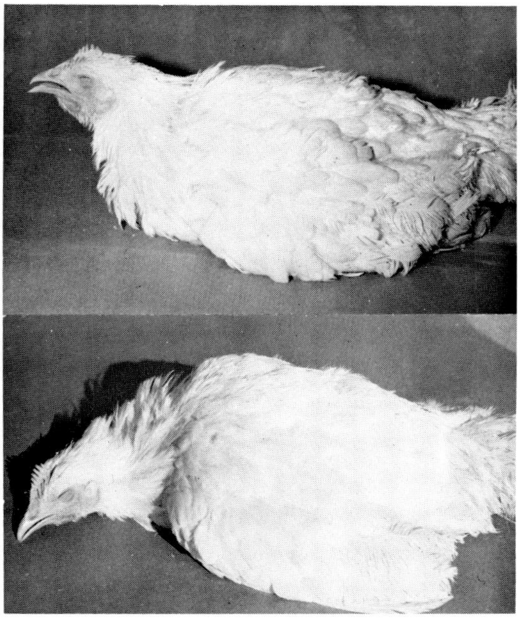

11.9. Botulism in chickens showing partial paralysis of wing and lower eyelid, difficult breathing caused by partial paralysis of respiratory muscles, and ruffled hackle feathers.

by ingestion of preformed toxin. Because the organism is widely distributed in the gut, dead birds provide conditions for *C. botulinum* growth and toxin production. Birds cannibalizing carcasses can obtain enough toxin to become diseased. Greater than 2000 minimum lethal doses (MLD) of type C toxin were found per gram of carcass tissue (3). Fly-blown carcasses may have maggots containing varying levels of botulinal toxin; maggots have been found to contain from 40,000–100,000 MLD of toxin (48). Maggots are readily devoured by chickens, pheasants, or ducks and can lead to explosive botulism outbreaks. In aquatic environments, small crustaceans and insect larvae may contain *C. botulinum* in their gut. If large numbers die due to oxygen depletion, toxin can be produced within these invertebrates. Ingestion of toxin-laden invertebrates has been proposed as the cause of type C botulism in ducks (42, 53). Lakes with shallow-sloping banks that experience dramatic fluctuations in water level have been associated with botulism outbreaks (25, 53).

Botulism caused by types A and E occur rarely and generally have been associated with consumption of spoiled human food products fed to backyard chicken flocks (31). Botulism in sea gulls, loons, and grebes was caused by eating dead or dying fish contaminated with type E toxin (33). A type A botulism case in broiler chickens was due to a contaminated feed source (7).

The pathogenesis of botulism was once exclusively thought to be due to ingestion of preformed toxin. There is growing evidence that *C. botulinum* type C elaborates toxin in vivo to cause disease (48). The term toxico-infection, originally used by Russian researchers, was adapted to describe this form of the disease in broiler chickens (39). In two cases of type C botulism in broiler chickens, carcasses were implicated as the toxin source (3, 21). However, in the majority of broiler chicken outbreaks, despite comprehensive searches, no toxin sources were identified (11, 19, 38, 44, 48). The disease pattern in many of these outbreaks was inconsistent with food or water as toxin sources. Dead carcasses could not account for intoxications.

Type C botulism was reproduced in leghorn chickens and pheasants fed botulism spores. Ceco-ligated chickens and pheasants had a lower incidence of disease after experimental spore challenge (34, 29), suggesting the cecum as the toxin production site. In pheasants, the crop supported toxin production (9). Although others have not been successful in reproducing the toxico-infectious form of botulism in broiler chickens (10, 29), Kurazono et al. (29) reported that toxin is produced in the cecum of broiler chickens but not at levels sufficient to kill the host. An environmental, bacterial, phage, and host interaction may be required to reproduce toxico-infectious botulism in broilers.

Immunity. Because the toxigenic dose is lower than the immunogenic dose, chickens and ducks recovering from botulism do not develop immunity (6, 18). However, carrion-eating crows and turkey vultures possessed antibodies to botulinal toxin (36). This may partly explain why vultures were resistant to experimental inoculations of botulism toxin (27).

DIAGNOSIS.

The differential diagnosis of botulism is based on clinical signs and lack of gross or microscopic lesions. Definitive diagnosis requires detection of toxin in serum, crop, or gastrointestinal washings from morbid birds (50).

Serum is the preferred diagnostic sample. Since *C. botulinum* is found in the gut of normal chickens, toxin can be produced in decaying body tissues; therefore, toxin found in tissues of dead birds does not confirm botulism.

The mouse bioassay is a sensitive and reliable method for confirming heat-labile toxin in serum (10). Groups of mice are inoculated with suspect serum samples. Other mice receive samples treated with type specific antiserum. If toxin is present in the sample, signs and death of mice given untreated samples usually occur within 48 hr. Mice inoculated with specific antitoxin will be protected. Other in vitro methods of detecting toxin have been reviewed (35).

In waterfowl and some poultry outbreaks, toxin levels in blood may be too low to produce disease in mice. Concentration of serum, or repeated inoculations of mice with suspect serum, may be required to demonstrate toxin in these cases (20).

In advanced stages of the disease, clinical signs are obvious; during mild intoxications only leg paralysis may be observed. The mild form of the disease must be differentiated from Marek's disease, drug and chemical toxicities, or appendicular skeletal problems. In these cases the mouse bioassay is particularly helpful in diagnosis. Botulism in waterfowl must be differentiated from fowl cholera and chemical toxicity. Lead poisoning of water birds is commonly confused with botulism (42).

Isolation of *C. botulinum* requires anaerobic culturing (23), and is of little help in diagnosis. The organism is widely distributed in gut, liver, and spleen of clinically normal chickens (11). However, detection of the organism in feed or environmental samples may prove useful in epizootiological studies. The organism can be demonstrated in samples inoculated into cooked meat medium and incubated anaerobically at 30 C (10). After 3–5 days incubation, toxin can be detected using the mouse bioassay with specific typing antitoxins. Other modifications of this procedure are available (23, 50). The organism can be detected using the fluorescent antibody technique (32).

TREATMENT. Many sick birds, if isolated and provided with water and feed, will recover. However, treatment of large numbers of morbid birds is difficult, and various protocols have been used but are not verified experimentally. The success of these treatments is hard to establish because of the difficultly in experimentally reproducing toxico-infectious botulism. The patterns of disease in untreated broiler houses can rise and fall during a given outbreak (11). Therefore, it is difficult to know if a particular treatment is effective, or, if by chance, treatment precedes a drop in mortality that would have occurred anyway. However, several treatments have been reported to be of benefit. Schettler (44) treated affected broiler flocks with sodium selenite, vitamins A, D_3, and E and reduced morality. The antibiotics bacitracin (100 g/ton in feed), streptomycin (1g/in water), or periodic chlortetracycline treatments reportedly reduced mortality (43). Page and Fletcher (38), found penicillin ineffective in controlling an outbreak, but others have found penicillin therapy reduced mortality (39). The in vitro susceptibility of *C. botulinum* to 13 antibiotics was reviewed (43).

Inoculation with specific antitoxin neutralizes only free and extracellularly bound toxin and might be considered when treating valuable birds in zoological collections. This is impractical in large poultry, duck, or pheasant outbreaks.

PREVENTION AND CONTROL. Management practices should emphasize removal of potential sources of the organism and its toxin from the environment. Prompt removal of dead birds and culling of sick birds is very important in prevention and control. In problem areas, removal of contaminated litter and thorough disinfection using calcium hypochlorite, iodophor, or formalin disinfectants may help reduce spore numbers in the environment (43). In houses with dirt floors, complete destruction of these spore-formers is difficult. Spores may be located in soil outside of the poultry facility and can be transported back into houses. Sato (43) recommends disinfection of areas around the poultry houses. Fly control may be another means of reducing the risk of toxic maggots in the environment. During outbreaks, it has been suggested feeding lower-energy diets reduces mortality caused by toxico-infectious botulism (44).

Immunization. Active immunization with inactivated bacterin-toxoids has been successfully used in pheasant operations (28). Similarly formulated toxoids protect chickens and ducks from experimental botulism (5, 13). However, vaccination of large numbers of broiler chickens is costly, and vaccination of wildfowl is not practical.

REFERENCES

1. Azuma, R., and T. Itoh. 1987. Botulism in waterfowl and distribution of C. botulinum type C in Japan. In M.W. Eklund and V.R. Dowell, Jr. (eds.), Avian Botulism: An International Perspective, pp. 167–187. Charles C Thomas, Springfield, IL.

2. Bengtson, I.A. 1922. Preliminary note on a toxin-producing anaerobe isolated from the larvae of Lucilia caesar. Public Health Rep 37:164–170.

3. Blandford, T.B., and T.A. Roberts. 1970. An outbreak of botulism in broiler chickens. Vet Rec 87:258–261.

4. Bonventre, P.F., and L.L. Kempe. 1960. Physiology of toxin production by Clostridium botulinum types A and B. I. Growth, autolysis, and toxin production. J Bacteriol 79:18–23.

5. Boroff, D.A., and J.R. Reilly. 1959. Studies of the toxin of Clostridium botulinum. V. Prophylactic immunization of pheasants and ducks against avian botulism. J Bacteriol 77:142– 146.

6. Clark, W.E. 1987. Avian botulism. In M.W. Eklund and V.R. Dowell, Jr. (eds.), Avian Botulism: An International Perspective, pp. 89–105. Charles C Thomas, Springfield, IL.

7. De Fagonde, A.P., and H.F. Sardi. 1967. Botulismo aviar, primer caso comprobado en la Republica Argentina. Bull Off Int Epiz 67:1479–1491.

8. Dickson, E.C. 1917. Botulism, a case of limberneck in chickens. 1917. J Am Vet Med Assoc 50:612–613.

9. Dinter, Z., and K.E. Kull. 1954. Uber einen ausbruch des botulismus bei frasanenkuken. Nord Veterinaermed 6:866–872.

10. Dohms, J.E. 1987. Laboratory investigation of botulism in poultry. In M.W. Eklund and V.R. Dowell, Jr. (eds.), Avian Botulism: An International Perspective, pp. 295–314. Charles C Thomas, Springfield, IL.
11. Dohms, J.E., and S.S. Cloud. 1982. Susceptibility of broiler chickens to Clostridium botulinum type C toxin. Avian Dis 26:89–96.
12. Dohms, J.E., P.H. Allen, and J.K. Rosenberger. 1982. Cases of type C botulism in broiler chickens. Avian Dis 26:204– 210.
13. Dohms, J.E., P.H. Allen, and S.S. Cloud. 1982. The immunization of broiler chickens against type C botulism. Avian Dis 26:340–345.
14. Egyed, M.N. 1987. Outbreaks of botulism in ruminants associated with ingestion of feed containing poultry waste. In M.W. Eklund and V.R. Dowell, Jr. (eds.), Avian Botulism: An International Perspective, pp. 371–380. Charles C Thomas, Springfield, IL.
15. Eklund, M.W., and V.R. Dowell Jr. 1987. Avian Botulism: An International Perspective. Charles C Thomas, Springfield, IL.
16. Eklund, M.E., F. Poysky, K. Oguma, H. Iida, and K. Inoue. 1987. Relationship of bacteriophages to toxin and hemagglutinin production by Clostridium botulinum types C and D and its significance in avian botulism outbreaks. In M.W. Eklund and V.R. Dowell Jr. (eds.), Avian Botulism: An International Perspective, pp. 191–222. Charles C Thomas, Springfield, IL.
17. Giltner, L.T., and J.F. Couch. 1930. Western duck sickness and botulism. Science 72:660.
18. Gross, W.B., and L.DS. Smith. 1971. Experimental botulism in gallinaceous birds. Avian Dis 15:716–722.
19. Haagsma, J. 1974. An outbreak of botulism in broiler chickens. Tijdschr Diergeneesk 99:1069–1070.
20. Haagsma, J. 1987. Laboratory investigation of botulism in wild birds. In M.E. Eklund and V.R. Dowell, Jr. (eds.), Avian Botulism: An International Perspective, pp. 283–293. Charles C Thomas, Springfield, IL.
21. Harrigan, K.E. 1980. Botulism in broiler chickens. Aust Vet J 56:603–605.
22. Holdeman, L.V. 1970. The ecology and natural history of Clostridium botulinum. J Wildl Dis 6:205–210.
23. Jansen, B.C. 1987. Clostridium botulinum type C, its isolation, identification, and taxonomic position. In M.W. Eklund and V.R. Dowell, Jr. (eds.), Avian Botulism: An International Perspective, pp. 123–132. Charles C Thomas, Springfield, IL.
24. Jensen, W.I., and R.M. Duncan. 1980. The susceptibility of the mallard duck (Anas platyrhynchos) to Clostridium botulinum C2 toxin. Jpn J Med Sci Biol 33:81–86.
25. Jensen, W.I., and J.I. Price. 1987. The global importance of type C botulism in wild birds. In M.W. Eklund and V.R. Dowell, Jr. (eds.), Avian Botulism: An International Perspective, pp. 33–54. Charles C Thomas, Springfield, IL.
26. Kalmbach, E.R. 1930. Western duck sickness produced experimentally. Science 72:658–660.
27. Kalmbach, E.R. 1939. American vultures and the toxin of Clostridium botulinum. J Am Vet Med Assoc 94:187–191.
28. Kurazono, H., K. Shimozawa, G. Sakaguchi, M. Takahashi, T. Shimizu, and H. Kondo. 1985. Botulism among penned pheasants and protection by vaccination with C1 toxoid. Res Vet Sci 38:104– 108.
29. Kurazono, H., K. Shimozawa, and G. Sakaguchi. 1987. Experimental botulism in pheasants. In M.W. Eklund and V.R. Dowell, Jr. (eds.), Avian Botulism: An International Perspective, pp. 267–281. Charles C Thomas, Springfield, IL.
30. Lamanna, C. 1959. The most poisonous poison. Science 130:763–772.
31. Levine, N.D. 1965. Botulism. In H.E. Biester and L.H. Schwarte (eds.), Diseases of Poultry, 5th Ed., pp. 456–461. Iowa State Univ Press, Ames.
32. Midura, T.F. 1987. Use of fluorescent antibody techniques in identification of Clostridium botulinum. In M.W. Eklund and V.R. Dowell, Jr. (eds.), Avian Botulism: An International Perspective, pp. 315–322. Charles C Thomas, Springfield, IL.
33. Mitchell, W.R., and S. Rosendal. 1987. Type C botulism: The agent, host susceptibility, and predisposing factors. In M.W. Eklund and V.R. Dowell, Jr. (eds.), Avian Botulism: An International Perspective, pp. 55–71. Charles C Thomas, Springfield, IL.
34. Miyazaki, S., and G. Sakaguchi. 1978. Experimental botulism in chickens: The cecum as the site of production and absorption of botulinal toxin. Jpn J Med Sci Biol 31:1–15.
35. Notermans, S., and S. Kozaki. 1987. In vitro techniques for detecting botulinal toxins. In M.W. Eklund and V.R. Dowell, Jr. (eds.), Avian Botulism: An International Perspective, pp. 323–336. Charles C Thomas, Springfield, IL.
36. Ohishi, I., and B.R. Dasgupta. 1987. Molecular structure and biological activities of Clostridium botulinum C2 toxin. In M.W. Eklund and V.R. Dowell, Jr. (eds.), Avian Botulism: An International Perspective, pp. 223–247. Charles C Thomas, Springfield, IL.
37. Ohishi, I., G. Sakaguchi, H. Riemann, D. Behymer, and B. Hurvell. 1979. Antibodies to Clostridium botulinum toxins in free-living birds and mammals. J Wildl Dis 15:3–9.
38. Page, R.K., and O.J. Fletcher. 1975. An outbreak of type C botulism in three-week-old broilers. Avian Dis 19:192–195.
39. Roberts, T.A., and I.D. Aitken. 1974. Botulism in birds and mammals in Great Britain and an assessment of the toxicity of Clostridium botulinum type C toxin in domestic fowl. In A.N. Barker, G.W. Gould, and J. Wolf (eds.), Spore Research 1973, pp. 1–9. Academic Press, London.
40. Roberts, T.A., and D.F. Collings. 1973. An outbreak of type-C botulism in broiler chickens. Avian Dis 17:650–658.
41. Roberts, T.A., A.I. Thomas, and R.J. Gilbert. 1973. A third outbreak of type C botulism in broiler chickens. Vet Rec 92:107–109.
42. Rosen, M.N. 1971. Botulism. In J.W. Davis, R.C. Anderson, L. Karstad, and D.O. Trainer (eds.), Infectious and Parasitic Diseases of Wild Birds, pp. 100–117. Iowa State Univ Press, Ames.
43. Sato, S. 1987. Control of botulism in poultry flocks. In M.W. Eklund and V.R. Dowell, Jr. (eds.), Avian Botulism: An International Perspective, pp. 349–356. Charles C Thomas, Springfield, IL.
44. Schettler, C.H. 1979. Clostridium botulinum type C toxin infection in broiler farms in North West Germany. Berl Muench Tierärztl Wochenschr 92:50–57.
45. Segner, W.P., and C.F. Schmidt. 1971. Heat resistance of spores of marine and terrestrial strains of Clostridium botulinum type C. Appl Microbiol 22:1030–1033.
46. Simpson, L.L. 1987. The pathophysiological actions of the binary toxin produced by Clostridium botulinum. In M.W. Eklund and V.R. Dowell, Jr. (eds.), Avian Botulism: An International Perspective, pp. 249–264. Charles C Thomas, Springfield, IL.
47. Smart, J.L., T.A. Roberts, K.G. McCullagh, V.M. Lucke, and H. Pearson. 1980. An outbreak of type C

botulism in captive monkeys. Vet Rec 107:445–446.
48. Smart, J.L., T.A. Roberts, and L. Underwood. 1987. Avian botulism in the British Isles. In M.W. Eklund and V.R. Dowell, Jr. (eds.), Avian Botulism: An International Perspective, pp. 111–122. Charles C Thomas, Springfield, IL.
49. Smith, L.DS. 1975. The Pathogenic Anaerobic Bacteria, 2nd Ed., pp. 203–229. Charles C Thomas, Springfield, IL.
50. Smith, G.R. 1987. Botulism in water birds and its relation to comparative medicine. In M.E. Eklund and V.R. Dowell, Jr. (eds.), Avian Botulism: and International Perspective, pp. 73–86. Charles C Thomas, Springfield, IL.
51. Syuto, B., and S. Kubo. 1981. Separation and characterization of heavy and light chains from Clostridium botulinum type C toxin and their reconstitution. J Biol Chem 256:3712–3717.
52. Wagenaar, R.O., G.M. Dack, and D.P. Mayer. 1953. Studies on mink food experimentally inoculated with toxin-free spores of Clostridium botulinum types A, B, C, and E. Am J Vet Res 14:479–483.
53. Wobeser, G.A. 1987. Control of botulism in wild birds. In M.W. Eklund and V.R. Dowell, Jr. (eds.), Avian Botulism: An International Perspective, pp. 339–348. Charles C Thomas, Springfield, IL.

12 BORDETELLOSIS (TURKEY CORYZA)

L.H. Arp and J.K. Skeeles

INTRODUCTION. Bordetellosis in poultry is a highly contagious upper respiratory tract disease caused by *Bordetella avium.* Colonization of ciliated epithelium by *B. avium* results in protracted inflammation and distortion of the respiratory mucosa. In young turkeys the disease is characterized by an abrupt onset of sneezing accompanied by clear, oculonasal discharge, mouth breathing, submandibular edema, altered voice, tracheal collapse, stunted growth, and predisposition to other infectious diseases. A careful analysis of the economic impact of bordetellosis has not been made; however, impaired growth and mortality resulting from secondary colisepticemia probably cause several million dollars in losses annually to the turkey industry in the USA.

The disease is still commonly referred to as turkey coryza. Other synonyms that have been largely abandoned are alcaligenes rhinotracheitis (ART), adenovirus-associated respiratory disease, acute respiratory disease syndrome, *Bordetella avium* rhinotracheitis (BART), and turkey rhinotracheitis. The numerous names used for this disease over the past decade reflect the confusion that has surrounded its etiology.

Members of the *Bordetella* genus are well known for their capacity to colonize ciliated epithelium and produce respiratory disease in vertebrates. However, despite similarities between whooping cough of humans (caused by *B. pertussis*) and bordetellosis of turkeys, there is no evidence that *B. avium* can either colonize or produce disease in humans (31).

HISTORY. Turkey rhinotracheitis (coryza) attributable to a bacterium of the genus *Bordetella* was first reported by Filion et al. (30) from Canada in 1967. Nearly a decade later a similar syndrome was recognized in W. Germany and in the USA where the causative agent was identified as *Bordetella bronchiseptica*-like (42) and *Alcaligenes faecalis* (85), respectively. The name *Bordetella avium* was eventually proposed and generally accepted (57).

Initial investigations into the cause of turkey rhinotracheitis in the USA focused on viruses. Adenoviruses were frequently associated with the disease (18), but attempts to reproduce it experimentally often failed (24, 82). The postmortem finding of bursal atrophy led to speculation that infectious bursal disease virus (IBDV) may have a role in turkey rhinotracheitis (69, 83). However, turkeys inoculated experimentally with IBDV failed to develop clinical disease or lesions, and concurrent inoculation with IBDV and *B. avium* failed to exacerbate experimental bordetellosis (48). Other infectious agents, including mycoplasmas, paramyxoviruses, Yucaipa virus, and chlamydia (2), have been considered in the etiology of turkey rhinotracheitis (59). In 1985, an acute, highly contagious upper respiratory disease of turkeys was recognized in England and Wales (3). The cause of that disease, which also has been called turkey rhinotracheitis, has been shown to be a pneumovirus (23) (see Avian Pneumovirus Infections, Chapter 29).

INCIDENCE AND DISTRIBUTION. Bordetellosis is an important disease in major turkey production regions of the USA, Canada (19), Australia (16), and W. Germany (42). However, the etiology of turkey rhinotracheitis in Great Britain, France, Israel, and South Africa may frequently include viruses and other bacteria in addition to *B. avium* (36, 59).

ETIOLOGY. Bordetellosis of turkeys is caused by *Bordetella avium* alone or in combination with environmental stresses and other respiratory pathogens. Experimental transmission (80) of the disease to susceptible poults by Simmons et al. (81) in the United States clearly established the etiologic agent as a small gram-negative bacillus. The bacterium, tentatively identified as *Alcaligenes faecalis,* closely resembled *Bordetella bronchiseptica* except for its failure to split urea. A systematic study by Kersters et al. (57) compared 28 pathogenic turkey isolates from diverse sources with 50 culture collection strains of closely related bacteria. Based on morphological, physiological, nutritional, serological, electrophoretic, and DNA-RNA hybridization, they concluded the bacterial cause of turkey rhinotracheitis represented a new species of *Bordetella;* the name *Bordetella avium* sp. nov. was proposed. Further molecular characterization of *B. avium* has confirmed its unique taxonomic position among species of the *Bordetella* and *Alcaligenes* genera (14, 41, 54, 68, 95).

Morphology and Growth. *Bordetella avium* is a gram-negative, nonfermentative, motile, strictly aerobic bacillus (53, 57) (Table 12.1). It grows readily on MacConkey's, Bordet-Gengou, veal infusion, trypticase-soy-blood agar, brain-heart infusion (BHI), and many other solid media (4), but not on minimal essential medium (53). Trypticase-soy and BHI broth support optimal growth when aeration is provided by agitation (10). Leyh et al. (58) have developed a defined minimal medium for growth of *B. avium* and detection of auxotrophic mutants. Biochemical properties of the organism are listed in Table 12.2.

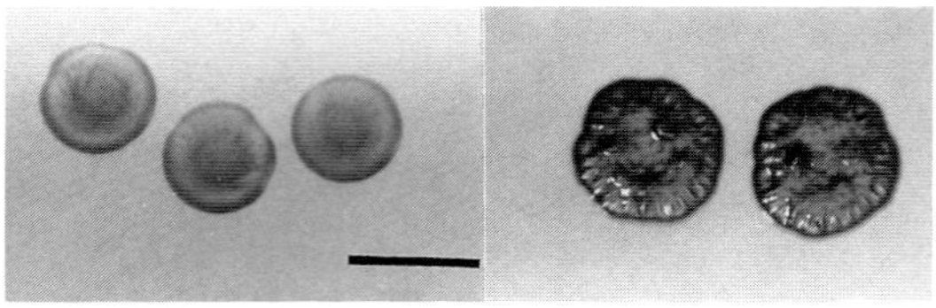

12.1. Colonies of *B. avium* strain 838 (*left*) and *B. avium*-like strain 007 (*right*) grown 48 hr at 35 C on MacConkey's. Note raised center in colonies of this *B. avium* strain. Bar = 1 mm.

Colony Morphology. Most strains of *B. avium* produce small, compact, translucent, pearl-like colonies (type I) with entire edges and glistening surfaces (57). Type I colonies are typically 0.2–1.0 mm in diameter after 24 hr of incubation and 1–2 mm in diameter after 48 hr of incubation. Many isolates develop a slightly raised brown-tinged center when grown 48 hr on MacConkey's agar (Fig. 12.1). A small percentage of strains dissociate into a larger colony type (type II). A third colony type, characterized by a serrated irregular edge, smooth surface, and larger size than type II colonies has been reported (41).

Resistance to Chemical and Physical Agents. Most commonly used disinfectants appear to kill *B. avium* when used according to manufacturer's recommendations. Survival of *B. avium* is prolonged by low temperatures, low humidities, and neutral pH (22). On simulated carrier materials such as dust and feces from turkey houses, the organism survived 25–33 days at 10 C and relative humidity 32–58%, whereas at 40 C with similar humidity the organism survived less than 2 days (22). Survival of the organism for at least 6 mo in undisturbed damp litter has been reported (11). In BHI broth culture, bacteria are killed within 24 hr at 45 C (10). Survival may be greatly prolonged at 10 C on smooth surfaces such as glass or aluminum (22). Fumigation of an uncleaned room with methyl bromide effectively stopped transmission of the disease to day-old susceptible poults (80).

Resistance to streptomycin, sulfonamides, and tetracycline by some strains of *B. avium* is encoded for on plasmids (60), however, most strains are sensitive in vitro to a large number of antibacterials. Treatment of *B. avium*-infected turkeys with oxytetracycline administered parenterally or by aerosol results in either no effect or a transient reduction in bacterial numbers (28, 87, 94).

Table 12.1. Physical properties of *B. avium*

Characteristic	References
Gram-negative rod (0.4-0.5 μm × 1–2 μm)	57, 85
Strict aerobe	57, 85
Motile (peritrichous flagella)	57, 85
Capsulated	57, 85
Fimbriated (2 nm diameter)	50
Colonies, 0.2–1 mm at 24 hr, round, glistening, covex (some strains dissociate to larger colonies)	41, 57
Hemagglutination of guinea pig erythrocytes	31, 53
Erythrocytes of other species	41, 75
Growth temperature, optimal at 35 C, killed at 45 C	10
Generation time, 35–40 min at 35 C	10
Strict tropism for ciliated epithelium	7, 34
Toxins	
Dermonecrotic (heat-liabile) toxin	31, 72, 73
Heat-stable toxin	78
Tracheal cytotoxin	31
Guanine + cytosine composition of DNA, 61.6–62.6 mol%	57

Table 12.2. Biochemical properties of *B. avium*

Biochemical Test	Results	References
Oxidase (Kovac's reagent)	Positive	57, 85, 95
Catalase	Positive	41, 85, 95
Urease	Negative	40, 57, 85
Nitrate reduced to nitrite	Negative	41, 57, 85
Growth on MacConkey's agar (lactose not fermented)	Positive	57, 85
Triple-sugar iron agar	Alkaline slant, no change in butt	14, 53, 85
Alkalinize amides and organic salts (Greenwood's low peptone)	Several positive	14, 16, 17, 41

Antigenic Structure. The antigenic structure of *B. avium* and related bacteria has been studied by agar-gel precipitation, cross-agglutination, and Western immunoblotting (10, 37, 51, 53, 57). All evidence to date suggests that *B. avium* isolates from various sources are closely related antigenically (57). Using antisera produced in rabbits, Kersters et al. (57) identified six different surface antigens, three of which were cross-reactive among three strains of *B. avium*. In addition they found two or three precipitation lines in common with *B. bronchiseptica*. Further antigenic relatedness was demonstrated with *Alcaligenes denitrificans* and *Achromobacter xylosoxidans* (57). Jackwood et al. (53) have demonstrated antigenic cross-reactivity between *B. avium* and *B. avium*-like (see later discussion) bacteria. Using convalescent serum and tracheal washings in immunoblotting procedures, Hellwig and Arp (37) have shown that infected turkeys recognize at least eight outer membrane proteins of *B. avium*. These proteins range in size from about 14 to about 116 kilodaltons (kD).

Potential Virulence Factors. Major virulence factors of *B. avium* can be divided into those involved in either adhesion, local mucosal injury, or systemic effects. Adhesion to cilia of respiratory epithelium is a consistent trait of *B. avium* and other species of *Bordetella*. The surface structures or molecules of *B. avium* responsible for adhesion have not been identified, but fimbriae (pili) and hemagglutinin may have roles (9, 50). Although fimbriae have been suggested as possible adhesive factors of *B. avium* (50), morphologically similar fimbriae are also common on adhesion-defective mutants and *B. avium*-like bacteria (38, 50). Hemagglutination (HA) of guinea pig erythrocytes correlates closely with virulence (31, 53), but appears to be unrelated to fimbriae (50). Two transposon-induced mutants selected for loss of HA activity had reduced adherence in vivo (9). Reversion of one mutant to HA-positive status resulted in reconstitution of adherence. As with other *Bordetella* species, it seems likely that more than one surface molecule is responsible for adhesion to cilia.

Several local effects have been attributed to toxins of *B. avium*. An acute cytotoxic and ciliostatic effect of *B. avium* on turkey tracheal organ cultures was reported by Gray et al. (33, 35) and others (61). Rimler (72) described a heat-labile toxin capable of killing mice and young turkeys. The toxin was later shown to produce necrotic and hemorrhagic lesions in the skin of turkeys and guinea pigs after intradermal injection and similar lesions in the liver and pancreas of turkeys following intraperitoneal injection (71, 73). Recent work has shown that *B. avium* produces a dermonecrotic toxin with physical, antigenic, and biologic properties comparable to those reported for the heat-labile toxin (31). The dermonecrotic toxin is a cell-associated, 155-kD protein with biological activity comparable to dermonecrotic toxins of *B. pertussis* and *B. bronchiseptica* (31). A role for the dermonecrotic toxin has not been established in the pathogenesis of bordetellosis in turkeys; the toxin appears not to be responsible for ciliostasis (73) or local epithelial damage (90).

Another toxin of *B. avium* implicated in local mucosal injury is the tracheal cytotoxin (TCT) isolated by Gentry-Weeks et al. (31). The TCT of *B. pertussis*, which is chemically identical to that produced by *B. avium*, has been shown to specifically damage ciliated epithelial cells leading to loss of epithelium and poor clearance of mucus (32). The TCT of *B. avium* is an anhydropeptidoglycan monomer with a mass of 921 daltons. Whether TCT is the mediator of cytotoxic activity reported earlier by Gray et al. (33, 35) remains to be determined.

Simmons et al. (78) have identified a *B. avium* heat-stable toxin capable of causing diarrhea and death in mice inoculated intraperitoneally; however, there is no evidence that the toxin produces adverse effects in poultry. Examination of several *B. avium* strains for the production of extracytoplasmic adenylate cyclase (31, 73) or pertussis toxin (31) failed to detect either one by immunologic and functional assays. Earlier studies by Simmons et al. (86) suggested that *B. avium* produces a histamine-sensitizing factor similar to that produced by other *Bordetella* species.

A number of systemic pathophysiologic effects have been attributed to *B. avium* infection. These include elevation of serum corticosterone (63), enhanced leukocyte migration (64), reduced body temperature (25), and reduced levels of monoamines in brain and lymphoid tissues (26, 27). Beginning with the original recognition of turkey rhinotracheitis in North Carolina, reports from flock caretakers have suggested defective immune function in affected poults (79). Vaccination of these poults with live vaccines resulted in unexpected deaths. This background, along with the observation of reduced bursa size in some poults with rhinotracheitis (83), lead to a series of experiments to determine effects of *B. avium* infection on immune function. Initially, depletion of thymic lymphocytes and decreased in vitro lymphocyte blastogenesis in response to the mitogen concanavalin A was described in poults infected with *B. avium* (79). However, subsequent studies of cell-mediated immunity in *B. avium*-infected poults revealed enhanced graft-vs-host and delayed hypersensitivity responses (65, 66); both are measures of cell-mediated immunity.

Pathogenicity and Strain Differences. Differences in pathogenicity have been reported among *B. avium* strains (75, 76). These differences, associated with colony morphology and hemagglutination, led to categorization of isolates into various groups or types (14, 53, 75). Continuing study of the molecular characteristics of *B. avium* and related bacteria has identified several differentiating features of *B. avium* (Table 12.3). Strains previously referred to as "group 1" (75) and "type 1" (53) should now be called *B. avium*. The term *B. avium*-like, as proposed by Jackwood et al. (54), will be reserved for nonpathogenic, avian isolates closely related to *B. avium*.

Studies of *B. avium* from various sources have revealed great similarity in electrophoretic patterns of outer-membrane proteins (38, 57). Furthermore, antigenic profiles examined by cross-agglutination, agar-gel precipitation, and Western immunoblotting, showed little variation among *B. avium* strains (37, 57). *Bordetella avium* shares several cross-reactive antigens with *B. avium*-like and other *Bordetella* species (37, 53). Despite the apparent genetic and molecular similarity among *B. avium* strains, differences have been noted in toxin production (72, 78), adherence to tracheal mucosa (9), plasmid profiles (52, 84), antibiotic sensitivity (52), pathogenicity (39, 76), and colony morphology (57).

PATHOGENESIS AND EPIZOOTIOLOGY

Natural and Experimental Hosts. The natural host of *B. avium* is the turkey, although isolations have also been made from chickens and other avian species (41, 77). Strains of *B. avium* isolated from avian species other than turkeys are pathogenic for day-old turkeys (41). A study of the prevalence of *B. avium* in North Carolina broiler flocks during the winter months revealed a 62% infection rate (12). Furthermore, there was a higher isolation rate from flocks with respiratory disease. Attempts to reproduce rhinotracheitis experimentally in chickens revealed that only two of eight *B. avium* strains colonized the trachea and produced disease (13); however, a later study (14) suggested the isolations from chickens may have included both *B. avium* and *B. avium*-like bacteria. It appears turkey and chicken strains of *B. avium* are similar (57), and cross-infection can occur between the species (77). Bordetellosis in chickens tends to be less severe than in turkeys (67, 77). A strain of *B. avium,* pathogenic for turkeys and Japanese quail, failed to produce clinical disease in guinea pigs, hamsters, and mice (62). Natural infection with *B. avium* is typically recognized in turkeys 2–6 wk old (19, 42, 70), although older turkeys and breeder flocks may also develop clinical disease (55, 56). Experimental inoculation of poults more than 1–2 wk old frequently results in colonization with only mild disease.

Transmission and Carriers. Bordetellosis is a highly contagious disease readily transmitted to susceptible poults through close contact with infected poults or through exposure to litter or water contaminated by infected poults (80). Infection is not transmitted between adjacent cages thus providing evidence against aerosol transmission (80). Litter contaminated by a flock infected with *B. avium* is likely to remain infective for 1–6 mo (11, 22). Although a carrier state has not been demonstrated in turkeys recovered from bordetellosis, the possibility seems likely.

Incubation Period. The incubation period is 7–10 days when susceptible poults are exposed to infected poults by close direct contact (80). Intranasal or intraocular inoculation of day-old poults with 10^5–10^7 colony-forming units of *B. avium* results in clinical signs (nasal exudate) of bordetellosis in 4–6 days (6, 34, 76).

Signs. An abrupt onset of sneezing (snick) in a high percentage of 2- to 6-wk-old turkeys over the course of a week is suggestive of bordetellosis. Older turkeys may also develop a dry cough (56). A clear nasal discharge can be expressed by placing gentle pressure over the bridge of the beak between the nostrils. During the first 2 wk of dis-

Table 12.3. Differentiation of *B. avium* and *B. avium*–like bacteria

Characteristic	*B. avium*	*B. avium*-like
Pathogenicity	Positive	Negative
In vivo adhesion[a]	Positive	Negative
Hemagglutination[b]	Positive	Negative
Growth on minimal essential medium agar[c]	Negative	Positive
Growth in 6.5% NaCl broth[c]	Few positive	Most positive
Other distinguishing features		
Outer membrane profiles on SDS-PAGE (38, 53)		
Cellular fatty-acid analyses (54, 68)		
Alkalinization of amides and organic acids (14, 15)		

[a]Adhesion to turkey tracheal mucosa (5, 9).
[b]Hemagglutination of guinea pig erythrocytes (53) may be weak or inconsistent with some strains or organisms grown in liquid medium.
[c](53).

ease, the nares and feathers of the head and wings become coated with wet, tenacious, brownish exudate (Fig. 12.2) and some birds develop submaxillary edema. Mouth breathing, dyspnea, and altered vocalization in the second week of clinical signs result when the nasal cavity and upper trachea become partially occluded with mucoid exudate. Tracheal softening can be palpated through the skin of the neck in some birds beginning in the second week of disease. Behavioral changes include reduced activity, huddling, and decreased consumption of feed and water. Concurrent infections and poor weight gains contribute to poor flock performance and numerous birds with stunted growth (10). Signs of disease begin to subside after a course of 2–4 wk (34, 70, 76, 93).

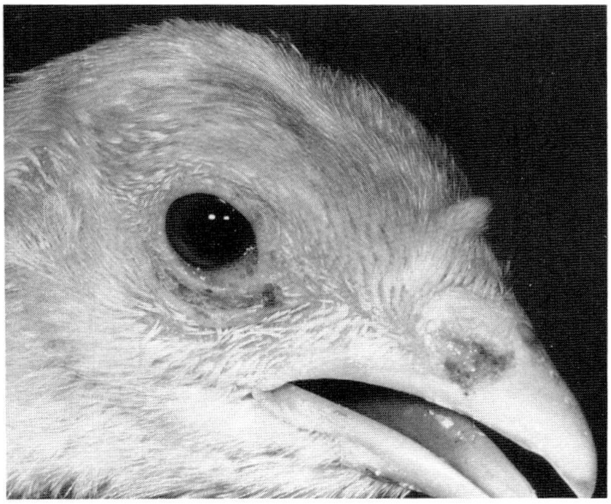

12.2. Clinical appearance of a poult with bordetellosis. Open-mouth breathing, dark stains around eye and nostril, and foamy exudate at the medial canthus of the eye.

Morbidity and Mortality. Bordetellosis in turkeys is typically characterized by high morbidity and low mortality. In turkeys 2–6 wk of age, morbidity reaches 80–100% (76), whereas the mortality rate is less than 10%. Infection of a breeder flock with *B. avium* resulted in only 20% morbidity with no mortality (56). High mortality rates (>40%) in young turkeys are frequently associated with concurrent isolation of *Escherichia coli* (19, 76). Experimental studies of concurrent *B. avium* and *E. coli* infections in 2- to 4-wk-old turkeys revealed defective clearance of *E. coli* from tracheas (29, 91) and increased severity of airsacculitis attributable to *E. coli* (92). Adverse environmental temperatures (10), high humidity (88), poor air quality, and concurrent respiratory pathogens may increase mortality rates (76).

Gross Lesions. Gross lesions are confined to the upper respiratory tract and vary with the duration of infection. Nasal and tracheal exudates change in character from serous initially to tenacious and mucoid during the course of disease. Tracheal lesions consisting of generalized softening and distortion of the cartilaginous rings, dorsal-ventral compression, and fibrinomucoid luminal exudate are highly suggestive of bordetellosis (6, 93). In isolated cases there is severe infolding of the dorsal tracheal wall into the lumen immediately below the larynx (Fig. 12.3) (6, 94). In cross-section, tracheal rings appear to have thick walls and a diminished lumen. Distortion of tracheal cartilages persists at least 53 days postinfection (6). Accumulation of mucoid exudate in an area of tracheal infolding frequently leads to death by suffocation (6). Hyperemia of the nasal and tracheal mucosae and edema of interstitial tissues of the head and neck are apparent during the first 2 wk of infection.

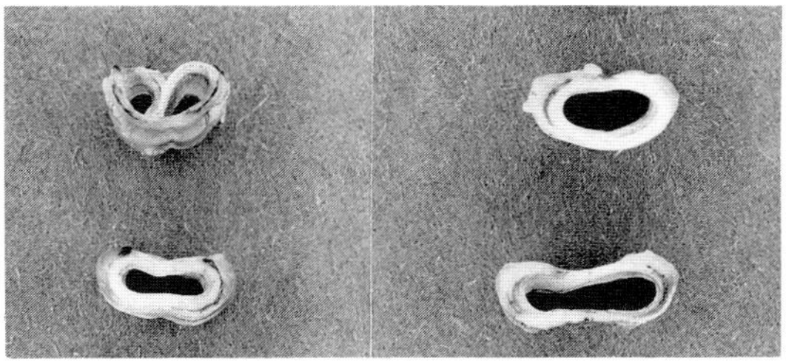

12.3. Cross sections of a collapsed trachea from a poult with bordetellosis. Section on top left, taken immediately below the larynx, has extreme dorsal-ventral infolding. Other sections were taken at 5-cm intervals along the trachea. (Am J Vet Res)

Histopathology. Cilia-associated bacterial colonies, progressive loss of ciliated epithelium, and depletion of mucus from goblet cells are distinctive characteristics of bordetellosis (6, 34). Colonization of ciliated epithelium begins on the nasal mucosa, progresses down the trachea, and into primary bronchi within 7–10 days. Bacteria adhere specifically to cilia and are never found attached to other cell types (7). As seen by scanning electron microscopy, surfaces of adherent bacteria are covered with numerous knoblike surface projections (Fig. 12.4). Colonized cells having increased eosinophilia of the apical cytoplasm may protrude slightly from the mucosa (94). Bacterial colonies (Fig. 12.5) are most apparent on the tracheal mucosa 1–2 wk after onset of clinical signs, before loss of ciliated cells is extensive (6, 7).

During the first 2 wk of signs, ciliated tracheal epithelium is gradually lost and replaced by nonciliated cuboidal epithelium (Fig. 12.6). These immature hyperplastic cells have basophilic cytoplasm with variable numbers of small mucous granules (6, 94). Late in the disease, squamous

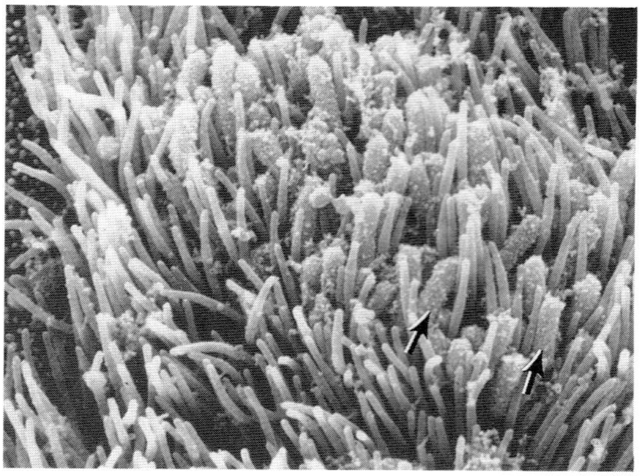

12.4. Numerous *B. avium* bacteria (*arrows*) intimately associated with cilia of tracheal epithelial cells. The bacterial surfaces are covered with irregularly shaped, knoblike projections, which may contribute to adhesion.

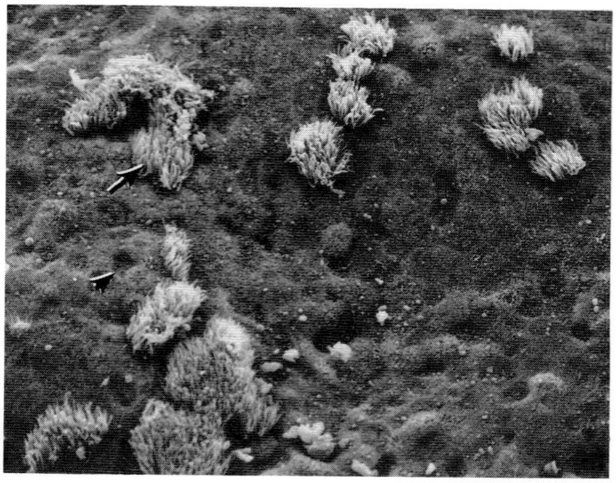

12.6. Loss of ciliated epithelium from the tracheal mucosal surface. Isolated clumps of ciliated cells (*arrow*) and dark pits left where ciliated cells have sloughed (*arrow head*).

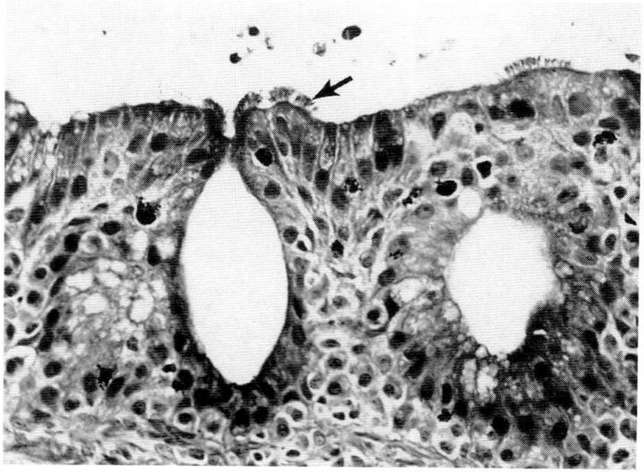

12.5. Trachea from a poult infected 3 wk previously with *B. avium*. Characteristic lesions of bordetellosis include cilia-associated bacterial colonies (*arrow*), loss of ciliated epithelium, dilated mucous glands depleted of mucus, and interstitial infiltration of plasma cells and lymphocytes.

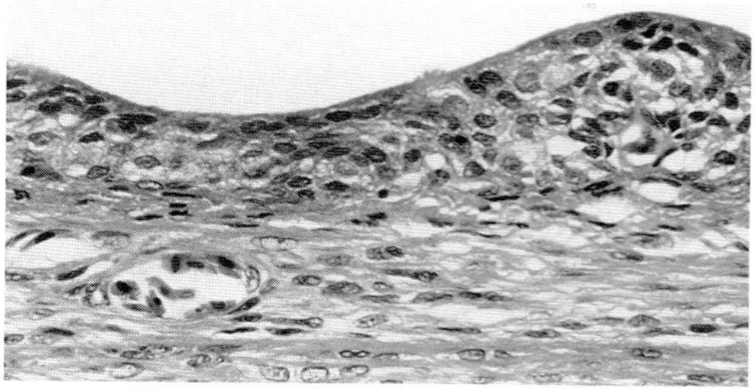

12.7. Squamous metaplasia of tracheal epithelium occurs in some poults late in the course of bordetellosis.

metaplasia of tracheal epithelium may occur (Fig. 12.7). Linear eosinophilic inclusions occur in the cytoplasm of tracheal epithelium during the first 3 wk of disease (6, 7). Ultrastructurally, these inclusions are proteinaceous crystals composed of parallel filaments surrounded by membrane (7). During the third and fourth week of disease, the tracheal mucosa becomes distorted by numerous folds and mounds of dysplastic epithelium. Depending on the severity of the disease, the tracheal epithelium returns to normal 4–6 wk after the onset of signs (6, 34), when *B. avium* can no longer be isolated.

Discharge of copious mucoid exudates from the upper respiratory tract is accompanied by depletion of mucus from isolated goblet cells and mucous glands along the mucosa (6, 94). Alveolar glands become cystic and lined by immature epithelium with small mucous granules (Fig. 12.5). Goblet cells remain largely depleted of mucous granules from the first through the third week of clinical disease. Mucosal surface exudates change from mucopurulent to fibrinopurulent after the first week of disease (7).

Cellular exudates in the tracheal lamina propria begin with multifocal infiltrates of heterophils and change to predominantly lymphocytes and plasma cells as clinical signs subside (6, 34). In the third through fifth week of disease, a diffuse increase in mucosal plasma cells is accompanied by multifocal lymphoid nodules in the submucosa.

Pulmonary lesions are restricted to primary bronchi and bronchus-associated lymphoid tissue (92, 93). In contrast to the tracheal mucosa, the bronchial mucosa maintains a near normal appearance, including ciliated columnar epithelium and goblet cells (93). Mild colonization of isolated ciliated cells by *B. avium* is accompanied by a mild infiltrate of heterophils. Bronchus-associated lymphoid tissue, normally found at the junction of primary and secondary bronchi, becomes grossly apparent, and lymphoid nodules protrude into the bronchial lumen (93). Other changes of lymphoid tissues include depletion of cortical lymphocytes from the thymus during the early disease (79).

In summary, distinctive microscopic lesions of diagnostic value include cilia-associated bacterial colonies, cytoplasmic inclusions, cystic mucosal glands, and generalized loss of ciliated epithelium.

Immunity. Most turkeys develop a humoral immune response to infection with *B. avium* (6, 47). Serum antibodies, detected by microtiter agglutination, appear within 2 wk after experimental exposure to *B. avium* and reach peak levels by 3–4 wk postexposure (6, 47). The period of peak antibody titer is followed within 1 wk by resolution of clinical disease and a decline in bacterial numbers in the trachea (6). This, combined with evidence for maternal immunity, suggests an important role for humoral immunity in prevention and recovery from infection (11, 43). Convalescent serum and tracheal secretions from turkeys infected with *B. avium* inhibit adherence of the bacteria to the tracheal mucosa in turkeys (8). Moreover, adherence of *B. avium* is inhibited whether convalescent serum is administered locally or parenterally. The passive administration of convalescent serum is believed to mimic many aspects of maternal immunity. Continuing studies of the immune response to *B. avium* using Western immunoblots have identified at least eight surface proteins recognized by antibody in serum and tracheal secretions during a 4-wk course of infection (37).

An active immune response is generated in most turkeys inoculated with live *B. avium* or various bacterins. The serum antibody response to a temperature-sensitive mutant of *B. avium* is variable depending on vaccination dosage, turkey age, and environmental factors affecting colonization (10, 21, 39, 44, 46, 49, 55). Recent studies have suggested that poults less than 3 wk of age respond poorly to *B. avium* vaccines (44, 49).

Infection with *B. avium* has been recognized as potentially immunosuppressive since Simmons et al. (79) reported thymic lesions and suppression of lymphocyte blastogenesis. Although subsequent tests have revealed no evidence for defects in cellular immunity (64–66), infection with *B. avium* apparently interferes with immunity to live *Pasteurella multocida* and hemorrhagic enteritis vaccines (74, 79). Reduced monoamine concentrations in brain and lymphoid tissues and elevated serum corticosterone have been recorded in turkeys infected with *B. avium* (26, 27, 63). Although such hormonal changes are probably not unique to bordetellosis, they may help explain the immunosuppression seen in the field.

Pathogenesis. Initial adhesion of bacteria to ciliated cells of the oronasal mucosa leads to progressive colonization from the upper trachea to the primary bronchi over the next week. Expansion of the bacterial population along the respiratory mucosa stimulates acute inflammation and release of mucus from goblet cells leading to sneezing, coughing, and nasal obstruction. Spread of infection against the flow of mucociliary clearance occurs as motile "swarmer" bacteria break free from microcolonies and move within the layer of mucin to other ciliated cells. Apparently, tracheal mucus does not contain receptor analogs to impede spread of the bacteria. During the next week, many of the cells colonized by *B. avium* slough into the tracheal lumen leaving large surfaces devoid of cilia.

How *B. avium* damages the tracheal mucosa and cartilage remains unknown, but the tracheal cytotoxin may be involved. The formation of cytoplasmic protein crystals and delayed restitution of normal mucosa are suggestive of a toxin that alters cell growth and differentiation. The molecular basis for softening and collapse of tracheal rings may result from abnormal connective tissue metabolism leading to qualitative and quantitative changes in collagen and elastin (96).

As ciliated cells are progressively lost, the flow of mucus and exudates becomes sluggish, particularly in the upper trachea and nasal cavity. Obstruction of nasolacrimal ducts causes foamy ocular exudate to accumulate at the medial canthus of the eye. Signs of bordetellosis result from local and systemic products of the inflammatory response, soluble bacterial toxins, and physical obstruction of large air passages.

Within a week of the onset of clinical signs, local and systemic immune responses develop to *B. avium* antigens. Antibody transported from serum and antibody produced by submucosal plasma cells accumulates in respiratory secretions. Local antibody interacts with free swarmer *B. avium* cells to inhibit their motility and prevent adhesion to other ciliated cells. Colonies of bacteria among the cilia are largely protected from host defenses; however, numerous bacteria are shed along with colonized epithelial cells. The bacterial population diminishes over the next several weeks as colonized cells are lost and newly formed ciliated cells are protected from colonization by antibody.

Some convalescent birds are probably slow to clear all *B. avium* from their respiratory tissues and serve as a source of infection for susceptible flocks. As mucosal immunity wanes over the next 4–8 wk, any residual population of *B. avium* in the nasal cavity or sinuses can again expand to produce clinical infection or be transmitted to susceptible birds.

DIAGNOSIS. The diagnosis of bordetellosis is currently based on clinical signs and lesions, isolation of *B. avium* from the respiratory tract, a positive serologic test, or some combination of these.

Isolation and Identification of Causative Agent. Bacterial isolation is accomplished on MacConkey's agar inoculated with a swab sample from the tracheal mucosa. Samples collected from the choanal opening and nostril, or by passing a swab into the trachea through the larynx, commonly yield large numbers of nonpathogenic bacteria (81, 89). When turkeys are available for necropsy examination, swab samples should be collected aseptically through an opening in the midcervical trachea. After 24 hr of incubation on MacConkey's agar, colonies of *B. avium* are clear and pinpoint in size. While most contaminating bacteria form large mucoid colonies (often lactose fermenters), which mask *B. avium* in the more concentrated streak pattern, the minute colonies of *B. avium* may be recognized in the more diluted streak pattern. By incubating culture plates up to 48 hr, *B. avium* colonies are more easily recognized and may develop a brownish raised center (Fig. 12.1). Early in the course of infection pure cultures can be obtained from the trachea, but in later stages *E. coli* and other opportunistic bacteria may be isolated (76). Physical and biochemical characteristics that serve to distinguish *B. avium* from closely related bacteria are presented in Tables 12.2 and 12.3.

Serology. Serologic testing has proven to be useful experimentally and in the natural disease for detection of serum antibodies to *B. avium*. Jackwood and Saif (47) developed a microagglutination test (MAT) using a killed, neotetrazolium chloride–stained *B. avium* antigen in a microtiter system. The MAT has been shown to correlate well with bacterial isolation. It seems likely that serologic tests remain positive for a period after *B. avium* can no longer be cultured. In a field study by Slavik et al. (89), flocks with a history of respiratory disease were more commonly positive serologically for *B. avium* even though bacteria were not isolated. In experimentally infected poults, antibody is detectable by the MAT from 2 wk postinoculation (PI) until at least 5–7 wk PI (6, 10, 47). Peak titers occur at about 3–4 wk PI. For each of the above tests, agglutination occurs at serum dilutions of from 1:320 to 1:512 (6, 47). Use of heterologous *B. avium* antigen has little effect on agglutination titers (10).

Hopkins et al. (45) developed an enzyme-linked immunosorbent assay (ELISA) for detection of serum antibodies to *B. avium* using a whole-bacteria antigen, a 1:200 serum dilution, and a 1:3200 dilution of commercially available antiturkey IgG conjugate. Serologic results obtained with the ELISA correlate well with those from the MAT, but ELISA may be more sensitive for detection of maternal antibody in day-old poults (45). Although *B. avium* has antigens in common with closely related *B. avium*–like bacteria, there is no evidence that these related bacteria cause a positive serologic reaction to *B. avium* in nature.

Differential Diagnosis. Bordetellosis must be differentiated from other primary and secondary causes of rhinotracheitis. Mycoplasmosis, chlamydiosis, and respiratory cryptosporidiosis may mimic or contribute to many of the clinical signs of bordetellosis (2, 56, 59). Of the viral agents, Newcastle disease virus, Yucaipa virus, adenovirus, influenza virus, and pneumovirus should be considered (23, 59). Although *B. avium* alone can produce all of the clinical signs and lesions of bordetellosis in the natural disease, *B. avium* is more frequently accompanied by Newcastle disease, *Mycoplasma* spp., and opportunistic bacteria such as *E. coli*.

Currently, the greatest diagnostic challenge is to differentiate *B. avium* from *B. avium*–like bacteria in primary cultures. Distinguishing characteristics of these closely related bacteria are presented in Table 12.3; however, pathogenicity testing in day-old poults is definitive. Intranasal inoculation of day-old poults with a 24-hr broth culture of *B. avium* is expected to produce clinical disease and nasal discharge in susceptible poults within 3–5 days.

TREATMENT. Treatment of bordetellosis with antibiotics administered in the water, by injection, or by aerosol has produced minimal clinical improvement in most cases. Treatment of an infected breeder flock with 1.8 g tetracycline-HCl and 2×10^6 I.U. potassium penicillin-G/gal of drinking water for 3 days produced clinical improvement within 24 hr (56). Treatment of bordetellosis in young turkeys with an aerosol of oxytetracycline-HCl reduced mortality associated with subsequent Newcastle disease vaccination compared with untreated flocks (28). Although these clinical testimonials suggest a favorable response to treatment, it remains unclear whether clinical improvement results from antibacterial effects against *B. avium* or to secondary pathogens such as *E. coli*.

In a group of experimentally infected poults, parenteral administration of long-acting oxytetracycline had no apparent effect on *B. avium* infection (87). Treatment of experimental bordetellosis with oxytetracycline-HCl administered by aerosol caused a transient reduction of bacterial numbers in the trachea and a delay in clinical signs and lesion development (94). However, by 4 days after treatment, bacterial numbers and disease severity were similar between treated and nontreated groups (94).

PREVENTION AND CONTROL

Management Procedures. *Bordetella avium* is highly contagious by direct contact and through contamination of water, feed, and litter. Strict biosecurity measures are required to prevent infection of clean flocks, and rigorous clean-up procedures are required to eliminate the organism from contaminated premises. A minimal clean-up procedure for contaminated premises should include complete removal of litter, thorough washing of all surfaces, disinfection of watering systems and feeders, and application of a disinfectant followed by either formaldehyde fumigation or by application of a dilute formaldehyde solution to all surfaces. *B. avium* is easily tracked from one facility to another, so the use of disinfectant foot baths, clean outer clothing, and even the requirement for showering between visits to different houses and locations is essential. Since the severity of bordetellosis is exacerbated by adverse environmental and infectious factors, attempts should be made to optimize temperature, humidity, and air quality while avoiding or delaying the use of live attenuated vaccines.

Immunization. Vaccines currently available commercially for prevention of bordetellosis in turkeys include a live temperature-sensitive (ts) mutant of *B. avium* (Art-Vax™, American Scientific Laboratories, Madison, WI) and a whole-cell bacterin (ADJUVAC-ART, Ceva Laboratories, Inc., Overland Park, KS). The live ts-mutant vaccine was induced by nitrosoguanidine mutation of a virulent *B. avium* isolate obtained from North Carolina (20). Original studies indicated the ts-mutant colonized the nasal mucosa and induced moderate levels of serum antibodies (20). Although subsequent use of the vaccine in Utah indicated substantial protection (21, 55), other controlled experiments indicated only moderate reduction in lesion severity or delayed onset of clinical disease (39, 44, 46, 49). The ts-mutant has the capacity to adhere to respiratory epithelium, but its slow growth rate may critically limit its ability to colonize and induce protective immunity (9, 10). Use of the ts-mutant vaccine according to label directions in day-old poults failed to prevent infection and disease, however, use of the vaccine in poults 3 wk of age and older prevented disease but not infection (44, 49). Concern exists that turkeys less than 3 wk of age may be unable to respond adequately to *B. avium* antigens or are unable to mount an adequate local immune response.

Houghten et al. (46) compared a spray method of vaccination with the method recommended by the manufacturer for the ts-mutant vaccine. Turkeys were immunized at 2 days of age using a spray cabinet followed 14 days later with another coarse spray exposure to the ts-mutant vaccine. Another group of turkeys was similarly immunized by eyedrop exposure followed 14 days later by oral exposure. The spray/eyedrop/oral methods of immunization were equally effective in reducing severity of tracheal lesions, but neither method prevented infection of the trachea by virulent challenge strains.

Two studies have indicated that breeder-hen vaccination may be useful for prevention of bordetellosis in progeny poults (11, 43). Vaccination of breeder hens with either heat-killed (43) or formalin-killed (11) adjuvanted bacterins delayed the onset and severity of clinical disease in challenge-exposed poults. Passive immunization of 3-wk-old poults with convalescent serum reduces adherence of *B. avium* to the tracheal mucosa in a dose- and time-dependent manner (8). Taken in total, these studies suggest that maternal antibody of the IgG class may confer temporary immunity to newly hatched poults. Additionally, vaccination of poults with purified pilus preparations and adjuvanted bacterins results in significant protection against *B. avium* colonization and clinical disease (1).

Since *B. avium* and *B. avium*-like bacteria are antigenically related, Jackwood and Saif (51) designed experiments to determine whether poults infected with nonpathogenic *B. avium*-like bacteria would develop immunity to *B. avium*. The *B. avium*-like bacteria failed to persist for a significant period in the respiratory tract and failed to induce either a serologic response or protection to *B. avium* challenge. Development of improved vaccines for bordetellosis requires better characterization of protective antigens of *B. avium* and an understanding of the turkey's immune response to them.

REFERENCES

1. Akeila, M.A., and Y.M. Saif. 1988. Protection of turkey poults from Bordetella avium infection and disease by pili and bacterins. Avian Dis 32:641–649.

2. Andral, B., C. Louzis, D. Trap, J.A. Newman, G. Bennejean, and R. Gaumont. 1985. Respiratory disease (rhinotracheitis) in turkeys in Brittany, France, 1981–1982. I. Field observations and serology. Avian Dis 29:26–34.

3. Anon. 1985. Turkey rhinotracheitis of unknown aetiology in England and Wales. A preliminary report from the British Veterinary Poultry Association. Vet Rec 117:653–654.

4. Arp, L.H. 1986. Adherence of Bordetella avium to turkey tracheal mucosa: Effects of culture conditions. Am J Vet Res 47:2618–2620.

5. Arp, L.H., and E.E. Brooks. 1986. An in vivo model for the study of Bordetella avium adherence to tracheal mucosa in turkeys. Am J Vet Res 47:2614–2617.

6. Arp, L.H., and N.F. Cheville. 1984. Tracheal lesions in young turkeys infected with Bordetella avium. Am J Vet Res 45:2196–2200.

7. Arp, L.H., and J.A. Fagerland. 1987. Ultrastructural pathology of Bordetella avium infection in turkeys. Vet Pathol 24:411–418.

8. Arp, L.H., and D.H. Hellwig. 1988. Passive im-

munization versus adhesion of Bordetella avium to the tracheal mucosa of turkeys. Avian Dis 32:494-500.

9. Arp, L.H., R.D. Leyh, and R.W. Griffith. 1988. Adherence of Bordetella avium to tracheal mucosa of turkeys: Correlation with hemagglutination. Am J Vet Res 49:693-696.

10. Arp, L.H., and S.M. McDonald. 1985. Influence of temperature on the growth of Bordetella avium in turkeys and in vitro. Avian Dis 29:1066-1077.

11. Barnes, H.J., and M.S. Hofstad. 1983. Susceptibility of turkey poults from vaccinated and unvaccinated hens to Alcaligenes rhinotracheitis (turkey coryza). Avian Dis 27:378-392.

12. Berkhoff, H.A., H.J. Barnes, S.I. Ambrus, M.D. Kopp, G.D. Riddle, and D.C. Kradel. 1984. Prevalence of Alcaligenes faecalis in North Carolina broiler flocks and its relationship to respiratory disease. Avian Dis 28:912-920.

13. Berkhoff, H.A., F.M. McCorkle, Jr., and T.T. Brown. 1983. Pathogenicity of various isolates of Alcaligenes faecalis for broilers. Avian Dis 27:707-713.

14. Berkhoff, H.A., and G.D. Riddle. 1984. Differentiation of Alcaligenes-like bacteria of avian origin and comparison with Alcaligenes spp. reference strains. J Clin Microbiol 19:477-481.

15. Blackall, P.J., and C.M. Doheny. 1987. Isolation and characterisation of Bordetella avium and related species and an evaluation of their role in respiratory disease in poultry. Aust Vet J 64:235-239.

16. Blackall, P.J., and J.G. Farrah. 1985. Isolation of Bordetella avium from poultry. Aust Vet J 62:370-372.

17. Blackall, P.J., and J.G. Farrah. 1986. An evaluation of two methods of substrate alkalinization for the identification of Bordetella avium and other similar organisms. Vet Microbiol 11:301-306.

18. Blalock, H.G., D.G. Simmons, K.E. Muse, J.G. Gray, and W.T. Derieux. 1975. Adenovirus respiratory infection in turkey poults. Avian Dis 19:707-716.

19. Boycott, B.R., H.R. Wyman, and F.C. Wong. 1984. Alcaligenes faecalis rhinotracheitis in Manitoba turkeys. Avian Dis 28:1110-1114.

20. Burke, D.S., and M.M. Jensen. 1980. Immunization against turkey coryza by colonization with mutants of Alcaligenes faecalis. Avian Dis 24:726-733.

21. Burke, D.S., and M.M. Jensen. 1981. Field vaccination trials against turkey coryza using a temperature-sensitive mutant of Alcaligenes faecalis. Avian Dis 25:96-103.

22. Cimiotti, W., G. Glünder, and K.-H. Hinz. 1982. Survival of the bacterial turkey coryza agent. Vet Rec 110:304-306.

23. Collins, M.S., and R.E. Gough. 1988. Characterization of a virus associated with turkey rhinotracheitis. J Gen Virol 69:909-916.

24. Dillman, R.C., and D.G. Simmons. 1977. Histopathology of a rhinotracheitis of turkey poults associated with adenoviruses. Avian Dis 21:481-491.

25. Edens, F.W., F.M. McCorkle, and D.G. Simmons. 1984. Body temperature response of turkey poults infected with Alcaligenes faecalis. Avian Pathol 13:787-795.

26. Edens, F.W., F.M. McCorkle, D.G. Simmons, and A.G. Yersin. 1987. Brain monoamine concentrations in turkey poults infected with Bordetella avium. Avian Dis 31:504-508.

27. Edens, F.W., F.M. McCorkle, D.G. Simmons, and A.G. Yersin. 1987. Effects of Bordetella avium on lymphoid tissue monoamine concentrations in turkey poults. Avian Dis 31:746-751.

28. Ficken, M.D. 1983. Antibiotic aerosolization for treatment of alcaligenes rhinotracheitis. Avian Dis 27:545-548.

29. Ficken, M.D., J.F. Edwards, and J.C. Lay. 1986. Clearance of bacteria in turkeys with Bordetella avium-induced tracheitis. Avian Dis 30:352-357.

30. Filion, P.R., S. Cloutier, E.R. Vrancken, and G. Bernier. 1967. Infection respiratoire du dindonneau causee par un microbe apparente au Bordetella bronchiseptica. Can J Comp Med Vet Sci 31:129-134.

31. Gentry-Weeks, C.R., B.T. Cookson, W.E. Goldman, R.B. Rimler, S.B. Porter, and R. Curtiss III. 1988. Dermonecrotic toxin and tracheal cytotoxin, putative virulence factors of Bordetella avium. Infect Immun 56:1698-1707.

32. Goldman, W.E. 1986. Bordetella pertussis tracheal cytotoxin: Damage to the respiratory epithelium. In L. Leive and P.F. Bonventre (eds.), Microbiology—1986, pp. 65-69. Am Soc Microbiol, Washington, DC.

33. Gray, J.G., J.F. Roberts, R.C. Dillman, and D.G. Simmons. 1981. Cytotoxic activity of pathogenic Alcaligenes faecalis in turkey tracheal organ cultures. Am J Vet Res 42:2184-2186.

34. Gray, J.G., J.F. Roberts, R.C. Dillman, and D.G. Simmons. 1983. Pathogenesis of change in the upper respiratory tracts of turkeys experimentally infected with an Alcaligenes faecalis isolate. Infect Immun 42:350-355.

35. Gray, J.G., J.F. Roberts, and D.G. Simmons. 1983. In vitro cytotoxicity of an Alcaligenes faecalis and its relationship in in vivo tracheal pathologic changes in turkeys. Avian Dis 27:1142-1150.

36. Heller, E.D., Y. Weisman, and A. Aharonovovitch. 1984. Experimental studies on turkey coryza. Avian Pathol 13:137-143.

37. Hellwig, D.H., and L.H. Arp. 1989. Identification of Bordetella avium antigens recognized during experimental infection in turkeys. Am J Vet Res. (In press).

38. Hellwig, D.H., L.H. Arp, and J.A. Fagerland. 1988. A comparison of outer membrane proteins and surface characteristics of adhesive and nonadhesive phenotypes of Bordetella avium. Avian Dis 32:787-792.

39. Herzog, M., M.F. Slavik, J.K. Skeeles, and J.N. Beasley. 1986. The efficacy of a temperature-sensitive mutant vaccine against Northwest Arkansas isolates of Alcaligenes faecalis. Avian Dis 30:112-116.

40. Hinz, K.-H., and G. Glünder. 1986. Identification of Bordetella avium sp. nov. by the API 20 NE system. Avian Pathol 15:611-614.

41. Hinz, K.-H., G. Glünder, and K.J. Römer. 1983. A comparative study of avian Bordetella-like strains, Bordetella bronchiseptica, Alcaligenes faecalis, and other related nonfermentable bacteria. Avian Pathol 12:263-276.

42. Hinz, K.-H., G. Glünder, and H. Lüders. 1978. Acute respiratory disease in turkey poults caused by Bordetella bronchiseptica-like bacteria. Vet Rec 103:262-263.

43. Hinz, K.-H., G. Korthas, H. Luders, B. Stiburek, G. Glunder, H.E. Brozeit, and T. Redmann. 1981. Passive immunisation of turkey poults against turkey coryza (Bordetellosis) by vaccination of parent breeders. Avian Pathol 10:441-447.

44. Hofstad, M.S., and E.L. Jeska. 1985. Immune response of poults following intranasal inoculation with Artvax™ vaccine and a formalin-inactivated Bordetella avium bacterin. Avian Dis 29:746-754.

45. Hopkins, B.A., J.K. Skeeles, G.E. Houghten, and J.D. Story. 1988. Development of an enzyme-linked immunosorbent assay for Bordetella avium. Avian Dis 32:353-361.

46. Houghten, G.E., J.K. Skeeles, M. Rosenstein, J.N. Beasley, and M.F. Slavik. 1987. Efficacy in turkeys of spray vaccination with a temperature-sensitive mutant of Bordetella avium (Art Vax™). Avian Dis 31:309–314.

47. Jackwood, D.J., and Y.M. Saif. 1980. Development and use of a microagglutination test to detect antibodies to Alcaligenes faecalis in turkeys. Avian Dis 24:685–701.

48. Jackwood, D.J., Y.M. Saif, P.D. Moorhead, and R.N. Dearth. 1982. Infectious bursal disease virus and Alcaligenes faecalis infections in turkeys. Avian Dis 26:365–374.

49. Jackwood, M.W., and Y.M. Saif. 1985. Efficacy of a commercial turkey coryza vaccine (Art-Vax™) in turkey poults. Avian Dis 29:1130–1139.

50. Jackwood, M.W., and Y.M. Saif. 1987. Pili of Bordetella avium: Expression, characterization, and role in in vitro adherence. Avian Dis 31:277–286.

51. Jackwood, M.W., and Y.M. Saif. 1987. Lack of protection against Bordetella avium in turkey poults exposed to B. avium-like bacteria. Avian Dis 31:597–600.

52. Jackwood, M.W., Y.M. Saif, and D.L. Coplin. 1987. Isolation and characterization of Bordetella avium plasmids. Avian Dis 31:782–786.

53. Jackwood, M.W., Y.M. Saif, P.D. Moorhead, and R.N. Dearth. 1985. Further characterization of the agent causing coryza in turkeys. Avian Dis 29:690–705.

54. Jackwood, M.W., M. Sasser, and Y.M. Saif. 1986. Contribution to the taxonomy of the turkey coryza agent: Cellular fatty acid analysis of the bacterium. Avian Dis 30:172–178.

55. Jensen, M.M., and M.S. Marshall. 1981. Control of turkey Alcaligenes rhinotracheitis in Utah with a live vaccine. Avian Dis 25:1053–1057.

56. Kelly, B.J., G.Y. Ghazikhanian, and B. Mayeda. 1986. Clinical outbreak of Bordetella avium infection in two turkey breeder flocks. Avian Dis 30:234–237.

57. Kersters, K., K.-H. Hinz, A. Hertle, P. Segers, A. Lievens, O. Siegmann, and J. De Ley. 1984. Bordetella avium sp. nov. isolated from the respiratory tracts of turkeys and other birds. Int J Syst Bacteriol 34:56–70.

58. Leyh, R.D., R.W. Griffith, and L.H. Arp. 1988. Transposon mutagenesis in Bordetella avium. Am J Vet Res 49:687–692.

59. Lister, S.A., and D.J. Alexander. 1986. Turkey rhinotracheitis: A review. Vet Bull 56:637–663.

60. Luginbuhl, G.H., D. Cutter, G. Campodonico, J. Peace, and D.G. Simmons. 1986. Plasmid DNA of virulent Alcaligenes faecalis. Am J Vet Res 47:619–621.

61. Marshall, D.R., D.G. Simmons, and J.G. Gray. 1984. Evidence for adherence-dependent cytotoxicity of Alcaligenes faecalis in turkey tracheal organ cultures. Avian Dis 28:1007–1015.

62. Marshall, D.R., D.G. Simmons, and J.G. Gray. 1985. An Alcaligenes faecalis isolate from turkeys: Pathogenicity in selected avian and mammalian species. Am J Vet Res 46:1181–1184.

63. McCorkle, F.M., F.W. Edens, and D.G. Simmons. 1985. Alcaligenes faecalis infection in turkeys: Effects on serum corticosterone and serum chemistry. Avian Dis 29:80–89.

64. McCorkle, F.M., and D.G. Simmons. 1984. In vitro cellular migration of leukocytes from turkey poults infected with Alcaligenes faecalis. Avian Dis 28:853–857.

65. McCorkle, F.M., D.G. Simmons, and G.H. Luginbuhl. 1982. Delayed hypersensitivity response in Alcaligenes faecalis-infected turkey poults. Avian Dis 26:782–786.

66. McCorkle, F.M., D.G. Simmons, and G.H. Luginbuhl. 1983. Graft-vs-host response in Alcaligenes faecalis-infected turkey poults. Am J Vet Res 44:1141–1142.

67. Montgomery, R.D., S.H. Kleven, and P. Villegas. 1983. Observations on the pathogenicity of Alcaligenes faecalis in chickens. Avian Dis 27:751–761.

68. Moore, C.J., H. Mawhinney, and P.J. Blackall. 1987. Differentiation of Bordetella avium and related species by cellular fatty acid analysis. J Clin Microbiol 25:1059–1062.

69. Page, R.K., O.J. Fletcher, P.D. Lukert, and R. Rimler. 1978. Rhinotracheitis in turkey poults. Avian Dis 22:529–534.

70. Panigrahy, B., L.C. Grumbles, R.J. Terry, D.L. Millar, and C.F. Hall. 1981. Bacterial coryza in turkeys in Texas. Poult Sci 60:107–113.

71. Rhoades, K.R., and R.B. Rimler. 1987. The effects of heat-labile Bordetella avium toxin on turkey poults. Avian Dis 31:345–350.

72. Rimler, R.B. 1985. Turkey coryza: Toxin production by Bordetella avium. Avian Dis 29:1043–1047.

73. Rimler, R.B., and K.R. Rhoades. 1986. Turkey coryza: Selected tests for detection and neutralization of Bordetella avium heat-labile toxin. Avian Dis 30:808–812.

74. Rimler, R.B., and K.R. Rhoades. 1986. Fowl cholera: Influence of Bordetella avium on vaccinal immunity of turkeys to Pasteurella multocida. Avian Dis 30:838–839.

75. Rimler, R.B., and D.G. Simmons. 1983. Differentiation among bacteria isolated from turkeys with coryza (rhinotracheitis). Avian Dis 27:491–500.

76. Saif, Y.M., P.D. Moorhead, R.N. Dearth, and D.J. Jackwood. 1980. Observations on Alcaligenes faecalis infection in turkeys. Avian Dis 24:665–684.

77. Simmons, D.G., D.E. Davis, L.P. Rose, J.G. Gray, and G.H. Luginbuhl. 1981. Alcaligenes faecalis-associated respiratory disease of chickens. Avian Dis 25:610–613.

78. Simmons, D.G., C. Dees, and L.P. Rose. 1986. A heat-stable toxin isolated from the turkey coryza agent, Bordetella avium. Avian Dis 30:761–765.

79. Simmons, D.G., A.R. Gore, and E.C. Hodgin. 1980. Altered immune function in turkey poults infected with Alcaligenes faecalis, the etiologic agent of turkey rhinotracheitis (coryza). Avian Dis 24:702–714.

80. Simmons, D.G., and J.G. Gray. 1979. Transmission of acute respiratory disease (rhinotracheitis) of turkeys. Avian Dis 23:132–138.

81. Simmons, D.G., J.G. Gray, L.P. Rose, R.C. Dillman, and S.E. Miller. 1979. Isolation of an etiologic agent of acute respiratory disease (rhinotracheitis) of turkey poults. Avian Dis 23:194–203.

82. Simmons, D.G., S.E. Miller, J.G. Gray, H.G. Blalock, and W. M. Colwell. 1976. Isolation and identification of a turkey respiratory adenovirus. Avian Dis 20:65–74.

83. Simmons, D.G., R.K. Page, P.V. Lukert, O.J. Fletcher, S.E. Miller, and R.C. Dillman. 1977. Bursal changes in turkey poults with acute respiratory disease. J Am Vet Med Assoc 171:1104–1105.

84. Simmons, D.G., L.P. Rose, F.J. Fuller, L.C. Maurer, and G.H. Luginbuhl. 1986. Turkey coryza: Lack of correlation between plasmids and pathogenicity of Bordetella avium. Avian Dis 30:593–597.

85. Simmons, D.G., L.P. Rose, and J.G. Gray. 1980. Some physical, biochemic, and pathologic properties of Alcaligenes faecalis, the bacterium causing rhinotracheitis (coryza) in turkey poults. Avian Dis 24:82–90.

86. Simmons, D.G., L.P. Rose, F.M. McCorkle, and

G.H. Luginbuhl. 1983. Histamine-sensitizing factor of Alcaligenes faecalis. Avian Dis 27:171–177.
87. Skeeles, J.K., W.S. Swafford, D.P. Wages, H.M. Hellwig, M.F. Slavik, J.N. Beasley, G.E. Houghten, P.J. Blore, and D. Crawford. 1983. Studies on the use of a long-acting oxytetracycline in turkeys: Efficacy against experimental infections with Alcaligenes faecalis and Pasteurella multocida. Avian Dis 27:1126–1130.
88. Slavik, M.F., J.K. Skeeles, J.N. Beasley, G.C. Harris, P. Roblee, and D. Hellwig. 1981. Effect of humidity on infection of turkeys with Alcaligenes faecalis. Avian Dis 25:936–942.
89. Slavik, M.F., J.K. Skeeles, C.F. Meinecke, and L. Holloway. 1981. The involvement of Alcaligenes faecalis in turkeys submitted for diagnosis as detected by bacterial isolation and microagglutination test. Avian Dis 25:761–763.
90. Van Alstine, W.G., and L.H. Arp. 1987. Effects of Bordetella avium toxin on turkey tracheal organ cultures as measured with a tetrazolium-reduction assay. Avian Dis 31:136–139.
91. Van Alstine, W.G., and L.H. Arp. 1987. Influence of Bordetella avium infection on association of Escherichia coli with turkey trachea. Am J Vet Res 48:1574–1576.
92. Van Alstine, W.G., and L.H. Arp. 1987. Effects of Bordetella avium infection on the pulmonary clearance of Escherichia coli in turkeys. Am J Vet Res 48:922–926.
93. Van Alstine, W.G., and L.H. Arp. 1988. Histologic evaluation of lung and bronchus-associated lymphoid tissue in young turkeys infected with Bordetella avium. Am J Vet Res 49:835–839.
94. Van Alstine, W.G., and M.S. Hofstad. 1985. Antibiotic aerosolization: The effect on experimentally induced alcaligenes rhinotracheitis in turkeys. Avian Dis 29:159–176.
95. Varley, J. 1986. The characterisation of Bordetella/Alcaligenes-like organisms and their effects on turkey poults and chicks. Avian Pathol 15:1–22.
96. Yersin, A.G. 1988. Personal communication.

13 MISCELLANEOUS BACTERIAL DISEASES

INTRODUCTION

H. John Barnes

Bacterial diseases continue to cause significant economic losses in the poultry industry. Those that are common, widespread, or of major public health significance are covered in subchapters or chapters elsewhere in this text. Bacterial diseases of more sporadic occurrence, limited distribution, or potential public health significance can be important when and where they occur. These, along with bacterial diseases of historical interest, are briefly discussed by etiology, disease, or pathologic lesion.

ACINETOBACTER. This organism has been recovered from ducks with arthritis (5).

ACTINOBACILLUS. *Actinobacillus* spp., distinct from *A. lignieresii* and *A. equuli,* have been isolated from a duck with septicemia and a goose with airsacculitis (18).

AEROBACTER. *Aerobacter* has been recovered occasionally from dead embryos (30).

AEROMONAS. *Aeromonas hydrophila,* either alone or in combination with other organisms, can cause localized and systemic infections in avian species including poultry (53). *A. formicans* has been isolated infrequently from arthritic lesions in ducks at slaughter (5).

ANTHRAX. Anthrax occurs rarely in birds where the disease is endemic. Chickens are highly resistant. Ostriches are moderately susceptible, often with high mortality, while ducks have occasionally developed the disease (54).

BACTEROIDES. *Bacteroides fragilis* has been occasionally isolated from salpingitis in laying hens (6).

BRUCELLA. Poultry can be experimentally and naturally infected with *Brucella* spp., and positive serological tests have been found when free-ranging birds in contact with livestock have been tested (54). There are no recent confirmed reports of *Brucella* infection in poultry; it is unlikely the organism has any importance in modern confinement poultry production.

CORYNEBACTERIUM. Recently, serious outbreaks of osteomyelitis caused by *Corynebacterium (Actinomyces) pyogenes* in commercial turkeys have resulted in considerable economic losses (15). At present little is known of the epidemiology or importance of the organism, but it should be considered an avian pathogen.

COXIELLA. There is serologic and cultural evidence of *Coxiella burnetii* infection in poultry, and chickens are susceptible to the organism following intraperitoneal inoculation (52).

FLAVOBACTERIUM. This organism has been recovered from ducks with arthritis (5).

FRANCISELLA. Birds are susceptible to tularemia. The disease has occurred in at least 25 avian species, primarily galliformes, including poultry, waterfowl, scavengers, and predatory wild birds. Major die-offs of blue grouse in the northwestern USA have resulted from tularemia, and *Francisella tularensis* has been isolated from them and infesting ticks (26). While a sporadic disease of significance in wild and free-ranging birds, which may play an important role in maintaining and disseminating the organism, tularemia is not known to occur or be important in commercial poultry.

KLEBSIELLA. *Klebsiella* is an environmental contaminant that occasionally causes embryo mortality and excess losses in young chickens and turkeys (43, 44, 50). Hygienic handling of hatching eggs and hatchery sanitation are necessary for prevention of losses.

LISTERIA. Outbreaks of listeriosis caused by *Listeria monocytogenes* occur sporadically in many avian species, including poultry (21). Typically the disease occurs as a septicemia with splenomegaly, necrotic areas in the liver and heart, and pericarditis. Emaciation and diarrhea are seen in affected birds (21). Less commonly, listeriosis occurs in an encephalitic form without grossly visible lesions; affected birds are depressed with incoordination and torticollis (11). Human infection can result from contact with affected birds (22) and the organism has been recovered from contaminated "oven-ready" carcasses (20).

L. monocytogenes is commonly found in feces and soil in temperate areas of the world. Infection can follow inhalation, ingestion, or wound contamination. Isolation of the organism may be difficult and require special procedures (4), although direct culture of brain stem was positive in 4 of 5 attempts in an outbreak of encephalitic listeriosis (11). Chicken embryos are readily infected and can be used for isolation.

Chickens (4) and turkeys (8) are relatively resistant but can be experimentally infected. The disease is more severe in young birds. *L. monocytogenes* has been used to study macrophage function in retrovirus infection (12) and cell-mediated responses in susceptible and resistant chickens exposed to Marek's disease virus (9).

Prevention of listeriosis depends on identifying and eliminating the source of infection. The organism is often resistant to most commonly used antibiotics; high levels of tetracyclines are usually recommended for treatment. Widespread use of antibiotics in feed may have prophylactic value in listeriosis prevention in poultry (22).

MORAXELLA. *Moraxella osloensis* caused a choleralike disease in commercial turkeys. Affected birds had at least one consolidated, pneumonic lung, multiple hemorrhages and inflammation of serous membranes, and abnormal spleens and livers. The organism could be distinguished from *Pasteurella multocida* by its growth on eosin methylene blue (EMB) and MacConkey's media. The disease was reproduced in experimentally inoculated turkeys (16).

Moraxella sp. has been recovered from salpingitis lesions in layers (6).

PROTEUS. *Proteus* was isolated from dead-in-shell chicken embryos (30, 43) and sick ducklings (48). Experimental inoculation of the organism from ducklings failed to cause disease. Septicemia has occurred in quail (49) and broilers suspected of having immunologic deficiency (45). *P. vulgaris* can occasionally produce arthritis in ducks (5). *P. mirabilis* has been recovered from a low percent of salpingitis lesions in layers (6).

PSEUDOMONAS. *Pseudomonas* can cause localized or systemic diseases in young and growing poultry, invade fertile eggs causing death of embryos and newly hatched birds, and reduce shelf life of contaminated meat. The organisms are ubiquitous, often associated with soil, water, and humid environments. *P. aeruginosa* is the most common cause of infection. However, *P. fluorescens* can cause turkey embryo mortality following dipping of eggs in contaminated antibiotic solutions (58), and pseudomonads are capable of digesting eggshell cuticle if the humidity is high (7). Lusis and Soltys (33) reviewed pseudomonas infections in domestic animals.

P. aeruginosa is a motile, gram-negative, nonspore-forming rod measuring 1.5–3 × 0.5–0.8 μm, occurring singly or in short chains. The organism is a strict aerobe that grows readily on common bacteriological media, usually producing a water-soluble green pigment composed of fluorescein and pyocyanin. A characteristic fruity odor can often be recognized. For a detailed account of characteristics and differentiation of pseudomonads, see Gilardi (19).

Pseudomonas is an opportunist producing septicemia and its sequelae when introduced into tissues of susceptible birds. Chickens (3, 14, 36), turkeys (24, 27), ducks (5, 48), and pheasants (25) have been affected. Although birds of any age can be infected, young birds are more susceptible to infection, as are severely stressed or immunodeficient birds. Concurrent infections with viruses and other bacteria occur and may also affect susceptibility to *Pseudomonas* (45). Morbidity and mortality are usually 2–10% but can be much higher, approaching 90%.

Clinical signs include lassitude; lameness; incoordination; ataxia; swelling of head, wattles, sinuses, hock joints, or foot pads; diarrhea; and conjunctivitis (14, 24, 39). Death usually occurs rapidly, often within 24–48 hr. Torticollis, indistinguishable from fowl cholera, occurs following *Pseudomonas* inoculation of turkeys via the eustachian tube (42).

Lesions are consistent with clinical findings and include subcutaneous edema and fibrin occasionally with hemorrhage; exudate in affected joints; inflammation of serous membranes mimicking lesions of colisepticemia (airsacculitis, pericarditis, perihepatitis); swelling and necrotic foci in liver, spleen, kidney, and brain; purulent conjunctivitis; and occasionally keratitis (14, 24, 39). Purulent exudate in the pharynx and pulmonary foci are present in respiratory infections of pheasants (25). Large numbers of bacteria, often in and around affected blood vessels within most tissues, including brain, are typically seen microscopically.

Pseudomonas is among a variety of bacteria often recovered from dead embryos and sick, newly hatched birds (30, 43, 48). With the exception of a respiratory outbreak in pheasants attributed to exploding contaminated eggs in the incubator, presence of *P. aeruginosa* in embryos is not considered a source for infection in older birds. Severe outbreaks have followed injection of large numbers of birds with contaminated vaccines (36, 57) and antibiotic solutions (59). In these cases, contamination resulted from poor hygiene during mixing and handling, and not the products themselves. Contact with infected birds (39) and intense, continuous broiler production with different ages being raised in the same facility (14) can result in spread of *Pseudomonas* infection. In some outbreaks, the source of the organism and how it spread could not be determined.

Diagnosis requires isolation and identification of the organism. Various methods including serological, phage, and aeruginocine-typing methods are available (47) and may be useful in epidemiological studies.

Prevention and control are based on identifying and eliminating the source of the organism. Good hygiene, especially in hatcheries and when birds are injected, is fundamental to *Pseudomonas* control. Reduction of stress and prevention of other viral and bacterial infections will aid in reducing susceptibility. Antibiotics can be useful in reducing losses if initiated early in the disease. Because of the organism's resistance to many antibiotics (47), sensitivity testing of available drugs is essential.

SHIGELLA. *Shigella boydii* has been isolated infrequently from poultry feces. Contamination of carcasses with shigella by infected food handlers can occur, but the likelihood of poultry serving as a source of shigellosis in man is considered negligible (41).

SPIROCHETES. Spirochetes other than *Borrelia anserina* have been recovered from livers of clinically normal hens by inoculation of chicken embryos (55), associated with cecal nodules (35), and identified as causing infectious typhlitis in chickens (13) and retarded growth and egg production in pullets (23). Infection is related to being on deep litter. The organisms resemble treponemes and sometimes will cross-react with *Treponema hyodysenteriae* in a fluorescent antibody test (13, 23). Broiler chicks can be experimentally infected with *T. hyodysenteriae* if given high numbers of the organism shortly after hatching (1). Preventing contact between swine and chickens would seem a prudent control measure until more is known about these organisms. Dimetridazole treatment resulted in clinical improvement of affected pullets (23).

STREPTOBACILLUS. *Streptobacillus moniliformis,* a gram-negative, often beaded, nonbranching, filamentous bacterium, can infect turkeys, usually following rat bites or exposure to infected rats. Polyarthritis and synovitis occur in infected birds; other tissues are usually normal. The disease can be reproduced in turkeys following experimental inoculation of the organism by intravenous, subcutaneous, and foot-pad routes, but not by oral administration. Diagnosis requires isolation and identification of the organism. Infection can be prevented through rodent control (37).

VIBRIO (CAMPYLOBACTER). Non-O1 *Vibrio cholerae* has been isolated from the liver of a goose that died following weight loss and lassitude of 2–3 days duration, and from nasal cavities of apparently healthy ducks. Individuals working with ill birds having contact with coastal waters and shellfish need to be aware that the birds could be a source of human *V. cholerae* infection (51).

Historically, a choleralike disease has been reported in poultry and zoo birds caused by *V. metschnikovii* (*metchnikovi*), and campylobacters have been implicated as the cause of hepatitis in chickens (see Chapter 9). Neither of these diseases have apparently been reported recently, but the former vibrio is still occasionally isolated from fowl (32).

DISEASES CAUSED BY OR ASSOCIATED WITH BACTERIA

Beak Necrosis. A gram-positive bacterium with affinity for keratin was associated with beak necrosis in a flock of broiler breeder hens. Nearly half of the flock was affected and mortality was 10% (10).

Goose Venereal Disease. Bacteria, especially *Neisseria* and *Mycoplasma* spp., and *Candida albicans* have been associated with a venereal disease affecting ganders. The disease has been reported from Eastern Europe, Russia, and the Middle East. Initially, the base of the phallus becomes swollen and inflamed; the process extending to the cloaca. Later, there is necrosis, ulceration, and eventually considerable scarring, making reproduction impossible. Morbidity ranges from 60 to 100% and newly introduced birds readily contract the disease. Increased infertility and gander mortality of approximately 5% are flock problems resulting from the disease (17, 56). Because of the significance of this disease, the normal phallus flora of the gander has been established (34).

Intracellular Infection in Ducks. Mortality in Muscovy ducks (*Cairina moschata*) caused by an intracellular organism primarily affecting endothelial cells in the lungs was initially attributed to *Haemoproteus* infection (28). However, subsequent examination of additional cases showed the organism was not a protozoan but probably a bacterium capable of forming spores, or an unidentified microorganism. Muscovy ducks appear most susceptible and can contract the infection from asymptomatic infected Pekin ducks. Experimental transmission is possible using blood from an infected bird. Lungs of affected ducks are dark red-purple color, slightly edematous, and firm. Microscopically, air capillaries are obliterated because of marked swelling of endothelial cells, which are often packed with intracellular organisms; interlobular septa are widened and contain inflammatory cells and edema. In tissue sections, organisms stain poorly with hematoxylin and eosin but are readily demonstrated with periodic acid-Schiff or silver stains (29, 46).

Liver Granulomas. Granulomas are occasionally seen in livers of turkeys at processing, requiring condemnation of the organ. The incidence may reach 50%. Lesions are grossly visible as firm, lobulated, roughly spherical, pale yellow to white masses ranging in size from a few millimeters to several centimeters. Advanced lesions have a rough appearance and may be "gritty" when cut. Bile stasis of adjacent normal hepatic tissue is often marked. A variety of bacteria, many of them anaerobes, have been recovered from liver granulomas. Lesions can be reproduced by *Eubacterium tortuosum.* Often mucosal ulcers in the lower intestinal tract can also be found in affected birds suggesting liver lesions develop from bacteria carried to the organ from the intestine via the blood stream (2, 31, 38). No causative organism was identified in similar lesions affecting the ceca and liver of older chickens from small flocks in Canada (40).

REFERENCES

1. Adachi, Y., M. Sueyoshi, E. Miyagawa, H. Minato, and S. Shoya. 1985. Experimental infection of young broiler chicks with Treponema hyodysenteriae. Microbiol Immunol 29:683-688.
2. Arp, L.H., I.M. Robinson, and A.E. Jensen. 1983. Pathology of liver granulomas in turkeys. Vet Pathol 20:80-89.
3. Bapat, J.A., V.B. Kulkarni, and D.V. Nimje. 1985. Mortality in chicks due to Pseudomonas aeruginosa. Indian J Anim Sci 55:538-539.
4. Basher, H.A., D.R. Fowler, F.G. Rodgers, A. Seaman, and M. Woodbine. 1984. Pathogenicity of natural and experimental listeriosis in newly hatched chicks. Res Vet Sci 36:76-80.
5. Bisgaard, M. 1981. Arthritis in ducks. I. Aetiology and public health aspects. Avian Pathol 10:11-21.
6. Bisgaard, M., and A. Dam. 1981. Salpingitis in poultry. II. Prevalence, bacteriology, and possible pathogenesis in egg-laying chickens. Nord Vet 33:81-89.
7. Board, R.G., S. Loseby, and V.R. Miles. 1979. A note on microbial growth on hen egg-shells. Br Poult Sci 20:413-420.
8. Bolin, F.M., and D.F. Eveleth. 1961. Experimental listeriosis of turkeys. Avian Dis 5:229-231.
9. Carpenter, S.L., and M. Sevoian. 1983. Cellular immune response to Marek's disease: Listeriosis as a model of study. Avian Dis 27:344-356.
10. Cheng, K.J., E.E. Gardiner, and J.W. Costerton. 1976. Bacteria associated with beak necrosis in broiler breeder hens. Vet Rec 99:503-504.
11. Cooper, G.L. 1989. An encephalitic form of listeriosis in broiler chickens. Avian Dis 33:182-185.
12. Cummins, T.J., I.M. Orme, and R.E. Smith. 1988. Reduced in vivo nonspecific resistance to Listeria monocytogenes infection during avian retrovirus-induced immunosuppression. Avian Dis 32:663-667.
13. Davelaar, F.G., H.F. Smit, K. Hovind-Hougen, R.M. Dwars, and P.C. van der Valk. 1986. Infectious typhlitis in chickens caused by spirochetes. Avian Pathol 15:247-258.
14. Devriese, L.A., N.J. Viaene, and G. De Medts. 1975. Pseudomonas aeruginosa infection on a broiler farm. Avian Pathol 4:233-237.
15. Edson, R. 1988. Personal communication.
16. Emerson, F.G., G.E. Kolb, and F.A. VanNatta. 1983. Chronic cholera-like lesions caused by Moraxella osloensis. Avian Dis 27:836-838.
17. Fadin, V.S., A.V. Kurilenko, S.M. Sherkevich, and N.V. Titov. 1976. Infektsionnaya bolezn organov razmnozheniya u gusei. Veterinariya, Moscow 8:85-87. [Poult Abstr 1977, # 1001].
18. Ganiere, J.P., P. Perreau, J. Brocas, and J. Chantal. 1982. Etude de deux souches "Actinobacillus species" d'origine aviaire. Revue Med Vet 133:125-128.
19. Gilardi, G.L. 1985. Pseudomonas. In E.H. Lennette, A. Balows, W.J. Hausler, Jr., and H.J. Shadomy (eds.), Manual of Clinical Microbiology, 4th Ed., pp. 350-372. Am Soc Microbiol, Washington, DC.
20. Gitter, M. 1976. Listeria monocytogenes in "oven-ready" poultry. Vet Rec 99:336.
21. Gray, M.L. 1958. Listeriosis in fowls—a review. Avian Dis 2:296-314.
22. Gray, M.L., and A.H. Killinger. 1966. Listeria monocytogenes and listeric infections. Bacteriol Rev 30:309-382.
23. Griffiths, I.B., B.W. Hunt, S.A. Lister, and M.H. Lamont. 1987. Retarded growth rate and delayed onset of egg production associated with spirochaete infection in pullets. Vet Rec 121:35-37.
24. Hafez, H.M., H. Woernle, and G. Heil. 1987. Pseudomonas-aeruginosa-infektionen bei Putenkuken und Behandlungsversuche mit Apramycin. Berl München Tierärztl Wochenschr 100:48-51.
25. Honich, M. 1972. Facancsibek jarvanyszeru Pseudomonas aeruginosa fertozottsege. Magyar Allatorvosok Lapja 27:329-335.
26. Jellison, W.L. 1974. Tularemia in North America, 1930-1974. Monogr, Univ Montana, Missoula.
27. Jones, J.C., and G.W. Anderson. 1948. Sulfamerazine in the treatment of a Pseudomonas infection of turkey poults. J Am Vet Med Assoc 113:458-459.
28. Julian, R.J., and D.E. Galt. 1980. Mortality in Muscovy ducks (Cairina moschata) caused by Haemoproteus infection. J Wildl Dis 16:39-44.
29. Julian, R.J., T.J. Beveridge, and D.E. Galt. 1985. Muscovy duck mortality not caused by Haemoproteus. J Wildl Dis 21:335-337.
30. Karim, M.R., and M.R. Ali. 1976. Survey of bacterial flora from chicken embryo and their effect on low hatchability. Bangladesh Vet J 10:15-18.
31. Langheinrich, K.A., and B. Schwab. 1972. Isolation of bacteria and histomorphology of turkey liver granulomas. Avian Dis 16:806-816.
32. Lee, J.V., T.J. Donovan, and A.L. Furniss. 1978. Characterization, taxonomy, and emended description of Vibrio metschnikovii. Int J Syst Bacteriol 28:99-111.
33. Lusis, P.I., and M.A. Soltys. 1971. Pseudomonas aeruginosa. Vet Bull 41:169-177.
34. Marius-Jestin, V., M. Le Menec, E. Thibault, J.C. Moisan, and R. L'Hospitalier. 1987. Normal phallus flora of the gander. J Vet Med B 34:67-78.
35. Mathey, W.J., and D.V. Zander. 1955. Spirochetes and cecal nodules in poultry. J Am Vet Med Assoc 126:475-477.
36. Mireles, V., and C. Alvarez. 1979. Pseudomonas aeruginosa infection due to contaminated vaccination equipment. Proc 28th West Poult Dis Conf, pp. 55-57.

37. Mohamed, Y.S., P.D. Moorhead, and E.H. Bohl. 1969. Natural Streptobacillus moniliformis infection of turkeys, and attempts to infect turkeys, sheep, and pigs. Avian Dis 13:379–385.

38. Moore, W.E.C., and W.B. Gross. 1968. Liver granulomas of turkeys–causative agents and mechanism of infection. Avian Dis 12:417–422.

39. Mosqueda, T., G. Moedano, and J. Moreno. 1976. Pseudomonas aeruginosa as a source of nervous signs and lesions in young chicks. Proc 25th West Poult Dis Conf, pp. 68–69.

40. Mutalib, A.A., and C. Riddell. 1982. Cecal and hepatic granulomas of unknown etiology in chickens. Avian Dis 26:732–740.

41. National Research Council. 1987. Poultry inspection. The basis for a risk-assessment approach, p. 72. National Academy Press, Washington, DC.

42. Olson, L.D. 1970. A comparison of the growth of various microorganisms in air spaces of the turkey head. Avian Dis 14:676–682.

43. Orajaka, L.J.E., and K. Mohan. 1985. Aerobic bacterial flora from dead-in-shell chicken embryos from Nigeria. Avian Dis 29:583–589.

44. Plesser, O., A. Even-Shoshan, and U. Bendheim. 1975. The isolation of Klebsiella pneumoniae from poultry and hatcheries. Refuah Vet 32:99–105.

45. Randall, C.J., W.G. Siller, A.S. Wallis, and K.S. Kirkpatrick. 1984. Multiple infections in young broilers. Vet Rec 114:270–271.

46. Randall, C.J., S. Lees, G.A. Pepin, and H.M. Ross. 1987. An unusual intracellular infection in ducks. Avian Pathol 16:479–491.

47. Sadasivan, P.R., V.A. Srinivasan, A.T. Venugopalan, and R.A. Balaprakasam. 1977. Aeruginocine typing and antibiotic sensitivity of Pseudomonas aeruginosa of poultry origin. Avian Dis 21:136–138.

48. Safwat, E.E.A., M.H. Awaad, A.M. Ammer, and A.A. El-Kinawy. 1984. Studies on Pseudomonas aeruginosa, Proteus vulgaris and S. typhimurium infection in ducklings. Egyptian J Anim Prod 24:287–294.

49. Sah, R.L., M.P. Mall, and G.C. Mohanty. 1983. Septicemic Proteus infection in Japanese quail chicks (Coturnix coturnix japonica). Avian Dis 27:296–300.

50. Sarakbi, T. 1989. Klebsiella–a killer in the hatchery. Int Hatch Pract 3:19–21.

51. Schlater, L.K., B.O. Blackburn, R. Harrington, Jr., D.J. Draper, J. Van Wagner, and B.R. Davis. 1981. A non-O1 Vibrio cholerae isolated from a goose. Avian Dis 25:199–201.

52. Sethi, M.S., B. Singh, and M.P. Yadev. 1978. Experimental infection of Coxiella burnetii in chicken: Clinical symptoms, serologic response, and transmission through egg. Avian Dis 22:391–395.

53. Shane, S.M., and D.H. Gifford. 1985. Prevalence and pathogenicity of Aeromonas hydrophila. Avian Dis 29:681–689.

54. Snoeyenbos, G.H. 1965. Brucellosis, anthrax, pseudotuberculosis, tetanus, vibrio infection, avian vibrionic hepatitis, and spirochetosis. In H.E. Beister and L.H. Schwarte (eds.), Diseases of Poultry, 5th Ed., pp. 427–450. Iowa State Univ Press, Ames.

55. Steinhaus, E.A., and L.E. Hughes. 1947. Isolation of an unidentified spirochete from hen's eggs after inoculation with liver tissue from hens. US Pub Health Rep 62:309–311.

56. Stipkovits, L., Z. Varga, G. Czifra, and M. Dobos-Kovacs. 1986. Occurrence of mycoplasmas in geese affected with inflammation of the cloaca and phallus. Avian Pathol 15:289–299.

57. Trenchi, H., M.T. Bellizzi, and C.G. de Sousa. 1981. Contaminacion en la vacunacion de Marek con Pseudomonas spp. (variedad acromogena). Gaceta Veterinaria 43:982–989.

58. Wages, D.P. 1988. Personal communication.

59. Williams, B.J., and H.L. Newkirk. 1966. Pseudomonas infection of one-day-old chicks resulting from contaminated antibiotic solutions. Avian Dis 10:353–356.

STAPHYLOCOCCOSIS

J.K. Skeeles

INTRODUCTION. *Staphylococcus aureus* infections (Table 13.1) are common in poultry; the most frequent sites being bones, tendon sheaths, and leg joints. Staphylococcus infections have also been reported in other locations including skin (35), sternal bursa (75), yolk sac (80), heart (5), vertebrae (8), eyelid (10), and as granulomas in liver and lungs (3, 54). Staphylococcal septicemia, affecting laying birds and causing acute death (6), seems to be prevalent in hot weather and resembles fowl cholera.

Economic and Public Health Significance. In addition to it being a major disease-producing

Table 13.1. Staphylococcal-related infections in poultry

Location	Age	Lesion	Usual Outcome
Bone	Any, usually older	Osteomyelitis	Lameness
Joint	Any, usually older	Athritis/synovitis	Lameness
Yolk sac	Chicks	Omphalitis	Death
Blood (septicemia)	Any	Generalized necrosis	Death
Skin	Young	Gangrenous dermatitis	Death
Feet	Mature	"Bumblefoot"	Lameness

organism for poultry, approximately 50% of typical and atypical *S. aureus* strains produce enterotoxins capable of causing food poisoning in humans (21, 25, 33, 62). Staphylococcal food poisoning has been associated with poultry (70). Enterotoxin-producing *S. aureus* strains, which contaminate poultry carcasses following processing, have their origin from either contaminated equipment or people in the processing plant (1, 60, 72). Currently, in the processing of turkeys, an association has been proposed between partial, green discolored livers observed at postmortem inspection and staphylococcal infections. The accuracy and validity of the proposed relationship have yet to be established.

HISTORY. Staphylococcosis in poultry and other avian species has been recognized for nearly 100 yr, most early reports describing it as the etiological agent of arthritis and synovitis (31, 36, 38, 47).

INCIDENCE AND DISTRIBUTION. *Staphylococcus* spp. are ubiquitous, normal inhabitants of skin and mucous membranes, and are common organisms in environments where poultry are hatched, reared, or processed. Most staphylococci species are considered to be normal flora, which help suppress other possible pathogens by their presence through interference or competitive exclusion. Some have the potential to be pathogenic and produce disease if allowed entry through skin or mucous membranes.

Staphylococcus spp. and staphylococcosis have been associated with poultry all over the world including the USA (37), Canada (55), UK (73), Australia (40), Argentina (71), W. Germany (44), E. Germany (43), Poland (82), Romania (51), Taiwan (76), India (61), Pakistan (74), Bulgaria (4), Japan (68), Belgium (13, 14), Hungary (27), China (9), Costa Rica (53), Italy (30), Netherlands (60) and France (79).

ETIOLOGY

Classification. The genus *Staphylococcus* contains approximately 20 species. It is the most important genus in the family Micrococcaceae. The term "staphylococcus" refers to the morphology of the microorganisms in stained smears, which resemble grapelike clusters. Other genera in the family are considered to be nonpathogenic and include *Micrococcus* and *Planococcus* (41).

Staphylococcus spp. isolated frequently from poultry include *S. aureus* and *S. epidermidis*. Recently a new species called *S. gallinarum* was described (18), which was isolated from processed poultry. Atypical strains of *S. aureus* are occasionally isolated from healthy and unhealthy fowl (21). Other *Staphylococcus* species, often encountered in humans and domestic animals and considered pathogenic for those species, have not been reported to be of any consequence in poultry.

Morphology and Staining. *S. aureus* is the only species of *Staphylococcus* found in poultry considered to be pathogenic. Typical pathogenic *S. aureus* strains are gram-positive, coccoid in shape, and found in clusters on solid media. In liquid media, they may be found in short chains. Cultures more than 24 hr old may stain gram-negative.

Growth Requirements. Staphylococci are readily isolated on 5% blood agar with growth evident in 18–24 hr.

Colony Morphology. *S. aureus* produces circular, smooth colonies, 1–3 mm in diameter within 24 hr, and are often pigmented white to orange when grown under aerobic conditions.

Biochemical Properties. *S. aureus* is aerobic, facultatively anaerobic, beta hemolytic, catalase-positive, fermentative for glucose and mannitol, and is gelatinase-positive.

Resistance to Chemical and Physical Agents. Staphylococci are extremely hardy and remain viable for long periods of time on solid media or in purulent exudate. Some strains are heat- and disinfectant-resistant (48). A resistance feature used to isolate *S. aureus* from heavily contaminated clinical material is its tolerance to high (7.5%) concentrations of NaCl (41).

Antigenic Structure and Toxins. The antigenic nature of *S. aureus* is complex involving, in some species, a capsule consisting of glucosaminouronic acid, manosaminouronic acid, lysine, glutamic acid, glycine, alanine, or glucosamine depending on the strain; polysaccharide-A consisting of linear ribitol teichoic acid, N-acetylglucosamine, and D-alanine; and Protein-A, a cell wall component that interacts nonspecifically with the Fc portion of immunoglobulin and may be a virulence factor. Other factors thought to play a role in both pathogenicity and virulence are a variety of enzymes and toxins including hyaluronidase (spreading factor), deoxyribonuclease, fibrinolysin, lipase, protease, hemolysins, leukocidin, dermonecrotoxin, hemolysins, exfoliative toxin, and enterotoxins (2, 52).

Strain Classification. Chicken *S. aureus* strains have been typed using phages, as have *S. aureus* strains from humans (26, 65–68). The ability to type with the International Series of *S. aureus* phages depends on where the organism was isolated. Strains isolated from diseased poultry are often untypable, while strains from processed poultry are more likely to be typable with the International Series. *S. aureus* strains from processed poultry are thought to be human strains endemic to the processing plant, or from the hands of workers in the plant (44). Phage sets isolated from poultry strains of *S. aureus* can be used to type strains of poultry origin (26, 65). These have been used in studies involving *S. aureus* of poultry origin from various locations around the world with varying results (40, 68, 73). Phages tend to be specific for *S. aureus* of poultry origin and cannot be used to type strains from other species (67).

Several biotyping schemes have been devised that divide *S. aureus* strains into species-specific ecovars. Poultry strains have been biotyped using these classification schemes (15, 32). Strains have also been classified using antibiotic susceptibility patterns and plasmid profiles (41).

Pathogenicity. Coagulase-positive isolates of *S. aureus* are considered to be pathogenic for poultry, while coagulase-negative strains are thought to be nonpathogenic.

PATHOGENESIS AND EPIZOOTIOLOGY

Natural and Experimental Hosts. All avian species are susceptible to staphylococcal infections.

Transmission, Carriers, Vectors. For infection to occur, a break in part of the defense mechanism of the host must occur (2). In most cases this would involve an environmental barrier such as a skin wound or damaged mucous membrane. *S. aureus* would enter through the breached barrier and travel to internal locations where a locus of infection (osteomyelitis) would be established, usually in the metaphyseal area of a nearby joint (57). In newly hatched chicks the open navel provides a site of entry leading to omphalitis and other types of infections. Minor surgical procedures (e.g., toe clipping, debeaking, desnooding, dubbing) of newly hatched birds may offer additional portals of entry for staphylococci.

Another type of host defense impairment occurs following infectious bursal disease (64) or possibly Marek's disease virus infection, where the bursa of Fabricius or the thymus is damaged and the immune system is compromised. Under these conditions septicemic staphylococcal infections can occur and often lead to acute death in the affected host. Gangrenous dermatitis (Chapter 11) caused by *S. aureus,* along with *Clostridium septicum,* can be seen following early infectious bursal disease virus infection (23, 63).

Incubation Period. The incubation period is short; in experimental chickens inoculated intravenously, clinical signs are evident within 48–72 hr postinfection. Experimentally, chickens can be readily infected only by the intravenous route, not by intratracheal or aerosol routes. Dosage of bacteria affects the ability to consistently produce experimental infection with 105 organisms/kg of body weight being required to produce signs of disease (55, 56).

Signs. Early clinical signs include ruffled feathers, reluctance to walk, and fever (55). This can be followed by severe depression and death. In birds that survive the acute disease, joints become swollen with most affected birds sitting on their hocks and keel bone (20, 55). Clinical signs of septicemic staphylococcal infection and gangrenous dermatitis are found in birds that die acutely while in good flesh (6, 23, 63).

Morbidity and Mortality. The morbidity and mortality from staphylococcosis is usually low, except when there has been massive contamination of chicks exposed to unusually high numbers of bacteria in a hatchery through environmental contamination, vaccination, or debeaking and detoeing procedures. Leg disorders are one of the most common problems observed in broilers and turkeys. With the advent of further processing and need for bigger broilers and turkeys with more breast meat, leg problems have become more prevalent. Several reports from diagnostic laboratories have indicated *S. aureus* to be the most common bacterial agent isolated from affected legs and joints (7, 39, 42).

Morbidity and mortality from septicemic staphylococcal infection are usually low. The number of chickens that develop gangrenous dermatitis is low, but usually all that develop lesions succumb to the infection (23, 42).

Gross Lesions. Gross lesions of osteomyelitis in bone consist of focal yellow areas of caseous exudate or lytic areas, which cause affected bones to be fragile. Bones and sites most frequently involved are the proximal tibiotarsus and proximal femur. In extensive cases, the proximal tarsometatarsus, distal femur, and tibiotarsus can be involved along with other bones. In affected birds, the femoral head often separates from the shaft by a fracture through the neck when the coxofemoral joint is disarticulated (femoral head necrosis) (55, 57).

Arthritis, periarthritis, and synovitis are common. Affected joints are swollen (Fig. 13.1) and filled with purulent exudate as the infection (osteomyelitis) extends from nearby metaphyseal areas (50, 57). Spondylitis involving articulating thoracolumbar vertebrae may cause lameness indirectly by pressure on the spinal cord from the lesion (8, 57).

Gross lesions of septicemic staphylococcal infection consist of necrosis and vascular conges-

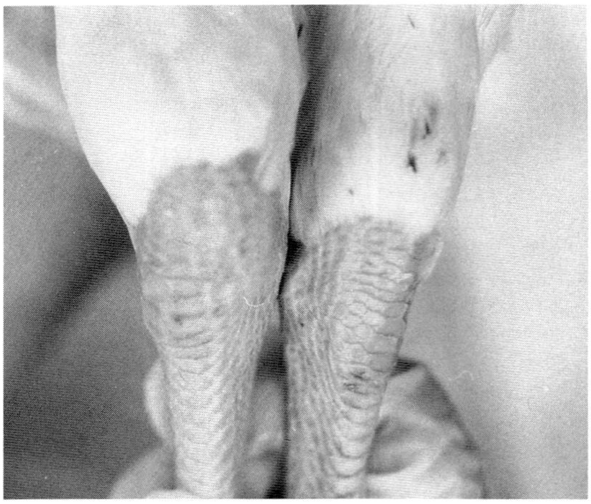

13.1. Swollen hock joint (tibiotarsal-tarsometatarsal) from *Staphylococcus aureus* infection. The leg on the left is swollen above the joint and the area is hot.

tion in internal organs including liver, spleen, kidneys, and lungs (6). Dark, moist areas under the skin covering the back and crepitation are seen in gangrenous dermatitis (6, 23).

Staphylococcal-related hatchery infections are common and can cause increased mortality within the first few days after hatching. Chicks have wet navel areas and deteriorate rapidly. Internally, yolk sacs are enlarged with the contents presenting an abnormal color and consistency.

Plantar abscess is a common infection seen in mature chickens ("bumblefoot"), an infection that leads to massive swelling of the foot and lameness.

Histopathology. Histologically, staphylococcal lesions consist of necrosis, presence of large numbers of coccoid bacteria, and heterophils (19, 28, 55).

Immunity. There is no evidence that active or passive immunity is important in preventing *S. aureus* infections in poultry. Several reports (22, 29) even imply that presence of specific antibody to *S. aureus* may promote development of *S. aureus*-related infections in chickens. Whole-cell vaccines and toxoids have not proven to be of any great benefit in other species (2, 52).

DIAGNOSIS

Isolation and Identification of Causative Agent. *S. aureus* is diagnosed by culturing suspected clinical material including exudate from joints, yolk material, and stab swabs of internal organs. The basic medium for growing staphylococci is blood agar (preferably sheep or bovine). The organisms grow well with colonies being 1–3 mm in diameter within 18–24 hr. Most strains of *S. aureus* are beta-hemolytic while most other *Staphylococcus* spp. are nonhemolytic. Heavily contaminated material should be streaked onto a selective medium such as mannitol-salt or phenylethyl alcohol agar, media inhibitory to gram-negative bacteria (41).

Colonies should be picked and Gram stained. Staphylococci are gram-positive cocci. Most *S. aureus* colonies will be pigmented. To differentiate pathogenic *S. aureus* from nonpathogenic *S. epidermidis,* coagulase and mannitol fermentation tests should be performed. *S. aureus* is positive on both tests while *S. epidermidis* is negative. Differential characteristics are listed in Table 13.2. There are several identification systems commercially available for identification of *Staphylococcus* species, but these are not routinely used for poultry isolates (41).

Table 13.2. Differentiation of *Staphylococcus aureus* and *S. epidermidis* from poultry

Characteristic	*S. aureus*	*S. epidermidis*
Colony pigment	+	–
Hemolysis	+	–
Coagulase	+	–
D-Mannitol fermentation	+	–

Serology. Serology is not routinely used for the diagnosis of staphylococcosis, but a microagglutination test has been described (22).

Differential Diagnosis. Staphylococcosis can resemble infection with *Escherichia coli, Pasteurella multocida, Salmonella gallinarum,* viral arthritis virus, *Mycoplasma synoviae,* and any other infection of the joints that is hatchery-related or causes septicemia.

TREATMENT. *S. aureus* infection can be successfully treated, but sensitivity tests should always be performed because antibiotic resistance is common (12, 14, 17, 69, 81). Drugs used successfully for treatment include penicillin, streptomycin, tetracyclines, erythromycin, novobiocin, sulfonamides, lincomycin, and spectinomycin. Staphylococcal dermatitis has also been associated with use of a sulfa drug in broiler breeder pullets (24).

PREVENTION AND CONTROL

Management Procedures. Any management procedure reducing damage to host defense mechanisms will help prevent staphylococcosis. Because wounds are a portal of entry for *S. aureus* into the body, anything reducing the chance of injury will help prevent infection. Sharp objects such as splinters, jagged rocks, or metal edges that cut or puncture feet should be eliminated from areas where poultry are reared. Maintenance of good litter quality will reduce footpad ulceration. Particular attention should be given to hatchery management and sanitation. *S. aureus* is found everywhere, and conditions in incubators and hatchers are ideal for bacterial growth. Recently hatched and hatching chicks with open navels and immature immune systems can be easily infected, leading to mortality and chronic infections very early after hatching. Prevention of early infectious bursal disease virus infection will also help prevent staphylococcosis (64).

Poultry under mild stress are actually more resistant to staphylococcosis than those not stressed and then experimentally infected (11, 34, 45, 55). This resistance is attributed to an increase in heterophil numbers, which occurs in birds under stress. The heterophil is thought to be the most important cell in controlling bacterial infections, particularly *S. aureus* (56).

Staphylococcal bacterins have been ineffective for preventing infections (2), but use of a live avirulent vaccine based on the principle of interference has shown promise. Avirulent *S. aureus* strain 502A has been utilized in humans in managing recurrent furunculosis and to abort nursery outbreaks (52). Devriese et al. (16) were able to show that one strain of staphylococcus would interfere with colonization of other strains of *S. aureus* in chickens.

Jensen et al. (37, 46, 49, 59, 78), using the principle of bacterial interference, have developed a vaccine for *S. aureus* for use in turkeys. They were able to isolate a coagulase-negative strain of *S. epidermidis,* strain 115, which colonizes cells and tissues in the respiratory tract and prevents adherence of virulent strains of *S. aureus. S. epidermidis,* strain 115, in addition to interfering with adherence of virulent *S. aureus,* also produces a bacteriocin, an extremely stable antibiotic-like substance capable of inhibiting and killing virulent *S. aureus.* Strain 115 has been used to vaccinate turkeys in the field with an apparent reduction in the number of turkeys with staphylococcosis and improved livability. The vaccine was administered by aerosol twice at 1–10 days and again at 4–6 wk of age. Another report described use of strain 115 in chickens with similar results (58).

Competitive gut exclusion using *Lactobacillus acidophilus* was attempted to exclude *S. aureus* from experimentally infected, germ-free chickens. The treatment was effective in reducing *S. aureus* counts in crop contents, but counts in the ceca and rectum were unaffected (77).

REFERENCES

1. Adams, B.W., and G.C. Mead. 1983. Incidence and properties of Staphylococcus aureus associated with turkeys during processing and further-processing operations. J Hyg 91:479–490.
2. Anderson, J.C. 1986. Staphylococcus. In C.L. Gyles and C.O. Thoen (eds.), Pathogenesis of Bacterial Infections in Animals, 1st Ed., pp 14–20. Iowa State Univ Press, Ames.
3. Arp, L.H., I.M. Robinson, and A.E. Jensen. 1983. Pathology of liver granulomas in turkeys. Vet Pathol 20:80–89.
4. Bajljosov, D., Z. Sachariev, and L. Georgiev. 1974. Characteristics of staphylococci isolated from slaughter fowl. Monatsh Veterinaermed 29:692–694.
5. Bergmann, V., B. Köhler, and K. Vogel. 1980. Staphylococcus aureus infection of fowls on industrialized poultry units. I. Types of infection. Arch Exp Vet 34:891–903.
6. Bickford, A.A., and A.S. Rosenwald. 1975. Staphylococcal infections in chickens. Poult Dig (July):285–287.
7. Bitay, Z., L. Quarini, R. Glavits, and R. Fischer. 1984. Staphylococcus infection in fowls. Magy Allatorv Lapja 39:86–91.
8. Carnaghan, R.B.A. 1966. Spinal cord compression in fowls due to spondylitis caused by Staphylococcus pyogenes. J Comp Pathol 76:9–14.
9. Chen, D.W., M.H. Gan, and R.P. Liu. 1984. Studies on staphylococcosis in chickens. III. Properties and pathogenicity of Staphylococcus aureus. Chin J Vet Med 10:6–8.
10. Cheville, N.F., J. Tappe, M. Ackermann, and A. Jensen. 1988. Acute fibrinopurulent blepharitis and conjunctivitis associated with Staphylococcus hyicus, Escherichia coli, and Streptococcus sp. in chickens and turkeys. Vet Pathol 25:369–375.
11. Coates, S.R., D.K. Buckner, and M.M. Jensen. 1977. The inhibitory effect of Corynebacterium parvum and Pasteurella multocida pretreatment on staphylococcal synovitis in turkeys. Avian Dis 21:319–322.
12. Devriese, L.A. 1976. In vitro susceptibility and resistance of animal staphylococci to macrolide antibiotics and related compounds. Ann Rech Vet 7:65–74.
13. Devriese, L.A. 1980. Pathogenic staphylococci in poultry. World Poult Sci 36:227–236.
14. Devriese, L.A. 1980. Sensitivity of staphylococci from farm animals to antibacterial agents used for growth promotion and therapy: A ten year study. Ann Rech Vet 11:399–408.
15. Devriese, L.A. 1984. A simplified system for biotyping Staphylococcus aureus strains isolated from different animal species. J Appl Bacteriol 56:215–220.
16. Devriese, L.A., A.H. Devos, and J. Beumer. 1972. Staphylococcus aureus colonization on poultry after experimental spray inoculations. Avian Dis 16:656–665.
17. Devriese, L.A., A.H. Devos, J. Beumer, and R. Moes. 1972. Characterization of staphylococci isolated from poultry. Poult Sci 51:389–397.
18. Devriese, L.A., B. Poutrel, R. Kilpper-Balz, and K.H. Schleifer. 1983. Staphylococcus gallinarium and Staphylococcus caprae, two new species from animals. Int J Syst Bacteriol 33:480–486.
19. Emslie, K.R., and S. Nade. 1985. Acute hematogenous staphylococcal osteomyelitis. Comp Pathol Bull 17:2–3.
20. Emslie, K.R., N.R. Ozanne, and S.M.L. Nade. 1983. Acute haemotogenous osteomyelitis: An experimental model. Pathology 141:157–167.
21. Evans, J.B., G.A. Ananaba, C.A. Pate, and M.S. Bergdoll. 1983. Enterotoxin production by atypical Staphylococcus aureus from poultry. J Appl Bacteriol 54:257–261.
22. Forget, A., L. Meunier, and A.G. Borduas. 1974. Enhancement activity of homologous antistaphylococcal sera in experimental staphylococcal synovitis of chicks:

A possible role of immune adherence antibodies. Infect Immun 9:641-644.

23. Frazier, M.N., W.J. Parizek, and E. Garner. 1964. Gangrenous dermatitis of chickens. Avian Dis 8:269-273.

24. Froyman, R., L. Deruyttere, and L.A. Devriese. 1982. The effect of antimicrobial agents on an outbreak of staphylococcal dermatitis in adult broiler breeders. Avian Pathol 11:521-525.

25. Gibbs, P.A., J.T. Patterson, and J. Harvey. 1978. Biochemical characteristics and enterotoxigenicity of Staphylococcus aureus strains isolated from poultry. J Appl Bacteriol 44:57-74.

26. Gibbs, P.A., J.T. Patterson, and J.K. Thompson. 1978. Characterization of poultry isolates of Staphylococcus aureus by a new set of poultry phages. J Appl Bacteriol 44:387-400.

27. Glavits, R., F. Ratz, T. Fehervari, and J. Povazsan. 1984. Pathological studies in chicken embryos and day-old chicks experimentally infected with Salmonella typhimurium and Staphylococcus aureus. Acta Vet Hung 32:39-49.

28. Griffiths, G.L., W.I. Hopkinson, and J. Lloyd. 1984. Staphylococcal necrosis of the head of the femur in broiler chickens. Aust Vet J 61:293.

29. Gross, W.G., P.B. Siegel, R.W. Hall, C.H. Domermuth, and R.T. Duboise. 1980. Production and persistence of antibodies in chickens to sheep erythrocytes. 2. Resistance to infectious diseases. Poult Sci 59:205-210.

30. Guarda, F., G. Cortellezzi, C. Cucco, and O. Massimino. 1979. Blindness due to Staphylococcus aureus in pullets. Clin Vet 102:315-324.

31. Gwatkin, R. 1940. An outbreak of staphylococcal infection in Barred Plymouth Rock males. Can J Comp Med 4:294-296.

32. Hajek, V., and E. Marsalek. 1971. The differentiation of pathogenic staphylococci and a suggestion for their taxonomic classification. Zentralbl Bakteriol 217(A):176-182.

33. Harvey, J., J.T. Patterson, and P.A. Gibbs. 1982. Enterotoxigenicity of Staphylococcus aureus strains isolated from poultry: Raw poultry carcasses as a potential food-poisoning hazard. J Appl Bacteriol 52:251-258.

34. Heller, E.D., D.B. Nathan, and M. Perek. 1979. Short heat stress as an immunostimulant in chicks. Avian Pathol 8:195-203.

35. Hoffman, H.A. 1939. Vesicular dermatitis in chickens. J Am Vet Med Assoc 48:329-332.

36. Hole, N., and H.S. Purchase. 1931. Arthritis and periostitis in pheasants caused by Staphylococcus pyogenes aureus. J Comp Pathol Ther 44:252-257.

37. Jensen, M.M., W.C. Downs, J.D. Morrey, T.R. Nicoll, S.D. LeFevre, and C.M. Meyers. 1987. Staphylococcosis of turkeys. 1. Portal of entry and tissue colonization. Avian Dis 31:64-69.

38. Jungherr, E. 1933. Staphylococcal arthritis in turkeys. J Am Vet Med Assoc 35:243-249.

39. Kibenge, F.S.B., M.D. Robertson, G.E. Wilcox, and D.A. Pass. 1982. Bacterial and viral agents associated with tenosynovitis in broiler breeders in Western Australia. Avian Pathol 11:351-359.

40. Kibenge, F.S.B., G.E. Wilcox, and D. Perret. 1982. Staphylococcus aureus isolated from poultry in Australia. I. Phage typing and cultural characteristics. Vet Microbiol 7: 471-483.

41. Kloos, W.E., and J.H. Jorgensen. 1985. Staphylococci. In E.H. Lenette, A. Balows, W.J. Hausler, Jr., and H.J. Shadomy (eds.), Manual of Clinical Microbiology, 4th Ed., pp. 143-153. Am Soc Microbiol, Washington, DC.

42. Köhler, B., V. Bergmann, W. Witte, R. Heiss, and K. Vogel. 1978. Dermatitis bei broilen durch Staphylococcus aureus. Monatsch Veterinaermed 33:22-28.

43. Köhler, B., H. Nattermann, W. Witte, F. Friedrichs, and E. Kunter. 1980. Staphylococcus aureus infection of fowls on industrialized poultry units. II. Microbiological tests for S. aureus and other pathogens. Arch Exp Veterinaermed 34:905-923.

44. Kusch, D. 1977. Biochemical characteristics and phage-typing of staphylococci isolated from poultry. Zentralbl Bakteriol Parasit Infekt Hyg [IB] 164:360-367.

45. Larson, C.T., W.B. Gross, and J.W. Davis. 1985. Social stress and resistance of chicken and swine to Staphylococcus aureus challenge infections. Can J Comp Med 49:208-210.

46. LeFevre, S.D., and M.M. Jensen. 1987. Staphylococcosis of turkeys. 2. Assay of protein A levels of staphylococci isolated from turkeys. Avian Dis 31:70-73.

47. Lucet, A. 1892. De l'ostèo-arthrite aigue infectieuse des jeunes oies. Ann Inst Past 6:841-850.

48. Mead, G.C., and B.W. Adams. 1986. Chlorine resistance of Staphylococcus aureus isolated from turkeys and turkey products. Appl Microbiol 3:131-133.

49. Meyers, C.M., and M.M. Jensen. 1987. Staphylococcosis of turkeys. 3. Bacterial interference as a possible means of control. Avian Dis 31:74-79.

50. Miner, M.L., R.A. Smart, and A.E. Olson. 1968. Pathogenesis of Staphylococcal synovitis in turkeys: Pathologic changes. Avian Dis 12:46-60.

51. Minzat, R.M., V. Volintir, S. Panaitescu, I. Javanescu, B. Kelciov, and E. Cretu. 1977. A peculiar form of staphylococcal infection in chickens. Lucr Stiint Inst Agron Timisoara, Ser Med Vet 14:141-144.

52. Morse, S.I. 1980. Staphylococci. In B.D. Davis, R. Dulbecco, H.N. Eisen, and H.S. Ginsberg (eds.), Microbiology, 3rd Ed., pp. 623-633. Harper and Row, Philadelphia.

53. Moya, S.F. 1986. Staphylococcus aureus as a potential contaminant of animal feeds. Ciencias Vet, Costa Rica 8:77-80.

54. Munger, L.L., and B.L. Kelly. 1973. Staphylococcal granulomas in a leghorn hen. Avian Dis 17:858-860.

55. Mutalib, A., C. Riddell, and A.D. Osborne. 1983. Studies on the pathogenesis of staphylococcal osteomyelitis in chickens. I. Effect of stress on experimentally induced osteomyelitis. Avian Dis 27:141-156.

56. Mutalib, A., C. Riddell, and A.D. Osborne. 1983. Studies on the pathogenesis of staphylococcal osteomyelitis in chickens. II. Role of the respiratory tract as a route of infection. Avian Dis 27:157-160.

57. Nairn, M.E. 1973. Bacterial osteomyelitis and synovitis of the turkey. Avian Dis 17:504-517.

58. Nicoll, T.R., and M.M. Jensen. 1987. Preliminary studies on bacterial interference of staphylococcosis of chickens. Avian Dis 31:140-144.

59. Nicoll, T.R., and M.M. Jensen. 1987. Staphylococcosis of turkeys. 5. Large-scale control programs using bacterial interference. Avian Dis 31:85-88.

60. Notermans, S., J. Dufrenne, and W.J. van Leeuwen. 1982. Contamination of broiler chickens by Staphylococcus aureus during processing: Incidence and origin. J Appl Bacteriol 52:275-280.

61. Rao, M.V.S., S.B. Kulshrestha, and S. Kumar. 1977. Biological properties and drug sensitivity reactions of intestinal staphylococci of poultry. Indian J Anim Sci 46:648-651.

62. Raska, K., V. Matejovska, D. Matejovska, M.S. Bergdoll, and P. Petrus. 1981. To the origin of contamination of foodstuffs by enterotoxigenic staphylococci. In J. Jeljaszewicz (ed.), Staphylococci and Staphylo-

coccal Infections, pp. 381-385. Gustav Fischer Verlag, Stuttgart.

63. Rosenberger, J.K., S. Klopp, R.J. Eckroade, and W.C. Krauss. 1975. The role of the infectious bursal agent and several avian adenoviruses in the hemorrhagic-aplastic-anemia syndrome and gangrenous dermatitis. Avian Dis 19:717-729.

64. Santivatr, D., S.K. Maheswaran, J.A. Newman, and B.S. Pomeroy. 1981. Effect of infectious bursal disease virus infection on the phagocytosis of Staphylococcus aureus by mononuclear phagocytic cells of susceptible and resistant strains of chickens. Avian Dis 25:303-311.

65. Shimizu, A. 1977. Establishment of a new bacteriophage set for typing avian staphylococci. Am J Vet Res 38:1601-1605.

66. Shimizu, A. 1977. Isolation and characteristics of bacteriophages from staphylococci of chicken origin. Am J Vet Res 38:1389-1392.

67. Shimizu, A. 1977. Bacteriophage typing of chicken staphylococci by adapted phages. Jpn J Vet Sci 39:7-13.

68. Shimizu, A. 1979. Phage-typing results of Staphylococcus aureus isolated from poultry in Japan and Europe. Avian Dis 23:39-46.

69. Takahashi, I., T. Yokoyama, T. Uehara, and T. Yoshida 1986. Susceptibility of S. aureus and Streptococcus isolates from diseased animals to commonly used antibacterial agents and nosiheptide. I. Susceptibility of S. aureus. Bull Nippon Vet Zootech No. 35:43-49.

70. Terayama, T., H. Ushioda, M. Shingaki, M. Inaba, A. Kai, and S. Sakai. 1977. Coagulase types of Staphylococcus aureus from food poisoning outbreaks and types of incriminated foods. Annu Rep Tokyo Metrop Res Lab Public Health 28:1-4.

71. Terzolo, H.R., J.A. Villar, A.S. Zamora, and A. Zoratti De Verona. 1978. Staphylococcus infection of fowls. Gaceta Vet 40:388-402.

72. Thompson, J.K., and J.T. Patterson. 1983. Staphylococcus aureus from a site of contamination in a broiler processing plant. Rec Agric Res 31:45-53.

73. Thompson, J.K., J.T. Patterson, and P.A. Gibbs. 1980. The use of a new phage set for typing poultry strains of Staphylococcus aureus obtained from seven countries. Br Poult Sci 21:95-102.

74. Vaid, M.Y., M.A. Muneer, M. Naeem, and H.A. Hashmi. 1979. A study on the incidence of Staphylococcus infections in poultry. Pak J Sci 31:155-158.

75. Van Ness, G. 1946. Staphylococcus citreus in the fowl. Poult Sci 25:647-648.

76. Wang, C.T., Y.C. Lee, and T.H. Fuh. 1977. Artificial infection of chicks with Staphylococcus aureus. J Chin Soc Vet Sci 3:1-6.

77. Watkins, B.A. and B.F. Miller. 1983. Competitive gut exclusion of avian pathogens by Lactobacillus acidophilus in gnotobiotic chicks. Poult Sci 62:1772-1779.

78. Wilkinson, D.M., and M.M. Jensen. 1987. Staphylococcosis of turkeys. 4. Characterization of a bacteriocin produced by an interfering staphylococcus. Avian Dis 31:80-84.

79. Willemart, J.P. 1980. Staphylococcal synovitis in poultry and its treatment with tiamulin. Bull Acad Vet Fr 53:209-213.

80. Williams, R.B., and L.L. Daines. 1942. The relationship of infectious omphalitis of poults and impetigo staphylogenes in man. J Am Vet Med Assoc 101:26-28.

81. Witte, W., and H. Kühn. 1978. Macrolide (antibiotic) resistance of Staphylococcus aureus strains from outbreaks of synovitis and dermatitis among chickens in large production units. Arch Exp Veterinaermed 32:105-114.

82. Wos, Z., and H. Jagodzinska. 1978. Characteristics of staphylococci found in chicken carcasses. Przem Spozyw 32:186-187.

STREPTOCOCCOSIS

Dennis P. Wages

INTRODUCTION. Streptococcosis in avian species is worldwide in distribution, occurring as both acute septicemic and chronic infections with mortality ranging from 0.5% to 50%. Infection is considered secondary, since streptococci form part of the normal intestinal flora of most avian species, including wild birds (4). Streptococci are ubiquitous in nature and commonly found in various poultry environments.

HISTORY. Acute streptococcal infections of poultry were first described in chickens in 1902 (24) and 1908 (22) as apoplectiform septicemia. Chronic streptococcosis caused 50% mortality in a flock over a 4-mo period (16) and was the cause of mortality due to salpingitis and peritonitis in chickens (10). Streptococcosis in turkeys was reported as early as 1932 (29). Bacterial or vegetative endocarditis associated with streptococci was first reported in 1927 (21), again in 1947 (26), and in 1971 (19). For a historical review see Peckham (25).

ETIOLOGY. The genus *Streptococcus* is composed of gram-positive, spherical bacteria, which are nonmotile, non-spore-forming, facultative anaerobes, occurring singly, in pairs, or in short chains. They are catalase-negative and ferment sugars, usually to lactic acid. Common avian isolates can be differentiated by their ability to ferment mannitol, sorbitol, and L-arabinose and by their growth on MacConkey's agar (Table 13.3). The relationship of these characteristics to pathogenicity is unknown. *Streptococcus* spp. isolated from avian species and associated with disease include *S. zooepidemicus* (occasionally referred to as *S. gallinarum*) from Lancefield antigenic serogroup C and *S. faecalis, S. faecium, S. durans,* and *S. avium* from Lancefield serogroup D (12). Lancefield serogroup D streptococci are commonly referred to as "fecal streps." It has been proposed that these streptococci should more appropriately be placed in the genus *Enterococcus* (6), but this has not been universally accepted. In this chapter, *S. faecalis* ssp. *faecalis, S. faecalis* ssp. *liquefaciens,* and *S. faecalis* ssp. *zymogenes* will all be considered *S. faecalis.* A new species, S.

pleomorphus, an obligate anaerobe in normal cecal contents of chickens, turkeys, and ducks has been described. Its possible role in disease for these species is undetermined (2). *S. mutans,* a common bacterium in the human oral cavity, has been associated with septicemia and mortality in geese; contaminated drinking water and poor quality litter were possible predisposing factors (17).

Bacterial endocarditis, commonly associated with streptococci, is caused by numerous bacteria in naturally occurring and experimental poultry infections. These include *S. faecalis* (7, 13, 19), *S. faecium* (7, 27), *S. durans* (7), *S. zooepidemicus* (25), *Staphylococcus aureus,* and *Pasteurella multocida* (13). Of streptococci isolated from naturally occurring infections, *S. faecalis* has been the most common isolate, and the one most consistent in producing bacterial endocarditis in experimental infections via the intravenous route.

PATHOGENESIS AND EPIZOOTIOLOGY. *Streptococcus zooepidemicus* occurs almost exclusively in mature chickens, but has been documented as a cause of mortality in wild birds (18). Experimentally, rabbits, mice, turkeys, pigeons, ducks, and geese are susceptible. *S. faecalis* affects species of all ages, the most serious disease occurring in embryos and young chicks from fecal contaminated eggs (1). *S. faecium* (27) and *S. mutans* (17) have been identified as causes of mortality in ducklings and goslings respectively.

Transmission of streptococci occurs most commonly via oral and aerosol routes (4). However, transmission can occur through skin injuries, especially in caged layers. Most antigenic serogroup D streptococci are pathogenic when administered intravenously. Aerosol transmission of *S. zooepidemicus* and *S. faecalis* results in acute septicemia in chickens (1). High mortality from acute septicemia and liver granulomas occur after experimental oral inoculation with *S. faecalis* (14), which has been incriminated as the cause of loss of intestinal epithelium integrity allowing bacteria, e.g., *Bacteroides* spp., *Catenabacterium* spp., *Eubacterium* spp., and *Streptococcus* spp., to produce liver granulomas in turkeys (23). These bacteria, and *Proprionibacterium* spp., *Corynebacterium* spp., *Staphylococcus* spp., and *Lactobacillus* spp. can often be isolated from turkey liver granulomas (23). Concurrent enteric infections, or any condition compromising the intestinal villous epithelium allowing penetration of resident serogroup D streptococci, can result in septicemia and/or bacterial endocarditis. Incubation periods range from 1 day to several weeks, with 5–21 days being most common.

Experimental bacterial endocarditis (vegetative or valvular) results from intravenous exposure. *S. faecalis* isolates from intestines of apparently normal birds are capable of producing endocarditis (13). Endocarditis occurs when septicemic streptococcal infection progresses to a subacute or chronic stage (19).

Signs. Streptococcal serogroup D infections in poultry can result in two distinct clinical forms of disease – acute and subacute/chronic. In the acute form, clinical signs are related to septicemia and include depression, lethargy, lassitude, pale comb and wattles, ruffled feathers, diarrhea, fine head tremors, and decrease or cessation of egg production. Often, only dead birds are found.

In the subacute/chronic form, depression, loss of body weight, lameness and head tremors may be observed. Streptococci enhance the severity of fibrinopurulent blepharitis and conjunctivitis in chickens (5). Chickens experimentally inoculated intravenously with *S. faecalis* develop leukocytosis 2–3 days post inoculation; highest values occur in birds that develop endocarditis (13). Heterophils predominate along with a slight monocytosis. Body temperatures are also elevated, and range from 108 to 110 F in birds with persistent bacteremia. Numbers of bacteria present in peripheral blood vary considerably. Clinically affected birds eventually die if not treated.

With *S. zooepidemicus* infections, clinical signs include lassitude, blood-stained tissue and feathers around the head, yellow droppings, emaciation, and pale combs and wattles.

Egg-transmission or fecal contamination of hatching eggs results in late embryo mortality, and increased number of chicks or poults unable to "pip," or penetrate through the shell at hatch.

Lesions. Gross lesions of *S. zooepidemicus* and serogroup D streptococci in acute disease are similar, characterized by splenomegaly, hepato-

Table 13.3. Lancefield antigenic serogroups C and D in poultry: differential characteristics

Species	Lancefield Antigenic Serogroup	Fermentation of mannitol	Fermentation of sorbitol	Fermentation of L-arabinose	Growth on MacConkey's
S. avium	D	+	+	+	+
S. durans	D	−	−	−	+
S. faecalis	D	+	+	−	+
S. faecium	D	+	−	+	+
S. zooepidemicus[a]	C		+		−

Source: (8, 11, 12).
[a]Fermentation of mannitol and L-arabinose are not considered useful in the differentiation of this species.

megaly (with or without miliary, to 1 cm red, tan, or white foci), enlarged kidneys, and congestion of subcutaneous tissue, with or without sanguineous pericardial or subcutaneous fluid, and peritonitis. Omphalitis is observed in chicks or poults infected at hatching.

Microscopically, liver has dilated sinusoids congested with red blood cells and increased heterophils. If foci are present grossly, there are multiple areas of necrosis and/or infarction with heterophil accumulation and thrombosis. Splenomegaly is characterized by congestion and reticuloendothelial hyperplasia (14).

Lesions of chronic streptococcal infections include fibrinous arthritis and/or tenosynovitis, salpingitis, fibrinous pericarditis and perihepatitis, necrotic myocarditis, and valvular endocarditis (Fig. 13.2). Vegetative valvular lesions are usually yellow, white, or tan small, raised rough areas on the valvular surface (Fig. 13.3). Valvular lesions are most consistently found on the mitral valve and less frequently on the aortic or right atrioventricular valves. Additional gross lesions associated with valvular endocarditis include

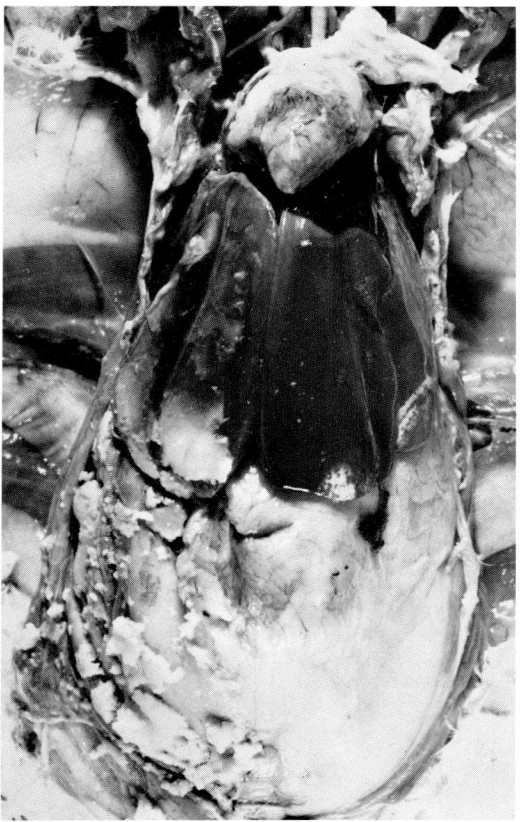

13.2. *Streptococcus zooepidemicus* infection showing perihepatitis and peritonitis. (25)

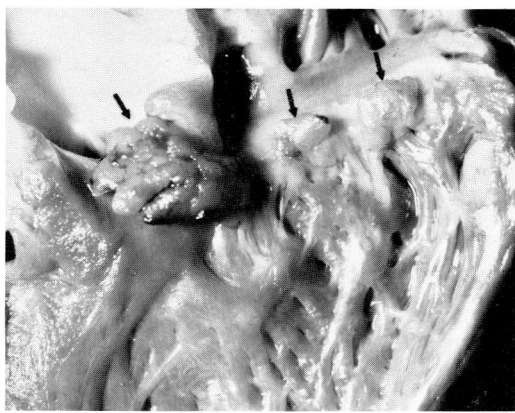

13.3. Bacterial endocarditis showing vegetations of mitral valve (*arrows*).

enlarged, pale, flaccid heart; pale to hemorrhagic areas in the myocardium, especially at the base of the valves, below the affected valve or apex of the heart; infarcts in the liver, spleen, or heart; and less commonly, infarcts in the lung, kidney, and brain. Infarcts can be light-colored or hemorrhagic with sharp margins. In the liver, infarcts are usually located near the ventral and posterior margins and are well demarcated extending beneath the capsule into the parenchyma (13) (Fig. 13.4). Lesions of longer duration tend to have a

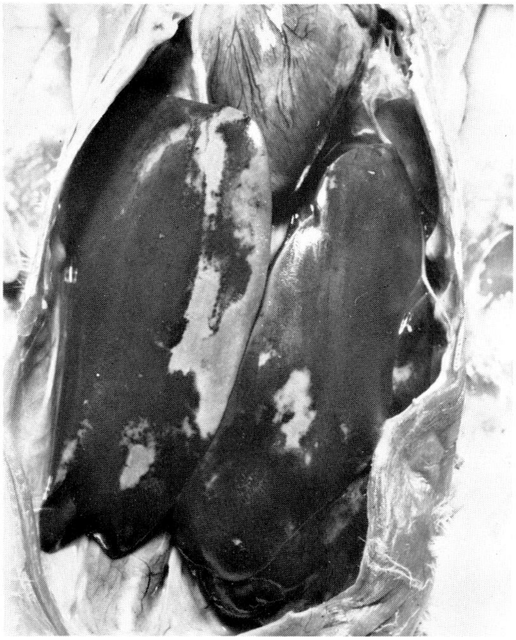

13.4. Bacterial endocarditis, showing infarcts of liver and myocardium.

sharp, narrow, lighter colored band just inside the infarct margin (19).

Microscopically, valvular lesions consist primarily of fibrin with bacteria, heterophils, macrophages, and fibroblasts. There is interstitial edema and infiltrative valvular distortion with focal deposition of platelets and fibrin and subsequent microbial growth (13, 19). Cardiac histiocytes (Anichkov's myocytes) are numerous in the fibrous portion of the valve. Events leading to the vegetative valvular lesion are 1) edema that loosens the valve surface epithelium, 2) fibrin deposition, and 3) bacterial attachment to the fibrin and colony formation. Other microscopic lesions related to endocarditis include cerebral vasculitis and infarcts, leptomeningitis, glomerulonephritis, and thrombosed pulmonary vessels (19). Cerebral lesions are usually confined to the corpus striatum. Focal granulomas can be found in virtually any tissue as a result of septic emboli. Liver infarcts are characterized by portal venous thrombosis followed by necrosis. Aggregates of bacteria are present throughout necrotic areas with a zone of heterophils just within the necrotic border, a characteristic feature of the lesion (Fig. 13.5). Gram-positive bacterial colonies are readily observed in thrombosed vessels and within necrotic foci with tissue Gram stains.

DIAGNOSIS. Demonstration of bacteria typical of streptococci in blood films (Fig. 13.6), impression smears of affected heart valves, or lesions from birds with typical signs and lesions will provide a presumptive diagnosis of streptococcosis.

Isolation of *S. zooepidemicus,* or any Lancefield serogroup D streptococci (without fecal contamination) from typical lesions in poultry with

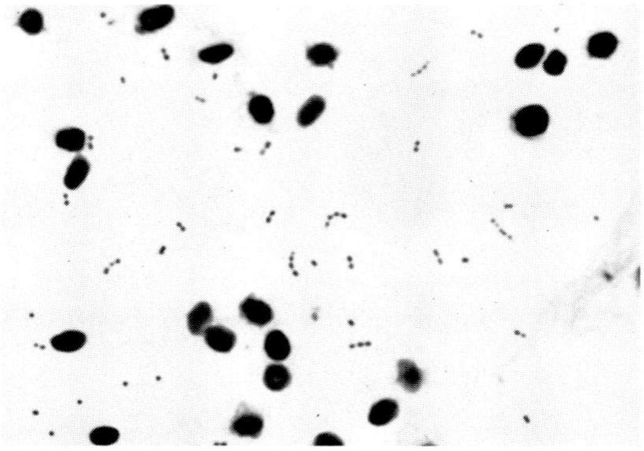

13.6. *Streptococcus zooepidemicus* in blood of naturally infected chicken. Gram, ×800. (25)

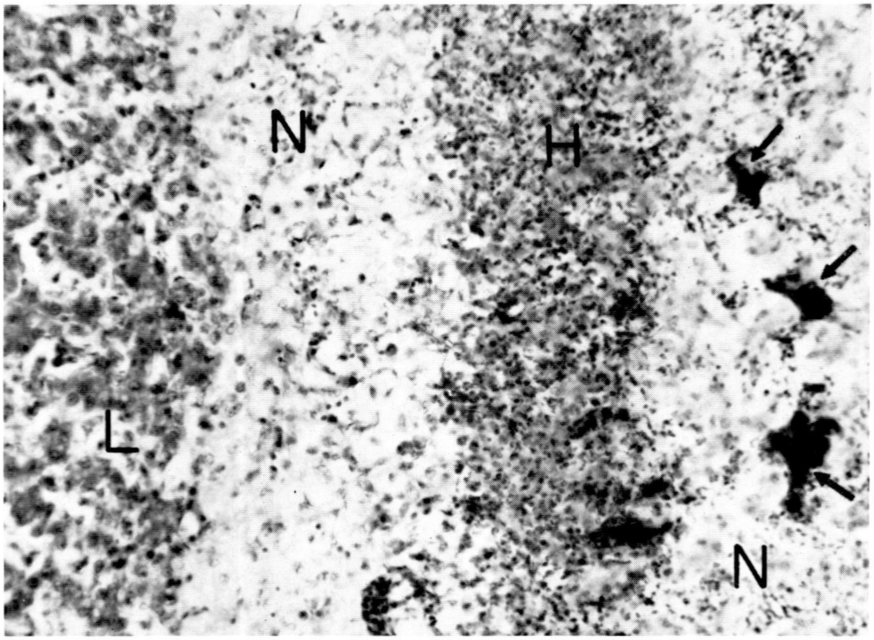

13.5. Margin of liver infarct associated with bacterial endocarditis, showing clumps of bacteria (*arrows*), necrotic area (*N*), zone of hecrotic heterophils (*H*), and relatively normal liver tissue (*L*). H & E, ×400.

appropriate clinical signs, will confirm streptococcosis. Streptococci are easily isolated on blood agar or more specific differential media (7), which should help differentiate species. Fermentation of mannitol, sorbitol, arabinose, and growth on MacConkey's agar can also aid in differentiation of streptococci in Lancefield serogroup D, and *S. zooepidemicus*. Preferred tissues for culture include liver, spleen, blood, yolk, embryo fluids, or any suspected lesion area. Diagnosis of bacterial endocarditis can be made based on valvular vegetations with secondary infarcts of myocardium, liver, and/or spleen. In suspected cases it is important to culture lesions to establish a definitive diagnosis and rule out other bacteria.

Differential diagnosis includes other bacterial septicemic diseases, e.g., staphylococcosis, colibacillosis, pasteurellosis, erysipelas, etc.

TREATMENT. Treatment includes use of antibiotics such as penicillin, erythromycin, novobiocin, oxytetracycline, chlortetracycline, tetracycline, or nitrofurans in acute and subacute infections. Clinically affected birds respond well early in the course of the disease. As the disease progresses within a flock, treatment efficacy decreases. Novobiocin has been found to be efficacious in ducks with *S. faecium* infection (27). Dietary bacitracin decreases the incidence of some strains of serogroup D streptococci in young chickens (3). Certain streptococcal strains can develop resistance after exposure to antibiotics such as tylosin, but treatment with such antibiotics may not shift the overall number of resistant organisms (15). Antibacterial sensitivity should be performed on bacterial isolates in any clinical cases of streptococcosis. Serogroup D streptococci vary in their resistance and susceptibility to growth-promoting agents (9). Environmental forces, feeding schedules, stress, interactions between different genotypes, and housing influence the response of chickens to streptococcal infections (20, 28). There is no treatment for poultry with bacterial endocarditis.

Prevention and control requires reducing stress and preventing immunodepressive diseases and conditions. Proper cleaning and disinfection can reduce environmental streptococcal resident flora to minimize external exposure.

REFERENCES

1. Agrimi, P. 1956. Studio sperimentale su alcuni focolai di streptococcosi nel pollo. Zooprofilassi 11:491-501.
2. Barnes, E.M., C.S. Impey, B.J.H. Stevens, and J.L. Peel. 1977. Streptococcus pleomorphus sp.nov.: An anaerobic streptococcus isolated mainly from the caeca of birds. J Gen Microbiol 102:45-53.
3. Barnes, E.M., G.C. Mead, C.S. Impey, and B.W. Adams. 1978. The effect of dietary bacitracin on the incidence of Streptococcus faecalis subspecies liquefaciens and related streptococci in the intestines of young chicks. Poult Sci 19:713-723.
4. Brittingham, M.C., S.A. Temple, and R.M. Duncan. 1988. A survey of the prevalence of selected bacteria in wild birds. J Wildl Dis 24:299-307.
5. Cheville, N.F., J. Tappe, M. Ackermann, and A. Jensen. 1988. Acute fibrinopurulent blepharitis and conjunctivitis associated with Staphylococcus hyicus, Escherichia coli, and Streptococcus sp. in chickens and turkeys. Vet Pathol 25:369-375.
6. Collins, M.D., D. Jones, J.A.E. Farrow, R. Kilpper-Balz, and K.H. Schleifer. 1984. Enterococcus avium nom. rev., comb. nov.; E. casseliflavus nom. rev., comb. nov.; E. durans nom. rev., comb. nov.; E. gallinarum comb. nov.; and E. malodoratus sp. nov. Int J System Bacteriol 34:220-223.
7. Domermuth, C.H., and W.B. Gross. 1969. A medium for isolation and tentative identification of fecal streptococci, and their role as avian pathogens. Avian Dis 13:394-399
8. Domermuth, C.H., and W.B. Gross. 1980. Streptococcosis, In S.B. Hitchner, C. H. Domermuth, H.G. Purchase, and J.E. Williams (eds.), Isolation and Identification of Avian Pathogens, 2nd Ed., pp. 31-32. Am Assoc Avian Pathol, Kennett Square, PA.
9. Dutta, G.N., and L.A. Devriese. 1982. Susceptibility of fecal streptococci of poultry origin to nine growth-promoting agents. Appl Environ Microbiol 44:832-837.
10. Edwards, P.R., and F.E. Hull. 1937. Hemolytic streptococci in chronic peritonitis and salpingitis of hens. J Am Vet Med Assoc 91:656-660.
11. Facklam, R.F., and R.B. Carey. 1985. Streptococci and aerococci. In E.H. Lennette, A. Balows, W.J. Hausler, Jr., and H.J. Shadomy (eds.), Manual of Clinical Microbiology, 4th Ed., pp. 154-175. Am Soc Micobiol, Washington, DC.
12. Farrow, J.A.E., D. Jones, B.A. Phillips, and M.D. Collins. 1983. Taxonomic studies on some group D streptococci. J Gen Microbiol 129:1423-1432.
13. Gross, W.B., and C.H. Domermuth. 1962. Bacterial endocarditis of poultry. Am J Vet Res 23:320-329.
14. Hernandez D.J., E.D. Roberts, L.G. Adams, and T. Vera. 1972. Pathogenesis of hepatic granulomas in turkeys infected with Streptococcus faecalis var. liquefaciens. Avian Dis 15:201-216.
15. Hinton, M., A. Kaukas, S.K. Lim, and A.H. Linton. 1986. Preliminary observations on the influence of antibiotics on the ecology of Escherichia coli and the enterococci in the faecal flora of healthy young chickens. J Antimicrob Chemother 18:165-173.
16. Hudson, C.B. 1933. A specific infectious disease of chickens due to a hemolytic streptococcus. J Am Vet Med Assoc 82:218-231.
17. Ivanics, E., Z. Bitay, and R. Glavits. 1984. Streptococcus mutans infection in geese. Magy Allatorv Lapja 39:92-95.
18. Jensen. W.I. 1979. An outbreak of streptococcosis in eared grebes (Podiceps nigricollis). Avian Dis 23:543-546.
19. Jortner, B.S., and C.F. Helmboldt. 1971. Streptococcal bacterial endocarditis in chickens. Vet Pathol 8:54-62.
20. Katanbaf, M.N., P.B. Siegel, and W.B. Gross. 1987. Prior experience and response of chickens to a streptococcal infection. Poult Sci 66:2053-2055.
21. Kernkamp, H.C.H. 1927. Idiopathic streptococcic peritonitis in poultry. J Am Vet Med Assoc 23:585-596.
22. Mack, W.B. 1908. Apoplectiform septicemia in chickens. Am Vet Rev 33:330-332.
23. Moore, W.E.C., and W.B. Gross. 1968. Liver granulomas of turkeys—causative agents and mechanism of infection. Avian Dis 12:417-422.
24. Nogaard, V.A., and J.R. Mohler. 1902. Apoplecti-

form septicemia in chickens. US Dep Agric BAI Bull 36.
25. Peckham M.C. 1966. An outbreak of streptococcosis (apoplectiform septicemia) in white rock chickens. Avian Dis 10:413-421.
26. Povar, M.L., and B. Brownstein. 1947. Valvular endocarditis in the fowl. Cornell Vet 37:49-54.
27. Sandhu, T.S. 1988. Fecal streptococcal infection of commercial White Pekin ducklings. Avian Dis 32:570-573.
28. Siegel, P.B., M.N. Katanbaf, N.B. Anthony, D.E. Jones, A. Martin, W.B. Gross, and E.A. Dunnington. 1987. Responses of chickens to Streptococcus faecalis: Genotype-housing interactions. Avian Dis 31:804-808.
29. Volkmar, F. 1932. Apoplectiform septicemia in turkeys. Poult Sci 11:297-300.

SPIROCHETOSIS

H. John Barnes

INTRODUCTION. Spirochetosis is a nonrelapsing, tick-borne borreliosis of avian species caused by the spirochete *Borrelia anserina.* It is usually an acute, septicemic disease characterized by marked illness, variable morbidity, and high mortality. In endemic areas, spirochetosis causes significant economic losses (61). Although closely related to *Borrelia* spp. causing disease in humans (6, 31), *B. anserina* is not known to infect humans or to be of public health significance. However, birds have been implicated in the spread of Lyme disease (4), a recently described borreliosis of humans caused by *B. burgdorferi,* and mallards can be experimentally infected with this spirochete (8). *B. burgdorferi* appears to be unique among borreliae in its ability to naturally infect both mammals and birds.

HISTORY. Spirochetosis was first described in 1891 by Sakharoff (57) as a severe septicemic disease of geese in Russia. In 1903, the disease was recognized in fowl in Brazil and the role of fowl ticks as primary vectors was identified (41). Subsequently, spirochetosis was recognized in many countries, often associated with ticks, which were considered the principle means of introduction. Many names for the spirochete were published by various authors resulting in numerous synonyms, and confusion with another tick-borne avian pathogen, *Aegyptianella pullorum,* led to considerable controversy about the spirochete's life cycle. Spirochetosis was first described in the USA among turkeys in California in 1946 (28). Although occasional additional outbreaks have been identified in the southwestern USA in fowl, turkeys, and pheasants, the disease has never been common.

INCIDENCE AND DISTRIBUTION. Spirochetosis occurs worldwide, most frequently in tropical and subtropical parts of the world where fowl ticks are common, and in extensive husbandry systems; occurrence in temperate areas or intensively managed flocks is uncommon (34). There have been no recent reports of the disease in the USA even though ticks and other vectors are present in southern states.

ETIOLOGY. The causative organism is *B. anserina.* Synonyms include *Spirochaeta anserina* (57), *S. gallinarum, S. anatis,* and *Treponema anserinum.* The organism belongs in the order Spirochaetales and family Spirochaetaceae (6). For additional information on *Borrelia* see Barbour and Hayes (6).

Morphology and Staining. *Borrellia anserina* is a highly motile, helical bacterium, with 5-8 spirals (Fig. 13.7) measuring about 6-30 × 0.3 μm. It will pass through a 0.45-μm-porosity membrane filter (7). Although possessing flagella, these are not free on the cell surface, but are in the periplasmic space beneath the outer cell membrane and are attached subterminally near the ends of the organism. Borreliae differ from treponemes and leptospires, staining readily with ordinary aniline dyes in addition to Romanowsky-type stains and silver impregnation (6). Spirochetes can be readily identified in wet smears of blood or tissues examined by dark-field or phase microscopy (Fig. 13.8).

Growth Requirements. Borreliae are microaerophilic, reproduce by binary fission, produce acid from glucose, and cannot be cultured on ordinary bacteriologic media. Recently, *B. anserina* has been successfully grown in Barbour-Stoenner-Kelly medium, but the organism lost its virulence within 12 passages (40). *B. anserina* is usually maintained in infected ticks, serially pas-

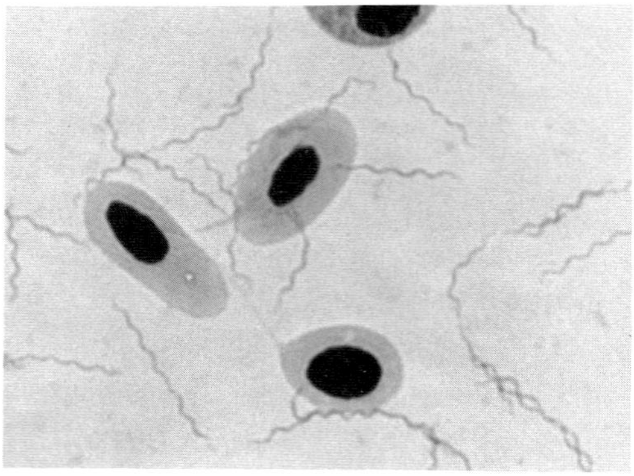

13.7. *Borrelia anserina* in blood film during acute stage of infection. Giemsa, ×1200.

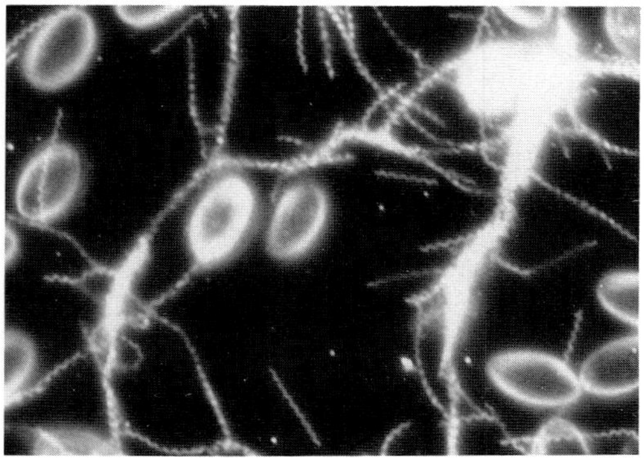

13.8. *Borrelia anserina* in plasma from infected chicken during terminal stages of spirochetosis. Note agglomeration of organisms. Dark-field, ×480.

saged by transfer of blood by any of several routes at 3- to 5-day intervals in chicks, or propagated in chicken embryos by yolk sac inoculation (43). The organism has also been cultivated in turkey embryos (44). Spirochetes are most numerous in embryo tissues, especially liver, blood, and membranes, with only few organisms in extraembryonic fluids uncontaminated by blood.

Resistance to Chemical and Physical Agents. *Borrelia anserina* is not resistant outside the host. Fowl ticks serve as the reservoir for the organism. The spirochete can survive in carcasses for up to 31 days at 0 C (44) and can be stored for as long as 3–4 wk in serum at 4 C. Strains can be maintained for extended periods at −70 C, especially if 10–15% glycerol or dimethylsulfoxide is added to infective blood (23).

Strain Classification. Immunologically distinct strains of *B. anserina* exist, but no formal serotype classification scheme has been developed (17, 35, 60). Differences in virulence also occur among strains (12).

Pathogenicity. *Borrelia anserina* is pathogenic for birds. Mammals are resistant to infection except for rabbits and mice, which may have transient infections. Attempts to adapt *B. anserina* to intact or splenectomized mice failed after the third passage (52). In chicks, intravenous (IV), intramuscular (IM), and subcutaneous inoculation give the shortest incubation periods and highest mortality (44). However, infection can be established by other routes including oral, ocular, nasal, and rectal. Virulent strains are capable of penetrating unbroken skin (33).

PATHOGENESIS AND EPIZOOTIOLOGY

Natural and Experimental Hosts. Chickens, turkeys, pheasants, ducks, geese, and canaries have been naturally infected with *B. anserina* (36, 42). A gray parrot (*Psittacus erithacus*) developed spirochetosis and died shortly after being imported from Ghana (19), and a *Borrelia* sp. was recovered from ticks collected from egret rookeries in South Africa (24). A wide variety of birds can be experimentally infected (44, 13). Pigeons and, to a lesser degree, guinea fowl are relatively resistant to experimental infection (36). Chicks <3 wk old are most susceptible; older birds tend to be more resistant (12). Infected day-old chicks experience a milder disease, lower mortality, and prolonged spirochetemia lasting 2–3 wk compared with 3–5 days in older birds (11).

Transmission, Vectors, Carriers. Spirochetosis can be transmitted by virtually any means whereby blood, excreta, or tissues from an infected live or recently dead bird comes in contact with a susceptible bird. Cannibalism, ingestion of blood or droppings, either directly or indirectly via contaminated feed and water, or use of syringes and needles for inoculation or sampling of multiple birds are all means by which the disease can be transmitted. A severe outbreak occurred in goslings injected with contaminated antiserum prepared for passive protection against viral hepatitis, even though the serum had been filtered to remove bacteria (7). Ornithophilic biting arthropods including mosquitoes (54, 56, 67) and fowl mites (*Dermanyssus*) (30) are capable of transmitting the spirochete.

Although a frequent means of spirochete transmission, especially among different groups of birds, soft ticks of the genus *Argas* serve in a much more important way as principle reservoirs of the organism (24). *B. anserina* is incapable of surviving in either the bird or environment for long periods; the organism must rely on the tick for its continued existence. Not all species of *Argas* function as biological vectors of the spirochete, and references to *A. persicus* in earlier literature may or may not have been that species (14).

A. persicus is an important vector. After it feeds on a heavily infected chicken, spirochetes are numerous in the gut lumen initially, decline in numbers during the next week, become immobile by days 15–20, and die by day 20. Within 2 hr of feeding, spirochetes penetrate the gut wall and are present in hemolymph, where they increase in numbers during the next 7 days. By day 7, organisms can be found in the tick's tissues, particularly the central nerve mass, salivary glands, and gonads where they remain at least 60 days (14). *B. anserina* survives transstadial molting from larva to adult and is transmitted transovarially from one generation to the next by suitable tick species (66). Infection rates in larvae from infected female ticks may be as high as 100% (66).

Ticks become infective 6–7 days after biting a host and can remain infective up to 488 days (36).

Larval ticks ("seed ticks," "fleas") remain attached to the bird and feed for 4–5 days in contrast to nymphs and adults, which are intermittent, nocturnal feeders spending most of their time in cracks and crevices in the poultry house or environment. Each stage can survive for months to years without feeding. Tick activity increases with increasing temperature and humidity and the spirochete develops most rapidly when ambient temperatures are >35 C. Although spirochete outbreaks are possible throughout the year, they are most common during warmer, humid seasons. Birds can become infected from saliva introduced by the tick when bitten, or by ingesting infected ticks or ova (36).

Recovered birds are not carriers (15, 36). Organisms disappear from tissues at or shortly after they disappear from the circulation (16).

Incubation Period. Incubation period depends on method of exposure, number of organisms in inoculum, and virulence of the *B. anserina* strain. Natural exposure via either tick bites or ingestion of infective blood or infected tick ova results in an incubation period of 3–12 days with 33–77% mortality. After IM or IV inoculation it may be as short as 24 hr with 100% mortality (36).

Signs. Birds infected with virulent strains of *B. anserina* are visibly sick with droopy, cyanotic heads, ruffled feathers, and a huddled-up appearance, have diarrhea, and are inactive and anorexic (Fig. 13.9). Characteristic findings in spirochetosis are an abrupt, marked elevation in body temperatures beginning shortly after infection, which, in turkeys, may reach or exceed 43 C (44), and a rapid loss of body weight that can exceed 20% during a 4- to 5-day course of illness. Body temperatures are elevated when spirochetes are in the circulation, even if their numbers are too low to detect by conventional methods. Affected birds pass fluid, green droppings containing excess bile and urates, probably resulting from anorexia, and have increased water consumption. Late in the disease, birds develop paresis or paralysis, become anemic, and are somnolent to comatose. Body temperatures are subnormal just prior to death. Birds recovering from the disease are often emaciated and have a temporary residual weakness or paralysis of one or both wings or legs. Infection with low virulent strains may be inapparent (12).

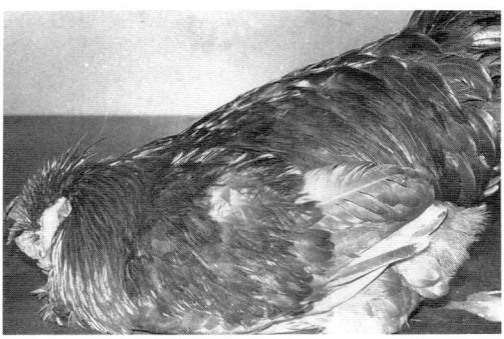

13.9. Typical clinical signs of spirochetosis in Rhode Island Red chicken experimentally infected with a virulent strain of *B. anserina*. Note fluid droppings containing excess urates.

Clinical Pathology. Anemia without intravascular hemolysis is a prominent and consistent finding in spirochetosis. Marked reductions in erythrocyte numbers, packed-cell volumes, and hemoglobin, along with an increased erythrocyte sedimentation rate occur. Peak anemia occurs after spirochetes have disappeared from the circulation. There are significant differences between infected normal and dwarf chickens in degree of anemia, its development, and erythrocyte fragility (32). Both cold agglutinins (37) and soluble immune complexes (38) have been identified and associated with anemia. It is postulated that these adhere to erythrocytes, enhancing their phagocytosis by macrophages in tissues, especially spleen.

Slight leucocytosis with increased mononuclear cells and decreased granulocytes, and an increase in coagulation time, have been found in chickens with experimental spirochetosis (58). Both qualitative and quantitative changes in serum proteins also occur (47, 48). Alterations in serum chemistries of chickens with spirochetosis include increases in total protein, globulins, uric acid, glutamate-oxalacetate transaminase, creatinine, creatine, urea, and bilirubin; and decreases in alkaline phosphatase, albumin, total lipids, cholesterol, inorganic phosphorus (slight), chloride, and iron. Blood glucose is either unchanged or decreased, and acid phosphatase unchanged (53, 58). Changes in the composition of blood from naturally infected ducks are similar to those in chickens (59).

Morbidity and Mortality. Morbidity and mortality are highly variable ranging from 1–2% to 100%. Lowest rates occur in closed flocks with constant exposure to infected ticks. Adults possess high immunity that is passively transferred to their progeny. When these chicks become exposed at a time when their resistance allows an attenuated infection, they subsequently develop active immunity, which is continually boosted, protecting them from clinical disease. Highest rates occur when either susceptible birds are mixed with tick-infected birds, or when tick-infested birds are mixed with susceptible birds. In either situation, explosive outbreaks may occur with high morbidity and mortality.

Gross Lesions. Marked enlargement and mottling of the spleen is the most characteristic lesion found in spirochetosis (Fig. 13.10). The liver may be enlarged and contain small hemorrhages and pale foci. Occasionally, marginal liver infarcts may be observed. Kidneys are swollen and pale with urates visible in ureters. A green mucoid enteritis is usually present, often with variable amounts of hemorrhage especially at the proventriculus-ventriculus junction. Occasionally there is mild, fibrinous pericarditis, but other serous membranes are not involved (44).

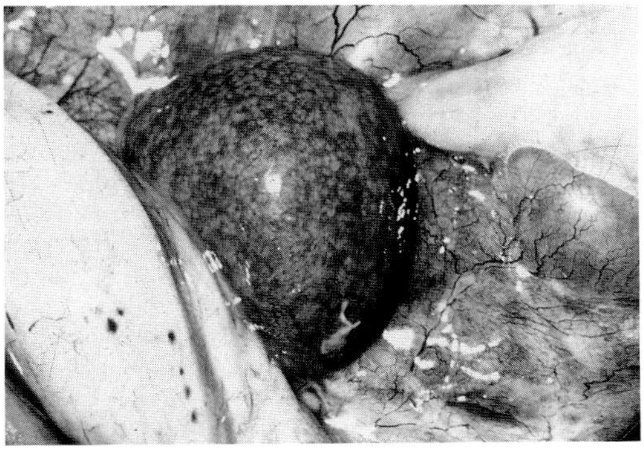

13.10. Mottled spleen in a chicken with spirochetosis. This lesion is characteristic of the disease. Splenic changes also occur in other avian species but may appear different from those in chickens depending on amount of necrosis and hemorrhage. There are also a few serosal hemorrhages on the proventriculus.

Histopathology. Splenic lesions result from an inflammatory reaction characterized by exaggerated macrophage response, mononuclear-phagocyte system (MPS) hyperplasia, erythrophagocytosis, and hemosiderin deposits (5). Central areas of MPS foci undergo hyalinization at times. Massive areas of hemorrhage may be present in some birds. Diffuse lymphatic tissue undergoes rapid growth. Cells consist of young large- and medium-sized lymphocytes and hemocytoblasts. Numerous mitotic figures are present. In poults, spirochetes occur in foci throughout the spleen but do not appear to be phagocytized by MPS cells.

Liver is congested with increased periportal infiltrates of mixed lymphocytes, hemocytoblasts, and phagocytic cells with vacuolated cytoplasm and extramedullary hematopoiesis is present. Silver stains reveal spirochetes in intercellular spaces and bile canaliculi. Organisms within hepatocytes are often fragmented or coiled forming small rings.

A mild to moderate lymphocytic meningoencephalitis is occasionally present (44).

Immunity. Long-lasting active immunity follows recovery from disease or immunization (20, 61). Active immunity is serotype specific; infection with other *B. anserina* serotypes can occur in recovered or vaccinated birds (45). Vaccines are best prepared from local strains where they are to be used (61). Passive maternal immunity capable of providing resistance to spirochetosis for as long as 5–6 wk was recognized as early as 1906 (39). Hyperimmune serum prepared in chickens or goats protected birds against challenge for up to 3 wk (46). Prior inoculation of chickens with *B. theileri,* a spirochete of ruminants, did not provide protection against *B. anserina* infection (65).

DIAGNOSIS. A clinical diagnosis of spirochetosis can be made on finding characteristic lesions in birds with signs consistent with the disease. Presence of larval ticks, most often found on the underside of wing webs, punctate hemorrhages from tick bites, especially on the shanks, or finding ticks in the bird's environment increase the likelihood of spirochetosis in severely ill birds.

Confirmation of spirochetosis requires demonstration of *B. anserina* or its antigen. During clinical illness, spirochetes can be found in stained blood or organ smears, wet mounts examined by dark-field or phase microscopy, or by immunofluorescence. Stained blood smears are best used when only a small quantity of blood is available, time between blood collection and examination will be long, specialized equipment and reagents for dark-field or fluorescent microscopy are unavailable, or a permanent specimen of the sample is needed. Giemsa stain is most often used, but the organism stains readily with most aniline and Romanowsky dyes. For demonstrating spirochetes in tissue sections, silver impregnation procedures are used (21).

Dark-field microscopy is the diagnostic method of choice because of its ease, rapidity, and accuracy. Autolysis produces background staining in tissue smears, which may obscure spirochetes, making wet mounts preferable for identifying the organism from carcasses. Early in the disease, spirochetemia may be so low detection of the organism is difficult. *B. anserina* can be concentrated in the buffy coat (27). Examination of buffy coat smears is useful in epidemiologic studies to identify early infections or infection with low virulent strains. A simple procedure used by the author (unpublished) is: fill microhematocrit tubes with blood, centrifuge for 5 min in a microhematocrit centrifuge, score tubes between packed red cells and buffy coat with a diamond-tipped pen, break the tube, expel buffy coat and plasma onto a slide leaving buffy coat intact, place cover slip on wet mount and gently press it over buffy coat pellet to spread pellet to about twice its original size, allow slide to sit at room temperature for at least 5 min, examine periphery of buffy coat for spirochetes using dark-field microscopy. If present, organisms move into the plasma from the buffy coat pellet and are easily recognized.

Spirochetes undergo agglomeration followed by lysis in the terminal stages of the disease and may no longer be recognizable in blood or tissues. In these cases spirochetal antigens can often be identified in liver or spleen by serological tests (1, 2, 62) or immunofluorescence (25, 64).

Spirochetes can be cultured by inoculating embryos or chicks with infective blood or organ suspensions. Six-day-old embryonated eggs from spirochete-free hens inoculated via the yolk sac are preferred for embryo culture. Live embryos are examined 6 days after inoculation; bleeding into chorioallantoic fluids is essential if spirochetes are to be found (43). Chicks free of spirochetal antibodies and less than 3 wk of age are most susceptible to infection. Bursectomy or dexamethasone treatment may be necessary for low-virulence strains to grow to detectable numbers (12).

Serology. Several serological tests have been developed to identify antibodies in immune birds including serum plate agglutination test (22), slide agglutination and immobilization tests (63), agar-gel precipitin test (9), and indirect fluorescent antibody test (49). Plate agglutination, tube agglutination, and spirochete immobilization tests have equal sensitivity when used for both hyperimmune and convalescent serums (10). Spirochetal antibodies can be readily detected in yolk of eggs laid by immune hens (3, 18).

Differential Diagnosis. Spirochetosis can resemble other poultry diseases characterized by acute septicemia including fowl typhoid, fowl cholera, and colisepticemia; acute viral diseases including viscerotropic, velogenic Newcastle disease, and highly virulent influenza; and Marek's disease. The characteristic lesions of spirochetosis; inability to culture *Salmonella, Pasteurella,* or *E. coli;* absence of respiratory disease and extensive hemorrhages in gastrointestinal tract and other tissues typical of virulent Newcastle disease and influenza infections; and absence of ocular, neural, or visceral tumors should allow distinction of spirochetosis from similar diseases.

TREATMENT. Initially a variety of arsenicals were used to treat birds affected with spirochetosis; antibiotics have superseded arsenicals as the treatment of choice. *B. anserina* is sensitive to most antibiotics including penicillin, chloramphenicol, kanamycin, streptomycin, tylosin, and tetracyclines (7, 29). In addition, numerous reports have been published concerning the value of locally available or experimental antimicrobials. Intramuscular injections of penicillin at 20,000 IU/bird given three times in 24 hr or 20 mg oxytetracycline given for 2 days represent currently used treatment regimens (61). Placing affected flocks on water containing approximately 1 g oxytetracycline/gal drinking water for 3 days, and treating severely affected birds with an intracrop gavage of 5 mg oxytetracycline in 5% glucose was found to be highly effective by the author.

PREVENTION AND CONTROL. Spirochetosis is best prevented in endemic areas by not introducing tick-infested birds into clean flocks or susceptible birds into infested flocks or housing where infected birds were once kept. Adult ticks can remain alive without feeding and carry the spirochete for as long as 3 yr.

Once the tick is present, it is extremely difficult to eradicate. The only complete success by the author resulted when houses were depopulated and burned. Larval ticks can be controlled on birds by dipping them in 0.5% malathion. Dipping is more effective than using insecticide dusts. Dusts are helpful when used in dusting baths. High-pressure spraying of the house and environment, paying particular attention to cracks, crevices, and other places where ticks hide, with 3% malathion at monthly intervals helps keep ticks at low levels. Insecticide-laced "paints" and "pastes" can control ticks if vigorously used (55). Attempts to tick proof roosts by suspending them from wire and keeping grease spread on the wire, or placing roost legs in oil-filled containers require almost constant attention to be effective. The same is true for tick proof houses surrounded by an oil-filled moat. If affected birds are roosting in trees, cutting and burning the trees while simultaneously dipping birds may be successful.

Immunization. Vaccination is practiced in areas where spirochetosis is prevalent. Birds are usually inoculated at 8–10 wk of age (61). Vaccines are inactivated with formalin or phenol and prepared from lysates of blood, tissues, or embryos infected with *B. anserina* (26, 50, 51); both lyophilized and liquid products are available. Immunity is type specific; polyvalent vaccines or autogenous vaccines may be necessary. Deliberate infection followed by antibiotic treatment has also been used to induce immunity.

REFERENCES

1. Al-Attar, M.A., and F.M. Jahanly. 1974. Demonstration by immunodiffusion agar-gel test of Borrelia anserina antigens in the organs of infected chickens. Avian Dis 18:463–466.

2. Al-Hilly, J.N.A. 1969. Immunodiffusion agar-gel test for demonstration of Borrelia anserina antigen produced by liver of infected chickens. Am J Vet Res 30:1877–1880.

3. Al-Hilly, J.N.A. 1971. Immobilization and immunodiffusion tests for determination of antibodies against spirochetosis in the yolk of convalescent fowls. Avian Dis 15:419–421.

4. Anderson, J.F., R.C. Johnson, L.A. Magnarelli, and F.W. Hyde. 1986. Involvement of birds in the epidemiology of the Lyme disease agent Borrelia burgdorferi. Infect Immun 51:394–396.

5. Bandopadhyay, A.C., and J.L. Vegad. 1983. Observations on the pathology of experimental avian spirochaetosis. Res Vet Sci 35:138–144.

6. Barbour, A.G., and S.F. Hayes. 1986. Biology of Borrelia species. Microbiol Rev 50:381–400.

7. Bok, R., Y. Samberg, M. Rubina, and A. Hadani. 1975. Studies on fowl spirochaetosis – survival of Borrelia anserina at various temperatures and its sensitivity to antibiotics. Refu Vet 32:147–153.

8. Burgess, E.C. 1989. Experimental inoculation of mallard ducks (Anas platyrhynchos platyrhynchos) with Borrelia burgdorferi. J Wildl Dis 25:99–102.

9. Chatterjee, A., and A.N. Sawhney. 1971. Diagnosis of fowl spirochaetosis by agar-gel-precipitation test. Indian J Anim Sci 41:727–730.

10. Chatterjee, A., and A.N. Sawhney. 1971. Serological studies on experimental fowl spirochaetosis. Indian J Anim Sci 41:1151–1153.

11. Choudhary, C.R., and K.N.P. Rao. 1985. Studies on clinicopathological changes in fowl spirochaetosis in young chicks. Indian Vet J 62:465–468.

12. DaMassa, A.J., and H.E. Adler. 1979. Avian spirochaetosis: Enhanced recognition of mild strains of Borrelia anserina with bursectomized and dexamethasone-treated chickens. J Comp Pathol 89:413–420.

13. DaMassa, A.J., and H.E. Adler. 1980. Avian spirochetosis: General comments and preliminary data on the experimental disease in budgerigars. Proc 29th West Poult Dis Conf, pp. 83–85.

14. Diab, F.M., and Z.R. Soliman. 1977. An experimental study of Borrelia anserina in four species of Argas ticks. 1. Spirochete localization and densities. Z Parasitenkd. 53:201–212.

15. Dickie, C.W., and J. Barrera. 1964. A study of the carrier state of avian spirochetosis in the chicken. Avian Dis 8:191–195.

16. Djankov, I., I. Soumrov, T. Lozeva, and P. Penev. 1970. Persistence and excretion of Treponema anserinum (Sakharoff, 1891) in hens. Zentralbl Veterinaermed [B] 17:544–548.

17. Djankov, I., I. Soumrov, and T. Lozeva. 1972. Use of the immunofluorescence method for the serotype identification of Borrelia anserina (Sakharoff, 1891) strains. Zentralbl Veterinaermed [B] 19:221–225.

18. Dutta, G.N., M.L. Mehta, and A.R. Muley. 1977. Studies on immunity in fowl spirochaetosis. Indian J Anim Sci 47:554–558.

19. Ehrsam, H. von. 1977. Borreliose (spirochaetose) bei einem graupapagei (Psittacus erithacus). Schweiz Arch Tierheilk 119:41–43.

20. El Dardiry, A.H. 1945. Studies on avian spirochetosis in Egypt. Min Egypt Tech Sci Serv Bull 243:1–78.

21. Felsenfeld, O. 1971. Borrelia strains, vectors, human and animal borreliosis. Warren H. Green, Inc., St. Louis, MO.

22. Garg, R.R., and O.P. Gautam. 1971. Serological diagnosis of fowl spirochetosis. Avian Dis 15:1–6.

23. Ginawi, M.A., and A.M. Shommein. 1980. Preservation of Borrelia anserina at different temperatures. Bull Anim Health Prod Afr 28:221–223.

24. Gothe, R., and W. Schrecke. 1972. Zur epizootiologischen bedeutung von Persicarges-zecken der huhner in Transvaal. Berl Muench Tierärztl Wochenschr 85:9–11.

25. Gross, W.M., and M.R. Ball. 1964. Use of fluorescein-labeled antibody to study Borrelia anserina infection (avian spirochetosis) in the chicken. Am J Vet Res 25:1734–1739.

26. Hart, L. 1963. Spirochaetosis in fowls: Studies on immunity. Aust Vet J 39:187–191.

27. Higgins, A.R. 1986. Demonstrating Borellia [sic] anserina: "A can of worms." Vet Rec 119:120.

28. Hoffman, H.A., and T.W. Jackson. 1946. Spirochetosis in turkeys. J Am Vet Med Assoc 109:481–486.

29. Hsiang, C.M., and A. Packchanian. 1951. A comparison of eleven antibiotics in the treatment of Borrelia anserina infection (spirochetosis) in young chicks. Tex Rep Biol Med 9:34–45.

30. Hungerford, T.G., and L. Hart. 1937. Fowl tick fever (spirochaetosis) also transmitted by common red mite. Agric Gaz 48:591–592.

31. Hyde, F.W., and R.C. Johnson. 1986. Genetic analysis of Borrelia. Zentralbl Bakteriol Hyg Abt 263:119–122.

32. Joshi, A.G., J.L. Soni, and A.G. Khan. 1980. Spirochaetosis anaemia and its influence on erythrocyte size in normal and dwarf chickens. Indian J Anim Sci 50:753–756.

33. Kapur, H.R. 1940. Transmission of spirochaetosis through agents other than Argas persicus. Indian J Vet Sci Anim Husb 10:354–360.

34. Kaschula, V.R. 1961. A comparison of the spectrum of disease in village and in modern poultry flocks in Nigeria. Bull Epizoot Dis Afr 9:397–407.

35. Kligler, I.J., D. Hermoni, and M. Perek. 1938. Studies on fowl spirochetosis. II. Presence of serologically differentiated types of spirochetes. J Comp Pathol Ther 51:206–212.

36. Knowles, R., B.M. Das Gupta, and B.C. Basu. 1932. Studies in avian spirochaetosis. Indian Med Res Mem 22:1–113.

37. Lad, P.L., and J.L. Soni. 1983. Role of cold agglutinin (CA) in anaemia production in acute avian spirochetosis. Indian J Anim Sci 53:937–943.

38. Lad, P.L., and J.L. Soni. 1983. Soluble spirochaete antigen-antibody immune complex in plasma of Borrelia anserina-infected chickens. Indian J Anim Sci 53:538–541.

39. Levaditi, C. 1906. La spirillose des embryons de poulet dans ses rapports avec la treponemose hereditaire de l'homme. Ann Inst Pasteur 20:924.

40. Levine, J.F. 1988. Personal communication.

41. Marchoux, E., and A. Salimbeni. 1903. La spirillose des poules. Ann Inst Pasteur 17:569–580.

42. Mathey, W.J., and P.J. Siddle. 1955. Spirochetosis in pheasants. J Am Vet Med Assoc 126:123–126.

43. McKercher, D.G. 1950. The propagation of Borrelia anserina in embryonated eggs employing the yolk sac technique. J Bacteriol 59:446–447.

44. McNeil, E., W.R. Hinshaw, and R.E. Kissling. 1949. A study of Borrelia anserina infection (spirochetosis) in turkeys. J Bact 57:191–206.

45. Mehta, M.L., and A.R. Muley. 1969. Efficacy of spirochaetosis vaccine prepared from the local (Jabalpur) strain of Borrelia gallinarum. Indian J Anim Sci 39:225–230.

46. Morcos, Z., O.A. Zaki, and R. Zaki. 1946. A concise investigation of fowl spirochetosis in Egypt. J Am Vet Med Assoc 109:112–116.

47. Pavlow, P., Y. Dumanov, Y. Denev, M. Kolev, R. Stoyanova, T. Loseva, and I. Djankov. 1973. A study of parasite-host immunological interrelations. IV. Investigation of the protein profiles in lambs, cats, and birds in experimental spirochetosis and leptospirosis. Zentralbl Veterinaermed [B] 20:230–240.

48. Perk, K., and I. Hort. 1966. Paper electrophoretic studies of the serum proteins of chicks during experimental spirochetosis. Avian Dis 10:208–215.

49. Prudovsky, S., A. Hadani, M. Rubina, and A. Sklair. 1978. The use of the indirect fluorescent anti-

body technique in avian spirochaetosis. Avian Pathol 7:421-425.

50. Rao, S.B.V. 1958. Spirochaetosis in poultry. Indian Council Agric Res, New Delhi, Res Ser No 18.

51. Rao, M.L.V., and J.L. Soni. 1982. Augmentation of haemo-tissue vaccine doses out-turn through blood transfusion in Borrelia anserina infected chickens. Zentralbl Veterinaermed [B] 29:408-410.

52. Rao, M.L.V., and J.L. Soni. 1986. Preliminary studies on murinization of Borrelia anserina. Indian J Anim Sci 56:1187-1189.

53. Rivetz, B., E. Bogin, Y. Weisman, J. Avidar, and A. Hadani. 1977. Changes in the biochemical composition of blood in chickens infected with Borrelia anserina. Avian Pathol 6:343-351.

54. Roberts, J.A. 1961. Experimental transmission of Borrelia anserina (Sakharoff, 1891) by Aedes aegypti. Nature 191:1225.

55. Rodey, M.V., and J.L. Soni. 1977. Epidemiology of spirochaetosis in chickens: Effective measures for control of ticks–Argas persicus. Poult Guide 14:35-37.

56. Rubina, M., Y. Braverman, and M. Malkinson. 1975. On the possible transmission of Borrelia anserina (Sakharoff, 1891) by mosquitoes. Refu Vet 32:16-18.

57. Sakharoff, M.N. 1891. Spirochaeta anserina et la septicemie des oies. Ann Inst Pasteur 5:564-566.

58. Soliman, M.K., A.A.S. Ahmed, S. El Amrousi, and I.H. Moustafa. 1966. Cytological and biochemical studies on the blood constituents of normal and spirochete-infected chickens. Avian Dis 10:394-400.

59. Soliman, M.K., S. El Amrousi, and A.A.S. Ahmed. 1966. Cytological and biochemical studies of the blood of normal and spirochaete-infected ducks. Zentralbl Veterinaermed [B] 13:82.

60. Soni, J.L., and A.G. Joshi. 1980. A note on strain variation in Akola and Jabalpur strains of Borrelia anserina. Zentralbl Veterinaermed [B] 27:70-72.

61. Supekar, P.G. 1989. Avian spirochaetosis is a perpetuating menace. Poultry 5:40-41.

62. Verma, K.C., and B.S. Malik. 1968. Diagnosis of spirochaetosis of poultry by gel diffusion test. Indian Vet J 45:460-462.

63. Verma, K.C., and B.S. Malik. 1968. Diagnosis of spirochaetosis of poultry by slide agglutination and spirochaete immobilization tests. Curr Sci 37:170-171.

64. Wadalkar, B.G., and J.L. Soni. 1982. Use of fluorescent antibody technique for the detection of spirochaete antigen in prepatent, peak and post-spirochaetemic phase organs. Indian J Anim Sci 52:776-781.

65. Wouda, W., Tj.W. Schillhorn van Veen, and H.J. Barnes. 1975. Borrelia anserina in chickens previously exposed to Borrelia theileri. Avian Dis 19:209-210.

66. Zaher, M.A., Z.R. Soliman, and F.M. Diab. 1977. An experimental study of Borrelia anserina in four species of Argas ticks. 2. Transstadial survival and transovarial transmission. Z Parasitenkd 53:213-223.

67. Zuelzer, M. 1936. Culex, a new vector of Spirochaeta gallinarum. J Trop Med Hyg 39:204.

14 CHLAMYDIOSIS (ORNITHOSIS)

James E. Grimes and Priscilla B. Wyrick

INTRODUCTION. Chlamydiosis, a naturally occurring contagious, systemic disease that is most likely to be fatal in younger birds, is caused by *Chlamydia psittaci.*

Chlamydiosis is a general term referring to an infection in birds, mammals, or other animals with organisms of the genus *Chlamydia.* The disease that was first recognized in humans as an infection contracted from psittacine birds was called psittacosis (37). Parrot fever, is a commonly used synonym. Ornithosis, a term first used in 1941 (33), was introduced to describe infections in humans contracted from nonpsittacine birds. Such a distinction between avian chlamydioses is purely artificial because the disease is essentially the same in humans and in all species of birds, except for epidemiological variations, and because strains of *C. psittaci* isolated from one kind of bird can produce experimental infections in other kinds of birds.

Avian chlamydiosis can be an economically devastating disease to producers because of carcass condemnation at slaughter, egg production decreases, and/or the expense of antibiotic treatment to reduce mortality and allow marketing of birds.

The public health significance of avian chlamydiosis is substantial. The disease in turkeys may cause infection of poultry processing-plant employees. Also at risk are turkey producers on the farm and poultry inspectors at processing plants. It now is known that personnel who are employed to further process turkey meat from infected birds can also become infected. Ducks present a potential threat similar to that from turkeys. Pigeons also may pose public health threats mainly to their producers. Chickens and pheasants are of lesser importance as potential public health hazards due to chlamydiosis.

This chapter will deal primarily with avian chlamydiosis as it occurs in turkeys, ducks, pigeons, geese, pheasants, and chickens. Chlamydioses and chlamydia in other species will be discussed when useful in describing avian chlamydiosis.

HISTORY. Previous editions of *Diseases of Poultry* (34, 47, 49, 51) contain detailed historical accounts of chlamydiosis in avian species.

Following worldwide investigations of psittacosis in humans and psittacine birds in the 1930s, a similar disease was observed in poultry. In the middle and late 1940s chlamydial epidemics in domestic ducks and turkeys caused numerous individual agricultural losses and human infections. Between 1951 and 1956 a widespread series of epidemics of unusual virulence caused such economic losses and so many human infections that the disease became a matter of national concern. Subsequent investigations focused on chlamydial microbiology, epizootiology, serology, pathogenesis, chemotherapy, and control. These studies formed the basis for recommendations and reforms in management of birds in areas of high incidence and for treatment, handling, and processing of birds suspected of having the disease.

During the 1960s the incidence of severe epidemics in poultry in the USA and Europe declined, although serologic surveys indicated that infection of reservoir hosts (pigeons, wild birds, mammals) was still prevalent.

INCIDENCE AND DISTRIBUTION. Chlamydial infections of avian species occur worldwide and are either epidemic or endemic depending upon the species and locale (51). The incidence of the disease is highly variable.

Reasons for the irregular cyclic occurrence of chlamydiosis in poultry are unknown. Perhaps the immune status of vectors or amplifying avian hosts influences the occurrence of outbreaks. The behavioral patterns of vector hosts could conceivably influence transmission from primary hosts to domestic turkeys or ducks. Mammalian chlamydial strains are probably not responsible for naturally occurring infections in birds.

Table 14.1 contains reported epidemics of chlamydiosis in poultry and pigeons in the USA from 1960 through 1987.

ETIOLOGY

Classification. The etiologic agent of avian chlamydiosis is an obligate intracellular bacterium, *Chlamydia psittaci,* in the family Chlamydiaceae, order Chlamydiales in the Rickettsias and Chlamydias, which compares to the class level of the bacterial kingdom Prokaryotae (38).

Table 14.1. Reports of epidemics of chlamydiosis in poultry in the USA, 1960–87

Year	State	Affected Species	Degree of Loss	Basis for Diagnosis	Investigator
1960	Oregon	Turkey	None reported	Agent isolation	E.M. Dickinson
1961	Texas	Turkey	Siginficant condemnation	Agent isolation	L. Passera
1964	Oregon	Chicken, pigeon, pheasant	No significant	Positive serology only	L.A. Page, K. Erickson
1965	Virginia	Turkey	20% mortality; severe condemnation	Agent isolation	W.S. Thompson, L.A. Page
1966	Virginia	Duck	10% mortality; severe condemnation	Agent isolation	E.C. Roukema, L.A. Page
	Texas	Turkey	Moderate	Agent isolation	L.C. Grumbles
1967	California	Turkey	Moderate with 3% mortality	Agent isolation	J.A. Newman
1968	Minnesota	Turkey (4 flocks)	None	Positive serology	B.S. Pomeroy
	Georgia	Turkey	High condemnations	Positive tissue antigen (FA and CF)	H.W. Yoder, L.A. Page
1969	South Carolina	Turkey	Mild condemnations	Positive serology	T.H. Eleazer, L.A. Page
	California	Turkey	Low mortality; moderate condemnations	Agent isolation	D.L. Bristow, G. Lucas
1973	South Carolina	Turkey	4.7% mortality	Agent isolation	L.A. Page, W.T. Derieux
1974	South Carolina	Turkey		Positive serology and tissue	L.A. Page, T.H. Eleazer
	Texas	Turkey (13 flocks)	0.5–30% mortality	Agent isolation and positive serology	J.E. Grimes, K. Hand, S. Glass
1975	Texas	Turkey (5 flocks)	0–25% mortality	Agent isolation and positive serology	J.E. Grimes, K. Hand, S. Glass
	Colorado	Turkey	2% increase in condemnations	Positive serology	D.D. King
1976	Texas	Turkey (1 flock)	Low mortality; moderate condemnation	Agent isolation; positive serology	J.E. Grimes
1980	South Carolina	Pigeon	Low mortality; increased condemnation	Agent isolation	J.E. Grimes
1981–82	California	Turkey	Low mortality	Agent isolation	R. Cooper
1981	Ohio	Turkey (presumed)	Unknown	Inferred from human infection following processing of turkeys	Centers for Disease Control, Atlanta, GA.
1984	Virginia	Turkey	High condemnation	Inferred from human infection following processing of turkeys	S.F. Wetterhall
1986–87	Minnesota	Turkey	Moderate condemnation	Agent isolation	J.A. Newman
1987	North Carolina	Turkey	None	Positive serology and agent isolation	D.V. Rives

Note: FA = fluorescent antibody, CF = complement fixation. All reports are personal communications to the authors.

Classification of the chlamydias took many years to become established in its present form and, undoubtedly, it will undergo further modification as better methods become available for determining taxonomic relationships among bacteria. It has been determined by studying the 16S ribosomal RNA (rRNA) that chlamydiae truly are eubacteria and that the organisms represent a hitherto unrecognized major eubacterial group possibly peripherally related to the planctomyces and relatives that also do not contain peptidoglycan in their cell walls (73).

There are only two recognized species (*C. psittaci, C. trachomatis*), but this is likely to change as more chlamydial isolations are made and as more precise methods of differentiation are used to distinguish between the many organisms now grouped together as either mammalian and avian chlamydias. The two species are differentiated mainly according to characteristics shown in Table 14.2 (38).

Many other characteristics are used to differen-

Table 14.2. Species differentiation in the genus *Chlamydia*

Characteristics	*C. trachomatis*	*C. psittaci*
Natural hosts	Humans, mice	Birds, mammals other than humans
Inclusion morphology		
Oval, vacuolar	+	–
Variable shape, dense	–	+
Glycogen in inclusions	+	–
Folate biosynthesis	+	–

tiate *C. trachomatis* into biovars and serovars and to differentiate this species from *C. psittaci*. Interested readers should consult a recent edition of *Bergey's Manual of Systematic Bacteriology* for details of chlamydia classification. The *C. psittaci* representatives of primary interest here are the various isolates that cause intestinal, respiratory, and systemic infections of turkeys, ducks, pigeons, geese, pheasants, and chickens. Of secondary interest, of course, should be those strains infecting psittacine and over 130 other bird species because some of those strains are likely to be epidemiologically involved in chlamydiosis of poultry.

Morphology and Biochemical Properties. There are two morphologically distinct forms of chlamydia, termed elementary body (EB) and reticulate body (RB) (Fig. 14.1). The EB is a small, dense, spherical body, about 0.2–0.3 μm in diameter, which rivals mycoplasma for the smallest of the prokaryotes. The EB is the infectious form of the organism, which attaches to target columnar epithelial cells and gains entry. Rigidity of the EB membrane is believed to be due more to disulfide bond cross-linking among the major outer membrane proteins than to an extensively cross-linked classical peptidoglycan matrix, since muramic acid is absent. The distribution of amino acids in chlamydial cell walls is similar to that of the cell walls of *Escherichia coli,* the wall content being largely protein (70%) and lipid (5.1%) with the remainder presumably carbohydrate (30). EBs are nonmotile, lacking flagella, and nonpiliated.

The RB is the intracellular, metabolically active form, which divides by binary fission. It is larger than the EB, about 0.6–1.5 μm in diameter, and is osmotically fragile. While DNA and RNA are found in both the EB and the RB, the ratio of RNA to DNA is greater in the RB. The RB forms synthesize their own DNA, RNA, and protein but some of their metabolic capabilities are limited when compared with free-living, colonizing bacteria. For example, they cannot complete the pentose cycle and do not utilize pyruvate by way of the tricarboxylic acid cycle. They can, however, catabolize pyruvic, aspartic, and glutamic acids, generating CO_2 and 2- and 4-carbon residues.

The chlamydial genome is a closed circular DNA molecule with a molecular weight of 6.6×10^8. A molecule of this size can provide information for about 600 different proteins, which is about one-fourth the amount provided by the *E. coli* genome. All strains of *C. trachomatis* and some strains of *C. psittaci* also possess plasmids, but their function has yet to be determined (23).

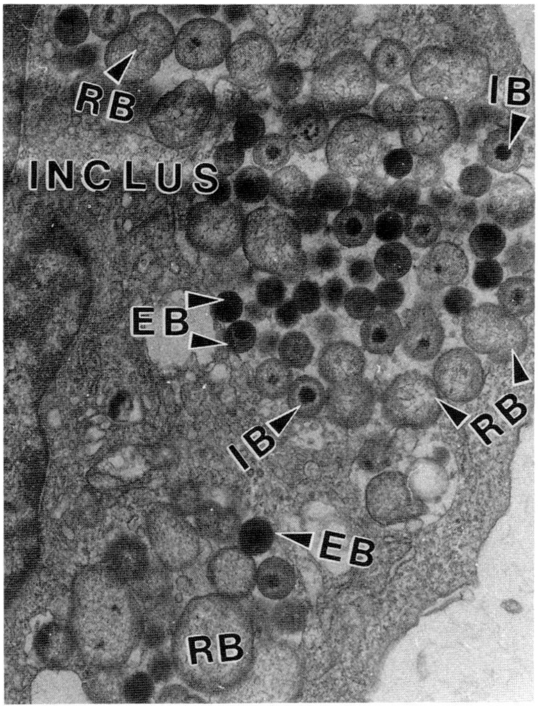

14.1. Transmission electron photomicrograph of a *C. psittaci* inclusion (*INCLUS*) in infected L929 cells. The various morphological forms of chlamydiae are present: elementary body (*EB*), reticulate body (*RB*), and intermediate body (*IB*). ×15,000.

Developmental Cycle. An unusual developmental cycle characterizes the growth of these obligate intracellular bacteria in their eucaryotic host cells. The cycle consists of essentially five major phases: 1) attachment and penetration by the EB, 2) transition of the metabolically inert EB into the metabolically active RB, 3) growth and division of the RB, producing many progeny, 4) maturation of the noninfectious RBs into infectious EBs, and 5) release of EBs from the host cell (39, 64).

The initial event in the infectious process begins with attachment of *C. psittaci* EBs to microvilli at the apical surface of a susceptible columnar epithelial cell. The EB travels down the microvilli and locates in indentions of the eukaryotic plasma membrane, some of which resemble coated pits (25). The EBs are subsequently internalized in invaginations of the plasma membrane. Thus uptake is akin to an endocytosislike process. *C. psittaci*-containing endocytic vesicles escape interaction with lysosomes and proceed to the nuclear hof area. The chlamydia remain surrounded and protected by the endosome membrane throughout their intracellular development.

Alterations in the EB cell wall occur and result in a spheroplastlike transition of the EB to the RB form. These changes primarily involve reduction in disulfide bond cross-linking among the major outer membrane proteins (22, 40). Synthesis of DNA, RNA, and protein are initiated, permitting growth of the RB and division by binary fission. The RB, however, cannot generate high-energy phosphate bonds. Thus, their adaptation to an intracellular habitat is due to their dependency on eukaryotic cells for energy. At some point, host cell mitochondria are positioned against the enlarging chlamydial endosome enabling the RB to parasitize mitochondrial ATP via a chlamydial ATP-ADP translocase. The ATP is broken down to ADP by a specific RB ATPase, and the resultant proton motive force helps drive the transport of nutrients (21). The chlamydiae possess unusual cylindrical surface projections, averaging 18 in number and arranged in a hexagonal array. These projections are anchored in the cytoplasmic membrane and protrude through holes in the envelope. Current evidence suggests that the projections penetrate the endosome membrane, which surrounds the developing chlamydial microcolony, permitting uptake of nutrients from the host cytoplasm (31).

The developing chlamydial microcolony is termed an "inclusion" and may contain anywhere from 100 to 500 progeny, depending on the species of chlamydia. In some cases, multiple inclusions can appear in *C. psittaci*-infected cells (Fig. 14.2). In contrast, *C. trachomatis*-containing endosomes seem to fuse with one another early in the developmental cycle, resulting in the eventual appearance of usually only one inclusion. By 48 hr, there is a marked increase in glycogen accumulation in the *C. trachomatis* inclusion. Presumably, when the nutrients have been depleted, the RB progeny mature and condense into EBs and are released. In the case of *C. psittaci,* the host cell is usually severely damaged and release of chlamydiae is by lysis within 48 hr after initial infection. Todd and Caldwell (72) reported the exocytosis of *C. trachomatis* inclusions between 72 and 96 hr postinfection in HeLa cells, followed by

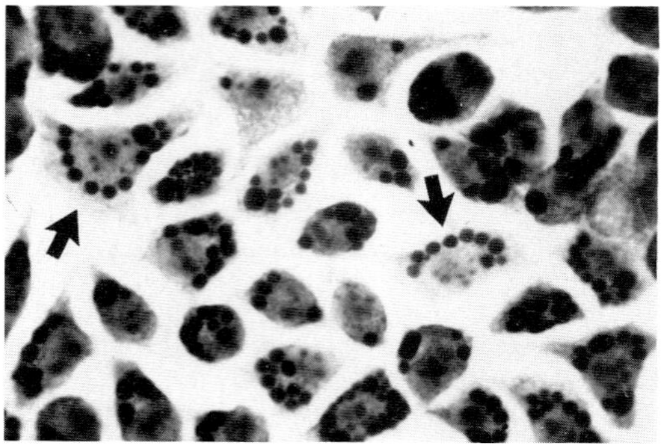

14.2. Multiple *C. psittaci* (Cal 10) inclusions in 24-hr infected L929 cells. ×450. (Hodinka, Infect Immun)

a "healing" or closing of the "open-cavern" structures where the inclusions had existed.

The pathology associated with human psittacosis includes inflammatory exudate within the alveoli in which polymorphonuclear leukocytes, and subsequently mononuclear phagocytes, are prominent. Opsonized EBs are rapidly engulfed by these cells and destroyed in the phagolysosomes. However, if the EBs are not coated by antibody and/or complement, they are still efficiently internalized by the professionally phagocytic cells, but their fate is different. The majority of the chlamydiae do not survive in the short-lived polymorphonuclear leukocytes, but *C. psittaci* do survive and grow in macrophages (56).

Chlamydia-specific lipopolysaccharide is exported to the surface of the infected eukaryotic host cell concomitant with active RB growth (57). The exoglycolipid is postulated to reduce plasma membrane fluidity thereby protecting the chlamydiae from cytotoxic T-cell onslaught. Whether or not this highly antigenic lipopolysaccharide plays a role in the perpetuation of disabling chlamydial disease via prolonged inflammatory response and immune-mediated pathology is at present a controversial issue (69, 70).

Staining Characteristics. The inclusion (or microcolony) of each chlamydial species can be distinguished by staining sections of infected tissues or monolayers of infected cell cultures with an alcoholic solution of 5% iodine and 10% potassium iodide. As indicated above, there is a marked increase in glycogen accumulation in the developing inclusion by 48 hr, which is specific for *C. trachomatis* (27). Iodine binds to the glycogen and stains *C. trachomatis* inclusions dark golden to reddish brown, whereas *C. psittaci* inclusions are devoid of accumulated glycogen and remain the same light tan color as the background after staining. The iodine technique, however, is the least sensitive cytological procedure and is not recommended for use with clinical specimens.

In wet mounts of impression smears of infected

tissues or exudates, intracellular chlamydiae are large enough to be seen at magnifications of ×800 or more in phase contrast microscopes (Fig. 14.3A). They are readily seen by dark-field illumination (Fig. 14.3B). With either technique, however, they cannot be distinguished from contaminating intracellular mycoplasma organisms. When only bright-field optics are available, chlamydiae may be seen in touch impressions of infected tissues by staining them with Giemsa, Castaneda, Macchiavello, or Gimenez methods after appropriate fixation. They appear dark purple with Giemsa, blue with Castaneda, and red with Macciavello and Gimenez stains against contrasting backgrounds. The Gimenez method (12) is preferred for staining chlamydiae in touch impressions of yolk sacs of infected chicken embryos, and has proved very useful in obtaining presumptive diagnoses in microscopic examination of touch impressions of diseased air sacs, spleens, and pericardia of naturally infected birds (13).

In infected cell cultures, chlamydiae stain well with Giemsa (Figs. 14.4E,F) and Gimenez (Fig. 14.4D) methods. All chlamydiae are gram-negative but the Gram stain is of no practical value in identifying intracellular organisms.

The development of monoclonal antibodies has revolutionized the detection of chlamydiae in clinical specimens (67). Direct (Fig. 14.4G) or indirect immunofluorescence and immunoenzymatic (29) methods are acceptable. While the antigen-detection approach is slightly less sensitive than culture, it is cheaper and faster. The major drawback to these kinds of immunoassays is the lack of specificity due to nonspecific staining that may occur in uninfected tissue or autofluorescence due to improper fixation. In situ DNA hybridization of chlamydiae in biopsied specimens may soon be a viable alternative for deep tissue infections (26).

Antibiotic Susceptibility. Multiplication of strains of *C. psittaci* and *C. trachomatis* (except for experimental mutants) is strongly inhibited by appropriate concentrations of tetracyclines, chloramphenicol, and erythromycin and less so by penicillin. Some strains of both species are inhibited by D-cycloserine. All strains of *C. trachomatis* are inhibited by sodium sulfadiazine. By varied mechanisms, tetracyclines, chloramphenicol, and erythromycin inhibit synthesis of protein on chlamydial ribosomes. Penicillin interferes with chlamydial cell wall synthesis, resulting in the interruption of RB binary fission and thus the formation of abnormally large RBs, which cannot mature into EBs; it does not prevent infection of cells by EBs, conversion of EBs to RBs, or metabolism of RBs. D-cycloserine acts similarly, but the drug's action can be reversed by the addition of alanine. Inhibition of multiplication by sodium sulfadiazine reflects the organism's ability to produce folic acid and this inhibition can be reversed by the addition of *p*-aminobenzoic acid. Certain antibiotics have little or no effect on the growth of chlamydiae and this fact can be useful in selecting for viable chlamydiae in suspensions containing contaminating bacteria. Concentrations of 1 mg/ml of streptomycin sulfate, vancomycin, and kanamycin sulfate may be used for this purpose. Chlamydiae are also unaffected by bacitracin, gentamicin, and neomycin.

Resistance to Chemical and Physical Agents. Chlamydiae are very susceptible to chemicals that affect their lipid content or the integrity of their cell walls. Even in a milieu of tissue debris they are rapidly inactivated by surface-active compounds such as quaternary ammonium compounds and lipid solvents. They are somewhat less susceptible to dilute solutions of protein denaturants, acids, and alkalies (methanol, ethanol, ammonium or zinc sulfate, phenol, hydrochloric acid, or sodium hydroxide). Infectivity is destroyed within minutes, however, by exposure to common disinfectants such as benzalkonium chloride (Roccal, Zephiran), alcoholic iodine solu-

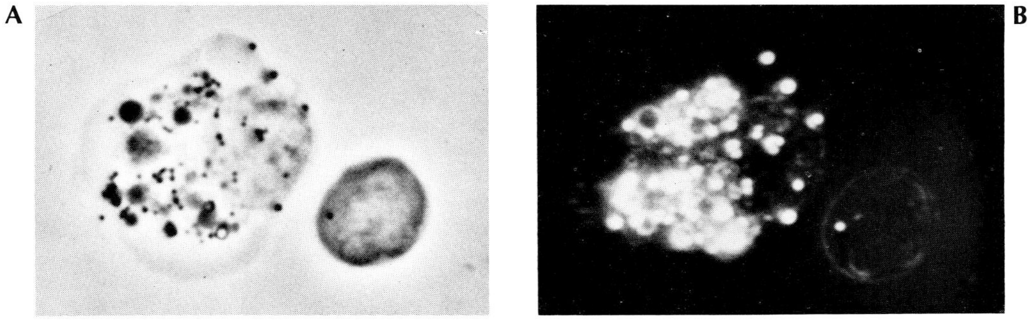

14.3. A. Phase contrast photomicrograph of chlamydiae-laden mononuclear cell in air sac exudate of turkey infected with *C. psittaci.* B. Dark-field photomicrograph of mononuclear cell in A. ×4000. (Page)

tion, 70% ethanol, 3% hydrogen peroxide, and silver nitrate; but they are resistant to cresyl compounds and lime (68). Dilute suspensions (20%) of infectious tissue homogenates are inactivated by incubation for 5 min at 56 C, 48 hr at 37 C, 12 days at 22 C, and 50 days at 4 C (43).

Infectious dense forms of the organisms in yolk sac membranes or mouse tissues may be preserved indefinitely at −20 C or below, although the initial freezing and subsequent thawing incurs a titer loss of 1–2 $\log_{10}$. Infectivity of the suspension is destroyed after six freeze-thaw cycles (43). Thin-walled, large forms of the organism are inactivated at −70 C.

Cell walls of the dense forms are disrupted by ultrasonification at frequencies above 100 kc or by treatment of intact organisms with sodium deoxycholate.

Antigenic Structure and Toxins. Chlamydiae are very complex antigenically. Principally, they consist of the immunodominant, genus-specific lipoglycoprotein and numerous proteins of varying molecular weights.

The lipoglycoprotein, which is common to all strains of both chlamydial species, contains an acidic polysaccharide, which is the antigenic determinant and it is thermostable (100 C, 30 min) and phenol (0.5%) stable. The immunodominant group is a 2-keto-deoxyoctanic acid. The antigen is soluble in ether or aqueous solutions of sodium laurylsulfate from which it can be precipitated with acid. The antigen is resistant to trypsin, chymotrypsin, and papain; but its reactivity is negated by oxidation with potassium periodate. This complex antigenic component can be purified and separated into several fractions by ion-exchange chromatography (60). Antibodies induced by this antigen in animals infected with any chlamydial organism apparently are not necessarily related to protective immunity.

Various proteinaceous components of chlamydia are best demonstrated and identified by sodium dodecyl sulfate-polyacrylamide gel electrophoresis. It has been shown that some proteins are shared by various chlamydial organisms (6, 62, 74). On the other hand, some proteins appear to be species specific whereas other proteins are subspecies specific. Winsor and Grimes (74) showed that a 29,000-molecular-weight protein was found in 10 avian isolates but not in 1 ovine isolate of *C. psittaci* or in 1 isolate of *C. trachomatis.*

The major outer membrane protein (MOMP) of chlamydia appears to be of great importance in determining antigenic grouping of these organisms. Caldwell and Schachter (5) demonstrated that various serovars of *C. trachomatis* fell into two serogroups according to antigenicity of their MOMPs. Similarly, Winsor and Grimes (74), by the use of immunoblotting, were able to demonstrate two serogroups of avian *C. psittaci* among 12 isolates studied and these serogroups coincided with their respective grouping according to high and low infectivity for cell cultures. Andersen and van Deusen (1), using monoclonal antibodies against 7 avian and 4 mammalian (3 ovine, 1 bovine) chlamydial isolates, have identified 2 avian serogroups and 1 mammalian serogroup using indirect immunofluorescence. Results of Winsor and Grimes (74) cannot be compared directly with those of Andersen and van Deusen (1) because different avian isolates were used and infectivity for cell cultures were not given in the latter study.

Toxigenicity of chlamydiae can be demonstrated by intravenous inoculation of mice with freshly harvested yolk sac cultures. It appears to be associated with cell wall components and is neutralizable by specific antiserum. Many cross-reactions have been demonstrated among the toxins of chlamydia from various birds and mammals.

Strain Classification. The *C. psittaci* species includes many diverse chlamydial strains, which infect a wide range of avian and mammalian hosts (35). Subspecies differentiation within the *C. psittaci* species has been attempted on the basis of inclusion morphology (61), plaque neutralization (59), micro-immunofluorescence (54), and more recently by restriction endonuclease analysis of chlamydial chromosomal DNA (32), the presence and properties of extrachromosomal agents (28), and with monoclonal antibodies (10).

A 7.5-Kb plasmid, which appears to be identical by restriction endonuclease analysis irrespective of avian host (24, 28), has been found in all avian strains examined to date. In contrast, feline, equine, and guinea pig inclusion conjunctivitis strains each contain a distinct plasmid, whereas other mammalian strains, i.e., ovine abortion of ewes and the nonzoonotic human *C. psittaci* strain, apparently do not possess plasmids (Table 14.3). The avian plasmid may therefore prove to be a useful taxonomic marker for avian *C. psittaci.*

The presence of a chlamydiophage may further identify one particular avian strain. This virus has been characterized as a unique single-stranded, circular DNA bacteriophage (63). It replicates within the RB to form crystalline arrays of virus within distended chlamydial forms (58). To date, this phage has only been detected in a few *C. psittaci* isolates recovered from domestic ducks, but since serolog evidence suggests infection may be cryptic (2), stringent DNA hybridization techniques are needed to absolutely exclude phage infection.

Immunotyping of strains by the degree of reactivity of monoclonal antibodies in indirect immunofluorescence may be possible based on studies

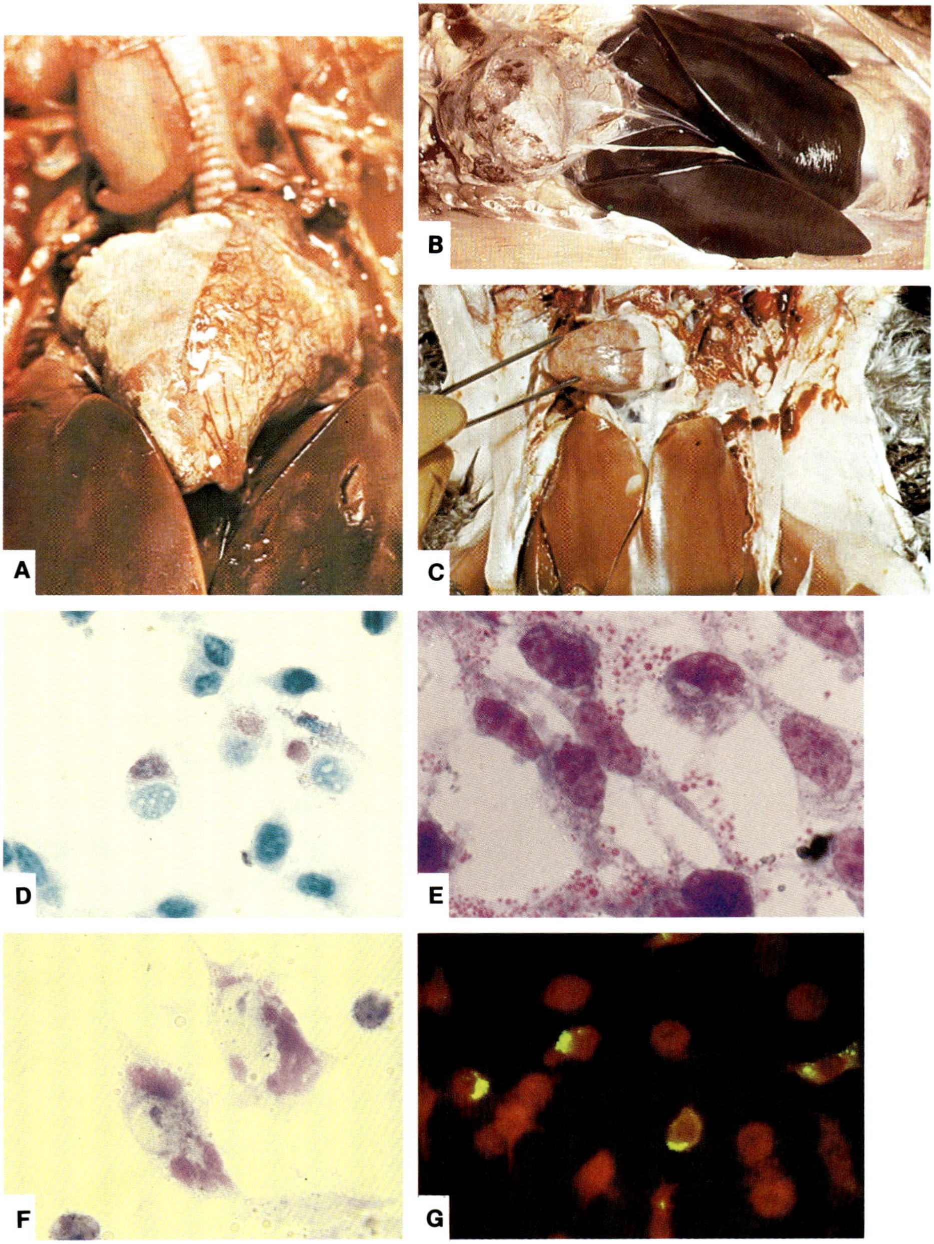

14.4. A. Gross lesions of acutely fatal chlamydiosis in young turkey infected by airborne route. Thickened, congested pericardial membrane has been partially removed to show severe pericarditis and epicardial encrustation. Cardiomegaly and hepatomegaly also are evident. (42). B. Gross lesions in turkey infected with virulent *C. psittaci* strain isolated from turkeys in South Carolina in 1973. Enlargement of heart and liver and severe pericarditis are the most prominent lesions. (Page). C. Field case of chlamydiosis caused by *C. psittaci* of low virulence. Arrows point to fibrin plaques on heart and the enlarged liver. (Page). D–G: Light photomicrographs of *Chlamydia* spp. inclusions in L929 cells. (Winsor, Nettum, and Grimes). D. Gimenez-stained *C. psittaci.* E. Giemsa-stained *C. trachomatis.* F. Giemsa-stained *C. psittaci*. G. Immunofluorescence-stained *C. psittaci.*

Table 14.3. Plasmids identified in the genus *Chlamydia*

Host	Strain	Plasmid	EcoR1 Fragments
C. psittaci			
Parakeet	6BC	+	6.2, 0.62
Duck	N352	+	0.47, 0.22
Duck	360	+	
Feline	Fpn Pring	+	7.45
Equine	N16	+	4.1, 1.3, 1.2, 0.4, 0.3, 0.15
Guinea Pig	GPIC	+	5, 1.52, 0.7, 0.25
?	Cal 10	−	
Human	10L207	−	
Ovine	A22	−	
	S26	−	
C. trachomatis			
Human	L2, 434	+	4.5, 2.5, 0.4

by Takahashi et al. (66), who studied avian strains only from pigeons and budgerigars. Therefore, as the authors state, this method needs further study to determine possible antigenic differences between isolates from various hosts.

Pathogenicity. In terms of natural pathogenicity for domestic fowl, strains of *C. psittaci* isolated from these hosts fall into two general categories: 1) Highly virulent strains that cause acute epidemics in which 5–30% of affected birds die. Strains of this type are isolated most often from turkeys and occasionally from unaffected wild birds. These strains are also labeled "toxigenic," because in natural and experimental hosts they produce rapidly fatal disease with lesions characterized by extensive vascular congestion and inflammation of vital organs. The toxigenicity of a strain can be measured experimentally by injecting large numbers of yolk sac–propagated chlamydiae intravenously into mice. The endpoint is lethal toxic shock within 48 hr postinoculation. Toxigenic strains have a broad spectrum of pathogenicity for laboratory animals. Most often such strains cause serious human infections (some fatal) in poultry handlers and laboratory research workers. 2) Strains of low virulence that cause slowly progressive epidemics with a mortality rate of less than 5% when uncomplicated by secondary bacterial or parasitic infection. Strains of this category have often been isolated from pigeons and ducks and occasionally from turkeys, sparrows, and other wild birds. Birds infected with these strains usually do not develop the severe vascular damage evident in birds infected with the virulent toxigenic strains, nor do they have such obvious clinical signs. Mouse toxigenicity titers of these strains are of much lower order than those of highly virulent toxigenic strains. Unless unusually high levels of exposure alter the balance between infection and resistance, humans are less susceptible to the strains commonly found in pigeons and ducks.

Chlamydiosis in pigeons and ducks may often be accompanied by concurrent infection with salmonellae. In such cases mortality rates among birds are high, chlamydiae are shed in very large numbers, and susceptible hosts in the immediate environment of infected birds are exposed to doses that can result in clinical disease.

Strains of both high and low virulence appear to have equal ability to spread rapidly through a flock, as determined by serologic tests. Such studies show that more than 90% of birds in any one enclosure have developed antibodies to the chlamydial group antigen by the time clinical signs of disease appear in the flock.

PATHOGENESIS AND EPIDEMIOLOGY

Natural and Experimental Hosts. In addition to the naturally occurring chlamydial infections in domesticated birds, Meyer (35) has listed over 120 wild avian species that are either transient or long-term hosts. Common reservoirs of chlamydia in the USA include wild and feral birds such as sea gulls, ducks, herons, egrets, pigeons, blackbirds, grackles, house sparrows, and killdeer, all of which freely intermingle with domestic birds. Highly virulent strains of *C. psittaci* are known to be carried by and excreted in large numbers by sea gulls and egrets without any apparent effect on these hosts.

Experimental hosts of avian chlamydia can include virtually any species of bird. However, the response of different species may vary in susceptibility with some being more or less refractory, whereas infections may be easily established in others. The length of time shedding may occur and the numbers of chlamydiae shed may vary considerably depending upon the avian species. Antibody production as a consequence of a chlamydial infection may also vary.

Mammalian laboratory hosts used for avian chlamydia are principally mice and occasionally guinea pigs. Both of these hosts can have naturally occurring chlamydial infections. Therefore, investigators using these animals should determine the chlamydial status of the breeding stock. Rabbits are refractory to clinical disease caused by avian chlamydia but they may be used to produce polyclonal antibodies (74).

Cell culture lines, such as McCoy, mouse L cells, HeLa, Vero, BHK 21, and others may be used to propagate chlamydia. Some avian strains are more infectious than others for mouse L cells (74), whereas Vero cells are reported to be superior for growing some strains (71).

Younger domestic birds are generally more susceptible than older birds to infection, clinical disease, and mortality. Therefore, infection in old turkeys such as spent breeder hens can go unnoticed unless birds are subjected to stressful conditions such as shipment to market on crowded trucks. Turkey toms also may have a higher mortality rate than turkey hens.

Transmission, Carriers, Vectors. The transmission of chlamydial strains to and from various wild and domestic avian hosts is probably intertwined, depending upon the species and their various habitats and behavioral patterns. It is possible that the continual interspecies transfer of chlamydiae has served to confound efforts to determine precisely the source(s) of these organisms for domestic poultry. An exception is the pigeon in which low-pathogenicity strains are known to be maintained. This does not mean, however, that pigeons can not be the source of spread of the highly pathogenic strains. Infection usually occurs via the respiratory route from airborne feces or respiratory exudates laden with chlamydiae. Infection may also occur through direct contact.

The principal vectors are undoubtedly birds, either inapparently infected carriers or secondarily infected species that serve to amplify the spread of chlamydia during migratory movements or feeding activities.

The role of arthropods in the transmission of chlamydiae is uncertain although it has been shown that homogenates of mites from turkey nests contained chlamydiae (9). Simulid flies are suspected of possibly transferring chlamydiae among turkeys in a South Carolina epidemic (52). Transovarial transmission of chlamydia in turkey eggs apparently does not occur (8, 50). Page and Grimes (51) provided additional information on this subject.

Incubation Period, Pathogenesis, Signs, Morbidity and Mortality, Gross Lesions, Histopathology

TURKEYS. Page (42) described the pathogenesis of experimental chlamydiosis when susceptible turkeys were exposed by the airborne route. Within 4 hr small numbers of organisms had penetrated the abdominal air sacs and mesentery with larger numbers present in the lungs and thoracic air sacs. Organisms had multiplied extensively by 24 hr and within 48 hr low numbers of chlamydiae were present in blood, spleen, and kidney. At 72 hr large numbers of chlamydia were present in the turbinates and colon contents. By 4 days large numbers were present on the heart. As organisms multiplied in the lung, air sacs, and pericardial membranes they were released into the blood stream and filtered out in the spleen, liver, and kidney or were returned to the environment via nasal and intestinal secretions. Tissues of birds that succumbed to acute chlamydiosis contained greater than 10^8 organisms per/g.

The incubation period of chlamydiosis in naturally infected birds varies, depending upon the numbers of chlamydiae inhaled and the virulence (toxigenicity) of the infecting strain. Experimentally, definitive disease signs in young turkeys receiving a virulent strain may be evident in 5–10 days. In birds naturally exposed to smaller doses or in older birds receiving greater exposures, the period may be longer. Strains of lower virulence, which cause less severe signs, may have indefinite incubation periods. Therefore, it may be 2–8 wk after exposure before signs are noticeable.

Signs of chlamydiosis in turkeys infected with virulent strains are cachexia, anorexia, and elevated body temperature. The birds excrete yellow-green, gelatinous droppings. Egg production of severely affected hens declines rapidly (60% production down to 10–20%) and may temporarily cease or remain at a very low rate until complete recovery. Disease signs in a flock infected with strains of low virulence are usually anorexia and loose, green droppings in some birds with less effects on egg production.

At the peak of disease in a flock infected with a virulent strain, 50–80% of the birds will show clinical signs whereas morbidity from less virulent strains is only 5–20%. Mortality caused by virulent chlamydia ranges from 10 to 30% and is only 1–4% with less virulent strains.

The less virulent strains cause gross lesions, which are similar to those caused by virulent strains; only they are less severe and extensive with the milder strains. In overwhelming infections with virulent strains, lungs show a diffuse congestion, and the pleural cavity may contain fibrinous exudate. In fatal cases a dark transudate may fill the thoracic cavity. The pericardial membrane is thickened, congested, and coated with fibrinous exudate. The heart may be enlarged and its surface may be covered with thick fibrin plaques or encrusted with yellowish flaky exudate (Fig. 14.4A, B). Severe damage to the lungs and heart undoubtedly is a major cause of death. The liver is enlarged and discolored and may be coated with thick fibrin. Air sacs are thickened and heavily coated with fibrinous exudate. The spleen is enlarged, dark, and soft, and may be covered with gray-white spots representing areas of focal cellular proliferation. The peritoneal serosa and mesentery show vascular congestion and may be coated with foamy, white fibrinous exudate. All these exudates contain large numbers of mononuclear cells in whose cytoplasm numerous microcolonies of chlamydial RBs may be seen. Fibrinous exudates found on all organs and tissues of the thoracic and peritoneal cavities reflect vascular damage as well as increasing inflammatory response caused by the continued multiplication of the organisms.

In birds that survive infection with a strain of low virulence, the lungs may not be seriously affected, however, multiplication of organisms on the epicardium may result in formation of one or more fibrin plaques on the heart (Fig. 14.4C).

Histopathologic changes occurring in turkeys of various ages injected intratracheally with the virulent TT strain of *C. psittaci* were described by Beasley et al. (3). They observed both necrotizing and proliferative changes comparable to those caused by other chlamydial strains in other species (with the exception of focal necrosis of the liver, which is prominent in parrots and mice). Specific cellular changes and corresponding organ damage were decidedly more severe and extensive in young turkeys than in older ones. A majority of the birds examined had tracheitis characterized by extensive infiltration of mononuclear cells, lymphocytes, and heterophils in the lamina propria and submucosa. Cilia were absent in severely affected areas. This extensive tracheal damage is not necessarily characteristic of naturally infected birds and may be a result of intratracheal inoculation of large numbers of organisms. Epithelioid pneumonitis in varying degrees was found in 80–100% of 10-wk-old birds but less often (10–20%) in mature birds. Lungs of severely affected birds were congested and had extensive infiltration of the tertiary bronchi and respiratory tubules with large mononuclear cells and fibrin. There was necrosis of individual cells and large areas of tissue; the parenchyma and stroma were equally affected.

Fibrinous to fibrinopurulent inflammatory exudates were present on respiratory and peritoneal surfaces and on the epicardium in a majority of infected turkeys. The pericardium and epicardium were thickened by swelling of congested vessels and an inflammatory exudate containing fibrin, large mononuclear cells, and varying numbers of lymphocytes and heterophils.

Infectious myocarditis was observed in more than half the infected birds, but arteritis was present in only 8%. Hepatitis was present in over 90% of the birds, and in severely affected individuals there was a diffuse dilation of sinusoids with infiltration of mononuclear cells, lymphocytes, and heterophils. Proliferated and swollen Kupffer cells were filled with debris and a yellowish pigment thought to be hemosiderin. Necrotic hepatic cells were scattered throughout the organ with little focal necrosis. Acutely sick turkeys had a catarrhal enteritis. Spleens of a majority of birds were altered with cellular proliferation and necrosis causing the enlarged and mottled appearance, which was more marked in younger than in older birds.

The organisms also caused orchitis and epididymitis seeming to have an affinity for the active germinal epithelium (4). Fibrin and inflammatory cells appeared in association with the desquamated and necrotic epithelium filling the seminiferous tubules with eosinophilic exudate. It was also observed that often the immediate cause of death in adult males was rupture of testicular blood vessels followed by massive internal bleeding. The brains of six infected birds examined were without significant changes.

The less virulent strains of *C. psittaci* also cause cellular proliferation and necrosis of major organs and vascular congestion in turkeys, but lesions are less extensive and severe (except in the air sacs) than those caused by more virulent strains. Pneumonitis is seen only in birds that succumb to the disease. Infections with strains of low virulence tend to produce chronic long-lasting infections with low mortality (11).

DUCKS. Chlamydiosis in domestic ducks is not an important disease in the USA but it is important both economically and as a public health hazard in Europe. The most severe epidemics occurred in Czechoslovakia between 1949 and 1963 and have been reviewed in detail by Strauss (65). Chlamydiosis in ducks is a severe, debilitating, often fatal disease in which young ducks develop trembling, imbalanced gait, and cachexia. They become anorexic with green, watery intestinal contents. They develop a serous or purulent discharge from the eyes and nostrils causing the feathers on the head to become encrusted with exudate. As the disease progresses, the ducks become emaciated and die in convulsions.

Morbidity ranges from 10 to 80% and mortality varies from 0 to 30% depending on age and the presence of concurrent infection with salmonellae.

Gross lesions (65) are lacrimation, conjunctivitis, rhinitis, occasionally panophthalmitis, bulbar atrophy, and inflammation of infraorbital sinuses. Atrophied pectoral muscles and a general polyserositis are evident at necropsy commonly accompanied by serous or serofibrinous pericarditis, hepatomegaly, perihepatitis, and splenomegaly. Some livers and spleens had grayish or yellowish necrotic foci.

PIGEONS. The incubation period for chlamydiosis in pigeons is not known. Infection is endemic and is believed to be perpetuated primarily by a parent-to-nestling transmission cycle (7, 36).

Signs of uncomplicated chlamydiosis in pigeons is variable but those that develop acute disease are anorexic, unthrifty, and diarrhetic. Some develop conjunctivitis, swollen eyelids, and rhinitis (Fig. 14.5). Respiratory difficulty is accompanied by rattling sounds. As disease progresses birds become weak and emaciated. Recovered birds become carriers without signs of disease. Some birds progress through an infection showing no signs or, at the most, transient diarrhea to become carriers. Salmonellosis or trichomoniasis exacerbates the illness in chlamydia-infected carrier birds resulting in signs and lesions of acute disease. Serologic surveys indicate that 30–90% of pigeons experience chlamydial infection with an active infection rate of 19.9% (34).

Gross lesions of uncomplicated chlamydiosis in pigeons are fibrinous exudates on thickened air sacs, the peritoneal serosa, and occasionally the epicardium. The liver is usually swollen, soft, and discolored. The spleen may be enlarged, soft, and dark. Higher than normal amounts of urates are seen in cloacal contents if catarrhal enteritis occurs. Less severe infections may involve only the liver or air sacs. Some heavily infected shedders have no lesions whatsoever (50).

CHICKENS. Epidemiologic and laboratory evidence indicates that chickens appear to be relatively resistant to disease caused by *C. psittaci.* While acute infection progresses to disease and mortality only in young birds, the incidence of actual epidemics is very low. Experimentally, even young birds are resistant to many strains of *C. psittaci.* Birds have fibrinous pericarditis and hepatomegaly in acute cases. Most natural infections in chickens are inapparent and transient but serologic surveys indicate that the incidence of infection is low.

GEESE. Incidental to studies of chlamydiosis in ducks, several investigators have observed the disease in geese and have isolated *C. psittaci* from diseased tissues (65). Clinical disease and necropsy findings were similar to those in ducks.

PHEASANTS. Chlamydiae of low virulence have been isolated from tissues of sick pheasants raised on pheasant farms, but no large-scale epidemics of chlamydiosis in this species have been reported (34). Serologic surveys of both wild and commercially raised pheasants in Illinois (34) and Iowa (44) indicate that incidence of infection with chlamydia is very low in the Midwest. Strauss (65), however, reported that humans have contracted psittacosis after contact with pheasants. It seems likely that both wild and domestic pheasants would be occasionally exposed to infectious chlamydia excreted by other hosts, but factors accounting for the lack of acute chlamydiosis in this species are not known.

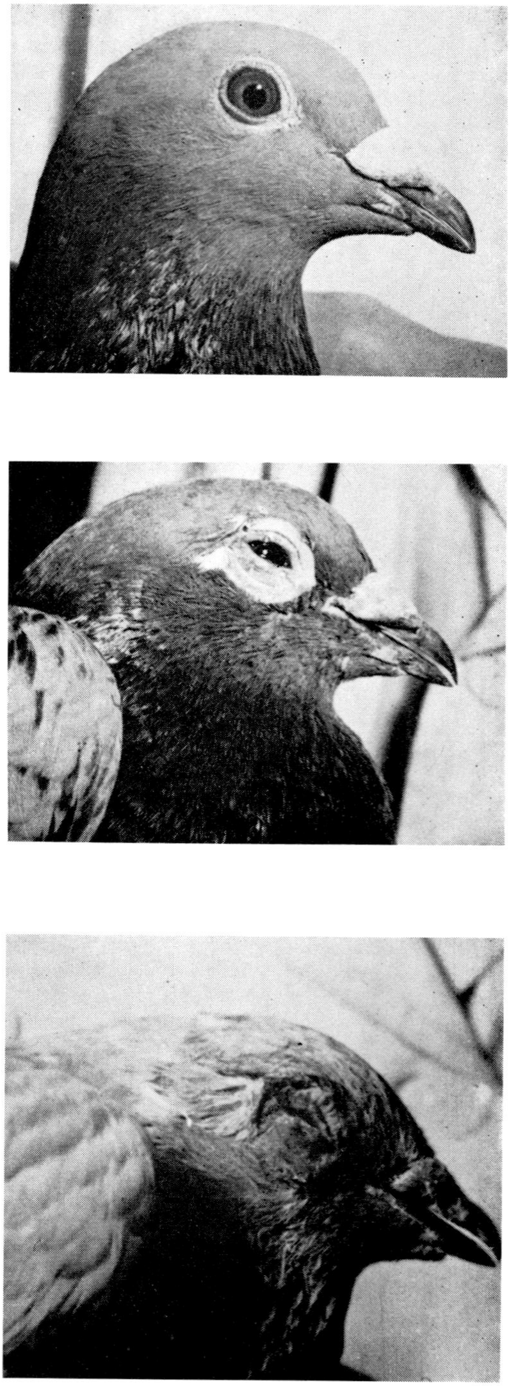

14.5. Pigeon with no signs of chlamydial infection (*top*), moderate chlamydial conjunctivitis (*middle*), and severe chlamydial conjunctivitis (*bottom*). (Jansen)

Immunity. Immunity to chlamydia is generally poor and short-lived. However, there is age-associated resistance to clinical disease as birds become older even though infection may occur. Indeed, some birds, notably pigeons, are refractory to disease-producing infection even with highly virulent strains.

In turkeys, a moderate degree of resistance to organ damage is present by the age of 15 wk (4) and it probably increases slightly with further aging. The degree of active immunity to reinfection induced in turkeys by natural infection has not been tested, nor has the resistance induced by experimental infection with organisms of low virulence been determined. That some postinfection immunity occurs in turkeys, however, was implied in experiments of Page (42). The progress of infection initiated by an oral dose of chlamydiae and then spread by natural means through a group of 19 turkeys was followed by isolation attempts from blood and clinical observations. At varying times over a period of 47 days, each bird developed chlamydemia, hyperthermia, and mild anorexia. The chlamydemia lasted up to 10 days in each bird but was followed by clinical normalcy and apparent resistance to further bloodstream infection in spite of environmental contamination sufficient to infect all unexposed birds and the caretaker who fed and watered the birds daily.

The resistance and immunity in ducks has not been sufficiently studied. However, pigeons are apparently innately resistant to many avian strains of *C. psittaci,* even the highly toxigenic ones, but they are very susceptible to isolates from pigeons and sparrows (34, 45).

Both antibodies and cell-mediated immunity are likely to be important in resistance to reinfection with chlamydia. One recent study of immunity to *C. trachomatis* in a guinea pig model indicates that serum IgG, secretory IgA, and cell-mediated immunity begins to wane by 30 days after infection and reinfection can readily occur. (55). Additionally, complete immunity to a third infection was not increased in duration after animals had recovered from two previous infections.

DIAGNOSIS

Isolation

SPECIMEN COLLECTION AND DIRECT EXAMINATION. Tissues and exudates from birds exhibiting signs and lesions of chlamydiosis should be collected aseptically and subjected to various examinations as indicated below. The tissues of choice are air sacs, spleen, pericardium, heart, liver, and kidney. From live birds, feces, cloacal swabs, heparinized blood (during febrile phase), conjunctival scrapings (if inflammation or exudate is present), and peritoneal fluid (if respiratory difficulty exists) may be collected for chlamydia isolation attempts or cytological examinations.

Touch impressions of tissues and wet mounts or dried fixed exudates may be examined directly using light microscopy ($\geq \times 800$) following use of appropriate procedures. Tentative identification of chlamydiae in cells in wet mounts can be made by an experienced chlamydiologist using phase contrast microscopy (Fig. 14.3A). Normal structures (usually few in number) that may resemble chlamydia have to be differentiated from the chlamydiae. The presence of numerous spherical bodies, 0.2–0.4 μm in diameter, especially when found in many of numerous mononuclear cells that are present, is indicative of a chlamydial infection provided mycoplasma organisms are absent.

Cytochemical staining, preferably by the Gimenez method but also by the Giemsa method can be used to obtain presumptive evidence of infection with chlamydia. Touch impressions should be made of spleen and liver surfaces and of air sacs, pericardium, and epicardium. These should be air-dried and lightly heat-fixed for the Gimenez method or fixed 5 min in methanol for the Giemsa method. Details of preparing reagents for these staining methods and the staining procedures have been published (19). With the Gimenez method, chlamydial EBs are red or reddish purple (Fig 14.4D) and the RBs are bluish green. Only EBs in inclusions are diagnostic because RBs could easily be mistaken for normal cellular structures and are not readily differentiated from the background coloration. Single EBs cannot be readily identified but the presence of EBs in intracytoplasmic inclusions are easily identified with experience. Ordinary bacteria that may be present can usually be recognized. Some bacteria stain red or reddish purple and others may be green or bluish green; but their size, shape, or location are unlike chlamydia in inclusions.

Acetone-fixed impressions of tissues or dried exudates may be made for microscopic examination following fluorescent antibody staining with a suitable conjugate. This procedure should identify the presence of chlamydia provided no bacterial antigen is present that could be cross-reactive with chlamydial antibody. Details of the procedure are available (19).

Other methods for detecting the presence of chlamydia are being developed but are not yet used extensively in avian medicine. Such methods include the use of enzyme-linked immunosorbent assays (ELISA) and peroxidase-antiperoxidase procedures.

Specimen Preparation and Inoculation. Isolation attempts may be made by the inoculation of properly processed specimens onto cell culture monolayers, into the yolk sac of 7-day-old chicken embryos, or into mice by the intraperitoneal route. A

20% (w/v) suspension of an appropriate specimen is made in a suitable diluent containing antibiotics to control ordinary bacteria but without effect on chlamydia (see Antibiotic Susceptibility). These diluents serve as transport media for the shipment of specimens whenever necessary. Details of their preparation are described (19). Specimen suspensions are centrifuged lightly (less than 800 × g) for 15–20 min prior to inoculation of the desired host system.

Cell Culture Inoculation. Monolayers of appropriate cells on glass coverslips (3 or 4/inoculum), in 24-well plates, or in screw-cap vials should be inoculated with 0.5–1.0 ml of specimen suspension. They are then centrifuged for 30 min at 1000–2000 × g. The excess inoculum is removed and fresh cell culture growth medium is added. After 72 hr coverslips are harvested, drained dry, placed cell side up, and fixed, stained, and examined microscopically. In some laboratories passage to second cell cultures is practiced in which case additional cells on coverslips must be inoculated so they can be removed and passaged.

Caution must be exercised when cell culture methods are used. It must be determined that fetal bovine serum used in the medium does not contain antibodies to chlamydia nor other factors or substances that may be chlamydiacidal. These are not common problems but they can be frustrating when they unexpectedly occur.

Chicken Embryo Inoculation. Fertile chicken eggs incubated 6 or 7 days at 39 C are inoculated with 0.2–0.5 ml/embryo via the yolk sac. Eggs for this use must be from chickens that are not consuming chlamydiastatic antibiotics in their feed. Inoculated embryos should be incubated at 39 C because that temperature significantly accelerates chlamydial growth (46). Vascular congestion in the yolk sac is the predominant lesion seen in embryos dying from *C. psittaci* infection. The yolk sacs are harvested from embryos that die 3–10 days after inoculation. Touch impressions are prepared for staining and microscopic examination as described above for direct impressions and cell cultures.

Mouse Inoculation. Mice, 3–4 wk old, may be inoculated intraperitoneally (most commonly used), intracerebrally, or intranasally; 4–6 mice are used for each specimen. Chlamydia in mice inoculated intraperitoneally multiply on the peritoneal serosa, producing inflammation that leads to an accumulation of fibrinous exudate in the cavity. Splenomegaly also commonly occurs in mice with peritoneal chlamydial infections. The exudate and the spleen contain numerous cells laden with chlamydiae that can be used for cytochemical or immunofluorescence staining as described above. Impressions of the meninges from mice inoculated intracerebrally and the lungs from mice inoculated intranasally are examined.

Identification. To be identified as *C. psittaci,* a pure chlamydial isolate must have typical microcolonies (inclusions) as indicated in Table 14.2, i.e., they must be dense and of variable shape. This is readily demonstrated in infected cell cultures that have been stained by Gimenez or Giemsa methods. Inclusions must not contain glycogen, which is detectable by appropriate iodine staining of organisms in cell cultures. Additionally, growth of the isolate must not be inhibited more than 10-fold (LD_{50}) in chicken embryos, which are also inoculated with 1 mg of sodium sulfadiazine/embryo when compared to embryos without the drug.

The presence of *Chlamydia* (genus-specific) antigen in infected cell cultures, chicken embryo yolk sacs, or mouse tissues or exudates also may be detected by appropriate complement-fixing antibodies to further identify the agent as a chlamydial isolate. Direct or indirect immunofluorescence, with appropriate fluorescein isothiocyanate–conjugated immunoglobulins may be used for the same purpose as can direct or indirect ELISA methods with appropriate enzyme-conjugated immunoglobulins.

Serology. The various serologic methods for detecting chlamydial antibodies have been reviewed recently (16). Therefore, only the most commonly used methods will be discussed here. Newer methods currently being evaluated will receive less discussion.

Complement fixation (CF) is a widely used method for detecting chlamydial antibodies. This is partly because the immunodominant carbohydrate-containing antigen of chlamydia readily induces complement-fixing antibodies. Such antibodies are no indication of immunity to reinfection with chlamydiae. They are useful, however, in detecting chlamydial infection, especially in a flock of birds. Generally, higher titers ($\geq$ 64 in poultry) are indicative of a current or recent infection. If low titers are obtained, it may be necessary to retest in about 10–14 days to detect any change in titer. A 4-fold or greater increase is considered to be diagnostic of a current chlamydial infection. Guinea pig serum as a source of complement for the test must come from chlamydia-free animals.

Direct CF. The use of antigen prepared from cell culture–propagated chlamydiae (18) has been used in a microprocedure to detect chlamydial antibodies in turkey serum (20), in wild bird sera (17), and in psittacine bird sera (13). Direct CF is a relatively sensitive method for detecting chlamydial antibody. Details of the microprocedure and for the method of antigen production are published (19).

Modified Direct CF. By the addition of fresh normal chicken serum at a level of 5% (v/v) to the complement, the sensitivity of the CF procedure is increased (17) so the procedure can be used to test sera from avian species whose antibodies do not normally fix guinea pig complement. (53).

Latex Agglutination. This method was developed for use with psittacine bird sera (15) but it has also been shown to be useful for screening turkey serum for antibodies (41) and for testing pigeon and dove sera (15). Its usefulness for testing sera of other domestic birds is not known. Primarily because of its usefulness for detecting chlamydia-infected psittacine birds now popular as pets, the antigen should soon be commercially available. The method is useful mainly because it detects IgM, which indicates that a current or recent chlamydial infection exists. Its main disadvantage is that it may not be suitable to test sera of all species and it is apparently not highly sensitive, a characteristic shared with other bacterial agglutination reactions.

Other Available Procedures. Older serological methods that are not widely used, e.g., rapid plate (or slide) and capillary tube agglutination, indirect complement fixation, passive hemagglutination, immunodiffusion, and others are described elsewhere (16).

Newer, but as yet not thoroughly proven or widely used, methods are indirect ELISA and competitive-inhibition ELISA. These highly sensitive methods need to be thoroughly researched and evaluated to ascertain their usefulness (16).

Differential Diagnosis. Suspected chlamydiosis may have to be differentiated from pasteurellosis, particularly in turkeys in which some signs and lesions may be similar. Pasteurellosis can be ruled out by appropriate culture procedures. Because of some similar signs and lesions, mycoplasmosis may need to be ruled out in turkeys suspected of having chlamydiosis. That can be accomplished by culturing and serologic testing for mycoplasmosis. Colibacillosis may mimic chlamydiosis to some extent; it can be excluded by the use of the appropriate coliform culturing procedures. Avian influenza may have to be ruled out in suspected chlamydiosis by virus isolation attempts and by serologic testing.

TREATMENT. Turkeys should be treated with chlortetracycline (CTC) at a concentration of 400 g/ton of pelleted feed. Care must be taken so that heat produced during the pelleting process does not destroy CTC and lower the effective concentration. The CTC-medicated feed must be given for 2 wk and then replaced by nonmedicated feed for 2 days prior to the birds being slaughtered for meat for human consumption. Calcium supplementation of CTC-medicated pellets must not be done because calcium ions chelate CTC and thus diminish its effectiveness. It is recommended that all turkeys on an infected premise be treated and sent for slaughter; reinfection can recur readily since resident wild birds may continue to harbor chlamydiae for some time. Also, complete chlamydial sterilization of some turkeys may not occur with the treatment outlined. Further discussion of treatment with CTC is discussed by Page and Grimes (51). Prior to turkeys being marketed, they should be examined by a veterinarian and 1–2% should be tested serologically. It may be advisable to also attempt isolations on tissues from birds randomly selected from those tested serologically.

Essentially the same treatment applies for treating other fowl infected with *C. psittaci.* In other birds, salmonellosis may often be a complicating factor so it may be necessary to use a combination of antibiotics.

Pigeons should be treated with CTC-medicated feed but the treatment may not be effective in eliminating the carrier state. Alternating periods of treatment and no treatment may be effective in eventually clearing the chronic infection (34).

PREVENTION AND CONTROL

Management Procedures. Ideally, birds should be reared in confinement without any contact with potentially contaminated equipment or premises. Contact with potential reservoirs or vectors such as wild and feral birds should also be prevented. General sanitation should be practiced diligently. Movement of people should be restricted so that visitors do not have free access to premises holding birds. That is perhaps easier to accomplish if birds are confined in houses. Additional discussion of management practices is given in Chapter 1 and by Page and Grimes (51).

Immunization. There are no commercial chlamydial vaccines that induce long- lasting protective immunity against chlamydia. In birds, Page (48) was successful in eliciting a cell-mediated response that protected >90% of turkeys against severe challenge. There was virtually no detectable humoral antibody response and two doses of vaccine had to be given 8 wk apart for best results. Additional discussion on vaccination and vaccines is given by Page and Grimes (51). The practicality of immunizing large numbers of birds that experience occasional epidemics of chlamydial infections is questionable.

State and Federal Regulations. State regulatory agencies may impose quarantine on intrastate movement of diseased flocks and may require antibiotic treatment of the flock prior to slaughter. Because regulations may vary from state to state, the appropriate public health and/or animal health agencies should be consulted as necessary.

According to USDA regulations, movement of poultry, carcasses, or offal from any premise is prohibited where the existence of chlamydiosis has been proved by isolation of a chlamydial agent. The Animal and Plant Health Inspection Service of the USDA and the U.S. Department of Health and Human Services forbid interstate movement of birds from infected flocks, but there is no restriction of movement of eggs from such flocks.

REFERENCES

1. Andersen, A.A., and R.A. van Deusen. 1988. Production and partial characterization of monoclonal antibodies to four Chlamydia psittaci isolates. Infect Immun 56:2075–2079.
2. Bacon, E.J., S.J. Richmond, D.J. Wood, P. Stirling, and B.J. Bevan. 1986. Serological detection of phage infection in Chlamydia psittaci recovered from ducks. Vet Rec 119:618–620.
3. Beasley, J.N., D.E. Davis, and L.C. Grumbles. 1959. Preliminary studies on the histopathology of experimental ornithosis in turkeys. Am J Vet Res 20:341–349.
4. Beasley, J.N., R.W. Moore, and J.R. Watkins. 1961. The histopathologic characteristics of diseases producing inflammation of the air sacs in turkeys: A comparative study of pleuropneumonia-like organisms and ornithosis in pure and mixed infections. Am J Vet Res 22:85–92.
5. Caldwell, H.D., and J. Schachter. 1982. Antigenic analysis of the major outer membrane protein of Chlamydia trachomatis. Infect Immun 35:1024–1031.
6. Caldwell, H.D., C.-C. Kuo, and G.E. Kenny. 1975. Antigenic analysis of Chlamydia by two-dimensional immunoelectrophoresis. I. Antigenic heterogenicity between C. trachomatis and C. psittaci. J Immunol 115:963–968.
7. Davis, D.J. 1955. Psittacosis in pigeons. In F.R. Beaudette (ed), Psittacosis: Diagnosis, Epidemiology and Control, pp. 66–73. Rutgers Univ Press, New Brunswick, NJ.
8. Davis, D.E., J.P. Delaplane, and J.R. Watkins. 1957. The role of turkey eggs in the transmission of ornithosis. Am J Vet Res 18:409–413.
9. Eddie, B., K.F. Meyer, F.L. Lambrecht, and D.P. Furman. 1962. Isolation of ornithosis bedsoniae from mites collected in turkey quarters and from chicken lice. J Infect Dis 110:231–237.
10. Fukushi, H., K. Nojiri, and K. Hirai. 1987. Monoclonal antibody typing of Chlamydia psittaci strains derived from avian and mammalian species. J Clin Microbiol 25:1978–1981.
11. Gale, C., V.L. Sanger, and B.S. Pomeroy. 1960. The gross and microscopic pathology of an ornithosis virus of low virulence for turkeys. Am J Vet Res 21:491–497.
12. Gimenez, D.F. 1964. Staining rickettsiae in yolk sac cultures. Stain Technol 39:135–140.
13. Grimes, J.E. 1985. Enigmatic psittacine chlamydiosis: Results of serotesting and isolation attempts, 1978 through 1983, and considertions for the future. Am J Vet Med Assoc 186:1075–1079.
14. Grimes, J.E. 1986. Chlamydia psittaci latex agglutination antigen for rapid detection of antibody activity in avian sera: Comparison with direct complement fixation and isolation results. Avian Dis 30:60–66.
15. Grimes, J.E. 1988. Unpublished data.
16. Grimes, J.E. 1989. Serodiagnosis of avian chlamydia infection. J Am Vet Med Assoc 195:1561–1564.
17. Grimes, J.E., and L.A. Page. 1978. Comparison of direct and modified direct complement-fixation and agar-gel precipitin methods in detecting chlamydial antibody in wild birds. Avian Dis 22:422–430.
18. Grimes, J.E., L.C. Grumbles, and R.W. Moore. 1970. Complement-fixation and hemagglutination antigens from a chlamydial (ornithosis) agent grown in cell cultures. Can J Comp Med 34:256–260.
19. Grimes, J.E., B.E. Daft, L.C. Grumbles, J.E. Pearson, and T.E. Vice. 1987. A manual of methods for laboratory diagnosis of avian chlamydiosis. Am Assoc Avian Pathol, Kennett Square, PA.
20. Hall, C.F., S.E. Glass, J.E. Grimes, and R.W. Moore. 1975. An epidemic of ornithosis in Texas turkeys in 1974. Southwest Vet 28:19–21.
21. Hatch, T.P., E. Al-Hossainy, and J.A. Silverman. 1982. Adenine nucleotide and lysine transport in C. psittaci. J Bacteriol 150:622–670.
22. Hatch, T.P., I. Allan, and J.H. Pearce. 1984. Structural and polypeptide differences between envelopes of infective and reproductive life cycle forms of Chlamydia spp. J Bacteriol 157:13–20.
23. Hatt, C., M.E. Ward, and I.N. Clark. 1988. Analysis of the entire nucleotide sequence of the cryptic plasmid of Chlamydia trachomatis serovar L1. Evidence for involvement in DNA replication. Nucleic Acids Res 16:4053–4067.
24. Herring, A.J., M. McClenaghan, and I.D. Aitken. 1986. Nucleic acid techniques for strain differentiations and detection of Chlamydia psittaci. In D. Oriel, G. Ridgeway, J. Schachter, D. Taylor-Robinson, and M. Ward (eds), Chlamydial Infections, pp. 578–580. Cambridge Univ Press, Cambridge.
25. Hodinka, R.L., and P.B. Wyrick. 1986. Ultrastructural study of mode of entry of C. psittaci into 929 cells. Infect Immun 54:855–863.
26. Horn, J.E., E.W. Kapus, S. Falkow, and T.C. Quinn. 1988. Diagnosis of Chlamydia trachomatis in biopsied tissue specimens by using in situ DNA hybridization. J Infect Dis 157:1249–1252.
27. Jenkin, H.M., and V.S.C. Fan. 1971. Contrast of glycogenesis of Chlamydia trachomatis and Chlamydia psittaci in Hela cells. In R.L. Nichols (ed.), Trachoma and Related Disorders Caused by Chlamydia Agents, pp. 52–59. Excerpta Medica Int Congr, Ser No. 223, Excerpta Medica, New York.
28. Lusher, M., C. Story, and S.J. Richmond. 1988. Characterization of plasmids from different Chlamydia psittaci strains. In R. Cevenini (ed.), First Conference of the European Society for Chlamydia Research, p. 63. Societa Editrice Esculapio, Bologna, Italy.
29. Mahony, J.B., J. Sellors, and M.A. Chernesky. 1987. Detection of chlamydial inclusions in cell culture or biopsy tissue by alkaline phosphatase-anti-alkaline phosphatase staining. J Clin Microbiol 25:1864–1867.
30. Manire, G.P., and A. Tamura. 1967. Preparation and chemical composition of the cell walls of mature infectious dense forms of meningopneumonitis organisms. J Bacteriol 94:1178–1183.
31. Matsumoto, A. 1981. Isolation and electron microscopic observations of intracycoplasmic inclusions containing C. psittaci. J Bacteriol 145:605–612.
32. McClenaghan, M., A.J. Herring, and I.D. Aitken. 1984. Comparison of Chlamydia psittaci isolates by DNA restriction endonuclease analysis. Infect Immun 45:384–389.
33. Meyer, K.F. 1941. Phagocytosis and immunity in psittacosis. Schweiz Med Wochenschr 71:436–438.

34. Meyer, K.F. 1965. Ornithosis. In H.E. Biester and L.H. Schwarte (eds), Diseases of Poultry, 5th Ed., pp. 675-770. Iowa State Univ Press, Ames.

35. Meyer, K.F. 1967. The host spectrum of psittacosis-lymphogranuloma venereum (PL) agents. Am J Ophthalmol 63: 1225- 1246.

36. Meyer, K.F., B. Eddie, and H.Y. Yanamura. 1942. Ornithosis (psittacosis) in pigeons and its relation to human pneumonitis. Proc Soc Exp Biol Med 49:609-615.

37. Morange A. 1895. De la psittacose, ou infection spéciale déterminée par des perruches. Thèse, Academie de Paris.

38. Moulder, J.W. 1984. Chlamydiales. In N.R. Kreig, (ed.), Bergey's Manual of Systematic Bacteriology, Vol. 1, pp. 729-739. Williams & Wilkins, Baltimore, MD.

39. Moulder, J.W. 1985. Comparative biology of intracellular parasitism. Microbiol Rev 49:298-337.

40. Newhall, W.J.V., and R.E. Jones. 1983. Disulfide-linked oligomers of MOMP of Chlamydia. J Bacteriol 154:998-1001.

41. Newman, J.A. 1988. Personal communication.

42. Page, L.A. 1959. Experimental ornithosis in turkeys. Avian Dis 3:51-66.

43. Page, L.A. 1959. Thermal inactivation studies on a turkey ornithosis virus. Avian Dis 3:67-79.

44. Page, L.A. 1964. Unpublished data.

45. Page, L.A. 1967. Comparison of "pathotypes" among chlamydial (psittacosis) strains recovered from diseased birds and mammals. Bull Wildl Dis Assoc 3:166-175.

46. Page, L.A. 1971. The influence of temperature upon the multiplication of chlamydiae in chicken embryos. Excerpta Med Proc Trachoma Conf, Int Conf Ser 223, pp. 40-51.

47. Page, L.A. 1972. Chlamydiosis (Ornithosis). In M.S. Hofstad, B.W. Calnek, C.F. Helmboldt, W.M. Reid, and H.W. Yoder, Jr. (eds.), Diseases of Poultry, 6th Ed., pp. 414-447. Iowa State Univ Press, Ames.

48. Page, L.A. 1975. Stimulation of cell-mediated immunity to chlamydiosis in turkeys by inoculation of chlamydial bacterin. Am J Vet Res 39:473-480.

49. Page, L.A. 1978. Avian Chlamydiosis (Ornithosis). In M.S. Hofstad, B.W. Calnek, C.F. Helmboldt, W.M. Reid, and H.W. Yoder, Jr. (eds.), Diseases of Poultry, 7th Ed., pp. 337-366. Iowa State Univ Press, Ames.

50. Page, L.A., and R.A. Bankowski. 1959. Investigation of a recent ornithosis epornitic in California turkeys. Am J Vet Res 20:941-945.

51. Page, L.A., and J.E. Grimes. 1984. Avian Chlamydiosis (Ornithosis). In M.S. Hofstad, H.J. Barnes, B.W. Calnek, W.M. Reid, and H.W. Yoder, Jr. (eds.), Diseases of Poultry, 8th Ed., pp. 283-308. Iowa State Univ Press, Ames.

52. Page, L.A., W.T. Derieux, and R.C. Cutlip. 1975. An epornitic of fatal chlamydiosis (ornithosis) in South Carolina turkeys. J Am Vet Med Assoc 166:175-178.

53. Pearson, J.E. 1988. Personal communication.

54. Perez-Martinez, J.A., and J. Storz. 1985. Antigenic diversity of Chlamydia psittaci of mammalian origin determined by microimmunofluorescence. Infect Immun 50:905-910.

55. Rank, R.G., B.E. Batteiger, and L.S.F. Soderberg. 1988. Susceptibility to reinfection after a primary chlamydial genital infection. Infect Immun 56:2243-2249.

56. Register, K.B., P.A. Morgan, and P.B. Wyrick. 1986. Interaction between Chlamydia spp and human polymorphonuclear leukocytes in vitro. Infect Immun 52:664-670.

57. Richmond, S.K., and P. Stirling. 1981. Localization of Chlamydial group antigen in McCoy cell monolayers infected with C. trachomatis or C. psittaci. Infect Immun 34:561-570.

58. Richmond, S.J., P. Stirling, and C.R. Ashley. 1982. Virus infecting the reticulate bodies of an avian strain of Chlamydia psittaci. FEMS Microbiol Lett 14:31-36.

59. Schachter, J., J. Banks, N. Sugg, M. Sung, J. Storz, and K.F. Meyer. 1974. Serotyping of Chlamydia. I. Isolates of ovine origin. Infect Immun 9:92-94.

60. Schmeer, N., and H. Krauss. 1982. Purification and genus-specific chlamydial antigen and its separation into several components by ion-exchange chromatography. J Clin Microbiol 15:830-834.

61. Spears, P., and J. Storz. 1979. Biotyping of Chlamydia psittaci based on inclusion morphology and response to DEAE-dextran and cycloheximide. Infect Immun 24:224-232.

62. Stephenson, E.H., and J. Storz. 1975. Protein profiles of dense-centered form of five chlamydial strains of animal origin. Am J Vet Res 36:881-887.

63. Storey, C.C., M. Lusher, and S.J. Richmond. 1988. Characterization of a bacteriophage recovered from an avian strain of Chlamydia psittaci. In R. Cevenini (ed.), First Conference of the European Society for Chlamydia Research, p. 94. Societa Editrice Esculapio, Bologna, Italy.

64. Storz, J., and P. Spears. 1977. Chlamydiales: Properties, cycle of development and effect on eukaryotic host cells. Curr Top Microbiol Immunol 76:167-214.

65. Strauss, J. 1967. Microbiologic and epidemiologic aspects of duck ornithosis in Czechoslovakia. Am J Ophthalmol 63:1246-1259.

66. Takahashi, T., I. Takashima, and N. Hashimoto. 1988. Immunotyping of Chlamydia psittaci by indirect immunofluorescence antibody test with monoclonal antibodies. Microbiol Immunol 32:251-263.

67. Tam, M.R., W.E. Stamm, H.H. Handsfield, R. Stephens, K.K. Holmes, K. Ditzenberger, M. Crieger, and R.C. Nowiniski. 1984. Culture-independent diagnosis of Chlamydia trachomatis using monoclonal antibodies. N Eng J Med 310:1146-1150.

68. Tarizzo, M.L., and B. Nabli. 1967. The effect of antibiotics on the growth of TRIC agents in embryonated eggs. Am J Ophthalmol 63:1550-1557.

69. Taylor, H.R., and R.A. Pendergrast. 1987. Attempted oral immunization with chlamydial lipopolysaccharide subunit vaccine. Invest. Ophthal Visual Sci 28:1722-1726.

70. Taylor, H.R. J. Schachter, and H.D. Caldwell. 1987. Pathogenesis of trachoma: The stimulus for inflammation. J Immunol 138:3023-3027.

71. Tessler, J. 1984. Growth of several strains of Chlamydia psittaci in Vero and McCoy cells in the presence of cytochalasin and cortisone. Can J Comp Med 48:290-293.

72. Todd, W.J., and H.D. Caldwell. 1985. The interaction of Chlamydia trachomatis with host cells: Ultrastructural studies of the mechanism of release of a biovar II strain from Hela 220 cells. J Infect Dis 151:1037-1044.

73. Weisburg, W.G., T.P. Hatch, and C.R. Woesc. 1986. Eubacterial origin of chlamydiae. J Bacteriol 167:570-574.

74. Winsor, D.K., Jr., and J.E. Grimes. 1988. Relationship between infectivity and cytopathology for L-929 cells, membrane proteins, and antigenicity of avian isolates of Chlamydia psittaci. Avian Dis 35:421-431.

15 FUNGAL INFECTIONS

INTRODUCTION

H.L. Chute and J.L. Richard

Advances and discoveries in the control and treatment of bacterial and virus diseases of birds has been outstanding over the past decade. However, little progress has been made in the control of fungal infections in birds. Fungal infections, while not the most economically important of the various poultry diseases, still have an impact on the health of birds.

Much research has transpired in relation to the growth and metabolism of the specific fungi, but no one has consolidated this data for the benefit of healthier flocks.

The chapter has been largely rewritten. Some of the older literature references have been removed and the section on favus has been deleted; previous editions of this book should be consulted for that information.

Fungal infections such as histoplasmosis and cryptococcosis are not common pathogens of domestic poultry, but are included because they are of public health significance. These pathogens occur widely in the environment and are more common in exotic birds.

ASPERGILLOSIS

J.L. Richard

INTRODUCTION. Aspergillosis is defined as any disease condition caused by a member of the fungal genus *Aspergillus.* However, when avian aspergillosis is mentioned it is usually in the context of pulmonary aspergillosis. Thus, synonyms such as mycotic pneumonia and brooder pneumonia will often appear in the literature. Although the primary target of the agent is the pulmonary system, other disease manifestations also occur in poultry.

HISTORY. Molds, likely belonging to the genus *Aspergillus,* were described in wild birds in the early 1800s, occurring in such species as the Scaup duck, jay, and swans (6, 50). However, the first time that an *Aspergillus* was described in a lesion was in 1842 when Rayer and Montagne (46) identified *A. candidus* from the air sac of a bullfinch. *A. fumigatus,* the most frequently observed agent of avian aspergillosis, was first found in the lungs of a bustard (*Otis tardaga*) in 1863, and the species name was attributed to Fresenius (11). He also applied the term "aspergillosis" to this respiratory disease. Interestingly, early investigators believed that fungi found in lesions of avian species were growing saprophytically on "morbid products" in the body (6). Aspergillosis is common in turkey poults, having been described by Lignieres and Petit (36). Hinshaw (27) described the disease in adult turkeys.

INCIDENCE AND DISTRIBUTION. Primarily two forms of aspergillosis occur in poultry. Acute aspergillosis is usually characterized by severe outbreaks in young birds and high morbidity and high mortality. Chronic aspergillosis occurs in adult breeder birds (particularly turkeys) or occasionally in an adult flock or aviary. The incidence of chronic disease is not as great, but in commercial poultry flocks there are significant economic losses when adult birds succumb to this disease. Aspergillosis appears to be more significant in confinement situations where stress factors may be involved or where moldy litter or grain are present.

Contaminated poultry litter is often the source of *Aspergillus* conidia (18). Pinello et al. (44) isolated 73 species of fungi from air, litter, or tissues in a confinement turkey house and *Aspergillus* was among the four major genera found. *Aspergillus* spp. were among the most common fungi found in other studies of air or litter flora of poultry houses (57, 37, 34, 61). Air flora density of the four major genera within the poultry house decreased when the windows were opened during the spring (54). Reducing the dust and improving ventilation in poultry houses resulted in a 75% decrease in the incidence of fungal disease (48). Outbreaks occur when the organism is present in sufficient quantities to establish disease or when the bird's resistance is impaired by factors such as environmental stresses, immunosuppressive compounds, or inadequate nutrition.

Chute et al. (14) observed that *A. fumigatus* is found frequently, yet is not always pathogenic in young broiler chicks. The following genera were found in lungs and air sacs: *Aspergillus, Penicillium, Paecilomyces, Cephalosporium, Trichoderma, Scopulariopsis,* and *Mucor.*

Aspergillosis can be one of the most frequently reported diseases and a source of considerable monetary loss in turkeys (43).

ETIOLOGY. The two major agents causing aspergillosis of poultry are *A. fumigatus* and *A. flavus.* Other organisms that may be involved are *A. terrus, A. glaucus, A. nidulans, A. niger, A. amstelodami,* and *A. nigrescens.* Both major organisms lack a sexual stage and, therefore, are classified in the Form Family Moniliaceae, Form Order Moniliales, and Form Class Fungi Imperfecti. These organisms are ubiquitous, commonly occurring in decaying vegetative matter, soil, and feed grains. Therefore, their reproductive structures (conidia) occur in the air flora of most environments. The organisms grow readily on most common laboratory media and the characteristics given below generally are obtained when *A. fumigatus* or *A. flavus* are grown on any of the three media mentioned.

A. FUMIGATUS FRESENIUS 1850

Colony Morphology. The organism grows rapidly on Sabouraud dextrose, Czapek's solution, or potato dextrose agar (25–37 C) with colonies having a diameter of approximately 3–4 cm in 7 days. The flat colonies are white at first, then bluish green as conidia begin to mature, especially near the center of the colony. As the colony matures, the conidial masses become gray-green while the colony edge remains white. The colony surface varies slightly among isolates, being either smooth and velvety to slightly floccose or folded. The colony reverse is usually colorless. A distinctive feature of *A. fumigatus* is the development of columnar masses of chains of conidia arising from the vesicle. The conidial chains may attain a length of up to 400 μm.

The organism is quite thermotolerant growing well at 45 C. The description presented here includes the most typical characteristics, but variations occur in colony color, both surface and reverse, and colony morphology.

Microscopic Morphology. The conidiophores of *A. fumigatus* are smooth, colorless to light green near the vesicle, up to 300 μm in length, and 5–8 μm in diameter (Fig. 15.1). The conidiophore gradually enlarges distally to form a flask-shaped vesicle. The vesicle is 20–30 μm in diameter with a single series of phialides (conidiogenous cells) over the distal half. The phialides (6–8 μm long) are arranged upward paralleling the axis of the conidiophore. The conidia, green in mass, are echinulate, globose to subglobose with a diameter of 2–3 μm.

A. FLAVUS LINK 1809

Colony Morphology. The organism grows very rapidly obtaining a colony diameter of 6–7

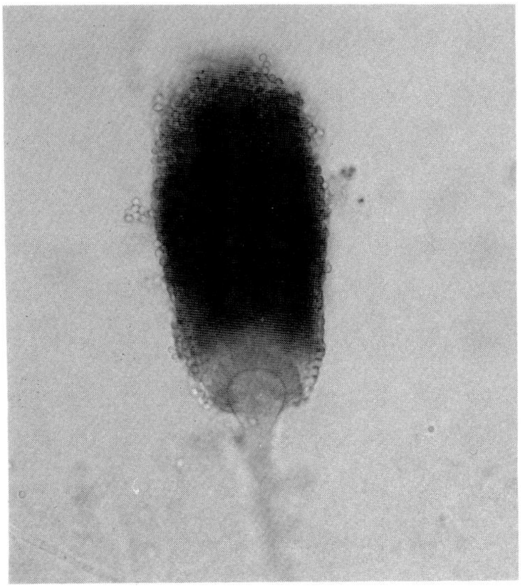

15.1. Conidiophore with flask-shaped vesicle, phialides, and columnar mass of chains of conidia of *Aspergillus fumigatus.* ×250.

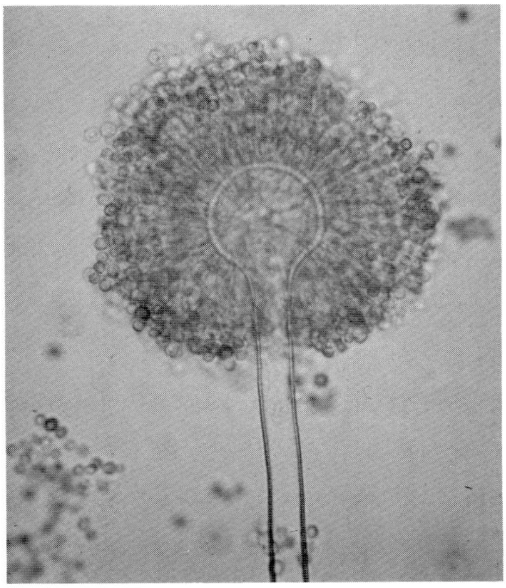

15.2. Conidiophore with globose vesicle, phialides, and radiate chains of conidia of *Aspergillus flavus.* ×250.

cm in 10 days at 25 C on Sabourand dextrose, Czapek's solution, or potato dextrose agar. Some isolates may be slower growing. The colony begins as a white, close-textured mycelium, turning yellowish to yellow-green in color with a white colony edge as conidia develop. Mature colonies may become somewhat olive green in color. The colony may be radially furrowed or flat. Brownish to black-brown sclerotia, which begin as white tufts of mycelia, may be more evident than conidial development in some isolates. The colony reverse varies from colorless to pinkish drab to brownish in sclerotial strains. The conidial heads of *A. flavus* are radiate with the chains of conidia splitting to form loose columns.

Microscopic Morphology. The conidiophores (up to 100 μm long and 10–65 μm in diameter) of *A. flavus* are thick-walled, rough, and colorless. The vesicles, although more elongated when young, are globose to subglobose (10–65 μm in diameter) with phialides usually in two series (biseriate or two-layered) on the entire surface of the vesicle (Fig. 15.2). Phialides may be one series (uniseriate) or, more rarely, each condition may be present in a single head. The conidia are globose to subglobose, echinulate, and between 3 and 6 μm in diameter (usually 3.5–4.5 μm).

Isolates vary considerably in color and number of sclerotia, if any are present. Because the majority of the fungi are identified using morphological criteria, biochemical properties are not used for this purpose. Some species of *Aspergillus* appear to be quite resistant to chemical agents and have been known to occur in "sanitizing" fluids, sulfuric acid, copper sulfate plating baths, and formalinized tissues for museum specimens (55).

Antigens prepared from *A. fumigatus* and *A. flavus* have been used in the detection of antibodies in experimentally exposed turkey poults (52). These were culture filtrate antigens produced on either a neopeptone dialysate medium or on Dorsett's medium (62).

Japanese workers (5) studied an allergic skin reaction in avian species against an alcoholic precipitate from a mycelial extract of *A. fumigatus*. Penguins showed severe and prolonged skin sensitivity, whereas pigeons and ducks were quite resistant. Zoo penguins frequently die from *A. fumigatus* infections.

TOXINS. *Aspergillus* spp. are among the three most common mycotoxigenic genera. Aflatoxins, along with other mycotoxins are discussed in detail in Chapter 35.

The significance of these toxins in the pathogenicity of the *Aspergillus* spp. is unknown except that Richard et al. (52) found no enhanced pathogenicity of aflatoxigenic strains of *A. flavus* in turkey poults. On the other hand, approximately 50% of poults died when aerosol-exposed to *A. fumigatus* conidia as compared to no deaths in those exposed to *A. flavus* conidia (52). Antibodies were found only in poults exposed to *A. fumigatus*.

PATHOGENESIS AND EPIZOOTIOLOGY

Disease Manifestations

PULMONARY ASPERGILLOSIS. Experimental pulmonary aspergillosis was readily produced by intrathoracic injection of fungal conidia as early as 1884 (63). In 1935, Durant and Tucker (17) produced the disease in a poult by feeding mash contaminated with *A. fumigatus*. Ghori and Edgar (22) found differences in susceptibility to *A. fumigatus* among Japanese quail, turkeys, and chickens, and also strain differences among three strains of chickens (23). Inbred strains were more susceptible than crossbred or outbred strains during an outbreak of aspergillosis in hatchery chicks (9).

Penguins appear to be extremely susceptible to aspergillosis (3), but the disease is significant primarily in captive penguins (33, 41).

The disease is known to occur in a wide variety of avian species and perhaps all birds, captive and free, domesticated and wild, should be considered as potential hosts susceptible to *Aspergillus* infection (1).

Vigorous healthy birds apparently can withstand considerable exposure to *Aspergillus* conidia under natural conditions. Inhalation of large numbers may occur when litter or feed are heavily contaminated with the organisms; infections may ensue. Approximately 50% of turkey poults died following a 10-min aerosol exposure to conidia of *A. fumigatus* resulting in 5×10^5 colony-forming units/gm of lung tissue (52). No deaths occurred in turkey poults similarly exposed to *A. flavus*, perhaps because the size of *A. flavus* conidia (3–6 μm) is considerably greater than that of *A. fumigatus* (2–3 μm), and thus they would not reach as deeply into the respiratory tract.

Walker (65) reported that 5- to 7-day-old ostriches succumbed in 2–8 days from pulmonary aspergillosis after conidia were aerosolized into the trachea. Turkey poults aerosol-exposed to 2.2×10^6 viable units of *A. fumigatus*/gm of lung tissue all died by day 5; lower doses (5.2×10^5 viable units) delayed and reduced mortality. Deaths began by 3–4 days post exposure.

SYSTEMIC ASPERGILLOSIS. Systemic aspergillosis in poults was reported by Witter and Chute (67). Chute et al. (13) also reported systemic aspergillosis infection in caponized 5-wk-old cockerels. The authors concluded that this resulted from a caponizing infection.

DERMATITIS. Necrotic granulomatous dermatitis

was described in chickens, and *A. fumigatus* was isolated from infected tissue (70). Lahaye (35) discussed cutaneous aspergillosis of pigeons. Otherwise cutaneous lesions as a manifestation of aspergillosis are rare in avian species.

OSTEOMYCOSIS. *Aspergillus fumigatus* infection in bone deformed vertebrae, resulting in partial paralysis of young chickens (8). Presumably, the infections were sequelae to lung disease with hematogenous dissemination of the organism.

OPHTHALMITIS. Ophthalmic lesions in birds due to *Aspergillus* have been reported since 1940 when Reis (49) recognized aspergillosis in the chicken eye. Similar lesions were described by Hudson (28) in young chicks and by Moore (40) in turkey poults. While these cases of ophthalmitis in avian species were similar in that the infection was unilateral, an important difference occured in these early reported cases. The first two cases had involvement primarily of the conjunctiva and external surfaces of the eye with the development of a cheesy exudate or plaque forming beneath the nictitating membrane. The fungus could be isolated readily from cultured plaque material. The eye infection described by Moore (40) involved turkey poults that had respiratory aspergillosis and the cornea of the eye was not involved. Most of the pathologic changes occurred in the posterior eye involving the vitreous humor and extending into adjacent tissue. Thus, the pathogenesis of the two conditions was apparently quite different; the keratitis and superficial infection probably resulted from exposure of conjunctival surfaces to viable fungal elements from environmental sources. However, the fungal ophthalmitis involving the posterior eye may have resulted from a hematogenous or lymph dissemination of the organism from a primary respiratory infection. Although not a frequent occurrence, the latter type of eye infection usually is apparent in birds with respiratory involvement.

Reis (49) was able to reproduce a superficial eye infection in chickens by introducing conidia of *A. fumigatus* into the eye. The yellow caseous plaque can become adherent to the cornea in the superficial type of infection (30). Because of swelling, this infection may resemble coryza or vitamin A deficiency in chicks (60). After Chute and O'Meara (12) injected conidia of *A. fumigatus* into the abdominal air sacs of chickens, one bird developed a plaque on the surface of one eye (Fig. 15.3). They did not speculate the route of infection.

Occasionally, turkeys experimentally exposed to aerosols of conidia developed a cloudy eye with retinitis and iridocyclitis with secondary involvement of the remainder of the eye (54). There was a cellular infiltration of heterophils and macrophages; cellular debris and fungal elements were

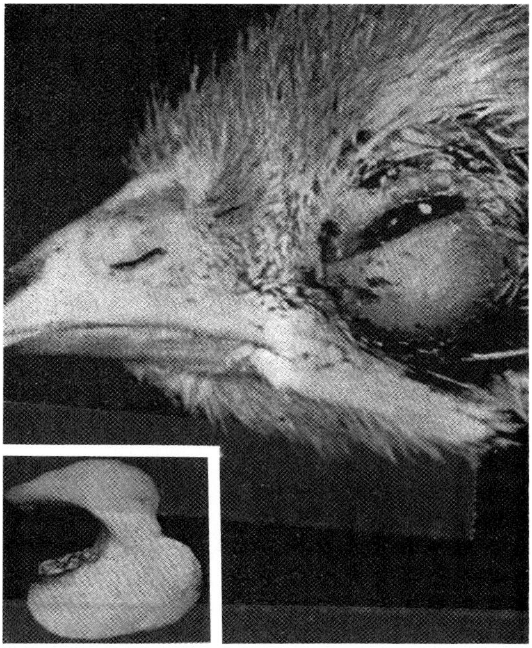

15.3. Plaque from eye of chick with aspergillosis involving the eye. ×2.

present in the chambers and retina. The pecten was severely involved with edema, heterophils, mononuclear cells, and fungal elements. In some turkeys the pecten contained granulomas.

Conidia of *A. fumigatus* may be disseminated by the hematogenous route. Richard and Thurston (51) isolated *A. fumigatus* from the blood of turkeys immediately after a 15-min aerosol exposure of conidia. At this time, respiratory macrophages contained numerous ingested conidia. This may be the route of dissemination resulting in the eye and brain lesions (54). Usually, by 24-hr postexposure the organism was cleared from the blood stream.

Following oculonasal vaccination against Newcastle disease, mortalities increased rapidly in chickens that had contracted superficial ocular aspergillosis in the hatchery (38). This type of ocular involvement was described by Moore (40) and occurred in five widely separated flocks of young poults and in three breeding flocks.

ENCEPHALITIS. Numerous reports have described encephalitic or meningoencephalitic aspergillosis in a variety of avian species. In turkeys, necrotic foci in the cerebrum or cerebellum were found to occur naturally (45). Richard et al. (53) found such foci in turkey poults experimentally exposed to aerosols of *A. fumigatus* conidia. Outbreaks of meningoencephalitis have occured in turkey poults, eider ducklings, and chickens (71). Others have described encephalitic aspergillosis in turkey poults and chickens occuring as caseous necrotic lesions of the cerebrum and cerebellum or as granulomatous encephalitis (2, 24).

Jungherr and Gifford (32) found fungal hyphae in the cerebellum of a poult that had exhibited nervous symptoms. In another outbreak in poults with pneumomycosis and nervous manifestations, they recovered *A. fumigatus, A. niger,* and *Penicillium varioti* from internal organs. *P. varioti* was also isolated from the brain of one poult, but since fungal hyphae could not be demonstrated and the culture proved nonpathogenic, it was concluded that the symptoms and brain lesions had a toxigenic origin. Bullis (10) recovered *A. fumigatus,* and later *Diplococcium* spp., from cerebrums of poults that showed incoordination. In most cases there was concurrent infection of the lungs and air sacs, and often the kidney and liver were involved.

Richard et al. (54) speculated that the brain lesions found after experimental aerosol exposure of turkeys may be the result of hematogenous dissemination as has been described in humans (56). Some experimentally exposed turkeys had a notable torticollis, and brain lesions were found at necropsy. Torticollis occurs also in natural infections of *A. fumigatus* in turkeys, geese, and chickens (64).

Transmission. A case of egg-borne aspergillosis was reported by Eggert and Barnhart (19). They suggested that the fungus had penetrated through the eggshell during incubation and recently hatched chicks were infected. Clark et al. (15) reported on other cases of aspergillosis that originated in hatcheries. From 21 ranches where 210,000 chicks were involved, there was mortality of 1–10%. Infection could not be traced to hatching eggs but was readily found in incubators, hatchers, incubator rooms, and intake ducts. Signs and lesions were noted in some day-old chicks, but generally, classic lesions were observed in chicks 5 days of age.

O'Meara and Chute (42) found that hatching chicks and up to 2-day-old chicks were easily infected with *A. fumigatus* spores by contaminating the forced-draft incubator with wheat seeded with *A. fumigatus.* Chicks older than 3 days were resistant to infection.

Egg embryos are quite susceptible to infection by *A. fumigatus* during incubation. Embryo contamination occurred when a petroleum jelly suspension of *A. fumigatus* conidia was applied to the surface of incubating eggs (68) and infections increased when the incubating eggs were dusted with *A. fumigatus* conidia (69). Within 8 days after the dusting application, the organism had penetrated the eggshell.

Signs. Dyspnea, gasping, and accelerated breathing may be present. When these signs are associated with other respiratory diseases such as infectious bronchitis and infectious laryngotracheitis, they are often accompanied by gurgling and rattling noises, whereas in aspergillosis there usually is no sound. Guberlet (25) ascribed somnolence, inappetence, emaciation, increased thirst, and pyrexia to aspergillosis. Cases under his observation emaciated rapidly and showed diarrhea in the later stages. Dysphagia was noted in cases in which esophageal mucosa was involved. Mortality was as high as 50% in confined birds on some farms, whereas birds running outdoors were more resistant or escaped infection entirely. According to Van Heelsbergen (63), some workers reported serous excretions from nasal and ocular mucosa. Extreme dyspnea was recorded in canaries by De Jong (16). Onset of signs did not occur before 48 hr in turkey poults experimentally infected with high doses of *A. fumigatus* or *A. flavus* (54). In an outbreak in captive wild poults, mortality totaling 75% began at 5 days, reached a peak at 15 days, and subsided at 3 wk of age (17). Some affected poults died in convulsions within 24 hr. Gauger (21) reported an outbreak in adult chickens in which about 10% of the flock had signs characteristic of laryngotracheitis and in which there was no abnormal mortality, but egg production was temporarely lowered.

Because torticollis and/or lack of equilibrium occurs in both experimental (53) and in natural infections by *Aspergillus* spp. (45, 64), this should be considered as a sign of avian aspergillosis. However, other infectious agents, including other genera of fungi, can cause similar signs.

Gross Lesions. Early lesions in experimental infections in turkey poults consisted of small white caseous nodules (approximately 1 mm in diameter) scattered throughout lung tissue, usually accompanied by similarly sized caseous plaques on thickened air sac membranes (54, 59) (Fig. 15.4). The caseous nodules consisted of inflammatory exudate and fungus tissue. Occasionally, red-tinged ascites was present. In more advanced cases, the plaques were larger and more numerous on greatly thickened air sac membranes; the plaques often coalesced to form aggregate lesions (54). In advanced cases of aspergillosis, the organism often sporulates on the surface of the caseous lesions and on the walls of the thickened air sacs (54, 59) as evidenced by visible greenish gray mold growth. Durant and Tucker (17) observed yellowish white nodules up to 5 × 8 mm in lungs of wild poults reared in captivity. Hyphae of the fungus also penetrated lung tissue, and there was involvement of adjacent air sacs.

In an outbreak of aspergillosis in chicks, no evidence of yellowish foci was found but the lungs were a diffuse grayish yellow (58). Mohler and Buckley (39) described lesions in a flamingo con-

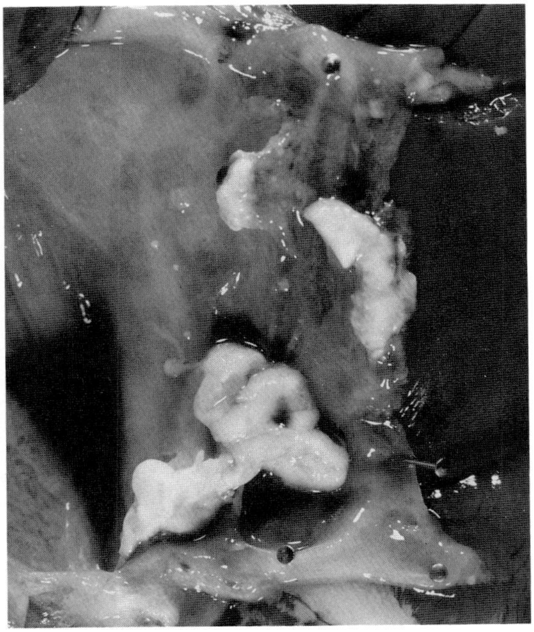

15.4. Caseous exudate on thickened air sac membranes in turkey poult with aspergillosis.

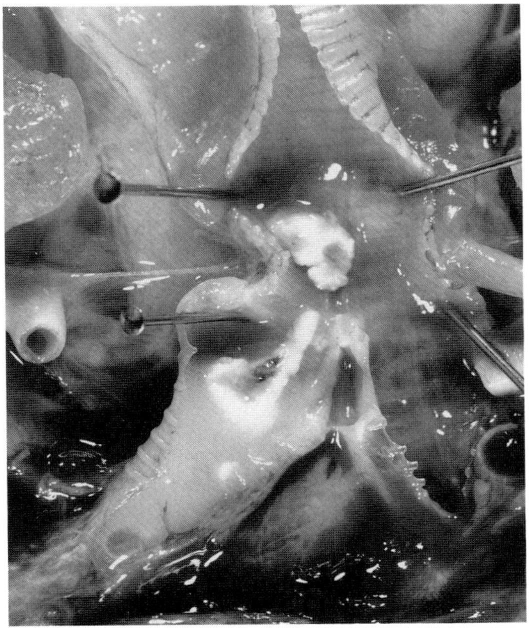

15.5. Caseous and mucopurulent exudate in syrinx of turkey poult with aspergillosis.

sisting of membranous masses of mycelia covering the bronchial mucosa in addition to lung nodules. Similarily, bronchiolar lesions of microcolonies of fungus were described in an ostrich (4). In another case in an ostrich, the lungs were covered with miliary foci (31).

Caseous exudate and mycelia, sometimes with mucopurulent to gelatinous exudate, may be present in the syrinx in infected birds (Fig. 15.5). Variations in lesions depend on the location.

Lesions in brain tissue were described by Richard et al. (54), as white to yellow circumscribed areas, usually visible on the brain surface. They were present either in the cerebellum or cerebrum or less frequently in both.

In canaries De Jong (16) observed small, whitish yellow, crusty coatings on the tongue, palate, and aditus laryngis and in the trachea and syrinx. Caseous foci in lungs and caseous coatings on the pleura and peritoneum were also observed. Lahaye (35) stated that *A. glaucus* may be the cause of a skin disease in pigeons, particularly in young birds, and that any part of the body may be affected with yellow scaly spots. Feathers in the affected areas were dry and easily broken.

Histopathology. Examination of lung tissues from turkey poults revealed no differences in histopathologic lesions caused by *A. fumigatus* or *A. flavus* (52). Early lesions were characterized by focal accumulations of lymphocytes, some macrophages, and a few giant cells. Later, lesions consisted of granulomas with a central area of necrosis containing heterophils surrounded by macrophages, giant cells, lymphocytes, and some fibrous tissue. By 8 wk postexposure, surviving poults had late granulomatous lesions consisting of a necrotic center surrounded by giant cells and a thick layer of fibrous tissue containing a few scattered heterophils. Using special stains for fungi, the organisms were seen within the necrotic areas of the lesions. In tissue sections of the well-oxygenated bronchi, bronchioles, and air sacs, the organism was sporulating asexually.

Brain lesions consisted of solitary abcesses with necrotic centers infiltrated with heterophils and surrounded by giant cells. Hyphae were seen in the central area of some lesions.

Eye lesions were characterized by edema of the pecten, which was heavily infiltrated with heterophils and mononuclear cells. Typical granulomas were found in the pecten. Fungal hyphae, heterophils, macrophages, and cellular debris were found in the chambers and retina of the eye. Edema and some heterophils were found in the sclera and surrounding tissues. In cases of ophthalmitis in turkeys described by Moore (40), primary involvement was in the vitreous humor and adjoining tissues. In one turkey he observed hyphae in the crystalline lens.

DIAGNOSIS

Isolation and Identification of Causative Agent. Aspergillosis is usually diagnosed at postmortem examination, often based upon observation of white caseous nodules in the lungs or air sacs of affected birds. Although it is sometimes possible to observe fungal growth and sporulation on the caseous nodules or plaques, especially in the air sacs, confirmation should be made by cultural isolation and identification of the causative fungus. Although *A. fumigatus* is the most likely agent of avian aspergillosis, other species of fungi can cause the disease. Therefore, isolates should be identified.

Because most agents of the mycoses are ubiquitous saprophytes, diagnostic samples should be carefully collected using aseptic technique. Samples so collected can be examined microscopically by placing a small portion of the nodule in 20% potassium hydroxide (KOH) on a microscope slide, teasing the material apart, and covering it with a glass coverslip. Following gentle heating of the slide over a flame, the specimen can be examined for presence of hyphae within the exudate. If the preparation is too thick, the slide should be incubated 12–24 hr in a moist chamber and reexamined. To aid in elucidating the fungus, the KOH can be mixed with ink dye (Ink blue pp or asb, Parker Pen Co., Janesville, WI). Hyphae of *Aspergillus* stained with the ink dye appear as blue-stained, septate, dichotomously branched structures 2–4 μm in diameter with hyphal walls generally parallel (Fig. 15.6).

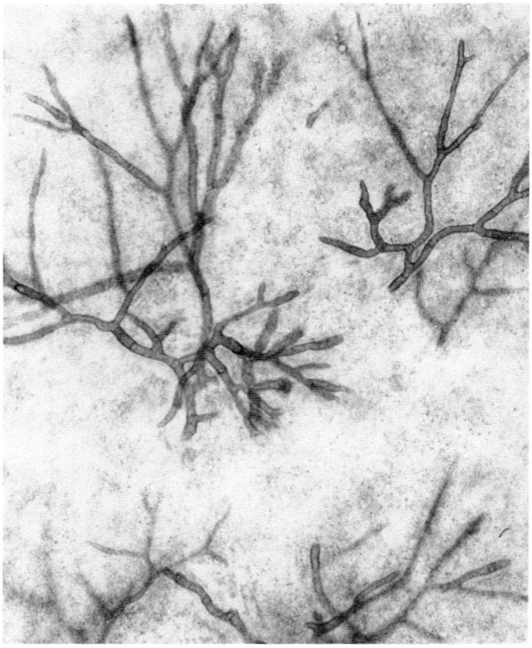

15.6. Hyphae of *Aspergillus fumigatus* in lesion material prepared as a wet mount in 20% KOH and ink dye. ×450.

Aseptically obtained specimens can be plated directly onto appropriate mycological media. Alternatively, specimens can be placed in saline solution, minced briefly in a tissue grinder, and then streaked onto the surfaces of mycological media. Replicate plates should be incubated at both 27 and 37 C. Collected fluids can be centrifuged and the sediment can be examined microscopically or cultured as above.

Satisfactory media for isolation and identification of most isolates from cases of aspergillosis include Sabouraud dextrose agar, Czapek's solution agar, and potato dextrose agar. All cultures should be examined daily and portions of fungal colonies should be transferred to fresh media.

For light microscopic examination, a small portion of the colony containing reproductive structures can be placed in a drop of suitable mounting medium (e.g., lactophenol blue) on a clear glass slide, teased apart, covered with a coverslip, and examined.

The major pathogens of aspergillosis can be identified based on specific characteristics of *A. fumigatus* or *A. flavus* (see Etiology).

Serology. Serologic tests are of limited value due to the nonspecific nature of the antigens. Agar-gel precipitin tests were used by Richard et al. (52) in comparisons of *A. fumigatus* and *A. flavus* infections in turkey poults. While most of the *A. fumigatus*-infected poults were positive for precipitating antibodies, poults infected with *A. flavus* were not. A direct enzyme-linked immunosorbent assay (ELISA) technique has been used in turkeys with a correlation occurring between exposure level and ELISA optical density (47). Perhaps the use of serologic methods for identifying poults with aspergillosis for culling procedures would be advantageous, but presently there is no legal or effective therapy for treating positive birds.

PREVENTION AND CONTROL. *Aspergillus fumigatus* infection in young chicks and poults has been somewhat controlled by hatchery sanitation. Sophisticated sampling equipment and media are available to monitor air in hatcheries. Moldy litter or feed and access to musty, moldy strawstacks should be avoided to prevent outbreaks of aspergillosis. Examination of premises or materials used for feed or litter will usually reveal the source of infection.

Areas around feed hoppers and watering places are fertile areas for growth of molds. Unless a permanent yard system is used, frequent moving of feed troughs and watering places is advisable. Placing feed containers and watering fountains on screened, elevated platforms helps to prevent turkeys from picking up molds that develop in such places. Drainage is advisable for areas where water is likely to stand after rains.

Daily cleaning and disinfection of feed and water utensils will aid in eliminating infection. Spraying the ground around containers with chemical solutions may be advisable if it is impossible to change feeding areas frequently. In outbreaks, a 1:2000 aqueous solution of copper sulfate for all drinking water may be used to aid in preventing the spread, though it should not be relied upon as a method to be used continually. Dyar et al. (18) reduced the mold count of contaminated litter and the mortalities of turkeys due to aspergillosis by treating the litter with nystatin and copper sulfate.

Wawrzkiewicz and Cygan (66) studied 64 strains of fungi of *Aspergillus,* 26 of *Rhizopus,* and 2 of *Mucor* from 56 lung tissue samples of poultry with aspergillosis. The most active fungistats against these in vitro were nystatin, amphotericin B, crystal violet, and brillant green.

Evidently, increased ventilation within poultry-rearing houses reduces the airborne mycoflora (54) suggesting that this could be used as a preventive measure in controlling aspergillosis. Natural ventilation appeared to be better than forced-air ventilation.

Generally, an effective means of therapy for avian aspergillosis is not available. While certain drugs (some are quite new) have been used for treatment of mammalian aspergillosis, they are apparently not cost-effective for poultry. Prevention is currently the preferred means of control. This usually involves eliminating the source of the organism, such as moldy feed and litter and treating the poultry houses and litter with antifungal compounds. In spite of precautions and preventive measures, outbreaks of aspergillosis frequently occur in some houses and at certain times of the year, particularly during the winter in closed rearing houses. Vaccines could be used, however, none are commercially available. Richard et al. (54) have reduced mortalities by 50% in turkey poults vaccinated with a germling (germinated conidia) vaccine prepared from *A. fumigatus* and subsequently challenge exposed to aerosols of *A. fumigatus* conidia. Viable spores of *A. fumigatus* administered to ducks provided some protection from death following challenge exposure (5). Hamycin in the drinking water was reportedly successful in controlling an outbreak of aspergillosis in young chicks (7). Miconazole was used successfully in the treatment of raptors with clinical aspergillosis (20). Infections in chick embryos have been controlled by use of amphotericin B (29) and phenylmercuric dinaphthylmethane-disulfonate (26).

REFERENCES

1. Ainsworth, G.C., and P.K. Austwick. 1973. Fungal diseases of animals. Farnham Royal, Slough, England.
2. Alexandrov, M., and A. Vesselinova. 1973. Durch Aspergillus fumigatus Fresenius bei truthuhnern verursachte Meningoenzephalitis. Zentralbl Veterinaermed [B] 20:204–309.
3. Appleby, E.C. 1962. Mycosis of the respiratory tract in penquins. Proc Zool Soc Lond 139:395–402.
4. Archibald, R.G. 1913. Aspergillosis in the Suda ostrich. J Comp Pathol Ther 26:171–173.
5. Asakura, A., S. Nakagawa, M. Masui, and J. Yasuda. 1962. Immunological studies of aspergillosis in birds. Mycopathol 18:249–256.
6. Austwick, P.K.C. 1965. Pathogenicity. In K.B. Raper and D.I. Fennell (eds.), The Genus Aspergillus, pp. 82–126, Williams & Wilkins Co., Baltimore, MD.
7. Babras, M.A., and C.V. Radhakrishnan. 1967. Aspergillosis in chicks and trial of hamycin in an outbreak. Hind Antibiot Bull 9:244–245.
8. Bergmann, V., G. Heider, and K. Vogel. 1980. Mycotic spondylitis as a cause of locomotor disorders in broiler chicken. Monatschefte Veterinaermed 35:349–351.
9. Brooksbank, N.H., and P.K. Austwick. 1955. Susceptibility of inbred and outbred chicks to aspergillosis. Br Vet J 111:64–67.
10. Bullis, K.L. 1950. Poultry disease control service. Univ Massachusetts Agric Exp Sta Annu Rep 459:85.
11. Castellani, A. 1928. Bronchomoniliasis fungi and fungus disease. Arch Dermatol Syph 17:61–97.
12. Chute, H.L., and D.C. O'Meara. 1958. Experimental fungous infections in chickens. Avian Dis 2:154–166.
13. Chute, H.L., J.F. Witter, J.L. Rountree, and D.C. O'Meara. 1955. The pathology of a fungous infection associated with a caponizing injury. J Am Vet Med Assoc 127:207–209.
14. Chute, H.L., D.C. O'Meara, H.D. Tresner, and E. Lacombe. 1956. The fungous flora of chickens with infections of the respiratory tract. Am J Vet Res 17:763–765.
15. Clark, D.S., E.E. Jones, W.B. Crowl, and F.K. Ross. 1954. Aspergillosis in newly hatched chicks. J Am Vet Med Assoc 124:116–117.
16. De Jong, D.A. 1912. Aspergillosis der Kanarienvögel (Aspergillosis in canaries). Zentralbl Bakteriol I Orig 66:390–393.
17. Durant, A.J., and C.M. Tucker. 1935. Aspergillosis of wild turkeys reared in captivity. J Am Vet Med Assoc 86:781–784.
18. Dyar, P.M., O.J. Fletcher, and R.K. Page. 1984. Aspergillosis in turkeys associated with use of contaminated litter. Avian Dis 28:250–255.
19. Eggert, M.J., and J.V. Barnhart. 1953. A case of egg-borne aspergillosis. J Am Vet Med Assoc 122:225.
20. Furley, C.W., and A.G. Greenwood. 1982. Treatment of aspergillosis in raptors (order Falconiformes) with miconazole. Vet Rec 111:584–585.
21. Gauger, H.C. 1941. Aspergillus fumigatus infection in adult chickens. Poult Sci 20:445–446.
22. Ghori, H.M., and S.A. Edgar. 1973. Comparative susceptibility of chickens, turkeys and Coturnix quail to aspergillosis. Poult Sci 52:2311–2315.
23. Ghori, H.M., and S.A. Edgar. 1979. Comparative susceptibility and effect of mild Aspergillus fumigatus infection on three strains of chickens. Poult Sci 58:14–17.
24. Guarda, F. 1974. Aspergillosi encefalica nei polli. Schweiz Arch Tierheilk 116:467–476.
25. Guberlet, J.E. 1923. An epizootic of aspergillosis in chickens. J Am Vet Med Assoc 63:612–622.

26. Harry, E.G., and D.M. Cooper. 1970. The treatment of hatching eggs for the control of egg transmitted aspergillosis. Br Poult Sci 11:269–272.
27. Hinshaw, W.R. 1937. Diseases turkeys. California Agric Exp Sta Bull 613.
28. Hudson, C.B. 1947. Aspergillus fumigatus infection in the eyes of baby chicks. Poult Sci 26:192–193.
29. Huhtanen, C.N., and J.M. Pensack. 1967. Effect of antifungal compounds on aspergillosis in hatching chick embryos. Appl Microbiol 15:102–109.
30. Itakura, C., and M. Goto. 1973. Pathological observation of fungal (Aspergillus fumigatus) ophthalmitis in chicks. Jpn J Vet Sci 35:473–479.
31. Jowett, W. 1913. Pulmonary mycosis in the ostrich. J Comp Pathol Ther 26:253–257.
32. Jungherr, E., and R. Gifford. 1944. Three hitherto unreported turkey diseases in Connecticutt: Erysipelas, hexamitiasis, mycotic encephalomalacia. Cornell Vet 34:214–226.
33. Kageruka, P. 1967. The mycotic flora of Antarctic Emperor and Adelia penguins. Acta Zool 44:87–99.
34. Katoch, R.C., K.B. Bhowmik, and B.S. Katoch. 1975. Preliminary studies on mycoflora of poultry feed and litter. Indian Vet J 52:759–762.
35. Lahaye, J. 1928. Maladies des pigeons et des poules, des oiseaux de basee-cour et de voliere (Diseases of pigeons and chickens, of birds in the farmyard and pigeon loft: Anatomy, hygiene, nutrition). Imprimerie Steinmetz-Haenen, Remouchamps.
36. Lignieres, J., and G. Petit. 1898. Péritonite aspergillaire des dindons (Aspergillus peritonitis of turkey toms). Rec Med Vet 5:145–148.
37. Lovett, J., J.W. Messer, and R.B. Read. 1971. The microflora of southern Ohio poultry litter. Poult Sci 50:746–751.
38. Milakovic-Novak, L., A. Nemanic, and A. Kostanjevac. 1977. Ocular aspergillosis in chicken (Aspergiloza ociju u pilica). Vet Arh 47:213–215.
39. Mohler, J.R., and J.S. Buckley. 1904. Pulmonary mycosis of birds with report of a case in a flamingo. USDA BAI Circ 58:122–136.
40. Moore, E.N. 1953. Aspergillus fumigatus as a cause of ophthalmitis in turkeys. Poult Sci 32:796–799.
41. Obendorf, D.L., and K. McColl. 1980. Mortality in little penguins (Eudyptula minor) along the coast of Victoria, Australia. J Wildl Dis 16:251–259.
42. O'Meara, D.C., and H.L. Chute. 1959. Aspergillosis experimentally produced in hatching chicks. Avian Dis 3:404–406.
43. Owings, W.J. 1986. Turkey health surveys, air quality study. Poult Newsl (Coop Ext Serv, Iowa State Univ, Summer, 1986), pp. 1–10.
44. Pinello, C.B., J.L. Richard, and L.H. Tiffany. 1977. Mycoflora of a turkey confinement brooder house. Poult Sci 56:1920–1926.
45. Raines, T.V., C.D. Kuzdas, F.H. Winkle, and B.S. Johnson. 1956. Encephalitic aspergillosis in turkeys a case report. J Am Vet Med Assoc 129:435–436.
46. Rayer and Montagne. 1842. Mycose aspergillaire dans les poches aeriennes d'un bouvreuil. J Inst Paris Muller's Arch 270. (Cited in Austwick, 1965).
47. Redig, P.T., G. Post, T. Concannon, and J. Dunnette. 1986. A direct ELISA for diagnosis of aspergillosis in turkeys. p. 30, Proc Conf Res Workers Anim Dis, 67th Meeting, Chicago, IL. (Abstract).
48. Reece, R.L., K. Taylor, D.B. Dickson, and P.J. Kerr. 1986. Mycosis of commercial japanese quail, ducks and turkeys. Aust Vet J 63:196–197.
49. Reis, J. 1940. Queratomicose aspergilica epizootica em pintos. Arch Inst Biol Sao Paulo 11:437–462.
50. Richard, J.L. 1975. Aspergillosis. In W.T. Hubbert, W.F. McCulloch, and P.R. Schnurrenberger (eds.), Diseases transmitted from animals to man, pp. 529–532. Charles C. Thomas, Springfield, IL.
51. Richard, J.L., and J.R. Thurston. 1983. Rapid hematogenous dissemination of Aspergillus fumigatus and A. flavus spores in turkey poults following aerosol exposure. Avian Dis 27:1025–1033.
52. Richard, J.L., R.C. Cutlip, J.R. Thurston, and J. Songer. 1981. Response of turkey poults to aerosolized spores of Aspergillus fumigatus and aflatoxigenic and nonaflatoxigenic strains of Aspergillus flavus. Avian Dis 25:53–67.
53. Richard, J.L., J.R. Thurston, R.C. Cutlip, and A.C. Pier. 1982. Vaccination studies of aspergillosis in turkeys: Subcutaneous inoculation with several vaccine preparations followed by aerosol challenge exposure. Am J Vet Res 43:488–492.
54. Richard, J.L., J.R. Thurston, W.M. Peden, and C. Pinello. 1984. Recent studies on aspergillosis in turkey poults. Mycopathologia 87:3–11.
55. Rippon, J.W. 1982. Medical mycology, the pathogenic fungi and the pathogenic actinomycetes. W.B. Saunders Co., Philadelphia.
56. Saravia-Gomez, J. 1978. Aspergillosis of the central nervous system. Handb Clin Neurol 35:395–400.
57. Sauter, E.A., C.F. Peterson, E.E. Steele, J.F. Parkinson, J.E. Dixon, and R.C. Stroh. 1981. The airborne microflora of poultry houses. Poult Sci 60:569–574.
58. Savage, A., and J.M. Isa. 1933. A note on mycotic pneumonia of chickens. Sci Agric 13:341.
59. Schlegel, M. 1918. Aspergillosis (pneumonomycosis aspergillina) bei Truthennen und Hühnern. Z Infektionskrankh Parasit Krankh Hyg Houstiere 19:333–334.
60. Sperling, F.G. 1953. Ophthalmic aspergillosis in chickens. Proc 25th Northeast Conf Lab Work Pullorum Dis Control, pp. 1–2.
61. Thi So, D., J.W. Dick, K.A. Holleman, and P. Labosky. 1978. Mold spore populations in bark residues used as broiler litter. Poult Sci 57:870–874.
62. Thurston, J.R., J.L. Richard, S.J. Cysewski, and R.E. Fichtner. 1975. Antibody formation in rabbits exposed to aerosols containing spores of Aspergillus fumigatus. Am J Vet Res 36:899– 901.
63. Van Heelsbergen, T. 1929. Handbuch der gelflüegelkrankheiten und der gelflüegelzucht, pp. 312–322. Ferdinand Enke, Stuttgart.
64. Veen, P.J. 1973. Torticollis and disease of the respiratory tract, caused by Aspergillus fumigatus in fowl. Neth J Vet Sci 5:132–133.
65. Walker, J. 1915. Aspergillosis in the ostrich chick. Union S Afr Dep Agric Annu Rep 3–4:535–574.
66. Wawrzkiewicz, K., and Z. Cygan. 1974. Wrazliwosc in vitro grzybow wyosobnionych z przypadkow grzybic ukladu oddechowego ptakow na fungistatyki. Pol Arch Weter 17:211–224.
67. Witter, J.F., and H.L. Chute. 1952. Aspergillosis in turkeys. J Am Vet Med Assoc 121:387–388.
68. Wright, M.L., G.W. Anderson, and N.A. Epps. 1960. Hatchery sanitation as a control measure for aspergillosis in fowl. Avian Dis 4:369–379.
69. Wright, M.L., G.W. Anderson, and J.D. McConachie. 1961. Transmission of aspergillosis during incubation. Poult Sci 40:727–731.
70. Yamada, S., S. Kamikawa, Y. Uchinuno, A. Tominaga, K. Matsuo, H. Fujikawa, and K. Takeuchi. 1977. Avian dermatitis caused by Aspergillus fumigatus. J Jpn Vet Med Assoc 30:200–202.
71. Zook, B.C., and G. Migaki. 1985. Aspergillosis in Animals. In Y. Al-Doory and G.E. Wagner (eds.), Aspergillosis, pp. 207–256. Charles C. Thomas, Springfield, IL.

THRUSH (MYCOSIS OF THE DIGESTIVE TRACT)

H.L. Chute

Stomatitis oidica, muguet, soor, moniliasis, oidiomycosis, candidiasis, and sour crop are other terms applied to mycotic infections of the digestive tract.

INCIDENCE. Mycosis of the digestive tract probably occurs rather frequently, but in many cases does not appear to be of sufficient significance to be considered seriously. Numerous general discussions of poultry diseases fail to mention this disorder, and the paucity of diagnoses in reports from diagnostic laboratories suggests that it may not be of great consequence. However, serious outbreaks have been reported in many species of birds. Animals and humans are also affected. Thrush has been observed in chickens, pigeons, geese, turkeys, pheasant, ruffed grouse, quail, peacocks, and parakeets.

Gierke (4) reported an outbreak of a thrushlike disease occurring in turkeys in California. Hart (5) reported the disease in turkeys and other fowl in New South Wales. A soluble endotoxin, toxic for mice, has been isolated from *Candida albicans*. A review on the disease in turkeys and chickens in California was recorded by Mayeda (13).

ETIOLOGY. The etiologic significance of yeastlike fungi in infections of the digestive tract of humans was recognized by Langenbeck in 1839. Questions relating to the validity of species described and their generic nomenclature have retarded proper understanding of this type of disease. Jungherr (8, 9) found *Monilia albicans, M. krusei,* and *Oidium pullorum* sp. nov. to be associated with cases of thrush but considered *M. krusei* to be of no etiologic significance. *Mucor* sp. and aspergillae were also found in association with some cases. Hinshaw (6) reported *M. albicans* was found in most cases of thrush in turkeys and chickens that came to his attention. Both investigators noted that the mycotic infections were apt to be associated with unhygienic conditions.

Studies of Benham (1), Worley and Stovall (19), Martin et al. (12), and others indicated the complexity of the problem. Stovall (14) presented a means of improving the present uncertain status, suggesting a specific set of environmental conditions under which biologic characteristics of the organism were constant and could be demonstrated. Jungherr (9) stated that *M. albicans* is of widespread occurrence in gallinaceous birds, pathogenic to birds and also to rabbits on intravenous (IV) injection, and indistinguishable from strains isolated from human sources. On Sabouraud's agar it produces a whitish, creamy, high-convex colony after incubation for 24–48 hr at 37 C. Young cultures consist of oval budding yeast cells about 5.5 × 3.5 μ. Older cultures show septate hyphae and occasionally spherical, swollen cells with thickened membranes, the so-called chlamydospores. In Dunham's peptone water containing 1% fermentable substance and 1% Andrade's indicator, the organism produces acid and gas in dextrose, levulose, maltose, and mannose; produce slight acid in galactose and sucrose; and does not attack dextrin (variable according to brand), inulin, lactose, and raffinose. Gelatin stab cultures show short villous to arborescent outgrowths without liquefaction of the medium.

The term "medical monilias" is frequently used in connection with the generic term *Monilia,* which is also used for a separate group of fungi. Most workers have accepted the decision of an informal group meeting at the Third International Microbiological Congress in 1939 and use *Candida* as a generic name to replace the familiar but invalid *Monilia. C. Albicans* is the most frequently isolated etiologic agent associated with the disturbance commonly referred to as moniliasis.

PATHOGENESIS AND EPIZOOTIOLOGY

Signs and Lesions. Signs are not particularly characteristic. Affected chicks show unsatisfactory growth, stunted appearance, listlessness, and roughness of feathers. Lesions occur most frequently in the crop and consist of thickening of the mucosa with whitish, circular raised ulcer formations, the surfaces of which tend to scale off. Pseudomembranous patches and easily removed necrotic material over the mucosa are not uncommon. The mouth and esophagus may show ulcerlike patches. When the proventriculus is involved, it is swollen, the serosa has a glossy appearance, and the mucosa is hemorrhagic and may be covered with catarrhal or necrotic exudate. Histologically, Jungherr (7) reported that crops showed extensive destruction of the stratified epithelium deep in the malpighian layer, and quite often walled-off ulcers or extensive diphtheroid to diphtheritic membranes were present. Lesions were characterized by absence of inflammatory reaction. Periportal focal necrosis in the liver in some cases suggested toxic action upon the system.

The frequent association of mycosis of the digestive tract with other debilitating conditions such as gizzard erosions and intestinal coccidiosis must be considered. Gizzard erosions, as such, probably are not directly related to thrush. Likewise, the thickened intestine with watery contents frequently noted in cases of thrush is probably due to coccidiosis or other protozoan infections.

In the case of thrush the esophagus, crop (Fig. 15.7), and proventriculus show an ulcerated and scaly condition. Spores and hyphae of what is termed *C. albicans* can readily be demonstrated in lesions. Diphtheroid lesions are noted in the proventriculus and small intestine. Abscess formations are present under pulpy, soft, grayish white to brownish red necrotic masses. Hinshaw (6) reported thrush in 12 flocks of turkeys, with lesions similar to those noted in chickens. Blaxland and Fincham (2) studied five serious outbreaks in young turkeys. Their observations supported previous conclusions that moniliasis is likely to be associated with unhygienic surroundings and other debilitating conditions, but spread of infection appeared definite in many instances. The disease has been described in pigeons and geese.

Tripathy (15) considered that vascular damage in infected turkeys may be associated with candida endotoxin. Atheromatous lesions were present on the intimal surface of the abdominal aorta in more than 50% of turkeys exposed to *C. albicans,* whereas there was only a 12.5% incidence of similar lesions in uninfected controls.

Young birds are more susceptible than older birds to mycosis of the digestive tract. Thus, as infected birds grow older they tend to overcome the infection. Jungherr (7) observed an outbreak in which losses amounted to 10,000 chicks out of 50,000 that were less than 60 days of age. He also reported (9) that turkeys under 4 wk of age succumbed rapidly to infection but that outbreaks in birds 3 mo of age resulted in high percentage of recoveries.

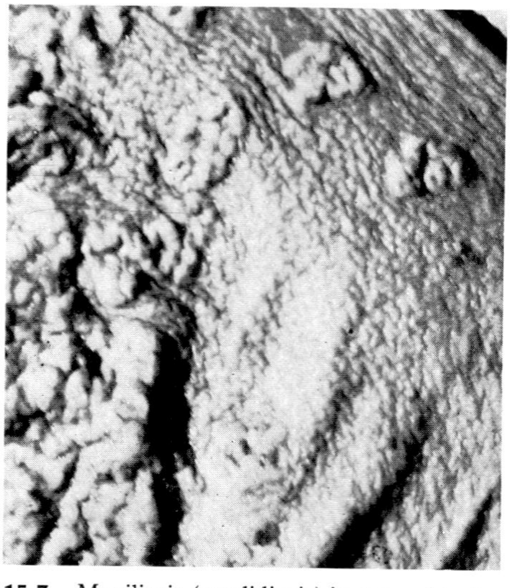

15.7. Moniliasis (candidiasis) in crop of turkey. Note raised, piled-up exudate that tends to form roselike masses. (Hinshaw)

Wyatt et al. (20) induced systemic candidiasis in 14-day-old broiler chickens with an IV injection of a suspension of *C. albicans* cells. Growth was severely retarded, with reddened livers and kidneys, pancreatitis, and neural disturbances.

DIAGNOSIS. Observation of characteristic proliferative, relatively noninflammatory lesions, with resultant heavy growth on primary cultures, serves to diagnose thrush. Because of the possibility of cultivation of *C. albicans* from apparently normal tissues, an original heavy growth is considered essential for diagnosis. Recognition of spores and more especially hyphae in fresh smear preparations is attended with some difficulty. Miliary abscesses are produced in kidneys of rabbits injected IV (1).

Underwood (16) described an instrument known as McCarthy's foroblique panendoscope that was used to diagnose experimental crop moniliasis. This instrument was equipped with a viewing lens and an independent light source. Birds were starved for 12 hr to empty the crop to allow a clear view of the mucosa. A normal crop appeared to be light pink, with a glistening smooth surface having numerous shallow convolutions, whereas a fungus-infected crop showed severe corrugations to mild whitish streaks, erosions or diphtheritic formations, and a deep red surrounding mucosa.

TREATMENT AND CONTROL. Since mycosis of the digestive tract is apt to be related to unhygienic, unsanitary, overcrowded conditions, they should not be allowed to exist or should be corrected. Jungherr (8) found that denatured alcohol and coal-tar derivatives were ineffective as disinfectants and suggested that iodine preparations be used. As a treatment he recommended that following an Epsom salt flush, 1 level teaspoon powdered bluestone ($CuSO_4$) be added to each 2 gal drinking water in nonmetal containers every other day for 1 wk. Hinshaw recommended that a 1:2000 solution of $CuSO_4$ for turkeys be used as the sole source of drinking water during the course of the outbreak. On the other hand, Underwood et al. (17) found $CuSO_4$ to be ineffective for treating or preventing the disease in chicks and poults with experimentally produced moniliasis. Affected birds should be segregated. Lesions in the mouth can be treated by local application of a suitable antiseptic. Appearance of the disease in very young chicks suggests the surface of the egg as a source of infection. Such a possibility could be removed by dipping eggs in an iodine preparation prior to incubation.

Kostin (11) found that *C. albicans* organisms mixed with poultry droppings and applied to wooden boards could be killed by exposure to 2%

formaldehyde or 1% sodium hydroxide solution for 1 hr. Treatment with a 5% solution of iodine monochloride in hydrochloric acid for 3 hr was also successful in disinfection.

Nystatin has been studied by Gentry et al. (3) and Kahn and Weisblatt (10). One group reported that 220 mg nystatin/kg diet was effective in eliminating moniliasis in a flock of turkeys. The other group found that in experimental infections with *C. albicans* in both chickens and turkeys, crop lesion severity appeared to be significantly reduced in the group fed the lowest level of nystatin (11 mg/kg). The highest level (110 mg/kg) showed very significant protection against mycotic infection.

Yacowitz et al. (21) reported successful prevention of candidiasis in chickens by addition of nystatin at a minimum level of 142 mg/kg ration for 4 wk. Kahn and Weisblatt (10) obtained similar results. Wind and Yacowitz (18) successfully treated crop mycosis with nystatin by dispersing it in drinking water at levels of 62.5–250 mg/L with sodium lauryl sulfate (7.8–25 mg/L) for 5 days.

Tripathy (15) found that addition of chlortetracycline (500 g/ton) to a vitamin A–deficient ration had no effect on incidence or severity of crop candidiasis but increased the cells being shed in feces. Turkeys fed nystatin (100 g/ton) had a higher average weight and milder crop lesions than untreated controls.

REFERENCES

1. Benham, R.W. 1931. Certain monilias parasitic on man. J Infect Dis 49:183–215.
2. Blaxland, J.D., and I.H. Fincham. 1950. Mycosis of the crop (moniliasis) in poultry, with particular reference to serious mortality occurring in young turkeys. Br Vet J 106:221- 231.
3. Gentry, R.F., G.R. Bubash, and H.L. Chute. 1960. Candida albicans in turkeys. 1. Treatment of crop infections with mycostatin. Poult Sci 39:1252.
4. Gierke, A.G. 1932. A preliminary report on a mycosis of turkeys. California Dept Agric Mon Bull 21:229–231.
5. Hart, L. 1947. Moniliasis in turkeys and fowls in New South Wales. Aust Vet J 23:191–192.
6. Hinshaw, W.R. 1933. Moniliasis (thrush) in turkeys and chickens. Proc 5th World's Poult Congr 3:190.
7. Jungherr, E.L. 1933. Observations on a severe outbreak of mycosis in chicks. J Agric 2:169–178.
8. Jungherr, E.L. 1933. Studies on yeast-like fungi from gallinaceous birds. Storrs Agric Exp Stn Bull 188.
9. Jungherr, E.L. 1934. Mycosis in fowl caused by yeast-like fungi. J Am Vet Med Assoc 3:500–506.
10. Kahn, S.G., and H. Weisblatt. 1963. A comparison of nystatin and copper sulfate in experimental moniliasis of chickens and turkeys. Avian Dis 3:304–309.
11. Kostin, V.V. 1966. Razrabotka rezhimov dezinfektsii pri kandidamikose Ptits. (Development of method for disinfection in candidasis of fowls.). Trudy Vses Inst Vet Sanit 26:157–162.
12. Martin, D.S., C.P. Jones, K.F. Yao, and L.E. Lee, Jr. 1937. A practical classification of the monilias. J Bacteriol 34:99.
13. Mayeda, B. 1961. Candidiasis in turkeys and chickens in the Sacramento Valley of California. Avian Dis 3:232–243.
14. Stovall, W.D. 1939. Classification and pathogenicity of species of Monilia. Microbiol 3rd Int Congr, p. 202.
15. Tripathy, S.B. 1965. Observations of changes in turkeys exposed to Candida albicans. Diss Abstr 6:3187.
16. Underwood, P.C. 1955. Detection of crop mycosis (moniliasis) in chickens and turkeys with a panendoscope. J Am Vet Med Assoc 127:229–231.
17. Underwood, P.C., J.H. Collins, C.G. Durgin, F.A. Hodges, and H.E. Zimmerman, Jr. 1956. Critical tests with copper sulphate for experimental moniliasis (crop mycosis) of chickens and turkeys. Poult Sci 3:599–605.
18. Wind, S., and H. Yacowitz. 1960. Use of mycostatin in the drinking water for the treatment of crop mycosis in turkeys. Poult Sci 39:904–905.
19. Worley, G., and N.D. Stovall. 1937. A study of milk coagulation by Monilia species. J Infect Dis 2:134.
20. Wyatt, R.D., D.C. Simmons, and P.B. Hamilton. 1975. Induced systemic candidiosis in young broiler chickens. Avian Dis 19:533–543.
21. Yacowitz, H., S. Wind, W.P. Jambor, N.P. Willett, and J.F. Pagano. 1959. Use of mycostatin for the prevention of moniliasis (crop mycosis) in chicks and turkeys. Poult Sci 3:653–660.

MISCELLANEOUS FUNGAL INFECTIONS

H.L. Chute

A number of rare fungal isolations from birds hâve been reported. These may not be of economic significance to the poultry industry but should be noted for diagnosticians and researchers.

HISTOPLASMOSIS

Histoplasmosis is an infectious but not contagious mycotic disease of human and lower animals. It has been reported commonly in zoo birds and occasionally in chicken and turkey populations. It occurs worldwide, especially in areas in the USA bordering the Missouri, Ohio, and Mississippi rivers where the disease appears to be indigenous.

The *Histoplasma capsulatum* organism grows readily in culture media and soil as a white to brown mold that bears spores of two types: 1) spherical, minutely spiny microconidia 3–4 μm in diameter and 2) spherical, or rarely clavate, macroconidia 8–12 μm in diameter, with evenly spaced fingerlike projections. The organism grows in the yeastlike phase but with difficulty. It requires a temperature of 37 C, a medium rich in protein, preferably blood, and high levels of humidity and carbon dioxide.

The mycelial phase grows on Sabouraud's medium, dextrose agar, potato, gelatin, or bread at any temperature. Colonies appear as white to brownish after 2 wk. The segmented branched hyphae are 2.5 μm wide and give rise to chlamydospores, often in chains with large round cells 20 μm in diameter.

Dodge (1) found the organism in samples from a starling roost in Italy and in soil samples from a schoolyard; a high proportion of the school children were histoplasmin-positive.

Diagnosis is based on three criteria: culture of the organism, histopathology, and histoplasmin sensitivity. The characteristic histopathology is an extensive proliferation of reticuloendothelial cells, many of which contain yeast forms.

Recognized cases of histoplasmosis in humans and animals have not been successfully treated. There is some evidence that the disease occurs in animals in a mild unrecognized form.

REFERENCE

1. Dodge, H.J. 1965. The association of a bird-roosting site with infection of school children by Histoplasma capsulatum. Am J Publ Health 55:1203–1211.

CRYPTOCOCCOSIS

Cryptococcosis is a disease of humans and animals. In humans, it is characterized by a meningitis. Synonyms are torulosis, torula, yeast meningitis, and European blastomycosis.

An encapsulated yeastlike fungus in human lesions was reported in 1894. Although it has not been diagnosed as a pathogen in birds, and epizootics have not occurred, its importance to public health and its occurrence in birds' environments warrant discussion.

The disease is widely distributed around the world and although not of economic significance in poultry, there are many sporadic reports from zoo birds.

The fungus belongs to the imperfect yeast group under the name of *Cryptococcus neoformans.* It reproduces by budding; cells are perfectly spherical and surrounded by a thick mucilaginous capsule. Cell diameter is 4–6 μm and the capsule is 1–2 μm thick. It grows well within 48 hr at 30 C on glucose agar.

Bisbocci (1) isolated cryptococci from a pheasant with enterohepatitis. Chickens were experimentally infected and developed the disease. Lesions consisted of granulomas and necrotic processes in liver, intestines, lungs, and spleen.

Emmons (3) shocked the public health world by isolating *C. neoformans* from 16 of 19 premises and 63 of 111 specimens of pigeon droppings. The organism was found in the dropping sites but was not isolated from 20 pigeons examined. It appeared to grow as a saprophyte. Bishop et al. (2) confirmed those findings by isolating *C. neoformans* from 6 of 13 samples of pigeon nests and droppings.

Staib (5) isolated cryptococci from 28 fecal samples obtained from 201 species of birds at zoological gardens and pet shops in Germany; 12 isolates were from canaries, 1 was from a wild pigeon, and the remainder were from psittacine and other birds. Fragner (4) isolated cryptococci from feces of 48 pigeons, 13 fowl, 7 pheasants, 10 house martins, 4 jackdaws, and 3 chaffinches.

Infections can be diagnosed by culturing the organism. Histopathology has proved extremely useful in diagnosis of cases in mammals. A significant feature is absence of an inflammatory reaction except in late stages, when compression effects end and a chronic inflammatory reaction is produced. Mucicarmine stain is specific; it shows many budding spores, with the thick capsule being darkly stained.

Prognosis is very grave for infected mammals, and no satisfactory treatment is known.

REFERENCES

1. Bisbocci, G. 1938. Infectious entero-hepatitis in fowls due to a cryptococcus. Nouvo Ercolani 43:290–314.

2. Bishop, R.H., R.K. Hamilton, and J.M. Slack. 1960. The isolation of cryptococcus neoformans from pigeon nests. Abstr W Va Bull 26:31–32.

3. Emmons, C.W. 1955. Saprophytic sources of cryptococcus neoformans associated with the pigeon (Columba livia). Am J Hyg 62:227–232.

4. Fragner, P. 1962. Isolation of cryptococcus from bird feces. Csl Epidem Mikrobiol Immunol 11:135–139.

5. Staib, F. 1961. C. neoformans in bird feces. Zbl Bakt 1, (orig.) 182:562–563.

OTHER FUNGAL INFECTIONS

Over the years there have been numerous reports of individual fungal isolations from all classes of birds. Many of these may have been opportunist infections. The most complete review of many of these infections is in a partially annotated bibliography of avian mycosis by Barden et al. (1). In another review (5), Wobeser and Saunders reported several cases of pulmonary oxalosis in humans and animals from an infection with *Aspergillus niger.* This fungus produced appreciable quantities of oxalix acid, which in turn caused tissue necrosis adjacent to the mycelial growth. A detailed description was given for a case in a great horned owl (*Bubo virginianus*).

Ranck et al. (3) described dactylariosis, a new fungal disease of chickens. A fatal encephalitis resulted from the thermophilic fungus *Dactylaria gallopava* in 200 birds from a flock of 65,000. The disease was experimentally reproduced by a spore suspension injected into the left posterior thoracic air sac, left maxillary sinus, and cerebrum. Brain lesions similar to those in the natural outbreak resulted. Georg et al. (2) described this thermophilic dematiaceous hyphomycete as the casual agent of encephalitis in poults, and Waldrip (4) reported an outbreak in 60,000 birds with a mortality rate of 3–5%. In the latter case, the organism was also isolated from litter samples of broiler houses. It was suggested that wood chips and sawdust litter might have introduced the organism.

Other rare fungal infections have included *Paecilomyces variota, Geotrichum candidum,* and *Trichophyton verrucosum.* Although apparently unimportant and rare, such cases should be reported. The diagnosis of fungal diseases is becoming very complex, particularly as it relates to mycotoxic effects on growth of birds.

REFERENCES

1. Barden, E.S., H.L. Chute, D.C. O'Meara, and H.T. Wheelwright. 1971. A bibliography of avian mycosis (partially annotated). College of Life Sciences and Agriculture. Univ of Maine, Orono, pp. 1–193.

2. Georg, L.K., B.W. Bierer, and W.B. Cooke. 1964. Encephalitis in turkey poults due to a new fungus species. Sabouraudia 3:239–244.

3. Ranck, F.M., Jr., K. Georg, and H. Wallace. 1974. Dactylariosis a newly recognized fungus disease of chickens. Avian Dis 18:4–20.

4. Waldrip, D.W., A.A. Padhye, L. Ajello, and M. Ajello. 1974. Isolation of Dactylaria gallopava from broiler-house litter. Avian Dis 18:445–451.

5. Wobeser, G., and J.R. Saunders. 1975. Pulmonary oxalosis in association with Aspergillus niger infection in a great horned owl (Bubo virginianus). Avian Dis 19:388–392.

16 NEOPLASTIC DISEASES

INTRODUCTION

B.W. Calnek

This chapter deals with a variety of related and unrelated conditions possessing a single common denominator: neoplastic character. Some have been extensively studied because of their considerable economic importance. Others have served as highly suitable models for studying various phenomena of neoplasia; indeed, medical research has found avian oncology an abundant resource. For this chapter, neoplasms are divided into two main categories, depending on whether the etiologic agent is known.

Virus-induced tumors are principally of mesodermal origin and are transmissible. Five diseases or disease complexes are described, each in a separate section because of its etiologic distinctness. The first, Marek's disease (MD), is a lymphoproliferative disease affecting the peripheral nervous system and, to a greater or lesser degree, other tissues and visceral organs. MD is caused by a herpesvirus.

Second is a group of leukoses, sarcomas, and related neoplasms induced by a number of closely related RNA retroviruses (now called the leukosis/sarcoma group). Prominent in this group is lymphoid leukosis, another lymphoproliferative disease, affecting primarily the bursa of Fabricius and visceral organs. Also included are other neoplasms of hematopoietic origin (erythroblastosis, myeloblastosis, myelocytomatosis, and certain related neoplasms such as nephroblastoma and osteopetrosis). These conditions, along with sarcomas and other connective tissue tumors, are etiologically related and discussed as a group.

A third section describes conditions associated with the reticuloendotheliosis virus (REV) group. Some members of this antigenically related group of RNA-containing retroviruses (unrelated to the leukosis/sarcoma group) cause nonneoplastic conditions in ducks, others apparently are the cause of lymphoid neoplasms in turkeys, and certain isolates induce reticuloendotheliosis in experimentally infected chickens.

The fourth section briefly describes a condition in turkeys called lymphoproliferative disease, which apparently is caused by yet another RNA retrovirus that is distinct from both the REV and leukosis/sarcoma groups.

Tumors of unknown etiology of necessity are described only on the basis of morphologic characteristics and are discussed in the final section. Included are a wide variety of benign and malignant neoplasms derived from muscle, epithelial, and nerve tissues; serous membranes; and pigmented cells.

Classification and nomenclature of the known transmissible neoplasms present a problem. The dilemma is largely due to two factors. First, many virus strains appear to have multipotent characteristics; i.e., they can sometimes induce a variety of neoplasms. Second, certain of the viruses induce some pathologic lesions difficult to distinguish from those induced by another unrelated virus. The two prevalent lymphomatotic diseases, now called lymphoid leukosis and Marek's disease, are particularly confusing with regard to the latter point. The problem is compounded by the fact that most flocks and many birds (sometimes including those employed for experimental purposes) are infected with more than one agent, and it is virtually impossible to examine one virus strain without often also observing effects of a second unrelated tumor virus. Prevalence of various unrelated (and related, but different) viruses in experimental birds used for passage of a given virus strain undoubtedly resulted in mixed virus populations in most cases (especially in earlier studies), a factor that must be considered in arguments of the multipotent character of some viruses.

In general, terminology evolved along with an understanding of the pathologic changes associated with a given condition. Thus while Marek (9) described a "polyneuritis," Pappenheimer et al. (10), who associated visceral lymphomata with the same disease, proposed the term "neurolymphomatosis gallinarum." Few workers could decide what terminology was appropriate for each kind of lesion, and there was soon an abundant supply of choices (see synonyms in the following sections).

Trying to resolve the classification and terminology problem, a committee proposed a pathologic nomenclature (8). Biggs (3) reviewed development of our present concepts and terminology and observed that not all persons accepted this "unitarian" theory and further that Campbell (5) had made a plea for clarification and a return to the earlier held concept of two groups of diseases. Ultimately, the World Veterinary Poultry Association (WVPA) adopted a classification and nomenclature scheme that clearly differentiated between the leukoses and MD (2). MD was classified as neural, visceral, or ocular and the leukoses were divided into lymphoid, erythroid, and myeloid types. It was soon obvious from studies on etiologic agents that this major division was warranted (1).

Choice of terminology for this chapter (Table 16.1) is based on that originally adopted by the WVPA and includes modifications in current use. The classification system accompanying this nomenclature is especially suited to the mode of presentation that follows, i.e., categorization of diseases or disease complexes by agent type instead of pathologic manifestation. Subdivision within agent-type diseases by pathologic expression has been employed where it seemed appropriate.

Incidence and importance of neoplasms in poultry can only be generally estimated. Feldman and Olson (6) quoted reports (1915–55) in which incidence of tumors, except neurolymphomatosis and osteopetrosis, varied from 3 to 19%. More recently we have had the advantage of data accumulated by the USDA from federally inspected slaughtered poultry. These data showed that incidence of "leukosis" in young chickens (probably nearly all MD) increased dramatically during a 10-yr period beginning in 1961.

There was a gradual rise in leukosis condemnations in young chickens from about 0.1% in 1961 to over 1.5% in 1968–70 (see 11). After 1970, the trend was reversed and condemnations of young birds returned to 1961 levels, undoubtedly the result of MD vaccination of broilers. However, during peak years over 40 million young birds (nearly 50% of all condemnations) were condemned for leukosis, and it was conceded that it was one of the most serious problems confronting the poultry industry.

Condemnations due to leukosis in mature birds were fairly consistent and much lower (less than 0.5 million birds, usually less than 10% of all condemnations). Condemnation rates with other tumors, many of which were leiomyomas of the mesosalpinx, were actually much higher (up to five times) than those from leukosis. Because most losses from leukotic diseases occur during growing and productive periods of layers, presence of gross lesions at slaughter is a poor index of their true incidence and importance. In 1967 annual losses in the USA and Great Britain were placed at more than $150 million and about $40 million, respectively (1, 3). The amount of present annual loss from neoplasms is not known, but the nearly universal use of MD vaccine since the early 1970s has certainly reduced it to a small fraction of the above figures. Purchase (11) estimated that benefits derived by the poultry industry in the USA as a result of MD vaccine totaled nearly $170 million annually. This included increased egg production and decreased losses from non-MD causes as indirect benefits as well as the direct effect of lowered MD mortality and condemnations. USDA data from 1975, summarized by Biggs (4), estimated all losses from neoplasms, including MD and lymphoid leukosis, to be $134 million; this was less than 10% of the total annual loss from all disease in the USA at that time. Lymphoid leukosis losses may be significant in some flocks, but mortality probably constitutes only a small portion of the economic loss from that disease. Studies by Gavora et al. (7) and Spencer et al. (12) have shown that lowered egg production and in-

Table 16.1. Transmissible neoplasms

Virus Type	Nucleic Acid Type	Virus Classification of Etiologic Agent	Neoplastic Diseases
Retrovirus	DNA	Leukosis/sarcoma group	Leukoses
			Lymphoid leukosis
			Erythroblastosis
			Myeloblastosis
			Sarcomas and other connective tissue tumors
			Fibrosarcoma, fibroma
			Myxosarcoma, myxoma
			Osteogenic sarcoma, osteoma
			Histiocytic sarcoma
			Related neoplasms
			Hemangioma
			Nephroblastoma
			Hepatocarcinoma
			Osteopetrosis
		Reticuloendotheliosis group	Reticuloendotheliosis
			Lymphoid leukosis
Herpesvirus	DNA	Marek's disease virus	Marek's disease

creased mortality from causes other than lymphoid leukosis are associated with infection by lymphoid leukosis virus, and the total economic impact from these could be extremely significant. Incidence of neoplasms other than lymphoid tumors appears to be low and of questionable economic significance.

REFERENCES

1. AAAP. 1967. Report of the AAAP-Sponsored Leukosis Workshop. Avian Dis 11:694-702.
2. Biggs, P.M. 1962. Some observations on the properties of cells from the lesions of Marek's disease and lymphoid leukosis. Proc 13th Symp Colston Res Soc, pp. 83-99.
3. Biggs, P.M. 1967. Marek's disease. Vet Rec 81:583-592.
4. Biggs, P.M. 1982. The world of poultry disease. Avian Pathol 11:281-300.
5. Campbell, J.G. 1954. Avian leucosis: A plea for clarification. Proc 10th World's Poult Congr, pp. 193-197.
6. Feldman, W.H., and C. Olson. 1965. Neoplastic diseases of the chicken. In H.E. Biester and L.H. Schwarte (eds.), Diseases of Poultry, 5th Ed., pp. 863-924. Iowa State Univ Press, Ames.
7. Gavora, J.S., J.L. Spencer, R.S. Gowe, and D.L. Harris. 1980. Lymphoid leukosis virus infection: Effects on production and mortality and consequences in selection for high egg production. Poult Sci 59:2165-2178.
8. Jungherr, E. 1941. Tentative pathologic nomenclature. Am J Vet Res 2:116.
9. Marek, J. 1907. Multiple Nervenentzuendung (polyneuritis) bei Hüehnern. Dtsch Tierärztl Wochenschr 15:417- 421.
10. Pappenheimer, A.M., L.C. Dunn, and V.C. Cone. 1926. A study of fowl paralysis (neuro-lymphomatosis gallinarum). Storrs Agric Exp Stn Bull 143:187-290.
11. Purchase, H.G. 1985. Clinical disease and its economic impact. In L.N. Payne (ed.), Marek's Disease. Developments in Veterinary Virology, pp. 17-42. Martinus Nijhoff Publishing, Boston.
12. Spencer, J.L., J.S. Gavora, and R.S. Gowe. 1980. Lymphoid leukosis virus: Natural transmission and nonneoplastic effects. Cold Spring Harbor Conf Cell Proliferation 7:553-564.

MAREK'S DISEASE

B.W. Calnek and R.L. Witter

INTRODUCTION. The most common of the lymphoproliferative diseases of chickens is Marek's disease (MD), which is characterized by a mononuclear infiltration of one or more of the following: peripheral nerves, gonad, iris, various viscera, muscle, and skin. MD is caused by a herpesvirus, is transmissible, and can be distinguished etiologically from other lymphoid neoplasms of birds.

Terminology has been confusing. The wide variety of clinical signs and pathologic expressions, depending primarily on the location of lesions, led to promulgation of an equally wide variety of terms to identify the conditions. Mononuclear infiltration of peripheral nerves results in gross enlargement and causes paralysis. The inflammatory character of some of the peripheral nerve lesions prompted Marek (260) to identify the disease as polyneuritis. Synonyms subsequently employed include neuritis, neurolymphomatosis gallinarum, and range paralysis. Mononuclear infiltration of the iris, which causes changes ranging from depigmentation to grayish opacity, is the basis for terms such as blindness, gray eye, iritis, uveitis, and ocular lymphomatosis. Leukotic lesions in various visceral organs and muscles were often referred to simply as visceral lymphomatosis, and those in the skin as skin leukosis. In 1961 Biggs (24) promoted the use of the term "Marek's disease" to clearly distinguish the condition from etiologically different lymphoproliferative diseases. This term is in common use.

Prior to use of vaccines, MD constituted a serious economic threat to the poultry industry because of heavy annual losses. Since vaccines are not 100% effective, losses still occur but they are no longer as serious a problem. Purchase (355) estimated that mortality and condemnation losses due to MD totalled about $12 million in the USA in 1984. However, when combined with economic loss from cost of vaccine and application and reduced egg production, the total was about $169 million in the USA and $943 million worldwide.

Purchase and Witter (359) have made a comprehensive review of the literature related to MD and human health concerns, particularly human cancer. They cite numerous reports of virologic, pathologic, serologic, and epidemiologic studies that support a conclusion that there is no etiologic relationship between MD virus (MDV) or any of the MD vaccine viruses and human cancer.

The literature on MD is voluminous and growing. Because it is increasingly difficult to cite all relevant publications and because a number of very comprehensive reviews on various aspects of MD are now available, literature citations for this chapter will be somewhat more selective than in previous editions. This will be especially true of older literature. Where possible, reference to reviews will substitute for many of the possible individual citations. A particularly useful source of information on Marek's disease is the multi-authored book: *Marek's Disease. Scientific Basis and Methods of Control,* edited by L. N. Payne (318).

HISTORY. Marek's 1907 report (260) of paresis in roosters owing to mononuclear infiltration of peripheral nerves and spinal nerve roots is probably the first account of the disease. Outbreaks dating to 1914 were reported in the USA; subsequent observations of the disease came from the Netherlands, Great Britain, and many other countries (26).

As observations were added to Marek's early description, it became apparent that lesions were not restricted to the spinal cord and peripheral nerves. It was learned that blindness was frequently accompanied by paralysis and that extraneural lesions included visceral lymphomata, particularly in the ovary, and infiltration of the iris and brain. Outbreaks of so-called acute MD with unusually high mortality and a preponderance of visceral lymphomas have been observed at least since 1949 and became quite common between 1960 and 1970.

Attempts to transmit the disease, often unsuccessful (306), along with descriptions of gross and microscopic lesions, accounted for much of the research effort during the 1920s and 1930s.

The importance of genetic constitution as it affected susceptibility to the disease was brought out by the classic work of Hutt and Cole (184). Their studies, which began in the 1930s, laid the foundation for efforts to control losses through genetic selection of breeding stocks.

During a 10-yr period beginning in the early 1960s, there was an exceptional succession of research findings that had a very profound effect on MD and, indeed, on cancer research in all species including humans. The first major breakthrough was the successful and regular experimental transmission of the disease (31, 400). The avid cell association of the agent (32) made identity of the agent elusive. It was not until 1967 that nearly simultaneous, but independent, research in Great Britain (104) and the USA (290, 444) uncovered a herpesvirus as the etiologic agent, following its successful propagation in cell cultures.

Virus culture and identification were followed by a veritable flood of data in which epizootiology, much of the pathogenesis, and many immunologic aspects of the disease were unraveled. A historic account of this work, which came from many laboratories, was provided by Witter (479). Perhaps the most important practical development was the attenuation of the virus and its successful application as a vaccine against MD (106, 107). Although superseded by other vaccines, it nonetheless was the first practical effective cancer vaccine in any species and should be recognized as a major advance in medical science.

The findings by Fabricant and coworkers (see 138) that MDV infection may lead to arteriosclerosis in chickens have profound implications as a model for the same condition in humans. This discovery, along with continuing studies on the oncogenic and immunologic features of MD as a model of oncogenic herpesvirus infection in other species and the need to develop alternative vaccines or other control methods for flocks with apparent vaccine failures, guarantees that research on the disease will continue.

Additional historical details can be found in a review by Payne (316).

INCIDENCE AND DISTRIBUTION.

MD exists in poultry-producing countries throughout the world, as reviewed by Purchase (355). Quite probably every flock of chickens raised in areas where poultry is prevalent experiences some loss, but reporting systems vary and it is difficult to determine the true incidence.

In the USA the incidence prior to the availability of vaccines was not uniform, largely because of repetitive, acute, explosive outbreaks in certain geographic areas. Losses were especially high in areas where poultry (broiler) raising was intensive. Such areas probably continue to have the greatest risk even in the face of vaccination. This uneven distribution may represent existence of a more virulent form of the disease that can occur as an epizootic in certain areas (25). Several reports lend credence to the implication of exceptionally virulent MDV isolates in vaccine failures on certain premises or in some areas (131, 508, 386, 340; see also 484).

Purchase (355) noted that there is a seasonal incidence in broiler flocks with losses higher during winter months, presumably because of lowered air circulation.

ETIOLOGY

Classification. MDV is characterized as a cell-associated herpesvirus (104, 290, 444). Proof that this herpesvirus was the etiologic agent of MD was acquired through circumstantial evidence (105, 498), reproduction of the disease with cell-free herpesvirus obtained from feather follicle epithelium (FFE) of infected chickens (68), and immunization of chickens against the disease with the attenuated MDV (107).

Two additional groups of nonpathogenic herpesviruses isolated from turkeys (219, 499) and chickens (30, 98), respectively, are considered part of the MDV group. The nonpathogenic chicken isolates are designated as MDVs, often with the modifying terms, nononcogenic or serotype 2. The turkey isolates are designated as turkey herpesviruses, although the common acronym, HVT, derives from an earlier terminology, herpesvirus of turkeys. These viruses, although clearly distinct from oncogenic MDV, are included in this chapter because they are commonly used to immunize chickens against MD and because they are not dealt with elsewhere.

Three serotypes are recognized: oncogenic MDVs are serotype 1, nononcogenic MDVs are serotype 2, and HVTs are serotype 3 (46, 47). Serotype designations are commonly used in conjunction with strain or group names (see also Strain Classification).

Morphology and Morphogenesis. The morphology and morphogenesis of MDV have been reviewed by Kato and Hirai (218) and Schat (379). Hexagonal naked particles or nucleocapsids, 85–100 nm, both with and without electron-dense nucleoids, were found usually in the nucleus and occasionally in the cytoplasm of infected tissue culture cells or in extracellular fluids. Enveloped particles 150–160 nm in diameter were seen occasionally and were principally associated with the nuclear membrane or nuclear vesicles but have been observed in the cytoplasm. Virus particles observed in negatively stained preparations of lysed FFE had envelopes measuring 273–400 nm and appeared as irregular amorphous structures (68). Thin-section preparations of the FFE revealed large numbers of cytoplasmic enveloped herpesvirus particles in keratinizing cells and cytoplasmic inclusion bodies composed of homogeneous amorphous material (Fig. 16.1). Smaller particles of 35 nm (281) or 70 nm (299) were observed in infected cells but were not shown to be structural components in the virion.

In negatively stained preparations the nucleocapsid was observed to have cubic, icosahedral symmetry and to possess 162 hollow-centered capsomeres, which are cylindric and measure 6 × 9 nm. The center-to-center distance between adjacent capsomeres is approximately 10 nm (282). Viral DNA appears to be wound around a central structure connecting two inner poles of the capsid, creating a nucleoid that varies from spherical to toroid (283) and consists of a pair of fibrils arranged in a cohelical configuration (303).

In general, morphology of HVT resembles that of MDV. In thin sections, however, nucleocapsids of HVT commonly show a unique crossed appearance (291). Three-dimensional electron microscopy (EM) revealed two crossed doughnutlike rings at right angles within the nucleocapsid, a finding that presumably explained the cross-shaped appearance in thin sections (302). Through computerized reconstruction of electron micrographs, Okada et al. (304) reported a core structure consisting of six round particles.

The morphology of nonpathogenic strains of MDV has not been studied in detail but typical particles have been visualized (382).

The morphology of MDV and HVT virions is shown in Fig. 16.2.

Viral DNA

PHYSICAL PROPERTIES. The DNA of MDV is a linear, double-stranded molecule that has a buoyant density of 1.706 g/ml, a base composition of 46% guanine plus cytosine ratio, and a molecular weight of 108–120 × 10^6 daltons (88, 169, 240), which is equivalent to a size of 166–184 kilobase pairs. The buoyant density and guanine plus cytosine ratio of HVT DNA is generally similar to that of MDV DNA (241); both are difficult to separate from host cell DNA, but preparative techniques have been described (210). Infectivity of MDV DNA has been demonstrated both in vitro and in vivo (208).

STRUCTURAL ORGANIZATION. The genome structure of MDV and HVT consists of a long unique re-

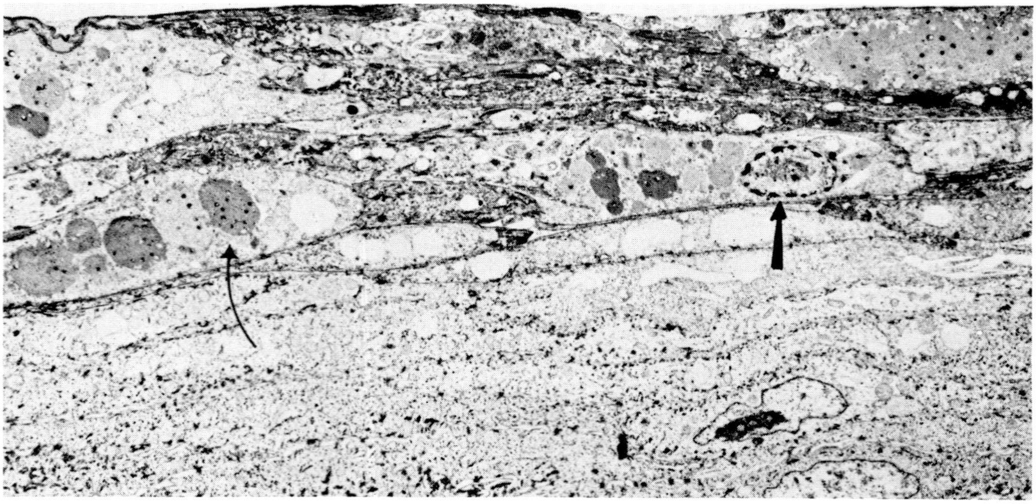

16.1. Thin section of FFE from chicken infected with MDV. These productively infected cells contain both intranuclear (*thick arrow*) and intracytoplasmic (*thin arrow*) inclusion bodies. Intracytoplasmic inclusions contain many enveloped virions. ×5000. (Nazerian)

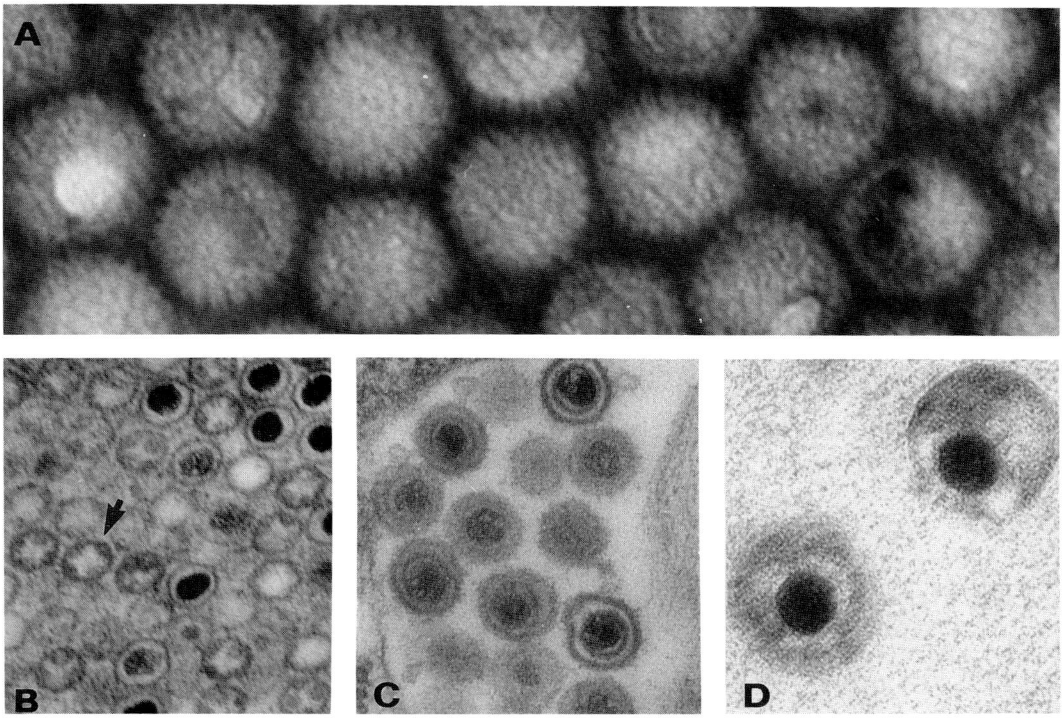

16.2. Electron micrographs of MDV and HVT. A. Negative-stained naked nucleocapsids of MDV showing typical hollow capsomeres. ×180,000. B. Thin section of cultured duck embryo fibroblast infected with HVT. Many nucleocapsids are seen with the typical cross-shaped internal structure (*arrow*). ×70,000. C. Thin section of cultured duck embryo fibroblast infected with MDV showing enveloped virions in a nuclear vesicle. ×60,000. D. Thin section of FFE of chicken infected with MDV showing enveloped virions within the cytoplasmic inclusions. Note difference in morphology compared with C. ×70,000. (Nazerian)

gion and a short unique region, each bounded by inverted repeats (88). Physical maps of restriction endonuclease fragments have been constructed for MDV (148) and HVT (186) but not yet for serotype 2 MDV. Based on cross hybridization of cloned DNA fragments, the genomes of MDV and HVT are similarly organized (186). The MDV genome more closely resembles that of alphaherpesviruses than that of gammaherpesviruses (44), although MDV has been classed as a gammaherpesvirus on the basis of biological criteria (368).

LOCALIZATION OF GENES. Efforts to identify and localize specific genes or genomic regions associated with certain biologic functions have begun to yield useful information. The gene encoding the A antigen of MDV has been localized to the central portion of the unique long region (201). More recently, the gene encoding the B antigen of MDV has been identified and mapped (440).

Efforts to identify genes associated with tumorigenicity have prompted comparisons of virulent and attenuated strains. Structural changes in DNA have been noted upon serial passage of MDV in cell cultures, including a lowered buoyant density (455) and loss of fragments obtained by restriction endonuclease digestion (172). A heterogenous expansion region containing multiple, tandem 132 base pair repeats has been identified in attenuated MDV and mapped to the inverted repeat region flanking the unique long portion of the genome (149, 258, 437). This region has been identified as a gene family containing three exons and is capable of forming five different messages (40). Usually, virulent strains have few copies and attenuated strains have multiple copies of the 132 base pair repeat, but the association of copy number with tumorigenicity is not firm (214, 372), and the function of this region requires further study. Amplification of an unrelated 178 base pair repeat region not associated with oncogenicity has also been described (162).

Random DNA sequencing of MDV and HVT with comparison to other herpesviruses by computer analysis has identified a number of gene homologues, including the DNA polymerase and ribonucleotide reductase (395). Genes for which no function is yet apparent have been tentatively identified by transcriptional analysis (43) or by screening of a genomic DNA library with monoclonal antibodies (239).

DIFFERENCES BETWEEN SEROTYPES. Minor but potentially important differences in the genomes of MDV and HVT have been observed. Compared to HVT, the MDV genome is slightly larger (88, 169) and has a lower buoyant density (169). All three serotypes differ substantially in their restriction endonuclease digestion patterns (375).

The DNAs of the three viral serotypes share limited homology (169, 173, 375). Although higher levels of homology have been demonstrated using less stringent methods (150) and regions of weak homology occur throughout the genome (174, 371), the DNAs of the three viral serotypes are distinguished more by their differences than their similarities.

The DNA of MDV lacks homology with most other herpesviruses (150, 173) but, interestingly, contains regions of homology with a human B-lymphotropic herpesvirus, human herpesvirus (HHV)-6 (223), and the proviral DNA of reticuloendotheliosis virus, an oncogenic avian retrovirus (233). Furthermore, several MDV and HVT genes have apparent homologues detectable by hybridization or by computer analysis of sequence data in other herpesviruses, including herpes simplex and varicella zoster (44, 116, 395). Thus, the relationship of the MDV genome with other herpesviruses may be closer than was originally apparent.

Viral Proteins and Antigens. As many as 46 virus-specific polypeptides have been identified (189, 464, 465), many by immunoprecipitation from extracts of cells infected with MDV or HVT. The functional characterization of antigens has been facilitated by the development of type-specific monoclonal antibodies (176, 190, 248). Thus far, at least six antigens and various other proteins have been characterized as noted in reviews by Kato and Hirai (218) and Ross (371). Nomenclature of MDV proteins has been confusing but the use of molecular weight preceded by the type of protein has gained the support of many workers and is used herein.

The A antigen, originally identified in the supernatant fluids of infected cell cultures by agar-gel precipitation (AGP) tests (106) has been characterized as a 57- to 65-kD molecular weight glycoprotein (gp57/65) (195, 200, 201). It is demonstrated on the cell surface and in the cytoplasm, is actively secreted by infected cells, does not appear related to oncogenicity, and is probably the antigen most readily detected by convalescent antisera in the AGP test. Production of A antigen decreases with serial passage of MDV in cell culture (106, 191), probably due to reduced transcription of the A antigen gene (466). The nucleotide sequence of this gene has been determined (116).

The B antigen, also identified originally by AGP tests as a nonsecreted antigen (106), is a complex of three glycoproteins with molecular weights of 100 kD, 60 kD, and 49 kD (gp100, gp60, gp49) (193, 199, 435). The proteins are derived from a 44-kD precursor polypeptide (436, 439). The antigen is located on both cell surface and in the cytoplasm (218), appears to induce neutralizing antibodies (307), and is believed to play a role in vaccinal immunity, although convincing evidence for this is not available.

Two antigens associated with the nucleus of productively-infected cells have been identified by immunoprecipitation with different monoclonal antibodies; one protein of 135 kD was capable of binding to DNA and another protein of 145–155kD lacked this property (279). These may be related to nuclear antigens detected by immunofluorescence in HVT-infected cells by heterologous MDV antiserum (499). Another 28kD protein that bound to cloned fragments of MDV DNA was recovered from nuclear extracts of latently infected tumor cells but not from productively infected cells (474).

A 92 kD polypeptide was designated as a major virus-specific protein because it reacted with a high proportion of monoclonal antibodies (192). It is located in the cytoplasm of productively infected cells and one of two epitopes was cross reactive with HVT (192).

A virus-specific phosphorylated protein complex containing polypeptides of 39–36 kD and 24 kD was demonstrated in the cytoplasm of MDV-transformed, latently infected lymphocytes as well as productively infected cells including the FFE (194, 278, 280). These antigens were unique to serotype 1 MDV and were demonstrated not only in latently infected cells following treatment with IUdR but also in a high proportion of tumor cells (197).

Virus-induced enzymes include a 100 kD DNA polymerase (39). An 87 kD thymidine kinase was induced in chicken embryo cells by HVT (226) and serotype 1 but not serotype 2 MDV (371, 390).

The possible incorporation of host cell antigens into the envelope of HVT virions is suggested by the ability of anticellular sera to neutralize the virus (270).

Viral membrane antigens and viral internal antigens of unspecified molecular characteristics have been demonstrated by fluorescent antibody (FA) tests (90, 353) and the viral membrane antigen in particular has been extensively studied (198, 267,269, 512).

Virus Replication. Replication of MDV and HVT is typical of other cell-associated herpesviruses, and has been reviewed by Kato and Hirai (218) and Ross (371). Enveloped virions enter the cell by conventional absorption and penetration, which occurs within 1 hr and is enhanced by chelators such as EDTA in the case of MDV (1). The time to appearance was 5 hr for viral antigens, 8 hr for DNA synthesis, 10 hr for nucleocapsid production, and 18 hr for enveloped virion production. Viral synthesis peaked at about 20 hr (170). The growth cycle of HVT required about 48 hr for completion, including a 10-hr eclipse phase (371). Viral DNA replication occurs during the S phase of cell replication (236). Replication rates vary with viral serotype.

More commonly, cells are infected by contact with other infected cells, but in this case temporal relationships are more difficult to define. Cell-to-cell transfer of infection in vitro is enhanced by cell fusion (177), is normally accomplished through formation of intracellular bridges (212), and is presumed to be the principal mode of virus spread, both in vitro and in vivo.

Three general types of virus-cell interactions are recognized: productive, latent, and transforming.

PRODUCTIVE INFECTION. Productive infection occurs mainly in nonlymphocytes but occasionally in lymphocytes. In productive infection, replication of viral DNA occurs, antigens are synthesized, and in some cases virus particles are produced. The number of genome copies per cell can exceed 1200 (216). There are two types of productive infection. Fully productive infection with MDV in the FFE of chickens results in development of large numbers of enveloped, fully infectious virions (68). In some lymphoid and epithelial cells in the chicken and in most cultured cells, a productive-restrictive infection occurs and antigens are produced, but most of the virions produced are nonenveloped and thus noninfectious. However, a variable number of the virions in cultured cells may be enveloped, and these can be recovered cell free and infectious by disruption of cells in distilled water (113) or an appropriate stabilizer (69, 96). A variant strain of HVT that releases large quantities of cell-free virus into the medium of infected cell cultures has been described (513).

Some B lymphocytes present in the bursa, spleen, and thymus during the first week after MDV exposure and a variable but small proportion of cells in some MD lymphomas and lymphoblastoid cell lines appear to be productively infected as evidenced by presence of antigens or virions. The proportion of antigen-containing lymphoid cells can be increased by in vitro culture (75) or treatment with IUdR (76, 126), probably representing a release from latency.

In all types of cells, productive infection is lytic and leads to intranuclear inclusion body formation, cell destruction, and in the chicken, frank necrobiotic lesion formation. Because of this, productive infection has been termed cytolytic and the terms are used synonymously (63). Polykaryocytosis is seen in cultured fibroblasts and is a major component of the viral plaques or foci frequently used as a marker in virus assays.

The antigens produced in productive infection are those described previously. Probably all viral antigens occur, at least in fully productive infections where enveloped virions are produced. It is presumed that productive infection proceeds similarly with all three viral serotypes, both in vitro and in vivo. However, reactions with biotinylated lectins have revealed differences attributed to viral glycoproteins in fibroblasts infected with the three viral serotypes (257).

In productively infected fibroblasts, most of the MDV DNA genome is transcribed and associated with polysomes (371, 438). Transcribed viral RNA can be detected in both nucleus and cytoplasm (371). Differences in transcripts between productive and nonproductive infection (175, 259, 462) and between productive infection with virulent and attenuated serotype 1 strains (38) have been described.

Productive infection in cell cultures is influenced by several factors. Arginine is required (268). The replicative process requires synthesis of a DNA polymerase (39) that can be inhibited by phosphonoacetate (243) and phosphonoformate (365). The effect of other inhibitors of MDV replication has been reviewed by Ross (371). Plaque size was increased or decreased by different doses of dimethylsulfoxide in the culture medium (266). Although interferon may be produced by at least some MDV and HVT strains (181, 211), its effect on virus replication appears slight (10). Growth rate of MDV and HVT in vitro is also influenced by virus strain, culture temperature, and cell type.

LATENT INFECTION. A second type of virus-cell interaction in MDV infection (latency) has been observed only in lymphocytes, predominantly in T cells, but also in some B cells (430). A possible exception is Schwann cells and satellite cells in spinal ganglia (328). Latent infections are nonproductive and can be detected only by hybridization with DNA probes or methods designed to activate the viral genome such as in vitro cultivation. Only about five copies of the viral genome are present (371). By definition, the viral genome is not expressed and, in practice, no virus- or tumor-associated antigens are found (75, 407). However, in vitro cultivation results in production of viral antigens and virus particles (75, 85,87) through a release from latency. A cytokine produced by concanavalin A–stimulated spleen cell cultures can help maintain latency in cultured lymphocytes (54). Latent infection has been demonstrated following infection of chickens with serotype 2 and 3 viruses (429).

TRANSFORMING INFECTION. A third type of interaction, transforming infection, is characteristic of most transformed cells from MD lymphomas and lymphoblastoid cell lines derived from such lymphomas. This type of infection occurs only in T lymphocytes of chickens and has been demonstrated only with virulent serotype 1 MDV. Presumably, a latent infection is a prerequisite to transformation. Unlike latent infection in which the viral genome is present but is not expressed, the transformed phenotype is characterized by limited expression of the MDV genome. Transformed cells contain about 5–15 copies of viral genome (371), although the mean number varies in different cell lines under different conditions, perhaps in relation to the proportion of productively infected cells in the population (171, 242, 292). Viral antigens (detectable by FA tests with convalescent sera) and virions are not observed, although a portion of the viral genome may be transcribed (438). A number of transcripts in transformed cells have been identified and mapped to selected regions of the viral genome; these transcripts differ from those in productively infected cells (175, 462), but these differences are best demonstrated in lines with a low proportion of antigen-positive cells (392).

The viral DNA of transformed cells is highly methylated whereas methylation was not detected in viral DNA from productively infected cells (215).

Of the several viral antigens, only the phosphorylated protein (pp36/39 and pp24) has been detected in transformed cells both in vitro and in vivo (197, 280). This antigen is induced by serotype 1 MDV but not by the nononcogenic serotype 2 and 3 viruses, thus suggesting it may play a possible role in the process of transformation.

Some transformed lymphocytes can be induced to produce viral antigens by treatment with iododeoxyuridine (126, 76) or by culture at suboptimal temperatures (9, 76). Some rare cells may spontaneously convert to a productive state, thus explaining the occasional antigen-positive cells observed in tumors and lymphoblastoid cell lines (5, 76). Although transformed cells induced into productive infection would be expected to produce the full range of viral antigens, there is some evidence for the absence of A antigen in such cells (373).

A number of nonviral antigens are associated with transformed cells.

A MD tumor-associated surface antigen (MATSA), was detected on cells from MD lymphomas and lymphoblastoid cell lines derived from lymphomas (344, 505). This antigen was not detected on the surface of productively infected cells (505). The MATSAs on different transformed cells were related but not identical (425, 505). Although initially it did not appear to be associated with most latently infected lymphocytes (75, 407), MATSA was also detected on lymphocytes from chickens vaccinated with HVT or nononcogenic strains of MDV (224, 341, 384); subsequent studies with monoclonal antibodies (249, 252) revealed MATSA to be present on activated T cells from uninfected chickens (265). Thus, MATSA is now considered to be a host antigen and is clearly not tumor specific. However, it still has importance in the differential diagnosis of MD.

Other nonviral antigens expressed on transformed cells include T cell (344) and other thymocyte antigens (230, 263), chicken fetal antigen (277), alpha fetoprotein (294), histocompatibility antigens (49), Ia-like antigen (387), a metastasis-specific antigen (428), a Hanganutziu and Deicher heterophile antigen (188), Forssman antigen (187), a chicken thrombocyte-associated antigen (165), and CD4, an antigen found on helper T cells (393). Functional roles for these antigens have not been determined.

INTEGRATION OF VIRAL DNA. Tanaka et al. (454) found no evidence for integration of viral DNA with the host cell genome. However, both integrated and free viral DNA has been demonstrated in nonproductively infected cells (217, 377), the nonintegrated DNA being in circular plasmid forms (377). The state of viral DNA integration seems to differ in different cell lines (218, 371). Viral DNA was associated with chromosomes of two size classes separated by density-gradient centrifugation (183) and with chromosome numbers 2 and 4 by in situ hybridization (218), further supporting the idea that some integration occurs. However, the nature of the association of viral and cellular DNA remains elusive.

DIFFERENCES BETWEEN SEROTYPES. In most reports, replication of MDV and HVT are similar. All three serotypes induce productive infection in permissive fibroblast cultures. Latent infection also occurs with all viruses. However, transforming infection has only been demonstrated with virulent MDV. Since HVT and serotype 2 MDV are nononcogenic (382, 499), no cell lines have been developed equivalent to those derived from MD lymphomas. However, a cell line has been derived from spleen cells of a chicken vaccinated with HVT (225) that has genomes of both MDV and HVT (171). The virus responsible for transformation is not clear, but the ability of both genomes to coexist in a single cell is of interest. Calnek et al. (71) also recovered infectious HVT and MDV from a single cell line.

VIRUS STOCK PRODUCTION. Productively infected cell cultures have been a common source of cell-associated virus stocks for all three viral serotypes and for cell-free HVT stocks. Cell-free virus from serotypes 1 and 2 is best obtained from FFE (low-passage virus) or infected cell cultures (high-passage virus) although small quantities of low-passage virus can be obtained from lysed infected cells in vitro. Techniques for the production and cryopreservation of virus stocks have been described (32, 69,446).

Stability and Disinfection. MDVs and HVT exist in either cell-associated or cell-free states, which have greatly different survival properties. Infectivity of cell-associated stocks of MDV or HVT is directly related to viability of the cells contained in these preparations.

Cell-free preparations of MDV obtained from skin of infected chickens were inactivated when treated for 10 min at pH 3 or 11 and stored for 2 wk at 4 C, 4 days at 25 C, 18 hr at 37 C, 30 min at 56 C, or 10 min at 60 C (65). Cell-free MDV from skin, and either MDV or HVT from infected cultured cells, can be stored at −70 C; with suitable stabilizers they can be lyophilized with minimal loss of infectivity (69).

Litter and feathers from infected chickens are infectious, and presumably contain cell-free virus from the FFE bound to cellular debris. The infectivity of such materials was retained for 4–8 mo at room temperature (179, 496) and for at least 10 yr at 4 C (59), but the virus was inactivated by a variety of common chemical disinfectants within a 10-min treatment period (67, 180). Survival of virus is adversely affected by increased humidity.

Influence of additives such as antibiotics on viability of cell-associated HVT vaccine has been investigated. Certain antibiotics (128) and other additives producing osmolality of 475 mOsm/kg (112) were highly detrimental, whereas other antibiotics appeared safe (130). Potency of both cell-associated and cell-free vaccines can be adversely affected by storage temperature, reconstitution technique, choice of diluent, and holding time and temperature after reconstitution (157, 297, 313, 434). Under ideal conditions the half-life of diluted, cell-associated vaccines may be 2–6 hr (460); however, it is prudent for vaccines to be administered within 1 hr to avoid unnecessary loss of titer (313).

Strain Classification

SEROTYPES. Bülow and Biggs (46, 47) first provided a serologic classification of the MDV-related herpesviruses. By AGP and FA tests three distinct virus groups were identified that correlated with biological properties. These groups were virulent MDVs, avirulent MDVs, and HVT. This serotypic classification has been confirmed through the use of type-specific monoclonal antibodies (190, 248).

Although distinguishable by serologic tests, the three serotypes also share many common antigens. Thus sera against one serotype will usually react with antigens of other serotypes, although somewhat less vigorously than with homologous antigens.

PATHOTYPES. Virulence or oncogenicity is associated only with serotype 1 MDVs. However, within this group a wide variation in pathogenic potential is recognized. Because this variation undoubtedly represents a continuum from nearly avirulent to maximally virulent, subclassifications are arbitrary at best. However, a need to distinguish strains that were well protected against by HVT vaccine from those that were not was recognized and prompted a pathotypic classification (482, 483) by which three classes of viruses and associated acronyms are designated as mild (mMDV), virulent (vMDV) or very virulent (vvMDV). Criteria have been presented, particularly for vMDVs and vvMDVs, that involve pathogenicity tests in vaccinated or unvaccinated chickens (487). Examples are the CU2 (441) strain of mMDV; the JM (400), GA (127), and HPRS-16 (356) strains of vMDVs; and the Md5 (508) and RB1B (388) strains of vvMDVs.

A pattern of evolution in the virulence of MDV strains is recognized. For many years MDVs induced a classical disease and were probably mMDVs. The vMDV strains were first noted in the late 1950s (23) and became the dominant type during the 1960s. The vvMDV strains were first noted in the late 1970s (131), mainly in HVT-vaccinated flocks with excessive MD losses. Selection pressure for increased virulence exists and may result in even more virulent pathotypes in the future.

BIOLOGICAL CHARACTERISTICS. Isolates of each serotype possess distinguishing biologic characteristics in vitro as first described by Biggs and Milne (30) and reviewed by Schat (379). Pathogenic serotype 1 viruses grow best in duck embryo fibroblast or chicken kidney cell cultures, grow slowly, and produce small plaques. Serotype 2 viruses grow best in chicken embryo fibroblasts, grow slowly, and produce medium plaques with some large syncytia. Serotype 3 viruses (HVT) grow best in chicken embryo fibroblasts, grow rapidly, and produce large plaques. More infectious virus can be extracted from HVT-infected cells than from cells infected with serotype 1 or 2 viruses. Also, a quail fibroblast cell line designated QT-35 (275) supported growth of HVT but was refractory to serotype 1 and 2 viruses (97), although Cowen and Braun (117) described limitêd replication of serotype 2 and 3 viruses in this line.

Shek et al. (429, 430) found that lymphocytes serving as primary targets for infection differed for the three serotypes. Whereas oncogenic MDV infected B cells, serotype 2 MDV and HVT infected two different cell populations that were neither B cells nor macrophages.

Serial passage in vitro results in attenuation of virulent isolates (106, 367, 481) with loss of certain antigens and a marked decrease in ability to infect and/or replicate in lymphocytes (391). Attenuated strains do not spread well by contact among chickens (121, 486). Some strains are incompletely attenuated and induce minor lesions in susceptible chickens (50, 332,486). Overattenuated strains do not replicate in or protect chickens (231, 492). The in vivo growth potential of attenuated serotype 1 isolates has been improved by back passage in chickens (122, 486), although in one case virulence was also increased (486). A temperature-sensitive mutant of MDV (492) and a mutant of HVT that was resistant to inhibition by phosphonoacetate (244) have been described. Thus, MDVs appear to be susceptible to mutation during replication both in vitro and in vivo.

Tumors in visceral organs, skin, and muscle are often induced by vMDVs, although other vMDVs and mMDVs may induce lesions principally in peripheral nerves and gonads. Enlargement of peripheral nerves is characteristic of infection induced by all MDV pathotypes. Since distribution of gross lesions varies greatly among different strains of host chickens, this criterion may be of less value than virulence in characterizing and classifying isolates.

The incidence of tumors induced by low-virulence strains of serotype 1 MDV is increased by infection in ovo or by immunosuppression (70, 74). Viruses of serotype 2 and 3 remained nononcogenic following similar treatments (74, 382).

Laboratory Host Systems. MDV has been propagated and assayed in newly hatched chicks, tissue cultures, and embryonated eggs. Lymphoblastoid cell lines from MD lymphomas and transplantable tumors are also important laboratory host systems.

CHICKENS. Newly hatched chicks inoculated with virulent serotype 1 MDV develop lesions that can be detected histologically in ganglia, nerves, and certain viscera after 2–4 wk. Response is greatly dependent on genetic susceptibility of the chicken and virulence of the MDV isolate. Presence of virus or antibody, which can be detected by in vitro tests, or presence of virus-associated antigen detected by FA tests on tissues, are also specific host responses of inoculated chickens to MD infection. All these responses are markedly enhanced in chicks lacking maternal antibodies against MDV (56). The induction of virus-specific lesions in the wing web (84) or the feather pulp (274) constitute alternate host systems that provide direct access to the site of lesion development.

CELL CULTURES. Cultured duck embryo fibroblasts or chicken kidney cells are suitable for propagation of virulent MDV isolates (104, 444). Attenuated MDV and serotype 2 and 3 viruses all grow well on chicken embryo fibroblast cultures (30, 382). Infected cultures usually develop discrete focal lesions, which consist of clusters of rounded, refractile degenerating cells when mature. These lesions are called foci or plaques (Fig. 16.3A-F). Lesions are usually less than 1 mm in diameter and of variable cell density. Affected cells may contain two or more nuclei, and type A intranuclear inclusion bodies are commonly seen. Despite release of rounded cells into the medium as plaques mature, large areas of cell lysis are not seen.

Serotype 1 plaques develop in 5–14 days on primary isolation and in 3–7 days after adaptation to culture and are usually enumerated by microscopic examination. Differences in development and morphology of serotype 1 plaques in chick and duck cells (445, 497) and in plaques induced by the three viral serotypes (30, 379) have been described. Other cell culture systems such as chick embryo skin (349) or tracheal explants (362) have been used also.

Serotype 1, but not serotype 2, MDVs can be grown in chicken splenic lymphocytes in vitro (77). Passages are made by the addition of fresh spleen cells to the suspension cell cultures every 2 days, and infection is monitored by immunofluorescence. HVT may be similarly grown in turkey spleen cell cultures, but viral antigen is seen rarely if at all.

EMBRYOS. Virus pocks (Fig. 16.4) develop on the chorioallantoic membrane (CAM) of chicken embryos following yolk sac inoculation with cellular MDV preparations (29, 45). Injection into the yolk sac usually obviates the nonspecific graft-vs-host pocks that are common when immunologically competent cells are inoculated directly onto the CAM. The sensitivity of this procedure for detecting virus in blood or buffy coat cells is about equal to that of cell culture assay (29). Embryos have also been used to study immune responses to MD vaccines. In this case, embryos inoculated in the amnionic sac on the 18th day are

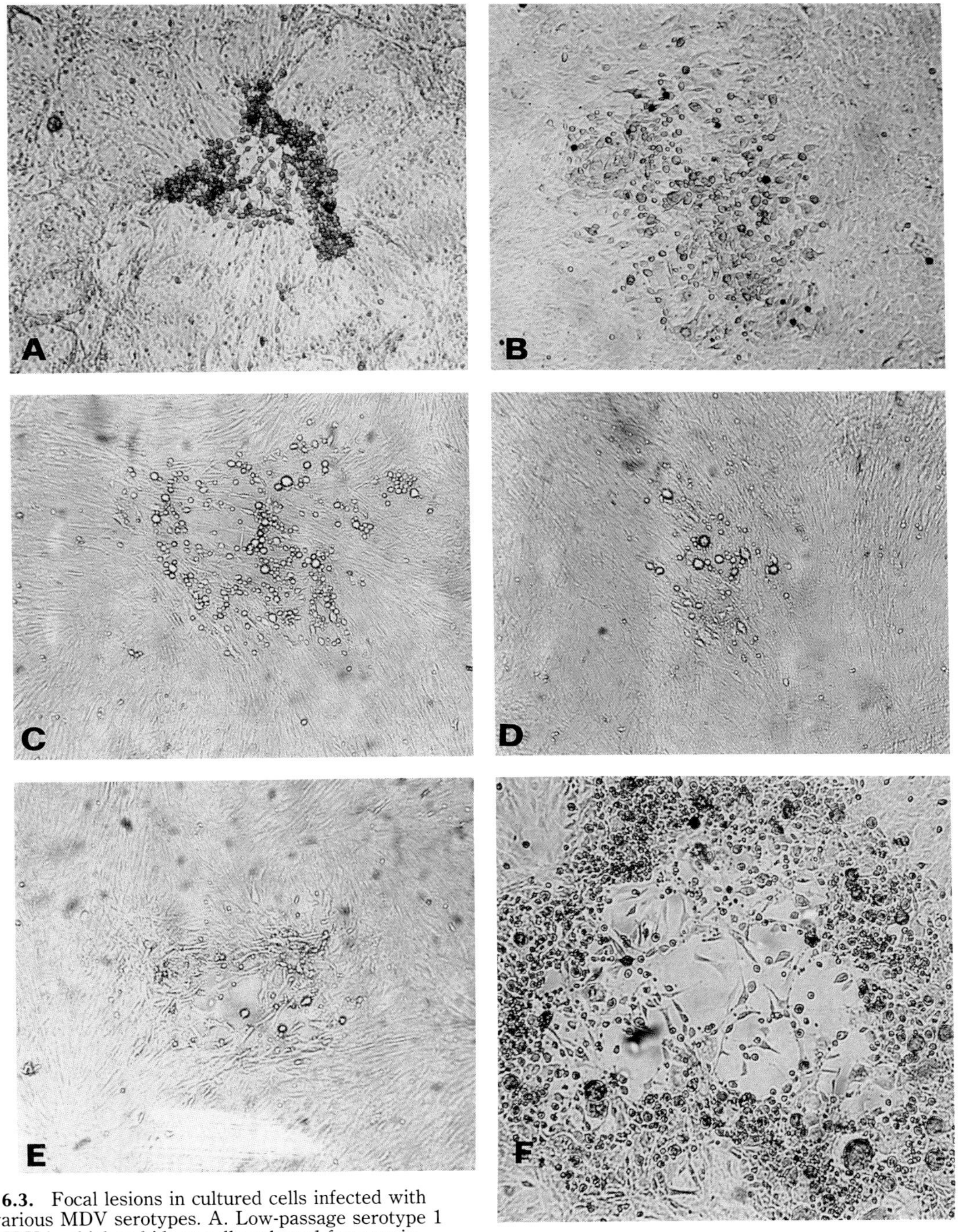

16.3. Focal lesions in cultured cells infected with various MDV serotypes. A. Low-passage serotype 1 MDV in chicken kidney cells cultured from an infected chicken, 9 days. B. Low-passage serotype 1 MDV in duck embryo fibroblasts (DEF), 5 days. C. High-passage, attenuated serotype 1 MDV in chicken embryo fibroblasts (CEF), 5 days. D. Low-passage serotype 2 MDV in CEF, 8 days. E. Low-passage serotype 3 HVT in CEF, 4 days. F. Low-pasage HVT in DEF, 12 days. All photos unstained, about ×40.

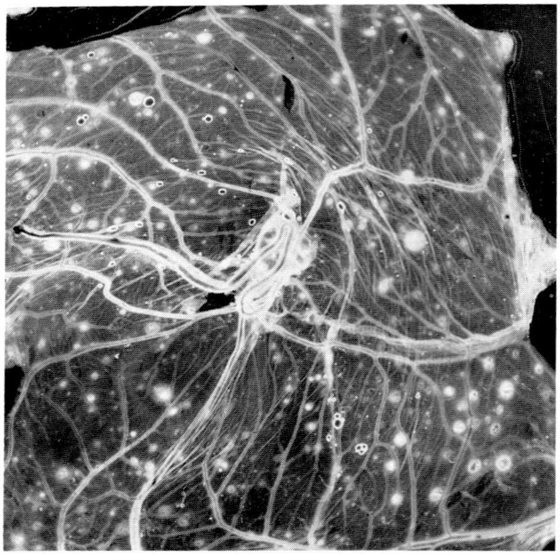

16.4. CAM from 19-day-old chicken embryo inoculated via yolk sac at 4 days with blood from chickens infected with JM isolate.

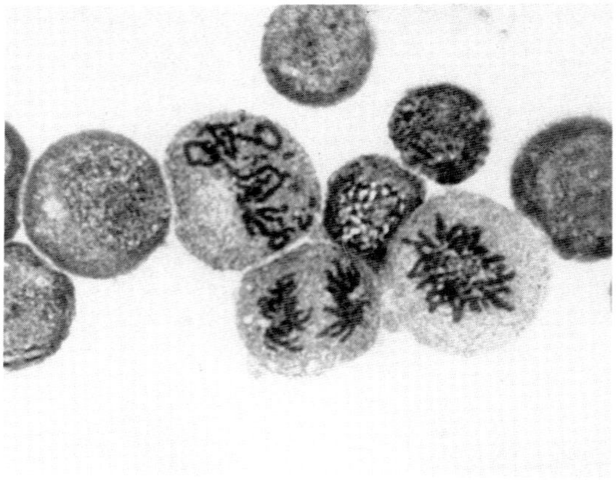

16.5. Smear from the MDCC-RP1 cell line. Note the characteristic lymphoblastoid morphology and the mitotic figures. Giemsa. (Nazerian)

protected earlier than those vaccinated at hatching (413). The growth potential of serotype 1 MDV is less than for serotypes 2 and 3 in 18-day embryos (411).

LYMPHOBLASTOID CELL LINES. Lymphoblastoid cell lines were first developed from MD lymphomas by Akiyama et al. (6) and subsequently by many other workers (see 64, 285). These grow continuously in cell culture without attachment to the culture vessel. They have T-cell markers and MATSA and most can be termed "producer" lines since a small proportion (1–2%) of the cells enter into productive infection (344). Virus can be readily recovered from most cell lines, although several nonproducer cell lines have been developed in which evidence of genome expression is limited or lacking (293, 326,454). In one such line (MDCC-RP1) the MDV genome may be incomplete because no virus can be rescued by in vitro or in vivo assays (293). Prolonged culture can result in reduced expression of the MDV genome (264).

Success rates for establishing cell lines from MD lymphomas have improved because of better methodology (76, 326). One cell line generated from in vitro infection has been reported (196). Many cell lines are now available (285) including several from MD lymphomas in turkeys. Cells of the MDCC-RP1 line are illustrated in Fig. 16.5.

TUMOR TRANSPLANTS. Somewhat like lymphoblastoid cell lines, transplantable lymphoid tumors derived from MD lymphomas serve as valuable laboratory host systems. Most transplantable tumors have been developed by rapid serial passage of tumor cells in chickens (203, 458,114). Such tumors may produce neoplastic growth at the site of inoculation or a generalized neoplastic disease, including lymphoblastic leukemia. The pathologic manifestations induced in inoculated chickens may vary with the transplant (143).

One such transplant, originally developed by Sevoian et al. (402) and designated JMV, has been used to challenge immunity of chickens inoculated with HVT (261, 399, 448) and as an experimental immunogen (431). JMV cells contain the MDV genome and express MATSA, but no productively infected cells were detected and chickens inoculated with this tumor did not show evidence of herpesvirus infection (451).

Other transplantable MD lymphomas have been developed; some from chickens homozygous at the Ea-B locus should be particularly useful (72, 110, 452).

PATHOGENESIS AND EPIZOOTIOLOGY

Natural and Experimental Hosts. The natural host range for MD is not well defined because reports of pathology characteristic of MD have usually lacked accompanying etiologic criteria. Nonetheless, it is clear that chickens are by far the most important natural host and that MD is very rare and probably of no real importance in other species, with the possible exception of quail.

Kenzy and Cho (221) isolated MDV from a mature quail that had ocular MD lesions. Pradhan et al. (347, 348) were able not only to isolate MDV from MD-affected Japanese quail raised on a poultry farm, but also to successfully transmit the disease to other quail and to chickens. Powell and Rennie (342) found chicken-quail hybrids to be susceptible to MD.

Turkeys hatched and held in strict isolation under experimental conditions were the source of an oncogenic MDV indistinguishable from chicken isolates (504), but there has been no confirmatory evidence that turkeys are a natural host for MDV. Lymphomas have been induced in turkeys following inoculation with oncogenic MDV (134, 346, 401).

Virus isolation attempts and serologic evidence have shown that red jungle fowl (*Gallus murghi*) and Ceylon jungle fowl (*Gallus gallus sonnerati*) can also be naturally infected (99, 473). Gross and microscopic lesions suggestive of MD have been observed in a variety of avian species including pheasants, pigeons, ducks, geese, canaries, budgerigars, swans, Japanese quail, and great horned owls (156, 205, 476). However, etiology of the lesions was not established. Morgan (273), Mohanty et al. (272), and Cho and Kenzy (99) failed to find virologic or serologic evidence of natural infection in apparently exposed zoo birds or free-ranging birds except for some genera (especially *Gallus*) of the order Galliformes.

Experimental transmission of MD was claimed for pheasants (161, 204). Sparrows were refractory to infection (221), whereas ducks became infected but without disease after MDV inoculation (20). Various mammalian species including hamsters, rats, marmosets, and monkeys (cynomolgus, rhesus, bonnet) were refractory to infection with virulent MDV (105, 178, 367, 421, 423).

Transmission. Direct or indirect contact between birds effects virus spread, apparently by the airborne route (see 28). The apparent paradox of these observations, considering the avid cell association of MDV, was solved when it was discovered that the virus replicates to the fully infectious state in FFE (68) (see Fig. 16.1). Affected follicular epithelial cells are in the keratinizing layer of stratified squamous epithelium; they slough off or detach with molted feathers to serve as a source of contamination to the environment. Virus associated with feathers and dander is infectious (21, 68, 207), and contaminated poultry house dust remains infectious for at least several months at 20–25 C and for years at 4 C (60).

Many apparently normal birds are carriers that can transmit the infection (221). Infection probably persists indefinitely; some birds were found to shed virus from skin as long as 76 wk (501). Continual shedding of virus by infected birds and hardiness of the virus (see Etiology) make prevalence of infection easy to understand.

Studies relating to transfer hosts for MDV were reviewed by Witter (480). Darkling beetles (*Alphitobius diaperinus*) were shown to passively carry the virus; however, free-living litter mites, mosquitoes, and coccidial oocysts could not be associated with transmission.

Witter and Solomon (494) noted that a preponderance of data argues strongly against egg transmission. It is now generally conceded that vertical transmission, if it occurs at all, is so rare as to be of no significance. Transmission from dam to progeny as the result of external egg contamination is also unlikely because of poor virus survival at temperature and humidity levels employed for incubation (67).

Experimental transmission is effected most consistently by inoculation of day-old, genetically susceptible chicks with blood, tumor suspensions, or cell-free virus or by direct or indirect contact with infected birds. Intratracheal instillation or inhalation exposure using cell-free virus is also effective for experimental transmission. With inoculation of tumor cell suspensions there is always the hazard of inducing tumors by cell transplantation; however, transplantation is not the usual cause of lesions in experimental birds (309).

The transmission of serotype 2 and 3 viruses is discussed under Turkey and Chicken Herpesviruses.

Incubation Period. The incubation period for experimentally induced MD is rather well established (see reviews 60, 324, 355). Chicks inoculated at 1 day of age excrete virus beginning at about 2 wk postinfection (PI) (220), with maximal shedding occurring between 3 and 5 wk (480). Cytolytic infections at 3–6 days PI are followed by degenerative lesions in lymphoid organs within 6–8 days PI. Mononuclear infiltrations may be found in nerves and other organs after about 2 wk (321). Clinical signs and gross lesions, however, generally do not appear until between 3 and 4 wk (319, 400).

While these figures represent the shortest incubation, there can be considerable variation. The same factors that influence incidence of disease also affect incubation period. These include virus strain, dosage, and route of infection as well as age, genetic strain, and sex of the host. Induction of tumors within 10–14 days after inoculation of cellular material is suggestive of a transplantation response, although death from an "early mortality syndrome" may occur as early as 8–12 days PI (508).

It is difficult to determine incubation period of the disease under field conditions. While outbreaks sometimes occur in birds as young as 3–4 wk, most serious cases begin after 8 or 9 wk, and it is usually impossible to determine the time and conditions of exposure. Purchase (355) noted that clinical signs in egg-type flocks are often not seen until 16–20 wk, and rarely as late as 24–30 wk. Nicholls (298) noted one outbreak as late as 60 wk. The transient paralysis that occasionally affects birds occurs at about 6–10 wk.

Signs. Signs associated with MD have been described by numerous workers as reviewed by

Biggs (26). In general, they are those associated with asymmetric progressive paresis and, later, complete paralysis of one or more of the extremities. Since any one or several nerves may be affected, signs vary from bird to bird. Wing involvement is characterized by drooping of the limb. If nerves controlling neck muscles are affected, the head may be held low and there may be some torticollis. Vagal involvement can result in paralysis and dilation of the crop and/or gasping. Because locomotor disturbances are easily recognized, incoordination or stilted gait may be the first observed sign. A particularly characteristic attitude is that in which the bird has one leg stretched forward and the other back as a result of unilateral paresis or paralysis of the leg.

A transient paralysis syndrome associated with MD has been described and reproduced (396). Affected birds display varying degrees of ataxia and partial or whole body paralysis lasting 1–2 days. Many affected birds may recover only to succumb a few weeks later from clinical MD. Electroencephalographic abnormalities during the period of clinical signs suggest that this syndrome is an inflammatory encephalopathy (232).

With acute outbreaks of MD the syndrome is much more explosive and initially is characterized by a high proportion of birds with severe depression. A few days later some but not all birds develop ataxia and subsequent unilateral or bilateral paralysis of extremities. Others may die without extensive clinical disease. Many birds become dehydrated, emaciated, and comatose.

Blindness may result from involvement of the iris. Affected eyes gradually lose their ability to accommodate to light intensity. Clinical examination also reveals changes varying from concentric annular or spotty depigmentation or diffuse bluish fading to diffuse grayish opacity of the iris (see Fig. 16.17C). The pupil at first becomes irregular and at advanced stages is only a small pinpoint opening.

Nonspecific signs such as weight loss, paleness, anorexia, and diarrhea may be observed, especially in birds in which the course is prolonged. Under commercial conditions death often results from starvation and dehydration because of inability to reach food and water or in many cases from trampling by penmates.

Morbidity and Mortality. Incidence of MD is quite variable. A few birds that develop signs may recover from the clinical disease (32), but in general, mortality is nearly equal to morbidity. Prior to use of vaccines, losses in affected flocks were estimated to range from a few birds to 25 or 30% and occasionally as high as 60%. Presently between 95 and 100% of egg-type chickens are vaccinated against MD, and this has reduced losses to less than 5% in most countries (355). Broiler flocks, which are vaccinated in some but not other countries, may experience losses of 0.1–0.5% and condemnations of 0.2% or more (355), although the average condemnation rate in the USA was 0.04% in 1987 (489).

MD occurs in chickens 3–4 wk of age or older and is most common between 12 and 30 wk of age although outbreaks at 60 wk have been described (298). Mortality builds gradually and generally persists for 4–10 weeks. Outbreaks occur in isolated flocks, or occasionally in several flocks in a region, or in succeeding flocks on a farm.

A number of factors influence the extent of losses in affected flocks. These deal with either the infective agent or host. Those specifically related to the agent are virus strain, dosage, and route of exposure. Strains of virus associated with acute outbreaks of MD are more virulent and cause a higher disease incidence than those associated with the so-called classic form of the disease (33, 356,379). The degree of pathogenicity (morbidity and mortality) thus depends in part on the virus strain. However, virulence of a given strain in turn depends in part on genetic constitution of the host (386, 442).

Dosage may be a factor under natural conditions, although the MD response in genetically susceptible birds given virulent virus was found to be maximal even when a limiting dilution of virus was inoculated (442). Dosage may be more significant in immunologically competent hosts (genetically resistant birds that have acquired age resistance) or with viruses of lower virulence. Route of exposure probably functions in the same manner; less efficient routes may effectively decrease the dose to the bird.

Influential host factors include sex, passive antibody, genetic constitution, and age. Biggs (27) cited several studies in which it was observed that females experienced higher losses than males; their greater susceptibility was manifested in a shorter latent period. The difference was apparently not due to sex hormones, was most pronounced with susceptible strains of chickens, and was apparent only in the case of infection with the more virulent virus isolates (vMDVs).

Passive antibody (see Immunity) reduces MD mortality (103) and clinical signs of transient paralysis and early mortality syndrome (312), probably by limiting spread of virus in tissues during the first few days postexposure (58).

Both genetic factors (see Prevention and Control) and age are important in determining the level of morbidity and mortality (see reviews 61, 109). It seems probable that host immune response to infection is the most significant event and that this forms a common basis to what has been called "genetic resistance" or "age resistance." Indeed, these two types are probably the same, since resistance associated with age could generally be associated with genetically resistant strains and to a much lesser degree with susceptible strains (7, 27, 58, 470, 503).

In studies comparing genetic strains (see reviews 60, 61, 337, 338, 396), resistance correlated with development of virus-neutralizing antibody (57, 418) and retention of cell-mediated immune functions (247, 385). This resulted from a sparing of immune competence in the case of resistant birds rather than from an inherent difference between strains (166, 167, 441). Lesion regression has been identified as the basis for age-related resistance (422); success of thymectomy and X-radiation (422) but failure of bursectomy (419) to circumvent resistance points to cellular immunity as the mediating factor.

Other resistance mechanisms that might conceivably influence incidence of MD morbidity and mortality include interferon production and natural killer (NK) cell activity. Settnes (396) offered a review of possible effects of interferon in MD. Interferon levels as an early response to MDV infection may be higher in resistant than susceptible birds (181), and there is a protective effect of interferon against the transplantable JMV tumor (467). However, since early pathogenesis is unaffected by age or genetic strain, a significant role for interferon in these resistance factors is unlikely.

NK cells (see reviews 337, 381) have been shown to be cytotoxic for MD tumor cells (234, 416). Sharma and Coulson (415) suggested a possible relationship between these cells and age-related MD resistance, and Sharma (406) subsequently reported that NK cell activity was greater in MD-resistant N-line than in MD-susceptible P-line chickens. Heller and Schat (163) were able to confirm the former (age) but not the latter (genetic) relationship.

Various environmental or other factors have been claimed to affect incidence of MD. Gross (152) observed increased incidence among chickens subjected to a high degree of social stress (or selected for high concentrations of plasma corticosterone), and Powell and Davison (339) showed that administration of corticosteroids to latently infected chickens precipitated the appearance of clinical MD. This could be related to a reactivation of infection, which has been shown to occur following immunosuppression (55). Reduced feed intake delayed and reduced incidence, and selection of chickens for fast growth rate seemed to correlate with increased susceptibility (158, 159).

Gross Lesions. Pathological changes in MD have been well summarized and reviewed (324, 317). Nerve lesions are the most constant findings in affected birds. Macroscopic changes are not seen in the brain, but gross lesions can usually be found in one or more peripheral nerves and spinal roots and root ganglia. Lesion distribution appears to be similar for natural and experimental diseases (311, 319). Goodchild (151) made detailed macroscopic examinations of 502 birds with MD and found that certain autonomic nerves, as well as the more obvious nerves and plexuses, were commonly affected. Ninety-nine percent of the cases could have been diagnosed by examining only the following: celiac, cranial mesenteric, brachial, and sciatic plexuses; nerve of Remak; and greater splanchnic nerve. The celiac plexus was most commonly involved; it was positive in 78% of the birds. Usually, plexuses of the sciatic and brachial nerves are more enlarged than the respective trunks. Sevoian et al. (400) found that dorsal root ganglia were consistently affected in chicks inoculated with JM strain.

Affected peripheral nerves are characterized by loss of cross-striations, gray or yellow discoloration, and sometimes an edematous appearance. Localized or diffuse enlargement causes the affected portion to be two to three times normal size, in some cases much more. Because lesions are often unilateral, it is especially helpful to compare opposite nerves in the case of slight changes. Careful examination of the various nerve ramifications may be necessary to expose gross lesions in some birds, since enlargement can vary in degree from one portion of an affected nerve to another. Figure 16.6 illustrates characteristic gross changes in nerves.

Pappenheimer et al. (311) described affected spinal root ganglia as enlarged, somewhat translucent, and of slightly yellowish tinge. Enlargement was rarely symmetric and lesions often extended into contiguous tissue of the spinal cord. Ganglia may be exposed by removal of the dorsal part of the vertebral column.

Lymphoid tumors may occur in one or more of a variety of organs. The gonad (especially the ovary) is most often affected, but lymphomatous lesions can also be found in lung, heart, mesen-

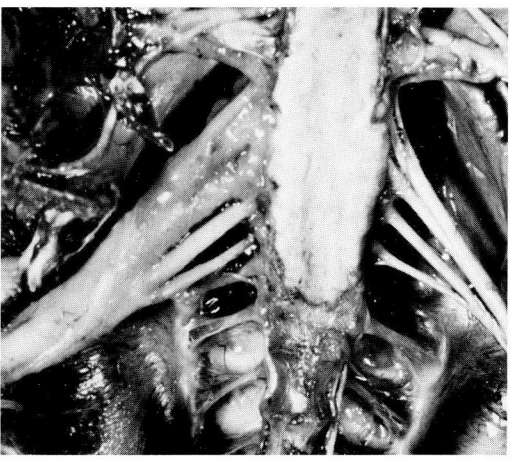

16.6. Leukotic sciatic plexus (*left*) and normal plexus (*right*). (Peckham)

tery, kidney, liver, spleen, bursa, thymus, adrenal gland, pancreas, proventriculus, intestine, iris, skeletal muscle, and skin. Probably no site is without occasional involvement. Visceral tumors are especially common in more acute forms of the disease and may be found in absence of gross nerve lesions. Virus isolates from severe outbreaks tested by Purchase and Biggs (356) induced visceral lesions in 62–89% of inoculated birds. In contrast, an isolate from a milder (classic) case of MD caused visceral lymphomata in only 5–7% of inoculated birds.

Macroscopic changes in affected viscera, with possible exception of the bursa of Fabricius, are indistinguishable from leukotic lesions induced by other agents (e.g., lymphoid leukosis virus). Enlargement of the organ, sometimes to several times normal size, is evident, and there is diffuse grayish discoloration. In some birds nodular tumorlike growths are found within and extending from the parenchyma of the organ. These are firm and smooth when cut. Involvement of the lung results in solidification (Fig. 16.7).

glands. These areas may be seen through the serosal surface or on section. Affected hearts are pale from diffuse infiltration or have single or multiple nodular tumors in the myocardium (Fig. 16.8). Skin lesions are usually associated with, but not limited to, feather follicles. They may coalesce. Distinct whitish nodules (Fig. 16.17A), especially evident in the dressed carcass, may become scablike with brownish crust formation in extreme cases (23). Lapen and Kenzy (235) found lesions in certain feather tracts more frequently than in others; highest incidences were in external and internal crural and dorsal cervical tracts. Muscle lesions may be in both superficial and deep layers and, according to Benton and Cover (23), are most common in pectoral muscles. Gross changes vary from tiny whitish streaks to nodular tumors. Affected areas are a lusterless whitish gray or may have a definite yellow-orange color (probably associated with necrosis). Muscle lesions can also include atrophic changes of neurogenic origin when nerve trunks are severely affected (256, 477).

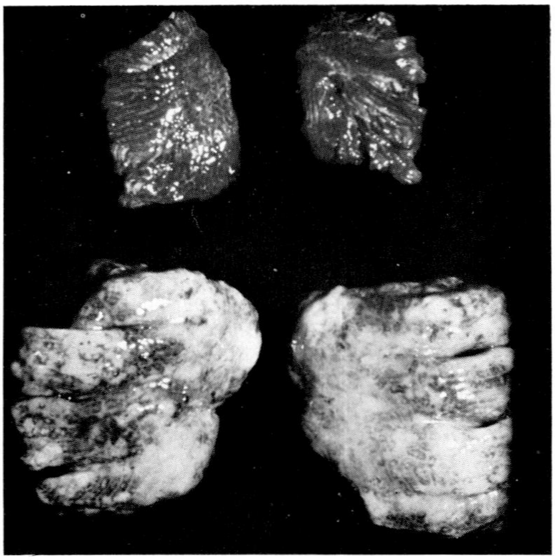

16.7. Normal lungs (*top*). Lungs severely affected with MD tumors and composed mostly of leukotic tumor cells (*bottom*). (Purchase)

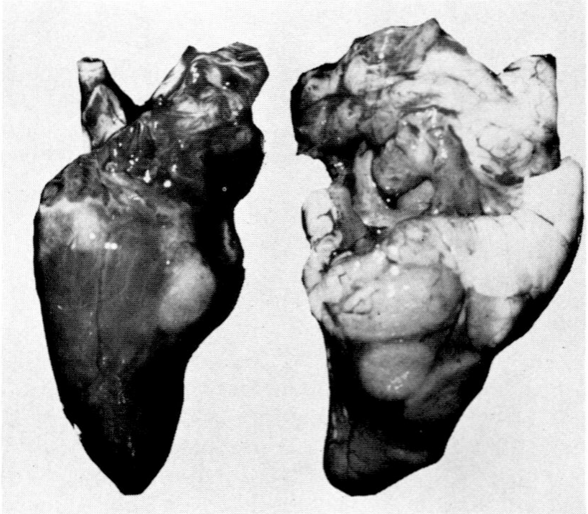

16.8. Tumors in hearts of birds inoculated with HPRS-16 isolate of MDV. (Purchase and Blackwell Scientific Publications)

Diffuse infiltration of the liver causes loss of normal lobule architecture and often gives the surface a coarse granular appearance. Lesions in the nonproducing ovary are observed as small to large grayish translucent areas (Fig. 16.17B). With large tumors the normal foliated appearance of the ovary is obliterated. Mature ovaries may retain function even though some follicles are tumorous. Marked involvement is indicated by a cauliflowerlike appearance. The proventriculus becomes thickened and firm as a result of small to large leukotic areas within and between the glands.

The bursa of Fabricius, while usually atrophic when affected (356), may (rarely) develop tumors that appear as diffuse thickening owing to interfollicular distribution of tumor cells. This lesion differs from the nodular tumor characteristic of lymphoid leukosis and may be easily differentiated histologically.

Nonneoplastic lesions of MD include severe atrophy of the bursa of Fabricius and thymus as well as degenerative lesions in the bone marrow and various visceral organs (202, 508). These are the result of intense cytolytic infections and they can result in death of chickens at an early age before lymphomas develop.

A discussion of MD pathology must include occlusive atherosclerosis following the discovery by Fabricant et al. (140) that such lesions may result from infection with MDV. Susceptible P-line chickens inoculated with the CU2 isolate of MDV developed grossly visible fatty atheromatous lesions in large coronary arteries, aortas and major aortic branches, and other arteries (Fig. 16.17D). These lesions were reputed as closely resembling those of chronic atherosclerosis in humans (271). A possible association between MDV and cholesterol-induced atherosclerosis in a susceptible strain of Japanese quail was reported by Shih et al. (432). They found DNA sequences complimentary to MDV DNA in the germline and suggested that there may be an interaction between the gene(s) and cholesterol in pathogenesis of atherosclerosis in the susceptible strain.

Histopathology. Histopathologic changes associated with MD have been described by numerous workers who were in general agreement about types of histologic lesions and cells involved (315, 324). However, significance and interpretation of some histologic changes have not been so universally agreed upon.

Various classifications were proposed, although the one suggested by Payne and Biggs (319), and used here, has been accepted by most workers. There has been controversy over the nature and sequence of lesions but fairly general agreement that there are two main types in peripheral nerves; these relate to whether the virus infection is productive (degenerative lesions) or nonproductive (proliferative lesions). One lesion response (type B) is essentially inflammatory and characterized by diffuse, light to moderate infiltration by small lymphocytes and plasma cells, usually with edema and sometimes with demyelination and Schwann cell proliferation. A few macrophages may be found; a mild version of type B is called type C. The other principal lesion (type A) is interpreted as neoplastic in character, consisting of masses of proliferating lymphoblastic cells; in some cases demyelination and Schwann cell proliferation are associated with this lesion also. Payne and Biggs (319) described an unusual cell, found in proliferative lesions, with very basophilic, pyroninophilic, and vacuolated cytoplasm and a nucleus with little or no detail. They called it a "Marek's disease cell" and thought it represented a degenerating blast-type cell, a conclusion consistent with electron microscopy (EM) observations in which MD cells were found with intranuclear herpesvirus particles (463).

These two lesion types may be observed in different nerves of the same bird or even in different areas of the same nerve. Payne and Biggs (319) studied the experimental disease sequentially and concluded that inflammatory lesions followed neoplastic changes. Lawn and Payne (237) substantially confirmed this conclusion in a chronologic study of ultrastructural changes in nerves in MD. They observed cellular infiltrations as early as 5 days, which gradually increased in intensity until 3 wk when severe proliferative type A lesions were seen in absence of paralysis or demyelination. Coincident with initial neurologic signs seen at 4 wk postinoculation, areas of widespread demyelination could be found within the proliferative type A lesions. Finally, characteristic type B lesions (edema, sparse infiltrations) appeared. Characteristic changes in nerves are illustrated in Figure 16.9.

Histopathologic changes in the brain were described by Pappenheimer et al. (311). Lesions were always focal in distribution and consisted of either compact perivascular cuffs of small densely staining lymphocytes (Fig. 16.10) or submiliary nodules composed of lymphocytes and paler elements. Jungherr and Hughes (206) stated that the latter were probably of glial origin. The spinal cord had, in addition to regional infiltrations, focal accumulations in white matter and occasionally in central gray matter. Root ganglia were intensely infiltrated but ganglion cells were intact. Wight (475) found the central nervous system (CNS) of affected birds often histologically normal or with only minimal lesions and concluded that MD is essentially a disease of peripheral nerves. Vickers et al. (468) injected chicks with the CONN-A isolate of virus and noted that CNS lesions, while apparent from 2 wk postinoculation, were most pronounced at 4–7 wk when clinical manifestations were most severe. They observed mostly immature lymphocytes, with only a few blast cells and no plasma cells.

According to Jungherr and Hughes (206), the most constant change in the eye is mononuclear infiltration of the iris (Fig. 16.11), but infiltrates may also be found in eye muscles, especially in rectus lateralis and ciliaris. Granular or amorphous material is sometimes present in the anterior chamber. Other but more rarely observed lesions involve the cornea (near Schlemm's canal), bulbar conjunctiva, pecten, and optic nerve. Sevoian and Chamberlain (397) and Smith et al. (443) reproduced ocular lesions experimentally. The latter reported that sequential changes included infiltration of proliferating lymphoreticular cells in optic and ciliary nerves and uvea followed by similar infiltrations throughout the eye.

Lymphomatous lesions in visceral organs are more uniformly proliferative in nature (Fig. 16.12). Cellular composition is much like the type A lesions described for nerves, consisting of diffusely proliferating small to medium lymphocytes, lymphoblasts, MD cells, and activated and primitive reticulum cells (319) (Fig. 16.13). Plasma cells are rarely present (356). The cellular composition of tumors is the same from one organ to another even though the gross pattern of in-

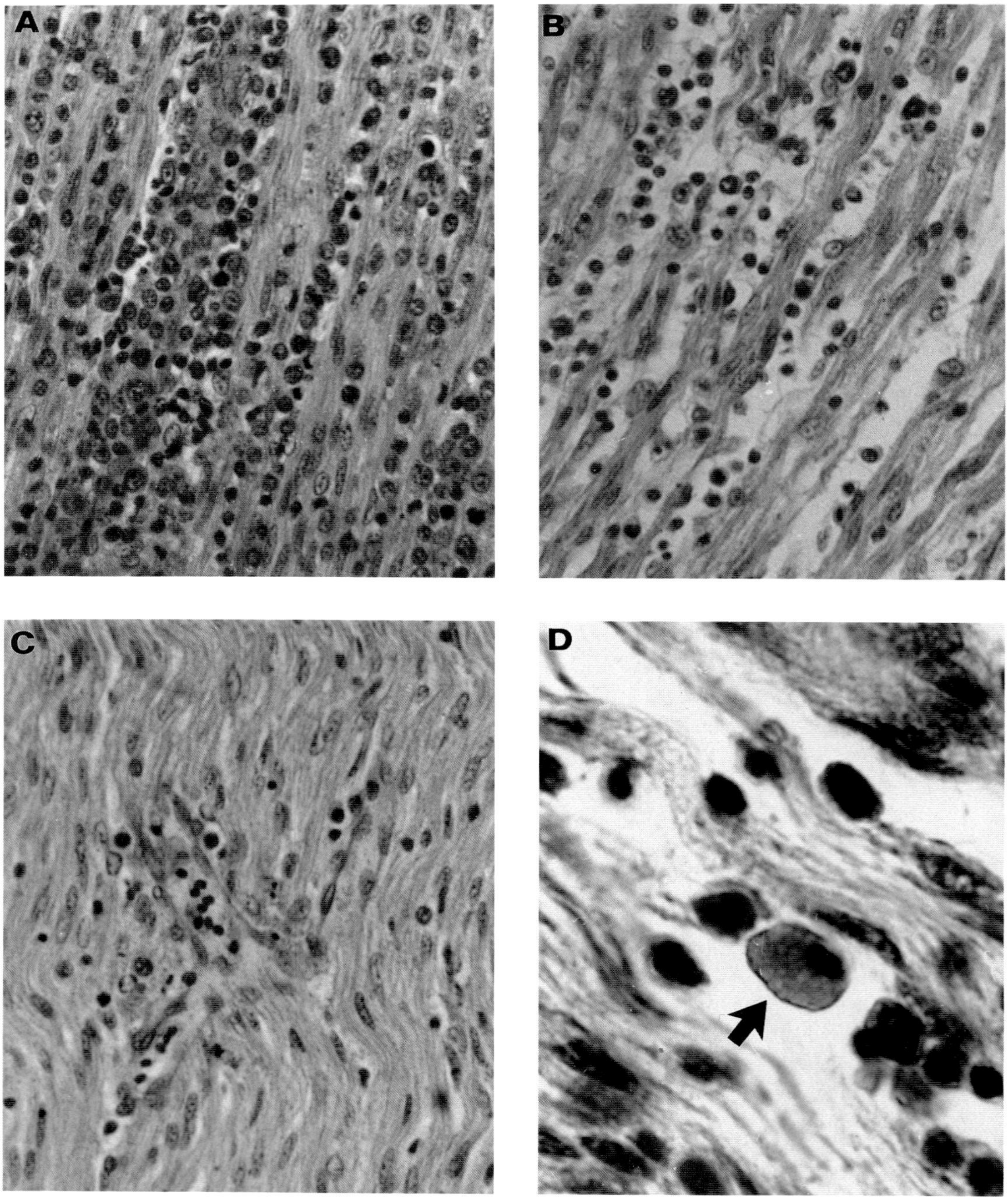

16.9. Microscopic lesions of MD in peripheral nerves. A. Type A lesion characterized by marked cellular infiltration, numerous proliferating lymphoblastic cells, and no edema. H & E, ×530. B. Type B lesions with edema, scattered infiltrating small and medium lymphocytes, plasma cells, and an occasional lymphoblast. H & E, ×530. C. Minimal nerve lesion considered diagnostic of MD. Note very light scattering of darkly stained mononuclear cells. H & E, ×530. D. "Marek's disease cell" (*arrow*) often seen in type A lesions. H & E, ×1600. (Helmboldt)

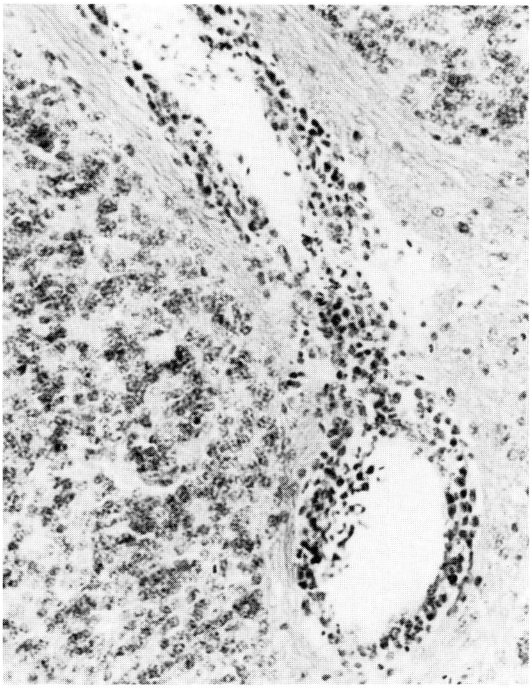

16.10. Perivascular cuff of lymphocytes in white matter of cerebellum of MDV-infected chicken. H & E, ×250. (Helmboldt)

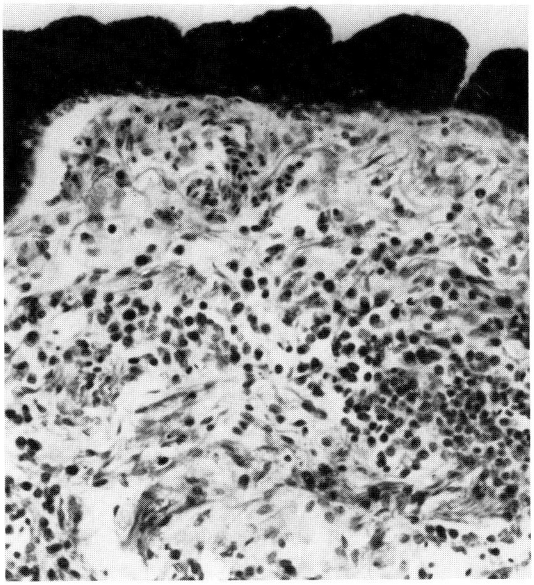

16.11. Lymphoid cell infiltration in iris of bird with ocular lesions of MD. H & E, ×250. (Helmboldt)

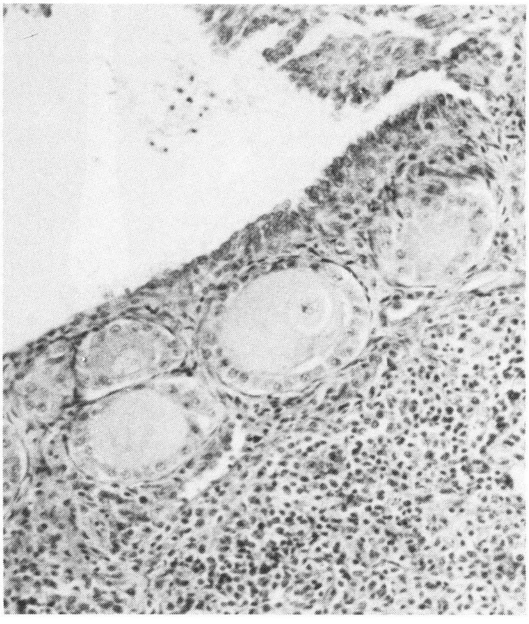

16.12. Lymphoid cell infiltration of ovary. Organ is largely composed of tumor cells, but a few ovarian follicles can be seen. H & E, ×210.

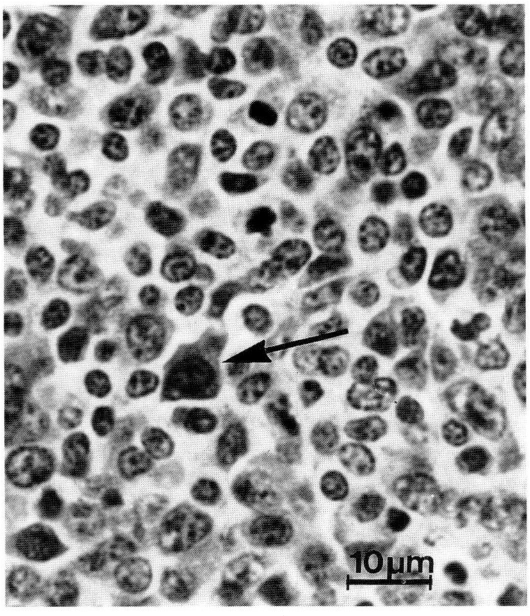

16.13. Higher magnification of ovarian lymphoma showing pleomorphic tumor cells. One MD cell is evident (*arrow*). H & E. (Payne)

volvement may vary. Doak et al. (123) examined visceral tumors by EM and found them to consist of only one cell type, an immature undifferentiated pleomorphic lymphocyte often with invaginations of the nuclear membrane. These lesions contrasted with neural lesions composed of a mixture of cell types. Ultrastructural features of tumor cells have been described by several workers (123, 145).

Lesions in the skin appear largely inflammatory but may also be lymphomatous. They are localized around infected feather follicles (Fig. 16.14). In addition to the sometimes massive accumulations of mononuclear cells around feather follicles, compact aggregates of proliferating cells, often perivascular, and a few plasma cells and histocytes are seen in the dermis (164, 319). With small lesions the architectural integrity of skin is maintained, but massive proliferative lesions may cause disruption of the epidermis, resulting in an ulcer. An unusual involvement of the comb was reported by Ekperigin et al. (132).

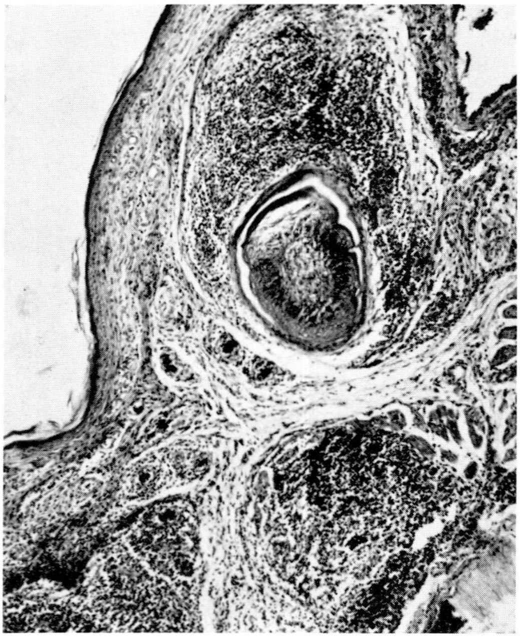

16.14. Dermal focal accumulations of mononuclear cells; note that one mass surrounds a feather shaft. H & E, ×100.

Productive herpesvirus replication in the bursa of Fabricius and thymus results in degenerative changes in these organs (see 60, 324). In experimental infections bursal lesions consisted of cortical and medullary atrophy, necrosis, cyst formation, and interfollicular lymphoid infiltration (Fig. 16.15). Atrophy of the thymus was sometimes severe and involved both cortex and medulla. In some cases there were areas of lymphoid proliferation in the thymus. Cowdry's type A intranuclear inclusions can sometimes be found in cells associated with degenerative lesions. Chicks infected in absence of maternal antibody may have aplastic bone marrow with accompanying anemia along with focal or generalized necrosis in a variety of organs, including the kidney (56, 144, 202).

Blood leukocytes may be elevated, largely because of increased numbers of large lymphocytes and lymphoblasts (137). Payne et al. (323) identified the majority of leukemic cells as T cells. The leukemic response is not consistent and may be absent or there may be only a mild leukocytosis (206, 398). Bone marrow changes in MD have variously been reported to include multiple tumor nodules (398) or aplasia (202), or changes were not observed (356). Productive viral infection of hematopoietic cells in bone marrow is the probable cause of anemia seen in some birds (137, 202), although the possibility of concurrent infection with chicken anemia agent (see Chapter 29, Infectious Anemia) would have to be considered.

Arterial lesions reported to be associated with MDV-induced atherosclerosis include proliferative and fatty proliferative changes in aortic, coronary, celiac, gastric, and mesenteric arteries (140, 271) (Fig. 16.16). Internal and medial foam cells, extracellular lipid, cholesterol clefts, and calcium deposits characterized the fatty proliferative lesions, and MD viral antigens could be detected by immunofluorescence adjacent to the arterial lesions. An altered lipid metabolism is suggested by the finding of Fabricant et al. (141) that MDV infection of arterial smooth muscle cells in vitro induced accumulation of phospholipids, free fatty acid, cholesterol, and cholesterol esters. In vivo studies supported this conclusion; Hajjar et al. (155) found that lipid accumulations in aortas resulted, in part, from altered cholesterol/cholesteryl ester metabolism during early stages of the disease.

Pathogenesis. Sequential events of MD have been extensively studied in many laboratories. Several comprehensive reviews have been published (27, 60, 62, 63, 284, 315, 324, 354, 380, 396, 380); these should be consulted for details of the large number of contributions that provide our current understanding of MD.

Four phases of infection in vivo can be delineated: 1) early productive-restrictive virus infection causing primarily degenerative changes, 2) latent infection, 3) a second phase of cytolytic infection coincident with permanent immunosuppression, and 4) a proliferative phase involving nonproductively infected lymphoid cells that may or may not progress to the point of lymphoma formation.

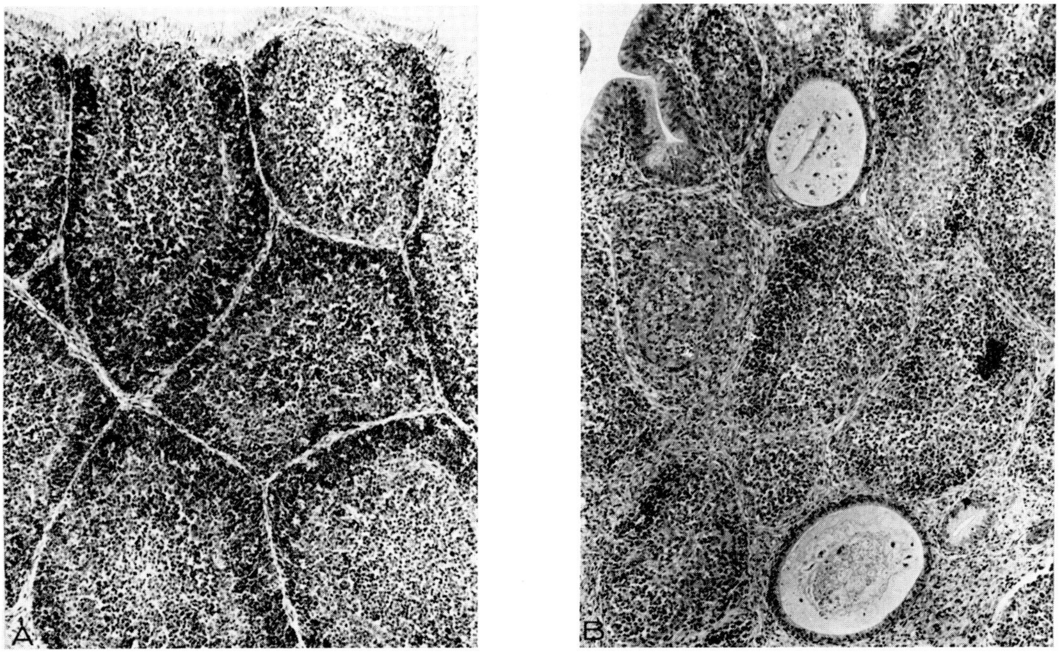

16.15. Changes in bursa of Fabricius associated with MD. A. Normal bursal follicles in chicken killed at 15 days of age; note uniform architecture. B. Cystic and necrotic follicles in atrophied bursa from chicken killed 28 days postinoculation with HPRS-16 isolate of MDV. H & E, ×50. (Purchase and Blackwell Scientific Publications)

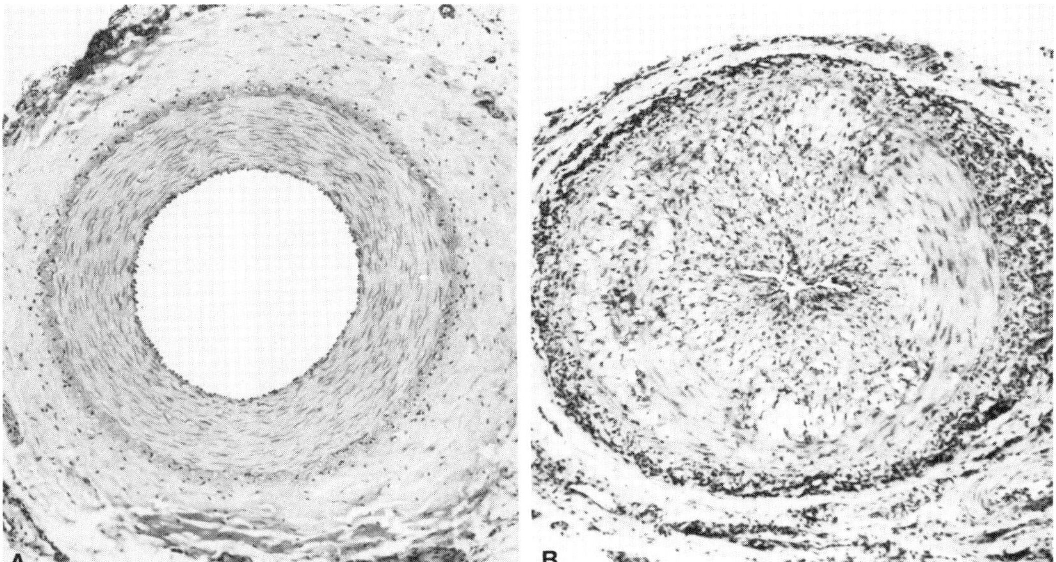

16.16. A. Gastric artery of normal chicken. B. Atherosclerotic artery in gizzard of chicken infected with CU2 isolate of MDV. Lumen is occluded by thickened intima and there are atheromatous changes deep in the intima and media. H & E, ×24. (C. Fabricant)

Virus gains entrance via the respiratory tract where it is probably picked up by phagocytic cells. Shortly thereafter, cytolytic infection can be detected in the spleen, bursa of Fabricius, and thymus, peaking at 3–6 days. Shek et al. (430) discovered that the primary target cells in all three organs are B cells although some activated T cells become infected and undergo degeneration as well. Resting T cells are refractory to infection (81). The necrotizing effects of this early infection provoke an acute inflammatory reaction with infiltration of various cells including macrophages, granulocytes, and both immunologically committed and uncommitted lymphocytes (322). A hyperplastic response in the spleen can follow, and at about 7 days a transient immunosuppression may occur due to the presence of suppressor macrophages (see Immunity). Ultimately there can be atrophy of the bursa and thymus. Chickens of susceptible and resistant strains of differing ages are equally susceptible to infection (58, 403, 503), and the level of infection in all birds is equally high in all cases during the early cytolytic period (139). However, the pathogenicity of the virus strain may affect the severity of early infection. Witter et al. (508) reported that more highly oncogenic MDV strains, like Md/5, can cause more severe lymphoid organ atrophy than do less oncogenic strains, and can cause an early death syndrome as the result of an especially marked cytolytic infection.

At about 6–7 days, the infection switches to latency coincident with the development of immune responses. Cell-mediated immunity (CMI) has been shown to be important in the switch (55), perhaps through a soluble mediator (54). Most latently infected cells are activated T cells, although B cells can also be involved (80, 430). The latent infection is persistent and can last for the lifetime of the bird (501). The extent to which nonlymphoid cells also are latently infected is not known, although apparent latent infection has been observed in Schwann cells and satellite cells in spinal ganglia (328).

Genetically resistant birds often do not progress past the second phase (latency) (58, 66, 247, 447). However, susceptible birds develop a second wave of cytolytic infections after 2 or 3 wk coincident with permanent immunosuppression. The lymphoid organs are again involved, and localized foci of infection can be found in tissues of epithelial origin in various visceral organs (e.g., kidney, pancreas, adrenal gland, proventriculus, etc.), especially in the skin, where a striking intion of the feather follicle epithelium occurs. The latter is unique in that it is the only known site of complete virus replication. There is focal necrosis, and inflammatory reactions develop around affected areas. The extent of infection during this phase (unlike that in the earlier phase in lymphoid organs) depends on factors known to govern incidence of tumors; the most susceptible birds develop the most widespread and intense infections.

The cause of inflammatory CNS lesions associated with MDV-induced transient paralysis is not clear, but it is known that the syndrome is under the control of genes of the major histocompatibility complex and that B cells are required for its induction (312, 394).

Lymphoproliferative changes constituting the ultimate response in the disease may progress to tumor development, although regression of lesions can and commonly does occur either before or after frank lymphomas are apparent (422). Death from lymphomas may occur at any time from about 3 wk onward.

The composition of lymphomas is complex, consisting of a mixture of neoplastic, inflammatory, and immunologically active cells. Both T and B cells are present, although the former predominate (182, 376).

The truly neoplastic cells have MDV DNA and can be grown as continuous lymphoblastoid cell lines in vitro (see 64 and ETIOLOGY). The infection in these cells is mostly nonproductive in vivo. Based on studies of a large number of cell lines, it appears that the usual target cells for transformation are T cells (262, 287, 344). Schat et al. (387) found them to possess Ia antigen signifying that they are activated. This is in keeping with the finding of Calnek et al. (81) that T cells are susceptible to infection only if activated. Several subpopulations of lymphocytes may be susceptible to transformation (289), but according to a report by Schat et al. (393), the principal target may be a helper T cell defined by the presence of CD4 antigen. On the other hand, there are some studies (52, 163, 457) that argue for tumor cells being suppressor T cells, based on their ability to suppress certain in vitro tests of CMI competence such as mitogenic stimulation of spleen cells and NK cell activity. McColl et al. (265) found MATSA (see ETIOLOGY) on at least some populations of noninfected, activated T cells. They concluded that MATSA may be a marker on transformation targets that continue to express it after transformation, hence its presence on MD tumor cell lines. MD lymphomas in some but not all chicken strains contain cells expressing chicken fetal antigen, indicating that the degree of dedifferentiation of tumor cells varies among strains (345). Some turkey MD lymphoblastoid cell lines (288) have been identified as B cells, others (346) as T cells. Further description of transformed cells can be found in the ETIOLOGY section.

Studies of graft-vs-host reactions in different genetic strains led Longenecker and Pazderka (254, 327) to suggest that low alloimmune competence and resistance to MD are very closely related through genetic linkage or functional dependence. That prompted speculation by Schat et al. (387) and Calnek (63) that the activation of T

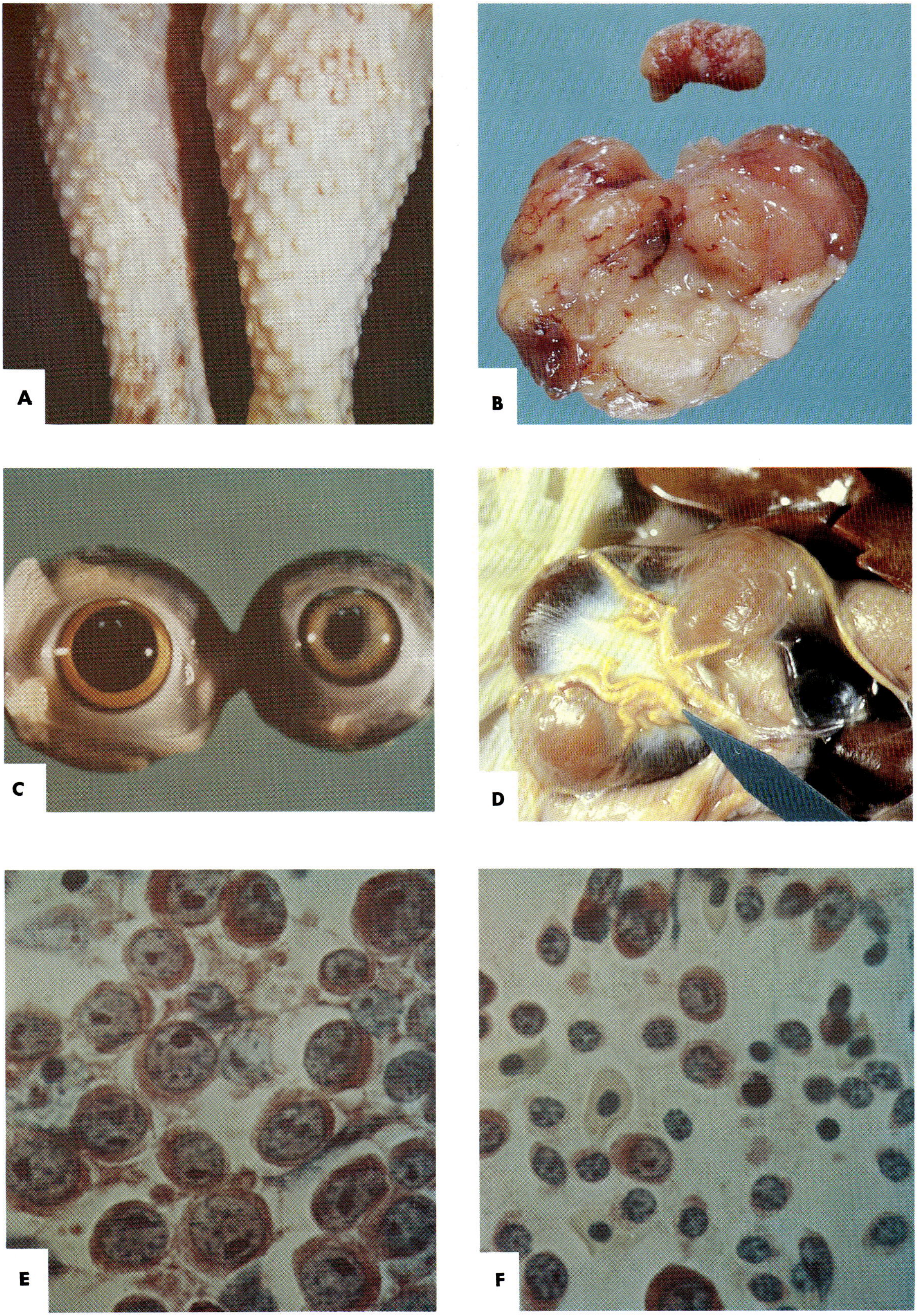
A
B
C
D
E
F

cells in response to the necrotizing infection of B cells is a very significant event in pathogenesis by providing an abundant supply of cells that are the usual target cells for transformation. This has been borne out by studies by Calnek showing that tumor induction at the site of inoculation with MDV is enhanced by provoking a CMI reaction against allogeneic cells at the site (83, 84). It is plausible that transformation requires 1) susceptibility to infection, 2) intrinsic or extrinsic control of virus replication (latency), 3) cell division to integrate virus genome, and 4) expression of viral oncogenes or activation of cellular oncogenes. Activated T cells infected at the time CMI responses cause a switch to latency could fit this model. Interestingly, cells present as early as 4 days after inoculation of MDV-infected allogeneic kidney cells can be grown in vitro as MD cell lines (83, 84). Thus, transformed cells, or at least transformation target cells, are present even during the early cytolytic phase of MD.

The pathogenesis of infection with oncogenic MDV that has become attenuated by passage in vitro has been studied by Bradley, Frazier, and Payne (quoted in 324) and by Schat et al. (391). Both groups found that attenuated virus failed to cause cytolytic infection of lymphoid organs and that cell-associated viremia levels were low. The latter authors further learned that attenuated virus was not infectious for lymphocytes in vitro, perhaps explaining the in vivo observations.

The actual mechanism(s) by which pathogenesis is altered in the case of host resistance in not clear. However, CMI is probably involved, and there is evidence (see Immunity) to suggest that immune responses of the host may be directed against either the early virologic events or the later proliferative phase and that an effective response at either stage might reduce the chance of overt disease. Both age and genetic resistance are dependent on immunological competence (58, 424). The availability of appropriate target cells is probably also important. If the hypothesis is correct that tumor development is enhanced by a strong T-cell response against the early cytolytic infection of B cells, then factors that limit that response should reduce tumor incidence. Vaccinal immunity and embryonal bursectomy both suppress the active viral infection (74, 388, 442), thereby obviating an inflammatory response; both reduce the incidence of tumors. Also, at least one genetic strain (line 6) is thought to be resistant to MD because of a paucity of T-cell targets (247). Interestingly, there is evidence (see 61, 82) that some genetic strains that have unusually strong CMI responses are especially susceptible to MD, although this is not true in all cases.

Virus strains differ in oncogenicity, but differences in pathogenesis associated with the strains are not well defined. All cause similar early cytolytic infections. Both the genetic strain and the virus strain are involved in determining the distribution as well as the incidence of lymphomas.

The immune response itself may be responsible for some lesions characteristic of MD. Nerve lesions have some characteristics suggestive of an autoimmune disease (366), and MD has been identified as a model for the Landry-Guillain-Barré syndrome (328).

The pathogenesis of atherosclerotic lesions is unknown.

16.17. A. Leukotic tumors involving feather follicles (skin leukosis). (Schmittle). B. Experimentally induced MD lymphoma in immature ovary (*bottom*) compared to normal ovary (*top*). C. Ocular lesions of MD. Note that normal eye (*left*) has a sharply defined pupil and well-pigmented iris. Affected eye (*right*) has a discolored iris and very irregular pupil as a result of mononuclear cell infiltration. (Peckham). D. Gizzard from a chicken infected with CU2 isolate of MDV. Note the grossly obvious atherosclerotic change in the arteries. (C. Fabricant). Microscopic changes from similar arteries are shown in Fig. 16.16B. E, F. Methyl green pyronin-stained smears of tumor cells from chickens with lymphoid leukosis (E) and MD (F). Lymphoid leukosis smear was from bursal tumor in bird inoculated 144 days earlier with RPL12 isolate of lymphoid leukosis virus. Note preponderance of uniformly large lymphoblastic cells (large nucleus, prominent nucleolus, abundant cytoplasm). Cells are characterized by red-staining (pyroninophilic, RNA-containing) cytoplasm. MD smear was from gonadal tumor in 6-wk-old bird infected with JM isolate of MDV. Note varied cell population: lymphoblasts, small and medium lymphocytes. Only a few cells are characterized by pyroninophilic cytoplasm. Both smears approx. ×700. (Siccardi)

Immunity. Importance of the immune response in MD cannot be overemphasized. The concern is fourfold: 1) MD can be immunosuppressive, 2) immunologic response is probably the basis to resistance in MD, 3) vaccinal immunity is the prime means of control, and 4) immunologic response may contribute to the cellular mass of the lymphoma (see Pathogenesis).

Immune responses and immunosuppressive features of MD have been well documented and reviewed. For details the various reviews (60, 324, 336–338, 380, 381, 396, 404) should be consulted.

IMMUNOSUPPRESSION. Impairment of the immune response might result directly from MDV infection through lytic infection of lymphocytes (see 324), or indirectly from activity of suppressor cell populations (245, 454). Probably both are important. Several reports (52, 163, 457) provided data from in vitro studies suggesting that the MD tumor cells themselves might have suppressor activity. This could be because they are true suppressor T cells or perhaps because they express chicken fetal antigen, which has been shown to have suppressor activity (301). Studies by Schat et al. (392) showing tumor cell lines to carry CD4 antigen, a marker for helper T cells, argues against the former, but direct evidence either way is lacking. Permanent immunosuppression tends to correlate with eventual tumor development (385) and may only be seen in birds that have already developed neoplasms (459); thus it is difficult to distinguish between cause and effect. Generally, the first appearance of permanent immunosuppression coincides with the second phase of cytolytic infection (see Pathogenesis). Because immunocompetence is required for latency to be maintained (55), it might be that immunosuppression associated with the appearance of transformed lymphoblasts results in the loss of additional B and T cells through cytolytic infection, thus compounding the situation and resulting in the bursal and thymic atrophy seen in birds destined to succumb to MD.

Both humoral and cell-mediated immunity can be depressed by MD; these are reflected by reduced antibody response to a variety of antigens and by alterations in T cell functions such as skin graft rejection, mitogen stimulation of lymphocytes, delayed hypersensitivity, reduced NK cell activity, and Rous sarcoma regression (see 324). MDV infection can increase susceptibility to primary and secondary infection with coccidia (34). It should be emphasized that while there may be depression, there is not a total loss of function.

A transient depression in cellular immunity, as measured by in vitro responsiveness to mitogens, is seen at about 7 days PI regardless of genetic constitution or virulence of the virus strain (see 381). This is apparently due to a population of suppressor macrophages (245.

IMMUNE RESPONSES. Both humoral and cell-mediated immunity develop in competent birds after infection with MDV. These can involve several types of responses and be directed against a variety of antigens. Those that are actually important in MD resistance are not yet determined, but several possibilities can be considered.

In spite of the lack of good in vitro correlates of MD immunity, known pathogenic aspects of the disease prompted Payne (315) to speculate that MD immunity could be either early against virus infection or later against transformed and proliferating lymphoid cells. Virus- or tumor-associated antigens would be respectively important. Payne's hypothesis was confirmed when it was shown in several laboratories that inactivated viral or tumor antigens can be used to immunize against MD (209, 250, 276, 333, 343). Inactivated antiviral vaccines protect against early cytolytic infections, latent infections, and tumor formation, whereas killed tumor cell vaccines only prevent the latter.

Humoral Immunity. Precipitating and virus-neutralizing (VN) antibodies can be detected within 1–2 wk; a transient immunoglobulin M (IgM) response is replaced by immunoglobulin G (IgG) (167). These antibodies generally persist throughout the life of the bird. Virus-neutralizing, but not virus-precipitating, antibodies correlate with survival of infected birds (57, 418). Probably this is an effect rather than a cause and may result from sparing of the bursa-dependent system in resistant birds (166, 167, 441). VN antibodies are probably directed against the B antigen, composed of three glycoproteins (see 380). Antibodies directed against a viral membrane antigen (VMA) detected on cells with productive-restrictive infections also are found in convalescent serum (90). These could be involved in complement lysis or antibody-dependent cell cytotoxicity reactions with infected cells (76, 227, 247).

A protective role for passively acquired humoral antibody has been observed in chicks (18, 102, and others); the effect of antibody is not to exclude but to reduce level of infection, perhaps by impeding spread. In vivo virus neutralization can occur (53); however, the exact mechanism is unknown. A humoral antibody response is not required for resistance to MD, since bursectomized birds may survive infection (419). This does not preclude a role for early antibody in suppressing destructive infection of immunologic organs required for subsequent resistance.

Cell-mediated Immunity (CMI). Since antibodies are not a required component of immune resistance to MD, it can be presumed that CMI is important. This conclusion is bolstered by the observation that functional T cells are required for resistance (70, 424) as well as vaccinal immunity (325).

A number of reports have suggested that spleen cells from MDV-infected chickens are suitable effector cells in in vitro tests for CMI. These have used MD lymphoblastoid cell lines or MDV latently infected lymphocytes as targets in chromium release assays (CRA) (3, 334, 414, and others) or plaque-inhibition tests (247, 370), respectively. Generally the studies on CRA have suffered from any evidence of major histocompatibility complex (MHC)-restriction; indeed, much of the activity could be shown to be not only non-MHC-restricted but in fact to be directed against alloantigens (389). Thus the effector cells in those tests are not likely to be cytotoxic T cells. Because most MD tumor cell lines express some VMA (76), that antigen should be considered a potential target in the CRA. Also, a phosphorylated protein common to infected chick kidney cultures and non-virus-producer MD cell lines

(194) is a candidate antigen. The plaque-inhibition tests may have detected responses against VMA since latently infected lymphocytes that serve as infectious centers when cultured with monolayer cells in in vitro assays generally "turn on" and produce viral antigens.

Vaccinal Immunity. Vaccinal immunity is almost certainly immunologic in nature. Not only does the protective effect of inactivated vaccines rule out the alternate possibility of viral interference, but vaccinal immunity can be abrogated by immunosuppressive treatments affecting CMI, such as cyclophosphamide treatment (358). Deletion of humoral immunity by bursectomy and X-radiation has no effect on protection conferred by attenuated MDV (136), although a similar treatment partially impairs vaccinal immunity from HVT (364).

Immunity from live virus vaccines including HVT, attenuated MDV, and low-virulence or nononcogenic MDV appears to be directed largely against viral antigens, but possibly also against tumor antigens. All protect against early replication of virulent viruses in the lymphoid organs of challenged birds and reduce the level of latent infection (74, 343, 361, 388, 442). The immunogen(s) important in antiviral immunity are not known, but glycoproteins associated with the B antigen (see ETIOLOGY) are likely candidates since they can be used to immunize chickens against MD (307). Evidence suggesting antitumor immunity comes from reports that attenuated MDV, HVT, and SB-1 can all immunize against transplantable MD tumors including the JMV transplant (261, 399, and others). The latter does not express any of the usual virus-associated antigens. However, a recently discovered phosphorylated protein found in both transformed and productively infected cells (194, 197, 280) could account for the ability of serotype 1 (but not 2 or 3) MD vaccines to immunize against challenge with transplantable MD tumor cells and, conversely, for the ability of nonproducer cells like JMV to induce immunity against MDV challenge. Other, yet undiscovered, immunogens may also be shared by tumor cells and productively infected cells. The existence of such a viral antigen(s) in transformed cells was predicted by Powell (335).

Macrophages may be involved in resistance by restricting virus replication directly (153, 168) or in concert with antibody (228, 238). Immune B cells and macrophages can interact to inactivate cell-free virus (383). Macrophages are also apparently involved in early transient immunosuppression following MDV infection (245, 246) and can inhibit DNA synthesis and proliferation by MD lymphoblastoid cell lines in vitro (245, 310, 405).

Finally, it should be noted that innate resistance in the form of NK cells could be important in MD; there is evidence of increased NK cell activity after vaccination with HVT or SB-1 (163, 406). Furthermore, Sharma (408) concluded that elevated levels of NK cells in regressive but not progressive tumors could indicate a role for intratumoral immunity in tumor regression.

DIAGNOSIS

Virus Isolation. Although not especially helpful in establishing a diagnosis of MD, the application of techniques for virus isolation has value in epizootiological and other virus characterization studies. Related techniques are used for the titration of MDV and its related vaccine viruses. Procedures have been reviewed by Sharma (410).

SOURCE OF VIRUS. MDV can be isolated from 1 or 2 days postinoculation (330) or 5 days after contact exposure (2) and throughout the life of the chicken. Intact viable cells are the preferred inoculum because in most cases infectivity is avidly cell associated, although cell-free preparations from skin, dander, or feather tips of infected chickens may contain virus (68). Inocula may consist of heparinized whole blood or suspensions containing blood lymphocytes or isolated tumor cells. Virus can often be recovered from infected cell suspensions following storage for 24 hr at 4 C, thus facilitating transport of samples (509).

CELL CULTURE TECHNIQUES. Probably the most widely used method for primary isolation of MDV is inoculation of susceptible tissue cultures with suspensions of buffy coat, spleen, or other lymphoid cells. Chicken kidney cell and duck embryo fibroblast cultures are commonly used as a substrate for serotype 1 MDV, but chicken embryo fibroblasts may be useful for isolation of viruses of serotypes 2 and 3. Cultures are inoculated with 10^6–10^7 cells although some inhibition may be encountered with doses over 8×10^6 cells for some viruses (78). After 24–48 hr, the inoculum is washed off and the culture maintained under liquid or agar medium, usually without subculture.

Development of typical plaques (see Fig. 16.3A–F) in inoculated cultures within 5–14 days and absence of such changes in comparable uninoculated control cultures is evidence for isolation of MDV. The plaques induced by serotype 1, 2, and 3 viruses can be distinguished, with practice, by morphologic criteria (379, 482). Optimal time for observation of plaques varies with the cell substrate and serotype of the virus. Known virus-infected inoculum may be used to determine susceptibility of the test cultures.

Direct cultivation of kidney (497) or lymphoid (75) cells from infected chickens is more sensitive than inoculation of monolayer cultures for demonstration of infection. The short-term lymphocyte culture technique followed by an FA test is an especially useful method to demonstrate virus (75) and presumably could also be used to recover virus if antigen-positive cultured lymphocytes were transferred to susceptible monolayer cultures. Cultured tissue explants have been examined by EM to demonstrate MDV (115).

OTHER ISOLATION METHODS. Methods for isolation of MDV by inoculation of embryos (29, 45) or chickens (32, 497) have been described. Because of the need to control the specificity of the responses measured and the labor-intensive nature of the tests, such procedures are infrequently used.

ISOLATE IDENTIFICATION. The identity and purity of a suspect isolate must be carefully ascertained. All three viral serotypes may coexist in the same chicken and are frequently isolated simultaneously. Procedures helpful in deriving serotypically pure MDV isolates include the use of inocula from nonvaccinated sentinel chickens placed in suspect flocks (to avoid contamination with serotype 3 viruses, which spread poorly by contact), the plaque purification or cloning of the isolate at the earliest possible passage, and the selective use of cell substrates (chicken and duck fibroblasts are relatively resistant to serotype 1 and 2 isolates, respectively) (487). Serotype identity and purity can be confirmed by immunofluorescent staining with serotype-specific monoclonal antibodies (248) or by analysis of restriction endonuclease patterns (375). Other distinguishing characteristics including oncogenicity for chickens may be determined. Oncogenic serotype 1 isolates may be typed as mild, virulent, or very virulent by inoculation of HVT-vaccinated chickens (487) (see ETIOLOGY). Freedom from other viruses is also critical, since contamination may alter the apparent pathogenicity of the isolate (51).

VIRUS ASSAY AND TITRATION. Viruses of serotypes 1, 2, and 3 can be quantitated by in vitro techniques similar to those described for virus isolation. Methods differ for different serotypes but all rely on plaque induction in susceptible cell cultures. Enumeration should be done as soon as plaques become mature, since secondary plaques may occur when cultures are maintained with liquid medium. Procedures for titration of vaccine viruses have been reviewed (460) and are not fundamentally different from those for pathogenic isolates.

Viral Markers in Tissues. It is often desirable to detect the presence of viral infection in chickens without isolating the virus in culture. Such infection markers also have value for the identification of putative MDV isolates in cell cultures.

DETECTION BY ANTIBODIES. Although polyclonal antibodies obtained from MDV-infected chickens have been applied to the detection of antigens in tissues, the availability of monoclonal antibodies directed to specific antigens or epitopes has greatly facilitated many of these tests. Monoclonal antibodies have been prepared against type-common and type-specific epitopes of all three MDV serotypes (248). Viral antigens can be detected in feather tips, tissues, or infected cell cultures with appropriate antibodies by FA tests (447), immunoperoxidase tests (86), AGP tests (154, 251), and enzyme-linked immunosorbent assays (ELISA) (119).

DNA PROBES. Methods utilizing DNA-DNA dot-blot hybridization with DNA probes for the detection of MDV DNA in feather tip extracts have been described (119). Furthermore, the localization of specific virus-infected cells has been accomplished by in situ hybridization (374).

ELECTRON MICROSCOPY. Herpesvirus particles can be detected in the FFE and other tissues of infected chickens and in productively infected cells in vitro (68, 281, 463). However, the particles must be differentiated from those of other avian herpesviruses by appropriate tests such as immunoferritin labeling (286).

Antibody Demonstration. Tests for identifying the presence of specific antibodies in chicken sera are useful in studies of viral pathogenesis and for monitoring specific-pathogen-free flocks. A number of procedures have been described. Thus far, however, none are capable of easily determining antibodies to a specific viral serotype in chickens exposed to multiple viral serotypes. Antigenic differences between serotypes have been reported (46, 47), but common antigens also appear to exist. The biologic significance of antibodies detected by different methods may vary (57).

AGAR-GEL PRECIPITATION TESTS. In the AGP test, serums are reacted with antigen in an agar medium containing 8% sodium chloride. The antigen is prepared by sonication or freezing and thawing of heavily infected tissue culture cells or skin or feather tip preparations from infected chickens. Development of single or multiple precipitin lines is evidence for presence of antibody in the test serum, but specificity should be determined by testing unknown serums in wells adjacent to a well containing a known positive serum. A line of identity should be seen.

IMMUNOFLUORESCENCE TESTS. In the indirect FA test a suitable antigen (coverslip-cultured cells containing MDV plaques) is reacted sequentially with test serum and fluorescein-conjugated antiserum directed against chicken Igs. Fluorescent staining of the cells of the focal lesions is evidence for antibody in the test serum provided the antigen does not autofluoresce and the chicken antiglobulin conjugate does not stain untreated antigen.

VIRUS-NEUTRALIZATION TESTS. Neutralization of cell-free virus obtained from the skin or feather tips of infected chickens is a further method for demonstrating antibody activity. One part of serum dilution may be added to four parts virus suspension and the mixture incubated at 37 C for 30 min before assay in tissue culture or other systems (65).

ENZYME IMMUNOASSAYS. ELISA using whole infected cell antigens (91) or cell extract antigens (48) have been described; both workers found their tests about 20-fold more sensitive than indirect FA tests.

Differential Diagnosis. Despite well established guidelines (357, 433), the clinical diagnosis of MD has been considered difficult in practice, probably because there is no truly pathognomonic gross lesion and because lesions can closely resemble those of lymphoid leukosis (LL) or reticuloendotheliosis (RE).

INFECTION CRITERIA. MDV is highly contagious and virtually ubiquitous among chickens. Only a small percentage of infected chickens develop clinical MD. Because of these factors, infection criteria have limited value in diagnosis of the disease. Diagnoses, therefore, must be based on disease-specific criteria such as epidemiology, pathology, and tumor-specific markers.

PATHOLOGY. Although enlarged peripheral nerves and visceral lymphomas are common in MD, neither lesion occurs consistently or is pathognomonic. Thus, other criteria such as age and lesion distribution must be considered in the postmortem diagnosis of MD. As a general guideline, chickens may be diagnosed positive for MD if at least one of the following conditions is met: (1) leukotic enlargement of peripheral nerves in the absence of RE virus (REV) infection; (2) lymphoid tumors in various tissues (liver, heart, gonad, skin, muscle, proventriculus) in birds under 16 wk of age; (3) visceral lymphoid tumors in birds 16 wk or older that lack neoplastic involvement of the bursa of Fabricius; or (4) iris discoloration and pupil irregularity, as in Figure 16.17C.

Some critical assumptions are the absence of bursal tumors in cases of MD in birds older than 16 wk, the consistent presence of gross bursal tumors in cases of LL, and the occurrence of LL or other unrelated tumors only in birds older than 16 wk. Although these assumptions may not be invariably correct, diagnostic errors on a flock basis should be infrequent if necropsies are done with care and several birds are examined. Proper examination of the bursa is particularly important and requires incision of the organ with close inspection of the epithelial surface.

Diagnostic accuracy may be enhanced by employment of histologic or cytologic procedures. A mixed population of small to large lymphocytes, lymphoblasts, plasma cells, and MD cells are found in MD tumors. These diagnostic features may be seen in routine histologic sections stained with hematoxylin and eosin. However, examination of touch preparations taken directly from lesions of freshly killed birds and stained with methyl green pyronin or Shorr's stain gives better cytologic detail and can be prepared in a few minutes. Pyroninophilia is observed infrequently in cells of MD tumors (433).

TUMOR-ASSOCIATED MARKERS. Even though MATSA is now recognized as a host antigen associated with activated T cells (265), this antigen and other host cell markers have diagnostic value. Membrane immunofluorescent staining for MATSA and IgM has proved particularly useful for the diagnosis of MD (295, 296): MD lymphomas have 5–40% of cells positive for MATSA, whereas IgM is present on less than 5% of cells from MD lymphomas. Similar findings have been reported on formalin-fixed, paraffin sections of tissues stained by the peroxidase-antiperoxidase method (124).

DIFFERENTIATION FROM OTHER DISEASES. LL is the principal disease to be considered in differential diagnosis of MD. However, LL may be differentiated from MD by the common involvement of the bursa of Fabricius, uniform blast morphology, pyroninophilia, and presence of B-cell markers and absence of MATSA on tumor cells (Table 16.2). Cytologic differences between MD and LL tumors are illustrated in Figure 16.17E, F.

Accidental or experimental inoculation of chickens with nondefective REV has caused clinical disease characterized by enlarged nerves, runting, and both bursal and nonbursal visceral lymphomas. Two types of REV-induced pathology closely resemble MD: nonbursal lymphomas that occur as early as 6 wk of age (510) and enlargements of peripheral nerves that occur both alone (500) and in the presence of lymphomas (510). Such lesions can be distinguished from MD by histopathologic and infection-related criteria (Table 16.2, Reticuloendotheliosis) but, thus far, are not commonly recognized in the field.

Other diseases that may present confusing gross lesions or paralytic signs are myeloblastosis, erythroblastosis, carcinoma of the ovary, other neoplasms, riboflavin deficiency, tuberculosis, histomoniasis, genetic gray eye, Newcastle disease, avian encephalomyelitis, perosis, and joint infections or injuries.

Table 16.2. Comparison of epizootiologic and pathologic features of Marek's disease (MD), lymphoid leukosis (LL), and nonbursal reticuloendotheliosis (RE)

Characteristic	MD	LL	RE[a]
Age of onset			
Peak time	2–7 mo	4–10 mo	2–6 mo
Limits	>1 mo	>3 mo	>1 mo
Clinical signs			
Paralysis	Common	Absent	Rare
Gross lesions			
Liver	Common	Common	Common
Nerves	Common	Absent	Common
Skin	Common	Rare	Rare
Bursa tumor	Rare	Common	Rare
Bursa atrophy	Common	Rare	Common
Intestine	Rare	Common	Common
Heart	Common	Rare	Common
Microlesions			
Pleomorphic cells	Yes	No	Yes
Uniform blast cells	No	Yes	No
Bursa tumor	Interfollicular	Intrafollicular	Rare
Surface antigens			
MATSA	5–40%	Absent	Absent
IgM	<5%	91–99%	Unknown
B cell	3–25%	91–99%	Rare
T cell	60–90%	Rare	Common

[a]Nonbursal form only. A bursal form also has been described with properties virtually identical to those of LL.

TREATMENT. There is no effective practical treatment for MD in either flocks or individual chickens. Some birds showing clinical signs of MD, however, spontaneously regress their lesions and recover under certain circumstances (319, 422).

PREVENTION AND CONTROL. Development of successful vaccines for control of MD (107, 305, 367) is a singular achievement both in agriculture (since MD prior to vaccination had become the most costly poultry disease) and basic cancer research (since this was the first time an important neoplastic disease had been so controlled in any species). Vaccination represents, for now and the foreseeable future, the central strategy for the prevention and control of MD. However, genetic resistance and isolation-rearing techniques are important as adjuncts to vaccination. Detailed reviews are available (313, 483).

Vaccination

TYPES OF VACCINES. Three classes of viruses are capable of protecting chickens against MD: attenuated serotype 1 MDV (107, 367), HVT (305), and naturally avirulent isolates of serotype 2 (382, 515). Polyvalent vaccines mainly composed of serotype 2 and 3 viruses (481) have been described. Although all vaccine types are protective, HVT has been most extensively used because it is economical to produce and cell-free virus extracted from infected cells may be lyophilized (69) for more convenient storage and handling. A cell-associated form of HVT requiring storage in liquid nitrogen has been most widely used, probably because it is more effective than cell-free virus in the presence of maternal antibodies (490). Only cell-associated vaccines of serotypes 1 and 2 are available.

FACTORS AFFECTING EFFICACY. Vaccine is usually administered at hatching. Both cell-associated and cell-free vaccines are given by parenteral inoculation at a dose usually in excess of 1000 plaque-forming units (PFU)/chick. The intramuscular route may be slightly more effective than the subcutaneous route (300), but this advantage was not observed by all workers (469).

Sharma and Burmester (413) found that vaccination of 18-day-old embryos accelerated development of protective immunity by several days and proposed this technique for controlling detrimental effects of early exposure to virulent MDV. Embryo vaccination was advantageous even in the presence of maternal antibodies (417) and with several types of vaccines (420). This procedure is just being commercially implemented and definitive results are not available.

The interval between vaccination and exposure to the virulent field virus (305) will affect vaccine efficacy. Early exposure is probably one of the most important causes of excessive MD in vaccinated flocks since up to 7 days is required for a solid immunity to be established (19) and since field exposure usually occurs very soon after placement of chickens (499).

The strain of chicken is also an important factor in MD vaccinal immunity (see Genetic Resistance). Schat et al. (388) found that HVT vaccine in a genetically resistant chicken provided better immunity than did the bivalent (HVT + SB-1) vaccine in a susceptible chicken.

In an effort to improve efficacy, increased vaccines doses (131, 482) or double vaccination (17) were tried with little or no success; however, in response to a perceived need, vaccine manufacturers have continued to increase recommended dosages. Many white leghorn chickens now receive up to 10,000 PFU of HVT at hatching.

Stress has long been suspected to interfere with the maintenance of vaccinal immunity. Apparent confirmation has been provided by Powell and Davison (339) who induced MD lesions and mortality by immunosuppressive treatment at 10 wk of age of vaccinated and previously challenged chickens. However, attempts to confirm this observation were unsuccessful (412).

Various other infections, including infectious bursal disease (409), REV (507), reovirus (369), and chicken anemia agent (308), have been reported to interfere with the induction of vaccinal immunity, although very specific conditions are sometimes required.

Natural infection with avirulent serotype 2 or low-virulence serotype 1 isolates may provide protection against subsequent exposure to virulent isolates (36, 37, 442) and may be an adjunct to vaccination. A role for natural exposure to virulent MDV strains in the maintenance of vaccinal immunity for long periods has also been proposed (469) but requires confirmation.

Proper handling of vaccine during thawing and reconstitution is crucial (157). Also, vaccination of breeders with a serotype 1 or 2 virus rather than HVT leaves progeny more susceptible to HVT (222); this technique to reduce the detrimental effect of homologous maternal antibody is in use in several parts of the world.

Outbreaks associated with vvMDV strains in flocks vaccinated with HVT can often be controlled by vaccination with polyvalent vaccines composed of all three viral serotypes, or of serotypes 2 and 3 (79, 481, 491). The improved efficacy of a bivalent vaccine against challenge with very virulent strains was confirmed by Schat et al. (388) and others (471).

The phenomenon through which two vaccines protect better than either alone has been termed protective synergism and is best demonstrated with viruses of serotypes 2 and 3 (486, 488), especially the FC126 strain of HVT coupled with either the SB-1 (388) or 301B/1 (486) strains of serotype 2 MDV. Attempts to achieve similar enhancement with serotypes 1 and 3 have been reported (340).

VACCINATION STRATEGIES. MD vaccines are unusually effective, often achieving over 90% protection under commercial conditions (484, 489). However, attention is often focused on an increasing number of flocks in which MD losses are perceived to be excessive (516). Causes for such "vaccine failures" are difficult to ascertain by retrospective analysis (483) but various strategies to minimize their occurrence have been developed.

The choice of vaccine type may be important. HVT is still widely used with excellent results but bivalent vaccination with serotypes 2 and 3 may help reduce MD losses in cases where HVT alone is not fully effective (79, 509). The original low-passage, partly attenuated serotype 1 strain CVI988 vaccine (367) is gaining in popularity (472) but has not yet been evaluated in the USA. However, the high-passage, completely attenuated CVI988 clone C vaccine (120) proved no more effective than HVT (486) and is infrequently used at present. The efficacy of some high-passage serotype 1 vaccine viruses may be improved by serial back-passage in chickens (122, 486).

The use of non-HVT-containing vaccines in parent stock in order to increase the efficacy of HVT in progeny chicks (222) has been practiced but the magnitude of the benefits achieved is difficult to estimate.

Vaccination by itself does not provide a complete control program for MD. High levels of sanitation to reduce early exposure and the presence of genetic resistance are highly useful adjuncts to a successful vaccination program (see next sections).

Genetic Resistance. Genetically controlled differences in MD susceptibility among lines of chickens has been reviewed by Calnek (61). Several lines of chickens with genetic resistance to MD have been selected and maintained experimentally (108, 185, 453). MD resistance appeared independent of genetic factors that control production traits (35), and variation of MD susceptibility in single-sire families indicated that there was sufficient heterogeneity to warrant selection for resistance in commercial chickens (35, 108).

SELECTION METHODS. Selection for resistance has historically utilized progeny testing (108) or reproduction from survivors of exposed breeding flocks (255). Resistant lines have been developed in which less than 5% were susceptible compared to 51% susceptibility of the unselected population (108).

An alternate selection method, based on blood

typing, relies on the close relationship between MD resistance and certain alleles, especially B^{21} (41, 160, 254), which are closely linked to the B-F region of the major histocompatibility (B) complex (42). Other *B* alleles are associated with susceptibility or with lesser degrees of resistance (13, 14). Such a selection procedure may simplify production of resistant stocks in populations containing a specific allele for resistance. In fact, Cole's dramatic success (108) may have been due in part to the fortuitous occurrence of B^{21} in his population.

Linkages between MD resistance and various other genetic loci such as Ly-4 and Th-1 (146) and IgG-1 (15), or traits such as immune response to GAT (329, 450) and graft-vs-host response (11) suggest additional criteria for the selection of resistant chickens.

Evidence that other factors may also be involved is provided by the observation that RPL line 6 and 7 chickens, which are both homozygous at the *B* locus for another allele (B^2) (327), differ markedly in MD susceptibility (118). Resistance has been considered dominant, although this varies to some extent, and in most cases resistance of crosses has been intermediate to that of the parent strains (61).

The mechanism(s) by which genetic constitution influences the incidence of MD is discussed elsewhere (see Pathogenesis).

APPLICATIONS. Since Spencer et al. (449) found genetically resistant chickens were protected by vaccination to a greater extent than more susceptible ones, breeding for genetic resistance may be a valuable adjunct to immunization for control of MD. Furthermore, genetic resistance might even obviate the need for measures such as bivalent vaccination, now needed to control challenge with very virulent strains (388). However, resistance of vaccinated and nonvaccinated chickens does not always vary in parallel, suggesting that selection should be performed in vaccinated stocks (12). In light of the selection tools available, the virtual absence of negative correlations, and the major benefits to be derived, it is surprising that breeders have not placed a higher priority on this approach.

Isolation and Sanitation. Isolation rearing and environmental sanitation have been advocated for control of MD, both as a primary control method and as an adjunct to vaccination. While useful for specific-pathogen-free flocks (469), application of these principles to commercial flocks has met with only limited success and has been infrequently used as a primary control method, probably because of the high cost of decontamination and prevention of reinfection, as well as the uncertainty of the results. The use of filtered-air, positive-pressure houses is generally required (8, 125).

However, good hygiene practice to limit the extent of early MDV exposure is a crucial and cost-effective adjunct to vaccination. Even partial protection such as the use of brooding paper to cover used litter has reduced MD losses (352). Other relevant sanitation principles have been reviewed (28, 313).

Chemoprophylaxis. Several drugs, including phosphonoacetate, phosphonoformate, ara-C, AUS, impacarzin, acyclovir, and FIAC, are reported to inhibit MDV replication in vitro (243, 365, 390), or to limit MD lymphoma induction (22, 89, 129, 213, 378). Various immunostimulants have been tested: levamisole had no consistent beneficial effect on MD (229, 320), but some protective effect has been reported for a purified extract residue from the bacterium *Progenitor cryptocides* (253), and a transfer-factor material (478). However, none of these have yet become established as useful in practical MD control programs.

NONONCOGENIC TURKEY AND CHICKEN HERPESVIRUSES. HVT and serotype 2 MDV are not recognized as pathogens in avian hosts. Interest in these viruses derives mainly from their use to immunize chickens against MD, reference to which is made earlier. However, both are naturally occurring viruses and it seems appropriate to also consider some aspects of their epizootiology and pathogenesis in their natural or alternate avian hosts since this has not been discussed elsewhere.

Turkey Herpesvirus (HVT). HVT was isolated from normal turkeys by Kawamura et al. (219) and Witter et al. (499). The virus is ubiquitous in domestic turkeys (493, 396) and isolations have also been reported from wild turkeys (111). In chickens, the virus has also become ubiquitous because of widespread vaccination of day-old chickens to prevent MD.

In turkeys the virus spreads rapidly through exposed flocks, presumably by contact exposure; virtually all individual turkeys become viremic and develop antibody within a few weeks (493). The virus appears to mature in the FFE, since cell-free skin extracts are infectious (502), although viral antigen was found only infrequently and at low levels in the FFE of infected turkeys (142). No vertical transmission has been demonstrated (314, 493). Virus may be transmitted from turkeys to chickens under experimental conditions (495), but such transmission is probably rare in the field. There is limited contact spread among chickens (101, 100), presumably because of maturation of virus in the FFE (92, 517). However, the virus appears to replicate less efficiently in skin than MDV (350).

Fabricant et al. (142) compared early pathogenesis of HVT infection in chickens and turkeys. Chickens had no cytolytic infections in lymphoid organs. In contrast, turkeys infected with HVT did have some viral antigen-positive cells at 4–14 days postexposure but no cytolytic infections in bursa or thymus were seen. In chickens, there was no depression of bursa or thymus size and NK cell activity was stimulated through at least 8 wk postinoculation (427). No adrenal-mediated stress response was detected through 3 wk postinoculation (147).

The virus is apparently nononcogenic in turkeys (499, 495), but the possibility of fertility problems in HVT-infected toms has been raised (4, 461). Evaluation of the effect of HVT on production characteristics of turkeys has been hampered by the difficulty in maintaining infection-free control flocks for long periods, but this deserves further study.

The virus generally causes no clinical disease in intact or immunodepressed chickens (426, 499) and is not detrimental to the immune response. In contrast, when chickens were infected with HVT in ovo and then hatched and raised, up to 19% developed clinical paralysis (74), and gross nerve enlargement due to B-type lesions was observed. HVT can be recovered from infected chickens for long periods and antibodies persist for life (360, 506).

No protection by HVT was noted in turkeys against MD lymphoma induction following challenge with oncogenic MDV (135, 288).

Serotype 2 Marek's Disease Virus. Viruses isolated from clinically normal chickens and originally described as apathogenic or low-pathogenic strains of MDV (30, 98) were subsequently grouped in a separate serotype (46, 47). The protective ability of such strains against MD was recognized early (30, 515). Other unique features of this virus group were further elucidated following the isolation of the SB-1 strain (382).

Epidemiological studies are meager, probably because virus isolation is more difficult than for other serotypes, and antibodies are usually masked by those of other serotypes. Witter (485) isolated serotype 2 virus from 34% of chicken flocks in seven states, suggesting the virus was reasonably prevalent but perhaps less so than serotype 1. The prevalence is further supported by early studies where 8 of 25 random MDV isolates were typed as avirulent (30). Similar viruses were considered prevalent in Australia (351).

The epidemiology in chickens has been complicated by the artificial distribution of the virus in the USA through a seeder chick program (514, 515) or through inoculation as a vaccine (79, 509).

Chickens appear to be the only natural host although apathogenic isolates that resembled the HN strain were isolated from Japanese silkies, red jungle fowl, and Ceylon jungle fowl reared in a zoo (94).

Viruses of this group spread readily by contact (382, 511) and are shed in the FFE (95) although perhaps at lower levels than serotype 1 MDV (363). Following inoculation of day-old chickens, virus can be first isolated 5–6 days postinoculation (73). Virus reaches peak titers at 2–4 wk and persists for long periods (73, 511). Antibodies are induced readily and persist.

The SB-1 strain produced no neoplastic lesions in immunocompetent or immunosuppressed chickens but because some cytolytic lesions were noted in immunosuppressed chickens, the virus was designated nononcogenic rather than apathogenic (382). Also, a variety of lesions were induced by in ovo inoculation of SB-1 but none were neoplastic (74). The absence of gross neoplastic lesions has been noted by other workers (30, 93, 511), but Pol et al. (331) described endoneural and visceral lymphomas in 2 of 48 chickens inoculated with the HPRS-24 strain.

A distinct splenomegaly was induced between 4–12 days after inoculation of chicks with SB-1 (73). No bursal atrophy and only occasional thymic atrophy was seen and there was no cytolytic infection of lymphoid organs. SB-1 did not cause suppression of humoral immunity (133).

Vaccination with serotype 2 viruses causes a pronounced enhancement of LL in certain genetic strains of chickens exposed to avian leukosis virus at an early age (16). However, most commercial strains are not susceptible to this phenomenon and problems in the field are relatively rare.

REFERENCES

1. Adldinger, H.K., and B.W. Calnek. 1972. Effect of chelators on the in vitro infection with Marek's disease virus. In P.M. Biggs, G. de Thé, and L.N. Payne (eds.), Oncogenesis and Herpesviruses, pp. 99–105. IARC, Lyons, France.

2. Adldinger, H.K., and B.W. Calnek. 1973. Pathogenesis of Marek's disease: Early distribution of virus and viral antigens in infected chickens. J Nat Cancer Inst 50:1287–1298.

3. Adldinger, H.K., and A.W. Confer. 1977. Personal communication.

4. Adldinger, H.K., R.J. Thurston, R.F. Solorzano, and H.V. Biellier. 1974. Herpesvirus–a possible cause of low fertility in male turkeys. Arch Gesamte Virusforsch 46:370–376.

5. Akiyama, Y., and S. Kato. 1974. Two cell lines from lymphomas of Marek's disease. Biken J 17:105–116.

6. Akiyama, Y., S. Kato, and N. Iwa. 1973. Cell surface antigen and viral antigen of Marek's disease virus in lymphoid cells of the spleen from chickens inoculated with virulent strains. Biken J 16:91–94.

7. Anderson, D.P., C.S. Eidson, and D.J. Richey. 1971. Age susceptibility of chickens to Marek's disease. Am J Vet Res 32:935–938.

8. Anderson, D.P., D.D. King, C.S. Eidson, and S.H. Kleven. 1972. Filtered-air positive-pressure (FAPP) brooding of broiler chickens. Avian Dis 16:20–26.

9. Arita, K., and S. Nii. 1979. Short communication–effect of culture temperature on the production of Marek's disease virus antigens in a chicken lymphoblastoid cell line. Biken J 22:31–34.

10. Ash, R.J., and J.D. Ware. 1972. Growth charac-

teristics of a herpesvirus of turkeys. Appl Microbiol 24:943–946.

11. Ashikaga, M., I. Okada, Y. Yamamoto, and H. Matsuda. 1984. Interaction of the GVHR-selected lines and the B genotypes in the genetic resistance to Marek's disease. Jpn Poult Sci 21:102–110.

12. Bacon, L. 1987. Influence of the major histocompatability complex on disease resistance and productivity. Poult Sci 66:802–811.

13. Bacon, L.D., R.L. Witter, L.B. Crittenden, A.M. Fadly, and J.V. Motta. 1981. B-haplotype influence on Marek's disease, Rous sarcoma, and lymphoid leukosis virus-induced tumors in chickens. Poult Sci 60:1132–1139.

14. Bacon, L.D., L.B. Crittenden, R.L. Witter, A.M. Fadly, and J. Motta. 1983. B5 and B15 associated with progressive Marek's disease, Rous sarcoma, and avian leukosis virus induced tumors in inbred 15I4 chickens. Poult Sci 62:573–578.

15. Bacon, L.D., L.K. Chang, J. Spencer, A.A. Benedict, A.M. Fadly, R.L. Witter, and L.B. Crittenden. 1986. Tests of association of immunoglobulin allotype genes and viral oncogenesis in chickens. Immunogenet 23:213–220.

16. Bacon, L.D., R.L. Witter, and A.M. Fadly. 1989. Augmentation of retrovirus-induced lymphoid leukosis by Marek's disease herpesviruses in white leghorn chickens. J Virol 63:504–512.

17. Ball, R.F., and J.F. Lyman. 1977. Revaccination of chicks for Marek's disease at twenty-one days old. Avian Dis 21:440–444.

18. Ball, R.F., J.F. Hill, J. Lyman, and A. Wyatt. 1971. The resistance to Marek's disease of chicks from immunized breeders. Poult Sci 50:1084–1090.

19. Basarab, O., and T. Hall. 1976. Comparisons of cell-free and cell-associated Marek's disease vaccines in maternally immune chicks. Vet Rec 99:4–6.

20. Baxendale, W. 1969. Preliminary observations on Marek's disease in ducks and other avian species. Vet Rec 85:341–342.

21. Beasley, J.N., L.T. Patterson, and D.H. McWade. 1970. Transmission of Marek's disease by poultry house dust and chicken dander. Am J Vet Res 31:339–344.

22. Benda, V. 1982. Inhibitory activity of cytosine arabinoside on Marek's disease virus. Folia Biologica 28:311–316.

23. Benton, W.J., and M.S. Cover. 1957. The increased incidence of visceral lymphomatosis in broiler and replacement birds. Avian Dis 1:320–327.

24. Biggs, P.M. 1961. A discussion on the classification of the avian leucosis complex and fowl paralysis. Br Vet J 117:326– 334.

25. Biggs, P.M. 1967. Marek's disease. Vet Rec 81:583–592.

26. Biggs, P.M. 1968. Marek's disease – current state of knowledge. Curr Top Microbiol Immunol 43:93–125.

27. Biggs, P.M. 1973. Marek's disease. In A.S. Kaplan (ed.), The Herpesviruses, pp. 557–594. Academic Press, New York.

28. Biggs, P.M. 1985. Spread of Marek's disease. In L.N. Payne (ed.), Marek's Disease, pp. 329–340. Martinus Nijhoff, Boston.

29. Biggs, P.M., and B.S. Milne. 1971. Use of the embryonating egg in studies on Marek's disease. Am J Vet Res 32:1795–1809.

30. Biggs, P.M., and B.S. Milne. 1972. Biological properties of a number of Marek's disease virus isolates. In P.M. Biggs, G. de Thé, and L.N. Payne (eds.), Oncogenesis and Herpesviruses, pp. 88–94. IARC, Lyons, France.

31. Biggs, P.M., and L.N. Payne. 1963. Transmission experiments with Marek's disease (fowl paralysis). Vet Rec 75:177–179.

32. Biggs, P.M., and L.N. Payne. 1967. Studies on Marek's disease. I. Experimental transmission. J Nat Cancer Inst 39:267– 280.

33. Biggs, P.M., H.G. Purchase, B.R. Bee, and P.J. Dalton. 1965. Preliminary report on acute Marek's disease (fowl paralysis) in Great Britain. Vet Rec 77:1339–1340.

34. Biggs, P.M., P.L. Long, S.G. Kenzy, and D.G. Rootes. 1968. Relationship between Marek's disease and coccidiosis. II. The effect of Marek's disease on the susceptibility of chickens to coccidial infection. Vet Rec 83:284–289.

35. Biggs, P.M., R.J. Thorpe, and L.N. Payne. 1968. Studies on genetic resistance to Marek's disease in the domestic chicken. Br Poult Sci 9:37–52.

36. Biggs, P.M., D.G. Powell, A.E. Churchill, and R.C. Chubb. 1972. The epizootiology of Marek's disease. I. Incidence of antibody, viraemia and Marek's disease in six flocks. Avian Pathol 1:5–25.

37. Biggs, P.M., C.A.W. Jackson, and D.G. Powell. 1973. The epizootiology of Marek's disease. II. The effect of supply flock, rearing house, and production house on the incidence of Marek's disease. Avian Pathol 2:127–134.

38. Binns, M.M., K.A. Schat, C.A. Sutton, P.A. Kitchen, and L.J.N. Ross. 1988. Personal communication.

39. Boezi, J.A., L.F. Lee, R.W. Blakesley, M. Koenig, and H.C. Towle. 1974. Marek's disease herpesvirus-induced DNA polymerase. J Virol 14:1209–1219.

40. Bradley, G., M. Hayashi, G. Lancz, A. Tanaka, and M. Nonoyama. 1989. Structure of the MDV BAMHI-H gene family: A gene potentially important for tumor induction. In S. Kato, T. Horiuchi, T. Mikami, and K. Hirai (eds.), Advances in Marek's Disease Research, pp. 69–75. Japanese Association on Marek's Disease, Osaka.

41. Briles, W.E., H.A. Stone, and R.K. Cole. 1977. Marek's disease: Effects of B histocompatibility alloalleles in resistant and susceptible chicken lines. Science 195:193–195.

42. Briles, W.E., R.W. Briles, R.E. Taffs, and H.A. Stone. 1983. Resistance to a malignant lymphoma in chickens is mapped to subregion of major histocompatibility (B) complex. Science 219:977–979.

43. Brunovskis, P., P.M. Coussens, and L.F. Velicer. 1988. Personal communication.

44. Buckmaster, A.E., S.D. Scott, M.J. Sanderson, M.E.G. Boursnell, L.J.N. Ross, and M.M. Binns. 1988. Gene sequence and mapping data from Marek's disease virus and herpesvirus of turkeys – implications for herpesvirus classification. J Gen Virol 69:2033–2042.

45. Bülow, V.v. 1971. Diagnosis and certain biological properties of the virus of Marek's disease. Am J Vet Res 32:1275–1288.

46. Bülow, V.v., and P.M. Biggs. 1975. Differentiation between strains of Marek's disease virus and turkey herpesvirus by immunofluorescence assays. Avian Pathol 4:133–146.

47. Bülow, V.v., and P.M. Biggs 1975. Precipitating antigens associated with Marek's disease viruses and a herpesvirus of turkeys. Avian Pathol 4:147–162.

48. Bülow, V.v., and M. Lesjak. 1987. Modifizierter ELISA zum machweis antiviraler antikorper in Hühnerseren unter einbeziehung vonvirusfreien Zellantigenen zur Spezifitatskontrolle. Zentralbl Veterinaermed Reihe [B] 34:655–669.

49. Bülow, V.v., and D.O. Schmid. 1979. Antigenic characteristics of Marek's disease tumour cells. Avian

Pathol 8:265–277.
50. Bülow, V.v. 1977. Further characterisation of the CVI 988 strain of Marek's disease virus. Avian Pathol 6:395–403.
51. Bülow, V.v., Fuchs, B., Vielitz, E., and H. Landgraf. 1983. Fruhsterblichkeitssyndrom bei Küken nach Doppelinfektion mit dem Virus der Marekshen Krankheit (MDV) und einem Anämie-Erreger (CAA). Zentralbl Veterinaermed Reihe [B] 30:742–750.
52. Bumstead, J.M., and L.N. Payne. 1987. Production of an immune suppressor factor by Marek's disease lymphoblastoid cell lines. Vet Immunol Immunopathol 16:47–66.
53. Burgoyne, G.H., and R.L. Witter. 1973. Effect of passively transferred immunoglobulins on Marek's disease. Avian Dis 17:824–837.
54. Buscaglia, C., and B.W. Calnek. 1988. Maintenance of Marek's disease herpesvirus latency in vitro by a factor found in conditioned medium. J Gen Virol 69:2809–2818.
55. Buscaglia, C., B.W. Calnek, and K.A. Schat. 1988. Effect of immunocompetence on the establishment and maintenance of latency with Marek's disease herpesvirus. J Gen Virol 69:1067–1077.
56. Calnek, B.W. 1972. Effects of passive antibody on early pathogenesis of Marek's disease. Infect Immun 6:193–198.
57. Calnek, B.W. 1972. Antibody development in chickens exposed to Marek's disease virus. In P.M. Biggs, G. de Thé, and L.N. Payne (eds.), Oncogenesis and Herpesviruses, pp. 129–136. IARC, Lyons, France.
58. Calnek, B.W. 1973. Influence of age at exposure on the pathogenesis of Marek's disease. J Nat Cancer Inst 51:929–939.
59. Calnek, B.W. 1979. Unpublished data.
60. Calnek, B.W. 1980. Marek's disease virus and lymphoma. In F. Rapp (ed.), Oncogenic Herpesviruses, pp. 103–143. CRC Press, Boca Raton, FL.
61. Calnek, B.W. 1985. Genetic Resistance. In L.N. Payne (ed.), Marek's disease, pp. 293–328. Martinus Nijhoff, Boston.
62. Calnek, B.W. 1985. Pathogenesis of Marek's disease – a review. In B.W. Calnek and J.L. Spencer (eds.), Proc Int Symp Marek's Dis, pp. 374–390. Am Assoc Avian Pathol, Kennett Square, PA.
63. Calnek, B.W. 1986. Marek's disease – a model for herpesvirus oncology. CRC Crit Rev Microbiol 12:293–320.
64. Calnek, B.W. 1987. Established cell lines of avian lymphocytes and their use. In A. Toivanen and P. Toivanen (eds.), Avian Immunology: Basis and Practice, Vol. II, pp. 57–70. CRC Press, Boca Raton, FL.
65. Calnek, B.W., and H.K. Adldinger. 1971. Some characteristics of cell-free preparations of Marek's disease virus. Avian Dis 15:508–517.
66. Calnek, B.W., and S.B. Hitchner. 1969. Localization of viral antigen in chickens infected with Marek's disease herpesvirus. J Nat Cancer Inst 43:935–949.
67. Calnek, B.W., and S.B. Hitchner. 1973. Survival and disinfection of Marek's disease virus and the effectiveness of filters in preventing airborne dissemination. Poult Sci 52:35–43.
68. Calnek, B.W., H.K. Adldinger, and D.E. Kahn. 1970. Feather follicle epithelium: A source of enveloped and infectious cell-free herpesvirus from Marek's disease. Avian Dis 14:219–233.
69. Calnek, B.W., S.B. Hitchner, and H.K. Adldinger. 1970. Lyophilization of cell-free Marek's disease herpesvirus and a herpesvirus from turkeys. Appl Microbiol 20:723–726.
70. Calnek, B.W., J. Fabricant, K.A. Schat, and K.K. Murthy. 1977. Pathogenicity of low-virulence Marek's disease viruses in normal versus immunologically compromised chickens. Avian Dis 21:346–358.
71. Calnek, B.W., K.K. Murthy, and K.A. Schat. 1978. Establishment of Marek's disease lymphoblastoid cell lines from transplantable versus primary lymphomas. Int J Cancer 21:100–107.
72. Calnek, B.W., J. Fabricant, K.A. Schat, and K.K. Murthy. 1978. Rejection of a transplantable Marek's disease lymphoma in normal versus immunologically deficient chickens. J Nat Cancer Inst 60:623–631.
73. Calnek, B.W., J.C. Carlisle, J. Fabricant, K.K. Murthy, and K.A. Schat. 1979. Comparative pathogenesis studies with oncogenic and nononcogenic Marek's disease viruses and turkey herpesvirus. Am J Vet Res 40:541–548.
74. Calnek, B.W., K.A. Schat, and J. Fabricant. 1980. Modification of Marek's disease pathogenesis by in ovo infection or prior vaccination. In M. Essex, G. Todaro, and H. zur Hausen (eds.), Viruses in Naturally Occurring Cancers, Vol. 7, pp. 185–197. Cold Spring Harbor, NY.
75. Calnek, B.W., W.R. Shek, and K.A. Schat. 1981. Latent infections with Marek's disease virus and turkey herpesvirus. J Nat Cancer Inst 66:585–590.
76. Calnek, B.W., W.R. Shek, and K.A. Schat. 1981. Spontaneous and induced herpesvirus genome expression in Marek's disease tumor cell lines. Infect Immun 34:483–491.
77. Calnek, B.W., K.A. Schat, W.R. Shek, and C.-L.H. Chen. 1982. In vitro infection of lymphocytes with Marek's disease virus. J Nat Cancer Inst 69:709–713.
78. Calnek, B.W., W.R. Shek, K.A. Schat, and J. Fabricant. 1982. Dose-dependent inhibition of virus rescue from lymphocytes latently infected with turkey herpesvirus or Marek's disease virus. Avian Dis 26:321–331.
79. Calnek, B.W., K.A. Schat, M.C. Peckham, and J. Fabricant. 1983. Research note – field trials with a bivalent vaccine (HVT and SB-1) against Marek's disease. Avian Dis 27:844–849.
80. Calnek, B.W., K.A. Schat, L.J.N. Ross, W.R. Shek, and C.-L.H. Chen. 1984. Further characterization of Marek's disease virus-infected lymphocytes. I. In vivo infection. Int J Cancer 33:289–398.
81. Calnek, B.W., K.A. Schat, E.D. Heller, and C. Buscaglia. 1985. In vitro infection of T-lymphoblasts with Marek's disease virus. In B.W. Calnek and J.L. Spencer (eds.), Proc Int Symp Marek's Dis, pp. 173–187. Am Assoc Avian Pathol, Kennett Square, PA.
82. Calnek, B.W., D.F. Adene, K.A. Schat, and H. Abplanalp. 1988. Immune response versus susceptibility to Marek's disease. Poult Sci 68:17–26.
83. Calnek, B.W., B. Lucio, and K.A. Schat. 1989. Pathogenesis of Marek's disease virus-induced local lesions. 2. Influence of virus strain and host genotype. In S. Kato, T. Horiuchi, T. Mikami, and K. Hirai (eds.), Advances in Marek's Disease Research, pp. 324–330. Japanese Association on Marek's Disease, Osaka.
84. Calnek, B.W., B. Lucio, K.A. Schat, and H.S. Lillehoj. 1989. Pathogenesis of Marek's disease virus-induced local lesions. 1. Lesion characterization and cell line establishment. Avian Dis 33:291–302.
85. Campbell, J.G., and G.N. Woode. 1969. Demonstration of a herpes-type virus in short-term cultured blood lymphocytes associated with Marek's disease. J Med Microbiol 3:463–473.
86. Cauchy, L. 1974. The detection of viral antigens in Marek's disease by immunoperoxidase. In E. Krustak and R. Morisett (eds.), Viral Immunodiagnosis, pp. 77–78. Academic Press, New York.

87. Cauchy, L., and F. Coudert. 1972. Virologie–Particules de type Herps de la maladie de Marek dans les lymphocytes infectes et maintenus in vitro. C R Acad Sci Paris 274:1864–1866.
88. Cebrian, J., C. Kaschka-Dierich, N. Berthelot, and P. Sheldrick. 1982. Inverted repeat nucleotide sequences in the genomes of Marek's disease virus and the herpesvirus of the turkey. Proc Nat Acad Sci, US 79:555–558.
89. Chang, T.S. 1984. AUS in the prevention of Marek's disease. Avian Dis 28:154–159.
90. Chen, J.H., and H.G. Purchase. 1970. Surface antigen on chick kidney cells infected with the herpesvirus of Marek's disease. Virology 40:410–412.
91. Cheng, Y.-Q., L.F. Lee, E.J. Smith, and R.L. Witter. 1984. An enzyme-linked immunosorbent assay for the detection of antibodies to Marek's disease virus. Avian Dis 28:900–911.
92. Cho, B.R. 1975. Horizontal transmission of turkey herpesvirus to chickens. IV. Viral maturation in the feather follicle epithelium. Avian Dis 19:136–141.
93. Cho, B.R. 1976. A possible association between plaque type and pathogenicity of Marek's disease herpesvirus. Avian Dis 20:324–331.
94. Cho, B.R. 1976. In vitro biological differences between the pathogenic and apathogenic Marek's disease herpesvirus. Avian Dis 20:242–252.
95. Cho, B.R. 1977. Dual virus maturation of both pathogenic and apathogenic Marek's disease herpesvirus (MDHV) in the feather follicles of dually infected chickens. Avian Dis 21:501–507.
96. Cho, B.R. 1978. An improved method for extracting cell-free herpesviruses of Marek's disease and turkeys from infected cell cultures. Avian Dis 22:170–176.
97. Cho, B.R. 1981. A simple in vitro differentiation between turkey herpesvirus and Marek's disease virus. Avian Dis 25:839–846.
98. Cho, B.R., and S.G. Kenzy. 1972. Isolation and characterization of an isolate (HN) of Marek's disease virus with low pathogenicity. Appl Microbiol 24:299–306.
99. Cho, B.R., and S.G. Kenzy. 1975. Virologic and serologic studies of zoo birds for Marek's disease virus infection. Infect Immun 11:809–814.
100. Cho, B.R., and S.G. Kenzy. 1975. Horizontal transmission of turkey herpesvirus to chickens. 3. Transmission in three different lines of chickens. Poult Sci 54:109–115.
101. Cho, B.R., S.G. Kenzy, and S.A. Haider. 1971. Horizontal transmission of turkey herpesvirus to chickens. 1. Preliminary observation. Poult Sci 50:881–887.
102. Chubb, R.C., and A.E. Churchill. 1968. Precipitating antibodies associated with Marek's disease. Vet Rec 83:4–7.
103. Chubb, R.C., and A.E. Churchill. 1969. Effect of maternal antibody on Marek's disease. Vet Rec 85:303–305.
104. Churchill, A.E., and P.M. Biggs. 1967. Agent of Marek's disease in tissue culture. Nature 215:528–530.
105. Churchill, A.E., and P.M. Biggs. 1968. Herpes-type virus isolated in cell culture from tumors of chickens with Marek's disease. II. Studies in vivo. J Nat Cancer Inst 41:951– 956.
106. Churchill, A.E., R.C. Chubb, and W. Baxendale. 1969. The attenuation, with loss of oncogenicity of the herpes-type virus of Marek's disease (strain HPRS-16) on passage in cell culture. J Gen Virol 4:557–564.
107. Churchill, A.E., L.N. Payne, and R.C. Chubb. 1969. Immunization against Marek's disease using a live attenuated virus. Nature 221:744–747.
108. Cole, R.K. 1968. Studies on genetic resistance to Marek's disease. Avian Dis 12:9–28.
109. Cole, R.K. 1985. Natural resistance to Marek's disease–a review. In B.W. Calnek and J.L. Spencer (eds.), Proc Int Symp Marek's Dis, pp. 318–329. Am Assoc Avian Pathol, Kennett Square, PA.
110. Coleman, R.M., and L.W. Schierman. 1982. Transplantable Marek's disease lymphomas. I. Growth characteristics during development in two inbred lines of chickens. Avian Dis 26:245– 256.
111. Colwell, W.M., C.F. Simpson, L.E. Williams, Jr., and D.J. Forrester. 1973. Isolation of a herpesvirus from wild turkeys in Florida. Avian Dis 17:1–11.
112. Colwell, W.M., D.G. Simmons, J.R. Harris, T.G. Fulp, J.H. Carrozza, and T.A. Maag. 1975. Influence of some physical factors on survival of Marek's disease vaccine virus. Avian Dis 19:781–790.
113. Cook, M.K., and J.F. Sears. 1970. Preparation of infectious cell-free herpes-type virus associated with Marek's disease. J Virol 5:258–261.
114. Cotter, P.F., R.M. Jakowski, T.N. Fredrickson, L.W. Schierman, and R.A. McBride. 1975. Marek's disease in immunosuppressed chickens: Growth of a transplantable lymphoma and development of the disease by natural exposure. J Nat Cancer Inst 54:969–973.
115. Coudert, F., and L. Cauchy. 1984. Ubiquity and persistence of Marek's disease virus in tumoral and nontumorous explants. Curr Top Vet Med Anim Sci 459–468.
116. Coussens, P.M., M.R. Wilson, H. Roehl, R.J. Isfort, and L.F. Velicer. 1989. Nucleotide sequence analysis of the MDHV strain GA and HVT strain FC126 gp 57–65 (A antigen) genes. In S. Kato, T. Horiuchi, T. Mikami, and K. Hirai (eds.), Advances in Marek's Disease Research, pp. 99–106. Japanese Association on Marek's Disease, Osaka.
117. Cowen, B.S., and M.O. Braune. 1988. The propagation of avian viruses in a continuous cell line (QT35) of Japanese quail origin. Avian Dis 32:282–297.
118. Crittenden, L.B., R. Muhm, and B.R. Burmester. 1972. Genetic control of susceptibility to the avian leukosis complex. Poult Sci 51:261–267.
119. Davidson, I., M. Malkinson, C. Strenger, and Y. Becker. 1988. An improved ELISA method, using a streptavidin-biotin complex, for detecting Marek's disease virus antigens in feather-tips of infected chickens. J Virol Methods 14:237–241.
120. de Boer, G.F., J.E. Groenendal, H.M. Boerrigter, G.L. Kok, and J.M.A. Pol. 1986. Protective efficacy of Marek's disease virus (MDV) CVI-988 CEF65 clone C against challenge infection with three very virulent MDV strains. Avian Dis 30:276–283.
121. de Boer, G.F., J. Pol, and H. Oei. 1987. Biological characteristics of Marek's disease vaccine CVI-988 clone Cl. Vet Q 9:16S-28S.
122. de Boer, G.F., J.M.A. Pol, and S.H.M. Jeurissen. 1989. Marek's disease vaccination strategies using vaccines made from three avian herpesvirus serotypes. In S. Kato, T. Horiuchi, T. Mikami, and K. Hirai (eds.), Advances in Marek's Disease Research, pp. 405–413. Japanese Association on Marek's Disease, Osaka.
123. Doak, R.L., J.F. Munnell, and W.L. Ragland. 1973. Ultrastructure of tumor cells in Marek's disease virus-infected chickens. Am J Vet Res 34:1063–1069.
124. Dren, C.N., and I. Nemeth. 1985. Differential diagnosis of Marek's disease and lymphoid leukosis on the basis of cell-surface antigens. Proc Int Symp Marek's Dis., pp. 196–213.
125. Drury, L.N., W.C. Patterson, and C.W. Beard. 1969. Ventilating poultry houses with filtered air under positive pressure to prevent airborne diseases. Poult Sci 48:1640–1646.
126. Dunn, K., and K. Nazerian. 1977. Induction of

Marek's disease virus antigens by IdUrd in a chicken lymphoblastoid cell line. J Gen Virol 34:413–419.

127. Eidson, C.S., and S.C. Schmittle. 1968. Studies on acute Marek's disease. I. Characteristics of isolate GA in chickens. Avian Dis 12:467–476.

128. Eidson, C.S., S.H. Kleven, and D.P. Anderson. 1973. Effect of antibiotics on turkey herpesvirus vaccine. Poult Sci 52:755–760.

129. Eidson, C.S., V.T. Than, and S.H. Kleven. 1974. The in vitro and in vivo effect of chemotherapeutic agents on the Marek's disease herpesvirus of chickens. Poult Sci 53:1533–1538.

130. Eidson, C.S., R.K. Page, and S.H. Kleven. 1978. In vivo and in vitro studies on the effect of gentamicin sulfate on the efficacy of the turkey herpesvirus vaccine. Poult Sci 52:1519–1525.

131. Eidson, C.S., R.K. Page, and S.H. Kleven. 1978. Effectiveness of cell-free or cell-associated turkey herpesvirus vaccine against Marek's disease in chickens as influenced by maternal antibody, vaccine dose, and time of exposure to Marek's disease virus. Avian Dis 22:583–597.

132. Ekperigin, H.E., A.M. Fadly, L.F. Lee, X. Liu, and R.H. McCapes. 1983. Comb lesions and mortality patterns in white leghorn layers affected by Marek's disease. Avian Dis 27:503–512.

133. Ellis, M.N., C.S. Eidson, J. Brown, O.J. Fletcher, and S.H. Kleven. 1981. Serological responses to mycoplasma synoviae in chickens infected with virulent or avirulent strains of Marek's disease virus. Poult Sci 60:1344–1347.

134. Elmubarak, A.K., J.M. Sharma, R.L. Witter, K. Nazerian, and V.L. Sanger. 1981. Induction of lymphomas and tumor antigen by Marek's disease virus in turkeys. Avian Dis 25:911–926.

135. Elmubarak, A.K., J.M. Sharma, R.L. Witter, and V.L. Sanger. 1982. Marek's disease in turkeys: Lack of protection by vaccination. Am J Vet Res 43:740–742.

136. Else, R.W. 1974. Vaccinal immunity to Marek's disease in bursectomized chickens. Vet Rec 95:182–187.

137. Evans, D.L., and L.T. Patterson. 1971. Serum lysozyme determinations in Marek's disease-infected chickens. Poult Sci 50:1575. (Abstr).

138. Fabricant, C.G. 1985. Atherosclerosis: The consequence of infection with a herpesvirus. Adv Vet Sci Comp Med 30:39–66.

139. Fabricant, J., M. Ianconescu, and B.W. Calnek. 1977. Comparative effects of host and viral factors on early pathogenesis of Marek's disease. Infect Immun 16:136–144.

140. Fabricant, C.G., J. Fabricant, M.M. Litrenta, and C.R. Minick. 1978. Virus-induced atherosclerosis. J Exp Med 148:335- 340.

141. Fabricant, C.G., D.P. Hajjar, C.R. Minick, and J. Fabricant. 1981. Herpesvirus infection enhances cholesterol and cholesteryl ester accumulation in cultured arterial smooth muscle cells. Am J Pathol 105:176–184.

142. Fabricant, J., B.W. Calnek, and K.A. Schat. 1982. The early pathogenesis of turkey herpesvirus infection in chickens and turkeys. Avian Dis 26:257–264.

143. Fletcher, O.J., and L.W. Schierman. 1985. Variation in histology and growth characteristics of transplantable Marek's disease lymphomas. Cancer Res 45:1762–1765.

144. Fletcher, O.J., Jr., C.S. Eidson, and R.K. Page. 1971. Pathogenesis of Marek's disease induced in chickens by contact exposure to GA isolate. Am J Vet Res 32:1407–1416.

145. Frazier, J.A. 1974. Ultrastructure of lymphoid tissue from chicks infected with Marek's disease virus. J Nat Cancer Inst 52:829–837.

146. Fredericksen, T.L., D.G. Gilmour, L.D. Bacon, R.L. Witter, and J. Motta. 1982. Tests of association of lymphocyte alloantigen genotypes with resistance to viral oncogenesis in chickens. 1. Marek's disease in F7 progeny derived from 6/3 x 15/1 crosses. Poult Sci 61:2322–2326.

147. Freeman, B.M., A.C.C. Manning, and R.S. Phillips. 1984. Failure to induce stress reactions following vaccination against Marek's disease or Newcastle disease. Res Vet Sci 36:247–250.

148. Fukuchi, K., M. Sudo, Y.S. Lee, A. Tanaka, and M. Nonoyama. 1984. Structure of Marek's disease virus DNA: Detailed restriction enzyme map. J Virol 51:102–109.

149. Fukuchi, K., M. Sudo, A. Tanaka, and M. Nonoyama. 1985. Map location of homologous regions between Marek's disease virus and herpesvirus of turkey and the absence of detectable homology in the putative tumor-inducing gene. J Virol 53:994–997.

150. Gibbs, C.P., K. Nazerian, L. Velicer, and H.-J. Kung. 1983. Extensive homology exists between Marek's disease herpesvirus and its vaccine virus, herpesvirus of turkeys. Proc Nat Acad Sci, US 81:3365–3369.

151. Goodchild, W.M. 1969. Some observations on Marek's disease (fowl paralysis). Vet Rec 84:87–89.

152. Gross, W.B. 1972. Effect of social stress on occurrence of Marek's disease in chickens. Am J Vet Res 33:2275–2279.

153. Haffer, K., M. Sevoian, and M. Wilder. 1979. The role of the macrophage in Marek's disease: In vitro and in vivo studies. Int J Cancer 23:648–656.

154. Haider, S.A., R.F. Lapen, and S.G. Kenzy. 1970. Use of feathers in a gel precipitation test for Marek's disease. Poult Sci 49:1654–1657.

155. Hajjar, D.P., C.G. Fabricant, C.R. Minick, and J. Fabricant. 1986. Virus-induced atherosclerosis. Am J Pathol 122:62–70.

156. Halliwell, W.H. 1971. Lesions of Marek's disease in a great horned owl. Avian Dis 15:49–55.

157. Halvorson, D.A., and D.O Mitchell. 1979. Loss of cell-associated Marek's disease vaccine titer during thawing, reconstitution, and use. Avian Dis 23:848–853.

158. Han, P.F.S., and J.R. Smyth, Jr. 1972. The influence of restricted feed intake on the response of chickens to Marek's disease. Poult Sci 51:986–991.

159. Han, P.F.S., and J.R. Smyth, Jr. 1972. The influence of growth rate on the development of Marek's disease. Poult Sci 51:975–985.

160. Hansen, M.P., J.N. Van Zandt, and G.R.J. Law. 1967. Differences in susceptibility to Marek's disease in chickens carrying two different B locus blood group alleles. Poult Sci 46:1268. (Abstr).

161. Harriss, S.T. 1939. Lymphomatosis (fowl paralysis) in the pheasant. Vet J 95:104–106.

162. Hayashi, M., J. Jessip, K. Fukuchi, M. Smith, A. Tanaka, and M. Nonoyama. 1988. The structure of Marek's disease virus DNA: Amplification of repeat sequence in IRs and TRs. Microbiol Immunol 32:265–274.

163. Heller, E.D., and K.A. Schat. 1985. Inhibition of natural killer activity in chickens by Marek's disease virus-transformed cell lines. In B.W. Calnek and J.L. Spencer (eds.), Proc Int Symp Marek's Dis, pp. 286–294. Am Assoc Avian Pathol, Kennett Square, PA.

164. Helmboldt, C.F., F.K. Wills, and M.N. Frazier. 1963. Field observations of the pathology of skin leukosis in Gallus gallus. Avian Dis 7:402–411.

165. Higashihara, T., T. Mikami, H. Kodama, H. Izawa, and H. Tamura. 1986. Detection of a new antigen associated with chicken thrombocytes on Marek's disease lymphoblastoid cell line. J Nat Cancer Inst 76:1085–1094.

166. Higgins, D.A., and B.W. Calnek. 1975. Fowl im-

munoglobulins: Quantitation in birds genetically resistant and susceptible to Marek's disease. Infect Immun 12:360–363.
167. Higgins, D.A., and B.W. Calnek. 1975. Fowl immunoglobulins: Quantitation and antibody activity during Marek's disease in genetically resistant and susceptible birds. Infect Immun 11:33–41.
168. Higgins, D.A., and B.W. Calnek. 1976. Some effects of silica treatment on Marek's disease. Infect Immun 13:1054–1060.
169. Hirai, K., K. Ikuta, and S. Kato. 1979. Comparative studies on Marek's disease virus and herpesvirus of turkey DNAs. J Gen Virol 45:119–131.
170. Hirai, K., K. Ikuta, and S. Kato. 1980. DNA synthesis in chicken embryo fibroblast cells replicating Marek's disease virus. Avian Dis 24:37–42.
171. Hirai, K., K. Ikuta, N. Kitamoto, and S. Kato. 1981. Latency of herpesvirus of turkey and Marek's disease virus genomes in a chicken T-lymphoblastoid cell line. J Gen Virol 53:133–143.
172. Hirai, K., K. Ikuta, N. Kitamoto, and S. Kato. 1981. Restriction endonuclease analysis of the genomes of virulent and avirulent Marek's disease viruses. Microbiol Immunol 25:671–681.
173. Hirai, K., K. Ikuta, K. Maotani, and S. Kato. 1984. Evaluation of DNA homology of Marek's disease virus, herpesvirus of turkeys and Epstein-Barr virus under varied stringent hybridization conditions. J Biochem 95:1215–1218.
174. Hirai, K., K. Nakajima, K. Ikuta, R. Kirisawa, Y. Kawakami, T. Mikami, and S. Kato. 1986. Similarities and dissimilarities in the structure and expression of viral genomes of various virus strains immunologically related to Marek's disease virus. Arch Virol 89:113–130.
175. Hirai, K., A. Kanamori, M. Niikura, K. Ikuta, and S. Kato. 1989. RNA transcribed from Marek's disease virus genomes in productively and latently infected cells. In S. Kato, T. Horiuchi, T. Mikami, and K. Hirai (eds.), Advances in Marek's Disease Research, pp. 140–147. Japanese Association on Marek's Disease, Osaka.
176. Hirose, H., M. Matsuda, M. Murata, and Y. Sekiya. 1986. Preparation of monoclonal antibodies against Marek's disease virus and herpesvirus of turkeys. Jpn J Vet Sci 48:1263–1266.
177. Hlozanek, I. 1970. The influence of ultraviolet-inactivated Sendai virus on Marek's disease virus infection in tissue culture. J Gen Virol 9:45–50.
178. Hlozanek, I., and V. Sovova. 1974. Lack of pathogenicity of Marek's disease herpesvirus and herpesvirus of turkeys for mammalian hosts and mammalian cell cultures. Folia Biol 20:51–58.
179. Hlozanek, I., O. Mach, and V. Jurajda. 1973. Cell-free preparations of Marek's disease virus from poultry dust (persisting infectivity/induction of tumours/temperature dependence/sucrose-density gradient and electron-microscopic characteristics). Folia Biol 19:118–123.
180. Hlozanek, I., V. Jurajda, and V. Benda. 1977. Disinfection of Marek's disease virus in poultry dust. Avian Pathol 6:241–250.
181. Hong, C.C., and M. Sevoian. 1971. Interferon production and host resistance to type II avian (Marek's) leukosis virus (JM strain). Appl Microbiol 22:818–820.
182. Hudson, L., and L.N. Payne. 1973. An analysis of the T and B cells of Marek's disease lymphomas of the chicken. Nature (New Biol) 241:52–53.
183. Hughes, S.K., E. Stubblefield, K. Nazerian, and H.E. Varmus. 1980. DNA of a chicken herpesvirus is associated with at least two chromosomes in a chicken lymphoblastoid cell line. Virology 105:234–240.
184. Hutt, F.B., and R.K. Cole. 1947. Genetic control of lymphomatosis in the fowl. Science 106:379–384.
185. Hutt, F.B., and R.K. Cole. 1948. The development of strains genetically resistant to avian lymphomatosis. Proc 8th World's Poult Congr, pp. 719–725.
186. Igarashi, T., M. Takagashi, J. Donovan, J. Jessip, M. Smith, K. Hirai, A. Tanaka, and M. Nonoyama. 1987. Restriction enzyme map of herpesvirus of turkey DNA and its collinear relationship with Marek's disease virus DNA. Virology 157:351–358.
187. Ikuta, K., N. Kitamoto, H. Shoji, S. Kato, and M. Naiki. 1981. Expression of Forssman antigen of avian lymphoblastoid cell lines transformed by Marek's disease virus or avian leukosis virus. J Gen Virol 52:145–151.
188. Ikuta, K., N. Kitamoto, H. Shoji, S. Kato, and M. Maidi. 1981. Hanganutziu and Deicher type heterophile antigen expressed on the cell surface of Marek's disease lymphoma derived cell lines. Biken J 24:23–37.
189. Ikuta, K., Y. Nishi, S. Kato, and K. Hirai. 1981. Immunoprecipitation of Marek's disease virus-specific polypeptides with chicken antibodies purified by affinity chromatography. Virology 114:277–281.
190. Ikuta, K., H. Honma, K. Maotani, S. Ueda, S. Kato, and K. Hirai. 1982. Monoclonal antibodies specific to and cross-reactive with Marek's disease virus and herpesvirus of turkeys. Biken J 25:171–175.
191. Ikuta, K., S. Ueda, S. Kato, and K. Hirai. 1983. Most virus-specific polypeptides in cells productively infected with Marek's disease virus or herpesvirus of turkeys possess cross-reactive determinants. J Gen Virol 64:961–965.
192. Ikuta, K., K. Nakajima, S. Ueda, S. Kato, and K. Hirai. 1984. Studies on the serological cross-reaction between Marek's disease virus and herpesvirus of turkeys using monoclonal antibodies to major virus-specific polypeptides. Arch Virol 81:337–343.
193. Ikuta, K., S. Ueda, S. Kato, and K. Hirai. 1984. Processing of glycoprotein gB related to neutralization of Marek's disease virus and herpesvirus of turkeys. Microbiol Immunol 28:923–933.
194. Ikuta, K., S. Ueda, S. Kato, K. Ono, S. Osafune, I. Yoshida, T. Naito, M. Naito, and K. Hirai. 1985. Identification of Marek's disease virus-specific antigens in Marek's disease lymphoblastoid cell lines using monoclonal antibody against virus-specific phosphorylated polypeptides. Int J Cancer 35:257– 264.
195. Ikuta, K., K. Nakajima, S. Ueda, S. Kato, and K. Hirai. 1985. Differences in the processing of secreted glycoprotein A induced by Marek's disease virus and herpesvirus of turkeys. J Gen Virol 66:1131–1137.
196. Ikuta, K., K. Nakajima, A. Kanamori, K. Maotani, J.S. Mah, S. Ueda, S. Kato, M. Yoshida, S. Nii, M. Naito, C. Nishida-Umehara, M. Saski, and K. Hirai. 1987. Establishment and characterization of a T-lymphoblastoid cell line MDCC-MTB1 derived from chick lymphocytes infected in vitro with Marek's disease serotype 1. Int J Cancer 39:514–520.
197. Ikuta, K., K. Nakajima, M. Naito, A. Kanamori, K. Hirai, and S. Kato. 1989. Expression of the antigen related to Marek's disease virus serotype 1-specific phosphorylated polypeptides in in vitro transformed cell line, MDCC-MTB-1. In S. Kato, T. Horiuchi, T. Mikami, and K. Hirai (eds.), Advances in Marek's Disease Research, pp. 135–139. Japanese Association on Marek's Disease, Osaka.
198. Inoue, M., T. Mikami, H. Kodama, M. Onuma, and H. Izawa. 1980. Antigenic difference between intracellular and membrane antigens induced by herpesvirus of turkeys. Arch Virol 63:23–30.
199. Isfort, R.J., I. Sithole, H.-J. Kung, and L.F. Veli-

cer. 1986. Molecular characterization of the Marek's disease herpesvirus B antigen. J Virol 59:411–419.
200. Isfort, R.J., R.A. Stringer, H.-J. Kung, and L.F. Velicer. 1986. Synthesis, processing, and secretion of the Marek's disease herpesvirus A antigen glycoprotein. J Virol 57:464–474.
201. Isfort, R., H. Kung, and L. Velicer. 1987. Identification of the gene encoding Marek's disease herpesvirus A antigen. J Virol 61:2614–2620.
202. Jakowski, R.M., T.N. Fredrickson, T.W. Chomiak, and R.E. Luginbuhl. 1970. Hematopoietic destruction in Marek's disease. Avian Dis 14:374–385.
203. Jakowski, R.M., T.N. Fredrickson, L.W. Schierman, and R.A. McBride. 1974. A transplantable lymphoma induced with Marek's disease virus. J Nat Cancer Inst 53:783–789.
204. Johnson, E.P. 1941. Fowl leukosis–manifestations, transmission, and etiological relationship of various forms. Virginia Agric Exp Stn Tech Bull 76.
205. Jungherr, E.L. 1939. Neurolymphomatosis phasianorum. J Am Vet Med Assoc 94:49–52.
206. Jungherr, E.L., and W.F. Hughes. 1965. The avian leukosis complex. In H.E. Biester and L.H. Schwarte (eds.), Diseases of Poultry, 5th Ed., pp. 512–567. Iowa State Univ Press, Ames.
207. Jurajda, V., and B. Klimes. 1970. Presence and survival of Marek's disease agent in dust. Avian Dis 14:188–190.
208. Kaaden, O.R. 1978. Transfection studies in vitro and in vivo with isolated Marek's disease virus DNA. In G. de Thé, W. Henle, F. Rapp (eds.), Oncogenesis and Herpesviruses III, pp. 627–634. IARC, Lyons, France.
209. Kaaden, O.R., B. Dietzschold, and S. Uberschar. 1974. Vaccination against Marek's disease: Immunizing effect of purified turkey herpesvirus and cellular membranes from infected cells. Med Microbiol Immunol 159:261–269.
210. Kaaden, O.R., A. Scholtz, A. BenZeev, and Y. Becker. 1977. Isolation of Marek's disease virus DNA from infected cells by electrophoresis on polyacrylamide gels. Arch Virol 54:75–84.
211. Kaleta, E.F., and R.A. Bankowski. 1972. Production of interferon by the Cal-l and turkey herpesvirus strains associated with Marek's disease. Am J Vet Res 33:567–571.
212. Kaleta, E.F., and U. Neumann. 1977. Investigations on the mode of transmission of the herpesvirus of turkeys in vitro. Avian Pathol 6:33–39.
213. Kaleta, E.F., K. Pressler, and O. Seigmann. 1984. Chemoprophylaxis of Marek's disease of the chicken by impacarzin. Fortschr Vet 35:310–318.
214. Kanamori, A., K. Nakajima, K. Ikuta, S. Ueda, S. Kato, and K. Hirai. 1986. Copy number of tandem direct repeats within the inverted repeats of Marek's disease virus DNA. Biken J 29:83– 89.
215. Kanamori, A., K. Ikuta, S. Ueda, S. Kato, and K. Hirai. 1987. Methylation of Marek's disease virus DNA in chicken T-lymphoblastoid cell lines. J Gen Virol 68:1485–1490.
216. Kaschka-Dierich, C., and R. Thomssen. 1979. Studies on the temperature-dependent DNA replication of the herpesvirus of the turkey in chicken embryo fibroblasts. J Gen Virol 45:253–261.
217. Kaschka-Dierich, C., K. Nazerian, and R. Thomssen. 1979. Intracellular state of Marek's disease virus DNA in two tumor-derived chicken cell lines. J Gen Virol 44:271–280.
218. Kato, S., and K. Hirai. 1985. Marek's disease virus. Adv Virus Res 30:225–277.
219. Kawamura, H., D.J. King, Jr., and D.P. Anderson. 1969. A herpesvirus isolated from kidney cell culture of normal turkeys. Avian Dis 13:853–863.
220. Kenzy, S.G., and P.M. Biggs. 1967. Excretion of the Marek's disease agent by infected chickens. Vet Rec 80:565–568.
221. Kenzy, S.G., and B.R. Cho. 1969. Transmission of classical Marek's disease by affected and carrier birds. Avian Dis 13:211–214.
222. King, D., D. Page, K.A. Schat, and B.W. Calnek. 1981. Difference between influences of homologous and heterologous maternal antibodies on response to serotype-2 and serotype-3 Marek's disease vaccines. Avian Dis 25:74–81.
223. Kishi, M., H. Harada, M. Takahashi, A. Tanaka, M. Hayashi, M. Nonoyama, S.F. Josephs, A. Buchbinder, F. Schacter, D.V. Ablashi, F. Wong-Staal, S.Z. Salahuddin, and R.C. Gallo. 1988. A repeat sequence, GGGTTA, is shared by DNA of human herpesvirus 6 and Marek's disease virus. J Virol 62:4824–4827.
224. Kitamoto, N., K. Ikuta, S. Kato, and K. Wataki. 1979. Demonstration of cells with Marek's disease tumor-associated surface antigen in chicks infected with herpesvirus of turkey, 01 strain. Biken J 22:137–142.
225. Kitamoto, N., K. Ikuta, and S. Kato. 1980. Persistence of genomes of both herpesvirus of turkeys and Marek's disease virus in a chicken T-lymphoblastoid cell line. Biken J 23:1–8.
226. Kit, S., G.N. Jorgensen, W.C. Leung, K. Trkula, and K.R. Dubbs. 1974. Thymidine kinases induced by avian and human herpesviruses. Intervirology 2:299–311.
227. Kodama, H., C. Sugimoto, F. Inage, and T. Mikami. 1979. Antiviral immunity against Marek's disease virus infected chicken kidney cells. Avian Pathol 8:33–44.
228. Kodama, H., T. Mikami, M. Inoue, and H. Izawa. 1979. Inhibitory effects of macrophages against Marek's disease virus plaque formation in chicken kidney cell cultures. J Nat Cancer Inst 63:1267–1271.
229. Kodama, H., T. Mikami, and H. Izawa. 1980. Effects of levamisole on pathogenesis on Marek's disease. J Nat Cancer Inst 65:155–159.
230. Kondo, T., T. Mikami, H. Kodama, and H. Izawa. 1988. Two distinct antigens on chicken thymocytes defined by monoclonal antibodies. Avian Pathol 17:589–600.
231. Konobe, T., T. Ishikawa, K. Takaku, K. Ikuta, N. Kitamoto, and S. Kato. 1979. Marek's disease virus and herpesvirus of turkey noninfective to chickens, obtained by repeated in vitro passages. Biken J 22:103–107.
232. Kornegay, J.N., E.J. Gorgacz, M.A. Parker, J. Brown, and L.W. Schierman. 1983. Marek's disease virus-induced transient paralysis: Clinical and electrophysiologic findings in susceptible and resistant lines of chickens. Am J Vet Res 44:1541–1544.
233. Kung, H.-J. 1989. Personal communication.
234. Lam, K.M., and T.J. Linna. 1979. Transfer of natural resistance to Marek's disease (JMV) with nonimmune spleen cells. I. Studies of cell population transferring resistance. Int J Cancer 24:662–667.
235. Lapen, R.F., and S.G. Kenzy. 1972. Distribution of gross cutaneous Marek's disease lesions. Poult Sci 51:334–336.
236. Lau, R.Y., and M. Nonoyama. 1980. Replication of the resident Marek's disease virus genome in synchronized nonproducer MKT-1 cells. J Virol 33:912–914.
237. Lawn, A.M., and L.N. Payne. 1979. Chronological study of ultrastructural changes in the peripheral nerves in Marek's disease. Neuropathol Appl Neurobiol 5:485–497.
238. Lee, L.F. 1979. Macrophage restriction of

Marek's disease virus replication and lymphoma cell proliferation. J Immunol 123:1088–1091.

239. Lee, L.F., and Z. Cui. 1989. Identification of Marek's disease virus genes in bacteriophage lambda gt11 with monoclonal antibodies. In S. Kato, T. Horiuchi, T. Mikami, and K. Hirai (eds.), Advances in Marek's Disease Research, pp. 56–61. Japanese Association on Marek's Disease, Osaka.

240. Lee, L.F., E.D. Kieff, S.L. Bachenheimer, B. Roizman, P.G. Spear, B.R. Burmester, and K. Nazerian. 1971. Size and composition of Marek's disease virus deoxyribonucleic acid. J Virol 7:289–294.

241. Lee, L.F., R.L. Armstrong, and K. Nazerian. 1972. Comparative studies of six avian herpesviruses. Avian Dis 16:799– 805.

242. Lee, L.F., K. Nazerian, and J.A. Boezi. 1975. Marek's disease virus DNA in a chicken lymphoblastoid cell line (MSB-1) and in virus-induced tumours. In G. de Thé, M.A. Epstein, and H. zur Hausen (eds.), Oncogenesis and Herpesviruses II, pp. 199–204, IARC, Lyons, France.

243. Lee, L.F., K. Nazerian, S.S. Leinbach, J.M. Reno, and J.A. Boezi. 1976. Effect of phosphonoacetate on Marek's disease virus replication. J Nat Cancer Inst 56:823–827.

244. Lee, L.F., K. Nazerian, R.L. Witter, S.S. Leinbach, and J.A. Boezi. 1978. A phosphonoacetate-resistant mutant of herpesvirus of turkeys. J Nat Cancer Inst 60:1141–1146.

245. Lee, L.F., J.M. Sharma, K. Nazerian, and R.L. Witter. 1978. Suppression of mitogen-induced proliferation of normal spleen cells by macrophages from chickens inoculated with Marek's disease virus. J Immunol 120:1554–1559.

246. Lee, Y.-S., A. Tanaka, S. Silver, M. Smith, and M. Nonoyama. 1979. Minor DNA homology between herpesvirus of turkey and Marek's disease virus? Virology 93:277–280.

247. Lee, L.F., P.C. Powell, M. Rennie, L.J.N. Ross, and L.N. Payne. 1981. Nature of genetic resistance to Marek's disease in chickens. J Nat Cancer Inst 66:789–796.

248. Lee, L.F., X. Liu, and R.L. Witter. 1983. Monoclonal antibodies with specificity for three different serotypes of Marek's disease viruses in chickens. J Immunol 130:1003–1006.

249. Lee, L.F., X. Liu, J.M. Sharma, K. Nazerian, and L.D. Bacon. 1983. A monoclonal antibody reactive with Marek's disease tumor-associated surface antigen. J Immunol 130:1007–1011.

250. Lesnik, F., and L.J.N. Ross. 1975. Immunization against Marek's disease using Marek's disease virus-specific antigens free from infectious virus. Int J Cancer 16:153–163.

251. Lesnik, F., D. Chudy, J. Bogdan, O.J. Vrtiak, and M. Rudic. 1978. Testing the immunogenicity of the dermal antigen of Marek's disease virus. Vet Med Praha 23:421–430.

252. Liu, X., and L.F. Lee. 1983. Development and characterization of monoclonal antibodies to Marek's disease tumor-associated surface antigen. Infect Immun 31:851–854.

253. Livingston-Wheeler, V., and J.J. Majnarick. 1983. Method for preparing a purified extraction residue fraction and its use in stimulating the immune response. U.S. Patent 4, 410,510.

254. Longenecker, B.M., F. Pazderka, J.S. Gavora, J.L. Spencer, and R.F. Ruth. 1976. Lymphoma induced by herpesvirus: Resistance associated with a major histocompatibility gene. Immunogenetics 3:401–407.

255. Maas, H.J.L., H.W. Antonisse, A.J. Van Der Zypp, J.E. Groenendal, and G.L. Kok. 1981. The development of two white plymouth rock lines resistant to Marek's disease by breeding from survivors. Avian Pathol 10:137–150.

256. Madarame, H., Y. Fujimoto, and R. Moriguchi. 1986. Ultrastructural studies on muscular atrophy in Marek's disease. II. Muscular lesions in spontaneous cases. Jpn J Vet Res 34:51– 75.

257. Malkinson, M., U. Orgad, and Y. Becker. 1986. Use of lectins to detect and differentiate subtypes of Marek's disease virus and turkey herpesvirus glycoproteins in tissue culture. J Virol Methods 13:129–133.

258. Maotani, K., A. Kanamori, K. Ikuta, S. Ueda, S. Kato, and K. Hirai. 1986. Amplification of a tandem direct repeat within inverted repeats of Marek's disease virus DNA during serial in vitro passage. J Virol 58:657–660.

259. Maray, T., M. Malkinson, and Y. Becker. 1988. RNA transcripts of Marek's disease virus (MDV) serotype-1 infected and transformed cells. Virus Genes 2:49–68.

260. Marek, J. 1907. Multiple Nervenentzuendung (Polyneuritis) bei Huehnern. Dtsch Tierärztl Wochenschr 15:417–421.

261. Mason, R.J., and K.E. Jensen. 1971. Marek's disease: Resistance of turkey herpesvirus-infected chicks against lethal JM-V agent. Am J Vet Res 32:1625–1627.

262. Matsuda, H., K. Ikuta, and S. Kato. 1976. Detection of T-cell surface determinants in three Marek's disease lymphoblastoid cell lines. Biken J 19:29–32.

263. Mazzella, O., L. Cauchy, F. Coudert, and J. Richard. 1986. Chicken thymocyte-specific antigens identified by monoclonal antibodies: Characterization and distribution in normal tissues and in tumoral tissues from Marek's disease chicken. Hybridoma 5:319–328.

264. McColl, K. 1988. Cellular and molecular studies on transformed cells in Marek's disease. PhD diss., Cornell Univ, Ithaca, NY.

265. McColl, K., B.W. Calnek, W.V. Harris, K.A. Schat, and L.F. Lee. 1987. Expression of a putative tumor-associated antigen on normal versus Marek's disease virus-transformed lymphocytes. J Nat Cancer Inst 79:991–1000.

266. Mikami, T., and R.A. Bankowski. 1971. Pathogenic and serologic studies of type 1 and type 2 plaque-producing agents derived from Cal-1 strain of Marek's disease virus. Am J Vet Res 32:303–317.

267. Mikami, T., M. Onuma, and T.T.A. Hayashi. 1973. Membrane antigens in arginine-deprived cultures infected with Marek's disease herpesvirus. Nature 246:211–212.

268. Mikami, T., M. Onuma, and T.T.A. Hayashi. 1974. Requirement of arginine for the replication of Marek's disease herpesvirus. J Gen Virol 22:115–128.

269. Mikami, T., M. Inoue, H. Kodama, F. Inage, M. Onuma, and H. Izawa. 1980. Relation between the neutralization of herpesvirus of turkeys and the antibody to late-appearing membrane antigen induced by the virus. J Gen Virol 47:221–226.

270. Mikami, T., T. Higashihara, M. Yasuda, K. Kunihiro, H. Kodama, H. Izawa, and I. Okada. 1985. Inhibition of turkey herpesvirus replication by anticellular serum. Avian Dis 29:250– 255.

271. Minick, C.R., C.G. Fabricant, J. Fabricant, and M.M. Litrenta. 1979. Atheroarteriosclerosis induced by infection with a herpesvirus. Am J Pathol 96:673–706.

272. Mohanty, G.C., L.N. Acharjyo, and B.S. Rajya. 1973. Epidemiology of Marek's disease (MD): Studies on the incidence of MD precipitins in some zoo birds. Poult Sci 52:963–966.

273. Morgan, H.R. 1971. Antibodies for Marek's disease virus in sera from domestic chickens and wild fowl in Kenya. Avian Dis 15:611-613.

274. Moriguchi, R., M. Oshima, F. Mori, I. Umezawa, and C. Itakura. 1989. Chronological change of feather pulp lesions during the course of Marek's disease virus-induced lymphoma formation in field chickens. In S. Kato, T. Horiuchi, T. Mikami, and K. Hirai (eds.), Advances in Marek's Disease Research, pp. 338-343. Japanese Association on Marek's Disease, Osaka.

275. Moscovici, C., M.G. Moscovici, and H. Jimenez. 1977. Continuous tissue culture cell lines derived from chemically induced tumors of Japanese quail. Cell 11:95-103.

276. Murthy, K.K., and B.W. Calnek. 1979. Pathogenesis of Marek's disease: Effect of immunization with inactivated viral and tumor-associated antigens. Infect Immun 26:547-553.

277. Murthy, K.I., R.R. Dietert, and B.W. Calnek. 1979. Demonstration of chicken fetal antigen (CFA) on normal splenic lymphocytes, Marek's disease lymphoblastoid cell lines and other neoplasms. Int J Cancer 24:349-354.

278. Naito, M., K. Nakajima, N. Iwa, K. Ono, I. Yoshida, T. Konobe, K. Ikuta, S. Ueda, S. Kato, and K. Hirai. 1986. Demonstration of a Marek's disease virus-specific antigen in tumour lesions of chickens with Marek's disease using monoclonal antibody against a virus phosphorylated protein. Avian Pathol 15:503-510.

279. Nakajima, K., K. Ikuta, S. Ueda, S. Kato, and K. Hirai. 1986. Identification with monoclonal antibodies of virus-specific DNA-binding proteins in the nuclei of cells infected with three serotypes of Marek's disease virus-related viruses. J Virol 59:154-158.

280. Nakajima, K., M. Ikuta, S. Naito, S. Ueda, S. Kato, and K. Hirai. 1987. Analysis of Marek's disease virus serotype-1 specific phosphorylated polypeptides in virus-infected cells and Marek's disease lymphoblastoid cells. J Gen Virol 68:1379-1390.

281. Nazerian, K. 1971. Further studies on the replication of Marek's disease virus in the chicken and in cell culture. J Nat Cancer Inst 47:207-217.

282. Nazerian, K. 1973. Marek's disease: A neoplastic disease of chickens caused by a herpesvirus. Adv Cancer Res 17:279-315.

283. Nazerian, K. 1974. DNA configuration in the core of Marek's disease virus. J Virol 13:1148-1150.

284. Nazerian, K. 1979. Marek's disease lymphoma of chicken and its causative herpesvirus. Biochim Biophys Acta 560:375-395.

285. Nazerian, K. 1987. An updated list of avian cell lines and transplantable tumours. Avian Pathol 16:527-544.

286. Nazerian, K., and H.G. Purchase. 1970. Combined fluorescent-antibody and electron microscopy study of Marek's disease virus-infected cell culture. J Virol 5:79-90.

287. Nazerian, K., and J.M. Sharma. 1975. Brief Communication: Detection of T-cell surface antigens in a Marek's disease lymphoblastoid cell line. J Nat Cancer Inst 54:277-279.

288. Nazerian, K., and J.M. Sharma. 1985. Pathogenesis of Marek's disease in turkeys. In B.W. Calnek and J.L. Spencer (eds.), Proc Int Symp Marek's Dis, pp. 262-267. Am Assoc Avian Pathol, Kennett Square, PA.

289. Nazerian, K., and R.F. Silva. 1988. Properties of producer and nonproducer clones of a Marek's disease turkey lymphoblastoid cell line. Avian Dis 32:486-493.

290. Nazerian, K., J.J. Solomon, R.L. Witter, and B.R. Burmester. 1968. Studies on the etiology of Marek's disease. II. Finding of a herpesvirus in cell culture. Proc Soc Exp Biol Med 127:177-182.

291. Nazerian, K., L.F. Lee, R.L. Witter, and B.R. Burmester. 1970. Ultrastructural studies of a herpesvirus of turkeys antigenically related to Marek's disease virus. Virology 43:442-452.

292. Nazerian, K., T. Lindahl, G. Klein, and L.F. Lee. 1973. Deoxyribonucleic acid of Marek's disease virus in virus-induced tumors. J Virol 12:841-846.

293. Nazerian, K., E.A. Stephens, J.M. Sharma, L.F. Lee, M. Gailitis, and R.L. Witter. 1977. A nonproducer T lymphoblastoid cell line from Marek's disease transplantable tumor (JMV). Avian Dis 21:69-76.

294. Neumann, U. 1980. Lack of serological homology between chicken alpha-foetoprotein, chicken foetal red blood cell antigen and Marek's disease tumour-associated surface antigen. Avian Pathol 9:597-601.

295. Neumann, U., and R.L. Witter. 1978. Differential diagnosis of lymphoid leukosis and Marek's disease by tumor-specific criteria. I. Studies on experimentally infected chickens. Avian Dis 23:417-425.

296. Neumann, U., and R.L. Witter. 1978. Differential diagnosis of lymphoid leukosis and Marek's disease by tumor- specific criteria. II. Studies on field cases. Avian Dis 23:426-433.

297. Nicholas, R.A.J., J.C. Muskett, and D.H. Thornton. 1979. A comparison of titration methods for Marek's disease vaccines. J Biol Stand 7:43-51.

298. Nicholls, T.J. 1984. Marek's disease in sixty week-old laying chickens. Aust Vet J 61:243.

299. Nii, S., I. Yasuda, and K. Ikuta. 1977. 70 nm particles detected in lymphoblastoid cell lines derived from Marek's disease tumors. Biken J 20:151-154.

300. Oei, H.L., and G.F. de Boer. 1986. Comparison of intramuscular and subcutaneous administration of Marek's disease vaccine. Avian Pathol 15:569-579.

301. Ohashi, K., T. Mikami, H. Kodama, and H. Izawa. 1987. Suppression of NK activity of spleen cells by chicken fetal antigen present on Marek's disease lymphoblastoid cell line cells. Int J Cancer 40:378-382.

302. Okada, K., Y. Fujimoto, K. Yonohama, M. Onuma, and T. Mikami. 1974. Three-dimensional observation of virion of turkey herpes. J Electron Microsc 23:133-135.

303. Okada, K., Y. Fujimoto, Y.H. Nakanishi, M. Onuma, and T. Mikami. 1980. Cohelical arrangement of the DNA strand in the core of Marek's disease virus particles. Arch Virol 64:81-85.

304. Okada, K., Y. Fujimoto, and N. Baba. 1980. Computerized reconstruction of the core of herpesvirus of turkeys. J Electron Microsc 29:401-402.

305. Okazaki, W., H.G. Purchase, and B.R. Burmester. 1970. Protection against Marek's disease by vaccination with a herpesvirus of turkeys. Avian Dis 14:413-429.

306. Olson, C. 1940. Transmissible fowl leukosis. A review of the literature. Massachusetts Agric Exp Stn Bull 370.

307. Ono, K., M. Takashima, T. Ishikawa, M. Hayashi, I. Yoshida, T. Konobe, K. Ikuta, K. Nakajima, S. Ueda, S. Kato, and K. Hirai. 1985. Partial protection against Marek's disease in chickens immunized with glycoproteins gB purified from turkey-herpesvirus-infected cells by affinity chromatography coupled with monoclonal antibodies. Avian Dis 29:533-539.

308. Otaki, Y., T. Nunoya, M. Tajima, A. Kato, and Y. Nomura. 1988. Depression of vaccinal immunity to Marek's disease by infection with chicken anaemia agent. Avian Pathol 17:333-347.

309. Owen, J.J.T., M.A.S. Moore, and P.M. Biggs. 1966. Chromosome studies in Marek's disease. J Nat Cancer Inst 37:199- 209.

310. Ozaki, K., H. Kodama, M. Onuma, H. Izawa, and T. Mikami. 1983. In vitro suppression of proliferation of Marek's disease lymphoma cell line (MDCC-MSB1) by peritoneal exudate cells from chickens infected with MDV or HVT. Zentralbl Veterinaermed [B] 30:223-231.

311. Pappenheimer, A.M., L.C. Dunn, and V. Cone. 1926. A study of fowl paralysis (neuro-lymphomatosis gallinarum). Storrs Agric Exp Stn Bull 143:187-290.

312. Parker, M.A., and L.W. Schierman. 1983. Suppression of humoral immunity in chickens prevents transient paralysis caused by a herpesvirus. J Immunol 130:2000-2001.

313. Pattison, M. 1985. Control of Marek's disease by the poultry industry: Practical considerations. In L.N. Payne (ed.), Marek's Disease, pp. 341-349. Martinus Nijhoff, Boston.

314. Paul, P., C.T. Larsen, M.C. Kumar, and B.S. Pomeroy. 1972. Preliminary observations on egg transmission of turkey herpesvirus (HVT) in turkeys. Avian Dis 16:27-33.

315. Payne, L.N. 1972. Pathogenesis of Marek's disease – a review. In P.M. Biggs, G. de Thé, and L.N. Payne (eds.), Oncogenesis and Herpesviruses, pp. 21-37. IARC, Lyons, France.

316. Payne, L.N. 1985. Historical review. In L.N. Payne (ed.), Marek's Disease, pp. 1-15. Martinus Nijhoff, Boston.

317. Payne, L.N. 1985. Pathology. In L.N. Payne (ed.), Marek's Disease, pp. 43-75. Martinus Nijhoff, Boston.

318. Payne, L.N. 1985. Marek's Disease. Scientific Basis and Control. Martinus Nijhoff, Boston.

319. Payne, L.N., and P.M. Biggs. 1967. Studies on Marek's disease. II. Pathogenesis. J Nat Cancer Inst 39:281-302.

320. Payne, L.N., and K. Howes. 1980. Lack of beneficial effect of levamisole on Marek's disease. Avian Pathol 9:525-529.

321. Payne, L.N., and M. Rennie. 1973. Pathogenesis of Marek's disease in chicks with and without maternal antibody. J Nat Cancer Inst 51:1559-1573.

322. Payne, L.N., and J. Roszkowski. 1973. The presence of immunologically uncommitted bursa and thymus dependent lymphoid cells in the lymphomas of Marek's disease. Avian Pathol 1:27-34.

323. Payne, L.N., P.C. Powell, and M. Rennie. 1974. Response of B and T lymphocytes and other blood leukocytes in chickens with Marek's disease. Cold Spring Harbor Symp Quant Biol 39:817- 826.

324. Payne, L.N., J.A. Frazier, and P.C. Powell. 1976. Pathogenesis of Marek's disease. Int Rev Exp Pathol 16:59-154.

325. Payne, L.N., M. Rennie, P.C. Powell, and J.G. Rowell. 1978. Transient effect of cyclophosphamide on vaccinal immunity to Marek's disease. Avian Pathol 7:295-304.

326. Payne, L.N., K. Howes, M. Rennie, J.M. Bumstead, and A.W. Kidd. 1981. Use of an agar culture technique for establishing lymphoid cell lines from Marek's disease lymphomas. Int J Cancer 28:757-766.

327. Pazderka, F., B.M. Longenecker, G.R.J. Law, H.A. Stone, W.E. Briles, and R.F. Ruth. 1974. Detection of identical B alleles in different strains of chickens: Association with resistance to Marek's disease. Anim Blood Groups Biochem Genet 5:18.

328. Pepose, J.S., J.G. Stevens, M.L. Cook, and P.W. Lampert. 1981. Marek's disease as a model for the Landry-Guillain-Barré Syndrome: Latent viral infection in nonneuronal cells is accompanied by specific immune responses to peripheral nerve and myelin. Am J Pathol 103:309-320.

329. Pevzner, I.Y., I. Kujdych, and A.W. Nordskog. 1981. Immune response and disease resistance in chickens. II. Marek's disease and immune response to GAT. Poult Sci 60:927-932.

330. Phillips, P.A., and P.M. Biggs. 1972. Course of infection in tissues of susceptible chickens after exposure to strains of Marek's disease virus and turkey herpesvirus. J Nat Cancer Inst 49:1367-1373.

331. Pol, J.M.A., Kok, G.L., and G.F. de Boer. 1985. Studies on the oncogenic properties of various Marek's disease virus strains. In B.W. Calnek and J.L. Spencer (eds.), Proc Int Symp Marek's Dis, pp. 469-479. Am Assoc Avian Pathol, Kennett Square, PA.

332. Pol, J.M.A., Kok, G.L., Oei, H.L., and G.F. de Boer. 1986. Pathogenicity studies with plaque-purified preparations of Marek's disease virus strain CVI-988. Avian Dis 30:271-275.

333. Powell, P.C. 1975. Immunity to Marek's disease induced by glutaraldehyde-treated cells of Marek's disease lymphoblastoid cell lines. Nature 257:684-685.

334. Powell, P.C. 1976. Studies on Marek's disease lymphoma-derived cell lines. Bibl Haematol 43:348-350.

335. Powell, P.C. 1978. Protection against the JMV Marek's disease-derived transplantable tumour by Marek's disease virus-specific antigens. Avian Pathol 7:305-309.

336. Powell, P.C. 1981. Immunity to Marek's disease. In M.E. Rose, L.N. Payne, and B.M. Freeman (eds.), Avian Immunology, pp. 263-283. Br Poult Sci, Edinburgh.

337. Powell, P.C. 1985. Immunity. In L.N. Payne (ed.), Marek's Disease, pp. 177-201. Martinus Nijhoff, Boston.

338. Powell, P.C. 1985. Host resistance factors: Immune responses – a review. In B.W. Calnek and J.L. Spencer (eds.), Proc Int Symp Marek's Dis, pp. 238-261. Am Assoc Avian Pathol, Kennett Square, PA.

339. Powell, P.C., and T.F. Davison. 1986. Induction of Marek's disease in vaccinated chickens by treatment with betamethasone or corticosterone. Isr J Vet Med 42:73-78.

340. Powell, P.C., and F. Lombardini. 1986. Isolation of very virulent pathotypes of Marek's disease virus from vaccinated chickens in Europe. Vet Rec 118:688-691.

341. Powell, P.C., and M. Rennie. 1980. Failure of attenuated Marek's disease virus and herpesvirus of turkey antigens to protect against the JMV Marek's disease derived transplantable tumour. Avian Pathol 9:193-200.

342. Powell, P.C., and M. Rennie. 1984. The expression of Marek's disease tumor-associated surface antigen in various avian species. Avian Pathol 13:345-349.

343. Powell, P.C., and J.G. Rowell. 1977. Dissociation of antiviral and antitumor immunity in resistance to Marek's disease. J Nat Cancer Inst 59:919-924.

344. Powell, P.C., L.N. Payne, J.A. Frazier, and M. Rennie. 1974. T lymphoblastoid cell lines from Marek's disease lymphomas. Nature 251:79-80.

345. Powell, P.C., K.J. Hartley, B.M. Mustill, and M. Rennie. 1983. The occurrence of chicken foetal antigen after infection with Marek's disease virus in three strains of chicken. Oncodev Biol Med 4:261-271.

346. Powell, P.C., K. Howes, A.M. Lawn, B.M. Mustill, L.N. Payne, M. Rennie, and M.A. Thompson. 1984. Marek's disease in turkeys: The induction of lesions and the establishment of lymphoid cell lines. Avian Pathol 13:201-214.

347. Pradhan, H.K., G.C. Mohanty, and A. Mukit. 1985. Marek's disease in Japanese quails (Coturnix coturnix japonica): A study of natural cases. Avian Dis

29:575-582.
348. Pradhan, H.K., C.G. Mohanty, A. Mukit, and B. Paattnaik. 1987. Experimental studies on Marek's disease in Japanese quail (Coturnix coturnix japonica). Avian Dis 31:225- 233.
349. Prasad, L.B.M., and P.B. Spradbrow. 1977. Multiplication of turkey herpes virus and Marek's disease virus in chick embryo skin cell cultures. J Comp Pathol 87:515-520.
350. Prasad, L.M.B., and P.B. Spradbrow. 1980. Ultrastructure and infectivity of tissue from normal and immunodepressed chickens inoculated with turkey herpesvirus. J Comp Pathol 90:47-56.
351. Prasad, L.B.M., Scott, J., and P.B. Spradbrow. 1977. Isolation of Marek's disease herpesvirus of low pathogenicity from commercial chickens. Aust Vet J 53:405-406.
352. Price, D.J. 1983. Use of brooding paper in relation to broiler performance. Proc 18th Nat Meet Poult Health Condemnations, pp. 102-103.
353. Purchase, H.G. 1969. Immunofluorescence in the study of Marek's disease. I. Detection of antigen in cell culture and an antigenic comparison of 8 isolates. J Virol 3:557-565.
354. Purchase, H.G. 1972. Recent advances in the knowledge of Marek's disease. Adv Vet Sci Comp Med 16:223-258.
355. Purchase, H.G. 1985. Clinical disease and its economic impact. In L.N. Payne (ed.), Marek's Disease, pp. 17-24. Martinus Nijhoff, Boston.
356. Purchase, H.G., and P.M. Biggs. 1967. Characterization of five isolates of Marek's disease. Res Vet Sci 8:440-449.
357. Purchase, H.G., and J.M. Sharma. 1970. The differential diagnosis of lymphoid leukosis and Marek's disease. Slide Study Set. Am Assoc Avian Pathol, Kennett Square, PA.
358. Purchase, H.G., and J.M. Sharma. 1974. Amelioration of Marek's disease and absence of vaccine protection in immunologically deficient chickens. Nature 248:419-421.
359. Purchase, H.G., and R.L. Witter. 1986. Public health concerns from human exposure to oncogenic avian herpesviruses. J Am Vet Med Assoc 189:1430-1436.
360. Purchase, H.G., W. Okazaki, and B.R. Burmester. 1972. Long term field trials with the herpesvirus of turkeys vaccine against Marek's disease. Avian Dis 16:57-71.
361. Purchase, H.G., W. Okazaki, and B.R. Burmester. 1972. The minimum protective dose of the herpesvirus turkeys vaccine against Marek's disease. Vet Rec 91:79-84.
362. Ramachandra, R.N., R. Raghavan, and B.S. Keshavamurthy. 1978. Propagation of Marek's disease virus in chicken tracheal explants. Indian J Anim Sci 48:525-528.
363. Rangga-Tabbu, C., and B.R. Cho. 1982. Marek's disease virus (MDV) antigens in the feather follicle epithelium: Difference between oncogenic and nononcogenic MDV. Avian Dis 26:907-917.
364. Rennie, M., P.C. Powell, and B.M. Mustill. 1980. The effect of bursectomy on vaccination against Marek's disease with the herpesvirus of turkeys. Avian Pathol 9:557-566.
365. Reno, J.M., L.F. Lee, and J.A. Boezi. 1978. Inhibition of herpesvirus replication and herpesvirus-induced deoxyribonucleic acid polymeraase by phosphonoformate. Antimicrob Agents Chemother 13:188-192.
366. Ringen, L.M., and A.S. Akhtar. 1968. Electrophoretic analysis of serum proteins from paralyzed and unparalyzed chickens exposed to Marek's disease. Avian Dis 12:4-9.
367. Rispens, B.H., H.J. VanVloten, N. Mastenbroek, H.J.L. Maas, and K.A. Schat. 1972. Control of Marek's disease in the Netherlands. I. Isolation of an avirulent Marek's disease virus (strain CVI988) and its use in laboratory vaccination trials. Avian Dis 16:108-125.
368. Roizman, B. 1978. Provisional classification of herpesviruses. In G. de Thé, W. Henle and F. Rapp (eds.), Oncogenesis and Herpesviruses III. Part 2, pp. 1079-1082. IARC, Lyons, France.
369. Rosenberger, J.K. 1983. Reovirus interference with Marek's disease vaccination. Proc 32nd West Poult Dis Conf, pp. 50-51.
370. Ross, L.J.N. 1977. Antiviral T-cell mediated immunity in Marek's disease. Nature 268:644-646.
371. Ross, L.J.N. 1985. Molecular biology of the virus. In L.N. Payne (ed.), Marek's Disease, pp. 113-150. Martinus Nijhoff, Boston.
372. Ross, N., and B. Milne. 1989. Manipulation of the genomes of MDV and HVT. In S. Kato, T. Horiuchi, T. Mikami, and K. Hirai (eds.), Advances in Marek's Disease Research, pp. 43-49. Japanese Association on Marek's Disease, Osaka.
373. Ross, L.J.N., Powell, P.C., Walker, D.J., Rennie, M., and L.N. Payne. 1977. Expression of virus-specific, thymus-specific and tumour-specific antigens in lymphoblastoid cell lines derived from Marek's disease lymphomas. J Gen Virol 35:219- 235.
374. Ross, L.J.N., W. Delorbe, H.E. Varmus, J.M. Bishop, and M. Brahic. 1981. Persistence and expression of Marek's disease virus DNA in tumour cells and peripheral nerves studied by in situ hybridization. J Gen Virol 57:285-296.
375. Ross, L.J.N., Milne, B., and P.M. Biggs. 1983. Restriction endonuclease analysis of Marek's disease virus DNA and homology between strains. J Gen Virol 64:2785-2790.
376. Rouse, B.T., R.J.H. Wells, and H.L. Warner. 1973. Proportion of T and B lymphocytes in lesions of Marek's disease: Theoretical implications for pathogenesis. J Immunol 110:534-539.
377. Rziha, H.J., and B. Bauer. 1982. Circular forms of viral DNA in Marek's disease virus-transformed lymphoblastoid cells. Arch Virol 72:211-216.
378. Samorek-Salamonowicz, E., A. Cakala, and T. Wijaszka. 1987. Effect of acyclovir on the replication of turkey herpesvirus and Marek's disease virus. Res Vet Sci 42:334-338.
379. Schat, K.A. 1985. Characteristics of the virus. In L.N. Payne (ed.), Marek's Disease, pp. 77-112. Martinus Nijhoff, Boston.
380. Schat, K.A. 1987. Marek's disease: A model for protection against herpesvirus-induced tumours. Cancer Surveys 6:1-37.
381. Schat, K.A. 1987. Immunity in Marek's disease and other tumors. In A. Toivanen and P. Toivanen (eds.), Avian Immunology: Basis and Practice, pp. 101-128. CRC Press, Boca Raton, FL.
382. Schat, K.A., and B.W. Calnek. 1978. Characterization of an apparently nononcogenic Marek's disease virus. J Nat Cancer Inst 60:1075-1082.
383. Schat, K.A., and B.W. Calnek. 1978. In vitro inactivation of cell-free Marek's disease herpesvirus by immune peripheral blood lymphocytes. Avian Dis 22:693-697.
384. Schat, K.A., and B.W. Calnek. 1978. Demonstration of Marek's disease tumor-associated surface antigen in chickens infected with nononcogenic Marek's disease virus and herpesvirus of turkeys. J Nat Cancer Inst 61:855-857.
385. Schat, K.A., R.D. Schultz, and B.W. Calnek.

1978. Marek's disease: Effect of virus pathogenicity and genetic susceptibility on response of peripheral blood lymphocytes to concanavalin-A. In P. Bentvelzen, J. Hilgers, and D.S. Yohn (eds.), Advances Comparative Leukosis Research, pp. 183-185. Elsevier, Amsterdam.

386. Schat, K.A., B.W. Calnek, and J. Fabricant. 1981. Influence of oncogenicity of Marek's disease virus on evaluation of genetic resistance. Poult Sci 60:2559-2566.

387. Schat, K.A., C.-L.H. Chen, W.R. Shek, and B.W. Calnek. 1982. Surface antigens on Marek's disease lymphoblastoid tumor cell lines. J Nat Cancer Inst 69:715-720.

388. Schat, K.A., B.W. Calnek, and J. Fabricant. 1982. Characterisation of two highly oncogenic strains of Marek's disease virus. Avian Pathol 11:593-605.

389. Schat, K.A., W.R. Shek, B.W. Calnek, and H. Abplanalp. 1982. Syngeneic and allogeneic cell-mediated cytotoxicity against Marek's disease lymphoblastoid tumor cell lines. Int J Cancer 29:187-194.

390. Schat, K.A., R.F. Schinazi, and B.W. Calnek. 1984. Cell-specific antiviral activity of 1-(2-fluoro-2-deoxy-alpha B-D-arabino-furanosyl)-5 iodocytosin (FIAC) against Marek's disease herpesvirus and turkey herpesvirus. Antiviral Res 4:259-270.

391. Schat, K.A., B.W. Calnek, J. Fabricant, and D.L. Graham. 1985. Pathogenesis of infection with attenuated Marek's disease virus strains. Avian Pathol 14:127-146.

392. Schat, K.A., A. Buckmaster, and L.J.N. Ross. 1989. Partial transcription map of Marek's disease herpesvirus in lytically infected cells and lymphoblastoid cell lines. Int J Cancer. (in press)

393. Schat, K.A., C.-L.H. Chen, H. Lillehoj, B.W. Calnek, and D. Weinstock. 1989. Characterization of Marek's disease cell lines with monoclonal antibodies specific for cytotoxic and helper T cells. In S. Kato, T. Horiuchi, T. Mikami, and K. Hirai (eds.), Advances in Marek's Disease Research, pp. 220-226. Japanese Association on Marek's Disease, Osaka.

394. Schierman, L.W., and O.J. Fletcher. 1980. Genetic control of Marek's disease virus-induced transient paralysis: Association with the major histocompatibility complex. In P.M. Biggs (ed.), Resistance and Immunity to Marek's Disease, pp. 429-442. Commission European Communities, Luxembourg.

395. Scott, S.D., A.E. Buckmaster, Sanderson, M.J., Boursnell, M.E.G., Ross, L.J.N., and M.W. Binns. 1989. Gene sequence and mapping data from MDV and HVT. In S. Kato, T. Horiuchi, T. Mikami, and K. Hirai (eds.), Advances in Marek's Disease Research, pp. 84-90. Japanese Association on Marek's Disease, Osaka.

396. Settnes, O.P. 1982. Marek's disease—a common naturally herpesvirus-induced lymphoma of the chicken. Nord Veterinaermed Suppl:11-132.

397. Sevoian, M., and D.M. Chamberlain. 1962. Avian lymphomatosis. II. Experimental reproduction of the ocular form. Vet Med 57:608-609.

398. Sevoian, M., and D.M. Chamberlain. 1964. Avian lymphomatosis. IV. Pathogenesis. Avian Dis 8:281-308.

399. Sevoian, M., and C.R. Weston. 1972. The effects of JM and JM-V leukosis strains on chicks vaccinated with herpes virus of turkeys (HVT). Poult Sci 51:513-516.

400. Sevoian, M., D.M. Chamberlain, and F.T. Counter. 1962. Avian lymphomatosis. I. Experimental reproduction of the neural and visceral forms. Vet Med 57:500-501.

401. Sevoian, M., D.M. Chamberlain, and R.N. Larose. 1963. Avian lymphomatosis. VII. New support for etiologic unity. Proc 17th World's Vet Congr 2:1475-1476.

402. Sevoian, M., R.N. Larose, and D.M. Chamberlain. 1964. Increased pathogenicity of JM virus. Proc 101st Annu Meet Am Vet Med Assoc, p. 342.

403. Sharma, J.M. 1973. Lack of a threshold of genetic resistance to Marek's disease and the incidence of humoral antibody. Avian Pathol 2:75-90.

404. Sharma, J.M. 1979. Immunosuppressive effects of lymphoproliferative neoplasms of chickens. Avian Dis 23:315-327.

405. Sharma, J.M. 1980. In vitro suppression of T-cell mitogenic response and tumor cell proliferation by spleen macrophages from normal chickens. Infect Immun 28:914-922.

406. Sharma, J.M. 1981. Natural killer cell activity in chickens exposed to Marek's disease virus: Inhibition of activity in susceptible chickens and enhancement of activity in resistant and vaccinated chickens. Avian Dis 25:882-893.

407. Sharma, J.M. 1981. Fractionation of Marek's disease virus induced lymphoma by velocity sedimentation and association of infectivity with cellular fractions with and without tumor antigen expression. Am Vet Res 42:483-486.

408. Sharma, J.M. 1983. Presence of adherent cytotoxic cells and nonadherent natural killer cells in progressive and regressive Marek's disease tumors. Vet Immunol Immunopathol 5:125-140.

409. Sharma, J.M. 1984. Effect of infectious bursal disease virus on protection against Marek's disease by turkey herpesvirus vaccine. Avian Dis 28:629-640.

410. Sharma, J.M. 1985. Laboratory diagnosis. In L.N. Payne (ed.), Marek's Disease, pp. 151-176. Martinus Nijhoff, Boston.

411. Sharma, J.M. 1987. Delayed replication of Marek's disease following in ovo inoculation during late stages of embryonal development. Avian Dis 31:570-576.

412. Sharma, J.M. 1987. Personal Communication.

413. Sharma, J.M., and B.R. Burmester. 1982. Resistance to Marek's disease at hatching in chickens vaccinated as embryos with the turkey herpesvirus. Avian Dis 26:134-149.

414. Sharma, J.M., and B.D. Coulson. 1977. Cell-mediated cytotoxic response to cells bearing Marek's disease tumor-associated surface antigen in chickens infected with Marek's disease virus. J Nat Cancer Inst 1647-1651.

415. Sharma, J.M., and B.D. Coulson. 1979. Presence of natural killer (NK) cells in specific pathogen free chickens. J Nat Cancer Inst 63:527-531.

416. Sharma, J.M., and B.D. Coulson. 1980. Natural immunity against Marek's disease tumour cells: Cytotoxicity of spleen cells from specific pathogen free chickens against MSB-1 target cells. In P.M. Biggs (ed.), Resistance and Immunity to Marek's Disease, pp. 223-229. Commission European Communities, Luxembourg.

417. Sharma, J.M., and C.K. Graham. 1982. Influence of maternal antibody on efficacy of embryo vaccination with cell-associated and cell-free MD vaccine. Avian Dis 26:860-870.

418. Sharma, J.M., and H.A. Stone. 1972. Genetic resistance to Marek's disease. Delineation of the response of genetically resistant chickens to Marek's disease virus infection. Avian Dis 16:894-906.

419. Sharma, J.M., and R.L. Witter. 1975. The effect of B-cell immunosuppression on age-related resistance of chickens to Marek's disease. Cancer Res 35:711-717.

420. Sharma, J.M., and R.L. Witter. 1983. Embryo vaccination against Marek's disease with serotypes 1, 2,

and 3 vaccines administered singly or in combination. Avian Dis 27:453-463.
421. Sharma, J.M., D. Burger, and S.G. Kenzy. 1972. Serological relationships among herpesviruses: Cross-reaction between Marek's disease virus and pseudorabies virus as detected by immunofluorescence. Infect Immun 5:406-411.
422. Sharma, J.M., R.L. Witter, and B.R. Burmester. 1973. Pathogenesis of Marek's disease in old chickens: Lesion regression as the basis for age-related resistance. Infect Immun 81:715-724.
423. Sharma, J.M., R.L. Witter, B.R. Burmester, and J.C. Landon. 1973. Public health implications of Marek's disease virus and herpesvirus of turkeys. Studies on human and sub-human primates. J Nat Cancer Inst 51:1123-1128.
424. Sharma, J.M., R.L. Witter, and H.G. Purchase. 1975. Absence of age-resistance in neonatally thymectomised chickens as evidence for cell-mediated immune surveillance in Marek's disease. Nature 253:477-479.
425. Sharma, J.M., K. Nazerian, and R.L. Witter. 1977. Reduced incidence of Marek's disesae gross lymphomas in T-cell-depleted chickens. J Nat Cancer Inst 58:689-692.
426. Sharma, J.M., L.F. Lee, and R.L. Witter. 1980. Effect of neonatal thymectomy on pathogenesis of herpesvirus of turkeys in chickens. Am J Vet Res 40:761-764.
427. Sharma, J.M., L.F. Lee, and P.S. Wakenell. 1984. Comparative viral, immunologic, and pathologic responses of chickens inoculated with herpesvirus of turkeys as embryos or a hatch. Am J Vet Res 45:1619-1623.
428. Shearman, P.J., W.M. Gallatin, and B.M. Longenecker. 1980. Detection of a cell-surface antigen correlated with organ-specific metastasis. Nature 286:267-269.
429. Shek, W.R., K.A. Schat, and B.W. Calnek. 1982. Characterization of nononcogenic Marek's disease virus-infected and turkey herpesvirus infected lymphocytes. J Gen Virol 63:333- 341.
430. Shek, W.R., B.W. Calnek, K.A. Schat, and C.-L.H. Chen. 1983. Characterization of Marek's disease virus-infected lymphocytes: Discrimination between cytolytically and latently infected cells. J Nat Cancer Inst 70:485-491.
431. Shieh, H.K., and M. Sevoian. 1975. Antibody response of genetically susceptible and resistant chickens to cell-free and attenuated JM-V leukosis strain and its influence on early type II (Marek's) leukosis infection. Poult Sci 54:69-77.
432. Shih, J.C.H., R. Pyrzak, and J.S. Guy. 1989. Discovery of noninfectious viral genes complementary to Marek's disease herpes virus in quail susceptible to cholesterol-induced atherosclerosis. J Nutr 119:294-298.
433. Siccardi, F.J., and B.R. Burmester. 1970. The differential diagnosis of lymphoid leukosis and Marek's disease. USDA Tech Bull 1412, Washington, DC.
434. Siegmann, O., E.F. Kaleta, and P. Schindler. 1980. Short- and long-term stability studies on four lyophilized and one cell-associated turkey herpesvirus vaccines against Marek's disease of chickens. Avian Pathol 9:21-32.
435. Silva, R.F., and L.F. Lee. 1984. Monoclonal antibody-mediated immunoprecipitation of proteins from cells infected with Marek's disease virus or turkey herpesvirus. Virology 136:307- 320.
436. Silva, R.F. and L.F. Lee. 1985. Isolation and partial characterization of three glycoproteins common to Marek's disease virus and turkey herpesvirus-infected cells. In B.W. Calnek and J.L. Spencer (eds.), Proc Int Symp on Marek's Disease, pp. 101-110. Am Assoc Avian Pathol, Kennett Square, PA.
437. Silva, R.F., and R.L. Witter. 1985. Genomic expansion of Marek's disease virus DNA is associated with serial in vitro passage. J Virol 54:690-696.
438. Silver, S., A. Tanaka, and M. Nonoyama. 1979. Transcription of the Marek's disease virus genome in a nonproductive chicken lymphoblastoid cell line. Virology 93:127- 133.
439. Sithole, I., L.F. Lee, and L.F. Velicer. 1988. Synthesis and processing of the Marek's disease herpesvirus B antigen glycoprotein complex. J Virol 62:4270-4279.
440. Sithole, I., P.M. Coussens, L.F. Lee, and L.F. Velicer. 1989. Identification of Marek's disease herpesvirus B antigen's precursor polypeptide and the gene encoding it. In S. Kato, T. Horiuchi, T. Mikami, and K. Hirai (eds.), Advances in Marek's Disease Research, pp. 148-154. Japanese Association on Marek's Disease, Osaka.
441. Smith, M.W., and B.W. Calnek. 1973. Effect of virus pathogenicity on antibody production in Marek's disease. Avian Dis 17:727-736.
442. Smith, M.W., and B.W. Calnek. 1974. High virulence Marek's disease virus infection in chickens previously infected with low-virulence virus. J Nat Cancer Inst 52:1595-1603.
443. Smith, T.W., D.M. Albert, N. Robinson, B.W. Calnek, and O. Schwabe. 1974. Ocular manifestations of Marek's disease. Invest Ophthalmol 13:586-592.
444. Solomon, J.J., R.L. Witter, K. Nazerian, and B.R. Burmester. 1968. Studies on the etiology of Marek's disease. I. Propagation of the agent in cell culture. Proc Soc Exp Biol Med 127:173-177.
445. Spencer, J.L. 1969. Marek's disease herpesvirus: In vivo and in vitro infection of kidney cells of different genetic strains of chickens. Avian Dis 13:753-761.
446. Spencer, J.L., and B.W. Calnek. 1967. Storage of cells infected with Rous sarcoma virus or JM strain of avian lymphomatosis agent. Avian Dis 11:274-287.
447. Spencer, J.L., and B.W. Calnek. 1970. Marek's disease: Application of immunofluorescence for detection of antigen and antibody. Am J Vet Res 31:345-358.
448. Spencer, J.L., J.S. Gavora, A.A. Grunder, and A. Robertson. 1973. Studies on the development of JM-V tumors (Marek's disease) in nonvaccinated or vaccinated chickens. Proc 5th Int Congr World Vet Poult Assoc, pp. 193-128.
449. Spencer, J.L., J.S. Gavora, A.A. Grunder, A. Robertson, and G.W. Speckman. 1974. Immunization against Marek's disease: Influence of strain of chickens, maternal antibody, and type of vaccine. Avian Dis 18:33-44.
450. Steadham, E.M., S.J. Lamont, I. Kujdych, and A.W. Nordskog. 1987. Association of Marek's disease with Ea-B and immune response genes in subline and F2 populations of the Iowa State S1 leghorn line. Poult Sci 66:571-575.
451. Stephens, E.A., R.L. Witter, L.F. Lee, J.M. Sharma, K. Nazerian, and B.M. Longenecker. 1976. Characteristics of JMV Marek's disease tumor: A nonproductively infected transplantable cell lacking in rescuable virus. J Nat Cancer Inst 57:865-874.
452. Stephens, E.A., R.L. Witter, K. Nazerian, and J.M. Sharma. 1980. Development and characterization of a Marek's disease transplantable tumor in inbred, Line 72 chickens homozygous at the major (B) histocompatibility locus. Avian Dis 24:358-374.
453. Stone, H.A. 1975. The usefulness and application of highly inbred chickens to research programs. USDA Tech Bull 1514. Washington, DC.
454. Tanaka, A., S. Silver, and M. Nonoyama. 1978.

Biochemical evidence of the nonintegrated status of Marek's disease virus DNA in virus-transformed lymphoblastoid cells of chickens. Virology 88:19-24.

455. Tanaka, A., Y.-S. Lee, and M. Nonoyama. 1980. Heterogeneous population of virus DNA in serially passaged Marek's disease virus preparation. Virology 103:510-513.

456. Theis, G.A. 1977. Effects of lymphocytes from Marek's disease-infected chickens on mitogen responses of syngeneic normal chicken spleen cells. J Immunol 118:887-894.

457. Theis, G.A. 1981. Subpopulations of suppressor cells in chickens infected with cells of a transplantable lymphoblastic leukemia. Infect Immun 34:526-534.

458. Theis, G.A., L.W. Schierman, and R.A. McBride. 1974. Transplantation of a Marek's disease lymphoma in syngeneic chickens. J Immunol 113:1710-1715.

459. Theis, G.A., R.A. McBride, and L.W. Schierman. 1975. Depression of in vitro responsiveness to phytohemagglutinin in spleen cells cultured from chickens with Marek's disease. J Immunol 115:848-853.

460. Thornton, D.H. 1985. Quality control and standardization of vaccines. In L.N. Payne (ed.), Marek's Disease, pp. 267-291. Martinus Nijhoff, Boston.

461. Thurston, T.J., R.A. Hess, H.K. Adldinger, R.F. Solorzano, and H.V. Biellier. 1975. Ultrastructural studies of semen abnormalities and herpesvirus associated with cultured testis cells from domestic turkeys. J Reprod Fertil 45:507-514.

462. Tillotson, J.K., Lee, L.F., and H.-J. Kung. 1989. Accumulation of viral transcripts coding for a DNA binding protein in Marek's disease tumor cells. In S. Kato, T. Horiuchi, T. Mikami, and K. Hirai (eds.), Advance in Marek's Disease Research, pp. 128-134. Japanese Association on Marek's Disease, Osaka.

463. Ubertini, T., and B.W. Calnek. 1970. Marek's disease herpesvirus in peripheral nerve lesions. J Nat Cancer Inst 45:507-514.

464. Van Zaane, D., J.M.A. Brinkhof, F. Westenbrink, and A.L.J. Gielkens. 1982. Molecular-biological characterization of Marek's disease virus. I. Identification of virus-specific polypeptides in infected cells. Virology 121:116-132.

465. Van Zaane, D., J.M.A. Brinkhof, F. Westenbrink, and A.L.J. Gielkens. 1982. Molecular-biological characterization of Marek's disease virus. II. Differentiation of various MDV and HVT strains. Virology 121:133-146.

466. Velicer, L.F., R.A. Stringer, L.L. Zalinskis, and P.M. Coussens. 1988. Personal communication.

467. Vengris, V.E., and C.J. Mare. 1973. Protection of chickens against Marek's disease virus JM-V strain with statolon and exogenous interferon. Avian Dis 17:758-767.

468. Vickers, J.H., C.F. Helmboldt, and R.E. Luginbuhl. 1967. Pathogenesis of Marek's disease (Connecticut A isolate). Avian Dis 11:531-545.

469. Vielitz, E. 1987. Recent problems and advances in the control of Marek's disease. Proc 10th Lat Am Poult Congr, Buenos Aires, Argentina, pp. 155-184.

470. Vielitz, E., and H. Landgraf. 1970. Beitrag zur Epidemiologie und Kontrolle der Marek'schen Krankheit. Dtsch Tierärztl Wochenschr 77:357-362.

471. Vielitz, E., and H. Landgraf. 1985. Experiences with monovalent and bivalent Marek's disease vaccines. In B.W. Calnek and J.L. Spencer (eds.), Proc Int Symp Marek's Dis, pp. 570-575. Am Assoc Avian Pathol, Kennett Square, PA.

472. Vielitz, E., and H. Landgraf. 1986. Protection against Marek's disease with different vaccines, determination of PD50 and duration of vaccinal immunity. Dtsch Tierärztl Wochenschr 93:53-55.

473. Weiss, R.A. and P.M. Biggs. 1972. Leukosis and Marek's disease virus of feral red jungle fowl and domestic fowl in Malaya. J Nat Cancer Inst 39:1713-1725.

474. Wen, L.-T., Tanaka, A., and M. Nonoyama. 1988. Identification of Marek's disease virus nuclear antigen in latently infected lymphoblastoid cells. J Virol 62:3764-3771.

475. Wight, P.A.L. 1962. The histopathology of the central nervous system in fowl paralysis. J Comp Pathol Ther 72:348-359.

476. Wight, P.A.L. 1963. Lymphoid leucosis and fowl paralysis in the quail. Vet Rec 75:685-687.

477. Wight, P.A.L. 1966. Histopathology of the skeletal muscles in fowl paralysis (Marek's disease). J Comp Pathol 76:333-339.

478. Wilson, G. 1986. Personal Communication.

479. Witter, R.L. 1971. Marek's disease research—History and perspectives. Poult Sci 50:333-342.

480. Witter, R.L. 1972. Epidemiology of Marek's disease—a review. In P.M. Biggs, G. de Thé, and L.N. Payne (eds.), Oncogenesis and Herpesviruses, pp. 111-122. IARC, Lyons, France.

481. Witter, R.L. 1982. Protection by attenuated and polyvalent vaccines against highly virulent strains of Marek's Disease virus. Avian Pathol 11:49-62.

482. Witter, R.L. 1983. Characteristics of Marek's disease viruses isolated from vaccinated commercial chicken flocks: Association of viral pathotype with lymphoma frequency. Avian Dis 27:113-132.

483. Witter, R.L. 1985. Principles of vaccination. In L.N. Payne (ed.), Marek's disease, pp. 203-250. Martinus Nijhoff, Boston.

484. Witter, R.L. 1985. Review: Vaccines and vaccination against Marek's disease. In B.W. Calnek and J.L. Spencer (eds.), Proc Int Symp Marek's Dis, pp. 482-500. Am Assoc Avian Pathol, Kennett Square, PA.

485. Witter, R.L. 1985. Association in broiler chickens between natural serotype 2 Marek's disease virus infection and leukosis condemnations. In B.W. Calnek and J.L. Spencer (eds.), Proc Int Symp Marek's Dis, pp. 545-554. Am Assoc Avian Pathol, Kennett Square, PA.

486. Witter, R.L. 1987. New serotype 2 and attenuated serotype 1 Marek's disease vaccine viruses: Comparative efficacy. Avian Dis 31:752-765.

487. Witter, R.L. 1989. Very virulent Marek's disease viruses: Importance and control. World's Poult Sci J 45:60-75.

488. Witter, R.L. 1989. Protective synergism among Marek's disease vaccine viruses. In S. Kato, T. Horiuchi, T. Mikami, and K. Hirai (eds.), Advances in Marek's Disease Research, pp. 398- 404. Japanese Association on Marek's Disease, Osaka.

489. Witter, R.L. 1989. Marek's disease: Prevention and control. In S. Kato, T. Horiuchi, T Mikami, and K. Hirai (eds.), Advances in Marek's Disease Research, pp. 389-397. Japanese Association on Marek's Disease, Osaka.

490. Witter, R.L., and B.R. Burmester. 1979. Differential effect of maternal antibodies on efficacy of cellular and cell-free Marek's disease vaccines. Avian Pathol 8:145-156.

491. Witter, R.L., and L.F. Lee. 1984. Polyvalent Marek's disease vaccines: Safety, efficacy, and protective synergism in chickens with maternal antibodies. Avian Pathol 13:75-92.

492. Witter, R.L., and L. Offenbecker. 1979. Nonprotective and temperature-sensitive variants of Marek's disease vaccine viruses. J Nat Cancer Inst 62:143-151.

493. Witter, R.L., and J.J. Solomon. 1971. Epidemiology of a herpesvirus of turkeys: Possible sources and

spread of infection in turkey flocks. Infect Immun 4:356-361.

494. Witter, R.L., and J.J. Solomon. 1972. Prospects for the control of Marek's disease through isolation rearing. Progr Immunobiol Stand 5:163-138.

495. Witter, R.L., and J.J. Solomon. 1972. Experimental infection of turkeys and chickens with a herpesvirus of turkeys (HVT). Avian Dis 16:34-44.

496. Witter, R.L., G.H. Burgoyne, and B.R. Burmester. 1968. Survival of Marek's disease agent in litter and droppings. Avian Dis 12:522-530.

497. Witter, R.L., J.J. Solomon, and G.H. Burgoyne. 1969. Cell culture techniques for primary isolation of Marek's disease-associated herpesvirus. Avian Dis 13:101-118.

498. Witter, R.L., G.H. Burgoyne, and J.J. Solomon. 1969. Evidence for a herpesvirus as an etiologic agent of Marek's disease. Avian Dis 13:171-184.

499. Witter, R.L., K. Nazerian, H.G. Purchase, and G.H. Burgoyne. 1970. Isolation from turkeys of a cell-associated herpesvirus antigenically related to Marek's disease virus. Am J Vet Res 31:525-538.

500. Witter, R.L., H.G. Purchase, and G.H. Burgoyne. 1970. Peripheral nerve lesions similar to those of Marek's disease in chickens inoculated with reticuloendotheliosis virus. J Nat Cancer Inst 45:567-577.

501. Witter, R.L., J.J. Solomon, L.R. Champion, and K. Nazerian. 1971. Long term studies of Marek's disease infection in individual chickens. Avian Dis 15:346-365.

502. Witter, R.L., K. Nazerian, and J.J. Solomon. 1972. Studies on the in vivo replication of turkey herpesvirus. J Nat Cancer Inst 49:1121-1130.

503. Witter, R.L., J.M. Sharma, J.J. Solomon, and L.R. Champion. 1973. An age-related resistance of chickens to Marek's disease: Some preliminary observations. Avian Pathol 2:43-54.

504. Witter, R.L., J.J. Solomon, and J.M. Sharma. 1974. Response of turkeys to infection with virulent Marek's disease viruses of turkey and chicken origins. Am J Vet Res 35:1325-1332.

505. Witter, R.L., E.A. Stephens, J.M. Sharma, and K. Nazerian. 1975. Demonstration of a tumor-associated surface antigen in Marek's disease. J Immunol 115:177-183.

506. Witter, R.L., J.M. Sharma, and L. Offenbecker. 1976. Turkey herpesvirus infection in chickens: Induction of lymphoproliferative lesions and characterization of vaccinal immunity against Marek's disease. Avian Dis 20:676-692.

507. Witter, R.L., B.W. Calnek, S. Kato, and P.C. Powell. 1979. A proposed method for designating avian cell lines and transplantable tumours. Avian Pathol 8:487-498.

508. Witter, R.L., J.M. Sharma, and A.M. Fadly. 1980. Pathogenicity of variant Marek's disease virus isolants in vaccinated and unvaccinated chickens. Avian Dis 24:210-232.

509. Witter, R.L., J.M. Sharma, L.F. Lee, H.M. Opitz, and C.W. Henry. 1984. Field trials to test the efficacy of polyvalent Marek's disease vaccines in broilers. Avian Dis 28:44-60.

510. Witter, R.L., Sharma, J.M., and A.M. Fadly. 1986. Nonbursal lymphomas induced by nondefective reticuloendotheliosis virus. Avian Pathol 15:467-486.

511. Witter, R., Silva, R., and L. Lee. 1987. New serotype 2 and attenuated serotype 1 Marek's disease vaccine viruses: Selected biological and molecular characteristics. Avian Dis 31:829-840.

512. Yachida, S., T. Mikami, M. Onuma, and H. Izawa. 1983. Comparative studies on antigens induced by turkey herpesvirus and Marek's disease virus. II. Immunofluorescent studies. Zentralbl Veterinaermed [B] 30:669-677.

513. Yachida, S., T. Kondo, K. Hirai, H. Izawa, and T. Mikami. 1986. Establishment of a variant type of turkey herpesvirus which releases cell-free virus into the culture medium in large quantities. Arch Virol 91:183-192.

514. Zander, D.V., and R.G. Raymond. 1985. Partial flock inoculation with a apathogenic strain (HN-1) of chicken herpesvirus of Marek's disease (MD) to immunize chicken flocks against pathogenic field strains of MD. In B.W. Calnek and J.L. Spencer (eds.), Proc Int Symp Marek's Dis, pp. 514-530. Am Assoc Avian Pathol, Kennett Square, PA.

515. Zander, D.V., R.W. Hill, R.G. Raymond, R.K. Balch, R.W. Mitchell, and J.W. Dunsing. 1972. The use of blood from selected chickens as an immunizing agent for Marek's disease. Avian Dis 16:163-178.

516. Zanella, A. 1982. Marek's disease—survey on vaccination failures. Dev Biol Stand 52:29-37.

517. Zygraich, N., and C. Huygelen. 1972. Inoculation of one-day-old chicks with different strains of turkey herpesvirus. II. Virus replication in tissues of inoculated animals. Avian Dis 16:793-798.

LEUKOSIS/SARCOMA GROUP

L.N. Payne and H.G. Purchase

INTRODUCTION. The avian leukosis/sarcoma viruses are grouped together because they share important characteristics. They induce in chickens, and to a much lesser extent in other birds, a variety of transmissible benign and malignant neoplasms. Under natural conditions by far the most common is lymphoid leukosis. The neoplasms and their synonyms are listed in Table 16.3. Viruses of the group, known as avian type C oncoviruses (197), have common physical and chemical characteristics and a common group-specific antigen.

Because of the relationships between these viruses, they are discussed as a group in most parts of this chapter. Sections reflecting the host response (Incubation Period, Signs, Gross Lesions, Histopathology, Ultrastructure, Hematology, Pathogenesis, Differential Diagnosis) are discussed under the pathological entities without regard for virologic properties of the inducing agent(s) other than their inclusion in the leukosis/sarcoma group.

HISTORY. Lymphoid leukosis appears to have been recognized for a long time. Roloff (270) reported a case of "lymphosarcomata" in 1868 and

Table 16.3. Neoplasms caused by viruses of leukosis/sarcoma group

Neoplasm	Synonyms (Reference Nos.)
Leukoses	
Lymphoid leukosis	Big liver disease, lymphatic leukosis (115), visceral lymphoma (229), lymphocytoma (130), lymphomatosis (142), visceral lymphomatosis (175), lymphoid leukosis (25, 56)
Erythroblastosis	Leukemia (329), intravascular lymphoid leukosis (116), erythroleukosis (117, 141), erythromyelosis (16), erythroblastosis (120), erythroid leukosis (25, 56)
Myeloblastosis	Leukemic myeloid leukosis (116), leukomyelose (183), myelomatosis (142), myeloblastosis (217), granuloblastosis (175), myeloid leukosis (97)
Myelocytoma (tosis)	Myelocytoma (241), aleukemic myeloid leukosis (115), leukochloroma (195), myelomatosis (142)
Connective tissue tumors	
Fibroma and fibrosarcoma	
Myxoma and myxosarcoma	
Histiocytic sarcoma	
Chondroma	
Osteoma and osteogenic sarcoma	
Epithelial tumors	
Nephroblastoma	Embryonal nephroma (131), renal adenocarcinoma (60), adenosarcoma (319), nephroblastoma (173, 327), cystadenoma (203)
Nephroma	Papillary cystadenoma, carcinoma of the kidney (20, 202)
Hepatocarcinoma (20, 202)	
Adenocarcinoma of the pancreas (20)	
Thecoma (20)	
Granulosa cell carcinoma (20)	
Seminoma	Adenocarcinoma of the testis (20)
Squamous cell carcinoma (20)	
Endothelial tumors	
Hemangioma	Hemangiomatosis, endothelioma (142), hemangioblastoma, hemangioendothelioma
Angiosarcoma (294, 178)	
Endothelioma (203)	
Mesothelioma (63, 20)	
Related tumors	
Osteopetrosis	Marble bone, thick leg disease, sporadic diffuse osteoperiostitis (252), osteopetrosis gallinarum (176)
Meningioma (20)	
Glioma (20)	

Caparini (59) described fowl leukemia in 1896. In 1905 Butterfield (52) made a diagnosis of "aleukemic lymphadenosis" in three hens in the USA. Ellermann (116) described three types of leukemia: erythroid ("intravascular Leukose"), myeloid ("myeloische Leukose"), and lymphoid ("lymphatische Leukose"). Comprehensive recent reviews of the conditions or their agents are those of Beard (20), Temin (313, 314), Hanafusa (161), Weiss (332), Weiss et al. (337, 338) and de Boer (98). Reviews of the history of avian retrovirus research are provided by Burmester and Purchase (44) and Dougherty (107).

LYMPHOID LEUKOSIS. Jungherr (175) termed the disease visceral lymphomatosis, but this nomenclature has been superseded by that of Biggs (25) and Campbell (56), and the disease is now called lymphoid leukosis (LL).

Furth (142) provided evidence for transmission of LL with filtrates, but proof of the filterability of the agent or agents awaited the work of Burmester and his associates (33, 39, 40).

ERYTHROBLASTOSIS. Ellermann and Bang (118) were the first to report experimental transmission of erythroblastosis. Subsequently, numerous strains were established, and the viral etiology and pathologic nature of the disease were characterized (17, 45, 49, 115).

MYELOBLASTOSIS. Myeloblastosis was transmitted by Schmeisser in 1915 (288); since then, Furth (141), Engelbreth-Holm and Rothe-Meyer (120), and Nyfeldt (217) have observed myeloblastosis in transmission experiments. Early passages of the BAI strain (BAI-A) virus (159) caused both erythroblastosis and myeloblastosis; however, passages derived by selection and cloning have induced a wide variety of tumors (20).

MYELOCYTOMATOSIS. The distinctive appearance and aleukemic character of this disease were first described by Pentimalli (241); later, Furth (141) described some leukemic cases. Most strains (isolates) causing myelocytoma also caused other neoplasms (20, 203).

CONNECTIVE TISSUE TUMORS. Fibrosarcomas and myxosarcomas were first transmitted with cell-free filtrates by Rous in 1911 (272). Ellermann and Bang (118) noticed this tumor in their early transmission studies.

NEPHROMAS AND NEPHROBLASTOMAS. Several viruses of the leukosis/sarcoma group have been found to induce kidney tumors, including nephromas and nephroblastomas; e.g., BAI-A (myeloblastosis), ES4 strain (erythroblastosis/sarcoma), MH2 strain (reticuloendothelioma), and MC29 strain (myelocytomatosis) (20, 49, 60, 61, 203).

OTHER EPITHELIAL TUMORS. Leukosis viruses were shown to cause other epithelial tumors, including hepatocarcinomas (190), adenocarcinomas of the pancreas (202), thecomas and granulosa cell tumors of the ovary, adenocarcinomas of the seminiferous tubules of the testes (seminoma), and squamous cell carcinomas of the skin (20).

ENDOTHELIAL TUMORS. Leukosis viruses were early recognized to cause a variety of tumors of the endothelium (142, 203) and have more recently been found to cause mesotheliomas (20, 63).

OSTEOPETROSIS. It is now apparent that the hypertrophic osteopathies of fowl described in the 1920s were probably osteopetrosis (252). Jungherr and Landauer (176) described the pathologic alterations and suggested the term "osteopetrosis gallinarum." They were the first to reproduce the disease and call attention to its frequent association with LL. For this reason they suggested its inclusion in the avian leukosis complex. Burmester and his associates (33, 135) also noticed that osteopetrosis was frequently associated with LL. Others have reproduced the disease without LL (57, 133, 167).

OTHER RELATED TUMORS. Viruses have been shown to cause meningiomas and gliomas in the brain (20).

INCIDENCE AND DISTRIBUTION.

With few exceptions, infection occurs in all chicken flocks; by sexual maturity most birds have been exposed. Nevertheless, the incidence of clinical disease is generally low.

Incidence of Disease.

LL only occasionally produces heavy losses, e.g., 23% in commercial breeder flocks (259), although sporadic cases occur in most flocks. De Boer (101) reported LL mortality in the Netherlands as 2.18% of 11,220 white layers and 0.57% of 7920 brown layers recorded in random sample tests over the period of 1973 to 1979. The incidence of LL in chickens may be reduced by the widespread occurrence of infectious bursal disease virus (83, 254). LL has been reported in many species of birds, but there is no assurance that such cases are not other types of lymphoid tumor.

Compared to LL, erythroblastosis occurs infrequently under field conditions (259). Exceptionally, it has been reported to occur in 5-wk-old birds as an epizootic (160). There are very few reports of natural occurrence of myeloblastosis, but cases occur sporadically.

Sporadic cases of myelocytomatosis occur among young adult birds (259). The disease was observed in about 1% of birds in two consecutive broiler flocks on one farm (196).

Of all tumors other than leukotic tumors, hemangiomas make up 25 and 19% and nephroblastomas 19 and 3–10% in broilers (58) and layers (259) respectively. Epizootic outbreaks of hemangiosarcomas have recently occurred in layers in Israel (51).

There is little information on incidence of connective tissue tumors, which are often not the primary cause of death; they make up about 20% of tumors other than leukosis in broilers (58). The incidence of connective tissue tumors in chickens is probably less than 1 in 1000 (259), but epizootics have occurred. Perek (242) reported an outbreak of histiocytic sarcomas in a flock of 600 1-yr-old hens. Tumors were found in 90% of 400 birds examined during a 4-mo period. Squamous cell carcinomas of the skin have been of concern at broiler-processing plants, though they make up less than 1% of the condemnations (263, 322); however, the viral etiology of these tumors has not been established.

Osteopetrosis occurs widely but much less frequently than LL, and epizootics occur sporadically in broilers. In all types of chicken, males are more frequently affected than females. It occurs very rarely in turkeys.

Incidence of Virus Infection. Leukosis/sarcoma viruses are almost ubiquitous. Subgroup A viruses are encountered more commonly than subgroup B. In one study (54) 1.6–12.5% of the embryos from eight commercial flocks representing a variety of sources contained subgroup A viruses, and there was significant shedding in every flock. Subgroup B viruses were relatively rare and were shed in eggs much less frequently than subgroup A. A similar preponderance of subgroup A viruses has been isolated from field outbreaks of LL.

Viruses representing subgroups A, B, C, and D have been isolated from commercial flocks in Finland; 5 of 10 flocks surveyed had antibody to all four subgroups (280).

Antibodies to subgroups A and B are common among wildfowl and domestic chickens in Kenya and Malaysia, and there was some evidence of antibody to subgroup D viruses in Kenya. Subgroup F viruses have been found in ring-necked and green pheasants and subgroup G viruses in Ghinghi, silver, and golden pheasants. Subgroup H virus has been isolated from Hungarian partridges and subgroup I virus from Gambel's quail (see VIRUS SUBGROUPS). Viruses that do not fit known subgroups have been isolated from Mongolian and Swinhoe pheasants, Chinese quail, and chickens. However, none was found in Japanese quail, pigeons, geese, and Pekin and Muscovy ducks (64).

Endogenous retroviral genomes, inherited in a Mendelian fashion, occur at distinct chromosomal loci in most vertebrate species. DNA sequences related to RAV-0, the endogenous avian retrovirus, occur in the germ lines of most domestic chickens and several species of galliform birds. For example, partridges, true pheasants, grouse, and jungle fowl contain sequences complementary to RAV-0, whereas guinea fowl, quail, peafowl, ruffed pheasants, gallo-pheasants, and turkeys do not (138).

ETIOLOGY

Classification. Viruses of the leukosis/sarcoma group are vernacularly termed avian type C oncoviruses and have been placed in a subgroup (as yet with no agreed international name) of the subfamily Oncovirinae of the family Retroviridae (197). Viruses of this family are characterized by possession of the enzyme reverse transcriptase, which is necessary for formation of a DNA provirus during viral replication, and include oncogenic type C RNA viruses of other animal species.

The avian leukosis/sarcoma viruses are closely related and cause, depending on their genetic makeup, a variety of neoplasms with short to long clinical latencies. Many, such as avian myeloblastosis virus (AMV), avian erythroblastosis virus (AEV), and the sarcoma viruses, carry specific oncogenes that cause rapid neoplastic transformation and tumor development within a few days or weeks. LL viruses (LLV) are exceptional in lacking transformation genes. They are slowly or weakly transforming, and tumor development takes many weeks or months; transformation is believed to be by viral activation of cellular genes homologous to virus-transforming genes (69).

VIRUS SUBGROUPS. Avian leukosis/sarcoma viruses that occur in chickens have been divided into 5 subgroups (A, B, C, D, and E) on the basis of their host range in chicken embryo fibroblasts of different genetic types, interference patterns with members of the same and different subgroups, and viral envelope antigens identified by virus and serum neutralization tests (337) (Table 16.4). These various properties are a reflection of the envelope glycoproteins present on the virus. Viruses of subgroups A and B occur as common exogenous viruses in the field (54). Subgroup C and D viruses have been reported in the field rarely (205, 280), and subgroup E viruses include the ubiquitous endogenous leukosis viruses of low pathogenicity (296).

Viruses of two additional subgroups (F and G) have been rescued from ring-necked pheasant (139, 162) and golden (139) and Lady Amherst pheasant (163). Subgroup G viruses are believed to belong to a virus species that differs from that of the chicken viruses (163). Endogenous virus of subgroup H has been isolated from Hungarian partridge (163) and of subgroup I from Gambel's quail (320).

Table 16.4. Common laboratory strains of avian leukosis/sarcoma viruses classified according to predominant neoplasm induced and virus subgroup

Virus Class According to Neoplasm	Virus Class According to Subgroup					No Subgroup (Defective Viruses)
	A	B	C	D	E	
Lymphoid leukosis virus (LLV)	RAV-1 RIF-1 MAV-1 RPL12 HPRS-F42	RAV-2 RAV-6 MAV-2	RAV-7 RAV-49	RAV-50 CZAV	RAV-60	
Avian erythroblastosis virus (AEV)						AEV-ES4 AEV-R
Avian myeloblastosis virus (AMV)						AMV-BAI-A E26
Avian sarcoma virus (ASV)	SR-RSV-A PR-RSV-A EH-RSV RSV29	SR-RSV-B PR-RSV-B HA-RSV	B77 PR-RSV-C	SR-RSV-D CZ-RSV	SR-RSV-E PR-RSV-E	BH-RSV BS-RSV FuSV PRCII PRCIV ESV Y73 UR1 UR2
Myelocytoma/endothelioma virus						MC29 MH2 CMII OK10
Endogenous virus (EV)					RAV-0 ILV	

A number of laboratory strains of avian leukosis/sarcoma viruses are genetically defective and lack the viral envelope (*env*) gene; their subgroup is that of the helper leukosis viruses used for their propagation.

VIRUS TYPES. Viruses within a subgroup cross-neutralize to varying extents, but with the exception of partial cross-neutralization between subgroups B and D, viruses of different subgroups do not. Antiserums raised against a particular strain of virus tend to neutralize the homologous virus more strongly than heterologous viruses of the same subgroup (66); viruses within a subgroup vary in ability to induce immunologic tolerance to other members of the subgroup (199). These findings indicate occurrence of varying antigenic types within subgroups; in general, subgroup B viruses appear to be more heterogenous than those of subgroup A.

Morphology

ULTRASTRUCTURE. Viruses of the avian leukosis/sarcoma group cannot be distinguished on the basis of their ultrastructural characteristics. In size, shape, and ultrastructural detail, particles from the various diseases studied are identical and similar to other type C oncoviruses (216, 313) (Fig. 16.18). Negatively stained preparations reveal essentially spheroidal particles that are readily distorted under certain conditions of drying (19). Characteristic knobbed spikes about 8 nm in diameter are present on the surface of the particles. The inner nucleoid of the virus appears to be less easily distorted than the outer part. Certain fixatives allow the interior nucleoprotein filaments to be visualized; these are approximately 3–5 nm in diameter, of undetermined length, and are probably in the form of an intricate coil (13, 216). Thin sections reveal an inner, centrally located electron-dense core about 35–45 nm in diameter, an intermediate membrane, and an outer membrane. This appearance typifies the C-type particle morphology. Overall diameter of the particle is 80–120 nm, with an average of 90 nm (19).

SIZE AND DENSITY. By filtration through membranes of graded pore size, ultracentrifugation, and electron microscopy, viruses have a diameter of 80–145 nm. The value of 1.15–1.17 g/ml for the buoyant density in sucrose is characteristic of oncoviruses (13, 267).

Chemical Composition. The overall composition of AMV, which has been studied extensively, is 30–35% lipid, 60–65% protein, 2.2% RNA, and a small amount of DNA, perhaps of cellular origin (13, 17).

VIRAL NUCLEIC ACIDS. The major size classes of RNA sediment at 60–70S, which is the viral genome, and at 4–5S, most of which is host tRNA,

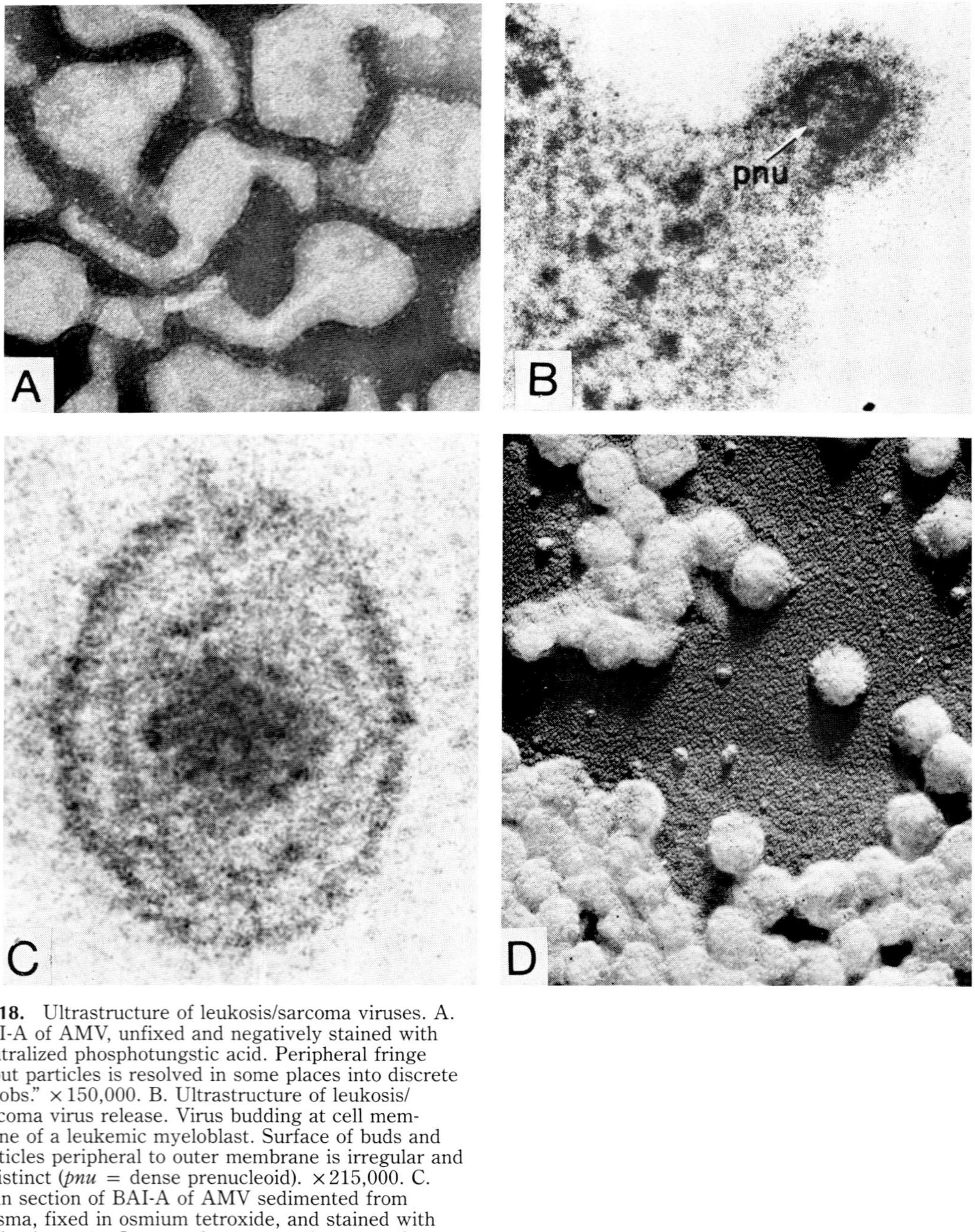

16.18. Ultrastructure of leukosis/sarcoma viruses. A. BAI-A of AMV, unfixed and negatively stained with neutralized phosphotungstic acid. Peripheral fringe about particles is resolved in some places into discrete "knobs." ×150,000. B. Ultrastructure of leukosis/sarcoma virus release. Virus budding at cell membrane of a leukemic myeloblast. Surface of buds and particles peripheral to outer membrane is irregular and indistinct (*pnu* = dense prenucleoid). ×215,000. C. Thin section of BAI-A of AMV sedimented from plasma, fixed in osmium tetroxide, and stained with lead subacetate. Inner and outer membranes and granular character of nucleoid can be seen. Impression of granules might be derived from sectioning of filaments. Some granules appear to be hollow. ×510,000. D. Purified BAI-A of AMV fixed and shadowed with chromium. ×50,000. (Bonar and de Thé)

were thought to be accidentally included in the virion and to play no role in viral replication. However, a tRNA primer associated with 70S RNA does occur and has a role in the viral life cycle. Small amounts of 18 and 28S ribosomal RNAs, viral and cellular mRNA, and DNA are also present. The 60–70S genomic RNA is a dimer and can be split into two subunits of about 34–38S, which are believed to represent a diploid genome. These subunits of genomic RNA are mRNAs, and their genes have been mapped for several avian retroviruses. The sequences of the structural genes of avian leukosis virus, from the 5′ end to the 3′ end of the RNA molecule, is *gag-pol-env;* these genes encode respectively the proteins of the virion group-specific (gs) antigens, RNA-dependent DNA polymerase (reverse transcriptase), and envelope glycoprotein. The structural genes are flanked by terminal genomic sequences concerned with organization of the replication and translation of viral RNA (165, 337). Acute transforming viruses possess additional genomic sequences concerned with oncogenic transformation. Nondefective Rous sarcoma virus (RSV) has the genetic composition *gag-pol-env-src.* The additional gene, *src,* responsible for sarcomatous transformation, is believed to have been acquired originally from a normal cellular gene, cellular *src.* The inclusion of this gene is responsible for the approximately 35S subunits of RSV being slightly larger than those of slowly transforming leukosis viruses. The gene *src* is an example of a number of host cell genes, termed *onc* genes, concerned with acute transformation (121, 328). Viral and cellular versions of *onc* genes, and of the specific varieties such as *src,* are distinguished by the prefixes v- and c-. Specific v-*onc* genes, with c-*onc* counterparts in normal cells, are present in other acute transforming viruses, e.g., *erb* (AEV), *myb* (AMV), *myc* (avian myelocytomatosis virus), *fps* (Fujinami and PRCII sarcoma viruses), *yes* (Y73 and Esh sarcoma viruses), and *ros* (UR2 virus). MH2 endothelioma virus has two oncogenes, *myc* and *mil.* Slow transformation, as in LL, is believed to be caused by an indirect mechanism independent of a v-*onc* but dependent on activation of a c-*onc,* namely c-*myc* in LL (185). Sequenced and cloned viral DNA is now available from many viruses of the leukosis/sarcoma group (338).

VIRAL LIPIDS. Viral lipids occur in the virion envelope and have a composition similar to that of the outer cell membrane from which the virion envelope is derived (13, 29).

VIRAL PROTEINS. The nature, location, and synthesis of proteins that constitute avian retroviruses have been extensively studied (337, 338). The virion core contains at least four nonglycosylated proteins encoded by the *gag* gene: $p27^{gag}$, the major gs antigen (27 kD) and believed to be a core shell component; $p19^{gag}$ and $p12^{gag}$, believed to be involved in RNA processing and packaging; and $p15^{gag}$, a protease involved in cleavage of protein precursors. Other minor polypeptides have also been reported. A variant form, $p27^{o}$, of $p27^{gag}$ has been reported in RAV-0 endogenous virus, but it is not characteristic of all endogenous viruses (171). The virion envelope contains two proteins encoded by the *env* gene: $gp85^{env}$, believed to be the knoblike structures that determine the subgroup specificity of the avian retroviruses; and $gp37^{env}$, representing the spikes that attach the knobs to the envelope. These two envelope proteins are linked to form a dimer, termed virion glycoprotein (VGP).

Virions contain a number of enzymic activities. Reverse transcriptase is present in the core and is encoded by the *pol* gene; it is a complex consisting of the beta subunit (92 kD) and the alpha subunit (58 kD) derived from it and has RNA- and DNA-dependent polymerase and DNA:RNA hybrid-specific ribonuclease H activities. Another virus-coded enzyme is $p32^{pol}$, an endonuclease related to the beta subunit. Other enzymic activities have been detected in virions and are believed to be cellular contaminants; these are ribonuclease, deoxyribonuclease, nucleoside triphosphate, nucleotide kinase, protein kinase, RNA-nucleoside triphosphate nucleotidyltransferase, RNA methylase, hexokinase, lactic dehydrogenase, and aminoacyl-tRNA synthetase (315). Of practical importance is the presence in AMV obtained from blood of infected chickens, or from myeloblast cultures, of adenosine triphosphatase derived from the cell membrane and incorporated into the virus particle envelope during maturation. This enzyme will dephosphorylate adenosine triphosphate, and this activity may be used for virus assay (22). Cells without enzyme activity on their surface release virus that is devoid of activity.

Virus Replication. As with other retroviruses, replication of avian leukosis/sarcoma viruses is characterized by formation of a DNA provirus, under the direction of reverse transcriptase, which becomes linearly integrated into the host cell genome. Subsequently, the proviral genes are transcribed into viral RNAs, which are translated to produce the precursor and mature proteins that constitute the virion. Great effort has been made since the 1970s to elucidate these events, the details of which are discussed by Weiss et al. (337, 338). Only an outline of the main events is provided here.

PENETRATION OF THE HOST CELL. Although adsorption of the virion to the cell membrane is nonspecific, occurring even in cells resistant to infection (244), penetration of cells is dependent on the occurrence, presumably in the cell membrane, of host gene-encoded receptors specific for each virus subgroup. Little is known of the nature of these receptors and the mechanism of penetration and virus uncoating. Dales and Hanafusa (96) observed virions taken into the cell in vacuoles and viral RNA in the nucleus within 120 min of attachment.

SYNTHESIS AND INTEGRATION OF VIRAL DNA. The unique features of avian and other retroviruses that characterize viral replication are the formation (under the influence of viral reverse transcriptase) of retroviral DNA from a template of viral RNA, integration of viral DNA (provirus) into the host cell genome, and formation of new viral RNA from the proviral DNA template. Major stages in formation of retroviral DNA are 1) synthesis of the first (minus) strand of viral DNA, probably forming an RNA:DNA hybrid; 2) removal of RNA from the hybrid by RNase-H and formation on the template of minus-strand DNA of second (plus) strands of viral DNA, giving rise to linear DNA duplexes (these duplex molecules are detectable in cytoplasm of the cell within a few hours of infection); and 3) migration of linear DNA to the cell nucleus and its conversion to a closed, circular form.

Circularized viral DNA becomes linearly integrated into the host DNA. This integration can occur at many sites, and infected cells can contain up to 20 copies of viral DNA. The proviral genes occur in the same order as their RNA copies occur in the virion, and they are flanked on either side by identical sequences of nucleotides – long terminal repeats (LTRs). These are composed of repeated sequences derived from terminal regions of viral RNA and act as promoters controlling transcription of viral DNA to RNA. LTRs may also cause abnormal transcription of host genes usually "downstream" of the proviral DNA, leading to oncogenesis.

TRANSCRIPTION. Formation of new virions in the infected cell is the result of transcription and translation of proviral DNA, the major events being 1) transcription of viral RNA on a template of proviral DNA under the influence of a host RNA polymerase. Viral RNA molecules may act as mRNA in association with polyribosomes, or they may serve as genomic RNA in the newly formed virions. New viral RNA is detectable within 24 hr of infection. 2) mRNA species, bound to polyribosomes, are translated to form the *gag, pol,* and *env* gene-coded proteins that compose the virion. The *gag* gene product is a precursor polyprotein (76 kD), Pr76^{gag}, that is cleaved to give rise to the virion core proteins described under viral proteins. The *pol* gene product is also a large protein precursor (180 kD) that also includes *gag* gene products, Pr180$^{gag\text{-}pol}$, which are cleaved to the viral polymerase and RNase activities described above. The *env* gene product is a precursor protein (90 kD), Pr90^{env}, from which the viral envelope proteins gp85^{env} and gp37^{env} are derived. The viral proteins localize at the plasma membrane of the cell, where crescent-shaped structures that develop into virions budded off from the cell may be visualized.

CELL TRANSFORMATION AND TUMOR FORMATION. Two main types of strategy are involved in oncogenesis by avian retrovirus (69). The acute transforming viruses carry differing *onc* genes (derived from normal cellular sequences), which are responsible for neoplastic transformation (207). RSV carries the *src* gene, which encodes a transformation-specific phosphoprotein (60 kD), pp60^{src}, in the infected cell, with protein kinase activity. Metabolic imbalance associated with high levels of pp60^{src} is believed to be responsible for the transformed state (165). The *onc* genes associated with other acute transforming viruses encode other transformation-associated proteins.

Slowly transforming viruses such as LLV do not possess an *onc* gene but transform cells indirectly by activation of a cellular *onc* gene. Molecular studies indicate that the LLV provirus becomes integrated within the host c-*myc* locus, which is then expressed under the influence of the viral LTR promoter sequence. Genetic deletions are a feature of the integrated provirus in lymphoma induction (148, 268). The enhanced expression of the c-*myc* gene by this "promoter insertion" is believed to initiate the lymphomagenic process, but multistep activation of other transforming genes such as *B-lym* may be necessary for the full development of LL (4, 69,165, 185).

DEFECTIVENESS AND PHENOTYPIC MIXING. A number of avian retroviruses have been shown to have defective genomes and arise either spontaneously or as a result of experimental mutagenesis (165, 337, 338). Some acutely transforming viruses, such as certain strains of RSV, have lost their *onc* gene and ability to transform rapidly: they are called transformation defective (*td*) mutants and have an oncogenic potential similar to that of nondefective leukosis viruses (27). Other viruses (acute leukemia viruses) are defective for genes required for replication – replication defective (*rd*) mutants. They will transform cells but require the presence of a helper virus to enable them to replicate; e.g., BH-RSV and AMV lack the *env* gene and AEV and MC29 lack the *pol* and *env* genes. *Td* and *rd* mutants are defective under all conditions (nonconditional mutants). Conditional mutants function under permissive conditions, not under nonpermissive conditions, and are exemplified by the temperature-sensitive (*ts*) mutants.

BH-RSV is the classic example of an *rd* mutant and is of practical importance in the nonproducer (NP) cell activation test for avian leukosis viruses (see DIAGNOSIS). On single infection of chicken embryo fibroblasts, the defective virus genome of BH-RSV functions to bring about replication of viral RNA, transformation of infected cells, and production of gs antigen, but only noninfectious progeny particles are produced, which are unable to enter new host cells because of an alteration in their envelope glycoproteins. The morphologically altered cells are called NP cells. A nondefective leukosis virus added to these cells acts as a helper virus by complementing the defective genome of BH-RSV and causes both infectious RSV and progeny leukosis virus to be produced simultaneously. Thus the presence of infectious RSV in the NP test denotes presence of leukosis virus in added test material. This RSV has envelope antigens identical to those of the helper virus, which thus determines infectivity and range of infectivity in genetically different cells, interference patterns among and between subgroups, and type-specific antigenicity. Stocks of *rd* mutant RSV must by their existence contain helper viruses; these were originally referred to as Rous-associated viruses (RAVs). Infectious RSVs formed in these circumstances are called pseudotypes, and their designation includes the helper virus when this is identified, e.g., BH-RSV (RAV-1) when RAV-1 strain leukosis helper virus is used. This phenomenon is an example of the phenotypic mixing (PM) (28) that occurs readily when two related viruses infect the same cell and in which virions with the genome of one virus may possess envelope and other structural proteins of the other parent, or both. The phenomenon of PM is also employed in the PM test for detection of leukosis viruses (see Diagnosis). Genetic recombination, in which exchanges of genes between two viruses (and consequent stable phenotypic changes) occur, are well recognized and must be distinguished from PM (335, 341). Use of defective strains of RSV allows tailor-made RSV to be made with envelope properties of the helper virus. Determinations of host range, interference pattern, and neutralization can be performed more easily with the appropriate pseudotype than with the leukosis virus, since the former can be readily quantified in cell culture by inoculation of the chorioallantoic membrane (CAM) of chick embryos or inoculation of chicks.

The above, notwithstanding, infectious RSV may be generated with BH-RSV and other *rd* mutants following solitary infections in absence of added helper viruses in certain types of chicken cells that carry endogenous leukosis virus genomes (see **ENDOGENOUS LEUKOSIS VIRUSES**). However, such RSV has the subgroup E host range of the endogenous viruses and may be distinguished from helper viruses of other subgroups when NP tests are conducted.

PM may also occur between unrelated viruses, such as vesicular stomatitis virus (VSV) and avian RNA tumor viruses (336), or between reticuloendotheliosis virus and RSV (285). VSV with avian RNA tumor virus envelope may be used in rapid interference, host range, and neutralization tests because it is rapidly cytopathic.

ENDOGENOUS LEUKOSIS VIRUSES. Virtually all normal chickens carry complete or defective DNA proviral genetic sequences of E subgroup leukosis viruses integrated in their cell genome (75, 76, 266, 296) (Fig. 16.19). These sites of integrated viral genes are endogenous viral (*ev*) loci, and some have now been located on particular chromosomes (318). They occur in somatic and germ line cells and are transmitted genetically in a Mendelian fashion to their progeny by both sexes (1, 88, 234). At least 29 *ev* loci have been identified (157, 296), but many more are believed to exist. On average each chicken carries about 5 *ev* loci (273). The phenotypic expressions of these loci vary, depending on the viral genes present and on as yet poorly understood control mechanisms (Tables 16.5 and 16.6). When the complete endogenous viral genome is present, subgroup E leukosis virus may be produced by the cell, either spontaneously or after induction by chemicals such as bromodeoxyuridine (BUDR). When the endogenous viral genome is incomplete (defective), genes present may be phenotypically expressed in the cells, but infectious virus is not produced because of absence of the complete set of genes needed for infectious virion production; e.g., the defective *ev*3 locus possesses the *gag* and *env* genes of subgroup E virus, and cells carrying this locus contain gs antigen and subgroup E viral envelope glycoproteins. However, the locus has a genetic deletion around the *gag-pol* junction and infectious virions are not formed. Presence of *ev* genes in such cells is responsible for their positive reactions in the ELISA test, the complement-fixation test for avian leukosis viruses (COFAL) and the chick helper factor (chf) test (see DIAGNOSIS), in which genetic defectiveness in the envelope of BH-RSV is complemented by endogenous envelope proteins resulting in an infectious form of RSV with subgroup E host range and other properties. Genetic characteristics of *ev* loci are described in detail by Weiss et al. (337, 338) and Smith (296). Expression of endogenous *ev* genes is responsible for a dominant form of genetic resistance of chicken cells to infection by subgroup E viruses from block of virus receptors by envelope protein (238, 269). Transmission of *ev* genes from parent to offspring has been called genetic transmission of leukosis virus, distinguishing it from vertical (congenital) and horizontal (contact) transmission of viruses in an infectious state. However, fully expressed infectious endogenous virus may sometimes also be transmitted vertically and horizontally (300). Related *ev* loci occur in several species of fowl other than domestic chick-

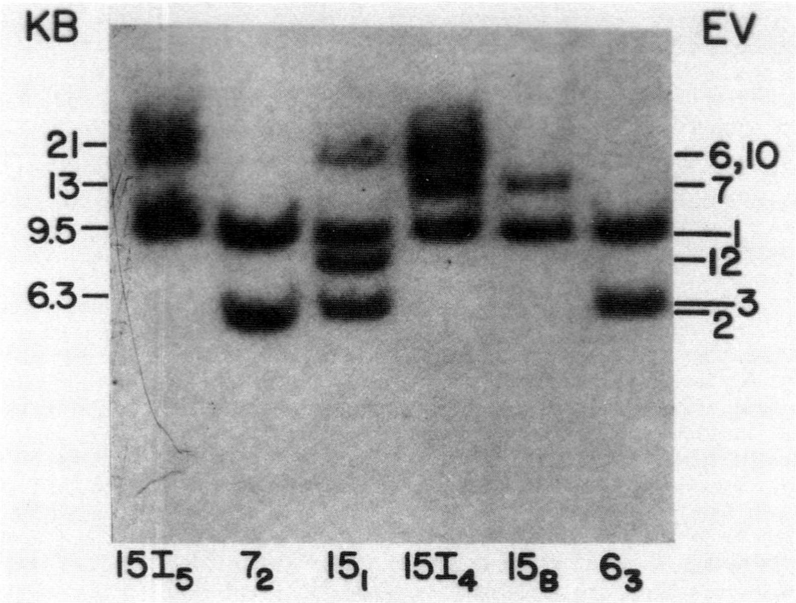

16.19. Endogenous viral (*ev*) loci detected in six inbred lines of white leghorns by restriction fragment polymorphisms generated after Sac-1 endonuclease digestion of red blood cell DNA and hybridized to ^{32}P-labelled RAV-2 genomic sequences. (Smith, Martinus Nijhoff)

Table 16.5. Phenotypic expression of representative endogenous viral (*ev*) genes in normal chicken cells

Phenotype	Symbol	*ev* locus
No detectable viral product	gs$^-$chf$^-$	1, 4, 5
Expression of subgroup E envelope antigen	gs$^-$chf$^+$	9
Coordinate expression of group-specific and envelope antigens	gs$^+$chf$^+$	3
Spontaneous production of subgroup E virus	V-E$^+$	2

Source: After (296).

ens, including red jungle fowl and some strains of pheasants, partridges, and grouse, but the distribution does not support a phylogenetic relationship (137). Rather, it is believed that the leukosis virus genomes have become incorporated at various loci relatively recently in the history of *Gallus* and independent of integration in other genera. It is not known whether endogenous viruses arise from exogenous LLV of other subgroups, from which they differ genomically at the *env* gene and in the LTR region, or vice versa.

Subgroup E LLV, typified by RAV-0, has little or no oncogenicity (211). Persistence of these viral loci suggests that birds carrying them are not at a great disadvantage and it is possible that they may be beneficial. Thus Crittenden et al. (90, 92) have shown that presence of *ev*2 or *ev*3 protects birds from a unique nonneoplastic syn-

Table 16.6. Phenotypes of endogenous retroviral (*ev*) genes in inbred and commercial lines of white leghorn chickens

ev	Phenotype	Line or Source[b]
1	gs$^-$chf$^-$	Most lines
2	V-E$^+$	RPRL-7_2
3	gs$^+$chf$^+$	RPRL-6_3
4	gs$^-$chf$^-$	SPAFAS
5	gs$^-$chf$^-$	SPAFAS
6	gs$^-$chf$^+$	RPRL-15I
7	V-E$^+$	RPRL-15B
8	gs$^-$chf$^-$	K-18
9	gs$^-$chf$^+$	K-18
10	V-E$^+$	RPRL-$15I_4$
11	V-E$^+$	RPRL-$15I_4$
12	V-E$^+$	RPRL-15I
14	V-E$^+$	H & N
15(C)	None	K-28 × K-16
16(D)	None	K-28 × K-16
17	gs$^-$chf$^-$	RC-P
18	V-E$^+$	RI
19	V-E$^+$(?)[a]	RW
20	V-E$^+$(?)[a]	RW
21	V-E$^+$	Hyline FP

Note: *Ev*13 is associated with the gs$^-$chf$^-$ phenotype but restriction fragments have not been characterized.

[a]The presence of five *ev* loci in Reaseheath line W birds precludes definitive assignment with the V-E$^+$ phenotype. Definitive association requires further segregation of *ev* genes. Hyline FP birds also carry *ev*1, *ev*3, and *ev*6.

[b]Not exclusive to line or source. K = Kimber; R = Reaseheath; H & N = Heisdorf and Nelson. For references see (296).

drome caused by infection with an exogenous subgroup A LLV. It is possible that endogenous viruses may have either beneficial or detrimental effects, perhaps by their induction of immunity or tolerance to tumor virus antigens, depending on when they are expressed. Embryonic infection with endogenous leukosis virus, RAV-0, caused more persistent viremia and more neoplasms following infection with exogenous LLV, apparently due to tolerant depression of specific humoral immunity (94). Endogenous viruses are not essential, since it has been possible to produce chickens free of *ev* genes (2). A line of such chickens has been produced, designated line 0 (77), and is of value in research studies where birds or cells free from *ev* loci are needed.

Of particular importance is the *ev*21 locus, which is tightly linked in White Leghorn stock to the dominant sex-linked gene, *K*, which regulates slow feathering. Some breeders have reported reduced egg production and higher mortality associated with an increased incidence of viremia with exogenous leukosis virus in female progeny from dams carrying the *K* gene. It appears that expression of the *ev*21 gene as infectious endogenous virus induces immunological tolerance and consequently increased susceptibility to infection by exogenous leukosis virus (9, 164).

Resistance to Chemical and Physical Agents

LIPID SOLVENTS AND DETERGENTS. Avian retroviruses have a high lipid content in the envelope, and their infectivity is abolished by ethyl ether (136). The detergent sodium dodecyl sulfate disrupts the virions and releases RNA and core proteins (267).

THERMAL INACTIVATION. The half-life of various leukosis/sarcoma viruses at 37 C varies from 100 to 540 min (avg. around 260 min), depending on medium in which the virus is suspended, tissue of origin, and virus strain (323). Avian tumor viruses are inactivated rapidly at high temperatures; the half-life for RSV at 50 C is 8.5 min and at 60 C, 0.7 min (106).

Thermal lability of infectivity of these viruses is a critical factor in storage. Even at −15 C the half-life of AMV is less than 1 wk (114); it is only at temperatures below −60 C that avian retroviruses can be stored for several years without loss of infectivity (32). Virus is degraded by freezing and thawing and the *gs* antigen is released.

pH STABILITY. There is little change in stability of viruses of this group between pH 5 and 9; outside this range inactivation rates are markedly increased.

ULTRAVIOLET IRRADIATION. RSV is 10 times more resistant to exposure to ultraviolet light than Newcastle disease virus, even though these viruses have similar size, structure, RNA content, and sensitivity to X rays (275). Similar resistance has been observed with certain field strains (136).

Strain Classification. Strains of avian leukosis/sarcoma viruses are classified according to the predominant pathological lesion they induce and the subgroup envelope they possess. Common laboratory strains of avian leukosis/sarcoma viruses are listed in Table 16.4 (337). They are given (by a convention based on common practice) a full and an abbreviated designation on the basis of the predominant neoplasm they induce, with an affix to indicate their origin with an individual, e.g., Rous sarcoma virus (RSV), or location, e.g., Regional Poultry Research Laboratory isolate 12 of LLV (RPL12-LLV). Substrains of RSV are designated according to individuals who studied them, e.g., the high-titer strain of Bryan (BH-RSV), or according to location, e.g., Prague (PR-RSV). Subgroups (e.g., A) may be designated also: PR-RSV-A.

Helper viruses isolated from stocks of other viruses, e.g., RAVs, have been designated numerically (e.g. RAV-1). Where a helper virus is used for replication of a defective virus, this is indicated also. Thus BH-RSV grown with RAV-1 as a helper is designated BH-RSV (RAV-1). Strains of LLV that act as resistance-inducing factors (see DIAGNOSIS) were designated RIFs.

Laboratory Host Systems

CHICK INOCULATION. RSV and other sarcoma viruses produce tumors when injected by the subcutaneous (SC), intramuscular (IM), or intraabdominal (IA) routes or by contact with inoculated chickens. SC injection into the wing web can be used for TD50 assays of stocks of RSV (31), and this route or IM inoculation is used for virus isolation and propagation (204, 257). Intracerebral (IC) inoculation of day-old chicks can be employed for detection of genetic resistance to the virus (156). Following wing-web injection with high doses of virus, tumors are first palpable at about 3 days; in susceptible chickens these may grow rapidly, ulcerate, and metastasize. With low doses of virus, tumors may occur as late as 35 days postinoculation. There are extensive reviews on methods and interpretation of results (31).

By injecting the RPL12 strain of LLV by the IA route into day-old susceptible line 15I chicks, Burmester and Gentry (42) were able to obtain a LL response in 200–270 days. This procedure was used by Burmester and Fredrickson (41) for initial isolation of virus from field cases. Time required for quantitative assay of certain strains passaged in the laboratory was shortened to 63 days by using the less sensitive erythroblastosis response (35). In these transmission experiments all sources of virus that caused LL also caused erythroblastosis. Osteopetrosis, hemangiomas, and fibrosarcomas were also observed in chickens of certain strains and passages. The host-virus interrelations were studied in detail by Burmester et al. (48, 50). AMV can be titrated in susceptible chicks by IV inoculation at 1–3 days of age (112, 113). AMV in chicken plasma can be assayed by its adenosine triphosphatase activity; this method is indispensable for routine and large-scale studies (22).

Osteopetrosis-inducing activity of some strains of virus can be examined by IV inoculation of day-old chicks (50) or by IM injection of infective material (168). Guinea fowl are particularly sensitive to osteopetrosis induced by MAV-2(0) (182).

EMBRYO INOCULATION. When RSV and other sarcoma viruses are inoculated onto the CAM of 11-day-old susceptible embryos, tumor pocks develop (Fig. 16.20), which can be counted 8 days later and are linearly related to virus dose (109). Tumors can also be produced by IV inoculation at 10–13 days of incubation and by yolk sac inoculation at 5–8 days incubation.

Leukosis viruses have been quantitated by their IV inoculation into 11-day-old susceptible chicken embryos. Within 2 wk of hatching, a high incidence of neoplasms occurs (mainly erythroblastosis), although hemorrhages and solid tumors can develop including fibrosarcomas, endothelial tumors, nephroblastomas, and chondromas. When chicks are held for a post inoculation period of 46 days, responses are higher by 1–2 $\log_{10}$ dilutions than those following chicken inoculation. Most chickens that survive the acute neoplasms develop LL after 100 days postinoculation (245).

AMV produces a myeloblastosis response within a few weeks when injected IV into susceptible embryos (12).

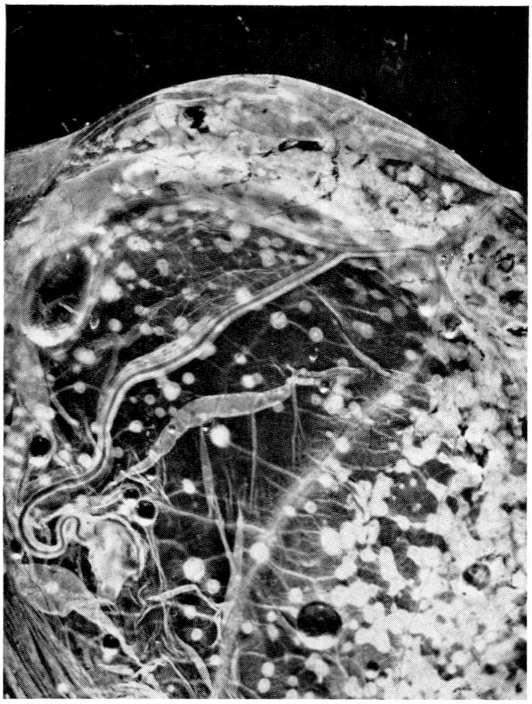

16.20. Pocks induced by BH-RSV on CAM of chicken embryo. (Piraino)

CELL CULTURE. RSV and other sarcoma viruses induce rapid neoplastic transformation of cells when inoculated onto monolayer cultures of chicken embryo fibroblasts. The transformed cells proliferate to produce within a few days discrete colonies or foci of transformed cells (Fig. 16.21), which can be used for quantitative assay of virus (316).

Most leukosis viruses replicate in fibroblast culture without producing any obvious cytopathic effect. Their presence can be detected by a variety of tests (see Diagnosis). Leukosis viruses of subgroups B and D may induce cytopathic plaques that may be used for virus assay (149). Morphologic alterations have also been reported after prolonged passage of leukosis virus-infected fibroblasts (53).

Defective leukemia viruses will transform hematopoietic cells in vitro (207). Yolk sac and bone marrow cells in culture are transformed to neoplastic myeloblasts on infection with AMV (209), and bone marrow cells transform to erythroblasts with AEV (150). Transformation of hematopoietic cells by MH2, MC29, and OK10 viruses was observed by Graf and Beug (151). In vitro transformation of B lymphocytes by nondefective LLV has not yet been reported.

Tumor cell lines derived from tumors induced in vivo by the avian retroviruses have been developed, including LL (220, 293), myeloblastosis (189), erythroblastosis (152), and myelocytoma (188).

The properties of leukosis/sarcoma viruses in cell culture are described in more detail under DIAGNOSIS.

Pathogenicity. Most strains of avian tumor virus under study were isolated from various types of neoplasms many years ago and have subsequently been passaged experimentally many times in chickens or cell culture. The strains may produce more than one type of neoplasm (Fig. 16.22). The oncogenic spectrum of each strain tends to be characteristic but often overlaps with responses to other strains, e.g., the RPL12 strain of LLV produces LL, erythroblastosis, fibrosarcomas, hemangiomas, and osteopetrosis; the BAI-A strain of AMV produces myeloblastosis, sarcomas, osteopetrosis, hemangiomas, LL, neph-

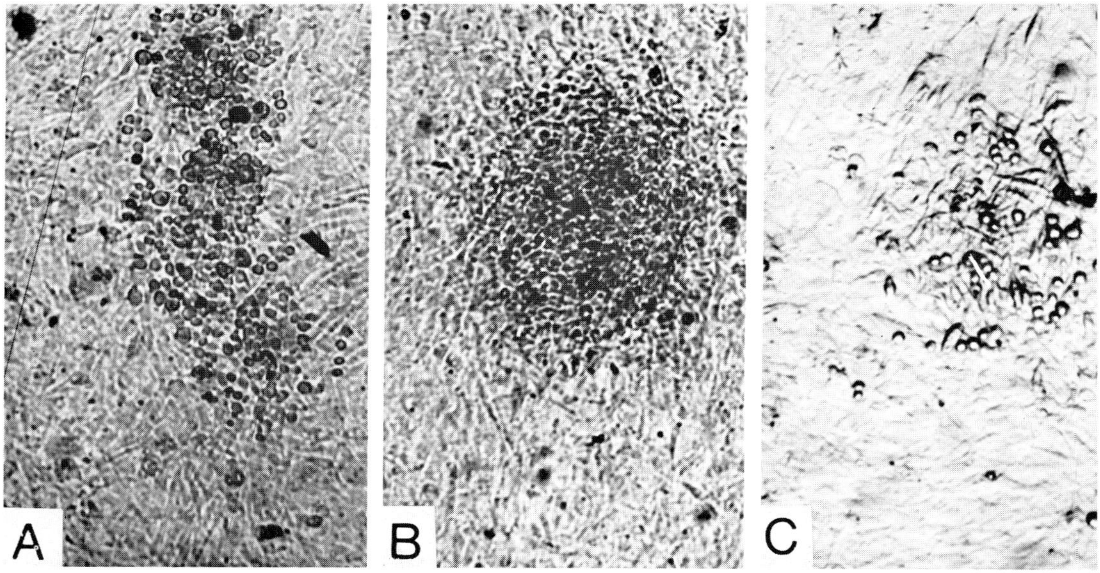

16.21. Foci induced by RSV in cell culture. A. Unstained focus of transformed spherical, refractile chicken embryo cells infected 6 days previously with Bryan's standard strain of RSV. ×100. B. Unstained focus of transformed, polygonal, opaque Rous sarcoma cells infected 6 days previously with Bryan's high-titer strain. ×100. C. Unstained focus of transformed round and fusiform cells infected 6 days previously with Popken's preparation of RSV. ×100.

roblastomas, thecomas, granulosa cell tumors, and epitheliomas (Fig. 16.22). As discussed below, the oncogenic patterns of different virus strains are influenced by viral and host factors such as origin; dose; route of inoculation; and age, genotype, and sex of the host. Most studies have been conducted with strains of virus that were not genetically purified, and an important question has been whether ability of a particular strain to cause several neoplasms was a result of presence in virus stocks of a mixture of virus types with differing oncogenic potentials or of pluripotential properties of a single genetic type. Studies show that both explanations can apply. Clone-purified strains of LLV can cause a variety of neoplasms in addition to LL, including erythroblastosis, osteopetrosis, and nephroblastomas (261). Other strains of virus consist of mixtures. This is best exemplified by the defective acute leukemia viruses, which require a nondefective helper virus for their replication. In this situation, oncogenic properties may originate from either the defective or helper virus. Even so, clone-purified strains of AEV can induce both erythroblastosis and sarcomas, irrespective of the helper virus (153). Varying degrees of relatedness between different pure strains of virus may be demonstrated by nucleic acid hybridization techniques, and the differences can be related to oncogenic properties. These differences may lie in the particular *onc* gene present in acute transforming viruses or in other parts of the viral genome in the slowly transforming viruses (165).

ORIGIN OF VIRUS. The strain of virus has a profound effect on the tumor response obtained. The tumor spectrum tends to be characteristic of the strain when it is handled under identical conditions but may be modified by changes in these conditions. Such differences are also seen in virus strains newly isolated from the field, as exemplified by tumor spectrums of RPL26, RPL27, and RPL28 isolates of LLV (135).

Within a particular strain, differences may be obtained that depend on type of neoplasm used for virus isolation. Thus, using viruses isolated from field cases, Fredrickson et al. (135) observed that serial transfer from donors with LL resulted primarily in LL, whereas virus from donors with erythroblastosis predominantly caused erythroblastosis. As will be explained later, this was almost certainly due to a dose effect. In another instance, selection of virus donors with hemangiomas resulted in a larger proportion of virus with this tumor than in the previous passage (48).

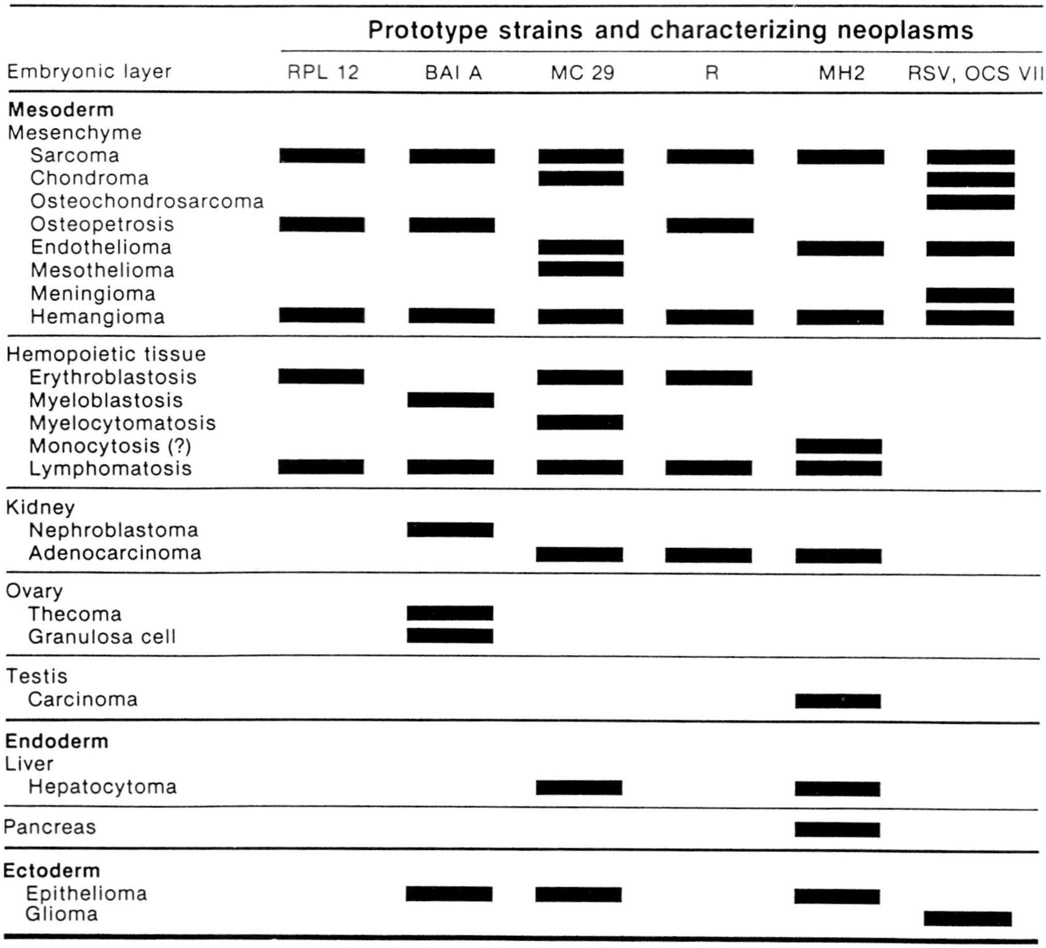

Prototype strains and characterizing neoplasms
Embryonic layer
RPL 12
BAI A
MC 29
R
MH2
RSV, OCS VII
Mesoderm
Mesenchyme
Sarcoma
Chondroma
Osteochondrosarcoma
Osteopetrosis
Endothelioma
Mesothelioma
Meningioma
Hemangioma
Hemopoietic tissue
Erythroblastosis
Myeloblastosis
Myelocytomatosis
Monocytosis (?)
Lymphomatosis
Kidney
Nephroblastoma
Adenocarcinoma
Ovary
Thecoma
Granulosa cell
Testis
Carcinoma
Endoderm
Liver
Hepatocytoma
Pancreas
Ectoderm
Epithelioma
Glioma

16.22. Oncogenic spectrum of selected avian leukosis viruses. Black bars represent a response of that type. (Beard, Raven Press)

VIRUS SUBGROUP. No relationship has been observed between virus subgroup and oncogenicity except for endogenous E subgroup LLVs, such as RAV-0, which have little or no oncogenicity (211). However, the low oncogenicity of RAV-0 is believed to be related to differences in the terminal region of the genome and not to the *env* gene.

VIRUS DOSE. High doses of RPL12-LLV mainly induced erythroblastosis, whereas doses close to the endpoint predominantly induced LL (48). Sarcomas, endotheliomas, and hemorrhages were also commoner with high virus doses. Occurrence of osteopetrosis showed no dependency on dose (134).

ROUTE OF INOCULATION. Responses obtained after virus administration by less efficient portals of entry into the host apparently reflect the decreased effective dose. Thus exposure of susceptible birds by contact with birds inoculated with a high dose of RPL12 virus resulted in a LL response similar to that expected with 1/1000 of the inoculated dose (48). IM inoculation of RPL26 virus favored sarcoma induction, whereas IV inoculation mainly produced erythroblastosis and hemorrhages (134). These differences may reflect variations in amounts of virus that reach the target cells by different routes.

AGE OF HOST. In general, resistance of birds to development of neoplasms of all types increases with age, the rate varying with route of inoculation. Resistance increases rapidly between 1 and 21 days of age with oral or nasal administration but relatively slowly when virus is inoculated intravenously (50). Types of tumors produced also reflect the decreased effective dose (48). However, the incidence of some tumors decreases more rapidly than expected from the dose effect alone; e.g., certain RPL12 virus preparations given intravenously at 1 day of age caused a high incidence of osteopetrosis; the proportion of chickens inoculated at 3 wk of age and developing osteopetrosis was only one-tenth that of chickens inoculated at 1 day of age (50).

An interesting exception is that very young birds are somewhat less susceptible to strain R of the AEV than older birds (23).

GENOTYPE AND SEX OF HOST. The genetic constitution of the host has a strong influence on response to leukosis/sarcoma viruses (see Pathogenesis and Epizootiology). Females are more susceptible to LL than males. Castration of both sexes increases incidence of this disease, and testosterone increases resistance of males and capons (43). These effects are probably a consequence of hormonal effects influencing regression and hence target cell numbers in the bursa of Fabricius.

Homotransplantation. Many of the tumors induced by viruses of the leukosis/sarcoma group are homotransplantable. In some instances transplanted tumors can be readily differentiated from primary virus-induced tumors. Thus transplanted LL tumors grow to a palpable size within 5–10 days and result in death shortly thereafter, whereas primary virus-induced tumors develop 4 mo after inoculation of day-old chicks. Other transplantable tumors also have a shorter incubation period than their virus-induced counterparts. Transplanted LL tumors and nephroblastomas generally appear at the site of inoculation instead of in their originating organs; e.g., in LL tumor transplants there is usually no bursal tumor (Fig. 16.23). Histologically, transplanted tumors are generally more uniform and more anaplastic than the tumors from which they originate (compare Figs. 16.24 and 16.29). Thus transplanted LL tumors are composed almost exclusively of large anaplastic lymphoblasts with a vesicular nucleus and several large nucleoli (Fig. 16.24).

Rous sarcomas can be serially transplanted; however, by the 2nd generation only 0.05% of these cells are of donor origin. Even in histocompatible chickens the proportion of donor cells falls rapidly until there are no mitotic donor cells 6

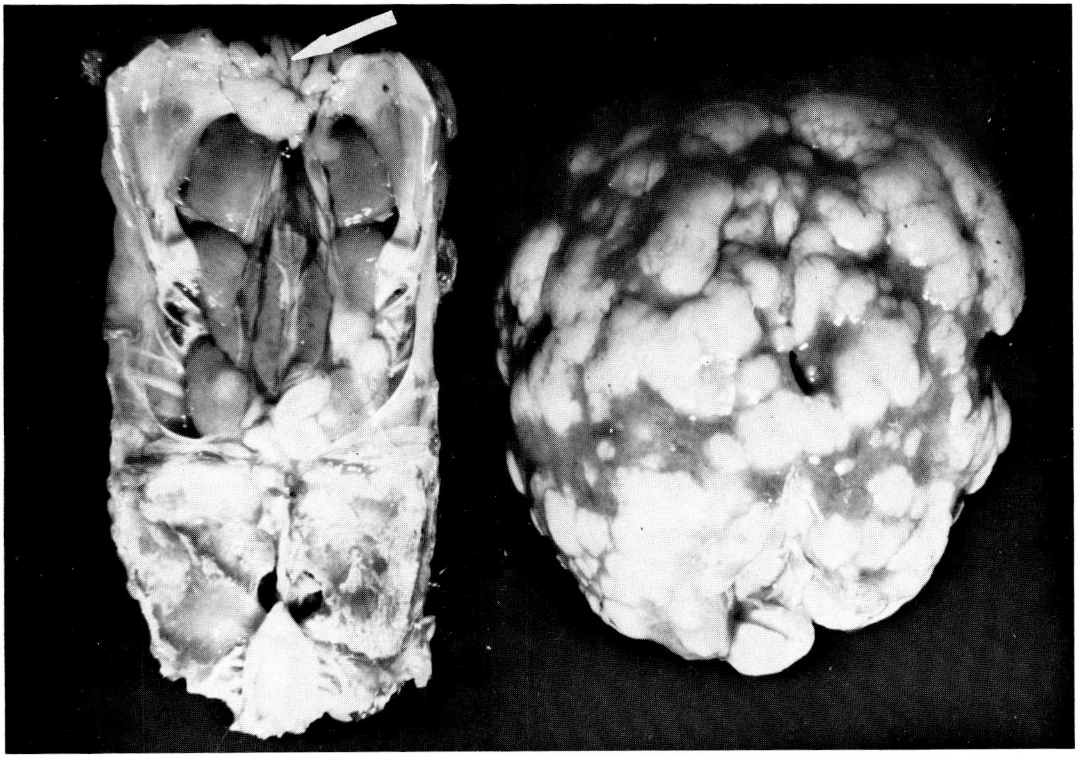

16.23. LL transplant. Bird died 14 days after inoculation at 1 day of age with suspension from LL tumor induced by HPRS-2 Rous-associated leukosis virus. A lymphoid tumor was also present in abdominal muscle at site of inoculation. Note metastases in liver, lung, and kidney and absence of tumor in bursa (*arrow*).

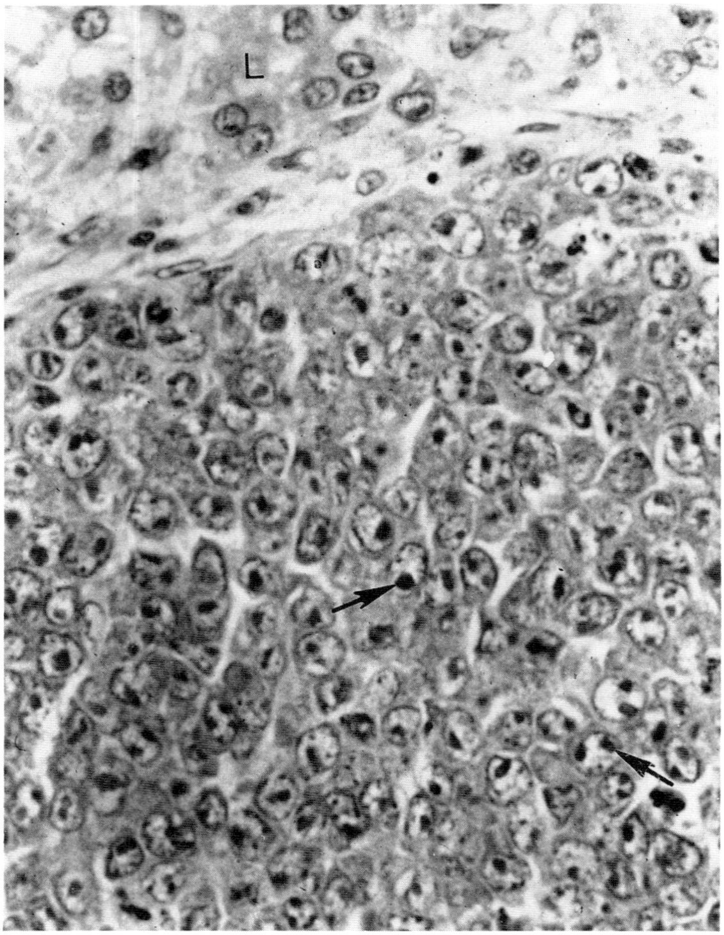

16.24. Microscopic appearance of tumor in Figure 16.23. Note homogenous large anaplastic lymphoblasts with prominent nucleoli (*arrows*) compressing the liver cells (*L*). Compare these cells with those in Figure 16.29 that resulted from infection with virus rather than cells. Cells from bird in Figure 16.29 were transplanted to induce tumors shown in Figures 16.23 and 16.24. ×700.

days after cell inoculation (247). Thus Rous sarcoma cells do not survive long in the recipient, and tumors in the recipient are formed largely from recruited virus-infected cells.

Leukemic myeloblasts from donor birds inoculated with AMV (BAI-A) failed to persist in the recipient when transplanted, and the leukemic cells had the karyotype of the recipient (10).

Erythroblasts from donor birds inoculated with strain R, on the other hand, persisted for longer periods in the recipient—in highly inbred chickens up to the 5th transplant generation (246).

Lymphoid cells from some LL tumors can be transplanted indefinitely. This is certainly true for the tumor from which the RPL12 strain of virus originated and for many other virus-induced LL tumors. However, some tumors are converted into neoplasms dominated by cells of recipient origin (248).

Several new LL transplantable tumors were described by Okazaki et al. (220).

Nephroblastomas induced by AMV (BAI-A) have been homotransplanted to the breast muscle (173, 327). In addition to tumors at the site of inoculation, recipients have metastatic tumors in the viscera and secondary tumors such as myeloblastosis and LL. Since typical renal growths occurred at the site of inoculation, there is not much doubt that these tumors were of donor origin. However, it is likely that the secondary neoplasms were induced by virus elaborated by the transplant.

Hepatomas induced by MC29 virus are readily transplantable (191, 190). A transplantable epithelial cell line was developed from a liver tumor of a bird infected with MC29 (188).

Investigations of tumor transplants have been of limited assistance in understanding virus-induced tumors; e.g., immunity and genetic resistance to tumors resulting directly from transplantation of neoplastic cells may have no relation to immunity or genetic resistance to virus infection or induction of tumors by virus.

PATHOGENESIS AND EPIZOOTIOLOGY

Natural and Experimental Hosts. Chickens are the natural hosts for all viruses of this group (232), and they have not been isolated from other avian species except pheasants, partridges, and quail, as described under VIRUS SUBGROUPS. However, experimentally, some viruses have a wide host range and can be adapted to grow in unusual hosts by passage in very young animals or induction of immunologic tolerance prior to inoculation of the virus. RSV has the widest host range. It will cause tumors in chickens, pheasants, guinea fowl, ducks, pigeons, Japanese quail, turkeys, and rock partridges. Some strains of sarcoma virus induce tumors in mammals (323), including monkeys (184). Osteopetrosis can be produced in turkeys by inoculation of fresh whole blood from affected chickens (168). RPL12 strain of LLV did not produce LL or erythroblastosis in Japanese quail (81, 262), and the virus did not multiply in quail. These birds are, however, susceptible to myeloblastosis.

Transmission. Exogenous LLVs are transmitted in two ways: vertically from hen to progeny through the egg and horizontally from bird to bird by direct or indirect contact (72, 277, 278) (Fig. 16.25). Although usually only a small minority of chicks are infected vertically, this route of transmission is important epizootiologically because it affords a means of maintaining the infection from one generation to the next. Most chickens become infected by close contact with congenitally infected birds. Although vertical transmission is important in maintenance of the infection, horizontal infection may also be necessary to maintain a rate of vertical transmission sufficient to

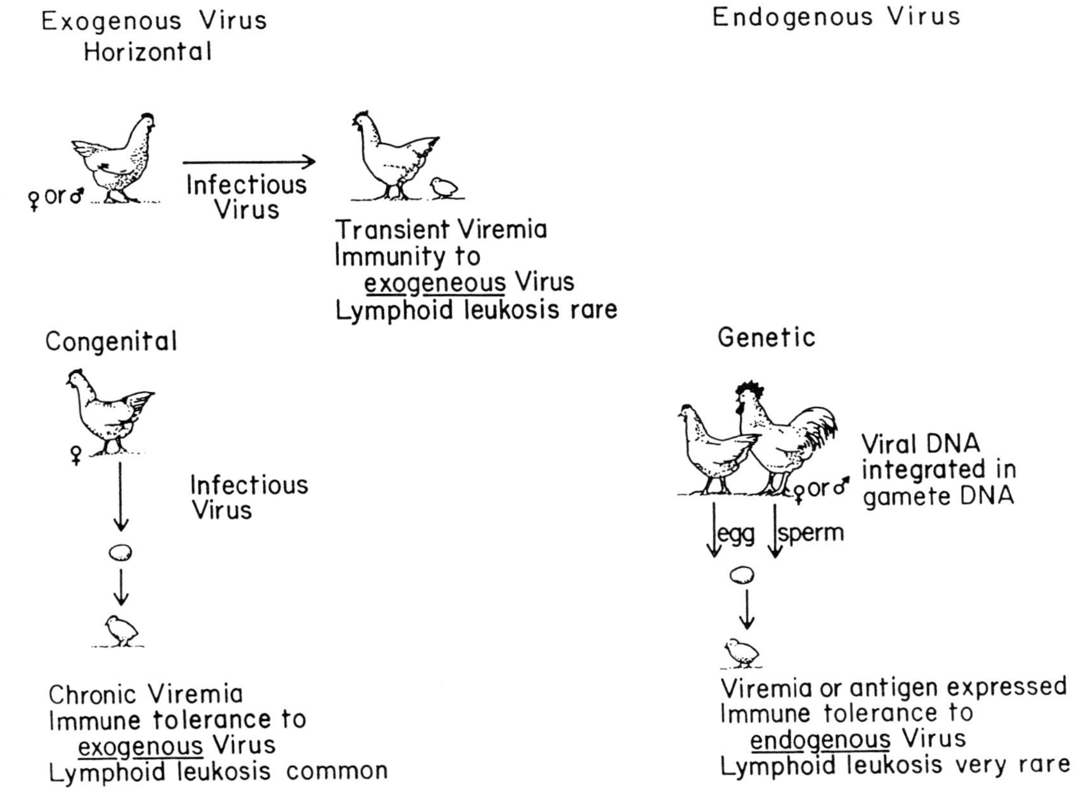

16.25. Horizontal and vertical transmission of exogenous LLV and genetic transmission of endogenous virus. (Crittenden, Avian Pathol)

prevent the infection from dying out (233). The infection does not spread readily from infected birds to birds in indirect contact (in separate pens or cages), probably because of the relatively short life of the virus outside the birds (see Thermal Inactivation).

Four serological classes occur in mature chickens in relation to LL infection: 1) no viremia, no antibody (V−A−); 2) no viremia, with antibody (V−A+); 3) with viremia, with antibody (V+A+); 4) with viremia, no antibody (V+A−) (277, 278). Birds in an infection-free flock and genetically resistant birds in a susceptible flock fall into the category V−A−. Genetically susceptible birds in an infected flock fall into one of the other three categories. Most are V−A+, and a minority, usually less than 10%, are V+A−. Most V+A− hens transmit leukosis virus to a varying but relatively high proportion of their progeny (239, 278). A small proportion of V−A+ hens transmit the virus congenitally and do so more intermittently. Congenitally infected embryos develop immunological tolerance to the virus and after hatching make up the V+A− class, with high levels of virus in the blood and tissues and an absence of antibodies. Older hens (2 or 3 yr of age) transmit virus in their eggs less consistently and at a lower level than birds under 18 mo (46). Infection of the cock apparently does not influence rate of congenital infection of progeny (277, 308). The genetics of the host and the strain of LLV influence shedding and congenital transmission after horizontal infection (92). With electron microscopy, virus budding has been seen on all structures of reproductive organs of cocks except germinal cells (104), indicating the virus does not multiply in germ cells. The cock, therefore, acts only as a virus carrier and source of contact or venereal infection to other birds (290, 308). Congenital infection of embryos is strongly associated with shedding by the hen of leukosis virus into egg albumen and with presence of virus in the vagina of hens (239, 307). These traits are also highly correlated with viremia.

Shedding of virus into egg albumen and transmission to the embryo is a consequence of virus production by albumen-secreting glands of the oviduct. Electron microscopy studies have revealed a high degree of virus replication in the magnum of the oviduct (103). Virus budding also occurs in various cell types in the ovary but not in the follicular cells or ovum, and transovarial infection does not seem to be important (239). Not all eggs that have leukosis virus in the albumen give rise to infected embryos or chicks; in the studies of Spencer et al. (307) and Payne et al. (239) only about 1/2–1/4 of embryos were infected from eggs with virus in the albumen. This intermittent congenital transmission may be a consequence of neutralization of virus by antibody in the yolk and of loss because of thermal inactivation.

Electron microscopy has revealed virus particles in many organs from infected chicken embryos, and virus has been observed to bud and accumulate in large amounts in pancreatic acinar cells of embryos (343). These particles, which are highly infectious, are shed in droppings of newly hatched chicks (36). Infectious virus is also present in saliva and feces of older birds that provide a source of horizontal infection to other birds (36).

Usually, only a minority of leukosis virus-infected birds develop LL; the others remain as carriers and shedders. Viremic-tolerant (V+A−) birds are reported to be several times more likely to die of LL than those with antibody (V−A+) (277). Incidence of leukosis decreases rapidly if infection by natural routes occurs after the first few weeks of age (50); there are well-established genetic differences in susceptibility to LL development in chickens that are equally susceptible to virus infection (86).

Endogenous leukosis viruses (see ETIOLOGY) are usually transmitted genetically in germ cells of both sexes (Fig. 16.25). Many are genetically defective and incapable of giving rise to infectious virions, but some are not and may be expressed in an infectious form in either embryos or hatched birds. In this form they are then transmitted similarly to exogenous viruses, although most chickens are genetically resistant to such exogenous infection. Endogenous viruses have little or no oncogenicity (211) but may influence response of the bird to infection by exogenous leukosis virus (90). Immunodepression induced by infectious bursal disease virus increased the rate of shedding of LL virus (129).

Pathology. One or more specific neoplasms induced by leukosis/sarcoma group viruses may occur in a given flock of chickens. Presence of a tumor similar to that produced under experimental conditions is only provisional evidence that the bird was infected with a virus of this group. Some tumors do not yield virus, so it has not been possible to show that all tumors of a given type are caused by a virus of this group. In this section the pathology of the different neoplasms will be discussed without regard for virological properties of the inducing agent(s). Only entities that have been reproduced with viruses of the leukosis/sarcoma group will be described. The strong promoters of gene expression in leukosis/sarcoma viruses can be integrated in many places in the host genome. They then have the capacity to increase expression of genes downstream from them. Depending on where they integrate, they can cause a whole variety of neoplasms and neoplastic processes or disturbances in the normal physiology of the host. Some viruses integrate more frequently in one location than another and thus tend to induce a particular neoplasm or physiological disturbance more frequently than other neoplasms or disturbances.

NONNEOPLASTIC CONDITIONS. Chickens, turkeys, and jungle fowl exposed to certain leukosis viruses (RAV-1, RAV-60, MAV-2[0], and viruses of subgroups B and D) when young develop anemia, hepatitis, immunodepression, and wasting: some may die (90, 301, 334). Chickens inoculated with RAV-7 develop neurological signs including ataxia, lethargy and imbalance resulting from a nonsuppurative meningoencephalomyelitis (339). Anemia is due to an aplastic crisis in the bone marrow in which erythrocytes fail to incorporate iron into hemoglobin and exhibit a decreased survival time (95). Administration of antiviral antibody will prevent anemia (251). The immunodepression may involve atrophy or aplasia of lymphoid organs, hypergammaglobulinemia, decreased mitogen-induced blastogenesis and decreased antibody response (301). The changes in the immune system are likely due to cessation of B-cell maturation and a block in development of suppressor T cells, possibly due to interference with the synthesis of functional interleukin-2 (167, 186). RAV-7 causes, in addition to stunting and atrophy of the lymphoid organs, obesity, high triglyceride and cholesterol levels, reduced thyroxine levels (hypothyroidism), and increased insulin levels (62). The frequent occurrence of stunting may relate to the virus's suppression of thyroid function. Although not examined extensively, leukosis viruses are likely to have similar physiological effects in the field. Subclinical physiological effects are likely to contribute to the decreased productivity described below.

Viral infection in the absence of overt disease can adversely affect productivity of egg-laying chickens. Hens that shed virus produced 20–35 fewer eggs per hen housed to 497 days of age; matured later sexually; and produced smaller eggs, at a lower rate, and with thinner shells compared to nonshedders. Mortality from causes other than neoplasms was 5–15% higher, fertility was 2.4% lower, and hatchability was 12.4% lower in shedders than nonshedders (144). These viruses have similar effects on broiler breeders and also caused a consistent though small (up to 5%) reduction in broiler growth rate (91, 145). Other studies on reduced productivity in chickens with LLV infections, and the genetic consequences, have been reviewed recently (143, 172, 305). The presence of LLV in semen was not associated with reduced semen production, but there is some evidence for an effect on semen quality and fertility (290).

LYMPHOID LEUKOSIS

Incubation period. After inoculation of susceptible embryos or 1- to 14-day-old susceptible chicks (e.g., line 15I) with a standard strain of virus RPL12 (48), B15, F42 (26), or RAV-1, LL appears between the 14th and 30th wk of age. Very rarely do cases occur in chickens under 14 wk. Certain laboratory recombinant viruses have been shown to cause lymphoid leukosis within 5–7 wk (178), though such short incubation periods are not found in field outbreaks. In field outbreaks, cases can occur any time after 14 wk of age; however, incidence is usually highest at about sexual maturity.

Signs. Outward signs of disease are not specific. The comb may be pale, shriveled, and occasionally cyanotic. Inappetence, emaciation, and weakness occur frequently. The abdomen is often enlarged and feathers are sometimes spotted with urates and bile pigments. Enlargement of liver, bursa of Fabricius, and/or kidneys can often be detected on palpation, and the nodular nature of liver tumors can at times be detected. Once clinical signs begin to develop, the course is usually rapid.

Gross lesions. Grossly visible tumors almost invariably involve liver (Fig. 16.26; see also Fig. 16.33A), spleen, and bursa of Fabricius (Fig. 16.27). Size of tumors is highly variable as are number of organs affected, which may include (in addition to liver and spleen) kidney, lung, gonad, heart, bone marrow, and mesentery.

Tumors are soft, smooth, and glistening; a cut surface appears slightly grayish to creamy white and seldom has areas of necrosis. Growth may be nodular (Fig. 16.26), miliary, or diffuse (see Fig. 16.33A), or a combination of these forms. In the nodular form lymphoid tumors vary from 0.5 mm to 5 cm in diameter and may occur singly or in large numbers. They are generally spherical but may be flattened when they are close to the surface of an organ. The granular or miliary form, which is most obvious in the liver, consists of numerous small nodules less than 2 mm in diameter and uniformly distributed throughout the parenchyma. In the diffuse form the organ is uniformly enlarged, slightly grayish in color, and usually very friable. Occasionally, the liver is firm, fibrous, and almost gritty.

Histopathology. Microscopically all tumors are focal and multicentric in origin. Even in organs appearing diffusely involved when examined grossly, the microscopic pattern is one of coalescing foci. As tumor cells proliferate, they displace and compress cells of the organ rather than infiltrate between them (Fig. 16.28). Nodules in the

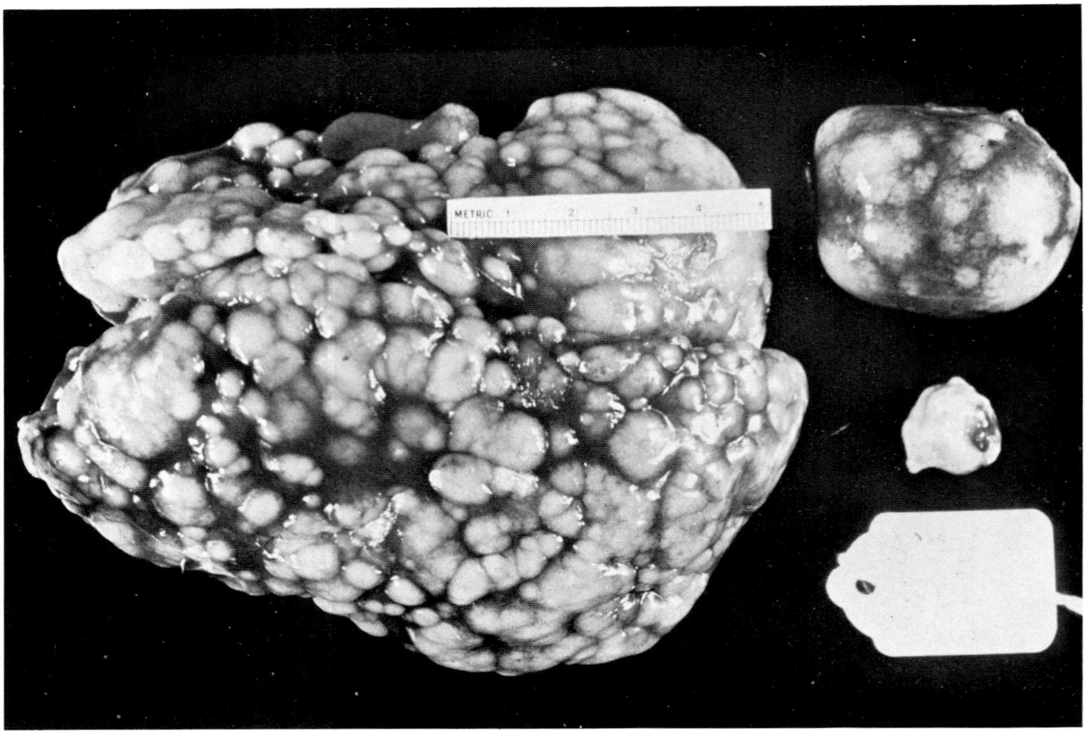

16.26. Nodular lesions in liver and spleen of bird with LL inoculated at 1 day of age with RPL12 virus. Bursa also has a small tumor.

liver are usually surrounded by a band of fibroblastlike cells that have been shown to be remnants of sinusoidal endothelial cells (155).

Tumors consist of aggregates of large lymphoid cells that may vary slightly in size but are all at the same primitive developmental stage. They have a poorly defined cytoplasmic membrane, much basophilic cytoplasm, and a vesicular nucleus in which there is margination and clumping of the chromatin and one or more conspicuous acidophilic nucleoli (Fig. 16.29).

The cytoplasm of most tumor cells contains a large amount of RNA, which stains red with methyl green pyronin, indicating that the cells are immature and rapidly dividing (70). The predominant cell is a lymphoblast. Characteristic features of the cell can best be seen in wet-fixed smears of fresh specimens that have been stained with May-Grünwald-Giemsa, methyl green pyronin, or other cytologic stains.

ULTRASTRUCTURE. Vacuoles are found infrequently in lymphoid cells of birds with LL, but some virus particles have been observed budding from the plasma membranes of lymphoblasts (105, 108). Intracytoplasmic viral matrix inclusion bodies have been observed in the myocardium of LLV-infected adult chickens (146, 212).

HEMATOLOGY. There are no consistent or significant changes in cellular elements of circulating blood. Rarely are there frank leukemic cases in which lymphoblasts predominate. Lymphoblasts are characterized by their large size, large eccentric nucleus with spongy chromatin, and moderate amount of intensely basophilic cytoplasm.

Pathogenesis. Calnek (55) infected day-old chicks and examined them 4–10 wk later. He observed no clinical signs of disease but found gross lesions in spleen, heart, and testis and microscopic lesions in liver and other visceral organs as well as dorsal root ganglia. The spleen was slightly or moderately enlarged and usually mottled; the testis and heart had one or more small (up to 1 mm diameter), grayish translucent areas. Microscopically, lesions were either small discrete foci or larger diffuse areas of lymphoblasts (Fig. 16.30). These lesions were transitory, since they were not grossly visible in birds over 10 wk of age, and microscopic accumulations were also markedly reduced. These lesions are most likely inflamma-

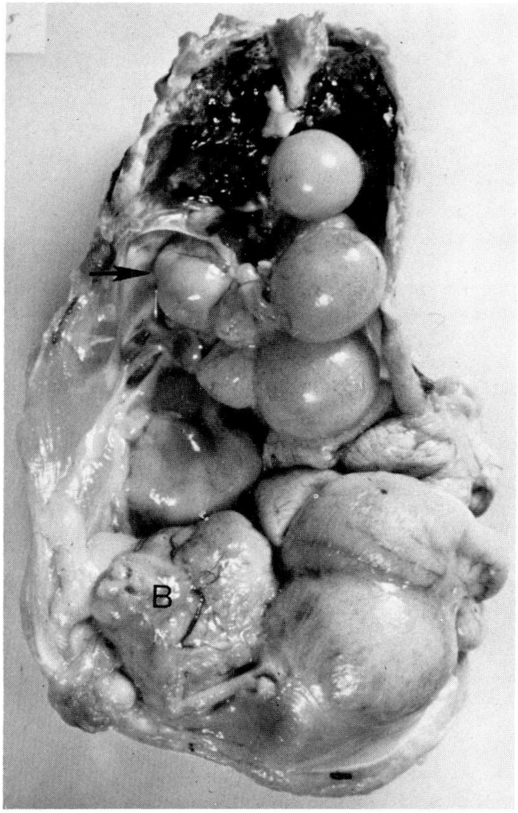

16.27. Large tumor of bursa of Fabricius (*B*) and kidneys (*arrow*) in naturally occurring case of LL in adult hen.

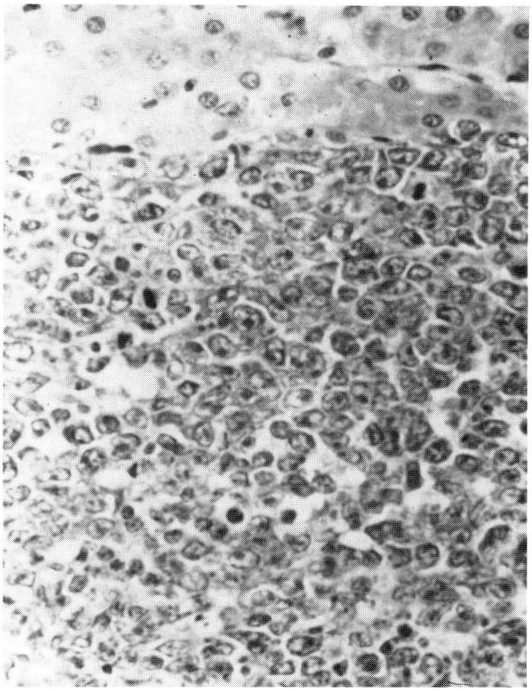

16.29. LL in liver of RPL12 virus-inoculated bird. Note compression of hepatic parenchyma by proliferation of extravascular, primitive lymphoid cells. ×500.

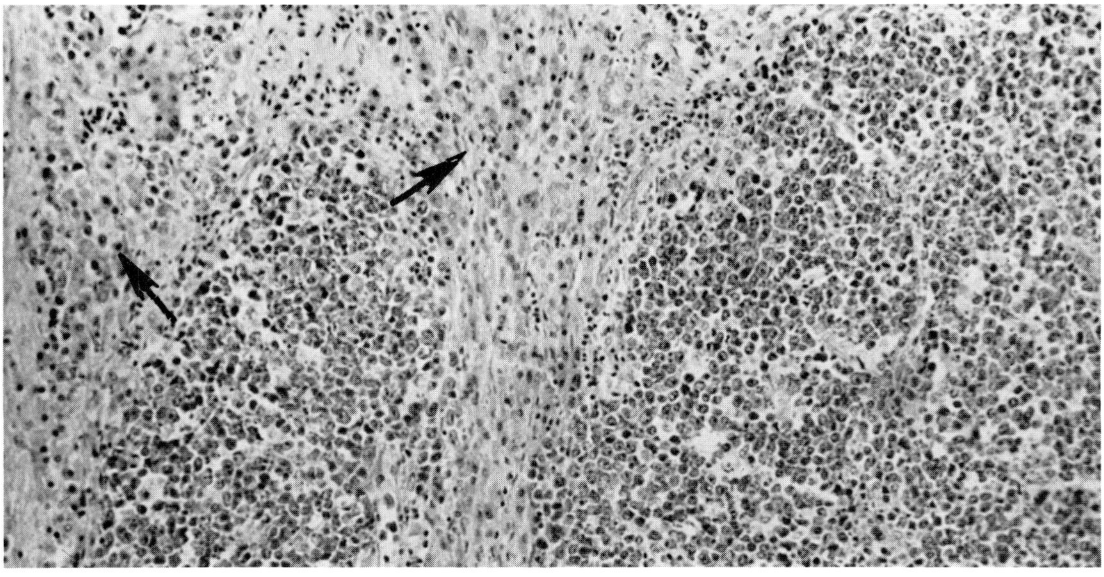

16.28. Liver tumor from bird that died from LL 207 days postinoculation at 1 day of age with HPRS-2 Rous-associated leukosis virus. Note displacement and compression of hepatic parenchyma (*arrows*). ×250.

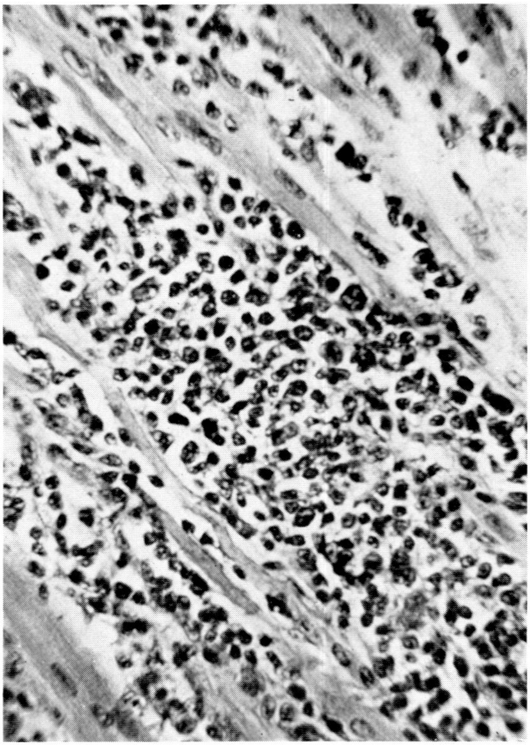

16.30. Lesions in young chickens induced by leukosis virus. Heart from 4-wk-old RIF3-infected chick. Diffuse accumulations of lymphoid cells among myocardial fibers. ×430. (Calnek)

tory and may relate to other nonneoplastic disease processes caused by leukosis viruses, e.g., anemia, hepatitis, and wasting (302, 334). Similar early lesions have been reported in LLV-infected turkeys (119).

Three lines of evidence indicate that LL is a malignancy of the bursa-dependent lymphoid system. The first is that removal of the bursa prevents LL and that it occurs in birds chemically bursectomized and transplanted with viable cells (256) from genetically susceptible chickens but not from chickens genetically resistant to tumor development (260). The following treatments applied to leukosis virus–infected birds effectively destroy the bursa of Fabricius and eliminate LL: surgical bursectomy between 1 day and 5 mo of age (243), treatment of embryos or hatched chicks with androgens either by inoculation or in feed (38), feeding of androgen analogs that have little or no androgenic effect (177), chemical bursectomy with cyclophosphamide (256), and infection with infectious bursal disease virus at 2 or 8 wk (254). Thymectomy has no effect on the course of the disease.

Histopathological examination of the bursa has provided the second line of evidence. Changes in isolated bursa follicles can be observed as early as 4 wk of age; by 7 wk abnormal follicles are present in the bursas of most infected chickens (Fig. 16.31) (213, 253). Most tumor nodules originate from transformation of a limited number of cells; i.e., they are clonal (78, 213). As transformed cells proliferate, affected follicles become engorged with uniform blastlike cells with a pyroninophilic cytoplasm, and there is a loss of distinction between the cortex and medulla. Abnormal follicles expand and displace adjacent normal bursal follicles until by 16–24 wk of age at the earliest a gross tumor of the bursa is visible (Fig. 16.32). Constituent cells of abnormal follicles are similar to those in LL tumors of the bursa and other visceral organs. Metastatic tumors in the viscera usually have the same DNA fragments as bursal tumors from the same birds, supporting the idea that they were of bursal origin (78). Autopsies performed on chickens dying with LL have revealed macroscopic tumors of the bursa in almost every case (38, 70, 102).

Immunofluorescence studies provide the third line of evidence. Cells of LL tumors, transplantable tumors, and lymphoid cell lines cultured in vitro have B-cell markers (71, 236) and IgM on their surface (214).

Although target cells may be transformed in the bursa of most birds, only a few develop LL (70). Thus some early tumors must regress. Other tumors enlarge, and cells burst into the vascular system and initiate metastatic foci in other visceral organs. At about the time of sexual maturity (16–24 wk of age), tumor involvement is so extensive that birds succumb.

Thus even though leukosis viruses multiply in most tissues and organs of the body (108), the infection persists longer in bursal lymphocytes than in other hematopoietic tissues (5) and cells of the bursa of Fabricius are the target cells that neoplastically transform. Medullary macrophages may be important in transmitting infection to the lymphoid cells (147). The target cells must have differentiated to some extent (i.e., they are not stem cells) because partial chemical bursectomy will destroy LL target cells before stem cells for the immune response (256). However, target cells must be resident in the bursa because bursectomy up to 5 mo of age will eliminate the disease (243).

Molecular biology studies indicate that a viral promoter gene activates a c-*myc* host gene in B cells and results simultaneously in neoplastic transformation and interference with the normal intraclonal switch of B-cell immunoglobulin production from IgM to IgG (78). The c-*myc* host gene is present in all animals and is the cell counterpart of a gene identified first in myelocytomatosis virus MC29. Promotion may be induced by other viruses such as reticuloendotheliosis viruses (see Reticuloendotheliosis) or occur spontaneously in certain virus-free flocks (78). Thus LL

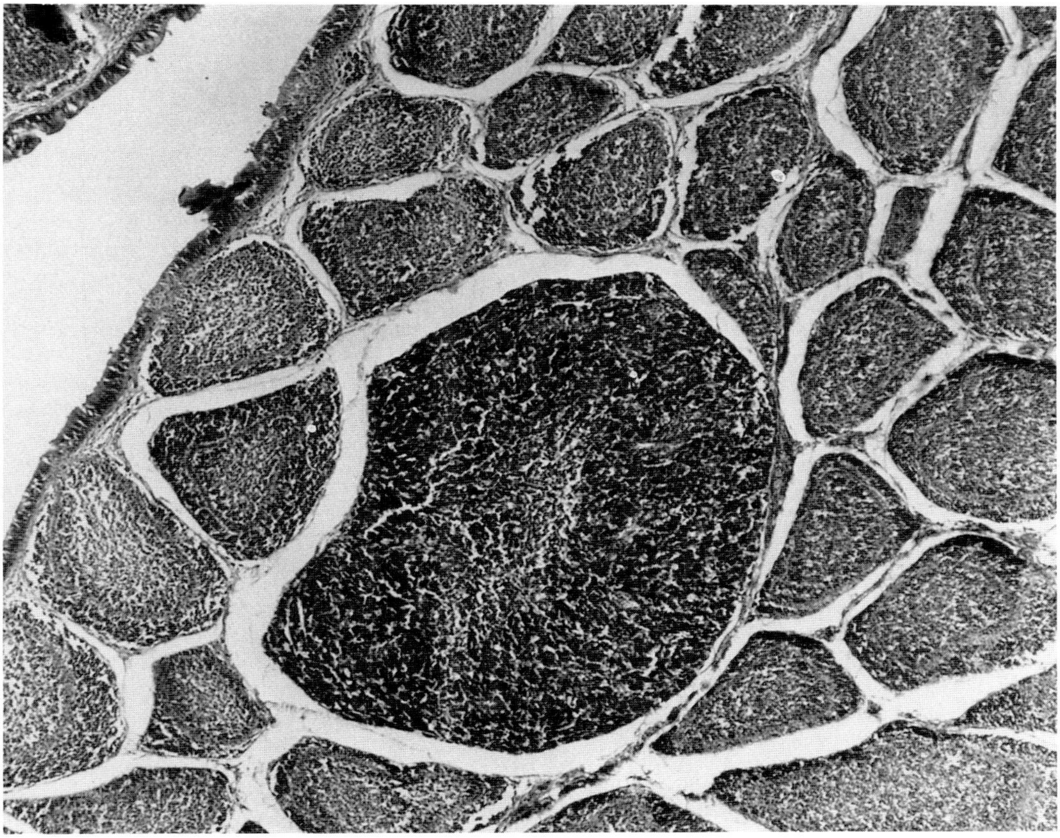

16.31. Lymphoblastic transformation in single bursal follicle in chicken with LL. All surrounding follicles are histologically normal in this and other sections from 16-day-old chicken infected with RPL12 virus at hatching. Methyl green pyronin, ×40. (Dent, J Nat Cancer Inst)

tumor cells have IgM on their surface and not IgG or IgA (71). The IgM may be heterogeneous and produced in excessive amounts, particularly late in the disease (298). In addition, subgroup B (but not subgroup A) viruses tested caused T-cell immunosuppression (279).

ERYTHROBLASTOSIS

Incubation period. The incubation period is influenced by the virus source, dose, and route of inoculation, and age and genetic constitution of the host. After IA inoculation of RPL12 strain virus into susceptible day-old chicks, the incubation period varies from 21 to 110 days (48). On IV

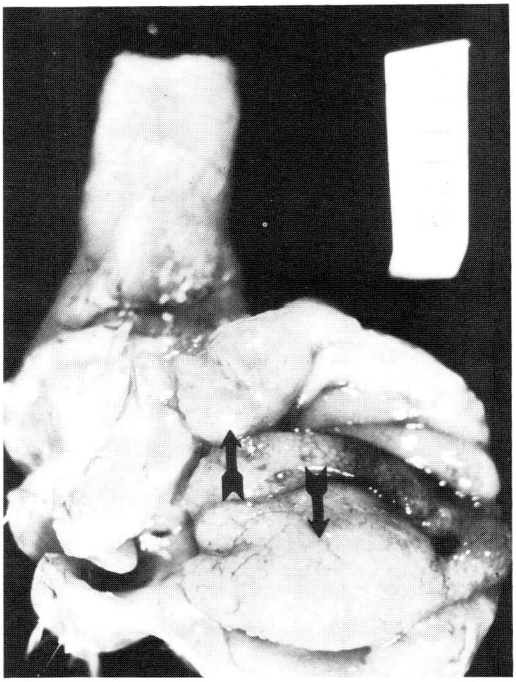

16.32. Earliest visible multiple LL tumors of bursa (*arrows*). (Siccardi)

inoculation of 11-day-old embryos, chicks have occasionally been found to have erythroblastosis on hatching. Strain R virus produces a much more rapid response, and in some experiments, birds inoculated with high doses have all died between 7 and 12 days postinoculation (17). Field strains and viruses passaged in cell culture induce erythroblastosis after a longer incubation period (41). Passage from donors with erythroblastosis greatly shortens the incubation period (135).

Other strains of virus that produce erythroblastosis include F42 (26), ES4, and strain 13 (17). Field cases usually occur in birds over 3 mo of age. Viruses such as RPL12 and F42 are nondefective, whereas ES4 and R are defective (151).

Signs. The earliest signs are lethargy, general weakness, and either slight paleness or cyanosis of the comb; as the condition advances, the paleness or cyanosis may increase. There are usually weakness, emaciation, and diarrhea, and there may be profuse hemorrhage from one or more feather follicles. The course varies from a few days to several months. With severe anemia, combs may become light yellow to almost white.

Gross lesions. In birds that die with either form of the disease there is usually a general anemia often accompanied by petechial hemorrhages in various organs such as muscles, subcutis, and viscera. Thrombosis, infarction, and rupture of the liver or spleen may be observed. There may be subcutaneous edema of lungs, hydropericardium, and ascites and a fibrinous clot on the ventral surface of the liver (Fig. 16.33B).

The most characteristic gross alteration is diffuse enlargement of liver and spleen and to a lesser extent kidneys (Fig. 16.33B). These organs are usually cherry red to dark mahogany and are soft and friable. The liver may be finely mottled from degeneration around the central veins of the lobules. The marrow is hyperplastic, very soft or watery, dark blood red or cherry red, and often has hemorrhages.

With severe anemia, visceral organs and organs of the immune system, particularly the spleen, usually atrophy.

Histopathology. Microscopic examination of the marrow in early cases reveals blood sinusoids filled with rapidly proliferating erythroblasts that fail to mature. In advanced cases, marrow consists of sheets of homogeneous erythroblasts with small islands of myelopoietic activity and little or no adipose tissue. With concurrent anemia the number of erythropoietic cells may be reduced.

Alterations in visceral organs are primarily due to hemostasis resulting in an accumulation of erythroblasts in the blood sinusoids and capillaries (Fig. 16.34). This results in dilation of the sinusoids, which is particularly evident in liver,

16.33. Comparison of leukoses. A. Lymphoid leukosis. Diffuse form affecting the liver; lesion is grossly indistinguishable from those in MD. B. Erythroblastosis. Enlarged cherry red liver and spleen; note the fibrinous exudate. C. Myeloblastosis. Note enlarged gray-red liver. D. Erythroblastosis. Note basophilic cytoplasm and perinuclear halo. Blood smear, Giemsa, ×1300. E. Myeloblastosis. Myeloblasts are slightly smaller than erythroblasts; cytoplasm is not as basophilic, nucleus is less vesicular, and nucleoli are not as frequent or conspicuous. Blood smear, Giemsa, ×1300. F. Myelocytomatosis. Note myelocytes packed with acidophilic granules. Section of tumor, Giemsa, ×1300. (Beard)

spleen, and bone marrow. As this process continues, the sinusoids become greatly distended, resulting in pressure atrophy of the parenchyma. In the liver there may also be a terminal degeneration and even a necrosis of the hepatic cells around the central veins caused by local anoxia. Even though accumulations of erythroblasts may be very extensive, they always remain entirely intravascular, unlike those in LL and myeloblastosis.

Varying degrees of anemia may occur. Sometimes there is no erythroblastosis and there may only be a severe anemia. Extramedullary erythropoiesis is common.

The primary cell involved is the erythroblast (Fig. 16.35). The cell has a large round nucleus with a very fine chromatin and one or two nucleoli and a large amount of cytoplasm that is basophilic. A perinuclear halo, vacuoles, and occasionally fine granules are present. The cell is irregular in shape and often has pseudopodia. Erythroblasts

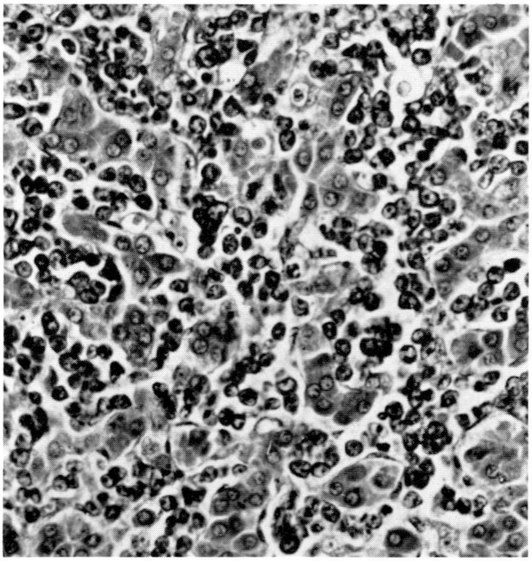

16.34. Erythroblastosis. Liver sinuses permeated with erythroblasts in bird 40 days after inoculation with strain MC29 leukosis virus. ×280. (Beard)

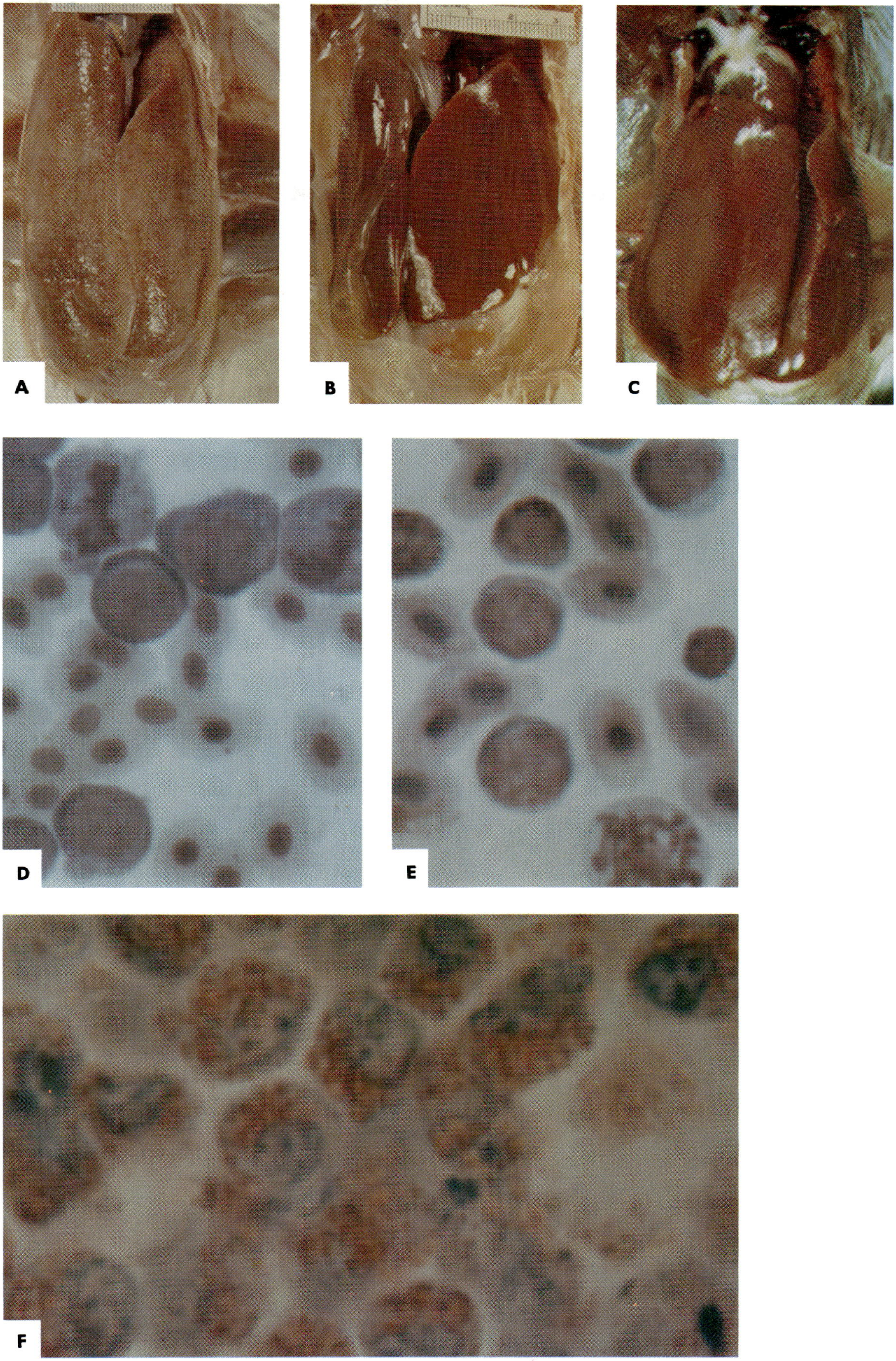
A
B
C
D
E
F

have physiological markers that identify them as members of the erythrocytic series (See Differential Diagnosis).

ULTRASTRUCTURE. Numerous studies have been made of the primitive cells in erythroblastosis induced by different strains of virus including R (17, 18) and RPL12 (105). Neoplastic erythroblasts in tissues, spleen, and bone marrow are for the most part indistinguishable from corresponding cells of the normal bird except that virus particles may be present in extracellular spaces and within vacuoles inside cells. In erythoblasts in the circulating blood, as in cell culture, there is a great increase in membrane activity, with vacuolization of the cytoplasm and budding of virus particles from the cell membrane. Only occasionally are aberrant structures seen in erythroblasts (105).

HEMATOLOGY. Changes in the blood reflect those occurring in other organs such as liver, spleen, and bone marrow and depend largely on the extent of anemia or leukemia. When there is severe anemia the blood is watery and light red and clots slowly. In contrast, acute cases may show no grossly apparent changes, though usually the blood appears dark red with a smoky overcast. Stained blood smears reveal a variable number of erythroblasts (see Fig. 16.33D). These vary in maturity from the early erythroblast, which is the predominant cell, to the various stages of polychrome erythrocytes. The more mature cells often appear early in the course of the disease or during remission, if and when it occurs.

The thrombocytic series of cells may be somewhat increased in number and immaturity. Similarly, in most naturally occurring cases, immature cells of the myelocytic series appear in the peripheral circulation. Occasionally, they are as prominent as the erythroblasts.

Pathogenesis. Defective erythroblastosis viruses contain the *erbB* gene specific for erythroblastosis viruses (v-*erbB*) and present in erythroblasts (c-*erbB*) and the tumor promoter gene common to avian tumor viruses. Some viruses may also contain another gene, v-*erbA*. On integration of the provirus into the host cell genome, erythroblastosis viruses induce transformation by blocking differentiation of erythroblasts. The block is a consequence of competitive inhibition of virus and cell products of the *erb* genes (78, 151, 154). Uncontrolled proliferation of erythroblasts causes erythroblastosis, which has a longer latency period and may also be induced by LLV by inserting a promoter gene adjacent to the cellular oncogene c-*erbB* (140, 185).

During the induction of erythroblastosis by LLV, new erythroblastosis virus possessing viral *erb* genes may be generated by recombination of host cell genes and LLV genes (166).

Many leukosis viruses, particularly those of subgroups B and D, may induce an anemia that may be independent of neoplasia; i.e., it may occur in absence of or concurrent with neoplastic proliferation (302). There is evidence that the anemia-inducing potential of these viruses is due to the nondefective helper viruses (154).

When birds are artificially exposed to a strain causing erythroblastosis, the first alterations are found in 3 days as foci of proliferating erythroblasts in bone marrow sinusoids. By the 7th day the primitive cells reach the circulating blood, and some foci of erythropoiesis are present in sinusoids of the liver and spleen. Erythroblasts continue to accumulate in hepatic sinusoids until death of the host. This may occur within a few days of appearance of erythroblasts in the blood, although in most naturally occurring cases the disease proceeds much more slowly (249).

MYELOBLASTOSIS

Incubation period. The most studied strain of virus that induces myeloblastosis predominantly is BAI-A. Virus stocks are defective and contain helper viruses of both A and B subgroups (174). After inoculation of susceptible day-old chicks with large doses of virus, changes in the blood can be observed in 10 days and birds die a few days thereafter. Mortality continues for about 1 mo, and only a few deaths occur after this (49, 113). The virus E26 (151) also predominantly induces myeloblastosis.

Signs. Signs are similar to those of erythroblastosis. At first there are lethargy, general weakness, and slight paleness of comb. As the condition develops, these signs become marked and inappetence, pronounced dehydration, emaciation, and diarrhea are seen. There may be hemorrhage from one or more of the feather follicles caused by blood clotting deficiency. The course is highly variable but is generally longer than that for erythroblastosis.

Gross lesions. There is usually an anemia. The parenchymatous organs are enlarged and friable, but in chronic cases the liver may be firm. Gray diffuse tumor nodules may occur in the liver and occasionally in other visceral organs. Bone marrow is usually firm and reddish gray to gray. In advanced cases liver, spleen, and kidneys have grayish infiltrations that are usually diffuse but often give the organ a mottled or even granular appearance (Fig. 16.33A).

Histopathology. Microscopic examination of parenchymatous organs reveals massive intravascular and extravascular accumulations of myeloblasts with a variable proportion of pro-

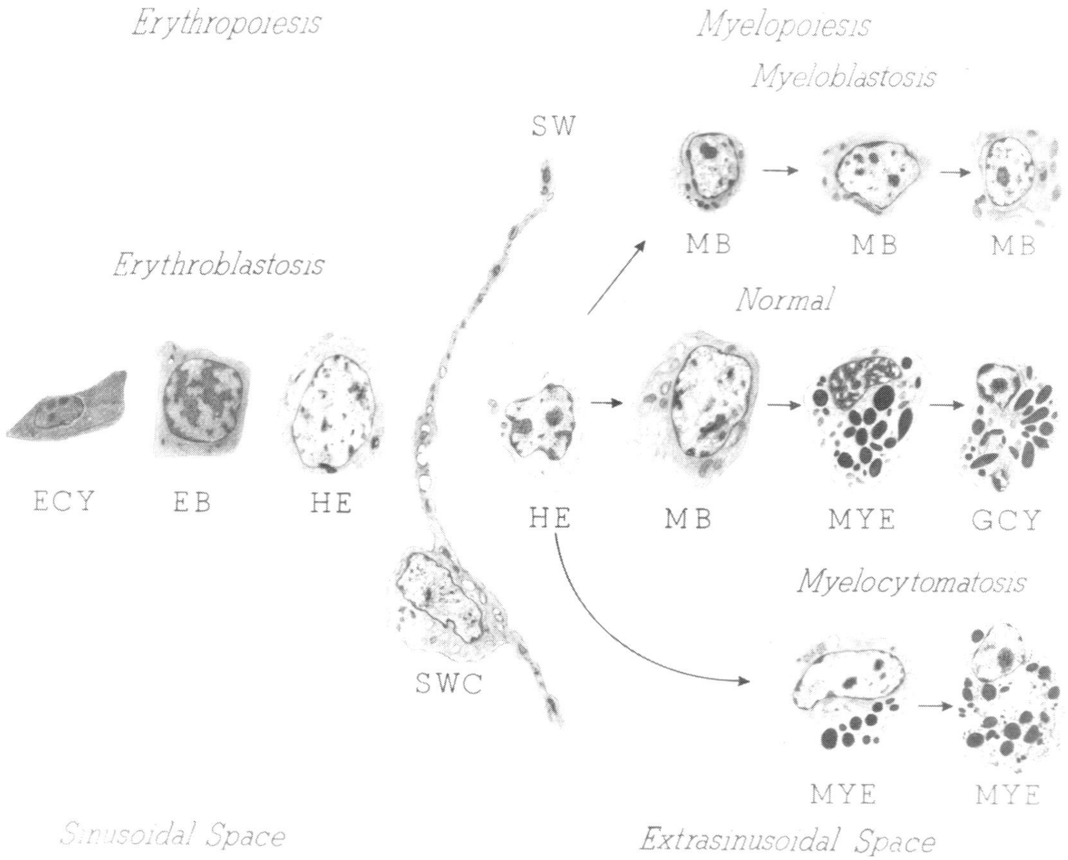

16.35. Semidiagrammatic illustration of normal and virus-induced neoplastic hemopoiesis in avian bone marrow. *SW* indicates sinus wall, and *SWC* indicates body and nucleus of the cell forming the wall. In normal erythropoiesis in the sinusoidal space, erythroblasts (*EB*) are derived from intrasinusoidal hemocytoblasts (*HE*) and mature to erythrocytes (*ECY*). The process in erythroblastosis begins in the same way, but in the fully developed disease differentiation does not progress beyond the *EB* stage. Normal myelopoiesis proceeds from the *HE* through the successive myeloblast (*MB*) and myelocyte (*MYE*) stages to the mature granulocyte (*GCY*). In myeloblastosis the primitive leukemia cell derived from the extrasinusoidal hemocytoblast is the *MB,* which proliferates without further differentiation. As in myeloblastosis, myelocytomatosis arises by infection and proliferation of the extrasinusoidal hemocytoblast. In contrast to myeloblastosis, however, differentiation of the *MYE* appears to bypass the stage typical of *MB* to attain the granulated, although not mature, granulocyte form. The first element derived from *HE* morphologically resembles *MB* but does not exhibit the attributes. (Beard, Beaudreau; Oregon State Univ Press)

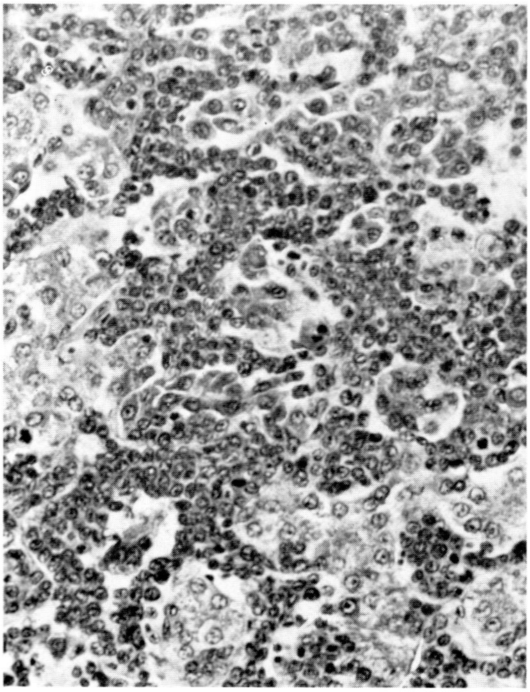

16.36. Myeloblastosis. Distribution of myeloblasts in liver of bird with myeloblastic leukemia 19 days after inoculation with BAI-A virus. ×280. (Langlois)

myelocytes (Fig. 16.35, 16.36). Infiltration and proliferation are particularly extensive outside the sinusoids and around the portal tracts in the liver lobules. There is, therefore, a marked replacement of original tissues by pathological cells in contrast to the fairly uniform intravascular leukostasis encountered in erythroblastosis. Intensive myeloblastic activity in bone marrow is confined to extrasinusoidal areas.

Pathological and hematological features of both erythroblastosis and myeloblastosis overlap in many naturally occurring cases.

ULTRASTRUCTURE. In circulating myeloblasts from birds with myeloblastosis induced by BAI-A, virus particles are only rarely found and then in small numbers in clear vacuoles (17, 105). However, reticular and phagocytic elements of the spleen and bone marrow are frequently packed with virus particles. When myeloblasts are transferred to cell culture, large numbers of lysosomes appear in the cytoplasm. After some time in cell culture, virus particles can be seen in lysosomes, in vacuoles, and budding at the cell membrane. No other changes can be observed in these cells.

HEMATOLOGY. Myeloblastosis is characterized by a spectacular leukemia (see Fig. 16.33E). Up to 2 million myeloblasts/mm^3 may be found in the peripheral blood. They may compose 75% of all blood cells; thus on centrifugation there may be more "buffy coat" than red cells. Myeloblasts are large cells with slightly basophilic clear cytoplasm and a large nucleus containing 1–4 acidophilic nucleoli, which do not usually stain prominently. Often promyelocytes and myelocytes are also present; they can easily be identified by their specific granulation, which in the early forms is primarily basophilic.

The disease may result in a secondary anemia. When this occurs, polychrome erythrocytes and reticulocytes are usually present. Such a secondary anemia is easily distinguished from the conditions in which erythroblastosis and myeloblastosis occur together, since in the latter case blast forms of both cell series are in the circulating blood.

Pathogenesis.

The *myb* gene of the virus plays a role in myeloblastosis similar to the role of the *erb* gene in erythroblastosis described earlier (121, 207). The target organ of the causative virus is bone marrow, and the first neoplastic alteration is in the form of multiple foci of proliferating myeloblasts in extrasinusoidal areas. These grow rapidly, overtake normal bone marrow elements, and spill over into the sinusoids. This is followed, perhaps within 1 day, by a leukemia and invasion of other organs by myeloblasts (187).

MYELOCYTOMATOSIS

Incubation period. Virus-induced myelocytomatosis generally has a longer incubation period than erythroblastosis and myeloblastosis but shorter than LL. On IV injection of MC29 into young chicks, myelocytomas were obtained in 3–11 wk (203). The incubation period in field cases is unknown, but most cases are observed in immature birds. Mathey (196) observed an outbreak in a 6-wk-old broiler flock. The virus CMII also induces myelocytomas (151).

Signs. General signs are similar to those of myeloblastosis. In addition, skeletal growth of myelocytes may result in abnormal protuberances of the head (Fig. 16.37), thorax, and shank. The course is highly variable and usually prolonged.

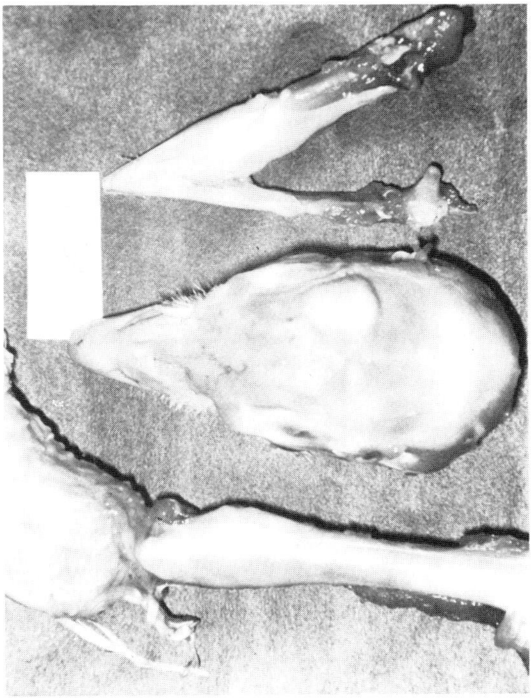

16.37. Myelocytoma of mandible, skull, and tibia of 8-wk-old chicken. (Mathey)

Gross lesions. Tumors are distinctive and can be recognized on gross examination with some degree of certainty. Characteristically they occur on the surface of bones in association with the periosteum and near cartilage, though any tissue or organ may be affected. Tumors often develop at the costochondral junctions of the ribs, posterior sternum, and cartilaginous bones of the mandible and nares. Flat bones of the skull are also often affected (Fig. 16.37). Myelocytomas are dull, yellow-white in color, soft and friable or cheesy, and diffuse or nodular. They sometimes have a thin layer of bone over them, which is easily broken. Multiple tumors are common and are usually bilaterally symmetrical.

Histopathology. Tumors consist of compact masses of strikingly uniform myelocytes with very little stroma (see Fig. 16.33F). Tumor cells are similar to the normal myelocytes found in bone marrow (see Fig. 16.35). Their nuclei are large, vesicular, and usually eccentrically located, and a distinct nucleolus is commonly present. The cytoplasm is tightly packed with acidophilic granules, which are usually spherical. When imprint preparations of fresh tumors are stained with May-Grünwald-Giemsa, granules appear brilliant red (see Fig. 16.33F) (203). In the liver, myelocytes crowd the sinuses, invade the acinar cords, and destroy and replace the hepatocytes. A principal attribute of the neoplastic myelocytes is formation of cohesive, organized, and invasive growths in parenchymatous organs (20).

ULTRASTRUCTURE. Ultrastructural features of myelocytoma and myelocytomatosis cells (203) vary from those of well-differentiated myelocytes to those of undifferentiated, nongranulated myelocytes. Myelocytes with granules staining red with May-Grünwald-Giemsa do not differ notably in ultrastructure from their normal myelocyte counterparts. Cells without granules exhibit primitive structure similar but not identical to that of the myeloid progenitor (hemocytoblast) cells. These myelocytes are essentially identical with cells originating in cultures of bone marrow treated with virus strain MC29. Principal features are a singular grainy appearance of the cytoplasm related to high ribosome, polysome, and protein content; sparse rough endoplasmic reticulum; relatively small nucleus with nucleoplasm containing some (but not predominantly) diffuse and dispersed chromatin; and a greatly enlarged nucleolus of usual structure. In structure and behavior these cells are very different from the myeloblasts induced by BAI-A virus.

HEMATOLOGY. The disease is essentially aleukemic but occasionally is associated with erythroblastosis. In some birds, especially in the laboratory disease, there may be a distinct leukemia of granulated or nongranulated myeloid cells (Fig. 16.38).

Pathogenesis. The *myc* gene of the virus plays a role in myelocytomatosis similar to those of *erb* and *myb* genes in erythroblastosis and myeloblastosis (121, 207). The earliest alterations occur in bone marrow in which there is crowding of intersinusoidal spaces, principally by myelocytes, and destruction of the sinusoid walls. Whereas in the normal bird the intersinusoidal spaces contain myeloid series cells in different stages of development, in myelocytomatosis the spaces contain essentially only two types of cells—the primitive hemocytoblast and the neoplastic cell (the myelocyte) (see Fig. 16.35). The latter appears to arise directly from the hemocytoblast, and differentiation is arrested most often at the nongranulated but also at the granulated myelocyte level (203). Nongranulated myelocytes are distinctly different from myeloblasts in morphology and in vitro growth potentials; myeloblasts proliferate enduringly in culture, but myelocytes persist only a few days. (Neoplasms composed of nongranulated myelocytes may be derived from neoplastic transformation of the common stem cell, which gives rise to granulocytes and macrophages; i.e., they may more accurately be called histiocytic sarcomas.) Myelocytes proliferate and soon overgrow the bone marrow. Tumors form by expansion of marrow growths, so that in some cases large neoplasms may crowd through the bone and extend through the periosteum. Extramedullary tumors may arise by metastasis. A transplantable myelocytoma has been developed (188).

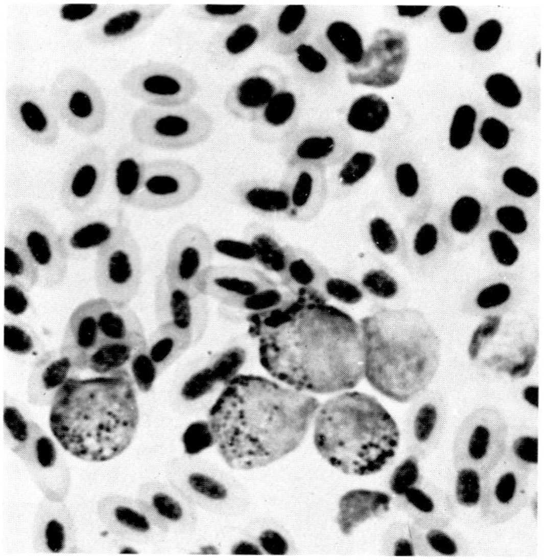

16.38. Myelocytomatosis. Granulated myelocytes in blood smear from bird 23 days after inoculation with strain MC29 leukosis virus. ×750. (Beard)

HEMANGIOMA

Incubation Period. After experimental inoculation of young chicks with field strains of virus (135), hemangiomas appeared in 3 wk to 4 mo. Most isolates or virus strains have been found to cause hemangiomas (33, 134). These tumors have been found in birds of various ages. In natural outbreaks, most mortality from hemangiosarcomas occurred at 6–9 mo (51). Induction of lung angiosarcomas by subgroup F avian leukosis viruses is reported (185, 294).

Signs. Hemangiomas usually occur singly in the skin, though primary multiplicity is not uncommon. When the wall ruptures, profuse hemorrhage ensues. Feathers near the tumor are blood-stained, and the bird may become pale and die of exsanguination.

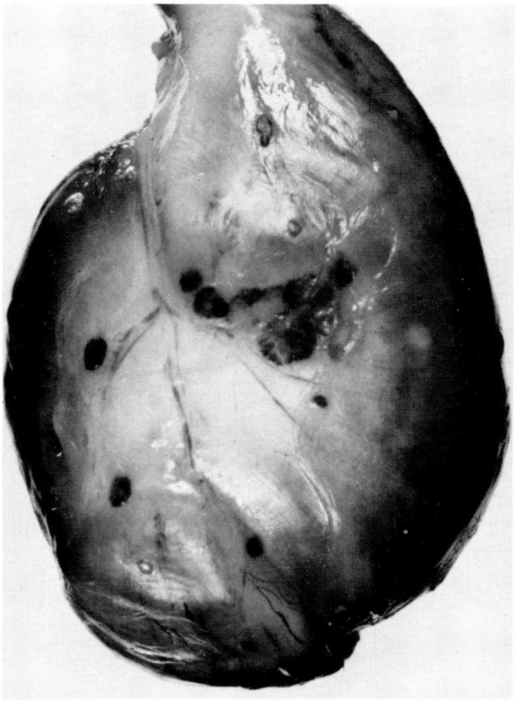

16.39. Hemangioma of gizzard serosa of RPL12 virus–inoculated bird. Note dark circumscribed and raised tumor nodules. (Gross, J Nat Cancer Inst)

Gross Lesions. Hemangiomas in the skin or on the surface of visceral organs can best be described as "blood blisters" (Fig. 16.39). Chickens with ruptured hemangiomas of the skin may be severely anemic. Blood clots are often found in visceral tumors.

Histopathology. The cavernous form is characterized by greatly distended blood spaces with thin walls composed of endothelial cells (Fig. 16.40). Capillary hemangiomas are solid masses varying from gray-pink to red. The endothelium may proliferate into dense masses (hemangioendothelioma), leaving mere clefts for blood channels (Fig. 16.41); develop into a lattice with capillary spaces; or grow into collagen-supported

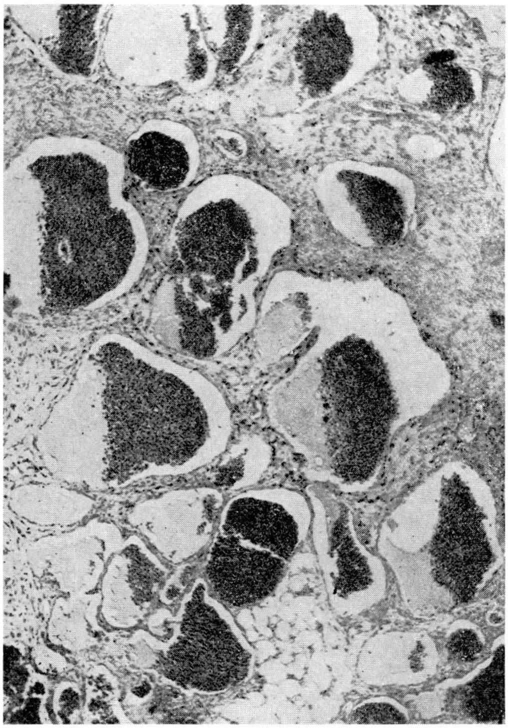

16.40. Cavernous hemangioendothelioma of mesentery. (Feldman and Olson)

chords with larger interspersed blood spaces. In general, skin tumors are more encapsulated and have more trabeculae than visceral tumors.

ULTRASTRUCTURE. There have been no reports of electron microscopy studies of hemangiomas.

HEMATOLOGY. The blood picture is normal in uncomplicated cases. When the tumor has ruptured, there may be signs of anemia. Hemangiomas often occur in conjunction with erythroblastosis and myeloblastosis.

Pathogenesis. Hemangiomas are tumors of the vascular system and as such usually involve all layers of blood vessels. In some instances the endothelium may proliferate more than the supporting tissue. Occasionally, the primitive anaplastic cells may differentiate to hemocytoblasts, so considerable erythropoiesis can occur in these growths.

NEPHROMA AND NEPHROBLASTOMA. Leukosis virus–induced tumors of the kidney are of two distinct kinds: nephroblastoma of the complex Wilm's tumor type and carcinomatous growths of widely varied morphology. In studies thus far described, nephroblastomas have been produced

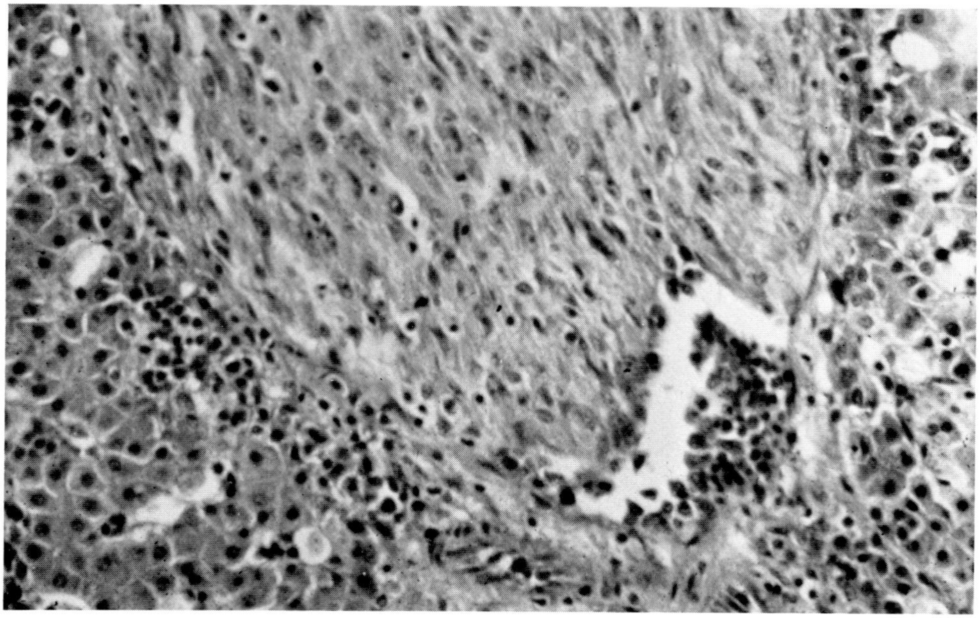

16.41. Endothelioma in liver of bird inoculated with RPL30 leukosis virus. Occlusion of portal vein by inward-growing spindle cells from blood vessel. ×250. (Frederickson, J Nat Cancer Inst)

experimentally only by BAI-A myeloblastosis virus (20, 49) and myeloblastosis-associated virus, MAV-2(N) (331), whereas only the relatively simple though extensive carcinomatous growths are associated with infection by all other virus strains: MC29 (20), ES4 (60), MH2 sarcoma virus (61), and Murray-Begg sarcoma virus and various field isolates (134).

Incubation period. Tumors are usually found at necropsy in birds dying or killed because of general aspects of disease. In the field, renal tumors are rarely seen in chickens older than 5 wk. Nephroblastomas induced by BAI-A may reach an incidence of 60–85% in birds not dying of myeloblastosis (49). Most cases are seen in birds between 2 and 6 mo of age.

Carcinomatous growth such as those produced by strain MC29 are found as soon as 18 days or as late as 7 wk after virus inoculation. Incidence in inoculated chickens may be 60% or more, but incidence in field flocks is not known.

Signs. In uncomplicated cases there are no signs while the tumors are small. As the tumor increases in size, emaciation and general debility are usually seen. Paralysis may result, when the tumor exerts pressure on the sciatic nerve.

Gross lesions. Nephroblastomas vary from small, pinkish gray nodules embedded in the kidney parenchyma to large, yellowish gray lobulated masses that replace most of the kidney tissue (Fig. 16.42). Tumors are often pedunculated and may be connected to the kidney by only a thin fibrous vascular stalk. Large tumors are often cystic and may involve both kidneys.

Histopathology. In nephroblastomas the histologic variation between different tumors or areas of the same tumor is striking (Fig. 16.43). There is usually neoplastic proliferation of both epithelial and mesenchymal elements, though their proportion and differentiation vary widely. Epithelial structures vary from enlarged tubules with invaginated epithelium and malformed glomeruli; through irregular masses of distorted tubules; to groups of large, irregular, cuboidal, undifferentiated cells with little tubular organization. Particularly in tumors induced by BAI-A avian myeloblastosis virus, epithelial growths may be embedded in loose mesenchyme or frank sarcomatous stroma. There may be islands of keratinizing stratified squamous epithelial structures (pearls), cartilage, or bone (173). Primary multiplicity of tumors may occur, but metastases are rare.

Carcinomatous growths or nephromas frequently involve both kidneys. Many are enveloped in single or multiple and massive cysts. They vary from a few small nodules to dozens of growths involving the entire organ.

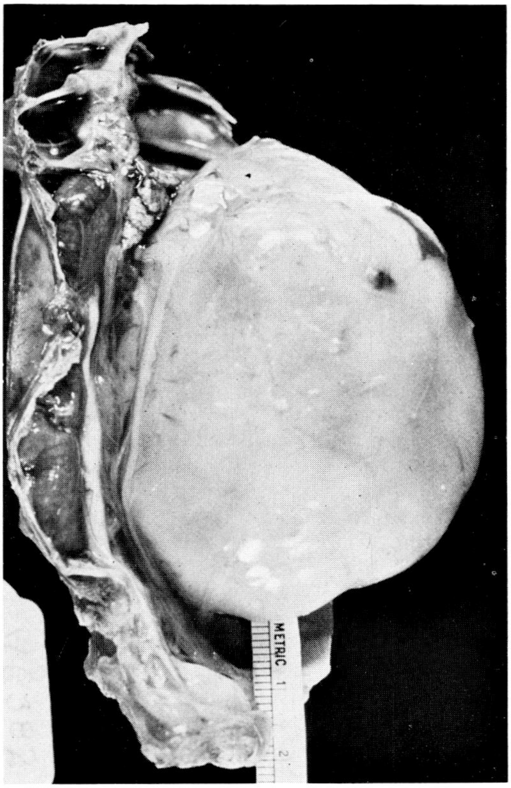

16.42. Nephroblastoma. Bird was inoculated at 1 day of age with AMV (BAI-A).

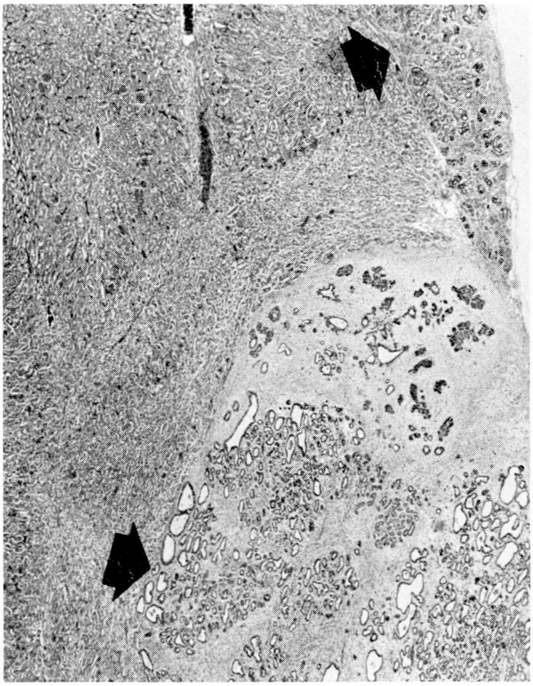

16.43. Nephroblastoma. Bird was inoculated at 1 day of age with cloned preparation of AVM (BAI-A). Note primary multiplicity of tumors of two distinct types in different areas (*arrows*). ×20

Tumors also vary greatly in microscopic appearance. In tubular adenocarcinomas, primitive abnormal glomeruli frequently occur in large numbers among abnormal tubules. Papillary cyst adenocarcinomas are frequent. At times, solid carcinomatous neoplasms with little evidence of renal tubules develop (21, 203). Rarely is there cartilage and never are there other mesenchymal tumor tissues. Hemangiomas and endotheliomas sometimes occur in nephromas.

ULTRASTRUCTURE. In the epithelial nephronic elements of nephroblastomas induced by BAI-A virus (17), cytoplasmic aberrant structures are occasionally seen in large or small aggregates. Virus particles bud from cell membranes of epithelial cells, fibroblastic elements of the stroma, and chondrocytes. Sarcomatous elements consist of cells similar in morphology to those in other avian sarcomas. Virus particles have been observed budding from epithelial cells in cystadenomas and adenocarcinomas induced by strain MC29 myelocytomatosis virus (203). Large accumulations of particles in spaces in the cysts and tubules were probably related to lack of tubule and glomerular drainage.

HEMATOLOGY. Uncomplicated cases are aleukemic.

Pathogenesis. Nephroblastomas originate from embryonic rests or nephrogenic buds in kidneys (173). These epithelial structures enlarge and become neoplastic. The supporting stroma of mesenchymal elements also proliferates and in turn may be altered. There is an extensive multiplication of tumor cells (usually convoluted tubules and/or stroma) and varying degrees of differentiation, some abnormal. In the most differentiated form, nephrogenic cells form glomeruli, tubules, or keratinized epithelium, whereas cells of the stroma form sarcomas, cartilage, and bone. Anaplasia of kidney cells can result in sheets of large epithelioid cells with almost no tubular organization. Malformed and blocked tubules result in cysts.

Carcinomatous growths originate only from the epithelial part of the embryonic rests and not from mesenchymal elements. Cartilage that occurs in a few growths originates from morphologically altered epithelial cells. Depending on degree of anaplasia of epithelial elements, tumors formed may be adenomas, adenocarcinomas, or solid carcinomas (21).

Hepatocarcinoma. In 18–100 days, the MC29 strain of leukosis virus (20, 190) caused a high incidence of primary tumors of the liver that arose by alteration of hepatocytes, principally in the portal regions. MH2 can also cause liver tumors but of a different type.

Tumors were elevated above the surface of the liver; varied in diameter from 0.5 to 10 mm or more; yellow-white, gray or reddish tan; and well circumscribed with scant stromal reaction.

Microscopic study revealed several distinct tumor patterns: trabecular, varying in structure from almost normal to markedly disarrayed cell masses; adenomatous or tubular; mosaic and giant cell arrays; hemorrhagic carcinoma complexes; and hepatobiliary cell processes. Within these patterns there were anaplastic and metaplastic changes, with some cartilage as well as osteoid and spindle-cell tumor formation. Infiltration and invasion of adjacent tissue; penetration of blood vessels; and metastasis to organs such as lung, kidney, and spleen were seen. Prominent features of the tumor cell morphology were very large nuclei of spheroidal and angular contours and large nucleoli ("bird's eye" appearance).

Hepatocarcinomas induced by MH2 are solid structureless masses of large altered liver cells (20) with irregular contours, vesicular nuclei, and large dense nucleoli. Hepatocarcinoma has not been observed under natural conditions.

Other Epithelial Tumors. Thecomas and granulosa cell growths of the ovary have been induced by BAI-A virus (20). A seminoma in the testes occurred in one bird inoculated with MH2. This tumor was an adenocarcinomatous growth of seminiferous tubules in which interstitial cells were not involved.

Adenocarcinomas of the pancreas have been induced in chickens by MC29 and MH2 viruses (20, 202). Spontaneous occurrence in nature is very rare.

Squamous cell carcinomas have been observed in a few chicks diseased with MC29 or MH2 (20). These tumors are occasionally encountered in broiler chickens in processing plants after feathers have been removed. No means has been found to reproduce these tumors by inoculation of virus or tumor extract from field cases.

Osteopetrosis

Incubation period. After experimental inoculation of day-old chicks with RPL12-L29 (282) or other viruses (167, 168, 251), osteopetrosis may develop anytime after 1 mo of age. It is most commonly seen in birds 8–12 wk of age. The disease probably has a similar incubation period in the field. MAV-2(0) virus will induce palpable osteopetrosis 7–10 days after hatching in chicks inoculated at 1 day of age or as 11- to 12-day-old embryos (133).

Signs. Long bones of the limbs are most commonly affected (Figs. 16.44, 16.45). There is uniform or irregular thickening of the diaphyseal or metaphyseal regions that can be detected by inspection or palpation. In active cases the affected areas are unusually warm. Birds with advanced disease have characteristic "bootlike" shanks. Affected chickens are usually stunted and pale and walk with a stilted gait or limp.

Gross lesions. The first grossly visible changes occur in the diaphysis of the tibia and/or tarsometatarsus. Alterations soon are seen in other long bones and bones of the pelvis, shoulder girdle, and ribs, but not the digits. Lesions are usually bilaterally symmetric; they first appear as distinct pale yellow foci against the gray-white translucent normal bone. The periosteum is thickened and the abnormal bone is spongy and at first easily cut. The lesion is commonly circumferential and advances to the metaphysis, giving the bone a fusiform appearance (Fig. 16.45). Occasionally the lesion remains focal or is eccentric. Severity of the lesion varies from a slight exostosis to a massive asymmetric enlargement with almost complete obliteration of the marrow cavity. In long-standing cases the periosteum is not as thickened as it was earlier; when it is removed, the porous irregular surface of the very hard osteopetrotic bone is revealed.

Osteopetrosis and LL frequently occur together in the same bird. Other tumors have also been described (56). There is an initial slight enlargement of the spleen followed, in birds not simultaneously affected with LL, with splenic atrophy that becomes very severe. There is also a premature atrophy of the bursa and thymus. Many of the other nonneoplastic conditions associated with leukosis/sarcoma viruses occur commonly in birds with osteopetrosis.

Histopathology. Microscopically, periosteum over the lesion is greatly thickened from an increase in number and size of basophilic osteoblasts. The number of osteoclasts per tibia increases but the density of osteoclasts (i.e., the number per unit volume of bone) decreases (289). Affected bones differ from normal bones in the following ways. Spongy bone converges centripetally toward the center of the shaft (Fig. 16.46). There is an increase in size and irregularity of the haversian canals and an increase in number and size and an alteration in position of lacunae (Fig. 16.47). Osteocytes are more numerous, large, and eosinophilic; the new bone is basophilic and fibrous.

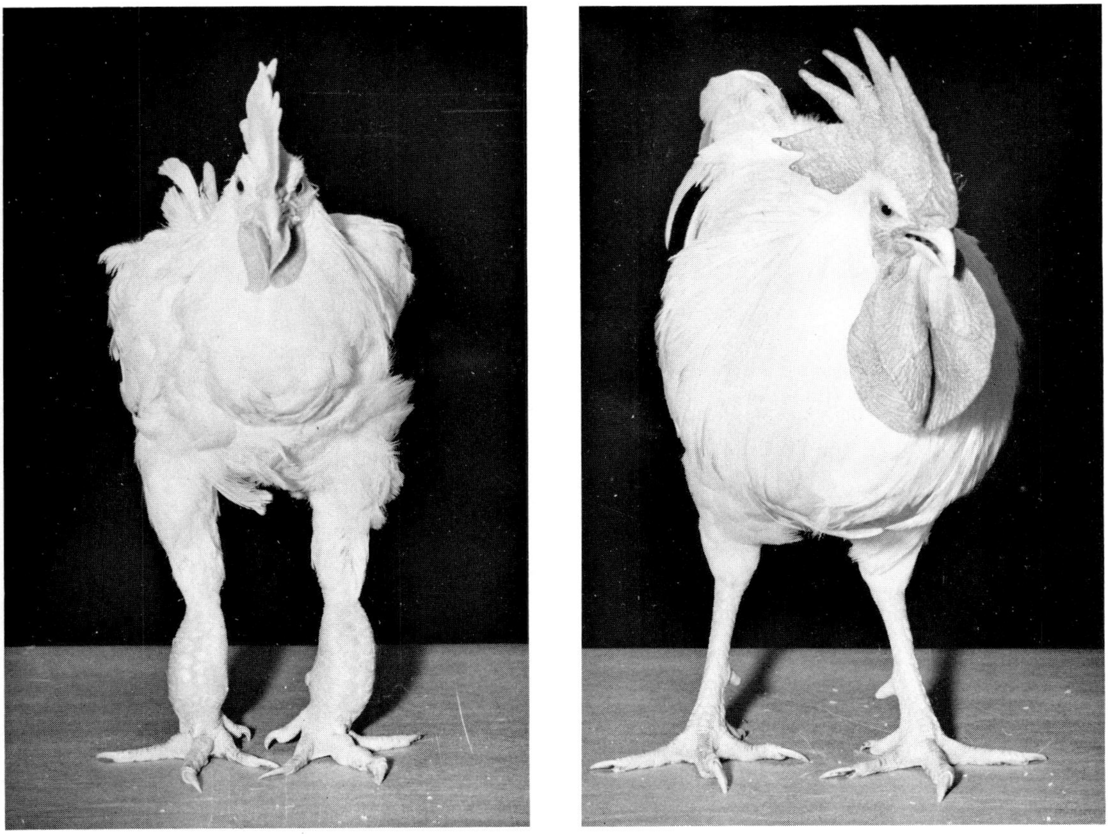

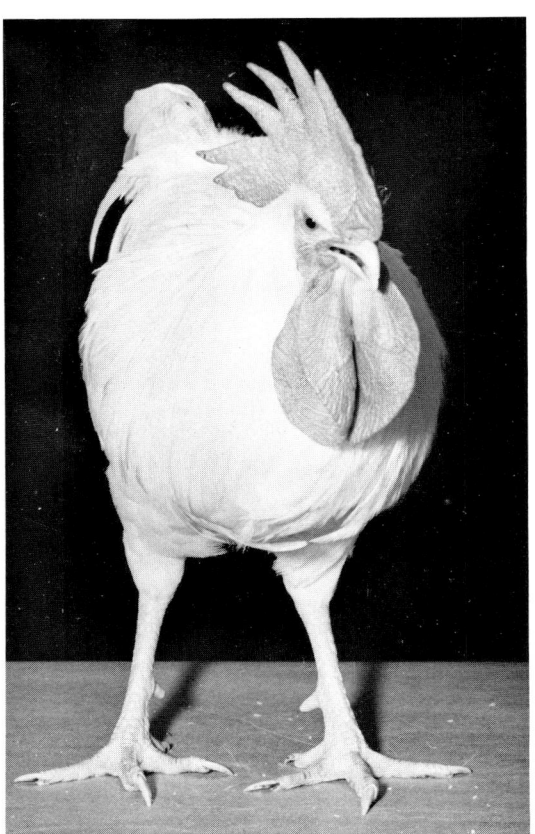

16.44. Osteopetrosis. Both birds at 24 wk old. Chicken injected with RPL12 at 1 day of age and has advanced osteopetrotic lesions of the shanks (*left*). Normal chicken (*right*). (Sanger)

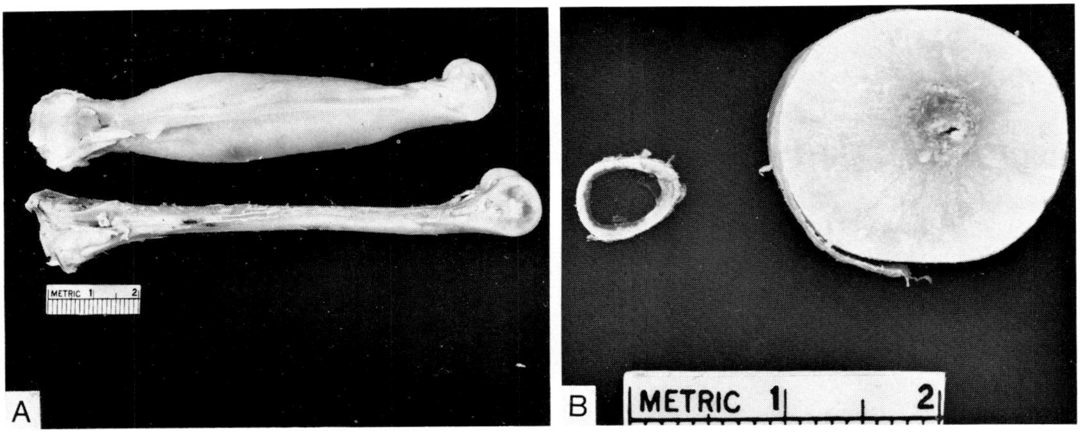

16.45. Osteopetrosis of tibia in 10-wk-old chicken. A. Shorter length of bone is due to reduced growth. Lower tibia is from control bird of same age. B. Cross section of middle of shaft of bones in A. (Sanger, Can J Comp Med Vet Sci)

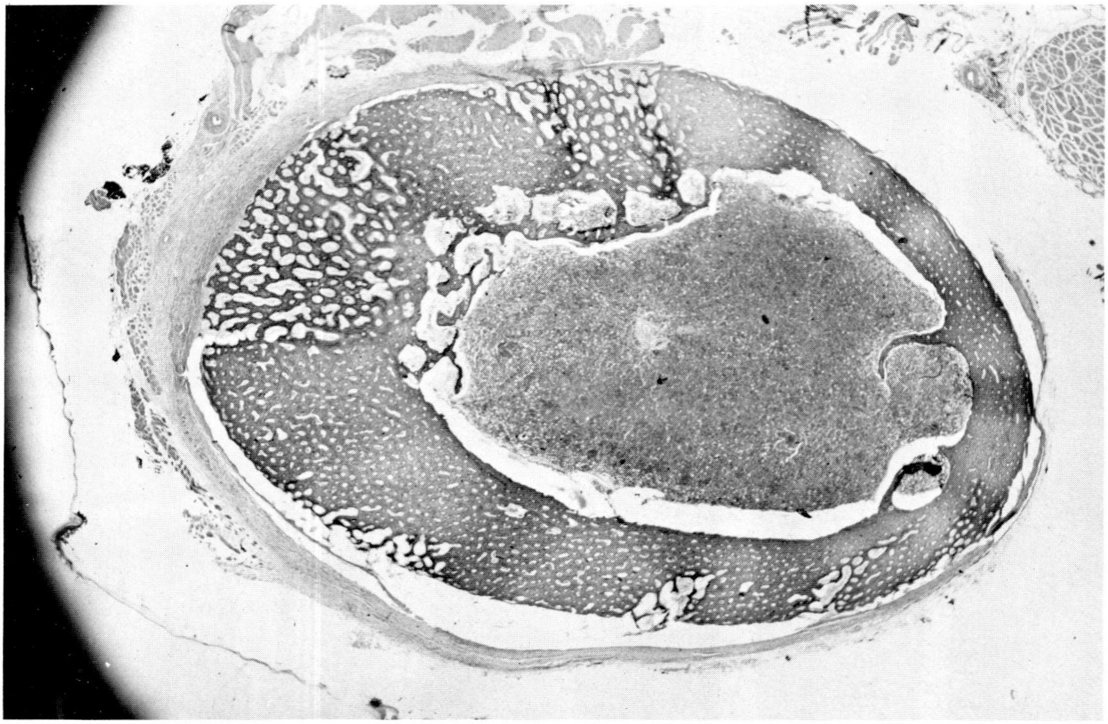

16.46. Osteopetrosis. Cross section of humerus from 8-wk-old chicken. Six separate osteopetrotic foci are present, two of which extend from endosteum to periosteum. ×18. (Sanger, Am J Vet Res)

ULTRASTRUCTURE. Virus particles bud transiently from osteoblasts and continuously from osteocytes and accumulate in the periosteocytic space. With calcification of the bone, the particles become incorporated in the bone trabeculae. No virus production is observed from osteoclasts (132).

HEMATOLOGY. The blood picture is ordinarily aleukemic and there is often a secondary anemia. There may be active erythropoiesis in remaining bone marrow and sometimes in focal areas of the liver, but immature stages are not observed in the peripheral blood. Experimentally, viruses that cause osteopetrosis can induce an aplastic anemia; and an increased corpuscular fragility (167, 251).

Pathogenesis. The osteopetrotic lesion is basically proliferative or hypertrophic (56, 282) and may be neoplastic (30, 289). Lesions of the lymphoid organs and bone marrow are degenerative or anaplastic (167). According to Shank et al. (291) the propensity for certain ALVs to induce osteopetrosis depends on sequences in the *gag-pol* region of the viral genome.

CONNECTIVE TISSUE TUMORS. This section deals with connective tissue tumors for which there is some evidence of transmissibility and viral etiology. They include fibroma and fibrosarcoma; myxoma and myxosarcoma; histiocytic sarcoma; osteoma and osteogenic sarcoma; and chondrosarcoma. All tumors of this group may occur as either benign or malignant growths. Benign tumors grow slowly, never invade surrounding tissues, and remain almost indefinitely strictly localized processes. Malignant forms grow more rapidly, infiltrate, and are capable of metastasis.

Most strains or isolates that induce tumors of the connective tissue are multipotent; i.e., they induce a variety of tumors. Examples are RSV (45) and ES4 (17), which also induce erythroblastosis and LL. Most strains of leukosis virus such as RPL12 (erythroblastosis and LL), BAI-A (myeloblastosis), and strain R (erythroblastosis) also cause one or more of the solid tumors listed

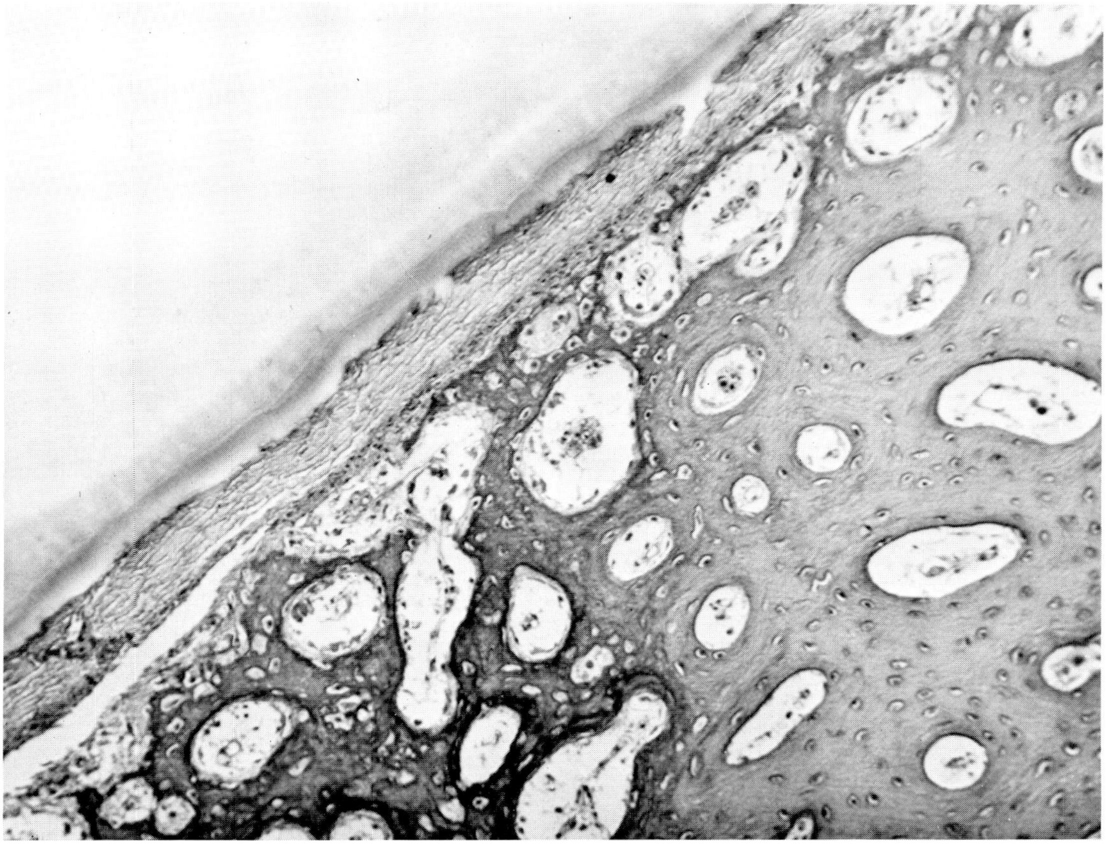

16.47. Osteopetrosis. Early lesion under periosteum (*top*). In more advanced part of lesion (*bottom left*), spaces are large and irregular, lacunae are large and scattered, and fibrous bone is stained basophilic. Normal compact bone (*right*). ×220. (Sanger, Am J Vet Res)

above. Even viruses isolated directly from field cases of LL have produced fibrosarcomas, myxosarcomas, and histiocytic sarcomas as well as hemangiomas and nephroblastomas (134, 135). For review and references see Beard (17, 20) and Vogt (323).

Incubation period. Tumors develop readily and are palpable within 3 days after inoculation of chicks with high doses of RSV. With leukosis viruses, sarcomas may occur anytime after inoculation but are most frequently observed in the first 2–3 mo. In field flocks, connective tissue tumors may occur in birds at any age.

Signs. Until tumors become extremely large, affect the function of an organ, ulcerate, or metastasize, they do not affect the well-being of the host. Some tumors of visceral organs and most of those affecting muscles or integument are palpable. Death may be from secondary bacterial infection, toxemia, hemorrhage, or dysfunction of an organ affected by the tumor. Benign tumors may never cause death, whereas malignant ones may follow a very rapid course, resulting in death within a few days.

Gross Lesions and Histopathology. The different connective tissues distributed throughout the body provide potential sources for a variety of tumors. Fibromas, myxomas, and sarcomas are most likely to arise in the integument or muscles; tumors composed of cartilage or bone or a mixture of these arise where the two tissues are normally found. Sometimes multipotent mesenchymal cells give rise to cartilage and bone where these tissues are not ordinarily present. Of all the connective tissue tumors, histiocytic sarcoma is capable of the widest distribution. Secondary metastatic foci of malignant tumors occur most frequently in lungs, liver, spleen, and intestinal serosa. Primary multiplicity may occur in both benign and malignant tumors; it is characteristic of histiocytic sarcomas.

Fibromas and fibrosarcomas are first noticed as firm lumps attached to the skin, in subcutaneous tissue, muscles, or occasionally other organs. As they grow, the overlying skin often undergoes necrosis and thus results in ulceration and secondary infection. When they are cut, their fibrous nature is apparent.

Fibromas in their simplest form consist of mature fibroblasts interspersed with collagen fibers arranged in wavy parallel bands or whorls. Slow-growing tumors are more differentiated and contain more collagen and fewer cells than those growing more rapidly. Some fibromas may have edematous areas and should not be confused with myxomas and myxosarcomas. If necrosis, ulceration, and secondary infection have occurred, various inflammatory and necrotic alterations may be observed in the tumor. Inflammatory changes may be so prominent that the tumor may be confused with a granuloma.

Fibrosarcomas are characterized by aggressive and destructive growth, their cellular composition, and the immaturity of constituent cells (Fig. 16.48). Large irregular and hyperchromic fibroblasts are abundant and mitosis is common. Tumors contain less collagen than fibromas, and this is concentrated in and near irregular septa that subdivide the tumor. Regions of necrosis often occur in rapidly growing tumors. Edema is sometimes present.

Myxomas and myxosarcomas are softer than fibromas and fibrosarcomas. They contain characteristic tenacious slimy material that pulls out into long strings.

Myxomas consist of stellate or spindle-shaped cells surrounded by a homogeneous, slightly basophilic, mucinous matrix. Long cytoplasmic processes may extend from stellate cells and become fused with sparse collagen fibrils. In the malignant form (myxosarcoma) the mucinous matrix is less abundant and fibroblasts are proportionately more numerous and more immature than in myxomas (Fig. 16.49). Histogenesis and structure of primary myxosarcomatous tumors are similar to those of fibroblastic tumors. The essential difference is that in myxomatous tumors, the fibroblastic cells are more specialized and capable of producing large amounts of mucin in addition to the usual products (collagen and elastic fibrils).

Histiocytic sarcomas are firm fleshy tumors consisting of a mixture of two or more cell types that, while morphologically dissimilar, are closely related histogenically. The most striking microscopic feature is the highly varied nature of the

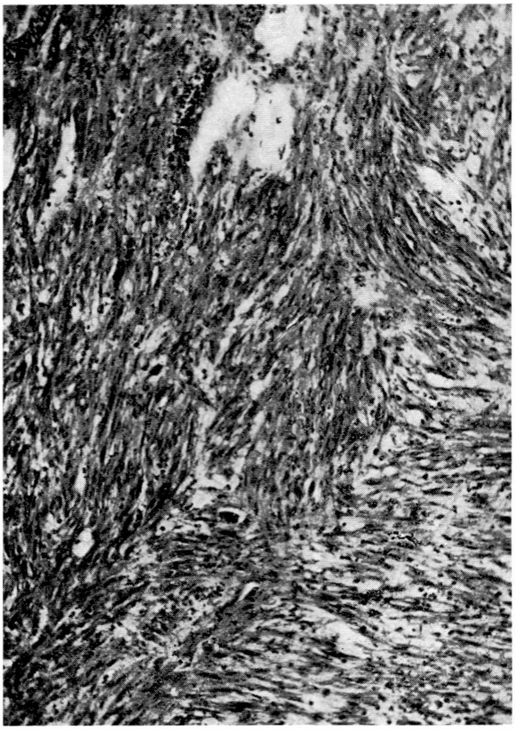

16.48. Fibrosarcoma in musculature of breast. ×120. (Feldman and Olson)

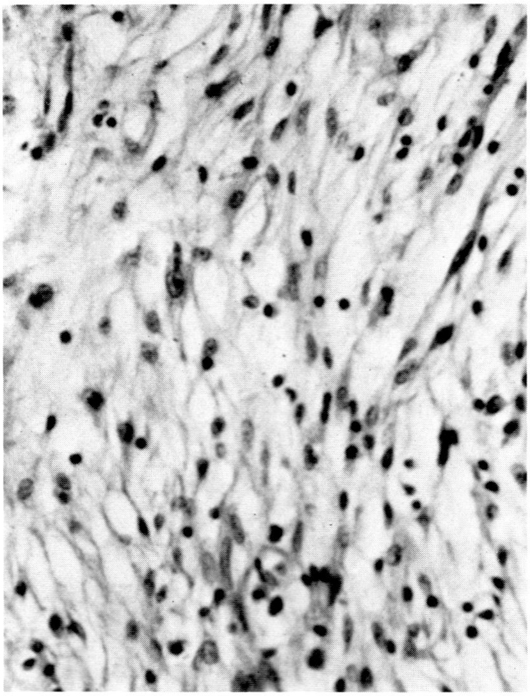

16.49. Myxosarcoma induced by RSV. ×240. (Helmboldt)

cellular constituents (Fig. 16.50). The cells may be spindle shaped, usually appearing in groups or bundles as in fibrosarcomas; stellate reticulum-producing elements (fixed histiocytes); and/or large phagocytic cells or macrophages (free histiocytes). In addition, there usually are numerous transitional forms, many of which are polymorphic. In primary tumors spindle-shaped cells usually predominate, whereas in metastatic foci primitive histiocytic forms are more numerous.

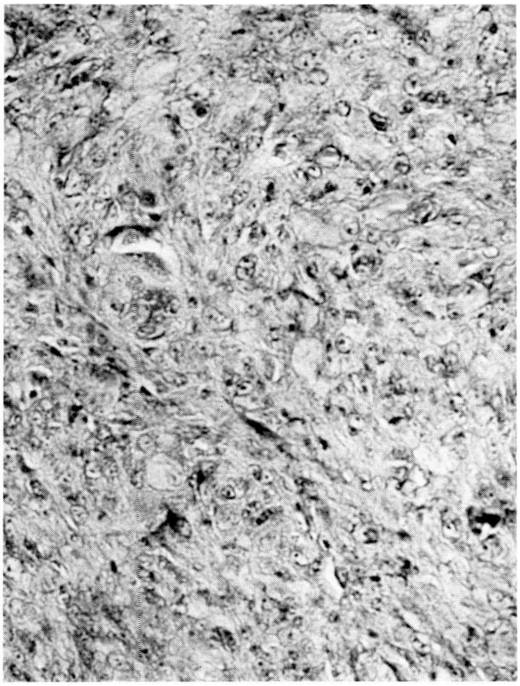

16.50. Histiocytic sarcoma of heart. Note varied character of cellular constituents. ×240. (Helmboldt)

Osteomas and osteogenic sarcomas are hard tumors that may arise from the periosteum of any bone. Osteomas are structurally similar to bone except that much of the inner histological details is lacking. They consist of a homogeneous acidophilic matrix of osseomucin containing collections of osteoblasts at irregular intervals. Osteogenic sarcomas are usually very cellular infiltrative growths that invade and destroy surrounding tissues. The cells are spindle shaped, ovoid, or polyhedral, and many are in mitosis. Nuclei are prominent and cytoplasm is basophilic. Multinucleated giant cells may be quite numerous. Although an osteogenic sarcoma is usually a rapidly growing, highly cellular neoplasm of mostly undifferentiated cells, there are usually areas in which there is sufficient differentiation for production of osseomucin. Presence of osseomucin is usually sufficient to identify these tumors.

Chondromas and chondrosarcomas rarely occur in chickens, although cartilage and bone are often found within fibrosarcomas or myxosarcomas. Such tumors may be designated as fibrochondroosteosarcomas. Microscopically, chondromas have a typical and unique structure, i.e., groups of two or more chondrocytes lying in a homogeneous matrix of chondromucin. Tumors may be separated into lobules by strands of fibrous connective tissue. In chondrosarcomas there is considerable cellular variation, ranging from the most immature to the fully mature chondrocyte. The former are undifferentiated and spindle shaped while the latter are spheroidal. Those in the intervening zone are polymorphic.

ULTRASTRUCTURE. Only the sarcomas produced by RSV have been examined in detail. Spindle-shaped cells, macrophagelike cells, and mast cells have been described (17, 158). It is possible that all these forms, as well as those seen in cultures of chick embryo cells treated with RSV, are originally derived from fibroblasts or connective tissue cells. Tumor cells (158) are similar to the cells in culture in showing numerous pseudopodia and pronounced cytoplasmic vacuolization. Some vacuoles may contain virus particles. Structures similar though not identical to the gray bodies in myeloblasts have been described, and "clusters" (158) (aberrant structures) may also occur in the cytoplasm. Cartilage and osteoid tissue occasionally occur in nephroblastomas, and their ultrastructure has been described. It is likely that chondrosarcomas and osteosarcomas will have many ultrastructural aspects in common with these tumors.

HEMATOLOGY. Anemia is common when tumors affect bone marrow or when they ulcerate and hemorrhage occurs.

Pathogenesis.

Several viral oncogenes have been associated with sarcoma induction, including *src, fps, yes,* and *ros* (121, 207, 328). The product of the v-*src* gene in an infected cell is a phosphoprotein with protein kinase activity that is believed to induce transformation by causing a metabolic imbalance within the cell. Growth of the tumor is by infection and transformation of adjoining cells and proliferation of transformed cells.

Connective tissue tumors probably originate from primitive mesenchymal cells of mesodermal origin. Their diverse structural forms reflect direction and extent of differentiation. Thus frequent occurrence of more than one tissue in a tumor is a reflection of the multipotency of precursor cells; e.g., chondrocytes are derived from primitive mesenchymal cells that have undergone a gradual process of change and maturation. Finally, mature chondrocytes, which produce chondromucin in addition to collagen and elastic fibrils, are evolved. An analogous differentiation occurs during ontogeny of osteoblasts and fibroblasts. The more anaplastic tumors are composed of cells in which maturation has been arrested at an earlier stage.

OTHER TUMORS. By introducing MC29 virus into the peritoneum, Beard (20) induced massive mesotheliomas of serosal cells, which became rounded or pear shaped, often forming solid papillary growths of round cells with large round nuclei and large nucleoli. The mesotheliomas were highly invasive into contiguous structures such as liver, intestine, ovary, and pancreas. Metaplasia to cartilage was common.

Immunity. Under natural conditions, most chicks become infected by exogenous leukosis virus from penmates or their surroundings and, after a transient viremia, develop virus-neutralizing (VN) antibodies that rise to a high titer and persist throughout the life of the bird (278, 303). These antibodies are passed via the yolk to progeny chicks and provide a passive immunity to infection that lasts for 3–4 wk. This passively acquired antibody delays infection by leukosis virus (340), reduces incidence of tumors (34), and reduces the incidence of viremia and shedding of LLV (124). Level and persistence of antibody in the chick is related to the titer of antibody in the dam's serum.

VN antibodies serve to restrict amounts of virus in the bird, which in turn may limit neoplasia, but they are generally considered to have little direct influence on tumor growth. Cytotoxic lymphocytes directed against viral envelope antigens also occur in birds infected with LLV or RSV (15). Birds infected with leukosis/sarcoma virus also produce antibodies to gs-antigens, but these are apparently not related to resistance to tumor growth (292).

Studies on Rous sarcomas reveal that the tumor-bearing host will also respond to tumor-associated cell surface antigens (TASAs), and this response serves to retard tumor growth or cause regression. TASAs may be viral structural antigens and be affected by antiviral responses, or they may be neoantigens arising on the tumor cell. Such neoantigens may be virus-directed and virus-specific or derepressed host antigens, such as embryonic antigens. TASAs may be designated as tumor-specific transplantation antigens (TSTA) when they induce tumor immunity in vivo or as transformation-specific cell surface antigens (TSSA) when demonstrated in in vitro tests only (14, 230, 325, 326). Little is known about antitumor immunity in LL. Immunosuppression can accompany LLV infection in some circumstances. However, Fadly et al. (127) observed that both B- and T-cell immune functions were normal during early and late stages of infection with RAV-1 LLV.

Genetically resistant chicks are resistant to infection and tumor induction by leukosis and sarcoma viruses of the subgroups concerned, and they usually fail to develop antibodies (74, 80). Genetic resistance to tumor development has been studied mainly with the Rous sarcoma, regression of which is determined by a dominant gene *R-RS-1* that lies within the major histocompatibility complex (*Ea-B* locus) of the chicken (68, 287). The *Ea-B* locus also influences incidence of erythroblastosis and to a lesser extent LL (7). Some influence of the lymphocyte antigen *Bu-1* locus on Rous sarcoma regression and of the *Th-1* locus on LL is reported (8).

Genetic resistance to LL tumor development, such as in RPL line 6, is conferred by bursal cells, not by other cellular elements of the immune system such as thymic or thymus-derived cells or nonlymphocytes. It appears as though the intrinsic inability of the bursal target cell to become infected or transformed is the major factor in resistance (260). No obvious difference in the pattern of bursal infection in susceptible and resistant lines was detected by Baba and Humphries (3).

Genetic Resistance. Two levels of genetic resistance to leukosis/sarcoma virus-induced tumors are recognized: cellular resistance to virus infection and resistance to tumor development (6, 74, 231).

Inheritance of cellular resistance to infection is of a simple Mendelian type (Table 16.7). Independent autosomal loci control responses to infec-

Table 16.7. Genes controlling cellular susceptibility to leukosis/sarcoma viruses

Virus Subgroup	Locus	Alleles	Dominant Trait
A	*Tv-A*	$Tv\text{-}A^{s}$, $tv\text{-}A^{r}$	Susceptibility
B and D	*Tv-B**	$Tv\text{-}B^{s1,s2,s3}$, $tv\text{-}B^{r}$	Susceptibility
C	*Tv-C*	$Tv\text{-}C^{s}$, $tv\text{-}C^{r}$	Susceptibility
E	*Tv-E**	$Tv\text{-}E^{s}$, $tv\text{-}E^{r}$	Susceptibility
	I-E	*I-E*, *i-E*	Resistance

Source: (304).
*Existence of independent *Tv-B* and *Tv-E* loci is not settled.

tion by leukosis/sarcoma viruses of subgroups A, B, and C and are designated *Tv-A* (tumor virus A subgroup), *Tv-B,* and *Tv-C* respectively. Gene designations given here are those recommended by Somes (304) and differ slightly from the original designations. The *Tv-B* locus also controls responses to subgroup D virus (225), and linkage occurs between *Tv-A* and *Tv-C* loci (235). At each *Tv* locus, alleles for susceptibility and resistance exist that are designated *Tv-A*^{s}, *tv-A*^{r}; *Tv-B*^{s}, *tv-B*^{r}; and *Tv-C*^{s}, *tv-C*^{r} respectively, and the susceptibility alleles are dominant over the resistance alleles. These genes are usually abbreviated to A^s, A^r, etc. It is probable that multiple alleles occur at each locus, encoding different levels of susceptibility, but this question has not been studied in detail.

Inheritance of resistance to E subgroup virus is more complex, with involvement and interaction of genes at two autosomal loci designated *Tv-E* and *I-E* (238). A dominant resistance gene, *I-E,* acting epistatically, blocks susceptibility conferred by presence of E^s allele. It has been reported, however, that susceptibility alleles at the *Tv-B* locus are required for susceptibility to E subgroup virus, and there is controversy about whether a separate *Tv-E* locus exists (87, 226, 227). Action of the *I-E* gene was ascribed to the control of endogenous virus production, which blocked E subgroup virus receptors. Studies suggest that the *I-E* locus is itself an *ev* locus (269). Susceptibility genes such as A^s code for presence of subgroup-specific virus receptor sites on the cell surface, which interact with viral envelope glycoprotein and allow viral penetration and infection of the cell. Little is known of the molecular events involved in this interaction (333). Cells resistant by virtue of presence of a resistance gene such as A^r in the homozygous state are believed to lack the specific receptor sites necessary for infection to occur, although nonspecific adsorption of virus to such cells can occur, but without infection being established.

Cellular susceptibility phenotypes associated with these genes are designated according to a convention that recognizes the virus subgroups to which the chicken (C) cell is resistant (/); e.g., C/AE denotes a cell resistant to A and E subgroups but susceptible to B, C, and D subgroups; C/0 denotes a cell resistant to no subgroup, i.e., susceptible to A, B, C, D, and E.

Resistance or susceptibility conferred by these genes is expressed by all cells, whether by cells cultured in vitro, such as chicken embryo fibroblasts; by chicken embryo cells, such as those of the CAM; or by chickens after hatching. These responses are applicable to leukosis or sarcoma viruses sharing the same envelope glycoproteins, and thus viral subgroup, but most genetic studies are undertaken with appropriate subgroups of RSV, since infection of the cell is expressed within a few days by visible growth of tumor cells. Thus the phenotype of an individual may be determined by inoculation of a standard dose of RSV into chicken embryo fibroblasts in culture, with production of foci of transformed cells in susceptible embryo cells but not in resistant cells (276). Similarly, RSV can be inoculated onto the CAM of the chicken embryo, with or without production of tumor pocks (84), or intracranially into day-old chicks, with death or survival as the response criterion (330) (see PREVENTION AND CONTROL). The phenotype of individual birds may be determined by culturing fibroblasts from plucked pin feather pulp and challenging these cultures with RSV (85, 240, 310).

Genetically resistant chicks are resistant to infection and tumor induction by leukosis and sarcoma viruses of the subgroups concerned, and they usually fail to develop antibodies (74, 80). Genetic resistance to tumor development has been studied mainly with the Rous sarcoma, regression of which is determined by a dominant gene *R-RS-1* that lies within the major histocompatibility complex (*Ea-B* locus) of the chicken (68, 287). The *Ea-B* locus also influences incidence of erythroblastosis and to a lesser extent LL (7). Some influence of the lymphocyte antigen *Bu-1* locus on Rous sarcoma regression and of the *Th-1* locus on LL is reported (8).

Genetic resistance to LL tumor development, such as in RPL line 6, is conferred by bursal cells, not by other cellular elements of the immune system such as thymic or thymus-derived cells or nonlymphocytes. It appears as though the intrinsic inability of the bursal target cell to become infected or transformed is the major factor in resistance (260). No obvious difference in the pattern of bursal infection in susceptible and resistant lines was detected by Baba and Humphries (3).

DIAGNOSIS

Isolation and Identification of Causative Agent. Plasma, serum, and tumor are the best materials for virus isolation (255). Virus can also be isolated from most soft organs of the body and from oral washings and feces (36, 277), from albumen of newly laid eggs or the 10 day-old embryo of eggs laid by hens that are transmitting virus vertically (307), from feather pulp (309), and from semen (290). All viruses of this group are very thermolabile and can be preserved for long periods only at temperatures below −60 C.

The first successful procedure developed for virus isolation was inoculation of susceptible chicks (see Laboratory Host Systems). Some viruses (e.g., RSV) produce pocks on the CAM of embryonated eggs. These procedures have been largely superseded by the more rapid and less expensive cell culture techniques described below.

than one occasion if necessary. Similarly, in the NP and PM tests, the supernatant fluid of cell cultures can be stored and tested for virus by the cell culture technique. Results are usually more clear-cut in the NP and PM tests than in the RIF, COFAL, or ELISA tests.

The subgroup of an infecting leukosis virus can be determined by any of the tests. In the RIF test, only RSV belonging to the same subgroup as the leukosis virus is subjected to interference. In COFAL and ELISA tests, genetically resistant cells can be used; thus a leukosis virus of subgroup A will not produce CF antigens in cells of the C/A phenotype (resistant to subgroup A viruses). In the NP test, genetically resistant NP cells can be prepared; and in the PM test, genetically resistant cells can be used in the mixing phase. In NP and PM tests, supernatant from the activation or mixing phase (which contains RSV of the same subgroup as the leukosis virus) can be placed on genetically resistant cells or embryos or used in an interference test with a leukosis virus of known subgroup.

Immunohistochemical Tests. Direct (180) and indirect (237) FA tests have been used to detect viral antigen in chicken embryo fibroblast cultures. When mammalian gs antiserums are used and cells are fixed in acetone, the test becomes analogous to the COFAL test. Avian serums are subgroup specific or even type specific (237). Other immunohistochemical techniques have also been described (110).

Enzyme Assays. AMV has on its surface an enzyme (ATPase) that dephosphorylates adenosine triphosphate. This activity can be used as a quantitative assay to determine amount of virus present in the plasma of infected chickens or in supernatants of myeloblast cultures (22).

All leukosis/sarcoma viruses contain reverse transcriptase (313). Detection of this enzyme, either directly when the correct template is used (181, 317) or indirectly when the radioimmunoassay is used (224), is an indication of presence of virus.

DETECTION OF VIRAL NUCLEIC ACIDS. Blot-hybridization analysis of viral DNA or RNA in cell extracts is used increasingly for detection of virus in avian tumor virus research (337, 338).

HEMATOPOIETIC TRANSFORMATION. AMV will infect cultures of avian hematopoietic tissue and induce focal transformation into myeloblasts. Assays are usually based on a quantal response in which individual cultures are scored as positive or negative (11, 206). Focus assays for myeloblastosis, erythroblastosis, and other defective leukemia viruses have been developed (150, 151, 209).

TRANSFORMATION OF FIBROBLASTS AND CYTOPATHOLOGY. In sensitive chicken embryo fibroblast cultures, sarcoma viruses produce foci of morphologically transformed cells, which can be seen microscopically after 4–5 days (Fig. 16.21) and grossly after about 10 days (316). The foci consist of rounded refractile cells that become multilayered. Morphology of the transformed cells and shape of the focus produced is characteristic of the infecting virus. Sarcoma viruses also activate NP cells, produce the complement-fixing gs antigen, and can be detected by the FA technique. A number of defective acute leukemia viruses can also transform chick fibroblasts (151).

Leukosis viruses of subgroups B and D induce cytopathic effects in cell culture (149, 179). Because this property is restricted to a few viruses, it cannot be used as an assay for field viruses.

Serology.

Serum or egg yolk is suitable for antibody determination, but heparinized plasma should not be used when tests are made in cell culture because of nonspecific effects.

TESTS. Neutralization of a RSV pseudotype is indicative of current or past infection with a leukosis or sarcoma virus of the same subgroup and the same or similar type. A virus of one subgroup will not be neutralized by antibodies provoked by a virus of a different subgroup (324). Usually, a 1:5 dilution of heat-inactivated (56 C for 30 min) serum is mixed with an equal quantity of a standard preparation of RSV of a known pseudotype; after incubation the residual virus is quantitated by any one of many procedures, the cell culture assay being most commonly used (278).

More recently, an indirect immunoperoxidase absorbance test (200) and ELISA tests (201, 299, 321) have been described for the detection of antibodies.

SEROTYPES. Viruses of the avian leukosis/sarcoma group occurring in chickens have been divided into five subgroups (A, B, C, D, E) on the basis of host range in genetically susceptible or resistant cells, interference spectrum, and viral envelope antigens (neutralizing antigens) (337).

Viruses of different subgroups can be distinguished by the ability of monovalent antiserums to neutralize them. However, even though there is usually some cross-neutralization between viruses belonging to the same subgroup, the kinetics of neutralization vary and slopes of curves for heterologous systems differ from those of homologous systems. There are no common neutralization antigens among viruses of different subgroups, except for a relationship between subgroups B and D. The diagnosis of infection by serological means requires that representatives of all serotypes be employed. Leukosis viruses themselves may be used, but more commonly,

RSV pseudotypes are employed in the neutralization tests.

Differential Diagnosis

Lymphoid Leukosis. LL and Marek's disease (MD) can be differentiated only with difficulty, because similar lymphoid tumors may occur in both diseases in the same visceral organs during the same age period. Visceral lesions of these two diseases cannot be distinguished by gross examination. Diagnosis is possible in most instances on careful microscopic examination; however, considerable experience is necessary. In coming to a decision, history, signs, gross and microscopic lesions, and cytology should all be considered. This section will describe points that should receive special attention (47, 123, 258) (see Table 16.2).

Ordinarily, LL does not occur before 14 wk of age, and most of the mortality occurs between 24 and 40 wk. MD, on the other hand, may occur as early as 4 wk, and the mortality peak varies from 10 to 20 wk. Occasionally, losses continue and may reach a peak after 20 wk.

Nodular tumors of the bursa can often be palpated through the cloaca in birds infected with LLV. Paralysis associated with gross lesions in autonomic and peripheral nervous systems and gross lesions of the iris ("gray eye") are specific for MD.

As stated above, the bursa of Fabricius plays a central role in development of LL. When distinct focal or nodular lymphoid tumors are present in the bursa, a diagnosis of LL can be made. Such tumors are sometimes quite small and may be overlooked. In some birds, MD induces a premature atrophy of the bursa. In others, the bursa may be tumorous, in which case the walls and plica may be thickened from interfollicular infiltration with pleomorphic lymphocytes. In contrast, intrafollicular tumors of the bursa consisting of uniform large lymphocytes are usual with LL.

Microscopic lymphoid infiltration in nerves, cuffing around small arterioles in white matter of the cerebellum, and follicular pattern of lymphoid cell infiltration in the skin, characteristic of MD, are not seen with LL.

Cytologically, LL tumors are generally composed of a homogeneous population of lymphoblasts (see Fig. 16.29). In contrast, tumors of MD usually contain lymphoid cells varying in size and maturity from lymphoblasts to small lymphocytes, and plasma cells may also be present. Special stains such as methyl green pyronin are helpful for cytology. Immature lymphoblasts characteristic of LL tumors are highly pyroninophilic, whereas the medium and small lymphocytes that predominate in tumors of MD do not stain with pyronin.

LL tumors are composed almost entirely of B cells and have surface IgM markers, whereas 60–90% of MD tumor cells are T cells that lack IgM markers and only about 3–25% are B cells. In addition, from 0.5 to 35% of MD tumor cells have a tumor-associated cell surface antigen (MATSA), which is absent from LL tumor cells (111, 214, 215, 250).

Other diseases that may be confused with LL are erythroblastosis, myeloblastosis, myelocytomatosis, pullorum disease, tuberculosis, enterohepatitis, Hjarre's disease, and fatty degeneration of the liver.

Erythroblastosis. Although gross lesions of liver, spleen, and bone marrow provide the basis for a presumptive diagnosis, a firm diagnosis must be based on finding large numbers of erythroblasts by microscopic examination of a blood smear and sections or smears of liver and bone marrow. Chickens in early stages of disease or without obvious signs may easily be missed unless microscopic examination is made.

Erythroblastosis with concurrent anemia is often difficult to differentiate from anemia resulting from nonneoplastic causes. In erythroblastosis there is usually a defect in maturation of erythroblasts, resulting in presence of large numbers of them and very few polychrome erythrocytes (see Fig. 16.35). In anemia the reverse usually occurs. Extramedullary erythropoiesis and stasis of erythroblasts in the sinusoids are usually more prominent in erythroblastosis than in anemia.

Erythroblastosis can be distinguished from myeloblastosis on the following grounds. In myeloblastosis the liver is usually pale red and the marrow is whitish, whereas in erythroblastosis the liver and marrow are usually cherry red (see Fig. 16.33B, C). In myeloblastosis the cells accumulate intravascularly and extravascularly, whereas in erythroblastosis they are always intravascular (see Fig. 16.35). The erythroblast and myeloblast may be difficult to distinguish. Erythroblasts have a basophilic cytoplasm and perinuclear halo; myeloblasts often have some granules (see Fig. 16.33D, E).

Erythroblasts are cells of the erythropoietic system and can be differentiated from cells of the myelopoietic system on the basis of presence of certain markers. Thus erythroblasts have erythroid markers including hemoglobin, chicken erythrocyte-specific histone H5, and chicken erythrocyte-specific cell surface antigens detected by immunofluorescence. Myeloblasts and myelocytes have myeloid markers including adherence and phagocytic capacity, Fc receptors as determined by rosette formation, macrophage- and granulocyte-specific cell surface antigen as detected by immunofluorescence, and dependence of colony formation on colony-stimulating factor (151, 208).

Erythroblastosis can be distinguished from LL

by the nature and distribution of lesions. Microscopically the cytoplasm of lymphoblasts is somewhat less basophilic than that of erythroblasts, and there is also a larger nuclear-cytoplasmic ratio than in the latter cells. Lymphoblasts are more variable in size and shape than erythroblasts, but they are all at the same primitive developmental stage. Lymphoblasts tend to have an ovoid rather than spherical nucleus and a finer, more delicate-looking chromatin network.

Myelocytomas are easily distinguished from erythroblastosis.

MYELOBLASTOSIS. As in erythroblastosis, a tentative diagnosis may be based on gross lesions; however, these are often so similar to those of lymphoid leukosis that specific diagnosis cannot be made without examination of a blood smear. Examination of liver or bone marrow sections is helpful when identity of the cell type is in doubt (see Fig. 16.35). The myeloblast is, on the average, smaller than the erythroblast or lymphoblast; its cytoplasm is more acidophilic and is polygonal or angular. The nucleus is less vesicular; the nucleolus, while present, is not nearly so frequently seen nor conspicuous as in the other two leukoses. Myeloblasts also have physiological markers that identify them as members of the myeloid series (see Differential Diagnosis, Erythroblastosis).

MYELOCYTOMATOSIS. The distinctive character and location of tumors provide the basis for diagnosis, which can be verified by examination of a stained smear or tumor section. Gross tumors must be differentiated from myeloblastosis, LL, osteopetrosis, and necrotic and/or purulent processes occurring in tuberculosis, pullorum disease, and mycotic infections.

HEMANGIOMA. Hemangiomas on the skin should be differentiated from wounds, bleeding feather follicles, and cannibalism. Those in the visceral organs should be differentiated from hemorrhages and sarcomas.

RENAL TUMORS. Renal tumors should be suspected when tumor nodules or large masses are found only in the kidney or are encountered suspended from the lumbar region. Diagnosis can be verified by microscopic examination. Tumors should be differentiated from other causes of kidney enlargement including hematomata, LL, and accumulation of urates.

OSTEOPETROSIS. Bone lesions of advanced cases are sufficiently distinctive to present no difficulty in diagnosis. Cross and longitudinal sectioning of long bones is helpful in detecting slight exostoses and endostoses, particularly in early stages.

Among other osteopathies, rickets and osteoporosis can be differentiated from osteopetrosis by their epiphyseal formation of osteoid or porous bone. In perosis there is twisting and flattening of the shank while the bone structure itself remains normal.

CONNECTIVE TISSUE TUMORS. These tumors are usually easy to distinguish from the leukoses. They should not be confused with granulomas (Hjarre's disease, tuberculosis, pullorum disease), results of trauma, myelocytomas, or leiomyomas.

TREATMENT. No practical therapeutic measures have been found for treatment of diseases of the avian leukosis complex. In evaluating potentially therapeutic agents, it must be remembered that temporary remissions of clinical signs may occur spontaneously. All attempts to treat virus-induced neoplasia have resulted in negative or nonreproducible results.

PREVENTION AND CONTROL

Eradication. Exogenous leukosis viruses can be eradicated from flocks. Until 1977, eradication was only applicable to experimental or special specific-pathogen-free flocks because methods used were long, complicated, and expensive. Since then, eradication from commercial flocks has become feasible using the techniques of Spencer et al. (307).

Eradication of leukosis virus infection depends on breaking the vertical transmission of virus from dam to progeny. To establish a leukosis-free flock it is necessary to hatch, rear, and maintain in isolation a group of chickens free from congenital infection. To achieve this, embryos must be obtained from dams that are not transmitting virus to their progeny. In earlier work on development of LLV-free flocks, several methods for selecting dams were used or recommended. The dams selected to produce the next and to be hoped virus-free generation were: 1) Immune, nonvirus-shedders. Hens with antibody were selected on the assumption that they were less likely than hens without antibody to shed virus. Chicks were hatched from those that did not transmit virus to their embryos, based on tests on at least three embryos/hen (169). 2) Nonimmune, nonvirus-shedders. Hens without antibody were selected on the assumption that they had not ever been infected and were less likely than hens with antibody to become intermittent shedders (193). 3) Nonviremic hens regardless of immune status. These were identified and used to provide replacements; however, up to four generations of testing were needed before flocks were free of viremics, and infection of nonviremics was not ruled out (342).

Application of eradication to commercial flocks

has depended on associations between virus infections in hens, eggs, embryos, and chicks (307): 1) Egg albumen may contain exogenous LLV and gs antigen, and both are usually present together. 2) There is a strong association between LLV or gs antigen in egg albumen and LLV in vaginal swabs. 3) There is an association between LLV in vaginal swabs or egg albumen and LLV in chicken embryos and newly hatched chicks. Consequently, hens with a low probability of producing infected embryos are hens negative for virus (or gs antigen) by the vaginal swab test or hens that produce eggs with albumen free from virus or gs antigen. Commonly, virus in vaginal or cloacal swabs may be detected by ELISA, NP, or PM tests, and in egg albumen by ELISA or direct CO-FAL tests. It is unlikely that a single test will detect all potential shedder hens. A problem that arises in applying the ELISA test to albumen or swabs is the need to differentiate positive reactions due to the presence of gs antigen derived from endogenous leukosis virus or loci from the reactions due to presence of exogenous LLV infection (170). Reactions due to the latter are usually markedly higher, but the setting of the boundary between endogenous and exogenous virus infections is sometimes difficult and somewhat arbitrary. High reactions due to exogenous virus are clearer with albumen samples than with swabs (82). There is a prospect that monoclonal antibodies developed against p27 protein will be used in ELISAs to differentiate between endogenous and exogenous infections (192).

A procedure for eradication of LLV involves: 1) selection of fertile eggs from hens negative in the egg albumen or vaginal swab test (2, 93, 125, 219, 239); 2) hatching of chicks in isolation in small groups (25–50) in wire-floored cages, avoidance of manual vent sexing (126), and vaccination with a common needle (100) to prevent mechanical spread of any residual infection; 3) testing of chicks for LLV by a biological assay on blood, discarding reactors and contact chicks (125, 126, 219, 222); and 4) rearing LLV-free groups in isolation. In practice, selection of hens with a low shedding rate is a simpler requirement to fulfill than the subsequent chick testing and isolation rearing needed to achieve complete eradication. Consequently, some commercial breeder organizations are concentrating only on reduction of infection rate by hen testing. Progress in reducing shedding rates was reported for many lines, although some responded poorly (222). Poor response to selection was not inherent in the lines but appeared to be related to environmental factors (128). For a review of these and other control methods, see Spencer (305) and de Boer (99).

Chicks are most susceptible to contact infection by leukosis viruses during the period immediately after hatching. Although congenitally infected hatchmates are likely to be the main source of such infection, there are several procedures that can reduce or eliminate infection remaining from previous populations. Incubators, hatchers, brooding houses, and all equipment should be thoroughly cleaned and disinfected between each use. Chick boxes should not be reused, and each farm should ideally have only one age group of chickens. The danger of introducing strains of virus not already present in the population can be eliminated if eggs or chicks from different sources are not mixed and chicks are reared under isolation conditions that will prevent cross-contamination of flocks.

Vaccination of chickens with virulent LLV at 8 wk of age is reported to prevent virus shedding to eggs and facilitate eradication of leukosis viruses (265), but this could not be confirmed by Okazaki et al. (221). Reports (194) indicated that while chicks vaccinated at 8 wk of age or older do not usually shed virus to their eggs, they may harbor it, particularly in white blood cells (WBC) and the spleen. Rarely, chickens inoculated for the first time at 71 wk of age may later harbor virus in WBC and the oviduct and therefore could potentially transmit virus to their progeny.

Selection for Genetic Resistance. The frequencies of the alleles that encode cellular susceptibility and resistance to infection by exogenous leukosis/sarcoma viruses (see Pathogenesis and Epizootiology) vary greatly among commercial lines of chickens (79, 210). In some lines high frequencies of a resistant allele may be found naturally. In others, frequencies of the resistant alleles can be increased by artificial selection. In practice, emphasis is placed on resistance to the predominating A subgroup virus and sometimes to B subgroup also.

In artificial selection, genotypes of unknown parents may be determined in a progeny test by mating them to recessive tester birds of the subgroup in question (e.g., A^rA^r for A subgroup virus (228). Depending on the segregation of susceptible and resistant progeny in a particular mating, the genotype of the unknown parent may be determined. The phenotypic identification of progeny in the test may be determined by inoculation of RSV onto the CAM, the embryo being scored as susceptible or resistant on the basis of pock count (84) or intracranial inoculation of RSV into hatched chicks, chicks being scored on the basis of death or survival (330). The former method is preferable and has many advantages.

Crittenden (73, 74) discussed some of the problems raised by this approach. Mutant viruses are more likely to overcome resistance from a single gene than that related to a multiple gene effect, and mutant subgroups may then be favored. In a host population resistant to virus penetration, there can be no effective selection for resistance to development of neoplasms; for this reason mutant viruses may take over. It is probable that past selection for host viability has increased the resistance of infected birds to development of neoplasms. This type of resistance is poorly defined but may be controlled by a number of genes and is consequently more difficult to overcome by viral mutation.

Immunization. Possible use of antiviral vaccines to increase host resistance is very attractive. However, in a series of attempts to inactivate leukosis viruses by various means, Burmester (37) demonstrated that ability of these virus preparations to induce antibody was destroyed almost concurrently with inactivation. Although some success has been obtained with inactivated virus, the procedures are not suitable for field application. Attempts to produce attenuated strains of virus that do not induce disease have failed (223).

Some success has been obtained in attempts to increase the resistance of the host to RSV by immunization with viral or cellular antigens (24, 230). Similar approaches to study of immunity to lymphoid leukosis are warranted.

Recently a recombinant leukosis virus with characteristics of RAV-0, yet expressing subgroup A envelope glycoproteins, has been produced that could have potential as a vaccine (198).

However, congenitally infected chicks are immunologically tolerant and thus cannot be immunized even if a suitable vaccine were available. Unfortunately, these chickens constitute the major source of virus transmission and are the most likely to develop neoplasms.

Removal of the Bursa of Fabricius. Since the bursa of Fabricius plays such a central role in pathogenesis of LL and LL is the most common of the diseases induced by this group of viruses, its removal offers some possibilities in control of the disease. In experimentally infected chickens, surgical removal of the bursa of Fabricius before 5 mo of age (243) or treatment of embryos or young chicks with testosterone or corticosteroids has resulted in elimination of the malignancy. Unfortunately, these procedures have had some undesirable side effects. In the cases of surgical bursectomy, there is a higher incidence of osteopetrosis and nonspecific deaths and a decrease in body weight. In addition to the increased nonspecific mortality and decrease in body weight caused by the hormones, testosterone also produces a masculinization of the chicken, which has a serious effect on egg production.

An androgen analog (Mibolerone) that will cause bursal atrophy if administered to chickens from the 1st to the 49th day post hatching will prevent LL (177, 271). The drug is anabolic and has no deleterious effects on egg production. Because the time between withdrawal (7th wk) and egg production (20th wk) is long, danger of residues is slight. It has little effect on the cycle of virus infection in a chicken. However, the drug is not used commercially to control LL.

Infectious bursal disease virus given at 2 or 8 wk of age to LL-susceptible, leukosis virus–infected birds will prevent LL (254). It should be noted that at 4–6 wk of age infectious bursal disease virus will cause heavy mortality among test chicks. Infectious bursal disease vaccines, which are relatively virulent and induce destruction of the bursa of Fabricius, prevent LL, whereas avirulent vaccines, which have no visible effect on bursal morphology, do not affect the occurrence of LL (65). The role of naturally occurring infectious bursal disease virus infection in the prevention of LL in the field is unknown.

REFERENCES

1. Astrin, S.M., H.L. Robinson, L.B. Crittenden, E.G. Buss, J. Wyban, and W.S. Hayward. 1979. Ten genetic loci in the chicken that contain structural genes for endogenous avian leukosis viruses. Cold Spring Harbor Symp Quant Biol 44:1105–1109.

2. Astrin, S.M., E.G. Buss, and W.S. Hayward. 1979. Endogenous viral genes are nonessential in the chicken. Nature 282:339–341.

3. Baba, T.W., and E.H. Humphries. 1984. Avian leukosis virus infection: Analysis of viremia and DNA integration in susceptible and resistant chicken lines. J Virol 51:123–130.

4. Baba, T.W., and E.H. Humphries. 1985. Formation of a transformed follicle is necessary but not sufficient for development of an avian leukosis virus–induced lymphoma. Proc Nat Acad Sci USA 82:213–216

5. Baba, T.W., and E.H. Humphries. 1986. Selective integration of avian leukosis virus in different hematopoietic tissues. Virology 155:557–566.

6. Bacon, L.D. 1987. Influence of the major histocompatability complex on disease resistance and productivity. Poult Sci 66:802–811.

7. Bacon, L.D., R.L. Witter, L.B. Crittenden, A. Fadly, and J. Motta. 1981. B-haplotype influence on Marek's disease, Rous sarcoma, and lymphoid leukosis virus–induced tumors in chickens. Poult Sci 60:1132–1139.

8. Bacon, L.D., T.L. Fredrickson, D.G. Gilmour, A.M. Fadly, and L.B. Crittenden. 1985. Tests of association of lymphocyte alloantigen genotypes with resistance to viral oncogenesis in chickens. 2. Rous sarcoma and lymphoid leukosis in progeny derived from 6_3 x 15I and 100 x 6_3 crosses. Poult Sci 64:39–47.

9. Bacon, L.D., E.J. Smith, L.B. Crittenden, and G.B. Havenstein. 1988. Association of the slow feathering (K) and an endogenous viral (ev 21) gene on the Z chromosome of chickens. Poult Sci 67:191–197.

10. Baluda, M.A. 1962. Properties of cells infected with avian myeloblastosis virus. Cold Spring Harbor Symp Quant Biol 27:415–425.

11. Baluda, M.A. 1963. Conversion of cells by avian myeloblastosis virus. Perspect Virol 3:118–137.

12. Baluda, M.A., and P.P. Jamieson. 1961. In vivo infectivity studies with avian myeloblastosis virus. Virology 14:33–45.

13. Bauer, H. 1974. Virion and tumor cell antigens of C-type RNA tumor viruses. Adv Cancer Res 20:275–341.

14. Bauer, H., and B. Fleischer. 1981. Immunobiology

of avian RNA tumor virus-induced cell surface antigens. In J.W. Blasecki (ed.), Mechanisms of Immunity to Virus-induced Tumors, pp. 69–118. Marcel Dekker, New York.

15. Bauer, H., R. Kirth, L. Rohrschneider, and H. Gelderblum. 1976. Immune response to oncornaviruses and tumor-associated antigens in the chicken. Cancer Res 36:598–602.

16. Bayon, H.P. 1929. The pathology of transmissible anaemia (erythromyelosis) in the fowl; its similarity to human hemopathies. Parasitology 21:339–374.

17. Beard, J.W. 1963. Avian virus growths and their etiological agents. Adv Cancer Res 7:1–127.

18. Beard, J.W. 1963. Viral tumors of chickens with particular reference to the leukosis complex. Ann NY Acad Sci 108:1057–1085.

19. Beard, J.W. 1973. Oncornaviruses. I. The avian tumor viruses. In A.J. Dalton and F. Haguenau (eds.), Ultrastructure in Biological Systems, Vol. 5. Ultrastructure of Animal Viruses and Bacteriophages, pp. 261–281. Academic Press, New York.

20. Beard, J.W. 1980. Biology of avian oncornaviruses. In G. Klein (ed.), Viral Oncology, pp. 55–87. Raven Press, New York.

21. Beard, J.W., J.F. Chabot, D. Beard, U. Heine, and G.E. Houts. 1976. Renal neoplastic response to leukosis virus strains BAI A (avian myeloblastosis virus) and MC29. Cancer Res 36:339–353.

22. Beaudreau, G.S., and C. Becker. 1958. Virus of avian myeloblastosis. X. Photometric microdetermination of adenosinetriphosphatase activity. J Nat Cancer Inst 20:339–349.

23. Beaudreau, G.S., R.A. Bonar, D. Beard, and J.W. Beard. 1956. Virus of avian erythroblastosis. II. Influence of host age and route of inoculation on dose-response. J Nat Cancer Inst 17:91–100.

24. Bennett, D.D., and S.E. Wright. 1987. Immunization with envelope glycoprotein of an avian RNA tumor virus protects against sarcoma virus tumor induction: Role of subgroup. Virus Res 8:73–77.

25. Biggs, P.M. 1961. A discussion on the classification of the avian leucosis complex and fowl paralysis. Br Vet J 117:326–334.

26. Biggs, P.M., and L.N. Payne. 1964. Relationship of Marek's disease (neural lymphomatosis) to lymphoid leukosis. Nat Cancer Inst Monogr 17:83–98.

27. Biggs, P.M., B.S. Milne, T. Graf, and H. Bauer. 1973. Oncogenicity of nontransforming mutants of avian sarcoma viruses. J Gen Virol 18:399–403.

28. Boettiger, D. 1979. Animal virus pseudotypes. Prog Med Virol 25:37–68.

29. Bolognesi, D.P. 1974. Structural components of RNA tumor viruses. Adv Virus Res 19:315–359.

30. Boyde, A., A.J. Banes, R.M. Dillaman, and G.L. Mechanic. 1978. Morphological study of an avian bone disorder caused by myeloblastosis-associated virus. Metab Bone Dis Relat Res 1:235–242.

31. Bryan, W.R. 1956. Biological studies on the Rous sarcoma virus. IV. Interpretation of tumour response data involving one inoculation site per chicken. J Nat Cancer Inst 16:843–863.

32. Bryan, W.R., J.B. Moloney, and D. Calnan. 1954. Stable standard preparations of the Rous sarcoma virus preserved by freezing and storage at low temperatures. J Nat Cancer Inst 15:315–329.

33. Burmester, B.R. 1947. Studies on the transmission of avian visceral lymphomatosis. II. Propagation of lymphomatosis with cellular and cell-free preparations. Cancer Res 7:786–797.

34. Burmester, B.R. 1955. Immunity to visceral lymphomatosis in chicks following injection of virus into dams. Proc Soc Exp Biol Med 88:153–155.

35. Burmester, B.R. 1956. Bioassay of the virus of visceral lymphomatosis. I. Use of short experimental period. J Nat Cancer Inst 16:1121–1127.

36. Burmester, B.R. 1956. The shedding of the virus of visceral lymphomatosis in the saliva and feces of individual normal and lymphomatous chickens. Poult Sci 35:1089–1099.

37. Burmester, B.R. 1968. Unpublished data.

38. Burmester, B.R. 1969. The prevention of lymphoid leukosis with androgens. Poult Sci 48:401–408.

39. Burmester, B.R., and G.E. Cottral. 1947. The propagation of filtrable agents producing lymphoid tumors and osteopetrosis by serial passage in chickens. Cancer Res 7:669–675.

40. Burmester, B.R., and E.M. Denington. 1947. Studies on the transmission of avian visceral lymphomatosis. I. Variation in transmissibility of naturally occurring cases. Cancer Res 7:779–785.

41. Burmester, B.R., and T.N. Fredrickson. 1964. Transmission of virus from field cases of avian lymphomatosis. I. Isolation of virus in line 15I chickens. J Nat Cancer Inst 32:37–63.

42. Burmester, B.R., and R.F. Gentry. 1956. The response of susceptible chickens to graded doses of the virus of visceral lymphomatosis. Poult Sci 35:17–26.

43. Burmester, B.R., and N.M. Nelson. 1945. The effect of castration and sex hormones upon the incidence of lymphomatosis in chickens. Poult Sci 24:509–515.

44. Burmester, B.R., and Purchase. 1979. The history of avian medicine in the United States. V. Insights into avian tumor virus research. Avian Dis 23:1–29.

45. Burmester, B.R., and W.G. Walter. 1961. Occurrence of visceral lymphomatosis in chickens inoculated with Rous sarcoma virus. J Nat Cancer Inst 26:511–518.

46. Burmester, B.R., and N.F. Waters. 1956. Variation in the presence of the virus of visceral lymphomatosis in the eggs of the same hens. Poult Sci 35:939–944.

47. Burmester, B.R., and Witter, R.L. 1971. An outline of the common neoplastic diseases of the chicken. USDA Prod Res Rep 129, pp. 8.

48. Burmester, B.R., M.A. Gross, W.G. Walter, and A.K. Fontes. 1959. Pathogenicity of a viral strain (RPL 12) causing avian visceral lymphomatosis and related neoplasms. II. Host-virus interrelations affecting response. J Nat Cancer Inst 22:103–127.

49. Burmester, B.R., W.G. Walter, M.A. Gross, and A.K. Fontes. 1959. The oncogenic spectrum of two 'pure' strains of avian leukosis. J Nat Cancer Inst 23:277–291.

50. Burmester, B.R., A.K. Fontes, and W.G. Walter. 1960. Pathogenicity of a viral strain (RPL 12) causing avian visceral lymphomatosis and related neoplasms. III. Influence of host age and route of inoculation. J Nat Cancer Inst 24:1423–1442.

51. Burstein, H., M. Gilead, U. Bendheim, and M. Kotler. 1984. Viral aetiology of haemangiosarcoma outbreaks among layer hens. Avian Pathol 13:715–726.

52. Butterfield, E.E. 1905. Aleukaemic lymphadenoid tumors of the hen. Folia Haematol 2:649–657.

53. Calnek, B.W. 1964. Morphological alteration of RIF-infected chick embryo fibroblasts. Nat Cancer Inst Monogr 17:425–447.

54. Calnek, B.W. 1968. Lymphoid leukosis virus: A survey of commercial breeding flocks for genetic resistance and incidence of embryo infection. Avian Dis 12:104–111.

55. Calnek, B.W. 1968. Lesions in young chickens induced by lymphoid leukosis virus. Avian Dis 12:111–129.

56. Campbell, J.G. 1961. A proposed classification of the leucosis complex and fowl paralysis. Br Vet J 117:316–325.

57. Campbell, J.G. 1963. Virus induced tumours in fowls. Proc R Soc Med 56:305–307.
58. Campbell, J.G., and E.C. Appleby. 1966. Tumours in young chickens bred for rapid body growth (broiler chickens): A study of 351 cases. J Pathol Bacteriol 92:77–90.
59. Caparini, U. 1896. Fetati leucemici nei polli. Clin Vet (Milan) 19:433–435.
60. Carr, J.G. 1956. Renal adenocarcinoma induced by fowl leukemia virus. Br J Cancer 10:379–383.
61. Carr, J.G. 1960. Kidney carcinomas of the fowl induced by the MH2 reticuloendothelioma virus. Br J Cancer 14:77–82.
62. Carter, J.K., and R.E. Smith. 1984. Specificity of avian leukosis virus-induced hyperlipidemia. J Virol 50:301–308.
63. Chabot, J.F., D. Beard, A.J. Langlois, and J.W. Beard. 1970. Mesotheliomas of peritoneum, epicardium, and pericardium induced by strain MC29 avian leukosis virus. Cancer Res 30:1287–1308.
64. Chen, Y.C., and P.K. Vogt. 1977. Endogenous leukosis viruses in the avian family Phasianidae. Virology 76:740–750.
65. Cheville, N.F., W. Okazaki, P.D. Lukert, and H.G. Purchase, 1978. Prevention of avian lymphoid leukosis by induction of bursal atrophy with infectious bursal disease viruses. Vet Pathol 15:376–382.
66. Chubb, R.C., and P.M. Biggs. 1968. The neutralization of Rous sarcoma virus. J Gen Virol 3:87–96.
67. Clark, D.P., and R.M. Dougherty. 1980. Detection of avian oncovirus group-specific antigens by the enzyme-linked immunosorbent assay. J Gen Virol 47:283–291.
68. Collins, W.H., W.E. Briles, R.M. Zsigray, W.R. Dunlop, A.C. Corbett, K.K. Clark, J.L. Marks, and T.P. McGrail. 1977. The B locus (MHC) in the chicken: Association with the fate of RSV-induced tumors. Immunogenetics 5:333–343.
69. Cooper, G.M. 1982. Cellular transforming genes. Science 217:801–806.
70. Cooper, M.D., L.N. Payne, P.B. Dent, B.R. Burmester, and R.A. Good. 1968. Pathogenesis of avian lymphoid leukosis. I. Histogenesis. J Nat Cancer Inst 41:373–389.
71. Cooper, M.D., H.G. Purchase, D.E. Bockman, and W.E. Gathings. 1974. Studies on the nature of the abnormality of B cell differentiation in avian lymphoid leukosis: Production of heterogeneous IgM by tumor cells. J Immunol 113:1210–1222.
72. Cottral, G.E., B.R. Burmester, and N.F. Waters. 1954. Egg transmission of avian lymphomatosis. Poult Sci 33:1174–1184.
73. Crittenden, L.B. 1968. Avian tumor viruses: Prospects for control. World's Poult Sci J 24:18–36.
74. Crittenden, L.B. 1975. Two levels of genetic resistance to lymphoid leukosis. Avian Dis 19:281–292.
75. Crittenden, L.B. 1981. Exogenous and endogenous leukosis virus genes—a review. Avian Pathol 10:101–112.
76. Crittenden, L.B., and S.M. Astrin. 1981. Genes, viruses and avian leukosis. Bioscience 31:305–310.
77. Crittenden, L.B., and A.M. Fadly. 1985. Response of chickens lacking or expressing endogenous avian leukosis virus genes to infection with exogenous virus. Poult Sci 64:454–463.
78. Crittenden, L.B., and H.-J. Kung. 1984. Mechanism of induction of lymphoid leukosis and related neoplasms by avian leukosis viruses. In J.M. Goldman and O. Jarrett (eds.), Mechanisms of Viral Leukaemogenesis, pp. 64–88. Churchill Livingstone, Edinburgh.
79. Crittenden, L.B., and J.V. Motta. 1969. A survey of genetic resistance to leukosis sarcoma viruses in commercial stocks of chickens. Poult Sci 48:1751–1757.
80. Crittenden, L.B., and W. Okazaki. 1966. Genetic influence of the Rs locus on susceptibility to avian tumor viruses. II. Rous sarcoma virus antibody production after strain RPL12 virus inoculation. J Nat Cancer Inst 36:299–303.
81. Crittenden, L.B., and H.G. Purchase, 1974. Unpublished data.
82. Crittenden, L.B., and Smith, E.J. 1984. A comparison of test materials for differentiating avian leukosis virus group-specific antigens of exogenous and endogenous origin. Avian Dis 28:1057–1070.
83. Crittenden, L.B., and R.L. Witter. 1978. Studies of flocks with high mortality from lymphoid leukosis. Avian Dis 22:16–23.
84. Crittenden, L.B., W. Okazaki, and R. Reamer. 1963. Genetic resistance to Rous sarcoma virus in embryo cell cultures and embryos. Virology 20:541–544.
85. Crittenden, L.B., E.J. Wendel, and D. Ratzsch. 1971. Genetic resistance to the avian leukosis-sarcoma virus group: Determining the phenotype of adult birds. Avian Dis 15:503–507.
86. Crittenden, L.B., H.G. Purchase, J.J. Solomon, W. Okazaki, and B.R. Burmester. 1972. Genetic control of susceptibility to the avian leukosis complex. I. The leukosis-sarcoma virus group. Poult Sci 51:242–267.
87. Crittenden, L.B., E.J. Wendel, and J.V. Motta. 1973. Interaction of genes controlling resistance to RSV(RAV-0). Virology 52:373–384.
88. Crittenden, L.B., J.V. Motta, and E.J. Smith. 1977. Genetic control of RAV-0 production in chickens. Virology 76:90–97.
89. Crittenden, L.B., D.A. Eagen, and F.A. Gulvas. 1979. Assays for endogenous and exogenous lymphoid leukosis viruses and chick helper factor with RSV(-) cell lines. Infect Immun 24:379–386.
90. Crittenden, L.B., A.M. Fadly, and E.J. Smith. 1982. Effect of endogenous leukosis virus genes on response to infection with avian leukosis and reticuloendotheliosis viruses. Avian Dis 26:279–294.
91. Crittenden, L.B., W. Okazaki, and E.J. Smith. 1983. Incidence of avian leukosis virus infection in broiler stocks and its effect on early growth. Poult Sci 62:2383–2386.
92. Crittenden, L.B., E.J. Smith, and A.M. Fadly. 1984. Influence of endogenous viral (ev) gene expression and strain of exogenous avian leukosis virus (ALV) on mortality and ALV infection and shedding in chickens. Avian Dis 28:1037–1056.
93. Crittenden, L.B., E.J. Smith, and W. Okazaki. 1984. Identification of broiler breeders congenitally transmitting avian leukosis virus by enzyme-linked immunosorbent assay. Poult Sci 63:492–496.
94. Crittenden, L.B., S. McMahon, M.S. Halpern, and A.M. Fadly. 1987. Embryonic infection with the endogenous avian leukosis virus Rous-associated virus-0 alters responses to exogenous avian leukosis virus infection. J Virol 612:722–725.
95. Cummins, T.J., and R.E. Smith. 1988. Analysis of hematopoietic and lymphopoietic tissue during a regenerative aplastic crisis induced by avian retrovirus MAV-2(0). Virology 163:452–461.
96. Dales, S., and H. Hanafusa. 1972. Penetration and intracellular release of the genomes of avian RNA tumor viruses. Virology 50:440–458.
97. Darcel, C. le Q. 1957. A note on the classification of the leucotic diseases of the fowl. Can J Comp Med 21:145–159.
98. de Boer, G.F. (ed.), 1987. Avian Leukosis, 292pp. Martinus Nijhoff, Boston.

99. de Boer, G.F. 1987. Approaches to control of avian lymphoid leukosis. In G.F. de Boer (ed.), Avian Leukosis, pp. 261-286. Martinus Nijhoff, Boston.

100. de Boer, G.F., J van Vloten, and D. van Zaane. 1980. Possible horizontal spread of lymphoid leukosis virus during vaccination against Marek's disease. In P.M. Biggs (ed.), Resistance and Immunity to Marek's Disease, pp. 552-565. C.E.C. Luxembourg.

101. de Boer, G.F., O.J.H. Devos, and H.J.L. Maas. 1981. The incidence of lymphoid leukosis in chickens in the Netherlands. Zootechnica Intern 10:32-35.

102. Dent, P.B., M.D. Cooper, L.N. Payne, R.A. Good, and B.R. Burmester. 1967. Characterization of avian lymphoid leukosis as a malignancy of the bursal lymphoid system. Perspect Virol 5:251-265.

103. DiStefano, H.S., and R.M. Dougherty. 1966. Mechanisms for congenital transmission of avian leukosis virus. J Nat Cancer Inst 37:869-883.

104. DiStefano, H.S., and R.M. Dougherty. 1968. Multiplication of avian leukosis virus in the reproductive system of the rooster. J Nat Cancer Inst 41:451-464.

105. Dmochowski, L., C.E. Grey, F. Padgett, P.L. Langford, and B.R. Burmester. 1964. Submicroscopic morphology of avian neoplasms. VI. Comparative studies on Rous sarcoma, visceral lymphomatosis, erythroblastosis, myeloblastosis, and nephroblastoma. Tex Rep Biol Med 22:20-60.

106. Dougherty, R.M. 1961. Heat inactivation of Rous sarcoma virus. Virology 14:371-372.

107. Dougherty, R.M. 1987. A historical review of avian retrovirus research. In G.F. de Boer (ed.), Avian Leukosis, pp. 1-27. Martinus Nijhoff, Boston.

108. Dougherty, R.M., and H.S. DiStefano. 1967. Sites of avian leukosis virus multiplication in congenitally infected chickens. Cancer Res 27:322-332.

109. Dougherty, R.M., J.A. Stewart, and H.R. Morgan. 1960. Quantitative studies of the relationships between infecting dose of Rous sarcoma virus, antiviral immune response, and tumor growth in chickens. Virology 11:349-370.

110. Dougherty, R.M., H.S. DiStefano, and A.A. Marucci. 1974. Application of soluble antigen-antibody complexes to the immune histochemical study of avian leukosis virus antigen. In E. Kurstak and R. Morisset (eds.), Viral Immunodiagnosis, pp. 88-99. Academic Press, New York, London.

111. Dren, Cs.N., and I. Nemeth. 1987. Demonstration of immunoglobulin M on avian lymphoid leukosis lymphoma cells by the unlabelled antibody peroxidase-antiperoxidase method. Avian Pathol 16:253-268.

112. Eckert, E.A., D. Beard, and J.W. Beard. 1953. Dose response relations in experimental transmission of avian myeloblastic leukosis. II. Host response to whole blood and to washed primitive cells. J Nat Cancer Inst 13:1167-1184.

113. Eckert, E.A., D. Beard, and J.W. Beard. 1954. Dose-response relations in experimental transmission of avian erythromyeloblastic leukosis III. Titration of the virus. J. Nat Cancer Inst. 14:1055-1066.

114. Eckert, E.A., I. Green, D.G. Sharp, D. Beard, and J.W. Beard. 1955. Virus of avian erythromyeloblastic leukosis. VII. Thermal stability of virus infectivity; of the virus particle; and of the enzyme dephosphorylating adenosinetriphosphate. J Nat Cancer Inst 16:153-161.

115. Ellermann, V. 1921. Histogenese der uebertragbaren Huehner leukose II. Die intravaskulere lymphoide leukose. Folia Haematol 26:165-175.

116. Ellermann, V. 1921. The Leucosis of Fowls and Leukemia Problems. Gyldendal, London.

117. Ellermann, V. 1923. Histogenese der uebertragbaren Huehnerleukose. IV. Zusammenfassende Betrachtungen. Folia Haematol 29:203-212.

118. Ellermann, V., and O. Bang. 1908. Experimentelle Leukamie bei Huhnern. Zentralbl Bakteriol Parasitenkd Infektionskr Hyg Abt J Orig 46:595-609.

119. Elmubarak, A.K., J.M. Sharma, R.L. Witter, L.B. Crittenden, and Sanger, V.L. 1983. Comparative response of turkeys and chickens to avian lymphoid leukosis virus. Avian Pathol 12:235-245.

120. Engelbreth-Holm, J., and A. Rothe-Meyer. 1932. II. Ueber den Zusammenhang zwischen den verschiedenen Huhnerleukosefornen (Anamie-erythroblastose-myelose). Acta Pathol Microbiol Scand 9:312-332.

121. Enrietto, P.J., and M.J. Hayman. 1987. Structure and virus-associated oncogenes of avian sarcoma and leukemia viruses. In G.F. de Boer (ed.), Avian Leukosis, pp. 29-46. Martinus Nijhoff, Boston.

122. Estola, T., K. Sandelin, A. Vaheri, E. Ruoslahti, and J. Suni. 1974. Radioimmunoassay for detecting group-specific avian RNA tumor virus antigens and antibodies. Dev Biol Stand 25:115-118.

123. Fadly, A.M. 1987. Differential diagnosis of lymphoid leukosis. In G.F de Boer (ed.), Avian Leukosis, pp. 197-211. Martinus Nijhoff, Boston.

124. Fadly, A.M. 1988. Avian leukosis virus (ALV) infection, shedding, and tumors in maternal ALV antibody-positive and -negative chickens exposed to virus at hatching. Avian Dis 32:89-95.

125. Fadly, A.M., W. Okazaki, E.J. Smith, and L.B. Crittenden. 1981. Relative efficiency of test procedures to detect lymphoid leukosis virus infection. Poult Sci 60:2037-2044.

126. Fadly, A.M., W. Okazaki, and R.L. Witter. 1981. Hatchery-related contact transmission and short-term small-group-rearing as related to lymphoid-leukosis-virus-eradication programs. Avian Dis 25:667-677.

127. Fadly, A.M., L.F. Lee, and L.D. Bacon. 1982. Immunocompetence of chickens during early and tumorigenic stages of Rous-associated virus-1 infection. Infect Immun 37:1156-1161.

128. Fadly, A.M., W. Okazaki, and L.B. Crittenden. 1983. Avian leukosis virus infection and congenital transmission in lines of chickens resisting selection for reduced shedding. Avian Dis 27:584-593.

129. Fadly, A.M., R.L. Witter, and L.F. Lee. 1985. Effects of chemically or virus-induced immunodepression on response of chickens to avian leukosis virus. Avian Dis 29:12-25.

130. Feldman, W.H. 1932. Neoplasms of Domesticated Animals. W.B. Saunders, Philadelphia.

131. Feldman, W.H., and C. Olson. 1933. Keratinizing embryonal nephroma of the kidneys of the chicken. Am J Cancer 19:47-55.

132. Frank, R.M., and R.M. Franklin. 1982. Electron microscopy of avian osteopetrosis induced by retrovirus MAV.2-0. Calcif Tissue Int 34:382-390.

133. Franklin, R.M., and M.T. Martin. 1980. In ovo tumorigenesis induced by avian osteopetrosis virus. Virology 105:245-249.

134. Fredrickson, T.N., H.G. Purchase, and B.R. Burmester. 1964. Transmission of virus from field cases of avian lymphomatosis. III. Variation in the oncogenic spectra of passaged virus isolates. Nat Cancer Inst Monogr 17:1-29.

135. Fredrickson, T.N., B.R. Burmester, and W. Okazaki. 1965. Transmission of virus from field cases of avian lymphomatosis. II. Development of strains by serial passage in line 15I chickens. Avian Dis 9:82-103.

136. Friesen, B., and H. Rubin. 1961. Some physicochemical and immunological properties of an avian

leucosis virus (RIF). Virology 15:387-396.
137. Frisby, D.P., R.A. Weiss, M. Roussel, and D. Stehelin. 1979. The distribution of endogenous chicken retrovirus sequences in the DNA of galliform birds does not coincide with avian phylogenetic relationships. Cell 17:623-634.
138. Frisby, D., R. MacCormick, and R. Weiss. 1980. Origin of RAV-0. The endogenous retrovirus of chickens. Cold Spring Harbor Conf on Cell Proliferation 7:509-517.
139. Fujita, D.J., Y.C. Chen, R.R. Friis, and P.K. Vogt. 1974. RNA tumor viruses of pheasants: Characterization of avian leukosis subgroups F and G. Virology 60:558-571.
140. Fung, Y.-K.T., W.G. Lewis, L.B. Crittenden, and H.-J. Kung. 1983. Activation of the cellular oncogene c-erbB by LTR insertion: Molecular basis of induction of erythroblastosis by avian leukosis virus. Cell 33:357-368.
141. Furth, J. 1931. Erythroleukosis and the anemias of the fowl. Arch Pathol 12:1-30.
142. Furth, J. 1933. Lymphomatosis, myelomatosis, and endothelioma of chickens caused by a filterable agent. J Exp Med 58:253-275.
143. Gavora, J.S. 1987. Influences of avian leukosis virus infection on production and mortality and the role of genetic selection in the control of lymphoid leukosis. In G.F. de Boer (ed.), Avian Leukosis, pp. 241-60. Martinus Nijhoff, Boston.
144. Gavora, J.S., J.L. Spencer, R.S. Gowe, and D.L. Harris. 1980. Lymphoid leukosis virus infection: Effects on production and mortality and consequences in selection for high egg production. Poult Sci 59:2165-2178.
145. Gavora, J., J. Spencer, and J. Chambers. 1982. Performance of meat-type chickens test-positive and -negative for lymphoid leukosis virus infection. Avian Pathol 11:29-38.
146. Gilka, F., and J.L. Spencer. 1985. Viral matrix inclusion bodies in myocardium of lymphoid leukosis virus-infected chickens. Amer J Vet Res 46:1953-1960.
147. Gilka, F., and J.L. Spencer. 1987. Importance of the medullary macrophage in the replication of lymphoid leukosis virus in the bursa of Fabricius of chickens. Am J Vet Res 48:613-620.
148. Goodenow, M.M., and W.S. Hayward. 1987. 5′ long terminal repeats of myc-associated proviruses appear structurally intact but are functionally impaired in tumors induced by avian leukosis viruses. J Virol 61:2489-2498.
149. Graf, T. 1972. A plaque assay for avian RNA tumor viruses. Virology 50:567-578.
150. Graf, T. 1975. In vitro transformation of chicken bone marrow cells with avian erythroblastosis virus. Z. Naturforsch 30:847-849.
151. Graf, T., and H. Beug. 1978. Avian leukemia viruses. Interaction with their target cells in vivo and in vitro. Biochim Biophys Acta 516:269-299.
152. Graf, T., B. Royer-Pokora, G.E. Schubert, and H. Beug. 1976. Evidence for the multiple oncogenic potential of cloned leukemia virus: In vitro and in vivo studies with avian erythroblastosis virus. Virology 71:423-433.
153. Graf, T., D. Fink, H. Beug, and B. Royer-Pokora. 1977. Oncornavirus-induced sarcoma formation obscured by rapid development of lethal leukemia. Cancer Res 37:59-63.
154. Graf, T., H. Beug, M. Roussel, S. Saule, D. Stehelin, and M.J. Hayman. 1980. Avian leukaemia viruses and haematopoietic cell differentiation. Br J Cancer 41:659-661.
155. Gross, M.A., B.R. Burmester, and W.G. Walter. 1959. Pathogenicity of a viral strain (RPL12) causing avian visceral lymphomatosis and related neoplasms. I. Nature of the lesions. J Nat Cancer Inst 22:83-101.
156. Groupé, V., F.J. Rauscher, A.S. Levine, and W.R. Bryan. 1956. The brain of newly hatched chicks as a host-virus system for biological studies on the Rous sarcoma virus (RSV). J Nat Cancer Inst 16:865-876.
157. Gudkov, A.V., E. Korec, M.V. Chernov, A.T. Tikhonenko, I.B. Obukh, and I. Hlozanek. 1986. Genetic structure of the endogenous proviruses and expression of the gag gene in Brown Leghorn chickens. Folia Biol (Praha) 32:65-72.
158. Haguenau, F., and J.W. Beard. 1962. The avian sarcoma-leukosis complex: Its biology and ultrastructure. In A.J. Dalton and F. Haguenau (eds.), Tumors Induced by Viruses, pp. 1-59. Academic Press, New York.
159. Hall, W.J., C.W. Bean, and M. Pollard. 1941. Transmission of fowl leucosis through chick embryos and young chicks. Am J Vet Res 2:272-279.
160. Hamilton, C.M., and C.E. Sawyer, 1939. Transmission of erythroleukosis in young chickens. Poult Sci 18:388-393.
161. Hanafusa, H. 1975. Avian RNA tumor viruses. In F.F. Becker (ed.), Cancer: A Comprehensive Treatise. Vol. 2: Etiology–Viral Carcinogenesis, pp. 49-90. Plenum, New York.
162. Hanafusa, T., and H. Hanafusa. 1973. Isolation of leukosis-type virus from pheasant embryo cells: Possible presence of viral genes in cells. Virology 51:247-251.
163. Hanafusa, T., H. Hanafusa, C.E. Metroka, W.S. Hayward, C.W. Rettemier, R.C. Sawyer, R.M. Dougherty, and H.S. DiStefano. 1976. Pheasant virus: New class of ribodeoxyvirus. Proc Nat Acad Sci USA 73:1333-1337.
164. Harris, D.L., V.A. Garwood, P.C. Lowe, P.Y. Hester, L.B. Crittenden, and A.M. Fadly. 1984. Influence of sex-linked feathering phenotypes of parents and progeny upon lymphoid leukosis virus infection status and egg production. Poult Sci 63:401-413.
165. Hayward, W.S., and B.G. Neel. 1981. Retroviral gene expression. Curr Top Microbiol Immunol 217-276.
166. Hihara, H., H. Yamamoto, H. Shimohira, K. Arai, and T. Shimizu. 1983. Avian erythroblastosis virus isolated from chick erythroblastosis induced by lymphatic leukemia virus subgroup A. J Nat Cancer Inst 70:891-897.
167. Hirota, Y., M.T. Martin, M. Viljanen, P. Toivanen, and R.M. Franklin. 1980. Immunopathology of chickens infected in ovo and at hatching with the avian osteopetrosis virus MAV 2-0. Eur J Immunol 10:929-936.
168. Holmes, J.R. 1964. Avian osteopetrosis. Nat Cancer Inst Monogr 17:63-79.
169. Hughes, W.F., D.H. Watanabe, and H. Rubin. 1963. The development of a chicken flock apparently free of leukosis virus. Avian Dis 7:154-165.
170. Ignjatovic J. 1986. Replication-competent endogenous avian leukosis virus in commercial lines of meat chickens. Avian Dis 30:264-270.
171. Ignjatovic J. 1988. Isolation of a variant endogenous avian leukosis virus: Non-productive exogenous infection with endogenous viruses containing p27 and p27o. J Gen Virol 69:641-649.
172. Ignjatovic J., R.A. Fraser, and T.J. Bagust. 1986. Effect of lymphoid leukosis virus on performance of layer hens and the identification of infected chickens by tests on meconia. Avian Pathol 15:63-74.
173. Ishiguro, H., D. Beard, J.R. Sommer, U. Heine, G. de Thé, and J.W. Beard. 1962. Multiplicity of cell

response to the BAI strain A (myeloblastosis) avian tumor virus. I. Nephroblastoma (Wilms' tumor): Gross and microscopic pathology. J Nat Cancer Inst 29:1-39.
174. Ishizaki, R., A.J. Langlois, and D.P. Bolognesi, 1975. Isolation of two subgroup-specific leukemogenic viruses from standard avian myeloblastosis virus. J Virol 15:906-12.
175. Jungherr, E.L. 1941. Tentative pathologic nomenclature for the disease complex variously designated as fowl leucemia, fowl leucosis, etc. Am J Vet Res 2:116.
176. Jungherr, E.L., and W. Landauer. 1938. Studies on fowl paralysis. III. A condition resembling osteopetrosis (marble bone) in the common fowl. Storrs Agric Exp Stn Bull 222.
177. Kakuk, T.J., F.R. Frank, T.E. Weddon, B.R. Burmester. H.G. Purchase, and C.H. Romero. 1977. Avian lymphoid leukosis prophylaxis with Mibolerone. Avian Dis 21:280-289.
178. Kanter, M.R., R.E. Smith, and W.S. Hayward. 1988. Rapid induction of B-cell lymphomas: Insertional activation of c-myb by avian leukosis virus. J Virol 62:1423-1432.
179. Kawai, S., and H. Hanafusa. 1972. Plaque assay for some strains of avian leukosis virus. Virology 48:126-135.
180. Kelloff, G., and P.K. Vogt. 1966. Localization of avian tumor virus group-specific antigen in cell and virus. Virology 29:377-384.
181. Kelloff, G., M. Hatanaka, and R.V. Gilden. 1972. Assay of C-type virus infectivity by measurement of RNA-dependent DNA polymerase activity. Virology 48:266-269.
182. Kirev, T.T. 1988. Neoplastic response of guinea fowl to osteopetrosis virus strain MAV-2(0). Avian Pathol 17:101-112.
183. Kitt, T. 1931. Die leukomyelose der Huehner. Mikrobiol Immunitaetsforsch Exp Ther 12:15-29.
184. Kumanishi, T., F. Ikuta, K. Nishida, K. Ueki, and T. Yamamoto. 1973. Brain tumors induced in adult monkeys by Schmidt-Ruppin strain of Rous sarcoma virus. Gann 64:641-643.
185. Kung, H.-J., and N.J. Maihle. 1987. Molecular basis of oncogenesis by nonacute avian retroviruses. In G.F. de Boer (ed.), Avian Leukosis, pp. 77-99. Martinus Nijhoff, Boston.
186. Labat, M.L. 1986. Retroviruses, immunosuppression and osteopetrosis. Biomed Pharm 40:85-90.
187. Lagerlof, B., and P. Sundelin. 1963. The histogenesis and haematology of virus-induced myeloid leukemia in the fowl. Acta Haematol 30:111-122.
188. Langlois, A.J., K. Lapis, R. Ishizaki, J.W. Beard, and D.P. Bolognesi. 1974. Isolation of a transplantable cell line induced by the MC29 avian leukosis virus. Cancer Res 34:1457-1464.
189. Langlois, A.M., R. Ishizaki, G.S. Beaudreau, J.F. Kummer, J.W. Beard, and D.P. Bolognesi. 1976. Virus infected avian cell lines established in vitro. Cancer Res 36:3894-3904.
190. Lapis, K. 1979. Histology and ultrastructural aspects of virus-induced primary liver cancer and transplantable hepatomas of viral origin in chickens. J Toxicol Environ Health 5:469-501.
191. Lapis, K., D. Beard, and J.W. Beard. 1975. Transplantation of hepatomas induced in the avian liver by MC29 leukosis virus. Cancer Res 35:132-138.
192. Lee, L.F., R.F. Silva, Y.-Q. Cheng, E.J. Smith, and L.B. Crittenden. 1986. Characterisation of monoclonal antibodies to avian leukosis viruses. Avian Dis 30:132-138.
193. Levine, S., and D. Nelsen. 1964. RIF infection in a commercial flock of chickens. Avian Dis 8:358-368.
194. Maas, H.J.L., G.F. de Boer, and J.E. Groenendal. 1982. Age related resistance to avian leukosis virus. III. Infectious virus, neutralising antibody, and tumours in chickens inoculated at various ages. Avian Pathol 11:309-327.
195. Mathews, F.P. 1929. Leukochloroma in the common fowl. Its relation to myelogenic leukemia and its analogies to chloroma in man. Arch Pathol 7:442-457.
196. Mathey, W.J. 1977. Personal communication.
197. Matthews, R.E.F. 1982. Fourth report of the international committee on taxonomy of viruses. Classification and nomenclature of viruses. Intervirology 17, Nos. 1-3.
198. McBride, M.A.T., and R.M. Shuman. 1988. Immune response of chickens inoculated with a recombinant avian leukosis virus. Avian Dis 32:96-102.
199. Meyers, P. 1976. Antibody response to related leukosis viruses induced in chickens tolerant to an avian leukosis virus. J Nat Cancer Inst 56:381-386.
200. Mizuno, Y., and H. Hatakeyama. 1983. Detection of antibodies against avian leukosis viruses with indirect immunoperoxidase absorbance test. Jpn J Vet Sci 45:31-37.
201. Mizuno, Y., and S. Itohara. 1986. Enzyme-linked immunosorbent assay to detect subgroup-specific antibodies to avian leukosis viruses. Amer J Vet Res 47:551-556.
202. Mladenov, Z. 1980. Comparative pathology of avian leukosis. In D.S. Yohn, B.A. Lapin, and J.R. Blakeslee (eds.), Advances in Comparative Leukemia Research, pp. 131-132. Elsevier/North Holland Biomedical Press, Amsterdam.
203. Mladenov, Z., U. Heine, D. Beard, and J.W. Beard. 1967. Strain MC29 avian leukosis virus. Myelocytoma, endothelioma, and renal growths: Pathomorphological and ultrastructural aspects. J Nat Cancer Inst 38:251-285.
204. Moloney, J.B. 1956. Biological studies on the Rous sarcoma virus. V. Preparation of improved standard lots of the virus for use in quantitative investigations. J Nat Cancer Inst 16:877-888.
205. Morgan, H.R. 1973. Avian leukosis-sarcoma virus antibodies in wildfowl, domestic chickens, and man in Kenya. Proc Soc Exp Biol Med 144:1-4.
206. Moscovici, C. 1975. Leukemic transformation with avian myeloblastosis virus: Present status. Curr Top Microbiol Immunol 71:79-101.
207. Moscovici, C., and L. Gazzolo. 1987. Virus-cell interactions of avian sarcoma and defective leukemia viruses. In G.F. de Boer (ed.), Avian Leukosis, pp. 151-169. Martinus Nijhoff, Boston.
208. Moscovici, M.G., and C. Moscovici. 1980. AMV-induced transformation of hemopoietic cells: Growth patterns of producers and nonproducers. In G.B. Rossi (ed.), In Vivo and In Vitro Erythropoiesis: The Friend System, pp. 503-514. Elsevier/North Holland Biomedical Press, Amsterdam.
209. Moscovici, C., L. Gazzolo, and M.G. Moscovici. 1975. Focus assay and defectiveness of avian myeloblastosis virus. Virology 68:173-181.
210. Motta, J.V., L.B. Crittenden, and W.O. Pollard. 1973. The inheritance of resistance to subgroup C leukosis-sarcoma viruses in New Hampshire chickens. Poult Sci 52:578-586.
211. Motta, J.V., L.B. Crittenden, H.G. Purchase, H.A. Stone, and R.L. Witter. 1975. Low oncogenic potential of avian endogenous RNA tumor virus infection or expression. J Nat Cancer Inst 55:685-689.
212. Nakamura, K., F. Abe, H. Hihara, and T. Taniguchi. 1988. Myocardial cytoplasmic inclusions in chick-

ens with haemangioma and lymphoid leukosis. Avian Pathol 17:3-10.

213. Neiman, P.E., L. Jordan, R.A. Weiss, and L.N. Payne. 1980. Malignant lymphoma of the bursa of Fabricius: Analysis of early transformation. Cold Spring Harbor Conf on Cell Proliferation 7:519-528.

214. Neumann, U., and R.L. Witter. 1979. Differential diagnosis of lymphoid leukosis and Marek's disease by tumor-associated criteria. I. Studies on experimentally infected chickens. Avian Dis 23:417-425.

215. Neumann, U., and R.L. Witter. 1979. Differential diagnosis of lymphoid leukosis and Marek's disease by tumor-associated criteria. II. Studies on field cases. Avian Dis 23:426-433.

216. Nowinski, R.C., E. Fleissner, and N.H. Sarkar. 1973. Structural and serological aspects of the oncornaviruses in Vol. 8 Persistent virus infections. Perspect Virol 8:31-60.

217. Nyfeldt, A. 1934. Etude sur les leucoses des poules. I. Une myeloblastose pure. Sang Biol Pathol 8:566-584.

218. Okazaki, W., H.G. Purchase, and B.R. Burmester. 1975. Phenotypic mixing test to detect and assay avian leukosis viruses. Avian Dis 19:311-317.

219. Okazaki, W., B.R. Burmester, A. Fadly, and W.B. Chase. 1979. An evaluation of methods for eradication of avian leukosis virus from a commercial breeder flock. Avian Dis 23:688-697.

220. Okazaki, W., R.L. Witter, C. Romero, K. Nazerian, J.M. Sharma, A. Fadly, and D. Ewart. 1980. Induction of lymphoid leukosis transplantable tumours and the establishment of lymphoblastoid cell lines. Avian Pathol 9:311-329.

221. Okazaki, W., A. Fadly, B.R. Burmester, W.B. Chase, and L.B. Crittenden. 1980. Shedding of lymphoid leukosis virus in chickens following contact exposure and vaccination. Avian Dis 24:474-480.

222. Okazaki, W., A.M. Fadly, L.B. Crittenden, and W.B. Chase. 1982. The effectiveness of selection for reduced avian leukosis virus shedding in different chicken strains. Avian Dis 26:612-617.

223. Okazaki, W., H.G. Purchase, and L.B. Crittenden. 1982. Pathogenicity of avian leukosis viruses. Avian Dis 26:553-559.

224. Panet, A., D. Baltimore, and T. Hanafusa. 1975. Quantitation of avian RNA tumor virus reverse transcriptase by radioimmunoassay. J Virol 16:146-152.

225. Pani, P.K. 1975. Genetic control of resistance of chick embryo cultures to RSV(RAV 50). J Gen Virol 27:163-172.

226. Pani, P.K. 1976. Further studies in genetic resistance of fowl to RSV(RAV-0): Evidence for interaction between independently segregating tumour virus B and tumour virus E genes. J Gen Virol 32:441-453.

227. Pani, P.K. 1977. Evidence for complementary action of tvb and tve genes that control susceptibility to subgroup E RNA tumour virus in chickens. J Gen Virol 37:639-646.

228. Pani, P.K., and P.M. Biggs, 1973. Genetic control of susceptibility to an A subgroup sarcoma virus in commercial chickens. Avian Pathol 2:27-41.

229. Pappenheimer, A.M., L.C. Dunn, and V. Cone. 1926. A study of fowl paralysis (neuro-lymphomatosis gallinarum). Storrs Agric Exp Stn Bull 143.

230. Payne, L.N. 1981. Immunity to lymphoid leukosis, Rous sarcoma, and reticuloendotheliosis. In M.E. Rose, L.N. Payne, and B.M. Freeman (eds), Avian Immunology, pp. 285-299. British Poultry Science, Edinburgh.

231. Payne, L.N. 1985. Genetics of cell receptors for avian retroviruses. In W.G. Hill, J.M. Manson, and D. Hewitt (eds.), Poultry Genetics and Breeding, pp. 1-16. British Poultry Science, Edinburgh.

232. Payne, L.N. 1987. Epizootiology of avian leukosis virus infections. In G.F. de Boer (ed.), Avian Leukosis, pp. 47-75, Martinus Nijhoff, Boston.

233. Payne, L.N., and N. Bumstead. 1982. Theoretical considerations on the relative importance of vertical and horizontal transmission for the maintenance of infection by exogenous avian lymphoid leukosis virus. Avian Pathol 11:547-553.

234. Payne, L.N., and R.C. Chubb. 1968. Studies on the nature and genetic control of an antigen in normal chick embryos which reacts in the COFAL test. J Gen Virol 3:379-391.

235. Payne, L.N., and P.K. Pani. 1971. Evidence of linkage between genetic loci controlling response of fowl to subgroup A and subgroup C sarcoma viruses. J Gen Virol 13:253-259.

236. Payne, L.N., and M. Rennie. 1975. B cell antigen markers on avian lymphoid leukosis tumour cells. Vet Rec 96:454-456.

237. Payne, F.E., J.J. Solomon, and H.G. Purchase. 1966. Immunofluorescent studies of group-specific antigen of the avian sarcoma-leukosis viruses. Proc Nat Acad Sci USA 55:341-349.

238. Payne, L.N., P.K. Pani, and R.A. Weiss. 1971. A dominant epistatic gene which inhibits cellular susceptibility to RSV(RAV-0). J Gen Virol 13:455-462.

239. Payne, L.N., A.E. Holmes, K. Howes, M. Pattison, D.L. Pollock, and D.E. Waters. 1982. Further studies on the eradication and epizootiology of lymphoid leukosis virus infection in a commercial strain of chickens. Avian Pathol 11:145-162.

240. Payne, L.N., K. Howes, and D.F. Adene. 1985. A modified feather pulp culture method for determining the genetic susceptibility of adult chickens to leukosis-sarcoma viruses. Avian Pathol 14:261-267.

241. Pentimalli, F. 1915. Ueber die Geschwuelste bei Huehnern. I. Mitteilung. Allgemeine Morphologie der spontanen und der transplantablen Huehnergeschwuelste. Z Krebsforsch 15:111-153.

242. Perek, M. 1960. An epizootic of histiocytic sarcomas in chickens induced by a cell-free agent. Avian Dis 4:85-94.

243. Peterson, R.D.A., H.G. Purchase, B.R. Burmester, M.D. Cooper, and R.A. Good. 1966. Relationships among visceral lymphomatosis, bursa of Fabricius, and bursa-dependent lymphoid tissue of the chicken. J Nat Cancer Inst 36:585-598.

244. Piraino, F. 1967. The mechanism of genetic resistance of chick embryo cells to infection by Rous sarcoma virus-Bryan strain (BS-RSV). Virology 32:700-707.

245. Piraino, F., W. Okazaki, B.R. Burmester, and T.N. Fredrickson. 1963. Bioassay of fowl leukosis virus in chickens by the inoculation of 11-day-old embryos. Virology 21:396-401.

246. Ponten, J. 1962. Transmission in vivo of chicken erythroblastosis by intact cells. J Cell Comp Physiol 60:209-215.

247. Ponten, J. 1964. The in vivo growth mechanism of avian Rous sarcoma. Nat Cancer Inst Monogr 17:131-145.

248. Ponten, J., and B.R. Burmester. 1967. Transplantability of primary tumors of RPL12 virus-induced lymphoid leukosis. J Nat Cancer Inst 38:505-513.

249. Ponten, J., and B. Thorell. 1957. The histogenesis of virus-induced chicken leukemia. J Nat Cancer Inst 18:443-454.

250. Powell, P.C., L.N. Payne, J.A. Frazier, and M. Rennie. 1974. T lymphoblastoid cell lines from Marek's

disease lymphomas. Nature 251:79-80.
251. Price, J.A., and R.E. Smith. 1981. Influence of bursectomy on bone growth and anemia induced by avian osteopetrosis viruses. Cancer Res 41:752-759.
252. Pugh, L.P. 1927. Sporadic diffuse osteoperiostitis in fowls. Vet Rev 7:189-190.
253. Purchase, H.G. 1987. The pathogenesis and pathology of neoplasms caused by avian leukosis viruses. In G.F. de Boer (ed.), Avian Leukosis, pp. 171-196. Martinus Nijhoff, Boston.
254. Purchase, H.G., and N.F. Cheville. 1975. Infectious bursal agent of chickens reduces the incidence of lymphoid leukosis. Avian Pathol 4:239-245.
255. Purchase, H.G., and A.M. Fadly. 1980. Leukosis and sarcomas. In S.B. Hitchner, C.H. Domermuth, H.G. Purchase, and J.E. Williams (eds.), Isolation and Identification of Avian Pathogens, pp. 54-58. Am Assoc Avian Pathol, Kennett Square, PA.
256. Purchase, H.G., and D.G. Gilmour. 1975. Lymphoid leukosis in chickens chemically bursectomized and subsequently inoculated with bursa cells. J Nat Cancer Inst 55:851-855.
257. Purchase, H.G., and W. Okazaki. 1964. Morphology of foci produced by standard preparations of Rous sarcoma virus. J Nat Cancer Inst 32:579-589.
258. Purchase, H.G., and J.M. Sharma. 1973. Slide Study Set 3. Am Assoc Avian Pathol, Kennett Square, PA.
259. Purchase, H.G., W. Okazaki, and B.R. Burmester. 1972. Long-term field trials with the herpesvirus of turkeys vaccine against Marek's disease. Avian Dis 16:57-71.
260. Purchase, H.G., D.G. Gilmour, C.H. Romero, and W. Okazaki. 1977. Post infection genetic resistance to avian lymphoid leukosis resides in a B target cell. Nature 270:61-62.
261. Purchase, H.G., W. Okazaki, P.K. Vogt, H. Hanafusa, B.R. Burmester, and L.B. Crittenden. 1977. Oncogenicity of avian leukosis viruses of different subgroups and of mutants of sarcoma viruses. Infect Immun 15:423-428.
262. Rauscher, F.J., J.A. Reyniers, and M.R. Sacksteder. 1964. Response or lack of response of apparently leukosis-free Japanese quail to avian tumor viruses. Nat Cancer Inst Monogr 17:211-229.
263. Riddell, C., and P.T. Shettigara. 1980. Dermal squamous cell carcinoma in broiler chickens in Saskatchewan. Can Vet J 21:287-289.
264. Rispens, B.H., P.A. Long, W. Okazaki, and B.R. Burmester. 1970. The NP activation test for assay of avian leukosis/sarcoma viruses. Avian Dis 14:738-751.
265. Rispens, B.H., G.F. de Boer, A. Hoogerbrugge, and J. Van Vloten. 1976. A method for the control of lymphoid leukosis in chickens. J Nat Cancer Inst 57:1151-1156.
266. Robinson, H. 1978. Inheritance and expression of chicken genes that are related to avian leukosis sarcoma virus genes. Curr Top Microbiol Immunol 83:1-36.
267. Robinson, W.S., and P.H. Duesberg. 1968. The chemistry of RNA tumor viruses. In H. Fraenkel-Conrat (ed.), Molecular Basis of Virology, pp. 306-331. Reinhold Book, New York.
268. Robinson, H.L., and G.C. Gagnon. 1986. Patterns of proviral insertion in avian leukosis virus induced lymphomas. J Virol 57:28-36.
269. Robinson, H.L., S.M. Astrin, A.M. Senior, and F.H. Salazar. 1981. Host susceptibility to endogenous viruses: Defective, glycoprotein-expressing proviruses interfere with infections. J Virol 40:745-751.
270. Roloff, F. 1868. Mag Ges Thierheilkd 34:190 (cited by Chubb, L.G. and R.F. Gordon. 1957). The avian leukosis complex—a review. Vet Rev Annotations 32:97-120.
271. Romero, C.H., H.G. Purchase, F. Frank, L.B. Crittenden, and T.S. Chang. 1978. The prevention of natural and experimental avian lymphoid leukosis with the androgen analogue Mibolerone. Avian Pathol 7:87-103.
272. Rous, P. 1911. A sarcoma of the fowl transmissible by an agent separable from tumor cells. J Exp Med 13:397-411.
273. Rovigatti, V.G., and S.M. Astrin. 1983. Avian endogenous viral genes. Curr Top Microbiol Immunol 103:1-22.
274. Rubin, H. 1960. A virus in chick embryos which induces resistance in vitro to infection with Rous sarcoma virus. Proc Nat Acad Sci USA 46:1105-1119.
275. Rubin, H. 1960. Growth of Rous sarcoma virus in chick embryo cells following irradiation of host cells or free virus. Virology 11:28-47.
276. Rubin, H. 1965. Genetic control of cellular susceptibility to pseudotypes of Rous sarcoma virus. Virology 26:270-276.
277. Rubin, H., A. Cornelius, and L. Fanshier. 1961. The pattern of congenital transmission of an avian leukosis virus. Proc Nat Acad Sci USA 47:1058-1060.
278. Rubin, H., L. Fanshier, A. Cornelius, and W.F. Hughes. 1962. Tolerance and immunity in chickens after congenital and contact infection with an avian leukosis virus. Virology 17:143-156.
279. Rup, B.J., J.D. Hoelzer, and H.R. Bose, Jr. 1982. Helper viruses associated with avian acute leukemia viruses inhibit the cellular immune response. Virology 116:61-71.
280. Sandelin, K., and T. Estola. 1974. Occurrence of different subgroups of avian leukosis virus in Finnish poultry. Avian Pathol 3:159-168.
281. Sandelin, K., T. Estola, S. Ristimaki, E. Ruoslahti, and A. Vaheri. 1974. Radio immunoassays of the group-specific antigen in detection of avian leukosis virus infection. J Gen Virol 25:415-420.
282. Sanger, V.L., T.N. Fredrickson, C.C. Morrill, and B.R. Burmester. 1966. Pathogenesis of osteopetrosis in chickens. Am J Vet Res 27:1735-1744.
283. Sarma, P.S., H.C. Turner, and R.J. Huebner. 1964. An avian leucosis group-specific complement fixation reaction. Application for the detection and assay noncytopathogenic leucosis viruses. Virology 23:313-321.
284. Sarma, P.S., T.S. Log, R.J. Huebner, and H.C. Turner. 1969. Studies of avian leukosis group-specific complement-fixing serum antibodies in pigeons. Virology 37:480-483.
285. Sawyer, R.C., and H. Hanafusa. 1977. Formation of reticuloendotheliosis virus pseudotypes of Rous sarcoma virus. J Virol 22:634-639.
286. Sazawa, H., T. Sugimori, Y. Miura, and T. Shimizu. 1966. Specific complement fixation test of Rous sarcoma with pigeon serum. Nat Inst Anim Health Q 6:208-215.
287. Schierman, L.W., D.H. Watanabe, and R.A. McBride. 1977. Genetic control of Rous sarcoma regression in chickens: Linkage with the major histocompatibility complex. Immunogenetics 5:325-332.
288. Schmeisser, H.C. 1915. Spontaneous and experimental leukemia of the fowl. J Exp Med 22:820-838.
289. Schmidt, E.V., J.D. Crapo, J.R. Harrelson, and R.L. Smith. 1981. A quantitative histologic study of avian osteopetrotic bone demonstrating normal osteoclast numbers and osteoblastic activity. Lab Invest 44:164-173.
290. Segura, J.C., J.S. Gavora, J.L. Spencer, R.W.

Fairfull, R.J. Gowe, and R.B. Buckland. 1988. Semen traits and fertility of White Leghorn males shown to be positive or negative for lymphoid leukosis virus in semen and feather pulp. Br Poult Sci 29:545–553.

291. Shank, P.R., P.J. Schatz, L.M. Jensen, P.N. Tsichlis, J.M. Coffin, and H.L. Robinson. 1985. Sequences in the gag-pol-5′env region of avian leukosis viruses confer the ability to induce osteopetrosis. Virology 145:94–104.

292. Sigel, M.M., P. Meyers, and H.T. Holden. 1971. Resistance to Rous sarcoma elicited by immunization with live virus. Proc Soc Exp Biol Med 137:142–146.

293. Siegfried, L.M., and C. Olson, Jrn. 1972. Characteristics of avian transmissible lymphoid tumor cells maintained in culture. J Nat Cancer Inst 48:791–796.

294. Simon, M.C., W.S. Neckameyer, W.S. Hayward, and R.E. Smith 1987. Genetic determinants of neoplastic diseases induced by a subgroup F avian leukosis virus. J Virol 61:1203–1212.

295. Smith, E.J. 1977. Preparation of antisera to group-specific antigens of avian leukosis-sarcoma viruses: An alternate approach. Avian Dis 21:290–299.

296. Smith, E. J. 1987. Endogenous avian leukemia viruses. In G.F. deBoer (ed.), Avian Leukosis, pp. 101–120. Martinus Nijhoff, Boston.

297. Smith, E.J., A. Fadly, and W. Okazaki. 1979. An enzyme-linked immunosorbent assay for detecting avian leukosis-sarcoma viruses. Avian Dis 23:698–707.

298. Smith, E.J., U. Neumann, and W. Okazaki. 1980. Immune response to avian leukosis virus infection in chickens: Sequential expression of serum immunoglobulins and viral antibodies. Comp Immunol Microbiol Infect Dis 2:519–529.

299. Smith, E.J., A.M. Fadly, and L.B. Crittenden. 1986. Observations on an enzyme-linked immunosorbent assay for the detection of antibodies against avian leukosis-sarcoma viruses. Avian Dis 30:488–493.

300. Smith, E.J., D.W. Salter, R.F. Silva, and L.B. Crittenden. 1986. Selective shedding and congenital transmission of endogenous avian leukosis viruses. J Virol 60:1050–1054.

301. Smith, R.E. 1987. Immunology of avian leukosis virus infections. In G.F. de Boer (ed.), Avian Leukosis, pp. 121–129. Martinus Nijhoff, Boston.

302. Smith, R.E., and E.V. Schmidt. 1982. Induction of anemia by avian leukosis viruses of five subgroups. Virology 117:516–518.

303. Solomon, T.J., B.R. Burmester, and R.N. Fredrickson. 1966. Investigations of lymphoid leukosis infection in genetically similar chicken populations. Avian Dis 10:477–484.

304. Somes, R.G. 1980. Alphabetical list of the genes of domestic fowl. J Hered 71:168–174.

305. Spencer, J.L. 1984. Progress towards eradication of lymphoid leukosis viruses–a review. Avian Pathol 13:599–619.

306. Spencer, J.L. 1987. Laboratory diagnostic procedures for detecting avian leukosis virus infections. In G.F. de Boer (ed.), Avian Leukosis, pp. 213–240. Martinus Nijhoff, Boston.

307. Spencer, J.L., L.B. Crittenden, B.R. Burmester. W. Okazaki, and R.L. Witter. 1977. Lymphoid leukosis: Interrelations among virus infections in hens, eggs, embryos, and chicks. Avian Dis 21:331–345.

308. Spencer, J.L., J.S. Gavora, and R.S Gowe. 1980. Lymphoid leukosis virus: Natural transmission and non-neoplastic effects. Cold Spring Harbor Conf on Cell Proliferation 7:553–564.

309. Spencer, J.L., F. Gilka, and J.S. Gavora. 1983. Detection of lymphoid leukosis virus infected chickens by testing for group specific antigen for virus in feather pulp. Avian Pathol 12:85–99.

310. Spencer, J.L., J.S. Gavora, and F. Gilka. 1987. Feather pulp organ cultures for assessing host resistance to infection with avian leukosis-sarcoma viruses. Avian Pathol 16:425–438.

311. Stephenson, J.R., R.E. Wilsnack, and S.A. Aaronson. 1973. Radioimmunoassay for avian C-type virus group-specific antigen: Detection in normal and virus-transformed cells. J Virol 11:893–899.

312. Stephenson, J.R., E.J. Smith, L.B. Crittenden, and S.A. Aaronson. 1975. Analysis of antigenic determinants of structural polypeptides of avian type C tumor viruses. J Virol 16:27–33.

313. Temin, H.M. 1974. The cellular and molecular biology of RNA tumor viruses, especially avian leukosis-sarcoma viruses, and their relatives. Adv Cancer Res 19:47–104.

314. Temin, H.M. 1974. On the origin of RNA tumor viruses. Annu Rev Genet 8:155–177.

315. Temin, H.M. 1974. The Bertner Foundation Memorial Award Lecture–from proviruses to protoviruses: RNA-directed DNA synthesis by RNA tumor viruses and cells. Molecular Studies in Viral Neoplasia, pp. 7–38. Williams & Wilkins, Baltimore, MD.

316. Temin, H.M., and H. Rubin. 1958. Characteristics of an assay for Rous sarcoma virus and Rous sarcoma cells in tissue culture. Virology 6:669–688.

317. Tereba, A., and K.G. Murti. 1977. A very sensitive biochemical assay for detecting and quantitating avian oncornaviruses. Virology 80:166–176.

318. Tereba, A., L.B. Crittenden, and S.M. Astrin. 1981. Chromosomal localization of three endogenous retrovirus loci associated with virus production in white leghorn chickens. J Virol 39:282–289.

319. Thorell, B. 1958. Induktion von Nierentumoren durch Leukaemievirus. Zentralbl Allg Pathol Pathol Anat 98:98–314.

320. Troesch, C.D., and P.K. Vogt. 1985. An endogenous virus from Lophortyx quail is the prototype for envelope subgroup I of avian retroviruses. Virology 143:595–602.

321. Tsukamoto, K., Y. Kono, and K Arai. 1985. An enzyme linked immunosorbent assay for detection of antibodies to exogenous avian leukosis virus. Avian Dis 29:1118–1129.

322. Turnquest, R.V. 1979. Dermal squamous cell carcinoma in young chickens. Am J Vet Res 40:1628–1633.

323. Vogt, P.K. 1965. Avian tumor viruses. Adv Virus Res 11:293–385.

324. Vogt, P.K., and R. Ishizaki. 1966. Criteria for the classification of avian-tumor viruses. In W.J. Burdett (ed.), Viruses Inducing Cancer, pp. 71–90. Univ Utah Press, Salt Lake City.

325. Wainberg, M.A., and M.S. Halpern. 1987. Avian sarcomas: Immune responsiveness and pathology. In G.F. de Boer (ed.), Avian Leukosis, pp. 131–152. Martinus Nijhoff, Boston.

326. Wainberg, M.A., and E.R. Phillips. 1976. Immunity against avian sarcomas–a review. Isr J Med Sci 12:388–406.

327. Walter, W.G., B.R. Burmester, and C.H. Cunningham. 1962. Studies on the transmission and pathology of a viral-induced avian nephroblastoma (embryonal nephroma). Avian Dis 6:455–477.

328. Wang, L.H., and H. Hanafusa. 1988. Avian sarcoma viruses. Virus Res 9:159–203.

329. Warthin, A.S. 1907. Leukemia of the common fowl. J Infect Dis 4:369–380.

330. Waters, N.F., and B.R. Burmester. 1961. Mode of inheritance of resistance to Rous sarcoma virus in chickens. J Nat Cancer Inst 27:655–661.

331. Watts, S.L., and R.E. Smith. 1980. Pathology of chickens infected with avian nephroblastoma virus MAV-2(N). Infect Immun 27:501-512.
332. Weiss, R.A. 1975. Genetic transmission of RNA tumor viruses. In M. Pollard (ed.), Perspect Virol 9:165-205.
333. Weiss, R.A. 1981. Retrovirus receptors. In K. Longberg-Holm and L. Philipson (eds.), Virus Receptors. Pt. 2: Receptors and Recognition, Ser. B, Vol. 8, pp. 187-202. Chapman and Hall, London.
334. Weiss, R.A., and D.P. Frisby. 1981. Are avian endogenous viruses pathogenic? In D.S. Yohn (ed.), 10th Int Symp for Comparative Research on Leukosis and Related Diseases. Elsevier/North Holland, New York.
335. Weiss, R.A., W.S. Mason, and P.K. Vogt. 1973. Genetic recombinants and heterozygotes derived from endogenous and exogenous avian RNA tumor viruses. Virology 52:535-552.
336. Weiss, R.A., D. Boettiger, and H.M. Murphy. 1977. Pseudotypes of avian sarcoma viruses with the envelope properties of vesicular stomatitis virus. Virology 76:808-825.
337. Weiss, R.A., N. Teich, H. Varmus, and J. Coffin (eds.). 1982. RNA Tumor Viruses, 2nd Ed. Cold Spring Harbor Laboratory, Cold Spring Harbor, NY
338. Weiss, R.A., N. Teich, H. Varmus, and J. Coffin (eds.). 1985. RNA Tumor Viruses, 2nd Ed. Supplements and Appendices. Cold Spring Harbor Laboratory, Cold Spring Harbor, NY.
339. Whalen, L.R., D.W. Wheeler, D.H. Gould, S.A. Fiscus, L.C. Boggie, and R.E. Smith. 1988. Functional and structural alterations of the nervous system induced by avian retrovirus RAV-7. Microbial Pathog 4:401-416.
340. Witter, R.L., B.W. Calnek, and P.P. Levine. 1966. Influence of naturally occurring parental antibody on visceral lymphomatosis virus infection in chickens. Avian Dis 10:43-56.
341. Wyke, J.A., J.G. Bell, and J.A. Beamand. 1975. Genetic recombination among temperature-sensitive mutants of Rous sarcoma virus. Cold Spring Harbor Symp Quant Biol 39:897-905.
342. Zander, D.V., R.G. Raymond, C.F. McClary, and K. Goodwin. 1975. Eradication of subgroups A and B lymphoid leukosis virus from commercial poultry breeding flocks. Avian Dis 19:408-423.
343. Ziegel, R.F. 1961. Morphological evidence of the association of virus particles with the pancreatic acinar cells of the chick. J Nat Cancer Inst 26:1011-1039.

RETICULOENDOTHELIOSIS

R.L. Witter

INTRODUCTION AND HISTORY. Reticuloendotheliosis (RE) designates a group of pathologic syndromes caused by retroviruses of the (REV) group. The disease syndromes include acute reticulum cell neoplasia, a runting disease syndrome, and chronic neoplasia of lymphoid and other tissues.

The initial REV isolate, strain T, was obtained in 1958 from a turkey with visceral lymphomas and was serially passaged over 300 times in turkeys and chickens (139). Although these authors obtained considerable experimental data on this virus during the period 1958-60, publication was unfortunately delayed because the unique nature of this viral isolate was not immediately recognized (22). Sevoian et al. (148) obtained this isolate from Twiehaus and found it acutely oncogenic, causing death of young chicks 6-21 days after inoculation. Theilen et al. (173) confirmed the acute oncogenicity of strain T for young chickens, turkeys, and Japanese quail; these authors were the first to designate the disease as a "reticuloendotheliosis" on the basis of the prominent cell in the neoplastic lesion.

Strain T is now known to be defective for replication in chicken fibroblast tissue cultures and to possess a unique oncogene of cellular origin (v-*rel*) that is responsible for its acute oncogenicity (67, 68). Stocks of strain T also contain a helper REV that replicates in chicken fibroblast cultures but lacks acute oncogenic properties (67). The helper virus has been variously designated as REV-A (67) or as nondefective strain T (202), sometimes accompanied by a further source designation (30).

Antigenic relationships between chick syncytial virus and strain T, first suggested by Cook (36), were confirmed by Witter et al. (200). Purchase et al. (132) found both strains antigenically related to duck infectious anemia (91) and spleen necrosis (178) viruses, and considered all these viruses as members of the REV group. The REV group now includes a large number of other isolates obtained from turkeys, chickens, ducks, pheasants, and geese (30).

Replication defectiveness and acute oncogenicity appear to be properties unique to strain T. All other strains, including strain T helper virus, are nondefective (replication-competent). The nondefective REVs are responsible for the runting disease and the chronic neoplastic disease, both of which occur in nature. The acute reticulum cell neoplasia induced by strain T is not known to occur in nature. Therefore, although strain T has long been recognized as the prototype REV, it is clearly atypical of the group.

RE has received uncommon attention by researchers considering that it is not and has not been a major economic problem. The acute and chronic neoplastic diseases represent (with Marek's disease and lymphoid leukosis) a third etiologically distinct group of avian viral neoplasms. The chronic neoplastic disease sporadically appears to cause significant death and condemnation loss in commercial turkey flocks. REV is a potential contaminant of poultry vaccines. Experimentally, REV causes various neoplastic syndromes in chickens that resemble both lymphoid leukosis and Marek's disease. RE is a model for the study of lymphoid leukosis and other retrovirus-induced neoplastic diseases. Recently, genetically engineered REVs (190) have been used as expression vectors designed to insert foreign genes into the chicken germline (153).

No public health hazard has been associated with REVs. Attempts to propagate the viruses in most mammalian cells and hosts have been unsuccessful but replication in dog and certain other mammalian cells has been reported. Molecular studies that have established a strong evolutionary link between REVs and various mammalian retroviruses have been reviewed by Moore and Bose (105).

INCIDENCE AND DISTRIBUTION. The chronic neoplastic form of RE appears to occur naturally, albeit sporadically, in the turkey. In addition to the original isolation by Robinson and Twiehaus (139), outbreaks of the disease were described in Minnesota (125), Virginia (161), Texas (197), and Pennsylvania (199). Cases of RE in turkeys have also been reported in England (97) and Israel (72). Chronic RE neoplastic disease has not frequently been recognized in chickens, although Ratnamohan et al. (134) reported a histiocytic lymphosarcoma in a single laying hen that was probably inoculated with REV-contaminated vaccine, and lymphomas presumably associated with REV have been reported in other flocks (72, 128). Chronic neoplasia associated with REV has also been observed in ducks (60, 124, 129), quail (24, 144, 185), pheasants (43), and geese (44).

A runting disease characterized by poor growth, abnormal feathering, proventriculitis, and immunodepression has been seen in chickens inoculated with strain T (117) or accidently vaccinated with REV-contaminated vaccines (76, 80, 208), and may have also occurred naturally in association with necrotic dermatitis in chickens (69). Acute reticulum cell neoplasia has not been observed in nature in association with REV infection. An epizootic of reticulum cell sarcomas in Japanese quail was reported (122) but a relationship to RE was not established.

The virus seems widely disseminated among avian species. Aulisio and Shelokov (2) found specific antibodies in yolks of eggs from 41 of 92 chicken flocks. Subsequent studies in several countries, reviewed by Witter (195), identified REV antibodies in 3–25% of chicken flocks that did not receive contaminated vaccines. Witter et al. (203) found REV antibodies in 21 of 101 layer flocks, 20 of 85 broiler and broiler breeder flocks, 1 of 43 backyard chicken flocks and 6 of 125 turkey flocks; most of the seropositive flocks were in Florida, Mississippi, and North Carolina. In a later study, 6 of 6 broiler breeder flocks in Mississippi seroconverted between 13 and 47 wk of age (198). No seropositive flock exhibited clinical evidence of disease.

Thus, on the basis of reported clinical disease, the economic importance of RE in turkeys is minor and in chickens is negligible. However, field isolates are highly immunodepressive and oncogenic under experimental conditions (198), and the possibility of subclinical immunosuppressive disease or the failure to differentiate chronic neoplastic disease from lymphoid leukosis in chickens warrants consideration (see DIAGNOSIS).

Accidental contamination of virus stocks with REV has been observed on a variety of occasions. Commercial vaccines have been contaminated with major economic consequences (76, 209). Certain stocks of avian myeloblastosis virus produced for biochemical purposes contained a low level of REV (203). Cross contamination of cultures in the laboratory has been observed. The occurrence of such problems points to a further mechanism for increasing the distribution of this virus in nature. Appropriate caution is advised.

ETIOLOGY

Classification. REVs are retroviruses immunologically, morphologically, and structurally distinct from the leukosis/sarcoma group of avian retroviruses (see review 195). Although cross protective immunity between RE and avian leukosis viruses has been described (10, 11), satisfactory explanations and confirmatory data are thus far lacking.

A relationship between REV and various mammalian retroviruses, especially those from old world primates, has been described on the basis of morphology, nucleic acid sequences, amino acid sequences of major polypeptides, and immunological determinants (see review 105). Although this may indicate an evolutionary link, no biological relationships are recognized and the host range of REV, except for certain mammalian cell cultures, remains largely restricted to avian species.

A number of REVs have been isolated. To simplify the nomenclature, Purchase and Witter (131) have proposed that all members of the REV group be termed strains of REV and be given appropriate strain designations.

Stability. Cell-free stocks of REV can be prepared from tissues of infected chickens or fluids from infected cell cultures and may be stored without loss of activity for long periods at −70 C.

The virus was relatively stable at 4 C but at 37 C 50% of the infectivity was lost in 20 min and 99% was lost after 1 hr (23). Infected cells may be stored indefinitely with dimethylsulfoxide at −196 C.

Morphology. Viral particles are about 100 nm in diameter (210), and are covered with surface projections about 6 nm long and 10 nm in diameter (79). Virions have a density of 1.16–1.18 g/ml in sucrose density gradients (9) but can be differentiated from avian leukosis/sarcoma viruses by morphology in thin sections (103, 210) and by density in cesium chloride gradients (94). The morphology of the viral particles is shown in Figure 16.51.

Chemical Composition

NUCLEIC ACID. Genomic single-stranded RNA of REVs consists of a 60–70S complex containing two 30–40S RNA subunits, each having a size of about 3.9 × 10⁶ daltons (12, 95). The nondefective REV has a genome of about 9.0 kilobases (kb), the replication-defective strain T genome is only about 5.7 kb due principally to a large deletion in the *gag-pol* region and a smaller deletion in the *env* region (see 34). Moreover, the replication-defective strain T genome contains a substitution of 0.8–1.5 kb in the *env* region that represents the transforming gene, identified as v-*rel* (29, 35, 205). The v-*rel* is not present in nondefective REVs or other avian or mammalian retroviruses. Related sequences (c-*rel*), probably conserved in many vertebrates, are present in the DNA of normal avian cells, including turkey cellular DNA from whence the oncogene was most likely derived (29, 193, 205) through transduction by a novel mechanism (194). The nucleotide sequence of the v-*rel* gene has been determined (162).

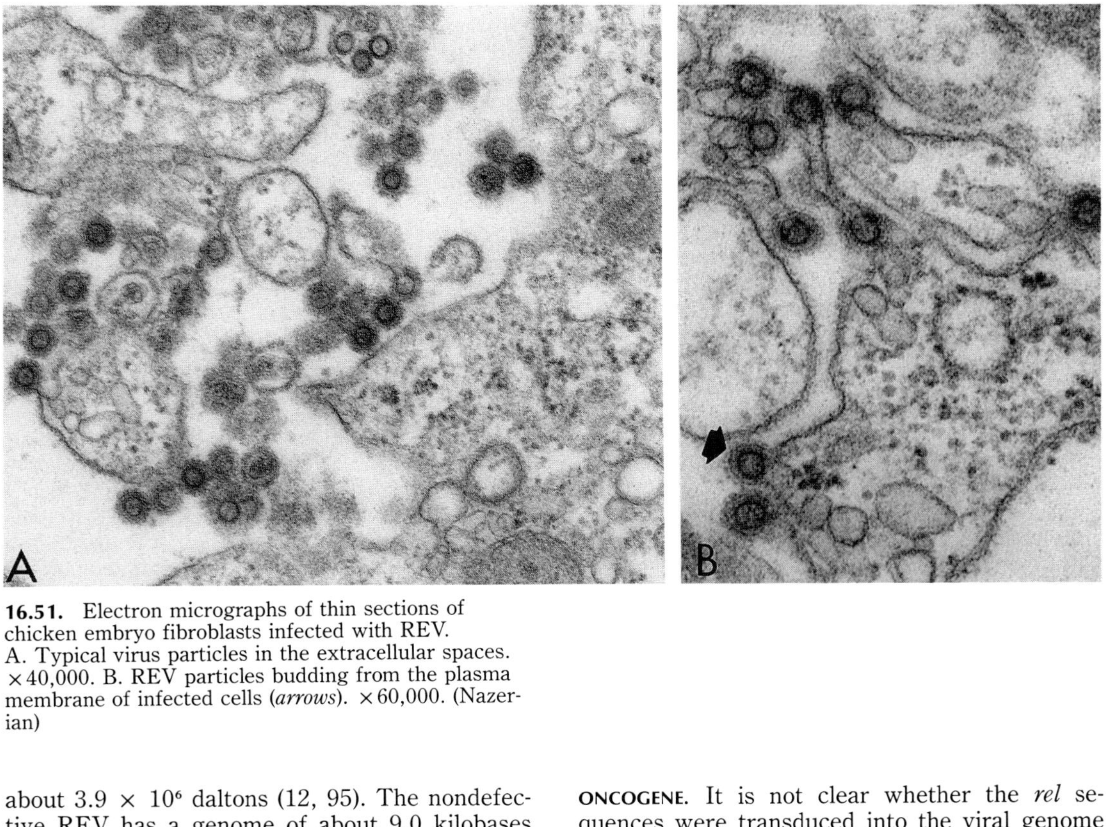

16.51. Electron micrographs of thin sections of chicken embryo fibroblasts infected with REV. A. Typical virus particles in the extracellular spaces. ×40,000. B. REV particles budding from the plasma membrane of infected cells (*arrows*). ×60,000. (Nazerian)

ONCOGENE. It is not clear whether the *rel* sequences were transduced into the viral genome prior to isolation of strain T in 1958 or during its subsequent extensive serial passage in chickens and turkeys (139). Prior transduction may have occurred, since on the first passage of the virus in chickens a mean survival time of 24.2 days was recorded (139), a much shorter interval than that reported by Paul et al. (126) and McDougall et al. (97) for their initial virus passages in turkeys.

The v-*rel* oncogene is transcribed (65) in strain T-transformed lymphoid cells and produces a phosphoprotein product identified as $pp59^{v\text{-}rel}$ (58, 59, 64, 137, 156), which has a protein kinase activity (66, 188) and is complexed to a 40-kD cellular phosphoprotein in the cytoplasm of transformed lymphoid cells (182) and to other proteins (155). The presence of $pp59^{v\text{-}rel}$ in the cytoplasm has been associated with its putative transforming activity (59, 104). However, other genomic alterations may also be required for acute oncogenicity (100, 101). Recombinant viruses where c-*rel* has replaced v-*rel* were also oncogenic, provided certain alterations in the amino terminus and mid-region were made (165). The nature of v-*rel* and its protein product has been reviewed by Moore and Bose (105).

In several cases, REV isolates other than strain T have induced neoplastic disease within very short latent periods (43, 44, 133, 135). Examination of such strains for viral oncogenes of cellular origin may be of interest.

Only limited sequence homology exists between the RNA of nondefective REV and the DNA of normal avian cells (77) and no endogenous REV sequences in host DNA have been recognized. The terminal regions of the viral genome, designated as the long terminal repeats (LTRs), consist of 569 base-pair repeats that appear structurally similar to bacterial transposable elements (152). A region responsible for the encapsidation of genomic RNA is located between the 5′ LTR and the initiation codon for the *gag* gene (189).

PROTEINS. REVs contain an RNA-directed DNA polymerase (reverse transcriptase) that differs structurally and immunologically from the comparable enzyme of leukosis/sarcoma viruses (8, 103). The preference of the REV-associated enzyme for Mn^{++} ions is a characteristic by which it can be differentiated from enzymes of other avian retroviruses (103, 145, 207). A nucleotidyl transferase activity associated with RE virions has also been described (102).

A variety of polypeptides have been isolated from REV including two *env* gene-encoded glycoproteins, gp90 and gp20 (179, 181), and five *gag* gene-encoded structural proteins, p12, pp18, pp20, p30 and p10 (180). The C-terminal epitope of gp90 is located on the surface of infected cells where it can participate in complement-mediated cytotoxicity reactions (179). The 30-kD (p30) protein constitutes the major group-specific antigen. Mosser et al. (107) located the two glycoproteins and two other proteins on the surface of the virions. Antiserum to p30 cross reacted with p30 of several other REVs, thus establishing this protein as group specific (96). Earlier reports described similar proteins, although with slightly different molecular weights (95, 206).

Replication

NONDEFECTIVE STRAINS. The nondefective REV replicates well in cells from several avian species. Fibroblast cultures from chickens, turkeys, and quail are most widely used for virus propagation. Replication of nondefective REV is by means of a chromosomally integrated DNA intermediate (37, 52) as is typical of other retroviruses (183). Following infection, the virion is assembled in the cytoplasm as a ribonucleoprotein complex and acquires an envelope by budding through the plasma membrane (210). About 20% of the released particles are immature; this indicates that nucleocapsid development occurs relatively slowly (103). Virus particle production was first noted at 24 hr (79) and maximum virus production occurred 2–4 days after infection (15, 52, 169).

DEFECTIVE STRAINS. The replication-defective strain T virus requires a nondefective RE helper virus for replication (67). Oncogenicity of this strain is maintained during passage in vivo (139) or during culture of infected hematopoietic cells (67) but is rapidly lost during passage in fibroblast cultures (23, 62, 85, 173, 200) and dog thymus cells (1). Breitman et al. (16) showed this apparent attenuation in chick embryo fibroblast cultures was due to the loss of the replication-defective, acutely oncogenic virus, which was completely absent after three passages; the helper REV continued to replicate. Franklin et al. (51) reported the persistence of acutely oncogenic strain T in a line of transformed chicken embryo fibroblasts, a cell type that has a limited susceptibility to transformation by strain T (104).

CYTOPATHOLOGY. In early studies, cytopathology was not regularly associated with infection of avian fibroblasts in vitro (173). However, syncytial cell formation has been noted in infected cultures (36, 127), and Temin and Kassner (169) reported that certain strains caused a mild, degenerative cytopathic change in several avian cell types. Temin et al. (171) proposed the following model. Infected cells synthesize unintegrated viral DNA, a part of which is integrated at multiple sites in the cellular genome. Progeny virus then superinfects the already infected cells leading to an accumulation of unintegrated viral DNA (28, 82, 192). Cells with large amounts of unintegrated DNA die, perhaps due to some toxic effect, while those cells able to prevent early superinfection have few copies of unintegrated viral DNA and survive.

The acute phase of cell killing (Fig. 16.52 A, B) lasts 2–10 days after infection and is followed by a state of chronic infection characterized by the disappearance of cytopathology and continued virus production (Fig. 16.52C) (169, 170). This cytopathic effect is the basis of a plaque assay (106, 169), but the method has not been widely used, perhaps because the cytopathology is somewhat inconsistent. Cho (32, 33) described a plaque assay in chemically transformed Japanese quail fibroblasts.

HOST RANGE. Cells from many or all avian species

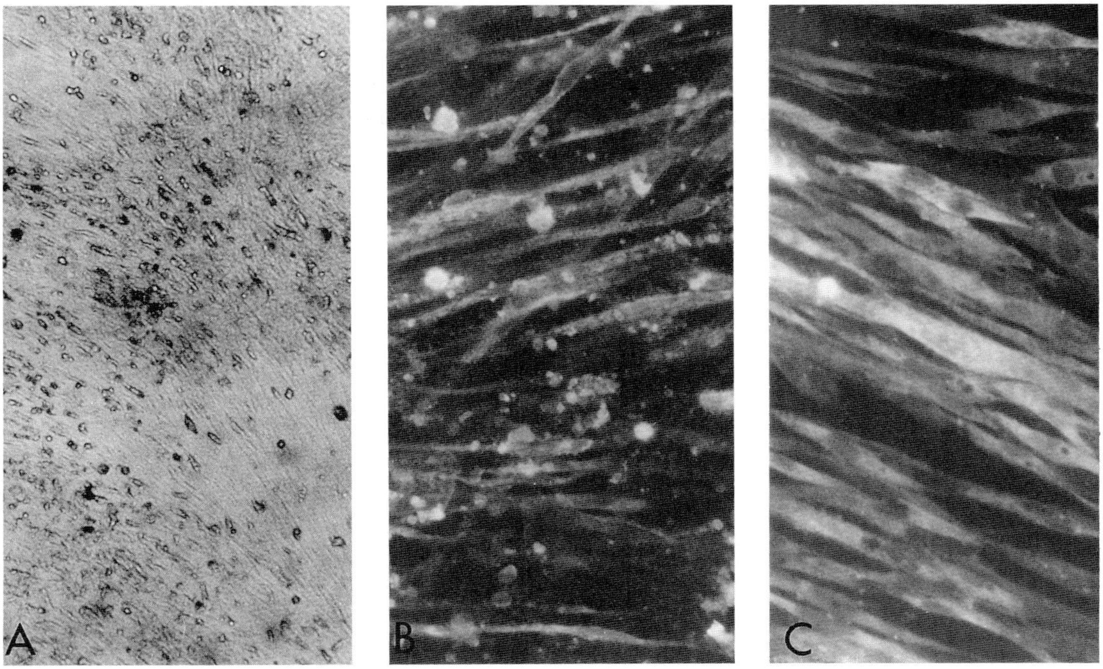

16.52. Acute (cytopathic) and chronic (noncytopathic) infection of chicken embryo fibroblasts inoculated with nondefective REV, strain T. A. Mild cytopathic changes 13 days after infection. Unstained, ×55. B. Cytopathic changes and viral antigens 13 days after infection. Indirect immunofluorescent staining. C. Chronically infected cultures 48 days after infection showing relatively normal-appearing cells, most of which contain cytoplasmic viral antigens. Immunofluorescent staining. ×360.

are susceptible to infection in vitro and are widely used for virus propagation and assay. However, certain mammalian cells support at least limited viral replication. Nondefective REV has also been grown in D17 dog sarcoma cells (6, 190), Cf2Th dog thymus cells (1, 154), normal rat kidney cells (82), and mink lung cells (1). D17 cells appear fully susceptible and constitute a useful host system for virus propagation (189, 190). Rat and mouse cells were only semipermissive for replication of REV, with blocks at different replication steps (45, 46). However, there is no evidence for in vivo replication of REV in nonavian species.

PSEUDOTYPES. The envelope component of nondefective REV forms pseudotypes with Rous sarcoma virus (143, 184) and with vesicular stomatitis virus (77). The pseudotype virus can be neutralized by antiserum to REV; Crittenden et al. (39) has used this principle to detect REV antibodies in test sera.

Strain Classification. The different isolates of REV are remarkably uniform in antigenicity (17, 132, 200) and appear to belong to a single serotype (30). The nondefective strains have similar structural and chemical properties (8, 79); however, differences in pathogenicity have been noted (132).

Definitive evidence for antigenic differences was provided by Cui et al. (40) who developed monoclonal antibodies that reacted with strain T but not with the chick syncytial strain; at least 3 different epitopes (A, B, and C) were identified. Chen et al. (30) grouped 26 isolates into 3 subtypes on the basis of neutralization tests and differential reactivity with monoclonal antibodies. Isolates of subtype 1 were considered to possess epitopes A, B, and C whereas subtype 2 contained epitope B, and subtype C contained epitopes A and B (30). However, viruses of subtype 1 and 2 could not be differentiated by receptor interference (49), thus confirming the absence of major subgroup differences.

RE viral isolates differ also in certain biological properties, including pathogenicity (131), but such differences have not been the basis for strain classification.

Laboratory Host Systems

CELL CULTURES. Fibroblasts from several avian species and certain cell lines, such as QT35 quail sarcoma cells (33, 38) and D17 dog osteosarcoma cells (6, 190), are susceptible to infection with nondefective REVs. In infected cultures, antigens (Fig. 16.52 B, C), virus particles, cytopathology, and reverse transcriptase may be detected and serve as criteria for virus assay. When the cultures are grown under agar, foci of cells containing immunofluorescent antigens can be localized and used as the basis for a quantitative fluorescent focus assay (132). However, chicken bone marrow-derived macrophages appear resistant to infection (19).

EMBRYOS AND BIRDS. Other laboratory host systems for REV include chicken embryos (149) and a variety of avian species including young chickens, Japanese quail, ducks, geese, turkeys, pheasants, and guinea fowl (133, 173). Embryos and animals may respond to infection by development of specific lesions, viremia, or antibodies.

CELL LINES. Cell lines consisting of cells transformed by REVs are further laboratory host systems of potential value. Lines of hematopoietic cells transformed in vivo (50, 81, 86) or in vitro (14, 88, 151, 191) by the replication-defective strain T have been described. A line of transformed chicken embryo fibroblasts has also been developed (51). Nonproducer clones can be isolated that produce pseudotypes when infected with nondefective REV strains (68). The cells possess surface viral antigens that co-cap with antigens of the major histocompatibility complex (92), and may also secrete growth factors (55, 56). The nondefective strains of REV induce chronic neoplasia (196) and a cell line with B determinants has been developed from chickens with this disease syndrome (119). At least 39 different REV-transformed cell lines have been described (118).

PATHOGENESIS AND EPIZOOTIOLOGY

Natural and Experimental Hosts. Natural hosts for REV infection include turkeys, chickens, ducks, geese, and Japanese quail; however, the turkey has most frequently been observed with evidence of disease. Disease is also recognized in chickens following inoculation with vaccines accidently contaminated with nondefective REV. Experimental hosts include all of the above species as well as pheasants and guinea fowl. Chickens and turkeys have been most frequently employed as experimental hosts.

Responses to Infection. Epizootiological studies have detailed some of the virological and serological responses of chickens and turkeys to infection with nondefective REVs. Tolerant infection, i.e., persistent viremia in the absence of antibody, is induced readily in chickens by embryo inoculation (72, 202). Tolerant infection occurs also after inoculation at hatching, but the rate of induction is variable (3, 80, 98, 202, 209) and is influenced by the strain of chicken (48). Some tolerantly infected chickens ultimately develop detectable antibody (110), which may indicate a release from tolerance.

More commonly, inoculated or contact-exposed birds develop a transient viremia followed by the development of antibodies (3, 201). Antibodies have been detected as early as 16–21 days after inoculation in chickens (17, 108) but 6–10 wk may be required in contact-exposed birds (72, 80, 87, 98). Precipitating and immunofluorescent antibodies may decline with age (3, 17, 202), but McDougall et al. (98) detected neutralizing antibodies at high frequency in experimentally infected turkeys through 40 wk. Antibodies can be detected in newly hatched chickens from exposed dams (198). Bagust and Grimes (3) described the persistence of noninfectious RE viral antigens in the blood for several weeks following the disappearance of infectious virus. A major histocompatibility complex (MHC)-restricted cell-mediated cytotoxicity response has been described in chickens within 7 days after inoculation with defective or nondefective RE viral strains (93, 191), which appears to be mediated by an Ia-positive T cell (191).

Factors influencing the susceptibility of avian hosts to infection have not been thoroughly studied. No genetic cellular resistance similar to that of avian leukosis viruses has been recognized. However, some differences in the pathologic response of lines or families has been recognized in chickens (48, 147, 150, 204) and quail (172). Although endogenous avian leukosis virus genes had no influence on tumor induction or antibody response following exposure of chickens to the chick syncytial strain, virus was isolated more frequently from chickens with *ev2* than from chickens lacking this gene (39). A cellular resistance (interference) due to viral envelope gene expression has been described in cultured D17 cells (42, 49) and suggests that similar resistance might be achieved in chickens modified to express envelope glycoproteins by transgenic technologies. An age-related resistance to clinical disease is apparent. Furthermore, maternal antibodies appear to limit susceptibility to infection (158).

Virus Transmission

HORIZONTAL TRANSMISSION. The virus is transmitted by contact with infected chickens and turkeys (87, 126). Virus has been isolated from feces and cloacal swabs (3, 130, 202, 209) as well as other body fluids (5) and litter from seropositive chicken flocks (198). Viral shedding probably occurs mainly during periods of active viremia. The efficiency of contact transmission may be influenced by the host species (132) and the virus strain (198, 209). Contact infection rarely results in clinical disease (130, 132, 198, 209) except perhaps in turkeys where lymphomas have been observed following contact exposure (98, 99, 126).

The role of insects in the transmission of REV has been studied. Although infection persisted in *Triatoma infestans* for 3 days and in *Ornithodoros moubata* for 7 days, an important role for these and other insects, including mosquitoes, in REV transmission was considered unlikely (175, 176). Attempts to propagate REV in cultures of *Aedes albopictus* were unsuccessful (136). However, Motha et al. (116) isolated virus from 7 of 39 batches of mosquitoes in contact with viremic chickens and demonstrated apparent transmission of the infection to recipient chickens exposed to *Culex annulirostris* that had previously fed on birds with persistent viremia. Mosquito transmission may explain seasonal variation in infection rates (116) or the prevalence of infection in Southern states (198, 203) and deserves further study.

VERTICAL TRANSMISSION. Vertical transmission of REV has been reported in both chickens and turkeys, usually at very low rates. McDougall et al. (98) isolated virus from 2 of 25 embryos from tolerantly infected turkey hens. Similar low rates of viral shedding and transmission were documented for tolerantly infected chickens (3, 5, 186, 202) although Motha and Egerton (114) reported transmission to over 50% of chicks in an experiment where eggs were incubated within 24 hr of lay. Albumen samples from tolerantly infected hens frequently contained RE viral gs antigen, although at low levels; infectious virus was rarely isolated (202). Vertical transmission from nontolerantly infected chickens is not common, but one exceptional antibody-positive, virus-positive, antigen-negative turkey hen transmitted virus to 6 of 21 progeny (199). Vertical transmission also occurs in ducks, since virus was isolated from embryos derived from tolerantly infected females (109).

Although semen from tolerantly infected turkeys contains infectious virus (98, 199), the role of the tom in vertical transmission is not clear. McDougall et al. (98) found that previously nonexposed turkey hens inseminated with infected semen produced infected progeny but, in contrast, Witter and Salter (199) found the frequency of vertical transmission was no greater from hens mated with viremic males than with hens mated with nonviremic males; however, the hens were from a previously exposed flock. Furthermore, they found no evidence in parents or congenitally infected progeny of clonal insertions of proviral DNA that would be indicative of genetic transmission (199). Male transmission has received less attention in chickens, but Salter et al. (142) found RE proviral DNA in 10 of 820 chicks from matings of viremic males and nonviremic females. Clearly, a role for the male in vertical transmission of REV has not been excluded and needs further study.

The relative role of horizontal and vertical transmission in the maintenance of infection in the field is still poorly understood. Neither mode of transmission appears highly efficient but horizontal exposure may be more common (197, 198). Since horizontal infection, especially at an older age, is less likely to induce clinical disease than vertical infection, this may account for the relative infrequency of clinical disease.

CONTAMINATED VACCINES. Artificial transmission by inoculation of chickens with REV-contaminated Marek's disease vaccine (76, 209) or inoculation of turkeys with presumptively contaminated fowl pox vaccine (13) has been reported. Such accidents often induce the runting disease or neoplasia at high rates since virtually all birds in a flock receive high doses of virus at a young age.

ACUTE RETICULUM CELL NEOPLASIA

Pathology. The pathology of the acute reticulum cell neoplasia (reticuloendotheliosis) caused by replication-defective strain T virus has been well described (117, 139, 148, 173). The incubation period can be as short as 3 days but death occurs more commonly 6–21 days after inoculation. Inoculation of newly hatched chickens or turkeys results in few clinical signs due to the rapid onset of the disease, and mortality rates often reach 100%.

The affected birds develop large livers and spleens with infiltrative focal or diffuse lesions. Lesions are also common in the pancreas, gonads, heart, and kidney. The blood shows a decrease in heterophils and an increase in lymphocytes (168), leading to a frank leukemia a few hours before death (150). The serum transferrin level is elevated (177) and Shen (150) reported elevated globulin and decreased albumin concentrations.

Histologic changes are generally characterized by the infiltration and proliferation of large vesicular cells variously described as mononuclear cells of the reticuloendothelial system (173) or primitive mesenchymal cells (139, 148). Some lesions are composed almost solely of such cells whereas others include also a moderate to heavy population of smaller lymphoid elements, probably indicating a host immunological response to the primary lesion. Areas of necrosis in association with the neoplastic lesions are also frequent. A typical liver lesion is shown in Fig. 16.53.

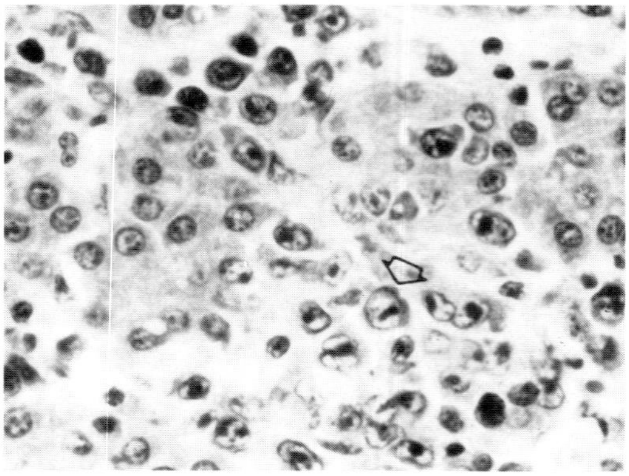

16.53. Microscopic lesions of acute reticulum cell neoplasia (RE) in the liver of a chicken inoculated with replication-defective, acutely transforming strain T REV. The liver is infiltrated with large primitive reticular cells (*arrow*).

Transformation. The identity of the target cell continues to be controversial. Cell lines developed from these tumors have been described as B lymphocytes (88, 151) or primitive cells with both B- and T-cell markers (14); two lines had immunoglobulin M (IgM) markers (81, 88). Chen et al. (31) found that the immunoglobulin genes of lymphoid cells transformed by v-*rel* were not expressed but showed various rearrangements. Neither neonatal bursectomy nor thymectomy conferred resistance to the disease (150, 174), indicating the target cells are not mature lymphocytes.

The difficulty in establishing the identity of the target cell may reflect either its highly undifferentiated state or the susceptibility of multiple cell types to transformation. In support of the latter possibility, Barth and Humphries (7) found strain T (v-*rel*) tumors induced in the presence of REV-A helper were negative for IgM whereas tumors induced in the presence of chick syncytial virus helper were nearly all positive for IgM. They suggest that highly immunosuppressive helper viruses such as REV-A may restrict the spectrum of target cells available for transformation and showed that B lymphocytes are clearly susceptible to transformation (7). Moreover, different cell lines transformed by replication-defective strain T expressed class I histocompatibility antigens of either type 2A (typical of bursal cells) or type 2B (typical of thymic cells), thus supporting the multiple target cell hypothesis (83).

Neoplastic transformation in acute reticulum cell neoplasia is mediated by the oncogene, v-*rel*, contained within the replication-defective strain T virus. No activation of a cellular oncogene is required. Furthermore, transformation does not require the presence of a helper virus (88). Lymphoid cells transformed by strain T in vitro but which produce no infectious virus will produce typical RE when transplanted into syngeneic recipients (88, 140).

Immunity. A protective immune response against the acute neoplasia induced by strain T has been described. Regression of strain T-induced wing-web tumors was partially abrogated by bursectomy, thymectomy, and bursectomy-thymectomy (90). Serum from hyperimmunized chickens was protective against tumor development even after absorption to remove antiviral antibodies (70), thus suggesting the existence of tumor-specific transplantation antigens on RE tumor cells. Chickens immunized with purified or inactivated preparations of nondefective strain T helper virus were resistant to challenge with acutely transforming strain T preparations (10).

RUNTING DISEASE SYNDROME. The runting disease syndrome is a term chosen to designate the several nonneoplastic lesions associated with infection with nondefective REV strains.

Pathology. The lesions include runting (117, 173, 200), atrophy of the thymus and bursa of Fabricius (117), enlarged peripheral nerves (200), abnormal feather development (84, 85), proventriculitis (76), enteritis (97), anemia (91, 80), and necrosis of the liver and spleen (131, 178). These are often accompanied by depression of cellular and humoral immune responses (17, 25, 72, 80).

Clinically, the birds may be notably stunted and pale. Stunted birds did not consume less food but had marked reduction of phosphoenolpyruvate carboxykinase, a key gluconeogenic enzyme in the liver (57). Weight depression in infected chicks can be detected as early as 6 days of age (110). Some chickens may have abnormal feather development ("Nakanuke"), i.e., wing feathers with adhesion of the barbs to a localized section of the shaft (84) that is apparently due to REV-induced necrosis of feather-forming cells early after injection (166). Lameness or paralysis is rare even in birds with gross nerve lesions. Affected birds are usually culled prior to death; a culling loss of over 50% between 5 and 8 wk was described in one flock (167). Acute hemorrhagic or chronic ulcerative proventriculitis has been observed (76), but could not be reproduced by Bagust et al. (4) with a similar isolate.

It is still unclear whether the proliferative lesions in enlarged peripheral nerves are neoplastic or inflammatory; however, nerve lesions often occur in the absence of other neoplasms (200). The infiltrating cells are shown in Fig. 16.54. Although lesions of the runting disease syndrome have been most extensively studied in chickens, at least parts of the syndrome occur in ducks inoculated with the spleen necrosis or duck infectious anemia strains of REV, and enlarged nerves

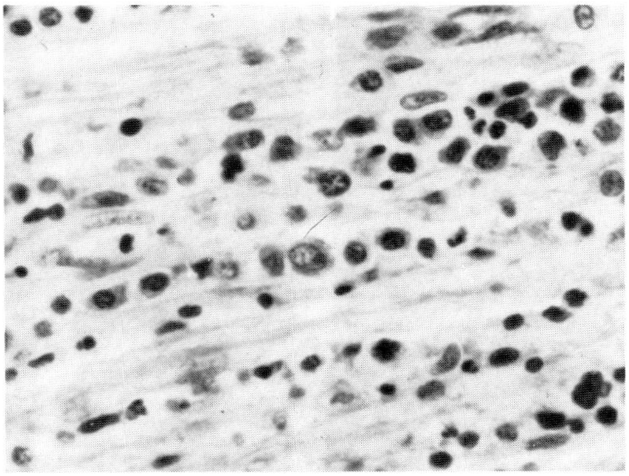

16.54. Microscopic lesions in a peripheral nerve of a chicken inoculated with nondefective strain T REV. Infiltrating cells consist of mature and immature lymphocytes and plasma cells.

(125) of enteritis (97) have been observed in turkeys with RE-related chronic lymphomas. Genetic differences in susceptibility have not yet been described; chicks from lines of different susceptibility to Marek's disease were equally susceptible to the development of nerve lesions following inoculation with REV (200).

IMMUNODEPRESSION. Humoral and cellular immune responses are frequently depressed in chickens infected with nondefective REV strains. Depressed antibody responses to Marek's disease virus and turkey herpesvirus (17, 80), Newcastle disease virus (72, 208), as well as sheep erythrocytes and *Brucella abortus* (201) are documented. The extent of depression is influenced by the dose and strain of virus, and primary responses are more severely affected than secondary (201). Barth and Humphries (7) found that different strains of nondefective REV varied in ability to induce bursal atrophy and in suppression of B-cell populations available for transformation by v-*rel.*

Spleen cells from chickens infected with replication-defective strain T were suppressed in their ability to respond to the mitogen, phytohemagglutinin (25, 146). This effect was subsequently associated with the nondefective helper virus in strain T stocks (26) and is mediated through a population of suppressor cells (27, 141). The suppressor cells could be demonstrated only through the 3rd wk after infection (140). Other cellular immune responses inhibited by REV infection include mixed lymphocyte reaction and allograft rejection (187).

Witter et al. (201, 202) found depression of humoral responses and mitogen responsiveness was transient following infection with the chick syncytial strain but persisted through 10–19 wk in chickens tolerantly infected with nondefective strain T. Infected chickens were more susceptible to the development of a Marek's disease tumor transplant (21), to reactions from infectious laryngotracheitis vaccine (108, 157), to natural fowl pox virus infection (115), to infectious bronchitis virus (157), and to mortality induced by *Eimeria tenella* (113) and *Salmonella typhimurium* (112) and may have been more susceptible to necrotic dermatitis (69) but no increase in susceptibility to Marek's disease virus was noted (18). Witter et al. (201) demonstrated interference by REV infection with immunity induced by turkey herpesvirus against Marek's disease in chickens. Humoral immunodepression was also seen in ducks infected with a field RE viral isolate (89).

These immunodepressive effects undoubtedly contribute to the nonneoplastic lesions described earlier and may also enhance the oncogenicity of these viruses. Indeed, immunodepression may be the most economically important consequence of infection with REV.

CHRONIC NEOPLASIA

CHICKEN BURSAL LYMPHOMA. Two types of chronic neoplastic disease caused by nondefective REV have been recognized in chickens. The first type includes bursal lymphomas induced after long latent periods in chickens. Witter and Crittenden (196) found chickens inoculated with the chick syncytial strain developed a high rate of lymphomas, involving principally the liver and bursa of Fabricius, that were indistinguishable from lymphoid leukosis (Fig. 16.55). Similar tumors were induced by nondefective strain T (202). A total of 25 lymphomas, 2 sarcomas, and 1 adenocarcinoma were induced by the two strains between 17 and 43 wk of age.

The frequent bursal involvement (92% of lymphoma cases) and surface IgM staining of the lymphoma cells suggested the tumors were bursa-dependent, B-cell lymphomas (202). Nazerian et al. (119) demonstrated specific B-cell but not T-cell antigens on the tumor cells and developed a lymphoblastoid cell line that produced IgM. The bursa dependency of this tumor was confirmed by the finding that chemically or surgically bursectomized chickens were refractory to tumor development (47).

Noori-Daloii et al. (123) found in REV-induced lymphomas that the DNA proviral genome of REV was integrated adjacent to c-*myc,* a cellular oncogene important in the induction of lymphoid leukosis by avian leukosis virus. The molecular mechanism by which c-*myc* is activated by insertion of proviral DNA has been studied (53, 138, 163). The proviral insert often contains major deletions that prevent the expression of infectious virus and apparently are important determinants for its oncogenic potential (164).

Avian leukosis proviral sequences are integrated adjacent to c-*myc* in the DNA of lymphoid leukosis tumors in the same fashion (54, 63) as described for RE viral sequences in chronic lymphomas. Therefore, these REV-induced lymphomas appear identical to those of lymphoid leukosis by both biological and molecular criteria. However, chickens of lines resistant and susceptible to lymphoid leukosis were uniformly less susceptible to lymphoma induction by REV than by avian leukosis virus (48). Grimes et al. (61) observed what may be similar lymphomas in two chickens at 22 and 24 wk after inoculation with a field strain of REV but no bursal involvement was reported.

CHICKEN NONBURSAL LYMPHOMA. Chronic nonbursal lymphomas have been described in chickens of certain genetic lines following infection with certain strains of nondefective REV (204). These lymphomas have latent periods as short as 6 wk and involve the thymus, heart, liver, and spleen but not the bursa of Fabricius (see Fig. 16.56). Nerve enlargements similar to those described with the runting disease syndrome can be seen. Thus, this neoplastic syndrome superficially resembles Marek's disease, but the tumor cells lack the tumor-associated surface antigen and the pleomorphic lymphocyte populations characteristics of Marek's disease (204). The cell type has not been defined, but no immunoglobulin or B-cell markers have been detected. The molecular mechanism of oncogenesis also involves insertional activation of c-*myc* but by a mechanism different from that in bursal lymphomas (75). Purchase et al. (132) described mortality within 7 wk due to RE-like lesions in visceral organs following inoculation with the spleen necrosis strain. These tumors may be similar to those described by Witter et al. (204) who also used the spleen necrosis strain.

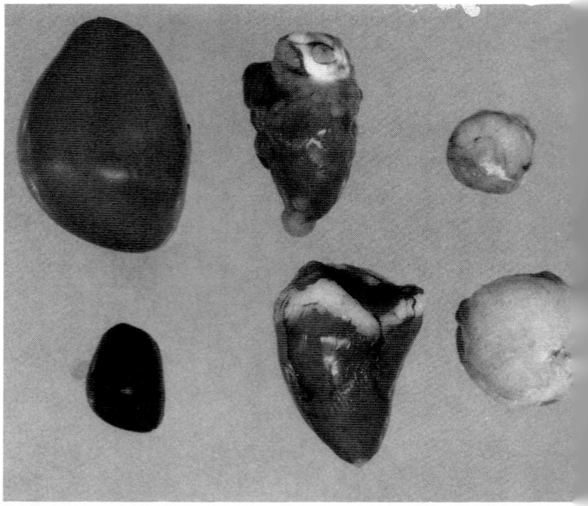

16.56. Nonbursal lymphoma in a chicken 48 days postinoculation with the nondefective spleen necrosis strain of REV. Note enlargement of spleen, nodular lymphomas on heart, and bursal atrophy of infected chicken (*top row*). Organs from age-matched control chicken (*bottom row*). (Courtesy of Avian Pathology)

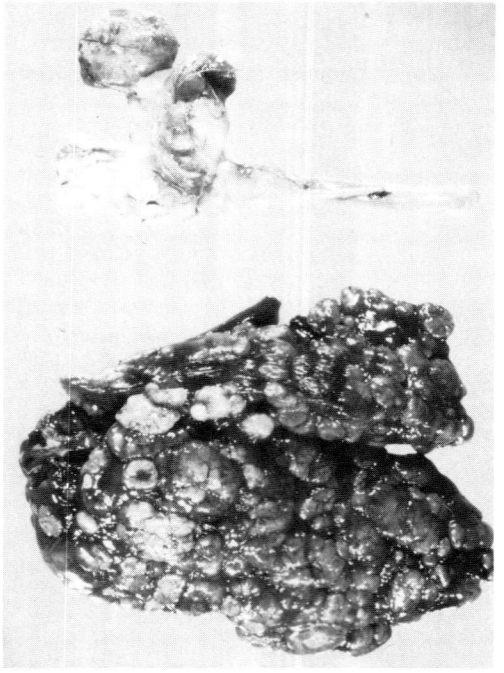

16.55. Bursal lymphoma in a chicken. Note gross lymphomas in the liver and bursa of a chicken 25 wk after inoculation with the nondefective chick syncytial strain of REV.

TURKEY LYMPHOMA. Natural infection with REV can result in lymphoma production in turkeys (97, 125) between 15 and 20 wk of age. In transmission studies, similar lymphomas were induced in 10–30% of turkey poults on the first passage after 8–11 wk (126) or 11–12 wk (97). Lesions typically included lymphomas in the liver and other visceral organs; Paul et al. (126) and McDougall et al. (97) both described lymphomatous lesions in the bursa but this lesion was apparently not very common. Critical comparisons between chronic lymphomas in turkeys and chickens have not been made and there is no evidence that a common mechanism of oncogenesis exists.

OTHER LYMPHOMAS. Chronic lymphomas of the spleen, liver, pancreas, and intestine have been described between 20 and 30 wk in the domestic goose (44); one of four spleen cell preparations when inoculated into chickens and geese induced lymphomas within 11–22 days, whereas the other preparations induced lymphomas after long latent periods. Naturally occurring lymphomas have been described in ducks at 20 wk (60) and at 4–10 wk (124). Perk et al. (129) described an outbreak characterized by generalized leukemia as well as lymphomas in visceral organs in 6-mo-old ducks. A virus isolate obtained from a duck of unknown age with nodular lymphoid tumors in the liver and spleen produced a high rate of lymphomas and other neoplasms between 8 and 24 wk; the frequency was not affected by age at infection or by embryonal bursectomy (89).

An REV-associated disease in pheasants characterized by cutaneous lesions on the head and mouth and nodular lymphomas in visceral organs occurred between 6 and 12 mo of age (43), and a tumor cell inoculum induced a high rate of lymphomas in pheasant chicks between 2–4 wk postinoculation.

Lymphomas occurring in Japanese quail between 2 and 7 mo of age have been associated with REV infection (24, 144). Lesions included lymphomas of the liver and spleen and nodular tumors of the intestine.

MULTIPLE SYNDROMES. Lesions of the different types can be observed in the same experiment, or even in the same bird. Nondefective REV strains may first induce lesions of the runting disease syndrome and lymphomas may occur later in the survivors. Chickens inoculated with replication-defective, acutely transforming strain T, especially those surviving the acute disease, may develop lesions associated with the nondefective strain T helper virus.

DIAGNOSIS.

A diagnosis of RE requires not only the presence of typical gross and microscopic lesions but also the demonstration of REV or its antibody. This virus, unlike avian leukosis and Marek's disease viruses, is not ubiquitous and its presence has diagnostic value.

Virus Isolation and Identification.

Viremia with REV is typically low titered and transient, except following congenital transmission or embryo inoculation that leads to tolerant infection. Birds with lesions are the best source of virus.

Virus may be isolated by inoculation of susceptible tissue cultures with tissue suspensions, whole blood, plasma, or other inocula. In general, cellular inocula are preferred over cell-free inocula, since the former usually contain higher titers of virus than the latter. The tissue cultures should be maintained through at least two blind 7-day passages and observed for cytopathic effects, but preferably for antigens by immunofluorescence (200), complement fixation (160), or enzyme immunoassay (41, 74) procedures using a specific antiserum against REV. In comparative studies, enzyme immunoassays were more sensitive than complement-fixation tests (41) and indirect immunofluorescence was more sensitive than indirect immunoperoxidase or immunoelectron microscopy (120). A convenient and sensitive indirect immunofluorescent assay conducted in 96-well plates (30) has been used for virus isolation from field samples (199).

Virus isolated by this procedure may be identified by reproduction of the typical disease in experimental animals and by further serologic analysis including neutralization tests. The production of C-type virus particles and the presence of reverse transcriptase by inoculated cultures may be of diagnostic value provided infection with leukosis/sarcoma group or lymphoproliferative disease viruses can be excluded. Some REVs may produce plaques in tissue culture and therefore can be further evaluated by plaque reduction tests with specific antiserum (33, 106).

Serology.

Confirmation of REV infection by serologic procedures involves the detection of antibodies or antigens in sera from chickens inoculated with suspect isolates or from chickens of field flocks. Antibodies are induced with various frequencies and persist for varied periods. Specific antibody may be detected in the serum or egg yolk from exposed birds by indirect immunofluorescence (2, 200), virus neutralization (98, 132), agar-gel precipitin (71, 111), enzyme immunoassay (20, 121, 159), and pseudotype neutralization (39) tests. Enzyme immunoassay kits are commercially available. The agar-gel precipitin test may also detect viral antigen in serum samples tested against an antibody-containing reference serum; in a survey of chicken and turkey flocks, 21 antigen-positive and 33 antibody-positive sera were detected (72). Witter et al. (203) found 46–100% of serum samples from 6 seropositive chicken and turkey flocks were positive; titers ranged from 80 to 2,560 (geometric mean 418) by the indirect immunofluorescent antibody test. Thus, pooled samples may be used in some cases. Antibody tests are particularly useful in ascertaining the absence of viral exposure in flocks, including those maintained as specific-pathogen-free.

The development of monoclonal antibodies to REV (40) has provided a powerful tool for the demonstration of viral antigens in tissues and cell cultures. A mixture of two monoclonal antibodies specifying different epitopes was used to develop an enzyme immunoassay (41), which was useful for detection of viral antigens in tissue samples, especially albumen (41, 199). An enzyme immunoassay based on rabbit anti-REV serum has also been described (74). Several of the monoclonal antibodies have also been used in indirect immunofluorescent assays for viral antigen (40), which recently has been adapted to 96-well plates (30). Antigen assays are an important part of biological assays for infectious virus, and are also useful for identifying hens that may shed infectious virus into eggs.

Differential Diagnosis. The differential diagnosis of REV-induced lesions from those of other diseases is difficult due to the lack of lesions pathognomonic for RE, the diverse types of lesions induced, and the similarity of the lesions to those caused by other organisms. As previously stated, diagnoses of RE should be supported by serologic or virologic evidence of infection with the virus. In addition, it may be helpful or necessary to reproduce the lesions experimentally with the REV recovered from the case material.

Some comparative features of RE, Marek's disease, and lymphoid leukosis are listed in Table 16.2.

The acute reticulum cell neoplasia syndrome, an experimentally induced disease, is unique because of its short latent period and lymphoreticular cell population. However, tumor transplants may also cause early death.

The runting disease syndrome must be distinguished from Marek's disease in the chicken, especially when nerve lesions are also present. Differences between REV- and Marek's disease virus–induced nerve lesions have been discussed (200, 201) but are not always easy to discern. Other immunodepressive diseases such as infectious bursal disease and infection with the chick anemia agent may also resemble the runting disease syndrome.

Chronic RE neoplasia in the turkey must be differentiated from lesions of lymphoproliferative disease of turkeys (73); differences in pathology and in properties of the viral reverse transcriptase can be helpful (145, 207).

Chronic neoplasia in the chicken where the tumors are of bursal origin cannot be differentiated from lymphoid leukosis on pathological criteria (196); virological or serological tests may help providing infection can be established for one virus and excluded for the other. However, RE or lymphoid leukosis tumors should contain proviral DNA sequences of the respective virus inserted near the c-*myc* gene, a characteristic that could permit differentiation of tumors by molecular hybridization; adaptation of such a procedure to routine field diagnosis has not been done but is worthy of study. Chronic neoplasia in the chicken where bursal tumors are lacking or where the latent period is too short for that of lymphoid leukosis must be differentiated from Marek's disease; good criteria are lacking.

In summary, naturally occurring RE lesions can be confused in the chicken with Marek's disease, lymphoid leukosis, and various immunodepressive conditions, and in the turkey with lymphoproliferative disease. Thus far, REV-induced lesions are not known to be common in chickens, but it is not known whether this is due to the absence of such lesions or their misdiagnosis. In view of the wide distribution of REV infection in commercial chickens (203), the prevalence of related lesions in this species may need reevaluation.

TREATMENT. No treatment for RE is known. Since immune responses are mounted to infection, it is possible that some affected birds may recover.

PREVENTION AND CONTROL. No procedures have been applied in commercial practice for the control of RE, mainly because the disease has been sporadic and self-limiting and has not been a problem in specific-pathogen-free flocks. However, studies by Witter and Salter (199) on a flock of naturally infected breeder turkeys showed that REV has the potential to be a major economic problem and provides an evaluation of some techniques for identification of shedder hens. Enzyme immunoassays to detect RE viral antigen in albumen samples seems to be the procedure of choice (74, 199). Presumably, it would be necessary to eliminate vertical transmission through removal of potential transmitter hens and to rear progeny under isolated conditions where horizontal infection could be precluded. Many of these principles have been applied to the control of avian leukosis virus in chickens. However, compared to avian leukosis virus, REV is likely to be vertically transmitted at lower rates, males may warrant greater consideration as potential transmitters, and horizontal infection seems more difficult to control. Such control procedures could be considered if the economic impact of RE in chickens or turkeys becomes more apparent.

REFERENCES

1. Allen, P.T., J.A. Mullins, C.L. Harris, A. Hellman, R.F. Garry, and M.R.F. Waite. 1979. Replication of reticuloendotheliosis virus in mammalian cells. Am Soc Microbiol Abst Annu Meet, No. SlOO, p. 256.

2. Aulisio, C.G., and A. Shelokov. 1969. Prevalence of reticuloendotheliosis in chickens: Immunofluorescence studies. Proc Soc Exp Biol Med 130:178–181.

3. Bagust, T.J., and T.M. Grimes. 1979. Experimental infection of chickens with an Australian strain of reticuloendotheliosis virus. 2. Serological responses and pathogenesis. Avian Pathol 8:375–389.

4. Bagust, T.J., T.M. Grimes, and D.P. Dennett. 1979. Infection studies on a reticuloendotheliosis virus contaminant of a commercial Marek's disease vaccine. Aust Vet J 55:153–157.

5. Bagust, T.J., T.M. Grimes, and N. Ratnamohan. 1981. Experimental infection of chickens with an Australian strain of reticuloendotheliosis virus. 3. Persistant infection and transmission by the adult hen. Avian Pathol 10:375–385.

6. Barbacid, M., E. Hunter, and S.A. Aaronson. 1979. Avian reticuloendotheliosis viruses: Evolutionary linkages with mammalian type C retroviruses. J Virol 30:508–514.

7. Barth, C.F., and E.H. Humphries. 1988. A nonimmunosuppressive helper virus allows high efficiency induction of B cell lymphomas by reticuloendotheliosis virus strain T. J Exp Med 167:89–108.

8. Bauer, G., and H.M. Temin. 1980. Specific anti-

genic relationships between the RNA-dependent DNA polymerases of avian reticuloendotheliosis viruses and mammalian type C retroviruses. J Virol 34:168–177.

9. Baxter-Gabbard, K.L., W.F. Campbell, F. Padgett, A. Raitano-Fenton, and A.S. Levine. 1971. Avian reticuloendotheliosis virus (strain T). II. Biochemical and biophysical properties. Avian Dis 15:850–862.

10. Baxter-Gabbard, K.L., D.A. Peterson, A.S. Levine, P. Meyers, and M.M. Sigel. 1973. Reticuloendotheliosis virus (strain T). VI. An immunogen versus reticuloendotheliosis and Rous sarcoma. Avian Dis 17:145–150.

11. Baxter-Gabbard, K.L., M.B. Seaward, and A.S. Levine. 1980. A survey of nonspecific cross-protective immunities induced by avian retroviruses. Avian Dis 24:1027–1037.

12. Beemon, K.L., A.J. Faras, A.T. Haase, P.H. Duesberg, and J.E. Maisel. 1976. Genomic complexities of murine leukemia and sarcoma, reticuloendotheliosis, and visna viruses. J Virol 17:525–537.

13. Bendheim, U. 1973. A neoplastic disease in turkeys following fowl pox vaccination. Refu Vet 30:35–41.

14. Beug, H., H. Muller, S. Grieser, G. Doederlein, and T. Graf. 1981. Hematopoietic cells transformed in vitro by REV-T avian reticuloendotheliosis virus express characteristics of very immature lymphoid cells. Virology 115:295–309.

15. Bose, H.R., and A.S. Levine. 1967. Replication of the reticuloendotheliosis virus (strain T) in chicken embryo cell culture. J Virol 1:1117–1121.

16. Breitman, M.L., M.M.C. Lai, and P.K. Vogt. 1980. Attenuation of avian reticuloendotheliosis virus: Loss of the defective transforming component during serial passage of oncogenic virus in fibroblasts. Virology 101:304–306.

17. Bülow, V. von. 1977. Immunological effects of reticuloendotheliosis virus as potential contaminant of Marek's disease vaccines. Avian Pathol 6:383–393.

18. Bülow, V. von. 1980. Effects of infectious bursal disease virus and reticuloendotheliosis virus infection of chickens on the incidence of Marek's disease and on local tumour development of the nonproducer JMV transplant. Avian Pathol 9:109–119.

19. Bülow, V. von, and A. Klasen. 1983. Effects of avian viruses on cultured chicken bone-marrow-derived macrophages. Avian Pathol 12:179–198.

20. Bülow, V. von, and M. Lesjak. 1987. A modified ELISA for the demonstration of antiviral antibodies in chicken sera which included the use of virus-free cellular antigens to control the specificity of assay results. J Vet Med [B] 34:655–669.

21. Bülow, V. von, and F. Weiland. 1980. Stimulation of local solid tumour development of the nonproducer Marek's disease tumour transplant JMV by virus-induced immunosuppression. Avian Pathol 9:93–108.

22. Burmester, B.R. 1964. Personal communication.

23. Campbell, W.F., K.L. Baxter-Gabbard, and A.S. Levine. 1971. Avian reticuloendotheliosis virus (strain T). I. Virological characterization. Avian Dis 15:837–849.

24. Carlson, H.C., G.L. Seawright, and J.R. Pettit. 1974. Reticuloendotheliosis in Japanese quail. Avian Pathol 3:169–175.

25. Carpenter, C.R., H.R. Bose, and A.S. Rubin. 1977. Contact-mediated suppression of mitogen-induced responsiveness by spleen cells in reticuloendotheliosis virus-induced tumorigenesis. Cell Immunol 33:392–401.

26. Carpenter, C.R., K.E. Kempf, H.R. Bose, and A.S. Rubin. 1978. Characterization of the interaction of reticuloendotheliosis virus with the avian lymphoid system. Cell Immunol 39:307–315.

27. Carpenter, C.R., A.S. Rubin, and H.R. Bose. 1978. Suppression of the mitogen-stimulated blastogenic response during reticuloendotheliosis virus-induced tumorigenesis: Investigations into the mechanism of action of the suppressor. J Immunol 120:1313–1320.

28. Chen, I.S.Y., and H.M. Temin. 1982. Establishment of infection by spleen necrosis virus: Inhibition in stationary cells and the role of secondary infection. J Virol 41:183–191.

29. Chen, I.S.Y., T.W. Mak, J.J. O'Rear, and H.M. Temin. 1981. Characterization of reticuloendotheliosis virus strain T DNA and isolation of a novel variant of reticuloendotheliosis virus strain T by molecular cloning. J Virol 40:800–811.

30. Chen, P.-Y., Z.-Z. Cui, L.F. Lee, and R.L. Witter. 1987. Serologic differences among nondefective reticuloendotheliosis viruses. Arch Virol 93:233–246.

31. Chen, L., M. Lim, H. Bose, and M. Bishop. 1988. Rearrangements of chicken immunoglobulin genes in lymphoid cells transformed by the avian retroviral oncogene v-rel. Proc Nat Acad Sci 85:549–553.

32. Cho, B.R. 1983. Cytopathic effects and focus formation by reticuloendotheliosis viruses in a quail fibroblast cell line. Avian Dis 27:261–270.

33. Cho, B.R. 1984. Improved focus assay of reticuloendotheliosis in a quail fibroblast cell line (QT35). Avian Dis 28:261–265.

34. Coffin, J.M. 1982. Structure of the retroviral genome. RNA tumor viruses. In R. Weiss, N. Teich, H. Varmus, and J. Coffin (eds.), Molecular Biology of Tumor Viruses, 2nd Ed., pp. 261–368. Cold Spring Harbor Laboratory, Cold Spring Harbor, NY.

35. Cohen, R.S., T.C. Wong, and M.M.C. Lai. 1981. Characterization of transformation and replication specific sequences of reticuloendotheliosis virus. Virology 113:672–685.

36. Cook, M.K. 1969. Cultivation of a filterable agent associated with Marek's disease. J Nat Cancer Inst 43:203–212.

37. Cooper, G.M., and H.M. Temin. 1974. Infectious Rous sarcoma virus and reticuloendotheliosis virus DNAs. J Virol 14:1132–1141.

38. Cowen, B.S., and M.O. Braune. 1988. The propagation of avian viruses in a continuous cell line (QT35) of Japanese quail origin. Avian Dis 32:282–297.

39. Crittenden, L.B., A.M. Fadly, and E.J. Smith. 1982. Effect of endogenous leukosis virus genes on response to infection with avian leukosis and reticuloendotheliosis virus. Avian Dis 26:279–294.

40. Cui, Z.-Z., L.F. Lee, R.F. Silva, and R.L. Witter. 1986. Monoclonal antibodies against avian reticuloendotheliosis virus: Identification of strain-specific and strain-common epitopes. J Immunol 136:4237–4242.

41. Cui, Z.-Z., L.F. Lee, R.F. Silva, R.L. Witter, and T.S. Chang. 1988. Monoclonal-antibody-mediated enzyme-linked immunosorbent assay for detection of reticuloendotheliosis viruses. Avian Dis 32:32–40.

42. Delwart, E.L., and A.T. Panganiban. 1989. Role of reticuloendotheliosis virus envelope glycoprotein in superinfection interference. J Virol 63:273–280.

43. Dren, C.N., E. Saghy, R. Glavits, F. Ratz, J. Ping, and V. Sztojkov. 1983. Lymphoreticular tumour in pen-raised pheasants associated with a RE-like virus infection. Avian Pathol 12:55–71.

44. Dren, C.N., I. Nemeth, I. Sari, F. Ratz, R. Glavits, and P. Somogyi. 1988. Isolation of a reticulendotheliosis-like virus from naturally occurring lymphoreticular tumours of domestic goose. Avian Pathol 17:259–277.

45. Embretson, J.E., and H.M. Temin. 1986. Pseudotyped retroviral vectors reveal restrictions to reticuloendotheliosis virus replication in rat cells. J Virol 60:662–668.

46. Embretson, J.E., and H.M. Temin. 1987. Tran-

scription from a spleen necrosis virus 5′ long terminal repeat is suppressed in mouse cells. J Virol 61:3454–3462.

47. Fadly, A.M., and R.L. Witter. 1983. Studies of reticuloendotheliosis virus induced lymphomagenesis in chickens. Avian Dis 27:271–282.

48. Fadly, A.M., and R.L. Witter. 1986. Resistance of Line 63 chickens to reticuloendotheliosis virus-induced bursa-associated lymphomas. Int J Cancer 38:139–143.

49. Federspiel, M.J., L.B. Crittenden, and S.H. Hughes. 1989. Expression of avian reticuloendotheliosis virus confers host resistance. Virology 173:167–177.

50. Franklin, R.B., R.L. Maldonado, and H.R. Bose. 1974. Isolation and characterization of reticuloendotheliosis virus transformed bone marrow cells. Intervirology 3:342–352.

51. Franklin, R.B., C.Y. Kang, K.M.M. Wan, and H.R. Bose. 1977. Transformation of chick embryo fibroblasts by reticuloendotheliosis virus. Virology 83:313–321.

52. Fritsch, E., and H.M. Temin. 1977. Formation and structure of infectious DNA of spleen necrosis virus. J Virol 21:119–130.

53. Fujita, D.J., R.A. Swift, A.A.G. Ridgway, and H.-J. Kung. 1984. Reticuloendotheliosis virus-induced B lymphomas in chickens: Characterization of a tumour cell DNA clone containing proviral and c-myc sequences. J Cell Biochem (Suppl 7, Pt B):12.

54. Fung, Y.K.T., A.M. Fadly, L.B. Crittenden, and H.-J. Kung. 1981. On the mechanism of retrovirus-induced avian lymphoid leukosis: Deletion and integration of the proviruses. Proc Nat Acad Sci 78:3418–3422.

55. Garry, R.F., and H.R. Bose. 1981. Secretion of a virus-regulated factor by clonal variants of reticuloendotheliosis virus-transformed hematopoietic cells. Virology 113:403–407.

56. Garry, R.F., and H.R. Bose. 1988. Autogenous growth factor production by reticuloendotheliosis virus-transformed hematopoietic cells. J Cell Biochem 37:327–338.

57. Garry, R.F., G.M. Shackleford, L.F. Berry, and H.R. Bose. 1985. Inhibition of hepatic phosphoenolpyruvate carboxykinase by avian reticuloendotheliosis viruses. Cancer Res 45:5020–5026.

58. Garson, K., and C.-Y. Kang. 1986. Identification of the v-rel protein in REV-T transformed chicken bone marrow cells and expression in Coxl cells. Biochem Biophys Res Commun 134:716–722.

59. Gilmore, T.D., and H.M. Temin. 1988. V-rel oncoproteins in the nucleus and in the cytoplasm transform chicken spleen cells. J Virol 62:703–714.

60. Grimes, T.M., and H.G. Purchase. 1973. Reticuloendotheliosis in a duck. Aust Vet J 49:466–471.

61. Grimes, T.M., T.J. Bagust, and C.K. Dimmock. 1979. Experimental infection of chickens with an Australian strain of reticuloendotheliosis virus. I. Clinical, pathological, and haematological effects. Avian Pathol 8:57–68.

62. Halpern, M.S., E. Wade, E. Rucker, K.L. Baxter-Gabbard, A.S. Levine, and R.R. Friis. 1973. A study of the relationship of reticuloendotheliosis virus to the avian leukosis-sarcoma complex of viruses. Virology 53:287–299.

63. Hayward, W.S., B.G. Neel, and S.M. Astrin. 1981. Activation of a cellular onc gene by promoter insertion in ALV-induced lymphoid leukosis. Nature 290:475–480.

64. Herzog, N.K., and H.R. Bose. 1986. Expression of the oncogene of avian reticuloendotheliosis virus in Escherichia coli and identification of the transforming protein in reticuloendotheliosis virus T-transformed cells. Proc Nat Acad Sci 83:812–816.

65. Herzog, N.K., W.J. Bergmann, and H.R. Bose. 1986. Oncogene expression in reticuloendotheliosis virus-transformed lymphoid cell lines and avian tissues. J Virol 57:371–375.

66. Herzog, N.K., D.S. Walro, J. Zhang, M.Y. Lin, and H.R. 1987. Bose. The transforming protein of avian reticuloendotheliosis virus is a soluble cytoplasmic protein which is associated with a protein kinase activity. Virology 160:433–444.

67. Hoelzer, J.D., R.B. Franklin, and H.R. Bose. 1979. Transformation by reticuloendotheliosis virus: Development of a focus assay and isolation of a non-transforming virus. Virology 93:20–30.

68. Hoelzer, J.D., R.B. Lewis, C.R. Wasmuth, and H.R. Bose. 1980. Hematopoietic cell transformation by reticuloendotheliosis virus: Characterization of the genetic defect. Virology 100:462–474.

69. Howell, L.J., R. Hunter, and T.J. Bagust. 1982. Necrotic dermatitis in chickens. NZ Vet J 30:87–88.

70. Hu, C.-P., and T.J. Linna. 1976. Serotherapy of avian reticuloendotheliosis virus-induced tumors. Ann NY Acad Sci 277:634–646.

71. Ianconescu, M. 1977. Reticuloendotheliosis antigen for the agar gel precipitation test. Avian Pathol 6:259–261.

72. Ianconescu, M., and A. Aharonovici. 1978. Persistant viraemia in chickens, subsequent to in ovo inoculation of reticuloendotheliosis virus. Avian Pathol 7:237–247.

73. Ianconescu, M., K. Perk, A. Zimber, and A. Yaniv. 1979. Reticuloendotheliosis and lymphoproliferative disease of turkeys. Refu Vet 36:2–12.

74. Ignjatovic, J., K.J. Fahey, and T.J. Bagust. 1987. An enzyme-linked immunosorbent assay for detection of reticuloendotheliosis virus infection in chickens. Avian Pathol 16:609–621.

75. Isfort, R., R.L. Witter, and H.-J. Kung. 1987. C-myc activation in an unusual retrovirus-induced avian T-lymphoma resembling Marek's disease: Proviral insertion 5′ of exon one enhances the expression of an intron promoter. Oncogene Res 2:81–94.

76. Jackson, C.A.W., S.E. Dunn, D.I. Smith, P.T. Gilchrist, and P.A. MacQueen. 1977. Proventriculitis, "Nakanuke," and reticuloendotheliosis in chickens following vaccination with herpesvirus of turkeys (HVT). Aust Vet J 53:457–458.

77. Kang, C.-Y., and H.M. Temin. 1974. Reticuloendotheliosis virus nucleic acid sequences in cellular DNA. J Virol 14:1179–1188.

78. Kang, C.-Y., and P. Lambright. 1977. Pseudotypes of vesicular stomatitis virus with the mixed coat of reticuloendotheliosis virus and vesicular stomatitis virus. J Virol 21:1252–1255.

79. Kang, C.-Y., T.C. Wong, and K.V. Holmes. 1975. Comparative ultrastructural study of four reticuloendotheliosis viruses. J Virol 16:1027–1038.

80. Kawamura, H., T. Wakabayashi, S. Yamaguchi, T. Taniguchi, N. Takayanagi, S. Sato, S. Sekiya, and T. Horiuchi. 1976. Inoculation experiment of Marek's disease vaccine contaminated with reticuloendotheliosis virus. Nat Inst Anim Health Q 16:135–140.

81. Keller, L.H., R. Rufner, and M. Sevoian. 1979. Isolation and development of a reticuloendotheliosis virus-transformed lymphoblastoid cell line from chicken spleen cells. Infect Immun 25:694–701.

82. Keshet, E., and H.M. Temin. 1979. Cell killing by spleen necrosis virus is correlated with a transient accumulation of spleen necrosis virus DNA. J Virol 31:376–388.

83. Kline, K., W.E. Briles, L.D. Bacon, and B.G.

Sanders. 1988. Characteristics of different B-F (MHC class I) molecules in the chicken. J Hered 79:239–248.
84. Koyama, H., Y. Suzuki, Y. Ohwada, and Y. Saito. 1976. Reticuloendotheliosis group virus pathogenic to chicken isolated from material infected with turkey herpesvirus (HVT). Avian Dis 20:429–434.
85. Koyama, H., T. Sasaki, Y. Ohwada, and Y. Saito. 1980. The relationship between feathering abnormalities ("Nakanuke") and tumour production in chickens inoculated with reticuloendotheliosis virus. Avian Pathol 9:331–340.
86. Koyama, H., T. Hodatsu, T. Sasaki, Y. Ohwada, Y. Saito, and H. Saito. 1981. Continuous cell culture from chick embryos inoculated with REV strain T. Avian Pathol 10:151–162.
87. Larose, R.N., and M. Sevoian. 1965. Avian lymphomatosis. IX. Mortality and serological response of chickens of various ages to graded doses of T strain. Avian Dis 9:604–610.
88. Lewis, R.B., J. McClure, B. Rup, D.W. Niesel, R.F. Garry, J.D. Hoelzer, K. Nazerian, and H.R. Bose. 1981. Avian reticuloendotheliosis virus: Identification of the hematopoietic target cell for transformation. Cell 25:421–431.
89. Li, J., B.W. Calnek, K.A. Schat, and D.L. Graham. 1983. Pathogenesis of reticuloendotheliosis virus infection in ducks. Avian Dis 27:1090–1105.
90. Linna, T.J., C. Hu, and K.D. Thompson. 1974. Development of systemic and local tumors induced by avian reticuloendotheliosis virus after thymectomy or bursectomy. J Nat Cancer Inst 53:847–854.
91. Ludford, C.G., H.G. Purchase, and H.W. Cox. 1972. Duck infections anemia virus associated with plasmodium louvers. Exp Parasitol 31:29–38.
92. Maccubbin, D., and L. Schierman. 1982. Evidence for association of viral and major histocompatibility complex antigens on reticuloendotheliosis virus transformed cells of chickens. Fed Proc 41(No. 2499):698.
93. Maccubbin, D., and L. Schierman. 1986. MHC-restricted cytotoxic response of chicken T cells: Expression, augmentation, and clonal characterization. J Immunol 136:12–16.
94. Maldonado, R.L., and H.R. Bose. 1971. Separation of reticuloendotheliosis virus from avian tumor viruses. J Virol 8:813–815.
95. Maldonado, R.L., and H.R. Bose. 1975. Polypeptide and RNA composition of the reticuloendotheliosis viruses. Intervirology 5:194–204.
96. Maldonado, R.L., and H.R. Bose. 1976. Group-specific antigen shared by the members of the reticuloendotheliosis virus complex. J Virol 17:983–990.
97. McDougall, J.S., P.M. Biggs, and R.W. Shilleto. 1978. A leukosis in turkeys associated with infection with reticuloendotheliosis virus. Avian Pathol 7:557–568.
98. McDougall, J.S., R.W. Shilleto, and P.M. Biggs. 1980. Experimental infection and vertical transmission of reticuloendotheliosis virus in the turkey. Avian Pathol 9:445–454.
99. McDougall, J.S., R.W. Shilleto, and P.M. Biggs. 1981. Further studies on vertical transmission of reticuloendotheliosis virus in turkeys. Avian Pathol 10:163–169.
100. Miller, C.K., and H M. Temin. 1986. Insertion of several different DNAs in reticuloendotheliosis virus strain T suppresses transformation by reducing the amount of subgenomic mRNA. J Virol 58:75–80.
101. Miller, C.K., J.E. Embretson, and H.M. Temin. 1988. Transforming viruses spontaneously arise from nontransforming reticuloendotheliosis virus strain T-derived viruses as a result of increased accumulation of spliced viral RNA. J Virol 62:1219–1226.
102. Mizutani, S., and H.M. Temin. 1976. RNA polymerase activity in purified virions of avian reticuloendotheliosis viruses. J Virol 19:610–619.
103. Moelling, K., H. Gelderblom, G. Pauli, R. Friis, and H. Bauer. 1975. A comparative study of the avian reticuloendotheliosis virus: Relationship to murine leukemia virus and viruses of the avian sarcoma-leukosis complex. Virology 65:546–557.
104. Moore, B.E., and H.R. Bose. 1988. Expression of the v-rel oncogene in reticuloendotheliosis virus-transformed fibroblasts. Virology 162:377–387.
105. Moore, B.E., and H.R. Bose. 1988. Transformation of avian lymphoid cells by reticuloendotheliosis virus. Mutation Res 195:79–90.
106. Moscovici, C., D. Chi, L. Gazzolo, and M.G. Moscovici. 1976. A study of plaque formation with avian RNA tumor viruses. Virology 73:181–189.
107. Mosser, A.G., R.C. Montelaro, and R.R. Rueckert. 1975. The polypeptide composition of spleen necrosis virus, a reticuloendotheliosis virus. J Virol 15:1088–1095.
108. Motha, M.X.J. 1982. Effects of reticuloendotheliosis virus on the response of chickens to infectious laryngotracheitis virus. Avian Pathol 11:475–486.
109. Motha, M.X.J. 1984. Distribution of virus and tumour formation in ducks experimentally infected with reticuloendotheliosis virus. Avian Pathol 13:303–320.
110. Motha, M.X.J. 1987. Clinical effects, virological and serological responses in chickens following in-ovo inoculation of reticuloendotheliosis virus. Vet Microbiol 14:411–417.
111. Motha, M.X.J. 1987. Demonstration of precipitating antibodies to reticuloendotheliosis virus in egg yolk. Aust Vet J 64:259–260.
112. Motha, M.X.J., and J.R. Egerton. 1983. Effect of reticuloendotheliosis virus on the response of chickens to Salmonella typhimurium infection. Res Vet Sci 34:188–192.
113. Motha, M.X.J., and J.R. Egerton. 1984. Influence of reticuloendotheliosis on the severity of Eimeria tenella infection in broiler chickens. Vet Microbiol 9:121–129.
114. Motha, M.X.J., and J.R. Egerton. 1987. Vertical transmission of reticuloendotheliosis virus in chickens. Avian Pathol 16:141–148.
115. Motha, M.X.J., and J.R. Egerton. 1987. Outbreak of atypical fowlpox in chickens with persistent reticuloendotheliosis viraemia. Avian Pathol 16:177–182.
116. Motha, M.X.J., J.R. Egerton, and A.W. Sweeney. 1984. Some evidence of mechanical transmission of reticuloendotheliosis virus by mosquitoes. Avian Dis 28:858–867.
117. Mussman, H.C., and M.J. Twiehaus. 1971. Pathogenesis of reticuloendotheliosis virus disease in chicks – an acute runting syndrome. Avian Dis 15:483–502.
118. Nazerian, K. 1987. An updated list of avian cell lines and transplantable tumours. Avian Pathol 16:527–544.
119. Nazerian, K., R.L. Witter, L.B. Crittenden, M.R. Noori-Daloii, and H.-J. Kung. 1982. An IgM-producing B lymphoblastoid cell line established from lymphomas induced by a nondefective reticuloendotheliosis virus. J Gen Virol 58:351–360.
120. Nicholas, R.A.J., and D.H. Thornton. 1983. Relative efficiency of techniques for detecting avian reticuloendotheliosis virus as a vaccine contaminant. Res Vet Sci 34:377–379.

121. Nicholas, R.A.J., and D.H. Thornton. 1987. An enzyme-linked immunosorbent assay for the detection of antibodies to avian reticuloendotheliosis virus using whole cell antigen. Res Vet Sci 43:403–404.
122. Nishimura, E.T., E. Ross, G. Leslie, H.-Y. Yang, and Y. Hokema. 1970. Epizootic reticulum cell sarcoma in a sequestered colony of Japanese quail. Cancer Res 30:2119–2126.
123. Noori-Daloii, M.R., R.A. Swift, H.J. Kung, L.B. Crittenden, and R.L. Witter. 1981. Specific integration of REV proviruses in avian bursal lymphomas. Nature 294:574–576.
124. Paul, P.S., and R.W. Werdin. 1978. Spontaneously occurring lymphoproliferative disease in ducks (case reports). Avian Dis 22:191–195.
125. Paul, P.S., K.A. Pomeroy, P.S. Sarma, K.H. Johnson, D.M. Barnes, M.C. Kumar, and B.S. Pomeroy. 1976. Brief communication: Naturally occuring reticuloendotheliosis in turkeys: Transmission. J Nat Cancer Inst 56:419–421.
126. Paul, P.S., K.H. Johnson, K.A. Pomeroy, B.S. Pomeroy, and P.S. Sarma. 1977. Experimental transmission of reticuloendotheliosis in turkeys with the cell-culture-propagated reticuloendotheliosis viruses of turkey origin. J Nat Cancer Inst 58:1819–1824.
127. Paul, P.S., K.A. Pomeroy, C.C. Muscoplat, B.S. Pomeroy, and P.S. Sarma. 1977. Characteristics of two new reticuloendotheliosis virus isolates of turkeys. Am J Vet Res 38:311–316.
128. Paul, I., O. Cotofan, and M. Boisteanu. 1986. The incidence of Marek's disease in anti-MD infected hens. Lucr Stiint Ser Zooteh Med Vet 30:95–96.
129. Perk, K., M. Malkinson, A. Gazit, A. Yaniv, and A. Zimber. 1981. Reappearance of an acute undifferentiated leukemia in a flock of Muscovy ducks. Proc 10th Int Symp Assoc for Comp Res Leukemia Related Dis, pp. 99–100.
130. Peterson, D.A., and A.S. Levine. 1971. Avian reticuloendotheliosis virus (strain T). IV. Infectivity and transmissibility in day-old cockerels. Avian Dis 15:874–883.
131. Purchase, H.G., and R.L. Witter. 1975. The reticuloendotheliosis viruses. Curr Top Microbiol Immunol 71:103–124.
132. Purchase H.G., C. Ludford, K. Nazerian, and H.W. Cox. 1973. A new group of oncogenic viruses: Reticuloendotheliosis, chick syncytial, duck infectious anemia, and spleen necrosis viruses. J Nat Cancer Inst 51:489–499.
133. Ratnamohan, N., T.J. Bagust, T.M. Grimes, and P.B. Spradbrow. 1979. Transmission of an Australian strain of reticuloendotheliosis virus to adult Japanese quail. Aust Vet J 55:506.
134. Ratnamohan, N., T.M. Grimes, T.J. Bagust, and P.B. Spradbrow. 1980. A transmissible chicken tumour associated with reticuloendotheliosis virus infection. Aust Vet J 56:34.
135. Ratnamohan, N., T. Bagust, and P.B. Spradbrow. 1982. Establishment of a chicken lymphoblastoid cell line infected with reticuloendotheliosis virus. J Comp Pathol 92:527–532.
136. Rehacek, J., T. Dolan, K. Thompson, R.G. Fischer, Z. Rehacek, and H. Johnson. 1971. Cultivation of oncogenic viruses in mosquito cells in vitro. Curr Top Microbiol Immunol 55:161–164.
137. Rice, N.R., T.D. Copeland, S. Simek, S. Oroszlan, and R.V. Gilden. 1986. Detection and characterization of the protein encoded by the v-rel oncogene. Virology 149:217–229.
138. Ridgway, A.A., R.A. Swift, H.-J. Kung, and D.J. Fujita. 1985. In vitro transcription analysis of the viral promoter involved in c-myc activation in chicken lymphomas: Detection and mapping for two RNA initiation sites with the reticuloendotheliosis virus long terminal repeat. J Virol 54:161–170.
139. Robinson, F.R., and M.J. Twiehaus. 1974. Isolation of the avian reticuloendothelial virus (strain T). Avian Dis 18:278–288.
140. Rup, B.J., J.L. Spence, J.D. Hoelzer, R.B. Lewis, C.R. Carpenter, A.S. Rubin, and H.R. Bose. 1979. Immunosuppression induced by avian reticuloendotheliosis virus: Mechanism of induction of the suppressor cell. J Immunol 123:1362–1370.
141. Rup, B.J., J.D. Hoelzer, and H.R. Bose. 1982. Helper viruses associated with avian acute leukemia viruses inhibit the cellular immune response. Virology 116:61–71.
142. Salter, D.W., E.J. Smith, S.H. Hughes, S.E. Wright, and L.B. Crittenden. 1986. Transgenic chickens: Insertion of retroviral genes into the chicken germ line. Virology 157:236–240.
143. Sawyer, R.C., and H. Hanafusa. 1977. Formation of reticuloendotheliosis virus pseudotypes of Rous sarcoma virus. J Virol 22:634–639.
144. Schat, K.A., J. Gonzales, A. Solorzano, E. Avila, and R.L. Witter. 1976. A lymphoproliferative disease in Japanese quail. Avian Dis 20:153–161.
145. Schwarzbard, Z., A. Yaniv, M. Ianconescu, K. Perk, and A. Zimber. 1980. A reverse transcriptase assay for the diagnosis of lymphoproliferative disease. Avian Pathol 9:481–487.
146. Scofield, V.L., and H.R. Bose. 1978. Depression of mitogen response in spleen cells from reticuloendotheliosis virus-infected chickens and their suppressive effect on normal lymphocyte response. J Immunol 120:1321–1325.
147. Scofield, V.L., J.L. Spence, W.E. Briles, and H.R. Bose. 1978. Differential mortality and lesion responses to reticuloendotheliosis virus infection in Marek's disease-resistant and susceptible chicken lines. Immunogenet 7:169–172.
148. Sevoian, M., R.N. Larose, and D.M. Chamberlain. 1964. Avian lymphomatosis. VI. A virus of unusual potency and pathogenicity. Avian Dis 3:336–347.
149. Sevoian, M., R.N. Larose, and D.M. Chamberlain. 1964. Avian lymphomatosis. VIII. Pathological response of the chicken embryo to T virus. J Nat Cancer Inst 17:99–119.
150. Shen, P.F.-L. 1981. Immunological, hematogical, pathological, and ultrastructural studies of chickens with reticuloendotheliosis. PhD diss, Univ of Arkansas.
151. Shibuya T., I. Chen, A. Howatson, and T.W. Mak. 1982. Morphological, immunological, and biochemical analyses of chicken spleen cells transformed in vitro by reticuloendotheliosis virus strain T. Cancer Res 42:2722–2728.
152. Shimotohno, K., S. Mizutani, and H.M. Temin. 1980. Sequence of retrovirus provirus resembles that of bacterial transposable elements. Nature 285:550–554.
153. Shuman, R.M., and R.N. Shoffner. 1986. Molecular approaches to poultry breeding: Gene transfer by avian retroviruses. Poult Sci 65:1437–1444.
154. Simek, S., and N.K. Rice. 1980. Analysis of the nucleic acid components in reticuloendotheliosis virus. J Virol 33:320–329.
155. Simek, S., and N.K. Rice. 1988. p59v-rel, the transforming protein of reticuloendotheliosis virus, is complexed with at least four other proteins in transformed chicken lymphoid cells. J Virol 62:4730–4736.
156. Simek, S.L., R.L. Stephens, and N.R. Rice. 1986. Localization of the v-rel protein in reticuloendotheliosis virus strain T-transformed lymphoid cells. J Virol 59:120–126.
157. Sinkovic, B. 1981. In vivo interactions between

reticuloendotheliosis virus and some other infectious agents of chickens. Proc 4th Aust Poult Stock Feed Conv, pp. 114–118.

158. Sinkovic, B., and C.O. Choi. 1979. Studies on reticuloendotheliosis maternal antibody. Proc 3rd Aust Poult Stock Feed Conv, pp. 119–122.

159. Smith, E.J., and R.L. Witter. 1983. Detection of antibodies against reticuloendotheliosis viruses by an enzyme-linked immunosorbent assay. Avian Dis 27:225–234.

160. Smith, E.J., J.J. Solomon, and R.L. Witter. 1977. Complement-fixation test for reticuloendotheliosis viruses. Limits of sensitivity in infected avian cells. Avian Dis 21:612–622.

161. Solomon, J.J., R.L. Witter, and K. Nazerian. 1976. Studies on the etiology of lymphomas in turkeys: Isolation of reticuloendotheliosis virus. Avian Dis 20:735–747.

162. Stephens, R.M., N.R. Rice, R.R. Hiebsch, H.R. Bose, and R.V. Gilden. 1983. Nucleotide sequence of v-rel: The oncogene of reticuloendotheliosis virus. Proc Nat Acad Sci, US 80:6229–6233.

163. Swift, R.A., E. Shaller, R.L. Witter, and H.-J. Kung. 1985. Insertional activation of c-myc by reticuloendotheliosis virus in chicken B lymphoma: Nonrandom distribution and orientation of the proviruses. J Virol 54:869–872.

164. Swift, R.A., C. Boerkoel, A. Ridgway, D.J. Fujita, J.B. Dodgson, and H.-J. Kung. 1987. B-lymphoma induction by reticuloendotheliosis virus: Characterization of a mutated chicken syncytial virus provirus involved in c-myc activation. J Virol 61:2084–2090.

165. Sylla, B.S., and H.M. Temin. 1986. Activation of oncogenicity of the c-rel proto-oncogene. Mol Cell Biol 6:4709–4716.

166. Tajima, M., T. Nunoya, and Y. Otaki. 1977. Pathogenesis of abnormal feathers in chickens inoculated with reticuloendotheliosis virus. Avian Dis 21:77–89.

167. Taniguchi, T., N. Yuasa, S. Sato, and T. Horiuchi. 1977. Pathological changes in chickens inoculated with reticuloendotheliosis-virus-contaminated Marek's disease vaccine. Nat Inst Anim Health Q 17:141–150.

168. Taylor, H.W., and L.D. Olson. 1973. Chronologic study of the T-virus in chicks. II. Development of hematologic changes. Avian Dis 17:794–802.

169. Temin, H.M., and V.K. Kassner. 1974. Replication of reticuloendotheliosis viruses in cell cultures: Acute infection. J Virol 13:291–297.

170. Temin, H.M., and V.K. Kassner. 1975. Replication of reticuloendotheliosis viruses in cell culture: Chronic infection. J Gen Virol 27:267–274.

171. Temin, H.M., E. Keshet, and S.K. Weller. 1980. Correlation of transient accumulation of linear unintegrated viral DNA and transient cell killing by avian leukosis and reticuloendotheliosis viruses. Cold Spring Harbor Symp 44:773–778.

172. Terada, N., T. Kuramoto, and T. Ino. 1977. Comparison of susceptibility to the T-strain of reticuloendotheliosis virus among families of Japanese quail. Jpn Poult Sci 14:259–265.

173. Theilen, G.H., R.F. Zeigel, and M.J. Twiehaus. 1966. Biological studies with REV (strain T) that induces reticuloendotheliosis in turkeys, chickens, and Japanese quail. J Nat Cancer Inst 37:731–743.

174. Thompson, K.D., and T.J. Linna. 1973. Bursa-dependent and thymus-dependent "surveillance" of a virus-induced tumor in the chicken. Nature New Biol 245:10–12.

175. Thompson, K.D., R.G. Fischer, and D.H. Luecke. 1968. Determination of the viremic period of avian reticuloendotheliosis virus (strain T) in chicks and virus viability in Triatoma infestans (KLUG) (Hemiptera:Reduviidae). Avian Dis 12:354–360.

176. Thompson, K.D., R.G. Fischer, and D.H. Luecke. 1971. Quantitative infectivity studies of avian reticuloendotheliosis virus (strain T) in certain hematophagous arthropods. J Med Entomol 8:486–490.

177. Torres-Medina, A., R.C. Mussman, M.B. Rhodes, and M.J. Twiehaus. 1973. Chicken transferrin: High levels in chickens with reticuloendothelial virus disease. Poult Sci 52:747–754.

178. Trager, W. 1959. A new virus of ducks interfering with development of malaria parasite (Plasmodium lophurae). Proc Soc Exp Biol Med 101:578–582.

179. Tsai, W.-P., and S. Oroszlan. 1988. Site-directed cytotoxic antibody against the C-terminal segment of the surface glycoprotein gp90 of avian reticuloendotheliosis virus. Virology 166:608–611.

180. Tsai, W.-P., T.D. Copeland, and S. Oroszlan. 1985. Purification and chemical and immunological characterization of avian reticuloendotheliosis virus gag-gene-encoded structural proteins. Virology 140:289–312.

181. Tsai, W.-P., T.D. Copeland, and S. Oroszlan. 1986. Biosynthesis and chemical and immunological characterization of avian reticuloendotheliosis virus env gene-encoded proteins. Virology 155:567–583.

182. Tung, H.Y.L., W.J. Bargmann, M.Y. Lim, and H.R. Bose. 1988. The v-rel oncogene product is complexed to a 40-KDA phosphoprotein in transformed lymphoid cells. Proc Nat Acad Sci 85:2479–2583.

183. Varmus, H., and R. Swanstrom. 1985. Replication of retroviruses. In R. Weiss, N. Teich, H. Varmus, and J. Coffin (eds.), RNA tumor viruses. Molecular Biology of Tumor Viruses, 2nd Ed., Supplements and Appendixes, pp. 75–134. Cold Spring Harbor Laboratory, Cold Spring Harbor, NY.

184. Vogt, P.K., J.L. Spencer, W. Okazaki, R.L. Witter, and L.B. Crittenden. 1977. Phenotypic mixing between reticuloendotheliosis virus and avian sarcoma viruses. Virology 80:127–135.

185. Von dem Hagen, D., and H.A. Loliger. 1978. Studies into epizootiology of quail leukosis. Monatsh Vet Med 33:591–593.

186. Wakabayashi, T., and H. Kawamura. 1975. Virus reticuloendotheliosis virus group: Persistent infection in chickens and viral transmission to fertile eggs. Proc 79th Annu Meet Jpn World Vet Poult Assoc, pp. 12–13.

187. Walker, M.H., B.J. Rup, A.S. Rubin, and H.R. Bose. 1983. Specificity in the immunosuppression induced by avian reticuloendotheliosis virus. Infect Immun 40:225–235.

188. Walro, D.S., N.K. Herzog, J. Zhang, M.Y. Lim, and H.R. Bose. 1987. The transforming protein of avian reticuloendotheliosis virus is a soluble cytoplasmic protein which is associated with a protein kinase activity. Virology 160:433–444.

189. Watanabe, S., and H.M. Temin. 1982. Encapsidation sequences for spleen necrosis virus and avian retrovirus, are between the 5′ long terminal repeat and the start of the gag gene. Proc Nat Acad Sci, US 79:5986–5990.

190. Watanabe, S., and H.M. Temin. 1983. Construction of a helper cell line for avian reticuloendotheliosis virus cloning vectors. Mol Cell Biol 3:2241–2249.

191. Weinstock, D., and K.A. Schat. 1987. Virus specific syngeneic killing of reticuloendotheliosis virus transformed cell line target cells by spleen cells. In W.T. Weber and D. Ewert (eds.), Avian Immunology, pp. 253–263. Alan R. Liss, Inc., New York.

192. Weller, S.K., and H.M. Temin. 1981. Cell killing by avian leukosis viruses. J Virol 39:713–721.

193. Wilhelmsen, K.C., and H.M. Temin. 1984. Structure and dimorphism of c-rel (turkey), the cellular homolog to the oncogene of reticuloendotheliosis virus strain T. J Virol 49:521–529.
194. Wilhelmsen, K.C., K. Eggleton, and H.M. Temin. 1984. Nucleic acid sequences of the oncogene v-rel in reticuloendotheliosis virus strain T and its cellular homolog the proto-oncogene c-rel. J Virol 52:172–182.
195. Witter, R.L. 1984. Reticuloendotheliosis. In M.S. Hofstad, H.J. Barnes, B.W. Calnek, W.M. Reid, and H.W. Yoder, Jr. (eds.), Diseases of Poultry, 8th Ed., pp 406–417. Iowa State Univ Press, Ames.
196. Witter, R.L., and L.B. Crittenden. 1979. Lymphomas resembling lymphoid leukosis in chickens inoculated with reticuloendotheliosis virus. Int J Cancer 23:673–678.
197. Witter, R.L., and S.W. Glass. 1984. Reticuloendotheliosis in breeder turkeys. Avian Dis 28:742–750.
198. Witter, R.L., and D.C. Johnson. 1985. Epidemiology of reticuloendotheliosis virus in broiler breeder flocks. Avian Dis 29:1140–1154.
199. Witter, R.L., and D.W. Salter. 1989. Vertical transmission of reticuloendotheliosis virus in breeder turkeys. Avian Dis 33:226–235.
200. Witter, R.L., H.G. Purchase, and G.H. Burgoyne. 1970. Peripheral nerve lesions similar to those of Marek's disease in chickens inoculated with reticuloendotheliosis virus. J Nat Cancer Inst 45:567–577.
201. Witter, R.L., L.F. Lee, L.D. Bacon, and E.J. Smith. 1979. Depression of vaccinal immunity to Marek's disease by infection with reticuloendotheliosis virus. Infect Immun 26:90–98.
202. Witter, R.L., E.J. Smith, and L.B. Crittenden. 1981. Tolerance, viral shedding, and neoplasia in chickens infected with nondefective reticuloendotheliosis viruses. Avian Dis 25:374–394.
203. Witter, R.L., I.L. Peterson, E.J. Smith, and D.C. Johnson. 1982. Serological evidence in commercial chicken and turkey flocks of infection with reticuloendotheliosis virus. Avian Dis 26:753–762.
204. Witter, R.L., J.M. Sharma, and A.M. Fadly. 1986. Nonbursal lymphomas by nondefective reticuloendotheliosis virus. Avian Pathol 15:467–486.
205. Wong, T.C., and M.M.C. Lai. 1981. Avian reticuloendotheliosis virus contains a new class of oncogene of turkey origin. Virology 111:289–293.
206. Wong, T.C., R.B. Lewis, H.R. Bose, Jr., and C.-Y. Kang. 1980. Assembly of avian reticuloendotheliosis virus: Association of the core precursor polypeptide with the intracellular ribonucleoprotein complex. J Virol 34:484.
207. Yaniv, A., A. Gazit, M. Ianconescu, K. Perk, B. Aizenberg, and A. Zimber. 1979. Biochemical characterization of the type C retrovirus associated with lymphoproliferative disease of turkeys. J Virol 30:351–357.
208. Yoshida, I., M. Sakata, K. Fujita, T. Noguchi, and N. Yuasa. 1981. Modification of low virulent Newcastle disease virus infection in chickens infected with reticuloendotheliosis virus. Nat Inst Anim Health Q 21:1–6.
209. Yuasa, N., I. Yoshida, and T. Taniguchi. 1976. Isolation of a reticuloendotheliosis virus from chickens inoculated with Marek's disease vaccine. Nat Inst Anim Health Q 16:141–151.
210. Zeigel, R.F., G.H. Theilen, and M.J. Twiehaus. 1966. Electron microscopic observations on REV (strain T) that induces reticuloendotheliosis in turkeys, chickens, and Japanese quail. J Nat Cancer Inst 37:709–729.

LYMPHOPROLIFERATIVE DISEASE OF TURKEYS

P.M. Biggs

INTRODUCTION, HISTORY, INCIDENCE, DISTRIBUTION. Lymphoproliferative disease (LPD) is a term used to describe a lymphoproliferative disorder of turkeys that was first recognized as a disease entity in 1972 in the UK (2, 3). In the same year a condition in turkeys described as similar to Marek's disease (MD) that closely resembled LPD was reported in the Netherlands (21). Since that time LPD has been reported in Israel (17) and recognized in several countries of Europe. It probably is not a new disease, because a retrospective examination of sections of tumors submitted for diagnosis in the past revealed a similarity between many of the lesions and those described for LPD (2, 3). In addition, lymphomatosis, leukosis, and MD-like disease have been reported in turkeys over the years (1, 4, 12, 20), and some of these cases could have been LPD. The disease may be endemic or sporadic in occurrence and some flocks may have a low incidence (3).

ETIOLOGY. Although Koch's postulates have not been fulfilled for the etiology of LPD because the agent has not been cultivated in vitro, strong circumstantial evidence suggests that it is a type C virus belonging to the family Retroviridae. Type C particles occur in tissues, lesions, and plasma pellets from birds with natural and experimentally produced disease, and preparations of these materials reproduce the disease when inoculated into poults (3, 11, 18). Type C particles, called LPD virus (LPDV), have been described as budding from cells in proliferative lesions. Mature particles measure 90–120 nm in diameter and have an electron-dense core with a less dense intermediate layer bounded by an outer envelope. Most particles are extracellular. Partially purified virus is infectious after filtration through a membrane filter with a pore diameter of 220 nm but not when the pore diameter is 100 nm; its infectivity is inactivated by lipid solvents (11). Density of the infectious particles is 1.16–1.18 g/cm³. The virus contains high molecular weight RNA, with a sediment coefficient of approximately 70S, and a RNA-dependent DNA polymerase (22). The reverse transcriptase of LPDV has a preference for Mg^{++} over Mn^{++} in both endogenous and exogenous reactions (19, 22).

LPDV is unrelated to other avian retroviruses serologically, and there is no nucleic acid sequence homology with them (11, 13, 14, 22). There has been difficulty in determining the structural polypeptides of LPDV. This is because of the lack of cell cultures susceptible to infection with LPDV and therefore an inability to use metabolic labelling techniques. Virus for study has had to be prepared from plasma collected from viremic turkeys. Preparations of virus from this source seem to be contaminated with host polypeptides, some of which are absorbed to the surface of the virus. Two groups have studied the LPDV polypeptides, which seem different from those of other retroviruses. Gazit et al. (7) described five structural polypeptides with molecular weights of 76, 31, 28, 20 and 15 kD. The 76-kD polypeptide is glycosylated and these authors suggested it was a major constituent of the virion envelope. They also suggested that p20 is a constituent of the envelope. They described p31 and p28 as the major structural polypeptides. Patel and Shilleto (15) described three major (p32, p26, and p22/21) and two minor (p41 and p12) structural polypeptides. They also suggested gp76 and a major doublet polypeptide p13.5/13 to be of viral origin. They concluded that gp76 is a surface protein and that p22/21 is probably intramembrane in location, whereas p32, p26, and p13.5/13 are in the viral core with p13.5/13 likely to be the ribonucleoprotein.

LPDV does not appear to be endogenous to turkeys because virus-specific sequences have not been found in the cell genome (5). Attempts to cultivate the virus in cell culture have been unsuccessful using embryo fibroblasts of chickens, turkeys, ducks, and quail, and kidney cells of chicks and turkeys (11).

PATHOGENESIS AND EPIZOOTIOLOGY. The disease has been described only in turkeys. Attempts to transmit the infection by parenteral inoculation were successful in chickens but unsuccessful in ducks and geese (10). Gross and microscopic lesions were produced in chickens but were less severe than in turkeys. The natural disease occurs in turkeys mainly between 7 and 18 wk of age, although it can occur sporadically in adults (2, 3, 8). Males may be more susceptible to the disease than females. Turkey hybrids differ in susceptibility to development of disease in response to inoculation with infectious material (11), and much of the disease in the field has been restricted to a few commercial hybrids. LPD can spread horizontally between poults in contact (11). Incubation period for the natural disease is not known. Field observations suggest it can be as short as 7 wk, and experimental transmission studies suggest it could be less than that in some individuals and more in others.

An unusual feature of the disease is that poults infected at 4 wk of age develop a higher incidence of disease than those infected at 1 day (2, 11). It does not appear that this is the result of a change in susceptibility to infection, because poults inoculated at 1 day of age do become infected (9, 11). It is possible that the presence of maternally derived antibody reduces probability of infection producing disease or, alternatively, that immune competence is required for development of disease. However, surgical or chemical bursectomy did not significantly influence the incidence or severity of experimentally produced disease (25).

The clinical course of the disease is rapid, with few if any premonitory signs; when clinical signs are noted, they are ruffled feathers, anorexia, and a disinclination to move. Poults showing signs die, and mortality may be as high as 25% of the flock.

The most consistent gross lesion is splenomegaly. Affected spleens can be as large as a chicken egg, and usually they are pale pink and marbled in appearance. The liver may be enlarged, but not greatly so, and it may contain miliary gray-white foci. Similar miliary or diffuse lesions may also occur in pancreas, thymus, kidneys, gonads, intestinal wall, lungs, and myocardium. In some birds, peripheral nerves are slightly enlarged (2, 3, 8). Anemia is frequently present; some affected birds have a leukocytosis, others are leukopenic and elevated IgG concentration has been recorded (23).

The characteristic lesion in all organs is lymphoproliferation of pleomorphic cells. Lesions consist of lymphocytes, lymphoblasts, reticulum cells, and plasma cells either scattered throughout the lesion or in some cases located around the periphery of small focal lesions. The proliferative lesions may be large and diffuse or small and focal. Rare lesions in peripheral nerves are similar to those of Marek's disease, but they tend to be focal and not diffuse throughout the nerve.

Development of the disease has been studied by McDougall et al. (11) and Zimber et al. (24). Specific lesions were first recognized in the spleen and thymus 14 days after inoculation of 4-wk-old poults. They referred to these as early lymphoid lesions that were small and consisted mainly of lymphocytes, although lymphoblasts, reticulum cells, and plasma cells were also present (11). In the spleen these lesions occurred as discrete foci in the red pulp. In the thymus there was atrophy of the cortex and loss of lymphocytes from the enlarged medulla, which were replaced by lymphoblasts and reticulum and plasma cells. By 21 days postinoculation the lesions in the spleen had enlarged and obliterated its normal architecture. In the thymus the cortex was almost completely atrophied. These enlarging lesions contained many mitotic figures and were characteristic of the tumors seen in the natural disease. At this time, numerous small focal lymphoproliferative lesions were seen in many other organs. A third type of lesion, which was small and focal and consisted of lymphocytes, was also noted; many of these lesions contained germinal centers. This type increases in frequency with time after inoculation, which suggests it is a regressing lesion. These observations are paralleled by appearance of LPDV-specific RNA sequences (6) and presence of virus particles (11). RNA sequences first appear in bone marrow 3 days postinfection; 2 and 7 days later they are present in the thymus and spleen, and bursa of Fabricius, respectively. By 15 days RNA sequences appear in many organs but at a lower level than in the lymphoid organs. Five days postinfection there is a viremia that increases in concentration at least until 6 wks postinfection. Over this period there was an increase in serum IgG (24). Up to 11 wk after infection a suppression in cell-mediated immunity but not humoral immunity has been described (23, 25). Using a competition enzyme-linked immunosorbent assay (ELISA) and radio immunoprecipitation, Patel and Shilleto (13) found turkeys do not respond to infection by producing antibodies.

DIAGNOSIS. Until recently the diagnosis of LPD depended on the appearance of the disease in a flock and gross and microscopic examination of lesions assisted by reverse transcriptase assays in plasma pellets where facilities for such a test are available. With the production of virus-specific antisera, serological tests for LPDV have been developed. Such virus-specific antibodies can be produced in chickens and rabbits by using bromelain-treated virus purified from plasma. This treatment removes all host components from the virus preparation (16). Using such antisera in an indirect immunofluorescence test, LPDV can be demonstrated in buffy coat cells and in frozen sections of spleen for up to 16 mo postinfection (14). An indirect ELISA using antiserum raised against bromelain-digested virus has been described for detecting virus in pellets derived from high-speed centrifugation of plasma from infected turkeys (13). Both tests correlate well with the reverse transcriptase test. Since antibodies could not be detected using a competition ELISA or a radio immunoprecipitation test in infected turkeys, tests for antibodies to LPDV for diagnostic purposes serve no purpose. The main disease with which LPD can be confused is reticuloendotheliosis (RE). The distinctive features of LPD are the characteristic splenomegaly and pleomorphic nature of the cellular composition of the tumors. A test has been described to aid in differential diagnosis of LPD and RE (19), which takes advantage of the common persistent viremia found in turkeys infected with these viruses and the difference in the cation requirements for the reverse transcriptase of LPDV and RE virus (REV) (22). REV reverse transcriptase prefers Mn^{++} over Mg^{++}, whereas the opposite is true for LPDV. The test requires that the exogenous reverse transcriptase test be done using pellets of plasma from the suspect flock in presence of 0.8 mM magnesium chloride and 0.08 mM manganese chloride (19). The divalent cation requirement index is calculated and defined as the ratio between the reverse transcriptase activity in presence of Mg^{++} and that in presence of Mn^{++}. An index above 2.0 is characteristic of LPDV and below 0.5 of REV. However, other tests are now available; for RE, there are virus isolation and serologic tests (see Reticuloendotheliosis) and for LPDV, the indirect immunofluorescence test and the indirect ELISA referred to above, which are specific for LPDV and show no cross reactions with REV or avian leukosis viruses (13, 14).

PREVENTION AND CONTROL. There is no information on prevention and control of LPD. Observed differences in susceptibility to LPD in experimental infections suggest that for the long term a selection for resistance to the disease is a possible approach to prevention. Where serious disease occurs, a change in breed or hybrid of turkey may be beneficial. As with all infectious disease, attention should be paid to management and hygiene procedures.

REFERENCES

1. Andrews, C.H., and R.E. Glover. 1939. A case of neurolymphomatosis in a turkey. Vet Rec 51:934–935.
2. Biggs, P.M., B.S. Milne, J.A. Frazier, J.S. McDougall, and J.C. Stuart. 1974. Lymphoproliferative disease in turkeys. Proc 15th World's Poult Congr, pp 55–56.
3. Biggs, P.M., J.S. McDougall, J.A. Frazier, and B.S. Milne. 1978. Lymphoproliferative disease of turkeys. 1. Clinical aspects. Avian Pathol 7:131–139.
4. Busch, R.H., and L.E. Williams, Jr. 1970. A Marek's disease-like condition in Florida turkeys. Avian Dis 14:550–554.
5. Gazit, A., A. Yaniv, M. Ianconescu, K. Perk, B. Aizenberg, and Z. Zimber. 1979. Molecular evidence for a type C retrovirus etiology of the lymphoproliferative disease of turkeys. J Virol 31:639–644.
6. Gazit, A., Z. Schwarzbard, A. Yaniv, M. Ianconescu, K. Perk, and A. Zimber. 1982. Organotropism of the lymphoproliferative disease virus (LPDV) of turkeys. Int J Cancer 29:599–604.
7. Gazit, A., R. Basri, M. Ianconescu, K. Perk, A. Zimber, and A. Yaniv. 1986. Analysis of structural polypeptides of the lymphoproliferative disease virus (LPDV) of turkeys. Int J Cancer 37:241–245.
8. Ianconescu, M., K. Perk, A. Zimber, and A. Yaniv. 1979. Reticuloendotheliosis and lymphoproliferative disease of turkeys. Refu Vet 36:2–12.

9. Ianconescu, M., A. Gazit, A. Yaniv, K. Perk, and A. Zimber. 1981. Comparative susceptibility of two turkey strains to lymphoproliferative disease virus. Avian Pathol 10:131–136.
10. Ianconescu, M., A. Yaniv, A. Gazit, K. Perk, and A. Zimber. 1983. Susceptibility of domestic birds to lymphoproliferative disease virus (LPDV) of turkeys. Avian Pathol 12:291–302.
11. McDougall, J.S., P.M. Biggs, R.W. Shilleto, and B.S. Milne. 1978. Lymphoproliferative disease of turkeys. II. Experimental transmission and aetiology. Avian Pathol 7:141–155.
12. McKee, G.S., A.M. Lucas, E.M. Denington, and F.C. Love. 1963. Separation of leukotic and nonleukotic lesions in turkeys on the inspection line. Avian Dis 7:19–30.
13. Patel, J.R., and R.W. Shilleto. 1987. Detection of lymphoproliferative disease virus by an enzyme-linked immunosorbent assay. Epidem Inf 99:711–722.
14. Patel, J.R., and R.W. Shilleto. 1987. Diagnosis of lymphoproliferative disease virus infection of turkeys by an indirect immunofluorescence test. Avian Pathol 16:367–376.
15. Patel, J.R., and R.W. Shilleto. 1987. Characterization of lymphoproliferative disease virus of turkeys. Structural polypeptides of the C-type particles. Arch Virol 95:159–176.
16. Patel, J.R., and R.W. Shilleto. 1987. Production of virus-specific antisera to lymphoproliferative disease virus of turkeys. Avian Pathol 16:699–705.
17. Perk, K., M. Ianconescu, A. Yaniv, and Z. Zimber. 1978. Lymphoproliferative disease in turkeys–structure, ultrastructure, and biochemistry. Refu Vet 35:29.
18. Perk, K., M. Ianconescu, A. Yaniv, and Z. Zimber. 1979. Morphologic characterization of proliferative cells and virus particles in turkeys with lymphoproliferative disease. J Nat Cancer Inst 62:1483–1485.
19. Schwarzbard, Z., A. Yaniv, M. Ianconescu, K. Perk, and A. Zimber. 1980. A reverse transcriptase assay for the diagnosis of lymphoproliferative disease (LPD) of turkeys. Avian Pathol 9:481–487.
20. Simpson, C.F., D.W. Anthony, and F. Young. 1957. Visceral lymphomatosis in a flock of turkeys. J Am Vet Med Assoc 130:93–96.
21. Voute, E.J., and A.E. Wagenaar-Schaafsma. 1974. Een op de ziekte van Marek lijkende afwijking bij mestkalkoenen in Nederland. Tijdschr Diergeneesk 99:166–169.
22. Yaniv, A., A. Gazit, M. Ianconescu, K. Perk, B. Aizenberg, and A. Zimber. 1979. Biochemical characterization of the type C retrovirus associated with lymphoproliferative disease of turkeys. J Virol 30:351–357.
23. Zimber, A., E.D. Heller, K. Perk, M. Ianconescu, and A. Yaniv. 1983. Effect of lymphoproliferative disease virus and of Niridazole on the in vitro blastogenic response of peripheral blood lymphocytes of turkeys. Avian Dis 27:1012–1024.
24. Zimber, A., K. Perk, M. Ianconescu, Y. Yegana, A. Gazit, and A. Yaniv. 1983. Lymphoproliferative disease of turkeys: Pathogenesis, viraemia and serum protein analysis following infection. Avian Pathol 12:101–116.
25. Zimber, A., K. Perk, M. Ianconescu, Z. Schwarzbard, and A. Yaniv. 1984. Lymphoproliferative disease of turkeys: Effect of chemical and surgical bursectomy on viraemia, pathogenesis and on the humoral immune response. Avian Pathol 13:277–287.

TUMORS OF UNKNOWN ETIOLOGY

T.N. Fredrickson and C.F. Helmboldt

INTRODUCTION. In the study of neoplastic diseases of poultry, attention has been focused on those of viral etiology, both from the standpoint of their economic importance and as a model applicable to cancer in humans. Neoplastic diseases of unknown etiology have not received much attention on either account for two main reasons. Perhaps the most obvious is that the average lifespan of commercially raised chickens and turkeys is generally less than that required for development of most nonvirally induced tumors. Secondly, there appears to be an appreciably lower incidence of tumors in chickens, even among aged birds, than in mammals. The reproductive tract is, however, an exception since carcinomas of the ovary and oviduct of the hen occur at an extremely high rate, possibly higher than in any other animal. It is estimated that they accounted for about 3/4 of the two million mature chickens condemned for tumors by the Inspection Service of the USDA in 1987 (39).

The restricted information available on the tumor incidence in older birds (the potential lifespan of chickens has been variably estimated as up to 35 yr but is generally considered to be around 15 yr) comes from four sources. The first is represented by long-term studies of flocks of aged chickens. The second is from diagnostic reports by poultry pathologists, particularly in countries where poultry are generally maintained for longer periods of time than in the USA (6, 18, 49, 53, 54). The third comes from zoos where various species of birds are maintained for natural lifespans and usually necropsied at death (9, 19, 42–44). These reports have provided useful information, albeit not directly applicable to poultry. Fourthly, with the same reservations as for zoo birds, reports of neoplastic diseases among pet birds have been of interest and Petrak and Gilmore (47) provide a detailed account of these.

Because of their importance, this chapter emphasizes tumors of the reproductive tract but also includes other neoplastic conditions, which have been described. In this respect much is owed to the accounts of poultry pathologists, including Jackson (36), Lesbouyries (40), Olson and Bullis (46), Guerin (30), Feldman and Olson (22) and particularly, Campbell (12). Personal observations are based on a study of spontaneous neoplasms in a flock of 466 white leghorn hens, many of which were allowed to live out their natural lifespan (24), as well as field cases submitted for necropsy. In the study flock, the following tumors were diagnosed: 142 ovarian, 40 oviductal, 1 pulmonary, 1 proventricular, 1 bile ductal, 7 pancreatic, 1 mesothelioma, and 1 hepatoma. No cases of Marek's disease were observed in the flock that was also free from infection with avian retroviruses and thus the tumors were not associated with known oncogenic viruses. However, it is uncertain how applicable these rates of spontaneous neoplasms are to other strains of chickens since there appears to be a genetic predisposition, at least for genital tumors, and a strain with a high incidence was used for the study. It is remarkable, however, how closely the distribution of types of epithelial tumors we found paralleled that reported by Goss (29) more than 40 yr ago.

REPRODUCTIVE SYSTEM

Ovary. Diagnosis of ovarian tumors in the hen has been somewhat complicated because of a tendency for investigators to apply to birds terms used in the diagnosis of mammalian and particularly human ovarian tumors. This ignores the dissimilarity between the histology and physiology of the mammalian and avian ovary, and in contrast to the numerous kinds of mammalian ovarian tumors, those in birds appear to be classifiable as granulosa cell tumors, Sertoli cell tumors, and adenocarcinomas (24). It is realized that this division of ovarian tumors may be an oversimplification of a complicated subject, but in view of the present stage of understanding, it appears warranted. As will be described, each tumor type has a distinct gross and histologic morphology and potential for invasive growth and, in the case of granulosa cell tumors, synthesis of estrogen has been established. By far the most common avian ovarian tumor is the ovarian adenocarcinoma, for which the cell of origin remains to be identified. All types of ovarian tumors are usually observed in hens over a year of age.

ADENOCARCINOMA. Early tumors may be detected as small, round, white, firm nodules on the ovarian surface that resemble atritic follicles. In advanced cases these coalesce into a cauliflowerlike mass that is firm and gray-white. Numerous transcoelomic implants are common at this stage, varying from small pearllike growths to massive nodular tumors on serosal surfaces of the pancreas, oviduct, mesentery, and intestines. Ascites usually develops when such cancerous growth is extensive, and the walls of affected intestines are thickened and adhered together so that they become blocked. Terminally, hens are extremely thin and assume an upright, penguinlike position. Usually there are no maturing follicles in advanced cases, and the oviducts are atrophied since most ovarian adenocarcinomas are not steroidogenic. The tumor appears to be multifocal in origin but grows fairly slowly over a period of months. Since the oviduct is so often involved, care must be taken to rule out a primary oviductal adenocarcinoma, which can grossly and histologically resemble ovarian adenocarcinoma. Failure to detect tumor growth in the mucosal lining of the oviduct indicates an ovarian, rather than an oviductal, primary. Histologically, the commonest structures composing the ovarian adenocarcinoma are acini formed by a single layer of low columnar or cuboidal epithelium. These nonciliated, eosinophilic cells, with basal, round nuclei are oriented around a lumen of variable size and shape, sometimes containing an intensely eosinophilic, homogeneous material that is periodic acid–Schiff (PAS)–positive and mucicarmine-negative (Fig. 16.57). Other tumors are more densely cellular; acinar structures are compressed, giving the impression of sheets of tumor cells, while in another variant the lumen may be enlarged with infolding of the neoplastic lining forming papillary structures (Fig. 16.58).

The tumor starts especially in the theca externa of smaller follicles but also in the interfollicular stroma and, in some cases, fairly deep in the ovarian stalk. Origin of the neoplastic cells remains unknown but may be from thecal glands (34), interstitial cells, remnants of embryonic sex cords, or the mesonephros. Mitotic figures are

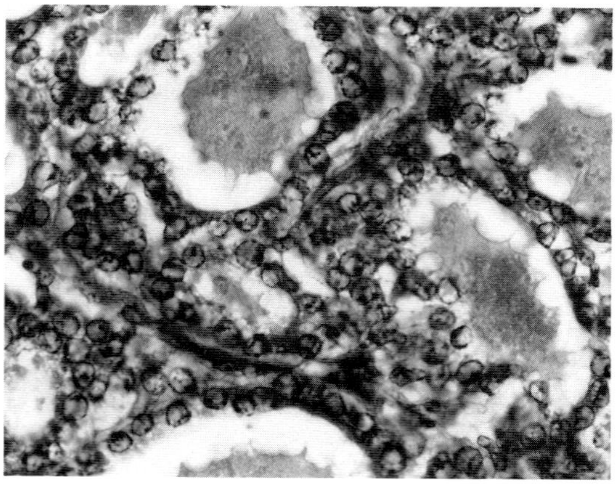

16.57. Acinar structures, typical of ovarian adenocarcinoma filled with eosinophilic material and lined by cuboidal cells containing round nuclei with condensed chromatin and sparse eosinophilic cytoplasm. H & E, ×600.

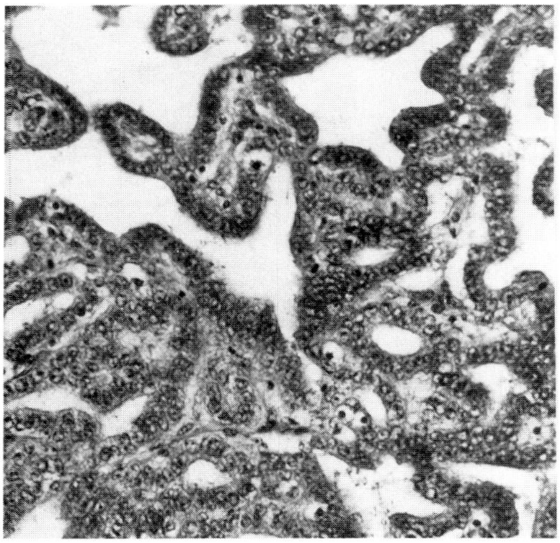

16.58. Ovarian adenocarcinoma with papillary structures projecting into dilated acini. ×160.

not a prominent feature of most tumors but in some the supporting stroma appears to be highly cellular, giving an impression of thecal cell tumors in mammals. However, this appears to be a reactive, not a primary neoplastic process since the connective tissue component does not metastasize (45). A similar reaction is seen when the ovarian tumor implants, producing an extensive proliferative response of smooth muscle in the muscularis of the intestine. Division of ovarian adenocarcinomas into medullary and scirrhous types seems unwarranted since tumor size appears to be the important factor in determining morphology. Generally, large tumors are scirrhous, composed of cuboidal epithelium forming small acini heavily interlaced with connective tissue (Figs. 16.59 and 16.60), whereas smaller tumors tend to have a reduced stromal component and are composed mainly of epithelial cells. Occasionally, ovarian adenocarcinomas are found in ovaries covered with grapelike clusters of follicles filled with yellow fluid. These cysts are not neoplastic growths, and thus entirely unrelated to ovarian cystadenocarcinomas of mammals, but appear to be the result of impaired lymphatic drainage. Ovarian adenocarcinomas similar to those seen in the chicken have been described in mature turkey hens (61).

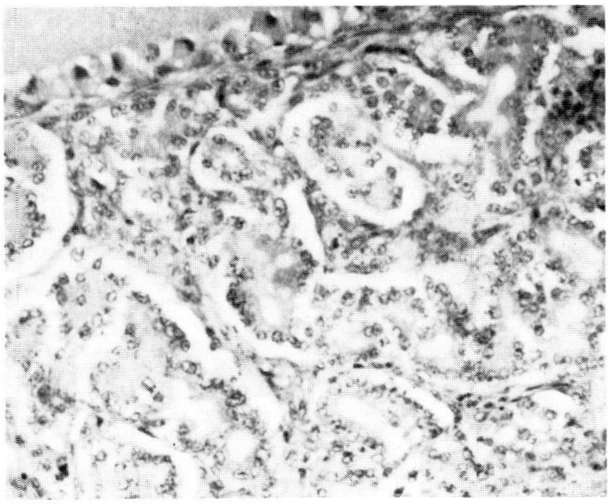

16.59. Ovarian adenocarcinoma in thecal region; a row of granulosa cells and the yolk material of a follicle (*upper left*). ×160.

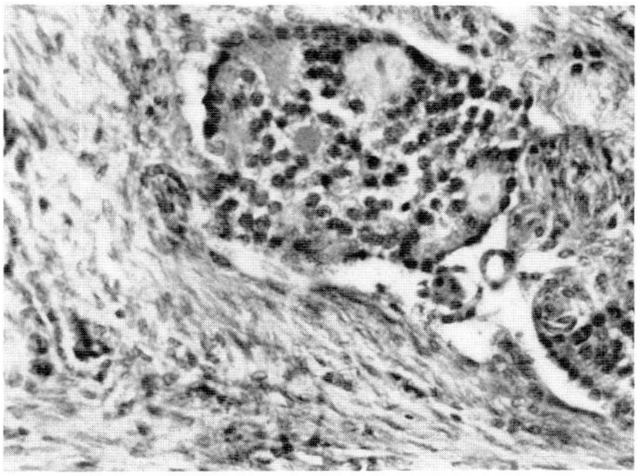

16.60. Another form of ovarian adenocarcinoma with dense bands of stromal cells enclosing clusters of neoplastic acinar cells intensely basophilic nuclei. H & E, ×160.

GRANULOSA CELL TUMOR. This tumor is yellow, round, and lobulated with an extremely friable consistency very different from the firm, cauliflowerlike adenocarcinoma. Granulosa cell tumors are encapsulated within a smooth, glistening membrane and because they are so friable, larger tumors have extensive areas of necrosis and hemorrhage. Transcoelomic metastases seldom occur, although tumors that are attached to the ovary only by a thin stalk may grow to enormous size. Histologically, the tumor is composed of pale, eosinophilic, polyhedral cells forming tubular or, less frequently, follicular structures (Fig. 16.61), separated by a delicate vascular stroma. The proportion of mitotic figures varies but tends to be low and the tumor appears to grow at a slow rate. The tumor cells have been identified as granulosa cells since they have an ultrastructural component called the transosome. This unique structure has heretofore been identified solely in follicular granulosa cells (34). Greatly elevated plasma levels of estrogen occur in hens with large granulosa cell tumors. The high levels are presumably the reason why the oviducts in such cases are similar in size to those of laying hens. Campbell's (12) description of ovarian thecal cell tumors is interpreted to be analogous to what we define as granulosa cell tumor.

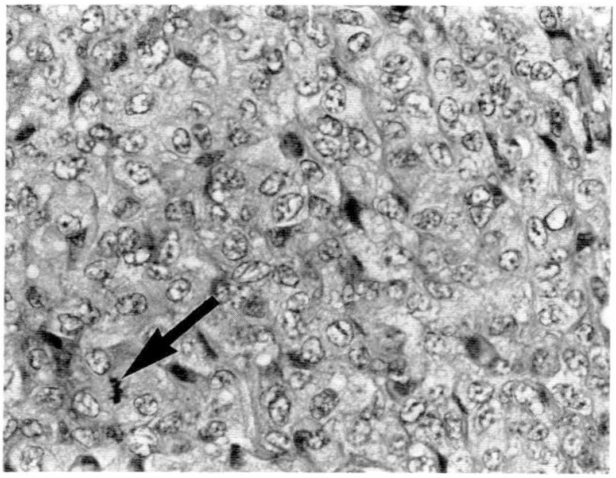

16.61. Ovarian granular cell tumor composed of a uniform population of tightly packed tumor cells with plentiful, pale eosinophilic cytoplasm and uniform, round vesicular nuclei. Note the mitotic figure at lower left corner (*arrow*). H & E, ×600.

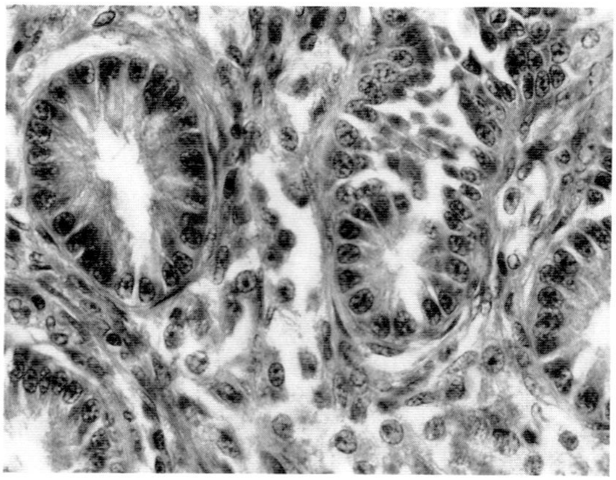

16.62. Arrhenoblastoma composed of well-defined seminiferous tubules, containing sertoli cells, interspersed with interstitial cells. H & E, ×600.

ARRHENOBLASTOMA. Arrhenoblastomas are characterized by growth of seminiferous tubules within the ovarian stroma. They have been associated with sex reversal in hens, and at least in one account, such a masculinized hen was able to successfully fertilize eggs (23). The tumors appear as white solid lobulated masses within the stroma of atrophic ovaries. Histologically they are somewhat variable but in most cases seminiferous tubules are clearly defined. In a case described by Gupta and Langham (31), seminiferous tubules were filled with vacuolated cells, and intertubular and interstitial cells were also present. The type of tumor associated with sex reversal features variable degrees of spermatogenesis within the tubules. Among five cases in our study obvious sex reversal was not apparent, the histology was much more of a Sertoli cell type with compact masses of tubules developing multifocally under the ovarian capsule. Interstitial cells were variably present and tubules were uniformly lined by a single layer of Sertoli cells (Fig. 16.62). Experimental induction of masculinizing arrhenoblastomas by injection of radioactive isotopes into the left ovary has been described (62).

DYSGERMINOMA. Wight (64) diagnosed two ovarian tumors as dysgerminomas occurring in pseudohermaphrodites, and it is thus unclear if tumors other than arrhenoblastomas can cause sex reversal in hens. However, at least one of the tumors Wight describes seems to be similar to a granulosa cell tumor.

Ovarian Ligament

LEIOMYOMA. Another common tumor of the female genital tract is the leiomyoma of the mesosalpinx. This tumor is usually a firm, encapsulated, round mass in the center of the ligament with a characteristic white, glistening appearance on cut surface. It is benign and composed entirely of bands of smooth muscle with fairly pyknotic nuclei and rare mitotic figures (Fig. 16.63). Hemorrhage and necrosis are rare, even though some tumors are several centimeters in diameter, and they appear to have little effect on the oviduct or its function. Occasionally similar leiomyomas can be seen on the peritoneal surface of the oviduct or growing in the mesentery.

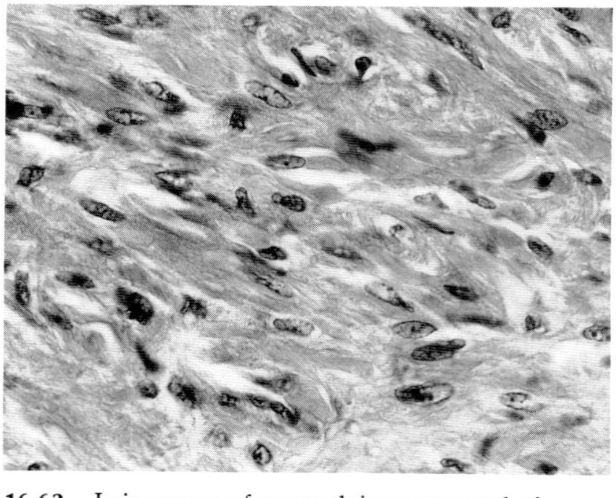

16.63. Leiomyoma of mesosalpinx composed of smooth muscle fibers arranged in compact whorls. Mitoses are absent and the nuclear/cytoplasmic ratio is low. H & E, ×600.

Oviduct

ADENOCARCINOMA. Adenocarcinomas of the oviduct may affect a very high percentage of hens in unusual flocks (26), and in the view of some diagnosticians they represent the majority of tumors of the reproductive tract. They generally occur in birds over a year of age.

Almost all oviductal tumors occur in the upper magnal portion of the oviduct with rare cases in the uterus and infundibulum. In their earliest stages of growth these tumors are observable as individual or clustered sessile growths that are gray in color and firm in consistency, which go on to coalesce, forming large, irregularly shaped tumors protruding into the oviductal lumen. These spread because oviductal adenocarcinomas are extremely malignant and even when the primary is quite small, tumor cells may penetrate through the muscularis to implant in the abdominal cavity. Such metastatic growths, generally composed of fairly anaplastic tumor cells, are similar, both grossly and histologically, to those produced by ovarian adenocarcinomas and the ovary itself is a frequent site of implantation. Histologically, it is evident that they originate from secretory cells (27, 58) and immunohistochemically they have been shown to contain ovalbumin (32). There is generally a distinct boundary between neoplastic and normal cells (Figs. 16.64 and 16.65). Malignant cells vary as to the degree they maintain the normal glandular architecture of the magnum and amount of acidophilic secretory granules within their cytoplasm. In some cases cells are agranular and grow in solid sheets. However, cytologic differences are not reflective of tumor invasiveness since implants may be found that are composed of well-differentiated cells. Ilchmann and Bergmann (35) described the ultrastructural aspects of such tumors. In the oviduct, penetration of the muscularis seems as active as lateral growth, and the invaded tissue becomes extremely hyperplastic, causing the oviduct wall to become greatly thickened. Similar hypertrophy occurs in the intestines, which have undergone implantation. Oviductal tumors, similar to those found in chickens, also have been described in turkeys (5).

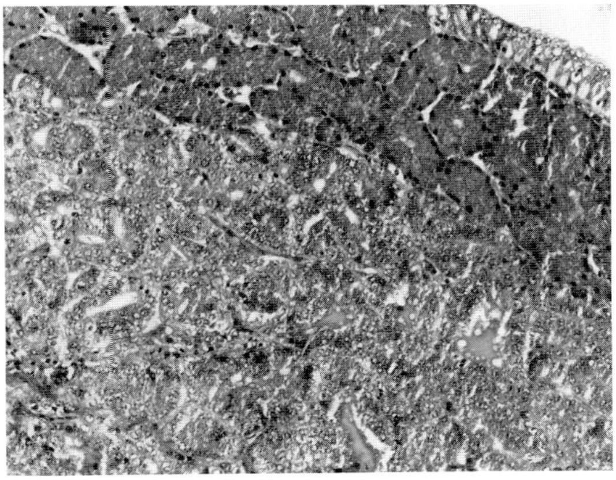

16.64. Oviductal adenocarcinoma with surface epithelium (*upper right*) above normal secretory cells with more lightly staining tumor cells (*below*). H & E, ×200.

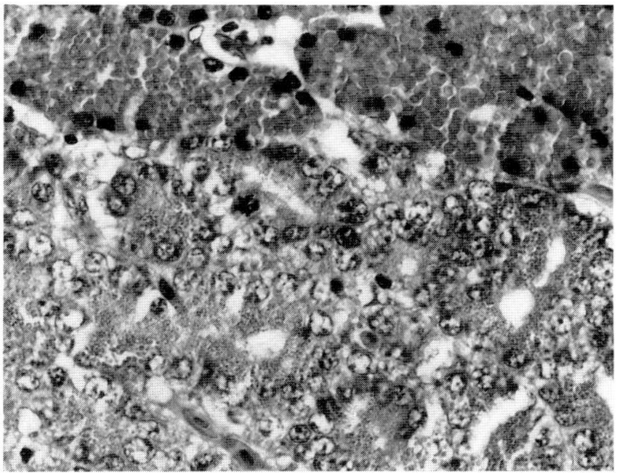

16.65. Same oviductal adenocarcinoma as in Fig. 16.64 showing the well-defined margin contrasting normal secretory tissue (*above*) with cellular cytoplasm containing eosinophilic granules of ovalbumen and very lightly granular tumor cells (*below*). H & E, ×600.

Testicle

TERATOMA. Tumors of embryonic origin have been mainly reported as occurring in the testicle, but they also have been described in the ovary (33, 46), and Guerin (30) and Campbell and Appleby (13) found them in a number of other sites. These are generally round, encapsulated firm masses that are yellow to white and sometimes contain cysts. Histologically, they are composed of variable embryonic tissues, including bone, cartilage, smooth muscle, nerves, fat, and melanocytes. The cysts are often lined with columnar ciliated epithelium that, along with cartilage and smooth muscle, forms tracheal structures. Additional structures and epithelial pearls formed by squamous epithelium may also be seen. Another type of teratoma that we have observed occasionally was described by Campbell and Appleby (13) as composed of a small fluid-filled sac containing fully formed feathers. They are always attached to the spinal column in the lumbar area. Histologically, the sac wall is composed of skin and arrector pili muscles.

SERTOLI CELL TUMOR. Sertoli cell tumors have been described in the testes of the chicken (52), Japanese quail (28), and the budgerigar (47). Grossly they appear as firm, smooth, rough masses with varying degrees of cyst formation. Histologically, they resemble seminiferous tubules lined with Sertoli cells, however, the definition of the tubules and number of interstitial cells between them is variable.

SEMINOMA. Seminomas have been described in two cockerels (11) as large abdominal masses composed of large, round cells containing a round to oval nucleus with prominent nucleoli. Mitotic figures were numerous and the tumor cells were generally arranged in sheets interspersed with a delicate stroma. Similar testicular tumors appear to be fairly common in budgerigars (47).

DIGESTIVE SYSTEM

Alimentary Tract. Tumors occurring in the alimentary tract of chickens are rarely observed. Perhaps the most striking exceptions are reports of pharyngeal and esophageal squamous cell carcinomas in chickens in northern China (14, 51). Humans in the same area also had a high incidence of esophageal carcinoma, indicating a common etiology. In addition there have been several reports of papillary adenomas of the crop, esophagus, and proventriculus (3, 13, 46). Campbell and Appleby (13) described an adenocarcinoma of the gizzard that was similar to tumors seen among slaughter chickens in the USA as shown in Fig. 16.66 (case kindly supplied by K. Langheinrich). Guerin (30) described five tumors of the small intestine and one of the ileocecal junction and cited several other reports of intestinal carcinomas in chickens. In these cases, gross examination revealed papillary projections of tumor tissue into the lumen of the affected organ sometimes with penetration of the muscularis by invading epithelial tissue, which formed acinar or cystic structures containing mucin. Cloacal papillomas of unknown etiology have been described in psittacine birds (57). Of 41 cases examined growth was benign in 40, consisting of proliferation of epithelial cells supported on a connective tissue stalk, but a single case diagnosed as carcinoma in situ was composed of undifferentiated cells showing numerous mitoses.

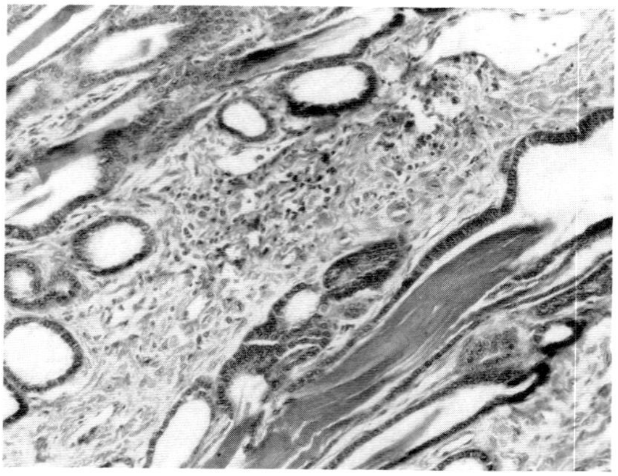

16.66. Adenocarcinoma of gizzard with growth of darkly staining cuboidal tumor cells downward into muscularis. The keratinous product of these cells is shown at lower right. H & E, ×200.

Liver

HEPATOMA. Spontaneous neoplasms of hepatocytes appear to be rare in chickens and only occasional reports of either benign trabecular hepatomas or anaplastic carcinomas have appeared (16). We observed one hepatic tumor that was growing in the hepatic parenchyma as a large, circumscribed, soft, yellow-gray mass. Microscopically, it was composed of eosinophilic hepatocytes, about twice normal size, forming thick, irregular hepatic cords unassociated with normal triad structures (Fig. 16.67). Mitotic figures were rare, and this appeared to be a benign tumor similar to three described by Olson and Bullis (46). Anaplastic hepatic carcinomas also have been described as composed of sheets of basophilic neoplastic cells smaller than in hepatomas and with numerous mitoses (49). Such tumors are similar to hepatocellular carcinomas induced with transforming avian retroviruses, most notably MC-29 (4). Hepatic tumors have also been reported in ducks (10) and they appear to be inducible in this species with aflatoxin (15). Also, hepatocellular carcinomas in ducks have been associated with duck hepatitis B virus (67).

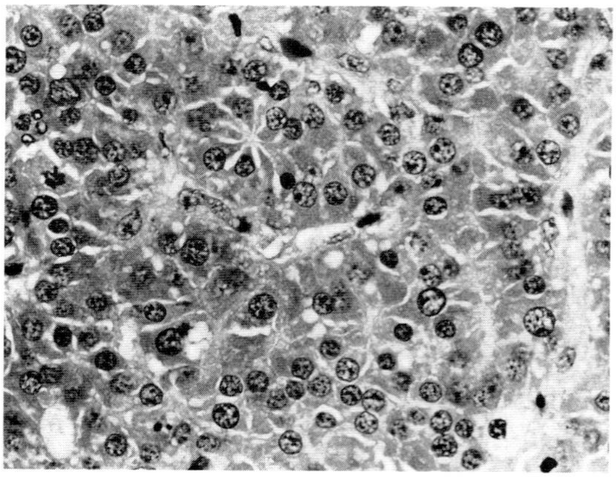

16.67. Hepatoma composed of large eosinophilic neoplastic cells, some in mitosis forming irregular plates. H & E, ×600.

CHOLANGIOMA. Tumors of the biliary system occur at a rate similar to those of hepatocytes. They are generally firm, demarcated from normal hepatic parenchyma, and yellow-gray in color. The histology varies according to the degree of malignancy. Adenomas composed of clearly recognizable but enlarged and distorted bile ducts, interspersed with fibrous connective tissue (Fig. 16.68), are similar to the case of Campbell and

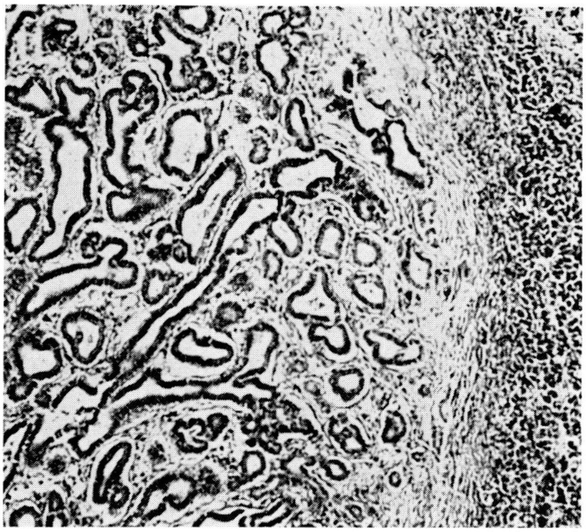

16.68. Bile duct adenoma composed of dilated ducts in a loose fibrocytic stroma. ×75.

Appleby (13). In bile duct adenocarcinomas, duct formation is much more irregular than in adenomas; the connective tissue is fibroblastic (Fig. 16.69), and diffuse infiltration into the rest of the liver is aggressive. Bile duct tumors have been described in pigeons (63) and captive wild birds (48, 60).

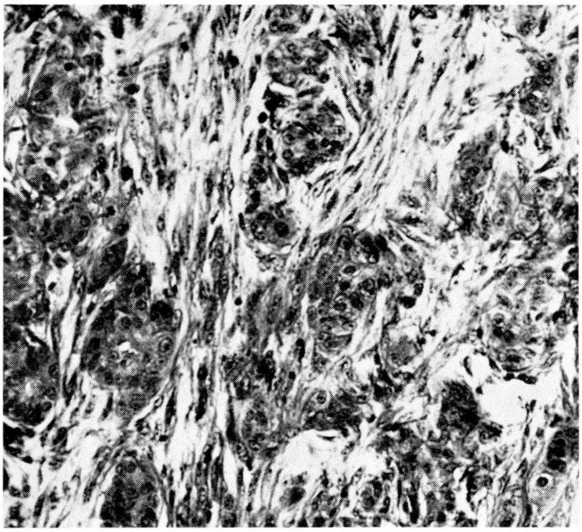

16.69. Bile duct adenocarcinoma composed of small clusters of epithelial cells in a fibroblastic stroma. ×190.

Pancreas

ADENOCARCINOMA. Tumors of the pancreas are difficult to diagnose because ovarian and oviductal adenocarcinomas, which spread so readily to the pancreas, often resemble pancreatic adenocarcinomas. There can be absolute certainty of a pancreatic primary tumor only in absence of ovarian or oviductal involvement. In one such case we observed the neoplastic cells were columnar, possible of ductal origin, and formed tubular structures (Fig. 16.70). The cytoplasm stained lightly basophilic and the basal nuclei were round to oval with large numbers of mitotic figures. Extensive metastatic implants were observed on the serosa of the duodenum and proventriculus and the hepatic capsule, but none were seen on the ovary. In another case it appeared that the tumor arose from exocrine tissue rather than ducts because a clearly defined transitional zone between normal acini and tumor tissue could be distinguished. The large neoplastic cells had extremely vesicular, round nuclei, and cytoplasm contained a variable number of the same deeply eosinophilic granules typical of normal acinar cells (Fig. 16.71).

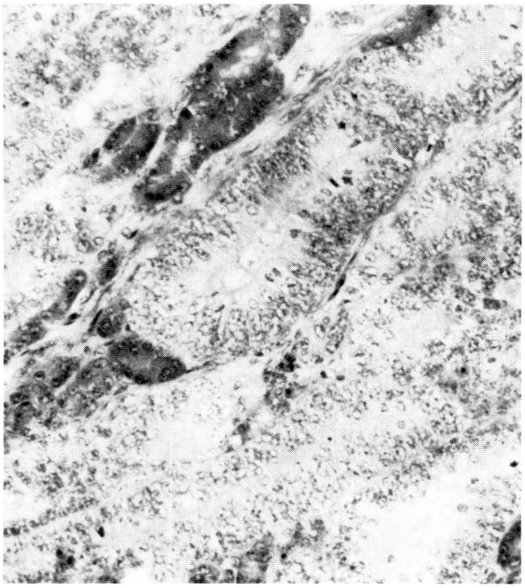

16.70. Pancreatic adenocarcinoma composed of columnar cells forming tubular structures among a few remnant acinar cells (*arrow*). ×160.

Peritoneum

MESOTHELIOMA. Mesotheliomas have been reported in chickens (30, 46), ducks (41), and a hawk (17). The single mesothelioma in the authors' series was in a hen that had about 200 ml of milky fluid in its abdominal cavity. The gross appearance was striking in that all serosal sur-

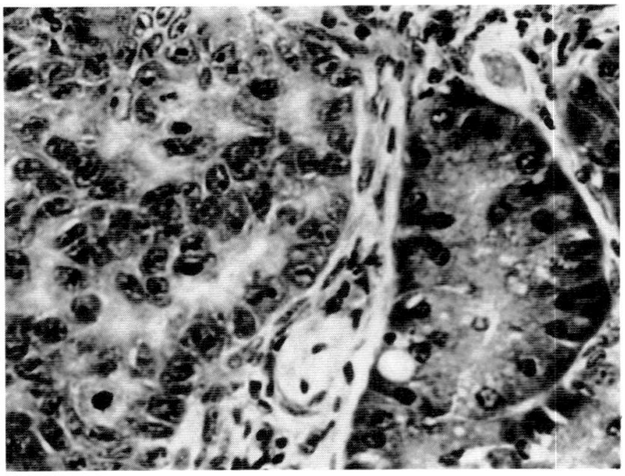

16.71. Pancreatic acinar cell adenocarcinoma with normal exocrine tissue (*right*) and agranular neoplastic cells (*left*). H & E, ×600.

faces were covered by glistening, gray cystic structures. Histologically, these appeared as papillary outgrowths of peritoneal cells supported by thick connective tissue stroma that formed the walls of the cysts into which the papillary structures projected (Fig. 16.72). Mitotic figures were rare but tumor growth was extensive.

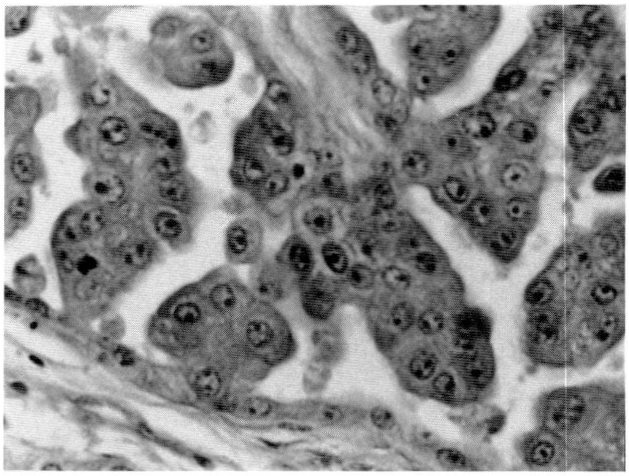

16.72. Mesothelioma with prominent neoplastic epithelial cells supported on a delicate stalk. H & E, ×600.

URINARY SYSTEM. Renal adenocarcinomas occur as spontaneous neoplasms in chickens but they are inducible with avian leukosis virus and this tumor is described elsewhere in this volume.

RESPIRATORY SYSTEM

Lung

ADENOCARCINOMA. Tumors of any part of this system are rare in birds, and the most complete description of avian pulmonary cancers remains that by Stewart (56) of 11 cases in zoo birds. The single case seen by the authors clearly arose multifocally from tertiary bronchi and resembled the papillary adenocarcinoma in a pigeon described by Stewart and a case described in a chicken (2). Cuboidal epithelium formed distorted bronchial tissue often containing eosinophilic material (Fig. 16.73). Widespread and distant metastases in the thorax and abdomen attested to the extreme malignancy of this tumor.

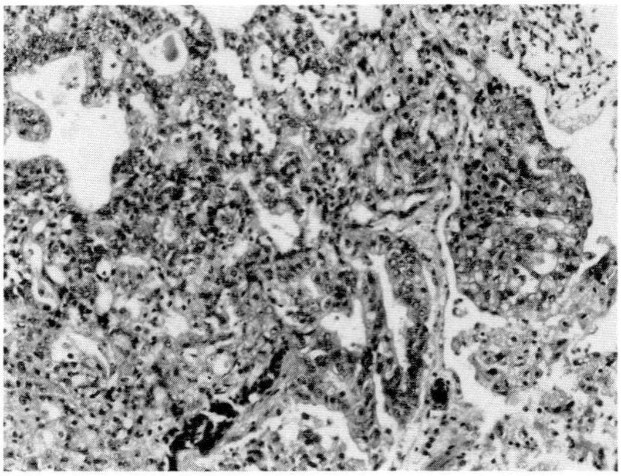

16.73. Adenocarcinoma of lung composed of papillary growth of epithelial cells that have replaced most of the normal lung. H & E, ×200.

NERVOUS SYSTEM

Central Nervous System

ASTROCYTOMA. Sporadic cases of astrocytoma have been described (8, 37, 38) but there is a report of an outbreak of epizootic proportions (66). Adult birds are usually affected and may show transitory torticollis, retropulsion, or incoordination. Although the tumor is small, usually no larger than 5 mm, it may be seen without difficulty, especially in fixed tissue, as a sharply delineated whitish mass. Those observed by Wight and Duff (66) always appeared at the base of the cerebellum; but in the authors' experience the neoplasm was always near the thalamus in the area of the third ventricle. These benign tumors were fibrillary astrocytomas and definitely not of ependymal origin, since they were covered by a single layer of ependymal cells. Demarcation from unaffected brain tissue was fairly sharp, with marked perivascular reaction of lymphocytes in the brain bordering the tumor, but without hemorrhage, giant cells, or areas of pressure necrosis. The neoplastic cells varied considerably in morphology but were mainly polygonal (Fig. 16.74). Fibrillar processes, compatible with

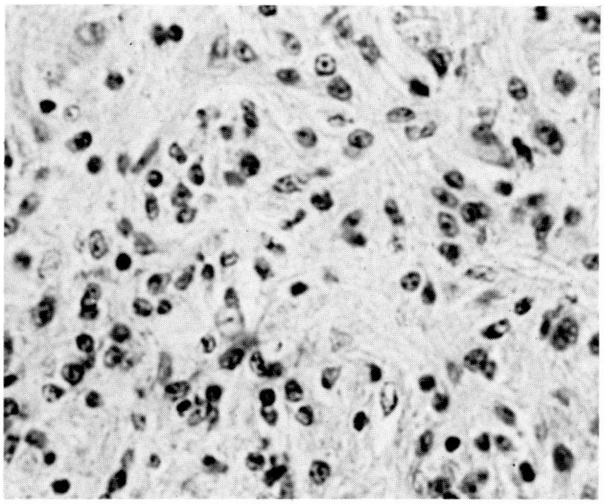

16.74. Astrocytoma uniformly composed of astrocytes that have extended cytoplasmic processes. ×190.

astrocytic origin, could be demonstrated.

Wight and Campbell (65) also reported an ependymoma and two meningiomas in chickens. The former was a growth in the lateral ventricle of palisaded or rosette-forming, vacuolated cells while the meningiomas were the angioblastic variety composed of vascular sinuses lined with plump endothelial cells associated with a dense network of reticulin.

Peripheral Nerves

NEUROFIBROMA. Campbell and Appleby (13) noted 39 tumors of the nerve sheath. They diagnosed them as either neurofibromas or neurilemomas; they also listed 17 described by other investigators who generally called them neurogenic sarcomas or Schwannomas. They are benign localized tumors forming white nodular or fusiform growths, most often in the region of the dorsal root ganglia. Campbell and Appleby (13) described tumor cells either forming whorls of Schwann cells or in a palisading arrangement and occasionally with Wagner-Meissner corpuscles. A neurofibrosarcoma has also been described by Anderson et al. (1). Neuromas developing from the stumps of the trigeminal nerve severed during debeaking have been described (25).

ENDOCRINE SYSTEM

Thymus. Five epithelial thymic tumors, true thymomas as distinct from thymic lymphomas, have been reported in chickens (13, 21,30, 46) and one in a budgerigar (68). They are characterized by replacement of the normal thymic architecture with sheets of large epithelial cells interspersed with variable numbers of lymphoid cells. The vesicular nucleus and abundant pale-staining cytoplasm of the epithelial cells contrast with lymphocytic morphology. No structural pattern is apparent and cytoplasmic borders of the neoplastic cells are indistinct, but Hassal's corpuscles, which are sometimes mixed among the tumor cells, help identify thymic epithelium.

Pituitary. Pituitary tumors occur fairly frequently among budgerigars and other pet birds (47). None were seen by the authors although pituitary glands were examined in several hundred aged hens.

Adrenal Gland. Campbell and Appleby (13) recorded a single case of an adenoma they felt was most likely derived from the adrenal gland.

Thyroid and Parathyroid. Guerin (30) described an adenoma arising in the parathyroid and pointed out that only one case of parathyroid carcinoma had been reported. Tumors of the thyroid in poultry also appear to be extremely rare; although goiters have been reported in chickens (30) and are fairly common in pet birds (47). Olson and Bullis (46) reported on a single adenoma of the thyroid.

INTEGUMENT

Subcutis

HEMANGIOPERICYTOMA. Two hemangiopericytomas in the subcutaneous tissue have been reported (53) and four cases have been observed by the authors. All of these benign tumors occurred as subcutaneous nodules of variable size, usually in the cervical region. They were dense, white, well delineated, and firmly embedded in the subcutis. The histologic appearance was of a spindle cell sarcoma but with a striking concentric arrangement around arterioles, which can be readily demonstrated by a silver stain (Fig. 16.75). The uniformly spindle-shaped cells have a fusiform nucleus and contain diffuse chromatin and abundant cytoplasm with indistinct cell borders.

Cutis

SQUAMOUS CELL CARCINOMA. Few cases of squamous cell carcinomas in chickens have been reported but it may be increasing in broilers in the USA (59), and a report from West Germany indicates that this is a widely distributed problem in broiler birds (7). In slaughter birds described by Turnquest (59), there were no sites of predilection for the round ulcerous lesions that were surrounded by a rim of thickened skin and dermis. Microscopically, there was downward growth of rete pegs into the dermis by normal-appearing cells of the basal layer and stratum corneum. Normal transition of deeply basophilic basal cells to

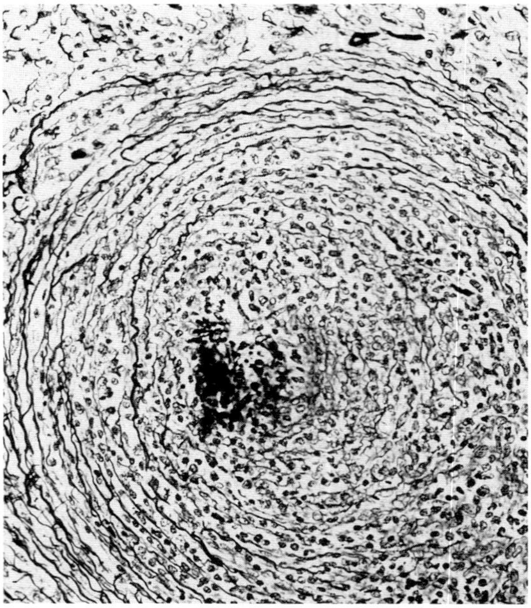

16.75. Hemangiopericytoma with concentric rings of pericytes clearly defined. Silver, ×190.

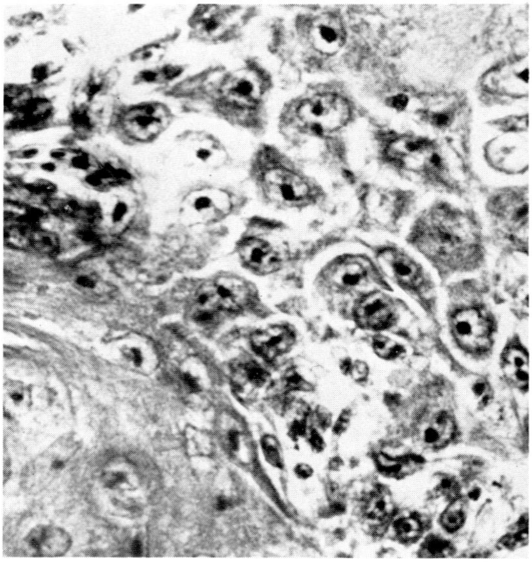

16.76. Squamous cell carcinoma with disorganized basal cells (*lower right*) and keratinized cells (*upper left*). ×480.

eosinophilic keratinized cells connected with cellular bridges and formation of keratin pearls characterized these cases. Penetration of the dermis and occasionally arrector muscle but not of skeletal muscle had occurred, but no distant metastases were observed. Since distant metastases and continued expansive growth are criteria in differentiating between a carcinoma and an acanthomatous reaction, Riddell and Shettigara (50) considered that skin lesions they observed may be keratoacanthomas rather than squamous cell carcinomas. In a case we observed, the tumors are quite anaplastic and appear to be unequivocal squamous cell carcinomas (Fig. 16.76).

LIPOMA AND LIPOSARCOMA. Lipoma associated with the cutis and subcutis are common tumors of budgerigars (47). They are generally encapsulated, benign tumors composed of mature fat cells with variable degrees of necrosis and hemorrhage. Malignant liposarcomas are considerably rarer and may be similar in histologic appearance to fibrosarcomas except for intracytoplasmic fat vacuoles within tumor cells. In others the tumor may be composed of obviously immature adipocytes. Multicentric liposarcomas have been described in the skeletal muscles of a Canada goose (20).

MUSCULOSKELETAL SYSTEM

LEIOMYOMA AND LEIOMYOSARCOMA. The most common muscle tumor in poultry appears to be the benign type of leiomyoma seen in the oviductal ligament (see above). There are a few reports of leiomyosarcomas associated with the musculature of the gut of the chicken (1) and the jejunum of a budgerigar (55).

RHABDOMYOSARCOMA. Rhabdomyosarcomas, with typical racquet- or star-shaped cells and multinucleated giant cells, but without cross striations, have been described (46, 13). They also have been described in budgerigars (47).

REFERENCES

1. Anderson, W.I., P.C. McCaskey, K.A. Langheinrich, and A.E. Dreesen. 1985. Neurofibrosarcoma and leiomyosarcoma in slaughterhouse broilers. Avian Dis 29:521–527.
2. Apperly, F.L. 1935. Primary carcinoma of the lung in the domestic fowl. Am J Cancer 23:556–557.
3. Baker, J.R. 1980. A proventricular adenoma in a Brazilian teal (Amazonetta brasiliensis). Vet Rec 107:63–64.
4. Beard, J.W., E.A. Hillman, D. Beard, K. Lapis, and U. Heine. 1975. Neoplastic response of the avian liver to host infection with strain MC-29 leukosis virus. Cancer Res 35:1603–1627.
5. Beasley, J.N., S. Klopp, and B. Terry. 1986. Neoplasms in the oviducts of turkeys. Avian Dis 30:433–437.
6. Bergmann, V., J. Scheer, A. Valentin, and P. Schwarz. 1984. Occurrence of neoplastic diseases in slaughter hens. Monatsh Veterinaermed 39:82–86.
7. Bergmann, V., A. Valentin, and J. Scheer. 1986. Skin carcinoma in broiler fowl. Monatsh Veterinaermed 41:815–817.
8. Biering-Sorensen, U. 1956. On disseminated, focal

gliomatosis ("multiple gliomas") and cerebral calcifications in hens. A study of pathogenesis. Nord Vet Med 8:887-901.
9. Blackmore, D.K. 1966. The clinical approach to tumours in cage birds. I. The pathology and incidence of neoplasia in cage birds. J Small Anim Pract 7:217-223.
10. Campbell, J.G. 1949. Spontaneous hepatocellular and cholangiocellular carcinoma in the duck. An experimental study. Br J Cancer 3:198-210.
11. Campbell, J.G. 1951. Some unusual gonadal tumours of the fowl. Br J Cancer 5:69-82.
12. Campbell, J.G. 1969. Tumors of the Fowl. Lippincott, Philadelphia.
13. Campbell, J.G., and E.C. Appleby. 1966. Tumours in young chickens bred for rapid body growth (broiler chickens). A study of 351 cases. J Pathol Bacteriol 92:77-90.
14. Cancer Institute, Chinese Academy Medical Sciences. 1973. The epidemiology of esophageal cancer in North China and preliminary results in the investigation of its etiological factors. Acta Zool Sinica 19:309-312.
15. Carnaghan, R.B.A. 1965. Hepatic tumours in ducks fed a low level of toxic groundnut meal. Nature (London) 208:308.
16. Christopher, J., J.V. Narayana, and G.A. Sastry. 1966. Primary neoplasms of the liver of the domestic fowl. Ceylon Vet J 14:61-64.
17. Cooper, J.E., and S.L. Pugsley. 1984. A mesothelioma in a ferruginous hawk (Buteo regalis). Avian Pathol 13:797-801.
18. Deka, B.C., and G.S. Grewal. 1982. Non-leucotic tumors in domestic fowl in the Punjab. Trop Anim Health and Prod 14:59-60.
19. Dillberger, J.E., S.B. Citino, and N.H. Altman. 1987. Four cases of neoplasia in captive wild birds. Avian Dis 31:206-213.
20. Doster, A.R., J.L. Johnson, G.E. Duhamel, T.W. Bargar, and G. Nason. 1987. Liposarcoma in a Canada goose (Branta canadensis). Avian Dis 31:918-920.
21. Feldman, W.H. 1936. Thymoma in a chicken (Gallus domesticus). Am J Cancer 26:576-580.
22. Feldman, W.H., and C. Olson. 1965. Neoplastic diseases of the chicken. In Diseases of Poultry, H.E. Biester and L.H. Schwarte (eds.), 5th Ed., Iowa State Univ Press, Ames, Iowa, pp. 863-924.
23. Fell, H.B. 1923. Histologic studies on the gonads of the fowl. I. The histologic basis of sex reversal. Br J Exp Biol 1:97-129.
24. Fredrickson, T.N. 1987. Ovarian tumors of the hen. Environ Health Persp 73:35-51.
25. Gentle, M.J. 1986. Neuroma formation following partial beak amputation (beak trimming) in the chicken. Res Vet Sci 41:383-85.
26. Goodchild, W.M. 1969. Adenocarcinoma of the oviduct in laying hens. Vet Rec 84:122.
27. Goodchild, W.M., and D.M. Cooper. 1968. Oviduct adenocarcinoma in laying hens. Vet Rec 82:389-390.
28. Gorham, S.L., and M.A. Ottinger. 1986. Sertoli cell tumors in Japanese quail. Avian Dis 30:337-339.
29. Goss, L.J. 1940. The incidence and classification of avian tumors. Cornell Vet 30:75-88.
30. Guerin, M. 1954. Tumeurs spontanees de la poule. In Tumeurs Spontanees des Animaux de Laboratoire, pp. 153-180. Legrand, Paris.
31. Gupta, B.N., and R.F. Langham. 1968. Arrhenoblastoma in an Indian Desi hen. Avian Dis 12:441-444.
32. Haritani, M., H. Kajigaya, T. Akashi, M. Kamemura, N. Tanahara, M. Umeda, M. Sugiyama, M. Isoda, and C. Kato. 1984. A study on the origin of adenocarcinoma in fowls using immunohistological technique. Avian Dis 28:1130-1134.
33. Helmboldt, C.F., G. Migaki, K.A. Langheinrich, and R.M. Jakowski. 1974. Case report–teratoma in domestic fowl (Gallus gallus). Avian Dis 18:142-148.
34. Hodges, R.D. 1974. The female reproductive tract. In The Histology of the Fowl, pp. 342-343. Academic Press, New York.
35. Ilchmann, G., and V. Bergmann. 1975. Histologische und elektronenmikroskopische Untersuchungen zu Adenokarzinomatose der Legehennen. Arch Exp Veterinaermed 29:897-907.
36. Jackson, C. 1936. The incidence and pathology of tumors of domesticated animals in South Africa. Onderstepoort J Vet Sci Anim Ind 6:1-460.
37. Jackson, C. 1954. Gliomas of the domestic fowl: Their pathology with special reference to histogenesis and pathogenesis and their relationship to other diseases. Onderstepoort J Vet Sci Anim Ind 26:501-592.
38. Jungherr, E.L., and A. Wolf. 1939. Gliomas in animals. A report of two astrocytomas in the common fowl. Am J Cancer 37:493-509.
39. Langheinrich, K. 1987. Personal communication.
40. Lesbouyries, C. 1941. Les processus tumoraux. In La Pathologie des Oiseaux, pp. 143-179. Vigot, Paris.
41. Ling, Y.S., and Y.Q. Guo. 1985. Pathological study of spontaneous mesothelioma in ducks. Chin J Vet Sci Technol 9:15-16.
42. Lombard, L.S., and E.J. Witte. 1959. Frequency and types of tumors in mammals and birds of the Philadelphia Zoological Garden. Cancer Res 19:127-141.
43. Loupal, G., and M. Reifinger. 1986. Tumors in zoo, companion, and wild birds. A review of 25 years (1960-1984). J Vet Med 33:180-192.
44. Montali, R.J. 1980. An overview of tumors in zoo animals. In R.J. Montali and G. Migaki (eds.), Comparative Pathology of Zoo Animals, pp. 531-542. Smithsonian Institute, Washington, DC.
45. Nobel, T.A., F. Neumann, and M.S. Dison. 1964. A histological study of peritoneal carcinomatosis in the laying hen. Avian Dis 8:513-522.
46. Olson, C., and K.L. Bullis. 1942. A survey of spontaneous neoplastic diseases in chickens. Massachusetts Agric Exp Sta Bull 391.
47. Petrak, M.L., and C.E. Gilmore. 1982. Neoplasms. In M.L. Petrak (ed.), Diseases of Cage and Aviary Birds, pp. 606-637. Lea & Febiger, Philadelphia.
48. Porter, K., T. Connor, and A.M. Gallina. 1983. Cholangiocarcinoma in a yellow-faced Amazon parrot (Amazona xanthops). Avian Dis 27:556-558.
49. Purvulov, B., and S. Bozhkov. 1984. Pathology of some spontaneous neoplasms of fowls. Obshcha i Stravnitelna Patologiya 16:55-58.
50. Riddell, C., and P.T. Shettigara. 1980. Dermal squamous cell carcinoma in broiler chickens in Saskatchewan. Can Vet J 21:287-289.
51. She, R.P. 1987. Epidemiology and pathology of oropharyngo-esophageal carcinoma in chickens from different areas in Zhongxian county, Hubei province. Acta Vet Zootech Sinica 18:195-200.
52. Siller, W.G. 1956. A Sertoli cell tumour causing feminization in a Brown Leghorn capon. J Endocrinol 14:197-203.
53. Sokkar, S.M., M.A. Mohammed, A.J. Zubaidy, and A. Mutalib. 1979. Study of some nonleukotic avian neoplasms. Avian Pathol 8:69-75.
54. Sriraman, P.K., S.R. Ahmed, N.R.G. Naidu, and P.R. Rao. 1981. Neoplasia in chickens and ducks. Indian J Poult Sci 16:436-437.
55. Steinberg, H. 1988. Leiomyosarcoma of the je-

junum in a budgerigar. Avian Dis 32:166–168.

56. Stewart, H.L. 1966. Pulmonary cancer and adenomatosis in captive wild mammals and birds from the Philadelphia Zoo. J Nat Cancer Inst 36:117–138.

57. Sundberg, J.P., R.E. Junge, M.K. O'Banion, E.J. Basgall, G. Harrison, G. Herron, and H.L. Shivaprasad. 1986. Cloacal papillomas in psittacines. Am J Vet Res 47:928–932.

58. Swarbrick, O., J.G. Campbell, and D.M. Berry. 1968. An outbreak of oviduct adenocarcinoma in laying hens. Vet Rec 82:57–59.

59. Turnquest, R.U. 1979. Dermal squamous cell carcinoma in young chickens. Am J Vet Res 40:1628–1633.

60. Wadsworth, P.F., S.K. Majeed, W.M. Brancker, and D.M. Jones. 1978. Some hepatic neoplasms in non-domesticated birds. Avian Pathol 7:551–555.

61. Walser, M.M., and P.S. Paul. 1979. Ovarian adenocarcinomas in domestic turkeys. Avian Pathol 8:335–339.

62. Warner, N.E., N.B. Friedman, E.J. Bomze, and F. Masin. 1960. Comparative pathology of experimental and spontaneous androblastomas and gynoblastomas of the gonads. Am J Obstet Gynecol 79:971–988.

63. Webster, W.S., B.C. Bullock, and R.W. Prichard. 1969. A report of three bile duct carcinomas occurring in pigeons. J Am Vet Med Assoc 155:1200–1205.

64. Wight, P.A.L. 1965. Neoplastic sequelae of gonadal maldevelopment in a flock of domestic fowls. Avian Dis 9:327–335.

65. Wight, P.A.L., and J.G. Campbell. 1976. Three unusual intracranial tumours of the domesticated fowl. Avian Pathol 5:201–214.

66. Wight, P.A.L., and R.H. Duff. 1964. The histopathology of epizootic gliosis and astrocytomata of the domestic fowl. J Comp Pathol 74:373–380.

67. Yokosuka, O., M. Omata, Y.-Z. Zhou, F. Imazeki, and K. Okuda. 1985. Duck hepatitis B virus DNA in liver and serum of Chinese ducks: Integration of viral DNA in a hepatocellular carcinoma. Proc Natl Acad Sci, USA 82:5180–5184.

68. Zubaidy, A.J. 1980. An epithelial thymoma in a budgerigar (Melopsittacus undulatus). Avian Pathol 9:575–581.

17 INFECTIOUS BRONCHITIS

D.J. King and David Cavanagh

INTRODUCTION

Definition and Synonyms. Infectious bronchitis (IB) is an acute, highly contagious viral respiratory disease of chickens characterized by tracheal rales, coughing, and sneezing. In addition, a nasal discharge may occur in young chicks, and in laying flocks there is usually a drop in egg production. Mortality may occur in young chicks due to respiratory or kidney manifestations of the infection.

IB is of economic importance because it is a cause of poor weight gain and feed efficiency, is a component of mixed infections that produce airsacculitis that may result in condemnations at processing of broilers, and is a cause of egg production and egg quality declines. The losses from production inefficiencies are usually of greater concern than losses from mortality. The highly transmissible nature of the disease and the confirmation that the etiology includes multiple serotypes of IB virus (IBV) have complicated and increased the cost of attempts to prevent the disease by immunization. The disease is also called avian infectious bronchitis.

Economic and Public Health Significance. IB appears to have no public health significance. Bronchitislike viruses isolated from humans were found to be morphologically similar but antigenically distinct from IBV (100, 134). Serums from individuals who were in contact with chickens by providing direct care or through handling poultry diagnostic accessions were found to have low neutralizing antibody titers against IBV (102), but the significance of the finding remains unknown.

HISTORY. A respiratory disease with mortality of chicks was first seen in the USA in North Dakota in 1930. A report by Schalk and Hawn in 1931 (114) of the clinical signs and preliminary laboratory studies of those cases is recognized as the first report of IB. Early reports by others also indicated that IB was primarily a disease of young chicks, however, it was later observed to be common in semimature and laying flocks. Although the morbidity rate was often high, the mortality rate was usually low in older chickens. Other manifestations of IB include egg production declines in laying flocks, noted following the typical respiratory disease in the 1940s, and kidney lesions observed in the 1960s. The prevalence and economic importance of the disease resulted in efforts to prevent IB in laying flocks by controlled exposure of chickens to IBV during the growing stage prior to the onset of egg production. This effort by Van Roekel et al. in 1941, which had some success, was the initial step toward the development of the immunization programs used today (130).

Other early milestones include the establishment of the virus etiology by Beach and Schalm in 1936 (6), the first cultivation of the virus in embryonated chicken eggs by Beaudette and Hudson in 1937 (7), and the report in 1956 by Jungherr et al. (81) that the Connecticut isolate of 1951 and the Massachusetts isolate of 1941 produced similar diseases but did not cross protect or cross neutralize. The latter report was the first demonstration that the etiology of IB included more than one serotype. Additional historical information can be found in the review by Cunningham (43) and earlier editions of this chapter by Hofstad (72).

INCIDENCE AND DISTRIBUTION. IB is distributed worldwide. A listing of the reported first identification of IB by country and year through 1966 was included in a review by Estola (60). In the USA, several serotypes in addition to the originally identified Massachusetts (Mass) type of IBV were identified beginning in the 1950s (75, 78). In contrast, the European isolates were considered to be primarily the Mass serotype until the late 1970s when new serotypes were frequently identified (25, 90). Outbreaks of IB still occur, even in vaccinated flocks, and virus strains isolated from those outbreaks are often found to be a serotype distinct from the vaccine type.

ETIOLOGY

Classification. IBV is a member of the family Coronaviridae, which comprises a single genus, *Coronavirus*. In addition to IBV, the genus includes turkey coronavirus (See Chapter 26) and at least nine species in mammals (116).

Morphology. IBV is pleomorphic but generally rounded. It possesses an envelope that is 90–200 nm in diameter with club-shaped surface projections (spikes) about 20 nm in length (Fig. 17.1). The spikes are not packed as closely as the rod-shaped spikes of paramyxoviruses (55). Smaller (7 nm) projections have also been observed (86). Ribonucleoprotein (RNP, core) structures released from spontaneously disrupted particles could be visualized by shadowing but not by negative staining (56). Mostly the RNP was observed as strands of only 1–2 nm in diameter, but coiled structures of 10–15 nm diameter were occasionally observed (56).

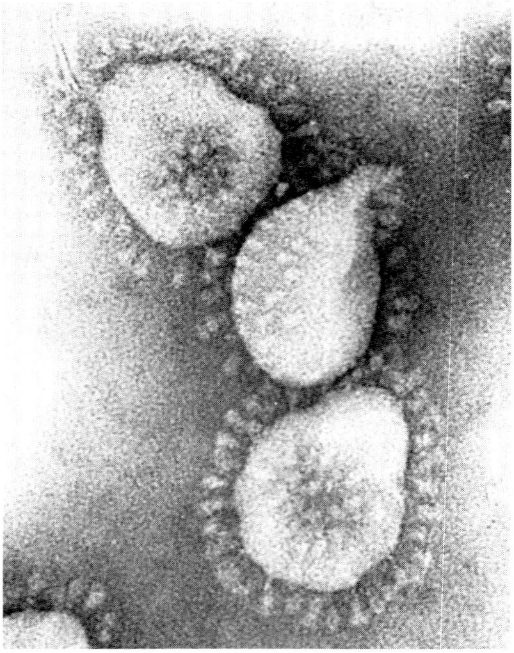

17.1. Virion of avian IBV illustrating club-shaped projections. Preparation negatively stained with phosphotungstic acid. ×300,000. (Berry and Almeida)

IBV strains differ in their density in sucrose gradients, peak density usually being in the range of 1.15–1.18 g/ml, but particles of lower (lacking RNP) and higher density can also be obtained. Centrifugation forces greater than 100,000 g's should be avoided as loss of spikes can occur. Those of IBV-Beaudette appear to be especially unstable; incubation at 37 C sometimes results in the loss of one of the spike components (122).

Chemical Composition. Several reviews on the composition of coronaviruses are available (115, 117, 120, 124), with one review devoted to IBV (10). IBV virions contain three virus-specific proteins: the large spike (S or E2), small matrix (M or E1) glycoproteins, the internal nucleocapsid (N) protein. The S protein comprises two or three copies of each of two glycopolypeptides, S1 and S2 (approximately 520 and 625 amino acids, respectively). Hemagglutination-inhibiting (HI) and most of the virus-neutralizing (VN) antibodies are induced by S1 (19, 20, 103, 128).

Most of the 225 amino acids of the M protein are either embedded in the virus membrane or at the inner membrane surface; only about 10% of the protein is exposed at the outer virus surface. The N protein is around the single piece of single-stranded, positive-sense, RNA genome (to form the RNP) that comprises 27,500 nucleotides, the whole of which has been cloned and sequenced (9). Preparations of purified virus always contain host cell polypeptides (15). The S2 protein can be difficult to detect (15, 16) and some N protein can be missing or degraded.

Virus Replication. IBV replicates in the cytoplasm, six messenger RNAs being produced by a discontinuous transcription mechanism that can generate recombinants (120). Virion formation occurs by a budding process at the membranes of the endoplasmic reticulum, not at the cell surface. Although the S protein can migrate through the reticulum to the cell surface (128), the M protein cannot. It is the localization of the M protein in the endoplasmic reticulum, which dictates that virion formation occurs there. The virions accumulate in smooth vesicles, but the mechanism of their release from the cell is unknown. New virus starts to appear 3–4 hr after infection with maximum output per cell being reached within 12 hr at 37 C.

Resistance to Chemical and Physical Agents

THERMOSTABILITY. Most strains of IBV are inactivated after 15 min at 56 C and after 90 min at 45 C (106). Storage of IBV at −20 C should be avoided but infectious allantoic fluid has remained viable after storage at −30 C for many years. Infected tissues stored in 50% glycerol are well preserved and tissues in this medium can be shipped to a laboratory for diagnosis without refrigeration (72).

Magnesium sulfate has a stabilizing effect on IBV (30). Satylganov (113) studied survival of IBV on artificially contaminated surfaces exposed to different temperatures and humidities during spring, summer, and winter. Outdoors, survival was up to 12 days in spring and 56 days in winter.

LYOPHILIZATION. Infectious allantoic fluid lyophilized, sealed under vacuum and stored in a refrigerator, has remained viable for at least 30 yr. Ten percent glucose gives a stabilizing effect to IBV in the lyophilized and frozen states. Lyophilized IBV is completely inactivated within 6 mo when stored at 37 C (72).

pH STABILITY. There is strain variation with respect to stability at pH 3. After 3 hr at 4 C the titer of some strains had decreased only 0.3 $\log_{10}$ whereas the titer of others was 1–2 $\log_{10}$ lower (106). In another survey the reduction in titer following a pH 3 treatment at room temperature for 4 hr varied from 1–2 $\log_{10}$, for most isolates, to 5 $\log_{10}$, for others (33). At 4 C virus inactivation at pH 11.0 was greater than at pH 3.0 (106). IBV in culture was more stable at pH 6.0 and 6.5 than at pH 7.0 to 8.0 (2).

CHEMICAL AGENTS. IBV is ether-labile but some virus survived 20% ether (4 C, 18 hr). All infectivity was destroyed by 50% chloroform (room temperature, 10 min) and 0.1% sodium deoxycholate (4 C, 18 hr) (106).

IBV is considered to be sensitive to the common disinfectants. Several have been compared for activity against another coronavirus, transmissible gastroenteritis virus of swine (12). An exposure of IBV to 10% ethylene oxide gas in carbon dioxide for 16 hr inactivated virus in either the moist state or after drying over anhydrous calcium chloride or dried state. However, lyophilized virus was not inactivated within this time (99). Treatment with a final concentration of 0.05% (27) or 0.1% beta-propiolactone (BPL) or 0.1% formalin (82) eliminated IBV infectivity. Only the BPL treatment had no adverse effect on IBV hemagglutination antigen activity.

Strain Classification. Strain classification of IBV has been based largely on VN tests in several systems. In the 1960s and 1970s several serotypes, distinct from the well-known Mass serotype, were described in the USA (75, 78). Since then extensive surveys in the Netherlands (54) and the UK (25, 26) have revealed many new serotypes of IBV. VN has been performed with chicken tracheal organ cultures (TOCs) (25, 26,50, 78), chicken kidney (CK) cells using plaque reduction (75), and chicken embryos (54).

Strain classification by HI tests has also been investigated. The HI antibody response following a single exposure and resulting infection can be highly strain specific, even differentiating the Holland from the M41 strains of the same (Mass) serotype (13, 84, 85). The specificity of the early response and the limited cross reactivity are the basis for a procedure for serotyping isolates by HI (85). In contrast, Cook et al. (28) compared the HI test with the VN test in TOCs and concluded that the HI test was subject to high and variable cross reactions and that IBV strains were more clearly differentiated by the VN test. The reason for the reported differences in cross reactivity is unknown. Both studies based the evaluations on the results from primary sera since it is known that secondary sera are much more broadly reactive (13, 63).

Other approaches used to study IBV variation include detection of fixed virus antigen in CK cells by an enzyme immunoassay (129), monoclonal antibodies (89), oligonucleotide fingerprinting (90), and nucleic acid sequencing (8, 17, 18, 91). Sequencing has revealed that while the S protein genes of some serotypes differ by 25–50%, other serotypes differ by only 2–3% of their amino acids. All methodologies used emphasize the great capacity of IBV to change and the difficulty of devising a simple system for classifying IBV strains and guiding the use of vaccines.

Laboratory Host Systems

CHICKEN EMBRYOS. IBV grows well in the developing chicken embryo. Dwarfing of a few embryos with survival of 90% through the 19th day of incubation is characteristic of IBV field material upon initial inoculation in 10- to 11-day-old embryonated chicken eggs. Embryo mortality and dwarfing increase as the number of serial passages increases, so that by the 10th passage most of the embryos are stunted, and up to 80% may die by the 20th day of incubation.

Characteristic embryo changes are seen several days after inoculation of the virus. Only slight movement of a dwarfed embryo may be observed during candling. Upon opening the air-cell end of the egg, the embryo is seen curled into a spherical form with feet deformed and compressed over the head and with the thickened amnion adhered to it (Fig. 17.2).

The yolk sac appears shrunken and the membrane ruptures easily. An increased volume of usually clear allantoic fluid is present. A consistent internal lesion of the IB-infected embryo is the persistence of the mesonephros containing urates. This lesion appears to be associated with the stunting of the embryo and is not specific for IB infection. Another lesion found in embryonated eggs inoculated with nonlethal isolates of IBV is the thickened amnion and adjacent layer of the allantois covering the stunted embryo. Evidence of this lesion can usually be detected on the 3rd day after inoculation. It likewise is not a pathognomonic lesion since it can also be observed following inoculation of eggs with lentogenic strains of NDV (72).

Microscopic lesions in the embryo infected with IBV-M41 strain have been studied by Loomis et al. (93). They found congestion with perivascular cuffing and some necrosis of the livers by the 6th day after inoculation. All lungs were pneumonic, characterized by congestion, cellular infiltration, and serous exudate in the bronchial sacs. In the kidneys there was interstitial nephritis with edema and distension of the

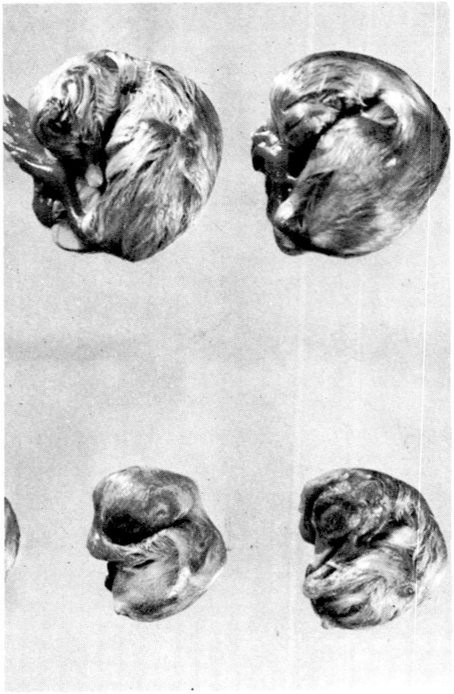

17.2. Comparison of normal 16-day-old embryos (*above*) and curled, dwarfed, infected embryos of the same age (*below*). (Hofstad and Bauriedel)

proximal convoluted tubules with casts. Glomeruli were not altered. The chorioallantoic membrane (CAM) and amniotic membrane were edematous. No inclusion bodies were found.

Optimum age of embryo and temperature and length of incubation, for maximum infectivity titer of IBV-Beaudette following allantoic cavity inoculation, have been thoroughly studied and reviewed (80). Following inoculation of approximately 10^7 embryo infective dose–50% (EID_{50}), similar peak titers in allantoic fluid (AF) of embryos inoculated at 10–11 days old were achieved after 12 and 24 hr at 37 C and 32 C, respectively. Virus titers of CAMs were higher than those of AFs. Virus-induced embryo death was first observed at 24 and 48 hr after incubation at 37 C and 32 C, respectively. Incubation at 42 C resulted in earlier mortality (12 hr) and lower titers. In a different study, a less egg-adapted strain (20–30 embryo passages) attained maximum titers after 24–30 hr at 37 C, irrespective of the inoculum dose (70). In general, inocula of about 10^3 TOC infectious doses or 10^4 EID_{50} should give near maximum titers by 36–40 hr at 37 C.

TURKEY EMBRYOS. IBV-Beaudette replicated in turkey embryos causing mortality (58). IBV-M41 required alternate passages in chicken and turkey embryos for adaptation to the latter (58). Although the viruses are serologically similar, the Beaudette strain inoculum was from high chicken embryo passage (>200), whereas the M41 inoculum was from the second embryo passage after isolation from chickens.

CELL CULTURES. When monolayer cell cultures have been required for IBV studies, chick embryo kidney (CEK) cells and CK cells have been used most successfully. Adaptation of IBV to CEK cells has been examined and reviewed by Gillette (66). The number of passages in CEK required to produce extensive cytopathic effect (CPE), evident in unstained cultures, and maximum titers varied among strains, although plaques, revealed by staining, could be seen after the first passage. Adaptation of some strains to CEK is facilitated by embryo passage. However, Wadey and Faragher (131) obtained plaque-forming virus on the second CEK passage although many of the isolates used had been passaged less than seven times in embryos. Plaque size and morphology vary among strains; plaque size of most strains was greater at 40 C than at 37 C (66).

The lag phase of IBV in CEK or CK cells is 3–4 hr (49, 94) with maximum titers in the culture medium being at 14–36 hr, depending on the multiplicity of infection (94, 49, 107). Chick embryo liver (CEL) cells produced titers of IBV similar to those from CEK cells (94). Titration of IBV in embryonated eggs gave higher titers (10- to 100-fold) than in CEK or CK cells (94, 49), which in turn were more sensitive than CEL cells (94). Maximum titers of IBV-Beaudette from CK cells were similar over the pH range 6–9. Virus was released more quickly but was also inactivated more rapidly with increasing pH (2). The optimum pH for maximum production of stable virus was pH 6.5.

IBV strains that had been passaged in embryos and many times in CK cells replicated in chicken embryo fibroblast cultures but to titers several $\log_{10}$ less than in CK cells (107). Plaques formed when trypsin was in the culture medium (105). IBV-Beaudette can grow, albeit poorly, in a number of primary kidney and embryo kidney cultures from various avian and mammalian species (29, 31). IBV-Beaudette (44) and the M41 and Iowa-97 strains (32) have been adapted to the mammalian Vero cell line. Of 10 strains examined, 2 and none replicated in BHK-21 and HeLa cells, respectively (107).

CK cells began to form syncytia 6 hr after inoculation with IBV-Beaudette (2). After 18–24 hr syncytia contained 20–40 or more nuclei, and became vacuolated. The nuclei were pycnotic. Syncytia in CK cultures quickly round up and detach from the substrate but syncytia in Vero cells infected with Vero cell–adapted IBV-Beaudette contain scores of nuclei and remain on the substrates longer (92).

ORGAN CULTURES. The propagation of IBV in organ cultures of trachea and other tissues has been reviewed by Darbyshire (45). Tracheal rings are prepared from 20-day-old embryos and maintained singly in roller tubes. Following infection with IBV, ciliostasis, easily observed by low-power microscopy, occurs within 3–4 days. Tracheal organ cultures have proved very successful for the isolation, titration, and serotyping of IBV (25, 26) because no adaptation of field strains is required for growth and induction of ciliostasis.

Pathogenicity.

IBV isolates, regardless of tissue of origin, readily infect the respiratory tract of chickens and produce characteristic lesions in the trachea. In many cases there is an unremarkable recovery unless the chickens are very young, airsacculitis develops because of a secondary bacterial infection, or kidney disease follows the respiratory phase. Cumming (41) enumerated some of the management factors that contribute to IB-related kidney disease in Australia. Greater mortality was seen in males where there was cold stress in certain breeds, and/or where animal products were the major component of high-protein diets. Some of these factors known to exacerbate the clinical disease have been used in experimental models to evaluate virulence differences among strains. A combination of cold stress plus *Mycoplasma synoviae* exposure 5 days after an IBV exposure (77) produces an airsacculitis that varies in incidence and severity with the virulence of the IBV strain. A combined intranasal inoculation of different IBV strains and *Escherichia coli* (27) produced mortality in young chickens; neither infection alone was lethal. Mortality ranged from 14 to 82% with different strains demonstrating that they did differ in virulence.

Other differences in virulence of IBV strains have been noted. Passage of IBV in chicken embryos gradually results in a decrease in virulence. The highly egg-adapted Beaudette strain is apathogenic, causes no detectable damage to the ciliated epithelium of the trachea, and replicates predominantly in the subepithelial cells. The immunogenicity of the strain is diminished as well (62). In contrast, the virulent M41 strain destroyed the ciliated epithelium prior to localization in the subepithelium. The Australian T strain is virulent and a known cause of mortality and kidney lesions. Viruses of other serotypes that are also known to be nephropathogenic, but of less severity than T strain, include Italian, the USA strains Gray and Holte (1), and the Mass-Holland strain (96).

Virulence for the reproductive tract may also differ among IBV strains. Different IBV strains can produce a range of effects in susceptible layers varying from shell pigment changes with no production drop (26) to production drops of 10–50% (76).

PATHOGENESIS AND EPIZOOTIOLOGY

Natural and Experimental Hosts.

Although susceptibility to disease varies among breeds or strains of chickens (41, 119), it is generally considered that the chicken is the only bird that is naturally infected by IBV and in which the virus causes disease. However, IBV has been isolated from pheasants in which breeding birds had respiratory signs and an associated depression in egg production and quality, and young birds had considerable respiratory distress (121). The source of the virus was probably a nearby chicken laying unit.

Experimental inoculation of turkeys with IBV by aerosol produced no response, but intravenous inoculation may produce a viremia for varying periods up to 48 hr (72). Ring-necked pheasants and starlings were resistant to intratracheal inoculation with IBV. Bronchial rales were detected in quail inoculated similarly but no virus was isolated or seroconversion detected (4). Suckling mice are susceptible by intracerebral inoculation to several but not all IBV strains (61). The limited host range is not unusual because coronaviruses such as IBV typically cause clinical disease only in the species from which they are isolated and they replicate predominantly in cultures derived from that host (134).

AGE OF HOST COMMONLY AFFECTED. All ages are susceptible, but the disease is most severe in baby chicks, causing some mortality (72). As age increases chickens become more resistant to the nephritogenic effects, oviduct lesions, and mortality due to infection (1, 37, 119).

Transmission, Carriers, Vectors.

IBV spreads rapidly among chickens in a flock. Susceptible birds placed in a room with infected chickens usually develop signs within 48 hr (43). Virus was isolated consistently from the trachea, lungs, kidney, and bursa of chickens at 24 hr and through the 7th day after aerosol exposure (73). The frequency of virus isolations declined with time and varied with the infecting strain, but IBV was isolated from the cecal tonsils at 14 wk and from feces 20 wk postinfection (3). Reexcretion of IBV has also been detected from hens that had been virus-negative for several weeks following recovery from inoculation at 1 day of age. Virus was isolated from tracheal and cloacal swabs collected at the point of lay, 19 wk of age (79). While there are reports of virus isolations from eggs up to 43 days after recovery, chickens have been hatched from infected flocks and reared free of IBV (43). The nature of the persistence of IBV infection remains undefined, but reports of extended and intermittent shedding are evidence of the potential risk of flock-to-flock transmission via contamination of personnel or equipment.

The frequency of airborne spread between flocks is unknown, but circumstantial evidence of transmission of IBV over a distance of 1200 yd was reported (42). Vectors do not appear to be a factor in the spread of IBV (72).

Incubation Period. The incubation period of IB is 18–36 hr, depending on dose and route of inoculation. Chickens exposed to an aerosol of undiluted infective egg fluid regularly have tracheal rales within 24 hr. Natural spread requires about 36 hr or more (72).

Signs. The characteristic respiratory signs of IB in chicks are gasping, coughing, sneezing, tracheal rales, and nasal discharge. Wet eyes may be observed and an occasional chick may have swollen sinuses. The chicks appear depressed, may be seen huddled under a heat source, and feed consumption and weight gain are significantly reduced. In chickens over 6 wk of age and in adult birds, the signs are similar to those in chicks, but nasal discharge does not occur as frequently and the disease may go unnoticed unless the flock is examined carefully by handling the birds or listening to them at night when the birds are normally quiet (43, 72).

Broiler chickens infected with one of the nephropathic viruses may appear to recover from the typical respiratory phase and then show signs of depression, ruffled feathers, wet droppings, and increased drinking (41, 135). When urolithiasis is associated with IB in layer flocks, there may be increased mortality but otherwise the flock appears healthy (34, 14).

In laying flocks, declines in egg production and quality are seen in addition to respiratory signs. However, IBV has been isolated from cloacal swabs or cecal tonsil samples from breeder or layer flocks with slight production drops and the production of pale shell eggs, but no respiratory signs (25, 26). The severity of the production declines may vary with the period of lay (59) and with the causative virus strain (26, 76). Six to 8 wk may elapse before production returns to the preinfection level, but in most cases this is never attained (43). In addition to production declines, the number of eggs unacceptable for setting is increased, hatchability is reduced, and soft-shelled, misshapen, and rough-shelled eggs are produced (Fig. 17.3).

Internal quality of eggs, as observed when breaking eggs on a flat surface, may be inferior. The albumen may be thin and watery without definite demarcation between the thick and thin albumen of the normal fresh egg (72) (Fig. 17.4).

IBV infection of 1-day-old chicks can produce permanent damage leading to reduced egg production and quality when the chickens come into lay. The severity of oviduct lesions was less in infections of older chickens and some serotypes failed to produce any pathological change even in infections of 1-day-old chicks (36, 37, 79).

Morbidity and Mortality. All birds in the flock become infected, but mortality is variable depending on virulence of the infecting serotype; age; status of immunity, either maternal or active; and stresses such as cold or secondary bacterial infections. Severe mortality has been noted with some of the nephropathic strains such as Australian T. Sex, breed, and nutrition are additional factors that contribute to the severity of kidney disease (41). Mortality may be as high as 25% or more in chickens less than 6 wk of age and is usually negligible in chickens over that age (72). Mortality in urolithiasis cases ranged from 0.5 to 1.0% per week (14, 34).

Gross Lesions. Infected chickens have serous, catarrhal, or caseous exudate in the trachea, nasal passages, and sinuses. Air sacs may appear cloudy or contain a yellow caseous exudate. A caseous plug may be found in the lower trachea or

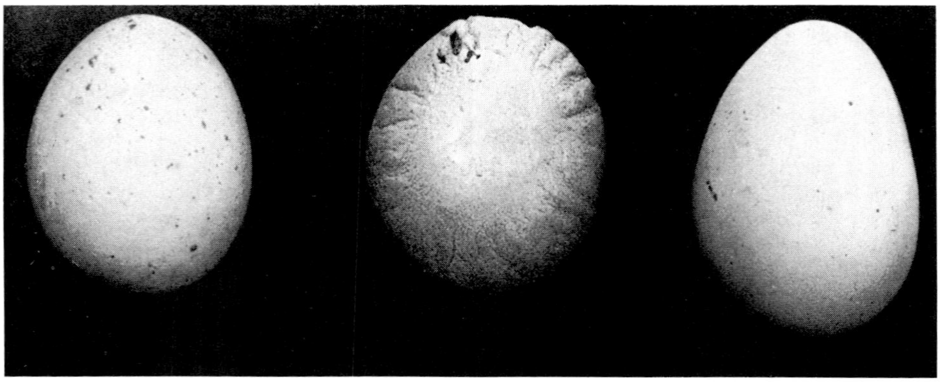

17.3. Thin-shelled, rough-shelled, and misshapen eggs laid by hens during an outbreak of IB. (Van Roekel)

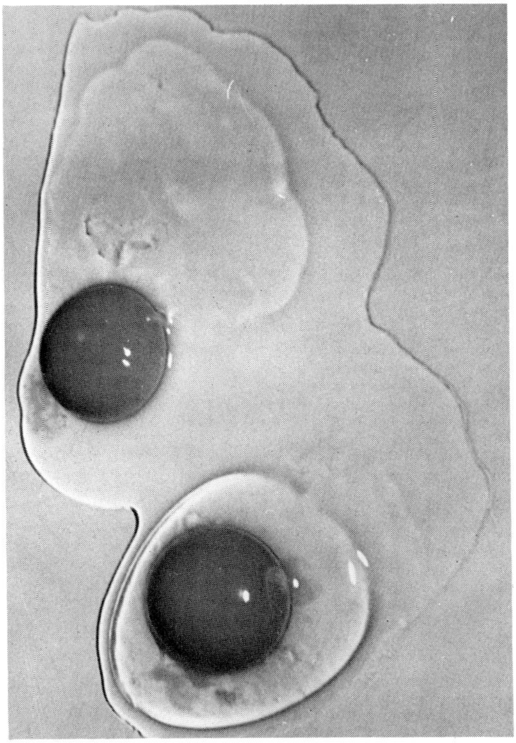

17.4. Contents of two eggs. Normal egg (*bottom*). Egg from chicken exposed to IBV at 1 day of age (*top*). Note watery albumen with yolk separated from thick albumen. (Hofstad)

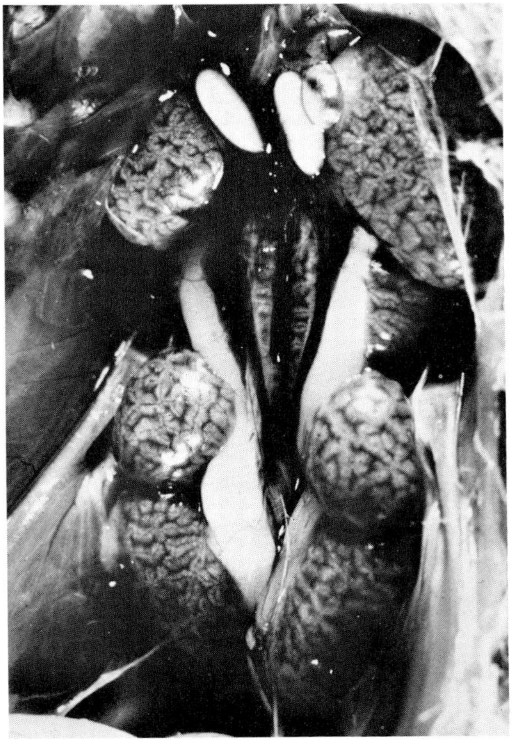

17.5. Kidney lesions associated with IB caused by T strain of virus. Note swollen kidneys with tubules and ureters distended with urates. (Cumming)

bronchi of chicks that die. Small areas of pneumonia may be observed around the large bronchi (72). Nephropathic infections produce swollen and pale kidneys with the tubules and ureters often distended with urates (40, 135) (Fig. 17.5).

Fluid yolk material may be found in the abdominal cavity of chickens that are in production, but this is also seen with other diseases that cause a marked drop in egg production. Permanent lesions in the oviduct may be a consequence of IBV infection of 1-day-old chicks and are a cause of nonlayers. The middle third of the oviduct is most severely affected and may be nonpatent and hypoglandular (38, 72).

Histopathology. The mucosa of the trachea of chickens with IB is edematous. There is a loss of cilia, rounding and sloughing of epithelial cells, and minor infiltration of heterophils and lymphocytes within 18 hr of infection. Regeneration of the epithelium starts within 48 hr. Hyperplasia is followed by massive infiltration of the lamina propria by lymphoid cells and a large number of germinal centers, which may be present after 7 days. If air sac involvement occurs, there is edema, epithelial cell desquamation, and some fibrinous exudate within 24 hr. Increased heterophils can be observed later with lymphoid nodules, fibroblast proliferation, and cuboidal epithelial regeneration (112).

The kidney lesions of IB are principally those of an interstitial nephritis. The virus causes granular degeneration, vacuolation and desquamation of the tubular epithelium, and massive infiltration of heterophils in the interstitium in acute stages of the disease. The lesions in tubules are most prominent in the medulla. Focal areas of necrosis may be seen as well as indications of attempted regeneration of the tubular epithelium. During recovery, the inflammatory cell population changes to lymphocytes and plasma cells. In some cases, degenerative changes may persist and result in severe atrophy of one or all of the divisions of the kidneys. In urolithiasis the ureters associated with atrophied kidneys are distended with urates and often contain large calculi composed mainly of urates (112).

Experimental IB infection of mature hens resulted in decreased height and loss of cilia from epithelial cells; dilation of the tubular glands; infiltration by lymphocytes, mononuclear cells, plasma cells, and heterophils; and edema and fibroplasia of the lamina propria of all regions of the oviduct (112). The histopathology of IB and comparisons with other diseases are given in detail in a book by Riddell (112) and a review of renal pathology by Siller (118).

Immunity

ACTIVE. Chickens just recovered from the natural disease are resistant to challenge with the same virus (homologous protection), but the extent of protection to challenge with other IBV strains (heterologous protection) varies. Factors that complicate studies of the mechanism and duration of immunity to IB are the multiple serotypes that are recognized (25, 75, 78, 90, 132), the variation in virulence observed among strains (see Pathogenicity), and the different manifestations of IBV infection for which protection may be needed (see Signs).

Respiratory protection is usually evaluated 3–4 wk after an IB infection or immunization and has been done in several different ways. In most cases an IBV challenge is given by a respiratory route. The failure to recover IBV from the trachea 4–5 days postchallenge has been used as a single criterion of immunity (71). More comprehensive evaluations have included two or more additional criteria of resistance to challenge including failure to isolate virus from the kidney and oviduct, no clinical signs of IB, no tracheal lesions, or the presence of tracheal ciliary activity (5, 47,136). Accumulating scores from the different criteria is used to indicate the range of protection from full to partial or none. An alternative approach is an evaluation of vaccinated chickens for protection against mortality from a challenge with a mixture of IBV and *Escherichia coli.* This method showed evidence of more vaccinal cross-protection than found with other assessments of tracheal immunity (27).

Protection against mortality from nephritis is important as evidence of satisfactory vaccinal immunity where nephritis is a major clinical problem, as in Australia (87, 111). The ability to reduce or prevent egg production declines from a challenge infection is evidence of IB protection in a laying flock (11).

Although there is evidence that the S1 glycopolypeptide is primarily responsible for the induction of VN and HI antibody and that the spike protein plays a major role in the induction of protective immunity (20), the knowledge of the mechanism of protection against clinical disease is incomplete. The local synthesis of neutralizing antibody into nasal secretions might prevent reinfection (74) and there is evidence for a contribution by the Harderian gland in the local response (51). The function of humoral immunity induced by an infection or immunization may be similar to that for passive antibody. However, antibody was not essential for resistance as demonstrated in chickens treated with cyclophosphamide and then vaccinated. Detectable antibodies were not produced, but the chickens did resist challenge (21). Evidence of cell-mediated immune responses to IBV are lymphocyte transformation assays of live and inactivated virus vaccinates (126, 127), cytotoxic lymphocyte activity (23), and delayed type hypersensitivity (24), but the role of these responses in immunity is not known. Interferon induction by IBV varies with the virus strain; however, there is no known role of interferon in resistance to IB (108). Immunity to IB and to other poultry diseases has been reviewed (109).

PASSIVE. Maternal antibody can reduce both the severity of vaccinal reaction and the efficacy of the vaccine if the vaccine is of the same type used in the breeder flock immunization (87, 88). Maternal antibody provided protection against challenge at 1 day and 1 wk but not at 2 wk of age (104).

DIAGNOSIS.

Diagnosis of IB is based on the clinical history, seroconversion or rising IBV antibody titers, IBV antigen detection by immunofluorescence in tissue sections or smears, and virus isolation. Virus isolation and serotypic characterization of the isolate are necessary for a definitive diagnosis.

Isolation and Identification of the Causative Agent. The trachea is a primary target for IBV and therefore is a preferred sampling site. Samples from the lung, kidney, oviduct, cecal tonsils, or cloaca should also be considered based on the clinical history of the disease. Cloacal swabs can be of particular value in cases where more than 1 wk may have elapsed since the start of infection, because IBV is cleared from the trachea sooner than from the intestinal tract. Tracheal and cloacal swabs are readily obtained from live or dead birds. Scrapings of the tracheal mucosa or tissue samples for homogenization for virus isolation can be collected during a postmortem examination. Sections or smears from the latter samples can be examined for IBV antigen by immunofluorescence (22, 69,95, 101). Sample selection from extremely large flocks can be a difficult problem. The placement of susceptible sentinel chickens in a problem flock has been successful when direct sampling methods in the flock had failed (64). Sentinels are removed for direct sampling after 1 wk of contact exposure.

Samples for virus isolation are inoculated into embryonated chicken eggs or tracheal organ cultures. Fluids should be harvested after 48–72 hr from either culture system for blind passage into another set of cultures. Each sample should receive at least four blind passages before being called negative, based on failure to cause typical embryo death or lesions or ciliostasis in the organ cultures. Inoculation of susceptible chicks intratracheally with the original samples or first-passage culture fluids will produce typical respiratory signs in 18–36 hr, if IBV is present. No further inoculations are given. Antiserum collected at 4 wk postinoculation should be suitable for use in two-way comparisons to determine the serotype of the isolate.

Isolates from positive cultures should have characteristics typical of a coronavirus as visualized by electron microscopy or determined by other procedures as described in etiology. Natural hemagglutination of IBV has been reported but is extremely rare (53). A greater concern is the differentiation from other viruses, such as avian adenoviruses, that can also cause embryo stunting and may frequently be isolated from similar samples. Serotypic classification of isolates should be done as described under Strain Classification. Type-specific antisera should be available in the diagnostic laboratory to determine if the isolate is similar to, or different from, any vaccine strains used in the infected flock. The details of identification of IBV isolates from respiratory and egg production problems (25), urolithiasis (35), and nephritis (95, 101) are described.

Serology. Serum antibody assays are routinely used to monitor the vaccinal response and to detect antibody titer increases attributable to field infection. The multiple IBV serotypes and the antigenic variation noted within the described types add complexity to the selection of an appropriate serological method and the analysis of test results. Antibody is produced to IBV antigens shared by all types, the group-specific antigens, and to the S1 glycopolypeptide, the type-specific antigen. The enzyme-linked immunosorbent assay (ELISA), immunofluorescence (IF), or immunodiffusion (ID) tests bind antibody to group- as well as type-specific antigens. Because of this dual binding characteristic, IBV types are not differentiated with these tests. Most of the primary antibody response to IBV infection appears to be type-specific and functions to differentiate types by VN or HI, which is similar to that reported for another coronavirus (97). However, as noted in Strain Classification, the secondary response to IBV is more broadly reactive even in VN and HI. Evidence of a broadly reactive serum in those two tests is an extensive reaction to more than one VN or HI antigen. Identification of the infecting strain can not be determined by serology when such cross reactivity exists and in such a case the differentiating capability of a VN or HI test is no better than a group reactive assay.

Routine serology is usually done with either VN, HI, or ELISA. Reviews of the methodologies for several serological procedures are available (43, 46, 72). VN tests are done with either a decreasing-virus, constant-serum or constant-virus, decreasing-serum method using embryonated eggs, tracheal organ cultures, or cell culture as the virus assay system. The emphasis on individual rather than pooled sample tests to get more complete information on antibody prevalence in a flock, and the application of microculture systems to conserve reagents and reduce costs, has resulted in a reduced use of embryonated eggs as an assay system. Different HI procedures have been used. A range of 4–8 hemagglutination (HA) units of antigen in serial dilutions of serum has been used and the results from the different procedures were compared (83). Antibody is detected earlier by HI than VN (67). Optimally, postvaccination serology by VN or HI should be conducted with test antigens homologous with each of the vaccine antigens employed in a flock. The ELISA method is used widely, and kits for conducting the procedure are commercially available. Antibody response can be detected earlier by ELISA than by VN (98). The procedures for IF have been either direct (39) or indirect (22, 39). Antibodies detected by the ID method have been found to be transient and the method has given variable results (67).

Differential Diagnosis. IB may resemble other acute respiratory diseases such as Newcastle disease (ND), laryngotracheitis (LT), and infectious coryza (IC). ND is generally more severe than IB. Nervous signs may be observed with virulent strains of ND, and in laying flocks drops in production may be greater than with IB. LT tends to spread more slowly in a flock, but respiratory signs may be more severe than with IB. IC can be differentiated on the basis of facial swelling that only rarely occurs in IB. Production declines and shell quality problems in flocks infected with the egg drop syndrome (EDS) adenovirus are similar to those seen with IB except that internal egg quality is not affected in the case of EDS (59).

TREATMENT.

There is no specific treatment for IB. Provision of additional heat to eliminate cold stress, elimination of overcrowding, and attempts to maintain feed consumption to prevent weight loss are flock management factors that may help reduce losses from IB. Treatment with appropriate antibacterials may be indicated to aid in reducing the losses from airsacculitis. Electrolyte replacers, supplied in the drinking water, are recommended and used in Australia to compensate for the acute loss of sodium and potassium and to thereby reduce losses from nephritis. The recommended concentration for treatment is 72 milliequivalents of sodium and/or potassium, with at least one-third in the citrate or bicarbonate salt form (41).

PREVENTION AND CONTROL

Management Procedures. Ideal management includes strict isolation and repopulation with only day-old chicks following the cleaning and disinfection of the poultry house. Airborne diseases can be prevented by ventilating houses with filtered air under positive pressure (57). Current production methods that include multiple ages in a house or multiple ages on a farm in a high-density poultry area make control more difficult and have necessitated the use of immunization to attempt to prevent production losses due to IB. Immunization is also used in isolated single-age laying flocks to prevent the heavy production losses that may result from an IBV infection of a susceptible flock during the laying cycle.

Immunization

TYPES OF VACCINE. Both live and inactivated virus vaccines are used in IB immunization. Live vaccines are used in broilers and for the initial vaccination of breeders and layers. Inactivated oil-emulsion vaccines (11, 123) are used primarily at point of lay in breeders and layers. IBV strains used for live vaccines are frequently attenuated by serial passage in embryonated chicken eggs (see Pathogenicity) (87). Extensive passage is avoided to prevent a reduction in immunogenicity as well. The degree and stability of such attenuation probably varies among vaccines. Evidence that some vaccines increased in virulence after back-passage in chickens (77) demonstrates the potential for enhancement of virulence of such vaccines by a cyclic infection in a flock.

Vaccine strains are selected to represent the antigenic spectrum of isolates in a particular country or region. The Massachusetts (M41) strain is used widely because initial isolates from many countries are of that serotype. New types are subsequently included when the prevalence of the new type is established. In the USA, M41, Holland, and Connecticut types are used widely and Florida, Arkansas, and JMK are used regionally with special license. In the Netherlands, strains Holland, D274, and D1466 are used. In Australia, strains of their B and C subtypes are used (87, 132).

APPLICATION METHODS. Live vaccine combinations of IBV with Newcastle disease virus (NDV) are used frequently. If the IBV component is in excess there may be an interference with the NDV response (68, 125). No similar interference with the IBV response has been reported.

Administration of live vaccine can be individually by eye-drop, intratracheal (5), or intranasal. An embryonal injection method has also been used experimentally (133). Mass application methods include coarse spray (5, 52), aerosol, and drinking water (110). Mass administration methods are popular because of convenience, but problems in attaining uniform vaccine application can occur and the aerosol method may cause more severe respiratory reactions. Vaccines applied by the drinking water method are susceptible to inactivation by sanitizers added to control bacterial and fungal contamination of the watering system. Removal of those sanitizers prior to vaccination and the incorporation of powdered skim milk at a 1:400 concentration has been shown to stabilize the virus titer during vaccine administration (65).

Inactivated vaccines require injection of individual birds. These vaccines are usually given after "priming" with live virus and are administered a few weeks before production commences. They may be given in combination with other inactivated vaccines

Two weeks of age is frequently used as the time for initial immunization (48), but vaccine may be successfully administered at 1 day of age (5, 52). Timing of initial immunization varies due to titer of maternal antibody in chicks and vaccination methods used. Schedules of subsequent immunization at 7–12 or 16–18 wk of age, and at point of lay, vary with flock management and needs for control of IB as well as other flock diseases.

REFERENCES

1. Albassam, M.A., R.W. Winterfield, and H.L. Thacker. 1986. Comparison of the nephropathogenicity of four strains of infectious bronchitis virus. Avian Dis 30:468–476.

2. Alexander, D.J., and M.S. Collins. 1975. Effect of pH on the growth and cytopathogenicity of avian infectious bronchitis virus in chick kidney cells. Arch Virol 49:339–348.

3. Alexander, D.J., and R.E. Gough. 1977. Isolation of avian infectious bronchitis virus from experimentally infected chickens. Res Vet Sci 23:344–347.

4. Allred, J.N., L.G. Raggi, and G.G. Lee. 1973. Susceptibility and resistance of pheasants, starlings, and quail to three respiratory diseases of chickens. Calif Fish Game 59:161–167.

5. Andrade, L.F., P. Villegas, and O.J. Fletcher. 1983. Vaccination of day-old broilers against infectious bronchitis: Effect of vaccine strain and route of administration. Avian Dis 27:178–187.

6. Beach, J.R., and O.W. Schalm. 1936. A filterable virus, distinct from that of laryngotracheitis, the cause of a respiratory disease of chicks. Poult Sci 15:199–206.

7. Beaudette, F.R., and C.B. Hudson. 1937. Cultivation of the virus of infectious bronchitis. J Am Vet Med Assoc 90:51–60.

8. Binns, M.M., M.E.G. Boursnell, F.M. Tomley, and T.D.K. Brown. 1986. Comparison of the spike precursor sequences of coronavirus IBV strains M41 and 6/82 with that of IBV Beaudette. J Gen Virol 67:2825–2831.

9. Boursnell, M.E.G., T.D.K. Brown, I.J. Foulds, P.F. Green, F.M. Tomley, and M.M. Binns. 1987. Completion of the sequence of the genome of the coronavirus avian infectious bronchitis virus. J Gen Virol 68:57–77.

10. Boursnell, M.E.G., M.M. Binns, T.D.K. Brown, D. Cavanagh, and F.M. Tomley. 1989. Molecular biology

of avian infectious bronchitis virus. Prog Vet Microbiol Immunol 5:65–82.

11. Box, P.G., H.C. Holmes, P.M. Finney, and R. Froymann. 1988. Infectious bronchitis in laying hens: The relationship between hemagglutination inhibition antibody levels and resistance to experimental challenge. Avian Pathol 17:349–361.

12. Brown, T.T., Jr. 1981. Laboratory evaluation of selected disinfectants as virucidal agents against porcine parvovirus, psuedorabies virus, and transmissible gastroenteritis virus. Am J Vet Res 42:1033–1036.

13. Brown, A.J., and C.D. Bracewell. 1988. Effect of repeated infections of chickens with infectious bronchitis viruses on the specificity of their antibody responses. Vet Rec 122:207–208.

14. Brown, T.P., J.R. Glisson, G. Rosales, P. Villegas, and R.B. Davis. 1987. Studies of avian urolithiasis associated with an infectious bronchitis virus. Avian Dis 31:629–636.

15. Cavanagh, D. 1984. Structural characterization of IBV glycoproteins. Adv Exp Med Biol 173:95–108.

16. Cavanagh, D., and P.J. Davis. 1987. Coronavirus IBV: Relationships among recent European isolates studied by limited proteolysis of the virion glycopolypeptides. Avian Pathol 16:1–13.

17. Cavanagh, D., and P.J. Davis. 1988. Evolution of avian coronavirus IBV: Sequence of the matrix glycoprotein gene and intergenic region of several serotypes. J Gen Virol 69:621–629.

18. Cavanagh, D., and P.J. Davis. 1988. Evolution of IBV studied by sequencing the spike and matrix glycoprotein genes. In E.F. Kaleta and U. Heffels-Redmann (eds.), Proc 1st Int Symp on Infectious Bronchitis, pp. 153–165. Giessen:Dtsch Veterinarmedizinische Gesellschaft e.V.

19. Cavanagh, D., J.H. Darbyshire, P. Davis, and R.W. Peters. 1984. Induction of humoral neutralizing and hemagglutination inhibiting antibody by the spike protein of avian infectious bronchitis virus. Avian Pathol 13:573–583.

20. Cavanagh, D., P.J. Davis, J.H. Darbyshire, and R.W. Peters. 1986. Coronavirus IBV: Virus retaining spike glycopolypeptide S2 but not S1 is unable to induce virus neutralizing or hemagglutination inhibiting antibody or induce chicken tracheal protection. J Gen Virol 67:1435–1442.

21. Chubb, R.C. 1974. The effect of the suppression of circulating antibody on resistance to the Australian avian infectious bronchitis virus. Res Vet Sci 17:169–173.

22. Chubb, R.C. 1986. The detection of antibody to avian infectious bronchitis virus by the use of immunofluorescence with tissue sections of nephritic kidneys. Aust Vet J 63:131–132.

23. Chubb, R.C., V. Huynh, and R. Law. 1987. The detection of cytotoxic lymphocyte activity in chickens infected with infectious bronchitis virus or fowl pox virus. Avian Pathol 16:395–405.

24. Chubb, R.C., V. Huynh, and R. Bradley. 1988. The induction and control of delayed type hypersensitivity reactions induced in chickens by infectious bronchitis virus. Avian Pathol 17:371–383.

25. Cook, J.K.A. 1984. The classification of new serotypes of infectious bronchitis virus isolated from poultry flocks in Britain between 1981 and 1983. Avian Pathol 13:733–741.

26. Cook, J.K.A., and M.B. Huggins. 1986. Newly isolated serotypes of infectious bronchitis virus: Their role in disease. Avian Pathol 15:129–138.

27. Cook, J.K.A., H.W. Smith, and M.B. Huggins. 1986. Infectious bronchitis immunity: Its study in chickens experimentally infected with mixtures of infectious bronchitis virus and Escherichia coli. J Gen Virol 67:1427–1434.

28. Cook, J.K.A., A.J. Brown, and C.D. Bracewell. 1987. Comparison of the hemagglutination inhibition test and the serum neutralization test in tracheal organ cultures for typing infectious bronchitis virus strains. Avian Pathol 16:505–511.

29. Coria, M.F. 1969. Intracellular avian infectious bronchitis virus: Detection by fluorescent antibody techniques in nonovarian kidney cell culture. Avian Dis 13:540–547.

30. Coria, M.F. 1972. Stabilizing effect of magnesium sulfate on avian infectious bronchitis virus propagated in chicken embryo kidney cells. Appl Microbiol 23:281–284.

31. Coria, M.F., and J.K. Peterson. 1971. Adaptation and propagation of avian infectious bronchitis virus in embryonic turkey kidney cell cultures. Avian Dis 15:22–27.

32. Coria, M.F., and A.E. Ritchie. 1973. Serial passage of 3 strains of avian infectious bronchitis virus in African green monkey kidney cells (VERO). Avian Dis 17:697–704.

33. Cowen, B.S., and S.B. Hitchner. 1975. pH stability studies with avian infectious bronchitis virus (Coronavirus) strains. J Virol 15:430–432.

34. Cowen, B.S., R.F. Wideman, H. Rothenbacher, and M.O. Braune. 1987. An outbreak of avian urolithiasis on a large commercial egg farm. Avian Dis 31:392–397.

35. Cowen, B.S., R.F. Wideman, M.O. Braune, and R.L. Owen. 1987. An infectious bronchitis virus isolated from chickens experiencing a urolithiasis outbreak. I. In vitro characterization studies. Avian Dis 31:878–883.

36. Crinion, R.A.P. 1972. Egg quality and production following infectious bronchitis virus exposure at one day old. Poult Sci 51:582–585.

37. Crinion, R.A.P., and M.S. Hofstad. 1972. Pathogenicity of four serotypes of avian infectious bronchitis virus for the oviduct of young chickens of various ages. Avian Dis 16:351–363.

38. Crinion, R.A.P., R.A. Ball, and M.S. Hofstad. 1971. Abnormalities in laying chickens following exposure to infectious bronchitis virus at one day old. Avian Dis 15:42–48.

39. Csermelyi, M., R. Thijssen, F. Orthel, A.G. Burger, B. Kouwenhoven, and D. Lutticken. 1988. Serological classification of recent infectious bronchitis virus isolates by the neutralization of immunofluorescent foci. Avian Pathol 17:139–148.

40. Cumming, R.B. 1963. Infectious avian nephrosis (uraemia) in Australia. Aust Vet J 39:145–147.

41. Cumming, R.B. 1969. The control of avian infectious bronchitis/nephrosis in Australia. Aust Vet J 45:200–203.

42. Cumming, R.B. 1970. Studies on Australian infectious bronchitis virus. IV. Apparent farm-to-farm airborne transmission of infectious bronchitis virus. Avian Dis 14:191–195.

43. Cunningham, C.H. 1970. Avian infectious bronchitis. Adv Vet Sci Comp Med 14:105–148.

44. Cunningham, C.H., M.P. Spring, and K. Nazerian. 1972. Replication of avian infectious bronchitis virus in African green monkey kidney cell line VERO. J Gen Virol 16:423–427.

45. Darbyshire, J.H. 1978. Organ culture in avian virology: A review. Avian Pathol 7:321–335.

46. Darbyshire, J.H. 1980. Immunity to avian infectious bronchitis virus. In M.E. Rose, L.N. Payne, and B.M. Freeman (eds.), Avian Immunology, pp. 205–226.

British Poultry Science Ltd., Edinburgh.
47. Darbyshire, J.H. 1985. A clearance test to assess protection in chickens vaccinated against avian infectious bronchitis virus. Avian Pathol 14:497–508.
48. Darbyshire, J.H., and R.W. Peters. 1985. Humoral antibody response and assessment of protection following primary vaccination of chicks with maternally derived antibody against avian infectious bronchitis virus. Res Vet Sci 38:14–21.
49. Darbyshire, J.H., J.K.A. Cook, and R.W. Peters. 1975. Comparative growth kinetic studies on avian infectious bronchitis virus in different systems. J Comp Pathol 85:623–630.
50. Darbyshire, J.H., J.G. Rowell, J.K.A. Cook, and R.W. Peters. 1979. Taxonomic studies on strains of avian infectious bronchitis virus using neutralization tests in tracheal organ cultures. Arch Virol 61:227–238.
51. Davelaar, F.G., and B. Kouwenhoven. 1976. Changes in the Harderian gland of the chicken following conjunctival and intranasal infection with infectious bronchitis virus in one- and 20-day old chickens. Avian Pathol 5:39–50.
52. Davelaar, F.G., and B. Kouwenhoven. 1980. Vaccination of 1-day-old broilers against infectious bronchitis by eye drop application or coarse droplet spray and the effect of revaccination by spray. Avian Pathol 9:499–510.
53. Davelaar, F.G., B. Kouwenhoven, and A.G. Burger. 1983. Experience with vaccination against infectious bronchitis in broilers and significance of and vaccination against infectious bronchitis variant viruses in breeders and layers in the Netherlands. Clinica Vet 106:7–11.
54. Davelaar, F.G., B. Kouwenhoven, and A.G. Burger. 1984. Occurrence and significance of infectious bronchitis virus variant strains in egg and broiler production in the Netherlands. Vet Q 6:114–120.
55. Davies, H.A., and M.R. Macnaughton. 1979. Comparison of the morphology of three coronaviruses. Arch Virol 59:25–33.
56. Davies, H.A., R.R. Dourmashkin, and M.R. Macnaughton. 1981. Ribonucleoprotein of avian infectious bronchitis virus. J Gen Virol 53:67–74.
57. Drury, L.N., W.C. Patterson, and C.W. Beard. 1969. Ventilating poultry houses with filtered air under positive pressure to prevent airborne diseases. Poult Sci 48:1640–1646.
58. DuBose, R.T. 1967. Adaptation of the Massachusetts strain of infectious bronchitis virus to turkey embryos. Avian Dis 11:28–38.
59. Eck, J.H.H. van. 1983. Effects of experimental infection of fowl with EDS'76 virus, infectious bronchitis virus, and/or fowl adenovirus on laying performance. Vet Q 5:11–25.
60. Estola, T. 1966. Studies on the infectious bronchitis virus of chickens isolated in Finland with reference to the serological survey of its occurrence. Acta Vet Scand (Suppl) 18:1–111.
61. Estola, T. 1967. Sensitivity of suckling mice to various strains of infectious bronchitis virus. Acta Vet Scand 8:86–87.
62. Geilhausen, H.E., F.B. Ligon, and P.D. Lukert. 1973. The pathogenesis of virulent and avirulent avian infectious bronchitis virus. Arch Gesamte Virusforsch 40:285–290.
63. Gelb, J., Jr., and S.L. Killian. 1987. Serum antibody responses of chickens following sequential inoculations with different infectious bronchitis virus serotypes. Avian Dis 31:513–522.
64. Gelb, J., Jr., P.A. Fries, C.K. Crary, Jr., J.P. Donahoe, and D.E. Roessler. 1987. Sentinel bird approach to isolating infectious bronchitis virus. J Am Vet Med Assoc 190:1628.
65. Gentry, R.F., and M.O. Braune. 1972. Prevention of virus inactivation during drinking water vaccination of poultry. Poult Sci 51:1450–1456.
66. Gillette, K.G. 1973. Plaque formation by infectious bronchitis virus in chicken embryo kidney cell cultures. Avian Dis 17:369–378.
67. Gough, R.E., and D.J. Alexander. 1978. Comparison of serological tests for the measurement of the primary immune response to avian infectious bronchitis virus vaccines. Vet Microbiol 2:289–301.
68. Hanson, L.E., F.H. White, and J.O. Alberts. 1956. Interference between Newcastle disease and infectious bronchitis viruses. Am J Vet Res 17:294–298.
69. Hawkes, R.A., J.H. Darbyshire, R.W. Peters, A.P.A. Mockett, and D. Cavanagh. 1983. Presence of viral antigens and antibody in the trachea of chickens infected with avian infectious bronchitis virus. Avian Pathol 12:331–340.
70. Hitchner, S.B., and P.G. White. 1955. Growth curve studies of chick embryo propagated infectious bronchitis virus. Poult Sci 34:590–594.
71. Hofstad, M.S. 1981. Cross-immunity in chickens using seven isolates of avian infectious bronchitis virus. Avian Dis 25:650–654.
72. Hofstad, M.S. 1984. Avian infectious bronchitis. In M.S. Hofstad, H.J. Barnes, B.W. Calnek, W.M. Reid, and H.W. Yoder, Jr., (eds.), Diseases of Poultry, 8th Ed., pp. 429–443. Iowa State Univ Press, Ames.
73. Hofstad, M.S., and H.W. Yoder, Jr. 1966. Avian infectious bronchitis–virus distribution in tissues of chicks. Avian Dis 10:230–239.
74. Holmes, H.C. 1973. Neutralizing antibody in nasal secretions of chickens following administration of avian infectious bronchitis virus. Arch Gesamte Virusforsch 43:235–241.
75. Hopkins, S.R. 1974. Serological comparisons of strains of infectious bronchitis virus using plaque purified isolants. Avian Dis 18:231–239.
76. Hopkins, S.R., and C.W. Beard. 1985. Studies on methods for determining the efficacy of oil emulsion vaccines against infectious bronchitis virus. J Am Vet Med Assoc 187:305.
77. Hopkins, S.R., and H.W. Yoder, Jr. 1986. Reversion to virulence of chicken passaged infectious bronchitis vaccine virus. Avian Dis 30:221–223.
78. Johnson, R.B., and W.W. Marquardt. 1975. The neutralizing characteristics of strains of infectious bronchitis virus as measured by the constant virus variable serum method in chicken tracheal cultures. Avian Dis 19:82–90.
79. Jones, R.C., and A.G. Ambali. 1987. Re-excretion of an enterotropic infectious bronchitis virus by hens at point of lay after experimental infection at day old. Vet Rec 120:617–620.
80. Jordan, F.T.W., and T.J. Nassar. 1973. The combined influence of age of embryo and temperature and duration of incubation on the replication and yield of avian infectious bronchitis (IB) virus in the developing chick embryo. Avian Pathol 2:279–294.
81. Jungherr, E.L., T.W. Chomiak, and R.E. Luginbuhl. 1956. Immunologic differences in strains of infectious bronchitis. Proc 60th Annu Meet US Livestock Sanit Assoc, pp. 203–209.
82. King, D.J. 1984. Observations on the preparation and stability of infectious bronchitis virus hemagglutination antigen from virus propagated in chicken embryos and chicken kidney cell cultures. Avian Dis 28:504–513.
83. King, D.J. 1988. A comparison of infectious bronchitis virus hemagglutination-inhibition test procedures.

Avian Dis 32:335-341.
84. King, D.J., and S.R. Hopkins. 1983. Evaluation of the hemagglutination inhibition test for measuring the response of chickens to avian infectious bronchitis virus vaccination. Avian Dis 27:100-112.
85. King, D.J., and S.R. Hopkins. 1984. Rapid serotyping of infectious bronchitis virus isolates with the hemagglutination inhibition test. Avian Dis 28:727-733.
86. Kjeldsberg, E. 1984. Demonstration of 7-nm projections on human and avian coronaviruses. Ultrastructural Pathol 7:201-205.
87. Klieve, A.V., and R.B. Cumming. 1988. Immunity and cross-protection to nephritis produced by Australian infectious bronchitis viruses used as vaccines. Avian Pathol 17:829-839.
88. Klieve, A.V., and R.B. Cumming. 1988. Infectious bronchitis: Safety and protection in chickens with maternal antibody. Aust Vet J 65:396-397.
89. Koch, G., L. Hartog, A. Kant, D. Van Roozelaar, and G.F. De Boer. 1986. Antigenic differentiation of avian infectious bronchitis virus variant strains employing monoclonal antibodies. Isr J Vet Med 42:89-97.
90. Kusters, J.G., H.G.M. Niesters, N.M.C. Bleumink-Pluym, F.G. Davelaar, M.C. Horzinek, and B.A.M. van der Zeijst. 1987. Molecular epidemiology of infectious bronchitis virus in the Netherlands. J Gen Virol 68:343-352.
91. Kusters, J.G., H.G.M. Niesters, J.A. Lenstra, W.J.M. Spaan, and B.A.M. van der Zeijst. 1988. Molecular epidemiology of infectious bronchitis virus. In E.F. Kaleta and U. Heffels-Redmann (eds.), Proc 1st Int Symp on Infectious Bronchitis, pp. 166-171. Giessen:Dtsch Veterinarmedizinische Gesellschaft e.V.
92. Li, D., and D. Cavanagh. 1988. Unpublished data.
93. Loomis, L.N., C.H. Cunningham, M.L. Gray, and F. Thorp, Jr. 1950. Pathology of the chicken embryo infected with infectious bronchitis virus. Am J Vet Res 11:245-251.
94. Lukert, P.D. 1965. Comparative sensitivities of embryonating chicken's eggs and primary chicken embryo kidney and liver cell cultures to infectious bronchitis virus. Avian Dis 9:308-316.
95. Lukert, P.D. 1980. Infectious bronchitis. In S.B. Hitchner, C.H. Domermuth, H.G. Purchase, and J.E. Williams (eds.), Isolation and Identification of Avian Pathogens, 2nd Ed., pp. 70-72. Am Assoc Avian Pathol, Kennett Square, PA.
96. Macdonald, J.W., and D.A. McMartin. 1976. Observations on the effects of the H52 and H120 vaccine strains of the infectious bronchitis virus in the domestic fowl. Avian Pathol 5:157-173.
97. Macnaughton, M.R., H.J. Hasony, M.H. Madge, and S.E. Reed. 1981. Antibody to virus components in volunteers experimentally infected with human coronavirus 229E group viruses. Infect Immun 31:845-849.
98. Marquardt, W.W., D.B. Snyder, and B.A. Schlotthober. 1981. Detection and quantification of antibodies to infectious bronchitis virus by enzyme-linked immunosorbent assay. Avian Dis 25:713-722.
99. Mathews, J., and M.S. Hofstad. 1953. The inactivation of certain animal viruses by ethylene oxide (carboxide). Cornell Vet 43:452-461.
100. McIntosh, K. 1974. Coronaviruses: A comparative review. Curr Top Microbiol Immunol 63:85-129.
101. Meulemans, G., M.C. Carlier, M. Gonze, P. Petit, and M. Vandenbroeck. 1987. Incidence, characterization, and prophylaxis of nephropathogenic avian infectious bronchitis viruses. Vet Rec 120:205-206.
102. Miller, L., and V.J. Yates. 1968. Neutralization of infectious bronchitis virus by human sera. Am J Epidemiol 88:406-409.
103. Mockett, A.P.A., D. Cavanagh, and T.D.K. Brown. 1984. Monoclonal antibodies to the S1 spike and membrane proteins of avian infectious bronchitis coronavirus strain Massachusetts M41. J Gen Virol 65:2281-2286.
104. Mockett, A.P.A., J.K.A. Cook, and M.B. Huggins. 1987. Maternally-derived antibody to infectious bronchitis virus: Its detection in chick trachea and serum and its role in protection. Avian Pathol 16:407-416.
105. Otsuki, K., and M. Tsubokura. 1981. Plaque formation by avian infectious bronchitis virus in primary chick embryo fibroblast cells in the presence of trypsin. Arch Virol 70:315-320.
106. Otsuki, K., H. Yamamoto, and M. Tsubokura. 1979. Studies on avian infectious bronchitis virus (IBV). 1. Resistance of IBV to chemical and physical treatments. Arch Virol 60:25-32.
107. Otsuki, K., K. Noro, H. Yamamoto, and M. Tsubokura. 1979. Studies on avian infectious bronchitis virus (IBV). 2. Propagation of IBV in several cultured cells. Arch Virol 60:115-122.
108. Otsuki, K., T. Nakamura, Y. Kawaoka, and M. Tsubokura. 1988. Interferon induction by several strains of avian infectious bronchitis virus, a coronavirus, in chickens. Acta Virol 32:55-59.
109. Powell, P.C. 1987. Immune mechanisms in infections of poultry. Vet Immunol Immunopathol 15:87-113.
110. Ratanasethakul, C., and R.B. Cumming. 1983. The effect of route of infection and strain of virus on the pathology of Australian infectious bronchitis. Aust Vet J 60:209-213.
111. Ratanasethakul, C., and R.B. Cumming. 1983. Immune response of chickens to various routes of administration of Australian infectious bronchitis vaccine. Aust Vet J 60:214-216.
112. Riddell, C. 1987. Avian Histopathology. Am Assoc Avian Pathol, Kennett Square, PA.
113. Satylganov, T.T. 1971. Survival of avian infectious bronchitis virus on artificially contaminated surfaces, in water and in air. Trudy Vsesoyuznogo Institut Veterinarnoi Sanitarii 38:27-34.
114. Schalk, A.F., and M.C. Hawn. 1931. An apparently new respiratory disease of baby chicks. J Am Vet Med Assoc 78:413-422.
115. Siddell, S., H. Wege, and V. ter Meulen. 1982. The structure and replication of coronaviruses. Curr Top Microbiol Immunol 99:131-163.
116. Siddell, S.G., R. Anderson, D. Cavanagh, K. Fujiwara, H.D. Klenk, M.R. Macnaughton, M. Pensaert, S.A. Stohlman, L. Sturman, and B.A.M. van der Zeijst. 1983. Coronaviridae. Intervirology 20:181-189.
117. Siddell, S., H. Wege, and V. ter Meulen. 1983. The biology of coronaviruses. J Gen Virol 64:761-776.
118. Siller, W.G. 1981. Renal pathology of the fowl—a review. Avian Pathol 10:187-262.
119. Smith, H.W, J.K.A. Cook, and Z.E. Parsell. 1985. The experimental infection of chickens with mixtures of infectious bronchitis virus and Escherichia coli. J Gen Virol 66:777-786.
120. Spaan, W., D. Cavanagh, and M.C. Horzinek. 1988. Coronaviruses: Structure and genome expression. J Gen Virol 69:2939-2952.
121. Spackman, D., and I.R.D. Cameron. 1983. Isolation of infectious bronchitis virus from pheasants. Vet Rec 113:354-355.
122. Stern, D.F., and B.M. Sefton. 1982. Coronavirus proteins: Biogenesis of avian infectious bronchitis virus virion proteins. J Virol 44:794-803.

123. Stone, H.D., M. Brugh, S.R. Hopkins, H.W. Yoder, and C.W. Beard. 1978. Preparation of inactivated oil-emulsion vaccines with avian viral or mycoplasma antigens. Avian Dis 22:666–674.
124. Sturman, L.S., and K.V. Holmes. 1983. The molecular biology of coronaviruses. Adv Virus Res 28:35–112.
125. Thornton, D.H., and J.C. Muskett. 1975. Effect of infectious bronchitis vaccination on the performance of live Newcastle disease vaccine. Vet Rec 96:467–468.
126. Timms, L.M., and C.D. Bracewell. 1981. Cell mediated and humoral immune response of chickens to live infectious bronchitis vaccines. Res Vet Sci 31:182–189.
127. Timms, L.M., and C.D. Bracewell. 1983. Cell mediated and humoral immune response of chickens to inactivated oil-emulsion infectious bronchitis vaccine. Res Vet Sci 34:224–230.
128. Tomley, F.M., A.P.A. Mockett, M.E.G. Boursnell, M.M. Binns, J.K.A. Cook, T.D.K. Brown, and G.L. Smith. 1987. Expression of the infectious bronchitis virus spike protein by recombinant vaccinia virus and induction of neutralizing antibodies in vaccinated mice. J Gen Virol 68:2291–2298.
129. Toro, H., B. Schemera, and E.F. Kaleta. 1987. Serological differentiation of avian infectious bronchitis field isolates using an enzyme immunoassay: Presence of Dutch strains in West Germany. Avian Dis 31:187–192.
130. Van Roekel, H., M.K. Clarke, K.L. Bullis, O.M. Olesiuk, and F.G. Sperling. 1951. Infectious bronchitis. Am J Vet Res 12:140–146.
131. Wadey, C.N., and J.T. Faragher. 1981. Australian infectious bronchitis viruses: Plaque formation and assay methods. Res Vet Sci 30:66–69.
132. Wadey, C.N., and J.T. Faragher. 1981. Australian infectious bronchitis viruses: Identification of nine subtypes by a neutralization test. Res Vet Sci 30:70–74.
133. Wakenell, P.S., and J.M. Sharma. 1986. Chicken embryonal vaccination with avian infectious bronchitis virus. Am J Vet Res 47:933–938.
134. Wege, H., St. Siddell, and V. ter Meulen. 1982. The biology and pathogenesis of coronaviruses. Curr Top Microbiol Immunol 99:165–200.
135. Winterfield, R.W., and S.B. Hitchner. 1962. Etiology of an infectious nephritis-nephrosis syndrome of chickens. Am J Vet Res 23:1273–1279.
136. Winterfield, R.W., A.M. Fadly, and A.A. Bickford. 1972. The immune response to infectious bronchitis virus determined by respiratory signs, virus infection, and histopathological lesions. Avian Dis 16:260–269.

18 LARYNGOTRACHEITIS

Lyle E. Hanson and Trevor J. Bagust

INTRODUCTION. Laryngotracheitis (LT) is an acute disease of chickens characterized by signs of respiratory depression, gasping, and expectoration of bloody exudate. Affected cells of the tracheal mucous membrane become swollen and edematous, resulting in erosion and hemorrhages. Intranuclear inclusions are present in early stages. LT is responsible for egg production losses and mortality.

HISTORY. The disease was first described in 1925 (84), but some reports indicate it may have existed earlier (7, 50). It has been identified as laryngotracheitis, infectious laryngotracheitis, and avian diphtheria. Some early investigators also referred to the disease as infectious bronchitis. The term laryngotracheitis was used as early as 1930 (8, 46) and the name infectious laryngotracheitis was adopted in 1931 by the Special Committee on Poultry Diseases of the American Veterinary Medical Association. The cause of LT was first shown to be a filterable virus by Beaudette (10).

INCIDENCE AND DISTRIBUTION. LT has been identified in most countries. It is a serious disease of chickens in areas of large concentrations of poultry in the USA, Europe, and Australia.

ETIOLOGY

Classification. LT virus (LTV) has all the characteristics of the herpes group. It is cuboidal, enveloped, ether-sensitive, and contains a core composed of DNA. LTV is classified as a member of the family Alphaherpesviridae with the virological nomenclature of Gallid herpesvirus 1 (103).

Morphology. Electron micrographs of LT-infected chicken embryo cell cultures contain icosahedral viral particles similar to the structure of herpes simplex virus. Watrach et al. (120) described the hexagonal virions to be 80–100 nm in diameter. The capsids have icosahedral symmetry and are composed of 162 elongated hollow capsomeres (Fig. 18.1) (33, 120). The complete virus particle, which has an irregular envelope surrounding the nucleocapsid, has a diameter of 195–250 nm. The surface of the envelope contains fine projections on the delimiting membrane.

Chemical Composition. The nucleic acid core of LTV is DNA, with a buoyant density of 1.704 g/ml, which is consistent with DNA values of some of the other herpesviruses (93). The molecular weight of LTV DNA is approximately 100×10^6, with the genome having two isomeric forms (79, 82). LTV DNA has been reported to have a guanine plus cytosine percentage of 45% (93), which is lower than that for many other animal herpesviruses. Four major envelope glycoproteins, of molecular weights 205, 115, 90, and 60 kD, respectively, and located both on the virus and on the surface of virus-infected cells, have been described by York et al. (127) and are considered to be the major immunogens of LTV.

Virus Replication. Replication of LTV appears to be similar to that of herpes simplex and pseudorabies viruses. Virus is adsorbed on the surface of the cell, and viral entry into the cell apparently occurs by pinocytosis. Rate of adsorption varies with volume of inoculum and cell system. Holmes and Watson (58) observed that enveloped particles of herpes simplex virus were more readily adsorbed than naked nucleocapsids.

The envelope and capsid are disrupted by host enzymes releasing DNA that migrates to the cell nucleus. The first evidence of new LTV components is observed in the nucleus in approximately 10–12 hr (99).

Completed nucleocapsids migrate through the nuclear membrane of the cell; the latter forms the envelope. Enveloped virus particles accumulate in a vacuolar membrane in the cytoplasm. Vacuoles containing viral particles migrate to the plasma membrane and release the virus at the surface through disruption of the cell wall (89). In the natural host, the greatest concentration of LTV occurs in the trachea (25).

Resistance to Chemical and Physical Agents. LTV particles are sensitive to lipolytic agents, heat, and various disinfectants. Fitzgerald and Hanson (40) reported LTV became noninfective after exposure to ether for 24 hr. Although

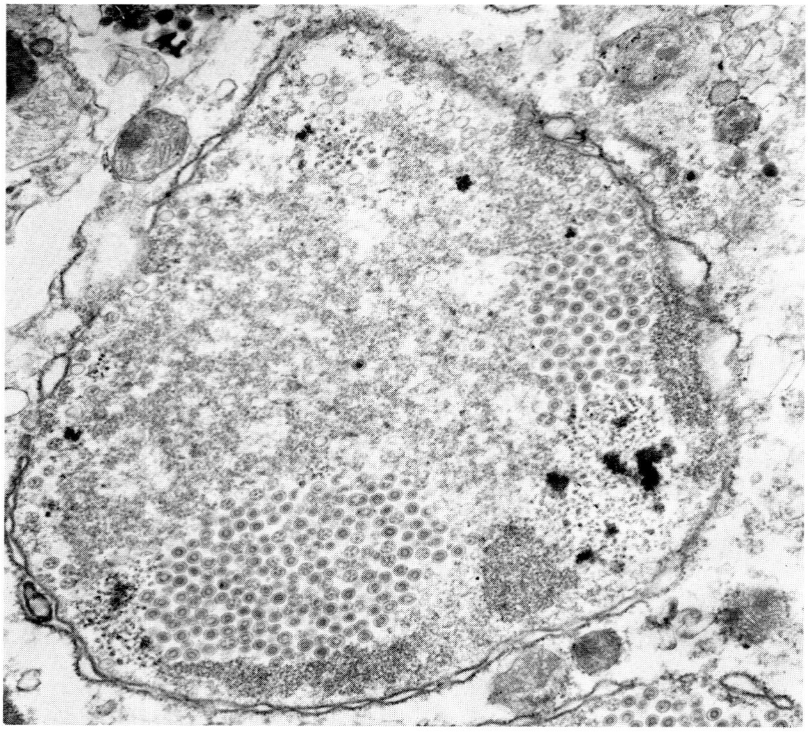

18.1. Electron micrograph of LTV. Aggregates of virus particles forming an inclusion body in nucleus of cultured chicken embryo kidney cell. Notice peripheral accumulations of chromatin and centrally located amorphous material; the latter forms part of the inclusion body. ×18,500. (Watrach)

LTV survived for extended periods when lyophilized or held at −20 to −60 C (45, 121), it was destroyed in 10–15 min at 55 C (108) and in 48 hr when held in broth at 38 C (15). However, Meulemans and Halen (86) reported some isolates were more resistant, since 1% of one strain was still viable after 60 min at 56 C. Virus in tracheal tissue of a chicken carcass was destroyed in 44 hr at 37 C or in the chorioallantoic membrane (CAM) in 5 hr at 25 C (30). On the other hand, Schalm and Beach (108) found that LTV associated with tracheas of chicken carcasses survived for 10 days at temperatures of 13–23 C. A solution of 3% cresol or 1% lye will inactivate LTV in less than 1 min.

Strain Classification. The many LTV strains of varying virulence that have been isolated throughout the world appear to be broadly antigenically homogeneous, based on virus-neutralization (VN) or immunofluorescence tests using reference-specific antiserum. Some strains, however, have been neutralized poorly by such antisera (23, 94, 95), and the question of minor antigenic variation among strains of LTV has also been suggested by other workers (105, 113).

Discrimination of LTV strains of varying pathogenicity, and particularly of field strains from vaccine strains, is a major practical problem. Currently, a biological system for assessment of mortality index in chicken embryos has been proposed (64). Alternatively, analysis of the DNA patterns with restriction endonucleases has been used with some success. Kotiw et al. (79) were able to identify an Australian vaccine strain by this method, and Leib et al. (81) were able to detect differences between American and European LTV strains and between an American field strain and a vaccine strain.

The use of cloned DNA fragments in reciprocal DNA:DNA hybridization also appears promising for differentiating LTV strains (80), but further testing of methodology for strain discrimination is required.

Laboratory Host Systems. LTV can be propagated in the embryonating chicken egg. It causes formation of opaque plaques on the CAM resulting from proliferative and necrotic lesions (Fig. 18.2). The plaques, which have opaque edges with depressed central areas of necrosis, are ob-

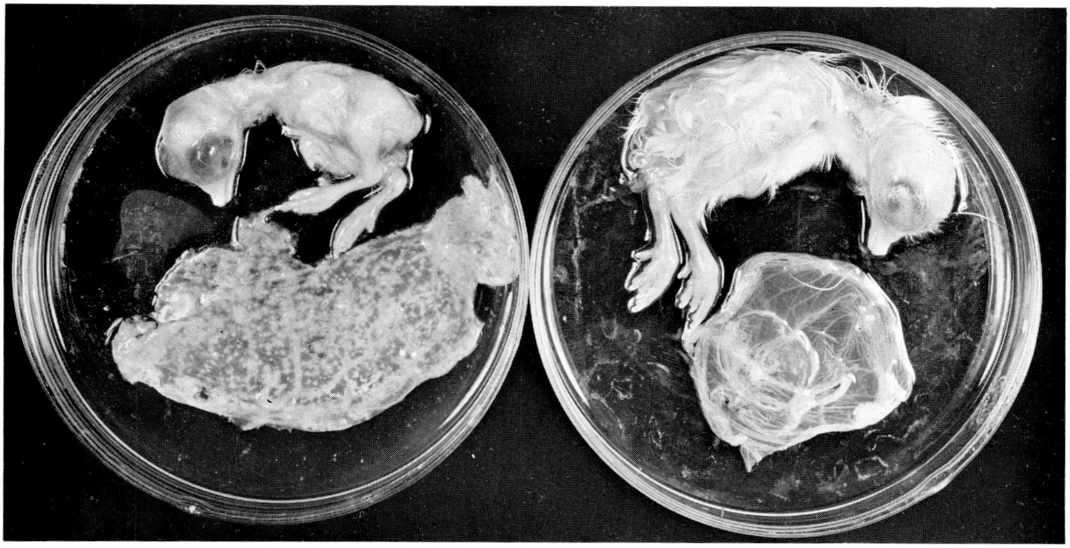

18.2. Chicken embryos at 14 days of age. Normal embryo and chorioallantoic membrane (CAM) (*right*). LTV-infected embryo is stunted, and CAM has numerous foci of proliferation (*left*).

served as early as 48 hr postinoculation (PI) and often extend linearly with increase in numbers and size. Embryo deaths occur in 2–12 days PI. Survival time of infected embryos decreases with additional egg passages (16, 18, 22).

LTV propagates in chicken embryonic liver (CEL), chicken embryo kidney (CEK), and chicken kidney (CK) cultures (3, 28, 85, 104). Recently, Hughes and Jones (60) reexamined the relative efficiency of several culture systems and CAM inoculation for LTV isolation and propagation. CEL and CK were found to be the preferred culture systems with CEK and chicken embryonic lung cultures and CAM being somewhat less sensitive. Chicken embryonic fibroblast cultures were contraindicated.

The first viral cytopathology in cell cultures, which can be observed as early as 4–6 hr PI with a high multiplicity of infection, are increased refractiveness and swelling of cells, chromatin displacement, and rounding of the nucleoli. Cytoplasmic fusion results in formation of multinucleated cells. Intranuclear inclusion bodies can be detected as early as 12 hr, with the highest concentration occurring 30–36 hr after inoculation (Fig. 18.3). Large cytoplasmic vesicles develop in the multinucleated cells and become more basophilic as cells degenerate (99).

LTV may also be grown in cultures of cells from the avian immune system. Chang et al. (26) first reported on the susceptibility of chicken buffy coat (leukocyte) cultures in vitro, while Bülow and Klasen (21) observed LTV growth in macrophages cultured from bone marrow and spleen.

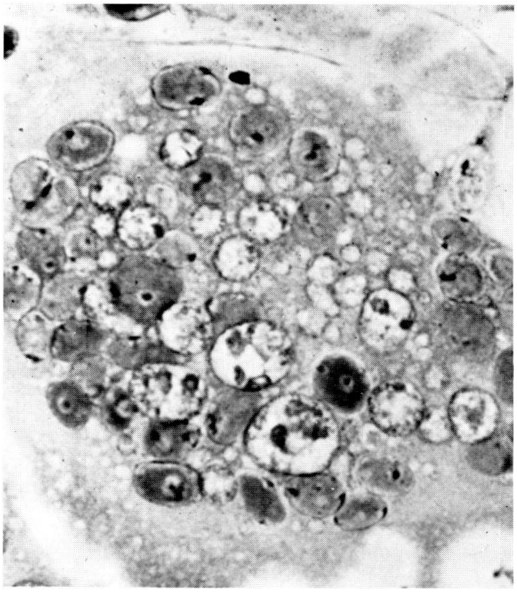

18.3. Chicken embryo kidney cell monolayer 72 hr after inoculation with LTV. Large giant cell with numerous nuclei containing inclusion bodies. May-Grünwald-Giemsa. ×320.

Calnek et al. (24) have subsequently confirmed and extended these earlier findings, determining that while macrophage cultures are as susceptible as CK cultures to infection, replication of most LTV strains tested was subsequently restricted to a variable extent depending on the genotype of both cells and the virus. Other cell types such as lymphocytes, thymocytes, buffy coat leukocytes, and activated T cells proved nearly or totally refractory to LTV infection.

PATHOGENESIS AND EPIZOOTIOLOGY

Natural and Experimental Hosts. The chicken is the primary natural host affected by LTV. Although the disease affects all ages, the most characteristic signs are observed in adult birds. Viral multiplication is limited to respiratory tissues, with little or no evidence of viremia normally occurring (5, 57).

Several workers described a form of LT in pheasants and pheasant-chicken crosses (32, 59, 76). Winterfield and So (123) were able to induce lesions in the upper respiratory tract of young turkeys. They also reported an isolation of LTV from the trachea of a peafowl. Previous failures to infect turkeys (17, 110) apparently indicated a definite age resistance. Starlings, sparrows, crows, doves, ducks, pigeons, and guinea fowl appeared to be refractory to LTV (9, 19, 110), although experimental infection of ducks producing subclinical disease and seroconversion, has been reported (124). Embryonated eggs of turkeys and chickens are susceptible to LTV, as are those of ducks to a lesser degree (71, 124), whereas eggs of guinea fowl and pigeons are not susceptible.

Transmission. Natural portals of entry of LTV are through the upper respiratory and ocular routes (10, 11). Ingestion can also be a mode of infection, although it may be that exposure of nasal epithelium following ingestion is required with this route (102). Transmission occurs more readily from acutely infected birds than through contact with clinically recovered carrier birds.

LTV infection of the upper respiratory tract of susceptible chickens is followed by intense viral replication. Several studies independently confirmed that infectious LTV is usually present in tracheal tissues and secretions for only 6–8 days PI (5, 57, 96, 102); no clear evidence exists for a viremic phase during or after this period. Extratracheal spread of LTV to the trigeminal ganglion 4–7 days after tracheal infection was detected (5) in 40% of chickens exposed to a virulent Australian LT strain. Reactivation of latent LTV from the trigeminal ganglion 15 mo after vaccination in a flock has since been reported from Germany (73). Hughes et al. (62) reported the reexcretion of LT virus from latently infected chicks following the stress of rehousing and the onset of reproduction.

Clinically inapparent LTV infection of the respiratory tract is a major feature of LT persistence. Pioneering observations by Komarov and Beaudette (78) and Gibbs (43), who collected laryngeal and tracheal swabs and inoculated susceptible chickens, indicated a "field" carrier rate of approximately 2% for periods up to 16 mo after a disease outbreak. In more recent studies with tracheal organ cultures explanted from chickens experimentally infected with Australian wild and vaccine LTV strains, latent tracheal infections were demonstrated for similar periods in 50% or more of infected chickens (4, 116). Repeated tracheal swabbing of small groups of chickens experimentally infected with a mildly pathogenic UK strain of LTV by Hughes et al. (61) detected intermittent and apparently spontaneous shedding of LTV between 7 and 20 wk after infection. Treatment with immunosuppressive drugs (e.g., cyclophosphamide, dexamethasone) has not yet proved successful in reactivation of latent LTV (4, 61).

Mechanical transmission can occur by use of contaminated equipment and litter (11, 37, 44, 77).

Egg transmission of virus contained in the interior or on the exterior of the egg has not been demonstrated. LTV-infected embryos die before hatching. LTV is inactivated in less than 24 hr at 37 C (71).

Incubation Period, Morbidity, and Mortality. Signs usually appear in 6–12 days following natural exposure (75, 109). Intratracheal exposure results in a shorter incubation period of 2–4 days (12, 69, 109).

The epizootic form of the disease, which spreads rapidly in susceptible chickens, affects up to 90–100% of the birds within the flock. Mortality varies from 5 to 70% (average 10–20%) (7, 51, 109). In the benign forms of the disease seen in more recent years in the USA, Australia, and the UK (34, 35), morbidity can be low or variable and mortalities very low (0.1–2%).

Signs. Characteristic signs of an acute infection are nasal discharge and moist rales followed by coughing and gasping (Fig. 18.4) (7, 76). Marked dyspnea and expectoration of blood-stained mucus is characteristic of severe forms of the disease (7, 50, 51, 68, 109).

Mild enzootic forms have been described by workers in Great Britain, Australia, the USA, and New Zealand (30, 95, 109, 121). In mild forms, signs are unthriftiness, reduction in egg production, watery eyes, conjunctivitis, swelling of infraorbital sinuses, persistent nasal discharge, and hemorrhagic conjunctivitis. Morbidity may be as low as 5% (98).

The course of the disease varies with severity of the lesions. Generally, most chickens recover in 10–14 days, but extremes of 1–4 wk have been reported (7, 51).

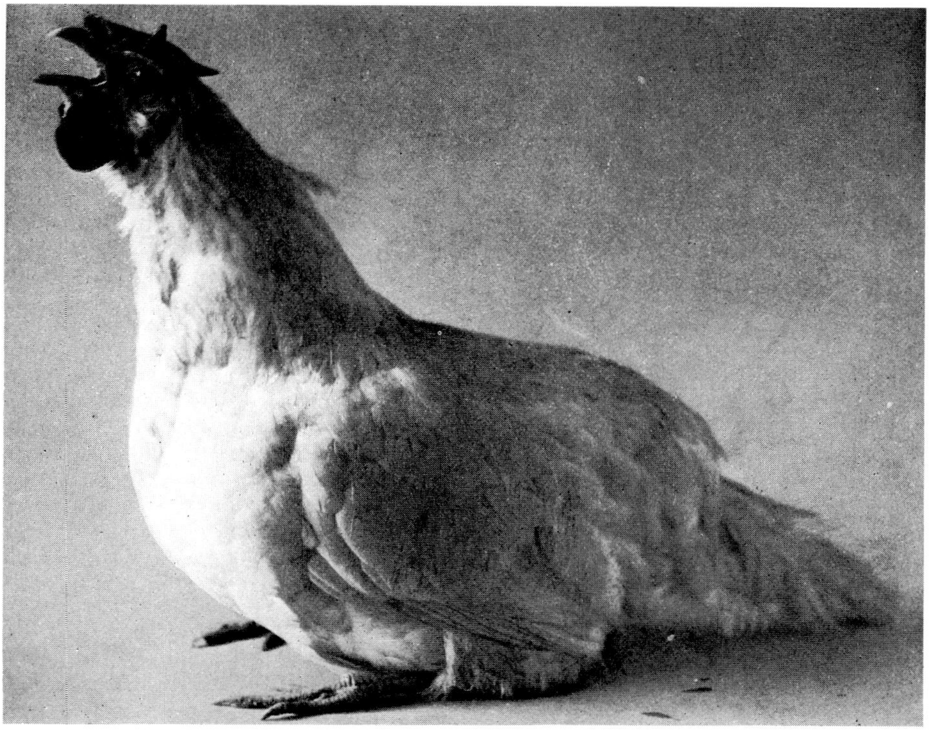

18.4. Chicken with LT, showing attitude during inspiration.

Gross Lesions. Lesions occur most consistently in tracheal and laryngeal tissues. Tissue changes vary from mucoid inflammation early in the disease to degeneration of the mucosa, resulting in necrosis and hemorrhages in later stages. Expulsion of desquamated epithelial tissue and blood clots may occur during violent coughing and convulsive respirations. Extension of inflammation down the bronchi into lungs and air sacs can occur. Edema and congestion of the epithelium of the conjunctiva and infraorbital sinuses may be the only lesion observed in some less pathogenic infections.

Histopathology. Microscopic changes vary with the stage of the disease. Electron microscopic studies indicate the first cellular change occurs in the nucleus of mucosal cells during formation of viral capsids. Following migration of virus through the nuclear membrane into the cytoplasm, the completely enveloped particles aggregate into large masses contained in a vacuolar structure. Large masses of viral particles in the cytoplasm result in the cloudy swelling observed in light microscopic studies of early cellular changes (99, 119).

As cellular changes progress, cells enlarge, lose cilia, and become edematous. Lymphocytes, histocytes, and plasma cells migrate into the mucosa and submucosa after 2–3 days. Later cellular destruction causes separation of the mucosa and submucosa, and hemorrhage ensues. As the disease progresses, cellular infiltration becomes more marked. Cellular infiltration and mucosal degeneration is most extensive in the trachea and larynx (47, 111).

Intranuclear inclusion bodies occur in epithelial cells as early as 12 hr PI. Cover and Benton (30) reported that the fixative is important in demonstration of inclusions (Fig. 18.5).

Immunity. Resistance of susceptible chicks to LTV is altered following natural infections or by vaccination. The apparent duration of resistance induced from a natural infection might appear to be a year or more, but this extended period of immunity could be the result of subclinical infection occurring within the flock from endemic carrier birds or from other sources.

Immunity induced by vaccination has been found to be of variable duration when vaccinated birds have been experimentally challenged by the infraorbital sinus or tracheal routes. Waning of LT immunity has been detected as early as 8–15 wk postvaccination (55), but generally substantial flock immunity has been observed for approxi-

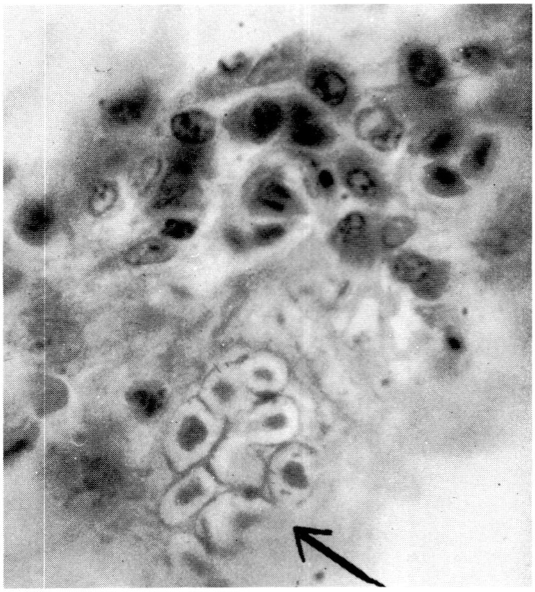

18.5. Tracheal mucosa from chick killed on 5th day following intratracheal inoculation. Group of nuclei containing inclusion bodies characteristic of LTV infection (*arrow*). ×1200.

mately 15–20 wk after vaccination (2, 42, 91). Although vaccine breaks in the field are most frequently observed after 15–20 wk postvaccination, the value of revaccination is questionable (72).

LTV infection readily induces the production of antibodies that can neutralize virus (23). These are detectable in the serum by 7 days after infection and peak around 21 days (56), coinciding with LTV-neutralizing activity appearing in tracheal washings (5). These humoral immune responses, although associated with infection, are not the primary mechanism of protection to LTV infection, and a poor correlation has generally been found between serum antibody titers and the immune status of flocks (72). Cell-mediated responses are the major mediators of LT resistance. Hence bursectomized, cyclophosphamide-treated chickens, which cannot mount humoral immune responses, can develop full immunity following LT vaccination (38, 100). Fahey et al. (39) demonstrated that LT resistance may be adoptively transferred in inbred chickens by transfer of immune spleen cells.

While maternal antibody to LTV is transmitted to offspring via the egg (13), the antibody does not confer protection to infection or interfere with vaccination in chickens (38, 114). Chickens less than 2 wk of age do not respond as well to vaccination as do older birds (2, 31, 42), although chickens can be successfully vaccinated as early as 1 day old (115).

Onset of immunity in chickens older than 2 wk is rapid, with partial protection occurring within 3–4 days and complete by 6–8 days after vaccination or field exposure to LTV (12, 41, 53).

Sinkovic (114) and Fahey et al. (38) found that susceptibility to LTV infection, and mortality resulting from infection, both decrease with age and are higher in males than females in meat-type chickens. They also reported that high environmental temperatures (35 C) cause higher mortality from LTV infection in heavy than in light adult breeds.

In his major review of immunity to LT, Jordan (72) stressed that valid comparisons of experimental studies require knowledge of the virulence of LTV strains used, the dose, the route of infection, and the age of the host.

DIAGNOSIS. LT cannot be reliably diagnosed by observation of signs and lesions. Although some acute signs of the disease are characteristic, many signs are similar to those of other respiratory diseases of poultry.

The acute disease, with typical coughing, expulsion of blood, and high mortality, can be readily identified as LT (36, 118). With all other forms, laboratory confirmation should be obtained prior to use of control procedures. Virus can be isolated from tracheal and lung tissue after chicken embryo inoculation, inoculation of trachea and infraorbital sinuses of susceptible chickens (54), and cell culture inoculation (27).

Demonstration of intranuclear inclusion bodies in tracheal or conjunctival tissues stained with Giemsa stain is also diagnostic of LTV (14, 30). Inclusion bodies can be consistently demonstrated in birds only in early stages (1–5 days) of the disease, as necrosis and desquamation destroy affected epithelial tissue. Use of a low-pH fixative is important in demonstration of inclusion bodies (30). The reliability of this procedure, as shown by Keller and Hebel (74), indicated that inclusion bodies could be observed in 57% of 60 specimens, while virus was isolated from 72% of the same specimens.

With a rapid diagnostic method developed by Pirozok et al. (92), tissues are embedded in Carbowax, sectioned and stained, and available for examination in 3 hr. Sevoian (112) developed a rapid procedure for identification of inclusion bodies in tissue by a simultaneous fixation and dehydration procedure.

Rapid identification of virus in tracheal tissue can be made with use of a fluorescent antibody (FA) test (20). Wilks and Kogan (122) were able to detect LTV in tracheal tissue from day 2 to day 14 PI using fluorescein-labeled anti-LTV globulins, although shorter periods (6–8 days PI) for successful detection of LT antigen in tracheal sections by FA test have been reported (5, 57).

Intratracheal inoculation of susceptible and immune chicks with tracheal exudate or tissue suspension from recently affected birds can provide a reliable diagnostic procedure (95). Rapid diagnosis may be made by direct electron microscopic examination of tracheal scrapings and recognition of herpesvirus particles (85, 117). Recently, an enzyme-linked immunosorbent assay (ELISA) using monoclonal antibodies was developed for rapid detection of LTV antigen in tracheal exudate. This system is reported to be as accurate but faster than virus isolation and more accurate than either the FA or gel precipitation tests (117) for detecting LTV antigen in tracheas.

For successful isolation of LTV from suspected clinical samples, it is imperative to obtain fresh material, i.e., within 6 days of infection (see Pathogenesis). Also, this material should be promptly transported to the laboratory on wet ice whenever possible.

Isolation of LTV is achieved by inoculation of suspensions of tracheal exudate, tracheal tissue, or lung tissue onto the CAM of 9- to 12-day-old embryonated eggs or into susceptible cell cultures (see Laboratory Host Systems). The CAM route, the most sensitive method of egg inoculation for LTV, results in titers 2 $\log_{10}$ or more higher than detected with other routes (54, 70). Of the cell cultures, chicken embryo liver cells and chicken kidney cells (60) are the laboratory systems of choice for the isolation of LTV. Two passages in such cultures are the maximum required for detection of LTV (4, 60).

Serology. VN has been used to demonstrate presence or absence of LT antibodies. Burnet (23) observed that VN could be measured by using the CAM pock-counting technique. VN antibodies are now usually detected by assay in cell culture using monolayers seeded in tubes, petri dishes, or microplates (28, 101, 104). More recently, various ELISA systems for the detection and assay of LTV antibody have been developed (87, 90, 125, 126). Direct comparison of the four serological tests most widely used for detection of antibody to LTV (1) indicates that ELISA, VN, and indirect FA tests are all valid systems for quantifying antibody levels, while ELISA is preferred for survey purposes. The agar-gel immunodiffusion test system used by these authors was less sensitive than ELISA, VN, and IFA but is still considered useful for detection of antibodies on a flock basis.

TREATMENT. No drug has been effective in reducing the severity of lesions or relieving disease signs. If a diagnosis of LT is obtained early in an outbreak, vaccination of the unaffected birds may induce adequate protection before they become infected.

PREVENTION AND CONTROL

Management Procedures. Since LTV infections often result in some carrier birds, it is extremely important to avoid mixing vaccinated or recovered chickens with susceptible ones. Special precautions should be taken to obtain a complete history when mixing breeding stock. Use of sound sanitation procedures will avoid exposing susceptible chickens via contaminated equipment or buildings.

The importance of site quarantine and hygiene in preventing the movement of (potentially contaminated) staff, service workers, other personnel, feed, equipment, and birds is central to successful prevention/control of LT. Rodent and dog control measures should also be in place (77). The persistent LT disease threat posed to commercial poultry operations by backyard and exhibition poultry flocks (83, 85) should be recognized and guarded against.

Cooperative control of LT outbreaks by collaboration between government and industry is most desirable. Correctly implemented (83), this approach may obviate the need for widespread use of LT vaccine. Where outbreaks have been contained, recovered flocks should be moved off-site under quarantine for processing as soon as is prudent. Experience with LT outbreaks in Pennsylvania (35) indicates that this interval can be as short as 2 wk after the last clinical signs of LT are observed on a site.

Immunization. Vaccination has provided a satisfactory method of developing resistance in susceptible chicken populations (see Immunity). Since vaccination can result in carrier birds, it is recommended for use only in geographic areas where the disease is endemic. The appropriate regulatory agency should be contacted to determine the approved vaccines and vaccine application procedures.

LTVs attenuated by passage in cell cultures (41, 66, 67) or embryonated eggs (106), or by feather follicle passage in chickens (63, 88), and selected mild enzootic strains (95) are capable of inducing acceptable protection in susceptible chickens. Availability of attenuated LT vaccines precludes use of virulent strains in most areas. Virulent strains of LT vaccines should be administered with caution, since carrier birds occur in most flocks where such vaccines are used.

Immunization of chickens was first accomplished by deliberate exposure through introduction of infected birds into susceptible flocks. Later, Brandly and Bushnell (19) recommended vaccination using unattenuated virus administered via the cloacal route, as it provided a more consistent immunity. Since then, effective vaccination of chickens has been accomplished by application of attenuated LT vaccine virus via infraorbital sinuses (113), intranasal instillation (12), feather follicle inoculation (88), eye-drop (115), and the oral administration through drinking water (48, 49, 107, 114). Robertson and Egerton (102) subsequently demonstrated that successful vaccination via the drinking water depends upon LTV contacting the epithelium of the nasal cavity during drinking.

While vaccine application by spray is highly desirable as a means of rapid mass application, if fine aerosols are generated there is the danger that they may penetrate deeply into the respiratory system. LT vaccine strains that are sufficiently mild and yet protective urgently need to be developed and licensed specifically for spray applications. The spray application of LT vaccine strains developed for use by other routes and in older chickens can result in unacceptable levels of adverse vaccine reaction and mortality in young chicks (29).

Careful attention must be given to procedures of vaccine administration with each technique to ensure adequate immunization. Although oral vaccination through drinking water provides the simplest method, it is the most susceptible to errors. Care must be taken to ensure that an adequate concentration of virus is maintained to provide effective vaccination of susceptible chickens (52).

Raggi and Lee (97) concluded that LT vaccine must contain more than 10^2 embryo plaque-forming units/ml to be capable of inducing satisfactory immunity when administered by other than the oral route. Hitchner (52) reported a virus concentration in the vaccine of 10^5 embryo infective dose-50% (EID_{50}) was necessary for satisfactory oral vaccination.

Great care must be taken in following the vaccine manufacturer's instructions for storage, diluting, resuspension, and application so as to ensure that an adequate dosage of infectious virus is delivered to each chick.

Caution may also be required when other live vaccines are administered at, or near, the same time as LTV. Studies in Japan indicated that while infectious bronchitis and LT vaccine could safely be administered together by eye-drop, Newcastle disease vaccine in chickens 5 wk old or younger markedly suppressed responses to LT vaccine if administered within 8 days of LT vaccination (65).

Although inactivated LT vaccines have been described (38, 6), they are still largely experimental. If developed and efficacious, however, inactivated vaccine could have potential for control of LT on sites that are persistently affected.

REFERENCES

1. Adair, B.M., D. Todd, E.R. McKillop, and K. Burns. 1985. Comparison of serological tests for detection of antibodies to infectious laryngotracheitis virus. Avian Pathol 14:461–469.

2. Alls, A.A., J.R. Ipson, and W.R. Vaughan. 1969. Studies on an ocular infectious laryngotracheitis vaccine. Avian Dis 13:36–45.

3. Atherton, J.G., and W. Anderson. 1957. Propagation in tissue culture of the virus of infectious laryngotracheitis of fowls. Aust J Exp Biol 35:335–346.

4. Bagust, T.J. 1986. Laryngotracheitis (Gallid-1) herpesvirus infection in the chicken. 4. Latency establishment by wild and vaccine strains of ILT virus. Avian Pathol 15:581–595.

5. Bagust, T.J., B.W. Calnek, and K.J. Fahey. 1986. Gallid-1 herpesvirus infection in the chicken. 3. Reinvestigation of the pathogenesis of infectious laryngotracheitis in acute and early post-acute respiratory disease. Avian Dis 30:179–190.

6. Barhoom, S., A. Forgacs, and F. Solyom. 1986. Development of an inactivated vaccine against infectious laryngotracheitis (ILT)–serological and protection studies. Avian Pathol 15:213–221.

7. Beach, J.R. 1926. Infectious bronchitis of fowls. J Am Vet Med Assoc 68:570–580.

8. Beach, J.R. 1930. The virus of laryngotracheitis of fowls. Science 72:633–634.

9. Beach, J.R. 1931. A filterable virus, the cause of infectious laryngotracheitis of chickens. J Exp Med 54:809–816.

10. Beaudette, F.R. 1930. Infectious bronchitis. New Jersey Agr Exp Stn Annu Rep 51:286.

11. Beaudette, F.R. 1937. Infectious laryngotracheitis. Poult Sci 16:103–105.

12. Benton, W.J., M.S. Cover, and L.M. Greene. 1958. The clinical and serological response of chickens to certain laryngotracheitis viruses. Avian Dis 2:383–396.

13. Benton, W.J., M.S. Cover, and W.C. Krauss. 1960. Studies on parental immunity to infectious laryngotracheitis of chickens. Avian Dis 4:491–499.

14. Beveridge, W.I.B., and F.M. Burnet. 1946. Med Res Council Spec Rep Ser London 256.

15. Brandly, C.A. 1934. Some studies on infectious laryngotracheitis–a preliminary report. J Am Vet Med Assoc 84:588–595.

16. Brandly, C.A. 1935. Some studies on infectious laryngotracheitis. The continued propagation of the virus upon the CAM of the hen's egg. J Infect Dis 57:201–206.

17. Brandly, C.A. 1936. Studies on the egg-propagated viruses of infectious laryngotracheitis and fowl pox. J Am Vet Med Assoc 88:587–599.

18. Brandly, C.A. 1937. Studies on certain filterable viruses. 1. Factors concerned with the egg propagation of fowl pox and infectious laryngotracheitis. J Am Vet Med Assoc 90:479–487.

19. Brandly, C.A., and J.D. Bushnell. 1934. A report of some investigations of infectious laryngotracheitis. Poult Sci 13:212–217.

20. Braune, M.O., and R.F. Gentry. 1965. Standardization of the fluorescent antibody technique for the detection of avian respiratory viruses. Avian Dis 9:535–545.

21. Bülow, V.v., and A. Klasen. 1983. Effects of avian viruses on cultured chicken bone-marrow-derived macrophages. Avian Pathol 12:179–198.

22. Burnet, F.M. 1934. The propagation of the virus of infectious laryngotracheitis on the CAM of the developing egg. Br J Exp Pathol 15:52–55.

23. Burnet, F.M. 1936. Immunological studies with the virus of infectious laryngotracheitis of fowls using the developing egg technique. J Exp Med 63:685–701.

24. Calnek, B.W., K.J. Fahey, and T.J. Bagust. 1986. In vitro infection studies with infectious laryngotrache-

itis virus. Avian Dis 30:327–336.

25. Chang, P.W., V. Jasty, D. Fry, and V.J. Yates. 1973. Replication of a cell-culture-modified infectious laryngotracheitis virus in experimentally infected chickens. Avian Dis 17:683–689.

26. Chang, P.W., F. Sculo, and V.J. Yates. 1977. An in vivo and in vitro study of infectious laryngotracheitis virus in chicken leukocytes. Avian Dis 21:492–500.

27. Chomiac, T.W., R.E. Luginbuhl, and C.F. Helmboldt. 1960. Tissue culture and chicken embryo techniques for infectious laryngotracheitis. Avian Dis 4:235–246.

28. Churchill, A.E. 1965. The use of chicken kidney tissue cultures in the study of the avian viruses of Newcastle disease, infectious laryngotracheitis, and infectious bronchitis. Res Vet Sci 6:162–169.

29. Clarke, J.K., G.M. Robertson, and D.A. Purcell. 1980. Spray vaccination of chickens using infectious laryngotracheitis virus. Aust Vet J 56:424–428.

30. Cover, M.S., and W.J. Benton. 1958. The biological variation of infectious laryngotracheitis virus. Avian Dis 2:375–383.

31. Cover, M.S., W.J. Benton, and W.C. Krauss. 1960. The effect of parenteral immunity and age on the response to infectious laryngotracheitis vaccination. Avian Dis 4:467–473.

32. Crawshaw, G.J., and B.R. Boycott. 1982. Infectious laryngotracheitis in peafowl and pheasants. Avian Dis 26:397–401.

33. Cruickshank, J.G., D.M. Berry, and B. Hay. 1963. The fine structure of infectious laryngotracheitis virus. Virology 20:376–378.

34. Curtis, P.E., and A.S. Wallis. 1983. Infectious laryngotracheitis. Vet Rec 112:486.

35. Davidson, S., and K. Miller. 1988. Recent laryngotracheitis outbreaks in Pennsylvania. Proc 37th West Poult Conf, pp. 135–136.

36. Delaplane, J.P. 1945. Differential diagnosis of respiratory diseases of fowl. J Am Vet Med Assoc 106:83.

37. Dobson, N. 1935. Infectious laryngotracheitis in poultry. Vet Rec 15:1467–1471.

38. Fahey, K.J., T.J. Bagust, and J.J. York. 1983. Laryngotracheitis herpesvirus infection in the chicken: The role of humoral antibody in immunity to a graded challenge infection. Avian Pathol 12:505–514.

39. Fahey, K.J., J.J. York, and T.J. Bagust. 1984. Laryngotracheitis herpesvirus infection in the chicken. 2. The adoptive transfer of resistance with immune spleen cells. Avian Pathol 13:265–275.

40. Fitzgerald, J.E., and L.E. Hanson. 1963. A comparison of some properties of laryngotracheitis and herpes simplex viruses. Am J Vet Res 24:1297–1303.

41. Gelenczei, E.F., and E.W. Marty. 1964. Studies on a tissue-culture modified infectious laryngotracheitis virus. Avian Dis 8:105–122.

42. Gelenczei, E.F., and E.W. Marty. 1965. Strain stability and immunologic characteristics of a tissue-culture modified infectious laryngotracheitis virus. Avian Dis 9:44–56.

43. Gibbs, C.S. 1933. The Massachusetts plan for the eradication and control of infectious laryngotracheitis. J Am Vet Med Assoc 83:214–217.

44. Gibbs, C.S. 1934. Infectious laryngotracheitis field experiments: Vaccination. Massachusetts Agr Exp Stn Bull 305:57–58.

45. Goldhaft, T.M. 1961. Viability of pox and laryngotracheitis vaccines. Avian Dis 5:196–200.

46. Graham, R.F., F. Throp, Jr., and W.A. James. 1930. Subacute or chronic infectious avian laryngotracheitis. J Infect Dis 47:87–91.

47. Hayashi, S., Y. Odagiri, T. Kotani, and T. Horiuchi. 1985. Pathological changes of tracheal mucosa in chickens infected with infectious laryngotracheitis virus. Avian Dis 29:943–950.

48. Hayles, L.B., W.C. Newby, H. Gasperdone, and E.W. Gilchrist. 1976. Immunization of broiler chickens with a commercial infectious laryngotracheitis vaccine in the drinking water. Can J Comp Med 40:129–134.

49. Hilbink, F., T.H. Smit, and H. Yadin. 1981. Drinking water vaccination against ILT. Can J Comp Med 45:120–123.

50. Hinshaw, W.R. 1931. A survey of infectious laryngotracheitis of fowls. California Agr Exp Stn Bull 520:1–36.

51. Hinshaw, W.R., E.C. Jones, and H.W. Graybill. 1931. A study of mortality and egg production in flocks affected with infectious laryngotracheitis. Poult Sci 10:375–382.

52. Hitchner, S.B. 1969. Virus concentration as a limiting factor in immunity response to laryngotracheitis vaccines. J Am Vet Med Assoc 154:1425. (Abstr).

53. Hitchner, S.B. 1975. Infectious laryngotracheitis: The virus and the immune response. Am J Vet Res 36:518–519.

54. Hitchner, S.B., and P.G. White. 1958. A comparison of embryo and bird infectivity using five strains of laryngotracheitis virus. Poult Sci 37:684–690.

55. Hitchner, S.B., and R.W. Winterfield. 1960. Revaccination procedures for infectious laryngotracheitis. Avian Dis 4:291–303.

56. Hitchner, S.B., C.A. Shea, and P.G. White. 1958. Studies on a serum neutralization test for the diagnosis of laryngotracheitis in chickens. Avian Dis 2:258–269.

57. Hitchner, S.B., J. Fabricant, and T.G. Bagust. 1977. A fluorescent-antibody study of the pathogenesis of infectious laryngotracheitis. Avian Dis 21:185–194.

58. Holmes, I.H., and D.H. Watson. 1963. An electron microscope study of the attachment and penetration of herpes virus in BHK 21 cells. Virology 21:112–123.

59. Hudson, C.B., and F.R. Beaudette. 1932. The susceptibility of pheasants and a pheasant bantam cross to the virus of infectious bronchitis. Cornell Vet 23:70–74.

60. Hughes, C.S., and R.C. Jones. 1988. Comparison of cultural methods for primary isolation of infectious laryngotracheitis virus from field material. Avian Pathol 17:295–303.

61. Hughes, C.S., R.C. Jones, R.M. Gaskell, F.T.W. Jordan, and J.M. Bradbury. 1987. Demonstration in live chickens of the carrier state in infectious laryngotracheitis. Res Vet Sci 42:407–410.

62. Hughes, C.S., R.M. Gaskell, R.C. Jones, J.M. Bradbury, and F.T.W. Jordan. 1989. Effects of certain stress factors on the re-excretion of infectious laryngotracheitis virus from latently infected carrier birds. Res Vet Sci 46:247–276.

63. Hunt, S. 1959. The feather follicle method of vaccinating baby chicks with laryngotracheitis vaccine. Proc Poult Sci Conv, pp. 29–30. Sydney, Australia.

64. Izuchi, T., and A. Hasegawa. 1982. Pathogenicity of infectious laryngotracheitis virus as measured by chicken embryo inoculation. Avian Dis 26:18–25.

65. Izuchi, T., and T. Miyamoto. 1984. Influence of Newcastle disease and infectious bronchitis live virus vaccines on immune response against infectious laryngotracheitis live virus vaccine in chickens. Jpn J Vet Sci 46:353–359.

66. Izuchi, T., A. Hasegawa, and T. Miyamoto. 1983. Studies on a live virus vaccine against infectious laryngotracheitis of chickens. I. Biological properties of attenuated strain C7. Avian Dis 27:918–926.

67. Izuchi, T., A. Hasegawa, and T. Miyamoto. 1984. Studies on the live virus vaccine against ILT of chickens. II. Evaluation of the tissue-culture-modified strain C7 in laboratory and field trials. Avian Dis 28:323–330.
68. Jordan, F.T.W. 1958. Some observations on infectious laryngotracheitis. Vet Rec 70:605–610.
69. Jordan, F.T.W. 1963. Further observations of the epidemiology of infectious laryngotracheitis of poultry. J Comp Pathol Ther 73:253–264.
70. Jordan, F.T.W. 1964. The control of infectious laryngotracheitis. Zentralbl Veterinaermed [B] 11:15–32.
71. Jordan, F.T.W. 1966. A review of the literature on infectious laryngotracheitis (ILT). Avian Dis 10:1–26.
72. Jordan, F.T.W. 1981. Immunity to infectious laryngotracheitis. In M.E. Ross, L.N. Payne, and B.M. Freeman (eds.), Avian Immunology, pp. 245–254. British Poultry Science Ltd., Edinburgh.
73. Kaleta, E.F., T.H. Redmann, U. Heffels-Redmann, and K. Frese. 1986. Zum Nachweis der Latenz des attenuierten Virus der infektiosen laryngotracheitis des Huhnes im trigeminus-ganglion. Dtsche Tierärztl Wochenschr 93:40–42.
74. Keller, K., and P. Hebel. 1962. Diagnostico de las inclusiones de laryngotraqueitis infecciosa en frotis y cortes histologicos. Zooiatria (Chile) 1:1.
75. Kernohan, G. 1931. Infectious laryngotracheitis of fowls. J Am Vet Med Assoc 78:196–202.
76. Kernohan, G. 1931. Infectious laryngotracheitis in pheasants. J Am Vet Med Assoc 78:553–555.
77. Kingsbury, F.W., and E.L. Jungherr. 1958. Indirect transmission of infectious laryngotracheitis in chickens. Avian Dis 2:54–63.
78. Komarov, A., and F.R. Beaudette. 1932. Carriers of infectious bronchitis. Poult Sci 11:335–338.
79. Kotiw, M., C.R. Wilks, and J.T. May. 1982. Differentiation of infectious laryngotracheitis virus strains using restriction endonucleases. Avian Dis 26:718–731.
80. Kotiw, M., M. Sheppard, J.T. May, and C.R. Wilks. 1986. Differentiation between virulent and avirulent strains of infectious laryngotracheitis virus by DNA:DNA hybridization using a cloned DNA marker. Vet Microbiol 11:319–330.
81. Leib, D.A., J.M. Bradbury, R.M. Gaskell, C.S. Hughes, and R.C. Jones. 1986. Restriction endonuclease patterns of some European and American isolates of avian infectious laryngotracheitis virus. Avian Dis 30:835–837.
82. Leib, D.A., J.M. Bradbury, C.A. Hart, and K. McCarthy. 1987. Genome isomerism in two alphaherpesviruses: Herpes saimiri-1 (herpesvirus tamaerinus) and avian infectious laryngotracheitis virus. Arch Virol 93:287–294.
83. Mallinson, E.T., K.F. Miller, and C.D. Murphy. 1981. Cooperative control of infectious laryngotracheitis. Avian Dis 25:723–729.
84. May, H.G., and R.P. Tittsler. 1925. Tracheo-laryngitis in poultry. J Am Vet Med Assoc 67:229–231.
85. McNulty, M.S., G.M. Allan, and R.M. McCracken. 1985. Infectious laryngotracheitis in Ireland. Ir Vet J 39:124–125.
86. Meulemans, G., and P. Halen. 1978. Some physico-chemical and biological properties of a Belgian strain (U 76/1035) of infectious laryngotracheitis virus. Avian Pathol 7:311–315.
87. Meulemans, G., and P. Halen. 1982. Enzyme-linked immunosorbent assay (ELISA) for detecting infectious laryngotracheitis viral antibodies in chicken serum. Avian Pathol 11:361–368.
88. Molgard, P.C., and J.W. Cavett. 1947. The feather follicle method of vaccinating with fowl laryngotracheitis vaccine. Poult Sci 26:263–267.
89. Nii, S., C. Morgan, and H.M. Rose. 1968. Electron microscopy of herpes simplex virus. II. Sequence of development. J Virol (Kyoto) 2:517–536.
90. Ohkubo, Y., K. Shibata, T. Mimura, and I. Taskashima. 1988. Labeled avidin-biotin enzyme-linked immunosorbent assay for detecting antibody to infectious laryngotracheitis virus in chickens. Avian Dis 32:24–31.
91. Picault, J.P., M. Guittet, and G. Bennejean. 1982. Innocuité et activité de différents vaccins de la laryngotracheite infectieuse aviaire. Avian Pathol 11:39–48.
92. Pirozok, R.P., C.F. Helmbolt, and E.L. Jungherr. 1957. A rapid histological technique for the diagnosis of infectious avian laryngotracheitis. J Am Vet Med Assoc 130:406–407.
93. Plummer, G., C.R. Goodheart, D. Henson, and C.P. Bowling. 1969. A comparative study of the DNA density and behavior in tissue culture of fourteen different herpesviruses. Virology 39:134–137.
94. Pulsford, M.F. 1953. Possible P-Q type variation in infectious laryngotracheitis virus. Nature 172:1193–1195.
95. Pulsford, M.F., and J. Stokes. 1953. Infectious laryngotracheitis in South Australia. Aust Vet J 29:8–12.
96. Purcell, D.A., and J.B. McFerran. 1969. Influence of method of infection on the pathogenesis of infectious laryngotracheitis. J Comp Pathol 79:285–291.
97. Raggi, L.G., and G.G. Lee. 1965. Infectious laryngotracheitis outbreaks following vaccination. Avian Dis 9:559–565.
98. Raggi, L.G., J.R. Brownell, and G.F. Stewart. 1961. Effect of infectious laryngotracheitis on egg production and quality. Poult Sci 40:134–140.
99. Reynolds, H.A., A.W. Watrach, and L.E. Hanson. 1968. Development of the nuclear inclusion bodies of infectious laryngotracheitis. Avian Dis 12:332–347.
100. Robertson, G.M. 1977. The role of bursa-dependent responses in immunity to infectious laryngotracheitis. Res Vet Sci 22:281–284.
101. Robertson, G.M., and J.R. Egerton. 1977. Micro-assay systems for infectious laryngotracheitis virus. Avian Dis 21:133–135.
102. Robertson, G.M., and J.R. Egerton. 1981. Replication of infectious laryngotracheitis virus in chickens following vaccination. Aust Vet J 57:119–123.
103. Roizman, B. 1982. The family Herpesviridae: General description, taxonomy and classification. In B. Roizman (ed.), The Herpesviruses, Vol. 1, p. 1–23. Plenum Press, New York.
104. Rossi, C.R., H.A. Reynolds, and A.M. Watrach. 1969. Studies of laryngotracheitis virus in avian tissue cultures. 1. Plaque assay in chicken embryo kidney tissue cultures. Arch für die Gesamte Virusforsch 28:219–228.
105. Russell, R.G., and A.J. Turner. 1983. Characterization of infectious laryngotracheitis viruses. 1. Antigenic comparison by kinetics of neutralization and immunization studies. Can J Comp Med 47:163–171.
106. Samberg, Y., and I. Aronovici. 1969. The development of a vaccine against avian infectious laryngotracheitis. 1. Modification of a laryngotracheitis virus. Refu Vet 26:54–59.
107. Samberg, Y., E. Cuperstein, U. Bendheim, and I. Aronovici. 1971. The development of a vaccine against avian infectious laryngotracheitis. IV. Immunization of chickens with a modified laryngotracheitis vaccine in the drinking water. Avian Dis 15:413–417.
108. Schalm, O.W., and J.R. Beach. 1935. The resistance of the virus of infectious laryngotracheitis to certain physical and chemical factors. J Infect Dis 56:210–223.
109. Seddon, H.R., and L. Hart. 1935. The occur-

rence of infectious laryngotracheitis in New South Wales. Aust Vet J 11:212-222.
110. Seddon, H.R., and L. Hart. 1936. Infectivity experiments with the virus of laryngotracheitis of fowls. Aust Vet J 12:13-16.
111. Seifried, O. 1931. Histopathology of infectious laryngotracheitis in chickens. J Exp Med 56:817-826.
112. Sevoian, M. 1960. A quick method for the diagnosis of avian pox and infectious laryngotracheitis. Avian Dis 4:474-777.
113. Shibley, G.P., R.E. Luginbuhl, and C.F. Hemboldt. 1962. A study of infectious laryngotracheitis. I. Comparison of serological and immunogenic properties. Avian Dis 6:59-71.
114. Sinkovic, B.S. 1974. Studies on the control of ILT in Australia. PhD diss, Univ of Sydney, Aust.
115. Sinkovic, B., and S. Hunt. 1968. Vaccination of day-old chickens against infectious laryngotracheitis by conjunctival instillation. Aust Vet J 44:55-57.
116. Turner, A.J. 1972. Persistence of virus in respiratory infections of chickens. Aust Vet J 48:361-363.
117. Van Kammen, A., and P.B. Spradbrow. 1976. Rapid diagnosis of some avian virus diseases. Avian Dis 20:748-751.
118. Van Roekel, H.V. 1955. Respiratory diseases of poultry. Adv Vet Sci 2:64-97.
119. Watrach, A.M., A.E. Vatter, L.E. Hanson, M.A. Watrook, and H.E. Rhoades. 1959. Electron microscopic studies of the virus of infectious laryngotracheitis. Am J Vet Res 20:537-544.
120. Watrach, A.M., L.E. Hanson, and M.A. Watrach. 1963. The structure of infectious laryngotracheitis virus. Virology 21:601-608.
121. Webster, R.G. 1959. Studies on infectious laryngotracheitis in New Zealand. NZ Vet J 7:67-71.
122. Wilks, C.R., and V.G. Kogan. 1979. Immunofluorescence diagnostic test for avian infectious laryngotracheitis. Aust Vet J 55:385-388.
123. Winterfield, R.W., and I.G. So. 1968. Susceptibility of turkeys to infectious laryngotracheitis. Avian Dis 12:191-202.
124. Yamada, S., K. Matsuo, T. Fukuda, and Y. Uchinuno. 1980. Susceptibility of ducks to the virus of infectious laryngotracheitis. Avian Dis 24:930-938.
125. York, J.J., and K.J. Fahey. 1988. Diagnosis of infectious laryngotracheitis using a monoclonal antibody ELISA. Avian Pathol 17:173-182.
126. York, J.J., K.J. Fahey, and T.J. Bagust. 1983. Development and evaluation of an ELISA for the detection of antibody to infectious laryngotracheitis virus in chickens. Avian Dis 27:409-421.
127. York, J.J., S. Sonza, and K.J. Fahey. 1987. Immunogenic glycoproteins of infectious laryngotracheitis herpesvirus. Virology 161:340-347.

19 NEWCASTLE DISEASE AND OTHER PARAMYXOVIRUS INFECTIONS

D. J. Alexander

INTRODUCTION. The virus family Paramyxoviridae consists of three genera: *Paramyxovirus, Morbillivirus,* and *Pneumovirus.* Turkey rhinotracheitis virus is a probable member of the *Pneumovirus* genus (see Chapter 29), but all other viruses of this family that have been isolated from avian species are in the *Paramyxovirus* genus along with Newcastle disease virus (NDV), the prototype for that genus. Nine serogroups of avian paramyxoviruses have been recognized: PMV-1 to PMV-9 (8). Of these, NDV (PMV-1) remains the most important pathogen for poultry, but PMV-2 and PMV-3 can be responsible for serious disease. The prototype viruses and the recognized natural hosts for each serogroup are shown in Table 19.1. Detailed descriptions of serotypes not shown to affect poultry and serotypes usually infecting feral waterfowl have been reviewed by Alexander (5, 6, 8, 10).

NDV may vary widely in the type and severity of the disease it produces. This has often caused some problems with nomenclature, usually when the disease was first recognized in a country. As a result Newcastle disease has been termed pseudofowl pest, pseudovogel pest, atypische Geflugelpest, pseudopoultry plague, avian pest, avian distemper, Ranikhet disease, Tetelo disease, Korean fowl plague, and avian pneumoencephalitis. There have been very few synonyms used for the other avian paramyxoviruses. The term "Yucaipa" viruses has been applied to PMV-2 viruses as the first isolate was PMV-2/chicken/California/Yucaipa/56, the prototype of the serogroup. Isolates of the PMV-5 serotype have occasionally been referred to as "Kunitachi" viruses, again after the prototype virus.

Newcastle disease is complicated in that different isolates and strains of the virus may induce enormous variation in the severity of disease, even in a given host such as the chicken. To simplify matters, division into forms of disease based on clinical signs in chickens has been made as summarized by Beard and Hanson (39): 1) Doyle's form (66), an acute, lethal infection of chickens of all ages. Hemorrhagic lesions of the digestive tract are frequently present and this form of disease has been termed viscerotropic velogenic Newcastle disease (VVND); 2) Beach's form (35), an acute, often lethal infection of chickens of all ages. Characteristically, respiratory and neurological signs are seen, hence the term neurotropic velogenic, (NVND); 3) Beaudette's form (42) appears to be a less pathogenic form of NVND in which deaths are usually seen only in young birds. Viruses causing this type of infection are of the mesogenic pathotype and may be used as secondary live vaccines; 4) Hitchner's form (108) is represented by mild or inapparent respiratory infections caused by viruses of the lentogenic pathotype, which are commonly used as live vaccines; and 5) Asymptomatic-enteric form (138), chiefly gut infections with lentogenic viruses causing no obvious disease.

HISTORY

NEWCASTLE DISEASE VIRUS (PMV-1). It is generally considered that the first outbreaks of Newcastle disease occurred in 1926, in Java, Indonesia (123) and Newcastle-upon-Tyne, England (66). There are reports of disease outbreaks in Central Europe similar to what we now recognize as Newcastle disease, which predate 1926 (93), and Levine (131), citing Ochi and Hashimoto, indicated that the disease may have been present in Korea as early as 1924. The name Newcastle disease was coined by Doyle as a temporary measure since he wished to avoid a descriptive name that might be confused with other diseases (67).

It later became clear that other less severe diseases were caused by viruses indistinguishable from NDV. In the USA a relatively mild respiratory disease, often with nervous signs, was first described in the 1930s and subsequently termed "pneumoencephalitis" (35). It was shown to be due to a virus indistinguishable from NDV in serological tests (36). Within a few years numerous NDV isolations that produced extremely mild or no disease in chickens were made around the world (29, 108, 139, 186).

Avian Paramyxovirus Type 2 (PMV-2). In 1956 Bankowski et al. (31) isolated a paramyxovirus (65) from a chicken suffering from infectious laryngotracheitis in Yucaipa, California. It was serologically distinct from NDV (Table 19.1) and caused only mild respiratory disease in chickens. Serological surveys of poultry in the USA indicated that this virus was widespread, more frequently infecting turkeys than chickens (32, 54). Subsequent investigations suggested that viruses of the same serotype were common in poultry around the world (8).

Testing during quarantine of imported caged birds since the early 1970s has frequently resulted in the isolation of PMV-2 viruses, primarily from passerines but also from psittacines (8, 184). Surveillance of wild birds during the 1970s often resulted in the isolation of PMV-2 viruses, most frequently from passerine species (8).

Avian Paramyxovirus Type 3 (PMV-3). Paramyxoviruses representing a third serotype were isolated from turkeys in Ontario in 1967 and Wisconsin in 1968 and later detected serologically in turkeys in other states of the USA (200). Serologically related viruses have now been reported from turkeys in several countries in Europe.

PMV-3 viruses are also frequently isolated from captive caged birds in most countries where quarantine is imposed, most often from psittacine species, although passerines are also susceptible (8). There is evidence that these viruses differ antigenically from the turkey PMV-3 viruses (27).

DISTRIBUTION

Newcastle Disease. Vaccination of poultry throughout the world makes assessment of the geographical distribution of Newcastle disease difficult. Nevertheless, international recording and reporting of Newcastle disease is carried out by the Food and Agriculture Organization of the United Nations (73), which formed the basis of several assessments of the geographical distribution of the disease (127, 128). Spradbrow (192), concluded that Newcastle disease is still widespread in many countries of Asia, Africa, and the Americas and confused in Europe, due to the presence of the variant virus in pigeons. Only the countries of Oceania appeared to have relative freedom from disease.

The distribution of Newcastle disease is dependent on the attempts at eradication and control made in different countries. The success of such measures is, in turn, dependent on the nature of the poultry industry, i.e., countries with mostly village chicken flocks have far greater problems than those with mostly large commercial flocks.

The nature of the spread of Newcastle disease also affects the distribution. Alexander (9) considered that three panzootics of Newcastle disease had occurred since the first recognition of the disease. The first represented the initial outbreaks of disease and appears to have arisen in Southeast Asia. Doyle (67) considered that the disease moved slowly through Asia to Europe and that isolated outbreaks, such as in England in 1926, were chance introductions ahead of the mainstream. This theory of panzootic spread of Newcastle disease would mean that virus that had apparently arisen in 1926 took over 30 years to spread worldwide and was still important in most countries in the early 1960s.

In marked contrast, the second panzootic appears to have begun in the Middle East in the late 1960s and to have reached most countries by 1973. The more rapid spread of the second panzootic could be because the poultry industry had undergone a major revolution in that it had developed into a major commercial industry with considerable international trade. In addition, the virus responsible for this panzootic appeared to be associated with imported caged psittacine species. The enormous trade in these birds, which involved rapid, airborne shipments, was considered to be a major factor in the spread of the disease (75, 204).

The serious effects of the second panzootic on the poultry industries of most countries led to the development of vaccines and regimens that provided significant protection to poultry. In addition, most countries imposed new control measures for the importation of exotic caged birds. However, another group of domesticated birds existed in large numbers in most countries which was generally ignored as a potential source of Newcastle disease. This group consisted of the pigeons and doves (*Columba livia*), which are kept for racing, show, or food purposes and in most European countries may represent several million birds. These were the birds primarily affected by the third panzootic of ND. The disease, which resembled the neurotropic form in chickens but without respiratory signs, apparently arose in the Middle East in the late 1970s (118). By 1981 it had reached Europe (46) and then spread rapidly to all parts of the world, largely as a result of contact between birds at races and shows and the large international trade in such birds. The variant nature of the virus enabled unequivocal demonstration of infection in 24 countries (21, 24, 166). Spread to chickens has occurred in several countries including Great Britain where 20 outbreaks in unvaccinated chickens occurred in 1984 as a result of feed that had been contaminated by infected pigeons (22).

Avian Paramyxovirus Type 2. Paramyxovirus type 2 viruses are found in feral birds, chiefly passerines and in European, Asian, African, and American countries (7, 86), probably accounting for their common isolation from imported caged birds (7). Isolations from domestic poultry have been rare although problems associated with such viruses have been recorded in USA, Canada, USSR, Japan, Italy, Israel, India, and France in chickens or turkeys (5, 7).

Avian Paramyxovirus Type 3. Paramyxovirus type 3 viruses have also been isolated from imported exotic birds, but unlike PMV-2 viruses, there have been no reports of PMV-3 viruses from feral birds (7). PMV-3 virus infections of domestic poultry have been restricted to turkeys in Canada and USA (200), Great Britain (135), France (28), and Germany (213). There have been no reports of natural infections of chickens with PMV-3 viruses, although they are fully susceptible.

ETIOLOGY

Classification. Members of the Paramyxoviridae family are RNA viruses showing helical capsid symmetry with a nonsegmented, single-stranded genome of negative polarity. They are enveloped, and this is formed from modified cell membrane as the virus is budded from the cell surface after capsid assembly in the cytoplasm (145).

The family consists of three genera. The genus *Morbillivirus* consists of measles, rinderpest and canine distemper viruses; no members have been isolated from avian species. The *Pneumovirus* genus consists of the mammalian respiratory syncytial viruses, mouse pneumonia virus, and an avian pneumovirus associated with turkey rhinotracheitis and swollen head syndrome of chickens (see Chapter 29). The third genus, *Paramyxovirus,* is formed from the mammalian parainfluenza viruses, mumps virus, and the avian paramyxoviruses. NDV is the prototype of the genus.

Members of the *Paramyxovirus* genus may be distinguished by the possession of neuraminidase activity, which is absent in the other viruses of the family.

CLASSIFICATION OF AVIAN PARAMYXOVIRUSES. Tumova et al. (201) suggested grouping avian paramyxoviruses on the basis of their antigenic relatedness in hemagglutination inhibition (HI) tests. The prefixes PMV-1, PMV-2, etc. were adopted to signify serotype, and the nomenclature proposed for naming influenza isolates (207) was used for the avian paramyxovirus isolates (Table 19.1).

There has been no attempt to make more specific definition of a serotype, and further, viruses have been grouped based on their relationships in HI tests. However, when neuraminidase inhibition (114, 120, 160, 200), serum neutralization (200), or agar-gel diffusion (2, 19, 114, 121) tests have been used similar groups have resulted.

Despite the consistency of the serological groupings there are some cross-relationships between viruses of the different serotypes (see 8). Usually these have been very minor, although Lipkind et al. (132, 134) considered them sufficient to suggest a phylogenic relationship between PMV-1, -3, -4, -7, -8, and -9 and between

Table 19.1. Representative strains of the avian paramyxovirus serotypes

Prototype Virus	Primary Host	Other Hosts	Related Disease in Poultry
PMV-1/Newcastle disease virus	Numerous avian hosts	See text	Spectrum of disease
PMV-2/chicken/Yucaipa/56	Passerines, turkeys	Chickens, psittacines, rails	Respiratory disease, egg production losses, serious if complicated
PMV-3/turkey/Wisconsin/68[a]	Turkeys	None	Egg production losses, respiratory disease
PMV-3/parakeet/Netherlands/75[a]	Psittacines	Passerines	No infections known
PMV-4/duck/Hong Kong/D3/75	Ducks	Geese, rails	Inapparent infections in commercial ducks
PMV-5/budgerigar/Japan/Kunitachi/75	Budgerigars	None	No infections known
PMV-6/duck/Hong Kong/199/77	Ducks, geese	Turkeys	Inapparent in ducks and geese, respiratory disease and egg losses in turkeys
PMV-7/dove/Tennessee/4/75	Pigeons, doves	None	No infections known
PMV-8/goose/Delaware/1053/75	Ducks, geese	None	No infections known
PMV-9/duck/New York/22/78	Ducks	None	Inapparent infections in commercial ducks

[a]Monoclonal antibodies allow host-related distinction between PMV-3 isolates.

PMV-2 and -6. However, the relationship between PMV-1 and -3 viruses appears to be closer and more important than the others.

Smit and Rondhuis (187) suggested there were low serological reactions between NDV and PMV-3/parakeet/Netherlands/75, which were later confirmed (14). In addition, prior infection of chickens with some PMV-3 viruses conferred protection against challenge with a virulent NDV strain (17). More recently, a monoclonal antibody against the pigeon variant PMV-1 inhibited PMV-3 viruses isolated from exotic birds in HI tests and bound to cells infected with these PMV-3 viruses (24, 61). However, since turkey PMV-3 isolates also show relationships with PMV-1 viruses and none could be demonstrated to react with this monoclonal antibody, other epitopes may be shared by the two serotypes.

Morphology. Negative contrast electron microscopy of members of the *Paramyxovirus* genus reveals very pleomorphic virus particles. Generally they are rounded and 100–500 nm in diameter, although filamentous forms of about 100 nm across and of variable length are often seen. The surface of the virus particle is covered with projections about 8 nm in length. In most electron micrographs of avian paramyxoviruses the "herring bone" nucleocapsid, about 18 nm across, may be seen either free or emerging from disrupted virus particles (Fig. 19.1).

Chemical Composition. Paramyxoviruses characteristically consist of a single molecule of single-stranded RNA of about 5×10^6-dalton molecular weight (122), which makes up about 5% by weight of the virus particle. Nucleotide sequencing of the NDV genome has shown it to consist of 15,156 nucleotides (152).

Virus particles have about 20–25% w/w lipid derived from the host cell and about 6% w/w carbohydrate. The overall molecular weight for an average virus particle is about 500×10^6 daltons with a density in sucrose of 1.18–1.20 g/ml.

VIRUS POLYPEPTIDES. Polyacrylamide gel electrophoresis (PAGE) of disrupted purified virus particles usually reveals a minimum of seven polypeptides for avian paramyxoviruses (15); however, one of these is the host protein actin, which is incorporated into the virus particle. The genome of NDV codes for six proteins (153), which have been described by Samson (180): L protein–RNA-directed RNA polymerase associated with the nucleocapsid; HN–responsible for the hemagglutinin and neuraminidase activities, forming the larger of the two types of projections seen on the surface of paramyxovirus particles; F–fusion protein, forming the smaller of the surface projections; NP–nucleocapsid protein; P–phosphorylated, nucleocapsid-associated; M–matrix. Comparable polypeptides have been seen for the other avian paramyxoviruses although minor variations in molecular weights has meant that PAGE profiles could be used to show similarities between isolates that coincide with the serogroups (15).

Biological Activities. Several biological activities are associated with paramyxoviruses that characterize the group.

HEMAGGLUTINATION (HA) ACTIVITY. The ability of NDV to agglutinate red blood cells (RBCs) is due to the binding of the HN protein to receptors on the surface of the RBCs. This property and the specific inhibition of agglutination by antisera (56) have proven powerful tools in the diagnosis of the disease.

Chicken RBCs are usually used in HA tests, but NDV will cause agglutination of all amphibian, reptilian, and avian cells (126). Winslow et al. (212) showed that human, mouse, and Guinea pig RBCs were agglutinated by all NDV strains tested but the ability to agglutinate cattle, goat, sheep, swine, and horse cells varied with the strain of NDV. Other avian paramyxoviruses also appear to be able to agglutinate a wide range of RBCs, but the exact range may vary with isolate as well as serotype. Paramyxoviruses will agglutinate cells other than RBCs if they possess the correct receptors.

NEURAMINIDASE ACTIVITY. The enzyme neuraminidase (mucopolysaccharide N-acetyl neuraminyl hydrolase EC 3.2.1.18) is also part of the HN molecule and present in all members of the *Paramyxovirus* genus. An obvious consequence of the possession of this enzyme is the gradual elution of agglutinated RBCs (4). However, the exact function of the neuraminidase in virus replication is unknown. Huang et al. (112) proposed that the enzyme acts at the receptor site enabling sufficient proximity for the F protein to bring about fusion of the virus and cell membranes.

CELL FUSION AND HEMOLYSIS. NDV and other paramyxoviruses may bring about hemolysis of RBCs or fusion of other cells by essentially the same mechanism. Attachment at the receptor site during replication is followed by fusion of the virus membrane with the cell membrane and this may result in the fusion of two or more cells (similar to the syncytial formation that occurs when virus particles are budded from cells). The rigid membrane of the RBCs usually results in lysis from the virus membrane fusion.

Virus Replication. The strategy for replication employed by paramyxoviruses is that of the negative strand viruses in general, as detailed by Peeples (167).

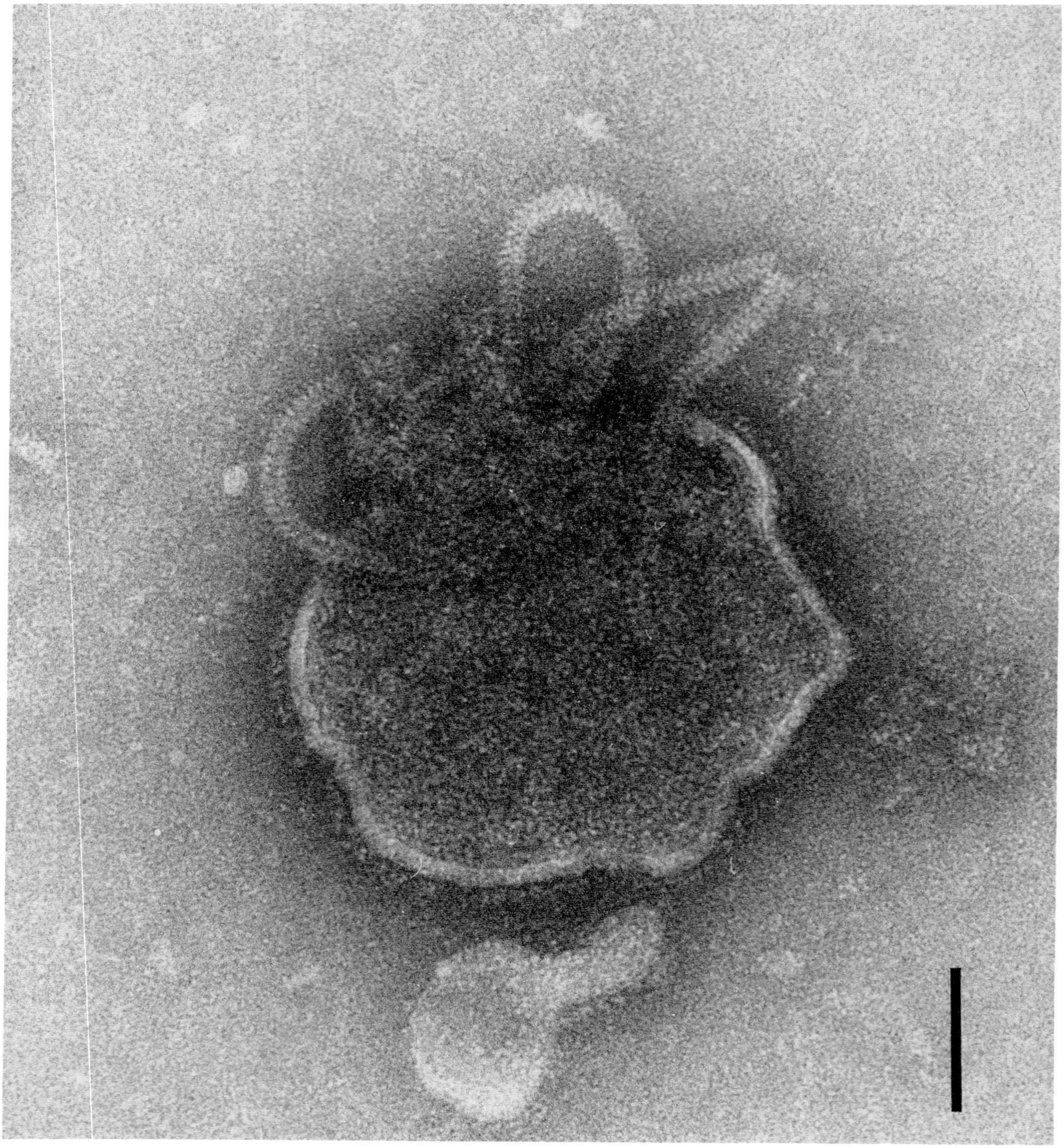

19.1. Negative-contrast electron micrograph of Newcastle disease virus strain Ulster 2C showing an intact and a disrupted particle with nucleocapsid emerging. ×202,000, bar = 100 nm. (Collins)

The initial step is attachment of the virus to cell receptors, mediated by the HN polypeptide. Fusion of the viral and cell membranes is brought about by action of the F protein, and thus the nucleocapsid complex enters the cell.

Intracellular virus replication takes place entirely within the cytoplasm. Because the virus RNA has negative sense it is necessary for the viral RNA-directed RNA polymerase (transcriptase) to produce complementary transcripts of positive sense that may act as messenger RNA and utilize the cell's mechanisms enabling translation into proteins and virus genomes. The F protein is synthesized as a nonfunctional precursor, F0, which requires cleavage to F1 and F2 by host proteases. The HN of some strains of NDV may also require posttranslational cleavage. The significance of this cleavage in the pathogenicity of

NDV strains is discussed below.

The viral proteins synthesized in an infected cell are transported to the cell membrane, which becomes modified by their incorporation. Following alignment of the nucleocapsid close to modified regions of the cell membrane, virus particles are budded from the cell surface.

Resistance to Agents. The infectivity of avian paramyxoviruses may be destroyed by physical and chemical treatments such as heat, irradiation (including light and ultraviolet rays), oxidation processes, pH effects, and various chemical compounds. The rate at which infectivity is destroyed depends on the strain of virus, the length of time of exposure, the quantity of virus, the nature of the suspending medium, and interactions between treatments. No one treatment can guarantee destruction of all virus, but may result in a low probability of infective virus remaining. Lancaster (126) and Beard and Hanson (39) provided detailed reviews.

Strain Classification

NEWCASTLE DISEASE VIRUS (PMV-1). The term strain is generally used to mean a well-characterized isolate of the virus. The important objective in characterizing viruses is to group similar viruses. For NDV isolates this has inevitably meant the distinction between viruses of high and low pathogenicity for chickens or perhaps more pertinently between enzootic and epizootic viruses.

Pathogenicity tests are useful markers and guides to the importance of the isolate. However, they give no further information and do not indicate epizootiological links between strains with the same virulence. Certain unrelated biological properties of viruses have been shown to vary with different strains and isolates, and these have been used to characterize and group isolates showing similar properties.

PATHOGENICITY TESTS. The first attempt to distinguish between, or group, isolates by a laboratory test was by assessment of virulence. Hanson and Brandly (98) suggested that strains of NDV could be conveniently grouped as velogenic, mesogenic, and lentogenic, based on chicken embryo mortality at <60 hr, 60–90 hr, and >90 hr respectively, after allantoic inoculation. The values obtained gave a guide to the disease produced in infected chickens. These terms have come to be applied to high-virulence, moderate-virulence and low-virulence viruses regardless of the method of assessment.

Other tests devised to distinguish between strains give a direct assessment of the clinical signs or deaths in infected birds. This enables quantification by designating scores according to the degree of severity and calculating a pathogenicity index. The most widely used tests are the intracerebral pathogenicity index in day-old chicks (ICPI) and the intravenous pathogenicity index in 6-wk-old chickens (IVPI).

PLAQUE FORMATION. Plaque formation, size, and morphology have been used to characterize viruses (95). NDVs of low virulence do not form plaques in cell cultures without the addition of diethylaminoethyl (DEAE) and magnesium (Mg^{++}) ions (34) or trypsin (176) to the agar overlay. Plaques may be of two morphological types, clear or red (182), and the size produced appears to be related to the virulence of the virus for chickens (171).

ELUTION. The rate of elution of chicken RBCs agglutinated by the virus has been used as a method of broadly grouping NDV isolates as rapid or slow eluters (191).

THERMOSTABILITY. The thermostability of the HA activity of NDV isolates varies (100) and has been used as a characterization test. This property has proven a useful tool in epizootiological studies (99) and a rapid method for distinguishing between some avirulent and virulent viruses.

STRUCTURAL POLYPEPTIDES. Variations and similarities of structural polypeptides between different strains have been reported (15, 156). Nagy and Lomniczi (159) used structural polypeptide analysis by PAGE after enzyme treatment to show close relationships between viruses isolated during the same epizootic but differences from other strains.

OLIGONUCLEOTIDE FINGERPRINTING. McMillan and Hanson (141, 142) used oligonucleotide fingerprinting of the genomic RNA to compare different strains and isolates of NDV. This approach demonstrated identity of viruses from the same source and differences from other isolates but it does not lend itself to routine diagnostic use.

LECTIN BINDING. McMillan et al. (143) demonstrated that different strains of NDV showed variation in lectin-binding profiles, which could be useful for differentiation and grouping.

ANTIGENICITY. Virus-neutralization (VN) or agar-gel diffusion techniques have shown minor antigenic variation between different strains and isolates of NDV (85, 168, 183). For all practical purposes, however, isolates of NDV have been considered to represent a single antigenically homogeneous group.

Monoclonal antibody (MAB) technology provided a new approach to antigenic differentiation of NDV strains and isolates (3, 21, 24, 68, 111,

114, 125, 149, 162, 179, 193).

MABs may detect slight variations in antigenicity, such as single amino acid changes at the epitope to which the antibody is directed. As a result they are capable of detecting differences not only between strains but between subpopulations of viruses (97). Some workers have used MABs to distinguish between specific viruses. For example, two groups have described MABs that distinguish between the common vaccine strains, Hitchner B1 and La Sota (68, 149), while other MABs can separate vaccine viruses from epizootic viruses in a given area (193).

The most comprehensive use of MAB for strain characterization and classification has been by Russell and Alexander (179) and Alexander et al. (21, 23, 24). They used MABs to place strains and isolates of NDV into groups on the basis of their ability to react with the different MABs. Viruses in the same MAB group shared biological and epizootiological properties.

MAB typing was also used to establish the uniqueness of the variant NDV responsible for the pigeon panzootic and to confirm its presence in many countries (21, 24, 166). During the epizootic of NDV in Great Britain in 1984, rapid identification of the pigeon variant enabled early tracing of the source of disease to contaminated feed ingredients, and subsequent control of the disease.

Avian Paramyxovirus Type 2. No attempt has been made to classify strains of PMV-2 viruses. Considerable antigenic and structural diversity has been recorded among these viruses (5, 15), but these have not been related to any epizootiological or biological properties.

Avian Paramyxovirus Type 3. PMV-3 virus isolates also show considerable diversity. There appears to be antigenic differentiation between those isolated from exotic birds and those from turkeys. This has been confirmed by MAB to PMV-3/turkey/England/MPH/81. Using these, Anderson et al. (27) showed that while some antibodies reacted with isolates from either source, others bound specifically to turkey viruses. Turkey isolates from the USA and Germany were distinguishable from turkey isolates from Great Britain and France and possibly more closely related to exotic bird isolates. This division of PMV-3 isolates into two groups was supported by studies with a MAB to a PMV-1 pigeon variant isolate, which was also able to react with PMV-3 isolates from exotic birds but not with those from turkeys (61).

Laboratory Host Systems

ANIMALS. NDV can infect and multiply in a range of nonavian (126) as well as avian (117) species following laboratory infection. However, the chicken remains the most readily available and frequently used laboratory animal as well as the most important natural host of the disease.

CHICKEN EMBRYOS. All avian paramyxoviruses replicate in embryonated chicken eggs. Because of their availability (especially from specific-pathogen-free sources), their sensitivity for virus growth, and the high titers to which viruses grow in them, they are generally used for virus isolation and propagation.

NDV strains and isolates vary in their capacity and time taken to kill chick embryos. Virus titers are also influenced by strain, with the highest titers obtainable by those causing slow or no death (89). With some strains, embryo death and virus growth is affected by the presence of maternal antibodies in the yolk (76).

The route of inoculation is also important (39). Inoculation of NDV via the yolk sac compared to the allantoic cavity produced rapider embryo deaths, and caused deaths by strains that do not consistently kill, by the latter route (71). For other avian paramyxoviruses, yolk sac or amniotic inoculation may be the route of choice for isolation or replication (88, 161).

CELL CULTURES. NDV strains can replicate in an enormous range of cells. For example, Lancaster (126) listed 18 primary cell types and 11 cell lines as susceptible. Many more have been added to the list since his 1966 report. Cytopathic effects (CPE) are usually the formation of syncytia and subsequent cell death, with the CPE having some relationship to the strain's virulence for chickens (171). Plaque formation in chick embryo cells is restricted to velogenic and mesogenic viruses unless Mg^{++} ions and DEAE (34) or trypsin (176) is added to the overlay.

Because of relatively poor growth of NDV in most cell culture systems, they are generally impracticable for virus propagation for most purposes.

Pathogenicity. The pathogenicity of NDV strains varies greatly with the host. Chickens are highly susceptible, but ducks and geese may be infected and show few or no clinical signs, even with strains lethal for chickens (104).

In chickens the pathogenicity of NDV is determined chiefly by the strain of virus, although dose, route of administration, age of the chicken, and environmental conditions all have an effect. In general, the younger the chicken the more acute the disease. With virulent viruses in the field, young chickens may experience sudden deaths without major clinical signs, while in older birds the disease may be more protracted and with characteristic clinical signs. Breed or genetic stock appears to have very little effect on the susceptibility of chickens to the disease (60). Natural routes of infection (nasal, oral, ocular) appear to emphasize the respiratory nature of the disease (38) while intramuscular, intravenous, and intracerebral routes appear to enhance the neurological signs (39).

MOLECULAR BASIS FOR PATHOGENICITY. During the replication of NDV it is necessary for the precursor glycoprotein F0 to be cleaved to F1 and F2 for the progeny virus particles to be infective (see 177). This posttranslation cleavage is mediated by host cell proteases (157). If cleavage fails to take place, noninfectious virus particles are produced. Trypsin is capable of cleaving F0 for all NDV strains and in vitro treatment of noninfectious virus will restore infectivity (158).

For a few strains of NDV the HN molecule is also produced as a precursor that requires cleavage to be biologically active (77).

The importance of F0 cleavage was easily demonstrated, since viruses normally unable to replicate or produce plaques in cell culture systems were able to do both if trypsin was added to the agar overlay or culture fluid. While all viruses could replicate and produce infectious progeny in the allantoic cavity, the viruses pathogenic for chickens could replicate in a wide range of cell types in vitro with or without added trypsin, whereas strains of low virulence could replicate only when trypsin was added (175, 176). Thus F0 molecules of virulent viruses can be cleaved by a wide range of proteases, but F0 molecules in viruses of low virulence were restricted in their sensitivity and these viruses can grow only in certain host cell types.

Amino acid sequencing of the F0 precursor has shown that low-virulence viruses have a single arginine plus another basic amino acid separated by two others at the site of cleavage, whereas the virulent viruses all possess additional basic amino acids, forming two pairs, at the site (57, 83, 140, 153, 199).

Thus it would appear that the mechanism controlling the pathogenicity of NDV is very similar to that described for influenza viruses (205). The presence of additional basic amino acids in virulent strains means that cleavage can be effected by a wide range of host proteases, but in lentogenic viruses, cleavage can occur only with proteases recognizing a single arginine, i.e., trypsin-like enzymes. Lentogenic viruses therefore only replicate in areas with trypsinlike enzymes, such as the respiratory and intestinal tracts, whereas virulent viruses can replicate in a range of tissues and organs resulting in a fatal systemic infection (175). An explanation for apparently refractory hosts such as ducks and geese would be that non-trypsinlike proteases are not capable of cleaving even those viruses possessing multiple basic amino acids at the cleavage site.

Garten et al. (77) indicated that proteolytic activation of the HN glycoprotein also played a role in virulence. Although there is less data than for F, the sequences of the HN for several strains have been determined. It appears the HN0 precursor seen for the avirulent strains Ulster 2C (155) and D26 (181) is never produced in more virulent strains. The lentogenic Hitchner B1 (116), mesogenic Beaudette C (154), and two velogenic strains, Australia Victoria (140) and Italien (206), have termination codons located before the end of the HN gene so that the HN0 protein is not produced and posttranslational cleavage is not required.

PATHOGENESIS AND EPIZOOTIOLOGY

Natural and Experimental Hosts. From the available literature Kaleta and Baldauf (117) concluded that, in addition to the domestic avian species, natural or experimental infection has been demonstrated in at least 236 species from 27 of the 50 orders of birds. These authors stressed the variation in severity of clinical signs, even with different species of a genus. Nevertheless, they considered it possible to make tentative groupings based on susceptibility to the disease. The most resistant species appear to be aquatic birds, while the most susceptible are gregarious birds forming temporary or permanent flocks. There is far less data available with other avian paramyxoviruses. The general groups of birds reported to be infected with the different serotypes are shown in Table 19.1 and in more detailed reviews (5, 8). Isolations of avian paramyxoviruses from different species have been rarely associated with specific disease episodes. PMV-3 viruses have been related to disease in certain psittacine species such as encephalitis with high mortality in parakeets of the *Neophoma* and *Psephotus* genera (187) and high mortality in lovebirds, *Agapornis roseicollis,* (107). PMV-5 viruses appear to have a very limited host range being isolated only from budgerigars, *Melopsittacus undulatus,* in which infection resulted in high mortality (160).

Transmission. In reviewing the modes of transmission of NDV between birds, Alexander (12) concluded that infection may take place by either inhalation or ingestion and that spread from one bird to another depends on the availability of the virus in an infectious form. It is tempting to assume that NDV is primarily transmitted by fine aerosols or large droplets that are inhaled by susceptible birds. However, experimental evidence to prove this conclusively is lacking. It is clear that infective virus may be present in aerosols and that birds placed in an atmosphere containing such aerosols become infected. This is the basis for mass application of live vaccines by spray and aerosol generators (146). In natural infections, large and small droplets containing virus will be liberated from infected birds as a result of replication in the respiratory tract or as a result of dust and other particles, including feces. These virus-laden particles may be inhaled or impinge upon the mucous membranes resulting in infection. However, the ability of such aerosols to form and support infectious virus for a sufficient period for transmission depends on many environmental factors.

During the course of infection of most birds with NDV, large amounts of virus are excreted in the feces. Ingestion of feces results in infection; this is likely to be the main method of bird-to-bird spread for avirulent enteric NDV and the pigeon variant virus (20), neither of which normally produces respiratory signs in infected birds.

Vertical transmission, i.e., passing of virus from parent to progeny via the embryo, is controversial. The true significance of such transmission in epizootics of Newcastle disease is not clear. Experimental assessment using virulent viruses is usually hampered by cessation of egg laying in infected birds. Infected embryos have been reported during natural infections of laying hens with virulent virus (39, 129), but this generally results in the death of the infected embryo during incubation. Cracked or broken infected eggs may serve as a source of virus for newly hatched chicks, as may virus-laden feces contaminating the outside of eggs. Virus may also penetrate the shell after laying (209), further complicating the assessment of true vertical or transovarian transmission. Infected chicks may be hatched from eggs infected with vaccinal or other lentogenic viruses that do not necessarily cause death of the embryo (62, 76). In natural infections it is not clear how the embryos become infected, although La Sota vaccine has been shown to be present in most of the reproductive organs after vaccination (170).

Spread. Lancaster and Alexander (12, 126, 129) reviewed the modes of spread of NDV. The following virus sources or methods have been implicated in various epizootics: 1) movement of live birds–feral birds, pet/exotic birds, game birds, racing pigeons, commercial poultry; 2) other animals; 3) movement of people and equipment; 4) movement of poultry products; 5) airborne spread; 6) contaminated poultry feed; 7) water; 8) vaccines.

The importance of any of these factors will depend on the situation in which the epizootic occurs. In countries where poultry are kept exclusively in birdproof housing, the ability of feral birds to invade affected flocks and transfer the disease will be minimal. Similarly, despite the huge international trade in exotic caged birds and the frequent isolation of virulent NDV from such birds (184), the threat of introduction and spread by this source (as in the California epizootic in 1971–72) (202) has been greatly reduced by strict importation quarantine procedures. However, smuggled birds or those removed prematurely from quarantine may still pose a threat (184). Airborne spread has been considered to be important in some epizootics, such as the 1970–71 outbreaks in England (113) but unimportant in others, such as the 1971–72 California outbreaks (202), even though the same virus appears to be involved.

In some cases more than one factor combines in the spread of the disease. For example, the 1984 outbreaks of Newcastle disease in Great Britain were considered to be spread by feed that had been contaminated by infected feral pigeons (22).

Without doubt the greatest potential for spread of NDV is by humans and their equipment. Humans may be infected in the conjunctival sac with NDV, which could pose a method of spread, but more probable is the mechanical transfer of infective material (most probably feces). Modern transportation enables personnel to travel rapidly to any country in the world, so spread by humans should not be treated as merely a local or national threat.

Vaccination crews moving from farm to farm have been implicated in the spread of NDV (202), as have incomplete inactivation (190) and contamination (41) of vaccines.

There is little information on the spread of other avian paramyxoviruses. For PMV-2 and PMV-3 serotypes, infection of poultry leads to shedding from the respiratory and intestinal tracts, so it is assumed that the methods of spread of NDV would also apply to these. PMV-2 viruses have been shown to infect feral passerines, which may invade poultry houses, but in the absence of any wild bird host for PMV-3 viruses it seems most likely that this subtype has been introduced into different countries by importation of infected poultry or by humans.

Incubation Period. The incubation period of ND after natural exposure has been reported to vary from 2 to 15 days (average 5–6). The speed with which signs appear, if at all, is variable depending on the infecting virus, the host species and its age and immune status, infection with other organisms, environmental conditions, the route of exposure, and the dose.

Clinical Signs, Morbidity, Mortality

Newcastle Disease. NDV isolates can be broadly grouped into pathotypes on the basis of clinical signs, which in turn are affected by the strain of virus. However, other factors also important in establishing the severity of the disease are the host species, age, immune status, co-infection with other organisms, environmental stress, social stress, route of exposure, and the virus dose (138).

With extremely virulent viruses the disease may appear suddenly, with high mortality occurring in the absence of other clinical signs. In outbreaks in chickens due to the VVND pathotype, clinical signs often begin with listlessness, increased respiration, and weakness, ending with prostration and death. During the panzootic caused by this type of virus in 1970–73, disease in some countries such as Great Britain (26) and Northern Ireland (138) was marked by severe respiratory signs, but in other countries these were absent. This type of ND may cause edema around the eyes and head. Green diarrhea is frequently seen in birds that do not die early in infection, and prior to death, muscular tremors, torticollis, paralysis of legs and wings, and opisthotonos may be apparent. Mortality frequently reaches 100% in flocks of fully susceptible chickens.

The neurotropic velogenic form of disease has been reported mainly from the USA. In chickens it is marked by sudden onset of severe respiratory disease, followed a day or two later by neurological signs. Egg production falls dramatically, but diarrhea is usually absent. Morbidity may reach 100%. Mortality is generally considerably lower, although up to 50% in adult birds and 90% in young chickens has been recorded.

Mesogenic strains of NDV usually cause respiratory disease in field infections. In adult birds there may be a marked drop in egg production that may last for several weeks. Nervous signs may occur but are not common. Mortality in fowl is usually low, except in very young susceptible birds, but may be considerably affected by exacerbating conditions.

Lentogenic viruses do not usually cause disease in adults. In young, fully susceptible birds, serious respiratory disease problems can be seen, often resulting in mortality, following infection with the more pathogenic La Sota strains with complicating infections. Vaccination or infection of broilers close to slaughter with these viruses can lead to colisepticemia or airsacculitis with resulting condemnation.

The virus responsible for the panzootic in pigeons during the 1980s induced clinical signs in field infections of pigeons (203) and chickens (22), unlike those from other viruses. In both species the predominant clinical features were diarrhea and nervous signs. In adult chickens precipitous falls in egg production were seen, while high mortality was recorded in younger birds. This virus did not induce respiratory signs in uncomplicated infections of pigeons or chickens.

The clinical signs produced by specific viruses in other hosts may differ widely from those seen in chickens. In general, turkeys are as susceptible as chickens to infection with NDV but clinical signs are usually less severe (50, 138). Although readily infected, ducks and geese are usually regarded as resistant, even to the strains of NDV most virulent for chickens. However, outbreaks of severe disease in ducks infected with NDV have been described (104). Outbreaks of virulent ND have been reported in most game bird species (126, 129) and the disease appears similar to that in chickens (44).

Avian Paramyxovirus Type 2. PMV-2 viruses have been associated with mild respiratory or inapparent diseases in chickens and turkeys (32, 54, 74). Unlike NDV, PMV-2 infections have been reported to be more severe in turkeys than chickens, and Lang et al. (130) reported severe respiratory disease, sinusitis, elevated mortality, and low egg production in turkey flocks infected with PMV-2 complicated by the presence of other organisms. PMV-2 viruses have been reported to be widespread in turkeys in Israel and associated with severe respiratory disease in complicated infections (133). In experiments conducted under field conditions, Bankowski et al. (33) demonstrated that PMV-2 infections of laying turkeys resulted in egg production losses with reduced hatchability and poult yield but fertility was unaffected.

Avian Paramyxovirus Type 3. PMV-3 virus infections of domestic poultry appear to have been restricted to turkeys. Clinical signs are usually egg production problems, although these have been occasionally preceded by mild respiratory disease (18, 28, 30, 135, 200). Egg production usually declined rapidly with a large number of white-shelled eggs, although hatchability and fertility were rarely affected.

Avian Paramyxovirus Type 6. PMV-6 isolates have also been obtained from turkeys showing mild respiratory disease and egg production problems. Viruses of this serotype have been isolated frequently from domestic ducks in which the virus appears to be apathogenic (137, 185).

Gross Lesions. As with clinical signs, the gross lesions and the organs affected in birds infected with NDV are dependent on the strain and pathotype of the infecting virus in addition to the host and all the other factors that may affect the severity of the disease. There are no pathognomonic lesions associated with any form of the disease. Gross lesions may also be absent.

Nevertheless, the presence of hemorrhagic lesions in the intestine of infected chickens has been used to distinguish VVND viruses from NVND viruses, a distinction of regulatory control importance in the diagnosis of ND in the USA (96, 101). These lesions are often particularly prominent in the proventriculus, ceca, and small intestine. They are markedly hemorrhagic and appear to result from necrosis of the intestinal wall or lymphoid foci, such as cecal tonsils.

Generally, gross lesions are not observed in the central nervous system of birds infected with NDV, regardless of the pathotype (138).

Gross pathological changes are not always present in the respiratory tract, but when observed they consist predominantly of hemorrhagic lesions and marked congestion of the trachea (13). Airsacculitis may be present even after infection with relatively mild strains and thickening of the air sacs with catarrhal or caseous exudates is often observed (39)

Chickens and turkeys infected in lay with velogenic viruses usually reveal egg yolk in the abdominal cavity. The ovarian follicles are often flaccid and degenerative. Hemorrhage and discoloration of the other reproductive organs may occur.

Histopathology. The histopathology of NDV infections is as varied as the clinical signs and gross lesions and can be greatly affected by the same parameters. In addition to the strain of virus and host, the method of infection may also be of paramount importance. For example, Beard and Easterday (38) were able to demonstrate similar histopathological changes in the tracheas of chickens infected with either lentogenic or velogenic viruses by the aerosol route. Most published descriptions of the histological changes following NDV infections are related to the virulent pathotypes, and several descriptive reports or reviews of the literature have covered the histological changes in the various organs during infection (38, 39, 138, 208). Briefly, the major changes are as follows.

VASCULAR SYSTEM. Hyperemia, edema, and hemorrhage are found in the blood vessels of many organs. Other changes that may be seen consist of hydropic degeneration of the media, hyalinization of capillaries and arterioles, development of hyaline thrombosis in small vessels, and necrosis of endothelial cells of the vessels.

LYMPHOID SYSTEM. A regressive change found in the lymphopoietic system consists of disappearance of lymphoid tissue. Hyperplasia of the reticulohistiocytic cells in various organs, especially the liver, may take place in subacute infections. Necrotic lesions are found throughout the spleen. Focal vacuolation and destruction of lymphocytes may be seen in the cortical areas and germinal centers of the spleen and thymus. Marked degeneration of the medullary region is seen in the bursa (194).

INTESTINAL TRACT. The hemorrhagic-necrotic lesions seen in the intestinal tract with infections of some virulent forms of ND appear to develop in lymphoid aggregates. Other lesions are related to changes in the vascular system.

RESPIRATORY TRACT. The effect of NDV infection on membranes of the upper respiratory tract may be severe and related to the degree of respiratory distress. Lesions may extend throughout the length of the trachea. Cilia may be lost within 2 days of infection. In the mucosa of the upper respiratory tract, congestion, edema, and dense cellular infiltration of lymphocytes and macrophages may be seen, particularly following aerosol exposure (38). The process appears to clear rapidly and birds examined as early as 6 days after infection may be free from inflammation.

Cheville et al. (58) infected birds with two US viscerotropic isolates, Texas 219 and Florida Largo. Marked lesions of the lung were seen with both viruses, the former producing hyperemia and edema of the parabronchi, the latter more extensive lesions consisting of hemorrhage and erythrophagocytosis in the alveolar areas of the parabronchi.

Edema, cell infiltration, and increased thickness and density of the air sacs may occur in chickens.

REPRODUCTIVE SYSTEM. Histopathological changes in the reproductive tract are extremely variable. Biswal and Morrill (47) reported the greatest functional damage was to the uterus or shell-forming portion of the oviduct. Changes in female reproductive organs included atresia of follicles with infiltration of inflammatory cells and formation of lymphoid aggregates. Similar aggregates were present in the oviduct.

OTHER ORGANS. Small focal areas of necrosis are seen in the liver and, sometimes with hemorrhage, in the gallbladder and heart. Lymphocyte infiltration has been reported in the pancreas. In infections with the viscerotropic velogenic viruses, hemorrhage and ulceration of the skin may occur; congestion and petechiae of the combs and wattle are common. Conjunctival lesions may be associated with hemorrhage.

Immunity

CELL-MEDIATED IMMUNITY. The initial immune response to infection with NDV is cell mediated and may be detectable as early as 2–3 days after infection with live vaccine strains (80, 198). This presumably explains the early protection against challenge that has been recorded in vaccinated birds before a measurable antibody response is seen (25, 87). The importance of cell-mediated immunity in protection conferred by vaccines is not clear and a strong secondary response to challenge similar to the antibody response does not seem to occur (198).

HUMORAL IMMUNITY. Antibodies capable of protecting the host can be measured in VN tests. However, since the VN response appears to parallel the HI response, the latter test is frequently used to assess protective response, especially after vaccination (26). Antibodies directed against either of the functional surface glycopolypeptides, the HN and F polypeptides, can neutralize NDVs (178). In fact, MABs specific for epitopes on the F polypeptide have been shown to induce greater neutralization than those directed against HN in in vitro and in vivo tests (148, 150). Therefore, the successful reliance on the simple HI test to assess protection up to now may have been fortuitous.

When chickens survive NDV infection long enough, antibodies are usually detectable in the serum within 6–10 days. The levels largely depend on the infecting strain, but generally, peak response is at about 3–4 wk. Decline in antibody titer varies with the titer achieved but is much slower than their development. HI antibodies may remain detectable for up to 1 yr in birds recovered from infection with mesogenic viruses or after a series of immunizations. Reinfection or immunization some weeks after the titer begins to decline produces a secondary response (26).

LOCAL IMMUNITY. Antibodies appear in secretions of the upper respiratory tract and intestinal tract of chickens at about the time humoral antibodies can be first detected. In the upper respiratory tract the immunoglobulins (Igs) appear to be chiefly IgA with some IgG (164). Similar excretions occur in the harderian gland following ocular but not parenteral infection (164, 169). Malkinson and Small (136) demonstrated effective local immunity when they found that birds may be susceptible to infection at one site but protected at another. The exact function of local immunity in protection is not clear, although a role in protection of the respiratory tract independent of humoral immunity has been proposed (110).

PASSIVE IMMUNITY. Hens with antibodies to NDV will pass these on to their progeny via the egg yolk (103). Levels of antibody in day-old chicks will be directly related to titers in the parent. Allan et al. (26) estimated that each two-fold decay in maternally derived HI titer takes about 4.5 days. Maternal immunity is protective and thus must be taken into account when timing primary vaccination of chicks.

IMMUNOSUPPRESSION. Suppression of the immune response has important effects on both the pathogenicity of infecting NDV strains and the protection levels achieved by vaccination. Under natural conditions immunosuppression may occur due to infection with other viruses such as infectious bursal disease virus. The subsequent immunodeficiency may result in a more severe disease caused by some NDV strains and a failure to respond adequately to vaccination (72, 82, 165, 174). More recently, immunosuppression from chicken anemia agent has been implicated in the failure of chickens to respond well to secondary inactivated NDV vaccine (53).

DIAGNOSIS.

The objective in the diagnosis of ND is to reach a decision on whether or not to impose control measures. None of the clinical signs or lesions of ND may be regarded as pathognomonic and the wide variation in disease with virus strain, host species and other factors means that, at best, these can only serve as a suggestion of ND. Similarly, the presence of lentogenic NDV strains in birds in most countries and the almost universal use of live vaccines means that mere demonstration of infection is rarely adequate cause for control measures to be imposed. Additionally, ND may cause such devastating epizootics and can have such far-reaching effects on trade in poultry products that control measures are usually defined at a national or international level.

Serology.

The presence of specific antibodies to NDV in the serum of a bird gives little information on the infecting strain of NDV and therefore has limited diagnostic value. Nevertheless, in certain circumstances the demonstration that infection has taken place is sufficient for the needs of the diagnostician. Postvaccinal serology can be used to confirm successful application of vaccine and an adequate immune response by the bird.

SEROLOGICAL TESTS FOR NDV ANTIBODIES. Antibodies to NDV may be detected in poultry sera by a variety of tests including single radial immunodiffusion (59), single radial hemolysis (102), agar-gel precipitin (78), VN in chick embryos (37), and plaque neutralization (39). Enzyme-linked immunosorbent assays, which lend themselves to semiautomated techniques, have become popular, especially as part of flock screening procedures (189), and a variety of such tests have been described (147, 152, 173, 188, 211). Conventionally, antibodies to NDV and the other avian paramyxoviruses have been detected and quantitated by the HI test. Many methods for HA and the HI tests have been described.

Sera from other species (including turkeys) may cause low-titer, nonspecific agglutination of chicken RBCs, complicating the test. Such agglutination may be removed by adsorption with chicken RBCs before testing.

HA and HI tests are not greatly affected by minor changes in the methodology although Brugh et al. (55) stressed the critical nature of the antigen/antiserum incubation period in test standardization. Surveys have not always reported good reproducibility in HI tests among different laboratories (40). An International Standard NDV Reference Antiserum is available from the International Laboratory for Biological Standards, Central Veterinary Laboratory, New Haw, Weybridge, Surrey, UK, which is intended for use in standardizing HI tests (195).

SEROLOGICAL TESTS FOR OTHER AVIAN PARAMYXOVIRUSES. The same serological tests used for NDV (PMV-1) can be used for the other avian paramyxoviruses with the exception of PMV-5 viruses, which do not hemagglutinate RBCs (160). HI antibodies to PMV-3 viruses may be detected in turkeys and chickens showing high vaccine-induced titers to NDV, and ND-vaccinated birds infected with PMV-3 viruses show a rise in HI titer to both viruses (18, 53).

Direct Detection of Viral Antigens. Immunohistological techniques offer a rapid method for the specific demonstration of the presence of virus or viral antigens in organs or tissues. Immunofluorescence techniques for thin sections of trachea (106) or impression smears (144) and an immunoperoxidase technique for thin sections (94) have been described and used in NDV infections.

Virus Isolation. At present, the only unequivocal method of ND diagnosis, which also allows characterization of the infecting strain, is virus isolation.

CULTURE SYSTEM. Virulent ND viruses can be propagated in many cell culture systems and viruses of low virulence can be induced to replicate in some of them. It is possible to use primary cell cultures or even cell lines for routine isolation of NDV. However, the embryonated chicken egg represents an extremely sensitive and convenient vehicle for the propagation of NDV and is used almost universally in diagnosis.

Embryonated chicken eggs should be obtained from a specific-pathogen-free (SPF) flock and incubated for 9–10 days at 37 C before use. If SPF eggs cannot be obtained, eggs from a flock free of NDV antibodies should be used. It is possible to propagate NDV strains in eggs containing yolk antibodies, but the virus titer is usually greatly reduced and such eggs should be avoided for diagnostic use.

SAMPLES. The two main sites of replication of NDV in infected poultry appear to be the respiratory and intestinal tracts so specimens taken should always include either feces, intestinal contents or cloacal swabs, and trachea or tracheal swabs, depending on the circumstances. Other specimens taken from carcasses should reflect the clinical signs prior to death and organs obviously affected.

NDV is relatively stable for long periods in nonputrefying tissues provided the ambient temperature is low (126). However, Gough et al. (91), considered the transport of samples in a frozen or chilled state as very important in virus isolation. Omojola and Hanson (163) suggested that bone marrow may be a useful sample in countries where transport is slow, temperatures high, and refrigeration not available, as they were able to isolate virus from this site after several days at 30 C.

ISOLATION METHOD. Ideally, each sample should be treated separately. However, it is common to pool organ and tissue samples although tracheal and fecal samples are best kept separate. Antibiotic media are used to make 20% w/v suspensions of feces or finely minced tissues and organs. Swabs are placed in sufficient antibiotic medium to ensure full immersion.

The suspensions are held at room temperature for 1–2 hr, then centrifuged at 1000 g's for 10 min. Each of five embryonated eggs should then be inoculated with 0.2 ml of the supernatant fluid into the allantoic cavity. The eggs are placed at 37 C and examined regularly.

Eggs dead or dying, or after a minimum of 4 days and a maximum of 7 days, should be chilled to 4 C and the allantoic/amniotic fluid harvested. The presence of virus can be detected by an HA test; nonhemagglutinating fluids should be passaged at least one more time. HA may be caused by bacteria and possible contamination should be assessed by culture. If bacteria are present the contaminated fluids can be passed through a 450-nm-membrane filter before repassaging in eggs.

ISOLATION OF OTHER AVIAN PARAMYXOVIRUSES. The samples taken and methods involved for the isolation of other avian paramyxoviruses are identical to those for NDV. However, inoculation of 6- to 7-day-old embryonated eggs via the yolk sac should also be considered, as greater success has been reported for this route with some viruses. PMV-5 viruses do not grow after inoculation into the allantoic cavity and require amniotic inoculation of embryonating eggs or propagation in primary cultures of chick embryo cells (160).

Differential Diagnosis. Viral HA activity may be due to any of the 9 avian paramyxovirus serotypes or any of the 13 influenza type A hemagglutinin subtypes that are known to infect birds. Demonstration that the virus is of a specific serotype can usually be carried out by a simple HI test with specific polyclonal antisera.

NDV (PMV-1) shows some cross-reaction in HI tests with several of the other avian paramyxovirus serotypes, especially PMV-3 psittacine isolates, using polyclonal antisera (10). While the potential for misdiagnosis can largely be eliminated by the use of control sera and antigens in conventional tests, the use of MABs in routine diagnosis can give an unequivocal result.

Virus Characterization. For ND, the widespread presence of lentogenic strains in feral birds and the use of such viruses as live vaccines means that isolation of NDV is rarely sufficient to confirm a diagnosis of disease. For such confirmation and to meet statutory requirements that may be in force (45), further virus characterization such as pathogenicity testing is necessary.

PATHOGENICITY TESTS. The importance and impact of an NDV isolate will be directly related to the virulence of that isolate. Since field disease may be an unreliable measure of the true virulence of the virus, it is necessary to carry out laboratory assessment of the pathogenicity of the virus. At present three in vivo tests are used for this purpose: 1) mean death time (MDT) in eggs, 2) ICPI, and 3) IVPI.

Examples of the values obtained in these three methods are shown for some well-characterized NDV strains in Table 19.2.

Some modifications of these tests have been made for specific purposes. For example, Hanson (96) used a method similar to the IVPI test, which involved swabbing the cloaca and conjunctiva of 8-wk-old chickens with undiluted allantoic fluid to distinguish between VVNDV and other velogenic viruses.

Although these pathogenicity tests have proved invaluable in distinguishing between vaccine, enzootic, and epizootic viruses during outbreaks, there are some drawbacks to the tests and difficulties in the interpretation of results. For example, Pearson et al. (166) reported 10 NDV isolates from pigeons to have ICPI values between 1.2 and 1.45 and a range of IVPI values of 0–1.3, suggesting the viruses to be at least mesogenic; however, the lowest MDT recorded was 98 hr, a characteristic of lentogenic viruses. In addition, work by Alexander and Parsons (16) on NDV (PMV-1) isolates from pigeons showed that both ICPI and IVPI values increased after passage through chickens or embryonated chicken eggs. This suggests that isolates from birds other than poultry may not show their potential virulence for chickens in conventional pathogenicity tests.

IN VITRO TESTS FOR PATHOGENICITY. Only NDVs possessing additional basic amino acids at the cleavage site of the fusion protein are rendered infectious by non-trypsinlike proteases. Rott (176) therefore suggested that the ability of NDV isolates to form plaques in cell culture systems in the absence of trypsin represents a simple in vitro method for the detection of virulent viruses.

VIRUS PROPERTY PROFILES. NDV isolates show a marked variation in biological and biochemical properties (see Etiology), and some workers used these properties to develop distinct profiles that allowed the grouping viruses for the purposes of diagnosis (39, 96). Under specific circumstances single properties of the virus may be sufficient to

Table 19.2. Examples of pathogenicity indices obtained for strains of NDV

Virus Strain	Pathotype	ICPI[a]	IVPI[b]	MDT[c]
Ulster 2C	Lentogenic	0.00	0.00	>150
Queensland V4	"	0.00	0.00	>150
Hitchner B1	"	0.20	0.00	120
F	"	0.25	0.00	119
La Sota	"	0.40	0.00	103
H	Mesogenic	1.20	0.00	48
Mukteswar	"	1.40	0.00	46
Roakin	"	1.45	0.00	68
Beaudette C	"	1.60	1.45	62
GB Texas	Velogenic	1.75	2.70	55
NY Parrott 70181 1972	"	1.80	2.60	51
Italian	"	1.85	2.80	50
Milano	"	1.90	2.80	50
Herts '33/56	"	2.00	2.70	48
Pigeon/England/561/83		1.50	0.00	120
Chicken/England/702/84		1.90	2.10	60

Note: Data from (11, 26).
[a]ICPI = intracerebral pathogenicity index in day-old chicks.
[b]IVPI = intravenous pathogenicity index in 6-wk-old chickens.
[c]MDT = mean death time (hr) for chicken embryos infected with one minimum lethal dose of virus.

distinguish between avirulent and virulent isolates and be usefully employed in diagnosis.

MONOCLONAL ANTIBODIES. In addition to their use in routine diagnosis, panels of MABs can be employêd to characterize and group isolates by establishing profiles. Such typing on an antigenic basis represents a powerful tool for the diagnostician and epizootiologist, allowing rapid grouping and differentiation of NDV isolates (24, 178).

PREVENTION AND CONTROL.

Regardless of whether control is applied at the international, national, or farm levels, the objective is to either prevent susceptible birds from becoming infected or to reduce the number of susceptible birds by vaccination. For the former strategy, each method of disease spread must be considered in prevention policies.

International Control Policies.

The raising of poultry and trade in their products is now organized on an international basis, frequently under the management of multinational companies. There is a desire to trade both poultry products and genetic stock. However, the threat of ND has proven a great restraint on such trade. Bennejean (45) considered that worldwide control of ND will be approached only if all countries report outbreaks within their borders to international agencies. International agreements on these and other points are not simple due to the enormous variation in the extent of disease surveillance in different countries.

A prerequisite to formulating control policies, particularly internationally, would be agreement on what constitutes disease and to what viruses control policies should apply. Some countries do not vaccinate and would not want any form of NDV introduced to their domestic poultry. Others allow only specific live vaccines and consider some vaccines to be unacceptably virulent. Yet other countries have the continued presence of circulating highly virulent virus, which is not seen as overt disease because of vaccination. Bennejean (45) suggested that any infection with virus having an ICPI greater than 0.7 should be reported as an outbreak of ND. Such a definition would probably be acceptable in countries where only lentogenic and inactivated vaccines are used, but completely unacceptable where mesogenic vaccines are used or where enzootic mesogenic viruses exist. Nevertheless this definition does not seem unreasonable and adoption of this definition may represent a goal for countries to achieve.

National Control Policies.

At the national level, control policies are directed at prevention of introduction of virus and prevention of spread within the country. To prevent the introduction of NDV, most countries have restrictions on trade in poultry products, eggs, and live poultry; these vary greatly.

Because of the link between exotic caged birds and the spread of ND during the 1970–74 panzootic (75, 204), and the known ability of psittacine birds to excrete NDV for many weeks after infection (69), most importing countries have established quarantine procedures for importations.

The panzootic of ND (PMV-1) in racing pigeons in the 1980s (203) produced a unique situation, in view of the potential spread to poultry (210). Due to the large number of international pigeon races that take place each year, national policies were created in some countries including banning of races, restricting races, or enforcing vaccination of participating pigeons.

In many countries legislation exists to control ND outbreaks that may occur. Some countries have adopted eradication policies with compulsory slaughter of infected birds, their contacts, and products. Such policies usually include restrictions of movement or marketing of birds within a defined quarantine area around the outbreak. Others require prophylactic vaccination of birds even in the absence of outbreaks, while some have a policy of "ring vaccination" around outbreaks to establish a buffer zone.

Higgins and Shortridge (105) stressed the importance of tailoring control policies to the country and warned against the dogmatic application of policies successful in one country to another that may differ socially, economically, and climatically.

Control and Prevention at the Farm Level.

Possibly the most important factors in preventing the introduction of NDV and its spread during outbreaks are the conditions under which the birds are reared and the degree of biosecurity practiced at the farm. Chapter 1 provides a comprehensive discussion of disease prevention through sanitation and security practices.

Control for Other Avian Paramyxoviruses.

Few, if any, countries have national control policies for the other avian paramyxoviruses, although in some, vaccination is permitted for PMV-3 viruses. Thus, despite the frequent isolation of PMV-2 and PMV-3 viruses from passerine and psittacine birds in quarantine (8), little is usually done to restrict the introduction of such birds.

At the farm level, birdproofing of poultry houses should greatly reduce the possibility of introduction of paramyxoviruses such as PMV-2 by feral birds. Other preventative measures taken for NDV will equally apply to the other PMV types. Lang et al. (130) suggested depopulation for turkey flocks infected with PMV-2 virus if complicated by other organisms.

Newcastle Disease Vaccination. Ideally, vaccination against ND would result in immunity against infection and replication of the virus. Realistically, ND vaccination usually protects the bird from the more serious consequences of disease, but virus replication and shedding may still occur, albeit at a reduced level.

Allan et al. (26) have produced a comprehensive description of all aspects of ND vaccination and vaccine production. More recently, detailed reviews have been published by Meulemans (146) on the use of vaccination in the control of ND, by Cross (64) on vaccine production, and by Thornton (197) on quality control of vaccines.

It should be emphasized that there are no circumstances in which vaccination can be regarded as an alternative to good management practice, biosecurity, or good hygiene in rearing domestic poultry.

HISTORICAL ASPECTS OF VACCINATION. Early studies demonstrated that inactivated infective material conferred protection on inoculated chickens, but problems in production and standardization discouraged its use on a large scale. Studies in the 1930s on the attenuation of virulent NDV strains by Haddow and Idmani and Iyer and Dobson (92, 115) led to the development of mesogenic vaccine strains that are still in use in some parts of the World.

The identification of ND in the USA led, initially, to the use of inactivated vaccines (109). The later observation that some of the enzootic viruses produced only mild disease resulted first in the development of the mesogenic live vaccine Roakin (43) and, subsequently, in the development of the milder Hitchner B1 (108) and La Sota (84) strains, which are now the most widely used vaccines.

Inactivated vaccines, usually with the virus adsorbed to aluminum hydroxide, were most widely used in Europe up to the 1970–74 panzootic, but their poor performance resulted in adoption of live vaccination with B1 and La Sota in most countries. However, this panzootic also supplied the impetus for the development of modern inactivated vaccines based on oil emulsions, which have proven highly effective.

VACCINATION POLICIES. Some governments have legislation affecting the use and quality control of vaccines. Policies vary enormously, in line with the enzootic status or perceived threat of ND. Some countries, such as Northern Ireland, ban the use of any vaccine, while others, e.g., the Netherlands, enforce vaccination of all poultry.

LIVE VACCINES

Virus Strains. It is convenient to divide live NDV vaccines into two groups, lentogenic and mesogenic, the mesogenic being suitable only for secondary vaccination of birds due to their greater virulence (Table 19.3). However, even within the lentogenic group there is a considerable range in virulence, as demonstrated by Borland and Allan (48), who developed a stress index test to assess the potential effects of vaccines on susceptible chickens. The immune response increases as the pathogenicity of the live vaccine increases (172). Therefore, to obtain the desired level of protection without serious reaction, vaccination programs are needed that involve sequential use of progressively more virulent viruses, or live virus followed by inactivated vaccine. Commonly used live vaccines and their pathogenicity indices for chickens are listed in Table 19.3.

Table 19.3. NDV viruses used as live vaccines

Virus	Pathotype	ICPI[a]	IVPI[b]	Derivation	Recommended Use in Chickens	Routes[c]
Strain H	Mesogenic	1.40	0.00	Laboratory attenuated by passage in eggs	Secondary	im, sc
Mukteswar	Mesogenic	1.40	0.00	Laboratory attenuated by passage in eggs	Secondary	im, sc
Komarov	Mesogenic	1.40	0.00	Laboratory attenuated by intracerebral passage in ducklings	Secondary	im, sc, io
Roakin	Mesogenic	1.45	0.00	Field isolate	Secondary	im, ww
La Sota	Lentogenic	0.40	0.00	Field isolate	Secondary	in, io, dw, sp, aer
F (Asplin)	Lentogenic	0.25	0.00	Field isolate	Primary	in, io, dw, sp, aer
Hitchner B1	Lentogenic	0.20	0.00	Field isolate	Primary	in, io, dw, sp, aer, bd
V4	Lentogenic	0.00	0.00	Field isolate	Primary	in, io, sp, aer, oral

[a]ICPI = intracerebral pathogenicity index in day-old chicks.
[b]IVPI = intravenous pathogenicity index in 6-wk-old chickens.
[c]Routes: im = intramuscular; sc = subcutaneous; in = intranasal; ww = wing web; io = intraocular; sp = coarse spray; dw = drinking water; aer = aerosol; bd = beak dipping; oral = in food.

Application of Live Vaccines. The objective of live vaccines is to establish an infection in the flock, preferably in each bird at the time of application. Individual bird treatments such as intranasal instillation, eyedropper, and beak dipping are often used for lentogenic vaccines. Mesogenic vaccines usually require inoculation by wing-web stabbing or intramuscular injection.

The main appeal of live vaccines is that they may be administered by inexpensive mass application techniques. Probably the most common method of application used worldwide is via the drinking water. Generally, water is withheld from the birds for a number of hours, and then vaccine is applied in fresh drinking water at concentrations carefully calculated to give each bird a sufficient dose. Addition of vaccine to header tanks has also been used successfully. Drinking water application must be carefully monitored, as the virus may be inactivated by excessive ambient heat, impurities in the water, and even the type of pipes or vessels used to distribute the water. To some extent virus viability can be stabilized by the addition of dried skim milk powder to the drinking water (79).

Mass application of live vaccines by sprays and aerosols is also very popular due to the ease with which large numbers of birds can be vaccinated in a short time. It is important to achieve the correct size of particles by controlling the conditions under which the aerosol is generated (26, 146). Aerosol application is usually limited to secondary vaccination to avoid severe vaccine reactions. Coarse sprays of large particles do not penetrate deeply into the respiratory tract of birds and give less reaction, so these may be more suitable for the mass application of vaccine to young birds. Coarse spraying of day-old chicks may result in the establishment of infection in the flock with the vaccinal virus despite maternally derived immunity. However, it is believed that in these circumstances infections are established by the nasal or ocular route as a result of head rubbing on the backs of other birds and not necessarily directly by the spray (146). Aerosol and coarse-spray generators are available commercially; in the USA a cabinet for coarse spraying of day-old chicks is widely used (81).

A vaccine, based on the Australian V4 virus, has been developed specifically for use in village flocks in tropical countries. The recommended method of administration of the vaccine is in coated, pelleted food, which is fed to the chickens. Laboratory and field trials suggest that this method is efficacious (63).

Advantages and Disadvantages of Live Virus Vaccination. Live vaccines are usually sold as freeze-dried allantoic fluid from infected embryonated eggs and are relatively inexpensive, easy to administer, and lend themselves to mass application. Local immunity is stimulated by infection with live viruses and protection occurs very soon after application. Vaccine viruses may spread from birds that have been successfully vaccinated to those that have not.

There are several disadvantages, the most important is that the vaccine may cause disease, depending upon environmental conditions and the presence of complicating infections. Because of this, it is important to use extremely mild virus for primary vaccination and, as a result, multiple applications of vaccine(s) are usually needed. Maternally derived immunity may prevent successful primary vaccination with live virus. Although the ability of vaccinal virus to spread may be an advantage within the flock, spread to susceptible flocks, especially on multiage sites, can cause severe disease problems. Live vaccines may be easily killed by chemicals and heat and, if not carefully controlled during production, can contain contaminating viruses.

INACTIVATED VACCINES

Production Methods. Inactivated vaccines are usually produced from infective allantoic fluid treated with betapropiolactone or formalin to kill the virus and mixed with a carrier adjuvant. Early inactivated vaccines used aluminum hydroxide adjuvants but the development of oil-emulsion-based vaccines proved a major advancement. Different oil-emulsion vaccines vary in their formulation of emulsifiers, antigen, and water-to-oil ratios; most now use mineral oil (64).

Various seed viruses used in the production of the oil-emulsion vaccines include Ulster 2C, B1, La Sota, Roakin, and several virulent viruses. The selection criterion should be the amount of antigen produced when the virus is grown in embryonated eggs. Apathogenic viruses grow to the highest titers (90); therefore, it would seem an unnecessary risk to use a virus virulent for chickens.

One or more other antigens may be incorporated into the emulsion with NDV, and bivalent or polyvalent vaccines may include infectious bronchitis virus, infectious bursal disease virus, egg drop syndrome virus, and reovirus (146).

Application of Inactivated Vaccines. Inactivated vaccines are administered by injection, either intramuscularly or subcutaneously.

Advantages and Disadvantages of Inactivated Vaccines. Inactivated vaccines are far easier to store than viable vaccines. They are expensive to produce and to apply because of the labor needed for their application; labor expense can be partly offset by the use of polyvalent vaccines. Inactivated oil-emulsion vaccines are not as adversely affected by maternal immunity as live vaccines and can be used in day-old chicks (51). Quality control of inactivated vaccines is often difficult and mineral oils may cause serious problems to the vaccinator if accidentally injected (196). The major advantages of inactivated vaccine are the very low level of adverse reactions in vaccinated birds, the ability to use them in situations unsuited for live vaccines, especially if complicating pathogens are present, and the extremely high levels of protective antibodies of long duration that can be achieved.

VACCINATION PROGRAMS. Vaccination programs and vaccines may be controlled by government policies. They should always be tailored to suit the prevailing disease situation and other factors, which include availability of vaccine, maternal immunity, use of other vaccines, presence of other organisms, size of flock, expected life of the flock, available labor, climatic conditions, past vaccination history, and cost.

Timing of vaccination of broiler chickens can be especially difficult due to the presence of maternal antibodies. Because of their short life, broiler chickens are sometimes not vaccinated in countries where there is a low risk of ND.

Vaccination of laying hens always requires more than one dose of vaccine to maintain immunity through their lives (26). Actual programs depend on local conditions. In many countries local customs or circumstances result in too little vaccination, over-vaccination, or mistiming of vaccination, all of which may have serious consequences. The problems and pressures that may face the poultry farmer in tropical developing countries can frequently result in what has been described as "vaccine abuse" (105).

INTERPRETATION OF VACCINE RESPONSE. For NDV the immune response is usually estimated by the HI titers obtained. Single vaccination with live lentogenic virus will produce a response in susceptible birds of about 2^4–2^6, but HI titers as high as 2^{11} or more may be obtained following a vaccination program involving oil-emulsion vaccine. The actual titers obtained and their relationship to the degree and duration of immunity for any given flock and program are difficult to predict. Allan et al. (26) presented predictions of the outcome of challenge of vaccinated young chickens with highly virulent NDV.

VACCINATION OF OTHER POULTRY. Although vaccines developed primarily for chickens may be used effectively in other species, some differences in response may be apparent. For example, turkeys generally show a lower response and, as a result, are often vaccinated first with La Sota followed by oil-emulsion vaccine (52). However, there is some evidence that La Sota may cause some reaction in the respiratory tract (146), and aerosol vaccination with lentogenic viruses causes pathological lesions of the trachea (1). There is still considerable investigation into vaccination programs, involving live and inactivated vaccines for use in turkeys (119, 124).

Guinea fowl and partridges have been vaccinated successfully with La Sota and/or oil-emulsion vaccines. Considerable investigation into the most suitable vaccines and regimens for pigeons has taken place due to the panzootic occurring in these birds during the 1980s (203).

FUTURE DEVELOPMENTS. Recently developed molecular biology technology has enabled a much greater understanding of the pathogenicity (177) and antigenicity (178) of NDV and has enabled cloning of the genes most closely involved (153). It is therefore possible to speculate on the use of cloned genes expressed in vectors or subunit vaccines for ND. Several groups are working along these lines of investigation at present. For example, Meulemans et al. (151) have demonstrated that chickens may be immunized by infection with recombinant vaccinia virus expressing NDV F glycoprotein. Subunit vaccines consisting of peptides of very few amino acids may be prepared synthetically to match very small areas of the polypeptide identified as immunologically important by MABs or predicted as such by computer analysis.

The capacity of MABs to detect antigenic variation in NDV isolates may have an important application in assessing antigenic relationships between field and vaccine viruses and ensuring close similarity between the two.

VACCINATION FOR OTHER AVIAN PARAMYXOVIRUSES. The other avian paramyxoviruses do not cause overt disease with high mortality and thus their economic impact is considerably less than NDV. Nevertheless, the egg production problems that have been associated with infections of turkeys by PMV-3 viruses can be sufficiently severe to warrant vaccination; for several years oil-emulsion vaccines to this serotype have been available in Great Britain and the USA (49, 70). They appear to be effective at preventing the serious egg production losses associated with PMV-3 infections in laying turkeys.

REFERENCES

1. Abdul-Aziz, T.A., and L.H. Arp. 1983. Pathology of the trachea in turkeys exposed by aerosol to lentogenic strains of Newcastle disease virus. Avian Dis 27:1002–1011.
2. Abenes, G.B., H. Kida, R. Yanagawa. 1983. Avian paramyxoviruses possessing antigenically related HN but distinct M proteins. Arch Virol 77:71–76.
3. Abenes, G.B., H. Kida, R. Yanagawa. 1986. Biological activities of monoclonal antibodies to the hemagglutinin-neuraminidase (HN) protein of Newcastle disease virus. Jpn J Vet Sci 48:353–362.

4. Ackerman, W.W. 1964. Cell surface phenomena of Newcastle disease virus. In R.P. Hanson (ed.), Newcastle Disease Virus An Evolving Pathogen, pp. 153-166. Univ Wisconsin Press, Madison.
5. Alexander, D.J. 1980. Avian Paramyxoviruses. Vet Bull 50:737-752.
6. Alexander, D.J. 1982. Avian paramyxoviruses—other than Newcastle disease virus. World Poult Sci J 38:97-104.
7. Alexander, D.J. 1985. Avian paramyxoviruses. Proc 34th West Poult Dis Conf, pp. 121-125.
8. Alexander, D.J. 1986. The classification, host range and distribution of avian paramyxoviruses. In J.B. McFerran and M.S. McNulty (eds.), Acute Virus Infections of Poultry, pp. 52-66. Martinus Nijhoff, Dordrecht, Neth.
9. Alexander, D.J. 1988. Historical Aspects. In D.J. Alexander (ed.), Newcastle Disease, pp. 1-10. Kluwer Academic Publ, Boston.
10. Alexander, D.J. 1988. Newcastle Disease Virus—An Avian Paramyxovirus. In D.J. Alexander (ed.), Newcastle Disease, pp. 11-22. Kluwer Academic Publ, Boston.
11. Alexander, D.J. 1988. Newcastle Disease Diagnosis. In D.J. Alexander (ed.), Newcastle Disease, pp. 147-160. Kluwer Academic Publ, Boston.
12. Alexander, D.J. 1988. Newcastle Disease: Methods of Spread. In D.J. Alexander (ed.), Newcastle Disease, pp. 256-272. Kluwer Academic Publ, Boston.
13. Alexander, D.J., and W.H. Allan. 1974. Newcastle disease virus pathotypes. Avian Pathol 3:269-278.
14. Alexander, D.J., and N.J. Chettle. 1978. Relationship of parakeet/Netherlands/449/75 virus to other avian paramyxoviruses. Res Vet Sci 25:105-106.
15. Alexander, D.J., and M.S. Collins. 1981. The structural polypeptides of avian paramyxoviruses. Arch Virol 67:309-323.
16. Alexander, D.J., and G. Parsons. 1986. Pathogenicity for chickens of avian paramyxovirus type 1 isolates obtained from pigeons in Great Britain during 1983-1985. Avian Pathol 15:487-493.
17. Alexander, D.J., N.J. Chettle, and G. Parsons. 1979. Resistance of chickens to challenge with the virulent Herts '33 strain of Newcastle disease virus induced by prior infection with serologically distinct avian paramyxoviruses. Res Vet Sci 26:198-201.
18. Alexander, D.J., M. Pattisson, and I. Macpherson. 1983. Avian paramyxoviruses of PMV-3 serotype in British turkeys. Avian Pathol 12:469-482.
19. Alexander, D.J., V.S. Hinshaw, M.S. Collins, and N. Yamane. 1983. Characterization of viruses which represent further distinct serotypes (PMV-8 and PMV-9) of avian paramyxoviruses. Arch Virol 78:29-36.
20. Alexander, D.J., G. Parsons, and R. Marshall. 1984. Infection of fowls with Newcastle disease virus by food contaminated with pigeon faeces. Vet Rec 115:601-602.
21. Alexander, D.J., P.H. Russell, G. Parsons, E.M.E. Abu Elzein, A. Ballough, K. Cernik, B. Engstrom, M. Fevereiro, H.J.A. Fleury, M. Guittet, E.F. Kaleta, U. Kihm, J. Kosters, B. Lomniczi, J. Meister, G. Meulemans, K. Nerome, M. Petek, S. Pokomunski, B. Polten, M. Prip, R. Richter, E. Saghy, Y. Samberg, L. Spanoghe, and B. Tumova. 1985. Antigenic and biological characterisation of avian paramyxovirus type 1 isolates from pigeons—an international collaborative study. Avian Pathol 14:365-376.
22. Alexander, D.J., G.W.C. Wilson, P.H. Russell, S.A. Lister, and G. Parsons. 1985. Newcastle disease outbreaks in fowl in Great Britain during 1984. Vet Rec 117:429-434.
23. Alexander, D.J., J.S. Mackenzie, and P.H. Russell. 1986. Two types of Newcastle disease virus isolated from feral birds in Western Australia detected by monoclonal antibodies. Aust Vet J 63:365-367.
24. Alexander, D.J., R.J. Manvell, P.A. Kemp, G. Parsons, M.S. Collins, S. Brockman, P.H. Russell, and S.A. Lister 1987. Use of monoclonal antibodies in the characterisation of avian paramyxovirus type 1 (Newcastle disease virus) isolates submitted to an international reference laboratory. Avian Pathol 16:553-565.
25. Allan, W.H., and R.E. Gough. 1976. A comparison between the haemagglutination inhibition and complement fixation tests for Newcastle disease. Res Vet Sci 20:101-103.
26. Allan, W.H., J.E. Lancaster, and B. Toth. 1978. Newcastle disease vaccines—their production and use. FAO Anim Prod Ser No. 10. FAO, Rome.
27. Anderson, C., R. Kearsley, D.J. Alexander, and P.H. Russell. 1987. Antigenic variation in avian paramyxovirus type 3 detected by mouse monoclonal antibodies. Avian Pathol 16:691-698.
28. Andral, B., and D. Toquin. 1984. Infectious a myxovirus: Chutes de ponte chez les dindes reproductrices I Infections par les paramyxovirus aviaires de type III. Recl Med Vet 160:43-48.
29. Asplin, F.D. 1952. Immunisation against Newcastle disease with a virus of low virulence (Strain F) and observations on subclinical infection in partially resistant fowls. Vet Rec 64:245-249.
30. Bahl, A.K., and M.L. Vickers. 1982. Egg drop syndrome in breeder turkeys associated with turkey para-influenza virus-3 (TPIV-3). Proc 31st West Poult Dis Conf, p. 113.
31. Bankowski, R.A., R.E. Corstvet, and G.T. Clark. 1960. Isolation of an unidentified agent from the respiratory tract of chickens. Science 132:292-293.
32. Bankowski, R.A., R.D. Conrad, and B. Reynolds. 1968. Avian influenza and paramyxoviruses complicating respiratory disease diagnosis in poultry. Avian Dis 12:259-278.
33. Bankowski, R.A., J. Almquist, and J. Dombrucki. 1981. Effect of paramyxovirus Yucaipa on fertility, hatchability and poult yield of turkeys. Avian Dis 25:517-520.
34. Barahona, H.H., and R.P. Hanson. 1968. Plaque enhancement of Newcastle disease virus (lentogenic strains) by magnesium and diethylaminoethyl dextran. Avian Dis 12:151-158.
35. Beach, J.R. 1942. Avian pneumoencephalitis. Proc Annu Meet US Livestock Sanit Assoc 46:203-223.
36. Beach, J.R. 1944. The neutralization in vitro of avian pneumoencephalitis virus by Newcastle disease immune serum. Science 100:361-362.
37. Beard, C.W. 1980. Serologic procedures. In S.B. Hitchner, C.H. Domermuth, H.G. Purchase, and J.E. Williams (eds), Isolation and Identification of Avian Pathogens, pp. 129-135. Am Assoc Avian Pathol, Kennett Square, PA.
38. Beard, C.W., and B.C. Easterday. 1967. The influence of route of administration of Newcastle disease virus on host response. J Infect Dis 117:55-70.
39. Beard, C.W., and R.P. Hanson. 1984. Newcastle disease. In M.S. Hofstad, H.J. Barnes, B.W. Calnek, W.M. Reid, H.W. Yoder (eds.), Diseases of Poultry, 8th Ed., pp. 452-470. Iowa State Univ Press, Ames.
40. Beard, C.W., and W.J. Wilkes. 1985. A comparison of Newcastle disease hemagglutination-inhibition test results from diagnostic laboratories in the southeastern United States. Avian Dis 29:1048-1056.
41. Beard, P.D., J. Spalatin, and R.P. Hanson. 1970. Strain identification of NDV in tissue culture. Avian Dis 14:636-645.
42. Beaudette, F.R., and J.J. Black. 1946. Newcastle

disease in New Jersey. Proc Annu Meet US Livest Sanit Assoc 49:49-58.
43. Beaudette, F.R., J.A. Bivins, and B.R. Miller. 1949. Newcastle disease immunization with live virus. Cornell Vet 39:302-334.
44. Beer, J.V. 1976. Newcastle disease in the pheasant, Phasianus colchicus, in Britain. In L.A. Page (ed.), Wildlife Diseases, pp. 423-430. Plenum Press, New York.
45. Bennejean, G. 1988. Newcastle disease: Control policies. In D.J. Alexander (ed.), Newcastle Disease, pp. 303-317. Kluwer Academic Publ, Boston.
46. Biancifiori, F., and A. Fioroni. 1983. An occurrence of Newcastle disease in pigeons: Virological and serological studies on the isolates. Comp Immunol Microbiol Infect Dis 6:247-252.
47. Biswal, G., and C.C. Morrill. 1954. The pathology of the reproductive tract of laying pullets affected with Newcastle disease. Poult Sci 33:880-897.
48. Borland, L.J., and W.H. Allan. 1980. Laboratory tests for comparing live lentogenic Newcastle disease vaccines. Avian Pathol 9:45-59.
49. Box, P. 1987. PMV3 disease of turkeys. Int Hatch Prac 2:4-7.
50. Box, P.G., B.I. Helliwell, and P.H. Halliwell. 1970. Newcastle disease in turkeys. Vet Rec 86:524-527.
51. Box, P.G., I.G.S. Furminger, W.W. Robertson, and D. Warden. 1976. The effect of Marek's disease vaccination on the immunisation of day-old chicks against Newcastle disease, using B1 and oil emulsion vaccine. Avian Pathol 5:299-305.
52. Box, P.G., I.G.S. Furminger, W.W. Robertson, and D. Warden. 1976. Immunisation of maternally immune turkey poults against Newcastle disease. Avian Pathol 5:307-314.
53. Box, P.G., H.C. Holmes, A.C. Bushell, and P.M. Finney. 1988. Impaired response to killed Newcastle disease vaccine in chicken possessing circulating antibody to chicken anaemia agent. Avian Pathol 17:713-723.
54. Bradshaw, G.L., and M.M. Jensen. 1979. The epidemiology of Yucaipa virus in relationship to the acute respiratory disease syndrome in turkeys. Avian Dis 23:539-542.
55. Brugh, M., C.W. Beard, and W.J. Wilkes. 1978. The influence of test conditions on Newcastle disease hemagglutination-inhibition titers. Avian Dis 22:320-328.
56. Burnet, F.M. 1942. The affinity of Newcastle disease virus to the influenza virus group. Aust J Exp Biol Med Sci 20:81-88.
57. Chambers, P., N.S. Millar, and P.T. Emmerson. 1986. Nucleotide sequence of the gene encoding the fusion glycoprotein of Newcastle disease virus. J Gen Virol 67:2685-2694.
58. Cheville, N.F., H. Stone, J. Riley, and A.E. Ritchie. 1972. Pathogenesis of virulent Newcastle disease in chickens. J Am Vet Med Assoc 161:169-179.
59. Chu, H.P., G. Snell, D.J. Alexander, and G.C. Schild. 1982. A single radial immunodiffusion test for antibodies to Newcastle disease virus. Avian Pathol 11:227-234.
60. Cole, R.K., and F.B. Hutt. 1961. Genetic differences in resistance to Newcastle disease. Avian Dis 5:205-214.
61. Collins, M.S., D.J. Alexander, S. Brockman, P.A. Kemp, and R.J. Manvell. 1989. Evaluation of mouse monoclonal antibodies raised against an isolate of the variant avian paramyxovirus type 1 responsible for the current panzootic in pigeons. Arch Virol 104:53-61.
62. Coman, I. 1963. Possibility of the elimination of strain F virus of Asplin (1949) in the eggs of inoculated hens. Lucr Inst Past Igiena Anim Buc 12:337-344.
63. Copland J.W. 1987. Newcastle disease in poultry. A new food pellet vaccine. Australian Centre for Int Agric Res Monogr No 5. ACIAR, Canberra.
64. Cross, G.M. 1988. Newcastle disease–vaccine production. In D.J. Alexander (ed.), Newcastle Disease, pp 333-346. Kluwer Academic Publ, Boston.
65. Dinter, Z., S. Hermodsson & L. Hermodsson. 1964. Studies on myxovirus Yucaipa: Its classification as a member of the paramyxovirus group. Virology 22:297-304.
66. Doyle, T.M. 1927. A hitherto unrecorded disease of fowls due to a filter-passing virus. J Comp Pathol Ther 40:144-169.
67. Doyle, T.M. 1935. Newcastle disease of fowls. J Comp Pathol Ther 48:1-20.
68. Erdei, J., J. Erdei, K. Bachir, E.F. Kaleta, K.F. Shortridge, and B. Lomniczi. 1987. Newcastle disease vaccine (La Sota) strain specific monoclonal antibody. Arch Virol 96:265-269.
69. Erickson, G.A. 1976. Viscerotropic velogenic Newcastle disease in six pet bird species: Clinical response and virus-host interactions. PhD Diss. Iowa State Univ, Ames.
70. Eskelund, K.H. 1988. Vaccination of turkey breeder hens against paramyxovirus type 3 infection. Proc 37th West Poult Dis Conf, pp. 43-45.
71. Estupinan, J., J. Spalatin, and R.P. Hanson. 1968. Use of yolk sac route of inoculation for titration of lentogenic strains of NDV. Avian Dis 12:135-138.
72. Faragher, J.T., W.H. Allan, and P.J. Wyeth. 1974. Immunosuppressive effect of infectious bursal disease agent in vaccination against Newcastle disease. Vet Rec 95:385-388.
73. Food and Agriculture Organisation. 1985. In M. Bellver-Gallent (ed.), Animal Health Yearbook, FAO Anim Prod Health Ser No. 25. FAO, Rome.
74. Franciosi, C., P.N. D'Aprile, and M. Petek. 1981. Isolamento di un paramixovirus Yucaipa dal tacchino. Boll Ist Sieroter Milan 60:225-228.
75. Francis, D.W. 1973. Newcastle and psittacines, 1970-71. Poult Dig 32:16-19.
76. French, E.L., T.D. St. George, and J.J. Percy. 1967. Infection of chicks with recently isolated Newcastle disease viruses of low virulence. Aust Vet J 43:404-409.
77. Garten, W., W. Berk, Y. Nagai, R. Rott, and H.-D. Klenk. 1980. Mutational changes of the protease susceptibility of glycoprotein F of Newcastle disease virus: Effects on pathogenicity. J Gen Virol 50:135-147.
78. Gelb, J., and C.G. Cianci. 1987. Detergent-treated Newcastle disease virus as an agar gel precipitin test antigen. Poult Sci 66:845-853.
79. Gentry, R.F., and M.O. Braune. 1972. Prevention of virus inactivation during drinking water vaccination of poultry. Poult Sci 51:1450-1456.
80. Ghumman, J.S., and R.A. Bankowski. 1975. In vitro DNA synthesis in lymphocytes from turkeys vaccinated with LaSota, TC and inactivated Newcastle disease vaccines. Avian Dis 20:18-31.
81. Giambrone J.J. 1985. Laboratory evaluation of Newcastle disease vaccination programs for broiler chickens. Avian Dis 29:479-487.
82. Giambrone, J.J., C.S. Eidson, R.K. Page, O.J. Fletcher, B.O. Barger, and S.H. Kleven. 1976. Effect of infectious bursal agent on the response of chickens to Newcastle disease and Marek's disease vaccination. Avian Dis 20:534-544.
83. Glickman, R.L., R.J. Syddall, R.M. Iorio, J.P. Sheehan, and M.A. Bratt. 1988. Quantitative basic residue requirements in the cleavage-activation site of the

fusion glycoprotein as a determinant of virulence for Newcastle disease virus. J Virol 62:354–356.
84. Goldhaft, T.M. 1980. Historical note on the origin of the La Sota strain of Newcastle disease virus. Avian Dis 24:297–301.
85. Gomez-Lillo, M., R.A. Bankowski, and A.D. Wiggins. 1974. Antigenic relationships among viscerotropic velogenic and domestic strains of Newcastle disease virus. Am J Vet Res 35:471–475.
86. Goodman, B.B., and R.P. Hanson. 1988. Isolation of avian paramyxovirus-2 from domestic and wild birds in Costa Rica. Avian Dis 32:713–717.
87. Gough, R.E., and D.J. Alexander. 1973. The speed of resistance to challenge induced in chickens vaccinated by different routes with a B1 strain of live NDV. Vet Rec 92:563–564.
88. Gough, R.E., and D.J. Alexander. 1983. Isolation and preliminary characterisation of a paramyxovirus from collared doves (Streptopelia decaocto). Avian Pathol 12:125–134.
89. Gough, R.E., W.H. Allan, D.J. Knight, and J.W.G. Leiper. 1974. The potentiating effect of an interferon inducer (BRL 5907) on oil-based inactivated Newcastle disease vaccine. Res Vet Sci 17:280–284.
90. Gough, R.E., W.H. Allan, and D. Nedelciu. 1977. Immune response to monovalent and bivalent Newcastle disease and infectious bronchitis inactivated vaccines. Avian Pathol 6:131–142.
91. Gough, R.E., D.J. Alexander, M.S. Collins, S.A. Lister, and W.J. Cox, 1988. Routine virus isolation or detection in the diagnosis of diseases of birds. Avian Pathol 17:893–907.
92. Haddow, J.R., and J.A. Idnani. 1946. Vaccination against Newcastle (Ranikhet) disease. Indian J Vet Sci 16:45–53.
93. Halasz, F. 1912. Contributions to the knowledge of fowlpest. Vet Doctoral Diss, Commun Hung Roy Vet Sch, pp. 1–36. Patria, Budapest.
94. Hamid, H., R.S.F. Campbell, C.M. Lamihhane, and R. Graydon. 1988. Indirect immunoperoxidase staining for Newcastle disease virus (NDV). Proc 2nd Asian/Pacific Poult Health Conf, pp. 425–427. Aust Vet Poult Assoc, Sydney.
95. Hanson, R.P. 1975. Newcastle disease. In S.B. Hitchner, C.H. Domermuth, H.G. Purchase, and J.E. Williams (eds.), Isolation and Identification of Avian Pathogens, pp. 160–173. Am Assoc Avian Pathol, Kennett Square, PA.
96. Hanson, R.P. 1980. Newcastle disease. In S.B. Hitchner, C.H. Domermuth, H.G. Purchase, and J.E. Williams (eds.), Isolation and Identification of Avian Pathogens, pp. 63–66a. Am Assoc Avian Pathol, Kennett Square, PA.
97. Hanson, R.P. 1988. Heterogeneity within strains of Newcastle disease virus: Key to survival. In D.J. Alexander (ed.), Newcastle Disease, pp. 113–130. Kluwer Academic Publ, Boston.
98. Hanson, R.P., and C.A. Brandly. 1955. Identification of vaccine strains of Newcastle disease virus. Science 122:156–157.
99. Hanson, R.P., and J. Spalatin. 1978. Thermostability of the hemagglutinin of Newcastle disease virus as a strain marker in epizootiological studies. Avian Dis 22:659–665.
100. Hanson, R.P., E. Upton, C.A. Brandly, and N.S. Wilson. 1949. Heat stability of hemagglutinin of various strains of Newcastle disease virus. Proc Soc Exp Biol Med 70:283–287.
101. Hanson, R.P., J. Spalatin, and G.S. Jacobson. 1973. The viscerotropic pathotype of Newcastle disease virus. Avian Dis 17:354–361.
102. Hari Babu, Y. 1986. The use of a single radial haemolysis technique for the measurement of antibodies to Newcastle disease virus. Indian Vet J 63:982–984.
103. Heller, E.D., D.B. Nathan, and M. Perek. 1977. The transfer of Newcastle serum antibody from the laying hen to the egg and chick. Res Vet Sci 22:376–379.
104. Higgins, D.A. 1971. Nine disease outbreaks associated with myxoviruses among ducks in Hong Kong. Trop Anim Health Prod 3:232–240.
105. Higgins, D.A., and K.F. Shortridge. 1988. Newcastle disease in tropical and developing countries. In D.J. Alexander (ed.), Newcastle Disease, pp. 273–302. Kluwer Academic Publ, Boston.
106. Hilbink, F., M. Vertommen, J.T.W. Van't Veer. 1982. The fluorescent antibody technique in the diagnosis of a number of poultry diseases: Manufacture of conjugates and use. Tijdschr Diergeneesk 107:167–173.
107. Hitchner, S.B., and K. Hirai. 1979. Isolation and growth characteristics of psittacine viruses in chicken embryos. Avian Dis 23:139–147.
108. Hitchner, S.B., and E.P. Johnson. 1948. A virus of low virulence for immunizing fowls against Newcastle disease (avian pneumoencephalitis). Vet Med 43:525–530.
109. Hofstad, M.S. 1953. Immunization of chickens against Newcastle disease by formalin-inactivated vaccine. Am J Vet Res 14:586–589.
110. Holmes, H.C. 1979. Resistance of the respiratory tract of the chicken to Newcastle disease virus infection following vaccination: The effect of passively acquired antibody on its development. J Comp Pathol 89:11–20.
111. Hoshi, S., T. Mikami, K. Nagata, M. Onuma, and H. Izawa. 1983. Monoclonal antibodies against a paramyxovirus isolated from Japanese sparrow-hawks (Accipter virugatus gularis). Arch Virol 76:145–151.
112. Huang, R.T.C., R. Rott, K. Wahn, H.-D. Klenk, and T. Kohama. 1980. The function of the neuraminidase in membrane fusion induced by myxoviruses. Virology 107:313–319.
113. Hugh-Jones, M., W.H. Allan, F.A. Dark, and G.J. Harper. 1973. The evidence for the airborne spread of Newcastle disease. J Hyg Camb 71:325–339.
114. Ishida, M., K. Nerome, M. Matsumoto, T. Mikami, and A. Oye. 1985. Characterization of reference strains of Newcastle disease virus (NDV) and NDV-like isolates by monoclonal antibodies to HN subunits. Arch Virol 85:109–121.
115. Iyer, S.G., and N. Dobson. 1940. A successful method of immunization against Newcastle disease of fowls. Vet Rec 52:889–894.
116. Jorgensen, E.D., P.L. Collins, and P.T. Lomedico. 1987. Cloning and nucleotide sequence of Newcastle disease virus hemagglutinin-neuraminidase mRNA: Identification of a putative sialic acid binding site. Virology 156:12–24.
117. Kaleta, E.F., and C. Baldauf. 1988. Newcastle disease in free-living and pet birds. In D.J. Alexander (ed.), Newcastle Disease, pp. 197–246. Kluwer Academic Publ, Boston.
118. Kaleta, E.F., D.J. Alexander, and P.H. Russell. 1985. The first isolation of the PMV-1 virus responsible for the current panzootic in pigeons? Avian Pathol 14:553–557.
119. Kelleher, C.J., D.A. Halvorson, and J.A. Newman. 1988. Efficacy of viable and inactivated Newcastle disease virus vaccines in turkeys. Avian Dis 32:342–346.
120. Kessler, N., M. Aymard, and A. Calvet. 1979. Study of a new strain of paramyxoviruses isolated from wild ducks: Antigenic and biological properties. J Gen Virol 43:273–282.
121. Kida, H., and R. Yanagawa. 1981. Classification

of avian paramyxoviruses by immunodiffusion on the basis of the antigenic specificity of their M protein antigens. J Gen Virol 52:103–111.

122. Kolakofsky, D., E. Boy de la Tour, and H. Delius. 1974. Molecular weight determination of Sendai and Newcastle disease virus RNA. J Virol 13:261–268.

123. Kraneveld, F.C. 1926. A poultry disease in the Dutch East Indies. Ned Indisch Bl Diergeneesk 38:448–450.

124. Kumar, M.C. 1988. New methods for immunizing turkeys against Newcastle disease. Turkey World (May-June):48–50.

125. Lana, D.P., D.B. Snyder, D.J. King, and W.W. Marquardt. 1988. Characterization of a battery of monoclonal antibodies for differentiation of Newcastle disease virus and pigeon paramyxovirus-1 strains. Avian Dis 32:273–281.

126. Lancaster, J.E. 1966. Newcastle disease–a review 1926–1964. Monogr No 3. Can Dep Agric, Ottawa.

127. Lancaster, J.E. 1977. Newcastle disease–a review of the geographical incidence and epizootiology. World Poult Sci J 33:155–165.

128. Lancaster, J.E. 1981. Newcastle disease. In E.P.J. Gibbs (ed.), Virus Diseases of Food Animals, Vol II, Disease Monographs, pp. 433–465. Academic Press, New York.

129. Lancaster, J.E., and D.J. Alexander. 1975. Newcastle disease: Virus and spread. Monogr No. 11, Can Dep Agric, Ottawa.

130. Lang, G., A. Gagnon, and J. Howell. 1975. Occurrence of paramyxovirus Yucaipa in Canadian poultry. Can Vet J 16:233–237.

131. Levine, P.P. 1964. World dissemination of Newcastle Disease. In R.P. Hanson (ed.), Newcastle Disease, an Evolving Pathogen, pp. 65–69. Univ Wisconsin Press, Madison.

132. Lipkind, M., and E. Shihmanter. 1986. Antigenic relationships between avian paramyxoviruses. I. Quantitative characteristics based on hemagglutination and neuraminidase inhibition tests. Arch Virol 89:89–111.

133. Lipkind, M., E. Shihmanter, Y. Weisman, A. Aronovici, and D. Shoham. 1982. Characterization of Yucaipa-like avian paramyxoviruses isolated in Israel from domesticated and wild birds. Ann Virol 133E:157–161.

134. Lipkind, M., D. Shoham, and E. Shihmanter. 1986. Isolation of a paramyxovirus from pigs in Israel and its antigenic relationships with avian paramyxoviruses. J Gen Virol 67:427–439.

135. Macpherson, I., R.G. Watt, and D.J. Alexander. 1983. Isolation of avian paramyxovirus, other than Newcastle disease virus, from commercial poultry in Great Britain. Vet Rec 112:479–480.

136. Malkinson, M., and P.A. Small. 1977. Local immunity against Newcastle disease virus in the newly hatched chicken's respiratory tract. Infect Immun 16:587–592.

137. Marius-Jestin, V., M. Cherbonnel, J.P. Picault, and G. Bennejean. 1987. Isolement chez des canards mulards d'une souche hypervirulente de virus de la peste du canard et d'un paramyxovirus aviaire de type 6. Comp Immunol Microbiol Infect Dis 10:173–186.

138. McFerran, J.B., and R.M. McCracken. 1988. Newcastle disease. In D.J. Alexander (ed.), Newcastle Disease, pp. 161–183. Kluwer Academic Publ, Boston.

139. McFerran, J.B., and R. Nelson. 1971. Some properties of an avirulent Newcastle disease virus. Archiv Ges Virusforsch 34:64–74.

140. McGinnes, L.W., and T.G. Morrison. 1986. Nucleotide sequence of the gene encoding the Newcastle disease virus fusion protein and comparisons of paramyxovirus fusion protein sequences. Virus Res 5:343–356.

141. McMillan, B.C., and R.P. Hanson. 1980. RNA oligonucleotide fingerprinting: A proposed method of identifying strains of Newcastle disease virus. Avian Dis 24:1016–1020.

142. McMillan, B.C., and R.P. Hanson. 1982. Differentiation of exotic strains of Newcastle disease virus by oligonucleotide fingerprinting. Avian Dis 26:332–339.

143. McMillan, B.C., S.F. Rehmani, and R.P. Hanson. 1986. Lectin binding and the carbohydrate moieties present on Newcastle disease virus strains. Avian Dis 30:340–344.

144. McNulty, M.S., and G.M. Allan. 1986. Application of immunofluorescence in veterinary viral diagnosis. In M.S. McNulty and J.B. McFerran (eds.), Recent Advances in Virus Diagnosis, pp. 15–26. Martinus Nijhoff, Dordrecht, Neth.

145. Melnick, J.L. 1982. Taxonomy and nomenclature of viruses, 1982. Prog Med Virol 28:208–221.

146. Meulemans, G. 1988. Control by vaccination. In D.J. Alexander (ed.), Newcastle Disease, pp. 318–332. Kluwer Academic Publ, Boston.

147. Meulemans, G., M.C. Carlier, M. Gonze, P. Petit, and P. Halen. 1984. Diagnostic serologique de la maladie de Newcastle par les tests d'inhibition de l'hemagglutination et Elisa. Zentralbl Veterinaermed [B] 31:690–700.

148. Meulemans, G., M. Gonze, M.C. Carlier, P. Petit, A. Burny, and Le Long. 1986. Protective effects of HN and F glycoprotein-specific monoclonal antibodies on experimental Newcastle disease. Avian Pathol 15:761–768.

149. Meulemans, G., M. Gonze, M.C. Carlier, P. Petit, A. Burny, and Le Long. 1987. Evaluation of the use of monoclonal antibodies to hemagglutination and fusion glycoproteins of Newcastle disease virus for virus identification and strain differentiation purposes. Arch Virol 92:55–62.

150. Meulemans, G., C. Letellier, D. Espion, Le Long, and A. Burny. 1988. Importance de la proteine F dans l'immunite au virus de la maladie de Newcastle. Bull Acad Vet France 61:51–62.

151. Meulemans, G., C. Letellier, M. Gonze, M.C. Carlier, and A. Burny. 1988. Newcastle disease virus F glycoprotein expressed from a recombinant vaccinia virus vector protects chickens against live virus challenge. Avian Pathol 17:821–827,

152. Miers, L.A., R.A. Bankowski, and Y.C. Zee. 1983. Optimizing the enzyme-linked immunosorbent assay for evaluating immunity in chickens to Newcastle disease. Avian Dis 27:1112–1125.

153. Millar, N.S., and P.T. Emmerson. 1988. Molecular cloning and nucleotide sequencing of Newcastle disease virus. In D.J. Alexander (ed.), Newcastle Disease, pp. 79–97. Kluwer Academic Publ, Boston.

154. Millar, N.S., P. Chambers, and P.T. Emmerson. 1986. Nucleotide sequence analysis of the haemagglutinin-neuraminidase gene of Newcastle disease virus. J Gen Virol 67:1917–1927.

155. Millar, N.S., P. Chambers, and P.T. Emmerson. 1988. Nucleotide sequence of the fusion and haemagglutinin-neuraminidase glycoprotein genes of Newcastle disease virus, strain Ulster: Molecular basis for variations in pathogenicity between strains. J Gen Virol 69:613–620.

156. Moore, N.F., and D.C. Burke. 1974. Characterization of the structural proteins of different strains of Newcastle disease virus. J Gen Virol 25:275–289.

157. Nagai, Y., H.-D. Klenk, and R. Rott. 1976. Proteolytic cleavage of the viral glycoproteins and its signif-

icance for the virulence of Newcastle disease virus. Virology 72:494-508.
158. Nagai, Y., H. Ogura, and H.-D. Klenk. 1976. Studies on the assembly of the envelope of Newcastle disease virus. Virology 69:523-538.
159. Nagy, E., and B. Lomniczi. 1984. Differentiation of Newcastle disease virus strains by one-dimensional peptide mapping. J Virol Methods 9:227-235.
160. Nerome, K., M. Nakayama, M. Ishida, H. Fukumi, and A. Morita. 1978. Isolation of a new avian paramyxovirus from a budgerigar. J Gen Virol 38:293-301.
161. Nerome, K., M. Ishida, A. Oya, and S. Bosshard. 1983. Genomic analysis of antigenically related avian paramyxoviruses. J Gen Virol 64:465-470.
162. Nishikawa, K., S. Isomura, S. Suzuki, E. Watanabe, M. Hamaguchi, T. Yoshida, and Y. Nagai. 1983. Monoclonal antibodies to the HN glycoprotein of Newcastle disease virus. Biological characterization and use for strain comparisons. Virology 130:318-330.
163. Omojola, E., and R.P. Hanson. 1986. Collection of diagnostic specimens from animals in remote areas. World Anim Rev 60:38-40.
164. Parry, S.H., and I.D. Aitken. 1977. Local immunity in the respiratory tract of the chicken. II. The secretory immune response to Newcastle disease virus and the role of IgA. Vet Microbiol 2:143-165.
165. Pattison, M., and W.H. Allan. 1974. Infection of chicks with infectious bursal disease and its effect on the carrier with Newcastle disease virus. Vet Rec 95:65-66.
166. Pearson, J.E., D.A. Senne, D.J. Alexander, W.D. Taylor, L.A. Peterson, and P.H. Russell. 1987. Characterization of Newcastle disease virus (avian paramyxovirus-1) isolated from pigeons. Avian Dis 31:105-111.
167. Peeples, M.E. 1988. Newcastle disease virus replication. In D.J. Alexander (ed.), Newcastle Disease, pp. 45-78. Kluwer Academic Publ, Boston.
168. Pennington, T.H. 1978. Antigenic differences between strains of NDV. Arch Virol 56:345-351.
169. Powell, J.R., I.D. Aitken, and B.D. Survashe. 1979. The response of the Harderian gland of the fowl to antigen given by the ocular route. II. Antibody production. Avian Pathol 8:363-373.
170. Raszewska, H. 1964. Occurence of the La Sota strain NDV in the reproductive tract of laying hens. Bull Vet Inst Pulawy 8:130-136.
171. Reeve, P., and G. Poste. 1971. Studies on the cytopathogenicity of Newcastle disease virus: Relationship between virulence, polykaryocytosis and plaque size. J Gen Virol 11:17-24.
172. Reeve, P., D.J. Alexander, and W.H. Allan. 1974. Derivation of an isolate of low virulence from the Essex '70 strain of Newcastle disease virus. Vet Rec 94:38-41.
173. Rivetz, B., Y. Weisman, M. Ritterband, F. Fish, and M. Herzberg. 1985. Evaluation of a novel rapid kit for the visual detection of Newcastle disease virus antibodies. Avian Dis 29:929-942.
174. Rosenberger, J.K., and J. Gelb. 1978. Response to several avian respiratory viruses as affected by infectious bursal disease virus. Avian Dis 22:95-105.
175. Rott, R. 1979. Molecular basis of infectivity and pathogenicity of myxoviruses. Arch Virol 59:285-298.
176. Rott, R. 1985. In vitro Differenzierung von pathogenen und apathogenen aviaren Influenzaviren. 1985. Berl Munch Tierärztl Wochenschr 98:37-39.
177. Rott, R., and H.-D. Klenk. 1988. Molecular basis of infectivity and pathogenicity of Newcastle disease virus. In D.J. Alexander (ed.), Newcastle Disease, pp. 98-112. Kluwer Academic Publ, Boston.
178. Russell, P.H. 1988. Monoclonal antibodies in research, diagnosis and epizootiology of Newcastle disease. In D.J. Alexander (ed.), Newcastle Disease, pp. 131-146. Kluwer Academic Publ, Boston.
179. Russell, P.H., and D.J. Alexander. 1983. Antigenic variation of Newcastle disease virus strains detected by monoclonal antibodies. Arch Virol 75:243-253.
180. Samson, A.C.R. 1988. Virus structure. In D.J. Alexander (ed.), Newcastle Disease, pp. 23-44. Kluwer Academic Publ, Boston.
181. Sato, H., M. Oh-Hira, N. Ishida, Y. Imamura, S. Hattori, and M. Kawakita. 1987. Molecular cloning and nucleotide sequence of P, M and F genes of Newcastle disease virus avirulent strain D26. Virus Res 7:241-255.
182. Schloer, G., and R.P. Hanson. 1968. Plaque morphology of Newcastle disease virus as influenced by cell type and environmental factors. Am J Vet Res 29:883-895.
183. Schloer, G., J. Spalatin, and R.P. Hanson. 1975. Newcastle disease virus antigens and strain variation. Am J Vet Res 36:505-508.
184. Senne, D.A., J.E. Pearson, L.D. Miller, and G.A. Gustafson. 1983. Virus isolations from pet birds submitted for importation into the United States. Avian Dis 27:731-744.
185. Shortridge, K.F., D.J. Alexander, and M.S. Collins. 1980. Isolation and properties of viruses from poultry in Hong Kong which represent a new (sixth) distinct group of avian paramyxoviruses. J Gen Virol 49:255-262.
186. Simmons, G.C. 1967. The isolation of Newcastle disease virus in Queensland. Aust Vet J 43:29-30.
187. Smit, T., and P.R. Rondhuis. 1976. Studies on a virus isolated from the brain of a parakeet (Neophema sp). Avian Pathol 5:21-30.
188. Snyder, D.B., W.W. Marquadt, E.T. Mallinson, and E. Russek. 1983. Rapid serological profiling by enzyme-linked immunosorbent assay. I. Measurement of antibody activity titer against Newcastle disease virus in a single dilution. Avian Dis 27:161-170.
189. Snyder, D.B., W.W. Marquadt, E.T. Mallinson, P.K. Savage, D.C. Allen. 1984. Rapid serological profiling by enzyme-linked immunosorbent assay. III. Simultaneous measurements of antibody titers to infectious bronchitis virus, infectious bursal disease and Newcastle disease virus in a single serum dilution. Avian Dis 28:12-24.
190. Spalatin, J.S., and R.P. Hanson. 1966. Recovery of a Newcastle disease virus strain indistinguishable from Texas GB. Avian Dis 10:372-374.
191. Spalatin, J., R.P. Hanson, and P.D. Beard. 1970. The hemagglutination-elution pattern as a marker in characterizing Newcastle disease virus. Avian Dis 14:542-549.
192. Spradbrow, P.B. 1988. Geographical distribution. In D.J. Alexander (ed.), Newcastle Disease, pp. 247-255. Kluwer Academic Publ, Boston.
193. Srinivasappa, G.B., D.B. Snyder, W.W. Marquardt, and D.J. King. 1986. Isolation of a monoclonal antibody with specificity for commonly employed vaccine strains of Newcastle disease virus. Avian Dis 30:562-567.
194. Stevens, J.G., R.M. Nakamura, M.L. Cook, and S.P. Wilczynski. 1976. Newcastle disease as a model for paramyxovirus-induced neurological syndromes: Pathogenesis of the respiratory disease and preliminary characterization of the ensuing encephalitis. Infect Immun 13:590-599.
195. Stewart, D.L., C.N. Hebert, and I. Davidson. 1968. International reference preparation of anti-Newcastle disease serum. Bull WHO 38:925-928.

196. Stones, P.B. 1979. Self injection of veterinary oil-emulsion vaccines. Br Med J 1:1627.
197. Thornton, D.H. 1988. Quality control of vaccines. In D.J. Alexander (ed.), Newcastle Disease, pp. 347-365. Kluwer Academic Publ, Boston.
198. Timms, L., and D.J. Alexander. 1977. Cell-mediated immune response of chickens to Newcastle disease vaccines. Avian Pathol 6:51-59.
199. Toyoda, T., T. Sakaguchi, K. Imai, N. Mendoza Inocencio, B. Gotoh, M. Hamaguchi, and Y. Nagai. 1987. Structural comparison of the cleavage-activation site of the fusion glycoprotein between virulent and avirulent strains of Newcastle disease virus. Virology 158:242-247.
200. Tumova, B., J.H. Robinson, and B.C. Easterday. 1979. A hitherto unreported paramyxovirus of turkeys. Res Vet Sci 27, 135-140.
201. Tumova, B., A. Stumpa, V. Janout, M. Uvizl, and J. Chmela. 1979. A further member of the Yucaipa group isolated from the common wren (Troglodytes troglodytes). Acta Virol 23:504-507.
202. Utterback, W.W., and J.H. Schwartz. 1973. Epizootiology of velogenic viscerotropic Newcastle disease in southern California, 1971-1973. J Am Vet Med Assoc 163:1080-1090.
203. Vindevogel, H., and J.P. Duchatel. 1988. Panzootic Newcastle disease virus in pigeons. In D.J. Alexander (ed.), Newcastle Disease, pp. 184-196. Kluwer Academic Publ, Boston.
204. Walker, J.W., B.R. Heron, and M.A. Mixson. 1973. Exotic Newcastle disease eradication program in the United States of America. Avian Dis 17:486-503.
205. Webster, R.G., and R. Rott. 1987. Influenza virus A pathogenicity: The pivotal role of hemagglutinin. Cell 50:665-666.
206. Wemers, C.D., S. de Henau, C. Neyt, D. Espion, C. Letellier, G. Meulemans, and A. Burny. 1987. The hemagglutinin-neuraminidase (HN) gene of Newcastle disease virus strain Italien (ndv Italien): Comparison with HNs of other strains and expression by a vaccinia recombinant. Arch Virol 97:101-113.
207. WHO Expert Committee. 1980. A revision of the system of nomenclature for influenza viruses: A WHO memorandum. Bull WHO 58:585-591.
208. Wilczynski, S.P., M.L. Cook, and J.G. Stevens. 1977. Newcastle disease as a model for paramyxovirus-induced neurologic syndromes. Am J Pathol 89:649-666.
209. Williams J.E., and L.H. Dillard. 1968. Penetration patterns of Mycoplasma gallisepticum and Newcastle disease virus through the outer structures of chicken eggs. Avian Dis 12:650-657.
210. Wilson, G.W.C. 1986. Newcastle disease and paramyxovirus 1 of pigeons in the European Community. World Poult Sci J 42:143-153,
211. Wilson, R.A., C. Perrotta, B. Frey, and R.J. Eckroade. 1984. An enzyme-linked immunosorbent assay that measures protective antibody levels to Newcastle disease virus in chickens. Avian Dis 28:1079-1085.
212. Winslow, N.S., R.P. Hanson, E. Upton, and C.A. Brandly. 1950. Agglutination of mammalian erythrocytes by Newcastle disease virus. Proc Soc Exp Biol 74:174-178.
213. Zeydanli, M.M., T. Redmann, E.F. Kaleta, and D.J. Alexander. 1988. Paramyxoviruses (PMV) isolated from turkeys with respiratory disease. Proc 37th West Poult Dis Conf, pp. 46-50.

20 AVIAN ENCEPHALOMYELITIS

B.W. CALNEK, R.E. LUGINBUHL, AND C.F. HELMBOLDT

INTRODUCTION. Avian encephalomyelitis (AE) is an infectious viral disease primarily affecting young chickens. It is characterized by ataxia and rapid tremors, especially of the head and neck; because of the latter, it was often called "epidemic tremor."

The disease was of great economic importance to the poultry industry prior to the widespread use of commercial vaccines in the early 1960s. No public health significance has been attached to this disease.

HISTORY. Jones (35, 36) first encountered AE in 1930 in 2-wk-old Rhode Island Red chicks from a commercial flock. Tremor but no ataxia was seen in this outbreak. In 1931 two additional outbreaks were observed in 1- and 4-wk-old chicks raised on different farms but originating from the same breeding flock; tremor and ataxia were noted. During the next 2 yr additional outbreaks were observed in Connecticut, Maine, Massachusetts, and New Hampshire, which led to AE being tagged "New England disease."

In 1934, Jones (36) first propagated the causative agent in susceptible chicks by intracerebral (IC) inoculation with brain material from spontaneous cases. However, it was not until the mid 1950s that Schaaf reported the first successful control of the disease by immunization (65). The epizootiology of AE was unraveled by Calnek et al. in 1960 (17). This was soon followed by the development of an orally administered vaccine (18) that forms the basis of modern day control of the infection in commercial flocks. Additional historical details are provided by van der Heide (78).

INCIDENCE AND DISTRIBUTION. AE has been reported from virtually all areas of the world where poultry are raised on a commercial basis (see 78). Nearly all flocks eventually become infected with the virus, but the incidence of clinical disease is very low unless a breeder flock is not vaccinated and becomes infected after egg production commences. When that happens, vertical transmission results in the infection of progeny which develop clinical disease.

ETIOLOGY

Characteristics of the Virus. AE virus (AEV) was first shown to be filterable by Jones (36) and was found by Olitsky and Bauer (58) to have a diameter of 20–30 nm. The small size was confirmed by filtration studies (12). By electron microscope (EM) examination of purified AEV, Gosting et al. (29) found the virions to have hexagonal profiles lacking envelopes and to be 24–32 nm in diameter; later EM studies by Tannock and Shafren (75) determined the mean diameter to be 26.1 ± 0.4 nm. Gosting et al. (29) further detected a fivefold symmetry with 32 or 42 capsomeres, in contrast to an earlier report by Krauss and Ueberschär (42), who proposed an icosahedral symmetry with only 12 capsomeres.

The virus has a buoyant density of 1.31–1.33 g/ml (12, 29, 75), and a sedimentation coefficient of 148 S (29). The virus is resistant to chloroform, acid, trypsin, pepsin, and DNase and is protected against effects of heat by divalent magnesium ions (7, 12). Based on these characteristics and resistance of AEV to DNase, Butterfield et al. (12) proposed that it be classified as an enterovirus belonging to the family Picornaviridae. Gosting et al. (29) cautioned that final classification should await definitive characterization of the viral nucleic acid. Tannock and Shafren (75) detected four virus-specific proteins (VP 1–4) with molecular weights of 43kD, 35kD, 33kD, and 14kD, respectively. They noted that these proteins were slightly larger than those reported for VPs 1–4 of Picornaviridae, and suggested that they could represent differences within that family of viruses.

Physical, chemical, and serologic tests demonstrate no significant differences between the Van Roekel laboratory strain of AEV and 19 field isolates of the virus (12).

Biologic Properties. Although no serologic differences have been detected between various isolates of AE, a distinction should be made between field strains and those that have been embryo-adapted.

NATURAL STRAINS (FIELD ISOLATES). Pathogenicity of field isolates varies. All are enterotropic; they infect young chicks readily via the oral route and are shed in feces. However, some tend to be more neurotropic than others and produce severe central nervous system (CNS) lesions, with signs in young chicks. Usually, field isolates are nonlethal for embryos until adapted to the embryo by rapid passage.

EMBRYO-ADAPTED STRAINS (VAN ROEKEL STRAIN). The Van Roekel strain is highly neurotropic and causes signs of disease in chickens of all ages by parenteral inoculation. It does not infect via the oral route except with very high dosage, and does not spread from bird to bird. This strain is pathogenic for embryos from nonimmune flocks and produces muscular dystrophy (Fig. 20.1) and decreased movement. Live embryos examined after 18 days of age may show a persistent heartbeat, but the voluntary muscles may be partially or completely immobilized (14, 39). Use of eggs from a susceptible flock is essential for isolation and propagation of the virus in embryos. The virus was detected in brains of inoculated embryos 3–4 days postinoculation (PI), and peak titers were found 6–9 days PI (9, 14). Histopathologic changes in embryos infected with egg-adapted virus have been described as uniform in character but variable in intensity and location and consist-

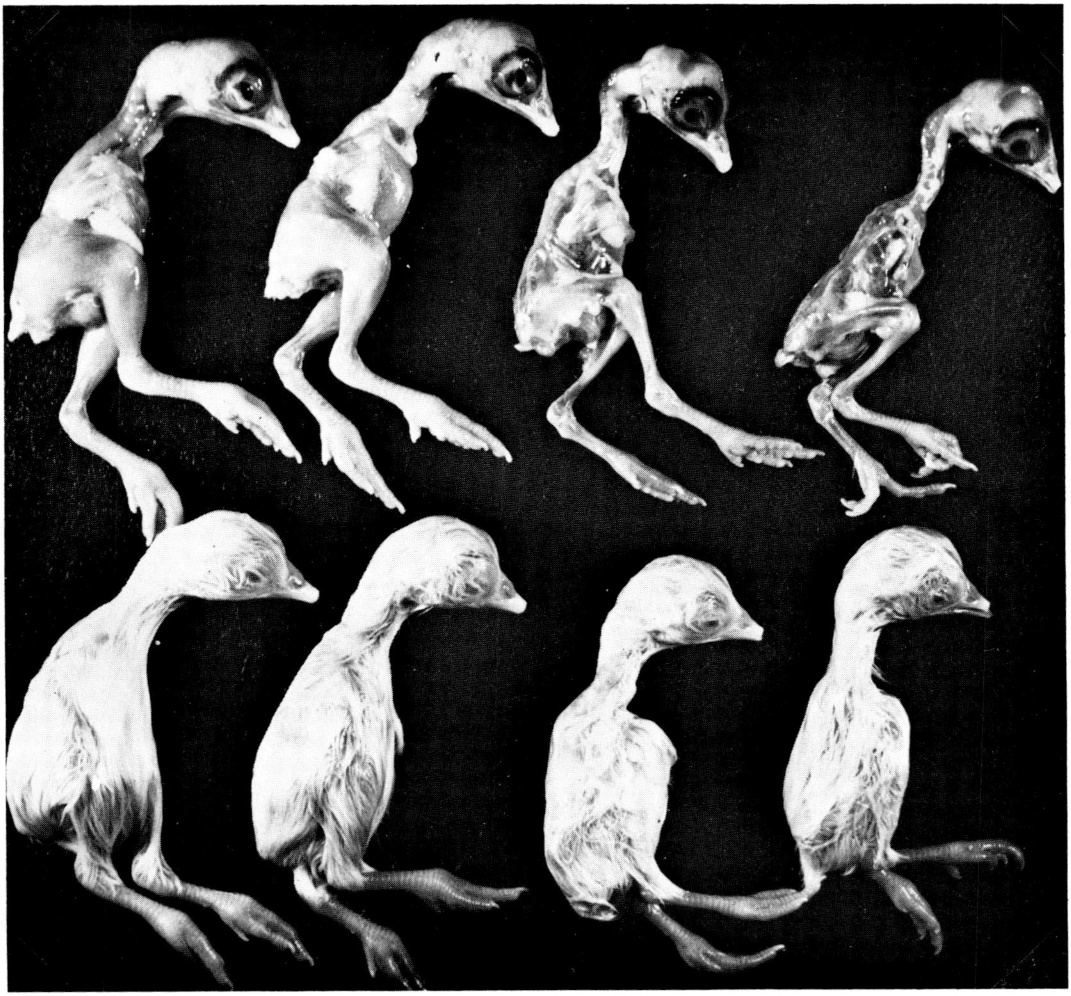

20.1. Embryos inoculated via yolk sac with Van Roekel strain of AE virus at 6 days incubation, and examined 12 days later. Embryos on top row have had the skin removed. Embryos on left of each row were uninoculated. Remaining six embryos (*left to right*) were inoculated with progressively greater doses of virus.

ing of encephalomalacia and muscular dystrophy (39). Muscular changes consisted primarily of eosinophilic swelling and necrosis, fragmentation, and loss of striations of affected fibers with rare sarcolemmal proliferation and heterophil infiltration (Fig. 20.2). Neural lesions were characterized by severe local edema, gliosis, vascular proliferation, and pyknosis (Fig. 20.3).

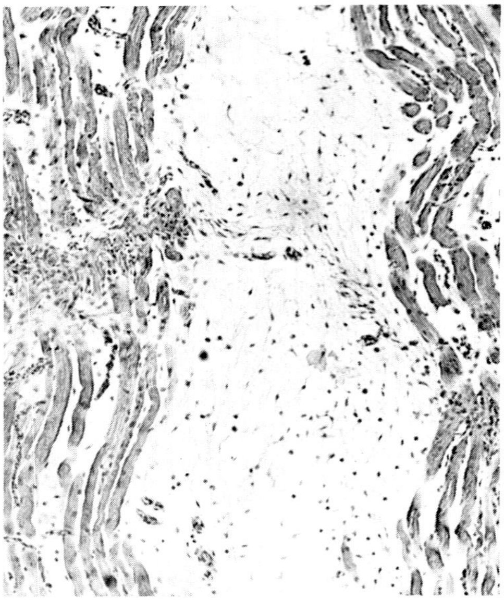

20.2. Bivicenter cervicis muscle of 18-day-old chicken embryo infected with AEV. Muscle fibers are fragmented and separated by edema. H & E, ×30.

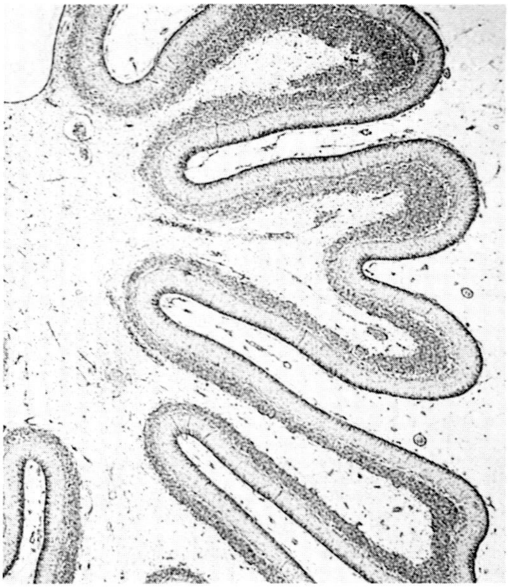

20.3. Cerebellum of infected 18-day-old chicken embryo, with marked lack of development of internal granular layer, cerebellar white matter, and nucleus cerebellaris. Brain should be almost complete at this stage. H & E, ×30.

Laboratory Host Systems. The baby chick, chicken embryos from susceptible flocks (39, 72, 82, 84, 90), cell cultures of neuroglial cells (2, 40, 47, 56, 64), chicken embryo kidney (49), chicken embryo fibroblast cells (48), and chicken embryo pancreatic cells (41) have been used to propagate the virus. It was successfully propagated in embryonating eggs inoculated via the yolk sac, allantoic sac, and intraocular routes (9, 39, 72, 90). The yolk sac route of inoculation for chicken embryos has been adopted by most investigators as the route of choice. Recent studies by Nicholas et al. (56) suggest that chicken embryo neuroglial cells may provide an excellent substrate for production of AEV antigen suitable for serological tests such as immunodiffusion (ID) and enzyme-linked immunosorbent assays (ELISA).

PATHOGENESIS AND EPIZOOTIOLOGY

Natural and Experimental Hosts. AEV appears to have a limited host range. Chickens, pheasants, coturnix quail, and turkeys have all succumbed to natural infection (see reviews 10, 78). Hill and Raymond (30) were able to produce clinical signs of AE in quail chicks inoculated at 1–14 days of age. Experimental chicks were maintained in the same room with adult breeding quail. Fifteen days after chicks were inoculated, the adult flock manifested a decline in egg production and hatchability. Clinical signs of AE and mortality were observed among the chicks hatched from eggs collected during the disease outbreak. Ducklings, poults, young pigeons, and guinea fowl have been infected experimentally. Mice, guinea pigs, rabbits, and monkeys were refractory to virus introduced intracerebrally (50, 55, 59, 82, 83). Van Steenis (85) found naturally occurring AEV antibodies in serums from partridges, pheasants, and turkeys, but not in serums from finches, sparrows, starlings, pigeons, jackdaws, rooks, doves, or ducks. The latter four species also failed to develop antibodies after oral exposure to AEV. Bodin et al. (3) compared adult pheasants and red and gray partridges for sensitivity to intramuscular or oral-nasal inoculation with the Van Roekel strain of virus. All became infected, but the severity of disease based on signs and lesions was greatest in gray partridges and least in pheasants. Embryonated eggs from the three species were also susceptible to infection.

Transmission. The IC route of inoculation has given the most consistent results in reproducing

AE in chickens. Other routes by which infection has been experimentally established are intraperitoneal, subcutaneous, intradermal, intravenous, intramuscular, intrasciatic, intraocular, oral, and intranasal inoculation (12, 17, 23, 38, 57, 67, 82).

Calnek et al. (17) suggested that under natural conditions, AE is essentially an enteric infection. Virus is shed in the feces for a period of several days, and because it is quite resistant to environmental conditions, it remains infectious for long periods of time. The period during which virus is excreted in feces is dependent in part on the age of the bird when infected. Very young chicks may excrete virus for more than 2 wk, whereas those infected after 3 wk of age may shed virus for only about 5 days (89). Infected litter is a source of virus that is easily transmitted horizontally by tracking or fomites. Infection spreads rapidly from bird to bird within a pen or house once introduced, and from pen to pen on farms in which no special precautions are taken to prevent spread. Birds in isolated flocks of a single age group were found to be less likely to have encountered infection than chickens on farms with multiple-age groups. Virus spread was found to be less rapid among birds in cages than in those on the floor (17, 24, 68).

Vertical transmission is a very important means of virus dissemination, based on both field evidence and experimental results (17, 38, 67, 77, 84). Taylor and Schelling (76) reported that 57% of breeder flocks tested in North America had been exposed to the virus by 5 mo of age; however, 96% were serologically positive by 13 mo. Although the source of infection for susceptible flocks is unknown, it is likely that it is carried from infected farms by people or fomites. When susceptible flocks are exposed after sexual maturity, the hens infect a variable proportion of their eggs. Calnek et al. (17) showed that infected embryos and chicks came from eggs laid during the period 5–13 days after experimental infection of susceptible breeders. Jungherr and Minard (38) reported that hatchability of eggs from an infected flock was not affected. On the contrary, Taylor et al. (77) observed a high embryo death pattern during the last 3 days of incubation. The percentage of embryos that hatched declined from a 78.6% preinfection level to 59.6% during the clinical stage and increased to 75.4% postinfection. Eggs produced just prior to and during the period of depressed egg production showed decreased hatchability and increased embryo mortality during the last 3 days of incubation. Furthermore, only chicks from the group with depressed hatchability showed signs of AE; chicks hatched prior to and after the affected hatch appeared normal. Similar observations have been reported by other workers (17, 62).

Calnek et al. (17) demonstrated that virus transmission can occur in the incubator. Chicks hatched from eggs inoculated at 6 days incubation manifested signs on the lst day of age; by the 6th day, 49 of 52 showed clinical evidence of AE. Chicks from uninoculated eggs hatched with the infected birds first manifested signs on the 10th day, and 15 of 18 chicks developed clinical signs. An isolated control group of 19 chicks remained negative.

The possibility of a carrier status is unknown. Richey (62) incriminated a ready-to-lay pullet flock housed in the same building, but in a separate pen, as the source of infection for outbreaks that occurred in several susceptible breeding flocks 45 wk of age. The pullet flock had experienced an acute outbreak of AE at 3 wk of age; it was suggested that a carrier existed in the flock. While certain aspects of transmission have been well established, other phases remain unknown.

Incubation Period. Studies conducted by Calnek et al. (17) demonstrated that the incubation period in chicks infected by embryo transmission was 1–7 days, whereas chicks infected by contact transmission or oral administration had a minimum incubation period of 11 days.

Signs. AE presents an interesting syndrome. In natural outbreaks it usually makes its appearance when chicks are 1–2 wk of age, although affected chicks have been observed at the time of hatching. Affected chicks first show a slightly dull expression of the eyes, followed by a progressive ataxia from incoordination of the muscles, which may be detected readily by exercising the chicks. As the ataxia grows more pronounced, chicks show an inclination to sit on their hocks. When disturbed, they may move about, exhibiting little control over speed and gait; finally, they come to rest or fall on their sides. Some may refuse to move or may walk on their hocks and shanks. The dull expression becomes more pronounced and is accompanied by a weakened cry. Fine tremors of the head and neck may become evident, the frequency and magnitude of which may vary. Exciting or disturbing the chicks may bring on the tremor, which may continue for variable periods and recur at irregular intervals. Ataxic signs usually but not always appear before the tremor. In some cases only tremor has been observed. Jungherr (37) found that 36.9% of histologically positive field cases showed ataxia, 18.3% showed tremor, and 35% showed both; 9.2% showed no clinical signs. Ataxia usually progresses until the chick is incapable of moving about, and this stage is followed by inanition, prostration, and finally death. Chicks with marked ataxia and prostration are frequently trampled by their penmates. Some chicks with definite signs of AE may survive and grow to maturity, and in some instances signs may disappear completely. Among 83 naturally infected chicks reared at the laboratory, only 24 survived after a period of 8 mo; 7 of these developed blindness as the result of an opacity or bluish discoloration of the lens of one or both eyes. As they became mature, a few progeny from these survivors developed an eye condition that resembled that observed in naturally infected dams. Gross pathology consisted of apparent enlargement of the eyeball, marked opacity of the lens, seemingly fixed pupil, and total blindness in some cases. No characteristic signs of AE were detected in these progeny (79, 80). Somewhat similar observations have been reported by other workers (6, 60).

There is a marked age resistance to clinical signs in birds exposed after they are 2–3 wk of age (see Pathogenesis). Mature birds may experience a temporary drop in egg production (5–10%) but do not develop neurologic signs.

Morbidity and Mortality. Morbidity from the natural disease has been observed only in young stock. The usual morbidity rate is 40–60% if all the chicks come from the infected flock. Mortality averages 25% and may exceed 50%. These rates are considerably lower if many of the chicks composing the flock originate from breeder flocks of immune birds.

Pathogenesis. Localization of viral antigen using virus isolation, immunodiffusion, and immunofluorescence techniques has been reported by Van der Heide (78), Braune and Gentry (5), Ikeda (33) and Miyamae (51–54). In young chicks exposed orally to field strains of AEV, primary infection of the alimentary tract, especially in the duodenum, is rapidly followed by a viremia and subsequent infection of the pancreas and other visceral organs (liver, heart, kidney, spleen) and skeletal muscle, and finally the CNS. Alimentary tract infections involve muscular layers, and pancreatic infections are found in both the acinar and islet cells, persisting more in the latter. Viral antigen is relatively abundant in the CNS where Purkinje cells and the molecular layer of the cerebellum are apparently favored sites of virus replication. Chicks with clinical signs at 10–30 days of age tend to have viral antigen mostly in the CNS and pancreas; lesser amounts of antigen have been seen in heart and kidney and only very small amounts in liver and spleen. Persistence of the virus infection is common in the CNS, alimentary tract, and pancreas. Interestingly, the CNS and the pancreas are the only sites uniformly infected by embryo-adapted strains of AEV.

Van der Heide (78) was unable to find viral antigen when tissues from experimentally infected mature birds were examined. However, Miyamae (53) did detect viral antigen in viscera and intestinal tract of 2-yr-old hens infected orally with field strains of AEV. In the intestinal tract, viral antigen was found in the epithelial tunica mucosa, circular muscle layer and/or muscularis mucosa, and in the tunica propria mucosa, but the detection rate was lower than has been reported for young chicks. No viral antigen was found in the CNS; presumably this lack of infection correlates with the absence of clinical disease in infected adults.

Cheville (19) and Westbury and Sinkovic (86–89) did much to clarify certain aspects of the pathogenesis of the natural or experimental disease. Age at exposure was especially important; Cheville noted that birds infected at 1 day of age generally died, whereas those infected at 8 days developed paresis but usually recovered, and infection at 28 days caused no clinical signs. Bursectomy but not thymectomy abrogated the age resistance. Westbury and Sinkovic also noted disease when infection was initiated at 14 or less days of age but not when it occurred at 20 or more days. They confirmed Cheville's conclusion that humoral immunity was the basis of age resistance. In their studies they correlated young age (thus immunologic incompetence) with extended viremia, persistence of virus in the brain, and development of clinical disease. Presumably, the immune response of an immunologically competent bird would stop the spread of infection before it reached the CNS. Age resistance was not expressed when experimental infection was induced by IC inoculation of virus. Interestingly, Calnek et al. (17) found clinical signs in contact-exposed young chicks to have a minimum incubation period of 10–11 days, the same time that virus-neutralizing (VN) antibodies can be detected in adult birds.

Gross Lesions. The only gross lesions associated with AE in chicks are whitish areas (due to masses of infiltrating lymphocytes) in the muscularis of the ventriculus. These are subtle changes and require favorable conditions to be discerned. No changes have been described for infected adult birds.

Histopathology. The principal changes are in the CNS and some viscera. The peripheral nervous system is not involved—a point of importance in differential diagnosis.

In the CNS the lesions are those of a disseminated, nonpurulent encephalomyelitis and a ganglionitis of the dorsal root ganglia. The most frequently encountered addition is a striking perivascular infiltrate seeming to occur in all portions of the brain and spinal cord (Figs. 20.4, 20.5) except the cerebellum, where it is confined to the nucleus (n.) cerebellaris. Infiltrating small lymphocytes may pile up several layers to form an impressive cuff.

Microgliosis occurs as diffuse and nodular aggregates. The glial lesion is seen chiefly in the cerebellar molecular layer, where it tends to be

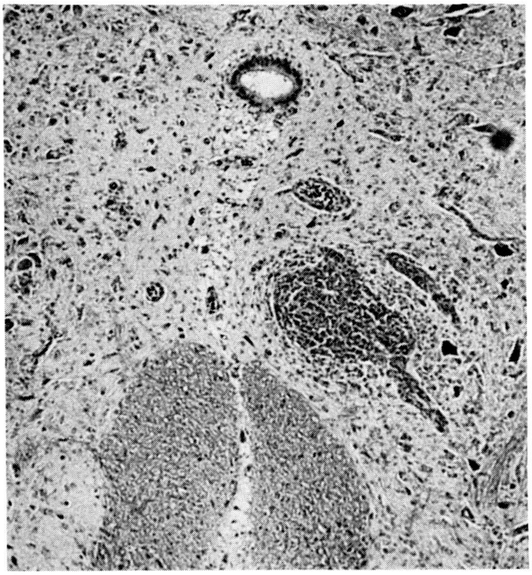

20.4. Spinal cord at lumbar level of chick. Large glial nodule and several perivascular infiltrates of lymphocytes are in gray matter. Central canal is at top. H & E, ×75.

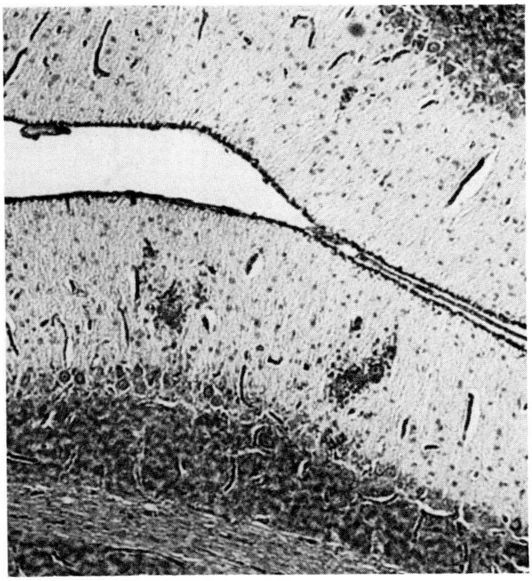

20.5. Perivascular infiltration and gliosis are seen in the nucleus cerebellaris. H & E, ×63. (Jakowski)

compact (Fig. 20.6). A loose gliosis is usually found in the n. cerebellaris, brain stem, midbrain, and optic lobes and less often in the corpus striata. In the midbrain, two nuclei–n. rotundus and n. ovoidalis–are invariably affected with a loose microgliosis that can be considered pathognomonic. Another lesion of pathognomonic significance is central chromatolysis (axonal reac-

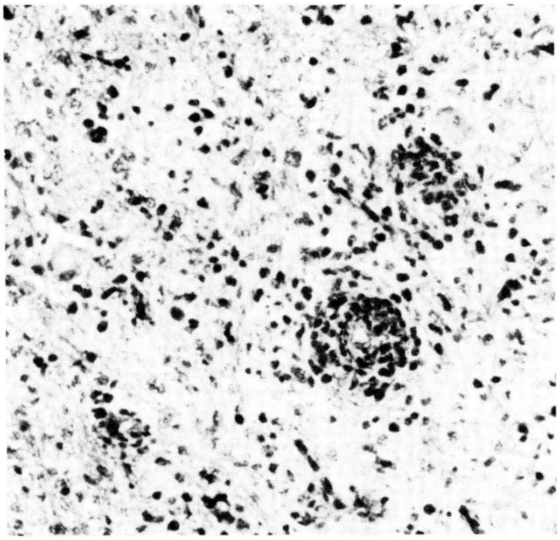

20.6. Cerebellum of chick. Glial foci common in AE are in the molecular layer. H & E, ×75.

tion) of the neurons in the nuclei of the brain stem, particularly those of the medulla oblongata (Fig. 20.7). If several sagittal sections are made, one can almost always find this alteration. The dying neuron is surrounded by satellite oligodendroglia and, later, microglia phagocytize the remains; the central chromatolysis is never seen without an attending cellular reaction.

Lesions in the spinal cord are identical to those of the brain. Although no detailed study of the spinal cord has been made, random sampling of various levels suggests that all are involved.

The dorsal root ganglia often contain rather tight aggregates of small lymphocytes amid the neurons. The lesion is always confined to the ganglion and never enters the nerves (Fig. 20.8).

In general, signs cannot be correlated with severity of lesions or distribution in the CNS.

Visceral lesions appear to be hyperplasia of the lymphocytic aggregates scattered in a random fashion throughout the bird. In the proventriculus there are normally a few small lymphocytes in the muscular wall; in AE these are obvious dense aggregates that are certainly pathognomonic (Fig. 20.9). Similar lesions occur in the ventriculus muscle, but unfortunately they also occur in Marek's disease. In the pancreas, circumscribed lymphocytic follicles are normal (43), but in AE the number increases several times (Fig. 20.10). In the myocardium and particularly the atrium there are aggregates of lymphocytes considered to be the result of AE (71). However, lymphocytes in the myocardium of young chicks are not unusual; one may consider them a lesion only if they are widespread and accompanied by previously noted alterations.

There appears to be an excellent correlation be-

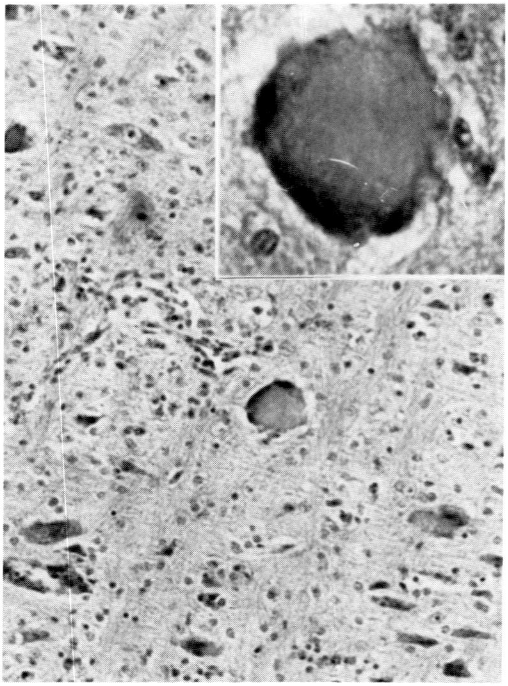

20.7. Medulla oblongata of chick. There is diffuse gliosis, and in the center a neuron is undergoing central chromatolysis. H & E, ×75. Inset shows tigrolysis and loss of nucleus, ×480.

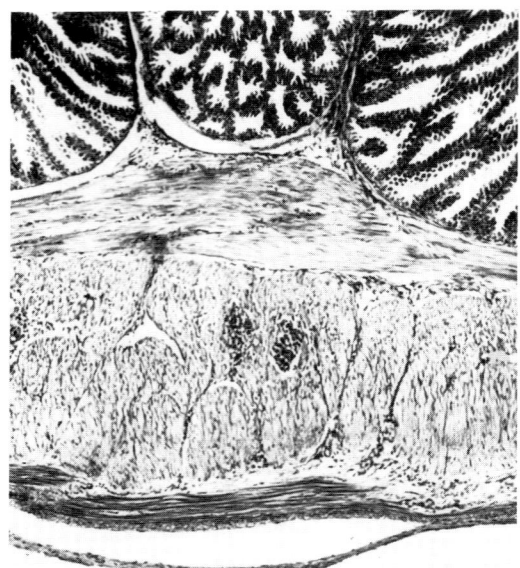

20.9. Proventriculus of chick. Dense lymphocytic foci are in muscular wall. This lesion is pathognomonic. H & E, ×30.

tween clinical signs and histologic lesions. In one study 11% had signs but no lesions, while 8% had lesions but no signs (38). Later, Jungherr believed that all birds with clinical signs had histologic lesions. This was based on more intensive research that in turn was based on multiple sections of

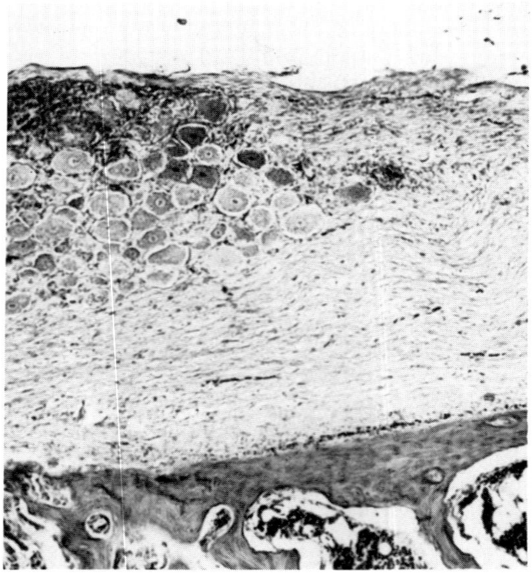

20.8. Dorsal root ganglion of lumbar level of chick. Dense infiltrate of lymphocytes is confined to ganglion. Sciatic nerve is unaffected. H & E, ×75.

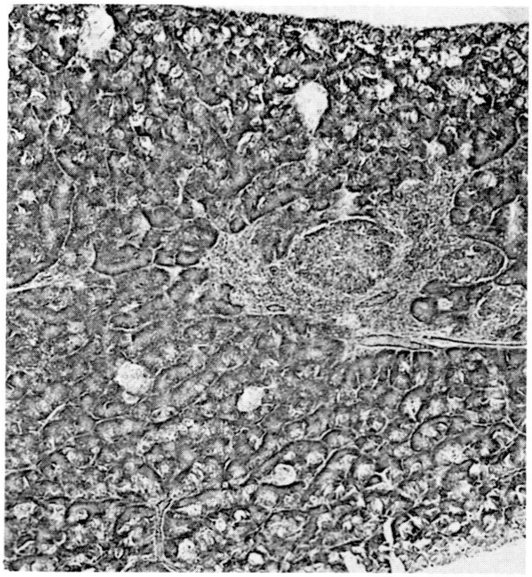

20.10. Pancreas of young chick. Several follicles of lymphocytes are present. This lesion is significant only when abnormal numbers of follicles are present. H & E, ×30.

brain and viscera. Experimentally inoculated chicks killed in sequential fashion invariably yield lesions 1–2 days before clinical signs. Recovered birds free from signs have CNS lesions for at least 1 wk and probably much longer.

Immunity. Birds recovered from natural and experimental infection develop circulating antibodies capable of neutralizing the virus (see reviews 10, 13). Antibodies also appear in yolks of eggs from immune hens and may render embryonating eggs resistant to virus inoculated via the yolk sac. In a flock survey for embryo susceptibility to the virus, Sumner et al. (73) found a wide range in titration endpoints of the AEV in eggs received from 119 flocks. Most tested flocks had no history of AE but produced embryos resistant to the virus, suggesting that they had undergone a mild infection. It was suggested that in an exposed flock not all hens become immune to a degree measurable by the test.

Cheville (19), and later Westbury and Sinkovic (87), clearly showed that humoral immunity, but not cellular, was important in curtailing infection. If the response is rapid, as is usual in birds over 21 days of age, the CNS infection apparently does not progress to the point where clinical signs may develop.

ACTIVE. When chickens are immunologically competent, the serologic response can be relatively rapid. Data from Calnek et al. (17) suggested that chicks from eggs laid as early as 11 days after exposure already carried passively acquired antibodies, since they were resistant to contact exposure after hatching. Also, positive VN tests can be found after 11–14 days PI (18, 88) and positive ID tests as early as 4–10 days PI (34).

Flocks of chickens containing birds with positive neutralization indices (NIs) or with positive embryo susceptibility tests rarely if ever have recurrent outbreaks of AE.

PASSIVE. Antibodies are transferred to progeny from the dam via the embryo and can be demonstrated in egg yolk (73). Birds from immune dams were not fully susceptible to oral inoculation until 8–10 wk of age, and antibodies were demonstrated in the serum until 4–6 wk of age (18). Passively acquired antibodies can prevent development of clinical disease (89) and prevent or reduce the period of virus excretion in feces (17, 89).

DIAGNOSIS

Isolation and Identification of Causative Agent. The brain is an excellent source of virus for isolation, although other tissues and organs induce the disease when injected into chicks (38, 81). Miyamae (54) found that in addition to the brain, the pancreas and duodenum were especially reliable sources of virus.

A sensitive system for assay of virus is to inoculate embryos (obtained from a susceptible flock) via the yolk sac when 5–7 days of age, allow these to hatch, and observe chicks for signs of disease during the first 10 days (8, 31). When clinical signs appear, brain, proventriculus, and pancreas should be examined for lesions as described under Histopathology. Additionally or alternatively, brain, pancreas, and duodenum from affected chicks can be examined for specific viral antigens by fluorescent antibody (FA) (4, 5, 51, 54, 78) or ID (33) tests.

Berger (2) infected chicken embryo brain cell cultures and then used indirect FA test to detect viral antigens. He found it to be more sensitive than the embryo inoculation method. Nicholas et al. (56) compared several methods for detection of AEV. Inoculation of brain cell cultures followed by indirect FA test was found to be convenient, but inoculation of 2-wk-old susceptible chicks followed by serological tests such as ELISA or ID was slightly more sensitive. They considered the latter be the method of choice for detection of AEV.

Serology. Chickens exposed to AEV develop antibodies that can be measured with the standard VN test (14, 73), the indirect FA test (20), the ID test (27, 34, 44), the ELISA (25, 69, 74), and the passive hemagglutination test (1).

The Van Roekel embryo-adapted strain is recommended to determine the neutralizing capacity of the serum or plasma. Six-day-old embryos inoculated via the yolk sac with virus dilutions mixed with serum are examined for characteristic lesions 10–12 days postinoculation. A NI of 1.1 or greater is considered as positive evidence of previous exposure to AEV. Among samples from a recently exposed flock, the NI may vary from 1.5 to 3.0. Antibodies may be detected as early as the 2nd wk after exposure and remain at significant levels for at least several months. Calnek and Jehnich (14) reported that in many instances birds having no detectable VN antibodies (NI less than 1.1) would resist IC challenge with an embryo infective dose–50% (EID_{50}) of virus of as many as 10,000.

Another method to determine immunity of a flock is the embryo susceptibility (ES) test (73). Fertile eggs from the flock to be tested are incubated, along with control eggs from a known susceptible flock. After 6 days, each embryo is inoculated via the yolk sac with 100 EID_{50} of egg-adapted virus. Embryos are examined 10–12 days PI for characteristic lesions. If 100% of embryos are affected, the flock is considered susceptible; less than 50% affected indicates immunity. Intermediate figures should be considered nondefinitive and may indicate recent exposure.

Titers in the indirect FA test appear to parallel those of the VN test. Choi and Miura (20), and Dovadola et al. (22) found the indirect FA test to be as useful as the ES test for assessing immunity in turkey breeder flocks.

Standard procedures for ID tests were first reported by Ikeda (33, 34), who used concentrated tissue extracts from infected embryos as the antigen. Antibodies could be found as early as 4–10 days postexposure, and these persisted for at least 28 mo. Rare false-positives and false-negatives were reported when the ID test was compared to the VN test. Girshick and Crary (27), who used a similar antigen, confirmed Ikeda's general results but did not find discrepancies between the ID and VN tests.

Ahmed et al. (1) described a passive hemagglutination test that they found to be more sensitive than the ID test and equal to the ES test in sensitivity.

An ELISA test using purified viral antigen compared well with the VN test and was found more suitable than the ID test for evaluation of immunity (25, 63, 74). Smart et al. (70) determined ELISA to correlate well with the ES test. They used ELISA to diagnose active infections with AEV by an increase in titer with sequential serum samples. Garrett et al. (26) were able to correlate ELISA titers in hens with the resistance of progeny embryos to challenge with AEV.

Differential Diagnosis. In spontaneous cases a tentative and frequently definite diagnosis of disease can be made when a complete history of the flock and typical specimens are provided for histopathology.

Histopathologic evidence of gliosis, lymphocytic perivascular infiltration, axonal type of neuronal degeneration in the CNS, and hyperplasia of the lymphoid follicles in certain visceral tissues usually can be considered as a basis for a positive diagnosis. Virus isolation or a rise in titer with serologic tests gives a more specific diagnosis.

AE should not be confused with other avian diseases manifesting similar clinical signs, such as Newcastle disease, equine encephalomyelitis infection, nutritional disturbances (rickets, encephalomalacia, riboflavin deficiency), and Marek's disease.

AE is predominantly a disease of 1- to 3-wk-old chicks. Since Newcastle disease may strike at this time, a problem of differential diagnosis can arise. Certain lesions are pecular to AE: central chromatolysis as opposed to peripheral chromatolysis of Newcastle disease, gliosis in the n. rotundus and n. ovoidalis that is not observed in Newcastle disease, lymphocytic foci in the muscular wall of the proventriculus, and circumscribed lymphocytic follicles in the pancreas. Newcastle disease rarely causes an interstitial pancreatitis.

Encephalomalacia generally appears 2-3 wk later than AE and from the standpoint of clinical history the signs should be no problem. Histologically it causes severe degenerative lesions in no way similar to AE.

Marek's disease, which occurs still later, presents little difficulty. The peripheral nerve invovlement and state of lymphomatosis of the viscera are two criteria not seen in AE.

PREVENTION AND CONTROL. No satisfactory treatment is known for acute outbreaks in young chicks. Removal and segregation of affected chicks may be indicated under certain conditions, but they generally will not develop into profitable stock. Once a flock has experienced an outbreak of AE no further evidence of it is likely to be observed (67).

Control of AE is achieved by vaccination of breeder flocks during the growing period to assure that they do not become infected after maturity, thereby preventing dissemination of the virus by the egg-borne route. Also, maternal antibodies protect progeny against contact to AEV during the critical first 2–3 wk. Vaccination may also be used with commercial egg-laying flocks to prevent a temporary drop in egg production associated with AE.

Inactivated vaccines have been developed (11, 16, 45, 66) and may be useful in flocks already in production or where the use of a live virus is contraindicated. However, most flocks are vaccinated with a live, embryo-propagated virus, such as strain 1143 (18), which can be administered by natural routes such as via drinking water or by spraying (8, 18, 24). Live virus vaccines, which can be stored frozen or after lyophilization (7, 61), are similar to field virus in that they spread readily within a flock. This allows for administration per os to a small percentage of the birds in a flock which then spread infection to others, although this method is generally unsatisfactory for birds in wire cages (24, 68). Vaccination by wing-web inoculation of AEV is also practiced in many flocks, but, as noted below, this method may carry some risk of clinical signs (28). Generally, vaccination is done after 8 wk of age and at least 4 wk before egg production.

It is very important that embryo adaptation of strains used for live virus vaccines does not occur: 1) adapted virus loses its ability to infect via the intestinal tract and therefore is no longer efficacious when administered by natural routes (18); 2) adapted virus, like field strains, can cause clinical disease when administered by the wing-web route (15). Glisson and Fletcher (28) observed clinical encephalitis in broiler breeder pullets given embryo-propagated AEV vaccine by the wing-web route, and concluded that the most probable explanation was that the vaccine virus was inadvertently adapted during manufacture.

Adaptation is detected by careful monitoring of inoculated embryos used in production of vaccine for characteristic signs (see ETIOLOGY), and any adapted virus can be eliminated from vaccine seed virus stocks by passage in susceptible chicks inoculated orally.

AE IN TURKEYS. In 1968, AE was encountered in turkey flocks in Minnesota (32). The disease in turkeys resembles AE in chickens. A drop in egg production occurs in laying flocks, which is of economic concern to the flock owner. In young poults the signs are primarily paralytic, and mortality and microscopic pathology are similar to that observed in chicks. The ELISA technique to detect antibodies is useful in turkeys (46), and vaccines used in controlling AE in chickens have been shown to be efficacious in turkeys as well (21).

REFERENCES

1. Ahmed, A.A.S., I.M. Abou El-Azm, N.N.K. Ayoub, and B.I.M. E.-Toukhi. 1982. Studies on the serological detection of antibodies to avian encephalomyelitis virus. Avian Pathol 11:253-262.
2. Berger, R.G. 1982. An in vitro assay for quantifying the virus of avian encephalomyelitis. Avian Dis 26:534-541.
3. Bodin, G., J.L. Pellerin, A. Milon, M.F. Geral, X. Berthelot, and R. Lautie. 1981. Etude de la contamination experimentale du gibier a plumes (faisnas, perdrix rouges, perdrix grises), par le virus de l'encephalomyelite infectieuse aviare. Rev Med Vet 132:805-816.
4. Braune, M.O., and R.F. Gentry. 1971. Avian encephalomyelitis virus. I. Pathogenesis in chicken embryos. Avian Dis 15:638-647.
5. Braune, M.O., and R.F. Gentry. 1971. Avian encephalomyelitis virus. II. Pathogenesis in chickens. Avian Dis 15:648-653.
6. Bridges, C.H., and A.I. Flowers. 1958. Iridocyclitis and cataracts associated with an encephalomyelitis in chickens. J Am Vet Med Assoc 132:79-84.
7. Bülow, V.v. 1964. Studies on the physico-chemical properties of the virus of avian encephalomyelitis (AE) with special reference to purification and preservation of virus suspensions. Zentralbl Veterinaermed [B] 11:674-686.
8. Bülow, V.v. 1965. Avian encephalomyelitis (AE). Cultivation, titration, and handling of the virus for live vaccines. Zentralbl Veterinaermed [B] 12:298-311.
9. Burke, C.N., H. Krauss, and R.E. Luginbuhl. 1965. The multiplication of avian encephalomyelitis virus in chicken embryo tissues. Avian Dis 9:104-108.
10. Butterfield, W.K. 1975. Avian encephalomyelitis: The virus and immune response. Am J Vet Res 36:557-559.
11. Butterfield, W.K., R.E. Luginbuhl, C.F. Helmboldt, and F.W. Sumner. 1961. Studies on avian encephalomyelitis. III. Immunization with an inactivated virus. Avian Dis 5:445-450.
12. Butterfield, W.K., C.F. Helmboldt, and R.E. Luginbuhl. 1969. Studies on avian encephalomyelitis. IV. Early incidence and longevity of histopathologic lesions in chickens. Avian Dis 13:53-57.
13. Calnek, B.W., and J. Fabricant. 1981. Immunity to infectious avian encephalomyelitis. In M.E. Rose, L.N. Payne, and B.M. Freeman (eds.), Avian Immunology, pp. 235-244. British Poultry Science, Ltd., Edinburgh.
14. Calnek, B.W., and H. Jehnich. 1959. Studies on avian encephalomyelitis. I. The use of a serum-neutralization test in the detection of immunity levels. Avian Dis 3:95-104.
15. Calnek, B.W., and H. Jehnich. 1959. Studies on avian encephalomyelitis. II. Immune responses to vaccination procedures. Avian Dis 3:225-239.
16. Calnek, B.W., and P.J. Taylor. 1960. Studies on avian encephalomyelitis. III. Immune response to beta-propiolactone inactivated virus. Avian Dis 4:116-122.
17. Calnek, B.W., P.J. Taylor, and M. Sevoian. 1960. Studies on avian encephalomyelitis. IV. Epizootiology. Avian Dis 4:325-347.
18. Calnek, B.W., P.J. Taylor, and M. Sevoian. 1961. Studies on avian encephalomyelitis. V. Development and application of an oral vaccine. Avian Dis 5:297-312.
19. Cheville, N.F. 1970. The influence of thymic and bursal lymphoid systems in the pathogenesis of avian encephalomyelitis. Am J Pathol 58:105-125.
20. Choi, W.P., and S. Miura. 1972. Research Note—indirect fluorescent antibody technique for the detection of avian encephalomyelitis antibody in chickens. Avian Dis 16:949-951.
21. Deshmukh, D.R., C.T. Larsen, T.A. Rude, and B.S. Pomeroy. 1973. Evaluation of live-virus vaccine against avian encephalomyelitis in turkey breeder hens. Am J Vet Res 34:863-867.
22. Dovadola, E., M. Petek, P. D'Aprile, and F. Cancellotti. 1973. Detection of avian encephalomyelitis virus antibodies in turkey breeder flocks by the embryo-susceptibility and immunofluorescence tests. Proc 5th Int Congr World Vet Poult Assoc, pp. 1501-1506.
23. Feibel, F., C.F. Helmboldt, E.L. Jungherr, and J.R. Carson. 1952. Avian encephalomyelitis—prevalence, pathogenicity of the virus, and breed susceptibility. Am J Vet Res 13:260-266.
24. Folkers, C., D. Jaspers, M.E.M. Stumpel, and E.A.E. Wittebrongel. 1976. Vaccination against avian encephalomyelitis with special reference to the spray method. Dev Biol Stand 33:364-369.
25. Garrett, J.K., R.B. Davis, and W.L. Ragland. 1984. Enzyme-linked immunosorbent assay for detection of antibody to avian encephalomyelitis virus in chickens. Avian Dis 28:117-130.
26. Garrett, J.K., R.B. Davis, and W.L. Ragland. 1985. Correlation of serum antibody titer for avian encephalomyelitis virus (AEV) in hens with the resistance of progeny embryos to AEV. Avian Dis 29:878-880.
27. Girshick, T., and C.K. Crary, Jr. 1982. Preparation of an agar-gel precipitating antigen for avian encephalomyelitis and its use in evaluating the antibody status of poultry. Avian Dis 26:798-804.
28. Glisson, J.R., and O.J. Fletcher. 1987. Clinical encephalitis following avian encephalomyelitis vaccination in broiler pullets. Avian Dis 31:383-385.
29. Gosting, L.H., B.W. Grinnell, and M. Matsumoto. 1980. Physico-chemical and morphological characteristics of avian encephalomyelitis virus. Vet Microbiol 5:87-100.
30. Hill, R.W., and R.G. Raymond. 1962. Apparent natural infection of Coturnix quail hens with the virus of avian encephalomyelitis. Case report. Avian Dis 6:226-227.
31. Hoekstra, J. 1964. Experiments with avian encephalomyelitis. Br Vet J 120:322-335.
32. Hohlstein, W.M., D.R. Deshmukh, C.T. Larsen, J.H. Sautter, B.S. Pomeroy, and J.R. McDowell. 1970. An epiornithic of avian encephalomyelitis in turkeys in Minnesota. Am J Vet Res 31:2233-2242.
33. Ikeda, S. 1977. Immunodiffusion tests in avian

encephalomyelitis. 1. Standardization of procedure and detection of antigen in infected chickens and embryos. Nat Inst Anim Health Q (Tokyo) 17:81-87.
34. Ikeda, S. 1977. Immunodiffusion tests in avian encephalomyelitis. II. Detection of precipitating antibody in infected chickens in comparison with neutralizing antibody. Nat Inst Anim Health Q (Tokyo) 17:88-94.
35. Jones, E.E. 1932. An encephalomyelitis in the chicken. Science 76:331-332.
36. Jones, E.E. 1934. Epidemic tremor, an encephalomyelitis affecting young chickens. J Exp Med 59:781-798.
37. Jungherr, E.L. 1939. Pathology of spontaneous and experimental cases of epidemic tremor. Poult Sci 18:406. (Abstr).
38. Jungherr, E., and E.L. Minard. 1942. The present status of avian encephalomyelitis. J Am Vet Med Assoc 100:38-46.
39. Jungherr, E.L., F. Sumner, and R.E. Luginbuhl. 1956. Pathology of egg-adapted avian encephalomyelitis. Science 124:80-81.
40. Kamada, M., G. Sato, and S. Miura. 1974. Characterization of multiplication of embryo-adapted avian encephalomyelitis virus in chick embryo brain cell cultures. Jpn J Vet Res 22:32-42.
41. Kodama, H., G. Sato, and S. Miura. 1975. Avian encephalomyelitis virus in chicken pancreatic cell cultures. Avian Dis 19:556-565.
42. Krauss, H., and S. Ueberschär. 1966. Zur Ultrastruktur des Virus der aviaeren Enzephalomyelitis. Berl Muench Tierärztl Wochenschr 79:480-482.
43. Lucas, A.M. 1951. Lymphoid tissue and its relationship to so-called normal lymphoid foci and to lymphomatosis. VI. A study of lymphoid areas in the pancreas of doves and chickens. Poult Sci 30:116-124.
44. Lukert, P.D., and R.B. Davis. 1971. New methods under investigation for the evaluation of the immune status of breeder hens to avian encephalomyelitis. II. Preliminary studies with an immunodiffusion test for avian encephalomyelitis antibodies. Avian Dis 15:935-938.
45. MacLeod, A.J. 1965. Vaccination against avian encephalomyelitis with a betapropiolactone inactivated vaccine. Vet Rec 77:335-338.
46. Malkinson, M., Y. Weisman, A. Stavinski, I. Davidson, U. Orgad, and M.S. Dison. 1986. Application of ELISA to study avian encephalomyelitis in a flock of turkeys. Vet Rec 119:503-504.
47. Mancini, I.O., and V.J. Yates. 1967. Cultivation of avian encephalomyelitis virus in vitro. I. In chick embryo neuroglial cell culture. Avian Dis 11:672-679.
48. Mancini, I.O., and V.J. Yates. 1968. Cultivation of avian encephalomyelitis virus in vitro. II. In chick embryo fibroblastic cell culture. Avian Dis 12:278-284.
49. Mancini, I.O., and V.J. Yates. 1968. Cultivation of avian encephalomyelitis virus in chicken embryo kidney cell culture. Avian Dis 12:686-688.
50. Mathey, W.J., Jr. 1955. Avian encephalomyelitis in pheasants. Cornell Vet 45:89-93.
51. Miyamae, T. 1974. Ecological survey by the immunofluorescent method of virus in enzootics of avian encephalomyelitis. Avian Dis 18:369-377.
52. Miyamae, T. 1977. Immunofluorescent study on egg-adapted avian encephalomyelitis virus infection in chickens. Am J Vet Res 38:2009-2012.
53. Miyamae, T. 1981. Localization of viral protein in avian-encephalomyelitis-virus-infected hens. Avian Dis 25:1065-1069.
54. Miyamae, T. 1983. Invasion of avian encephalomyelitis virus from the gastrointestinal tract to the central nervous system in young chickens. Am J Vet Res 44:508-510.
55. Mohanty, G.C., and J.L. West. 1968. Some observations on experimental avian encephalomyelitis. Avian Dis 12:689-693.
56. Nicholas, R.A.J., A.J. Ream, and D.H. Thornton. 1987. Replication of avian encephalomyelitis virus in chick embryo neuroglial cell cultures. Arch Virol 96:283-287.
57. Olitsky, P.K. 1939. Experimental studies on the virus of infectious avian encephalomyelitis. J Exp Med 70:565-582.
58. Olitsky, P.K., and J.H. Bauer. 1939. Ultrafiltration of the virus of infectious avian encephalomyelitis. Proc Soc Exp Biol Med 42:634-636.
59. Olitsky, P.K., and H. Van Roekel. 1952. Avian encephalomyelitis (epidemic tremor). In H.E. Biester and L.H. Schwarte (eds.), Diseases of Poultry, 3rd Ed., pp. 619-628. Iowa State Univ Press, Ames.
60. Peckham, M.C. 1957. Lens opacities in fowls possibly associated with epidemic tremors. Case report. Avian Dis 1:247-255.
61. Polewaczyk, D.E., Z. Zolli, Jr., and W.D. Vaughn. 1972. Efficacy studies for a freeze-dried avian encephalomyelitis vaccine. Poult Sci 51:1851.
62. Richey, D.J. 1962. Avian encephalomyelitis (epidemic tremor). Southeast Vet 13:55-57.
63. Richter, V.R., J. Kosters, and S. Kuhavanta-Kalkosol. 1985. Vergleichende untersuchungen zur anwendung eines enzyme-linked-immunosorbent-assay (ELISA) zum antikorpernachweis gegen den erreger der aviaren encephalomyelitis. Zentralbl Veterinaermed [B] 32:116-127.
64. Sato, G., M. Kamada, T. Miyamae, and S. Miura. 1971. Propagation of non-egg-adapted avian encephalomyelitis virus in chick embryo brain cell culture. Avian Dis 15:326-333.
65. Schaaf, K. 1958. Immunization for the control of avian encephalomyelitis. Avian Dis 2:279-289.
66. Schaaf, K. 1959. Avian encephalomyelitis immunization with inactivated virus. Avian Dis 3:245-256.
67. Schaaf, K., and W.F. Lamoreaux. 1955. Control of avian encephalomyelitis by vaccination. Am J Vet Res 16:627-633.
68. Schneider, T. 1967. Beobachtungen ueber die Durchseuchung von Zuchthuehnerbestaenden nach Lebendvaccination mit dem Virus der aviaeren Encephalomyelitis (AE) der Huehner. Arch Gefluegelkd 31:342-348.
69. Smart, I.J., and D.C. Grix. 1985. Measurement of antibodies to infectious avian encephalomyelitis virus by ELISA. Avian Pathol 14:341-352.
70. Smart, I.J., D.C. Grix, and D.A. Barr. 1986. The application of the ELISA to the diagnosis and control of avian encephalomyelitis. Aust Vet J 63:297-299.
71. Springer, W.T., and S.C. Schmittle. 1968. Avian encephalomyelitis. A chronological study of the histopathogenesis in selected tissues. Avian Dis 12:229-239.
72. Sumner, F.W., E.L. Jungherr, and R.E. Luginbuhl. 1957. Studies on avian encephalomyelitis. I. Egg adaption of the virus. Am J Vet Res 18:717-723.
73. Sumner, F.W., R.E. Luginbuhl, and E.L. Jungherr. 1957. Studies on avian encephalomyelitis. II. Flock survey for embryo susceptibility to the virus. Am J Vet Res 18:720-723.
74. Sytuo, B., and M. Matsumoto. 1981. Detection of chicken antibodies against avian encephalomyelitis virus by an enzyme-linked immunoassay. Poult Sci 60:1742.
75. Tannock, G.A., and D.R. Shafren. 1985. A rapid procedure for the purification of avian encephalomyelitis viruses. Avian Dis 29:312-321.
76. Taylor, J.R.E., and E.P. Schelling. 1960. The distribution of avian encephalomyelitis in North America

as indicated by an immunity test. Avian Dis 4:122–133.
77. Taylor, L.W., D.C. Lowry, and L.G. Raggi. 1955. Effects of an outbreak of avian encephalomyelitis (epidemic tremor) in a breeding flock. Poult Sci 34:1036–1045.
78. Van der Heide, L. 1970. The fluorescent antibody technique in the diagnosis of avian encephalomyelitis. Univ Maine Tech Bull 44:1–79.
79. Van Roekel, H., K.L. Bullis, O.S. Flint, and M.K. Clarke. 1936. "Epidemic tremors" in chickens. Massachusetts Agric Exp Stn Annu Rep Bull 327:75.
80. Van Roekel, H., K.L. Bullis, O.S. Flint, and M.K. Clarke. 1932. "Epidemic tremors" in chicks. Massachusetts Agric Exp Stn Annu Rep Bull 369:389.
81. Van Roekel, H., K.L. Bullis, and M.K. Clarke. 1938. Preliminary report on infectious avian encephalomyelitis. J Am Vet Med Assoc 93:372–375.
82. Van Roekel, H., K.L. Bullis, and M.K. Clarke. 1939. Infectious avian encephalomyelitis. Vet Med 34:754–755.
83. Van Roekel, H., K.L. Bullis, O.S. Flint, and M.K. Clarke. 1940. Avian encephalomyelitis. Massachusetts Agric Exp Stn Annu Rep Bull 369:94.
84. Van Roekel, H., K.L. Bullis, and M.K. Clarke. 1941. Transmission of avian encephalomyelitis. J Am Vet Med Assoc 99:220.
85. Van Steenis, G. 1971. Survey of various avian species for neutralizing antibody and susceptibility to avian encephalomyelitis virus. Res Vet Sci 12:308–311.
86. Westbury, H.A., and B. Sinkovic. 1978. The pathogenesis of infectious avian encephalomyelitis. I. The effect of the age of the chicken and the route of administration of the virus. Aust Vet J 54:68–71.
87. Westbury, H.A., and B. Sinkovic. 1978. The pathogenesis of infectious avian encephalomyelitis. II. The effect of immunosuppression on the disease. Aust Vet J 54:72–75.
88. Westbury, H.A., and B. Sinkovic. 1978. The pathogenesis of infectious avian encephalomyelitis. III. The relationship between viraemia, invasion of the brain by the virus, and the development of specific serum neutralising antibody. Aust Vet J 54:76–80.
89. Westbury, H.A., and B. Sinkovic. 1978. The pathogenesis of infectious avian encephalomyelitis. IV. The effect of maternal antibody on the development of the disease. Aust Vet J 54:81–85.
90. Wills, F.K., and I.M. Moulthrop. 1956. Propagation of avian encephalomyelitis virus in the chick embryo. Southwest Vet 10:39–42.

21 INFLUENZA

B.C. Easterday and V.S. Hinshaw

INTRODUCTION. Influenza is an infection and/or disease syndrome caused by any type A influenza virus, a member of the Orthomyxoviridae family. Influenza A viruses are responsible for major disease problems in birds, as well as humans and lower mammals (45, 64, 92, 115). Literally thousands of viruses, belonging to many different antigenic subtypes based on hemagglutinin (HA) and neuraminidase (NA) surface antigens, have been recovered from domestic and wild avian species throughout the world. Infections among domestic or confined birds have been associated with a variety of disease syndromes, ranging from subclinical to mild upper respiratory disease to loss of egg production to acute, generalized fatal disease.

In domestic species, influenza viruses have caused considerable economic losses. The U.S. government expended over $60 million in 1983–84 to eradicate a highly pathogenic H5N2 virus in poultry in the Pennsylvania-Virginia-New Jersey outbreak. The potential cost of the disease without the eradication program was estimated to be many times higher (102). The $60 million included the cost of eradication (diagnosis, quarantine, flock disposal, clean-up, decontamination, epidemiologic investigation, and other regulatory procedures) and indemnity payments to flock owners. Consumers paid an estimated additional $349 million to cover losses passed on by the producers (102). More limited outbreaks of avian influenza are also quite costly. For example, on one chicken farm in Australia in 1985, an outbreak involving a highly pathogenic virus cost over $2 million to eradicate (40).

The economic impact is not limited to chickens; losses have been suffered by turkey producers for many years in several countries in Europe and in the USA, Israel, and Great Britain (10, 110, 130, 158, 170). An epidemic in Minnesota in 1978 cost turkey producers in excess of $5 million (131); the estimated cost of outbreaks in Minnesota since 1977 totaled more than $10 million (130).

In most cases, losses cannot be predicted when an influenza outbreak appears because many factors influence the outcome of infection. These factors include the variation in the biological characteristics of the virus, intercurrent infection, environmental stresses, age and sex of the bird, etc., with the result being that the morbidity and mortality rates range from negligible to near 100%. Any calculation of economic impact must include all of those factors that impinge on the cost of production, e.g., medication, extra feed, extra care, quarantine measures, vaccines, decreased carcass quality, cleaning and sanitizing, and loss of local and international trade. Unfortunately, there are insufficient data to provide a reasonable estimate of avian influenza losses on a nationwide basis for any country.

In contrast to domestic or confined birds, free-flying birds typically do not experience significant disease problems due to influenza viruses; yet, these infections are widespread in many of these birds (64, 72). Influenza viruses are readily recovered from migratory waterfowl, particularly ducks, throughout the world. There is considerable speculation about the epidemiologic significance of this very large reservoir of viruses in wild birds: that this reservoir can serve as a source of viruses for other species, including humans, lower mammals, and birds, and that such a high rate of infection provides the opportunity for the maintenance and emergence of "new" and potentially highly pathogenic strains through the process of mutation and/or genetic reassortment. The genetic diversity of avian influenza viruses in the wildlife reservoirs may be important in the overall survival of these viruses in nature.

Because of the significant losses from avian influenza, international symposia were convened in 1981 and 1986 to exchange information on this virus; the first (133) focused on definition of highly pathogenic strains and identification of sources of the virus, and the second (134) on the virus and on the problems and possible solutions in outbreaks involving highly pathogenic influenza viruses in chickens and turkeys. Influenza is an international problem so solutions will require international efforts and cooperation.

HISTORY. Fowl plague, now known to be caused by highly pathogenic strains of avian influenza viruses, was described by Perroncito as a serious disease of chickens in Italy in 1878 and caused by a "filterable" agent (virus) by Centanni and Savunozzi in 1901 (156). However, it was not until 1955 that it was demonstrated that fowl plague viruses were actually type A influenza viruses (143). Viruses related to the original "fowl plague" isolates (surface antigens H7N1 and H7N7) caused high mortality among chickens, turkeys, and other species. Disease outbreaks involving these particular strains have been reported in many areas of the world during this century, including North and South America, North Africa, the Middle and Far East, Europe, Great Britain, and the USSR. Highly pathogenic strains belonging to the H5 subtype were detected in chickens in Scotland, chick/Scot/59 (H5N1) and common terns, tern/S.A./61 (H5N3); both species suffered severe disease problems. These isolations led to the speculation that all H7 and H5 viruses were highly pathogenic but this was not found true. As an example, a virus, avirulent for chickens, with an H7 hemagglutinin was recovered from turkeys in Oregon in 1971 (21, 22). Since that time, many other viruses with the H5 and H7 hemagglutinins have been isolated from domestic and wild birds in various areas of the world and many of these are avirulent for any species (5, 64). It should be mentioned, however, that, historically, the most severe disease problems have been due to viruses of the H5 and H7 subtypes.

From 1950–60, the discoveries that the fowl plague virus was an influenza A virus and that influenza viruses could be recovered from many different domestic and wild avian species initiated increased efforts to understand avian influenza viruses. Since detailed histories of the isolation of influenza viruses in this century are available (5, 45, 64), only more recent events will be described here.

Reports of severe disease outbreaks involving highly pathogenic influenza A viruses during the past 20 yr have, fortunately, been rare. Alexander (6) listed five substantiated outbreaks since 1975; these occurred in Australia (1975 and 1985), England (1979), USA (1983–84), and Ireland (1983–84). In the USA, the only severe outbreaks were reported in 1929 (156) and 1983–84, indicating the infrequency of such events. Much information on the outbreak in Pennsylvania in 1983–84 is presented in the *Proceedings of the 2nd Symposium on Avian Influenza* (134) but some specific aspects (46) will be mentioned here. The first isolates were obtained in April 1983, from chickens experiencing acute respiratory disease with 0–15% mortality and declining egg production. The viruses were identified as H5N2 and, based on chicken inoculation, were not classified as being highly pathogenic. This problem continued at a low level with about six infected flocks present at any given time until October 1983 when mortality increased to 50–89% with the birds experiencing severe depression, tremor, and a complete cessation of egg production. Viruses isolated from these birds were also H5N2 but were designated as highly pathogenic based on chicken inoculation. This apparent change in the disease led the U.S. Department of Agriculture to declare an "extraordinary emergency" with the goal of eradication. The eradication effort included strict quarantine; total poultry population surveillance with destruction of all flocks with clinical, serologic, or virologic evidence of H5N2 influenza; environmental clean-up followed by decontamination; and intensive education on biosecurity (51). Over the next 2 yr, this effort had to include, not only poultry farms, but also live-bird markets in metropolitan areas such as New York City because these markets were found to be involved in the maintenance of the virus and exposure of poultry flocks (55). The highly pathogenic strain was successfully eliminated; however, avirulent H5N2 viruses have since been recovered from farms and live-bird markets in several states.

Since the first influenza isolates from turkeys in North America in 1963 (97), these viruses have frequently caused disease problems. Viruses found in turkeys on open range are often thought to have been introduced by migratory waterfowl (59, 64). An interesting situation in turkeys has developed during the last decade in that H1N1 viruses typically associated with pigs have been responsible for outbreaks in turkeys (69) characterized by respiratory disease and diminished egg production (112). This swine-turkey connection was the first indication that mammalian viruses could be responsible for infection and disease in birds. Studies on H1N1 isolates from pigs and birds throughout the world (12, 13, 70) suggest that swine viruses are being transmitted to turkeys and, in addition, H1N1 viruses from ducks are being transmitted to pigs in some areas of the world.

Although evidence for the infection of wild birds existed prior to the 1970's, it was not until then that the high infection rate among migratory waterfowl was recognized. Surveillance studies revealed the widespread distribution of influenza viruses in these birds, particularly ducks (63, 66) and, more recently, in shorebirds (88). Such studies (64, 67) have shown that virtually all known antigenic subtypes of type A influenza viruses and combinations of H and N surface antigens exist in the avian wildlife reservoir; the viruses are typically avirulent for the hosts; the viruses possess broad host ranges, including other birds and mammals; genetic reassortment between their viruses occurs in the natural setting; and intestinal replication of the viruses in these birds may be an important factor in the efficient transmission of these viruses among waterfowl and potentially to other species. This reservoir in wildlife occupies an important role in the ecology of influenza.

During the last 10 yr, viruses typically found in

avian species have been recovered from outbreaks of disease in mammals, such as seals (71, 101, 166) and mink (48, 95), and have been detected in whales (73). These findings suggest that the association between birds and mammals in the natural setting may lead to transmission of avian viruses, resulting in significant disease problems.

INCIDENCE AND DISTRIBUTION. Avian influenza viruses are distributed throughout the world in many domestic birds, including turkeys, chickens, guinea fowl, chukars, quail, pheasants, geese, and ducks, and in wild species, including ducks, geese, sandpipers, sanderlings, ruddy turnstones, terns, swans, shearwaters, herons, guillemots, puffins, and gulls (see 5, 7, 10, 45, 64, 115). Migratory waterfowl, particularly ducks, have yielded more viruses than any other group while domestic turkeys and chickens have experienced the most substantial disease problems due to influenza. Influenza viruses have also been isolated from cage birds, including mynahs, parakeets, parrots, cockatoos, weaverbirds, finches, hawks (4, 81, 147, 151, 152). These birds were often being held in quarantine and the significance of infection in these birds is not yet clear. Passerine birds have yielded relatively few influenza viruses, particularly in view of the size of this bird population. There have been some isolations from passerine birds in contact with sick domestic birds, e.g., starlings in Israel (104) and Australia (40). Studies on the Australian isolate, A/starling/Victoria/5156/85 (H7N7) (122) led the authors to suggest that highly pathogenic viruses were transmitted between domestic poultry and passerine birds.

Precise distribution and prevalence of influenza viruses are difficult to determine because of the sampling anomalies. The World Health Organization has encouraged and supported surveillance programs to increase the available data on the prevalence and distribution. Even so, most surveillance efforts are conducted by investigators who have a specific interest in avian influenza and/or the ecology of influenza.

Distribution data on avian influenza are clearly influenced by the distribution of both domestic and wild species, the locality of poultry production, migratory routes, season, and disease-reporting systems. Prevalence is also influenced by some of the same factors. Accurate prevalence rates are difficult to determine because of the variety of surveillance systems and procedures employed. For any one episode of avian influenza in a domestic species, a reasonable prevalence rate can be determined; however, the prevalence and distribution are not predictable. For example, in turkeys in Minnesota, the prevalence has been very high some years and nearly nonexistent during others (130). The absence is not due to residual immunity but rather to an unexplained absence of the viruses. Waterfowl have been viewed as a significant source of viruses for turkeys on open range and this may be important in areas such as Minnesota and Wisconsin, which are located along a major flyway. Investigators there (59, 60) have recovered many influenza viruses from free-flying and sentinel ducks during the fall migration and have established that the outbreaks in turkeys coincide with the presence of the migratory ducks. Even so, it is difficult to predict which virus will appear and cause problems in the turkeys at any time.

Surveillance of migratory waterfowl in North America has indicated that up to 60% of juvenile birds may be infected as they congregate in marshalling areas prior to migration (66, 72). As the birds migrate, the rate of virus recovery drops precipitously. Since ducks have been shown to excrete virus for as long as 30 days (165), this means that few cycles of transmission would be required to maintain the viruses. It seems possible that the viruses are maintained in the wild duck population by passage to susceptible birds, even at a low level, throughout the year until the next breeding season results in a new group of susceptible juveniles. Transmission can readily occur due to the excretion of high quantities of the virus in the feces, resulting in heavily contaminated lake or pond water (65). Recent studies (88) on shorebirds (such as sanderlings, ruddy turnstones and sandpipers) and gulls suggested that they constitute a significant reservoir of viruses. The involvement of wild birds, particularly waterfowl, with influenza viruses, underlines the need for producers of domestic, commercial birds to provide separation between domestic and wild bird populations.

There have been only three incidents of influenza viruses in chickens in North America since the last fowl plague outbreak in 1929: Alabama in 1975 (78, 79), Minnesota in 1979 (58), and Pennsylvania in 1983–84 (47). There are reports of influenza infections in chickens in several other countries including Belgium, Scotland, Italy, USSR, Australia, Hong Kong, Belgium, France, and Israel (5, 110). Influenza infections of domestic ducks have been detected in many areas of the world, including North America (142). Influenza in turkeys has also been reported in many countries, including Hungary, France, Holland, Italy, Ireland, England, Canada, USA, and Israel (5, 6). Alexander (5), Hinshaw et al. (67), and the symposia proceedings (133, 134) provide information and tabulations of the countries, years, and subtypes of viruses in wild waterfowl, chickens, domestic ducks, and turkeys.

In considering the prevalence and distribution of influenza viruses in avian species, it becomes clear that many viruses circulate in birds throughout the world. In view of that, it is puzzling that avian influenza viruses are not responsible for more extensive poultry disease problems.

ETIOLOGY

Classification. Avian influenza viruses, along with all other influenza viruses, constitute the virus family Orthomyxoviridae (92, 115). These are medium-sized, pleomorphic RNA viruses with helical symmetry and glycoprotein projections from the envelope that have hemagglutinating and neuraminidase activity. There are three antigenically distinct types of influenza viruses: A, B, and C. The type specificity is determined by the antigenic nature of the nucleoprotein (NP) and matrix (M) antigens, which are closely related among all influenza A viruses. Types B and C are typically found only in humans. Type A influenza viruses are found in humans; swine; horses; occasionally other mammals such as mink, seals, and whales; and many avian species.

CLASSIFICATION BASED ON THE HEMAGGLUTININ AND NEURAMINIDASE. Type A viruses are divided into subtypes according to the antigenic nature of the HA and NA. There are currently 13 distinct HAs and 9 distinct NAs. A standard system of nomenclature for influenza viruses was proposed in 1971 (171) and revised in 1980 (172). The name of an influenza virus includes the type (A, B, or C), host of origin (except human), geographic origin, strain number (if any), and year of isolation followed by the antigenic description of the HA (H) and NA (N) in parentheses. For example, a type A influenza virus isolated from turkeys in Wisconsin in 1968 and classified as H8N4 is designated A/turkey/Wisconsin/1/68 (H8N4). The H and N subtype designations, which include the previous and current descriptions, are listed in Table 21.1.

CLASSIFICATION BASED ON PATHOGENICITY. The term "fowl plague" was often used to refer either to the clinical disease or the virus involved in outbreaks with high mortality. It had become clear that a definition of fowl plague based on antigenic characteristics (presence of H7) was inadequate because antigenically similar, if not identical, viruses were frequently isolated from avian species and they were avirulent (21). Therefore, it was important to develop recommendations for a uniform terminology for the highly pathogenic avian influenza viruses, especially fowl plague (16). Unfortunately, most, if not all, disease regulations for the control of fowl plague were based on the H7 surface antigen requirement.

Participants at an international symposium recommended that the term "fowl plague" be discarded, except for historical purposes and proposed criteria for defining "highly pathogenic" influenza viruses (133). One recommendation was that 75% mortality in experimentally inoculated birds be considered as one criterion for highly pathogenic strains (16). Unfortunately, the initial H5N2 isolates from chickens in the Pennsylvania outbreak failed to produce 75% mortality and did not qualify as a "highly pathogenic" virus (126). In view of this, the U.S. Animal Health Association Committee on Transmissible Diseases of Poultry and Other Avian Species (135) has revised the original recommendations for determining if an avian influenza isolate should be classified as highly pathogenic and, therefore, must be considered for eradication. These recommendations are:

a. Any influenza virus that is lethal for 6, 7, or 8 of eight 4- to 6-wk-old susceptible chickens within 10 days following intravenous inoculation with 0.2 ml of a 1:10 dilution of a bacteria-free, infectious allantoic fluid.

b. After the above criterion is met for an isolate, any additional flocks may be declared positive for influenza and treated appropriately based only upon disease signs, isolation of the virus of the same hemagglutinin subtype, demonstration of antibody, and/or epidemiologic evidence connected with other avian influenza-infected flocks.

Table 21.1. Type A influenza subtypes according to WHO system of nomenclature

Hemagglutinin		Neuraminidase	
1980–(Current)	Previous	1980–(Current)	Previous
H1	H0, H1, Hsw1	N1	N1
H2	H2	N2	N2
H3	H3, Heq2, Hav7	N3	Nav2, Nav3
H4	Hav4	N4	Nav4
H5	Hav5	N5	Nav5
H6	Hav6	N6	Nav1
H7	Hav1, Heq1	N7	Neq1
H8	Hav8	N8	Neq2
H9	Hav9	N9	Nav6
H10	Hav2		
H11	Hav3		
H12	Hav10		
H13	Hav11		

Source: (172).

c. Further tests and evaluation will be required for any virus that kills 1–5 of 8 chickens in the pathotype test or has a hemagglutinin that is H5 or H7.

d. If an avian influenza virus is isolated that kills 1–5 of 8 inoculated chickens and shows evidence of growth in cell culture with cytopathic effect or plaque formation in the absence of trypsin, an amino acid sequence of the connecting peptide of the HA must be determined before declaring that the isolate is not highly pathogenic.

As of October, 1988, no regulatory agency has officially adopted these recommendations; however, the recent experiences of several countries with highly pathogenic influenza viruses necessitates guidelines for dealing with these viruses when they occur.

Morphology. The morphology and arrangement of the components in the influenza virion have been reviewed (92, 115). Virions are roughly spherical with a diameter of 80–120 nm; however; there are often filamentous forms of the same diameter with varying lengths. The surface of the virion is covered with closely spaced spikes or projections 10–12 nm long. A helical nucleocapsid is enclosed within the viral envelope. The surface spikes with two different shapes are the HA, which is a rod-shaped trimer, and the NA, which is a mushroom-shaped tetramer. The virion may be disrupted with detergents, resulting in the release of the spikes that retain their respective activities. The HA is responsible for the attachment of the virion to cell surface receptors (sialyloligosaccharides) and is responsible for the hemagglutinating activity of the virus. Antibodies against the HA are very important in neutralization of the virus and protection against infection. NA enzyme activity is responsible for the release of new virus from the cell by its action on the neuraminic acid in the receptors. Antibodies to NA are also important in protection, apparently by restricting the spread of virus from infected cells. The 3-dimensional structures of the H3 hemagglutinin (173) and the N2 (38) and N9 neuraminidases (15) have now been determined and important antigenic domains, or epitopes, have been defined.

The HA and NA, in addition to a small protein called M2, are embedded in a lipid envelope derived from the plasma membrane of the host cell. Underneath the viral envelope is the major structural protein M1 that surrounds the RNA molecules in association with the NP and three large proteins (PB1, PB2, and PA), which are responsible for RNA replication and transcription.

The viral genome is composed of eight segments of single-stranded RNA of a negative sense. Those eight segments code for ten viral proteins, eight of which are constituents of the virions (HA, NA, NP, M1, M2, PB1, PB2, and PA). The RNA segment with the smallest molecular weight codes for two nonstructural (NS) proteins, NS1 and NS2. These can be detected in the infected cell and NS1 has been associated with inclusions in the cytoplasm; however, the functions of NS1 and NS2 are not yet defined.

The eight RNA segments, all with different molecular weights, can be isolated from the virus particles; the coding function for each segment is known. The RNA segments of a virus can be separated by polyacrylamide gel electrophoresis. Comparison of the migration patterns of the RNAs of different viruses, particularly reassortants (see section on antigenic shift), has been used to examine the source of viral genes. In addition, the RNAs of closely related influenza viruses can be compared by oligonucleotide mapping to determine the degree of differences between strains–a sensitive method to detect mutations. This approach was used initially for comparing isolates of high and low pathogenicity from chickens in Pennsylvania (17). There has been a dramatic increase in information on RNA sequences of influenza viral genes during the last 10 yr. The genetic sequence information is significant and includes partial sequence data and, in some cases, complete data on all of the eight viral genes. Specific information on genes of avian viruses is also available; for example, the sequences of the HA genes of several avian subtypes, including H3 (49, 91), H5 (85, 87), and H7 (117, 129), are known in their entirety and partial sequence data on all 13 hemagglutinins are available (2). The available information is increasing at a rapid rate and should prove valuable in permitting determination of the genetic basis for important biological properties such as pathogenicity, tissue tropism, and host range.

Chemical Composition. The approximate composition of influenza virions is reported as 0.8–1.1% RNA, 70–75% protein, 20–24% lipid, and 5–8% carbohydrate (37). The lipids are located in the viral membrane; most are phospholipids with smaller amounts of cholesterol and glycolipid. Several carbohydrates (94) including ribose (in the RNA), galactose, mannose, fucose, and glucosamine are present in the virion mainly as glycoproteins or glycolipids. The virion proteins, as well as potential glycosylation sites, are all specified by the viral genome, but the composition of the lipid and carbohydrate chains linked to glycoproteins or glycolipids of the viral membrane are determined by the host cell.

Virus Replication. Replication of influenza viruses has been studied by many investigators and the process described in detail (93). Briefly, as described by Fenner et al. (50), the virus adsorbs to glycoprotein receptors containing sialic acid on the cell surface. The virus then enters the cell by receptor-mediated endocytosis. This includes exposure to a low pH in the endosome, resulting in a conformational change in the HA, which mediates membrane fusion. The nucleocapsid thus enters the cytoplasm and migrates to the nucleus. Influenza virus utilizes a unique mechanism to initiate transcription in that a viral endonuclease cleaves the 5′ cap from cellular mRNAs and uses this as a primer for transcription by the viral transcriptase. Six monocistronic mRNAs are produced and translated into the HA, NA, NP, and the three polymerases (PB1, PB2, and PA). The mRNAs for NS and M genes undergo splicing and each yields two mRNAs, which are translated in different reading frames and thus produce the NS1, NS2, M1, and M2 proteins. The HA and NA are glycosylated in the rough endoplasmic reticulum, trimmed in the Golgi, and transported to the surface where they remain embedded in the cell membrane. An important requirement for the HA is cleavage by host cell proteases into HA1 and HA2, which remain linked by disulfide bonds; cleavage is required for production of infectious virus. After production and assembly of viral proteins and RNA, the virus exits the cell by budding from the plasma membrane.

Antigenic Variation. The frequency of antigenic variation among influenza viruses is high and occurs in two ways, drift and shift (115). Antigenic drift involves minor antigenic changes in the HA and/or NA, whereas antigenic shift involves major antigenic changes in the HA and/or NA.

ANTIGENIC DRIFT. Antigenic drift is due to point mutations in the genes coding for the HA and/or NA proteins and is a reflection of selection of variants in an immune population. Antigenic drift has been most elegantly defined with influenza viruses from humans but is also known to occur with avian strains (12, 70, 77, 91). These studies have suggested that avian viruses show less antigenic drift than mammalian strains; the reason for this is not clear but could include lack of immunologic pressure in short-lived birds.

In defining the mechanisms of antigenic drift of human strains, four antigenic sites on the 3-dimensional structure of the H3 hemagglutinin of a human virus have been defined (173). This was based on sequence data from naturally occurring variants and variants selected with monoclonal antibodies. In essence, a single-point mutation can alter the structure of the surface protein (HA or NA) and therefore its antigenic and/or immunologic properties, resulting in an antigenic variant.

ANTIGENIC SHIFT. The segmented nature of the viral genome (8 segments of RNA) allows segments to reassort when a cell is infected with two different influenza viruses, potentially yielding 256 genetically different progeny viruses. That activity is called genetic reassortment. Genetic reassortment was initially demonstrated by antigenic analyses of the viruses produced during mixed infections (163). Antigenic reassortant viruses, i.e., those with combinations of HA and NA of the parental viruses, were readily detected when a cell, embryo, or susceptible host was infected with two antigenically distinct viruses. Those exchanges that are detected by antigenic analysis involve only the segments that code for the HA and NA surface proteins (antigens); however, genetic exchanges can certainly involve genes other than those. In addition, viruses from different species also readily exchange genes.

It has been demonstrated "that mixed infections occur reasonably frequently in nature" (64). In such cases two or more antigenically distinct influenza viruses have been recovered from cloacal samples of free-flying ducks. Experimentally, genetic reassortment takes place when ducks are infected with two antigenically distinct viruses. Thus, it is not surprising that viruses with almost every possible combination of antigenic subtypes have been recovered from ducks in nature.

Genetic reassortment between human and avian viruses is suggested as the mechanism by which "new" human pandemic strains arise (163). Thus, avian viruses may play a role in the influenza viruses in people by contributing genes to human strains.

Biological Properties. The biological property of pathogenicity of the avian influenza viruses is extremely variable and cannot be predicted based on the host of origin or antigenic subtype (HA) of the virus. Avian viruses of the H5 and H7 subtypes have been associated with severe disease in chickens, turkeys, ducks, and terns; e.g., chicken/Scotland/59 (H5N1), chicken/Penn/83 (H5N2), turkey/Ontario/7732/66 (H5N6), Tern/South Africa/61 (H5N3), and the fowl plague viruses (H7N1 and H7N7) (6). However, there are many examples of H5 and H7 virus isolates that are not pathogenic so antigenic configuration alone does not determine pathogenicity.

As with any virus, pathogenicity is a property of the interaction of the host and virus. An influenza virus that is pathogenic for one avian species will not necessarily be pathogenic for another avian species (9). For example, turkey/Ontario/7732/66 virus is highly pathogenic (100% mortality) for turkeys and chickens and at the same time nonpathogenic (no mortality) for other species, such as ducks (150). The tissue tropism of a virus may well be involved in its pathogenicity; for example, viruses restricted to the respiratory or intestinal tract will produce quite a different disease problem than a virus that becomes systemic and reaches vital organs. The basis for tissue tropism is not yet defined, but receptor specificities of human, equine, and avian viruses differ (137, 138). Studies (118) indicate that mutations in the receptor binding site of the viral HA can alter the ability of viruses to infect different hosts. It seems possible that receptor recognition is an important factor in both host range and tissue tropism, as well as pathogenicity. Since there is as yet no cellular receptor identified for influenza viruses, the role of virus-receptor interactions in disease is unclear.

The molecular basis for pathogenicity is not totally defined. Rott and Scholtissek (139) suggested that pathogenicity is polygenic and can be disassociated from the HA and NA. On the other hand, there is substantial evidence (164) that the HA gene is extremely important in pathogenicity. The feature that is particularly relevant is the cleavability of the HA (28, 164).

As mentioned earlier, highly pathogenic viruses possess HAs that are readily cleaved in a variety of cells in vivo and in vitro. The ability of proteases in the host cell to accomplish this cleavage is considered important in determining the extent of replication. For example, the highly pathogenic viruses possess HAs that are cleaved in a number of different cells so infectious virus would be produced. However, the HAs of low to moderately pathogenic influenza viruses are typically not cleaved in many cells so no infectious virus is produced. The highly pathogenic viruses have a series of basic amino acids at the carboxy-terminus of HA1, whereas avirulent viruses have a single basic amino acid at that site. It seems likely that the basic amino acids are involved in protease recognition and cleavage of the HA of highly pathogenic viruses.

Studies (84–86, 169) on both low and highly pathogenic H5N2 viruses from chickens in Pennsylvania suggested that this group of viruses all possessed the cleavage site sequence associated with highly pathogenic viruses; however, the HA of the early less pathogenic isolates had a glycosylation site in the cleavage region and the presence of this may have blocked efficient cleavage. A single mutation removing that glycosylation site resulted in a highly pathogenic strain. Thus, in this case, determination of the sequence around the cleavage site of the HAs would have indicated the dangerous nature of these particular viruses. Studies with another highly pathogenic H5 virus, turkey/Ontario/7732/66 (128), revealed that changes in neutralizing epitopes on the HA alter the virulence of the virus; thus, there may be different means by which changes on the HA alter the outcome of the viral infection.

In addition to assessing viruses for their in vivo pathogenicity, in vitro analyses provide useful information for evaluating virulence. Senne et al. (148) have compared in vitro and in vivo activities of H5N2 isolates from Pennsylvania and determined that chicken inoculations were inadequate to evaluate the virulence of these viruses. As mentioned above, cleavage of the HA is an important marker for highly pathogenic viruses and this can be measured in vitro. The ability of influenza viruses to produce plaques in tissue culture cells as chick embryo fibroblasts (CEF) and Madin-Darby canine kidney (MDCK) cells in the absence of trypsin correlates with pathogenicity because it indicates that the HA of that strain is readily cleaved by cell proteases. In contrast, low to moderately pathogenic viruses cannot form plaques in the absence of trypsin because the HA remains uncleaved. The addition of trypsin to the cells will accomplish the cleavage and allow plaquing (28). Trypsin requirements correlate well with pathogenicity; however, there are exceptions. For example, mixed virus populations may be present and limit the usefulness of the procedure in predicting the pathogenicity of influenza isolates (29). In recent studies (127), highly pathogenic variants of turkey/Ont/7732/66 plaqued without trypsin in CEF but required trypsin to plaque in MDCK. This suggested that CEF may prove more reliable for evaluating this aspect. Another assay is analysis of HA cleavage by radioimmunoprecipitation of HA from tissue culture cells as described by Senne et al. (148).

The in vivo and in vitro analyses can identify a typical highly pathogenic strain. However, the presence of several basic amino acids at the carboxy-terminus of HA1 is probably the most reliable indicator that the virus has the potential to be highly pathogenic (164). Thus, this is the reason for the recommendation (135) that the sequence at the cleavage site in the HA be determined in evaluating pathogenicity of isolates.

Resistance to Chemical and Physical Agents. Avian influenza A viruses are enveloped viruses and thus are relatively sensitive to inactivation by lipid solvents, such as detergents. Infectivity is also rapidly destroyed by formalin, beta-propiolactone, oxidizing agents, dilute acids, ether, sodium desoxycholate, hydroxylamine, sodium dodecylsulfate, and ammonium ions (54, 103). Avian influenza viruses are not endowed with unusual stability so inactivation of the viruses themselves is not difficult. They are inactivated by heat, extremes of pH, nonisotonic conditions, and dryness.

LABORATORY SITUATIONS. Influenza viruses are generally grown in embryonated chicken eggs and are very stable in the allantoic fluid because the presence of protein protects the viruses. Infectivity, as well as hemagglutinating and neuraminidase activities of egg-grown virus, can be maintained for several weeks at 4 C. However, to maintain infectivity for the long term, storage at

−70 C or lyophilization is required. It should be mentioned that hemagglutinating and neuraminidase activities can be maintained even if the virus is no longer infectious. Formalin and beta-propiolactone have been used to eliminate infectivity, yet retain hemagglutinating and neuraminidase activities. Inactivation of these viruses in the laboratory situation can be accomplished with many common detergents and disinfectants (such as phenolic disinfectants or sodium hypochlorite).

FIELD SITUATIONS. In the field situation, influenza viruses are often released in nasal secretions and feces of infected birds so that the viruses are protected by the presence of organic material. This greatly increases their resistance to inactivation. To disinfect contaminated premises, the organic material needs to be removed and/or reduced by cleaning with detergent. The premises can then be decontaminated with heat, sodium hypochorite solution, formalin, or One-Stroke Environ to decontaminate (53, 57).

Heavily contaminated manure represents a special problem in efforts to control influenza (51, 57). Litter and manure can be disposed of by burial, composting in a pile covered with plastic, or rototilling. It should be emphasized that influenza viruses can survive for long periods of time in the environment, particularly under cool and moist conditions. To exemplify this, infectious virus could be recovered from liquid manure for 105 days after depopulation during the influenza outbreak in chickens in Pennsylvania (51). Infectivity was retained in fecal material for as long as 30–35 days at 4 C and for 7 days at 20 C (23, 165). Influenza viruses have been recovered from lake and pond water where there were large concentrations of waterfowl, but not after the birds had left, suggesting that the viruses are not readily inactivated in the environment but may not survive for long periods (65). During disease outbreaks in domestic birds, recovery of virus from water troughs contaminated by secretions and feces is not unusual, but it it not known how long virus can survive in these areas.

Strain Classification. Strain classification of the avian influenza viruses is based on the HA and NA subtype. There are currently 13 hemagglutinins and 9 neuraminidases, all of which have been identified in various combinations in avian isolates. To identify the HA and NA of a virus, the isolate is tested in hemagglutination-inhibition (HI) and neuraminidase-inhibition (NI) tests, using a panel of antisera specific for the different subtypes. These procedures have been described in detail in a Centers for Disease Control manual entitled "Concepts and Procedures for Laboratory-Based Influenza Surveillance" (35) and by Kendal (89).

Comparison of viruses belonging to the same subtype is often accomplished by using postinfection sera from chickens and ferrets and monoclonal antibodies. The use of monoclonal antibodies has enabled more detailed comparisons of related viruses appearing in the same or different species. For example, monoclonal antibodies to the H1 hemagglutinin of H1N1 viruses present in turkeys and pigs have been used to establish the level of antigenic relatedness of their hemagglutinins (12, 70). Comparisons of viruses with these reagents are typically accomplished by HI, enzyme-linked immunosorbent assays (ELISA), and/or neutralization. Additional information on classification is given under "Virus Identification".

Laboratory Host Systems

CHICKEN EMBRYOS. All strains of avian influenza viruses grow readily in 9- to 11-day-old embryonated chicken eggs, making this the most universally used method. The viruses grow to high levels in the egg and have a cleaved hemagglutinin. Additional information is provided in the section on "Isolation and Identification of Causative Agent." Cultivation of influenza viruses in eggs is also used for vaccine production and for preparation of large quantities of virus for laboratory studies.

CELL CULTURE. Avian influenza viruses replicate in a limited number of cell cultures; CEF are those most commonly used primary cultures whereas the most frequently used continuous cell line is the MDCK. Few influenza viruses will grow and produce plaques in cell cultures unless trypsin is added to the agar overlay to cleave the HA molecule for production of infectious virus. Using trypsin in the culture medium allows plaque assays with many strains in CEF or MDCK.

LABORATORY ANIMALS. Chickens, turkeys, and ducks have been the most commonly used species for laboratory studies because they have been the most commonly infected species under natural conditions. Generally, because of the considerable variation between species, it is advisable to use the natural avian host, preferably of the same age and species for laboratory studies. Avian viruses also replicate in a number of experimentally inoculated mammals, such as ferrets, cats, hamsters, mice, monkeys, mink, and pigs (92).

Pathogenicity. There is a wide range of pathogenicity among the avian influenza viruses. Infections with these viruses may be inapparent or result in disease that ranges from mild, transient syndromes to 100% morbidity and/or mortality. The signs of disease may be evident as respiratory, enteric, or reproductive and will vary with virus, species, age, intercurrent infections, environment, and immune status of the host.

Given the very large number of influenza viruses that have been isolated from avian species, the number known to be highly pathogenic is extraordinarily small; however, there is a large number of viruses classified as low to moderately pathogenic. The method for detecting such strains has been described under "Classification." Viruses isolated from free-flying waterfowl typically are nonpathogenic, especially for the species from which they were isolated.

There are many situations in which influenza viruses produce marked morbidity and mortality under field conditions yet appear to produce no disease in experimentally inoculated birds. Studies by Toshiro et al. (157) have suggested that the concurrent bacterial infections play a major role in disease related to the low to moderately pathogenic influenza viruses. This could occur because the bacteria provide enzymes capable of cleaving the HA of these low or moderately virulent influenza viruses, allowing them to replicate and spread to a greater extent in that host. This is an interesting explanation for the ability of some strains to cause significant disease problems in the field, but not in experimentally inoculated birds.

PATHOGENESIS AND EPIZOOTIOLOGY

Natural and Experimental Hosts. Many avian species, domestic or wild, can be infected with influenza viruses that may or may not cause disease. More influenza viruses have been isolated from ducks than any other species. Other avian species from which the viruses have been isolated include guinea fowl, domestic geese, quail (*Coturnix japonica*), pheasants, partridge, mynah birds, passerines, psittacines, budgerigars, gulls, shorebirds, and seabirds.

Among the domestic avian species, turkeys have been the most frequently involved in disease outbreaks of influenza, whereas chickens have been less frequently involved.

Influenza A viruses, antigenically and genetically most closely related to avian viruses, have been isolated from two disease outbreaks in harbor seals (*Phoca vitulina*) in the USA (70). The infected experienced pneumonia and significant morbidity and mortality was produced. During studies on infected seals in the laboratory, an individual developed conjunctivitis due to the seal virus, A/Seal/Mass/1/80 (H7N7); several field workers had experienced the same problem (167). The infection was limited to conjunctivitis and cleared with no sequelae. There have been two reports of influenza virus isolates most related to avian viruses from whales (73); whether these viruses are involved in a disease process in these animals is not yet known.

The H1N1 viruses typically found in pigs have also been detected in turkeys in the USA during the last decade. Antigenic and genetic comparisons of these viruses (70, 145, 13, 12) indicate that the turkey viruses are very closely related to those continually circulating in pigs and thus are of swine origin. It has been suggested that the viruses from pigs were introduced either by direct or indirect contact with pigs or by people infected with these viruses.

Scholtissek and Naylor (144) have raised an interesting suggestion that pigs represent a "mixing vessel" for viruses from avian and mammalian species. Thus, close contact between these groups, as in coculture of fish, ducks, and pigs, might facilitate the emergence of "new" strains.

Avian influenza viruses have also been responsible for disease outbreaks in mink (48, 95).

Experimentally, pigs, ferrets, cats, mink, monkeys, and humans (25, 68, 92) can be infected with influenza viruses originating from avian species.

Transmission and Carriers. Infected birds excrete virus from the respiratory tract, conjunctiva, and feces; thus, likely modes of transmission include both direct contact between infected and susceptible birds and indirect contact including aerosol (droplets) or exposure to virus-contaminated fomites. Since infected birds can excrete high levels of virus in their feces, spread is readily accomplished by virtually anything contaminated with fecal material, e.g., birds and mammals, feed, water, equipment, supplies, cages, clothes, delivery vehicles, insects, etc. Thereby, the viruses are readily transported to other areas by people and equipment shared in support and marketing services.

Alexander (5) categorized the sources of primary introduction of infection for domestic poultry as 1) other species of domestic poultry, 2) exotic captive birds, 3) wild birds, and 4) other animals. In category 1, there are examples of spread from one domestic species to another on the same or adjacent farms, e.g., ducks to chickens, or turkeys to chickens, guinea fowl, and pheasants. It is likely that most are due to mechanical transmission as described above. In category 2, while the potential for such spread appears to be real, there are no known introductions of influenza viruses into domestic poultry by infected exotic cage birds, as has been observed for Newcastle disease virus.

Category 3 is a commonly considered source for infection in domestic poultry, i.e., wild birds, particularly migratory waterfowl. There is no conclusive evidence, however, to incriminate wild birds for the introduction of influenza into domestic poultry flocks. However, turkeys and migratory waterfowl are frequently spatially and temporally related. Studies in Minnesota (59, 82) have indicated that influenza viruses appear in the turkeys, concurrently with the arrival of migratory birds. Given the high frequency of influenza viruses in duck feces, such sources should remain suspect. In addition, feces introduced into water supplies could serve as a source of virus for fecal-oral transmission to other birds.

In the Pennsylvania outbreak, surveillance studies (73, 123) demonstrated that many viruses, including a nonpathogenic H5N2 isolate, were present in wild birds in the area, However, there was no evidence that wild birds were disseminating the highly pathogenic virus. In addition, experimental studies (175) showed that ducks and gulls were poor hosts for this virus. The possibility that wild birds were involved in the initial introduction cannot be excluded. During the recent outbreak in turkeys in Ireland involving the highly pathogenic turkey/Ireland/1378/83 (H5N8) strain, a virus of the same subtype was isolated from healthy domestic ducks on an adjacent farm (113). Genetic studies (87) indicated that these viruses were closely related and replicated in ducks and chickens but only produced disease in chickens. Surveillance studies (113) suggested that the initial outbreak in domestic ducks may have occurred through contact with wild birds. Although much of the evidence implicating wild birds as a source is circumstantial, it is sufficient to view these birds as a real source. Wild birds have also been considered important in the influenza problems in seals, in that birds and seals frequently share habitats.

In category 4, there is evidence that turkeys may become infected with viruses from pigs; how frequently this might occur is difficult to estimate. As indicated previously, viruses of swine origin have been detected in turkeys and were presumably transmitted from pigs to turkeys, either mechanically or by people infected with the virus.

There is ample evidence for horizontal transmission of influenza viruses but little evidence to indicate that the viruses can be transmitted vertically. It should be noted, however, that virus can be present within or on the surface of eggs when the hen is infected, as demonstrated by the isolation of H5N2 viruses from chicken eggs during the Pennsylvania outbreak (34). After experimental infection of hens with the H5N2 virus from Pennsylvania, almost all eggs laid on postinfection days 3 and 4 contained virus (23).

Successful experimental routes of exposure include aerosol, intranasal, intrasinus, intratracheal, oral, conjunctival, intramuscular, intraperitoneal, intracaudal air sac, intravenous, cloacal, and intracranial administration of the various viruses.

Incubation Period. The incubation periods for the various diseases caused by these viruses range from as short as a few hours to 3 days. The incubation period is dependent on the dose of virus, the route of exposure, and the species exposed.

Signs. The signs of disease are extremely variable and depend on the species affected, age, sex, concurrent infections, virus, environmental factors, etc. Signs may reflect abnormalities of the respiratory, enteric, reproductive, or nervous systems. The signs most commonly reported include decreased activity; decreased feed consumption and emaciation; increased broodiness of hens and decreased egg production; mild to severe respiratory signs including coughing, sneezing, rales, and excessive lacrimation; huddling; ruffled feathers; edema of head and face; cyanosis of unfeathered skin; nervous disorder; and diarrhea. Any of these signs may occur singly or in various combinations.

In some cases, the disease is rapidly fulminating and birds are found dead without previous signs. Some viruses cause severe disease in one species and inapparent infections in others under experimental conditions. Similarly, viruses that are identical antigenically may have quite different biological characteristics, with one producing severe disease in a given species and the other being an inapparent infection (9, 150). In the recent situation of H5N8 viruses in turkeys and ducks in Ireland (113), there were significant disease problems in the turkeys and none in the ducks; thus, the species involved is quite significant. In all but the case of the mass mortality among common terns (26), influenza virus infections in wild birds have been inapparent with no obvious signs of disease.

In the outbreak in chickens in Pennsylvania (1, 46), initially there was an acute respiratory disease with increasing mortality and declining egg production. However, when the virus became highly pathogenic, there were other problems, including high mortality (50–89%), significant declines in feed and water consumption and egg production. Respiratory signs were less prominent but the birds were severely depressed and some had tremors or unusual attitudes of the head.

Morbidity and Mortality. Morbidity and mortality rates are as variable as the signs and are dependent on the species and virus, as well as age, environment, and intercurrent infections. The more frequent observation is one of high morbidity and low mortality. Morbidity rates generally are poorly defined, largely because of the very large size of flocks involved and the ill-defined signs of disease in many of the outbreaks. On the other hand, in the case of highly pathogenic viruses, the morbidity and mortality can reach 100%.

Gross Lesions. The gross lesions observed in several avian species have been extremely varied with regard to their location and severity, depending greatly on the species and the pathogenicity of the infecting virus. The gross lesions that have been described generally are from observations in chickens and turkeys with natural or experimental infections (45). There are a few descriptions of lesions in terns, domestic ducks, reared quail, partridges, and pheasants.

In many cases, there are few striking lesions because the disease is mild. Mild lesions may be observed in the sinuses, characterized by catarrhal, fibrinous, serofibrinous, mucopurulent, or caseous inflammation. There may be edema of the tracheal mucosa with an exudate that varies from serous to caseous. Air sacs may be thickened and have a fibrinous or caseous exudate. Catarrhal to fibrinous peritonitis and "egg peritonitis" may be observed. Catarrhal to fibrinous enteritis may be observed in the ceca and/or intestine, especially in turkeys. Exudates may be found in the oviducts of laying birds.

In the case of highly pathogenic viruses, there may be no prominent lesions because the birds die very quickly before gross lesions can develop. However, a variety of congestive, hemorrhagic, transudative, and necrobiotic changes have been described with highly pathogenic viruses such as fowl plague virus (H7N7), tern/S.A./61 (H5N3), chicken/Scotland/59 (H5N1), turkey/Ontario/7732/66 (H5N9), turkey/Ontario/6213/65 (H5N1) and chicken/Pennsylvania/83 (H5N2). With these viruses, initial changes may include edema of the head with swollen sinuses and cyanotic, congested, and hemorrhagic wattles and combs. Congestion and hemorrhage may also be seen on the legs. As the disease progresses, internal lesions vary greatly. Necrotic foci were frequently observed in the liver, spleen, kidneys, and lungs in chickens experimentally infected with fowl plague virus (80), but similar lesions were not observed in terns experiencing infection with tern/S.A./61 (141). Congestive and hemorrhagic lesions were common in birds infected with the pathogenic strains, turkey/Ontario/7732/66 and turkey/Ontario/6213/65 (98, 99, 120, 121, 140). Descriptions of lesions observed in a number of individual outbreaks have been described in detail previously (45).

Gross lesions in chickens in the Pennsylvania outbreak, as described by Acland et al. (1), were characterized by severe swelling of the comb and wattles, with periorbital edema. Lesions of the comb were dramatic, ranging from vesicles to severe swelling and cyanosis, ecchymosis, and frank necrosis. Sometimes there was swelling of the feet with ecchymotic discoloration. Visceral lesions included petechial hemorrhage of various serosal and mucosal surfaces, particularly the mucosal surface of the proventriculus near the junction with the ventriculus. The pancreas often had blotchy light yellow and dark red areas along its length. In some birds, gross lesions were limited to dehydration. The lesions were very similar to those described for fowl plague by Stubbs and Beaudette in the 1920's (156).

Not all the highly pathogenic strains produce the same gross lesions. In recent studies by Van Campen et al. (60) chickens infected with the virus turkey/Ontario/7732/66 (H5N9) indicated that this virus causes severe necrosis of lymphoid tissues that is evident grossly by the mottled appearance of the spleen. However, natural and experimental infections of chickens with other virulent strains, such as tern/S.A./61 and chicken/Penn/83, did not cause lymphoid necrosis. The basis for the differences among these viruses is unknown.

When examining birds for gross lesions, an important consideration is that influenza virus infection may be accompanied by bacterial involvement, so lesions may reflect the effects of both virus and bacteria.

Histopathology. Histopathologic descriptions of avian influenza infection have been limited primarily to those conditions with severe overt disease and obvious gross changes, involving highly pathogenic viruses.

Classic fowl plague, as described in 1926 (56) was characterized by edema, hyperemia, hemorrhages, and foci of perivascular lymphoid cuffing, chiefly in the myocardium, spleen, lungs, brain, wattles, and, to a lesser extent, liver and kidney. Parenchymal degeneration and necrosis were present in spleen, liver and kidney. Brain lesions (52, 146) included foci of necrosis, perivascular lymphoid cuffing, glial foci, vascular proliferation, and neuronal changes. Chickens dying after intravenous inoculation of highly virulent fowl plaque virus have widespread edema, hyperemia and hemorrhage, and also foci of necrosis in the spleen, liver, lung, kidney, intestine, and pancreas in decreasing order of frequency (80). Brain lesions were similar to those described earlier (146, 52).

The histologic changes caused by other highly pathogenic influenza viruses in various species, particularly chickens and turkeys, have some similarities, as well as differences, to the changes caused by fowl plague viruses.

In chickens inoculated with tern/S.A./61 (H5N3) (27), foci of necrosis and lymphoid infiltration were seen in spleen, myocardium, brain, eyes, ocular muscles, comb, and skeletal muscle. Splenic lesions were chiefly proliferation of reticular cells in the red pulp accompanied by heterophil accumulation. Severe myocarditis with focal areas of necrotic muscle was also evident. Despite high virus titers, there were no lesions in the lung (and no respiratory signs). After 5 or 6 days, a diffuse encephalitis developed in both the cerebrum and cerebellum, characterized by widespread perivascular cuffing with mononuclear cells, necrosis of neuronal cells, edema and a diffuse cellularity, and some hemorrhage. In contrast to the extensive lesions observed with tern/S.A./61, lesions in chickens infected with another highly pathogenic virus, chicken/Scot/59 (H5N1), were much less severe. Distinguishing features between the lesions caused by these two viruses were degree of cardiac, brain, ocular, and cutaneous involvement, being less severe or absent with chicken/Scot/59.

One of the most striking lesions observed in turkeys infected with turkey/Ont/6213/66 (H5N1) or turkey/Ont/7732/66 (H5N9) was pancreatitis with extensive necrosis of acinar cells (121, 140). Degenerative and necrotic changes were observed in other organs including the liver, brain and meninges, myocardium, and cutaneous tissues (97, 121). Progressive myocardial necrosis and myocarditis accompanied by marked alterations in the myocardial ultrastructure have been described in detail (108). These changes coincided with high levels of virus in myocardial tissue, the maximum levels of serum glutamic-oxalacetic transaminase and lactic dehydrogenase, and cardiac arrhythmias. Resende (136) described necrotic depletion of lymphoid centers in turkeys infected with turkey/Ont/7732/66. Recent studies (160) indicate that turkey/Ont/7732/66 also produces severe lymphoid necrosis in experimentally inoculated chickens; this necrosis was evident in lymphoid cells present in the spleen, thymus, bursa, intestinal tract, and lung. A prominent feature in these birds was necrosis of lymphoid nodules present in the lamina propria of the bronchioles whereas the respiratory epithelium of the airways was relatively spared and no respiratory disease was evident.

Histopathological examination of chickens naturally infected during the Pennsylvania outbreak have been very well described by Acland et al. (1). They defined the major microscopic lesions as mild to severe diffuse, nonsuppurative encephalitis; very mild to severe diffuse, necrotizing pancreatitis; and very mild to severe subacute, necrotizing myositis involving numerous skeletal muscles and most severe in the external ocular muscles and limbs. They also noted that the microscopic lesions were more severe in broilers than in layers; possible explanations include variable age or strain of bird, virus pathogenicity, or stage of disease.

There has been little examination of tissues from wild birds, such as ducks, which become infected with influenza viruses, but typically develop disease. Cooley et al. (39) described pneumonic lesions in mallards experimentally infected with the highly pathogenic virus, turkey/Ont/7732/66. These lesions were characterized by rapid infiltration of lymphocytes and macrophages. There were no obvious clinical signs in these birds suggesting that, although healthy in appearance, ducks may experience damage to the respiratory tract during infection. There are currently no reports of lesions in naturally infected waterfowl, so whether this occurs during natural infection is not known.

In summary, the lesions caused by at least six influenza viruses considered to be highly pathogenic share some similarities but have some distinctive features. For example, multiple focal lymphoid necrosis was characteristic of infection with turkey/Ont/7732/66 but not with turkey/Ont/6213/66 or chicken/Penn/83, whereas pancreatic necrosis was a noteworthy lesion with the latter two viruses. Myocarditis, as described with tern/S.A./61 infection, was not observed in the chicken/Scot/59 infection but was found with the turkey/Ont/7732/66 and chicken/Penn/83 infections. Skeletal muscle lesions, along with brain and comb lesions, were observed in birds infected with chicken/Penn/83 or tern/S.A./61, but infection with tern/S.A./61 did not produce pancreatic lesions. The basis for differences is not yet understood.

DIAGNOSIS. A definitive diagnosis of influenza A virus infection is dependent on the isolation and identification of the virus. Since clinical symptoms can vary dramatically, clinical diagnosis is considered presumptive, except in an epizootic.

Isolation and Identification of Causative Agent. Viruses are recovered commonly from the trachea and/or cloaca of either live or dead birds, because the viruses typically replicate in the respiratory and/or intestinal tracts. Tissues, secretions, or excretions from these tracts are appropriate for virus isolation. In the case of systemic infections produced by highly pathogenic viruses, virtually every organ can yield virus because of the high levels of viremia.

Dry cotton, dacron, or alginate swabs of various sizes may be used to swab the trachea and/or cloaca. A nasopharyngeal swab may be used for collecting materials from the trachea and cloaca of very small birds. The swabs should be placed in a sterile transport medium (1–2 ml) containing high levels of antibiotics to reduce bacterial growth. Organs can be collected and placed into sterile plastic tubes or bags. In the examination of organs for virus, efforts should be made to collect and store internal organs from the respiratory and intestinal tract tissues separately because isolation of virus from internal organs, generally an indication of systemic spread, is more often associated with the highly pathogenic viruses.

It is very important to keep samples for virus

isolation cold (4 C) and moist prior to processing. If the samples for virus isolation can be tested within 48 hr after collection, they may be kept at 4 C; however, if the samples must be held for additional time, storage at −70 C is recommended. Freezing at −20 C is not usually advisable, but storage in liquid nitrogen or with dry ice is satisfactory. Before processing, tissues can be ground as a 10% suspension in the transport medium and clarified by low-speed centrifugation.

Methods for the isolation and identification of influenza viruses have been described in detail (19, 35, 124). Embryonated chicken eggs are most commonly used for virus isolation because avian influenza viruses grow very well in them. Chicken embryos, 10–11 days old, are inoculated via the allantoic cavity with approximately 0.1 ml of sample. To increase the probability of growth of virus, both the allantoic and amniotic routes may be used on the same egg.

The death of inoculated embryos within 24 hr after inoculation usually results from bacterial contamination and these eggs should be discarded. A few viruses may grow rapidly and kill the embryos by 48 hr; however, in most cases the embryos will not die. After 72 hr, or at death, the eggs should be removed from the incubator, chilled, and allantoic fluids collected. Viral replication is demonstrated by chicken erythrocyte hemagglutinating activity in the allantoic fluid.

Generally, if there is virus present in the samples, there will be sufficient growth in the first passage to result in hemagglutination. If no hemagglutinating activity is detected, a sample of the collected egg fluids may be injected into eggs (2nd passage) and the procedure repeated. However, repeated passage of samples is laborious and increases the risk of laboratory contamination; thus, these concerns must be considered when using multiple passage.

Long-term storage of viruses should be done at −70 C. Lyophilization of viruses is also appropriate for long-term storage; however, these stocks should be tested periodically to ensure infectivity.

Virus Identification. Standard methods for testing the egg fluids for the presence of hemagglutinating activity using chicken erythrocytes by macro- or microtechniques are employed (19, 35, 124). Allantoic fluid positive for hemagglutination is used for virus identification.

It is important to determine whether the hemagglutinating activity detected in the allantoic fluid is due to influenza virus or other hemagglutinating viruses, such as paramyxoviruses like Newcastle disease virus (NDV). Thus, the isolate is tested in HI assays against Newcastle disease antiserum. If negative, the virus is then tested for the presence of the Type A NP to establish that an influenza A virus is present. The type-specific NP or matrix protein (MP) may be detected by the double immunodiffusion test (18, 43) or the single radial-hemolysis test (43). More recently, monoclonal antibodies which react with the NP or MPs have proven useful in identifying these antigens in ELISA (162).

The next step in the identification procedure is to determine the antigenic subtype of the surface antigens, HA, and NA. The HA is identified in the HI test (35) using a panel of antisera prepared against the 13 distinct hemagglutinins. Typing is facilitated by using antisera against the isolated HA or against reassortant viruses with irrelevant NAs; this helps avoid steric inhibition due to antibodies against the NA (89). An influenza virus with a new HA would not be detected in tests utilizing antisera to the known HA subtypes. Therefore, it is important that a procedure be used to determine that the unknown hemagglutinating agent is an influenza virus, usually by testing for the type-specific antigens (NP or MP) as described above.

The NA subtype is usually identified by NI assays with antisera prepared against the nine known neuraminidases (35, 124). A micro-NI assay (161) has been developed to assist in the processing of large numbers of isolates and to economize on reagents and handling.

If laboratories are unfamiliar with the techniques or do not have the necessary antisera, final identification can be accomplished by state, federal, or World Health Organization–designated influenza reference laboratories.

Serology. Serological tests are used to demonstrate the presence of antibodies that may be detected as early as 7–10 days after infection. Several techniques are used for serologic surveillance and diagnosis. The most commonly used are the HI test to detect antibodies to the HA and double immunodiffusion to detect antibodies to the NP. Other serologic tests (18, 19, 43, 92, 124) to detect antibodies include virus neutralization, complement fixation (generally unsatisfactory for avian serum), neuraminidase-inhibition, and single radial-hemolysis. More recently, ELISA assays have been developed to detect antibodies to avian influenza viruses (111, 153). In serologic surveillance programs, a test for the detection of anti-NP antibody is frequently used, since this detects antibodies to a cross-reactive antigen shared by all influenza A viruses.

In serological assays, it is important to be aware that there is considerable variation in the immune response among the various avian species. For example, antibodies to the NP are generally prominent in turkeys and pheasants but may be undetectable in ducks known to have been infected (150). In addition, antibodies may be induced in ducks, as well as other species, but fail to be detected in conventional HI tests performed with intact virus (90, 106).

For serologic diagnosis, it is important that acute and convalescent sera be collected. The acute serum sample is collected from affected birds as soon as possible after the onset of the disease. A convalescent phase serum should be collected 14–28 days after onset (75). Paired acute and convalescent serum samples are used to compare the levels of antibodies before and after infection. For example, the sera can be tested in HI assays for antibodies to a suspected virus a fourfold rise in antibody titer in a convalescent serum would be indicative of recent infection with that particular influenza virus. Serum should be kept frozen (−20 C) until tested. Sodium azide (0.01%) may be added to the serum as a preservative.

The sera of many species contain nonspecific inhibitors that may interfere with the specificity of the HI and other tests. Since these inhibitors are especially active against certain viruses, they present a very practical problem in serologic testing and the identification of viruses. Therefore, sera should be treated to reduce or destroy such activity, although it should be recognized that some treatments may lower specific antibody levels. The two most commonly used treatments for these inhibitors have been receptor-destroying enzyme (RDE) and potassium periodate (35, 43). In addition to the nonspecific inhibitors of hemagglutination, sera from other birds, such as turkey and goose, may cause agglutination of the chicken erythrocytes used in the HI test. This may mask low levels of HI activity. Such hemagglutinating activity can be removed by pretreatment of the serum with chicken erythrocytes (119). This problem may sometimes be avoided by using erythrocytes in the HI test of the same species as the serum being tested.

The direct demonstration of influenza viruses or viral proteins in samples from animals is not routinely used for diagnosis at this time. However, immunofluorescence techniques have been used for rapid diagnosis of influenza in humans (3, 62, 105, 109). Skeeles et al. (149) described the use of fluorescent antibody tests for rapid detection of avian influenza virus in tissue samples during the Pennsylvania disease outbreak. Also, ELISA designed to detect viral antigens in samples should become feasible within the near future. At this time, monoclonal antibodies are proving quite useful for localizing viral antigen in tissues by immunoperoxidase staining (160) and radiolabelled gene probes for in situ hybridization can locate cells involved in viral replication in tissues of infected birds (159). These tools are not yet applicable in routine situations; however, their use in the future is a realistic consideration.

Differential Diagnosis. Because of the broad spectrum of signs and lesions reported with infections of avian influenza viruses in several species, a definitive diagnosis must be made by virologic and serologic methods. Other infections that must be considered in the differential diagnosis include Newcastle disease virus and other paramyxoviruses, chlamydia, mycoplasma, and other bacteria. Concurrent infections with influenza viruses and mycoplasma or other bacteria have been commonly observed (45).

TREATMENT. Presently there is no practical specific treatment for avian influenza virus infections. Amantadine hydrochloride and rimantadine hydrochloride are effective in the prophylaxis of human influenza infections (42). Amantadine has also been shown to be effective against influenza A virus infection of quail (44), turkeys (100), and chickens (24, 168). The results of these studies are similar in several aspects. Rinaldi used amantadine for treatment of infection in a large flock of Japanese quail in Italy and the mortality rate was reduced by approximately 50%, but the rate of infection was unaffected. Similarly the severity of disease caused by the turkey/Ont/7732/66, under experimental conditions, was markedly reduced when the turkeys were treated with amantadine hydrochloride. In recent studies in chickens (24, 168), amantadine and rimantadine administered in the drinking water reduced the mortality; however, the birds were still infected and shed virus. Additionally, there was a rapid emergence of amantadine-resistant viruses that killed hens receiving the drug. Amantadine was present in serum, muscle, and liver of treated birds. After withdrawal of the drug, the levels in serum and tissue fell to virtually zero within 24 hr; however, the level in the albumin and yolk of eggs was maintained at least 3 days. At this time, this drug is not approved for use in birds for consumption.

All other treatments used have been of a supportive nature to relieve respiratory distress. Antibiotic treatment has been employed to reduce the effects of concurrent mycoplasma and bacterial infections.

PREVENTION AND CONTROL. Methods for prevention and control of influenza virus infection center on preventing the initial introduction of the viruse and controlling spread if it is introduced. One critical aspect in reaching the goal of prevention and control is the education of the poultry industry regarding how the viruses are introduced, how they spread, and how such events can be prevented.

Prevention. The most likely source of virus for birds is other infected birds, so the basic means for the prevention of infection of poultry with influenza viruses is the separation of susceptible birds from infected birds and their secretions and excretions. "Biosecurity," as it applies to any infectious disease, should be the first line of defense (see Chapter 1). Transmission can occur when susceptible and infected birds are in close contact or when infectious material from infected birds is introduced into the environment of susceptible birds. Such introductions take place by the contamination of equipment, footwear and clothing, vehicles, insemination equipment, feed, water, etc. The presence of virus in fecal material is a likely means for movement of the virus by equipment and people. Another consideration is that there should be no contact with recovered birds because the length of time they shed virus is not clearly defined.

The reservoir of influenza viruses in wild birds should be considered as a potential source for domestic birds, particularly those on open range, so it is important to reduce the contact between these two groups. Swine may serve as a source of virus for turkeys with the virus tranmitted mechanically or by infected people or pigs (69).

Control. In the case of most influenza outbreaks in birds involving viruses of low to moderately high pathogenicity, efforts focus on containing the original disease problem. Control programs in Minnesota (57, 132) and Pennsylvania (30) provide information on measures that have been used by poultry producers to handle their influenza problems. Recommendations and responsibilities for containing influenza outbreaks have been described (51).

In the face of a highly pathogenic influenza virus like chicken/Penn/83, eradication procedures (quarantine, slaughter, disposal, and cleanup) are employed. The decision to eradicate is based on the nature and dimension of the problem and the biological properties of the virus. During the 1983–84 eradication effort in Pennsylvania, more than 17 million birds were destroyed. Area quarantines were essential to prevent spread and to accomplish eradication. Epidemiological surveillance requiring field personnel and laboratory support (125, 126) was critical to detect new outbreaks and contain them. In Pennsylvania, surveillance efforts revealed that live-bird markets were a source of virus, and elimination of that source, as well as infected farms, had to be accomplished (55).

The legal authority to conduct an emergency disease eradication program is shared by the state and federal government, the state being responsible for intrastate quarantine regulation and the federal government being responsible for interstate and international regulations.

VACCINES. Inactivated vaccines against influenza in birds are used in some outbreaks. Considerations that influence decisions on vaccination have been discussed by Beard (20). Vaccination has been prohibited in outbreaks involving highly pathogenic viruses, when eradication is the goal. This was the case in Pennsylvania. When vaccination is practiced, serological surveillance is impeded and viral infection and maintenance can occur in the absence of disease. In the case of viruses of low to moderate pathogenicity that do not fit the category of highly pathogenic (there are many of these), vaccination has been allowed using inactivated viral vaccines with adjuvants administered individually. There are currently no fully licensed influenza vaccines for birds in the USA although vaccines under limited licensure are used, particularly in turkeys (61, 107). Numerous experimental studies (8, 11,14, 31–33, 83, 154, 155, 168, 174) have demonstrated that inactivated monovalent and polyvalent virus vaccines, with adjuvants, are capable of inducing antibody and providing protection against mortality, morbidity, and egg production declines. It should also be noted that, upon challenge, these vaccinated birds often become infected and excrete virus although they show no disease signs. Such vaccines could potentially reduce the severity of disease and the spread of virus in the field situation, but the virus would not be eliminated from the population.

Approaches other than use of inactivated virus vaccines are currently being evaluated; several have been discussed by Murphy and Kendall (114). The use of genetic engineering has been applied to isolate the hemagglutinin genes, particularly H5 and H7, and place them into alternate viral vectors, such as vaccinia virus (36, 41), baculovirus (96) and retrovirus (76). These have been used successfully to immunize and protect birds. Thus, opportunities to develop a variety of effective vaccines clearly exists; the debate (20) centers on the role they should play in controlling influenza viruses of varying pathogenicity in different domestic bird populations.

An interesting application of avian influenza viruses has been their use as gene donors for making live attenuated vaccines for potential use in humans (116). Whether these vaccines will be used is not yet known.

Based on the multitude of influenza A viruses in birds, it seems likely that the future, like the past, will include avian disease problems involving influenza viruses.

ROLE OF AVIAN SPECIES IN MAMMALIAN INFLUENZA.

Avian influenza viruses may play a role in the evolution of new human strains by contributing viral genes to human strains via genetic reassortment (163). Antigenic and genetic evidence supports the suggestion that the hemagglutinin gene in the virus responsible for the 1968 pandemic in humans originated from a virus circulating in ducks. Direct transmission of viruses between birds and humans does not generally occur, however. The harbor seal isolate that resulted in conjunctivitis in a laboratory worker demonstrates, however, that a virus similar to avian viruses was infectious for mammals, including humans. Furthermore, there is evidence to suggest that the H1N1 viruses present in pigs, turkeys, and ducks may be involved in interspecies transmission (70), so a swine-avian-human connection could conceivably have public health significance. In experimental infections of humans, some avian influenza viruses have been shown to replicate to a limited extent (25). Therefore, the evidence suggests that avian influenza viruses have the potential to infect mammals, including humans. On the other hand, there are no reports of avian viruses producing disease outbreaks in human populations; thus, the potential public health concern is based primarily on circumstantial evidence and not actual events. Although the interspecies exchange of these viruses may well be an infrequent event, potential of interspecies transmission must not be excluded.

REFERENCES

1. Acland, H.M., L.A. Silverman-Bachin, and R.J. Eckroade. 1984. Lesions in broiler and layer chickens in an outbreak of highly pathogenic avian influenza virus infection. Vet Pathol 21:564-569.
2. Air, G.M. 1981. Sequence relationships among the hemagglutinin genes of 12 subtypes of influenza A virus. Proc Nat Acad Sci US 78:7639-7643.
3. Al-Attar, M., K. Nielsen, and W.R. Mitchell. 1981. The application of the soluble antigen fluorescent antibody test for the diagnosis of avian influenza. Can J Comp Med 45:140-146.
4. Alexander, D.J. 1981. Isolation of influenza A viruses from exotic birds in Great Britain. In R.A. Bankowski (ed.), Proc 1st Int Symp Avian Influenza, pp. 79-92. Carter Comp. Corp., Richmond, VA.
5. Alexander, D.J. 1982. Avian Influenza: Recent developments. Vet Bull 52:341-359.
6. Alexander, D.J. 1987. Criteria for the definition of pathogenicity of avian influenza viruses. Proc 2nd Int Symp Avian Influenza, pp. 228-245. US Anim Health Assoc, Athens, GA.
7. Alexander, D.J., and R.E. Gough. 1986. Isolations of avian influenza virus from birds in Great Britain. Vet Rec 118:537-538.
8. Alexander, D.J., and G. Parsons. 1980. Protection of chickens against challenge with virulent influenza A viruses of Hav5 subtype conferred by prior infection with influenza A viruses of Hsw1 subtype. Arch Virol 66:265-269.
9. Alexander, D.J., G. Parsons, and R.J. Manvell. 1986. Experimental assessment of the pathogenicity of eight avian influenza A viruses of H5 subtype for chickens, turkeys, ducks, and quail. Avian Pathol 15:647-662.
10. Alexander, D.J., T.M. Murphy, and M.S. McNulty. 1987. Avian influenza in the British Isles during 1981 to 1985. Proc 2nd Int Symp Avian Influenza, pp. 70-78. US Anim Health Assoc, Athens, GA.
11. Allan, W.H., C.R. Madeley, and A.P. Kendal. 1971. Studies with avian influenza A viruses: Cross protection experiments in chickens. J Gen Virol 12:79-84.
12. Austin, F.J., and R.G. Webster. 1986. Antigenic mapping of an avian H1 influenza virus hemagglutinin and interrelationships of H1 viruses from humans, pigs, and birds. J Gen Virol 67:983-992.
13. Aymard, M., A.R. Douglas, M. Fontaine, J.M. Gourreau, C. Kaiser, J. Million, and J.J. Skehel. 1985. Antigenic characterization of influenza A (H1N1) viruses recently isolated from pigs and turkeys in France. Bull WHO 63:537-542.
14. Bahl, A.K., and B.S. Pomeroy. 1977. Efficacy of avian influenza oil-emulsion vaccine in breeder turkeys. J Am Vet Med Assoc 171:1105.
15. Baker, A.T., J.N. Varghese, W.G. Laver, G.M. Air, and P.M. Colman. 1987. Three-dimensional structure of neuraminidase of subtype N9 from an avian influenza virus. Proteins 2:111-117.
16. Bankowski, R.A. 1981. Introduction and objectives of the symposium. In R.A. Bankowski (ed.), Proc 1st Int Symp Avian Influenza, pp. vi-xiv. Carter Comp. Corp., Richmond, VA.
17. Bean, W.J., Y. Kawaoka, J.M. Wood, J.E. Pearson, and R.G. Webster. 1985. Characterization of virulent and avirulent A/Chicken/Pennsylvania/83 influenza A viruses: Potential role of defective interfering RNAs in nature. J Virol 54:151-160.
18. Beard, C.W. 1970. Avian influenza antibody detection by immunodiffusion. Bull WHO 42:799-86.
19. Beard, C.W. 1980. Isolation and Identification of Avian Pathogens. In S.B. Hitchner, C.H. Domermuth, H.G. Purchase, and J.E. Williams, (eds.), pp. 67-69. Am Assoc Avian Pathol, Kennett Square, PA.
20. Beard, C.W. 1987. To vaccinate or not to vaccinate. Proc 2nd Int Symp Avian Influenza, pp. 258-263. US Anim Health Assoc, Athens, GA.
21. Beard, C.W., and B.C. Easterday. 1973. A/turkey/Oregon/71, an avirulent influenza isolate with the hemagglutinin of fowl plague virus. Avian Dis 17:173-181.
22. Beard C.W., and D.H. Helfer. 1972. Isolation of two turkey influenza viruses in Oregon. Avian Dis 16:1133-1136.
23. Beard, C.W., M. Brugh, and D. C. Johnson. 1984. Laboratory studies with the Pennsylvania avian influenza viruses (H5N2). Proc 88th Meet US Anim Health Assoc, pp. 462-473.
24. Beard, C.W., M. Brugh, and R.G. Webster. 1987. Emergence of amantadine-resistant H5N2 avian influenza virus during a simulated layer flock treatment program. Avian Dis 31:533-537.
25. Beare, A.S. 1982. Personal communication.
26. Becker, W.B. 1966. The isolation and classification of tern virus: Influenza virus A/tern/South Africa/1961. J Hyg 64:309-320.
27. Becker, W.B., and C.J. Uys. 1967. Experimental infection of chickens with influenza A/tern/South Africa/1961 and chicken/Scotland/1959 viruses. J Comp Pathol 77:159-165.
28. Bosch, F.X., W. Garten, H.-D. Klenk, and R. Rott. 1981. Proteolytic cleavage of influenza virus haemagglutinins: Primary structure of the connecting peptide between HA1 and HA2 determines proteolytic cleavability and pathogenicity of avian influenza viruses. Virology 113:725-735.
29. Brugh, M. 1987. Highly pathogenic virus recovered from mildly or nonpathogenic H4N8 and H5N2 avian influenza virus isolates. Proc 2nd Int Symp Avian Influenza, pp. 309-313. US Anim Health Assoc, Athens, GA.
30. Brugh, M., and D.C. Johnson. 1987. Epidemiology of avian influenza in domestic poultry. Proc 2nd Int Symp Avian Influenza, pp. 177-186. US Anim Health Assoc, Athens, GA.
31. Brugh, M., and H.D. Stone. 1987. Immunization of chickens against influenza with hemagglutinin-specific (H5) oil emulsion vaccine. Proc 2nd Int Symp Avian Influenza, pp. 283-292. US Anim Health Assoc, Athens, GA.
32. Brugh, M., C.W. Beard, and H.D. Stone. 1979.

Immunization of chickens and turkeys against avian influenza with monovalent and polyvalent oil emulsion vaccines. Am J Vet Res 40:165-169.

33. Butterfield, W.K., and C.H. Campbell. 1979. Vaccination of chickens with influenza A/turkey/Oregon/71 virus and immunity challenge exposure to five strains of fowl plague virus. Vet Microbiol 4:101-107.

34. Cappucci, D.T., D.C. Johnson, M. Brugh, T.M. Smith, C.F. Jackson, J.E. Pearson, and D.A. Senne. 1985. Isolation of avian influenza virus (subtype H5N2) from chicken eggs during a natural outbreak. Avian Dis 29:1195-1200.

35. Centers for Disease Control. 1982. Concepts and procedures for laboratory based influenza surveillance. Centers for Disease Control, US Dep of Health and Human Serv, Washington, DC.

36. Chambers, T., Y. Kawaoka, and R.G. Webster. 1988. Protection of chickens from lethal influenza infection by vaccinia expressed hemagglutinin. Virology 167:414-421.

37. Choppin, P.W., and R.W. Compans. 1975. The structure of influenza virus. In E.D. Kilbourne (ed.), The Influenza Viruses and Influenza, pp. 15-47. Academic Press, New York.

38. Colman, P.M., J.N. Varghese, and W.G. Laver. 1983. Structure of the catalytic and antigenic sites in influenza virus neuraminidase. Nature 303:41-44.

39. Cooley, J., H. Van Campen, M.S. Philpott, B.C. Easterday, and V.S. Hinshaw. 1989. Pathological lesions in the lungs of ducks infected with influenza A viruses. Vet Pathol 26:1-5.

40. Cross, G.M. 1987. The status of avian influenza in poultry in Australia. Proc 2nd Int Symp Avian Influenza, pp. 96-103. US Anim Health Assoc, Athens, GA.

41. De, B.K., M.W. Shaw, P.A. Rota, M.W. Harmon, J.J. Esposito, R. Rott, N.J. Cox, and A.P. Kendal. 1988. Protection against virulent H5 avian influenza virus infection in chickens by an inactiviated vaccine produced with recombinant vaccinia virus. Vaccine 6:257-261.

42. Dolin, R., R.C. Reichman, H.P. Madore, R. Maynard, P.N. Linton, and J. Webber-Jones. 1982. A controlled trial of amantadine and rimantadine in the prophylaxis of influenza A infection. N Engl J Med 307:580-584.

43. Dowdle, W.R., and G.C. Schild. 1975. Laboratory propagation of human influenza viruses, experimental host range, and isolation from clinical materials. In E.D. Kilbourne (ed.), The Influenza Viruses and Influenza, pp. 243-268. Academic Press, New York.

44. Easterday, B.C. 1975. Animal influenza. In E.D. Kilbourne (ed.), The Influenza Viruses and Influenza, pp. 449-481. Academic Press, New York.

45. Easterday, B.C., and C.W. Beard. 1984. Avian Influenza. In M.S. Hofstad, H.J. Barnes, B.W. Calnek, W.M. Reid, and H.W. Yoder (eds.), Diseases of Poultry, 8th Ed., pp. 482-496. Iowa State Univ Press, Ames.

46. Eckroade, R.J., and L.A. Silverman-Bachin. 1987. Avian influenza in Pennsylvania. The beginning. Proc 2nd Int Symp Avian Influenza, pp. 22-32. US Anim Health Assoc, Athens, GA.

47. Eckroade, R.J., L.A. Silverman, and H.M. Acland. 1984. Avian influenza in Pennsylvania. Proc 33rd West Poult Dis Conf, pp. 1-2.

48. Englund, L., and B. Klingeborn. 1986. Avian influenza A virus causing an outbreak of contagious interstitial pneumonia in mink. Acta Vet Scand 27:497-504.

49. Fang, R., W. Min Jou, D. Huylebroeck, R. Devos, and W. Fiers. 1981. Complete structure of A/Duck/Ukraine/63 influenza hemagglutinin gene: Animal virus as progenitor of human H3 Hong Kong 1968 influenza hemagglutinin. Cell 25:315-323.

50. Fenner, F., P.A. Bachmann, E.P.J. Gibbs, F.A. Murphy, M.J. Studdert, and D.O. White (eds.). 1987. Veterinary Virology, pp. 473-484. Academic Press, New York.

51. Fichtner, G.J. 1987. The Pennsylvania/Virginia experience in eradication of avian influenza (H5N2). Proc 2nd Int Symp Avian Influenza, pp. 33-38. US Anim Health Assoc, Athens, GA.

52. Findlay, G.M., R.D. MacKenzie, and R.O. Stern. 1937. The histopathology of fowl pest. J Pathol Bacteriol. 45:589-96.

53. Foreign Animal Disease Report. 1987. Approved Disinfectants, p. 143. US Dep Agric, Washington, DC.

54. Franklin, R.M., and E. Wecker. 1959. Inactivation of some animal viruses by hydroxylamine and the structure of ribonucleic acid. Nature 84:343-345.

55. Garnett, W. H. 1987. Status of avian influenza in poultry: 1981-1986. Proc 2nd Int Symp Avian Influenza, pp. 61-66. US Anim Health Assoc, Athens, GA.

56. Gerlach, F., and J. Michalka. 1926. Ueber die in Jahre 1925 in Oesterreich beobachtete Gefluegelpest. Dtsche Tierärztl Wochenschr 34:897-902.

57. Halvorson, D.A. 1987. Avian influenza: A Minnesota cooperative control program. Proc 2nd Int Symp Avian Influenza, pp. 327-336. US Anim Health Assoc, Athens, GA.

58. Halvorson, D.A., D. Karunakaran, and J.A. Newman. 1980. Avian influenza in caged laying chickens. Avian Dis 288-294.

59. Halvorson, D.A., D. Karunakaran, D. Senne, C. Zelleher, C. Bailey, A. Abraham, V. Hinshaw, and J. Newman. 1983. Epizootiology of avian influenza–simultaneous monitoring of sentinel ducks and turkeys in Minnesota. Avian Dis 27:77-85.

60. Halvorson, D.A., C.J. Kelleher, D.A. Senne. 1985. Epizootiology of avian influenza: Effect of season on incidence in sentinel ducks and domestic turkeys in Minnesota. Appl Environ Microbiol 49:914-919.

61. Halvorson, D.A., D. Karunakaran, A.S. Abraham, J.A. Newman, V. Sivanandan, and P.E. Poss. 1987. Efficacy of vaccine in the control of avian influenza. Proc 2nd Int Symp Avian Influenza, pp. 264-270. US Anim Health Assoc, Athens, GA.

62. Hers, J.F.P. 1962. Fluorescent antibody technique in respiratory viral disease. Am Rev Respir Dis 88:316-332.

63. Hinshaw, V.S. 1987. The nature of avian influenza in migratory waterfowl, including interspecies transmission. Proc 2nd Int Symp Avian Influenza, pp. 133-141. US Anim Health Assoc, Athens, GA.

64. Hinshaw, V.S., and R.G. Webster. 1982. The natural history of influenza A viruses. In A.S. Beare (ed.), Basic and Applied Influenza Research, pp. 79-104. CRC Press, Inc., Boca Raton, FL.

65. Hinshaw, V.S., R.G. Webster, and B. Turner. 1979. Waterborne transmission of influenza A viruses. Intervirology 11:66-68.

66. Hinshaw, V.S., R.G. Webster, and B. Turner. 1980. The perpetuation of orthomyxoviruses and paramyxoviruses in Canadian waterfowl. Can J Microbiol 26:622-629.

67. Hinshaw, V.S., R.G. Webster, and R.G. Rodriquez. 1981. Influenza Viruses: Combinations of hemagglutinin and neuraminidase subtypes isolated from animals and other sources. Arch Virol 67:191-201.

68. Hinshaw, V.S., R.G. Webster, B.C. Easterday, and W.J. Bean. 1981. Replication of avian influenza A viruses in mammals. Infect Immun 34:354-361.

69. Hinshaw, V.S., R.G. Webster, W.J. Bean, J. Downie, and D.A. Senne. 1983. Swine influenza-like viruses in turkeys: A potential source of virus for humans? Science 220:206-208.

70. Hinshaw, V.S., D.J. Alexander, M. Aymard, P.A. Bachmann, B.C. Easterday, C. Hannoun, H. Kida, M. Lipkind, J.S. MacKenzie, K. Nerome, G.C. Schild, C. Scholtissek, D.A. Senne, K.F. Shortridge, J.J. Skehel, and R.G. Webster. 1984. Antigenic comparisons of swine-influenza-like H1N1 isolates from pigs, birds, and humans: An international collaborative study. Bull WHO 62:871-878.

71. Hinshaw, V.S., W.J. Bean, R.G. Webster, J.E. Rehg, P. Fiorelli, G. Early, J.R. Geraci, and D.J. St. Aubin. 1984. Are seals frequently infected with avian influenza viruses? J Virol 51:863-865.

72. Hinshaw, V.S., J.M. Wood, R.G. Webster, R. Deibel, and B. Turner. 1985. Circulation of influenza viruses and paramyxoviruses in waterfowl originating from two different areas of North America. Bull WHO 63:711-791.

73. Hinshaw, V.S., V.F. Nettles, L.F. Schorr, J.M. Wood, and R.G. Webster. 1986. Influenza virus surveillance in waterfowl in Pennsylvania after the H5N2 avian outbreak. Avian Dis 30:207-212.

74. Hinshaw, V.S., W.J. Bean, J. Geraci, P. Fiorelli, G. Early, and R.G. Webster. 1986. Characterization of two influenza A viruses from a pilot whale. J Virol 58:655-656.

75. Homme, P.J., and B.C. Easterday. 1970. Antibody response in turkeys to influenza A/turkey/Wisconsin/1966 virus. Avian Dis 14:277-284.

76. Hunt, L.A., D.W. Brown, H.L. Robinson, C.W. Naeve, and R.G. Webster. 1988. Retrovirus-expressed hemagglutinin protects against lethal influenza virus infections. J Virol 62:3014-3019.

77. Ito, T., H. Kida, and R. Yanagawa. 1985. Antigenic analysis of H4 influenza isolates using monoclonal antibodies to defined antigenic sites on the hemagglutinin of A/Budgerigar/Hokkaido/1/77 strain. Arch Virol 84:251-259.

78. Johnson, D.C., and B.G. Maxfield. 1976. An occurrence of avian influenza virus infection in laying chickens. Avian Dis 20:422-424.

79. Johnson, D.C., B.G. Maxfield, and J.I. Moulthrop. 1977. Epidemiologic studies of the 1975 avian influenza outbreak in chickens in Alabama. Avian Dis 21:167-177.

80. Jungherr, E.L., E.E. Tyzzer, C.A. Brandly, and H.E. Moses. 1946. The comparative pathology of fowl plague and Newcastle disease. Am J Vet Res 7:250-288.

81. Kaleta, E.F. 1987. The epidemiology of avian influenza in pet birds and free living birds other than migratory waterfowl. Proc 2nd Int Symp Avian Influenza, pp. 142-149. US Anim Health Assoc, Athens, GA.

82. Karunakaran, D., V.S. Hinshaw, P. Poss, J. Newman, and D. Halvorson. 1983. Influenza A outbreaks in Minnesota turkeys due to subtype H10N7 and possible transmission by waterfowl. Avian Dis 27:357-366.

83. Karunakaran., D., J.A. Newman, D.A. Halvorson, and A. Abraham. 1987. Evaluation of inactivated influenza vaccines in market turkeys. Avian Dis 31:498-503.

84. Kawaoka, Y., and R.G. Webster. 1985. Evolution of the A/Chicken/Pennsylvania/83 (H5N2) influenza virus. Virology 146:130-137.

85. Kawaoka, Y., C.W. Naeve, and R.G. Webster. 1984. Is virulence of H5N2 influenza viruses in chickens associated with loss of carbohydrate from the hemagglutinin? Virology 139:303-316.

86. Kawaoka, Y., W.J. Bean, and R.G. Webster. 1987. Molecular characterization of the A/Chicken/Pennsylvania/83 (H5N2) influenza viruses. Proc 2nd Int Symp Avian Influenza, pp. 197-206. US Anim Health Assoc, Athens, GA.

87. Kawaoka, Y., A. Nestorowicz, D.J. Alexander, and R.G. Webster. 1987. Molecular analyses of the hemagglutinin genes of H5 influenza viruses: Origin of a virulent turkey strain. Virology 158:218-227.

88. Kawaoka, Y., T.M. Chambers, W.L. Sladen, and R.G. Webster. 1988. Is the gene pool of influenza viruses in shorebirds and gulls different from that in wild ducks? Virology 163:247-250.

89. Kendal, A.P. 1982. Newer techniques in antigenic analysis with influenza viruses. In A.S. Beare (ed.), Basic and Applied Influenza Research, pp. 51-78. CRC Press, Inc. Boca Raton, FL.

90. Kida, H., R. Yanagawa, and Y. Matsuoka. 1980. Duck influenza lacking evidence of disease signs and immune response. Infect Immun 30:547-553.

91. Kida, H., Y. Kawaoka, C.W. Naeve, and R.G. Webster. 1987. Antigenic and genetic conservation of H3 influenza virus in wild ducks. Virology 159:109-119.

92. Kilbourne, E.D. 1987. Influenza. Plenum Press, New York.

93. Kingsbury, D. 1985. Orthomyxo- and paramyxoviruses and their replication. In B. Fields (ed.), Virology, pp. 1157-1178. Raven Press, New York.

94. Klenk, H.-D., W. Keil, H. Niemann, R. Geyer, and R.T. Schwarz. 1983. The characterization of influenza A viruses by carbohydrate analysis. Curr Top Microbiol Immunol 104:247-257.

95. Klingeborn, B., L. Englund, R. Rott, N. Juntti, and G. Rockborn. 1985. An avian influenza A virus killing a mammalian species–the mink. Arch Virol 86:347-351.

96. Kuroda, K., C. Hauser, R. Rott, H.-D. Klenk, and W. Doerfler. 1986. Expression of the influenza virus hemagglutinin in insect cells by a baculovirus vector. EMBO 5:1359-1365.

97. Lang, G., A.E. Ferguson, M.C. Connell, and C.G. Wills. 1965. Isolation of an unidentified hemagglutinating virus from the respiratory tract of turkeys. Avian Dis 9:495-504.

98. Lang, G., B.T. Rouse, O. Narayan, A.E. Ferguson, and M.C. Connell. 1968. A new influenza virus infection in turkeys. I. Isolation and characterization of virus 6213. Can Vet J 9:22-29.

99. Lang, G., O. Narayan, B.T. Rouse, A.E. Ferguson, and M.C. Connell. 1968. A new influenza A virus infection in turkeys. II. A highly pathogenic variant, A/turkey/Ontario/7732/66. Can Vet J 9:151-160.

100. Lang. G., O. Narayan, and B.T. Rouse. 1970. Prevention of malignant avian influenza by 1-adamantanamine hydrochloride. Arch Gesamte Virusforsch 32:171-184.

101. Lang, G., A. Gagnon, J.R. Geraci. 1981. Isolation of influenza A virus from seals. Arch Virol 68:189-195.

102. Lasley, F.A. 1987. Economics of avian influenza: Control vs noncontrol. Proc 2nd Int Symp Avian Influenza, pp. 390-399. US Anim Health Assoc, Athens, GA.

103. Laver, W.G. 1963. The structure of influenza viruses. II. Disruption of the virus particle and separation of neuraminidase activity. Virology 20:251-262.

104. Lipkind, M., Y. Weisman, E. Shihmanter, and D. Shoham. 1981. Studies on the ecology of avian influenza viruses in Israel. In R.A. Bankowski (ed.), Proc 1st Int Symp Avian Influenza, p. 30. Carter Comp. Corp., Richmond, VA.

105. Liu, C. 1961. Diagnosis of influenza infection by means of fluorescent antibody staining. Am Rev Respir Dis 83:130-132.

106. Lu, B.L., R.G. Webster, and V.S. Hinshaw. 1982. Failure to detect hemagglutination-inhibiting antibodies with intact avian influenza virions. Infect Immun 38:530-535.

107. McCapes, R.H., and R.A. Bankowski. 1987.

Use of avian influenza vaccines in California turkey breeders–medical rationale. Proc 2nd Int Symp Avian Influenza, pp. 271–278. US Anim Health Assoc, Athens, GA.

108. McKenzie, B.E., B.C. Easterday, and J.A. Will. 1972. Light and electron microscopic changes in the myocardium of influenza-infected turkeys. Am J Pathol 69:239–254.

109. McQuillin, J., C.R. Madeley, and A.P. Kendal. 1985. Monoclonal antibodies for the rapid diagnosis of influenza A and B virus infections by immunofluorescence. Lancet 2:911–914.

110. Meulemans, G. 1987. Status of Avian Influenza in Western Europe: 1981–1987. Proc 2nd Int Symp Avian Influenza, pp. 77–83. US Anim Health Assoc, Athens, GA.

111. Meulemans, G., M.C. Carlier, M. Gonze, P. Petit. 1987. Comparison of hemagglutination-inhibition, agar gel precipitin and enzyme-linked immunosorbent assay for measuring antibodies against influenza viruses in chickens. Avian Dis 31:560–563.

112. Mohan, R., Y.M. Saif, G.A. Erickson, G.A. Gustafson, and B.C. Easterday. 1981. Serologic and epidemiologic evidence of infection in turkeys with an agent related to the swine influenza virus. Avian Dis 25:11–16.

113. Murphy, T.M. 1987. The control of avian influenza in Ireland. Proc 2nd Int Symp Avian Influenza, pp. 39–50. US Anim Health Assoc, Athens, GA.

114. Murphy, F.A., and A.P. Kendal. 1987. Biotechnology and modern vaccine development. Proc 2nd Int Symp Avian Influenza, pp. 434–443. US Anim Health Assoc, Athens, GA.

115. Murphy, B.R., and R.G. Webster. 1985. Influenza viruses. In B. Fields (ed.), Virology, pp. 1179–1140. Raven Press, New York.

116. Murphy, B.R., A.J. Buckler-White, W.T. London, J. Harper, E.L. Tierney, N.T. Miller, L.J. Reck, R.M. Chanock, and V.A Hinshaw. 1984. Avian-human reassortant influenza A viruses derived by mating avian and human influenza A viruses. J Infect Dis 150:841–50.

117. Naeve, C.W., and R.G. Webster. 1983. Sequence of the hemagglutinin gene from influenza virus A/Seal/Mass/1/80. Virology 129:298–308.

118. Naeve, C.W., R.G. Webster, and V.S. Hinshaw. 1984. Mutations in the hemagglutinin receptor-binding site can change the biological properties of an influenza virus. J Virol 51:567–569.

119. Nakamura, R.M., and B.C. Easterday. 1967. Serological studies of influenza in animals. Bull WHO 37:559–567.

120. Narayan, O., G. Lang, and B.T. Rouse. 1969. A new influenza A virus infection in turkeys. IV. Experimental susceptibility of domestic birds to virus strain Turkey/Ontario/7732/1966. Arch Gesamte Virusforsch 26:149–165.

121. Narayan, O., G. Lang, and B.T. Rouse. 1969. A new influenza A virus infection in turkeys. V. Pathology of the experimental disease by strain Turkey/Ontario/7732/1966. Arch Gesamte Virusforsch 26:166–182.

122. Nestorowicz, A., Y. Kawaoka, W.J. Bean, and R.G. Webster. 1987. Molecular analysis of the hemagglutinin genes of Australian H7N7 influenza viruses: Role of passerine birds in maintenance or transmission? Virology 160:411–418.

123. Nettles, V.F., J.M. Wood, and R.G. Webster. 1985. Wildlife surveillance associated with an outbreak of lethal H5N2 avian influenza in domestic poultry. Avian Dis 29:733–741.

124. Palmer, D.F., M.T. Coleman, W.R. Dowdle, and G.C. Schild. 1975. Advanced Laboratory Techniques for Influenza Diagnosis. US Dep Health, Educ Welfare Immunol Ser No. 6, Procedure Guide. Center for Disease Control, Atlanta, GA.

125. Pearson, J.E., and D.A. Senne. 1987. Diagnostic procedures for avian influenza. Proc 2nd Int Symp Avian Influenza, pp. 222–227. US Anim Health Assoc, Athens, GA.

126. Pearson, J.E., D.A. Senne, E.A. Carbrey, G.A. Gustafson, J.G. Landgraf, D.R. Cassidy, and G.A. Erickson. 1987. Laboratory support for the Pennsylvania/Virginia avian influenza outbreak. Proc 2nd Int Symp Avian Influenza, pp. 39–50. US Anim Health Assoc, Athens, GA.

127. Philpott, M.S., B.C. Easterday, and V.S. Hinshaw. 1989. Antigenic and phenotypic variants of a virulent avian influenza virus selected during replication in ducks. J Wildl Dis 25:507–513.

128. Philpott, M.S., B.C. Easterday, and V.S. Hinshaw. 1989. Neutralizing epitopes of the H5 hemagglutinin of a virulent avian influenza virus and their relationship to pathogenicity. J Virol 63:3453–3489.

129. Porter, A.G., C. Barber, N.H. Carey, R.A. Hallewell, G. Threlfall, and J.S. Emtage. 1979. Complete nucleotide sequence of an influenza virus hemagglutinin gene from cloned DNA. Nature 282:471–477.

130. Poss, P.E., and D.A. Halvorson. 1987. The nature of avian influenza in turkeys in Minnesota. Proc 2nd Int Symp Avian Influenza, pp. 112–117. US Anim Health Assoc, Athens, GA.

131. Poss, P.E., D.A. Halvorson, D. Karunakaran. 1981. Economic impact of avian influenza in domestic fowl in the United States. In R.A. Bankowski (ed.), Proc 1st Int Symp Avian Influenza, pp. 100–11. Carter Comp. Corp., Richmond, VA.

132. Poss, P.E., K.A. Friendshuh, and L.T Ausherman. 1987. The control of avian influenza. Proc 2nd Int Symp Avian Influenza, pp. 318–326. US Anim Health Assoc, Athens, GA.

133. Proceedings 1st International Symposium on Avian Influenza. 1981. Carter Comp. Corp., Richmond, VA.

134. Proceedings 2nd International Symposium on Avian Influenza. 1987. US Anim Health Assoc, Athens, GA.

135. Proceedings 91st Annual Meeting, US Anim Health Association. 1987. Report of the committee on transmissible diseases of poultry and other avian species, pp. 374–398. Lewis Printing Co., Richmond, VA.

136. Resende, M. 1980. Comparative pathogenesis of virulent and avirulent avian influenza viruses in turkeys. PhD diss, University of Wisconsin-Madison, Madison.

137 Rogers, G.N., and J.C. Paulson. 1983. Receptor determinants of human and animal influenza virus isolates: Differences in receptor specificity of the H3 hemagglutinin based on species of origin. Virology 127:361–373.

138. Rogers, G.N., T.J. Pritchett, J.L. Lane, and J.C. Paulson. 1983. Differential sensitivity of human, avian, and equine influenza A viruses to a glycoprotein inhibitor of infection: Selection of receptor specific variants. Virology. 131:394–408.

139. Rott, R., and C. Scholtissek, 1982. The molecular basis of biological properties of influenza viruses. In A.S. Beare (ed.), Basic and Applied Influenza Research, pp. 189–210. CRC Press, Inc., Boca Raton, FL.

140. Rouse, B.T., G. Lang, and O. Narayan. 1968. A new influenza A virus infection in turkeys. J Comp Pathol Ther 78:525–533.

141. Rowan, M.K. 1962. Mass mortality among European common terns in South Africa in April-May 1961. Br Birds 55:103–114.

142. Sandhu, T.S., and V.S. Hinshaw. 1981. Influenza A virus infection in domestic ducks. In R.A. Bankowski (ed.), Proc 1st Int Symp Avian Influenza, pp. 93-99. Carter Comp. Corp., Richmond, VA.
143. Schafer, W. 1955. Vergleichende sero-immunologische Untersuchungen uber die viren der influenza und klassichen Geflugelpest Z Naturforsch 10b:81-91.
144. Scholtissek, C., and E. Naylor. 1988. Fish farming and influenza pandemics. Nature 331:215.
145. Scholtissek, C., H. Burger, P.A. Bachmann, and C. Hannoun. 1983. Genetic relatedness of hemagglutinins of the H1 subtype of influenza A viruses isolated from swine and birds. Virology 129:521-523.
146. Seifried, O. 1931. Gefluegelpest-Encephalitis. Pathologische Histologic. Lubarsch-Ostertag Ergebnisse der allgemeinen Pathologic und Pathologischen. Anat Menschen Tiere 24:661-65.
147. Senne, D.A., J.E. Pearson, L.D. Miller, and G.A. Gustafson. 1983. Virus isolations from pet birds submitted for importation into the United States. Avian Dis 27:731-744.
148. Senne, D.A., J.E. Pearson, Y. Kawaoka, E.A. Carbrey, and R.G. Webster. 1987. Alternative methods for evaluation of pathogenicity of chicken Pennsylvania H5N2 viruses. Proc 2nd Int Symp Avian Influenza, pp. 246-257. US Anim Health Assoc, Athens, GA.
149. Skeeles, J.K., R.L. Morrissey, A. Nagy, F. Helm, T.O. Bunn, M.J. Langford, R.E. Long, and R.O. Apple. 1984. The use of fluorescent antibody (FA) techniques for the rapid diagnosis of avian influenza (H5N2) associated with the Pennsylvania outbreak of 1983/1984. Proc 35th N Central Avian Dis Conf, p. 32.
150. Slemons, R.D., and B.C. Easterday. 1972. Host response differences among five avian species to an influenza virus A/turkey/Ontario/7732/66 (Hav5 N?). Bull WHO 47:521-525.
151. Slemons, R.D., R.S. Cooper, and J.S. Orsborn. 1973. Isolation of type A influenza viruses from imported exotic birds. Avian Dis 17:746-751.
152. Slemons, R.D., D.C. Johnson, and T. G. Malone. 1973. Influenza type A isolated from imported exotic birds. Avian Dis 17:458-459.
153. Snyder, D.B., W.W. Marquardt, F.S. Yancey, and P.K. Savage. 1985. An enzyme-linked immunosorbent assay for the detection of antibody against avian influenza virus. Avian Dis 29:136-44.
154. Stone, H.A. 1987. Efficacy of avian influenza oil-emulsion vaccines in chickens of various ages. Avian Dis 31:483-490.
155. Stone, H.D. 1988. Optimization of hydrophilic-lipophil balance for improved efficacy of Newcastle disease and avian influenza oil-emulsion vaccine. Avian Dis 32:68-73.
156. Stubbs, E.L. 1965. Fowl plague. In H.E. Biester and L.H. Schwarte (eds.), Diseases of Poultry, 5th Ed., pp. 813-822. Iowa State Univ Press, Ames.
157. Tashiro, M., P. Ciborowski, H.-D. Klenk, G. Pulverer, R. Rott. 1987. Role of Staphylococcus protease in the development of influenza pneumonia. Nature 325:536-537.
158. Tumova, B. 1987. Avian influenza and paramyxoviruses in central and eastern Europe: A review. 2nd Int Symp Avian Influenza, pp. 84-89. US Anim Health Assoc, Athens, GA.
159. Van Campen, H., B.C. Easterday, and V.S. Hinshaw. 1989. Virulent influenza A viruses: Their effect on avian lymphocytes and macrophages in vivo and in vitro. J Gen Virol 70:2887-2895.
160. Van Campen, H., B.C. Easterday, and V.S. Hinshaw. 1989. Pathogenesis of a virulent avian influenza A virus: Lymphoid infection and destruction. J Gen Virol 70:467-472.
161. Van Deusen, R.A., V.S. Hinshaw, D.A. Senne, and D. Pellacani. 1983. Micro neuraminidase-inhibition assay for classification of influenza A virus neuraminidases. Avian Dis 27:745-750.
162. Walls, H.H., M.W. Harmon, J.J. Slagle, C. Stocksdale, and A.P. Kendal. 1986. Characterization and evaluation of monoclonal antibodies developed for typing influenza A and influenza B viruses. J Clin Microbiol 23:240-245.
163. Webster, R.G., and W.G. Laver. 1975. Antigenic variation of influenza viruses. In E.D. Kilbourne (ed.), The Influenza Viruses and Influenza, pp 270-314. Academic Press, New York.
164. Webster, R.G., and R. Rott. 1987. Influenza virus A pathogenicity: The pivotal role of hemagglutinin. Cell 50:665-666.
165. Webster, R.G., M. Yakhno, V.S. Hinshaw, W.J. Bean, and K.G. Murti. 1978. Intestinal influenza: Replication and characterization of influenza viruses in ducks. Virology 84:268-278.
166. Webster, R.G., V.S. Hinshaw, W.J. Bean, K.L. van Wyke, J.R. Geraci, D.J. St. Aubin, and G. Petursson. 1981. Characterization of an influenza A virus from seals. Virology 113:712-724.
167. Webster, R.G., J.R. Petursson, and K. Skirnisson. 1981. Conjunctivitis in human beings caused by influenza A virus of seals. N Engl J Med 304:911.
168. Webster, R.G., Y. Kawaoka., W.J. Bean, C.W. Beard, and M. Brugh. 1985. Chemotherapy and vaccination: A possible strategy for the control of highly virulent influenza virus. J Virol 55:173-176.
169. Webster, R.G., Y. Kawaoka, and W.J. Bean, Jr. 1986. Molecular changes in A/Chicken/Pennsylvania/83 (H5N2) influenza virus associated with acquisition of virulence. Virology 149:165-173.
170. Weisman, Y., M. Lipkind, E. Shihmanter, and A. Aronovici. 1987. Current situation on avian influenza in Israel from 1981-1986. 2nd Int Symp Avian Influenza, pp. 90-95. US Anim Health Assoc, Athens, GA.
171. WHO Expert Committee. 1971. A revised system of nomenclature for influenza viruses. Bull WHO 45:119-124.
172. WHO Expert Committee. 1980. A revision of the system of nomenclature for influenza viruses: A WHO memorandum. Bull WHO 58:585-591.
173. Wiley, D.C., I.A. Wilson, and J.J. Skehel. 1981. Structural identification of the antibody-binding sites of Hong Kong influenza hemagglutinin and their involvement in antigenic variation. Nature 289:373-378.
174. Wood, J.M., Y. Kawaoka, L.A. Newberry, E. Bordwell, and R.G. Webster. 1985. Standardization of inactivated H5N2 influenza vaccine and efficacy against lethal A/Chicken/Pennsylvania/1370/83 infection. Avian Dis 29:867-872.
175. Wood, J.M., R.G. Webster, and V.F. Nettles. 1985. Host range of A/chicken/Pennsylvania/83 (H5N2) influenza virus. Avian Dis 29:198-207.

22 ADENOVIRUS INFECTIONS

INTRODUCTION

J.B. McFerran

The first adenovirus isolated was the virus of infectious canine hepatitis (ICH) (12), although Cowdrey and Scott (2) predicted that the intranuclear inclusions they saw in ICH cases would be found to be due to a filterable agent.

The first avian adenovirus was isolated when material from a case of lumpy skin disease in cattle was inoculated into embryonated hens' eggs (14). Other early unintentional isolates of fowl adenoviruses were the chicken embryo lethal orphan (CELO) isolates made in embryonated eggs (16) and the gallus adenolike (GAL) viruses from chicken cell cultures (1). The first isolate of an avian adenovirus from diseased birds was from an outbreak of respiratory disease in bobwhite quail (*Colinus virginianus*) by Olson (10).

Human adenoviruses were isolated during investigations of respiratory disease (5) and were initially called adenoidal-pharyngeal-conjunctival viruses, but the name adenoviruses was subsequently adopted (4).

The general properties required for classifying an isolate have been laid down by a number of international committees (9, 11, 15). They recognize the family Adenoviridae with two genera, *Mastadenovirus* and *Aviadenovirus,* with human adenovirus type 2 and the CELO virus as the respective type species. One of the features distinguishing these two genera is that they do not share the same group antigen (13).

The second report on Adenoviridae (15) suggested the substitution of species for type and defined a species on the basis of its quantitative neutralization with animal antisera. A species has either no cross-reaction with others or shows a homologous-to-heterologous titer ratio of >16 in both directions. If neutralization shows cross-reactivity in either or both directions (titer ratio 8 to 16), distinctiveness of species is assumed if the hemagglutinins are unrelated or if substantial biophysical/biochemical differences of DNAs exist. It should be noted however that the majority of avian adenoviruses do not hemagglutinate.

It is possible to subdivide the present avian adenoviruses into three groups. The first includes the conventional group I adenovirus, or avian adenovirus group I isolates from chickens, turkeys, geese, and other species that share a common group antigen (6, 7, 17). The second group includes the viruses of turkey hemorrhagic enteritis, marble spleen disease, and avian adenovirus group II splenomegaly virus of chickens. These viruses share a common group antigen that is distinct from the group I viruses (3). The third group is the viruses associated with egg drop syndrome 1976 and similar viruses from ducks, which only partially share the group I common antigen (8).

REFERENCES

1. Burmester, B.R., G.R. Sharpless, and A.K. Fontes. 1960. Virus isolated from avian lymphomas unrelated to lymphomatosis virus. J Nat Cancer Inst 24:1443–1447.

2. Cowdry, E.V., and G.H. Scott. 1930. A comparison of certain intranuclear inclusions found in the livers of dogs without history of infection with intranuclear inclusions characteristic of the action of filterable viruses. Arch Pathol 9:1184–1196.

3. Domermuth, C.H., C.R. Weston, B.S. Cowen, W.M. Colwell, W.B. Gross, and R.T DuBose. 1980. Incidence and distribution of avian adenovirus group II splenomegaly of chickens. Avian Dis 24:591–594.

4. Enders, J.F., J.A. Bell, J.H. Dingle, T. Francis, H.R. Hilleman, R.J. Huebner, and A.M. Payne. 1956. Adenoviruses: Group name proposed for new respiratory-tract virus. Science 124:119–120.

5. Huebner, R.J, W.P. Rowe, T.G. Ward, R.J. Parrott and J.A. Bell. 1954. Adenoidal-pharyngeal-conjunctival agents. New Engl J Med 257:1077–1086.

6. Kawamura, H., F. Shimizu, and H. Tsubahara. 1964. Avian adenovirus: Its properties and serological classification. Nat Inst Anim Health Q (Tokyo) 4:183–193.

7. McFerran, J.B., B. Adair, and T.J. Connor. 1975. Adenoviral antigens (CELO, QBV, GAL). Am J Vet Res 36:527–529.

8. McFerran, J.B., T.J. Connor, and B.M. Adair. 1978. Studies on the antigenic relationship between an isolate (127) from the egg drop syndrome 1976 and a fowl adenovirus. Avian Pathol 7:629–636.

9. Norrby, E., A. Bartha, P. Boulanger, R.S. Dreizin, H.S. Ginsberg, S.S. Kalter, H. Kawamura, W.P. Rowe, W.C. Russell, R.W. Schlesinger, and R. Wigand. 1976. Adenoviridae. Intervirology 7:117–125.

10. Olson, N.O. 1950. A respiratory disease (bronchitis) of quail caused by a virus. Proc 54th Annu Meet US Livestock Sanit Assoc, pp. 171–174.

11. Pereira, H.G., R.J. Huebner, H.S. Ginsberg, and J. Van der Veen. 1963. A short description of the adenovirus group. Virology 20:613–620.
12. Rubarth, S. 1947. An acute virus disease with liver lesions in dogs (hepatitis contagiosa canis). A pathologico-anatomical and etiological investigation. Acta Pathol Microbiol Scand 24 (Suppl No.69):1–222.
13. Sharpless, G.R. 1962. GAL virus. Ann NY Acad Sci 101:515–519.
14. Van den Ende, M.P., P.A. Don, and A. Kipps. 1949. The isolation in eggs of a new filterable agent which may be the cause of bovine lumpy skin disease. J Gen Microbiol 3:174–182.
15. Wigand, R., A. Bartha, R.S. Dreizin, H. Esche, H.S. Ginsberg, M. Green, J.C. Hierholzer, S.S. Kalter, J.B. McFerran, U. Pettersson, W.C. Russell, and G. Waddell. 1982. Adenoviridae: Second report. Intervirology 18:169–176.
16. Yates, V.J., and D.E. Fry. 1957. Observations on a chicken embryo lethal orphan (CELO) virus. Am J Vet Res 18:657–660.
17. Zsak, L. and J. Kisary. 1984. Characterisation of adenoviruses isolated from geese. Avian Pathol 13:253–264.

ADENOVIRUS (GROUP I) INFECTIONS OF CHICKENS

J.B. McFerran

INTRODUCTION. In contrast with the clear association with disease of the group II and egg drop syndrome viruses, the role of the group I avian adenoviruses as pathogens is not well defined. There is conflicting evidence for their role as primary pathogens in nature, but there is growing evidence for their role as secondary pathogens associated with other viruses such as chicken anemia agent and infectious bursal disease. It is not possible to assess their economic importance until their role is better delineated. They have no known public health importance. Several reviews are available (4, 57, 59).

INCIDENCE AND DISTRIBUTION. Group I avian adenoviruses are widely distributed throughout the world. Domestic avian species of all ages are susceptible and other avian species appear to be susceptible to infection with chicken serotypes and probably also serotypes of their own, but this has not been fully investigated.

ETIOLOGY

Morphology and Physical Properties. Details have been reviewed by McFerran (57). The adenovirus virion is an unenveloped icosahedral structure 70–90 nm in diameter, composed of 252 capsomeres, surrounding a core 60–65 nm in diameter. The capsomeres are arranged in triangular faces with 6 capsomeres along each edge. There are 240 nonvertex capsomeres (hexons) of 8–9.5 nm diameter and 12 vertex capsomeres (penton bases). The vertex capsomeres carry projections called fibers (82). The mammalian adenoviruses have one fiber on each penton base. The Phelps strains of fowl adenovirus serotype 1 (F1) was reported to have two fibers, one of 42.5 nm and the other of 8.5 nm, but other workers only reported one fiber. In a study of 11 fowl serotypes, Gelderblom and Maichle-Laupper (36) found that they all had two fibers on the penton bases and it was possible to show a relationship between the fiber length and the antigenic properties. Thus, different serotypes that showed some relationship in the serum neutralization test had fibers of similar length.

In thin-section studies, particles of approximately 70 nm diameter with a central nucleoid of approximately 40 nm can be seen in the nucleus of infected cells (Fig. 22.1).

Densities between 1.32 and 1.37 gm/ml in cesium chloride (CsCl) have been estimated for fowl adenoviruses. Similar differences in density have been found in the human adenoviruses and these have been attributed to differences in DNA content and base composition in different isolates.

Chemical Composition. The nucleic acid is double-stranded DNA and this is reported to account for 11.3–13.5% of the virion with the remainder being protein. However, others have reported 17.3% DNA in F1 and estimated the guanine-cytosine (G-C) content of DNA at 54%, intermediate between the G-C content of highly oncogenic human viruses (47–49%) and the nononcogenic serotypes (57–59%). There are between 11 and 14 structural polypeptides in F1.

Virus Replication. Adenoviruses replicate in the nucleus, producing basophilic inclusions (Fig. 22.2 and 22.3). Human adenoviruses have been classified into subgroups A and B based on their cytopathology, and it has been possible to classify the avian viruses into similar subgroups with F1, F2, F4, F5 (340), and F8 (H6 and TR59) belonging to subgroup A and F3, F5 (TR22), F6, F7, F8 (784), F9, and turkey adenovirus serotype 1 (T1) and serotype 2 (T2) belonging to subgroup B (1).

These divisions appear to have wider implica-

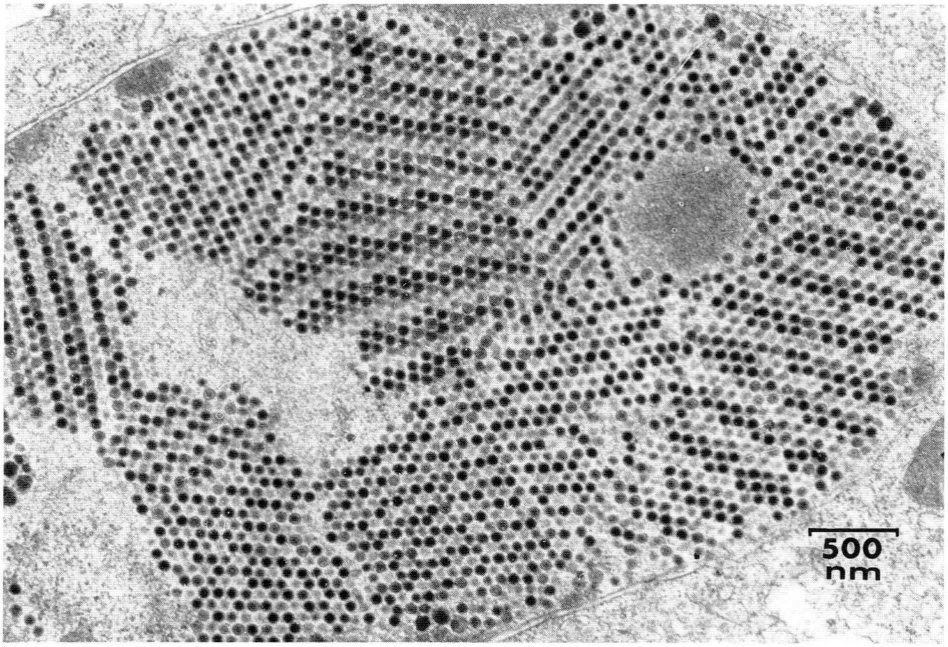

22.1. Adenovirus-infected chick liver cell (48 hr postinfection). Adenovirus particles almost fill the nucleus. (Adair)

tions. Thus subgroup A viruses tend to cause sporadic outbreaks of disease in humans and persist in the tonsils, whereas subgroup B cause epidemics and do not normally persist in the tonsils. There also appears to be a relationship with human adenoviruses between cytopathology and the G-C content, the hemagglutinating characteristics, and oncogenicity of the subgroups (57).

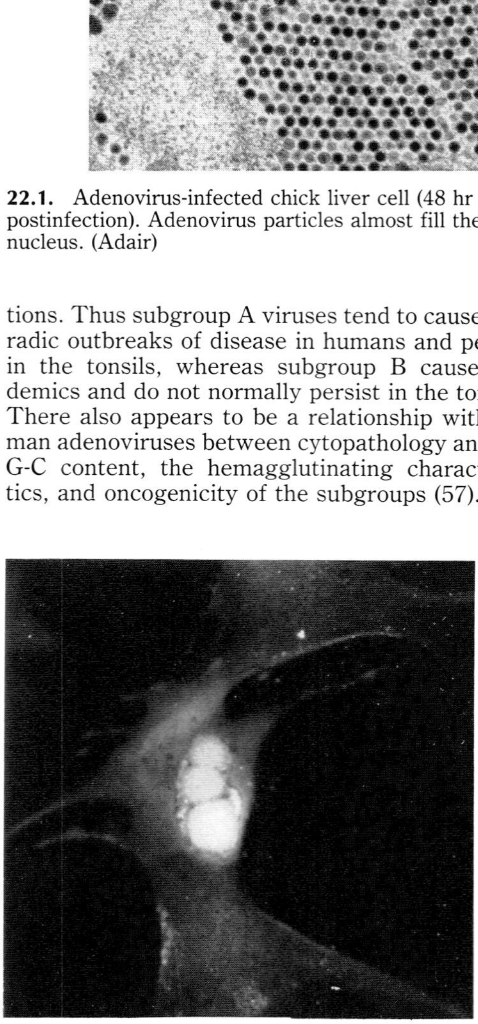

22.2. Growth of F8 (764) in chick kidney cell cultures. Intranuclear inclusions stained by fluorescein isothiocyamate-labelled antibody. (Adair)

Subgroup A produced refractile pearllike inclusions, which progressed into a central basophilic inclusion surrounded by a clear halo. Immunofluorescence staining demonstrated peripheral accumulation of antigen in the area corresponding to the halo. In subgroup B the first signs are the development of nonrefractile irregular eosinophilic inclusions that increase in size to fill the nucleus. Large circular bodies, probably corresponding to eosinophilic inclusions, are revealed by immunofluorescent staining. In the cases of F5 and F8, different isolates fell into different subgroups. However these are strains of broad antigenicity and their type of replication may aid classification (1).

Ultrastructurally, virus particles, some with electron-dense and some with electron-lucent cores, accumulate in the nucleus, often forming crystalline lattices. Four types of inclusions composed of viral protein and some with viral DNA, differing in density and morphology, were demonstrated, as were large protein paracrystals with a well-defined morphology. These inclusions correspond to those described for human adenoviruses (2).

Resistance to Physical and Chemical Agents. All the avian adenoviruses tested have shown typical adenovirus properties (see reviews 4, 57, 59). Thus they are resistant to lipid solvents such as ether and chloroform, sodium deoxycholate, tryp-

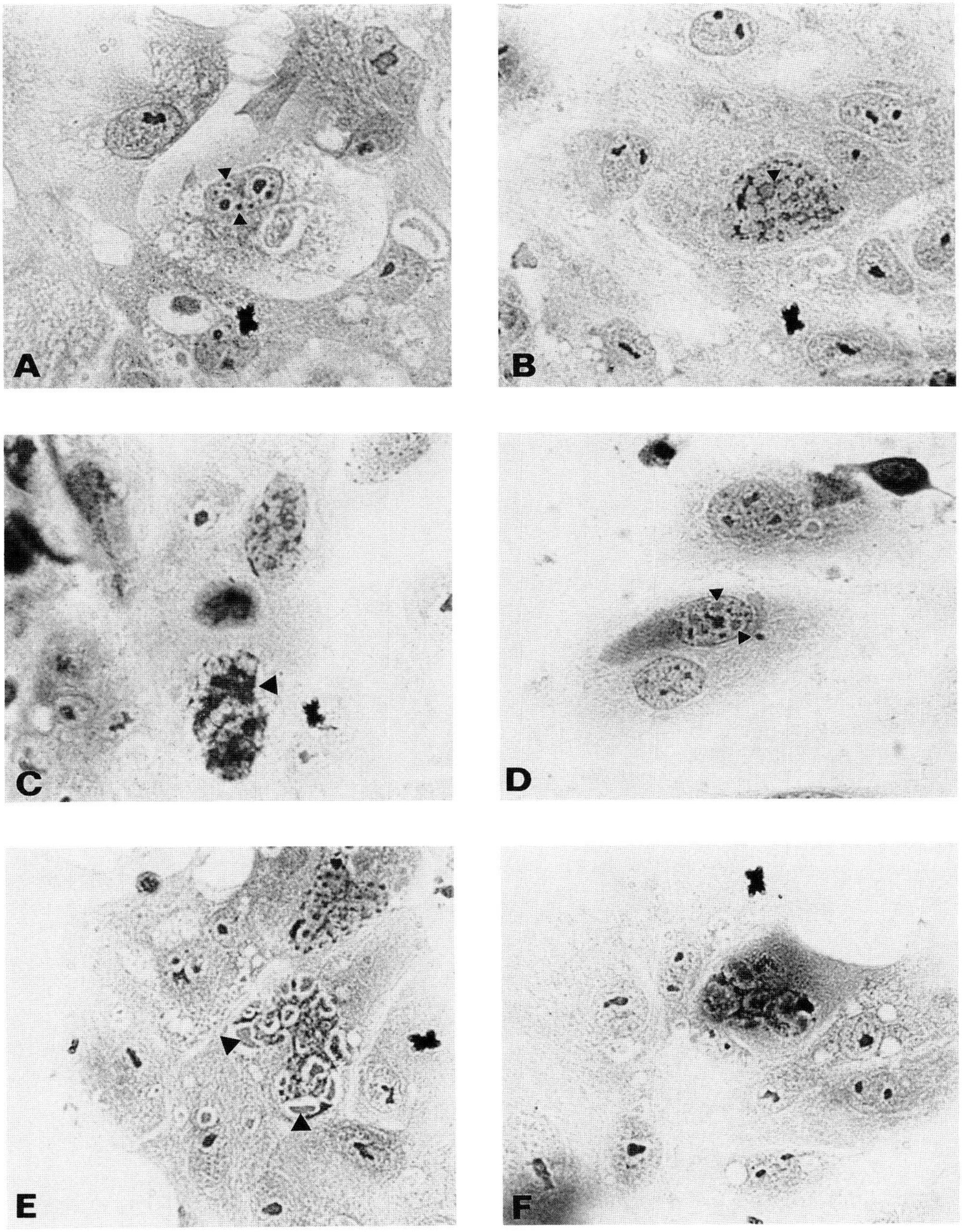

22.3. Cytopathic effects of avian adenoviruses on chick kidney cell cultures. A–C: Effect of group I. F1, F2, F4, F5 (340), F8 (H6 and TR59). A. Early stage – refractile inclusions in nucleus. B. Middle stage – formation of basophilic aggregation around refactile inclusions. C. Late stage – concentration of basophilic material in nucleus. D–E: Effect of group II. F3, F5 (TR22), F6, F7, F8 (784), T1, and T2. D. Early stage – irregular eosinophilic bodies in nucleus. E. Middle stage – formation of multiple eosinophilic inclusion bodies surrounded by granular basophilic material. F. Late stage – condensation to form large nuclear inclusions. (Adair)

sin, 2% phenol, and 50% alcohol. They are resistant to variations in pH between pH 3 and 9. They are inactivated by a 1:1000 concentration of formaldehyde and inhibited by the DNA inhibitors IuDR and BuDR.

Although it is accepted that adenoviruses in general are inactivated in aqueous solution by 56 C for 30 min, and that the heat stability is reduced by divalent ions, the avian adenoviruses show more variability and are apparently more heat resistant. Thus some strains appear to survive 60 C and even 70 C for 30 min. One F1 virus fell rapidly in titer after 180 min at 56 C, while another F1 strain apparently survived 18 hr at 56 C. Even strains tested in the same laboratory have shown differences in thermostability, suggesting these differences were not just a matter of technique. Although most workers found that divalent cations destabilize adenoviruses some workers found no effect. These divergent results may be due to technique and it is important to standardize suspending media and pH.

Hemagglutination. Hemagglutination has been reviewed by McFerran (57). F1 virus hemagglutinates rat cells. Optimal agglutination of erythrocytes occurs between pH 6 and pH 9 at temperatures between 20 and 45 C. The hemagglutinin is stable to treatment with trypsin, RNase, DNase, and neuraminidase. It is inactivated by 15 min at 56 C, and 0.2% formaldehyde reduces its titer eightfold. F1 has not agglutinated a wide range of other erythrocytes. Although a number of strains of F1 were found not to hemagglutinate sheep cells, the Indiana C strain did, suggesting variation within serotypes. There is no evidence for any of the other fowl serotypes, or turkey or duck isolates hemagglutinating cells (8).

Strain Classification. Avian adenoviruses have been classified by their serological relationships, on their growth in cell culture (1, 2), and on their nucleic acid characteristics (89).

A number of workers have compared the strains by neutralization tests. (13, 38, 49–51, 60, 62). There is agreement over the number of serotypes (or species), but some disagreement over the serotype designations (Table 22.1). Twelve fowl serotypes have been recognized but there are undoubtably more isolated but not yet classified.

A major problem has been the discovery of prime strains and strains of broad antigenicity (23, 63). As more strains are tested, two apparently unrelated serotypes can be shown to be related by isolates partly sharing antigens. If the need arises at any time for identification of field isolates, it is important that antiserums are chosen that give as clear-cut differentiation as possible. Monoclonal typing antibody may solve this problem and nucleic acid analysis may prove helpful (6, 89). However, whereas Zsak and Kisary (89) classified 7 and 8 as group E and 10 as group D, Barr and Scott (6) classified their 7, 8, and 10 isolates as group E.

Turkey isolates are not included in Table 22.1 because they have not been compared. Two sero-

Table 22.1. Serological classification of group I avian adenoviruses

Serotype No. European	Serotype No. American	Proposed Type Strain	Japan (49)	Northern Ireland (60, 62)	USA	Hungary (51)	Restriction Patterns
Chicken							
1	1	CELO (Phelps) (84)	OTE	112	QBV (67) Phelps (84)	H1	A12
2	2	GAL1 (11)	SR48	685	P7 (13)	H3	D
3	3	SR49 (49)	SR49	75	–	H5	D
4	4	KR5 (49)	KR5	506	J2 (13)	H2	C
5	8	340 (62)	TR22	340	M2 (13) Tipton (32)	–	B
6	5	CR119 (49)	CR119	168	–	–	E
7	11	YR36 (11)/X11 (13)	YR36	122	X11 (13)	–	E
8	6	TR59 (49)	TR59	58	T8 (13)	H6	E
9	7	764 (62)	–	764	B3 (13)	–	E
10	9	A2 (13)	–	93	A2 (13)	–	D
11	10	C2B (13)	–	–	C2B (13)	–	C
12	12	380 (59)	–	380	–	–	D
Duck							
1		GR (8)	–	–	–	–	NR[a]
Goose							
1		HA (88)	–	–	–	–	NR
2		N1 (88)	–	–	–	–	NR
3		569 (88)	–	–	–	–	NR

Note: The group II avian adenoviruses and the egg drop syndrome virus are not included in this table.
[a]NR = not reported.

types of adenovirus in turkeys exist in Northern Ireland (63) and three serotypes have been described in the USA (31), but these have not been compared.

Laboratory Host Systems. Most chicken isolates have been made in chick kidney (CK) or in chicken embryo liver (CEL) cells. Although it has been claimed that CEL cells are more sensitive, there appears to be little difference when examining clinical material. However, CEL cells are preferable for diagnostic work because of their greater sensitivity to other viruses. Fowl adenoviruses form plaques in CK. Chicken tracheal organ cultures and chicken embryo fibroblasts are not sensitive (see review 59).

Adenoviruses have been isolated from turkeys and a variety of other birds including ducks (8), guinea fowl (68), pigeons, budgerigars, and mallard ducks (64), using chicken cell cultures. However, there are viruses in turkeys that grow in turkey cells and do not grow or only grow poorly in chicken cells (77). It may be that if other avian species are examined using the homologous cell systems, an extended range of viruses will be recognized.

Although it is probable that all avian adenoviruses multiply in the embryonated egg, not all chicken or turkey isolates cause recognizable lesions. Kawamura et al. (49) found that the chorioallantoic membrane route of inoculation was more sensitive than the allantoic cavity. High virus titers of all prototype strains except SR49-killed embryos, but when low titers were used only OTE-killed embryos. Using material from natural infections Burke et al. (10) made only 3 isolations in embryonated eggs compared to 45 in cell culture. The majority of adenovirus isolates made in eggs reported in the literature have been serotype 1 or serotype 5, which are not the most prevalent isolates when either serological surveys (40) or virus isolation studies (25, 85) are undertaken. However, Cowen (22) has shown that inoculations into the yolk sac and to a lesser degree onto the chorioallantoic membrane permits the growth of 11 recognized serotypes. The signs and lesions produced in the embryo are death, stunting, curling, hepatitis, splenomegaly, congestion, and hemorrhage of body parts and urate formation in the kidneys. There are basophilic or eosinophilic intranuclear inclusion bodies in the hepatocytes.

Pathogenicity. Because the role of group I adenoviruses as primary pathogens is not clearly established, the factors determining pathogenicity are not clear. There are indications that different serotypes, and even strains with the same serotype, can vary in their ability to produce illness and death (9, 20), respiratory disease (29), or to grow and persist in embryo tendon explants (37). However Barr and Scott (6) could find no relationship between genotype, serotype, and virulence. Although F1 will produce a range of tumors when inoculated into hamsters and will transform human and hamster cells (57), attempts to demonstrate oncogenicity with other avian serotypes have been unsuccessful (33).

In many studies the route of inoculation has been extremely important, with many isolates failing to cause disease when given by natural routes or by direct spread, but being highly pathogenic when given by parenteral injection. This suggests that many adenoviruses are potential pathogens and require some other agent to allow them to cause disease. The age of the bird is also important. Thus it has been possible to produce mortality (20) in day-old chicks by injection, but not in 10-day-old birds. Virulence could be associated with strain of virus, age of bird, and titer, with the minimum of lethal dose ranging from >300,000 to 4 tissue culture infective dose–50% (6).

Infectious bursal disease enhances the pathogenicity of avian adenoviruses (34, 75), and the ability of avian adenoviruses to cause hepatitis and death was considerably enhanced by the presence of chicken anemia agent (CAA) (9). In contrast the presence of an adenovirus-associated parvovirus may reduce the growth of the adenovirus in cell cultures as well as pathogenicity and oncogenicity (see 57).

PATHOGENESIS AND EPIZOOTIOLOGY

Natural and Experimental Hosts. The chicken adenovirus is ubiquitous in fowl as demonstrated by many antibody surveys (40, 85) and from the high isolation rates of adenoviruses from specimens taken from normal and sick birds (25, 49, 51, 61). In addition to infecting chickens, fowl adenovirus serotypes have been recovered from turkeys, pigeons, budgerigars, and a mallard duck (15, 64), and probable fowl isolates have come from guinea fowl (68) and from pheasants (12).

Particles that are probably adenoviruses have been seen in thin sections of tissue taken from kestrels (79), herring gulls (53), peach-faced lovebirds (81), cockatiels (78), and tawny frogmouths (70).

In addition to being infected with chicken serotypes, turkeys are also infected with adenoviruses that grow in cells of turkey origin but either do not grow or only grow poorly in cells of fowl origin (77). Antibody to these viruses is widespread.

Adenoviruses have been isolated from geese and antibody is widespread. These viruses are unrelated to the recognized fowl serotypes, but they grow in cells of both goose and fowl origin (88). A group I adenovirus has been isolated from a Muscovy duck (8). This virus is unrelated to recognized fowl or turkey serotypes, but does grow in chicken as well as duck cells.

Attempts to grow avian adenoviruses in mammals have met with very limited success. F1 has produced fibrosarcomas, hepatomas, ependymomas, and adenocarcinomas when injected into hamsters (57), and another isolate has produced hepatitis in hamsters (33).

Transmission. Vertical transmission is very important. Adenoviruses are transmitted through the embryonated egg and are often unmasked in cell cultures prepared from embryos and young chicks from infected flocks (59). This has been one of the strongest motivations for establishing specific-pathogen-free (SPF) flocks. There is evidence that adenovirus infection can remain latent and undetected by the double immunodiffusion test for at least one generation in a SPF flock (35).

Although adenoviruses can be isolated from the first day of life, viruses are normally excreted from 3 wk onward. In broilers, peak excretion was found from 4–6 wk of life (57). In layer replacements virus excretion was at maximum from 5–9 wk but was still at 70% after 14 wk. There were six serotypes isolated from four farms (85). Cowen et al. (25) in a study beginning with 8-wk-old birds found excretion continued at a high level until 14 wk. In their cases eight serotypes were found on seven farms. It is not uncommon to isolate two or even three serotypes from one bird suggesting that there is little cross-protection. Certainly birds can excrete one serotype in spite of high levels of neutralizing antibody to other serotypes. There is a second period, around peak egg production when adenoviruses are often present. Presumably the stress of egg production or high levels of sex hormones cause reactivation of virus. This of course would ensure maximum egg transmission to the next generation.

Horizontal spread is also important. Virus is present in the feces, in the tracheal and nasal mucosa, and in the kidneys. Therefore, virus could be transmitted in all excretions, but the highest titers are found in the feces. There is a juvenile and adult pattern of excretion. Thus a 35-day-old bird showing the adult pattern has a lower peak titer of fecal virus, with an earlier decline in virus titer, and it excretes for a shorter time than a newly hatched chick, which exhibits the juvenile pattern (17). Horizontal spread appears to be mainly by direct fecal contact but also by aerial contact over short distances, with a slow spread taking weeks (19). This pattern has also been seen in experimentally infected and in adventitiously infected SPF flocks and contrasts markedly with the normal patterns usually found around in commercial flocks, when most birds in a flock are often excreting adenoviruses. In these circumstances it is probable that there are many foci of infection due to reactivation of latent viruses. In commercial flocks often derived from a number of parent flocks, each with their own range of serotypes, there is considerable mixing of serotypes and birds may be infected concurrently with more than one virus. Aerial spread between farms does not appear to be important, but spread by fomites, personnel, and transport can be very important.

Incubation Period and Signs in Fowl. Although adenoviruses have been associated with a number of clinical conditions, the evidence for them being primary pathogens is conflicting. The incubation period for adenoviruses is short (24–48 hr) following infection by natural routes.

EFFECT ON EGG PRODUCTION. Some workers have reported that adenovirus infection caused a 10% fall in egg production (18) or affected eggshell quality (83). In another such study, experimental infection of birds with four strains did not produce any effect on egg quality and only one strain had a minimal effect on egg numbers (24). Adenoviruses can be isolated from commercial flocks, even when there are exceptionally high levels of production and fertility, and adenovirus infections of SPF flocks in lay are often associated with no or only minimal effect on egg production and shell quality.

EFFECT ON FOOD CONVERSION AND GROWTH. There have been reports of adenovirus infection resulting in decreased food consumption (24). Although birds injected with adenovirus may have depressed body weights and even high mortality (20, 39), there is little evidence to suggest that natural infection causes either reduced food conversion or growth.

INCLUSION BODY HEPATITIS (IBH). There have been many different serotypes associated with natural outbreaks of IBH. Among those recorded are F1 (83); F2, F3, and F4 (38, 65); F5 (32, 64); F6, F7, and F8 (50); F7 and F10 (6); F8 (41, 54, 65); and F9 (42).

Some workers have been successful in reproducing liver lesions with basophilic intranuclear inclusions following parenteral inoculation of very young chicks (41, 55, 74) (see Fig. 22.4A) and Rinaldi et al. (73) induced both liver and pancreatic lesions. Kawamura and Horiuchi (47) were unable to produce signs but did produce degeneration, necrosis and a cellular response in livers and mild response in the trachea and lungs of 12-mo-old birds injected intravenously with a F1 virus. One group reproduced liver lesions using natural routes of infection in older birds (32). However other groups could not reproduce the disease even with unnatural routes (54, 56). Barr and Scott (6) were able to reproduce the disease using isolates from affected flocks up to 18 days old, but not with isolates from birds 27–30 days of age, suggesting that another undetected agent may be present in the younger birds.

Immunosuppression produced by infectious bursal disease (IBD) was found to aid the adenoviruses in producing IBH (34, 75). However, in Northern Ireland IBH occurred in chickens before IBD was present in the country (58), and IBH has occurred spontaneously in SPF birds without IBD (71). When birds are infected with both CAA and adenovirus, there is increased incidence of hepatitis and death (9).

Inclusion body hepatitis is characterized by a sudden onset of mortality peaking after 3–4 days and usually stopping on the 5th day, but occasionally continuing for 2–3 wk. Morbidity is low, and sick birds adopt a crouching position with ruffled feathers and die within 48 hr or recover (43, 54, 65). Mortality may reach 10% and occasionally up to 30% (6). It is normally seen in meat-producing birds 3–7 wk of age, but it has been reported in birds as young as 7 days old (6) and as old as 20 wk (50). There is evidence that in an integrated broiler operation disease occurs in chickens from certain breeder flocks (54).

RESPIRATORY DISEASE. Adenoviruses have been frequently isolated from both the upper and lower respiratory tract of birds with respiratory disease (48, 61, 73). Experimental infection produced equivocal results. Using aerosol exposure mild respiratory disease was produced (5). Following intratracheal inoculation, Cox (26) reported no signs but others reproduced disease (18, 56).

A survey of records of virus isolations and clinical and autopsy findings over a 20-yr period, involving the isolation of hundreds of adenoviruses, indicated no primary role for adenoviruses in fowl respiratory disease. However, before infectious bronchitis was controlled and *Mycoplasma gallisepticum* and *Mycoplasma synoviae* were eradicated, respiratory disease outbreaks were considerably more severe when adenoviruses were isolated from the respiratory tract (58). Schmidt et al. (76) recorded similar findings when mixed infectious bronchitis mycoplasma and adenovirus infections mimicked infectious laryngotracheitis. Dhillon and Kibenge (28) studied 13 outbreaks and found catarrhal tracheitis and multifocal pneumonic lesions similar to lesions they had found with experimental adenovirus infections and concluded that adenoviruses were a significant cause of respiratory disease.

TENOSYNOVITIS. Adenoviruses have been isolated from chickens with tenosynovitis, but experimental work has not confirmed that they are involved (46).

Signs in Turkeys. Adenoviruses have been isolated from clinical outbreaks of respiratory disease, diarrhea, and depressed egg production, but attempts to reproduce disease have been generally unsuccessful (58, 80).

Signs in Geese and Ducks. Zsak and Kisary (88) isolated three serotypes from geese but could not reproduce disease in goslings. In outbreaks of high mortality associated with hepatitis, adenoviruslike particles were seen in the liver (72).

A diphtheroid stenotizing tracheitis and sometimes bronchitis and pneumonia were seen in up to 10% of 7- to 21-day-old muscovy ducks. The epithelial cells of the trachea contained large numbers of adenoviruses (7).

Signs in Guinea Fowl. Two strains of adenovirus were isolated from natural outbreaks of pancreatitis in guinea fowl. One strain induced severe disease and death with respiratory and pancreatic lesions after oral and nasal infection of day-old guinea fowl (68). Foci of necrosis with large basophilic and smaller eosinophilic inclusion bodies were seen in guinea fowl suffering from necrotic pancreatitis (69).

Lesions

RESPIRATORY DISEASE. In natural outbreaks gross lesions were found. These were mild to moderate catarrhal tracheitis with excess mucus production (28). Hyperemia of the lungs, cloudy air sacs and petechial hemorrhages in the pharynx and larynx were described after experimental infection (5).

Microscopically the main lesions were loss of cilia, necrosis of some epithelial cells, intranuclear inclusion bodies, and infiltration of mononuclear cells into the lamina propria. Multifocal or occasionally a diffuse interstitial pneumonia was found (5, 28, 29).

Following aerosol exposure epithelial hyperplasia, edema, and infiltration by mononuclear cells were seen in air sacs (5).

INCLUSION BODY HEPATITIS. In the literature there are several descriptions of a disease primarily affecting the liver and also one where the primary lesions appeared to be in the hemopoietic system. It is probable that the aplastic anemia described was due to infection with CAA (87) (see Chapter 29).

The main lesions are pale, friable, swollen livers. Petechial or ecchymotic hemorrhages may be present in the liver and skeletal muscles (43, 54, 65).

There are inclusion bodies in the hepatocytes. These inclusions can be eosinophilic, large, and round or irregularly shaped with clear pale (43, 44) or occasionally basophilic inclusions (45, 65) (Fig. 22.4A, B). In Australia, basophilic inclusions predominate (6, 50). Itakura et al. (45) found that virus particles were detected only in the cells with the basophilic inclusions and the eosinophilic inclusions were of fibrella granular material.

Immunity. Group I fowl adenoviruses have a common group antigen and this antigen is distinct from that of human adenoviruses (49, 63). There are differences in the degree of sharing between these antigens. Thus F1 gave a strong reaction with its own antiserum but failed to detect antibody to F2 and F4 (49). A microtiter fluorescent test (3) confirmed these differences in titer.

The turkey adenoviruses of group I share a line of identify with F1 in double immunodiffusion tests, and this distinguishes them from the group II (turkey hemorrhagic enteritis) virus (30, 63). The isolate from a muscovy duck also shares an antigen with F1 (8).

Following infection, birds rapidly develop neutralizing antibody detectable after 1 wk and reaching peak titers at 3 wk (86). They may develop transient precipitating antibody (18) or they may fail to do so (63, 86). This apparent failure is probably due to the insensitivity of the double immunodiffusion test, since an antibody response can be detected using the immunofluorescent test (3).

This development of serum neutralizing antibody coincides with the cessation of virus excretion. The young chick excretes longer because of slower development of neutralizing antibody (17).

Clemmer (16) found that birds were resistant to reinfection with the same serotype 45 days after the primary infection. Serum neutralizing antibody, induced by an inactivated vaccine, had no effect on the excretion of virus in the feces, but did reduce pharyngeal excretion, possibly by preventing spread of virus from the intestine to the pharynx in the blood. Yates et al. (86) were able to reinfect birds after 8 wk with the same strain, eliciting a secondary response of both neutralizing and precipitating antibodies, and virus excretion occurred despite humoral antibody. Khanna (52) found peaks of virus excretion when they were 2.5, 4.5, and 7.5 mo of age, giving support to the conclusion that a local immunity lasts about 8 wk, but then regresses and allows virus to replicate once again on the mucosal surfaces. It is therefore possible that the immunity found by Clemmer is due to short-lived local immunity, and the circulating antibody only protects against invasion of the internal organs. The apparent correlation between the development of circulating antibody and ending of excretion is due to the concurrent development of both local immunity (which is short-lived) and the longer lasting general serum-based immunity. Support for this comes from the finding that maternal antibody does not protect against natural routes of infection (16) but does protect against intra-abdominal infection (32, 39).

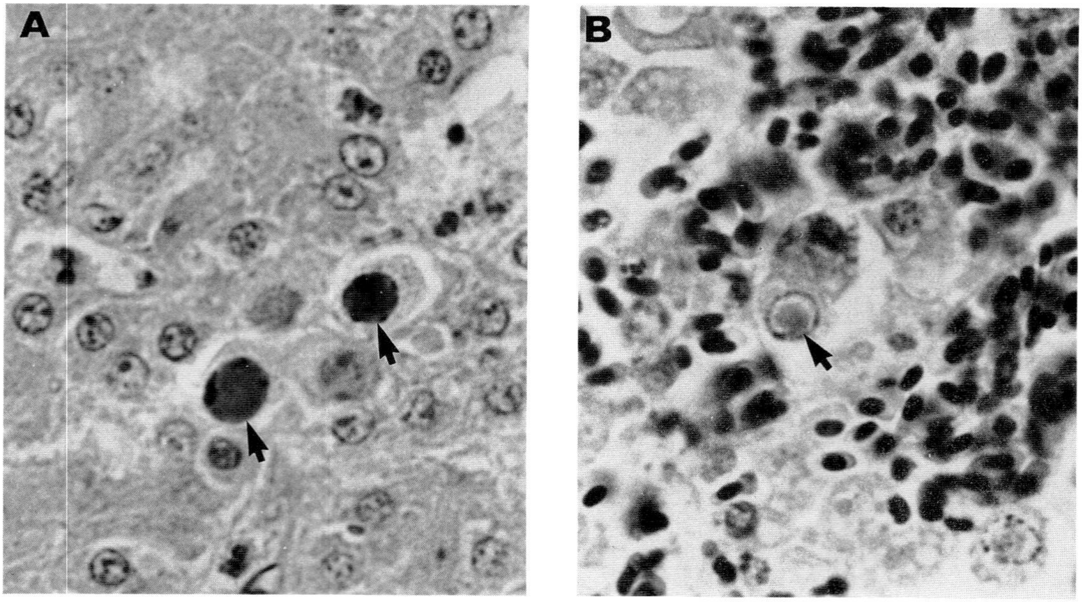

22.4. A. Large basophilic intranuclear inclusion bodies in liver of a chicken experimentally infected with F8. B. Eosinophilic intranuclear inclusion body in hepatocyte of a chicken with naturally occurring inclusion body hepatitis.

DIAGNOSIS

Isolation and Identification of Virus. The specimens of choice are feces, pharynx, kidneys, and affected organs (e.g., livers in cases of inclusion body hepatitis). These should be made into a 10% suspension and, in the case of chickens, inoculated onto either chick embryo liver cells or chick kidney cells. Chick embryo fibroblasts and tracheal organ cultures are not sensitive. Although three passages have been used (10, 25), generally two blind passages of 7 days duration each are sufficient. If attempting to isolate adenoviruses from other avian species, it is preferable to use cells from the avian species being investigated although fowl cells can be used. However, there are turkey isolates that either grow only poorly or not at all in chick cell cultures (77). Embryonated eggs are insensitive for primary isolation of most serotypes of adenoviruses, although Cowen (22) has showed that the yolk sac is a sensitive route for isolating laboratory strains representative of 10 serotypes. It remains to be shown if this route is equally sensitive with field material, but it clearly should be tried in laboratories lacking cell culture technology.

Once an agent is isolated in cell cultures, the easiest method to confirm that it is an adenovirus is to stain the cells with an antiserum labelled with a fluorescent dye. Direct examination of cell lysate in the electron microscope also gives a quick and positive answer and has the added advantage that parvoviruses can also be detailed if present. If these techniques are not available, then hematoxylin and eosin staining of the monolayers will demonstrate the presence of intranuclear basophilic inclusions. To identify a serotype it is necessary to conduct virus neutralization tests with the isolate against standard reference antiserums of all known serotypes. This labor-intensive process can be reduced by using the "antiserum pool" modification (25).

Serology. Antibody to the group antigen can be detected using the double immunodiffusion (DID) test, but its apparent sensitivity in natural outbreaks is often due to multiple infection with adenovirus serotypes and it cannot be relied upon to detect infection in SPF flocks (18, 35, 63). However, Cowen (21) has shown that if a trivalent antigen incorporating three adenovirus serotypes is used, the DID test is sensitive. The indirect immunofluorescent test is much more sensitive, rapid, and inexpensive (3). However, it requires skill to interpret it. The enzyme-linked immunosorbent assay (ELISA) has been used to detect group antibodies and it is cheap and sensitive (14, 27, 66).

Type-specific antibody has normally been detected using the serum neutralization test, but it can also be detected using the ELISA (66).

The main problem with any serological test for adenoviruses is interpreting the results, because antibodies are so widespread in both healthy and diseased birds, and so many birds are infected with a number of serotypes. Furthermore, the presence of antibody gives no indication of the state of local immunity at the mucosal surfaces.

PREVENTION AND CONTROL. As both IBD and CAA have been shown to potentiate the pathogenicity of adenoviruses, the first step must be to control or eliminate these two viruses.

Adenoviruses are resistant and although it is possible to eliminate them from most environmentally controlled houses that have impervious floors and walls and that can be made airtight, the value of attempted eradication of adenovirus from commercial flocks is questionable. This is because the virus is so effectively spread vertically through the embryonated egg that the viruses would be introduced in the next flock, and therefore control would have to start at primary breeder level. Furthermore, experience with SPF flocks has indicated that horizontal spread would be a major problem and it would be exceedingly difficult to keep a commercial flock from being infected.

On current knowledge, it is not possible to identify a primary role for adenoviruses in disease; therefore, the need for a vaccine does not exist at present.

REFERENCES

1. Adair, B.M. 1978. Studies on the development of avian adenoviruses in cell cultures. Avian Pathol 7:541–550.

2. Adair, B.M., W.L. Curran, and J.B. McFerran. 1979. Ultrastructural studies of the replication of fowl adenoviruses in primary cell cultures. Avian Pathol 8:133–144.

3. Adair, B.M., J.B. McFerran, and V.M. Calvert. 1980. Development of a microtitre fluorescent antibody test for serological detection of adenovirus infection in birds. Avian Pathol 9:291–300.

4. Aghakhan, S.M. 1974. Avian adenoviruses. Vet Bull 44:531–552.

5. Aghakhan, S.M., and M. Pattison. 1974. Pathogenesis and pathology of infections with two strains of avian adenovirus. J Comp Pathol 84:495–503.

6. Barr, D.A., and P. Scott. 1988. Adenoviruses and IBH. Proc 2nd Asian/Pacific Poult Health Conf, Proc 112, pp. 323–326. Post Graduate Comm Vet Sci, Univ Sydney, Aust.

7. Bergmann, Von V., R. Heidrich, and E. Kinder. 1985. Pathomorphologische und Elektronenmikroskopische Feststellung einer Adenovirus-tracheitis bei Moschusenten (Cairina moschata). Mh-Vet Med 40:313–315.

8. Bouquet, J.F., Y. Moreau, J.B. McFerran, and T.J. Connor. 1982. Isolation and characterisation of an adenovirus isolated from muscovy ducks. Avian Pathol 11:301–307.

9. Bülow V.v., R. Rudolph, and B. Fuchs. 1986. Folgen der Doppelinfektion von Kuken mit adenovirus oder Reovirus und dem Erreger der aviaren infektiosen

Anamie (CAA). Zentralbl Veterinaermed [B] 33:717-726.
10. Burke, C.N., R.E. Luginbuhl, and E.L. Jungherr. 1959. Avian enteric cytopathogenic viruses. I. Isolation. Avian Dis 3:412-419.
11. Burmester, B.R., G.R. Sharpless, and A.K. Fontes. 1960. Virus isolated from avian lymphomas unrelated to lymphomatosis virus. J Nat Cancer Inst 24:1443-1447.
12. Cakala, A. 1966. Szczep wirusa CELO wyosobniony z bazantow. Med Wet 22:261-264.
13. Calnek, B.W., and B.S. Cowen. 1975. Adenoviruses of chickens: Serologic groups. Avian Dis 19:91-103.
14. Calnek, B.W., W.R. Shek, N.A. Menendez, and P. Stiube. 1982. Serological cross-reactivity of avian adenovirus serotypes in an enzyme-linked immunosorbent assay. Avian Dis 26:897-906.
15. Cho, B.R. 1976. An adenovirus from a turkey pathogenic to both chicks and turkey poults. Avian Dis 20:714-723.
16. Clemmer, D.L. 1965. Experimental enteric infection of chickens with an avian adenovirus (strain 93). Proc Soc Exp Biol Med 118:943-948.
17. Clemmer, D.I. 1972. Age-associated changes in fecal excretion patterns of strain 93 chick embryo lethal orphan virus in chicks. Infect Immun 5:60-64.
18. Cook, J.K.A. 1972. Avian adenovirus alone or followed by infectious bronchitis virus in laying hens. J Comp Pathol 82:119-128.
19. Cook, J.K.A. 1974. Spread of an avian adenovirus (CELO virus) to uninoculated fowls. Res Vet Sci 16:156-161.
20. Cook, J.K.A. 1974. Pathogenicity of avian adenoviruses for day-old chicks. J Comp Pathol 84:505-515.
21. Cowen, B.S. 1987. A trivalent antigen for the detection of type 1 avian adenovirus precipitin. Avian Dis 31:351-354.
22. Cowen, B.S. 1988. Chicken embryo propagation of type I avian adenoviruses. Avian Dis 32:347-352.
23. Cowen, B., B.W. Calnek, and S.B. Hitchner. 1977. Broad antigenicity exhibited by some isolates of avian adenovirus. Am J Vet Res 38:959-962.
24. Cowen, B., B.W. Calnek, N.A. Menendez, and R.F. Ball. 1978. Avian Adenoviruses–effect on egg production, shell quality, and feed consumption. Avian Dis 22:459-470.
25. Cowen, B., G.B. Mitchell, and B.W. Calnek. 1978. An adenovirus survey of poultry flocks during the growing and laying periods. Avian Dis 22:115-121.
26. Cox, J.C. 1966. An avian adenovirus isolated in Australia. Aust Vet J 42:482.
27. Dawson, G.J., L.N. Orsi, V.J. Yates, P.W. Chang, and A.D. Pronovost. 1980. An enzyme-linked immunosorbent assay for detection of antibodies to avian adenovirus and avian adenovirus-associated virus in chickens. Avian Dis 24:393-402.
28. Dhillon, A.S., and F.S.B. Kibenge. 1987. Adenovirus infection associated with respiratory disease in commercial chickens. Avian Dis 31:654-657.
29. Dhillon, A.S., and R.W. Winterfield. 1984. Pathogenicity of various adenovirus serotypes in the presence of Escherichia coli in chickens. Avian Dis 28:147-153.
30. Domermuth, C.H., J.R. Harris, W.B. Gross, and R.T. DuBose. 1979. A naturally occurring infection of chickens with a hemorrhagic enteritis/marble spleen disease. Avian Dis 23:479-484.
31. Easton, G.D., and D.G. Simmons. 1977. Antigenic analysis of several turkey respiratory adenoviruses by reciprocal-neutralization kinetics. Avian Dis 21:605-611.
32. Fadly, A.M., and R.W. Winterfield. 1973. Isolation and some characteristics of an agent associated with inclusion body hepatitis, hemorrhages, and aplastic anaemia in chickens. Avian Dis 17:182-193.
33. Fadly, A.M., R.W. Winterfield, and H.J. Olander. 1976. The oncogenic potential of some avian adenoviruses causing diseases in chickens. Avian Dis 20:139-145.
34. Fadly, A.M., R.W. Winterfield, and H.J. Olander. 1976. Role of the bursa of Fabricius in the pathogenicity of inclusion body hepatitis and infectious bursal disease viruses. Avian Dis 20:467-472.
35. Fadly, A.M., B.J. Riegle, K. Nazerian, and E.A. Stephens. 1980. Some observations on an adenovirus isolated from specific pathogen-free chickens. Poult Sci 59:21-27.
36. Gelderblom, H., and I. Maichle-Laupper. 1982. The fibers of fowl adenoviruses. Arch Virol 72:289-298.
37. Georgiou, K., R.C. Jones, and J.R.M. Guneratne. 1983. Organ cultures studies on adenoviruses isolated from tenosynovitis in chickens. Avian Pathol 12:199-212.
38. Grimes, T.M., and D.J. King. 1977. Serotyping avian adenoviruses by a microneutralization procedure. Am J Ves Res 38:317-321.
39. Grimes, T.M., and D.J. King. 1977. Effect of maternal antibody on experimental infections of chickens with a type 8 avian adenovirus. Avian Dis 21:97-112.
40. Grimes, T.M., D.H. Culver, and D.J. King. 1977. Virus-neutralizing antibody titers against 8 avian adenovirus serotypes in breeder hens in Georgia by a microneutralization procedure. Avian Dis 21:220-229.
41. Grimes, T.M., D.J. King, S.H. Kleven, and O.J. Fletcher. 1977. Involvement of a type-8 avian adenovirus in the etiology of inclusion body hepatitis. Avian Dis 21:25-38.
42. Grimes, T.M., D.J. King, O.J. Fletcher, and R.K. Page. 1978. Serologic and pathogenicity studies of avian adenovirus isolated from chickens with inclusion body hepatitis. Avian Dis 22:177-180.
43. Howell, J., B.W. McDonald, and R.G. Christian. 1970. Inclusion body hepatitis in chickens. Can Vet J 11:99-101.
44. Itakura, C., M. Yasuba, and M. Goto. 1974. Histopathological studies on inclusion body hepatitis in broiler chickens. Jpn J Vet Sci 36:329-340.
45. Itakura, C., S. Matsushita, and M. Goto. 1977. Fine structure of inclusion bodies in hepatic cells of chickens naturally affected with inclusion body hepatitis. Avian Pathol 6:19-32.
46. Jones, R.C., and K. Georgiou. 1984. Experimental infection of chickens with adenoviruses isolated from tenosynovitis. Avian Pathol 13:13-23.
47. Kawamura, H., and T. Horiuchi. 1964. Pathological changes in chickens inoculated with Celo virus. Nat Inst Anim Health Q (Tokyo) 4:31-39.
48. Kawamura, H., T. Sato, H. Tsubahara, and S. Isogai. 1963. Isolation of celo virus from chicken trachea. Nat Inst Anim Health Q (Tokyo) 3:1-10.
49. Kawamura, H., F. Shimizu, and H. Tsubahara. 1964. Avian adenovirus:Its properties and serological classification. Nat Inst Anim Health Q (Tokyo) 4:183-193.
50. Kefford, B., R. Borland, J.F. Slattery, and D.C. Grix. 1980. Serological identification of avian adenoviruses isolated from cases of inclusion body hepatitis in Victoria, Australia. Avian Dis 24:998-1006.
51. Khanna, P.N. 1964. Studies on cytopathogenic avian enteroviruses. I. Their isolation and serological classification. Avian Dis 8:632-637.
52. Khanna, P.N. 1965. Studies on cytopathogenic avian enteroviruses. II. Influence of age on virus excre-

tion and incidence of certain serotypes in a colony of chicks. Avian Dis 9:27-32.

53. Leighton, F.A. 1984. Adenovirus-like agent in the bursa of Fabricius of Herring gulls (Larus argentatus pontoppidan) from Newfoundland, Canada. J Wildl Dis 20:226-230.

54. Macpherson, I., J.S. McDougall, and A.P. Laursen-Jones. 1974. Inclusion body hepatitis in a broiler integration. Vet Rec 95:286-289.

55. McCracken, R.M., J.B. McFerran, R.T. Evans, and T.J. Connor. 1976. Experimental studies on the aetiology of inclusion body hepatitis. Avian Pathol 5:325-339.

56. McDougall, J.S., and R.W. Peters. 1974. Avian adenoviruses. A study of 8 field isolates. Res Vet Sci 16:12-18.

57. McFerran, J.B. 1981. Adenoviruses of vertebrate animals. In E. Kurstak and C. Kurstak (eds.), Comparative Diagnosis of Viral Diseases III, pp. 102-165. Academic Press, New York.

58. McFerran, J.B. 1988. Unpublished observations.

59. McFerran, J.B., and B.M. Adair. 1977. Avian adenoviruses—a review. Avian Pathol 6:189-217.

60. McFerran, J.B., and T.J. Connor. 1977. Further studies on the classification of fowl adenovirus. Avian Dis 21:585-595.

61. McFerran, J.B., W.A.M. Gordon, S.M. Taylor, and P.J. McParland. 1971. Isolation of viruses from 94 flocks of fowl with respiratory disease. Res Vet Sci 12:565-569.

62. McFerran, J.B., J.K. Clarke, and T.J. Connor. 1972. Serological classification of avian adenoviruses. Archiv Virusforsch 39:132-139.

63. McFerran, J.B., B. Adair, and T.J. Connor. 1975. Adenoviral antigens (CELO, QBV, GAL). Am J Vet Res 36:527-529.

64. McFerran, J.B., T.J. Connor, and R.M. McCracken. 1976. Isolation of adenoviruses and reoviruses from avian species other than domestic fowl. Avian Dis 20:519-524.

65. McFerran, J.B., R.M. McCracken, T.J. Connor, and R.T. Evans. 1976. Isolation of viruses from clinical outbreaks of inclusion body hepatitis. Avian Pathol 5:315-324.

66. Mockett, A.P.A., and J.K.A. Cook. 1983. The use of an enzyme-linked immunosorbent assay to detect IgG antibodies to serotype-specific and group-specific antigens of fowl adenovirus serotypes 2, 3 and 4. J Virol Methods 7:327-335.

67. Olson, N.O. 1950. A respiratory disease (bronchitis) of quail caused by a virus. Proc 54th Annu Meet US Livest Sanit Assoc, pp. 171-174.

68. Pascucci, S., A. Rinaldi, and A. Prati. 1973. Celo virus in guinea-fowl: Characterization of two isolates. Proc 5th Int Conf World Vet Poult Assoc, pp. 1524-1531.

69. Reece, R.L., and D.A. Pass. 1986. Inclusion body pancreatitis in guinea fowl (Numida meleagris). Aust Vet J 63:26-27.

70. Reece, R.L., D.A. Pass, and R. Butler. 1985. Inclusion body hepatitis in a tawny frogmouth (Podargus strigoides: Caprimulgiformes). Aust Vet J 62:426.

71. Reece, R.L., D.C. Grix, and D.A. Barr. 1986. An unusual case of inclusion body hepatitis in a cockerel. Avian Dis 30:224-227.

72. Riddell, C. 1984. Virus hepatitis in domestic geese in Saskatchewan. Avian Dis 28:774-782.

73. Rinaldi, A., G Mandelli, D. Cessi., A. Valeri, and G. Cervio. 1968. Proprieta di un ceppo di virus CELO isolato dal Pollo in Italia. Clinica Vet (Milan) 91:382-404.

74. Rosenberger, J.K., R.J. Eckroade, S. Klopp, and W.C. Krauss. 1974. Characterization of several viruses isolated from chickens with inclusion body hepatitis and aplastic anaemia. Avian Dis 18:399-409.

75. Rosenberger, J.K., S. Klopp, R.J. Eckroade, and W.C. Krauss. 1975. The role of the infectious bursal agent and several avian adenoviruses in the hemorrhagic-aplastic-anaemia syndrome and gangrenous dermatitis. Avian Dis 19:717-729.

76. Schmidt, U., H. Hantschel, P. Schulze, and H. Linsert. 1970. Untersuchungen uber eine Mischinfektion von aviarem. Adenovirus und dem virus der infektiosen bronchitis. Arch Exp Veterinaermed 24:587-607.

77. Scott, M., and J. B. McFerran. 1972. Isolation of adenoviruses from turkeys. Avian Dis 16:413-420.

78. Scott, P.C., R.J. Condron, and R.L. Reece. 1986. Inclusion body hepatitis associated with adenovirus-like particles in a cockatiel (Psittaciformes:Nymphicus hollandicus). Aust Vet J 63:337-338.

79. Sileo, L., J.C. Franson, D.L. Graham, C.H. Domermuth., B.A. Rattner, and O.H. Patee. 1983. Hemorrhagic enteritis in captive American Kestrels (Falco Sparverius). J Wildlife Dis 19:244-247.

80. Sutjipto, S., S.E. Miller, D.G. Simmons, and R.C. Dillman. 1977. Physicochemical characterization and pathogenicity studies of two turkey adenovirus isolants. Avian Dis 21:549-556.

81. Wallner-Pendleton, E., D.H. Helfer, J.A. Schmitz, and L. Lowenstine. 1983. An inclusion body pancreatitis in Agapornis. Proc 32nd West Poult Dis Conf, p. 99.

82. Wigand, R., A. Bartha, R.S. Dreizin, H. Esche, H. S. Ginsberg, M. Green, J.C. Hierholzer, S.S. Kalter, J.B. McFerran, U. Pettersson, W.C. Russell, and G. Wadell. 1982. Adenoviridae: Second report. Intervirology 18:169-176.

83. Winterfield, R.W., A.M. Fadly, and A.M. Gallina. 1973. Adenovirus infection and disease. I. Some characteristics of an isolate from chickens in Indiana. Avian Dis 17:334-342.

84. Yates, V.J., and D.E. Fry. 1957. Observations on a chicken embryo lethal orphal (CELO) virus. J Vet Res 18:657-660.

85. Yates, V.J., Y.-O. Rhee, D.E. Fry, A.M. El Mishad, and K.J. McCormick. 1976. The presence of avian adenoviruses and adenovirus associated viruses in healthy chickens. Avian Dis 20:146-152.

86. Yates, V.J., Y.-O. Rhee, and D.E. Fry. 1977. Serological response of chickens exposed to a type 1 avian adenovirus alone or in combination with the adeno associated virus. Avian Dis 21:408-414.

87. Yuasa, N., T. Taniguchi, and I. Yoshida. 1979. Isolation and some characteristics of an agent inducing anaemia in chicks. Avian Dis 23:366-385.

88. Zsak, L., and J. Kisary. 1984. Characterisation of adenoviruses isolated from geese. Avian Pathol 13:253-264.

89. Zsak, L., and J. Kisary. 1984. Grouping of fowl adenoviruses based upon the restriction patterns of DNA generated by BAM HI and Hind III. Intervirology 22:110-114.

QUAIL BRONCHITIS

R.W. Winterfield and R.T. DuBose

INTRODUCTION. Quail bronchitis (QB) is an acute, highly contagious respiratory disease of bobwhite quail (*Colinus virginianus*). Until recently, the disease has been recognized only in captive quail, but evidence now suggests that it is also present in wild quail (11). QB and its etiologic agent, QB virus (QBV), have been reviewed in detail by DuBose (2, 3) and were also included in an extensive review on avian adenoviruses by Aghakhan (1).

After comparing chicken embryo lethal orphan (CELO) virus, isolated from endogenously infected chicken embryos by Yates and Fry (17), and QBV, isolated from quail with bronchitis, DuBose and Grumbles (5) considered QBV and CELO virus to be the same agent. Both viruses are now included in avian adenovirus serotype 1. Most of the agents designated in the literature as CELO or avian adenovirus serotype type 1 have not been tested for pathogenicity in bobwhite quail and were isolated from other species. To distinguish other adenoviruses isolated within serotype 1, the term "quail bronchitis virus" will be used in this section. General information applicable to all avian adenoviruses is of serotype 1 is included in the preceding section on avian adenoviruses.

HISTORY, INCIDENCE, DISTRIBUTION. QB was first described by Olson (12) from a 1949 outbreak in West Virginia. Subsequent descriptions were from occurrences in Texas in 1956–57 (6, 7) and Virginia in 1959 (2). Circumstantial evidence indicated transmission of QBV from inapparently infected chickens or captive game birds other than quail to the affected bobwhite quail. The disease was reproduced in quail by experimental infection with QBV (5, 12) and CELO (5, 16). QBV and CELO were shown to be similar to infectious bronchitis virus (IBV) of chickens in their effect on inoculated chicken embryos and inability to agglutinate chicken red blood cells; they were differentiated from IBV by virus-neutralization (VN) tests and their greater resistance to heat.

Since 1960, diagnostic reports from many states in which bobwhite quail are raised in captivity have noted at least sporadic incidence of the disease. Incidence and distribution in wild quail are not known, however, but high mortality in young quail and immunity in survivors suggest that the disease is self limiting.

ETIOLOGY. Classification of QBV as an avian adenovirus by Wilner (13) was supported by its morphology (8) and indistinguishability by the VN test (17) from the Phelps strain of CELO, the type strain for serotype 1 of the avian adenoviruses. Although not investigated as extensively, QBV isolates have not been found to differ significantly in their physicochemical and biologic properties from the type strain (1). As with other adenoviruses, avian adeno-associated virus (AAAV) may be isolated along with QBV (20). The principal feature of QBV remains its causation of an acute disease resulting in very high mortality in young bobwhite quail.

Laboratory Hosts and Pathogenicity. QBV usually is isolated and propagated in embryonating chicken eggs or cell cultures as described for CELO or serotype 1 in the section on avian adenovirus infections of chickens. Some isolates may require several blind passages in embryos before typical lesions and mortality patterns are observed. Propagation of QBV may be interfered with by concurrent AAAV infection (20) or by maternal antibodies in the yolk of embryonating eggs (18, 19).

DuBose and Grumbles (5) propagated viruses QB, CELO, and infectious bronchitis by inoculating chicken embryos via the chorioallantoic sac (CAS) but could not differentiate the viruses by gross lesions or mortality patterns in infected embryos.

PATHOGENESIS AND EPIZOOTIOLOGY

Natural and Experimental Hosts. Because bobwhite quail are naturally infected and develop a recognized disease (5, 12), and because inapparent infections in chickens are widespread (16, 17), we may for practical purposes consider them both as natural hosts for QBV or CELO virus. If overt signs of the disease occur in infected bobwhite quail, they usually appear before 8 wk of age. The incidence of mild forms or possible inapparent infections is not known (2, 3). Evidence for inapparent infections in captive young quail is noted under Treatment, Prevention, Control.

Chickens and turkeys were susceptible to experimental infections with QBV (12). Either no clinical signs or relatively mild respiratory signs resulted, but virus was reisolated from both species.

Transmission, Carriers, Vectors. QB is apparently highly contagious (2, 3, 12). Signs are usually seen in all susceptible young quail in contact with each other within 3–7 days of first notice of signs; transmission from pen to pen is rapid, and unless stringent precautions are taken, the disease occurs in succeeding hatches during the year on the same game-bird farm. Although not proved experimentally, airborne transmission is probable in addition to mechanical transmission. Circumstantial evidence indicates that QBV may be transmitted to bobwhite quail from a variety of other avian species not showing overt signs of disease.

Incubation Period, Signs, Morbidity, Mortality. The incubation period of 2–7 days in experimentally infected quail (5, 12) is consistent with rapid onset of signs noted in natural outbreaks (2, 6). In quail under 4 wk of age, tracheal rales, coughing, and sneezing are characteristic, sometimes accompanied by huddling and depressed attitudes. Lacrimation and conjunctivitis may be observed, but nasal exudate is not a usual feature. Neural signs are infrequent but have appeared in both natural and experimental infections. The course of the disease is 1–3 wk and morbidity may be 100%, with mortality ranging from 10 to 100% and frequently over 50%. Rapidity of spread and severity of disease may be markedly less in older quail. In an experimental infection, mortality following intraperitoneal (IP) or intratracheal (IT) infection occurred from 4–12 or 2–9 days postinoculation (PI), respectively, peaking at 5 days PI in both cases (9). Losses were 66 and 87%, respectively.

Gross Lesions and Histopathology. Excess mucus in the trachea or bronchi and cloudy air sac membranes, sometimes with mucoid exudate, have been observed (2, 6, 12). Cloudy corneas, conjunctivitis, and congestion of nasal passages or infraorbital sinuses may occur. A few young quail may be infected but present no signs or gross lesions. Jack et al. (10) reported an outbreak of QB in captive-raised bobwhite quail in which over 60% died without signs. The principle lesions were 1–2 mm pale foci in the liver. Histologically, the foci were seen as areas of hepatocellular necrosis, many with infiltrating inflammatory cells and occasional heterophils. Hepatocytes adjacent to necrotic foci often had large basophilic intranuclear inclusions. Virus isolated from affected livers had group-specific antigen(s) of group I avian adenovirus. Thus, it appears that adenovirus-induced inclusion body hepatitis can occur in quail as it does in chickens.

Following IP or IT inoculation of 1-wk-old quail, the predominant lesions were in the respiratory tract, liver, and spleen (9). Tracheas had opaque white areas that were thickened and sometimes filled with blood; occasionally the trachea was thin walled and translucent. Lungs were reddened and had consolidated zones. Liver lesions consisted of pale foci scattered widely but sometimes coalesced, and spleens were swollen and mottled. Histologically, the tracheal and bronchial lesions included deciliation and moderate hyperplasia of the mucosal epithelium, occasionally infiltrated by leukocytes and the presence of intranuclear inclusions in epithelial cells. Bronchial lesions also included edema and necrotic cellular debris in the lumen. Severely affected lungs had inflammatory lesions extending into the parenchyma. Hepatic lesions were as seen in the field case of inclusion body hepatitis in quail (10). Spleens showed histiocytic hyperplasia and fibrinoid necrosis; lymphocytes were depleted. The bursa of Fabricius had lesions consisting of lymphoid necrosis, lymphocyte depletion, and atrophy. Inclusion bodies were observed in mucosal epithelium.

Immunity. In QB, duration of immunity is not known, but survivors of both natural and experimental infections were refractory to challenge with QBV for at least 6 mo, and significant antibody levels developed in serum of quail following infection (2, 5, 12). DuBose (3) suggested a procedure for determining degree and duration of immunity and demonstrating possible inapparent infections in adult quail.

DIAGNOSIS. Criteria for diagnosis have been reviewed by DuBose (2, 3). In quail chicks sudden onset of rales, sneezing, or coughing that spreads rapidly through the group and results in mortality suggests QB. Excess mucus in the trachea, bronchi, and air sacs is added evidence of the disease. Severity of signs, rapidity of spread, and presence of lesions probably would be less marked in older quail. Isolation and identification of an agent indistinguishable from QBV (or CELO virus) would confirm the diagnosis. Inoculation of 9- to 11-day embryonating chicken eggs via the CAS with suspensions of aqueous humor, trachea, air sacs, or lungs has been used for isolation of the agent. As other sources of the virus, Yates et al. (20) recommended suspensions of fecal samples or homogenates of the posterior small intestine (ileum) or colon, and he described their processing. Three to five blind passages are made with allantoamniotic fluid harvested from chilled eggs up to 6 days or more postinoculation or earlier from embryos that die 24 hr postinoculation or later or that exhibit signs of stunting in daily candling. According to Yates et al. (20), a few strains seem to require inoculation via the yolk sac in 5- to 7-day-old embryos.

Embryo mortality (increasing with the number of passages), stunting, thickening of the amnion, necrotic foci or mottling of the liver, and accumulation of urates in the mesonephros are typical changes caused by QBV or CELO virus. Neutralization of the isolated virus by specific QBV or CELO virus antiserum would confirm identification of the virus and the diagnosis.

In general, information in regard to isolation, propagation, and identification of CELO or adenovirus serotype 1 in the section Avian Adenoviruses should be applicable to QBV. Yates et al. (20) noted preference for chick embryo kidney or chick kidney cell cultures and gave details on methods and identification criteria. The agar-gel precipitin (AGP) test may be used to place isolated virus in the avian adenovirus group but does not identify the serotype. In the absence of virus isolation facilities or with failure to isolate a virus, the AGP test using stock antigen on paired sets of serum samples may be of value. A markedly higher percentage of positive precipitin tests among samples collected during convalescence (2.5–4 wk after initial signs) than among serums collected during the acute phase (first few days of signs) should add weight to a presumptive diagnosis of QB otherwise based only on clinical observations.

Pulmonary aspergillosis may be differentiated from QB by presence of caseous nodules in lungs or deposits in air sacs, with pockets of grayish or greenish spore accumulations. Although bacterial infections might complicate the disease, none is known to cause rapid development signs, lesions, and mortality of QB. DuBose (2) suggested that Newcastle disease might present a clinical picture similar in part to QB, but clinical Newcastle disease has not been described in bobwhite quail.

TREATMENT, PREVENTION, CONTROL. There is no specific treatment for QB. Prevention and control were described in detail by DuBose (2, 3).

Slightly increased warmth in the brooder or house, adequate ventilation but no drafts, and avoidance of crowding are suggested supportive measures during an outbreak. Prevention is based on protecting susceptible quail from all possible sources of QBV or CELO virus. In addition to the usual sanitation procedures and measures to prevent entry of infectious agents onto the premises, care should be taken to keep adult quail, as well as other avian species, away from young quail. Control measures on a farm should be started immediately when even a tentative diagnosis of QB is made. In addition to general measures to prevent transmission from group to group, hatching operations may be deferred until 2 wk after signs have disappeared to provide a break in the presence of highly susceptible young quail.

An attempt by DuBose (4) to eradicate QBV from bobwhite quail on a large game-bird farm was unsuccessful but may have been responsible for preventing losses and clinical QB over a 2.5-yr period. In 1-yr hatches of 10,000 quail, 80% had died from the disease. In addition to most measures described above and elsewhere (3), older quail were marketed, and only survivors from hatches that had been affected at less than 4 wk of age were kept for breeders. VN antibody at a high level was detected in 3.5-mo-old quail hatched 2 yr later, but no signs of QB were detected in the intervening period or up to the time the farm closed the following winter. Winterfield and Dhillon (14) employed a type 1 adenovirus serotype in quail chicks as a vaccine against QB. The isolate, designated Indiana C virus, was isolated from chickens (15). It proved apathogenic for quail in a laboratory trial and was subsequently used on a farm where QB was endemic and losses were extensive. The owner of the quail farm reported that the disease quickly subsided. More observations on using a QB vaccine under these circumstances are needed, however, along with laboratory studies.

REFERENCES

1. Aghakhan, S.M. 1974. Avian adenoviruses. Vet Bull 44:531–552.
2. DuBose, R.T. 1967. Quail bronchitis. Bull Wildl Dis Assoc 3:10–13.
3. DuBose, R.T. 1971. Quail bronchitis. In J.W. Davis, R.C. Anderson, L. Karstad, and D.O. Trainer (eds.), Infectious and Parasitic Diseases of Wild Birds, pp. 42–47. Iowa State Univ Press, Ames.
4. DuBose, R.T. 1977. Unpublished data.
5. DuBose, R.T., and L.C. Grumbles. 1959. The relationship between quail bronchitis virus and chicken embryo lethal orphan virus. Avian Dis 3:321–344.
6. Dubose, R.T., L.C. Grumbles, and A.I. Flowers. 1958. The isolation of a nonbacterial agent from quail with a respiratory disease. Poult Sci 37:654–658.
7. DuBose, R.T., L.C. Grumbles, and A.I. Flowers. 1960. Differentiation of quail bronchitis virus and infectious bronchitis virus by heat stability. Am J Vet Res 21:740–743.
8. Dutta, S.K., and B.S. Pomeroy. 1967. Electron microscopic studies of quail bronchitis virus. Am J Vet Res 28:296–299.
9. Jack, S.W., and W.M. Reed. 1988. Pathology of quail bronchitis. Proc 37th West Poult Dis Conf, pp. 161–162.
10. Jack, S.W., W.M. Reed, and T.A. Bryan. 1987. Inclusion body hepatitis in bobwhite quail (Colinus virginianus). Avian Dis 31:662–665.
11. King, D.J., S.R. Pursglove, Jr., and W.R. Davidson. 1981. Adenovirus isolation and serology from wild bobwhite quail (Colinus virginianus). Avian Dis 25:678–682.
12. Olson, N.O. 1950. A respiratory disease (bronchitis) of quail caused by a virus. Proc 54th Annu Meet US Livest Sanit Assoc, pp. 171–174.
13. Wilner, B.I. 1969. A Classification of the Major Groups of Human and Other Animal Viruses, 4th Ed., Burgess Publ. Co., Minneapolis.
14. Winterfield, R.W., and A.S. Dhillon. 1980. Unpublished data.
15. Winterfield, R.W., A.M. Fadly, and A.M. Gallina. 1973. Adenovirus infection and disease. I. Some characteristics of an isolate from chickens in Indiana. Avian Dis 17:334–342.
16. Yates, V.J. 1960. Characterization of the chicken-embryo-lethal-orphan (CELO) virus. PhD diss., Univ Wisconsin, Madison.
17. Yates, V.J., and D.E. Fry. 1957. Observations on a chicken embryo lethal orphan (CELO) virus. Am J Vet Res 18:657–660.
18. Yates, V.J., P.W. Chang, A.H. Dardiri, and D.E. Fry. 1960. A study in the epizootiology of the CELO virus. Avian Dis 4:500–505.
19. Yates, V.J., D.V. Ablashi, P.W. Chang, and D.E. Fry. 1962. The chicken-embryo-lethal-orphan (CELO) virus as a tissue-culture contaminant. Avian Dis 6:406–411.
20. Yates, V.J., Y.-O. Rhee, and D.E. Fry. 1975. Comments on adenoviral antignes (CELO, QBV, GAL). Am J Vet Res 36:530–531.

HEMORRHAGIC ENTERITIS AND RELATED INFECTIONS

C.H. Domermuth and W.B. Gross

INTRODUCTION. Hemorrhagic enteritis (HE) is an acute disease of 4-wk-old or older turkeys. It is characterized by depression, bloody droppings, and sudden death. Signs and mortality occur in individuals within 24 hr. The disease persists in flocks 7–10 days. The infection causes immunosuppression (see Immunity)

Complete records of losses from the disease have not been kept; however, estimates of losses within states totaled in excess of $3 million per year prior to development of a vaccine. There is no evidence of transmission of the disease to humans or other animals.

Because of the relatedness of the etiologic agents (see ETIOLOGY), two other conditions are described here, marble spleen disease (MSD) of pheasants and the recently described avian adenovirus group II splenomegaly (AAS) of chickens (also sometimes referred to as "marble spleen" disease).

HISTORY. HE was first observed by Pomeroy and Fenstermacher (48) in Minnesota and later by Gale and Wyne (26) in Ohio. The disease reached epidemic proportions in Texas in the early 1960s. It reached Virginia in the mid-1960s (29), where it also assumed epidemic proportions. It has occurred in confined and range flocks and exhibits a strong tendency to infect successive flocks on the same premises. Information developed on HE prior to 1984 has been reviewed (10, 47).

INCIDENCE AND DISTRIBUTION. HE has been a serious problem in at least 10 states and has been observed throughout the world where turkeys are raised. Variations that produce insignificant or no mortality are known (15). Seroconversion studies performed by the authors suggest that almost all flocks of adult turkeys have been infected by HE virus (HEV). Similarly, a high incidence of antibody in mature chickens suggests that most flocks have been infected with AAS virus (AASV) (9).

ETIOLOGY. HE was first transmitted with both filtered and unfiltered intestinal contents obtained from turkeys that had died of the disease (29). It was later transmitted by intravenous (IV) inoculation of filtered serum (6), and the causative virus was found to be in highest concentration in the spleen (11).

Evidence indicates that the causative viruses of HE of turkeys, MSD of pheasant, and AAS of chickens belong to a new group of avian adenoviruses.

Classification

VIRUS GROUP. Morphologic (4, 35, 51), histologic (4, 25, 28), immunologic (8, 14, 33), and chloroform resistance (12) studies indicate that the causative agent of HE of turkeys is an adenovirus. Convalescent HE turkey antiserum protects pheasants against MSD (14). Furthermore, viruses respectively associated with MSD of pheasants and AAS of chickens are indistinguishable from HEV in agar-gel double diffusion tests (8, 14, 18–20, 33) and all are unrelated to chicken embryo lethal orphan (CELO) virus (19, 38) or to four isolates of turkey adenoviruses (38). This indicates that they constitute an immunologically distinct group of adenoviruses, which has been designated avian adenovirus group II (19) to distinguish it from the large group of adenoviruses (CELO and others) that share a different group antigen and are classified as avian adenovirus group I. Recently, members of avian adenovirus group II have been distinguished from each other by restriction endonuclease fingerprinting (58) and from each other and from members of adenovirus group I by monoclonal antibodies (54).

Morphology

ULTRASTRUCTURE, SIZE, SYMMETRY. HE and MSD virions are nonenveloped and icosohedral and reportedly vary in diameter between 70–80 nm and 70–90 nm, respectively (3, 32, 35, 51). Differences in size are probably within the limits of experimental error. HEV readily passed filters with porosities of 220 and 100 nm but not 10 nm (6, 12, 29). In thin section preparations examined by electron microscopy, virions associated with both infections ranged from empty to dense and from loosely packed to crystalline arrays; the total capsomere count was 252 (4, 25, 35, 51).

DENSITY. Sucrose gradient density studies reported for HEV revealed a density of 1.34 g/ml (4). MSD virus (MSDV) produces a band in equilibrium cesium chloride density gradient centrifugation at a density corresponding to 1.32–1.33 g/ml (31).

Chemical Composition. Nucleic acid of density gradient–purified MSDV was obtained by phenol extraction, assayed for deoxyribose by direct colorimetric diphenylamine reaction, and determined to be DNA (31). The exclusively intranuclear location of HEV also strongly suggests that it is a DNA virus.

Virus Replication. Electron micrographs suggest that HEV and MSDV are replicated intranuclearly in cells of the reticuloendothelial system, primarily in the spleen (3, 4, 25, 31, 35, 51, 57). These findings are supported by immunodiffusion studies, which indicate that viral antigen is concentrated in the spleen (11, 38), is barely discernible in a small percentage of liver and serum samples, and is not detectable in thymus, bursa of Fabricius, intestinal wall, or muscle. The more sensitive immunofluorescence and enzyme-linked immunosorbent assay (ELISA) test results have detected viral antigen in small amounts in many tissues (23, 49).

Resistance to Chemical and Physical Agents. Infectivity of HEV was destroyed by heating at 70 C for 1 hr (12); drying at 37 or 25 C for 1 wk (6); or by treatment with 0.0086% sodium hypochlorite (7), 1.0% sodium lauryl sulfate, 0.4% Chlorocide, 0.4% Phenocide, 0.4% Wescodyne, or 1.0% Lysol (6). Infectivity was not destroyed by heating at 65 C for 1 hr; storage for 6 mo at 4 C, 4 yr at −40 C, or 4 wk at 37 C; maintenance at pH 3.0 at 25 C for 30 min; or by treatment with 50% chloroform or 50% ethyl ether (12).

Strain Classification. HEV, AASV, and MSDV have been classified only as to source (turkeys, chickens, pheasants).

Laboratory Host Systems. Early attempts at propagating HEV strains in chicken and turkey embryos and in cell cultures were unsuccessful (4, 12, 32, 33, 57). There have been several attempts to infect lymphocytes. Perrin et al. (45) inoculated spleen cells with HEV and were subsequently able to recover virus, but they did not show that it was other than the inoculum virus itself. Fasina and Fabricant (24) demonstrated in vitro infection of chicken, turkey, and pheasant spleen cells by immunofluorescence, but no demonstrable virus release occurred. Successful serial passage of HEV in vitro in a turkey cell line of lymphoblastoid B cells derived from a Marek's disease tumor was reported by Nazerian and Fadly (43), and in normal turkey leukocytes by van den Hurk (52).

Pathogenicity. Mortality in field outbreaks of HE has varied from over 60% (29) to less than 0.1%. In experiments where spleen size and presence of precipitating antigen indicated 100% infection, mortality varied between 80% for the most pathogenic strain to 0% for the least. All strains produced virtually 100% infection under laboratory conditions. Present information suggests that the ability of a given strain to produce mortality is a fairly stable characteristic.

PATHOGENESIS AND EPIZOOTIOLOGY

Natural and Experimental Hosts. Turkeys, pheasants, and chickens are the only known natural hosts of members of the HE-MSD-AAS group of viruses. Antibodies have not been detected in serums of wild birds (16). Laboratory experiments indicate that pheasant MSDV isolates will infect turkeys (17, 34) and turkey HEV isolates will infect pheasants. Similarly, chicken isolates will infect turkeys (18–20). In addition, isolates from HE have produced spleen swelling and lesions in all avian species where infection has been attempted (golden pheasants, peafowl, chickens, chukars). Death has not occurred in experimentally infected species other than the natural host.

AGE OF HOST MOST COMMONLY AFFECTED. In the first reported outbreaks, HE occurred in 6- to 11-wk-old poults (26, 48). More recently it has occurred most frequently in 7- to 9-wk-old birds, although in one instance a spontaneous infection was reported in 2½-wk-old poults (30). The disease has been artificially transmitted to birds as old as 52 wk of age. Unless free of maternal HEV antibody, poults younger than 3½–4 wk are refractory to the disease. When free of maternal antibody they have been somewhat (21) to fully susceptible.

MSD in pheasants usually occurs in 3- to 8-mo-old birds (2, 3, 31). The disease has been reproduced experimentally in mature pheasants (14). In chickens with AAS, field infection is observed as splenomegaly of market-age or younger broilers (18, 30) or as splenomegaly with pulmonary congestion and edema in mature birds (20).

Transmission, Carriers, Vectors. HEV has several features in common with group I avian adenoviruses. It can be transmitted orally or cloacally by inoculation of infectious feces (29, 37). The causative virus remains infectious for several weeks at 37 C in carcasses protected from drying and in broth suspensions of infectious feces. HEV has been recovered from litter contaminated by HEV-infected flocks. The disease reoccurs in houses where it has appeared before. Unlike the situation with group I adenoviruses, there is no epidemiologic evidence for egg transmission. Carriers and vectors have not been implicated in transmission of HEV. These observations strongly indicate that HEV is usually transmitted to subsequent flocks by HEV-contaminated litter and that transmission between flocks can occur as a result of direct transportation of infectious virus to susceptible flocks.

Incubation Period. HE mortality occurs about 3–4 days after IV inoculation or 5–6 days after oral or cloacal inoculation of dilute extract of infectious spleen (11). In a naturally infected flock, all signs of disease usually subside within 6–10 days after the first observation of bloody droppings. Mortality in experimentally induced MSD occurred in pheasants 6 days after oral inoculation of pheasant-derived virus (14). Mortality has not been produced in chickens inoculated with AASV, but spleens were enlarged at 5, 6, and 7 days after oral inoculation (18) and pulmonary congestion and edema resembling field lesions has been reproduced (55).

Signs. HE is characterized by rapid onset; all signs in individuals usually occur within 24 hr (9, 10, 47). Signs of HE include depression, bloody droppings, and death. Dark red to brownish blood is frequently present on the skin and feathers around the vents of dead or dying birds. Blood may be forced from the vents of such birds if moderate pressure is applied to the abdominal area. Death of pheasants infected with MSDV and of chickens infected with AASV is rapid and due to asphyxia; therefore, signs are generally believed to be nonexistent.

Morbidity and Mortality. Depressed poults usually die in a few hours or appear to recover completely. Field mortality has ranged from less than 1 to slightly over 60%, with the average in the 10–15% range. Mortality of 80% often occurs in laboratory experiments in which 100% infection is usually achieved (28). In field outbreaks all or nearly all birds are infected, as indicated by seroconversion (11) and resistance to experimental challenge.

Mortality in MSDV-infected, pen-reared pheasants has been reported to be 2–3% (3, 38), but it may reach 10–15%. In mature chickens with AAS, an 8.9% mortality has been reported (20).

Gross Lesions. Dead poults appear pale due to anemia, but they are in good flesh and usually have feed in the crop unless otherwise debilitated. Intestines are distended, dark in color, and filled with red to brownish blood. The jejunal mucosa is red and highly congested. In some individuals, fibrin and necrotic epithelium form a loose yellow covering over the mucosa. Spleens of infected birds are characteristically enlarged, friable, and marbled or mottled; however, enlarged spleens of dead poults tend to be smaller and less marbled. Usually, lungs are congested and vascular organs are pale. Enlarged livers and petechial hemorrhages in various tissues of dead poults have been reported but are too inconsistent to be of diagnostic significance (4, 25, 26, 27, 34, 48).

Gross lesions in pheasants infected by MSDV consist of enlarged spleens, with characteristic mottling resembling marbling, and edema and congestion of the lungs (2, 3, 40, 57). In broiler chickens infected by AASV, gross splenic lesions resemble those of MSD of pheasants (18), as do the gross lung and splenic lesions found in mature chickens (20).

Histopathology. The pathologic changes that characterize HE are most evident in the reticuloendothelial (RE) system and intestine. The spleen seems to be most severely affected, and most of the virus appears to be produced in cells described either as "reticular or reticuloendothelial cells" (36, 51). Death is caused by bleeding into the intestinal lumen through damaged capillaries located in the tips of the villi, and poults that die of HE invariably exhibit characteristic intestinal lesions.

Lesions of the small intestine include severe congestion of the mucosa, degeneration of epithelial cells covering tips of villi, and sloughing of epithelial cells and tips of the villi, followed by hemorrhage into the lumen from broken capillaries. Increased numbers of reticular cells, plasma cells, and heterophils occur in the lamina propria, and intranuclear inclusion bodies are present in some of the RE cells. Histopathologic changes are most pronounced in the duodenum just posterior to the pancreatic ducts (Fig. 22.5). Similar but

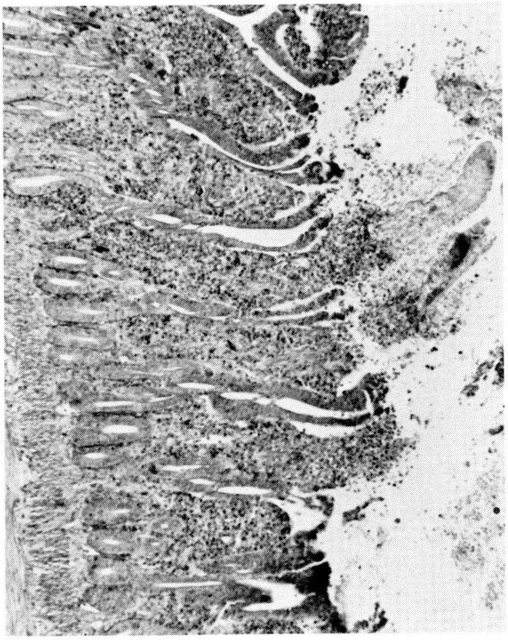

22.5. Section of small intestine of turkey affected with HE. Lesions include severe congestion of the mucosa, degeneration of epithelial cells covering tips of villi, sloughing of epithelial cells and tips of villi, and hemorrhage into the lumen. H & E, ×550.

less severe lesions may also occur in the proventriculus, gizzard, large intestine, ceca, cecal tonsils, and bursa of Fabricius (4, 25, 27, 36, 48).

Splenic lesions present at death of poults (Fig. 22.6) include hyperplasia of white pulp and necrosis of lymphoid cells, proliferation of enlarged RE cells, and presence of a few intranuclear inclusion bodies (4, 25, 28, 36). Inclusions are much more numerous in spleens of individuals killed when death is imminent. A sequential study of splenic changes associated with HE has been reported (28), and RE cell changes and other minor lesions of liver, thymus, bone marrow, kidney, lung, pancreas, and brain have also been observed (4, 25, 36, 56). Characteristic histologic lesions in field MSDV infections include splenic RE cell hyperplasia and necrosis with intranuclear inclusions and congestion and edema of lungs (2, 3, 40, 57). In AASV-infected chickens, spleens are also characterized by RE cell hyperplasia and intranuclear inclusions, and lungs by pulmonary congestion and edema (20, 55). It should be noted that "reticuloendothelial" cells referred to above are now considered to be macrophages derived from monocytes and part of the mononuclear phagocytic system; however, the precise identity of all HEV target cells remains to be fully elucidated.

Immunity

ACTIVE. Poults that have recovered from natural outbreaks of HE have not become reinfected.

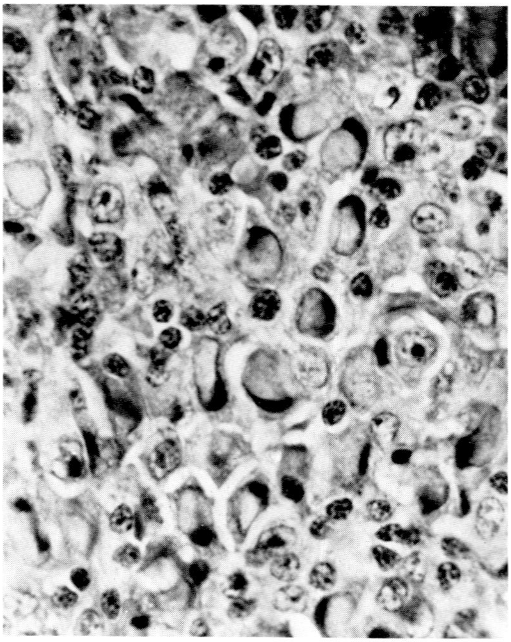

22.6. Section of spleen of turkey affected with HE. Nuclei of reticular cells contain characteristic inclusions. H & E, ×550.

Poults that recovered from laboratory-induced HE were similarly refractory to reinfection. Antibodies persist. In one flock studied for 4 yr, incidence of antibody gradually fell from 100% at 4 wk postinfection to 83% at 40 mo postinfection. Protection does not seem to be virus strain-specific. Strains that cause less than 1% or no mortality induce immunity that prevents infection upon subsequent challenge with pathogenic strains that normally produce greater mortality (15). Birds remain resistant for life.

PASSIVE. Immunity can be conferred by injection of convalescent antiserum obtained from recovered flocks. In laboratory experiments, 0.5–1.0 ml antiserum prevented all gross lesions, and as little as 0.1–0.25 ml prevented intestinal but not splenic lesions (8).

IMMUNOSUPPRESSION. Lymphocyte function tests have indicated that HEV infection is followed by low-level transient immunosuppression (41, 42). Colibacillosis (39, 50) and rhinotracheitis, caused secondarily by paramyxovirus type II or chlamydia (1), have been reported as significant sequelae to HEV infection. Thus, it appears that immunosuppression results from HEV infection. This is not surprising since lymphocytes and RE cells (probably macrophages) are target cells of HEV.

DIAGNOSIS

Isolation and Identification of Causative Agent.

The causative virus of HE can be recovered from sanguinous intestinal contents (29) or minced splenic tissue from dead or moribund poults. Isolations of HEV can be made in susceptible poults reared in isolation. Poults, preferably 5–10 wk old, should be inoculated orally or cloacally with crude sanguinous intestinal contents. Alternatively, they may be inoculated IV with a crude saline extract of minced spleen. Death should occur about 3 days after IV inoculation and 5–6 days after oral or cloacal inoculation. Poults that do not die of HE may have enlarged, marbled, infected spleens. Serum obtained at these times is also infectious (11). Lymphoblastoid B cell cultures derived from a Marek's disease tumor may also be used to isolate and propagate HEV (43, 44).

Serology

AGAR-GEL PRECIPITIN (AGP) TESTS. Antigen characteristically associated with HE can be identified in extracts of spleen, and antibody can be detected in blood plasma or serum of infected flocks by AGP tests (11, 13). For diagnostic purposes, a positive HE precipitin test obtained with antigen from spleens of dead turkeys can be regarded as proof of HEV infection in the flock. Antibody can be detected 2 wk postinfection. At 4 wk postinfection the incidence of precipitin in flocks has varied from 100 to less than 10% and there may be direct relationship between pathogenicity and precipitin incidence. All isolates of HEV tested to date have been indistinguishable from one another and from MSDV in precipitin tests. Chicken AASV and antibody are also indistinguishable from HEV and MSDV and antibody (9).

ENZYME-LINKED IMMUNOSORBENT ASSAY (ELISA). ELISA tests have been developed to detect HEV and HEV antibody (5, 44, 53). These tests are more sensitive than AGP and therefore more useful in quantitation of antibody, but probably not in detecting infected flocks.

Differential Diagnosis. In turkeys, if a marbled enlarged spleen occurs without intestinal bleeding, and if precipitating antigen cannot be demonstrated in the spleen, one should consider other diseases such as reticuloendotheliosis or leukosis (see Chapter 16). Acute bacterial infections, toxic fungi, and toxic drugs or other chemicals may produce intestinal bleeding resembling that in HE. Pheasants that die of acute asphyxia with accompanying pulmonary edema and congestion, splenomegaly, and demonstrable MSDV antigen may be considered to have died of MSDV infection. Similarly, chickens exhibiting splenomegaly with demonstrable AASV antigen may be considered to have died of AASV infection, but antigen is rarely present in sufficient quantity to make such a diagnosis. In this case, histopathologic examination should be used to distinguish between leukotic and nonleukotic hyperplastic tissue reactions.

TREATMENT. HE can be treated by injection of convalescent antiserum, which is obtained from healthy flocks and usually collected at slaughter (8). Treatment has not been described for MSD of pheasants or AAS of chickens.

PREVENTION AND CONTROL

Management Procedures. Prevention of HE can probably be accomplished by preventing transportation of infected litter or feces from flock to flock. This may not be possible in areas where potential vectors may exist; however, vector transmission has not been reported.

Immunization. To control HE, avirulent isolates can be successfully used as live, water-administered vaccines (15, 22). If flocks are less than 100% protected by vaccination they are subsequently protected by lateral transmission of vaccine virus within 2-3 wk (46). A live, avirulent, water-administered vaccine may also be used to control MSD of pheasants (17). A similar vaccine has not been developed to control AAS of chickens nor is its use currently indicated.

REFERENCES

1. Andral, B., M. Metz, D. Toquin, J. LeCoz, and J. Newman. 1985. Respiratory disease (rhinotracheitis) of turkeys in Brittany, France. III. Interaction of multiple infecting agents. Avian Dis 29:233-243.

2. Bygrave, A.C., and M. Pattison. 1973. Marble spleen disease in pheasants (Phasianus colchicus). Vet Rec 92:534-535.

3. Carlson, H.C., J.R. Pettit, R.V. Hemsley, and W.R. Mitchell. 1973. Marble spleen disease of pheasants in Ontario. Can J Comp Med 37:281-286.

4. Carlson, H.C., F. Al-Sheikhly, J.R. Pettit, and G.L. Seawright. 1974. Virus particles in spleens and intestines of turkeys with hemorrhagic enteritis. Avian Dis 18:67-73.

5. Davidson, I., A. Aronovici, Y. Weisman, and M. Malkinson. 1985. Enzyme immunoassay studies on the serological response of turkeys to hemorrhagic enteritis virus. Avian Dis 29:43-52.

6. Domermuth, C.H., and W.B. Gross. 1971. Effect of disinfectants and drying on the virus of hemorrhagic enteritis of turkeys. Avian Dis 15:94-97.

7. Domermuth, C.H., and W.B. Gross. 1972. Effect of chlorine on the virus of hemorrhagic enteritis of turkeys. Avian Dis 16:952-953.

8. Domermuth, C.H., and W.B. Gross. 1975. Hemorrhagic enteritis of turkeys. Antiserum–efficacy, preparation, and use. Avian Dis 19:657-665.

9. Domermuth, C.H., and W.B. Gross. 1980. Hemorrhagic enteritis of turkeys. In S.B. Hitchner, C.H. Domermuth, H.G. Purchase, and J.E. Williams (eds.), Isolation and Identification of Avian Pathogens, 2nd Ed., pp. 106-107. Am Assoc Avian Pathol, Kennett Square, PA.

10. Domermuth, C.H., and W.B. Gross. 1984. Hemorrhagic enteritis and related infections. In M.S. Hofstad, H.J. Barnes, B.W. Calnek, W.M. Reid, and H.W. Yoder, Jr. (eds.), Diseases of Poultry, 8th Ed., pp. 511-516. Iowa State Univ Press, Ames.

11. Domermuth, C.H., W.B. Gross, R.T. DuBose, C.S. Douglass, and C.B. Reubush, Jr. 1972. Agar gel diffusion precipitin test for hemorrhagic enteritis of turkeys. Avian Dis 16:852-857.

12. Domermuth, C.H., W.B. Gross, R.T. DuBose, D.F. Watson, and S.A. Tolin. 1972. Hemorrhagic enteritis of turkeys. 3. Characterization of the causative virus. Proc 44th Northeast Conf Avian Dis. (Abstr).

13. Domermuth, C.H., W.B. Gross, and R.T. DuBose. 1973. Microimmunodiffusion test for hemorrhagic enteritis of turkeys. Avian Dis 17:439-444.

14. Domermuth, C.H., W.B. Gross, R.T. DuBose, and E.T. Mallinson. 1975. Experimental reproduction and antibody inhibition of marble spleen disease of pheasants. J Wildl Dis 11:338-342.

15. Domermuth, C.H., W.B. Gross, C.S. Douglass, R.T. DuBose, J.R. Harris, and R.B. Davis. 1977. Vaccination for hemorrhagic enteritis of turkeys. Avian Dis 21:557-565.

16. Domermuth, C.H., D.J. Forrester, D.O. Trainer, and W.J. Bigler. 1977. Serologic examination of wild birds for hemorrhagic enteritis of turkey and marble spleen disease of pheasants. J Wildl Dis 13:405-408.

17. Domermuth, C.H., W.B. Gross, L.D. Schwartz, E.T. Mallinson, and R. Britt. 1979. Vaccination of ring-necked pheasant for marble-spleen disease. Avian Dis 23:30-38.

18. Domermuth, C.H., J.R. Harris, W.B. Gross, and R.T. DuBose. 1979. A naturally occurring infection of

chickens with a hemorrhagic enteritis/marble spleen disease type of virus. Avian Dis 23:479–484.
19. Domermuth, C.H., C.R. Weston, B.S. Cowen, W.M. Colwell, W.B. Gross, and R.T. DuBose. 1980. Incidence and distribution of "avian adenovirus group II splenomegaly of chickens." Avian Dis 24:591–594.
20. Domermuth, C.H., L. van der Heide, and G.P. Faddoul. 1982. Pulmonary congestion and edema (marble spleen disease) of chickens produced by group II avian adenovirus. Avian Dis 26:629–633.
21. Fadly, A.M., and K. Nazerian. 1982. Evidence for bursal involvement in the pathogenesis of hemorrhagic enteritis of turkeys. Avian Dis 26:525–533.
22. Fadly, A.M., K. Nazerian, K. Nagaraja, and G. Below. 1985. Field vaccination against hemorrhagic enteritis of turkeys by a cell-culture live-virus vaccine. Avian Dis 29:768–777.
23. Fasina, S.O., and J. Fabricant. 1982. In vitro studies of hemorrhagic enteritis virus with immunofluorescent antibody technique. Avian Dis 26:150–157.
24. Fasina, S.O., and J. Fabricant. 1982. Immunofluorescence studies on the early pathogenesis of hemorrhagic enteritis virus infection in turkeys and chickens. Avian Dis 26:158–163.
25. Fujiwara, H., S. Tanaami, M. Yamaguchi, and T. Yoshino. 1975. Histopathology of hemorrhagic enteritis in turkeys. Nat Inst Anim Health Q (Tokyo) 15:68–75.
26. Gale, C., and J.W. Wyne. 1957. Preliminary observations on hemorrhagic enteritis of turkeys. Poult Sci 36:1267–1270.
27. Gross, W.B. 1967. Lesions of hemorrhagic enteritis. Avian Dis 11:684–693.
28. Gross, W.B., and C.H. Domermuth. 1976. Spleen lesions of hemorrhagic enteritis of turkeys. Avian Dis 20:455–466.
29. Gross, W.B., and W.E.C. Moore. 1967. Hemorrhagic enteritis of turkeys. Avian Dis 11:296–307.
30. Harris, J.R., and C.H. Domermuth. 1977. Hemorrhagic enteritis in two-and-one-half-week-old turkey poults. Avian Dis 21:120–122.
31. Iltis, J.P. 1976. Experimental transmission of marble spleen disease in turkeys and pheasants with demonstration, characterization and classification of the causative virus. Diss Abstr 36:4890–B.
32. Iltis, J.P., and D.S. Wyand. 1974. Indications of a viral etiology for marble spleen disease in pheasants. J Wildl Dis 10:272–278.
33. Iltis, J.P., R.M. Jakowski, and D.S. Wyand. 1975. Transmission of marble spleen disease in turkeys and pheasants. Am J Vet Res 36:97–101.
34. Iltis, J.P., R.M. Jakowski, and D.S. Wyand. 1975. Experimentally transmitted marble spleen disease in pen-raised wild turkeys. J Wildl Dis 11:484–485.
35. Itakura, C., and H.C. Carlson. 1975. Electron microscopic findings of cells with inclusion bodies in experimental hemorrhagic enteritis of turkeys. Can J Comp Med 39:299–304.
36. Itakura, C., and H.C. Carlson. 1975. Pathology of spontaneous hemorrhagic enteritis of turkeys. Can J Comp Med 39:310–315.
37. Itakura, C., H.C. Carlson, and G.N. Lang. 1974. Experimental transmission of hemorrhagic enteritis of turkeys. Avian Pathol 3:279–292.
38. Jakowski, R.M., and D.S. Wyand. 1972. Marble spleen disease in ring-necked pheasants: Demonstration of agar gel precipitin antibody in pheasants from an infected flock. J Wildl Dis 8:261–263.
39. Larsen, C.T., C.H. Domermuth, D.P. Sponenberg, and W.B. Gross. 1985. Colibacillosis of turkeys exacerbated by hemorrhagic enteritis virus. Laboratory studies. Avian Dis 29:729–732.
40. Mandelli, G., A. Rinaldi, and G. Cervio. 1966. A disease involving the spleen and lungs in pheasants: Epidemiology, symptoms, and lesions. Clin Vet (Milano) 89:129–138.
41. Nagaraja, K.V., D.J. Emery, B.L. Patel, B.S. Pomeroy, and J.A. Newman. 1982. In vitro evaluation of B-lymphocyte function in turkeys infected with hemorrhagic enteritis virus. Am J Vet Res 43:502–504.
42. Nagaraja, K.V., B.L. Patel, D.A. Emery, B.S. Pomeroy, and J.A. Newman. 1982. In vitro depression of the mitogenic response of lymphocytes from turkeys infected with hemorrhagic enteritis virus. Am J Vet Res 43:134–136.
43. Nazerian, K., and A. Fadly. 1982. Propagation of virulent and avirulent turkey hemorrhagic enteritis virus in cell culture. Avian Dis 26:816–827.
44. Nazerian, K., and A.M. Fadly. 1987. Further studies on in vitro and in vivo assays of hemorrhagic enteritis virus (HEV). Avian Dis 31:234–240.
45. Perrin, G., C. Louzis, and D. Toquin. 1981. L'enterite hemorragique du dindon: Culture du virus in vitro. Bull Acad Vet Fr 54:231–235.
46. Pierson, F.W., C.H. Domermuth, and D.W. Byrd. 1988. Lateral transmission of hemorrhagic enteritis virus. Proc South Conf Avian Dis. (Abstr).
47. Pomeroy, B.S. 1972. Hemorrhagic enteritis. In M.S. Hofstad, B.W. Calnek, C.F. Helmboldt, W.M. Reid, and H.W. Yoder, Jr. (eds.), Diseases of Poultry, 6th Ed., pp. 253–255. Iowa State Univ Press, Ames.
48. Pomeroy, B.S., and R. Fenstermacher. 1937. Hemorrhagic enteritis in turkeys. Poult Sci 16:378–382.
49. Silim, A., and J. Thorsen. 1981. Hemorrhagic enteritis: Virus distribution and sequential development of antibody in turkeys. Avian Dis 25:444–453.
50. Sponenberg, D.P., C.H. Domermuth, and C.T. Larsen. 1985. Field outbreaks of colibacillosis of turkeys associated with hemorrhagic enteritis virus. Avian Dis 29:838–842.
51. Tolin, S.A., and C.H. Domermuth. 1975. Hemorrhagic enteritis of turkeys. Electron microscopy of the causal virus. Avian Dis 19:118–125.
52. van den Hurk, J. 1985. Propagation of hemorrhagic enteritis virus in normal (nontumor derived) cell culture. J Am Vet Med Assoc 187:307.
53. van den Hurk, J. 1988. Characterization of group II avian adenoviruses using a panel of monoclonal antibodies. Can J Vet Res 52:458–467.
54. van den Hurk, J.V. 1986. Quantitation of hemorrhagic enteritis virus antigen and antibody using enzyme-linked immunosorbent assays. Avian Dis 30:662–671.
55. Veit, H.P., C.H. Domermuth, and W.B. Gross. 1981. Histopathology of avian adenovirus group II splenomegaly of chickens. Avian Dis 25:866–873.
56. Wilcock, B.P., and H.L. Thacker. 1976. Focal hepatic necrosis in turkeys with hemorrhagic enteritis. Avian Dis 20:205–208.
57. Wyand, D.S., R.M. Jakowski, and C.N. Berke. 1972. Marble spleen disease in ring-necked pheasants: Histology and ultrastructure. Avian Dis 16:319–329.
58. Zhang, C., and Nagaraja, K.V. 1988. Differentiation of avian adenovirus type II strains by restriction endonuclease fingerprinting. J Am Vet Med Assoc 192:1240.

EGG DROP SYNDROME

J.B. McFerran

INTRODUCTION. Since the initial description (53), egg drop syndrome 1976 (EDS 76) has become a major cause of loss of egg production throughout the world. It is caused by an adenovirus, probably introduced into chickens through a contaminated vaccine. EDS 76 is characterized by otherwise healthy birds producing thin-shelled or shell-less eggs. Once established in a breeding organization, the condition is more often seen as a failure to achieve production targets, and eggshell changes are less apparent, although still present. Since its initial recognition, it has become apparent that sporadic outbreaks of EDS 76 occur as a result of fowl becoming infected through direct or indirect contact with infected wild or domestic waterfowl.

The virus affects only avian species and therefore has no public health significance.

HISTORY. A condition of laying hens was described by Dutch workers in 1976 (53) and hemagglutinating adenoviruses were isolated (34). Using serologic studies with one of these isolates and flock records it was possible to establish the disease pattern (34, 36). It appeared that the virus was transmitted vertically and that horizontal transmission between flocks was not a feature; the virus often remained latent until birds were approaching peak egg production. Because of absence of antibody to the virus in chickens prior to 1974 and failure of the virus to grow in mammalian cells as well as its poor growth in turkey cells and optimal growth in duck cells, it was suggested that this was probably a duck adenovirus. This suggestion was quickly confirmed by isolation of EDS 76 virus from normal ducks and demonstration of antibody in many duck flocks (9, 12).

INCIDENCE AND DISTRIBUTION. EDS 76 virus has been isolated from chickens in Australia (17), Belgium (37), France (41), Great Britain (9), Hungary (60), India (38), Italy (59), Japan (57), Northern Ireland (36), Singapore (44), South Africa (22), and Taiwan (29). Serologic evidence of infection has been found in chickens in Brazil (24), Denmark (5), Mexico (42), New Zealand (23), and Nigeria (39).

ETIOLOGY

Classification. EDS 76 virus is classified as an adenovirus on the basis of its morphology, replication, and chemical composition. While the avian adenovirus group antigen is not detected by immunodiffusion or immunofluorescence, if birds infected with another avian adenovirus are kept until antibody to this virus is no longer detectable and are then infected with EDS 76 virus, they develop antibody to both the adenovirus and EDS 76, indicating there is a shared antigen (35). EDS 76 is not related to 11 fowl and 2 turkey prototype adenoviruses using serum neutralization (SN) or hemagglutination inhibition (HI) tests (3).

Morphology. The size of EDS 76 virus observed in negatively stained preparations has been reported as ranging from 76 nm (36) to 80 ± 5 nm (27). These sizes are within those acceptable for adenoviruses (56).

Using preparations made from a cesium chloride (CsCl) gradient, Kraft et al. (27) were able to demonstrate typical adenovirus morphology, with triangular faces with six capsomeres on the edge and a single 25-nm fiber projecting from each vertex. In normal preparations this structure is not obvious (36, 57); although EDS 76 particles are clearly adenoviruses with well-defined capsomeres with hollow centers, it is possible to distinguish them from conventional adenoviruses (Fig. 22.7). In thin sections of infected chick embryo liver cells, virus particles of 70–75 nm are seen in the nucleus (3). Particles of 68–80 nm diameter have been described in nuclei of epithelial cells of oviduct mucosa (50).

Density in CsCl. There are differences in the reported density of EDS 76 virus in CsCl. Todd

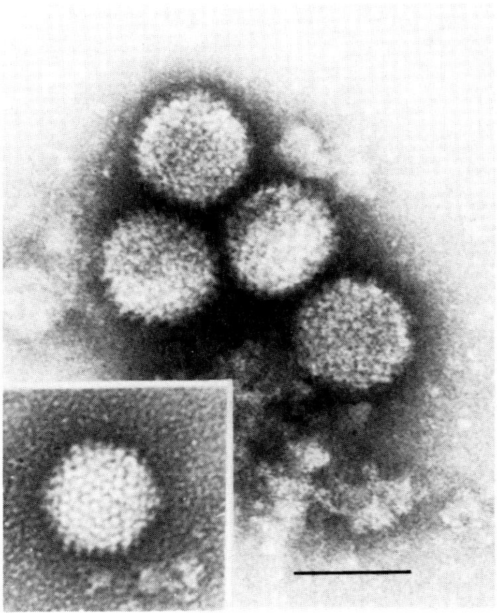

22.7. Four particles of EDS 76 virus. Although individual capsomeres are well resolved, typical adenovirus morphology is not apparent. *Inset:* Type 8 fowl adenovirus particle showing well-defined, triangular faces. Bar = 80 nm.

and McNulty (51) found that infectious virus particles banded at densities of 1.32 and 1.30 g/ml. However, the heavier particles did not agglutinate chicken erythrocytes and appeared by electron microscopy to be slightly damaged. Particles with a density of 1.30 g/ml hemagglutinated and appeared undamaged. A band of empty, disrupted, noninfectious hemagglutinating particles was present at a density of 1.28 g/ml. In contrast, Kraft et al. (27) reported presence of two bands of infectious hemagglutinating particles at 1.32 g/ml, with noninfectious disrupted particles banding at 1.30 g/ml. Yamaguchi et al. (57) reported hemagglutinating particles banding at 1.30 g/ml and infectious particles with a density of 1.33 g/ml, while Takai et al. (49) found infectivity and hemagglutinin associated with a band at 1.33 g/ml and hemagglutinin also in a band at 1.29. This discrepancy was explained, at least in part, by Zsak and Kisary (60), who reported that density and hemagglutinating ability of EDS 76 particles depended on the method used for virus purification and whether the virus was grown in cell cultures or embryonated eggs.

Chemical Composition. From studies using labelling with 3H-thymidine and inhibition with iododeoxyuridine, EDS 76 virus was shown to contain DNA (3, 27, 51, 57). The molecular weight of the DNA is estimated at 22.6×10^6 daltons compared to 28.9×10^6 daltons for fowl adenovirus type 1 (Phelps), and restriction endonuclease patterns indicate no relationship between these two viruses (60). The EDS 76 virus has 13 structural polypeptides, and at least 7 of these correspond with polypeptides of fowl adenovirus type 1 (51).

Hemagglutination. EDS 76 virus agglutinates erythrocytes of chickens, ducks, turkeys, geese, pigeons, and peacocks, but does not agglutinate rat, rabbit, horse, sheep, cattle, goat, or pig erythrocytes (3, 29).

The hemagglutinin (HA) is resistant. At 56 C there is an initial fourfold fall in titer after 16 hr but the titer remained stable for 4 days and is finally undetectable after 8 days. It survived 60 C but is destroyed by 70 C for 30 min. It retains its activity for long periods at 4 C (3, 37). It is resistant to trypsin, 2-mercaptoethanol, EDTA, papain, ficin, and 0.5% formaldehyde at 37 C for 1 hr, but the titer is greatly reduced by potassium periodate and 0.5% glutaraldehyde (49). The purified soluble HA, however, is destroyed by trypsin (51). Alpha-chymotrypsin destroyed the receptor for the virus on chicken erythrocytes whereas trypsin and neuraminidase had no effect (49).

Virus Replication. EDS 76 virus replicates in the nucleus in a similar fashion to avian adenoviruses belonging to subgroup A (1, 2, 3). Intranuclear inclusions are seen in hematoxylin- and eosin-stained preparations in infected cell cultures (3); in epithelial cells of the infundibulum, tubular shell gland, pouch shell gland, isthmus, and nasal mucosa; and in spleen of experimentally infected fowl (47, 50). In ultrathin sections, virus particles and type I–IV inclusions are obvious in the nucleus similar to other avian adenoviruses (2, 3).

Resistance to Chemical and Physical Agents. EDS 76 virus is stable to treatment with chloroform and variations in pH between 3 and 10. It is inactivated by heating for 30 min at 60 C, survives for 3 hr at 56 C, and is stable in monovalent but not divalent cations (3, 57). Infectivity was not demonstrated after treating with 0.5% formaldehyde or 0.5% glutaraldehyde (49).

Strain Classification. Only one serotype has been recognized (16, 57). However, using restriction endonuclease analysis it has been possible to divide a number of isolates into three genotypes (52). One includes isolates made over an 11-yr period from infected European chickens. A second group are viruses isolated from ducks in the UK. One virus isolated from chickens in Australia forms the third group.

Laboratory Host Systems. EDS 76 virus grows to highest titers in duck kidney, duck embryo liver, and duck embryo fibroblast cells. It also grows well in chick embryo liver cells, less well in chick kidney cells, and rather poorly in chicken embryo fibroblast cultures. There is poor growth in turkey cells, and no replication could be detected in a range of mammalian cells (3). The virus grows to high titers in goose cell cultures (60). In chick liver cells, peak virus and intracellular HA titers are reached after 48 hr, and peak extracellular HA titers were seen at 72 hr (57).

The virus grows to very high titers when inoculated into the allantoic sac of embryonated duck and goose eggs and produces titers of 1/16,000–1/32,000. No growth has been detected in embryonated chicken eggs (3, 61).

Pathogenicity. While all chicken isolates appear to be of similar virulence, isolates made from ducks in the USA produced no effect on egg production (54) or only affected the egg size (11) when chickens were infected. Isolates from ducks and chickens in Europe behaved identically in chickens (7).

PATHOGENESIS AND EPIZOOTIOLOGY

Natural and Experimental Hosts. Although the disease outbreaks have been in laying hens, it is probable that the natural hosts are ducks and geese. Antibody is widespread in domesticated ducks (5, 8, 9, 12, 17, 30, 31) and domestic geese (8, 61). In a study of ducks in the Atlantic flyway in the USA, antibody was found in ruddy ducks, ring-necked ducks, wood ducks, bufflehead ducks, lesser scaups, mergansers, mallards, gadwalls, and northern shovelers in addition to coots and grobes (20). Antibody has also been detected in Muscovy ducks and cattle egrets (31), Canada geese and mallards (43), herring gulls (8), owls, a stork, and a swan (25).

Virus has been isolated from healthy domestic ducks (9, 54). Virus has also been recovered from diseased ducks (18) but the disease could not be reproduced using the isolate. Bartha (6) isolated a virus from ducks with a fall in egg production and a severe diarrhea, and Liu (28) considered that EDS may cause rough and thin shells and falls in production in ducks.

Infection is common in geese (25, 30, 61). Experimentally infected goslings and geese showed neither illness nor an a change in egg production (61).

There has been no evidence of natural infection of turkeys or pheasants, but they can be experimentally infected (8, 40, 59). Guinea fowl may be infected naturally or experimentally (19) and soft-shelled eggs may be produced. However, Watanabe and Ohmi (55) infected but could not reproduce disease in guinea fowl with a fowl isolate.

Because EDS 76 virus was initially primarily transmitted vertically, there was often an apparent breed association in chickens. However, a wide range of breeds are equally susceptible to experimental infection, although analysis of natural outbreaks suggests that broiler breeders and heavy breeds producing brown eggs are more severely affected than white-egg producers (33). Higashihara et al. (21) infected two brown and one white-egg-layer strain and found that although egg production was depressed in the white layer strain, little depression occurred in the brown layers even though they produced more eggs with shell defects. There were differences in the response between the two-brown-egg-laying strains with one brown-egg-producing strain laying almost three times as many affected eggs as the white-egg-laying strain.

Birds of all ages are susceptible to infection, and if EDS 76 virus is introduced onto a site, effects on egg production can be seen in all ages of laying hens. However, when birds apparently become infected around peak egg production (36), this may be due to reactivation of latent virus.

Pathogenesis. Following experimental oral infection of adult hens there is a limited virus replication in the nasal mucosa and a viremia (47). At 3–4 days postinfection virus replication occurs in lymphoid tissue throughout the body, especially in the spleen and thymus. In addition, the infundibulum is consistently affected. At 7–20 days postinfection there is a massive replication in the pouch shell gland (Fig. 22.8) and to a much lesser extent in other parts of the oviduct. This replication is associated with a pronounced inflammatory response in the pouch shell gland, and the production of abnormally shelled eggs (45, 50, 58).

Unlike conventional adenoviruses, EDS does not replicate in the intestinal mucosa and the presence of virus in the feces is probably due to contamination with the oviduct exudate (47).

Transmission. It is now possible to divide EDS outbreaks into three types. In the initially observed classical form, where primary breeders were infected, the main method of spread was vertically through the embryonated egg (36). Although the number of infected embryos is probably low with this type (10), spread is very efficient. In many cases chicks infected in ovo do not excrete virus or develop HI antibody until the flock has achieved between 50% and peak egg

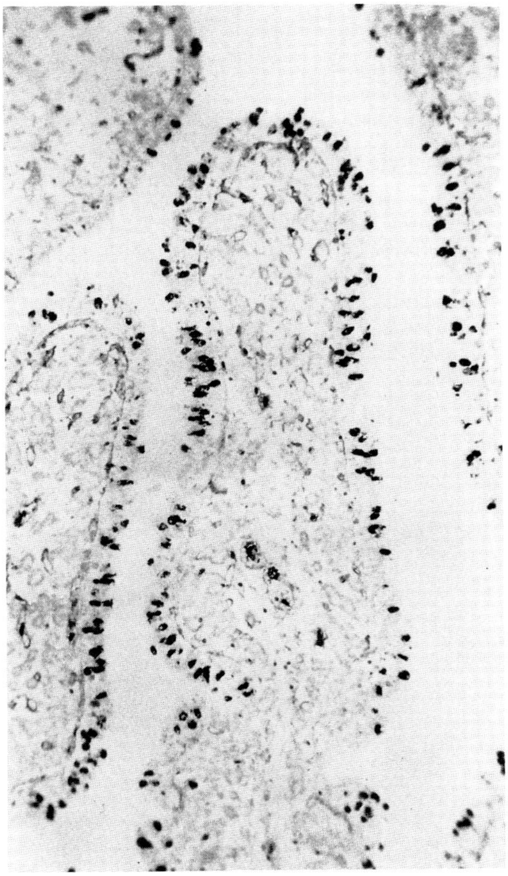

22.8. Pouch shell gland from hen experimentally infected with EDS virus. Note the viral nucleic acid in surface epithelial layer, demonstrated by a biotinylated purified virus genome probe. (Allan)

production. At this stage the virus is unmasked and excreted, resulting in an apparently rapid spread of virus due to multiple foci of infection.

Probably arising from the classical form, virus has become established in some areas in commercial egg-laying flocks. This endemic form is often associated with a common egg-packing station. Both normal- and abnormal-shelled eggs laid during the period of virus growth in the pouch shell gland contain virus, both on their exterior and interior (46). This leads to contamination of egg trays. Droppings also contain virus, but this excretion is intermittent often of low titer (14), and in the adult bird may result from contamination of the feces by oviduct exudate (47). Apart from direct spread between birds, there is evidence that spread can occur when birds are transported in inadequately cleaned trucks or when unused food has been taken from one site to another. There is also evidence that needles or blades used for vaccination or bleeding of viremic birds, if not properly sterilized, can transmit infection. Lateral spread is slow and intermittent, taking up to 11 wk to spread through a cage house; in one case, spread to an adjoining pen was prevented by a wire fence. Spread between birds on litter is usually faster (14, 53).

Spread from both domestic or wild ducks, geese, and possibly other wild birds to hens through drinking water contaminated by droppings appears to give rise to a third type of outbreak. This type is very important in some areas. These cases tend to be sporadic, but there is always the danger of it producing an endemic situation.

Following experimental infection most workers have found the first signs after 7–9 days (15, 32), but in some experiments not until 17 days postinfection (37).

Signs. The first sign is loss of color in pigmented eggs. This is quickly followed by production of thin-shelled, soft-shelled, or shell-less eggs (Fig. 22.9). The thin-shelled eggs often have a rough, sandpaperlike texture or a granular roughening of the shell at one end. If obviously affected eggs are discarded, there is no effect on fertility or hatchability and no long-term effect on egg quality. If birds are infected in late production, forced molting of the flock will restore egg production to normal. The fall in production can be very rapid or extend over weeks. Outbreaks

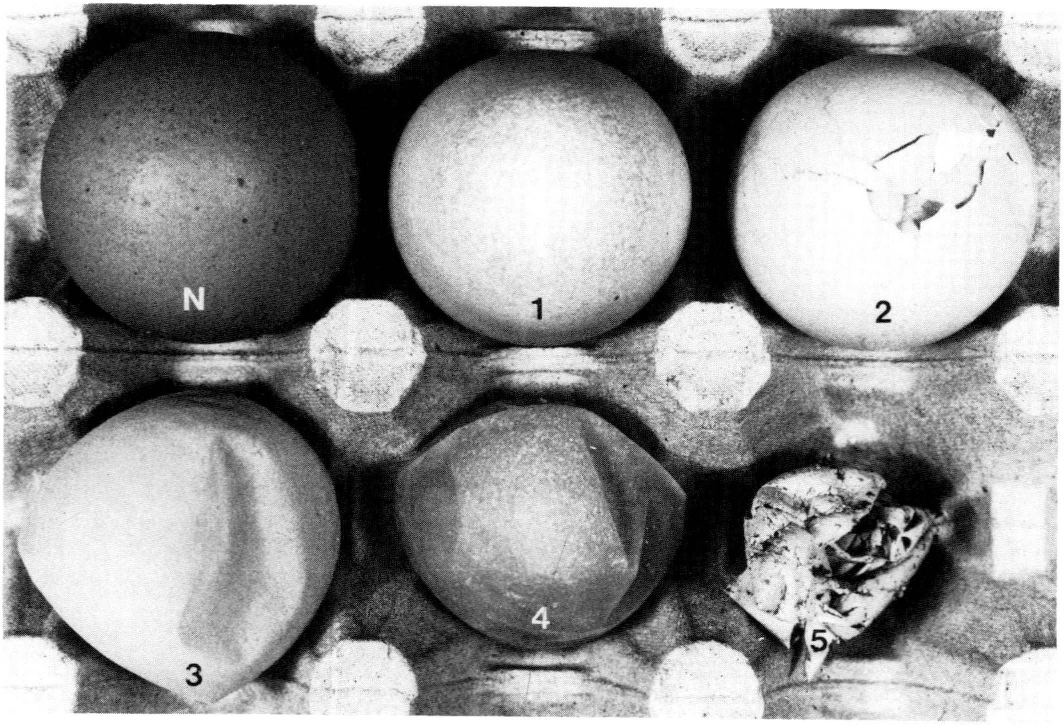

22.9. Eggs from hens infected with EDS 76 virus. Changes range from normal brown egg (*N*), to loss of shell pigment (*1* and *2*), thinning at the pole (*1*), thin-shelled (*2*), soft-shelled (*3*), and shell-less eggs (*4*). Eggs may be eaten or broken, but many membranes (*5*) may be found.

usually last 4–10 wk, and egg production can be reduced by up to 40%; however, there is usually compensation later in lay, so that the total number lost is usually 10–16 eggs/bird. If the disease is due to reactivation of latent virus, the fall usually occurs when production is between 50% and peak level. Small eggs have been described in natural outbreaks (36), but no effect on egg size was found in experimental infections (32). Watery albumen has been described (37, 53), although no effect on albumen has been seen by other workers (16, 32, 58). However, age of infection may be important; Cook and Darbyshire (15) found that birds infected at 1 day of age subsequently laid apparently normal eggs except for impaired quality of albumen and smaller size.

If some birds have acquired antibody before the latent virus is unmasked, an apparently different clinical syndrome is seen. There is failure to achieve predicted egg production, and onset of lay may be delayed. If a careful examination is made, it can usually be established that there is a series of small clinical episodes of classical EDS. Presumably, birds with antibody slow down spread of virus. A similar picture is often seen in birds in cage units, where spread can be slow and EDS not suspected.

The affected birds remain otherwise healthy. Although inappetence and dullness have been described in some affected flocks, these are not consistent findings. The transient diarrhea described by some authors is probably due to the exudate from the oviduct (47). Most workers agree that EDS 76 virus does not cause disease in growing chickens in the field. Oral infection of susceptible day-old chicks resulted in increased mortality in the 1st wk of life (15), but there was no increase in mortality in many flocks of chickens produced by infected parent flocks (33).

Gross Lesions. In naturally occurring outbreaks inactive ovaries and atrophied oviducts are often the only recognized lesions and these are not consistently present. In one outbreak uterine edema has been described (29). The absence of lesions may be a reflection on the difficulty in selecting birds undergoing acute disease.

Following experimental infection, edema of the uterine folds and presence of exudate in the pouch shell gland commonly occurs within 9–14 days (50, 45). There is also mild splenomegaly, flaccid ovules, and eggs in various stages of formation in the abdominal cavity (45, 50).

Histopathology. The major pathological changes occur in the pouch shell gland. Virus replication in the nuclei of the surface epithelial cells, producing intranuclear inclusion bodies, occurs from 7 days postinfection onward (45, 50). Many affected cells are sloughed into the lumen and there is a rapid and severe inflammatory response involving macrophages, plasma cells, and lymphocytes, together with variable numbers of heterophils invading the lamina propria and epithelium. Inclusion bodies are not seen after the 3rd day of abnormal egg production, but viral antigen persists for up to 1 wk (45). Characteristic histological lesions in the uterus are shown in Fig. 22.10.

Immunity. After experimental infection, antibody can be detected by indirect fluorescent antibody (IFA), enzyme-linked immunosorbent assay (ELISA), SN and HI tests in 5 days, and double immunodiffusion (DID) tests in 7 days (4). They reach a peak in about 4–5 wk. Immunoprecipitating antibodies are more transient than others.

Birds still excrete virus even in the presence of high HI antibody, but some birds that excrete virus fail to develop antibody (15).

Antibody is transferred through the yolk sac, and chicks have high HI titers (geometric mean titers, 6–9 $\log_2$). This antibody has a half-life of 3 days (16). Active antibody production is not stimulated until chicks are 4–5 wk of age and maternal antibody is nearly undetectable (16). When the disease was being eradicated it was found that some flocks, although 100% free from detectable antibody on 2 or 3 occasions, nevertheless suddenly developed EDS. The assumption made is that some of the chicks infected in ovo failed to develop antibody until they came into egg production and then excreted virus. It is not known if they developed antibody at this point, but it is possible they did not, because less than 100% of birds in infected flocks have antibody (33).

If a flock as a whole develops antibody to EDS 76 virus before coming into lay, egg production will not be affected (10).

DIAGNOSIS

Isolation and Identification of Causative Agent. The most sensitive indicator system is either embryonated duck or goose eggs from a flock free of EDS 76 virus infection, or duck or goose cell cultures. If these are not available, chicken cells should be used. Chicken embryo liver cells are more sensitive than chicken kidney cells, and chicken embryo fibroblasts are insensitive (3). Embryonating chicken eggs are not suitable. Not only are duck or goose cells or embryonated duck or goose eggs more sensitive, they also have the advantage that many chicken viruses do not grow in these systems.

It is not sufficient to rely on embryo death or cytopathic effects with EDS 76 viruses. The allantoic fluid from goose or duck eggs or cell culture supernatant should be checked after each passage for presence of HAs for avian erythrocytes (0.8% chick erythrocyte suspension is suitable). Alternatively, immunofluorescence using a labelled

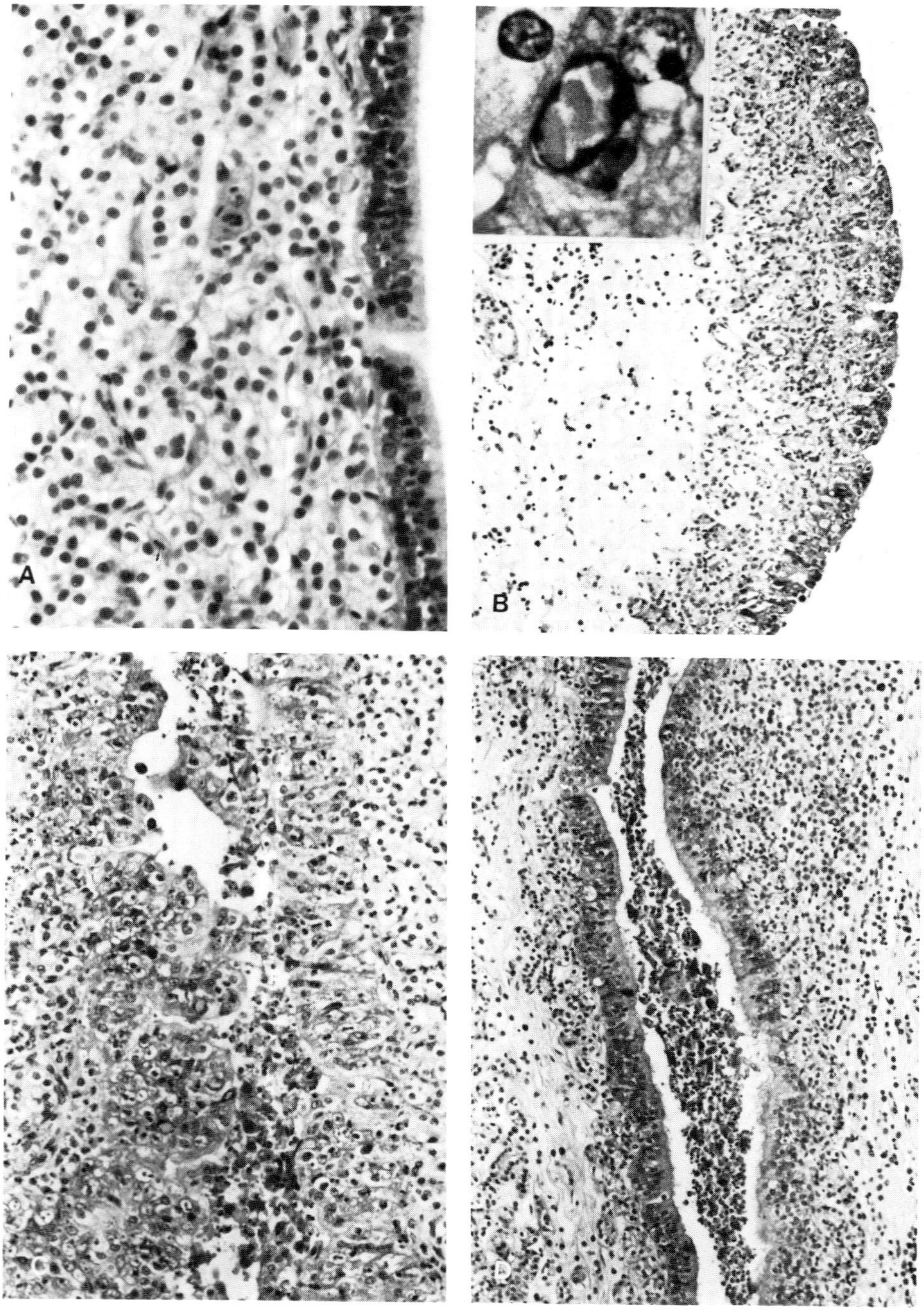

22.10. A. Normal uterine mucosa. Surface epithelium consists of a single layer of columnar cells, many of which are ciliated; underlying these are tubular glands. B. Pronounced edema of uterine submucosa, atrophy of tubular glands, and infiltration of entire mucosa by mononuclear cells are present at 8 days postinoculation (PI). *Inset:* Intranuclear inclusion body in superficial epithelial cell. Note margination of nuclear chromatin and three eosinophilic inclusions in the nucleus. C. Uterine surface epithelium is markedly hyperplastic 11 days PI; there is complete loss of cilia. D. Exudate in uterine lumen consists of degenerating epithelial cells and heterophils mixed with mucus. Epithelium is devoid of cilia, tubular glands are almost absent, and uterine wall is infiltrated with lymphocytes and heterophils.

23 POX

Deoki N. Tripathy

INTRODUCTION. Pox is a common viral disease of domestic birds (chickens, turkeys, pigeons, and canaries) and has been reported in more than 60 species of wild birds representing 20 families. It is a slow-spreading disease characterized by the development of discrete, nodular, proliferative skin lesions on the unfeathered parts of the body (cutaneous form) or fibrino-necrotic and proliferative lesions in the mucous membrane of the upper respiratory tract, mouth, and esophagus (diphtheritic form).

In the mild cutaneous form of the disease, flock mortality is usually low but it may be high with generalized infection, when in diphtheritic form, or when the disease is complicated by other infections or poor environmental conditions.

Avian pox is not of public health significance. It does not generally affect mammals, however, a poxvirus isolated from a rhinoceros (50) was characterized as fowl poxvirus.

HISTORY. Pox has long been observed in several avian species. The term "fowl pox" initially included all poxvirus infections of birds, but now it is often used to refer to the disease of commercial poultry, e.g., chickens and turkeys. Woodruff and Goodpasture (104–106) presented evidence that the virus particles (Borrell bodies) within the inclusion bodies (Bollinger bodies) were the etiologic agent of the disease. Ledingham and Aberd (45) demonstrated that antisera produced against fowl poxvirus after immunization or following recovery agglutinated a suspension of elementary bodies of fowl poxvirus.

INCIDENCE AND DISTRIBUTION. Avian poxviruses infect birds of all ages, sexes, and breeds. Natural poxvirus infections have been reported in approximately 60 species of wild birds, representing about 20 families (40). The disease is worldwide in distribution (64).

ETIOLOGY. Avian poxviruses (fowl, turkey, pigeon, canary, junco, quail, sparrow, and starling) are members of the genus Avipoxvirus of the family Poxviridae (47, 94). Cross-protection studies indicate that psittacine poxvirus and mynah poxvirus are perhaps different members of the genus (12, 70). Fowl poxvirus is the type species of the genus.

Morphology. Like other genera of the Poxviridae family, all avian poxviruses show identical morphology. The mature virus (elementary body) is brick shaped and measures about 250 × 354 nm. It consists of an electron dense, centrally located biconcave core or nucleoid and two lateral bodies in each concavity and envelope (Fig. 23.1). The outer coat is composed of random arrangements of surface tubules (17) (Fig. 23.2).

Chemical Composition. The main components of the virus are protein, DNA, and lipid. The virus has a particle weight of 2.04×10^{-14} g, and contains 7.51×10^{-15} g protein, 4.03×10^{-16} g DNA, and 5.54×10^{-15} g lipid (68). Nearly one-third of fowl poxvirus is lipid (99). Squalene as a major lipid component and elevation of cholesterol esters was detected in virus preparation from infected chick scalp epithelium (46, 99). The average weight of the inclusion body is about 6.1×10^{-7} mg, 50% of which is extractable lipids. The protein content per inclusion body is 7.69×10^{-8} mg and the average weight of DNA per inclusion is 6.64×10^{-9} mg (67).

Hemagglutinin has been detected in some strains of pigeon pox (32, 82) and in a strain of fowl poxvirus (96).

VIRAL GENOME. Electron microscopic studies of contour length measurements revealed that the fowl poxvirus genome was a single linear, double-stranded DNA molecule of approximately 200×10^6 daltons (38). However, sedimentation analyses in neutral and alkaline sucrose gradients (31) and summation of the molecular weights of the DNA fragments obtained after restriction endonuclease digestion indicated the molecular weight of fowl poxvirus genome to be approximately 160–185 × 10^6 daltons (62). The guanine-cytosine (G-C) content of fowl poxvirus DNA is about 35%.

The electrophoretic profiles of restriction enzyme–digested fowl poxvirus and vaccinia virus DNAs are distinct (62, 73). In spite of this apparent lack of genomic similarity, at least some conservation has been maintained at the nu-

Contributions of Dr. Charles H. Cunningham to this chapter in previous editions are gratefully acknowledged.

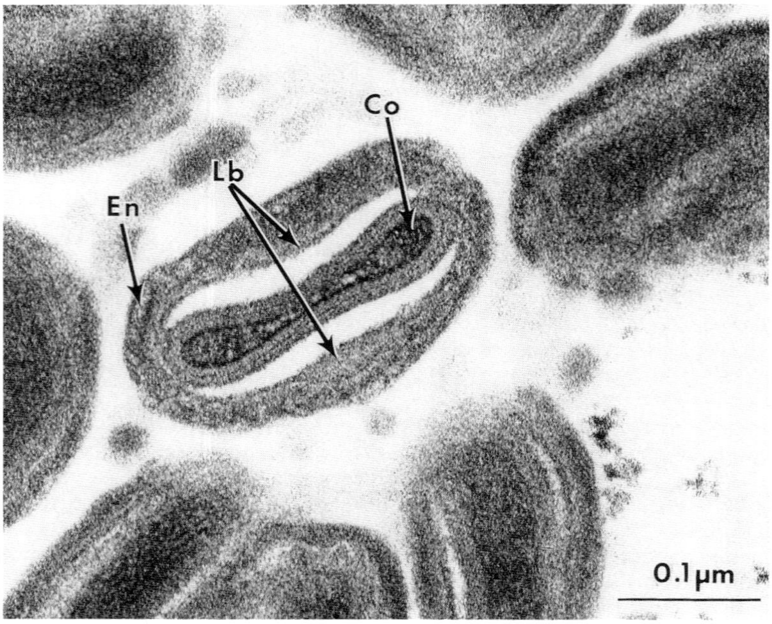

23.1. Ultrathin section of an avian poxvirus from cutaneous eyelid lesion in a dove. *Co* = core; *Lb* = lateral bodies; *En* = envelope. (Basgall)

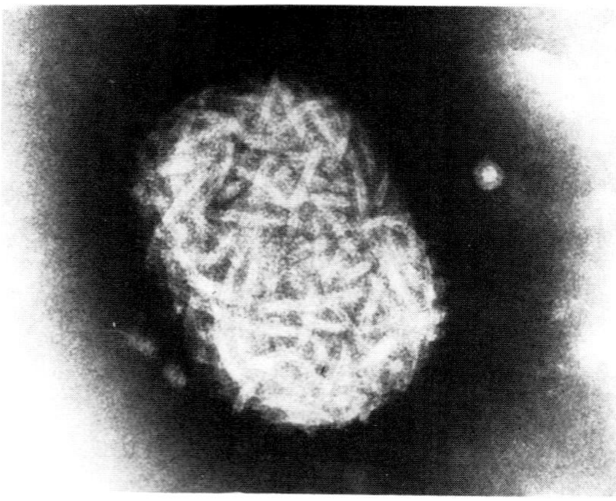

23.2. Negatively stained fowl poxvirus showing random distribution of surface tubules. (17)

cleotide and amino acid level. A 3.1 kb fowl poxvirus DNA fragment, which hybridizes to vaccinia virus HindIII J fragment, contains six open reading frames similar in size, sequence, and relative positions to those contained in the corresponding DNA fragments in vaccinia virus (25). However, the fowl poxvirus counterpart to the internally located vaccinia virus thymidine kinase (TK) gene is located elsewhere. Similar observations have been made by Binns et al. (11). The TK gene of fowl poxvirus has been identified and sequenced (13, 15). It has an open reading frame of 183 codons, which is homologous at the nucleotide and deduced amino acid levels with the vaccinia virus TK gene. The DNA fragment containing quail poxvirus TK gene has been cloned and identified (74). It shows homology to the fowl poxvirus TK gene. Even though fowl and quail poxviruses belong to the same genus, their genomic profiles are markedly different. It appears that fowl and quail poxvirus TK genes may be confined to different loci of their genomes.

Recently, the nucleotide sequence of the DNA polymerase gene of fowl poxvirus was reported (10). When the DNA sequence of fowl poxvirus enzyme is compared with that of vaccinia virus DNA polymerase, only approximately 60% of the nucleotides are conserved. However, a strong homology is observed when amino acid sequences of fowl poxvirus and vaccinia virus DNA polymerases are compared.

POLYPEPTIDES. Twenty-eight polypeptides were detected in purified fowl poxvirus by Obijeski et al. (63). Mockett et al. (55) observed about 30 structural polypeptides in fowl poxvirus, most of which were immunogenic. Twenty-one fowl poxvirus-coded polypeptides were resolved by ^{35}S methionine pulse labeling, and 57 major structural polypeptides were identified in purified fowl poxvirus preparations (66). Several major and minor immunogenic polypeptides of fowl poxvirus strains have been resolved by immunoblotting (73).

Replication. The cytoplasmic site of DNA synthesis and packaging within the infectious virus particle is characteristic of poxviruses. Noteworthy information on replication of poxviruses has been reviewed by Moss (60). Replication of avian poxviruses appears to be similar in dermal or follicular epithelium of chicken, ectodermal cells of the chorioallantoic membrane (CAM), and embryo skin cells. However, differences in the host cell and virus strain may reflect in the time scale and virus output.

Biosynthesis of fowl poxvirus in dermal epithelium involves two distinct phases: a host response characterized by marked cellular hyperplasia during the first 72 hr and synthesis of infectious virus from 72 to 96 hr (18, 19).

The replication of viral DNA in dermal epithelium begins between 12 and 24 hr postinfection (PI) and is followed by the first appearance of infectious virus at 22–24 hr. Epithelial hyperplasia between 36 and 48 hr ends in a 2.5-fold increase in cell number at 72 hr. The rate of viral DNA synthesis is low during the first 60 hr of infection. Enhancement in the rate of viral DNA synthesis occurs between 60 and 72 hr, concomitantly with a sharp decline of cellular DNA synthesis. Between 72 and 96 hr, the synthesis of viral DNA becomes progressively more prominent, and no further hyperplasia is observed (18, 19). Swallen (80) demonstrated by autoradiography that chicken epidermis infected for 48 hr with fowl poxvirus shows a threefold higher percentage of labeled nuclei as compared to controls, indicating that infection is associated with an increased incidence of intranuclear DNA synthesis. Both viral RNA and DNA were detected by hybridization in the nucleus of infected cells from 24 to 72 hr PI (30).

Infection of chicken embryo skin cell culture involves an increase in virus titer at 16 hr after infection with evidence of cytopathic effects (CPE). Although the viral titer continues to increase for up to 36 hr, the rate of titer increase declines between 36 and 48 hr PI. A total increase in fowl poxvirus titer of 100-fold is observed over the growth period. Fowl poxvirus DNA replication occurs between 12 and 16 hr PI, which continues up to 48 hr PI (66).

Ultrastructural studies have been made on the morphogenesis of the virus in various developmental stages that lead to mature virions (4, 5, 20, 71). After adsorption to and penetration of the cell membrane by fowl poxvirus, 1 hr PI of dermal epithelium (5) and 2 hr PI of CAM (4), there is uncoating of the virus before synthesis of new virus from the precursor material. At 48 hr, areas of viroplasm with incomplete membranes around them are present in the cytoplasm. Inclusion bodies are present at 72 hr PI of dermal epithelium (5) and at 96 hr PI of the CAM (4). The type A inclusions may contain virions within or toward the periphery. Similar inclusions have been observed in fowl, canary, and pigeon poxviruses and perhaps occur in all avian poxviruses. Fowl poxvirus emerges from cells of the CAM by a budding process, with acquisition of an additional outer membrane obtained from the cell membrane (Fig. 23.3).

An avian poxvirus isolated from *Junco hyemalis* produced nuclear inclusions in addition to cytoplasmic inclusions (9). However, the intranuclear inclusions are devoid of viral particles.

Although poxviruses are assembled exclusively in the cytoplasm of infected cells, Gafford and Randall (30) found that the nucleus participates in the complexities of fowl poxvirus replication,

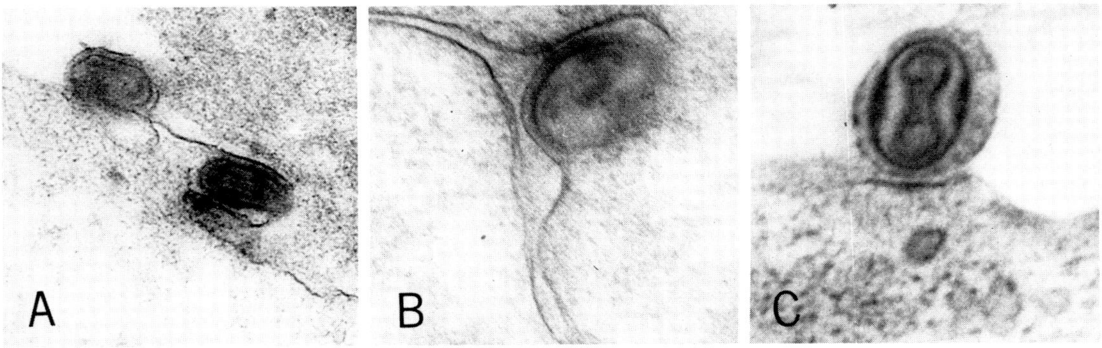

23.3. Emergence of fowl poxvirus from cells of CAM. A, B. Particles appear to be budding from surface, and cell membrane appears to surround virus. C. Virus is separated from cell and completely enclosed by outer layer obtained from cell membrane. A. ×43,000; B, C. ×62,000. (4)

since viral RNA and DNA were detected in the nucleus of infected cells from 24–72 hr PI.

Resistance to Chemical and Physical Agents. Resistance to ether treatment is listed as one of the taxonomic criterion for poxviruses (47). While some authors (68) stated that the virus was sensitive to both ether and chloroform, others (82) reported that a pigeon poxvirus and its two mutants were resistant to both chloroform and ether. A poxvirus isolate from a peacock was ether-resistant but chloroform-sensitive (2). Fowl poxvirus is known to withstand 1% phenol and 1:1000 formalin for 9 days, but is inactivated by 1% caustic potash when freed from its matrix. Heating at 50 C for 30 min or 60 C for 8 min also inactivates the virus (3). Trypsin is without effect on the DNA or whole virus (69). When desiccated the virus shows marked resistance. It can survive in dried scabs for months or even years.

Strain Classification. A nucleoprotein precipitinogen is common to all poxviruses (103). Avian poxviruses are antigenically and immunologically distinguishable from each other, but varying degrees of cross-relationships do exist. Attempts have been made to differentiate strains by immunological methods, e.g., complement-fixation, passive hemagglutination, agar-gel precipitation, immunoperoxidase, virus neutralization, and immunofluorescence. Genomic characterization by restriction endonuclease analysis of DNA and antigenic characterization of immunogenic proteins by immunoblotting has been useful to some extent in detecting minor differences among the strains tested (73). While fowl, pigeon, and junco poxvirus DNAs have similar genomic profiles, restriction endonuclease analysis of quail, canary, and mynah poxvirus DNA reveal marked differences from fowl poxvirus. Similarly, quail poxvirus shows distinct antigenic differences from fowl poxvirus by immunoblotting although some common proteins are also detected (34).

Laboratory Host Systems

BIRDS. Avian poxviruses affect a wide range of birds of various families by natural or artificial infection. Chickens commonly used to determine the pathogenicity of new avian poxvirus isolates may not be suitable hosts because of their lack of susceptibility.

A substantial degree of host specificity exists among some avian poxviruses, especially those that infect wild birds. A poxvirus from a flicker (*Colaptes auratus*) (41) revealed strict host specificity when several species of wild and domestic birds were tested for susceptibility (42). Avian poxvirus strains isolated from various species of thrushes (*Turdidae*) did not protect chickens against fowl poxvirus (43). Differences in host susceptibility were also observed when a poxvirus isolated from parrots was inoculated into susceptible parrots and chickens. Although it was more pathogenic for parrots than chickens, it did not provide protection against fowl poxvirus. Further, vaccination of chickens with either fowl or pigeon poxvirus vaccine did not provide protection against the psittacine poxvirus (12). A poxvirus from a Canada goose (*Branta canadensis*) was transmissible to domestic geese, but not to chickens or to domestic ducks (23). Sparrows and canaries were highly susceptible to a poxvirus isolated during an outbreak from sparrows, but produced mild, local cutaneous reaction in chickens, turkeys, and pigeons (35). Chickens and pigeons were found refractory to infection with an avian poxvirus isolated from a buzzard (*Accipiter nisus*) by Tantwai et al. (83). In an aviary housing over 100 birds of a variety of species, only Rothchild's mynahs (*Leucospar rothchildii*) were infected with an avian poxvirus. The virus, however, was pathogenic for starlings in the surroundings, but did not infect chickens. Mynahs and starlings are members of the family Sturnidae and starling pox has been reported specific for that family (44). Poxvirus strains from magpies (*Pica pica*) and great tits (*Parus major*) did not infect young chickens (37); however, an avian poxvirus isolated from a black-backed magpie produced lesions in chickens, but was related more closely to pigeon than fowl poxvirus (22). Poxvirus strains from various species of grouse immunized chickens against fowl poxvirus challenge (42). High pathogenicity for chickens of a virus isolated from captive peacocks (*Pavo cristatus*) in a zoological park indicated a close relationship of this virus to fowl poxvirus (2). The peacocks had been vaccinated with a fowl poxvirus vaccine, but were the only birds affected among other wild and domestic birds in the aviary. An isolate of poxvirus from previously vaccinated turkeys was antigenically different from fowl poxvirus (102).

Studies on differentiation of fowl, canary, turkey, and pigeon poxviruses based on pathogenicity for chickens, turkeys, pigeons, ducks, and canaries (33, 48) have been summarized (87). Canaries are highly susceptible to canary poxvirus, but show resistance to turkey, fowl, and pigeon poxviruses. The pigeon poxvirus produces milder infection in chickens and turkeys, but is more pathogenic for pigeons. Susceptibility of ducks to turkey poxvirus and not to fowl poxvirus has been suggested for differentiation of these two closely related viruses.

AVIAN EMBRYOS. Developing chicken embryos are commonly employed for propagation of avian poxvirus on the CAM (24, 106). Duck and turkey embryos have been used as well as other species of avian embryos. Typically, infection of chicken embryo CAM results in compact, proliferative pock lesions that may be focal or diffuse (Fig. 23.4).

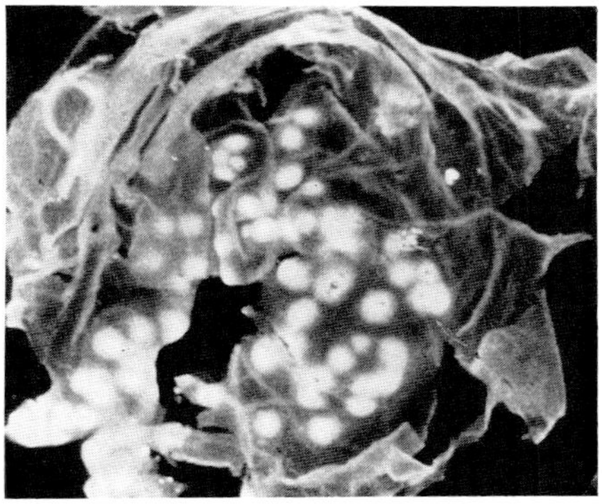

23.4. Fowl pox lesions on the CAM.

Macroscopic lesions considered to be characteristic for some avian poxviruses have been described (48). Occasionally, isolates from wild birds fail to grow on the CAM of chicken embryos.

Quantitative assay of viral infectivity may be by the embryo infective dose-50% (EID_{50}) method or by the "pock-counting-enumerative-dose" response (24).

CELL CULTURE. Avian poxviruses can be propagated in cell cultures of avian origin, e.g., chicken embryo fibroblasts, chicken embryo dermis and kidney cells, and duck embryo fibroblasts. A permanent cell line "QT 35" (59) of Japanese quail origin will support growth of some avian poxviruses after adaptation. However, some isolates, especially from turkeys, fail to grow in this cell line even after repeated passages (86).

Cytopathic Effects. Characteristic CPE produced by the avian poxviruses in chicken embryo fibroblasts are an initial phase of rounding of the cells followed by a second phase of degeneration and necrosis. The time sequence of these events and the variations observed with different viruses have been reported (48). Quantitative assay is by the cell culture dose-50% method based on CPE (24).

Plaque Formation. Differences in the plaque-forming ability of avian poxviruses have been observed. Adaptation of the virus in cell culture is necessary, since not all strains produce plaques (7, 57, 82). Plaque formation in monolayers of chicken embryo fibroblast cell cultures by some avian poxviruses has been shown sufficiently characteristic to be considered as an aid in differentiation (48). Plaques are evident in quail cells by 3–4 days PI with certain avian poxviruses, after adaptation (73).

PATHOGENESIS AND EPIZOOTIOLOGY

Natural and Experimental Hosts. Fowl and turkey poxvirus infections are economically important diseases in domestic poultry. Among companion birds, avian poxvirus infections most often occur in large aviaries of canaries and the disease is likely to be enzootic because of intimate contact. Canary pox is, therefore, of special significance for aviculturists as this infection can result in high losses in a short time. Severe outbreaks of quail pox in pen-raised quails have been reported. As natural infection has been reported in approximately 60 species of wild birds representing about 20 families, as well as in caged birds (40, 65), it seems that all avian species are susceptible to avian poxviruses. The infection can occur in susceptible birds of any age.

Pathogenesis of fowl poxvirus infection in chickens inoculated intradermally or intratracheally was similar with only minor differences. In chickens infected intradermally, the virus was first detected in the skin at the inoculation site on day 2 and in lungs on day 4, followed by detectable viremia on day 5. In chickens infected intratracheally, the virus was first detected in the lungs on day 2, followed by viremia on day 4. The virus was recovered from liver, spleen, kidney, and brain of birds of both groups (79).

Transmission. Poxvirus infection occurs through mechanical transmission of the virus to the injured or lacerated skin. Insects mechanically carrying the virus may deposit it in the eye. The virus may reach the laryngeal region via the lacrimal duct to cause infection of the upper respiratory tract (28). In a contaminated environment the aerosol generated by feathers and dried scabs containing poxvirus particles provide suitable condition for both cutaneous and respiratory infection. Cells of the mucosa of the upper respiratory tract and mouth appear to be highly susceptible to the virus, as initiation of infection may occur in the absence of apparent trauma or injury.

Mosquitoes have been shown to be capable of infecting a number of different birds after a single feeding on a bird infected with avian poxvirus. Eleven species of Diptera have been reported as vectors of avian poxvirus (1). The mite, *Dermanyss gallinae,* has been implicated in the spread of fowl poxvirus (77). Mechanical transmission of fowl poxvirus from infected toms to turkey hens through artificial insemination has been reported (53).

In some flocks, the virus may exist as a latent infection (88). Duran-Reynals and Bryan (26) showed that cutaneous treatment of chickens and pigeons with methylcholanthrene activated a latent fowl poxvirus infection. Kirmse (41) observed persistent cutaneous lesions of avian poxvirus infection in a yellow-shafted flicker over a period of 13 mo during which intracytoplasmic inclusions were demonstrable in the lesion.

Incubation Period. Incubation period of the natural disease varies from about 4–10 days in chickens, turkeys, and pigeons and is about 4 days in canaries.

Signs. The disease may occur in one of the two forms, cutaneous or diphtheritic, or both. The signs vary depending upon the susceptibility of the host, virulence of the virus, distribution of the lesions, and other complicating factors. The cutaneous form of the disease is characterized by appearance of nodular lesions on the comb, wattle, eyelids, and other unfeathered areas of the body. In the diphtheritic form (wet pox), cankers or diphtheritic yellowish lesions occur on the mucous membrane of mouth, esophagus, or trachea with accompanying coryzalike mild or severe respiratory signs when lesions involve the trachea.

Morbidity and Mortality. Morbidity rate of pox in chickens and turkeys varies from a few birds being infected to involvement of the entire flock if a virulent virus is present and no control measures are taken. Birds affected with the cutaneous form of the disease are more likely to recover than those with the diphtheritic form involving the respiratory tract.

Effects of pox in chickens usually involve emaciation and poor weight gain; egg production is temporarily retarded if layers are infected. The course of the disease is about 3–4 wk, but if complications are present, duration may be considerably longer.

In turkeys, retardation of growth development of market birds is of greater financial importance than mortality. Blindness due to cutaneous eye lesions and starvation cause most of the losses. If pox occurs in breeding birds, decreased egg production and impaired fertility may result. In uncomplicated mild infections the course of the disease in a flock may be 2–3 wk. Severe outbreaks often last 6, 7, or even 8 wk.

Flock mortality in chickens and turkeys is usually low, but in severe cases it may be as high as 50%. In pigeons morbidity and mortality rates are similar to those in chickens. Pox in canaries can cause mortality as high as 80–100%. Significant mortality has been observed in quail infected with quail poxvirus.

Gross Lesions. The characteristic lesion of the cutaneous form of pox in chickens is a local epithelial hyperplasia involving epidermis and underlying feather follicles, with formation of nodules that first appear as small white foci and then rapidly increase in size and become yellow. In chickens infected intradermally, few primary lesions appear by the 4th day. Papules are formed by the 5th or 6th day. This is followed by the vesicular stage, with formation of extensive thick lesions (54). Adjoining lesions may coalesce (Fig. 23.5) and become rough and gray or dark brown. After about 2 wk, sometimes sooner, lesions have areas of inflammation at the base and become hemorrhagic. Formation of a scab, which may last for another 1–2 wk, ends with desquamation of the degenerated epithelial layer. If the scab is removed early in its development, there is a moist, seropurulent exudate underneath covering a hemorrhagic granulating surface. When the scab drops off naturally, a smooth scar may be present; in mild cases there may be no noticeable scar.

In the diphtheritic form, slightly elevated, white opaque nodules develop on the mucous membranes. Nodules rapidly increase in size and often coalesce to become a yellow, cheesy, necrotic, pseudodiphtheritic, or diphtheritic membrane (Fig. 23.6). If the membranes are removed they leave bleeding erosions. The inflammatory process may extend into sinuses, particularly the infraorbital sinus (resulting in swelling) and also into the pharynx and larynx (resulting in respiratory disturbances) and esophagus.

The first indication of pox in turkeys is seen as minute yellowish eruptions on the dewlap, snood, and other head parts. These eruptions are soft

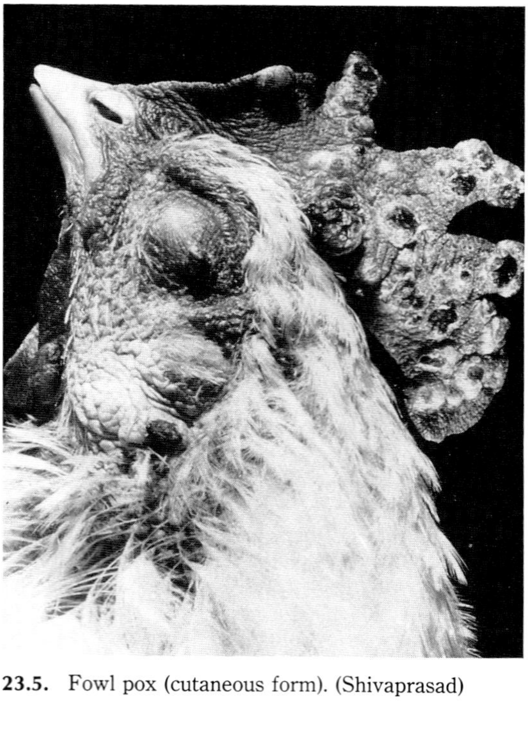

23.5. Fowl pox (cutaneous form). (Shivaprasad)

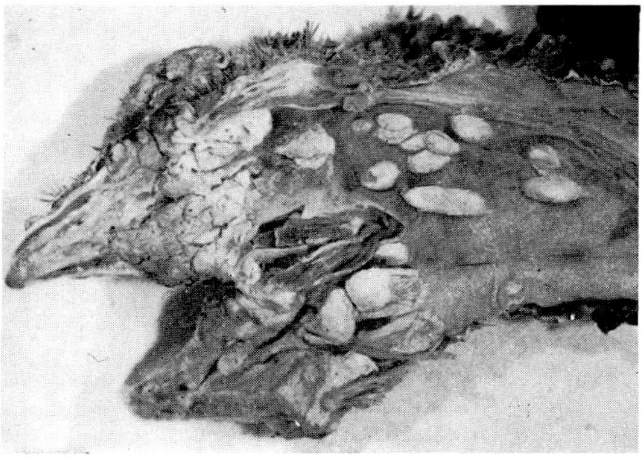

23.6. Fowl pox lesions in mouth and esophagus of turkey. (Hinshaw)

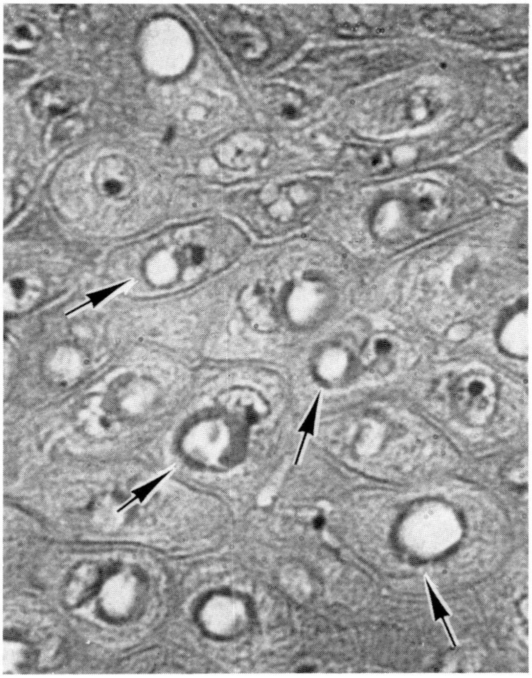

23.7. Cutaneous epithelium infected with fowl poxvirus. Infected cells are enlarged and contain cytoplasmic inclusion bodies (*arrows*).

and easily removed in this pustular stage, leaving an inflamed area covered with a sticky serous exudate. The corners of the mouth, eyelids, and oral membranes are commonly affected. Lesions enlarge and become covered with a dry scab or a yellow-red or brown wartlike mass. In young poults the head, legs, and feet may be completely covered with lesions. The disease may even spread to the feathered parts of the body. In an unusual outbreak of pox in breeding turkeys, proliferative lesions occurred in the oviduct, cloaca, and skin surrounding the vent (53).

Histopathology. The most important feature of infection (whether the lesion is cutaneous, diphtheritic, or from the infected CAM) is hyperplasia of the epithelium and enlargement of cells, with associated inflammatory changes. Characteristic eosinophilic A-type cytoplasmic inclusion bodies (Bollinger bodies) are observable by light microscopy (Fig. 23.7).

Histopathological changes of tracheal mucosa include initial hypertrophy and hyperplasia of mucus-producing cells with subsequent enlargement of epithelial cells, which contain eosinophilic cytoplasmic inclusion bodies. Often clusters of epithelial cells resemble a papilloma (81). Inclusion bodies may be present in various stages of development, depending on the time after infection. The inclusion body may occupy almost the entire cytoplasm, with resulting cell necrosis.

Immunity. Actively acquired immunity against avian poxviruses results from recovery from natural infection or vaccination. Cell-mediated and humoral immunity following vaccination or natural infection provide protection (8, 56, 88). Cell-mediated immunity develops earlier than the humoral antibody response.

DIAGNOSIS. Methods for diagnosis, prevention, and control are also available in other publications (24, 90, 94).

Clinical. Cutaneous lesions typical of avian pox (Fig. 23.5) must be confirmed by either histopathology (presence of cytoplasmic inclusions) or virus isolation. The diphtheritic form of the disease (Fig. 23.6) in chickens with associated respiratory signs must be differentiated from infectious laryngotracheitis, an infection caused by a herpesvirus.

Lesions caused by pantothenic acid or biotin deficiency in young chicks (6) or by T-2 toxin (21, 108) could be mistaken for pox lesions. Diphtheritic pox lesions in doves and pigeons may be mistaken for lesions caused by *Trichomonas gallinae,* which are diagnosed by microscopic examination of smears or by culture.

Microscopy. Elementary bodies (Borrel bodies) of fowl poxvirus can be detected in smears prepared from lesions and stained with Wright's stain or by the Gimenez method (89). Tissue sections from cutaneous (Fig. 23.7) or diphtheritic lesions may be processed by conventional methods (18) or by using a solution that fixes and dehydrates tissues simultaneously (75) for detection of cytoplasmic inclusions. Various histochemical and histopathological techniques are described by Thompson and Hunt (84).

Electron microscopy can be employed for demonstration of virus particles in lesions and exudate by negative staining or in ultrathin sections of the infected tissues (52, 71, 98). Type A inclusions with virions around the periphery or virus-filled inclusions may be observed on electron microscopic examination.

Isolation and Identification of Virus

BIRD INOCULATION. Avian poxviruses can be transmitted by applying a suspension of the lesion material from infected to susceptible birds by scarification of the comb or by the wing-web stick and feather follicle methods. Fowl poxvirus can be transmitted readily from chicken to chicken, with typical cutaneous lesions developing in 5–7 days (Fig. 23.5). In atypical cases, microscopy of lesion specimens may be advisable as well as bird inoculation.

EMBRYO INOCULATION. A suspension of specimen from a dermal or diphtheritic lesion is inoculated on the CAM of 9- to 12-day-old developing chicken embryos from a specific-pathogen-free flock; 5–7 days PI the CAM is examined for pox lesions (Fig. 23.4). Occasionally, some isolates fail to grow on the CAM of chicken embryos (23, 41).

CELL CULTURE. Cell cultures are not generally employed for initial isolation of avian poxviruses. Adaptation of the virus to this host system is sometimes necessary, since not all strains produce CPE on initial inoculation.

IMMUNOLOGY AND SEROLOGY

Protection Tests. Protection tests are generally used to determine immunogenicity of fowl and pigeon pox vaccines. At least five susceptible birds are vaccinated according to directions of the manufacturer. An additional five nonvaccinated and isolated birds of the same source and age are kept as controls. At least 10 days after vaccination, vaccinated and control birds are challenged with a different strain of fowl poxvirus capable of causing clinical signs of pox in at least 80% of the control birds. The challenge virus may be applied on the comb or by the wing-web or feather follicle method at a site opposite that used for vaccination. The birds should be examined for takes (see Immunization). For satisfactory immunization, at least 80% of the controls should have lesions of fowl pox and at least 80% of the vaccinated birds should not.

Cross-protection tests for the antigenic relationship of the avian poxviruses are not generally practical for routine diagnosis but may be necessary for their antigenic characterization (70, 101).

Immunodiffusion. Immunodiffusion may be used for differential identification of fowl and pigeon poxviruses or antibody from those of other avian viral diseases (39, 95).

As precipitating antibodies are detectable for only a short duration after infection, serum must be collected at the appropriate time, usually 15–20 days after known infection.

Passive Hemagglutination. A passive hemagglutination test detects antibodies in serum of chickens earlier than the immunodiffusion test (22, 92).

Neutralization. Virus neutralization in cell culture (58) or chicken embryos (7) may be used. However, this procedure is not practical as a routine diagnostic test.

Fluorescent Antibody and ELISA Tests. An indirect fluorescent antibody, immunoperoxidase, or enzyme-linked immunosorbent assay (ELISA) test can be used to detect antibody (16, 55, 93).

Immunoblotting. Immunogenic proteins of vaccine and field strains of fowl poxvirus can be compared by immunoblotting. Common antigens are detected among strains (Fig. 23.8A). However, the strains can be differentiated by unique proteins of differing electrophoretic mobilities (73).

Restriction Endonuclease Analysis of Avian Poxvirus DNA. Restriction endonuclease analysis is among the most sensitive methods for comparing closely related DNA genomes, since a single base change in recognition sequence may cause a change in restriction endonuclease profile. Müller et al. (62) reported differences of fowl poxvirus from vaccinia virus by the examination of the pattern of DNA fragments by their relative mobilities. Recently, genomes of fowl, pigeon, and junco poxviruses were compared by restriction enzyme analysis using BamHI and HindIII endonuclease digestion and subsequent agarose gel electrophoresis (73). The genetic profiles of these strains were similar, with a high proportion of comigrating fragments, although most strains could still be distinguished by presence or absence of one or two DNA fragments (Fig. 23.8B). The characteristic electrophoretic profile of restriction endonuclease–digested DNA has facilitated comparison of other members of the *Avipoxvirus* genus. Genomic profiles of quail, canary, and mynah poxviruses are different from the profile of fowl poxvirus (86).

TREATMENT, PREVENTION, CONTROL.

There is no specific treatment for birds infected with avian poxviruses. Proper husbandry should be practiced to alleviate environmental stress.

Immunization. Two types of live virus vaccines are used for immunization of birds against pox: fowl pox and pigeon pox vaccines. These should

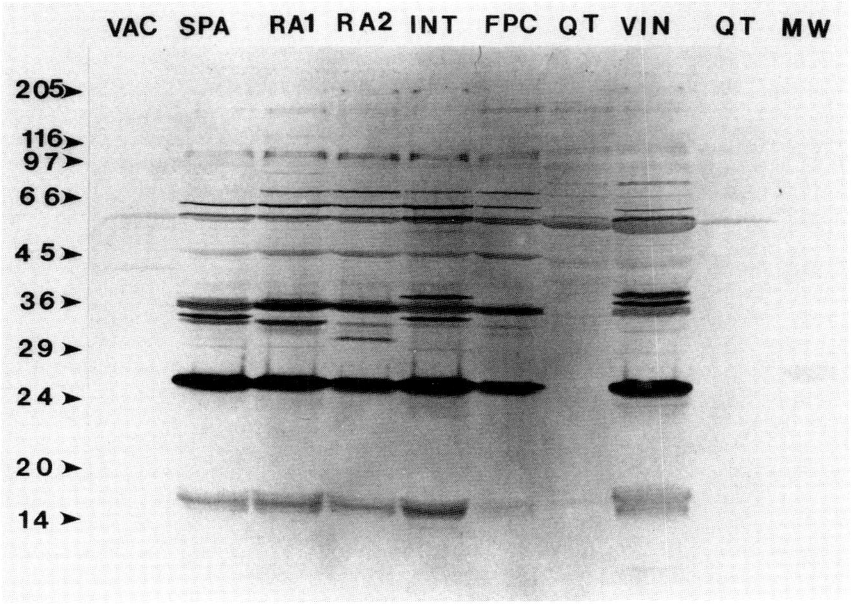

A

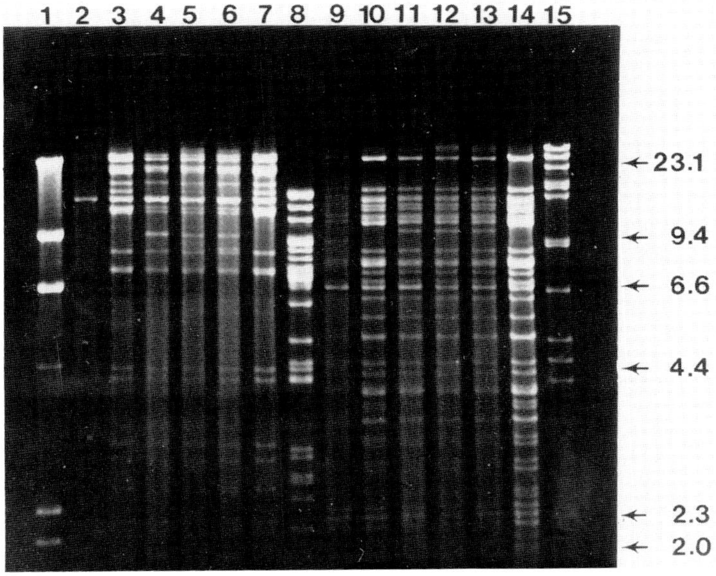

B

23.8. Strain variation in antigenic and DNA composition. A. Immunoblotting of soluble antigens of avian poxviruses. Antigens prepared from uninfected cells (*QT*) or cells infected with vaccinia (*VAC*) or fowl poxvirus strains Spafas (*SPA*), Randall-1 (*RA1*), Randall-2 (*RA2*), Intervet (*INT*), C (*FPC*), and Vineland (*VIN*). Proteins were separated by SDS-PAGE and transferred to nitrocellulose. Viral antigens were detected by reaction with chicken antifowl poxvirus serum. (73). B. Agarose gel electrophoresis analysis of avian poxvirus DNA from strains FPC (lanes *2* and *9*), Vineland (lanes *3* and *10*), UI (lanes *4* and *11*), Sterwin (lanes *5* and *12*), Salsbury (lanes *6* and *13*), CEVA (lanes *7* and *14*), and vaccinia (lanes *8* and *15*), after cleavage with BamHI (lanes *2–8*) or HindIII (lanes *9–15*). Lane *1* is a HindIII digestion profile of lambda phage DNA, and the size (kb) of its fragments are shown on the right-hand side of the gel. (73)

contain a minimum concentration of 10^5 EID_{50}/ml (33, 100) to establish satisfactory takes for good immunity. Fowl pox and pigeon pox vaccines labeled "chicken embryo origin" are prepared from the infected CAM. Fowl pox vaccine labeled "tissue culture origin" is prepared from chicken embryo fibroblast cultures. A fowl poxvirus vaccine strain adapted to chicken embryo dermis cell cultures was more economical with more uniformity than conventional vaccine prepared on the CAM of chicken embryos (29).

Success of a vaccination program depends on potency and purity of the vaccine and its application under conditions for which it is specifically intended. Vaccination essentially produces a mild form of the disease. Directions for use of vaccine as supplied by the producer should be followed explicitly. Vaccine should not be used in a flock affected with other diseases or in generally poor condition. All birds within a house should be vaccinated on the same day. Other susceptible birds on the premises should be isolated from those being vaccinated. If pox appears in a flock in an initial outbreak, with only a few birds affected, nonaffected birds should be vaccinated.

A vaccine vial should be opened immediately before use. Only one vial should be opened at a time, and the entire contents should be used within 2 hr. After vaccine is prepared, vaccinator's hands should be washed thoroughly. Vaccine should contact the bird only at the site for vaccination. Extreme precautions should be taken not to contaminate other parts of the bird, the premises, or miscellaneous equipment.

All contaminated vaccine equipment, unused vaccine, empty vials, etc., should be decontaminated, preferably by incineration. No prepared vaccine should be saved for later use.

FOWL POX VACCINE. The vaccine of chick embryo origin contains live, nonattenuated fowl poxvirus capable of producing serious disease in a flock if used improperly.

Fowl pox vaccine is applied by the wing-web method to 4-wk-old chickens and to pullets about 1–2 mo before egg production is expected to start. It is also used to revaccinate chickens held for the 2nd yr of egg production. The vaccine is not to be used on hens while they are laying.

Attenuated fowl poxvirus vaccines of cell culture origin can be used effectively on chicks as young as 1 day of age and have been used at times in combination with Marek's disease vaccine (27, 78).

Oral vaccination with an attenuated cell culture vaccine has been reported effective in Germany (49). Comparative immunogenicity of fowl pox vaccines administered by intramuscular, feather follicle, oral, and intranasal routes in chickens of different age groups was recently evaluated by Sharma and Sharma (76). They reported oral vaccination did not provide protection over 50% while other methods provided 80–100% protection.

Turkeys may be vaccinated by the wing-web method, but the virus may spread and infect the head region. The site of choice for vaccination is about midway on the thigh. Initially, turkeys are vaccinated when they are 2–3 mo old, but those to be used as breeders should be revaccinated before production. Revaccination at 3- to 4-mo intervals during the laying season might be of some advantage, depending on the level of risk.

Fowl pox vaccine is not to be used on pigeons.

PIGEON POX VACCINE. Pigeon pox vaccine contains live, nonattenuated, natural poxvirus for pigeons. If used improperly, the vaccine can cause a severe reaction in these birds. The virus is less pathogenic for chickens and turkeys.

Pigeon pox vaccine has been commonly applied by brush to denuded feather follicles on the leg. However, recently developed vaccines may be applied by the wing-web method and can be used on chickens of any age. It is generally used, however, on 4-wk-old chickens and about 1 mo before egg production is expected to start. When birds younger than 4 wk are vaccinated, they should be revaccinated before start of production. Birds held for the 2nd yr of production should be revaccinated.

Turkeys can be vaccinated at any age by the wing-web or thigh stick methods. Day-old poults can be vaccinated if necessary, but it is better to wait until they are about 8 wk old for a better immune response. Revaccination may be necessary and advisable during the growing period. Turkeys retained as breeders should be revaccinated.

Pigeons can be vaccinated by the wing-web method. The vaccine can be applied by the feather follicle method, but this is not generally employed. Differences in the immunizing properties of pigeon pox vaccines have been observed (107).

CANARY POX VACCINE. A live chicken embryo-attenuated canary pox vaccine has been used effectively in canaries under experimental conditions (36, 51). Canary pox vaccine is currently available commercially in the USA.

QUAIL POX VACCINE. A live vaccine of quail poxvirus origin is available commercially for use in quail. It does not provide protection against fowl poxvirus infection (101).

VACCINE TAKES. The flock should be examined about 7–10 days after vaccination for evidence of "takes." A take consists of swelling of the skin or a scab at the site where vaccine was applied and is evidence of successful vaccination. Immunity will normally develop in 10–14 days after vaccination. If the vaccine is properly applied to susceptible birds, the majority should have takes. In large flocks at least 10% of the birds should be examined for takes.

The lack of a take could be the result of vaccine being applied to an immune bird, use of a vaccine of inadequate potency (after the expiration date or subjected to deleterious influences), or improper application.

PROPHYLACTIC VACCINATION. Immunization against pox consists of vaccinating susceptible birds prior to the time the disease is likely to occur. This is usually done during spring and summer in areas where the disease occurs in fall and winter. In tropical climates where the disease may occur throughout the year, vaccination may be done at any time when warranted, without regard to the season.

Vaccination is indicated under three conditions: 1) When a flock on the premises was infected the previous year. All young stock produced on the premises or introduced from other sources should receive fowl pox vaccine. 2) If pox was present the previous year and pigeon pox vaccine was used, birds should be revaccinated with fowl pox vaccine, because immunity from pigeon pox vaccine is not of long duration. 3) In areas where pox is prevalent, fowl pox vaccine should be used for protection against infection from neighboring flocks.

RECOMBINANT VACCINES

Fowl Poxvirus as Cloning and Expression Vector. Fowl poxvirus has one of the largest genomes and, like vaccinia virus perhaps, can accommodate significant amounts of foreign DNA while maintaining its infectivity. Since the first demonstration in 1982 of the insertion and expression of the herpes simplex virus TK gene, a large variety of genes from specific pathogens representing genetic elements responsible for specific immune responses have been inserted into vaccinia virus (61). Thus, recombinant DNA studies on vaccinia virus have provided great impetus toward development of fowl poxvirus as an expression vector for genes from poultry pathogens.

In order to develop fowl poxvirus as an expression vector, the following are required: (a) a nonessential region in the fowl poxvirus genome, (b) the foreign gene(s) of interest, and (c) the promoter(s) that will regulate the expression of the foreign gene(s). Since TK gene is not required for fowl poxvirus multiplication, it provides a convenient region for insertion of a foreign gene. Initially, the fowl poxvirus TK gene is cloned in a convenient vector, e.g., plasmid pBR 322. The foreign gene of interest ligated to the promoter, is then inserted into the TK gene such that TK sequences flank the foreign gene. In order to facilitate the selection of the recombinant progeny virus, often a marker gene, e.g., beta-galactosidase or *Escherichia coli* xanthine phosphoribosyl transferase (Ecogpt), ligated to another promoter is also cloned in the same plasmid. The donor plasmid containing the foreign gene is introduced by transfection in cells that have been infected with fowl poxvirus. When replicating DNA from the infecting fowl poxvirus comes in contact with donor DNA, in vivo recombination takes place in the cytoplasm between the homologous TK sequences of replicating fowl poxvirus and the homologous TK sequences flanking the foreign gene. The resulting recombinant progeny virus containing the foreign gene is identified either by hybridization with a specific probe or through expression of the marker gene. The major steps that have taken place in this direction are briefly described below.

Thymidine Kinase Gene. Boyle and Couper (13) first identified the fowl poxvirus TK gene by marker rescue using vaccinia virus as a selection and cloning vehicle. The TK gene of a field strain of fowl poxvirus has been cloned and identified by restriction mapping and by sequencing part of the gene using a synthetic oligonucleotide primer (86). Identification of the TK gene of fowl poxvirus and quail poxvirus has been accomplished by hybridization (74) with an end-labeled degenerate oligonucleotide probe, representing a consensus sequence (97) of three TK genes. Nucleotide sequence of fowl pox TK has been reported (11, 15).

Regulatory Sequences (Promoter) of Fowl Poxvirus. Initial studies of Boyle and Couper (13) suggested that the vaccinia virus RNA polymerase was able to recognize the fowl poxvirus promoter sequences of fowl poxvirus TK gene, indicating that vaccinia virus promoter sequences might be able to operate in fowl poxvirus, although perhaps with reduced efficiency. Tripathy and Wittek (91) confirmed this in a transient assay in which fowl poxvirus–infected cells were transfected with a plasmid DNA containing chloramphenicol acetyltransferase (CAT) gene ligated to a vaccinia virus promoter. The CAT activity was observed only in cells infected with fowl poxvirus that had been transfected with plasmid DNA containing vaccinia virus promoter ligated to CAT gene and not in uninfected cells or fowl poxvirus–infected cells. Subsequently, a bacterial gene, beta-galactosidase, has been inserted and expressed in recombinant fowl poxvirus under the control of vaccinia virus promoters (72). Recently, the hemagglutinin gene of avian influenza (14) has been inserted in fowl poxvirus and has been expressed. Although currently vaccinia virus promoters are being used in fowl poxvirus recombinants, the sequences immediately upstream of open reading frames of fowl poxvirus genome show similarity to vaccinia virus early gene promoters (85).

REFERENCES

1. Akey, B.L., J.K. Nayar, and D.J. Forrester. 1981. Avian pox in Florida wild turkeys: Culex nigripalpus and Wyeomyia vanduzeei as experimental vectors. J Wildl Dis 17:597-599.
2. Al Falluji, M.M., H.H. Tantawi, A. Albana, and S. Al Sheikhly. 1979. Pox infection among captive peacocks. J Wildl Dis 15:597-600.
3. Andrews, C., H.G. Pereira, and P. Wildy. 1978. Viruses of Vertebrates, 4th Ed., pp. 356-389. Bailliere Tindall, London.
4. Arhelger, R.B., and C.C. Randall. 1964. Electron microscopic observations on the development of fowlpox virus in chorioallantoic membrane. Virology 22:59-66.
5. Arhelger, R.B., R.W. Darlington, L.G. Gafford, and C.C. Randall. 1962. An electron microscopic study of fowlpox infection in chick scalps. Lab Invest 11:814-825.
6. Austic, R.E., and M.L. Scott. 1984. Nutritional deficiency diseases. In M.S. Hofstad, B.W. Calnek, W.M. Reid, and H.W. Yoder, Jr. (eds.), Diseases of Poultry, 8th Ed., pp. 38-64. Iowa State Univ Press, Ames.
7. Baxendale, W. 1971. Studies of three avian pox viruses and the development of an improved fowlpox vaccine. Vet Rec 88:5-10.
8. Baxendale, W. 1981. Immunity to fowlpox. In M.E. Rose, L.N. Payne, and B.M. Freeman (eds.), Avian Immunology, pp. 255-261. Edinburgh, British Poultry Science Ltd.
9. Beaver, D.L., and W.J. Cheatham. 1963. Electron microscopy of juncopox. Am J Pathol 42:23-40.
10. Binns, M.M., L. Stenzler, F.M. Tomley, J. Campbell, and M.E.G. Boursnell. 1987. Identification by a random sequencing strategy of fowlpoxvirus DNA polymerase gene, its nucleotide sequence and comparison with other viral DNA polymerases. Nucleic Acids Res 15:6563-6573.
11. Binns, M.M., F.M. Tomley, J. Campbell, and M.E.G. Boursnell. 1988. Comparison of a conserve region in fowlpox virus and vaccinia virus genomes and the translocation of the fowlpox virus thymidine kinase gene. J Gen Virol 69:1275-1283.
12. Boosinger, T.R., R.W. Winterfield, D.S. Feldman, and A.S. Dhillon. 1982. Psittacine poxvirus: Virus isolation and identification, transmission and cross-challenge studies in parrots and chickens. Avian Dis 26:437-444.
13. Boyle, D.B., and B.E.H. Couper. 1986. Identification and cloning of the fowlpox virus thymidine kinase gene using vaccinia virus. J Gen Virol 67:1591-1600.
14. Boyle, D.B., and B.E.H. Couper. 1988. Construction of recombinant fowlpox viruses as vectors for poultry vaccines. Virus Res 10:343-356.
15. Boyle, D.B., B.E.H. Couper, A.J. Gibbs, L.J. Seigman, and G.W. Both. 1987. Fowlpox virus thymidine kinase: Nucleotide sequence and relationships to other thymidine kinases. Virology 156:355-365.
16. Buscaglia, C., R.A. Bankowski, and L. Miers. 1985. Cell-culture virus-neutralization test and enzyme-linked immunoabsorbent assay for evaluation of immunity in chickens against fowl pox. Avian Dis 29:672-680.
17. Carter, J.K.Y., and N.F. Cheville. 1981. Isolation of surface tubules of fowlpox virus. Avian Dis 25:454-462.
18. Cheevers, W.P., and C.C. Randall. 1968. Viral and cellular growth and sequential increase of protein and DNA during fowlpox infection in vivo. Proc Soc Exp Biol Med 127:401-405.
19. Cheevers, W.P., D.J. O'Callaghan, and C.C. Randall. 1968. Biosynthesis of host and viral deoxyribonucleic acid during hyperplastic fowlpox infection in vivo. J Virol 2:421-429.
20. Cheville, N.F. 1966. Cytopathic changes in fowlpox (turkey origin) inclusion body formation. Am J Pathol 49:723-737.
21. Chi, M.S., and C.J. Mirocha. 1978. Necrotic oral lesions in chickens fed diacetoxyscirpenol, T-2 toxin, and crotocin. Poult Sci 57:807-808.
22. Chung, Y.S., and P.B. Spradbrow. 1977. Studies on poxvirus isolated from a magpie in Queensland. Aust Vet J 53:334-336.
23. Cox, W.R. 1980. Avian pox infection in a Canada goose (Branta canadensis). J Wildl Dis 16:623-626.
24. Cunningham, C.H. 1973. A Laboratory Guide in Virology, 7th Ed. Burgess, Minneapolis.
25. Drillien, R., D. Spehner, D. Villeval, and J.P. Lecocq. 1987. Similar genetic organization between a region of fowlpox virus DNA and the vaccinia virus HindIII J fragment despite divergent location of the thymidine kinase gene. Virology 160:203-209.
26. Duran-Reynals, F., and E. Bryan. 1952. Studies on the combined effects of fowl poxvirus and methylcholanthrene in chickens. Ann NY Acad Sci 54:977-991.
27. Eidson, C.S., P. Villegas, and S.H. Kleven. 1975. Efficacy of turkey herpesvirus vaccine when administered simultaneously with fowl pox vaccine. Poult Sci 54:1975-1981.
28. Eleazer, T.H., J.S. Harrel, and H.G. Blalock. 1983. Transmission studies involving a wet fowl pox isolate. Avian Dis 27:542-544.
29. El-Zein, A., S. Nehme, V. Ghoraib, S. Hasbani, and B. Toth. 1974. Preparation of fowlpox vaccine on chicken-embryo-dermis cell culture. Avian Dis 18:495-506.
30. Gafford, L.G., and C.C. Randall. 1976. Virus-specific RNA and DNA in nuclei of cells infected with fowlpox virus. Virology 69:1-14.
31. Gafford, L.G., B.E. Mitchell, Jr., and C.C. Randall. 1978. Sedimentation characteristics and molecular weights of three poxvirus DNAs. Virology 89:229-239.
32. Garg, S.K., M.S. Sethi, and S.K. Negi. 1967. Hemagglutinating property of pigeonpox virus strains. Indian J Microbiol 7:101-102.
33. Gelenczei, E.F., and H.N. Lasher. 1968. Comparative studies of cell-culture-propagated avian poxviruses in chickens and turkeys. Avian Dis 12:142-150.
34. Ghildyal, N., W. Schnitzlein, and D.N. Tripathy. 1989. Genetic and antigenic differences between fowlpox and quailpox viruses. Arch Virol 106:85-92.
35. Giddens, W.E., L.J. Swago, J.D. Handerson, Jr., R.A. Lewis, D.S. Farner, A. Carlos, and W.C. Dolowy. 1971. Canary pox in sparrows and canaries (Fringillidae) and in Weavers (Ploceidae). Vet Pathol 8:260-280.
36. Hitchner, S.B. 1981. Canary pox vaccination with live embryo-attenuated virus. Avian Dis 25:874-881.
37. Holt, G., and J. Krogsrud. 1973. Pox in wild birds. Acta Vet Scand 14:201-203.
38. Hyde, J.M., L.G. Gafford, and C.C. Randall. 1967. Molecular weight determination of fowl poxvirus DNA by electron microscopy. Virology 33:112-120.
39. Jordan, F.T.W., and R.C. Chubb. 1962. The agar gel diffusion technique in the diagnosis of infectious laryngotracheitis (ILT) and its differentiation from fowlpox. Res Vet Sci 3:245-255.
40. Karstad, L. 1971. Pox. In J.W. Davis, R.C. Ander-

son, L. Karstad, and D.O. Trainer (eds.), Infectious and Parasitic Diseases of Wild Birds, pp. 34–41. Iowa State Univ Press, Ames.

41. Kirmse, P. 1967. Host specificity and long persistence of pox infection in the flicker (Colaptes auratus). Bull Wildl Dis Assoc 3:14–20.

42. Kirmse, P. 1969. Host specificity and pathogenicity of pox viruses from wild birds. Bull Wildl Dis Assoc 5:376–386.

43. Kirmse, P., and H. Loftin. 1969. Avian pox in migrant and native birds in Panama. Bull Wildl Dis Assoc 5:103–107.

44. Landolt, M., and R.M. Kocan. 1976. Transmission of avian pox from starlings to rothchild's mynahs. J Wildl Dis 12:353–356.

45. Ledingham, J.C.G., and M.B. Aberd. 1931. The aetiological importance of the elementary bodies in vaccinia and fowlpox. Lancet 221:525–526.

46. Lyles, D.S., C.C. Randall, L.G. Gafford, and H.B. White, Jr. 1976. Cellular fatty acids during fowlpox virus infection of three different host systems. Virology 70:227–229.

47. Matthews, R.E.F. 1982. Classification and nomenclature of viruses. Intervirology 17:42–46.

48. Mayr, A. 1963. Neue Verfahren für die Differenzierung der Geflügelpokenviren. Berl Muench Tierärztl Wochenschr 76:316–324.

49. Mayr, A., and K. Danner. 1976. Oral immunization against pox. Studies on fowlpox as a model. 14th Congr Int Assoc Biol Stand Dev Bio Stand 33:249–259.

50. Mayr, A., and H. Mahnel. 1970. Charakteisierung eines Vom Rhinozeros isolierten Hühnerpockenvirus. Arch Gesamte Virusforsch 31:51–60.

51. Mayr, A., F. Hartig, and I. Bayr. 1965. Entwicklung eines Impfstoffes gegen die Kanarienpocken auf der Basis eines attenuierten Kanarienpocken-Kulturvirus. Zentralbl Veterinaermed. Reihe [B] 12:41–49.

52. McFerran, J.B., J.K. Clarke, and W.L. Curran. 1971. The application of negative contrast electron microscopy to routine veterinary virus diagnosis. Res Vet Sci 12:253–257.

53. Metz, A.L., L. Hatcher, J.A. Newman, and D.A. Halvorson. 1985. Venereal pox in breeder turkeys in Minnesota. Avian Dis 29:850–853.

54. Minbay, A., and J.P. Kreier. 1973. An experimental study of the pathogenesis of fowlpox infection in chickens. Avian Dis 17:532–539.

55. Mockett, A.P.A., D.J. Southee, F.M. Tomley, and A. Deuter. 1987. Fowlpox virus: Its structural proteins and immunogens and the detection of viral-specific antibodies by ELISA. Avian Pathol 16:493–504.

56. Morita, C. 1973. Role of humoral and cell-mediated immunity on the recovery of chickens from fowl poxvirus infection. J Immunol 111:1495–1501.

57. Morita, C. 1973. Studies on fowlpox viruses. I. Plaque formation of fowlpox virus on chick embryo cell culture. Avian Dis 17:87–92.

58. Morita, C. 1973. Studies on fowlpox viruses. II. Plaque-neutralization test. Avian Dis 17:93–98.

59. Moscovici, C., M.G. Moscovici, H. Jimenez, M.M.C. Lai, M.J. Hayman, and P.K. Vogt. 1977. Continuous tissue culture cell lines derived from chemically induced tumors of Japanese quail. Cell 11:95–103.

60. Moss, B. 1985. Replication of poxviruses. In B.N. Fields, D.N. Knipe, R.M. Chanock, J.L. Melnick, B. Roizman, and R.E. Shope (eds.), Virology, pp. 685–703. Raven Press, New York.

61. Moss, B., and C. Flexner. 1987. Vaccinia virus expression vectors. Annu Rev Immunol 5:305–324.

62. Müller, H.K., R. Wittek, W. Schaffner, D. Schümperli, A. Menna, and R. Wyler. 1977. Comparison of five poxvirus genomes by analysis with restriction endonucleases Hind III, Bam HI and Eco RI. J Gen Virol 38:135–147.

63. Obijeski, J.F., E.L. Palmer, L.G. Gafford, and C.C. Randall. 1973. Polyacrylamide gel electrophoresis of fowlpox and vaccinia virus proteins. Virology 51:512–516.

64. Odend'hal, S. 1983. The Geographical Distribution of Animal Viral Diseases. Academic Press, NY.

65. Petrak, M.L. 1982. Diseases of Cage and Aviary Birds. Lea & Febiger, Philadelphia.

66. Prideaux, C.T., and D.B. Boyle. 1987. Fowlpox virus polypeptides: Sequential appearance and virion associated polypeptides. Arch Virol 96:185–199.

67. Randall, C.C., and L.G. Gafford. 1962. Histochemical and biochemical studies of isolated viral inclusions. Am J Pathol 40:51–62.

68. Randall, C.C., L.G. Gafford, R.W. Darlington, and J. Hyde. 1964. Composition of fowlpox virus and inclusion matrix. J Bacteriol 87:939–944.

69. Randall, C.C., L.G. Gafford, R.L. Soehner, and J.M. Hyde. 1966. Physiochemical properties of fowlpox virus deoxyribonucleic acid and its anomalous infectious behavior. J Bacteriol 91:95–100.

70. Reed, W. 1988. Pathogenicity and immunologic relationship of quail and mynah pox viruses to fowl and pigeon pox viruses. Proc 37th West Poult Dis Conf, pp. 5–8.

71. Sadasiv, E.C., P.W. Chang, and G. Gluka. 1985. Morphogenesis of canary poxvirus and its entrance into inclusion bodies. Am J Vet Res 46:529–535.

72. Schnitzlein, W.M., and D.N. Tripathy. 1988. Recognition of a vaccinia virus promoter by a recombinant fowl poxvirus. Proc Conf Vector-based Vaccines. (Abstr).

73. Schnitzlein, W.M., N. Ghildyal, and D.N. Tripathy. 1988. Genomic and antigenic characterization of avipoxviruses. Virus Res 10:65–76.

74. Schnitzlein, W.M., N. Ghildyal, and D.N. Tripathy. 1988. A rapid method for identifying the thymidine kinase genes of avipoxviruses. J Virol Meth 20:341–352.

75. Sevoian, M. 1960. A quick method for the diagnosis of avian pox and infectious laryngotracheitis. Avian Dis 4:474–477.

76. Sharma, D.K., and S.N. Sharma. 1988. Comparative immunity of fowl pox virus vaccines. J Vet Med B 35:19–23.

77. Shirinov, F.B., A.I. Ibragimova, and Z.G. Misirov. 1972. Spread of fowl poxvirus by the mite Dermanyssus gallinae. Veterinariya (Moscow) 4:48–49 (Vet Bull 42:5206).

78. Siccardi, F.J. 1975. The addition of fowlpox and pigeonpox vaccine to Marek's vaccine in broilers. Avian Dis 19:362–365.

79. Singh, G.K., N.P. Singh, and S.K. Garg. 1987. Studies on pathogenesis of fowlpox: Virological study. Acta Virol 31:417–423.

80. Swallen, T.O. 1963. A radioautographic study of the lesions of fowlpox using thymidine-H^3. Am J Pathol 42:485–491.

81. Tanizaki, E., T. Kotani, and Y. Odagiri. 1986. Pathological changes of tracheal mucosa in chickens infected with fowlpox virus. Avian Dis 31:169–175.

82. Tantwai, H.H., M.M. Al Falluji, and M.O. Shony. 1979. Heat-selected mutants of pigeon poxvirus. Acta Virol 23:249–252.

83. Tantwai, H.H., S. Al Sheikhly, and F.K. Hussain. 1981. Avian pox in buzzard (Accipiter nisus) in Iraq. J Wildl Dis 17:145–146.

84. Thompson, S.W., and R.D. Hunt. 1966. Selected

Histochemical and Histopathological Methods, pp. 885–887. Charles C. Thomas, Springfield, IL.
85. Tomley, F., M. Binns, J. Campbell, and M. Boursnell. 1988. Sequence analysis of an 11.2 kilobase, near-terminal BamHI fragment of fowlpox virus. J Gen Virol 69:1025–1040.
86. Tripathy, D.N. 1988. Unpublished data.
87. Tripathy, D.N., and C.H. Cunningham. 1984. Avian pox. In M.S. Hofstad, H.J. Barnes, B.W. Calnek, W.M. Reid, and H.W. Yoder, Jr. (eds.), Diseases of Poultry, 8th Ed., pp. 524–534. Iowa State Univ Press, Ames.
88. Tripathy, D.N., and L.E. Hanson. 1975. Immunity to fowlpox. Am J Vet Res 36:541–544.
89. Tripathy, D.N., and L.E. Hanson. 1976. A smear technique for staining elementary bodies of fowlpox. Avian Dis 20:609–610.
90. Tripathy, D.N., and L.E. Hanson. 1980. Avian pox. In S.B. Hitchner, C.H. Domermuth, H.G. Purchase, and J.E. Williams (eds.), Isolation and Identification of Avian Pathogens, pp. 109–111. Am Assoc Avian Pathol, Kennett Square, PA.
91. Tripathy, D.N., and R. Wittek. 1987. Foreign gene regulation in fowlpox virus by a vaccinia virus promoter. Proc 68th Annu Meet Conf Res Work Anim Dis, p. 63. (Abstr).
92. Tripathy, D.N., L.E. Hanson, and W.L. Myers. 1970. Passive hemagglutination test with fowlpox virus. Avian Dis 14:29–38.
93. Tripathy, D.N., L.E. Hanson, and A.H. Killinger. 1973. Immunoperoxidase technique for detection of fowlpox antigen. Avian Dis 17:274–278.
94. Tripathy, D.N., L.E. Hanson, and R.A. Crandell. 1981. Poxviruses of veterinary importance; diagnosis of infections, Chap. 6. In E. Kurstak and C. Kurstak (eds.), Comparative Diagnosis of Viral Diseases, Vol. III, pp. 267–346. Academic Press, New York.
95. Uppal, P.K., and P.R. Nilakantan. 1970. Studies on the serological relationships between avianpox, sheep pox, goat pox and vaccinia viruses. J Hyg Camb 68:349–358.
96. Uppal, P.K., and P.R. Nilakantan. 1974. Hemagglutination by fowlpox, sheep pox and vaccinia viruses. Indian Vet J 51:451–456.
97. Upton, C., and G. McFadden. 1986. Identification and nucleotide sequence of the thymidine kinase gene of shope fibroma virus. J Virol 60:920–927.
98. Van Kammen, A., and P.B. Spradbrow. 1976. Rapid diagnosis of some avian virus diseases. Avian Dis 20:748–751.
99. White, H.B., S.S. Powell, L.G. Gafford, and C.C. Randall. 1968. The occurrence of squalene in lipid of fowlpox virus. J Biol Chem 243:4517–4525.
100. Winterfield, R.W., and S.B. Hitchner. 1965. The response of chickens to vaccination with different concentrations of pigeon pox and fowl pox viruses. Avian Dis 9:237–241.
101. Winterfield, R.W., and W. Reed. 1985. Avian pox: Infection and immunity with quail, psittacine, fowl, and pigeon pox viruses. Poult Sci 64:65–70.
102. Winterfield, R.W., W.M. Reed, and H.L. Thacker. 1985. Infection and immunity with a virus isolate from turkeys. Poult Sci 64:2076–2080.
103. Woodroofe, G.M., and F. Fenner. 1962. Serological relationship within the poxvirus group: An antigen common to all members of the group. Virology 16:334–341.
104. Woodruff, A.M., and E.W. Goodpasture. 1931. The susceptibility of the chorio-allantoic membrane of chick embryo to infection with the fowlpox virus. Am J Pathol 7:209–222.
105. Woodruff, C.E., and E.W. Goodpasture. 1929. The infectivity of isolated inclusion bodies of fowlpox. Am J Pathol 5:1–10.
106. Woodruff, C.E., and E.W. Goodpasture. 1930. The relation of the virus of fowl-pox to the specific cellular inclusions of the disease. Am J Pathol 6:713–720.
107. Woodward, H., and D.C. Tudor. 1973. The immunizing effect of commercial pigeon pox vaccines on pigeons. Poult Sci 52:1463–1468.
108. Wyatt, R.D., B.A. Weeks, P.B. Hamilton, and H.R. Brumeister. 1972. Severe oral lesions in chickens caused by ingestion of dietary fusariotoxin T-2. Appl Microbiol 24:251–257.

24 DUCK VIRUS HEPATITIS

P.R. Woolcock and J. Fabricant

INTRODUCTION. Duck hepatitis (DH) is a highly fatal, rapidly spreading viral infection of young ducklings characterized primarily by hepatitis. It can be caused by any of three different viruses, namely duck hepatitis virus (DHV) types 1, 2, and 3. DHV types 2 and 3 were first recognized as separate entities because they induced hepatitis in DHV type 1–immune ducklings. DH is of economic importance to all duck-growing farms because of the high potential mortality if not controlled. The three virus types are not known to have any public health significance.

HISTORY AND DISTRIBUTION

Duck Hepatitis Virus Type 1. An acute disease of ducklings, characterized by enlarged livers mottled with hemorrhages, was observed in 1945 by Levine and Hofstad (70). The disease affected ducklings during the 1st wk of age, and death was rapid after signs were observed. While the disease could be transmitted in ducklings, no agent was isolated. During the spring of 1949, Levine and Fabricant (69) studied a highly fatal disease in young White Pekin ducks on Long Island, NY. The disease spread rapidly; before the summer was over, practically all 70-odd duck farms in the area had suffered losses. At first, ducks 2–3 wk old were succumbing. On severely affected farms, mortalities up to 95% were not uncommon in some broods. Successive lots of ducks almost invariably became infected. Later, occasional broods would escape with little mortality. It is estimated that 15% of the total number of ducklings started for that year died from the disease–a total of 750,000 birds. In the USA the disease has also been diagnosed in other duck-raising areas. The disease is worldwide in distribution (103); the most recent reports of new isolations include China (46) and Korea (86).

Duck Hepatitis Virus Type 2. A disease outbreak in ducklings vaccinated with attenuated DHV type 1 was reported in Norfolk, England, in 1965 (7). The agent isolated was shown, by cross-protection studies in ducklings, to be different from DHV type 1 and was named DHV type 2 (7). The disease disappeared from commercial flocks by 1969 but reappeared in 1983/84 on three farms in Norfolk, England. Losses between 10–25% in 3- to 6-wk-old birds and up to 50% in 6- to 14-day-old birds were recorded (45). Outbreaks on affected farms were often sporadic, affecting some batches of ducks and not others. There are no reports of the disease occurring outside of East Anglia, England.

Duck Hepatitis Virus Type 3. A disease, causing mortality and morbidity in ducklings immune to DHV type 1, on Long Island, was first reported by Toth (105). The disease was less severe than DHV type 1 infection and mortality rarely exceeded 30%. Haider and Calnek (49) characterized and named the agent DHV type 3. The disease is only known to have occurred in the USA.

ETIOLOGY

Duck Hepatitis Virus Type 1. DHV type 1 was first isolated in chicken embryos by Levine and Fabricant (69). No serologic relationship was demonstrated between this virus and that causing duck plague; likewise, no neutralization of the DHV type 1 occurred when tested with convalescent serum from cases of human and canine virus hepatitis (26). It bears no relationship to the duck hepatitis B virus described by Mason et al. (78) that has been found in domestic ducks in China and the USA. DHV type 1 contains RNA and has been classified as a picornavirus (102).

Morphology. DHV type 1 has been estimated to be 20–40 nm in size (92). Richter et al. (94) observed 30-nm particles in thin liver sections by electron microscopy (EM). Tauraso et al. (102) confirmed the size to be less than 50 nm by filtration studies.

Biologic Properties. Fitzgerald and Hanson (29) were unable to demonstrate hemagglutination of chicken, duck, sheep, horse, guinea pig, mouse, snake, swine, and rabbit red blood cells (RBCs) with use of cell-cultured DHV type 1.

Cell cultures infected with DHV type 1 failed to hemadsorb green and rhesus monkey, hamster, mouse, rat, rabbit, guinea pig, human O, goose, duck, and day-old chicken RBCs. High-titered virus suspensions would not hemagglutinate RBCs of the same species when tested at a pH range of 6.8–7.4 and at temperatures of 4, 24, and 37 C (102).

Resistance to Chemical and Physical Agents. DHV type 1 is resistant to ether and chloroform, relatively heat stable, and capable of survival for long periods under environmental conditions.

DHV type 1 resisted treatment with ether or fluorocarbon (87), chloroform, pH 3 and trypsin (102), and 30% methanol or ammonium sulfate (51). Using cell culture-grown virus Davis (18) reported that DHV type 1 resisted pH 3 for 9 hr, but longer exposure (48 hr) reduced virus titer. The virus was not inactivated by 2% lysol or 0.1% formalin (6); 15% creolin, naphthalysol, xylonaphtha; or 20% anhydrous sodium carbonate (88). Complete inactivation was reported with 1% formaldehyde or 2% caustic soda within 2 hr at 15–20 C, 2% calcium hypochlorite within 3 hr at 15–20 C (88), 3% chloramine in 5 hr, or 0.2% formalin in 2 hr (25). Haider (47) reported complete virus inactivation with 5% phenol, undiluted Wescodyne (an inorganic iodine solution), and undiluted Clorox (sodium hypochlorite solution).

Heating the virus at 50 C for 1 hr had no effect on virus titer (102). Most of the virus was inactivated at 56 C after 30 min (51). However, Asplin (6) reported it would survive at 56 C for 60 min but not at 62 C for 30 min. Dvorakova and Kosusnik (25) reported that 23 hr were required for complete inactivation at 56 C. DHV type 1 survived for 21 days at 37 C (87). Heat stability was unaffected by 1 M divalent cation (Mg^{++}) (106). Davis (18), using cell culture-grown virus, showed that the type 1 virus had a half-life of 48 min at 50 C, but the presence of molar NaCl, Na_2SO_4, $MgCl_2$, or $MgSO_4$ protected the virus from inactivation at 50 C.

Under more natural environmental conditions virus survived at least 10 wk in uncleaned infected brooders and for longer than 37 days in moist feces stored in a cool shed (6). At 4 C virus survived over 2 yr (6, 25) and at −20 C for as long as 9 yr (51).

Variability. Viruses differing from or serologically distinct from DHV type 1 have been recognized as causes of hepatitis in ducklings and have been reported from India (91) and Egypt (100). The Indian isolate is known to be distinct from DHV type l, but its relationship to the other DHV types is unknown.

An apparent serologic variant (Barnhardt strain) of DHV type I has been recognized (98). This strain, so far identified on only one duck farm, gives partial cross-neutralization with DHV type 1. However, immunization with type 1 vaccine does not provide effective protection against challenge with this variant isolate. Using a 50% plaque reduction assay in primary duck embryo kidney cells to monitor neutralizing antibodies, Woolcock (113) found that antisera prepared in ducks to both DHV type 1 and the variant Barnhardt virus had high titers (>1/100,000) against homologous virus, but against heterologous virus, the titers in both cases were 1/1000 or less. Antiserum to the variant virus may have a slightly greater neutralizing effect on type 1 virus than antiserum to the type 1 virus has on the variant.

Laboratory Host Systems

EMBRYOS. Levine and Fabricant (69) were the first to propagate the virus in the allantoic sac of 9-day-old chicken embryos. From 10 to 60% of the embryos died by the 5th or 6th day and were stunted or edematous (Fig. 24.1A). Hwang and Dougherty (60) passaged a DHV type 1 strain as two lines in 10-day-old chicken embryos. The serially passaged lines became nonpathogenic for newly hatched ducklings at the 20th and 26th transfers. The virus titer in chicken embryos was 1–3 $\log_{10}$ lower than when grown in ducklings.

Hwang (52) developed a chicken embryo lethal strain of DHV type 1 by embryo serial passages. Using a homogenate of dead embryos and chorioallantoic membrane (CAM) in embryonic fluid, mortality reached 100% at the 63rd passage. More consistent results were obtained when 5- to 7-day-old embryos were inoculated via the yolk sac.

Toth (104) found titers of 80th-passage-adapted virus to be highest at about 53 hr after inoculation: embryo, $10^{7.50}$; CAM, $10^{5.79}$; and amnioallantoic fluid, $10^{3.62}$. A high-titer live vaccine could be harvested from all these parts 53–69 hr postinoculation (PI). Essentially similar results were reported by Pan (83).

Mason et al. (77) noted a somewhat higher titer of attenuated DHV type in chicken embryos that reached a peak (10^8) in 48 hr. The latent period was between 6 and 24 hr.

Goose embryos were found to be susceptible to the virus, and embryo deaths occurred 2–3 days after allantoic inoculation (4).

CELL CULTURES. Various attempts to grow and assay DHV type 1 in cell cultures of duck and chicken embryo origin have been described (29, 30, 54, 62, 77, 87). Maiboroda (72) followed development of DHV type 1 in monolayers of duck kidney cells with a direct fluorescent antibody (FA) technique. Fluorescence was observed after 8 hr, reached a maximum after 2–4 days, and was confined to the cytoplasm. Cytopathic effects (CPE) (rounding of cells) and maximum virus titers occurred after 2 days. Maiboroda and Kontrimavichus (73) produced growth and CPE in goose embryo kidney cells. Kurilenko and Strelnikov (68) reported similar results in piglet kidney cell culture. Davis and Woolcock (21) showed that attenuated DHV type 1 grew in embryo cell cultures of goose, turkey, quail, pheasant, guinea fowl, and chicken origin, while virulent virus strains grew to varying degrees in only guinea fowl, quail, and turkey embryo cells. Golubnichi et al. (39) reported successful growth and a high level of cytopathogenicity in duck embryo fibroblasts inoculated with chick embryo-adapted DHV type 1. They recommended this procedure for vaccine production and virus neutralization (VN) tests.

Woolcock et al. (116) described a plaque assay for attenuated DHV type 1 in primary monolayers of duck embryo kidney (DEK) cells. The concentration of fetal calf serum in the overlay medium affected plaque size. Subsequently Chalmers and Woolcock (15) demonstrated that several mammalian sera had an inhibitory effect on the virus, which was nonspecific and only occurred when the serum was in direct contact with the virus. The virus-inhibitory substance in fetal calf serum appeared to be present in the albumin fraction. There was no or minimal inhibitory effect in sera from ducks or chickens. Woolcock (112) reported plaque assays for both virulent and attenuated DHV type 1 in primary duck embryo liver (DEL) cells and compared the results of in vitro assays with those obtained in ovo and in vivo. Kaleta (63) described a microneutralization assay using attenuated DHV type 1 in primary DEK cells.

Pathogenicity. Asplin (5) and Reuss (93) reported loss of pathogenicity for ducklings after chicken embryo passages. Hwang (52) found one virus strain to have lost its pathogenicity for ducklings after 20 or more passages in chicken embryos. He also found that the same strain had lost its pathogenicity for ducklings after 6 passages in duck embryo fibroblasts, but the virus retained its pathogenicity for chicken embryos (53).

Hwang and Dougherty (60) reported chicken embryo-passaged strains, while nonpathogenic for ducklings, did multiply in the tissues but at a lower titer than field strains. Field strains were found in fairly high concentrations in duckling brain; chicken embryo-passaged strains could not be detected or were present in low concentrations in the brain.

A similar attenuation of pathogenicity has been reported when DHV type 1 was passaged in duck embryos (11). Embryo passage-attenuated DHV type 1 strains are still capable of causing very mild and transitory histologic changes after inoculation (97, 101), and reversion to virulence occurs after back passage in young ducklings (114, 115).

When Kapp et al. (64) encountered heavy losses from DH type 1 in several flocks of ducklings 3-4 wk old, they suspected inadequate rations as contributory causes. This was borne out experimentally when eight of nine 3-wk-old ducks fed the farm ration died after virus exposure. No mortality occurred in controls on normal feed. It was concluded that faulty diet had impaired liver function, which predisposed ducklings to hepatitis at an unusually advanced age.

Friend and Trainer (32, 34, 35) fed low levels of polychlorinated biphenyl, DDT, and dieldrin to mallard ducklings for 10 days; 5 days later birds were infected with DHV type 1. Birds receiving toxic substances had significantly higher mortality than controls not previously fed the chemicals. It appears that inadequate diet or ingestion of toxic substances exacerbates pathogenic effects of the virus.

Duck Hepatitis Virus Type 2. DHV type 2 has been classified as an astrovirus, and it has been suggested that it should be renamed duck astrovirus (40). It has been compared with astrovirus isolates from chickens and turkeys by cross-protection and transmission studies, and found to be antigenically distinct (41).

Morphology. Virus particles, with astrovirus-like morphology and a diameter between 28-30 nm, have been shown by EM using negative staining (44). Aggregates containing more than 1000 virus particles have been observed in liver suspensions.

Resistance to Chemical and Physical Agents. The virus is resistant to chloroform, pH 3.0, and trypsin treatment. Infectivity is unaffected following heating at 50 C for 60 min. Formaldehyde fumigation and standard disinfection procedures have eliminated the infection from contaminated premises (41).

Laboratory Host Systems

EMBRYOS. Replication of DHV type 2 was demonstrated in embryonated chicken eggs following several blind passages in the amniotic sac. Few embryos died in less than 7 days, but infected embryos appeared stunted and had greenish necrotic livers in which astroviruslike particles could be demonstrated by EM (45).

CELL CULTURES. Virus growth has not been demonstrated following passage in various duck and chicken cell cultures (45, 112).

Pathogenicity. Attenuation of pathogenicity of DHV type 2 has been effected by serial passage in embryonated chicken eggs (45).

Duck Hepatitis Virus Type 3. Haider and Calnek (49) reported that DHV type 3 contained RNA, based on insensitivity to IUdR. On the basis of this and other findings they suggested that DHV type 3 be classified as a picornavirus unrelated to type 1 virus; no common antigens could be demonstrated in VN and FA tests.

Morphology. EM of cultured duck kidney (DK) cells infected with the virus revealed crystalline arrays containing particles about 30 nm in diameter in the cytoplasm (49).

Resistance to Chemical and Physical Agents. The virus resisted treatment with chloroform and pH 3.0 but was sensitive to 50 C irrespective of the presence of 1*M* $MgCl_2$ (49).

Laboratory Host Systems. Nine- to 10-day-old duck embryos inoculated onto the CAM were susceptible to the virus. During the first passages embryo death was erratic and did not occur until 8 or 9 days PI, but this was reduced with higher passages. In severely affected embryos, the CAMs were discolored and the surface of the affected areas had a dry crusty or cheesy appearance. Underneath, the CAM was edematous and thickened up to 10 times normal. Embryo lesions included stunting, edema, skin hemorrhages, flaccid appearance, gelatinous fluid accumulations and enlargement of liver, kidneys, and spleen. Chicken embryos were not susceptible to inoculation with DHV type 3 (49).

Liver and kidney cell cultures of duck embryo or duckling origin were shown to support replication of the virus. This was demonstrated by a direct FA test to show foci of positively infected cells (49). Woolcock (112) reported that the type 3 virus failed to produce plaques in primary DEK and DEL cell monolayers.

Pathogenicity. DHV type 3 has a low pathogenicity for ducklings experimentally infected. Mortality and virus yields from liver could be increased if ducklings received two or three doses of cyclophosphamide (2 mg/dose) on days 1–3 and were challenged with virus at 6 days of age (14). Attenuation of pathogenicity for ducklings has been achieved by serial passage in embryonated duck eggs inoculated by the CAM route. This has increased the pathogenicity of the virus for duck embryos.

PATHOGENESIS AND EPIZOOTIOLOGY

Duck Hepatitis Virus Type 1

Natural and Experimental Hosts. In outbreaks, DH type 1 occurred only in young ducklings. Adult breeders on infected premises did not become clinically ill and continued in full production. Field observations indicated that chickens and turkeys were resistant. However, Rahn (90) found that day-old and week-old poults exposed to DHV type 1 developed signs, lesions, and neutralizing antibody. Poults, after either oral or intraperitoneal exposure, had mottled livers and enlarged gall bladders and spleens. DHV type 1 was isolated from livers up to 17 days after oral exposure of day-old poults. Schoop et al. (99) and Reuss (92) failed to infect chickens experimentally. Reuss could not transmit the disease to rabbits, guinea pigs, white mice, or dogs. Asplin (6) reported that young chickens can contract an inapparent infection and pass it on by contact with other chicks. Experimental infections in goslings (4) and mallard ducklings (33) have been reported. In experimentally exposed birds, no mortality occurred in chicks, muscovy ducklings, or pigeon squabs; low mortality occurred in young turkeys and quail, while high mortality occurred in young pheasants, geese, and guinea fowl. All exposed birds became infected with DHV type 1 (58).

Transmission, Carriers, Vectors. Under field conditions the disease spreads rapidly to all susceptible ducklings in the flock. Although high mortality and rapid spread of the disease on farms indicates extreme contagiousness, occasional exceptions have been observed. In one pen 65% of the ducks died, while in an adjoining pen, separated only by a 14-in. curb, mortality was negligible.

The first efforts to transmit the disease to small groups of three or four caged ducklings by injection and feeding of egg-propagated virus were not successful. In another experiment, with tissues from a natural outbreak, some ducklings became infected. Transmission was most easily accomplished by intramuscular (IM) injection and feeding egg-propagated virus and infected organs to larger groups of ducklings (10–20) kept on litter under a hover. The incubation period was 24 hr in most experiments, and nearly all deaths took place by the 4th day. Uninoculated ducklings placed in the same pens with inoculated birds contracted the disease and died somewhat later than injected ducks.

Egg transmission presumably does not take place. Newly hatched ducklings produced by breeders on infected premises remained well when taken where no ducks were being kept. Asplin (5) confirmed this finding.

Priz (89) found that aerosol infection of ducklings with Yagotinski strain of DHV type 1 was lethal.

Hanson and Tripathy (50) reported successful infection with attenuated DHV type 1 by the oral route, although Toth and Norcross (107) suggested that in this case the portal of entry was really the pharynx or upper respiratory tract, since the virus administered in a capsule failed to produce infection.

Recovered ducks may excrete virus in feces for

up to 8 wk PI (92). Asplin (6) stated that there is strong field evidence to incriminate wild birds as mechanical carriers of the virus over short distances. He also suggested the possibility that an unknown host acting as a healthy carrier might be responsible for new outbreaks at great distances. However, Asplin (8) found no serologic evidence of DH type 1 in VN tests of sera from 520 wild aquatic fowl of six species. These negative results were fortified by failure of Ulbrich (109) to find VN antibodies in 36 wild ducks (four species) taken from ponds where DH type 1 had occurred in domestic ducks. In addition, all 153 wild duck embryonated eggs from an infected area were susceptible to experimental infection.

Of possible significance in epizootiology of the disease is the report of Demakov et al. (22) indicating that brown rats (*Rattus norvegicus*) could act as a reservoir host of DHV type 1. Ingested virus remained alive in the body up to 35 days and the virus was excreted 18–22 days PI. Serum antibodies were also present 12–24 days PI.

Vectors are not known to be a factor in transmission of the disease.

Signs. Onset and spread of the disease are very rapid, with practically all mortality occurring within 3–4 days. Affected ducklings at first fail to keep up with the brood. Within a short time they stop moving and squat down with eyes partially closed. Birds fall on their sides, kick spasmodically with both legs, and die with heads drawn back (Fig. 24.1B). Death occurs within an hour or so after signs are noted. During the height of severe outbreaks, the rapidity with which ducklings die is astonishing.

Farmer et al. (27, 28) described duck fatty kidney syndrome and focal pancreatic necrosis, which they considered aspects of DVH. Between 1978 and 1983 losses up to 30% were recorded on certain duck-rearing farms in the UK. Two age groups, 1–2 wk and 4–6 wk old, were affected despite routine vaccination with type 1 vaccine. Gross lesions were characterized by pale swollen livers and kidneys and swollen mottled spleens. Histological evidence was indicative of DHV type 1. Despite vaccination and the age of the older group of birds, the authors suggested that this syndrome was a manifestation of DHV type 1. However, they acknowledged that DHV type 2, which was subsequently diagnosed in East Anglia (44, 45), may have played a role in this syndrome.

Morbidity and Mortality. Morbidity is 100% and mortality is variable in young ducklings. In some broods less than 1 wk old mortality may reach 95%. In ducklings 1–3 wk of age mortality may be 50% or less. In ducklings 4–5 wk of age morbidity and mortality are low or negligible.

Gross Lesions. Principal lesions are found in the liver, which is enlarged and contains punctate or ecchymotic hemorrhages (Fig. 24.1C). Frequent reddish discoloration or mottling of the liver surface is seen. The spleen is sometimes enlarged and mottled. In numerous cases the kidneys are swollen and renal blood vessels congested.

Histopathology. Microscopic changes in uncomplicated, experimentally induced infections have been studied (26). Primary changes in the acute disease consisted of necrosis of hepatic cells (Fig. 24.1D); survivors with more chronic lesions showed widespread bile duct hyperplasia (Fig. 24.1E). Varying degrees of inflammatory cell response and hemorrhage occurred. Regeneration of liver parenchyma was observed in ducklings that did not die. Ten day-old chicken embryos inoculated with DHV type 1 were killed and examined histologically at 12-hr intervals for periods up to 10 days PI (31). Histologic changes included proliferation of granulocytes in various organs, focal necrosis of the liver, bile duct hyperplasia, and subcutaneous edema. Inclusion bodies were not found. Six-day-old ducklings were infected intranasally and intramuscularly with DHV type 1 and killed 14–24 hr later. Their livers were examined by EM. One hour after infection there was an occasional breakup of glycogen within the liver cells. Spherical particles 100–300 nm in diameter and of unknown origin were visible. Changes seen in peracute cases were degenerative, and there was extensive cell necrosis after 24 hr. Viruslike particles were detected at 1 hr and 18–20 hr PI (1).

Adamiker (2) examined spleen and muscle of ducks infected with DHV type 1 by EM. The spleen showed regressive changes from the 6th hr PI and became necrotic by the 24th hr. There were degenerative changes in the nuclei of plasma cells that may have been caused by the virus. Virus particles were not identified. Only slight changes were seen in muscles.

Biochemical Effects. Ahmed et al. (3) reported that in clinical cases of DH type 1 there were lower serum levels of total protein and albumen and elevated levels of alkaline phosphatase, glutamic pyruvic transaminase (GPT), bilirubin, and creatinine. Mennella and Mandelli (79) noted that serum levels of GPT and glutamic oxaloacetic transaminase were increased in relation to severity of infection. Buynitzky et al. (12, 13) indicated that even in clinically inapparent DHV type 1 infection in mallards, liver enzyme patterns were altered, with a consequent alteration in metabolism of DDT. This may partially explain the interrelationship between chlorinated hydrocarbons and DH type 1 (32, 34, 35).

Immunity. Recovery from the disease results in solid immunity and VN antibodies in the serum. Active immunity can be induced in adult ducks by injection of certain strains of virus (6). Some strains require repeated injections to obtain high levels of antibody (93). Passive immunity can be conferred to ducklings by injection of serum from recovered or immunized birds. Passive antibodies may also be transferred through yolk to hatched ducklings to protect them. Malinovskaya (75) investigating the antibody response to DHV type 1 vaccine in breeder ducks and 7-day-old ducklings showed by a passive hemagglutination (HA) test that duck serum contained more 7S antibodies (cysteine-sensitive) than 19S antibodies (cysteine-resistant). Decline of the 7S antibodies halved the hemagglutination-inhibition titers in 43% of serum samples taken 3–7 days PI. In ducklings experimentally infected between 3 and 21 days of age the main type of antibody response was 19S during the ensuing 20 days; in ducklings infected at 30 days of age, 19S antibody was formed first but 7S antibody began to appear after 15 days. Davis and Hannant (20) reported that VN antibody was present 4 days postvaccination of 2-day-old ducklings. The antibodies were shown to be in the macroglobulin and 7S fractions by Sephadex G200 chromatography and had Ÿ or β_2 mobility by immunoelectrophoresis.

Duck Hepatitis Virus Type 2

Natural and Experimental Hosts. Ducks appear to be the only species affected and no wildlife reservoirs or vectors have been detected. All recorded outbreaks have initially involved ducks kept on open fields; therefore, wildfowl, gulls, and other wild birds have been suspected as being vectors (40).

Transmission. Virus entry appears to be by both oral and cloacal routes and deaths occur within 1–4 days, depending on the age of the ducks. Survivors excrete virus for at least 1 wk after infection (41).

Subcutaneous (SC) inoculation of 20 ducklings with an infected liver suspension resulted in deaths of five birds 2–4 days PI (45).

Signs. Ducks usually die in good condition within 1–2 hr of appearing sick. Death may be preceded by convulsions and acute opisthotonos. Polydypsia with loose droppings and excessive urate excretion is often seen. Survivors rear normally with little evidence of retarded growth (45).

Morbidity and Mortality. Birds showing signs of sickness usually die. Mortality ranged from 10–50% depending upon age of ducklings; mature ducks were refractory to the disease (45).

Gross Lesions. The target organs appear to be liver and kidneys. Significantly more virus is present in the liver. In the liver, which is usually pale pink, multiple, small punctate hemorrhages, often forming confluent bands can be seen. The spleen is invariably enlarged and "sago-like" in appearance due to scattered pale foci. Kidneys are often swollen with blood vessels injected and standing out from the pale kidney substance. The alimentary tract is usually devoid of food. Occasionally small hemorrhages are seen in the intestinal wall and on the heart fat (45).

Histopathology. Microscopic changes in the acute disease are characterized by extensive necrosis of the hepatocyte cytoplasm, and bile duct hyperplasia is usually present and widespread (45).

Immunity. Survivors were immune to further infection. Detectable antibody levels were low following infection, using a varying virus-constant serum neutralization test in embryonated chicken eggs. The virus used in this test was a chick embryo–adapted strain (41).

Duck Hepatitis Virus Type 3

Natural and Experimental Hosts. Ducklings appear to be the only species affected.

Signs. Ducklings dying from DHV type 3 infection showed the typical appearance of type 1 infection, i.e., outstretched legs and opisthotonus (105).

Morbidity and Mortality. The disease was observed to be less severe than DHV type 1 and mortality rarely exceeded 30% (105).

Gross Lesions. The gross pathological changes are similar to those caused by DHV type 1.

Immunity. An active immune response can be stimulated in adult ducks by inoculation of attenuated virus. This immunity may be passively transferred, via the yolk, to progeny.

DIAGNOSIS

Duck Hepatitis Virus Type 1

Virus Isolation and Identification. The virus may be isolated by inoculating infective liver suspensions or blood into the allantoic sac of 8- to 10-day-old chicken embryos. In embryos that die 5–8 days PI, gross lesions consist of cutaneous hemorrhage and edema, dwarfing, and enlarged greenish livers with necrotic foci. On subsequent passages the proportion of embryos that die with specific lesions tends to increase.

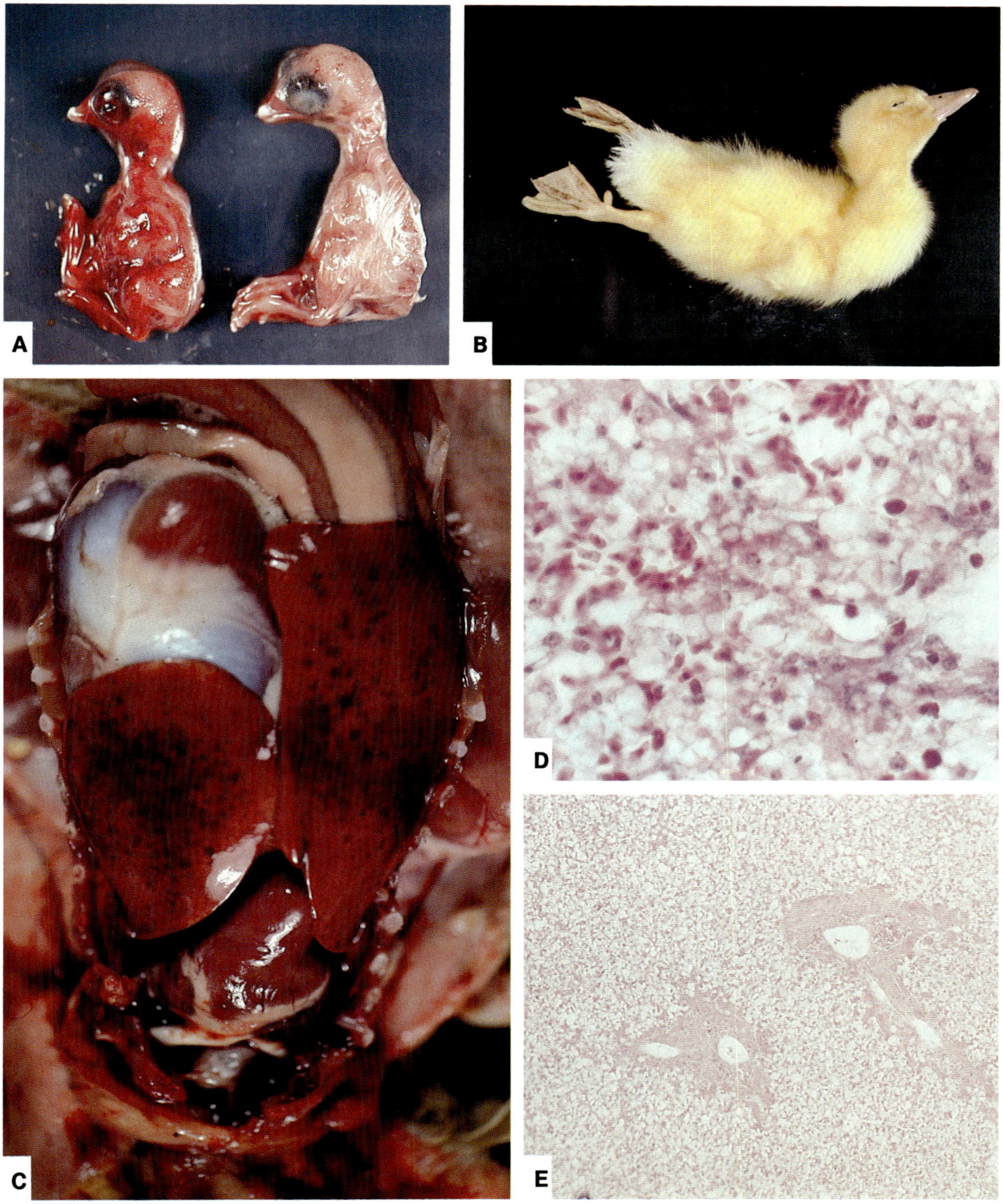

24.1. A. Normal 15-day-old chick embryo (*right*); 15-day-old chick embryo inoculated with DHV type 1, 6 days previously (*left*). Note small size, hemorrhage, and edema. B. Duckling dead from infection with DHV type 1. Note typical opisthotonos. C. Liver with hemorrhagic lesions caused by DHV type 1 infection. D. Microscopic lesions in liver of duckling 24 hr after infection. Note massive liver cell necrosis and hemorrhage. H & E, ×1000. E. Microscopic lesions in liver of duckling 7 days after infection. Note extensive bile duct proliferation. H & E, ×250.

If available, 10- to 14-day-old duck embryos from susceptible breeder ducks are preferable to chicken embryos, since embryo mortality and lesions occur sooner after inoculation and at earlier embryo passages (47, 106). A still more sensitive and reliable method of virus diagnosis is reproduction of typical signs and lesions of DHV type 1 by inoculation of virus-susceptible 1- to 7- day-old ducklings.

A rapid and accurate diagnosis of DH type 1 can be made using the direct FA technique on livers of natural cases or inoculated duck embryos (72, 110).

Primary DEL cells were shown to be particularly sensitive to the virulent field strain Quodling (Q), of DHV type 1; CPE was best detected as plaques in cultures overlaid with agarose (112).

Serology. Serologic tests have not been useful in diagnosing acute outbreaks of the disease. However, from the time the virus was first recognized (69), the VN test has been used for other purposes: virus identification, titration of serologic response to vaccination, and epidemiologic surveys.

Hwang (55) described an accurate, reproducible DHV type 1 neutralization test in chicken embryos. Modifications of this procedure were described (42, 107). Haider (47) described several modified VN tests in duck embryos or ducklings, and Golubnichi et al. (39) described a VN test with virus adapted to tissue culture. Malinovskaya (74) reported that a passive HA test was more sensitive than the VN test. Ivashhenko (61) examined the use of an indirect HA test for the diagnosis of DHV type 1 and showed a 90% correspondence between indirect HA and VN results.

Murty and Hanson (80) described the use of an agar-gel diffusion precipitin test for identification of DHV type 1. Later studies by Wachendörfer (111) and Toth and Norcross (107) claimed that reactions seen by Murty and Hanson were not specific or related to DHV type 1 or antibodies.

Woolcock et al. (116) first described a plaque-reduction test for VN antibody. This assay was considerably more sensitive than VN assays in eggs. Chalmers and Woolcock (15) showed that sera collected from 16 uninfected ducks had 50% plaque reduction titers (SN_{50}) ranging between 1/12 and 1/250 with an average of 1/59. They suggested that the maximum SN_{50} titer for negative control serum should be taken as 1/250. Woolcock (112) reported a plaque reduction assay in DEL cells and showed that type 1 virus was only neutralized by type 1 antiserum and not by antisera to type 2 or type 3. He also reported that an SN_{50} of 1/64 in embryonated chicken eggs was equivalent to an SN_{50} in excess of 1/3200 in DEK cells. Kaleta (63) described a microneutralization assay for DHV type 1 in DEK cells. He claimed the assay to be more practical, rapid, and economical than alternative tests but considered the plaque reduction assay more sensitive.

Differential Diagnosis. Sudden onset, rapid spread, and acute course of this disease are characteristic. Hemorrhagic lesions in livers of ducklings up to 3 wk of age are practically pathognomonic. Occurrence of similar disease outbreaks, caused by serologic variants or type 2 and 3 viruses, offer the main problem in differential diagnosis.

Chalmers et al. (16) reported an outbreak of DHV type 1 associated with *Chlamydia psittaci* in 4- to 6-wk-old birds and suggested a possible synergistic effect as the cause of the persistent 15% mortalities recorded. Gough and Wallis (43) reported DHV type 1 associated with influenza virus in 2- to 5-wk-old mallard ducks reared on a game farm. The DHV type 1 isolated was of low virulence, and it is suggested that the influenza virus may have exacerbated the hepatitis infection.

Other potential causes of acute mortality in ducklings include salmonellosis and aflatoxicosis. The latter disease may cause ataxia, convulsions, and opisthotonus as well as microscopic lesions of bile duct hyperplasia suggestive of DH but does not cause the same characteristic liver hemorrhages. None of the other common lethal diseases of ducks occur frequently in this young age group.

Duck Hepatitis Virus Type 2

Virus Isolation and Identification. The most reliable diagnostic method is EM examination of liver homogenates for the detection of astrovirus-like particles. The virus can be isolated, with difficulty, following repeated passage in the amniotic sac of embryonated chicken or duck eggs. The response in susceptible ducklings to challenge with type 2 virus is variable. Mortality up to 20% may occur within 2–4 days PI (45).

Serology. Convalescent serum samples have low antibody levels, as shown by a variable virus-constant serum neutralization test in embryonated chicken eggs and a chick embryo–adapted strain of virus (40).

Differential Diagnosis. Similar to that described for type 1 virus.

Duck Hepatitis Virus Type 3

Virus Isolation and Identification. SC or IM inoculation of liver homogenate from infected ducklings into susceptible day-old ducklings is unreliable. Intravenous inoculation may increase the effectiveness. An effective method to detect

DHV type 3 is by inoculation onto the CAM of 10-day-old embryonated duck eggs. Initially the response is erratic but some embryo mortality occurs within 7–10 days. The membranes have a dry crusty appearance over the area of the "dropped" CAM and beneath this they are edematous. Embryos may be stunted and edematous with skin hemorrhages (49). Alternatively, virus may be isolated and identified in DK or DEK cultures examined by FA test 48–72 hr PI.

Serology. A direct FA test in duckling livers and DEK or DK cells has been described (49). A serum neutralization test in embryonated duck eggs is possible.

Differential Diagnosis. Differential diagnosis is similar to that described for type 1 virus.

TREATMENT

Duck Hepatitis Virus Type 1. As soon as the cause and nature of DH type 1 were recognized by Levine and Fabricant (69) it became apparent that ducklings might be protected by administration of serum from immune ducks. This procedure proved to be highly successful in laboratory experiments and in the field. For many years the Duck Research Laboratory at Eastport, Long Island, NY, kept a bank of antiserum processed from blood collected at the time of slaughter from recovered birds. IM injection of 0.5 ml DHV type 1 antiserum into each duckling of a brood at the time of the first deaths in an outbreak was an effective control method.

Rispens (96) suggested passive immunization by injection of yolk from eggs produced by hyperimmune breeder ducks. This procedure was modified (48) by substituting yolk from eggs produced by hyperimmunized specific-pathogen-free chickens.

Duck Hepatitis Virus Type 2. Inoculation of susceptible ducklings with convalescent serum obtained from DHV type 2–infected ducks has been used successfully in the field (41).

Duck Hepatitis Virus Type 3. Convalescent sera obtained from infected ducks has been used effectively in the field to control outbreaks (98).

PREVENTION AND CONTROL

Duck Hepatitis Virus Type 1

Management Procedures. DH type 1 can be prevented by strict isolation, particularly during the first 4–5 wk. However, in areas where the disease is prevalent, it is very difficult to obtain the necessary degree of isolation.

Panikar (84) and Kaszanyitzky and Tanyi (65) demonstrated the feasibility of eradicating DH type 1 in selected areas where isolation can be achieved. In both studies, vaccination of breeder ducks was used as part of the program.

Immunization. Resistance against DH type 1 may be conferred to ducklings by three methods: injection of immune serum or yolk as described under Treatment; immunization of breeding stock to ensure high levels of passively transferred antibody in the hatched ducklings; and direct active immunization of ducklings with live avirulent strains of DHV type 1.

Attenuated DHV type 1 strains suitable for vaccine use have been produced by passage in chicken embryos (5, 36, 37, 39, 59, 99) or duck embryos (96). Up to this time various strains of chicken embryo–passaged DHV type 1 have been used most frequently as vaccines.

Davis (19) reported that triple-plaque-purified strains of DHV type 1 vaccines could revert to virulence as readily as noncloned virus. This finding has been confirmed with various egg-passage levels of DHV type 1 (113). Davis suggested rapid passage as a method to increase genetic stability.

BREEDERS. Asplin (5) developed a chicken embryo–attenuated strain of virus that was used to immunize breeders. The method was to inoculate 0.5 ml undiluted egg-propagated virus IM 2–4 wk before collecting hatching eggs. Reuss (93) found it necessary with the strain of virus he used to make repeated injections in breeders to obtain sufficient antibody levels to protect hatched ducklings against challenge with virulent virus. The optimum age, dosage, route of inoculation, strain of virus, and interval between initial and subsequent vaccinations are not known (6).

Rispens (96) recommended two doses of attenuated virus vaccine administered to breeders at least 6 wk apart. Passive immunity is transmitted to progeny for about 9 mo after the 2nd vaccination.

Hwang (56), Rinaldi et al. (95), Nikitin and Panikar (81), and Doroshko and Bezrukavaya (24) all confirmed that two or three doses of attenuated virus vaccine were necessary to secure satisfactory levels of protection of progeny. Bezrukavaya (11) secured effective protection by vaccination of breeders with duck embryo–attenuated vaccine. Demakov et al. (23) reported that effectiveness of the chicken embryo–attenuated strain was improved by aluminum hydroxide adsorption and a saponin adjuvant. Malinovskaya (76) looked at the effect of chemical stimulators on postvaccinal immunity against DHV type 1 by assaying for passive HA and VN antibodies. Dibazol had no effect but saponin, methyluracil, and ascorbic acid promoted an accelerated antibody response, which was particularly pronounced 15 days postvaccination.

Gough and Spackman (42) reported that effective levels of duckling protection can be secured by administering three doses of inactivated DHV type 1 oil-emulsion vaccine. These workers also reported that live DHV type 1 vaccine at 2-3 days of age followed by inactivated vaccine at 22 wk produced significantly higher VN antibody levels than three doses of inactivated vaccine. Finally, they reported that inactivated vaccine prepared from virus grown in duck eggs gave a better antibody response than virus grown in chicken eggs.

Golubnichi and Malinovskaya (38) monitored the immune response, following up to three immunizations, over a 3-mo period by assaying HA and VN antibody. The titers of laying ducks necessary to protect their offspring was 1/64 for HA and 1/32 for VN antibodies.

DUCKLINGS. Asplin (5) used his chicken embryo-attenuated strain of DHV type 1 to vaccinate ducklings by the foot-web-stick method. Reuss (93) also reported successful immunization experiments with an attenuated strain.

Newly hatched ducklings injected IM with an attenuated DHV type 1 developed resistance in 3 days (57). Oral exposure required up to 6 days for protection to occur. There was evidence that vaccination would be of benefit even at the start of an outbreak.

Lyophilized, attenuated strains of DHV type 1 induced a considerable degree of protection in day-old ducklings inoculated by the IM, intranasal, or foot-web route (117). Crighton and Woolcock (17) and Gazdzinski (37) also reported successful immunization of ducklings by the IM route with chicken embryo-passaged DHV type 1. Golubnichi et al. (39) used tissue culture-passaged DHV type 1 for duckling immunization. Effective mass vaccination of ducklings by the aerosol and drinking water routes have been reported (50, 66, 67, 82, 85, 108). Ducklings vaccinated orally at 2-3 days of age did not show an increased immune response when revaccinated at 17 days (9). Balla et al. (10) examined administration in the field of DHV type 1 vaccine by SC and drinking water routes. They reported that two doses given in the drinking water at 2-3 days of age were as effective as one dose given orally at 2 days of age.

Balla and Veress (9) examined the antibody response of ducklings of different immune status to SC and oral vaccination with live attenuated DHV type 1. They found that susceptible ducklings and those hatched with maternally derived immunity both responded to vaccination with 1600-9600 EID_{50} given during the first 3 wk of life. The maternally immune birds responded only marginally less. They also showed that a dose of 300-600 EID_{50}/duckling between 2 and 21 days and 100 EID_{50} at 35 days was sufficient for seroconversion to occur irrespective of the ducklings immune status. Exposure to an aerosol vaccine for 5-6 min at 2-5 days of age produced a good response in susceptible birds but not in maternally immune ducklings; 30 min exposure to aerosol vaccine gave good response, which was not boosted by reexposure at 16 days. They did not report any results covering challenge of any of these ducklings with virulent virus. Luff and Hopkins (71) also looked at the effect of maternally derived immunity on vaccination of ducklings with live attenuated DHV type 1. Ducklings were vaccinated when about 12 hr old and were challenged with virulent DHV type 1 at 24 hr, 3 and 6 days. Their results suggested that partially protective levels of maternally derived antibody did not adversely affect either the speed of onset or the extent of protection afforded by the currently available live vaccine. This data is unfortunately limited to the first 6 days of life.

Despite these more recent results, field experience has indicated that successful practical duckling vaccination is dependent on the absence of maternal antibodies and is influenced by time and severity of exposure to virulent virus. Vaccination is also less effective when ducklings are exposed to virulent virus early in life, especially in endemic areas and on heavily infected premises. Judicious application of proper hygiene and sanitation methods could do much to solve this problem.

REFERENCES

1. Adamiker, D. 1969. Elektronenmikroskopische Untersuchungen zur Virushepatitis der Entenküken. Zentralbl Veterinaermed [B] 16:620-636.
2. Adamiker, D. 1970. Die Virushepatitis der Entenk ken im elektronenmikroskopischen Bild. Teil II: Befunde an der Milz und am Muskel. Zentralbl Veterinaermed [B] 17:880-889.
3. Ahmed, A.A.S., Y.Z. El-Abdin, S. Hamza, and F.E. Saad. 1975. Effect of experimental duck virus hepatitis infection on some biochemical constituents and enzymes in the serum of White Pekin ducklings. Avian Dis 19:305-310.
4. Akulov, A.V., L.M. Kontrimavichus, and A.D. Maiboroda. 1972. [Susceptibility of geese to duck hepatitis virus]. Veterinariya 3:47. (Abstr Vet Bull 42:4629).
5. Asplin, F.D. 1958. An attenuated strain of duck hepatitis virus. Vet Rec 70:1226-1230.
6. Asplin, F.D. 1961. Notes on epidemiology and vaccination for virus hepatitis of ducks. Off Int Epizoot Bull 56:793-800.
7. Asplin, F.D. 1965. Duck hepatitis: Vaccination against two serological types. Vet Rec 77:1529-1530.
8. Asplin, F.D. 1970. Examination of sera from wildfowl for antibodies against the viruses of duck plague, duck hepatitis and duck influenza. Vet Rec 87:182-183.
9. Balla, L., and T. Veress. 1984. [Immunization experiments with a duck virus hepatitis vaccine. I. Antibody response of ducklings of different immune status after subcutaneous, oral and aerosol vaccination]. Magy Allatorv Lapja 39:395-400. (Abstr Vet Bull 1985:100).
10. Balla, L., T. Veress, E. Horvath, and G. Hegedus. 1984. [Immunization experiments with a duck virus hep-

atitis vaccine. II. Efficacy of vaccination by drinking water in large duckling flocks]. Magy Allatorv Lapja 39:401-404. (Abstr Vet Bull 1985:100).

11. Bezrukavaya, I.J. 1978. [Vaccine against duck virus hepatitis from strain ZM]. Sborn Rab Puti Ob Vet Blago Prom Zivot (Kiev), pp.90-95. (Abstr Landwirtsch Zentralbl Abt IV 1981:1061).

12. Buynitzky, S.J., G.J. Tritz, and W.L. Ragland. 1977. Correlation of induced drug metabolism with titer of duck hepatitis virus in chickens. Res Commun Chem Pathol Pharmacol 17:275-282.

13. Buynitzky, S.J., G.O. Ware, and W.L. Ragland. 1978. Effect of viral infection on drug metabolism and pesticide disposition in ducks. Toxicol Appl Pharmacol 46:267-278.

14. Calnek, B.W. 1988. Personal communication.

15. Chalmers, W.S.K., and P.R. Woolcock. 1984. The effect of animal sera on duck hepatitis virus. Avian Pathol 13:727-732.

16. Chalmers, W.S.K., H. Farmer, and P.R. Woolcock. 1985. Duck hepatitis virus and Chlamydia psittaci outbreak. Vet Rec 116:223.

17. Crighton, G.W., and P.R. Woolcock. 1978. Active immunisation of ducklings against duck virus hepatitis. Vet Rec 102:358-361.

18. Davis, D. 1987. Temperature and pH stability of duck hepatitis virus. Avian Pathol 16:21-30.

19. Davis, D. 1987. Triple plaque purified strains of duck hepatitis virus and their potential as vaccines. Res Vet Sci 43:44-48.

20. Davis, D., and D. Hannant. 1987. Fractionation of neutralising antibodies in serum of ducklings vaccinated with live duck hepatitis virus vaccine. Res Vet Sci 43:276-277.

21. Davis, D., and P.R. Woolcock. 1986. Passage of duck hepatitis virus in cell cultures derived from avian embryos of different species. Res Vet Sci 41:133-134.

22. Demakov, G.P., S.N. Ostashev, V.N. Ogorodnikova, and M.A. Shilov. 1975. [Infection of brown rats with duck hepatitis virus]. Veterinariya 3:57-58. (Abstr Vet Bull 45:4375).

23. Demakov, G.P., V.N. Ogorodnikova, A.P. Semenovykh, and F.A. Nabatov. 1979. [Improvement of prophylaxis of duck viral hepatitis]. Vestn Skh Nauki 10:85-87.

24. Doroshko, I.N., and I. Yu. Bezrukavaya. 1975. [Field trials of duck viral hepatitis vaccine]. Veterinariya 1:52-53. (Abstr Vet Bull 45:2458).

25. Dvorakova, D., and Z. Kozusnik. 1970. The influence of temperature and some disinfectants on duck hepatitis virus. Acta Vet Brno 39:151-156.

26. Fabricant, J., C.G. Rickard, and P.P. Levine. 1957. The pathology of duck virus hepatitis. Avian Dis 1:256-275.

27. Farmer, H., W.S.K. Chalmers, and P.R. Woolcock. 1986. Recent advances in duck viral hepatitis. In J.B. McFerran and M.S. McNulty (eds.), Acute Virus Infections of Poultry, pp. 213-222. Martinus Nijhoff, Dordrecht, Neth.

28. Farmer, F., W.S.K. Chalmers, and P.R. Woolcock. 1987. The duck fatty kidney syndrome–an aspect of duck viral hepatitis. Avian Pathol 16:227-236.

29. Fitzgerald, J.E., and L.E. Hanson. 1966. Certain properties of a cell-culture-modified duck hepatitis virus. Avian Dis 10:157-161.

30. Fitzgerald, J.E., L.E. Hanson, and M. Wingard. 1963. Cytopathic effects of duck hepatitis virus in duck embryo kidney cell cultures. Proc Soc Exp Biol Med 114:814-816.

31. Fitzgerald, J.E., L.E. Hanson, and J. Simon. 1969. Histopathologic changes induced with duck hepatitis virus in the developing chicken embryo. Avian Dis 13:147-157.

32. Friend, M., and D.O. Trainer. 1970. Polychlorinated biphenyl: Interaction with duck hepatitis virus. Science 170:1314-1316.

33. Friend, M., and D.O. Trainer. 1972. Experimental duck virus hepatitis in the mallard. Avian Dis 16:692-699.

34. Friend, M., and D.O. Trainer. 1974. Experimental DDT–duck hepatitis virus interaction studies in mallards. J Wildl Manage 38:887-895.

35. Friend, M., and D.O. Trainer. 1974. Experimental dieldrin–duck hepatitis virus interaction studies in mallards. J Wildl Manage 38:896-902.

36. Gazdzinski, P. 1979. Attenuation of duck hepatitis virus and evaluation of its usefulness for duckling immunization. I. Studies on attenuation of the virus. Bull Vet Inst Pulawy 23:80-89.

37. Gazdzinski, P. 1979. Attenuation of duck hepatitis virus and evaluation of its usefulness for duckling immunization. II. Studies on application of the attenuated strain of DVH for vaccination of ducklings. Bull Vet Inst Pulawy 23:89-98.

38. Golubnichi, V.P., and G.V. Malinovskaya. 1984. [Dynamics of postvaccinal antibodies in blood serum against duck hepatitis virus]. Vet Nauk Proiz (Minsk) 22:72-75. (Abstr Agro Selekt 1985:1973).

39. Golubnichi, V.P., G.P. Tishchenko, and V.I. Korolkov. 1976. [Preparation of tissue culture antigens of duck hepatitis virus]. Vet Nauk Proiz Tr (Minsk) 14:88-90. (Abstr Landwirtsch Zentralbl Abt IV 1977:2251).

40. Gough, R.E. 1986. Duck hepatitis type 2 associated with an astrovirus. In J.B. McFerran and M.S. McNulty (eds.), Acute Virus Infections of Poultry, pp. 223-230. Martinus Nijhoff, Dordrecht, Neth.

41. Gough, R.E. 1988. Personal communication.

42. Gough, R.E., and D. Spackman. 1981. Studies with inactivated duck virus hepatitis vaccines in breeder ducks. Avian Pathol 10:471-479.

43. Gough, R.E., and A.S. Wallis. 1986. Duck hepatitis type I and influenza in mallard ducks (Anas platyrhynchos). Vet Rec 119:602.

44. Gough, R.E., M.S. Collins, E. Borland, and L.F. Keymer. 1984. Astrovirus-like particles associated with hepatitis in ducklings. Vet Rec 114:279.

45. Gough, R.E., E.D. Borland, I.F. Keymer, and J.C. Stuart. 1985. An outbreak of duck hepatitis type II in commercial ducks. Avian Pathol 14:227-236.

46. Guo, Y.P., and W.S. Pan. 1984. [Preliminary identifications of the duck hepatitis virus serotypes isolated in Beijing, China]. Chin J Vet Med 10:2-3. (Abstr Vet Bull 1986:378).

47. Haider, S.A. 1980. Duck virus hepatitis. In S.B. Hitchner, C.H. Domermuth, H.G. Purchase, and J.E. Williams (eds.). Isolation and Identification of Avian Pathogens, 2nd Ed., pp. 75-76. Am Assoc Avian Pathol, Kennett Square, PA.

48. Haider, S.A. 1982. Personal communication.

49. Haider, S.A., and B.W. Calnek. 1979. In vitro isolation, propagation, and characterization of duck hepatitis virus type III. Avian Dis 23:715-729.

50. Hanson, L.E., and D.N. Tripathy. 1976. Oral immunization of ducklings with attenuated duck hepatitis virus. Dev Biol Stand 33:357-363.

51. Hanson, L.E., H.E. Rhoades, and R.L. Schricker. 1964. Properties of duck hepatitis virus. Avian Dis 8:196-202.

52. Hwang, J. 1965. A chicken-embryo-lethal strain of duck hepatitis virus. Avian Dis 9:417-422.

53. Hwang, J. 1965. Duck hepatitis virus in duck em-

bryo fibroblast cultures. Avian Dis 9:285–290.
54. Hwang, J. 1966. Duck hepatitis virus in duck embryo liver cell cultures. Avian Dis 10:508–512.
55. Hwang, J. 1969. Duck hepatitis virus-neutralization test in chicken embryos. Am J Vet Res 30:861–864.
56. Hwang, J. 1970. Immunizing breeder ducks with chicken embryo-propagated duck hepatitis virus for production of parental immunity in their progenies. Am J Vet Res 31:805–807.
57. Hwang, J. 1972. Active immunization against duck hepatitis virus. Am J Vet Res 33:2539–2544.
58. Hwang, J. 1974. Susceptibility of poultry to duck hepatitis viral infection. Am J Vet Res 35:477–479.
59. Hwang, J., and E. Dougherty III. 1962. Serial passage of duck hepatitis virus in chicken embryos. Avian Dis 6:435–440.
60. Hwang, J., and E. Dougherty III. 1964. Distribution and concentration of duck hepatitis virus in inoculated ducklings and chicken embryos. Avian Dis 8:264–268.
61. Ivashhenko, V. 1982. [The use of indirect hemagglutination reaction for the diagnosis of virus hepatitis of ducklings]. Eksp Inf Inst Ptits 109:32–34. (Abstr Landwirtsch Zentralbl Abt IV 1983:174).
62. Kaeberle, M.L., J.W. Drake, and L.E. Hanson. 1961. Cultivation of duck hepatitis virus in tissue culture. Proc Soc Exp Biol Med 106:755–757.
63. Kaleta, E. F. 1988. Duck viral hepatitis type I vaccination: Monitoring of the immune response with a microneutralization test in Pekin duck embryo kidney cell culture. Avian Pathol 17:325–332.
64. Kapp, P., F. Karsai, and I. Weiner. 1969. [On the pathogenesis of virus hepatitis of ducks]. Magy Allatorv Lapja 24:289–294. (Abstr Vet Bull 40:112).
65. Kaszanyitzky, E.J., and J. Tanyi. 1980. [Studies on the laboratory diagnosis and epizootiology of duck virus hepatitis]. Magy Allatorv Lapja 35:808–814.
66. Korolkov, V.I., and G.P. Tishchenko. 1975. [Laboratory trials of a duck hepatitis vaccine]. Tr Beloruss NI Vet Inst 13:79–83.
67. Korolkov, V.I., and V.P. Golubnichi, P.S. Khandogin, and M.A. Karvus. 1979. [Aerosol vaccination method for virus hepatitis in ducklings]. Vet Nauk Proiz Tr (Minsk) 17:82–83. (Abstr Landwirtsch Zentralbl Abt IV 1980:2235).
68. Kurilenko, A.N., and A.P. Strelnikov. 1976. [Cytopathic effect of duck hepatitis virus in transplantable piglet kidney cell culture]. Sb Nauk Trud Moscow Vet Akad 85:122–124. (Abstr Vet Bull 1978:317).
69. Levine, P.P., and J. Fabricant. 1950. A hithertoundescribed virus disease of ducks in North America. Cornell Vet 40:71–86.
70. Levine, P.P., and M.S. Hofstad. 1945. Duck disease investigation. Annu Rep New York State Vet Coll, Ithaca, pp. 55–56.
71. Luff, P.R., and I.G. Hopkins. 1986. Live duck virus hepatitis vaccination of maternally immune ducklings. Vet Rec 119:502–503.
72. Maiboroda, A.D. 1972. [Formation of duck hepatitis virus in culture cells]. Veterinariya (8):50–52. (Abstr Vet Bull 42:6905).
73. Maiboroda, A.D., and L.M. Kontrimavichus. 1968. [Propagation of duck hepatitis virus in goose-embryo cells]. Byull Vses Inst Eksp Vet 4:5–7.
74. Malinovskaya, G.V. 1980. [Use of passive hemagglutination reaction to determine antibodies in hyperimmune serum against virus hepatitis of ducklings]. Tr Beloruss Inst Eksp Vet Minsk 18:54–56. (Abstr Landwirtsch Zentralbl Abt IV 1981:1796).
75. Malinovskaya, G.V. 1982. [Formation of 19S and 7S antibodies during immunogenesis and pathogenesis of duck viral hepatitis]. Vet Nauk Proiz (Minsk) 19:68–70. (Abstr Vet Bull 53:3209).
76. Malinovskaya, G.V. 1984. [Influence of chemical stimulators on postvaccinal immunity against duck viral hepatitis]. Vet Nauk Proiz (Minsk) 22:75–78. (Abstr Agro Selekt 1985:1973).
77. Mason, R.A., N.M. Tauraso, and R.K. Ginn. 1972. Growth of duck hepatitis virus in chicken embryos and in cell cultures derived from infected embryos. Avian Dis 16:973–979.
78. Mason, W.S., G. Seal, and J. Summers. 1980. Virus of Pekin ducks with structural and biological relatedness to human hepatitis B virus. J Virol 36:829–836.
79. Mennella, G.R., and G. Mandelli. 1977. [Glutamic-oxaloacetic (GOT) and glutamic-pyruvic (GPT) transaminases in the blood serum in experimental viral hepatitis of ducklings]. Arch Vet Ital 28:187–190.
80. Murty, D.K., and L.E. Hanson. 1961. A modified microgel diffusion method and its application in the study of the virus of duck hepatitis. Am J Vet Res 22:274–278.
81. Nikitin, M.G., and I.I. Panikar. 1974. [Specific prophylaxis of duck virus hepatitis]. Veterinariya 8:51–53. (Abstr Vet Bull 45:692).
82. Nikitin, M.G., I.I. Panikar, and V.V. Garkavaya. 1976. [Aerosol immunization against duck virus hepatitis]. Vestn Skh Nauki 1:124–26.
83. Pan, W.S. 1981. [Growth curve and distribution of chick-embryo-adapted duck hepatitis virus in embryonated chicken eggs]. Acta Vet Zootech Sin 12:259–262. (Abstr Vet Bull 1982:494).
84. Panikar, I.I. 1979. [Eradicating duck hepatitis virus from flocks]. Veterinariya 4:35–36.
85. Panikar, I., and V. Gostrik. 1981. [Aerosol vaccination of ducklings against duck virus hepatitis]. Ptitsevodstvo 11:35. (Abstr Landwirtsch Zentralbl Abt IV 1982:1475).
86. Park, N.Y. 1985. [Occurrence of duck virus hepatitis in Korea]. Korean J Vet Res 25:171–174.
87. Pollard, M., and T.J. Starr. 1959. Propagation of duck hepatitis virus in tissue culture. Proc Soc Exp Biol Med 101:521–524.
88. Polyakov, A.A., and G.D. Volkovsky. 1969. [Survival of duckling hepatitis virus outside the host and methods of disinfection]. Vses Inst Vet Sanit 34:278–290. (Abstr Vet Bull 40:4843).
89. Priz, N.N. 1973. [Comparative study of virus hepatitis in animals (dogs and ducks) using different routes of influence]. Vopr Virusol 6:696–700. (Abstr Vet Bull 44:2746).
90. Rahn, D.P. 1962. Susceptibility of turkeys to duck hepatitis virus and turkey hepatitis virus. MS thesis, Univ Illinois.
91. Rao, S.B.V., and B.R. Gupta. 1967. Studies on a filterable agent causing hepatitis in ducklings, and biliary cirrhosis and blood dyscrasia in adults. Indian J Poult Sci 2:18–30.
92. Reuss, U. 1959. Virusbiologische Untersuchungen bei der Entenhepatitis. Zentralbl Veterinaermed 6:209–248.
93. Reuss, U. 1959. Versuche zur aktiven und passiven Immunisierung bei der Virushepatitis der Entenküken. Zentralbl Veterinaermed 6:808–815.
94. Richter, W.R., E.J. Rozok, and S.M. Moize. 1964. Electron microscopy of virus like particles associated with duck viral hepatitis. Virology 24:114–116.
95. Rinaldi, A., G. Mandelli, G. Cervio, and A. Valeri. 1970. [Immunization of the duck against viral hepatitis]. Atti Soc Ital Sci Vet 24:663–665.
96. Rispens, B.H. 1969. Some aspects of control of infectious hepatitis in ducklings. Avian Dis 13:417–426.

97. Roszkowski, J., W. Kozaczynski, and P. Gazdzinski. 1980. Effect of attenuation on the pathogenicity of duck hepatitis virus, histopathological study. Bull Vet Inst Pulawy 24:41–48.
98. Sandhu, T. 1988. Personal communication.
99. Schoop, G., H. Staub, and K. Erguney. 1959. [Virus hepatitis of ducks. V. Attempted adaptation of the virus to chicken embryos]. Monatsh Tierheilkd 11:99–106.
100. Shalaby, M.A., M.N.K. Ayoub, and I.M. Reda. 1978. A study on a new isolate of duck hepatitis virus and its relationship to other duck hepatitis virus strains. Vet Med J Cairo Univ 26:215–221.
101. Syurin, V.N., I.I. Panikar, and I.M. Shchetinskii. 1977. [Immunogenesis and pathogenesis of viral hepatitis of ducks]. Veterinariya 8:53–55.
102. Tauraso, N.M., G.E. Coghill, and M.J. Klutch. 1969. Properties of the attenuated vaccine strain of duck hepatitis virus. Avian Dis 13:321–329.
103. Tempel, E., and J. Beer. 1968. Die virushepatitis der enten. In H. Rohrer (ed.), Handbuch der Virusinfektionen bei Tieren, Vol. 3, pp. 1019–1032. Gustav Fischer, Jena.
104. Toth, T.E. 1969. Chicken-embryo-adapted duck hepatitis virus growth curve in embryonated chicken eggs. Avian Dis 13:535–539.
105. Toth, T.E. 1969. Studies of an agent causing mortality among ducklings immune to duck virus hepatitis. Avian Dis 13:834–846.
106. Toth, T.E. 1975. Duck virus hepatitis. In S.B. Hitchner, C.H. Domermuth, H.G. Purchase, and J.E. Williams (eds.), Isolation and Identification of Avian Pathogens, pp. 192–196. Am Assoc Avian Pathol, College Station, TX.
107. Toth, T.E., and N.L. Norcross. 1981. Humoral immune response of the duck to duck hepatitis virus: Virus-neutralizing vs. virus-precipitating antibodies. Avian Dis 25:17–28.
108. Tripathy, D.N., and L.E. Hanson. 1986. Impact of oral immunization against duck viral hepatitis in passively immune ducklings. Prevent Vet Med 4:355–360.
109. Ulbrich, F. 1971. [Significance of wild ducks in the transmission of duck viral hepatitis]. Monatsh Veterinaermed 26:629–631.
110. Vertinskii, K.I., B.F. Bessarabov, A.N. Kurilenko, A.P. Strelnikov, and P.M. Makhno. 1968. [Pathogenesis and diagnosis of duck viral hepatitis]. Veterinariya 7:27–30. (Abstr Vet Bull 39:2074).
111. Wachendörfer, G. 1965. Das Agar-präzipitationsverfahren bei der Entenhepatitis, der Newcastle-Krankheit und besonders der klassischen Schweinepest-Seine Leistungsfähigkeit und Grenzen in der Virusdiagnostik. Zentralbl Veterinaermed 12:55–66.
112. Woolcock, P.R. 1986. An assay for duck hepatitis virus type I in duck embryo liver cells and a comparison with other assays. Avian Pathol 15:75–82.
113. Woolcock, P.R. 1988. Unpublished data.
114. Woolcock, P.R., and G.W. Crighton. 1979. Duck virus hepatitis: Serial passage of attenuated virus in ducklings. Vet Rec 105:30–32.
115. Woolcock, P.R. and Crighton, G.W. 1981. Duck virus hepatitis: The effect of attenuation on virus stability in ducklings. Avian Pathol 10:113–119.
116. Woolcock, P.R., W.S.K. Chalmers, and D. Davis. 1982. A plaque assay for duck hepatitis virus. Avian Pathol 11:607–610.
117. Zubtsova, R.A. 1971. [Laboratory trial of live vaccine against duck hepatitis containing GNKI attenuated strains]. Tr Gos Nauchn-Kontrol Inst Vet Prep 17:127–132. (Abstr Vet Bull 42:1870).

25 DUCK VIRUS ENTERITIS (DUCK PLAGUE)

Louis Leibovitz

INTRODUCTION. Duck virus enteritis (DVE) is an acute, contagious herpesvirus infection of ducks, geese, and swans, characterized by vascular damage, with tissue hemorrhages and free blood in body cavities, digestive mucosal eruptions, lesions of lymphoid organs, and degenerative changes in parenchymatous organs.

Synonyms for the disease are duck plague, eendenpest (Dutch), peste du canard (French), entenpest (German), and DVE (58). Although Bos (3) first used the term duck plague, it was proposed as the official name by Jansen and Kunst in 1949 (30). Subsequently, DVE, based on principal features of the disease and to distinguish it from fowl plague, has become the preferred term.

In duck-producing areas of the world where the disease has been reported, DVE has produced significant economic losses. When severe outbreaks occur in breeders, associated loss of egg production and replacement ducklings may halt production. If the disease occurs at marketing, high carcass condemnation can be expected. DVE has caused losses in excess of $1 million during a 1-yr period for the small, but concentrated, duck-producing area of Long Island, NY (41).

Since the first reports of DVE in free-flying anseriforms (ducks, geese, and swans) (36, 42), serious outbreaks in migratory waterfowl with high mortality have occurred (18). Outbreaks in zoos and game farm flocks have also been reported (24, 40, 48). Although the virus has been adapted to grow in embryonating chicken eggs and chicks under 2 wk of age (29), natural infection has been limited to anseriforms. Infection has not been reported in other avian species, mammals, or humans.

Prior to the 1973 massive outbreak in migratory waterfowl in the Mississippi flyway, the USDA considered the disease exotic; however, DVE is now considered enzootic because of its wide geographic distribution in North America. For a review of the disease in North American waterfowl see Brand (4).

HISTORY. Baudet (1923) (2) reported an outbreak of an acute, hemorrhagic disease of domestic ducks in the Netherlands. Bacterial cultures were negative, and the disease was experimentally reproduced in domestic ducks by injection of sterile filtered liver suspensions. Although presented as a previously unknown viral infection of ducks not infecting chickens, it was concluded the disease was due to a specific duck-adapted strain of fowl plague (influenza) virus. Subsequently, similar outbreaks were reported in the Netherlands. DeZeeuw (17) substantiated Baudet's findings and again indicated specificity of the virus for ducks. Although chickens, pigeons, and rabbits were refractory to experimental infection, DeZeeuw believed the agent to be a specific duck-adapted strain of fowl plague virus and suspected wild waterfowl were carriers of the disease, as they were found within outbreak areas.

Bos (3) reexamined findings of the above workers and observed new outbreaks. He further characterized lesions, clinical course, and immune response of ducks by experimental study and was unable to experimentally infect chickens, pigeons, rabbits, guinea pigs, rats, or mice. He concluded the disease was not due to fowl plague virus, but was a new distinct viral disease of ducks, which he termed "duck plague." This conclusion was based on the high degree of specificity of the agent for ducks, both in experimental and natural infections, persistence of the disease as a uniform entity in the Netherlands, and longer incubation period. He differentiated it from Newcastle disease. These observations have been further supported by more detailed studies on virus propagation, incidence and distribution, pathology, and immunity (25–32).

INCIDENCE AND DISTRIBUTION. In addition to the Netherlands, DVE has been suspected in China (31) and confirmed in France (19, 46), Belgium (16), India (50, 51), Thailand (52), England (1, 20), and Canada (21, 61).

In 1967 the first reported outbreak on the American continent was observed in White Pekin ducks in the concentrated duck-producing area of Long Island (41). In addition, outbreaks in wild, free-flying waterfowl on Long Island have occurred at seven different locations (36, 42). The disease has been repeatedly detected in New York, Pennsylvania (23), Maryland (49), and California (55). An extensive survey for DVE virus in North American wild waterfowl failed to detect the virus, indicating the disease is not enzootic in them (5).

Concentrated large numbers of susceptible domestic ducks and geese enhance the probability of disease detection. In contrast, lack of information on DVE in wild waterfowl, small domestic flocks, ornamental-bird collections, and zoos results from limited surveillance and inadequate sampling. Accordingly, the reported incidence of DVE in domestic ducks may be misleading when compared to its natural occurrence in other anseriformes.

In the Netherlands a higher incidence of DVE was noted in the spring (26); however, on Long Island, no seasonal increase was noted. In contrast, a higher incidence of DVE in wild, free-flying anseriforms on Long Island was observed in the fall of 1967 (36).

ETIOLOGY. The causative agent of DVE is a herpesvirus.

Morphology. Electron microscopy of virus-infected cell cultures 48 hr postinoculation revealed virus particles in both the nucleus and cytoplasm of the cell (6). Two types of particles were present in the nucleus: one approximately 91 nm in diameter with a core approximately 48 nm, and the other a small, dense particle approximately 32 nm in diameter. Larger particles, approximately 181 nm in diameter with densely stained 74-nm cores were observed in the cytoplasm (Fig. 25.1). These had a less densely stained envelope. Capsid structure of the virion has not been resolved (6). Estimated size of the virus has also been determined by filtration studies. Virus suspensions passed through membrane filters of 220 nm porosity, but infectious virus was retained by 100-nm-porosity membranes (22).

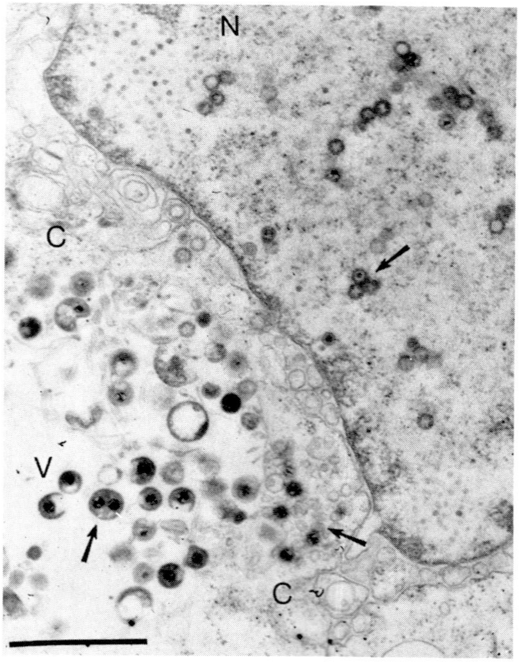

25.1. Thin section of Epon-embedded cells infected 48 hr with Long Island isolate of DVE virus. Virus particles (*arrows*) appear in several forms in the nucleus (*N*). Bar = 1 μm. (Breese and Dardiri)

Biologic Properties. DVE virus is nonhemagglutinating (25) and nonhemadsorbing (14). It causes intranuclear inclusions in infected chicken and duck embryo cell cultures (22) (Fig. 25.2). The virus has the ability to form plaques in cell cultures (14). In the presence of complement, antibodies to DVE virus are capable of lysing infected duck embryo fibroblasts (35).

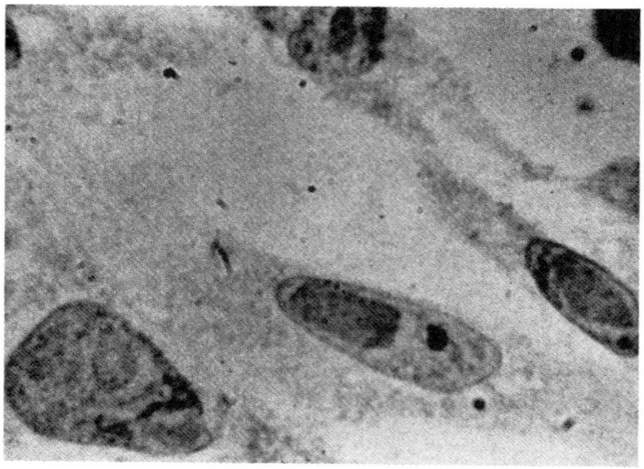
25.2. Inclusion bodies in duck embryo fibroblasts infected with DVE virus. ×10,000. (Plum Island Anim Dis Lab)

Chemical Composition. The virion contains DNA (6). RNase had no effect on ultrastructural morphology of the virus, while exposure to DNase led to removal of the central core without affecting the envelope. Fluorescence of intranuclear inclusion bodies in cell cultures stained with acridine orange was also consistent with presence of DNA (22). Inactivation by pancreatic lipase indicates virions contain an essential lipid (22).

Replication. Development of the virus in cell cultures was studied by electron microscopy and growth curves of intracellular and extracellular virus. Examination of thin sections revealed development forms only in the nucleus 12 hr postinoculation. By 24 hr, in addition to viral forms in the nucleus, larger particles with an envelope were observed in the cytoplasm. Virus titrations of similar cell cultures demonstrated new cell-associated virus 4 hr postinoculation, with maximum titer at 48 hr. Extracellular virus was first detected 6–8 hr postinoculation and reached maximum titer at 60 hr (6). Increased incubation temperatures of tissue cultures (39.5–41.5 C) favored viral replication, especially less-virulent strains (7).

Resistance to Chemical and Physical Agents The virus was found to be sensitive to ether and chloroform (22). Exposing virus for 18 hr at 37 C to trypsin, chymotrypsin, and pancreatic lipase markedly reduced or inactivated it, while papain, lysozyme, cellulase, DNase, and RNase had no effect.

Thermal inactivation studies (22) revealed that infectivity was destroyed after heating for 10 min at 56 C or 90–120 min at 50 C. At room temperature (22 C), infectivity was lost after 30 days. Drying over calcium chloride at 22 C resulted in inactivation after 9 days.

Exposure of virus for 6 hr at pH 7, 8, and 9 resulted in no loss of titer, but a measurable titer reduction was noted at pH 5, 6, and 10. At pH 3 and 11, virus was rapidly inactivated. A marked difference in inactivation rates was noted between pH 10 and 10.5 (22).

Strain Classification. While differences in virulence among DVE virus strains have been noted, all appear immunologically identical (22, 29, 56). The virus is immunologically distinct from other avian viruses, including fowl plague, Newcastle disease, duck hepatitis viruses (3, 14, 30, 43), and herpesviruses (54).

Laboratory Host Systems. Primary isolation of virus can best be obtained by propagation in duck embryo fibroblast tissue culture (63) incubated at 39.5–41.5 C (7), or on the chorioallantoic membrane (CAM) of 9–14 day old embryonating duck eggs (25). Virus can be adapted to grow in embryonating chicken eggs (25); however, they are unsatisfactory for primary isolation. It has been propagated in chicken embryo cell cultures (14) and Muscovy duck fibroblasts (33).

A cytopathic effect occurs in cell cultures (34); a cell culture plaque assay method for titrating DVE virus concentrations and plaque inhibition by neutralizing antisera have been developed (14).

PATHOGENESIS AND EPIZOOTOLOGY

Natural and Experimental Hosts. Natural susceptibility to DVE has been limited to members of the family Anatidae (ducks, geese, swans) of the order Anseriformes. The fact that the virus can be adapted by serial passage to grow in embryonating chicken eggs and chickens up to 2 wk of age (28, 29) suggests a wider host range may exist than is currently known. Natural outbreaks have occurred in a variety of domestic ducks (*Anas platyrhynchos*), including White Pekin, Khaki Campbell, Indian runner, hybrids, and native ducks of mixed breeding. Outbreaks have been noted in muscovy ducks (*Cairina moschata*) (25, 42) and domestic geese (*Anser anser*) (32). Grey call ducks have been found resistant to lethal infection (59). Outbreaks of DVE in domestic ducks are frequently associated with aquatic environments cohabited by wild waterfowl (17, 42).

Susceptibility of various species of anseriforms to experimental DVE has been studied (59). In addition to domesticated species, they found mallards (*A. platyrhynchos*), Garganey teals (*A. querquedula*), gadwalls (*A. strepera*), European widgeons (*A. penelope*), wood ducks (*Aix sponsa*), shovelers (*Spatula clypeata*), common pochards (*Aythya ferina*), common eiders (*Somateria mollissima*), white-fronted geese (*Anser albifrons*), bean geese (*Anser fabalis*), and mute swans (*Cygnus olor*) susceptible to lethal infection. European teals (*A. crecca*) and pintails (*A. acuta*) were resistant to lethal effects but produced antibodies against DVE as a result of experimental exposure. Mallards were more resistant to lethal effects, and were considered a possible natural reservoir of infection. A recent experimental study (60) showed blue-winged teals (*A. discors*) and Canada geese were extremely susceptible to DVE and experienced high mortalities. Blue-winged teals had few gross lesions at necropsy.

Of the order Charadriiformes, herring gulls (*Larus argentatus*) and black-headed gulls (*L. ridibundus*) were not susceptible to experimental infection and failed to produce antibodies against DVE (59).

The first reported outbreaks of spontaneous DVE in wild waterfowl were diagnosed on Long Island, NY (36, 41). It was detected in mallards, black ducks (*A. rubripes*), a Canada goose (*Branta canadensis*), a bufflehead (*Bucephala albeola*), a greater scaup (*Aythya marila*), and a mute swan. In addition, it has been detected in domestic muscovy ducks and wild mute swans in central New York, in Canada geese and Egyptian geese (*Alopochen aegyptiacus*) in Pennsylvania, and in a black duck in Maryland.

A major epornitic of DVE occurred at Lake Andes, SD, in 1973, with an estimated loss of 43,000 ducks and geese out of a total population of 100,000 (18). DVE was diagnosed in black ducks, mallards, pintail-mallard hybrids, redheads (*Aythya americana*), common mergansers, common goldeneyes (*Bucephala clangula*), canvasbacks (*Aythya valisineria*), American widgeons (*Mareca americana*), wood ducks, and Canada geese.

Transmission. DVE can be transmitted by direct contact between infected and susceptible birds, or indirectly by contact with a contaminated environment. Since waterfowl are dependent on an aquatic medium to provide a common vehicle for feeding, drinking, and body support, water appears to be the natural means of virus transmission from infected to susceptible individuals. Support for this concept is found in the history of new outbreaks in domestic ducks, which have been limited to birds having access to open bodies of water cohabited by free-flying waterfowl. Once infection is established, it can be maintained in the absence of open water or infected birds if susceptible populations are moved onto recently contaminated premises.

New foci of infection may be established by movement of infected waterfowl into susceptible flocks or onto bodies of water previously free of virus contamination. Once virus dispersion occurs, environmental contamination can be increased and sustained by recycling of infection through new susceptible populations that arrive at infected aquatic premises. Accordingly, course and direction of the infection are defined by population densities and rate of transmission between infected and susceptible waterfowl. Population densities in concentrated duck-producing areas encourage rapid spread of DVE with high mortality. Breeder ducks are usually selected and placed in a defined area and maintained in the same location for the balance of their productive life. Once a breeder population is exposed, DVE is self-limiting. In contrast, market ducks are progressively moved as they mature and relocated in areas formerly occupied by the next oldest age group. Infection in market ducklings tends to be a continuous recycling as susceptible birds are sequentially moved to contaminated environments.

Experimentally, DVE can be transmitted via oral, intranasal, intravenous, intraperitoneal, intramuscular, and cloacal routes. Potential transmission by bloodsucking arthropods may be possible during viremia. While virus has been recovered from an egg removed from the cloaca of an infected domestic duck (28), it has not been recovered from eggs laid during a natural outbreak. Experimental vertical transmission has been reported in persistently infected waterfowl (8).

A carrier state has been suspected in wild ducks (11, 17, 59). Contact between domestic and wild anseriforms is common and frequently mediated by use of open bodies of water for duck production. Experimentally stressed carrier mallards shed more virus (10).

Incubation Period and Age. In domestic ducks, the incubation period ranges from 3–7 days. Once overt signs appear, death usually follows within 1–5 days. Natural infection has been observed in ages ranging from 7-day-old ducklings to mature breeder ducks.

Signs. In domestic breeders, sudden, high, persistent flock mortality is often the first observation. Mature ducks die in good flesh. Prolapse of the penis may be evident in dead mature male breeders. In laying flocks, a drop in egg production of 25–40% may be noted during the period of greatest mortality.

As DVE progresses within a flock, more signs are observed. Photophobia, associated with half-closed, pasted eyelids, inappetence, extreme thirst, droopiness, ataxia, ruffled feathers, nasal discharge, soiled vents, and watery diarrhea appear. Affected ducks are unable to stand; they maintain a posture with drooping outstretched wings and head down, suggesting weakness and depression. Sick ducks forced to move may have tremors of head, neck, and body.

Young market ducklings 2–7 wk of age show dehydration, loss of weight, blue beaks, and often a bloodstained vent.

Mortality. Total mortality in domestic ducks has ranged from 5–100%. Morbidity, based on the observation that sick birds usually die, closely approaches mortality. Adult breeder ducks tend to experience greater mortality than young ducks. No differences in mortality rates were found in mallards and White Pekin ducks infected with DVE and *Pasteurella anatipestifer,* indicating these organisms do not act synergistically (47).

Gross Lesions. The specific pathologic response to DVE virus is dependent on species affected (36); age, sex, and susceptibility of the affected host; stage of infection; and virulence and intensity of virus exposure (41, 42).

Lesions of DVE are those of vascular damage (tissue hemorrhages and free blood in body cavities), eruptions at specific locations on the mucosal surface of the gastrointestinal tract, lesions of lymphoid organs, and degenerative sequelae in parenchymatous organs. These collective lesions, when present, are diagnostic of DVE.

Petechial, ecchymotic, or larger extravasations of blood may be found on or in the myocardium and other visceral organs and their supporting structures, including the mesentery and serous membranes. On the visceral pericardium of the heart, especially within coronary grooves, closely packed petechiae give the surface a red "paintbrush" appearance. The latter lesion is observed more frequently in mature breeder ducks than in young market ducklings. When heart chambers are exposed, endocardial mural and valvular hemorrhages may also be observed.

Surfaces of liver, pancreas, intestine, lungs, and kidney may be covered with petechiae. In mature laying females, hemorrhages may be observed in deformed, discolored ovarian follicles, and massive hemorrhage from the ovary may fill the abdominal cavity. Lumina of intestines and gizzard are often filled with blood. The esophageal-proventricular sphincter appears as a hemorrhagic ring.

Specific digestive mucosal lesions are found in the oral cavity (11), esophagus (Fig. 25.3), ceca, rectum, and cloaca (Fig. 25.4). Each of these lesions undergoes progressive alterations during

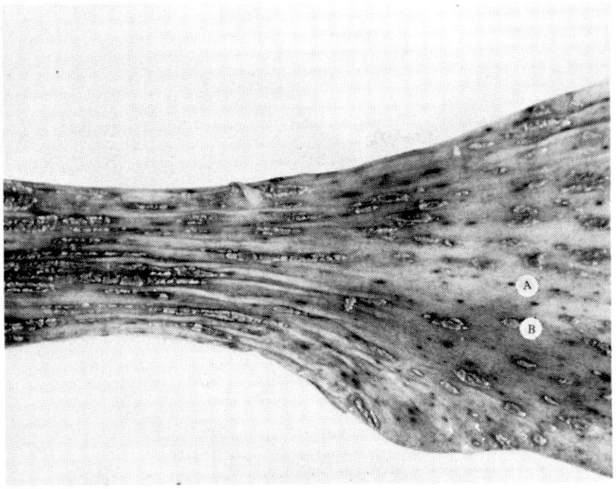

25.3. Mucosal lesions on longitudinal folds of esophagus of mature White Pekin duck with DVE. Hemorrhagic macular lesions (*A*). Supplemental crusty necrotic plaques appearing later in course of disease (*B*).

the course of the disease. Initially, macular surface hemorrhages appear, which are later covered by elevated yellow-white crusty plaques. Subsequently the lesion becomes organized into a green superficial scab devoid of its former hemorrhagic base. Lesions range in size from approximately 1–10 mm in length. In the esophagus and cloaca, lesions may become confluent; however, close inspection will often reveal their composite structure. In the esophagus, macules occur parallel to longitudinal folds. When macular concentrations are numerous, small lesions may merge to form larger ones, suggesting a patchy diphtheritic

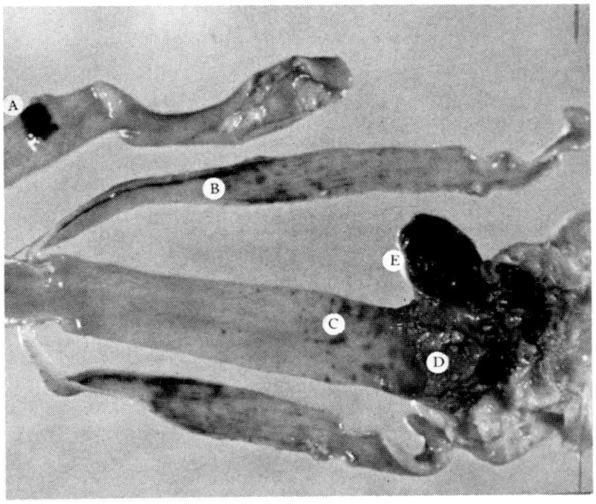

25.4. Mucosal lesions of posterior digestive tract of 4-wk-old White Pekin duckling with DVE. Dark (red) posterior ileal annular band (*A*). Hemorrhagic macular cecal lesions (*B*). Hemorrhagic macular rectal lesions (*C*). Cloacal lesions composed of dark (green), closely packed, crusty plaques (*D*). Thin-walled, dark (red) bursa of Fabricius (*E*).

membrane. In young ducklings individual lesions in the esophagus are less frequent; sloughing of the entire mucosa is more common, and the lumen becomes lined with a thick yellow-white membrane. Oral erosions can be found at openings of sublingual salivary gland ducts in chronically infected waterfowl (11). Meckel's diverticulum may be hemorrhagic and contain a fibrinous core (53).

In ceca, macular lesions are singular, separated, and well defined between mucosal folds. The external surface of affected ceca often presents a barred, congested appearance.

Rectal lesions are usually few in number with greatest concentration at the posterior portion of the rectum, adjacent to the cloaca.

In the cloaca (Fig. 25.4) macular lesions are densely packed; initially the entire mucosa appears reddened. Later, individual plaquelike elevations become green and form a continuous scalelike band lining the lumen of the organ.

All lymphoid organs are affected. The spleen tends to be normal or smaller in size, dark, and mottled (Fig. 25.5). The thymus has multiple petechiae and yellow focal areas on the surface and

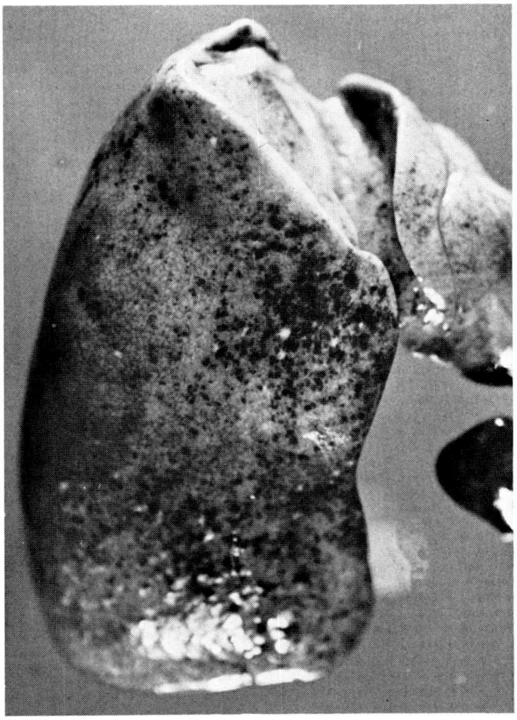

25.5. Liver and spleen of 5-wk-old White Pekin duckling with DVE. Note pale (copper) liver surface marked by pinpoint to larger hemorrhages and irregular white foci representative of early stages of infection. Spleen is slightly smaller than normal with dark mottling.

cut section, and is surrounded by clear yellow fluid that infiltrates and discolors subcutaneous tissues of the adjacent cervical region from the thoracic inlet to the upper third of the neck. The latter lesion is of importance in meat inspection and is easily detected when the opened neck of the carcass is observed on the processing line. The bursa of Fabricius is intensely reddened during early infection (Fig. 25.4). The exterior becomes surrounded by clear yellow fluid that discolors adjacent tissue of the pelvic cavity. When the lumen of the bursa is opened, pinpoint yellow areas are found in an intensely reddened surface. Later, walls of the bursa become thin and dark, and the bursal lumen is filled with white coagulated exudate. Intestinal annular bands (Fig.25.6) appear as intensely reddened rings visible from external and internal surfaces. Yellow pinpoint areas can be observed on the mucosal surface. Later, the entire band becomes dark brown and tends to separate at its margins from the mucosal surface.

During early stages of infection, the entire liver surface is a pale copper color with an admixture of irregularly distributed pinpoint hemorrhages and white foci, giving it a heterogeneous, speckled appearance (Fig. 25.5). Late stages of infection are characterized by dark bronze or bile-stained livers without hemorrhages; the white foci are larger and appear more distinct on the darker background.

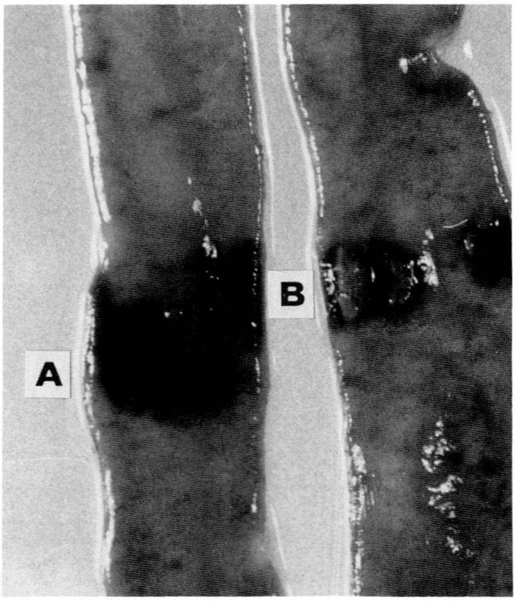

25.6. Lesions of intestinal annular bands of 4-wk-old White Pekin duckling infected with DVE virus. Anterior jejunal annular bands (*A*). Posterior jejunal annular band (*B*). Note dark (red) bands with lighter (yellow) plaques and pinpoint hemorrhages on intestinal mucosa.

Although the above lesions are representative, each age group responds distinctively. In ducklings, tissue hemorrhages are less pronounced and lymphoid lesions are more prominent. In mature domestic ducks with naturally regressed bursa of Fabricius and thymus, tissue hemorrhages and reproductive tract lesions predominate.

In geese, intestinal lymphoid disks (38) are analogous to annular bands in ducks. In a single Canada goose, lesions of the intestinal lymphoid disks resembled "buttonlike ulcers" (37). Similar intestinal lesions have been observed in an outbreak of DVE in Canada and Egyptian geese.

Histopathology. The initial lesion occurs in the walls of blood vessels. Smaller blood vessels, venules, and capillaries, instead of larger blood vessels, are more markedly involved. The endothelial lining is disrupted, and connective tissue of the wall becomes less compact, with visible separations at points where extravasations of blood pass from the lumen through the thin ruptured wall into surrounding tissues.

Hemorrhages are especially pronounced in certain locations: interlobular venules of the proventriculus, hepatic and portal venules at the margins of liver lobules, venules in the spaces between lung parabronchi, capillaries within intestinal villi, and star-shaped intralobular renal hemorrhages.

As a result of vascular damage, affected tissues undergo progressive degenerative changes. Microscopic changes can be found in any visceral organs including those without gross lesions.

Digestive lesions appear initially as hemorrhages of capillary arcades of submucosal papillae or folds. Hemorrhages become larger and confluent, elevating and separating the overlying mucosa. The affected epithelium above the hemorrhage becomes edematous, necrotic, and raised into the lumen above normal adjacent mucosal surfaces. Later, margins of necrotic epithelium separate to define the borders of elevated plaques (Fig. 25.7).

Hemorrhage from venules and capillaries fills lymphoid tissue within intestinal annular bands or lymphoid disks and lymphoid tissue of the esophageal-proventricular sphincter and spleen. Lymphocytes undergo karyorrhexis and pyknosis. Fragments of lymphocytes appear everywhere and are engulfed by phagocytes. In addition to cellular debris and hemorrhage within lymphoid follicles, there is marked swelling of reticulum cells, and their cytoplasm becomes subdivided and condensed into spherical and oval pale-staining bodies. Reticulum cells rupture and discharge their cytoplasmic contents into tissue spaces. An intranuclear inclusion body and delicate nuclear membrane and cell wall are remaining vestiges of reticulum cells.

Intestinal lymphoid lesions become large hem-

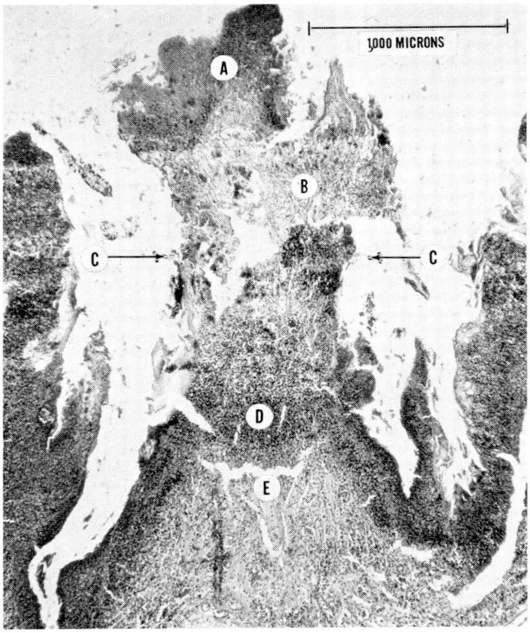

25.7. Late stage of esophageal mucosal lesion of White Pekin duckling 96 hr after inoculation. Calcified necrotic plaque on luminal surface with admixture of bacterial and cellular debris (*A*). Coagulative necrotic epithelial base of plaque (*B*). Separative margins of plaque (*C*). Hemorrhagic zone beneath plaque (*D*). Blood vessels of esophageal fold (*E*).

orrhagic infarcts. A layer of free blood separates lymphoid tissue from the mucosa, which undergoes coagulation necrosis. The necrotic mucosa forms a pseudomembrane higher than adjacent normal intestinal mucosa (Fig. 25.8).

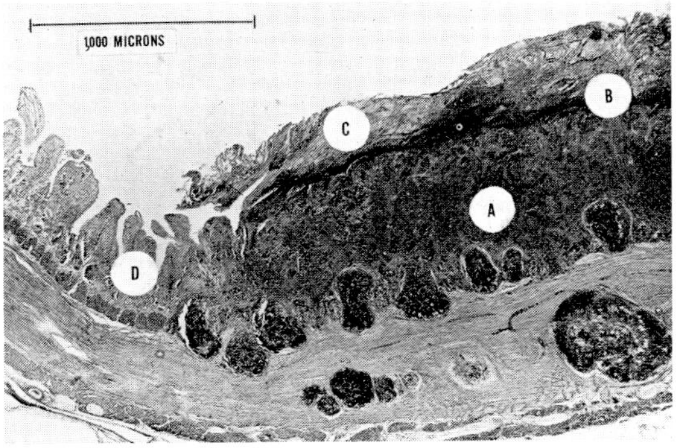

25.8. Portions of intestinal lymphoid disk and ileum of young adult Canada goose naturally infected with DVE virus. Hemorrhage and necrosis of lymphoid tissue within disk (*A*). Hemorrhagic layer (*B*) separating elevated coagulated necrotic mucosa from deeper lymphoid structures (*C*). Slightly affected adjacent ileum (*D*). Notice deeper separated lymphoid follicles in muscular layer.

In the small intestines, sheets of epithelial cells are displaced from the surface of villi, many of which are broken and cast into the lumen. Abundant blood and cellular debris fill the lumen.

Within the bursa of Fabricius, submucosal and interfollicular capillary hemorrhages are found. There is a severe depletion of lymphocytes in the follicles, many of which have empty hollow cavities in the medulla. Corticomedullary epithelial cells, capillary networks, and large phagocytic cells containing fragmented lymphocytes form the circumference around these cavities.

In the thymus, free blood fills interfollicular spaces. Coagulation necrosis of central medullary reticulum cells and destruction of cortical lymphocytes are pronounced.

In mature female breeder ducks, congestive, hemorrhagic, and necrotic alterations occur in the oviduct. Follicles may be misshapen and blood-stained. In the ovary of immature female breeder ducks, focal intestinal hemorrhages from capillaries and venules may be found.

In mature breeder drakes, focal capillary hemorrhages occur in interstitial tissues between seminiferous tubules. In parenchymatous organs such as liver, pancreas, and kidneys, hemorrhages and focal necrosis are found surrounding blood vessels.

Within necrotic foci in the liver, hepatic cords show a variety of changes including detachment and disassociation of hepatocytes from each other and their surrounding structure. A few necrotic liver cells become swollen or subdivided and discharge their cytoplasmic contents through a ruptured cell surface and are represented only by intranuclear inclusion bodies (Fig. 25.9). Similar but more limited changes occur in pancreas and kidney (39).

Immunity. Field observations suggest recovered birds are immune to reinfection by DVE virus. In an experimental study (9), superinfection of persistently infected mallard ducks resulted in death, indicating protection against mortality was dependent on route of exposure, strain of the initial virus, and strain of superinfecting virus. Active immunity has been demonstrated following use of a modified live virus vaccine (28). Parental (egg-transmitted) immunity occurs in ducklings and may interfere with response to live virus vaccines.

DIAGNOSIS. Gross lesions are diagnostic of DVE. Histopathological studies can further support these findings. Isolation and identification of DVE virus provide confirmation, even in the absence of diagnostic morphologic alterations. Isolation of a virus that fails to infect chicken embryos, but grows in duck embryo fibroblasts or on the CAM of 9- to 14-day-old embryonating duck eggs, and produces characteristic lesions and mortality

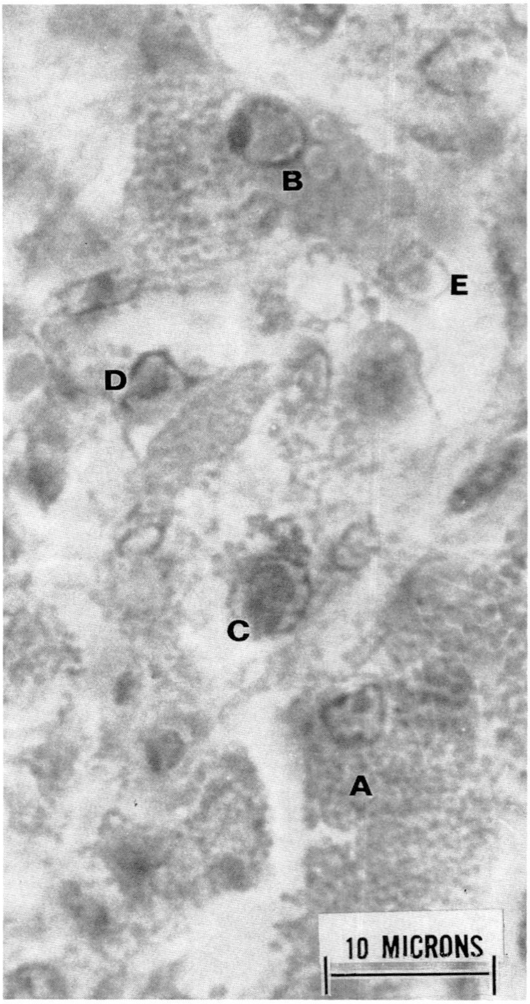

25.9. Lesions of liver of 3-wk-old White Pekin duckling 96 hr after inoculation. Nearly normal hepatic cell (*A*). Hepatic cell with intranuclear inclusion bodies and spherical bodies within the cytoplasm (*B*). Swollen hepatic cell with intranuclear inclusion body and disrupted cytoplasm (*C*). Hepatic cell with intranuclear inclusion body and devoid of cytoplasmic contents that were discharged (*D*). Empty hepatic cell with transposed intranuclear inclusion body and vestige of cell wall (*E*).

when injected into susceptible day-old ducklings is highly suggestive of DVE. Neutralization of such an isolate by known antiserum will confirm identification. Increase in virus-neutralization (VN) titers following convalescence from DVE will demonstrate progress of the disease within a flock. A VN index of 1.75 or more indicates infection with DVE virus (13). A VN index of 0–1.5 has been found in sera of domestic and wild waterfowl not exposed to the disease. Use of chicken embryo–adapted virus in chicken eggs for VN studies would be safer and more convenient than use of field strain viruses inoculated onto the CAM of duck eggs (13). Other serologic procedures for detecting antibodies include a microtiter isolation and neutralization test using duck embryo fibroblasts (62), and a reverse passive hemagglutination test (15).

Differential diagnosis requires consideration of other diseases producing hemorrhagic and necrotic lesions in anseriforms. In domestic ducks common diseases producing such changes are duck virus hepatitis, pasteurellosis, necrotic and hemorrhagic enteritis, trauma, drake damage, and specific intoxications. While Newcastle disease, fowl pox, and fowl plague are reported to produce similar changes in anseriforms, these diseases have been infrequently reported.

PREVENTION AND CONTROL. There is no specific treatment for DVE. Prevention is achieved by maintaining susceptible birds in environments free from exposure to the virus. These measures include addition of stock known to be free from infection and avoiding direct and indirect contact with possibly contaminated material. Introduction of the disease by free-flying anseriforms and contaminated aquatic environments must be prevented. Once DVE has been introduced, control can be effected by depopulation, removal of birds from the contaminated environments, sanitation, and disinfection. All possible measures should be taken to prevent dissemination of virus by free-flowing water. If authorized by government agencies, all susceptible ducklings should be vaccinated with a chicken embryo–adapted DVE vaccine.

If the disease is not enzootic and is truly exotic, measures should be taken to further prevent entry and dissemination into geographic areas known to be free from DVE. This would include specific examination to prevent importation of infected anseriforms. Accordingly, there would be surveillance of ornamental-bird collectors, zoos, and domestic growers of anseriforms. Efforts should be made to increase efficiency of detection of DVE virus by laboratory workers and waterfowl specialists so that its presence, status, and importance can be better defined.

Immunization. Immunization has been used as a preventive measure and also for controlling disease outbreaks.

The effectiveness of inactivated vaccine has been studied (12). Field experience suggests currently employed inactivated vaccines are not as efficacious as modified live virus vaccines.

A chicken embryo–adapted DVE virus strain, avirulent for domestic ducks, has been developed and used extensively with good success in the Netherlands (28). This vaccine strain has also been used to control DVE outbreaks on commercial duck farms on Long Island. An interference phenomenon following vaccination has been reported (27). Vaccinated birds acquired resistance to infection as early as one day after vaccination. In outbreaks on commercial farms on Long Island, protection afforded by the interference phenomenon has not been as dramatic, and persistent field infections have been observed in vaccinated flocks. An apathogenic, immunogenic strain of DVE virus has recently been isolated and reported to be successful for active and passive immunization of ducks (44, 45).

The modified chicken embryo-adapted vaccine for use in domestic ducks has not been authorized for use in wild or captive waterfowl in the USA.

The vaccine is administered in 0.5-ml doses by subcutaneous or intramuscular routes in domestic ducklings over 2 wk of age. The vaccine strain does not spread among contacts. Apparently, vaccinated ducklings do not excrete inoculated virus to a degree that would be sufficient to bring about contact immunization (29, 57).

REFERENCES

1. Asplin, F. 1970. Examination of sera from wildfowl for antibodies against the viruses of duck plague, duck hepatitis and duck influenza. Vet Rec 87:182–183.
2. Baudet, A.E.R.F. 1923. Mortality in ducks in the Netherlands caused by a filtrable virus; fowl plague. Tijdschr Diergeneeskd 50:455–459.
3. Bos, A. 1942. Some new cases of duck plague. Tijdschr Diergeneeskd 69:372–381.
4. Brand, C.J. 1987. Duck plague. In M. Friend (ed.), Chap. 11, Field Guide to Wildlife Diseases (General Field Procedures and Disease of Migratory Birds), US Dep Int Fish and Wildl Serv Resour Publ 167.
5. Brand, C.J., and D.E. Docherty. 1984. A survey of North American migratory waterfowl for duck plague (duck virus enteritis) virus. J Wildl Dis 20:261–266.
6. Breese, S.S., Jr., and A.H. Dardiri. 1968. Electron microscopic characterization of duck plague virus. Virology 34:160–169.
7. Burgess, E.C., and T.M. Yuill. 1981. Increased cell culture incubation temperatures for duck plague virus isolation. Avian Dis 25:222–224.
8. Burgess, E.C., and T.M. Yuill. 1981. Vertical transmission of duck plague virus (DPV) by apparently healthy DPV carrier waterfowl. Avian Dis 25:795–800.
9. Burgess, E.C., and T.M. Yuill. 1982. Superinfection in ducks persistently infected with duck plague virus. Avian Dis 26:40–46.
10. Burgess, E.C., and T.M. Yuill. 1983. The influence of seven environmental and physiological factors on duck plague virus shedding by carrier mallards. J Wildl Dis 19: 77–81.
11. Burgess, E.C., J.Ossa, and T.M. Yuill. 1979. Duck plague: A carrier state in waterfowl. Avian Dis 23:940–949.
12. Butterfield, W.K., and A.H. Dardiri. 1969. Serologic and immunologic response of ducks to inactivated and attenuated duck plague virus. Avian Dis 13:876–887.
13. Dardiri, A.H., and W.R. Hess. 1967. The incidence of neutralizing antibodies to duck plague virus in serums from domestic ducks and wild waterfowl in the United States of America. Proc 71st Annu Meet US Livest Sanit Assoc, pp. 225–237.
14. Dardiri, A.H., and W.R. Hess. 1968. A plaque assay for duck plague virus. Can J Comp Med Vet Sci 32:505–510.
15. Deng, M.Y., E.C. Burgess, and T.M. Yuill. 1984. Detection of duck plague virus by reverse passive hemagglutination test. Avian Dis 28:616–628.
16. Devos, A., N. Viaene, and H. Staelens. 1964. Duck plague in Belgium. Vlaams Diergeneeskd Tijdschr 33:260–266.
17. DeZeeuw, F.A. 1930. Nieuwe gevallen van eendenpest en de specificiteit van het virus. Tijdschr Diergeneeskd 57:1095–1098.
18. Friend, M., and G.L. Pearson. 1973. Duck plague (duck virus enteritis) in wild waterfowl. US Dep Int Bur Sport Fish Wildl Bull. Washington, DC.
19. Gaudry, D., P. Precausta, G. de Saint-Aubert, J. Fontaine, J. Janson, R. Wemmenhove, and H. Kunst. 1970. Mise en evidence d'agents infectieux dans un elevage de Canards de Barbarie. Rev Med Vet 121:317–331.
20. Hall, S.A., and J.R. Simmons. 1972. Duck plague (duck virus enteritis) in Britain. Vet Rec 90:691.
21. Hanson, J.A., and N.G. Willis. 1976. An outbreak of duck virus enteritis (duck plague) in Alberta. J Wildl Dis 12:258–262.
22. Hess, W.R., and A.H. Dardiri. 1968. Some properties of the virus of duck plague. Arch Gesamte Virusforsch 24:148–153.
23. Hwang, J., E.T. Mallinson, and R.E. Yoxheimer. 1975. Occurrence of duck virus enteritis (duck plague) in Pennsylvania, 1968–74. Avian Dis 19:382–384.
24. Jacobsen, G.S., J.E. Pearson, and T.M. Yuill. 1976. An epornitic of duck plague on a Wisconsin game farm. J Wildl Dis 12:20–26.
25. Jansen, J. 1961. Duck plague. Br Vet J 117:349–356.
26. Jansen, J. 1963. The incidence of duck plague. Tijdschr Diergeneeskd 88:1341–1343.
27. Jansen, J. 1964. The interference phenomenon in the development of resistance against duck plague. J Comp Pathol Ther 74:3–7.
28. Jansen, J. 1964. Duck plague (a concise survey). Indian Vet J 41:309–316.
29. Jansen, J. 1968. Duck plague. J Am Vet Med Assoc 152:1009–1016.
30. Jansen, J., and H. Kunst. 1949. Is duck plague related to Newcastle disease or to fowl plague? Proc 14th Int Vet Congr 2:363–365.
31. Jansen, J., and H. Kunst. 1964. The reported incidence of duck plague in Europe and Asia. Tijdschr Diergeneeskd 89:765–769.
32. Jansen, J., and R. Wemmenhove. 1965. Duck plague in domesticated geese (Anser anser). Tijdschr Diergeneeskd 90:811–815.
33. Kocan, R.M. 1976. Duck plague virus replication in Muscovy duck fibroblast cells. Avian Dis 20:574–580.
34. Kunst, H. 1967. Isolation of duck plague virus in tissue cultures. Tijdschr Diergeneeskd 92:713–714.
35. Lam, K.M. 1984. Antibody- and complement-mediated cytolysis against duck-enteritis-virus-infected cells. Avian Dis 28:1125–1129.
36. Leibovitz, L. 1968. Progress report: Duck plague surveillance of American Anseriformes. Bull Wildl Dis Assoc 4:87–90.
37. Leibovitz, L. 1969. The comparative pathology of duck plague in wild Anseriformes. J Wild Manage 33:294–303.
38. Leibovitz, L. 1969. Duck plague. In J.W. Davis, R.C. Anderson, L. Karstad, and D.O. Trainer (eds.), Infectious and Parasitic Diseases of Wild Birds, pp. 22–33. Iowa State Univ Press, Ames.
39. Leibovitz, L. 1971. Gross and histopathologic

changes of duck plague (duck plague enteritis). Am J Vet Res 32:275–290.
40. Leibovitz, L. 1973. Necrotic enteritis of breeder ducks. Am J Vet Res 34:1053–1061.
41. Leibovitz, L., and J. Hwang. 1968. Duck plague on the American continent. Avian Dis 12:361–378.
42. Leibovitz, L., and J. Hwang. 1968. Duck plague in American Anseriformes. Bull Wildl Dis Assoc 4:13–14.
43. Levine, P.P., and J. Fabricant. 1950. A hitherto-undescribed virus disease of ducks in North America. Cornell Vet 40:71–86.
44. Lin, W., K.M. Lam, and W.E. Clark. 1984. Active and passive immunization of ducks against duck viral enteritis. Avian Dis 28:968–977.
45. Lin, W., K.M. Lam, and W.E. Clark. 1984. Isolation of an apathogenic immunogenic strain of duck enteritis virus from waterfowl in California. Avian Dis 28:641–650.
46. Lucam, F. 1949. La peste aviare en France. Proc 14th Int Vet Congr 2:380–382.
47. Mo, C.L., and E.C. Burgess. 1987. Infection of duck plague carriers with Pasteurella multocida and P. anatipestifer. Avian Dis 31:197–201.
48. Montali, R.J., M. Bush, and G.A. Greenwell. 1976. An epornitic of duck viral enteritis in a zoological park. J Am Vet Med Assoc 169:954–958.
49. Montgomery, R.D., G. Stein, Jr., M.N. Novilla, S.S. Hurley, and R.J. Fink. 1981. An outbreak of duck virus enteritis (duck plague) in a captive flock of mixed waterfowl. Avian Dis 25:207–213.
50. Mukerji, A., M.S. Das, B.B. Ghosh, and J.L. Ganguly. 1963. Duck plague in West Bengal. I and II. Indian Vet J 40:457–462.
51. Mukerji, A., M.S. Das, B.B. Ghosh, and J.L. Ganguly. 1965. Duck plague in West Bengal. III. Indian Vet J 42:811–815.
52. Poomvises, P. 1976. Personal communication.
53. Proctor, S.J., G.L. Pearson, and L. Leibovitz. 1975. A color atlas of wildlife pathology. 2. Duck plague in free-flying water-fowl. Wildl Dis Color Fiche 67.
54. Roizman, B., L.E. Carmicheal, F. Deinhardt, G. de Thé, A.J. Nahmias, et al. 1981. Herpesviridae: Definition, provisional nomenclature, and taxonomy. Intervirology 16:201–217.
55. Snyder, S.B., J.G. Fox, L.H. Campbell, K.F. Tam, and A.O. Soave. 1973. An epornitic of duck virus enteritis (duck plague) in California. J Am Vet Med Assoc 163:647–652.
56. Spieker, J.O. 1977. Virulence assay and other studies of six North American strains of duck plague virus tested in wild and domestic waterfowl. PhD Diss. Univ Wisconsin, Madison.
57. Toth, T.E. 1971. Active immunization of White Pekin ducks against duck virus enteritis (duck plague) with modified-live virus vaccine: Serologic and immunologic response of breeder ducks. Am J Vet Res 32:75–81.
58. USDA. 1967. Duck virus enteritis. Fed Regist 32:7012–7013.
59. Van Dorssen, C.A., and H. Kunst. 1955. Susceptibility of ducks and various other waterfowl to duck plague virus. Tijdschr Diergeneeskd 80:1286–1295.
60. Wobeser, G. 1987. Experimental duck plague in blue-winged teal and Canada geese. J Wildl Dis 23:368–375.
61. Wobeser, G., and D.E. Docherty. 1987. A solitary case of duck plague in a wild mallard. J Wildl Dis 23:479–482.
62. Wolf, K., C.N. Burke, and M.C. Quimby. 1974. Duck viral enteritis: Microtiter plate isolation and neutralization test using the duck embryo fibroblast cell line. Avian Dis 18:427–434.
63. Wolf, K., C.N. Burke, and M.C. Quimby. 1976. Duck viral enteritis: A comparison of replication by CCL-141 and primary cultures of duck embryo fibroblasts. Avian Dis 20:447–454.

virus-infected turkey embryo intestine cell cultures; a test with potential value for rapid identification of TCV (9).

PATHOGENESIS AND EPIZOOTIOLOGY

Hosts. CE affects turkeys of all ages. Chickens (23, 39, 46), pheasants (23), seagulls (23), coturnix quail (22), and hamsters (22) are refractory to infection.

Transmission. CE is readily transmitted by unfiltered and filtered intestinal material by oral or rectal routes. Filtrates given intraperitoneally reproduce the disease, but intramuscular and subcutaneous inoculation fail to infect poults. Suspensions of heart, liver, spleen, kidney, and pancreas from infected turkeys did not cause CE when administered orally to day-old poults. Cell-free filtrates of the bursa of Fabricius from infected birds were pathogenic for adult turkeys (28).

Under natural conditions CE spreads rapidly through a flock and from flock to flock on the same farm. Circumstantial evidence indicates CE is spread from farm to farm by personnel, equipment, and vehicles. Free-flying birds may serve as mechanical vectors.

There is no evidence CE is egg transmitted, but infection may be introduced into poults in a hatchery from contamination.

TCV is eliminated in droppings of turkeys recovered from CE for several months, and remains viable in intestinal tracts stored at −20 C or lower for over 5 yr. TCV is readily destroyed by cleaning and sanitizing. In the field it can only be eliminated in buildings that can be thoroughly cleaned and disinfected, and allowed to remain empty for at least 3–4 wk before reintroducing birds. TCV may survive in pole barns, yards, and ranges from year to year even though depopulated of turkeys (39).

Incubation Period. The typical incubation period is 2–3 days, but may vary from 1 to 5 days; clinical signs usually develop within 48 hr.

Signs. In young poults and growing turkeys, CE appears suddenly; there is depression, subnormal body temperature, a drop in feed and water consumption, loss of body weight, and frothy or watery droppings. Poults constantly chirp, huddle together, and seek additional heat. In growing turkeys, the flock is depressed and sick birds show darkening of the head and skin accompanied by drooping of wings, arched back, and retracted head (Fig. 26.2). Droppings may be green to brown and contain mucus threads and casts. As the disease progresses, droppings contain mostly urates. When breeder hens in production are affected, a pattern of disease similar to that seen in growing turkeys occurs along with a rapid drop in egg production and chalky eggshells (39).

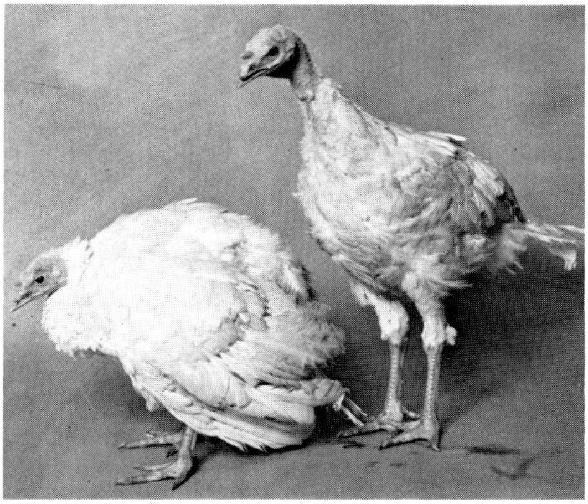

26.2. Turkey with signs of transmissible CE (*left*) compared with healthy turkey (*right*).

During experimental CE in medium white 8- to 10-wk-old turkeys, reductions in body weight, ingestion and excretion of dry matter and water, and rectal temperature were comparable to those seen in control-fasted turkeys (16). The clinical course of CE often extends over a period of 10–14 days. Birds may require several weeks to regain lost weight. In mature birds, particularly males, some never regain satisfactory weight, and there is general unevenness in the flock.

Morbidity and Mortality. Morbidity approaching 100% with weight loss depending on the degree birds go off feed and water is typical of CE. Morbidity loss may be high because of weight loss, stunted birds, and an inability of the flock to grow at a normal rate. Experimentally, losses in young poults range from 50 to 100%. In older birds (6–8 wk) mortality may approach 50%. In naturally occurring CE, losses range from 5 to 50% or occasionally even higher. In young turkeys 4–8 wk old, mortality can be kept minimal if supplemental heat is provided. In range turkeys 8 wk or older, loss may be low but is dependent on environmental conditions. In adverse weather, losses may be as high as 25–50%.

Infected poults have increased numbers of coliforms, clostridia, and non-lactose-fermenting bacteria (27). Gnotobiotic poults suffered only mild weight retardation, while conventional poults inoculated with intestinal filtrates from them suffered severe disease. Gnotobiotes inoculated with intestinal filtrates and common enteric bacteria also suffered heavier losses than those inoculated with filtrate alone (23).

Gross Lesions. Gross lesions are seen primarily in the intestinal tract. Contents of the duodenum, jejunum, and ceca are watery and gaseous. There may be gelatinous mucus and occasionally casts. Ceca are distended and filled with watery, yellow-brown contents having a fetid odor. Small petechial hemorrhages may be seen on the intestinal mucosa.

Breast muscle is usually dark and dehydrated, and the carcass generally emaciated (Fig. 26.3). Usually, internal organs are normal, but abnormalities are occasionally noted. The pancreas may have a chalky appearance with numerous white foci. Urate deposits are occasionally present in kidneys and ureters. Spleen is frequently smaller than normal (39).

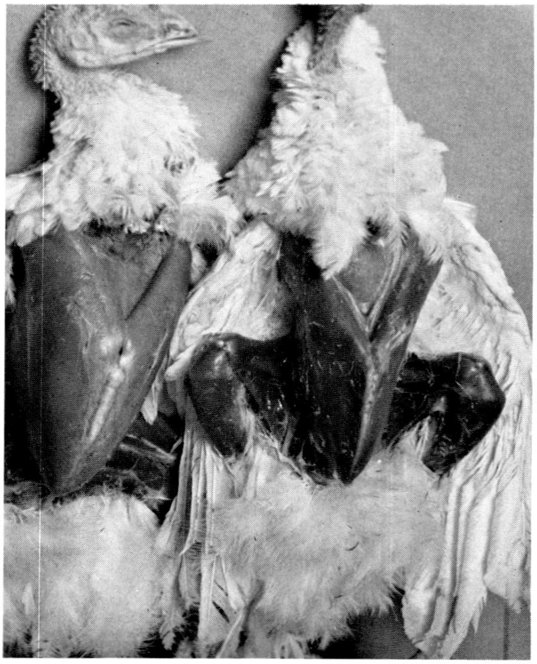

26.3. Exposed breast of normal turkey (*left*). Breast from turkey affected with CE shows dehydration and loss of flesh (*right*).

Histopathology. Intraluminal mononuclear cell exudate is present in the duodeno-jejunal area of experimentally and spontaneously infected turkeys (21). Histopathologic studies of 18-day-old poults experimentally infected with more purified virus preparations showed at 2 days postinfection, prominent concentrations of goblet cells on villi tips, cuboidal epithelial cells without microvilli, infiltration of lamina propria with mononuclear cells, and separation of epithelium from lamina propria; at 3 days, nearly all goblet cells had disappeared, and epithelial cells were "washed out" (2). A diminished cross-sectional intestinal diameter occurred along with a significantly decreased villus-to-crypt ratio (20). Lesions were most distinct in the jejunum but also seen in duodenum, ileum, and cecum. Over the following 2 wk goblet cells reappeared, epithelial cells regained their microvilli and normal density, and infiltration of lamina propria gradually subsided. Argentaffin cell numbers decreased gradually until the 7th day, returning to normal by 21 days.

Fasting produced similar signs and gross lesions in the intestinal tract (16), but not histopathologic changes (2, 13).

Transmission EM from infected poults corroborated histopathologic findings, but also showed damaged mitochondria, disrupted mucin production, and virus replication (3). Ultrastructural alterations are confined to epithelial cells (41).

Changes in the intestines of infected young turkeys, detected with scanning EM, began 1 day postinfection, progressed through the 3rd day, and regressed on the 4th and 5th days. Tissues at 10 days were similar to controls. Diapedesis and catarrhal enteritis presented a striking picture with scanning EM compared to the equivocal lesions seen with light microscopy (20).

In combined immunofluorescence and transmission EM studies of sequential intestinal samples from turkey embryos and poults infected with TCV (41), coronavirus antigens were first detected at 12 hr in a few cells at the base of villi. By 24 hr villi were markedly shortened and immunofluorescent cells were observed over the entire villi. By 120 hr villi had returned to normal, but specific fluorescence persisted in small groups of cells randomly located on villi and in crypts until 336 hr postinfection. Virus particles were detected from 24 to 96 hr postinoculation.

Hematology. Hematologic changes in CE have been described, but are not consistent except for heterophilia (21, 43). Both lymphopenia and lymphocytosis, with and without monocytosis, were found by different investigators. Other changes in hematologic parameters (hypoproteinemia, hypoalbuminemia, hemoconcentration) apparently result from fasting rather than infection. In recovered turkeys, levels of alpha and gamma globulins are increased (40).

Immunity

ACTIVE. Turkeys that had recovered from experimental CE, challenged 3–4 wk later, or longer, resisted challenge (45). Turkeys surviving experimental infection at 4 days of age and challenged at 11 and 22 wk showed no clinical signs. Gross lesions were observed and fluorescent antibody (FA) tests on intestinal sections collected at 3 and 7 days postinfection were positive in control groups but negative in immune groups (40). Field observations indicated flocks that had recovered from CE previously were resistant to subsequent attacks (39). IgM and IgG were present in the acute phase and IgA fraction at 14 days, but at 21 days only IgG was present (7).

Intestinal secretions and bile from affected birds contained secretory IgA against coronaviral antigen for at least 6 mo (24). Tissue localization of secretory antibodies in intestines of recovered birds was demonstrated by immunofluorescence (26).

Cell-mediated immune responses in turkeys infected with TCV may be important in determining immunity against infection (25).

PASSIVE. Poults given serum from recovered birds subcutaneously and subsequently exposed to experimental infection were not protected (39). When poults from recovered and susceptible breeding flocks were challenged with filtrates or infective intestinal material, they had little or no protection (49).

DIAGNOSIS. In turkeys of any age, typical signs with characteristic gross and microscopic lesions are suggestive of CE, but not diagnostic. Intestinal material from the small intestine, ceca, and bursa of Fabricius may be passed through a membrane filter of 220 or 300 nm porosity and injected into embryonating turkey eggs (>15 days) or 1- to 4-day-old poults for infectivity tests. The former has been used for routine cultivation of field isolates (31). Sections of intestinal tract from field cases and inoculated poults or embryos may be used for the direct FA test.

Immunology and Serology

FLUORESCENT ANTIBODY PROCEDURE. The direct FA test is highly useful for detecting TCV in intestinal epithelium from 1 to 28 days postinfection from field cases, infected turkey embryos, and poults. The indirect FA test will detect antibodies in serum from 9 to at least 160 days postinfection. These tests permit detection of clinically affected, recovered, and carrier flocks (31–34).

VIRUS NEUTRALIZATION. Virus-neutralizing (VN) tests may be done using turkey embryo intestinal homogenate as a source of virus, 1- to 4-day-old poults, and the suspected serum sample. The virus usually has a titer of 5 $\log_{10}$ poult-infective doses (PID)/ml. Pooled serum samples from recovered turkeys usually have a neutralizing index (NI) of 2–3 $\log_{10}$ PID. Pooled serum samples from susceptible turkeys usually have an NI of 0–1 $\log_{10}$ (38, 40).

Electron microscopy. Examination of intestinal contents by negative-staining direct EM may provide a preliminary diagnosis of CE or identification of other enteric viruses. Particles resembling coronaviruses, presumably cell debris, are often seen especially when whole intestine is prepared for examination. This, along with the pleomorphic nature of the virus, can make definitive morphological recognition of TCV difficult. Coronavirus was more easily recognized by direct EM following precipitation with polyethylene glycol than by ultracentrifugation (8). Failure to identify coronaviruses on EM does not rule out the possibility of CE. A final diagnosis of CE must be made by FA or VN procedures.

Differential Diagnosis. In young poults CE must be differentiated from inanition (starve-outs); water deprivation; and intestinal viral, bacterial, and protozoal infections. Medicated flocks may have secondary candidiasis. In growing and mature birds, increased numbers of trichomonads are found in contents of the ceca and rectum. Their role in natural outbreaks is unknown. The possibility of known specific infections such as erysipelas, fowl cholera, and enterohepatitis must be eliminated by appropriate diagnostic methods.

TREATMENT. No treatment regimen has been found completely effective in preventing CE. Antibiotics and other drugs help reduce mortality, most likely by controlling secondary infections. Individual oral treatment of turkeys with penicillin, chlortetracycline, and oxytetracycline (35) and treatment with penicillin, chlortetracycline, oxytetracycline, and streptomycin in feed or drinking water were effective in reducing death loss, but had little effect on morbidity (36, 37, 39, 47). Three nitrofurans had prophylactic value in experimental infections, reducing mortality but having no effect on morbidity (50).

Force-feeding birds under laboratory conditions produced no beneficial effect (14, 15), nor did use of milk replacer, electrolytes, and glucose (17).

Treatment commonly used in outbreaks includes:

1. In the brooder house, provide additional heat until birds are comfortable, then decrease gradually as flock improves. Birds on range need protection from adverse weather.
2. Calf milk replacer, 25 lb/100 gal drinking water, is commonly used and mixed fresh each day.
3. Potassium chloride (KCl), 450 g/100 gal drinking water, is added to milk suspension.
4. An antibiotic is added to drinking water at the highest recommended level. Neomycin, oxytetracycline, chlortetracycline, streptomycin, penicillin, or bacitracin may be used.
5. Because secondary intestinal mycosis usually follows high levels of antibiotics, mycostatin may be used in feed.
6. Medicated drinking water is used 4–5 days,

then untreated water is given 1 day and medication repeated an additional 4–5 days. It is usually about 10 days before the flock improves feed and water consumption.

PREVENTION AND CONTROL

Management Procedures. Prevention is the only means to achieve control of CE. The Minnesota turkey industry eliminated CE by controlled depopulation and decontamination of turkey buildings and surrounding areas with a rest period before restocking (34).

Farms that have had flocks with CE need to be completely depopulated of all turkeys and other fowl, followed by cleanup and disinfection of houses, equipment, and area around permanent buildings. A period of depopulation for 3–4 wk is highly desirable before repopulation, since feces from carrier birds remain the primary source of infection. Die-off of virus in feces and litter probably occurs faster in summer than winter.

CE may be introduced onto a turkey farm from outside sources. Observations point to processing trucks, loaders, equipment, and personnel that move from one farm to another without proper precautions. Other vectors may also be involved in transmission from active infections to new flocks in the area.

Immunization. Turkeys that recover from CE are immune to challenge but remain carriers for life. No licensed vaccine is available. Attempts to live with CE have been tried on some farms. To be successful, the disease must be prevented in the brooding period to avoid serious losses. This requires strict isolation between brooder house and grow-out (range) houses with prevention of backtracking from older to younger birds on the farm.

Following brooding, an exposure program may be used as follows: Poults 5–6 wk of age are transferred to a growing barn equipped with supplemental heat and controlled environment. Birds from a flock on the same farm that have gone through CE are placed in an adjacent pen to provide exposure. As soon as the susceptible flock contracts CE (usually within 1 wk), place exposed birds on treatment.

An exposure program is recommended only after all other methods of control have failed, and only on farms and in areas where CE is a continual problem.

REFERENCES

1. Adams, N.R. and M.S. Hofstad. 1971. Isolation of transmissible enteritis agent of turkeys in avian embryos. Avian Dis 15:426–433.

2. Adams, N.R., R.A. Ball, and M.S. Hofstad. 1970. Intestinal lesions in transmissible enteritis of turkeys. Avian Dis 14:392–399.

3. Adams, N.R., R.A. Ball, C.L. Annis, and M.S. Hofstad. 1972. Ultrastructural changes in the intestines of turkey poults and embryos affected with transmissible enteritis. J Comp Pathol 82:187–192.

4. Adams, N.R., M.S. Hofstad, and M.L. Frey. 1972. Growth of transmissible enteritis virus of turkeys in intestinal organ cultures. Arch Gesamte Virusforsch 38:97–99.

5. Anon. 1986. Minnesota turkey death losses and causes in 1985. Minnesota Agric Stat Serv, pp. 1–4. St. Paul.

6. Boyer, C.I., Jr. 1953. Personal communication.

7. Carson, C.A., S.A. Naqi, and C.F. Hall. 1972. Serologic response of turkeys to an agent associated with infectious enteritis (bluecomb). Appl Microbiol 23:903–907.

8. Dea, S., G. Marsolais, J. Beaubien, and R. Ruppanner. 1986. Coronaviruses associated with outbreaks of transmissible enteritis of turkeys in Quebec: Hemagglutination properties and cell cultivation. Avian Dis 30:319–326.

9. Deshmukh, D.R., and B.S. Pomeroy. 1974. In vitro test for the detection of turkey bluecomb coronavirus interference against Newcastle disease virus. Am J Vet Res 35:1553–1556.

10. Deshmukh, D.R., and B.S. Pomeroy. 1974. Physicochemical characterization of a bluecomb coronavirus of turkeys. Am J Vet Res 35:1549–1552.

11. Deshmukh, D.R., C.T. Larsen, S.K. Dutta, and B.S. Pomeroy. 1969. Characterization of pathogenic filtrate and viruses isolated from turkeys with bluecomb. Am J Vet Res 30:1019–1025.

12. Deshmukh, D.R., C.T. Larsen, and B.S. Pomeroy. 1973. Survival of bluecomb agent in embryonating turkey eggs and cell cultures. Am J Vet Res 34:673–675.

13. Deshmukh, D.R., J.H. Sautter, B.L. Patel, and B.S. Pomeroy. 1976. Histopathology of fasting and bluecomb disease in turkey poults and embryos experimentally infected with bluecomb disease coronavirus. Avian Dis 20:631–640.

14. Duke, G.E., H.E. Dziuk, O.A. Evanson, and D.E. Nelson. 1970. Food metabolizability in normal and bluecomb diseased turkeys. Poult Sci 49:1037–1042.

15. Dziuk, H.E., G.E. Duke, O.A. Evanson, D.E. Nelson, and P.N. Schultz. 1969. Force-feeding turkeys during bluecomb disease. Poult Sci 48:843–846.

16. Dziuk, H.E., O.A. Evanson, and C.T. Larsen. 1969. Physiologic effects of fasting and bluecomb in turkeys. Am J Vet Res 30:1045–1056.

17. Dziuk, H.E., G.E. Duke, and O.A. Evanson. 1970. Milk replacer, electrolytes, and glucose for treating bluecomb in turkeys. Poult Sci 49:226–229.

18. Ferguson, A.E. 1961. Bluecomb-transmissible enteritis in turkeys. Can Poult Rev 85:74–76.

19. Fujisaki, Y., H. Kawamura, and D.P. Anderson. 1969. Reoviruses isolated from turkeys with bluecomb. Am J Vet Res 30:1035–1043.

20. Gonder, E., B.L. Patel, and B.S. Pomeroy. 1976. Scanning electron, light, and immunofluorescent microscopy of coronaviral enteritis of turkeys (bluecomb). Am J Vet Res 37:1435–1439.

21. Hilton, F.E. 1954. The pathology of bluecomb of turkeys. MS thesis. Univ Minnesota, Minneapolis–St. Paul.

22. Hofstad, M.S., N. Adams, and M.L. Frey. 1969. Studies on filterable agent associated with infectious enteritis (bluecomb) of turkeys. Avian Dis 13:386–393.

23. Larsen, C.T. 1979. The etiology of bluecomb disease of turkeys. PhD diss. Univ Minnesota, Minneapolis–St. Paul.

24. Nagaraja, K.V., and B.S. Pomeroy. 1978. Secretory antibodies against turkey coronaviral enteritis. Am

J Vet Res 39:1463–1465.
25. Nagaraja, K.V., and B.S. Pomeroy. 1980. Cell-mediated immunity against turkey coronaviral enteritis (bluecomb). Am J Vet Res 41:915–917.
26. Nagaraja, K.V., and B.S. Pomeroy. 1980. Immunofluorescent studies on localization of secretory immunoglobulins in the intestines of turkeys recovered from turkey coronaviral enteritis. Am J Vet Res 41:1283–1284.
27. Naqi, S.A., C.F. Hall, and D.H. Lewis. 1971. The intestinal microflora of turkeys: Comparison of apparently healthy and bluecomb-infected turkey poults. Avian Dis 15:14–21.
28. Naqi, S.A., B. Panigrahy, and C.F. Hall. 1972. Bursa of Fabricius, a source of bluecomb infectious agent. Avian Dis 16:937–939.
29. Naqi, S.A., B. Panigrahy, and C.F. Hall. 1975. Purification and concentration of viruses associated with transmissible (coronaviral) enteritis of turkeys (bluecomb). Am J Vet Res 36:548–552.
30. Panigrahy, B., S.A. Naqi, and C.F. Hall. 1973. Isolation and characterization of viruses associated with transmissible enteritis (bluecomb) of turkeys. Avian Dis 17:430–438.
31. Patel, B.L. 1975. Studies on immunofluorescent techniques for the diagnosis of turkey bluecomb disease (coronaviral enteritis). MS thesis. Univ Minnesota, Minneapolis–St. Paul.
32. Patel, B.L., D.R. Deshmukh, and B.S. Pomeroy. 1975. Fluorescent antibody test for rapid diagnosis of coronaviral enteritis of turkeys (bluecomb). Am J Vet Res 36:1265–1267
33. Patel, B.L., B.S. Pomeroy, E. Gonder, and C.E. Cronkite. 1976. Indirect fluorescent antibody test for the diagnosis of coronaviral enteritis of turkeys (bluecomb). Am J Vet Res 37:1111–1112.
34. Patel, B.L., E. Gonder, and B.S. Pomeroy. 1977. Detection of turkey coronaviral enteritis (bluecomb) in field epiornithics, using the direct and indirect fluorescent antibody tests. Am J Vet Res 38:1407–1411.
35. Peterson, E.H., and T.A. Hymas. 1951. Antibiotics in the treatment of an unfamiliar turkey disease. Poult Sci 30:466–468.
36. Pomeroy, B.S. 1956. High level use of antibiotics. Proc 1st Int Conf Antibiot Agric. Nat Acad Sci Res Counc Publ 397, pp. 56–67.
37. Pomeroy, B.S. 1956. Use of furazolidone and antibiotics in bluecomb disease of turkeys. Proc 1st Nat Symp Nitrofurans Agric, pp. 75–78.
38. Pomeroy, B.S. 1980 Coronaviral enteritis of turkeys. In S.B. Hitchner, C.H. Domermuth, H.G. Purchase, and J.E. Williams (eds.), Isolation and Identification of Avian Pathogens, pp. 73–74. Am Assoc Avian Pathol, Kennett Square, PA.
39. Pomeroy, B.S., and J.M. Sieburth. 1953. Bluecomb disease of turkeys. Proc 90th Annu Meet Am Vet Med Assoc, pp. 321–328.
40. Pomeroy, B.S., C.T. Larsen, D.R. Deshmukh, and B.L. Patel. 1975. Immunity to transmissible (coronaviral) enteritis of turkeys (bluecomb). Am J Vet Res 36:553–555.
41. Pomeroy, K.A., B.L. Patel, C.T. Larsen, and B.S. Pomeroy. 1978. Combined immunofluorescence and transmission electron microscopic studies of sequential intestinal samples from turkey embryos and poults infected with turkey enteritis coronavirus. Am J Vet Res 39:1348–1354.
42. Ritchie, A.E., D.R. Deshmukh, C.T. Larsen, and B.S. Pomeroy. 1973. Electron microscopy of coronavirus-like particles characteristic of turkey bluecomb disease. Avian Dis 17:546–558.
43. Schultz, P.N., D.E. Nelson, H.E. Dziuk, G.E. Duke, and C.T. Larsen. 1970. Hemic studies in normal and bluecomb diseased turkeys. Poult Sci 49:136–145.
44. Sharma, T.S. 1968. Characterization and comparative studies of vibrios associated with bluecomb disease (transmissible enteritis) of turkeys. PhD diss. Univ Minnesota, Minneapolis–St. Paul.
45. Sieburth, J.M. 1954. Bluecomb disease of turkeys. Antibiotic prophylactic and etiology. PhD diss. Univ Minnesota, Minneapolis–St. Paul.
46. Sieburth, J.M., and E.P. Johnson. 1957. Transmissible enteritis of turkeys (bluecomb disease). I. Preliminary studies. Poult Sci 36:256–261.
47. Sieburth, J.M., and B.S. Pomeroy. 1956. Bluecomb disease of turkeys. II. Antibiotic treatment of poults. J Am Vet Med Assoc 128:509–513.
48. Truscott, R.B. 1968. Transmissible enteritis of turkeys – disease reproduction. Avian Dis 12:239–245.
49. Tumlin, J.T., and B.S. Pomeroy. 1958. Bluecomb disease of turkeys. V. Preliminary studies on parental immunity and serum neutralization. Am J Vet Res 19:725–728.
50. Tumlin, J.T., and B.S. Pomeroy. 1958. The prophylactic effect of nitrofurans in feed on bluecomb disease, mortality, and weight gains in day-old poults. Proc 2nd Nat Symp Nitrofurans Agric, p. 144.
51. Tumlin, J.T., B.S. Pomeroy, and R.K. Lindorfer. 1957. Bluecomb disease of turkeys. IV. Demonstration of a filterable agent. J Am Vet Med Assoc 130:360–365.
52. Wooley, R.E. 1973. Serological comparison of the Georgia and Minnesota strains of infectious enteritis in turkeys. Avian Dis 17:150–154.
53. Wooley, R.E., T.A. Dees, A.S. Cromack, and J.B. Gratzek. 1972. Infectious enteritis of turkeys: Characterization of two reoviruses isolated by sucrose density gradient centrifugation from turkeys with infectious enteritis. Am J Vet Res 33:157–164.

ROTAVIRUS INFECTIONS

M.S. McNulty

INTRODUCTION. Rotaviruses are now established as a major cause of enteritis and diarrhea in a wide range of mammalian species, including humans (51). Rotavirus infection in avian species was first reported in 1977 by Bergeland et al. (2), who found particles morphologically indistinguishable from rotaviruses in intestinal contents of poults with watery droppings and increased mortality. Since then it has become apparent rotaviruses infect many species of domesticated birds.

As in mammals, rotavirus infection in avian species is frequently associated with outbreaks of diarrhea. The economic significance of rotaviral enteritis to the poultry industry has not yet been defined, but by analogy with the situation in mammals, it is likely to be significant. While some mammalian rotaviruses have limited ability to infect other mammalian species, and rotaviruses from turkeys and pheasants can infect chickens (54), there is no evidence avian rotaviruses infect mammals or vice versa.

In this section, the term rotavirus includes those viruses described as atypical rotaviruses and rotaviruslike viruses.

INCIDENCE AND DISTRIBUTION. Rotaviral enteritis has been described in poults in the UK (12, 21, 22), USA (2, 39, 53), and France (1). Rotavirus isolation from chicken feces has been documented in the UK (22, 24, 25), Belgium (29), and USA (53), and neutralizing antibody to rotavirus has been reported in chickens in Japan (40). Rotavirus was detected in feces of guinea fowl with transmissible enteritis in Italy, but their etiological role is uncertain (33). Rotaviruses have been found in feces of diseased pheasant chicks in the UK (8, 9) and USA (36, 53), and were isolated from feces of apparently healthy ducks (43) and pigeons (31) in Japan. Antibody to rotavirus was found in ducks in the UK (22) and pigeons in Belgium (52). A chicken embryo lethal rotavirus was isolated from liver and small intestine of a lovebird in England (10). This evidence suggests rotaviruses have a worldwide distribution in a wide variety of avian species.

ETIOLOGY

Classification. Rotaviruses are classified as a genus in the family Reoviridae.

Morphology. Intact rotavirus particles have a double-shelled capsid and are approximately 70 nm in diameter. They have been described as reoviruslike, but can be distinguished from reoviruses by their more clearly defined smooth outer edge (Fig. 26.4). The outer capsid shell may be lost producing noninfectious or poorly infectious single-shelled particles (4) that resemble orbiviruses and are about 10 nm smaller than intact virions (Fig.26.4). Double- and single-shelled particles of turkey rotavirus have densities in cesium chloride of 1.34 and 1.36 g/ml respectively (18). There is disagreement about the precise arrangement of capsomeres in rotaviruses. Models involving icosahedral arrangement of 32 (32), 180 (42), 320 (6), and 132 (38) capsomeres in the inner capsid shell have been proposed.

Chemical Composition. Like their mammalian counterparts, avian rotaviruses possess a double-stranded RNA genome consisting of 11 segments ranging from about 0.2×10^6 to 2.1×10^6 in molecular weight (8, 9, 10, 25, 28, 31, 39, 49, 50, 53).

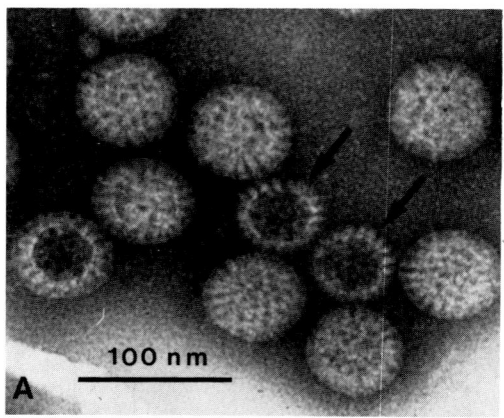

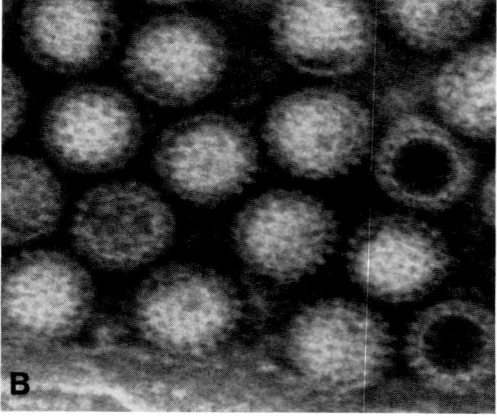

26.4. A. Rotavirus particles in chicken feces showing intact particles with smooth outer edge and particles with serrated edges (*arrows*), lacking outer capsid shell. B. Reovirus isolated from guinea fowl feces. Intact rotavirus and reovirus particles can be differentiated by the more distinct, smooth outer margin of rotavirus. Methylamine tungstate.

Ten major virus polypeptides were detected in MA104 cells infected with a turkey rotavirus. Three polypeptides, designated VP1, VP2, and VP6 with approximate molecular weights of 125 kD, 100 kD and 45 kD, were associated with the inner capsid. Polypeptides VP3, VP4, VP5s and VP7 with molecular weights of 90 kD, 88 kD, 54–55 kD, and 37 kD formed part of the outer capsid shell. The 37-kD polypeptide was glycosylated and two nonstructural polypeptides (30 kD and 28 kD) were also identified as glycoproteins (17).

Virus Replication. The morphogenesis of turkey and chicken rotaviruses has been investigated by thin section electron microscopy (19, 25). Virus replication occurs in the cytoplasm. Both in cell cultures and in vivo, virus cores are formed within granular matrices of viral precursor material (viroplasm), which lies free in the cytoplasm. Developing virus particles are liberated into dilated cisternae of rough endoplasmic reticulum. Some particles appear to bud through ribosome-free areas of endoplasmic reticulum, acquiring an envelope in the process (Fig. 26.5). Virus is released by cell lysis.

Resistance to Chemical and Physical Agents. There is little published information about resistance of avian rotaviruses to chemical and physical inactivation. Two isolates of turkey rotavirus were stable to treatment with chloroform for 30 min and to pH 3 for 2 hr. Heating at 56 C for 30 min decreased infectivity of both viruses 100-fold, both in the presence and absence of magnesium ions (18). Similarly, a pigeon rotavirus was stable to ether, chloroform, and sodium deoxycholate treatment (31).

Strain Classification. The vast majority of mammalian rotaviruses share a group antigen. These have been termed group A or conventional rotaviruses to distinguish them from so-called atypical rotaviruses, which do not have this antigen. Atypical rotaviruses have been further divided into groups B, C, D, and E, based on possession of different group antigens and by terminal finger-printing analysis of viral RNA (34, 35).

Some avian rotaviruses show antigenic relationship with mammalian group A rotaviruses by cross-immunofluorescence using hyperimmune or

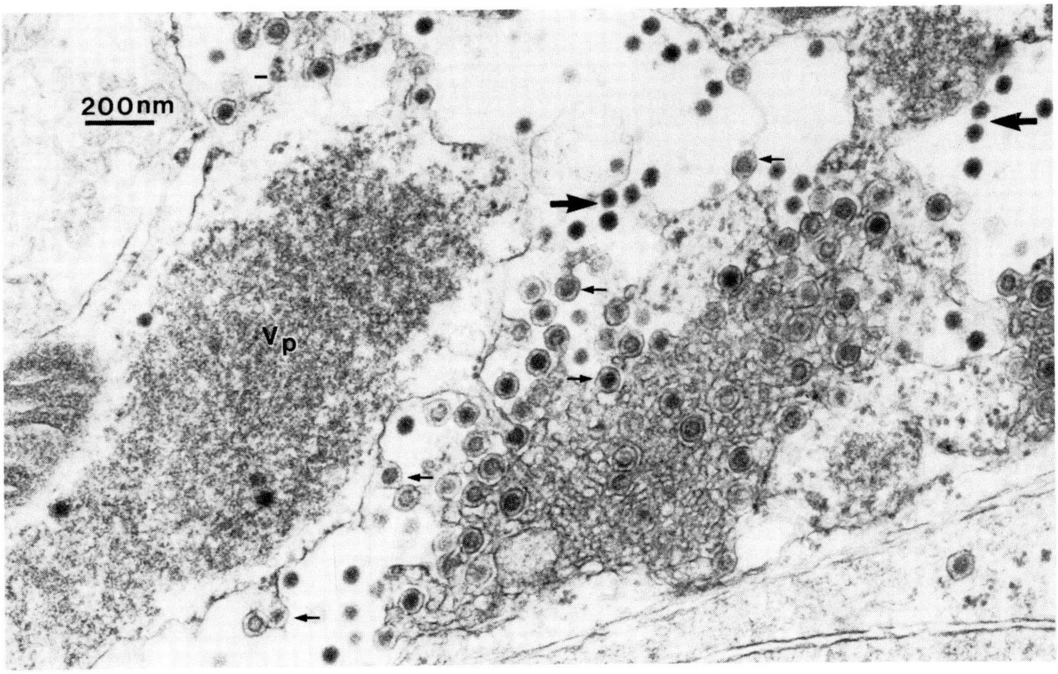

26.5. Electron micrograph of chicken embryo liver cell culture 48 hr postinfection with turkey rotavirus. Part of the cytoplasm of an infected cell is shown, with viroplasm (*Vp*) containing virus cores and virus particles gaining envelopes by budding (*small arrows*) from rough endoplasmic reticulum and from type 2 inclusion material. Nonenveloped virus particles (*large arrows*) are also present.

convalescent antisera (22, 24, 46, 53). This relationship was originally assumed to occur through sharing the mammalian rotavirus group A antigen, but more recent work, using monoclonal antibodies, suggests a determinant other than group A antigen may be involved (7, 13). Those avian rotaviruses antigenically related to mammalian group A rotaviruses are referred to as group A avian rotaviruses.

In addition to group A avian rotaviruses, three other antigenically distinct serogroups of rotavirus have been identified in chickens (28). The prototype virus of one of these groups, the 132 chicken isolate, has been classified as a group D rotavirus (35). So far group D rotaviruses have been identified only in avian species. Rotavirus-like viruses of turkeys (39, 46, 47) are antigenically related by cross-immunofluorescence to the 132 chicken rotavirus isolate (20) and should also be regarded as group D rotaviruses. The antigenic relationship of the other two chicken serogroups to mammalian rotavirus groups B, C, and E has not yet been investigated. It is possible they represent two new groups. An avian serogroup antigenically distinct from groups A and D, designated atypical rotavirus, has been identified in turkeys in the USA (47).

Limited information exists about avian rotavirus-type antigens. Using a fluorescent focus-neutralization test, three serotypes were identified in a collection of six turkey and two chicken isolates of group A avian rotavirus (24). However, using a more sensitive plaque-reduction test, two of the viruses classified as different serotypes had a prime strain relationship (13). Given the serotypic diversity of group A mammalian rotaviruses (13), it is anticipated similar diversity of serotypes will be identified among avian rotaviruses.

Analysis of the pattern of migration of genome segments, especially segment 5; the triplet consisting of segments 7, 8, and 9; and doublet of segments 10 and 11, following polyacrylamide gel electrophoresis, has been extremely useful, both in preliminary characterization of avian rotaviruses and in investigating their epidemiology. An important advantage of this technique is that it does not require isolation and propagation of virus in cell cultures, but can be carried out on virus in intestinal contents or feces. Five major types of RNA profiles, termed electropherogroups, were recognized when turkey and chicken rotavirus RNAs were electrophoresed (49) (Fig. 26.6). Rotaviruses belonging to electropherogroups 1, 2, 3, and 4 were detected in chickens, while electropherogroups 1, 2, 3, and 5 were found in turkeys.

Interestingly, four representative isolates, each belonging to different chicken electropherogroups, were also found to belong to different serogroups (28). Furthermore, turkey rotavirus-like viruses from the USA, antigenically related

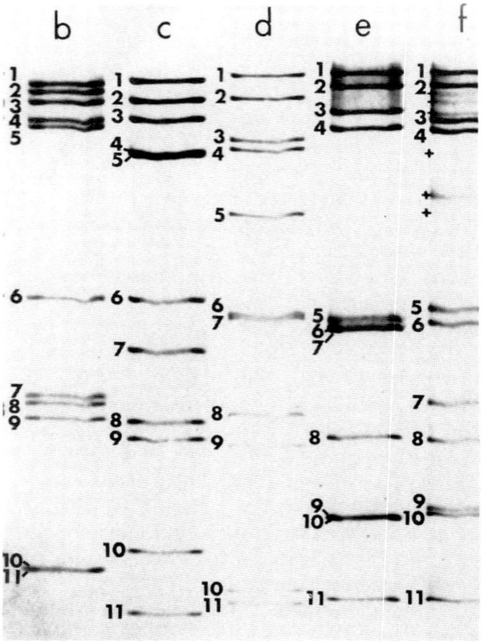

26.6. Genome profiles following electrophoresis of rotavirus RNAs in 5% polyacrylamide gel, showing profiles typical of avian electropherogroups 1 (lane *b*), 2 (lane *c*), 3 (lane *d*), 4 (lane *f*) and 5 (lane *e*). Genome segments are numbered 1–11, + indicates unidentified, contaminating bands. (Avian Pathol)

to chicken group D rotavirus (20), have a similar pattern of migration of RNA segments to group D chicken virus (25, 28, 47, 49). This suggests electropherogrouping may be a useful indicator of group antigenic differences. It will be interesting to see if turkey viruses from the USA with genome profiles similar to those of electropherogroup 3 (15, 47), i.e., so-called atypical rotaviruses, are antigenically related to chicken rotaviruses from the UK with similar profiles.

Within each electropherogroup, minor variations, termed electropherotypes, were described in turkey and chicken rotaviruses from the UK (49). Similar variations have also been described in turkey rotaviruses in the USA (15, 48). These variations may be useful for classifying rotavirus strains, although minor electrophoretic differences do not necessarily imply serotypic differences (18).

Some group A avian rotaviruses agglutinate erythrocytes, particularly human O or guinea pig (11, 18, 31). Hemagglutination and hemagglutination-inhibition tests may also provide a means of strain classification.

Laboratory Host Systems. Isolations of turkey and chicken rotaviruses were first made in primary chick kidney or chick embryo liver cell cultures (22, 24, 25). Since then, rotaviruses from chickens, turkeys, pheasants (53), and ducks (43) have been isolated in chick kidney cells. Primary isolation of turkey (16, 46) and pigeon (31) rotaviruses has been achieved in a continuous line of fetal rhesus monkey kidney cells (MA104). The pigeon isolate also replicated to a higher titer in Madin–Darby bovine kidney (MDBK) cells than in chick embryo kidney cell cultures (31). Some group A rotaviruses are capable of infecting both nonstimulated avian splenic lymphocytes and transformed avian lymphoblastoid cell lines (41).

Serial propagation of rotaviruses in cell culture usually requires trypsin treatment of virus inoculum. Most isolates are noncytopathic on primary isolation; several passages in cell cultures are required before a cytopathic effect is seen. With the exception of the 132 chicken rotavirus isolate (25), rotaviruses isolated to date in cell cultures have all been group A avian rotaviruses.

A rotavirus from lovebirds was lethal for chick embryos following yolk sac inoculation. Passage of the virus in 6- to 8-day-old embryos resulted in death 4–6 days after inoculation (10). So far there is no information concerning replication of other avian rotaviruses in embryos.

Accounts of experimental propagation of avian rotaviruses in their natural hosts are numerous (26, 30, 33, 54–57). Some group A avian rotaviruses are also capable of infecting avian species other than their natural hosts (53, 54, 55, 57).

PATHOGENESIS AND EPIZOOTIOLOGY

Natural and Experimental Hosts. As discussed above, turkeys, chickens, pheasants, ducks, guinea fowl, pigeons, and lovebirds are naturally infected with rotaviruses, and some have been experimentally infected. Most naturally occurring infections in turkeys, chickens, pheasants, and ducks involve birds <6 wk old. Paradoxically, older chickens (56–119 days) and turkeys (112 days) were more susceptible to experimental infection than birds in the first few weeks of life (54, 56). While this observation is interesting, its relevance to the field situation is questionable, because available evidence indicates most turkeys and chickens will have been infected and presumably have developed immunity well before this age. However, lack of age resistance to infection is illustrated by an outbreak of diarrhea associated with rotavirus infection in commercial laying hens between 32 and 92 wk of age (14).

Longitudinal surveys have shown flocks of broilers and turkeys frequently experience simultaneous or sequential infections with different rotavirus electropherogroups (28, 37, 45, 49).

Transmission, Carriers, Vectors. Rotaviruses are excreted in feces in very large numbers (56). No data is available concerning survival of avian rotaviruses in feces, but by extrapolation from mammals, environmental contamination is likely to be persistent. Horizontal transmission occurs readily between birds in direct and indirect contact. Egg transmission of rotaviruses has not been demonstrated, but rotavirus detection in 3-day-old turkey poults prompted speculation that transmission occurs either in or on the egg (45). There is no evidence for a carrier state in birds or biologic vectors.

Incubation Period, Signs, Morbidity, Mortality. The incubation period is short. In experimentally infected turkeys, watery droppings were passed 2–5 days postinfection. Gross lesions at this time consisted of intestinal tract pallor and ceca distended with liquid contents. Rotavirus infection caused significant impairment of D-xylose absorption from the intestinal tract at 2 and 4 days postinfection (55). Mild (26) or no clinical signs (30, 54) were observed following experimental infection of chickens. When signs occurred, their onset coincided with peak virus excretion about 3 days postinfection. Birds passed increased quantities of cecal droppings, and at necropsy, ceca were abnormally distended with fluid and gas (26). No mortality occurred in experimentally infected turkeys or chickens. Laying hens experimentally infected with rotavirus showed a drop in egg production from 4 to 9 days postinfection (56). Rotavirus was detected in feces of experimentally infected chickens and turkeys from 24 hr postinfection, and, in some birds, excretion continued for more than 16 days (26, 54, 55, 56).

Under field conditions, clinical signs associated with rotavirus infection in broilers have varied from subclinical infections to outbreaks of diarrhea severe enough to warrant attention to the litter, with associated dehydration, poor weight gains, and increased mortality (22, 24). In poults variations in severity of clinical signs have also been observed, including a very mild scour in the 1st wk of life, which caused mortality only if vent pecking occurred (12); a more severe disease in 12- to 21-day-old poults characterized by restlessness, litter eating, and watery droppings with mortality between about 4 and 7% (2); and profuse scouring in 2- to 5-wk-old poults with affected birds huddling together, mortalities from suffocation, and stunting of survivors (21). In other outbreaks, predominant signs have been diarrhea and wet litter.

Pheasant chicks 2–3 wk old in the USA had diarrhea and increased mortality associated with rotavirus infection (36). In the UK, rotavirus infection was associated with stunting and increased mortality in pheasant chicks in the 1st wk of life (8, 9). Six of 20 2-day-old pheasants inoculated with intestinal contents containing rotaviruses from naturally occurring cases died 5–6 days postinfection. At necropsy, ceca were distended with frothy, ochre-colored material. Hemorrhages were present in cecal walls of several chicks, and intestinal contents were fluid (9).

Variations in severity of clinical signs associated with rotavirus infections could be due to genuine differences in virulence of avian rotavirus strains, as has been shown for bovine rotavirus (3, 5), and/or interaction of rotavirus with other factors such as other infectious agents or environmental stress.

Morbidity is high. Most fecal specimens taken randomly from birds in affected flocks will contain rotaviruses.

Gross Lesions. The most common finding at necropsy is presence of abnormal amounts of fluid and gas in the intestinal tract and ceca. Secondary findings include dehydration, inflamed vents, anemia due to vent pecking, litter in the gizzard, and inflammation and encrustation with droppings on plantar surfaces of the feet (2, 12, 24, 26).

Histopathology. Immunofluorescence (IF) studies using chickens and turkeys experimentally infected with rotavirus have demonstrated the principal site of virus replication to be cytoplasm of mature villous absorptive epithelial cells in the small intestine. Infected cells were more numerous in the distal third of villi (Fig. 26.7). Small numbers of infected cells were also detected in colon epithelium, ceca, and lamina propria of some villi. No IF was observed in proventriculus, gizzard, spleen, liver, or kidney (26, 30, 54–56). Within the small intestine different rotavirus strains may show preference for specific areas. A group A rotavirus grew best in the duodenum, while a group D rotavirus favored the jejunum and ileum (26). In general, experimental infections using chickens and turkeys of differing ages showed increasing amounts of viral antigen synthesized in birds of increasing age (56).

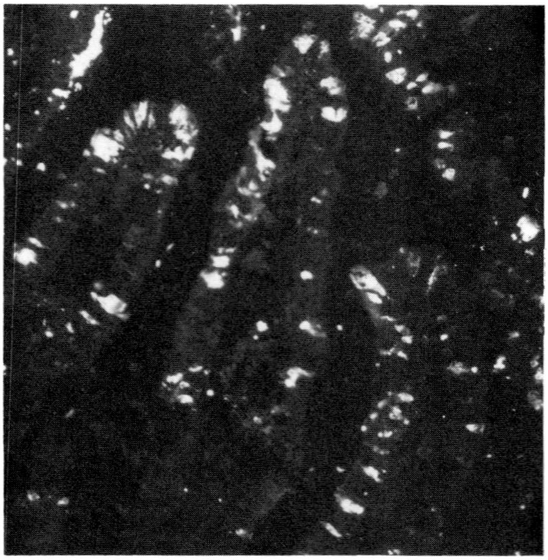

26.7. Immunofluorescent staining of duodenum of specific-pathogen-free chicken infected with rotavirus at 14 days of age and killed 3 days postinfection; rotavirus antigen is seen in villous epithelial cells. ×96. (Avian Pathol)

Histopathologic lesions in experimentally infected turkeys consisted of basal vacuolation of enterocytes, separation of enterocytes from the lamina propria with subsequent desquamation, villus atrophy and enlargement of the lamina propria, scalloping of the villus surface, fusion of villi, and leukocytic infiltration of the lamina propria. In general, mean villus lengths were decreased and crypt depths increased following experimental infection, resulting in significantly decreased villus-to-crypt ratios (57). In experimentally infected chickens, only minimal leukocytic infiltration of the lamina propria was found in one study (57). However, moderate villus atrophy, mainly in the ileum, in experimentally infected chickens has also been described (30). Changes observed in experimentally infected chickens in this laboratory are shown in Fig. 26.8.

No histopathological changes were observed in poults with naturally acquired rotavirus infection (12). However, degeneration and inflammation of villi of the duodenum and jejunum have also been reported in poults with rotaviral enteritis (2). Lesions were not found in ileum, cecum, colon, cloaca, or other organs.

Immunity. Chickens and turkeys inoculated orally with rotaviruses showed serum antibody responses as early as 4–6 days postinfection measured by indirect IF. In general, older birds developed higher antibody titers and responded faster than younger birds (54–56). Nothing is known about development or duration of immunity to rotaviruses following infection of birds. However, by analogy with mammals, serum antibody alone is unlikely to be protective. Local immunity is probably very important in determining susceptibility. Maternally derived antibodies to rotavirus are passively transferred to the avian embryo through the egg yolk. They progressively decline in titer and are undetectable at 3–4 wk of age (19, 55). Presence of maternal antibody had no apparent affect on susceptibility of chickens and turkeys to experimental rotavirus infection (30, 55).

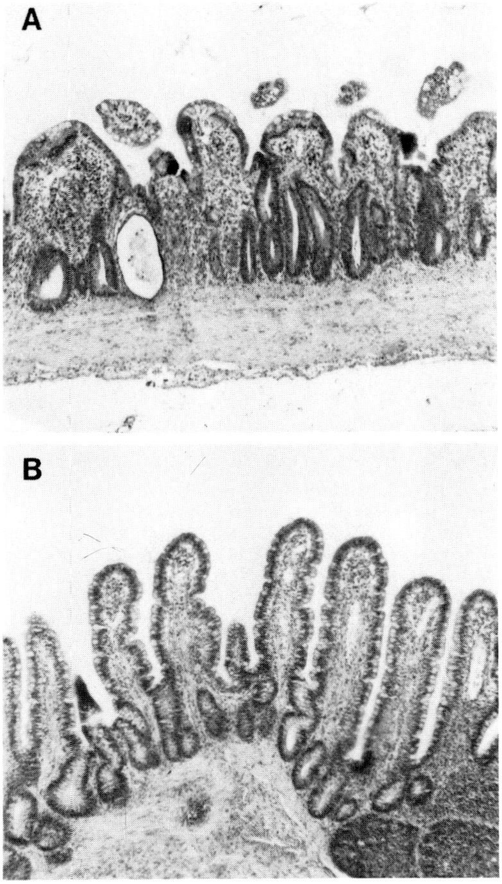

26.8. A. Jejunum from chicken killed 6 days after oral inoculation with rotavirus a 1 day of age. B. Compare blunting and thickening of villi and crypt dilation with uninfected control. H & E stain, ×60. (Pearson)

DIAGNOSIS

Isolation and Identification of Causative Agent. The classical way to diagnose rotavirus infections in the laboratory is to identify the virus in feces or intestinal contents by direct electron microscopy. This technique is relatively sensitive and detects rotaviruses of all serogroups. Material can be prepared in a variety of ways (23). The standard method is to extract an approximately 15% suspension of feces made in phosphate buffered saline with an equal volume of fluorocarbon. Following centrifugation at 3000 g's for 15–30 min to separate aqueous and fluorocarbon phases, the aqueous phase is removed and centrifuged at approximately 12,000 g's for 15 min using an Ependorf 5414 bench centrifuge. This pelleting procedure gives similar results to those obtained by ultracentrifugation, but is quicker and simpler. The pellet is resuspended in a few drops of water and examined. Some workers use immune electron microscopy. While this technique requires availability of specific antisera, it allows rotaviruses of different serogroups to be distinguished (39, 47). The morphology of rotavirus is sufficiently distinct that experienced electron microscopists should have little difficulty identifying the virus with certainty. However, rotaviruses can be confused with reoviruses, which are also frequently found in avian feces. The main distinguishing feature is the more clearly defined outer capsid shell of rotavirus (Fig. 26.4).

Detection of rotavirus RNA in intestinal contents or feces provides an alternate means of diagnosis. Following extraction of RNA, electrophoresis on polyacrylamide gels, and silver staining; rotavirus RNA can be identified by the pattern of migration of the 11 genome segments. This technique is almost as sensitive as electron microscopic techniques (28, 44, 47), and provides a convenient means of distinguishing between different isolates. At present this technique is used mostly by those interested in rotavirus epidemiology and classification.

Diagnosis of rotavirus infection by virus isolation in cell cultures is useful only for group A avian rotaviruses. It has proved extremely difficult to isolate other rotavirus serogroups in cell cultures (16, 28, 46). As infections with other serogroups constitute the majority of rotavirus infections in chickens (28, 49) and turkeys (37, 45), virus isolation in cell cultures cannot be recommended as a diagnostic technique. Even with group A avian rotaviruses, in most cases, serial passage can be achieved only by activation of virus infectivity with proteolytic enzymes such as trypsin. Furthermore, not all group A avian rotaviruses detected by electron microscopy grow in cell cultures. Those that do are often noncytopathic on primary isolation requiring IF to detect virus growth. For isolation of group A avian rotaviruses, the MA104 cell line or primary cultures of chick embryo liver or chick kidney cells, trypsin treatment and centrifugation of inoculum onto the cell monolayer are recommended (16, 22, 29, 31, 43, 46, 53).

Serology. Serological diagnosis of rotavirus infections is difficult and not recommended. The high prevalence of antibody (27, 31) makes results difficult to interpret. Few laboratories offer serological tests for avian rotaviruses on a routine basis. Furthermore, the inability to adapt some avian serogroups to cell culture means there are gaps in the available battery of antigens.

Differential Diagnosis. Rotavirus infection must be differentiated from other conditions causing diarrhea. Since the clinical signs and pathology of rotavirus infection are not pathognomonic, laboratory diagnosis is necessary. However, it is important to remember rotavirus infection does not necessarily result in disease.

TREATMENT, PREVENTION, CONTROL.

The ubiquity of rotavirus infections in turkeys and chickens indicates it is not practical to keep commercial flocks free from infection. At present there is no specific treatment or means of control. The effect of diarrhea on the litter can be minimized by increasing ventilation rate and temperature and adding fresh litter. In those countries where litter is reused several times, infection will build up and problems are likely to be more severe than when houses are cleaned and fumigated and fresh litter is used for each batch of birds. If severe problems arise, it is recommended that litter be removed and the house and equipment be thoroughly cleaned and fumigated with formaldehyde before restocking with a new flock.

Vaccines have not yet been developed. Given the number of serogroups and difficulty in growing some rotaviruses in cell culture, there are obvious problems in vaccine development. Available knowledge of immunity to avian rotavirus suggests live attenuated vaccines given orally might be more effective than parenterally administered inactivated vaccines.

REFERENCES

1. Andral, B., and D. Toquin. 1984. Observations au microscope electronique a partir de prelevements de dindes presentant des troubles pathologiques. Avian Pathol 13:389-417.

2. Bergeland, M.E., J.P. McAdaragh, and I. Stotz. 1977. Rotaviral enteritis in turkey poults. Proc 26th West Poult Dis Conf, pp. 129-130.

3. Bridger, J.C., and D.H. Pocock. 1986. Variation in virulence of bovine rotaviruses. J Hyg 96:257-264.

4. Bridger, J.C., and G.N. Woode. 1976. Characterization of two particle types of calf rotavirus. J Gen Virol 31:245-250.

5. Carpio, M., J.E.C. Bellamy, and L.A. Babiuk. 1981. Comparative virulence of different bovine rotavirus isolates. Can J Comp Med 45:38-42.

6. Esparza, J., and F. Gil. 1978. A study on the ultrastructure of human rotavirus. Virology 91:141-150.

7. Gary, G.W., Jr., R. Black, and E. Palmer. 1982. Monoclonal IgG to the inner capsid of human rotavirus. Arch Virol 72:223-227.

8. Gough, R.E., G.W. Wood, M.S. Collins, D. Spackman, J. Kemp, and L.A.C. Gibson. 1985. Rotavirus infection in pheasant poults. Vet Rec 116:295.

9. Gough, R.E., G.W. Wood, and D. Spackman. 1986. Studies with an atypical avian rotavirus from pheasants. Vet Rec 118:611-612.

10. Gough, R.E., M.S. Collins, G.W. Wood, and S.A. Lister. 1988. Isolation of a chicken embryo-lethal rotavirus from a lovebird (Agapornis species). Vet Rec 122:363-364.

11. Hancock, K., G.W. Gary, Jr., and E.L. Palmer. 1983. Adaptation of two avian rotaviruses to mammalian cells and characterization by haemagglutination and RNA electrophoresis. J Gen Virol 64:853-861.

12. Horrox, N.E. 1980. Some observations and comments on rotaviruses in turkey poults. Proc 29th West Poult Dis Conf, pp. 162-164.

13. Hoshino, Y., R.G. Wyatt, H.B. Greenberg, J. Flores, and A.Z. Kapikian. 1984. Serotypic similarity and diversity of rotaviruses of mammalian and avian origin as studied by plaque-reduction neutralization. J Infect Dis 149:694-702.

14. Jones, R.C., C.S. Hughes, and R.R. Henry. 1979. Rotavirus infection in commercial laying hens. Vet Rec 104:22.

15. Kang, S.Y., K.V. Nagaraja, and J.A. Newman. 1986. Electropherotypic analysis of rotaviruses isolated from turkeys. Avian Dis 30:794-801.

16. Kang, S.Y., K.V. Nagaraja, and J.A. Newman. 1986. Primary isolation and identification of avian rotaviruses from turkeys exhibiting signs of clinical enteritis in a continuous MA104 cell line. Avian Dis 30:494-499.

17. Kang, S.Y., K.V. Nagaraja, and J.A. Newman. 1987. Characterization of viral polypeptides from avian rotavirus. Avian Dis 31:607-621. 1987.

18. Kang, S.Y., K.V. Nagaraja, and J.A. Newman. 1988. Physical, chemical, and serological characterization of avian rotaviruses. Avian Dis 32:195-203.

19. McNulty, M.S. 1980. Morphology and chemical composition of rotaviruses. In F. Bricout and R. Scherrer (eds.), Viral Enteritis in Humans and Animals, pp. 111-140. INSERM, Paris.

20. McNulty, M.S. 1988. Unpublished data.

21. McNulty, M.S., G.M. Allan, and J.C. Stuart. 1978. Rotavirus infection in avian species. Vet Rec 103:319-320.

22. McNulty, M.S., G.M. Allan, D. Todd, and J.B. McFerran. 1979. Isolation and cell culture propagation of rotaviruses from turkeys and chickens. Arch Virol 61:13-21.

23. McNulty, M.S., W.L. Curran, D. Todd, and J.B. McFerran. 1979. Detection of viruses in avian faeces by direct electron microscopy. Avian Pathol 8:239-247.

24. McNulty, M.S., G.M. Allan, D. Todd, J.B. McFerran, E.R. McKillop, D.S. Collins, and R.M. McCracken. 1980. Isolation of rotaviruses from turkeys and chickens: Demonstration of distinct serotypes and RNA electropherotypes. Avian Pathol 9:363-375.

25. McNulty, M.S., G.M. Allan, D. Todd, J.B. McFerran, and R.M. McCracken. 1981. Isolation from chickens of a rotavirus lacking the rotavirus group antigen. J Gen Virol 55:405-413.

26. McNulty, M.S., G.M. Allan, and R.M. McCracken. 1983. Experimental infection of chickens with rotaviruses: Clinical and virological findings. Avian Pathol 12:45-54.

27. McNulty, M.S., G.M. Allan, and J.B. McFerran. 1984. Prevalence of antibody to conventional and atypical rotaviruses in chickens. Vet Rec 114:219.

28. McNulty, M.S., D. Todd, G.M. Allan, J.B. McFerran, and J.A. Greene. 1984. Epidemiology of rotavirus infection in broiler chickens: Recognition of four serogroups. Arch Virol 81:113-121.

29. Meulemans, G., G. Charlier, and P. Halen. 1985. Détection de rotavirus aviaire et adaptation a la culture céllulaire. Ann Med Vet 127:43-48.

30. Meulemans, G., J.E. Peeters, and P. Halen. 1985. Experimental infection of broiler chickens with rotavirus. Br Vet J 141:69-73.

31. Minamoto, N., K. Oki, M. Tomita, T. Kinjo, and Y. Suzuki. 1988. Isolation and characterization of rotavirus from feral pigeon in mammalian cell cultures. Epidemiol Infect 100:481-492.

32. Palmer, E.L., M.L. Martin, and F.A. Murphy. 1977. Morphology and stability of infantile gastroen-

teritis virus: Comparison with reovirus and bluetongue virus. J Gen Virol 35: 403-414.
33. Pascucci, S., M.E. Misciattelli, and L. Giovanetti. 1981. Transmissible enteritis of guinea fowl; electron microscopic studies and isolation of a rotavirus strain. Proc 8th Int Congr World Vet Poult Assoc pp. 57. (Abstr).
34. Pedley, S., J.C. Bridger, J.F. Brown, and M.A. McCrae. 1983. Molecular characterization of rotaviruses with distinct group antigens. J Gen Virol 64:2093-2101.
35. Pedley, S., J.C. Bridger, D. Chasey, and M.A. McCrae. 1986. Definition of two new groups of atypical rotaviruses. J Gen Virol 67:131-137.
36. Reynolds, D.L., K.W. Theil, and Y.M. Saif. 1987. Demonstration of rotavirus and rotavirus-like virus in the intestinal contents of diarrheic pheasant chicks. Avian Dis 31: 376-379.
37. Reynolds, D.L., Y.M. Saif, and K.W. Theil. 1987. A survey of enteric viruses of turkey poults. Avian Dis 31:89-98.
38. Roseto, A., J. Escaig, E. Delain, J. Cohen, and R. Scherrer. 1979. Structure of rotaviruses as studied by the freeze-drying technique. Virology 98:471-475.
39. Saif, L.J., Y.M. Saif, and K.W. Theil. 1985. Enteric viruses in diarrheic turkey poults. Avian Dis 29:798-811.
40. Sato, K., Y. Inaba, T. Shinozaki, and M. Matumoto. 1981. Neutralizing antibody to bovine rotavirus in various animal species. Vet Microbiol 6:259-261.
41. Schat, K.A., and T.J. Myers. 1987. Cultivation of avian rotaviruses in chicken lymphocytes and lymphoblastoid cell lines. Arch Virol 94:205-213.
42. Stannard, L.M., and B.D. Schoub. 1977. Observations on the morphology of two rotaviruses. J Gen Virol 37:435-439.
43. Takase, K., F. Nonaka, M. Sakaguchi, and S. Yamada. 1986. Cytopathic avian rotavirus isolated from duck faeces in chicken kidney cell cultures. Avian Pathol 15:719-730.
44. Theil, K.W. 1987. A modified genome electropherotyping procedure for detecting turkey rotaviruses in small volumes of intestinal contents. Avian Dis 31:899-903.
45. Theil, K.W., and Y.M. Saif. 1987. Age-related infections with rotavirus, rotavirus-like virus, and atypical rotavirus in turkey flocks. J Clin Microbiol 25:333-337.
46. Theil, K.W., D.L. Reynolds, and Y.M. Saif. 1986. Isolation and serial propagation of turkey rotaviruses in a fetal rhesus monkey kidney (MA104) cell line. Avian Dis 30:93-104.
47. Theil, K.W., D.L. Reynolds, and Y.M. Saif. 1986. Comparison of immune electron microscopy and genome electropherotyping techniques for detection of turkey rotaviruses and rotavirus-like viruses in intestinal contents. J Clin Microbiol 23:695-699.
48. Theil, K.W., D.L. Reynolds, and Y.M. Saif. 1986. Genomic variation among avian rotavirus-like viruses detected by polyacrylamide gel electrophoresis. Avian Dis 30:829-834.
49. Todd, D., and M.S. McNulty. 1986. Electrophoretic variation of avian rotavirus RNA in polyacrylamide gels. Avian Pathol 15:149-159.
50. Todd, D., M.S. McNulty, and G.M. Allan. 1980. Polyacrylamide gel electrophoresis of avian rotavirus RNA. Arch Virol 63:87-97.
51. Tzipori, S. 1985. The relative importance of enteric pathogens affecting neonates of domestic animals. Adv Vet Sci Comp Med 29:103-206.
52. Vindevogel, H., L. Dagenais, B. Lansival, and P.P. Pastoret. 1981. Incidence of rotavirus, adenovirus, and herpesvirus in pigeons. Vet Rec 109:285-286.
53. Yason, C.V., and K.A. Schat. 1985. Isolation and characterization of avian rotaviruses. Avian Dis 29:499-508.
54. Yason, C.V., and K.A. Schat. 1986. Experimental infection of specific-pathogen-free chickens with avian rotaviruses. Avian Dis 30:551-556.
55. Yason, C.V., and K.A. Schat. 1986. Pathogenesis of rotavirus infection in turkey poults. Avian Pathol 15:421-435.
56. Yason, C.V., and K.A. Schat. 1987. Pathogenesis of rotavirus infection in various age groups of chickens and turkeys: Clinical signs and virology. Am J Vet Res 48:977-983.
57. Yason, C.V., B.A. Summers, and K.A. Schat. 1987. Pathogenesis of rotavirus infection in various age groups of chickens and turkeys: Pathology. Am J Vet Res 48:927-938.

ASTROVIRUS INFECTIONS

D.L. Reynolds

INTRODUCTION. Astroviruses have been identified in cases of diarrhea and gastroenteritis in human infants (3), calves (10), lambs (9), and piglets (1). More recently, they have been detected in birds with enteric disease. The economic impact of astrovirus infections on the poultry industry has yet to be determined. Whether or not avian astroviruses can infect other animal species, including humans, constituting a public health concern, is also unknown.

HISTORY. Astroviruses were first identified in 1980 by McNulty et al. (4) from intestinal contents of 11-day-old turkey poults with diarrhea and increased mortality. Subsequently astroviruses in flocks of young turkeys were reported in the USA in 1985 (8) and 1986 (5).

Avian astroviruses have not been propagated in vitro. Perhaps because of this their presence in feces and intestinal contents of birds has eluded investigators until recently. Astroviruses have only been detected by direct or immune electron microscopy (EM, IEM).

INCIDENCE AND DISTRIBUTION.

Astrovirus infections are geographically widespread and usually the most prevalent virus infection, other than rotavirus infection, in poults 1–5 wk of age with enteric disease (5, 6, 8). In one study, astrovirus infections occurred in nearly 80% of affected flocks, and was the most prevalent virus detected (6). Astroviruses have also been detected in normal healthy flocks, but far less frequently (<30%). Astroviruses are seldom the only virus detected in flocks with enteric disease. Generally, they occur in combination with other enteric viruses, especially rotaviruslike virus (group D rotaviruses) (6).

Astrovirus infections usually occur within the first 4 wk of life, and are rare in older turkeys (7). Although they have been detected as early as 3 days of age, astrovirus infections are more common after 7 days (7). When flocks were continuously monitored for enteric viral infections from 1 day of age until market, the first samples positive for viruses always contained astroviruses, either alone or with other viruses (7).

ETIOLOGY.

Avian astroviruses have been classified and named solely on the basis of size and morphology determined by EM. Initially, they were reported to be 28–31 nm (mean 30.1 nm) in diameter with about 10% of virus particles displaying a 5- or 6-pointed star shape (4). Later, astroviruses were described as having an average diameter of 31 nm with a few particles having a 5-pointed star shape (8). Subsequently, in the USA, only a small percentage of astroviruses had 5- or 6-pointed star-shaped morphology with an average diameter of 29.6 nm (5) (Fig. 26.9). Avian astroviruses have not yet been classified into a viral taxon.

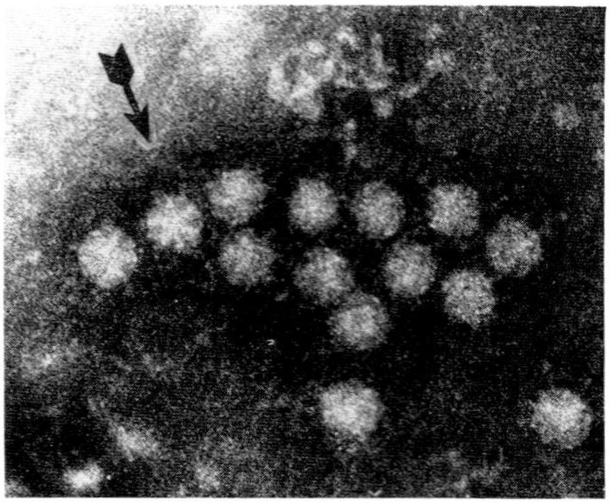

26.9. A star-shaped astrovirus particle (*arrow*) among an aggregate of astroviruses from intestinal samples of experimentally infected diarrheic poults, detected by immune electron microscopy.

PATHOGENESIS AND EPIZOOTIOLOGY.

Turkeys appear to be the only avian species naturally infected by astroviruses, except possibly for astroviruslike particles identified from ducklings with hepatitis (2) (see Chapter 24). Astroviruses have been observed from turkey poults experiencing viral enteritis (see Introduction). Clinical signs of the disease usually develop between 1 and 3 wk of age, and generally last 10–14 days. They vary somewhat, but typically include diarrhea, listlessness, litter eating, and nervousness. Severity ranges from mild to moderate with only slight mortality. Morbidity, occurring as decreased growth (stunting), is of greatest concern. Rarely are astroviruses the only enteric virus identified from viral enteritis in poults.

Experimental studies have shown astroviruses can cause enteric disease in turkey poults (5). When specific-pathogen-free (SPF) poults were given an inoculum containing only astrovirus, they gained significantly less weight and absorbed significantly less D-xylose compared to uninoculated control poults. Astrovirus-inoculated poults had watery to frothy, yellow-brown droppings. At necropsy, characteristic pathologic changes were dilated ceca containing yellow, frothy contents; gaseous fluid; and loss of tone (gut thinness) of the intestinal tract (Fig. 26.10). Astroviruses were detected in intestinal contents of poults prior to the onset of clinical disease and gross pathologic changes. It was suggested that this phenomenon may explain why astroviruses are sometimes detected from poults appearing normal and healthy, when in fact these poults could be in an early stage of the disease. In addition, it was shown that the shedding of astroviruses into the intestinal tract wanes before clinical signs and pathologic changes abate. Therefore, poults in the later stages of astrovirus disease may display clinical signs and gross pathologic changes but may not have detectable levels of astrovirus present in their intestinal tract.

Astrovirus and group D rotavirus frequently occur together in naturally infected turkey poults (7). SPF poults, experimentally inoculated with this combination, shed astrovirus into their intestinal tract (detected by IEM) prior to shedding detectable levels of group D rotavirus. Also, they developed more pronounced clinical disease than that produced by astrovirus alone. Interactions between astroviruses and other viruses have not been reported.

It is assumed the mode of transmission for astroviruses is fecal-oral. Experimentally, poults inoculated orally with astrovirus developed infection (5). Studies on natural transmission of astroviruses have not been reported.

No reports specifically address astrovirus immunity in poultry. However, SPF poults infected with astroviruses ceased intestinal shedding by 14 days postinfection and convalescent sera ag-

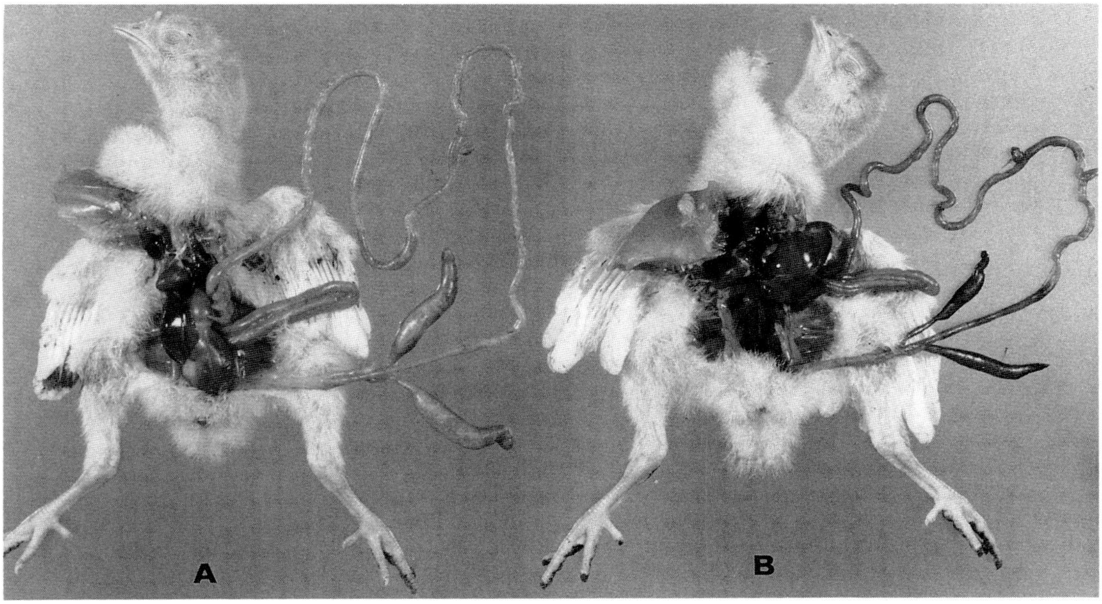

26.10. Pathologic changes produced by astrovirus infection in an SPF turkey poult inoculated orally at 1 day of age and necropsied at 7 days postinoculation (*left*). Note dilated light-colored ceca and intestinal tract. Uninoculated control poult from same hatch (*right*).

gregated astrovirus particles when used for IEM, indicating astrovirus-specific antibodies (5). Whether convalescent birds are protected from further astrovirus infection has not been determined. However, this appears likely to be true in naturally infected turkeys since astroviruses were rarely detected beyond 5 wk of age when commercial turkey flocks were monitored until market age (7). The effect of maternal antibodies on astrovirus infections is unknown.

DIAGNOSIS. IEM is the preferred method for identifying astroviruses from fecal and/or intestinal samples. This procedure is done by diluting the fecal/intestinal sample with sterile diluent such as phosphate-buffered saline (pH 7.2) to make a working solution. The diluted sample is thoroughly mixed using a homogenizer or vortex mixer and sonicated. Particulate matter and bacteria are removed by centrifugation at 500 g's for 20 min, and filtering the resulting supernatant fluid through a 450-nm-porosity membrane filter. The filtrate is incubated with an appropriate dilution of antiserum containing astrovirus antibodies. Following incubation, the sample is pelleted by ultracentrifugation, negatively stained with phosphotungstic acid, and observed by EM. Aggregates of astrovirus can be easily observed at ×30,000 and ×50,000 magnification. Although astroviruses have star-shaped morphology, only a small percentage of particles display this characteristic. It is quite difficult to accurately diagnose astrovirus infections without IEM. A definitive diagnosis of astrovirus infection is made by recognizing aggregates of typical astrovirus particles in the IEM preparation. In the author's experience, turkey astroviruses do not display nonspecific agglutination; therefore, one must rely on IEM for aggregation of particles (Fig. 26.9).

The differential diagnosis of astrovirus infections in turkey poults needs to include infectious, parasitic, and noninfectious agents that can cause enteric disease. Cultures for enteropathogenic bacteria such as *Salmonella* spp. should be done. Smears or tissue sections will demonstrate protozoa. Other enteric viruses need to be excluded including coronavirus and rotavirus. The latter needs to be highly considered and a method to detect rotavirus infections should be employed. There is evidence astroviruses and rotaviruses often occur together and may be involved in the same disease entity (6).

TREATMENT, PREVENTION, CONTROL. There are no vaccines, chemotherapeutics, or other measures reported to be efficacious for control and/or prevention of astrovirus infections. Generally, good management practices emphasizing cleaning, disinfecting, litter management, and resting of facilities between flocks are recommended. However, astrovirus infections have continued to be problems for some producers with modern facilities employing high standards of management, suggesting contemporary management practices may not have been entirely effective.

REFERENCES

1. Bridger, J.C. 1980. Detection by electron microscopy of caliciviruses, astroviruses and rotavirus-like particles in the faeces of piglets with diarrhoea. Vet Rec 107:532–533.

2. Gough, R.E., M.S. Collins, E. Borland, and L.F. Keymer. 1984. Astrovirus-like particles associated with hepatitis in ducklings. Vet Rec 114:279.

3. Kurtz, J.B., T.W. Lee, and D. Pickering. 1977. Astrovirus associated gastroenteritis in a children's ward. J. Clin Pathol 30:948–952.

4. McNulty, M.S., W.L. Curran, and J.B. McFerran. 1980. Detection of astroviruses in turkey faeces by direct electron microscopy. Vet Rec 106:561.

5. Reynolds, D.L., and Y.M. Saif. 1986. Astrovirus: A cause of an enteric disease in turkey poults. Avian Dis 30:728–735.

6. Reynolds, D.L., Y.M. Saif, and K.W. Theil. 1987. A survey of enteric viruses of turkey poults. Avian Dis 31:89–98.

7. Reynolds, D.L., Y.M. Saif, and K.W. Theil. 1987. Enteric viral infections of turkey poults: Incidence of infection. Avian Dis 31:272–276.

8. Saif, L.J., Y.M. Saif, and K.W. Theil. 1985. Enteric viruses in diarrheic turkey poults. Avian Dis 29:798–811.

9. Snodgrass, D.R., and E.W. Gray. 1977. Detection and transmission of 30 nm virus particles (astroviruses) in faeces of lambs with diarrhaea. Arch Virol 55:287–291.

10. Woode, G.N., and J.C. Bridger. 1978. Isolation of small viruses resembling astroviruses and caliciviruses from acute enteritis of calves. J Med Microbiol 11:441–452.

27 REOVIRUS INFECTIONS

J.K. Rosenberger and N.O. Olson

INTRODUCTION. Viruses that are members of the genus *Reovirus* can be separated into two subdivisions based on their mammalian or avian origins (25, 36). These two subdivisions are further differentiated by antigenic configuration, growth in cell culture, host specificity, and ability to induce hemagglutination in vitro.

Reoviruses have been isolated from a variety of tissues in chickens affected by assorted disease conditions including viral arthritis/tenosynovitis, stunting syndrome, respiratory disease, enteric disease, and a so-called malabsorption syndrome. They have frequently been found in chickens that were clinically normal (57). The nature of the disease that occurs following reovirus infection is very much dependent upon host age, virus pathotype, and route of exposure.

Economic losses caused by reovirus infections are frequently the result of crippling (viral arthritis/tenosynovitis) and a general lack of performance including diminished weight gains, poor feed conversion, and a reduced marketability of affected birds.

HISTORY. In 1954 Fahey and Crawley (9) made what was later confirmed by Petek et al. (50) to be the initial isolation of avian reovirus from the respiratory tract of chickens with chronic respiratory disease. The Fahey-Crawley virus, when inoculated into susceptible chickens, produced a moderate respiratory disease, liver necrosis, and an inflammation of the tendons and synovial membranes.

Olson et al. in 1957 (46) described a naturally occurring synovitis in chickens from which they were able to isolate an agent insensitive to chlortetracycline and furazolidone and serologically unrelated to either *Mycoplasma gallisepticum* or *Mycoplasma synoviae*. This agent, later named the "viral arthritis agent" by Olson and Kerr (42), was eventually identified as a reovirus by Walker et al. in 1972 (82). Dalton and Henry (4) used the term tenosynovitis to define the changes in the tendons and tendon sheaths associated with a condition they considered different from that caused by *M. synoviae*. This difference was substantiated by Olson and Solomon (44) when they reported tenosynovitis in commercially produced chickens that had been derived from *M. synoviae*-free broiler chickens. An isolate obtained from these birds had characteristics identical to those described for the viral arthritis agent and was shown to be antigenically similar to the Fahey-Crawley virus (45). Since the first reports of tenosynovitis in the USA and England, the disease has been described in many other countries. Several reviews document the incidence of reovirus-induced tenosynovitis (29, 56, 74).

Reoviruses have been associated with other disease conditions including ruptured gastrocnemius tendons, pericarditis, myocarditis, hydropericardium, cloacal pasting, early mortality in poults, and most recently malabsorption syndrome. In the case of the latter condition, the etiologic picture is not clear-cut. In addition to reoviruses, several other viruses as well as bacteria and noninfectious agents have been claimed to be involved. Thus, although this chapter will briefly discuss malabsorption syndrome, a more thorough treatment of the subject can be found in the section on infectious stunting syndrome in Chapter 34.

INCIDENCE AND DISTRIBUTION. Reovirus infections are prevalent worldwide in chickens, turkeys, and other avian species. Viral arthritis/tenosynovitis is found primarily in meat-type chickens but has been diagnosed in egg-type birds (67) and turkeys (48). Reovirus-associated malabsorption syndrome has been reported in the USA, Europe, and Australia, but many of these associations are tenuous and need confirmation. Reoviruses are commonly found in the digestive and respiratory tracts of clinically normal chickens and turkeys (26, 50, 68, 87) and have been identified as contaminants in Marek's disease vaccine (85).

ETIOLOGY. As a group, reoviruses are nonenveloped with an icosahedral symmetry and a double capsid structure. Intact virus particles have a diameter of approximately 75 nm and a density in cesium chloride of 1.36–1.37 g/ml (12, 65, 66, 70). The viral genome consists of dsRNA that is segmented and can be further segregated into at least three size classes, which contain a total of ten discrete molecular species (13, 14, 70).

Reoviruses are heat-resistant, being able to withstand 60 C for 8–10 hr, 56 C for 22–24 hr, 37 C for 15–16 wk, 22 C for 48–51 wk, 4 C for over 3 yr, −20 C for over 4 yr, and −63 C for over 10 yr (41). The titer of semipurified virus at 60 C is reduced but not completely inactivated in 5 hr. Heat treatment in the presence of magnesium chloride results in increased titers.

Reoviruses are not sensitive to ether but are slightly sensitive to chloroform. They are resistant to pH 3; hydrogen peroxide when incubated for 1 hr at room temperature; 2% Lysol; 3% formalin; and the DNA metabolic inhibitors actinomycin D, cytosine arabinoside, and 5-fluoro-2-deoxyuridine. They are inactivated by 70% ethanol and 0.5% organic iodine (38).

Attempts to demonstrate hemagglutination by avian reovirus have been generally unsuccessful (56) with two exceptions (5, 11).

Strain Classification. Reoviruses can be classified using serological procedures or grouped according to their relative pathogenicity for chickens. Kawamura et al. (25, 26) identified 5 serotypes of reovirus from 77 isolates originally obtained from feces, cloacal swabs, and tracheas. Sahu and Olson (64) found 4 serotypes from intestines, respiratory tract, and synovial isolates. Wood et al. (86) calculated the relatedness of reoviruses originating from the USA, UK, Germany, and Japan and found at least 11 serotypes, although there was considerable cross-neutralization among heterologous types. Hieronymus et al. (17) grouped 5 malabsorption syndrome isolates into 3 serotypes while Robertson and Wilcox (55) assigned 10 Australian isolates into three groups with considerable cross-reactivity. It is apparent that reoviruses frequently exist as antigenic subtypes rather than distinct serotypes.

Rosenberger (60) inoculated specific-pathogen-free (SPF) chickens by various routes with plaque-purified, antigenically similar viruses and demonstrated clear strain differences based on relative pathogenicity and virus persistence.

Laboratory Host Systems. Reoviruses grow readily in the embryonating chicken egg following inoculation via yolk sac or chorioallantoic membrane (CAM). The yolk sac is preferred for original isolation and generally results in embryo mortality 3–5 days after inoculation with affected embryos exhibiting a purplish discoloration due to massive subcutaneous hemorrhage. Mortality in CAM-inoculated embryos usually occurs 7–8 days postinoculation; embryos are slightly dwarfed with occasional enlargement of the liver and spleen. Necrotic foci may occur in both the liver and spleen, particularly in embryos that survive longer than 7 days postinoculation. Small, discrete, slightly raised white lesions may be found on the CAM. Histologically, areas of necrosis of the ectoderm with only moderate stimulation of the epithelial cells are seen. Mesoderm adjacent to the lesion is edematous and contains numerous inflammatory cells. Edema alone may be found. Embryo mortality is less consistent following inoculation via the chorioallantoic sac.

The virus grows in primary chicken cell cultures of embryo, lung, kidney, liver, macrophages, and testicle. Primary chicken kidney cells from 2- to 6-wk-old chickens are satisfactory, but for plaques and isolation, primary embryo liver cells are preferred (1, 16). Chicken embryo fibroblasts are suitable for reovirus growth but the virus often requires adaptation (1). Chicken-origin cell cultures infected with reoviruses are characterized by the formation of syncytia, which may occur as early as 24–48 hr followed by degeneration leaving holes in the monolayer and giant cells floating in the medium. Infected cells exhibit intracytoplasmic inclusions, which may appear either eosinophilic or basophilic (56). Of many established cell lines tested, virus has been grown on Vero (64), baby hampster kidney (BHK) 21/13, feline kidney (CRFK), Georgia bovine kidney (GBK), rabbit kidney (RK), and porcine kidney (PK) cells (1).

Pathogenicity. Although normally associated with arthritis/tenosynovitis, reoviruses have been identified as the etiology of other disease conditions as well, including growth retardation, pericarditis, myocarditis, hydropericardium, enteritis, hepatitis, bursal and thymic atrophy, osteoporosis, and acute and chronic respiratory syndromes (56). The pathogenicity of selected reovirus isolates was enhanced by co-infection with *Eimeria tenella* or *Eimeria maxima* (62, 63). Exposure to infectious bursal disease virus or particular dietary regimes increased the severity of tenosynovitis resulting from infections with the WVU 2937 isolate (2, 3, 71). Reoviruses may also exacerbate disease conditions caused by other pathogens, including chicken anemia agent (8), *Escherichia coli,* and Newcastle disease virus (61). The increased susceptibility to other infectious agents following or concomitant with reovirus exposure may result from immune system compromise (54).

PATHOGENESIS AND EPIZOOTIOLOGY

Natural and Experimental Hosts. Although reoviruses have been found in many avian species, chickens and turkeys are the only recognized natural or experimental hosts for reovirus-induced arthritis/tenosynovitis. Reoviruses have been isolated from turkeys with arthritis (48) and Van der Heide et al. (79) found a turkey isolate to be pathogenic for chickens. The turkey isolate was neutralized by chicken reovirus S1133 antiserum. High mortality in turkey poults has also been associated with reovirus (68). McFerran et al. (37) identified a reovirus in turkey feces that shared the group-specific antigen with chicken isolates but was not neutralized by available reference antiserum.

Reoviruses were found in clinically affected ducks, pigeons, geese, and psittacines but a firm etiological relationship was not always established (56). A disease in Muscovy ducks characterized by a general malaise, diarrhea, and stunted growth has been reported in several countries (10, 24, 34) and reproduced experimentally with isolated reoviruses (10, 34). Attempts to establish active infection in the canary, pigeon, guinea pig, rat, mouse, hamster, and rabbit failed; however, Phillips et al. (51) reported liver lesions in neonatal mice after oral and nasal infection, and Nersessian et al. (40) produced stunted growth and incoordination in suckling mice inoculated intracerebrally with several turkey isolates.

Age-associated Resistance. Kerr and Olson (27) were the first to report on age-related resistance to reovirus-induced arthritis/tenosynovitis. The disease can be readily reproduced in 1-day-old chickens free of maternal antibody (20, 78), whereas older chickens are infected, but the disease is generally less severe and the incubation period longer. Similar results were reported by Rosenberger (60) with reoviruses isolated from birds with an apparent stunting or malabsorption syndrome. Jones and Georgiou (20) suggested the age-associated susceptibility may be related to the inability of young birds to develop an effective immune response.

Transmission. Horizontal transmission of reovirus has been extensively documented (56, 74). There is considerable variation, however, among strains of virus in their ability to spread laterally. Although reovirus may be excreted from both the intestinal and respiratory tracts for at least 10 days postinoculation, virus generally appears to be shed from the intestine for longer periods suggesting fecal contamination as a primary source of contact infection (22, 33). Roessler (58) demonstrated that 1-day-old chickens are more susceptible to reovirus introduced via the respiratory route than orally. Virus may persist for long periods in the cecal tonsils and hock joints, particularly in birds infected at a young age (21, 35), implicating carrier birds as potential sources of infection for penmates.

Menendez et al. (38) and Van der Heide and Kalbac (75) have clearly demonstrated avian reoviruses can be vertically transmitted. Menendez et al. showed that following oral, tracheal, and nasal inoculation of 15-mo-old breeders, virus was present in chicks from eggs laid 17, 18, and 19 days postinfection. Egg-transmission rate was low (1.7%). Reoviruses were also isolated from chicken embryo fibroblast cell cultures prepared from embryonated eggs derived from experimentally infected hens (75).

Incubation Period. The incubation period differs depending upon virus pathotype, age of host, and route of exposure (56, 74). For inoculated 2-wk-old chickens the incubation period varied from 1 day (footpad inoculation) to 11 days (intramuscular, intravenous, intrasinus inoculation). The incubation period following intratracheal inoculation and contact exposure was 9 and 13 days, respectively (44).

Often, infections are inapparent and demonstrable only by serology or virus isolations. Mature birds inoculated by oral and respiratory routes with the FDO isolate had virus in all organs tested at 4 days postinfection. The number of virus isolations was greatly reduced by 2 wk and no virus was present 20 days postinfection. There was frequent localization of virus in the flexor and extensor tendons of the pelvic limb, although gross lesions were not evident (39). Many reoviruses cause microscopic inflammatory changes in the digital flexor and metatarsal extensor tendons without development of gross lesions (43).

When disease (viral arthritis/tenosynovitis) does occur from natural infection, it is usually seen in young birds 4–7 wk old but may be seen in much older chickens as well (74). Morbidity can be as high as 100% while mortality is generally less than 6%.

Signs

VIRAL ARTHRITIS/TENOSYNOVITIS. In acute infections, lameness is present and some chickens are stunted. With chronic infection, lameness is more pronounced, and in a small percentage of infected chickens the hock joint is immobilized. In a flock of 36,000 broilers the infection, first diagnosed as infectious synovitis, appeared in 8 of 16 pens when the chicks were 3–4 wk old. Approximately 550 birds died or were removed because of lameness by 7–8 wk. Another 4,500 birds were stunted.

In another flock of approximately 15,000 broilers, no clinical signs of viral arthritis/tenosynovitis were observed, but approximately 5% of the birds had enlargement in the area of the gastrocnemius or digital flexor tendons when observed at slaughter. At 9 wk, birds from this flock had an average weight of only 3.66 lb, feed conversion was 2.45, mortality totaled 5%, and the condemnation rate was 2.6%. Virus was isolated from two birds condemned for toxemia; of 80 serum samples obtained from this flock, 89% had reovirus antibodies detected in a precipitin test. This inapparent infection probably caused the poor performance of these broilers.

Similar observations have been made by other workers (12, 19). Rupture of the gastrocnemius tendon, especially in male roaster birds 12–16 wk old, is often associated with reovirus infection (19, 23). A similar lesion has been seen in 5- to 8-wk-old turkeys (48). The typical uneven gait in bilateral rupture of the tendon results from inability of the bird to immobilize the metatarsus. The latter is often accompanied by ruptured blood vessels.

MALABSORPTION SYNDROME. Malabsorption syndrome in chickens is characterized by uneven growth, poor pigmentation, abnormal feathering, skeletal abnormalities, and increased mortality. Undigested feed in the feces and diarrhea have also been reported (31, 32, 47). The disease affects young 1- to 3-wk-old meat-type chickens and has been observed in the USA (47, 60), Europe (31), and Australia (49, 53).

Gross Lesions

VIRAL ARTHRITIS/TENOSYNOVITIS. Gross lesions in naturally infected chickens are observed as swellings of digital flexor and metatarsal extensor tendons. The latter lesion is evident by palpation just above the hock and may be readily observed when feathers are removed (Fig. 27.1).

Swellings of the foot pad and hock joint are less frequent. The hock usually contains a small amount of straw-colored or blood-tinted exudate; in a few cases there is a considerable amount of purulent exudate resembling that seen with infectious synovitis. Early in the infection there is marked edema of the tarsal and metatarsal tendon sheaths (Fig. 27.2). Petechial hemorrhages are frequent in the synovial membranes above the hock (Fig. 27.3B).

Inflammation of tendon areas progresses to a

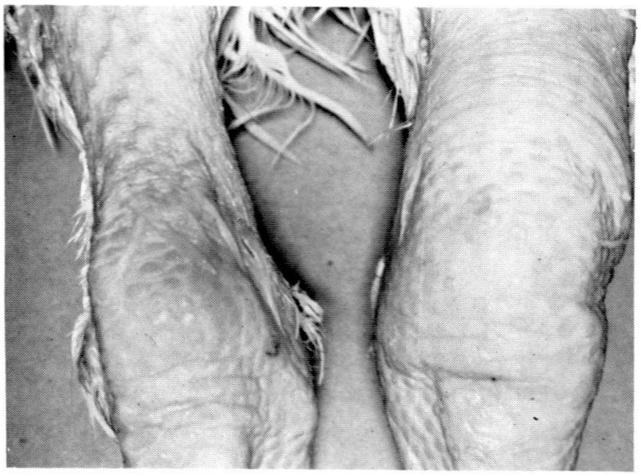

27.1. An 8-wk-old broiler showing marked swelling of digital flexor and metatarsal extensor tendons. Diagnosis can frequently be made on the basis of the bilateral swelling of these tendons.

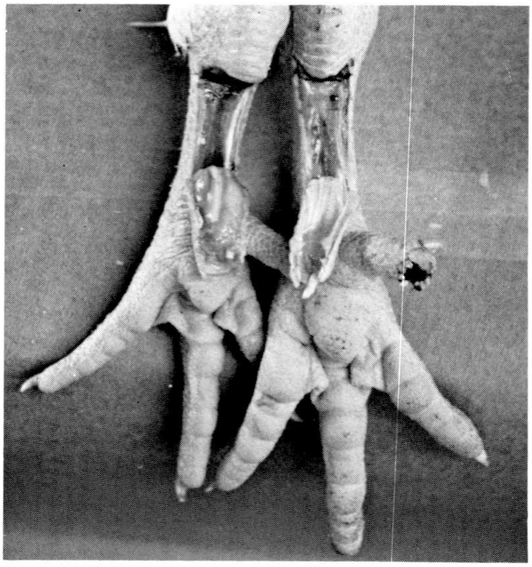

27.2. Marked edema of digital flexor tendon sheaths (*left*); normal (*right*).

chronic-type lesion characterized by hardening and fusion of tendon sheaths. Small pitted erosions develop in the articular cartilage of the distal tibiotarsus. These erosions enlarge, coalesce, and extend into underlying bone (Fig. 27.3 B, C). An overgrowth of fibrocartilaginous pannus develops on the articular surface. Condyles and epicondyles are frequently involved (28). In experimentally inoculated chickens, the diaphysis of the proximal metatarsal of the affected limb is enlarged.

MALABSORPTION SYNDROME. Although reoviruses have frequently been isolated from birds with malabsorption syndrome, etiological relationships are not unequivocally established. The most common lesions reported are an enlarged proventriculus, which may be hemorrhagic or necrotic, and a catarrhal enteritis. In addition there may be an apparent lameness associated with arthritis and osteoporosis (56). Rosenberger (60) isolated several reoviruses of varying pathogenicity from birds exhibiting signs of malabsorption syndrome. The virulent isolates induced a transient malabsorption in broilers that was associated with a degeneration of the intestinal villi. These same isolates were capable of producing lesions in other tissues as well including bursal atrophy, hepatic necrosis, and inflammation of the gastrocnemius tendon. Page et al. (47) identified reoviruses of varying pathogenicity from birds with malabsorption syndrome and reproduced the condition by oral inoculation. Van der Heide (80) isolated a reovirus that induced osteoporosis and feather defects but no other lesions.

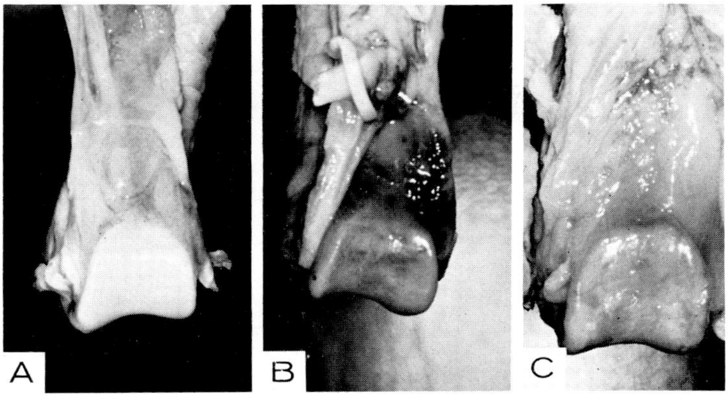

27.3. Viral arthritis lesions in distal posterior tibia of inoculated chickens. A. Normal. B. Cartilage erosions and hemorrhages of synovial membrane 35 days postinoculation. C. Erosions of cartilage and marked thickening of synovial membrane 212 days postinoculation.

Histopathology

VIRAL ARTHRITIS/TENOSYNOVITIS. Histologic changes have been described by Kerr and Olson (28). In general, they are the same for natural and experimental infections. During the acute phase (7–15 days following foot-pad inoculation), edema, coagulation necrosis, heterophil accumulation, and perivascular infiltration are seen. There also are hypertrophy and hyperplasia of synovial cells, infiltration of lymphocytes and macrophages, and a proliferation of reticular cells. These last lesions cause parietal and visceral layers of the tendon sheaths to become markedly thickened. The synovial cavity is filled with heterophils, macrophages, and sloughed synovial cells. Periostitis characterized by increased osteoclasts develops. During the chronic phase (starting by 15 days postinfection) the synovial membrane develops villous processes, and lymphoid nodules are seen. After 30 days inflammatory changes become more chronic. There is an increase in the amount of fibrous connective tissue and a pronounced infiltration or proliferation of reticular cells, lymphocytes, macrophages, and plasma cells.

The same general inflammatory changes develop in the tarsometatarsal and hock joint areas. Development of sesamoid bones in the tendon of the affected limb is inhibited. Some tendons are completely replaced by irregular granulation tissue, and large villi form on the synovial membrane.

At 54 days postinfection, orally infected birds showed chronic fibrosis of tendon sheaths, with fibrous tissues invading tendons and resulting in ankylosis and immobility (77).

Linear growth of cartilage cells in the proximal tarsometatarsal bone becomes narrow and irregular. Erosions on the hock joint cartilage are accompanied by a granulation pannus. Osteoblasts become active and lay down a thickened layer of bone beneath the erosion. Osteoblastic activity is present on the condyles, epicondyles, and accessory tibia, producing osteoneogenesis and subsequent exostosis (28).

Lesions found in the heart have been described in detail (28, 44). An infiltration of heterophils between myocardial fibers is a constant finding. In some cases it is accompanied by proliferating mononuclear cells, probably reticular cells. The pathogenicity of avian reoviruses for day-old chicks revealed the arthrogenic potential for all strains and marked hepatic necrosis (15).

Erythrocyte, hematocrit, and total leukocyte determinations are generally within the normal range, although there may be a rise in the heterophil percentage and a decrease in the lymphocyte percentage.

MALABSORPTION SYNDROME. Histopathological changes include proventriculitis with focal necrosis, myocarditis, atrophy of the bursa of Fabricius, catarrhal enteritis, and pancreatitis. There are transverse and vertical clefts in the femur growth plate with necrosis of cartilage and fragmentation of bone bark (47). Atrophic intestinal villi with associated lymphocyte infiltration have also been observed (60).

Immunity. Avian reoviruses possess a group-specific antigen discernable with gel diffusion techniques and a serotype-specific antigen demonstrable with neutralizing antibody in plaque-reduction or chicken embryo assays (56, 74). Neutralizing antibodies can be detected 7–10 days following infection and precipitating antibodies at approximately 2 wk. Neutralizing antibody appears to persist longer than precipitating antibody, but this may simply be a reflection of assay sensitivity. The importance of antibody in establishing protection is not well understood since birds may become persistently infected in the presence of high levels of circulating antibody. It is apparent, however, that maternal antibody can afford a degree of protection to 1-day-old chickens against natural and experimental challenges (76, 78). Relative protection afforded by antibody appears to be as much related to serotype homogeneity, virus virulence, and host age as to antibody titer (52, 60, 78).

Interferon induction by avian reoviruses has been demonstrated in vitro and in vivo. The S1133 attenuated strain induced interferon in chick embryo cell cultures while in vivo interferon was detected in the lungs but not in other tissues (6, 7, 83). A more pathogenic reovirus did elicit the production of interferon detectable in serum samples (6, 7).

DIAGNOSIS

VIRAL ARTHRITIS/TENOSYNOVITIS. A presumptive diagnosis of viral arthritis may be made on the basis of signs and lesions. Involvement of primarily the metatarsal extensor and digital flexor tendons (Fig. 27.2) and heterophil infiltration in the heart assist in differentiating the infection from bacterial and mycoplasmal synovitis. Demonstration of reoviruses in the tendon sheaths by fluorescent antibody techniques (56) or virus isolation in chicken embryos or chicken embryo liver cells provides further evidence (56, 74). The relative pathogenicity of a reovirus obtained from an affected joint can be confirmed by inoculation into the foot pad of susceptible day-old chickens. If pathogenic, the virus will induce a pronounced inflammation of the foot pad within 72 hr postinoculation.

Reoviruses can be readily differentiated from other viruses by their typical physicochemical characteristics and the presence of a group-specific antigen demonstrable with the agar-gel precipitin test. For preparation of the antigen, 9- to 11-day-old embryonating chicken eggs are inoculated by the CAM route and CAMs are harvested from dead or affected embryos within 7 days postinoculation. The CAMs are then homogenized and used as antigen (45). The precipitin test can be utilized to identify isolates as reovirus if known positive antiserum is available or it can be used as an indication of antibody status in affected flocks.

MALABSORPTION SYNDROME. Although reoviruses are frequently isolated from affected birds they cannot always be identified as the sole etiology of malabsorption syndrome. Signs and lesions associated with malabsorption syndrome such as stunted growth, proventriculitis, and feathering abnormalities may be induced by other agents including reticuloendotheliosis virus (84) and mycotoxins (72). Parvoviruslike agents (30) and calicivirus (88) have also been found in birds with signs of malabsorption . Reoviruses, when isolated from birds with malabsorption syndrome, can be propagated and identified using techniques described for the arthrotropic isolates.

Serology. Reovirus group-specific antibody can be readily detected with the agar-gel precipitin test (25, 45) or indirect fluorescent antibody (IFA) assay (18). The IFA test is more sensitive and therefore better suited for quantitative evaluations. Virus neutralization, based on plaque-reduction in chicken kidney or chicken embryo liver cell cultures, has been routinely utilized for determining serotype differences with rabbit or chicken antiserum (56, 74). Although several serotypes have been described, there is considerable heterogeneity among reovirus isolates, with many being classified as antigenic subtypes rather than distinct serotypes.

Slaght et al. (69) were the first to describe an enzyme-linked immunosorbent assay (ELISA) for detecting avian reovirus antibody. The S1133 strain was used as antigen and found to react with antibodies to the Reo-25 and WVU 2937 isolates; homologous antibody gave the highest titer. ELISA systems now available from commercial sources are apparently suitable for assessing reovirus antibody levels on a flock basis (73).

PREVENTION AND CONTROL.

The ubiquitous nature of the avian reoviruses and their inherent stability coupled with modern, high-density confinement-rearing practices suggests that elimination of virus exposure may be difficult. The virus can be transmitted both vertically and horizontally, and because of its resistance to inactivation may in addition be frequently carried by mechanical means. Thorough cleaning of a poultry house appears to prevent infection with pathogenic virus in subsequent groups following removal of an infected flock from the premises. Common disinfectants have not been adequately tested, but lye and 0.5% organic iodine solutions are thought to be effective inactivating agents.

Chickens are most susceptible to pathogenic reoviruses at 1 day of age and then develop an age-associated resistance beginning as early as 2 wk. Because of this enhanced period of susceptibility, vaccines and vaccination programs have evolved that are directed at providing protection at 1 day of age. Active immunization can be achieved by vaccination with viable attenuated reovirus, which is normally applied by the subcutaneous route (81). Protection from subsequent challenge can be demonstrated, but the S1133-

derived reovirus vaccines may interfere with Marek's disease vaccination if administered simultaneously (59). Reovirus vaccination of breeding stock can be done with viable or inactivated vaccines or combinations of both. The advantages of this type of immunization program includes immediate protection of 1-day-old progeny provided by maternal antibody and a limitation of the potential for transovarian transmission. Vaccination of breeders is an efficacious method of controlling viral arthritis/tenosynovitis and other pathogenic reoviruses, but it should be recognized that protection is assured against homologous serotypes only (52).

REFERENCES

1. Barta, V., W.T. Springer, and D.L. Miller, 1984. A comparison of avian and mammalian cell cultures for the propagation of avian reovirus WVU 2937. Avian Dis 28:216–223.

2. Cook, M.E., W.T. Springer, K.M. Kerr, and J.A. Herbert. 1984. Severity of tenosynovitis in reovirus-infected chickens fed various dietary levels of choline, folic acid, manganese, biotin, or niacin. Avian Dis 28:562–573.

3. Cook, M.E., W.T. Springer, and J.A. Herbert. 1984. Enhanced incidence of leg abnormalities in reovirus WVU 2937-infected chickens fed various dietary levels of selected vitamins. Avian Dis 28:548–561.

4. Dalton, P.J., and R. Henry. 1967. Tenosynovitis in poultry. Vet Rec 80:638.

5. Dutta, S.K., and B.S. Pomeroy. 1967. Isolation and characterization of an enterovirus from baby chicks having an enteric infection. I. Isolation and pathogenicity. Avian Dis 11:1–9.

6. Ellis, M.N., C.S. Eidson, J. Brown, and S.H. Kleven. 1983. Studies on interferon induction and interferon sensitivity of avian reoviruses. Avian Dis 27:927–936.

7. Ellis, M.N., C.S. Eidson, O.J. Fletcher, and S.H. Kleven. 1983. Viral tissue tropisms and interferon production in White Leghorn chickens infected with two reovirus strains. Avian Dis 27:644–651.

8. Engstrom, B.E., O. Fossum, and Margaretha Luthman. 1988. Blue wing disease of chickens: Experimental infection with Swedish isolate of chicken anemia agent and an avian reovirus. Avian Pathol 17:33–50.

9. Fahey, J.E., and J.F. Crawley. 1954. Studies on chronic respiratory disease of chickens. II. Isolation of a virus. Can J Comp Med 18:13–21.

10. Gaudry, D., J. Tektoff, and J.M. Charles. 1972. A-propos d'un nouveau virus isole chez le canard de Barbarie. Bull Soc Sci Vet Med Comparée de Lyon. 74:137–143.

11. Gershowitz, A., and R.E. Wooley. 1973. Characterization of two reoviruses isolated from turkeys with infectious enteritis. Avian Dis 17:406–414.

12. Glass, S.E., S.A. Naqi, C.F. Hall, and K.M. Kerr. 1973. Isolation and characterization of a virus associated with arthritis of chickens. Avian Dis 17:415–424.

13. Gouvea, V.S., and T.J. Schnitzer. 1982. Polymorphism of the genomic RNAs among the avian reoviruses. J Gen Virol 61:87–91.

14. Gouvea, V.S., and T.J. Schnitzer. 1982. Polymorphism of the migration of double-stranded RNA genome segments of avian reoviruses. J Virol 43:465–471.

15. Gouvea, V., and T.J. Schnitzer. 1982. Pathogenicity of avian reoviruses: Examination of six isolates and a vaccine strain. Infect Immun 38:731–738.

16. Guneratne, J.R.M., R.C. Jones, and K. Georgiou. 1982. Some observations on the isolation and cultivation of avian reoviruses. Avian Pathol 11:453–462.

17. Hieronymus, D.R.K., P. Villegas, and S.H. Kleven. 1983. Identification and serological differentiation of several reovirus strains isolated from chickens with suspected malabsorption syndrome. Avian Dis 27:246–254.

18. Ide, P.R. 1982. Avian reovirus antibody assay by indirect immunofluorescence using plastic microculture plates. Can J Comp Med 46:39–42.

19. Johnson, D.C., and L. Van der Heide. 1971. Incidence of tenosynovitis in Maine broilers. Avian Dis 15:829–834.

20. Jones R.C., and K. Georgiou. 1984. Reovirus-induced tenosynovitis in chickens: The influence of age at infection. Avian Pathol 13:441–457.

21. Jones, R.C., and F.S.B. Kibenge. 1984. Reovirus-induced tenosynovitis in chickens: The effect of breed. Avian Pathol 13:511–528.

22. Jones, R.C., and O. Onunkwo. 1978. Studies on experimental tenosynovitis in light hybrid chickens. Avian Pathol 7:171–181.

23. Jones, R.C., F.T.W. Jordan, and S. Lioupis. 1975. Characteristics of reovirus isolated from ruptured gastrocnemius tendons of chickens. Vet Rec 96:153–154.

24. Kaschula, V.R. 1950. A new virus disease of the Muscovy duck (Cairina moschata) present in Natal. J S Afr Vet Med Assoc 21:18–26.

25. Kawamura, H., and H. Tsubahara. 1966. Common antigenicity of avian reoviruses. Nat Inst Anim Health Q (Tokyo) 6:187–193.

26. Kawamura, H., F. Shimizu, M. Maeda, and H. Tsubahara. 1965. Avian reovirus: Its properties and serological classification. Nat Inst Anim Health Q (Tokyo) 5:115–124.

27. Kerr, K.M., and N.O. Olson. 1964. Control of infectious synovitis. The effect of age of chickens on the susceptibility to three agents. Avian Dis 8:256–263.

28. Kerr, K.M., and N.O. Olson. 1969. Pathology of chickens experimentally inoculated or contact-infected with an arthritis-producing virus. Avian Dis 13:729–745.

29. Kibenge, F.S.B., and G.E. Wilcox. 1983. Tenosynovitis in chickens. Vet Bull 53:431–444.

30. Kisary, J., B. Nagy, and Z. Bitay. 1984. Presence of parvoviruses in the intestine of chickens showing stunting syndrome. Avian Pathol 13:339–343.

31. Kouwenhoven, B., M. Vertommen, and J.H.H. van Eck. 1978. Runting and leg weakness in broilers: Involvement of infectious factors. Vet Sci Comm 2:253–259.

32. Kouwenhoven, B., F.G. Davelaar, and J. van Walsum. 1978. Infectious proventriculitis causing runting in broilers. Avian Pathol 7:183–187.

33. Macdonald, J.W., C.J. Randall, M.D. Dagless, and D.A. McMartin. 1978. Observations on viral tenosynovitis (viral arthritis) in Scotland. Avian Pathol 7:471–482.

34. Malkinson, M., K. Perk, and Y. Weisman. 1981. Reovirus infection of young Muscovy ducks (Cairina moschata). Avian Pathol 10:433–440.

35. Marquardt, J., W. Herrmanns, L.C. Schulz, and W. Leibold. 1983. A persistent reovirus infection of chickens as a possible model of human rheumatoid arthritis (RA). Zentralbl Veterinaermed [B] 30:274–282.

36. Mathews, R.E.F. 1982. Classification and nomenclature of viruses. Intervirology 17:1–200.

37. McFerran, J.B., T.J. Connor, and R.M. McCracken. 1976. Isolation of adenoviruses and reoviruses from avian species other than domestic fowl. Avian Dis 20:519–524.

38. Menendez, N.A., B.W. Calnek, and B.S. Cowen. 1975. Experimental egg-transmission of avian reovirus. Avian Dis 19:104–111.
39. Menendez, N.A., B.W. Calnek, and B.S. Cowen. 1975. Localization of avian reovirus (FDO isolate) in tissues of mature chickens. Avian Dis 19:112–117.
40. Nersessian, B.N., M.A. Godwin, S.H. Kleven, and D. Pesti. 1985. Studies on orthoreoviruses isolated from young turkeys. I. Isolation and characterization. Avian Dis 29:755–767.
41. Olson, N.O., and K.M. Kerr. 1966. Some characteristics of an avian arthritis viral agent. Avian Dis 10:470–476.
42. Olson, N.O., and K.M. Kerr. 1967. The duration and distribution of synovitis-producing agents in chickens. Avian Dis 11:578–585.
43. Olson, N.O., and M.A. Khan. 1972. The effect of intranasal exposure of chickens to the Fahey-Crawley virus on the development of synovial lesions. Avian Dis 16:1073–1078.
44. Olson, N.O., and D.P. Solomon. 1968. A natural outbreak of synovitis caused by the viral arthritis agent. Avian Dis 12:311–316.
45. Olson, N.O., and R. Weiss. 1972. Similarity between arthritis virus and Fahey-Crawley virus. Avian Dis 16:535–540.
46. Olson, N.O., D.C. Shelton, and D.A. Munro. 1957. Infectious synovitis control by medication-effect of strain differences and pleuropneumonia-like organisms. Am J Vet Res 18:735–739.
47. Page, R.K., O.J. Fletcher, G.N. Rowland, D. Gaudry, and P. Villegas. 1982. Malabsorption syndrome in chickens. Avian Dis 26:618–624.
48. Page, R.K., O.J. Fletcher, and P. Villegas. 1982. Infectious tenosynovitis in young turkeys. Avian Dis 26:924–927.
49. Pass, D.A., M.D. Robertson, and G.E. Wilcox. 1982. Runting syndrome in broiler chickens in Australia. Vet Rec 110:386–387.
50. Petek, M., B. Felluga, G. Borghi, and A. Baroni. 1967. The Crawley agent: An avian reovirus. Arch Gesamte Virusforsch 21:413–424.
51. Phillips, P.A., N.F. Stanley, and M. Walters. 1970. Murine disease induced by avian reovirus. Aust J Exp Biol Med Sci 48:277–284.
52. Rau, W.E., L. Van der Heide, M. Kalbac, and T. Girshick. 1980. Onset of progeny immunity against viral arthritis/tenosynovitis after experimental vaccination of parent breeder chickens and cross immunity against six reovirus isolates. Avian Dis 24:648–657.
53. Reece, R.L., P.T. Hooper, S.H. Tate, V.D. Beddome, W. M. Forsyth, P.C. Scott, and S.D.A. Barr. 1984. Field, clinical and pathological observations of a runting and stunting syndrome in broilers. Vet Rec 115:483–485.
54. Rinehart, C.L., and J.K. Rosenberger. 1983. Effects of avian reoviruses on the immune responses of chickens. Poult Sci 62:1488–1489.
55. Robertson, M.D., and G.E. Wilcox. 1984. Serological characteristics of avian reoviruses of Australian origin. Avian Pathol 13:585–594.
56. Robertson, M.D., and G.E. Wilcox. 1986. Avian reovirus. Vet Bull 56:155–174.
57. Robertson, M.D., G.E. Wilcox, and F.S.B. Kibenge. 1984. Prevalence of reoviruses in commercial chickens. Aust Vet J 61:319–322.
58. Roessler, D.E. 1986. Studies on the pathogenicity and persistence of avian reovirus pathotypes in relation to age resistance and immunosuppression. PhD diss. Univ Delaware, Newark.
59. Rosenberger, J.K. 1983. Reovirus interference with Marek's disease vaccination. Proc 32nd West Poult Dis Conf, pp. 50–51.
60. Rosenberger, J.K. 1983. Characterization of reoviruses associated with runting syndrome in chickens. Proc No 66, pp. 141–152. Int Union Immunol Soc, Sydney, Aust.
61. Rosenberger, J.K., P.A. Fries, S.S. Cloud, and R.A. Wilson. 1985. In vitro and in vivo characterization of Escherichia coli. II. Factors associated with pathogenicity. Avian Dis 29:1094–1107.
62. Ruff, M.D., and J.K. Rosenberger. 1985. Concurrent infections with reoviruses and coccidia in broilers. Avian Dis 29:465–478.
63. Ruff, M.D., and J.K. Rosenberger. 1985. Interaction of low-pathogenicity reoviruses and low levels of infection with several coccidia species. Avian Dis 29:1057–1065.
64. Sahu, S.P., and N.O. Olson. 1975. Comparison of the characteristics of avian reoviruses isolated from the digestive and respiratory tract, with viruses isolated from the synovia. Am J Vet Res 36:847–850.
65. Schnitzer, T.J., T. Ramos, and V. Gouvea. 1982. Avian reovirus polypeptides: Analysis of intracellular virus-specified products, virions, top component, and cores. J Virol 43:1006–1014.
66. Schnitzer, T.J., J. Rosenberger, D.D. Huang, V. Gouvea, T. Ramos, and K. Hassett. 1983. Molecular biology and pathogenicity of avian reoviruses. In R.W. Compons and D.H. Bishop (eds.), Double-stranded RNA Viruses, pp. 383–390. Elsevier, New York.
67. Schwartz, L.D., R.F. Gentry, H. Rothenbacher, and L. Van der Heide. 1976. Infectious tenosynovitis in commercial white leghorn chickens. Avian Dis 20:769–773.
68. Simmons, D.G., W.M. Colwell, K.E. Muse, and C.E. Brewer. 1972. Isolation and characterization of an enteric reovirus causing high mortality in turkey poults. Avian Dis 16:1094–1102.
69. Slaght, S.S., T.J. Yang, L. Van der Heide, and T.N. Fredrickson. 1978. An enzyme-linked immunosorbent assay (ELISA) for detecting chicken anti-reovirus antibody at high sensitivity. Avian Dis 22:802–805.
70. Spandidos, D.A., and A.F. Graham. 1976. Physical and chemical characterization of an avian reovirus. J Virol 19:968–976.
71. Springer, W.T., N.O. Olson, K.M. Kerr, and C.J. Fabacher. 1983. Responses of specific-pathogen-free chicks to concomitant infections of reovirus (WVU-2937) and infectious bursal disease virus. Avian Dis 27:911–917.
72. Stuart, B.P., R.J. Cole, E.R. Waller, and R.E. Vesonder. 1986. Proventricular hyperplasia (malabsorption syndrome) in broiler chickens. J Environ Pathol Toxicol Oncol 6:369–385.
73. Thayer, S.G., P. Villegas, and O.J. Fletcher. 1987. Comparison of two commercial enzyme-linked immunosorbent assays and conventional methods for avian serology. Avian Dis 31:120–124.
74. Van der Heide, L. 1977. Viral arthritis/tenosynovitis: A review. Avian Pathol 6:271–284.
75. Van der Heide, L., and M. Kalbac. 1975. Infectious tenosynovitis (viral arthritis): Characterization of a Connecticut viral isolant as a reovirus and evidence of viral egg transmission by reovirus-infected broiler breeders. Avian Dis 19:653–658.
76. Van der Heide, L., and R.K. Page. 1980. Field experiments with viral arthritis/tenosynovitis vaccination of breeder chickens. Avian Dis 24:493–497.
77. Van der Heide, L., J. Geissler, and E.S. Bryant. 1974. Infectious tenosynovitis: Serologic and histopathologic response after experimental infection with a

Connecticut isolate. Avian Dis 18:289–296.

78. Van der Heide, L., M. Kalbac, and W.C. Hall. 1976. Infectious tenosynovitis (viral arthritis): Influence of maternal antibodies on the development of tenosynovitis lesions after experimental infection by day-old chickens with tenosynovitis virus. Avian Dis 20:641–648.

79. Van der Heide, L., M. Kalbac, M. Brustolon, and M.G. Lawson. 1980. Pathogenicity for chickens of a reovirus isolated from turkeys. Avian Dis 24:989–997.

80. Van der Heide, L., D. Lütticken, and M. Horzinek. 1981. Isolation of avian reovirus as a possible etiologic agent of osteoporosis ("brittle bone disease": "femoral head necrosis") in broiler chickens. Avian Dis 25:847–856.

81. Van der Heide, L., M. Kalbac, and M. Brustolon. 1983. Development of an attenuated apathogenic reovirus vaccine against viral arthritis/tenosynovitis. Avian Dis 27:698–706.

82. Walker, E.R., M.H. Friedman, and N.O. Olson. 1972. Electron microscopic study of an avian reovirus that causes arthritis. J Ultrastruct Res 41:67–79.

83. Winship, T.R., and P.I. Marcus. 1980. Interferon induction by viruses. VI. Reovirus: Virion genome dsRNA as the interferon inducer in aged chick embryo cells. J Interferon Res 1:155–167.

84. Witter, R.L. 1984. Reticuloendotheliosis. In M.S. Hofstad, H.J. Barnes, B.W. Calnek, W.M. Reid, and H.W. Yoder, Jr. (eds.), Diseases of Poultry, 8th Ed., pp. 406–417. Iowa State Univ Press, Ames.

85. Woernle, H., A. Brunner, and K.F. Kussaul. 1974. Nachweis aviären Reo-Viren im Agar-Gel-Präzipitationstest. Tierärztl Umsch 29:307–312.

86. Wood, G.W., R.A.J. Nicholas, C.N. Hebert, and D.H. Thornton. 1980. Serological comparisons of avian reoviruses. J Comp Pathol 90:29–38.

87. Wooley, R.E., T.A. Dees, A.S. Cromack, and J.B. Gratzek. 1972. Infectious enteritis of turkeys: Characterization of two reoviruses isolated by sucrose density gradient centrifugation from turkeys with infectious enteritis. Am J Vet Res 33:157–164.

88. Wyeth, P.J., N.T. Chettle, and J. Labramo. 1981. Avian calicivirus. Vet Rec 109:477.

28 INFECTIOUS BURSAL DISEASE

P.D. Lukert and Y.M. Saif

INTRODUCTION. Infectious bursal disease (IBD) is an acute, highly contagious viral infection of young chickens that has lymphoid tissue as its primary target with a special predilection for the bursa of Fabricius. It was first recognized as a specific disease entity by Cosgrove (19) in 1962 and was referred to as "avian nephrosis" because of the extreme kidney damage found in birds that succumbed to infection. Since the first outbreaks occurred in the area of Gumboro, Del., "Gumboro disease" was a synonym for this disease and is still frequently used. The economic importance of this disease is manifested in two ways. First, some virus strains may cause up to 20% mortality in chickens 3 wk of age and older. The second, and more important, manifestation is a severe, prolonged immunosuppression of chickens infected at an early age. Sequelae that have been associated with immunosuppression induced by the virus include gangrenous dermatitis, inclusion body hepatitis-anemia syndrome, *E. coli* infections, and vaccination failures. The virus does not affect humans and has no public health significance.

HISTORY. Early studies to identify the etiologic agent of IBD (avian nephrosis) were clouded by the presence of infectious bronchitis virus in the kidneys of field cases. Winterfield and Hitchner (139) described a virus isolate (Gray) that came from a field case of nephrosis not unlike the newly reported syndrome. Because of the similarity between kidney lesions induced by Gray virus and those seen in avian nephrosis as described by Cosgrove (19), it was believed that Gray virus was the causative agent. Later studies, however, revealed that birds immune to Gray virus could still be infected with the IBD agent and would develop changes in the cloacal bursa specific for the disease. In subsequent studies with IBD, Winterfield et al. (140) succeeded in isolating an agent in embryonating eggs. The mortality pattern was irregular and the agent was difficult to maintain in serial passage. The isolate was referred to as "infectious bursal agent" and was identified as the true cause of IBD; Gray virus was identified as an isolate of infectious bronchitis virus with nephrotoxic tendencies. Hitchner (40) subsequently proposed the term infectious bursal disease as the name of the disease causing specific pathognomonic lesions of the cloacal bursa.

In 1972, Allan et al. (1) reported that IBD virus (IBDV) infections at an early age were immunosuppressive. The recognition of the immunosuppressive capability of IBDV infections greatly increased the interest in the control of these infections. The existence of a second serotype was reported in 1980 (80). Control of IBD viral infections has been complicated by the recognition of "variant" strains of serotype 1 IBDV that were found in the Delmarva poultry-producing area (106, 112). These strains were breaking through maternal immunity against "standard" strains, and they also differed from standard strains in their biological properties (110, 111). Variants, or subtypes, were either already present in nature but unrecognized, or are new mutants that have arisen, possibly due to immune pressure.

INCIDENCE AND DISTRIBUTION. Infections with serotype 1 IBDV are of worldwide distribution, occurring in all major poultry-producing areas. The incidence of infection in these areas is high; essentially all flocks are exposed to the virus during the early stages of life. One exception to the ubiquitous nature of IBDV is New Zealand. It has been reported (60, 141) that there is no evidence of IBDV infections in that country. Because of vaccination programs carried out by most producers, all chickens eventually become seropositive to IBDV. However, clinical cases are very rare because infections are either modified by maternal antibody or are due to variant strains that do not cause obvious clinical disease but only induce immunosuppression.

In the USA, it was shown that antibodies to serotype 2 IBDV were widespread in chicken (51, 112) and turkey flocks (5, 14, 53), indicating the common prevalence of the infection.

ETIOLOGY

Classification. IBDV is a member of the Birnaviridae family (12, 23, 87). The family has one genus, *Birnavirus,* and the prototype is infectious pancreatic necrosis virus of fish. Other viruses in that family include tellina virus of bivalve mollusks and drosophila x virus of the fruit fly (23). Viruses in that family have genomes consisting of two segments of double-stranded (ds)RNA (76, 87, 133), hence the name birnaviruses. Before the recognition of the Birnaviridae family and before there was adequate information on morphology and physicochemical characteristics of IBDV, it was placed at times in the Picornaviridae (16, 75) or the Reoviridae families (34, 65, 71, 99).

Morphology. The virus is a single-shelled, nonenveloped virion with icosahedral symmetry and a diameter varying from 55 to 65 nm (37, 92, 95) (Fig. 28.1). The capsid symmetry is askew, with a triangulation number T = 13 and a dextrohandedness (95).

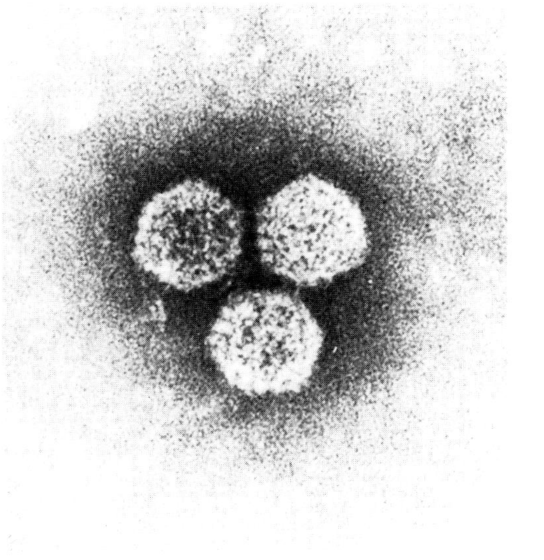

28.1. Electron micrograph of negatively stained IBD viral particles. ×200,000. (Reed)

Buoyant density of complete particles in cesium chloride gradients has been reported to range from 1.31 to 1.34 g/ml (7, 28, 53, 86, 92, 99, 136). Lower density values were reported for incomplete virus particles.

Chemical Composition. The dsRNA of the IBDV genome has two segments (7, 23, 54, 87) as shown by polyacrylamide gel electrophoresis. Jackwood et al. (54) reported that the two segments of five serotype 1 viruses migrated similarly when coelectrophoresed. The RNA segments from serotype 2 viruses migrated similarly but were different from serotype 1 viruses when coelectrophoresed, suggesting that RNA migration patterns could be used to differentiate IBDV isolates that differ serotypically. Becht et al. (8) reported similar results when comparing isolates of each serotype.

It is currently recognized that the virus has four viral proteins designated VP1, VP2, VP3, and VP4 (7, 22, 23, 92, 136). The above designations are not used universally. The approximate molecular weights of the four proteins are 90 kD, 41 kD, 32 kD and 28 kD, respectively. Additional proteins, such as VPX, have been observed and are thought to have a precursor-product relationship (22). Jackwood et al. (54) reported that two serotype 2 viruses had VPX and no VP2, but Kibenge et al. (64) detected VP2 in the same strains. The discrepancy seems to be a matter of terminology, since the molecular weight ranges reported by both groups were comparable. Becht et al. (8) compared isolates of serotype 1 and 2 and reported viral proteins with molecular weights in the same range as those observed by Jackwood et al. and Kibenge et al. (54, 64). VP2 and VP3 are the major proteins of IBDV. In serotype 1 viruses they constitute 51 and 40% of the virus proteins, respectively (23), whereas VP1 (3%) and VP4 (6%) are minor proteins. VP1 is presumed to be the viral RNA polymerase and it is speculated that VP4 is a viral protease (44, 89, 132). The small segment of the IBDV genome (B) codes for VP1, whereas the large segment (A) encodes the rest of the viral proteins (3, 44, 84).

A conformational dependent (discontinuous) neutralizing epitope was detected on VP2 and a conformational independent (continuous) epitope on VP3. Antibodies to these epitopes were found to passively protect chickens (4). It was reported earlier (29) that VP3 had the antigenic determinants for serotype specificity but later studies indicated that these determinants were on VP2 (4, 8). According to Becht et al. (8), monoclonal antibodies to VP2 differentiated between the two serotypes of the virus, whereas monoclonal antibodies to VP3 recognized a group-specific antigen from both serotypes. Snyder et al. (129) developed a monoclonal antibody to VP2 that neutralized both serotypes of the virus, indicating the existence of multiple epitopes on VP2.

The chemistry of the virus has been reviewed in detail by Kibenge et al. (62).

Virus Replication. Kibenge et al. (62) has reviewed this subject. In general, little is known about the biochemical events associated with replication of birnaviruses. Several laboratory hosts for IBDV are described later in this chapter. The virus was shown to attach to chicken embryo kidney cells maximally 75 min after inoculation (71). The multiplication cycle in chicken embryo cells is 10–36 hr and the latent period is 4–6 hr (7, 54, 71, 92). In Vero and baby grivet monkey (BGM)-70 cells, a longer (48-hr) multiplication cycle was described (57, 63, 74). Viral polypeptides were detected in chicken bursal lymphoid cells grown in vitro and in their culture media at 90 min and 6 hr postinfection, respectively (86). The cell receptor recognition site on the virus is not known.

The mechanism of viral RNA synthesis has not been clearly determined. A dsRNA-dependent RNA polymerase thought to be VP1 was described (132). Genome-linked proteins have been demonstrated, indicating that the virus replicates its nucleic acid by a strand displacement mechanism. RNA polymerase activity could be demonstrated without pretreatment of the virus, indicating that transcription and replication occur following cell penetration without uncoating of the virus (132).

Becht (7) reported that synthesis of host proteins is not shut off in chicken embryo fibroblasts infected with IBDV.

Resistance to Chemical and Physical Agents. Studies have indicated that IBDV is very stable. Benton et al. (9) found that IBDV resisted treatment with ether and chloroform, was inactivated at pH 12 but unaffected by pH 2, and was still viable after 5 hr at 56 C. The virus was unaffected by exposure to 0.5% phenol and 0.125% thimerosal for 1 hr at 30 C. There was a marked reduction in virus infectivity when exposed to 0.5% formalin for 6 hr. The virus was also treated with various concentrations of three disinfectants (an iodine complex, a phenolic derivative, a quaternary ammonium compound) for a period of 2 min at 23 C. Only the iodine complex had any deleterious effects. Landgraf et al. (66) found that the virus survived 60 C but not 70 C for 30 min, and 0.5% chloramine killed the virus after 10 min.

Certainly, the hardy nature of this virus is one reason for its long, persistent survival in poultry houses even when thorough cleaning and disinfection procedures are followed.

Strain Classification. McFerran et al. (80), in N. Ireland, were the first to report antigenic variations among IBDV isolates of European origin. They presented evidence for the presence of two serotypes designated 1 and 2, and showed only 30% relatedness between several strains of serotype 1 and the designated prototype of that serotype. Similar results were observed in the USA (53, 70), and the American serotypes were designated I and II. Later studies (81) indicated the relatedness of the European and American isolates of the second serotype and use of the Arabic numerals 1 and 2 to describe the two serotypes of IBDV was proposed. Antigenic relatedness of only 33% between two strains of serotype 2 was reported (81), indicating an antigenic diversity similar to that of serotype 1 viruses.

The two serotypes are differentiated by virus-neutralization (VN) tests, but they are not distinguishable by fluorescent antibody tests or enzyme-linked immunosorbent assay (ELISA). Immunization against serotype 2 does not protect against serotype 1. The reverse situation cannot be tested because there are no virulent serotype 2 viruses for challenge (45, 56). The first isolates of serotype 2 (53) originated from turkeys and it was thought that this serotype was host specific. However, later studies showed that viruses of serotype 2 could be isolated from chickens (46), and antibodies to serotype 2 IBDVs are common in both chickens and turkeys (51, 112).

Variant viruses of serotype 1 were described (107, 112). Vaccine strains available at the time they were isolated did not protect against the variants, which are antigenically different from the standard serotype 1 isolates.

Jackwood and Saif (52) conducted a cross-neutralization study of 8 serotype 1 commercial vaccine strains, 5 serotype 1 field strains, and 2 serotype 2 field strains. Six subtypes were distinguished among the 13 serotype 1 strains studied. One of the subtypes included all of the variant isolates. Snyder et al. (130), using monoclonal antibodies, suggested that a major antigenic shift in serotype 1 viruses had occurred in the field.

Laboratory Host Systems

CHICKEN EMBRYOS. Initially, most workers had difficulty in isolating virus or, if successful, in serially transferring virus using chicken embryos. Landgraf et al. (66) reported a typical experience using the allantoic sac route of inoculation. On the first passage all inoculated embryos died, on the second, 30% died, and on the third, there was no embryo mortality.

Continued studies (40) uncovered three factors that could explain these difficulties: 1) Embryonating eggs that originated from flocks recovered from the disease were highly resistant to growth of the virus. 2) In early virus passage, the allantoamnionic fluid (AAF) had a very low virus content while the chorioallantoic membrane (CAM) and embryo each had a much higher and nearly equal virus content. 3) Comparison of the allantoic sac, yolk sac, and CAM as routes of inoculation showed the allantoic sac to be the least desirable, yielding embryo infective dose-50% (EID_{50}) virus titers of 1.5–2.0 $\log_{10}$ lower than by the CAM route. The yolk sac route gave titers that were intermediate.

Winterfield (138) increased virus concentration in the AAF by serial passage in embryonating eggs. Hitchner (40) used isolate 2512, obtained from Winterfield in the 46th embryo passage, to perform a multistep growth curve study. He found that virus concentration reached a peak 72 hr postinoculation.

Injection of the virus into 10-day-old embryonating eggs resulted in embryo mortality from the 3–5 days postinoculation. Gross lesions observed in the embryo were edematous distention of the abdominal region; cutaneous congestion and petechial hemorrhages, particularly along feather tracts; occasional hemorrhages on toe joints and in the cerebral region; mottled-appearing necrosis and ecchymotic hemorrhages in the liver (latter stages); pale "parboiled" appearance of the heart; congestion and some mottled necrosis of kidneys; extreme congestion of lungs; and pale spleen, occasionally with small necrotic foci. The CAM had no plaques, but small hemorrhagic areas were observed at times. Lesions induced in embryos by IBDV variants differ from those induced by standard isolates. Splenomegaly and liver necrosis are characteristic of the lesions induced by the variants, but there is little mortality (110).

CELL CULTURE. Many strains of IBDV have been adapted to cell cultures of chicken embryo origin and cytopathic effects have been observed. Cell culture–adapted virus may be quantified by plaque assay or microtiter techniques. Rinaldi et al. (105) and Petek et al. (102) were able to culture egg-adapted strains of IBDV in chicken embryo fibroblasts, which proved more sensitive to the virus than either embryonating eggs or suckling mice. Most laboratories now use these cells for culture propagation of the virus.

Lukert and Davis (71) successfully adapted wild-type virus from infected bursas in cells derived from the chicken embryo bursa. After four serial passages in chicken embryo bursa cells the virus grew in chicken embryo kidney cells and produced plaques under agar. This virus was subsequently propagated in chicken embryo fibroblasts and used as an attenuated live virus vaccine (122). Cells susceptible to the virus other than cells of chicken origin include turkey and duck embryo cells (82), mammalian cell lines derived from rabbit kidneys (RK-13) (105), monkey kidneys (Vero) (74, 63) and baby grivet monkey kidney cells (BGM-70) (57).

Jackwood et al. (57) compared three mammalian cell lines (MA-104, Vero, and BGM-70) for their ability to support several strains of IBDV serotypes 1 and 2, including serotype 1 variants. The viruses replicated in the three cell lines but the cytopathic effect was most pronounced in the BGM-70 cells. The growth curve of one strain tested in BGM-70 cells was similar to that in chicken embryo fibroblasts, and VN titers in BGM-70 cultures compared well with those in chicken embryo fibroblasts. The BGM-70 cells are used routinely for serology by one of the authors (113).

A continuous fibroblast cell line of Japanese quail origin was found to support the replication of IBDV and several other viral pathogens of poultry (20). These viruses, already adapted to tissue culture, produced a cytopathic effect in the quail cells.

Hirai and Calnek (36) propagated virulent IBDV in normal chicken lymphocytes and in a lymphoblastoid B-cell line derived from an avian leukosis virus-induced tumor. The virus would not replicate in six T-cell lymphoblastoid cell lines initiated from Marek's disease tumors. Their work showed that IgM-bearing B lymphocytes were the probable target cells of IBDV. This was subsequently verified in a study on normal lymphocytes of chickens (90). Lymphocytes from the cloacal bursa and thymus were purified and separated into T cells, B cells, and null cells. The B cells bearing surface IgM were susceptible to IBDV but the T cells and null cells were not.

Müller (85) enriched Ig-bearing cells by rosetting and cell sorting and observed that IBDV replicated preferentially in a population of proliferating cells and that susceptibility did not correlate with expression of immunoglobulins on their surface.

Isolation of IBDV from field cases of the disease may be difficult. McFerran et al. (80) found it very difficult to isolate and serially propagate the virus in cell cultures of chicken embryo origin. Lee and Lukert (67) attempted isolations of IBDV from several field cases in turkeys and chickens as well as challenge strains received from other laboratories. Turkey strains (five of five) were readily adapted to chicken embryo fibroblast cells after 3–10 blind passages. Only two of nine chicken strains could be adapted to chicken embryo fibroblast cells; the other seven strains could be grown only in chicken embryo bursal cells, even after 20 bursal cell passages.

BGM-70 cells were used successfully for isolation of IBDV from the bursas of naturally infected chickens (113). Usually a cytopathic effect was detected after two or three blind passages.

One aspect that should be considered concerning in vitro replication of the virus is the possibility of development of defective particles. Müller et al. (88) reported that serial passages of undiluted virus in chicken embryo cells resulted in fluctuations in infectivity and the development of a stable small plaque–forming virus that interfered with the replication of the standard virus and favored the generation of defective particles. The defective particles had lost the large segment of dsRNA.

Pathogenicity. Chickens are the only animals known to develop clinical disease and distinct lesions when exposed to IBDV. Field viruses exhibit different degrees of pathogenicity in chickens. Vaccine viruses also have varying pathogenic potential in chickens as discussed later in this chapter.

There has been considerable interest in studying the potential pathogenicity of viruses belonging to serotype 2 in chickens and turkeys. Jackwood et al. (56) reported a lack of clinical signs, and either gross or microscopic lesions in chickens inoculated with a serotype 2 isolate. However,

Sivanandan et al. (121) observed typical IBDV lesions in chickens inoculated with the same isolate. In later studies (46), five isolates of serotype 2, three of chicken origin, and two of turkey origin (including the isolate studied by Jackwood et al. and Sivanandan et al.) were found nonpathogenic in chickens.

In turkey poults inoculated at 1–8 days of age, an isolate of serotype 2 from turkeys failed to cause disease, gross or microscopic lesions in the cloacal bursa, thymus, or spleen (55). However, the virus was infectious and the poults responded serologically to the infection. Nusbaum et al. (93) studied experimental infection in day-old poults with isolates representing serotypes 1 and 2 that originated from turkeys. Virus-infected cells were detected by immunofluorescence in the bursa, thymus, spleen, and the gland of Harder of infected birds; no clinical disease resulted, only slight gross changes were observed, and no histologic differences were seen between infected and noninfected birds. In general, the distribution of fluorescing cells (infected) from the above tissues seemed to indicate that the majority were not lymphocytes. However, the number of plasma cells in the gland of Harder was reduced at 28 days of age.

PATHOGENESIS AND EPIZOOTIOLOGY

Natural and Experimental Hosts. For many years the chicken was considered the only species in which natural infection occurred. All breeds were affected and it was observed by many that white leghorns exhibited the most severe reactions and had the highest mortality rate. However, Meroz (83) found no difference in mortality between heavy and light breeds in a survey of 700 outbreaks of the disease.

The period of greatest susceptibility is between 3 and 6 wk of age. Susceptible chickens younger than 3 wk do not exhibit clinical signs but have subclinical infections that are economically important because the result can be severe immunosuppression of the chicken. This immunosuppressive effect of IBDV was first recognized by Allan et al. (1) and Faragher et al. (30) and is discussed later in this chapter.

The reason for the apparent age susceptibility of chickens to IBD has been the subject of several research publications regarding the pathogenesis of IBDV infections. Fadley et al. (27) treated 3-day-old chicks with cyclophosphamide and found they were refractory to clinical signs and lesions when challenged at 4 wk of age. Kaufer and Weiss (61) found similar results with birds surgically bursectomized at 4 wk of age. When they were challenged immediately or 1 wk later, there was no clinical disease, whereas 100% of control nonbursectomized chickens died. Bursectomized chickens challenged with virulent virus produced 1000 times less virus than control birds, produced VN antibodies by the 5th day, and had only very discrete and transient necrosis of lymphatic tissues. In contrast, Schat et al. (114) performed embryonal bursectomy of chickens and then challenged them at 2 and 6 wk of age. These birds developed typical hemorrhagic lesions of IBD, were clinically ill, and some died of the infection.

Skeeles et al. (123) attempted to show that lesions were a result of formation of immune complexes, as proposed by Ivanyi and Morris (49). Histologic lesions in the cloacal bursa resemble an Arthus reaction (necrosis, hemorrhage, large numbers of polymorphonuclear cells). This reaction is a type of localized immunologic injury induced by antigen-antibody complexes and complement. The hypothesis is that either antibody or complement is deficient early in the life of the chicken and therefore the Arthus reaction would not occur. They demonstrated that 2-wk-old chicks produced antibody just as fast as 8-wk-old chicks; however, the former had very little complement. They also showed that complement was depleted in IBDV-infected chickens 3, 5, and 7 days postinfection. However, Skeeles et al. (126) could not substantiate depletion of complement at 3 days postinfection. The report by Schat et al. (114) demonstrated formation of lesions in embryonally bursectomized chickens that did not produce IBDV antibodies. These findings also would not support an Arthus reaction.

Kosters et al. (65) and Skeeles et al. (123, 126) found increased clotting times in IBDV-infected chickens and suggested that such coagulopathies would contribute to the hemorrhagic lesions observed with this disease. Skeeles et al. (126) found that 17-day-old chickens did not exhibit clotting defects, but at 42 days they had greatly increased clotting times and became clinically ill; 4 of 11 died. The key to the pathogenesis of IBDV in birds of different ages may lie with the factors involved in the clotting of blood and not with an immunologic response.

Natural infections of turkeys and ducks have been recorded (59, 80, 82, 96). Serologic evidence and isolation of IBDV from these species indicate that natural infections do occur. McNulty et al. (82) examined turkey serums from several flocks and could not detect IBDV antibodies prior to 1978, suggesting that IBDV infections of turkeys were a relatively new occurrence.

Giambrone et al. (32) found that experimental IBDV infections of turkeys were subclinical in 3- to 6-wk-old poults, producing microscopic lesions in the bursa. Virus-infected cells in the bursa were detected by immunofluorescence. Neutralizing antibody was detected 12 days postinfection, and the virus could be reisolated after five serial passages in chicken embryos. Weisman and Hitchner (137) could not reisolate virus from their 6- to 8-wk-old IBDV-infected poults, but they observed an increase in VN antibody. Infection was subclinical and no damage to the bursa was evident. These authors were not able to infect Coturnix quail with a chicken strain of IBDV.

Transmission, Carriers, Vectors. IBD is highly contagious and the virus is persistent in the environment of a poultry house. Benton et al. (10) found that houses from which infected birds were removed were still infective for other birds 54 and 122 days later. They also demonstrated that water, feed, and droppings taken from infected pens were infectious after 52 days.

There is no evidence that IBDV is transmitted through the egg or that a true carrier state exists in recovered birds. Resistance of the virus to heat and disinfectants is sufficient to account for virus survival in the environment between outbreaks. Snedeker et al. (127) demonstrated that the lesser mealworm (*Alphitobius diaperinus*), taken from a house 8 wk after an outbreak, was infectious for susceptible chickens when fed as a ground suspension. It was not determined whether it acted as a biologic or mechanical vector.

Howie and Thorsen (42) isolated IBDV from mosquitoes (*Aedes vexans*) that were trapped in an area where chickens were being raised in Southern Ontario. The isolate was nonpathogenic for chickens. If IBDV were found to be arthropod-borne, the methods of control would be drastically altered.

Okoye and Uche (94) detected IBDV antigens by the agar-gel precipitation (AGP) test in 6 of 23 tissue samples from rats caught dead from four poultry farms that had a history of IBDV infection. Further observations are needed on the possible role of rodents in transmission of the disease.

Incubation Period and Signs. The incubation period is very short and clinical signs of the disease are seen in 2–3 days. Helmboldt and Garner (35) detected histologic evidence of infection in the cloacal bursa within 24 hr. Müller et al. (87), using immunofluorescence techniques, observed infected gut-associated macrophages and lymphoid cells within 4–5 hr after oral exposure to IBDV. Virus-infected cells were present in the cloacal bursa by 11 hr after oral exposure and 6 hr after direct application of virus to the bursa.

One of the earliest signs of infection in a flock is the tendency for some birds to pick at their own vents. Cosgrove (19), in his original report, described soiled vent feathers, whitish or watery diarrhea, anorexia, depression, ruffled feathers, trembling, severe prostration, and finally death. Affected birds became dehydrated and, in terminal stages of the disease, had a subnormal temperature.

Morbidity and Mortality. In fully susceptible flocks, the disease appears suddenly and there is a high morbidity rate, usually approaching 100%. Mortality usually begins on the 3rd day postinfection and will peak and recede in a period of 5–7 days. Actual mortality may be nil but can be as high as 20–30%. Striking features of this disease are the sudden and high morbidity rate, spiking death curve, and rapid flock recovery.

Initial outbreaks on a farm are usually the most acute. Recurrent outbreaks in succeeding broods are less severe and frequently go undetected. Many infections are silent, owing to age of birds (less than 3 wk), infection with avirulent field strains, or infection in presence of maternal antibody.

Gross Lesions. Birds that succumb to the infection are dehydrated, with darkened discoloration of pectoral muscles. Frequently, hemorrhages are present in the thigh and pectoral muscles (Fig. 28.2). There is increased mucus in the intestine, and renal changes (19) may be prominent in birds that die or are in advanced stages of the disease. Such lesions are most probably a consequence of severe dehydration. In birds killed and examined during the course of infection, kidneys appear normal.

The cloacal bursa appears to be the primary target organ of the virus. Cheville (13) made a detailed study of bursal weights for 12 days postinfection. It is important that the sequence of changes be understood when examining birds for

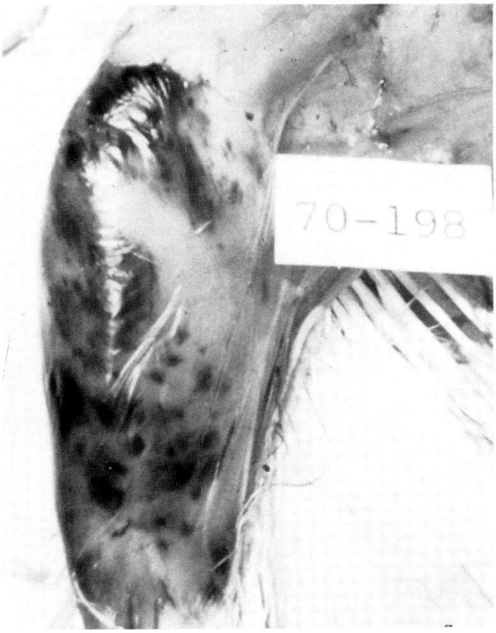

28.2. Hemorrhages of leg muscle typical in IBD.

diagnosis. By the 2nd or 3rd day postinfection, the bursa has a gelatinous yellowish transudate covering the serosal surface. Longitudinal striations on the surface become prominent, and the normal white color turns to cream. The transudate disappears as the bursa returns to its normal size and becomes gray during and following the period of atrophy. On the 3rd day postinfection the bursa begins to increase in size and weight because of edema and hyperemia (Fig. 28.3). By the 4th day it usually is double its normal weight and then it begins to recede in size. By the 5th day it has returned to normal weight, but the bursa continues to atrophy and from the 8th day on it is approximately one-third its original weight.

Variant isolates of IBDV were reported not to induce an inflammatory response (107, 117). Hence, the initial enlargement of the bursa and the gelatinous yellowish transudate might not be observed.

The infected bursa often shows necrotic foci and at times petechial or ecchymotic hemorrhages on the mucosal surface. Occasionally, extensive hemorrhage throughout the entire bursa has been observed (Fig. 28.3); in these cases birds may void blood in droppings.

The spleen may be slightly enlarged and very often has small gray foci uniformly dispersed on the surface (104). Occasionally, hemorrhages are observed in the mucosa at the juncture of the proventriculus and gizzard.

Histopathology. Histologic lesions of IBD occur primarily in the lymphoid structures–cloacal bursa, spleen, thymus, harderian gland, and cecal tonsil. Histopathology at the level of light microscopy has been studied by Helmboldt and Garner (35), Cheville (13), Mandelli et al. (78), and Peters (103). Changes were most severe in the cloacal bursa. As early as 1 day postinfection there was degeneration and necrosis of lymphocytes in the medullary area of the bursal follicles. Lymphocytes were soon replaced by heterophils, pyknotic debris, and hyperplastic reticuloendothelial cells. Hemorrhages often appeared but were not a consistent lesion. All lymphoid follicles were affected by 3 or 4 days postinfection. Increase of bursal weight at this time was caused by severe edema, hyperemia, and marked accumulation of heterophils. As the inflammatory reaction declined, cystic cavities developed in medullary areas of follicles, necrosis and phagocytosis of heterophils and plasma cells occurred, and there was a fibroplasia in interfollicular connective tissue (13). Proliferation of the bursal epithelial layer produced a glandular structure of columnar epithelial cells containing globules of mucin. During the suppurative stage, scattered foci of lymphocytes appeared but did not form healthy follicles during the observation period of 18 days postinoculation (35). Some of the histologic changes observed in the cloacal bursa are shown in Figure 28.4. One of the recent isolates (variant A) of IBDV was reported to cause extensive lesions in the cloacal bursa but the inflammatory response was lacking (117).

The spleen had hyperplasia of reticuloendothelial cells around the adenoid sheath arteries in early stages of infection. By the 3rd day there was lymphoid necrosis in the germinal follicles and periarteriolar lymphoid sheath. The spleen recovered from the infection rather rapidly, with no sustained damage to the germinal follicles.

The thymus and cecal tonsils exhibited some cellular reaction in the lymphoid tissues in early stages of infection, but as in the spleen the damage was less extensive than in the bursa and recovery was more rapid. A variant virus (A) was reported to cause milder lesions in the thymus than a standard isolate (IM) (117).

Survashe et al. (134) and Dohms et al. (25) found that the harderian gland was severely af-

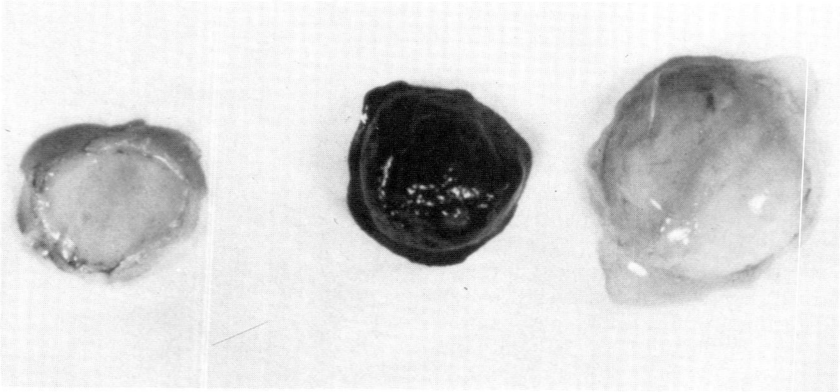

28.3. Edematous (*right*) and hemorrhagic (*center*) cloacal bursas typical in acute IBD at 3–4 days postinfection. Normal bursa (*left*).

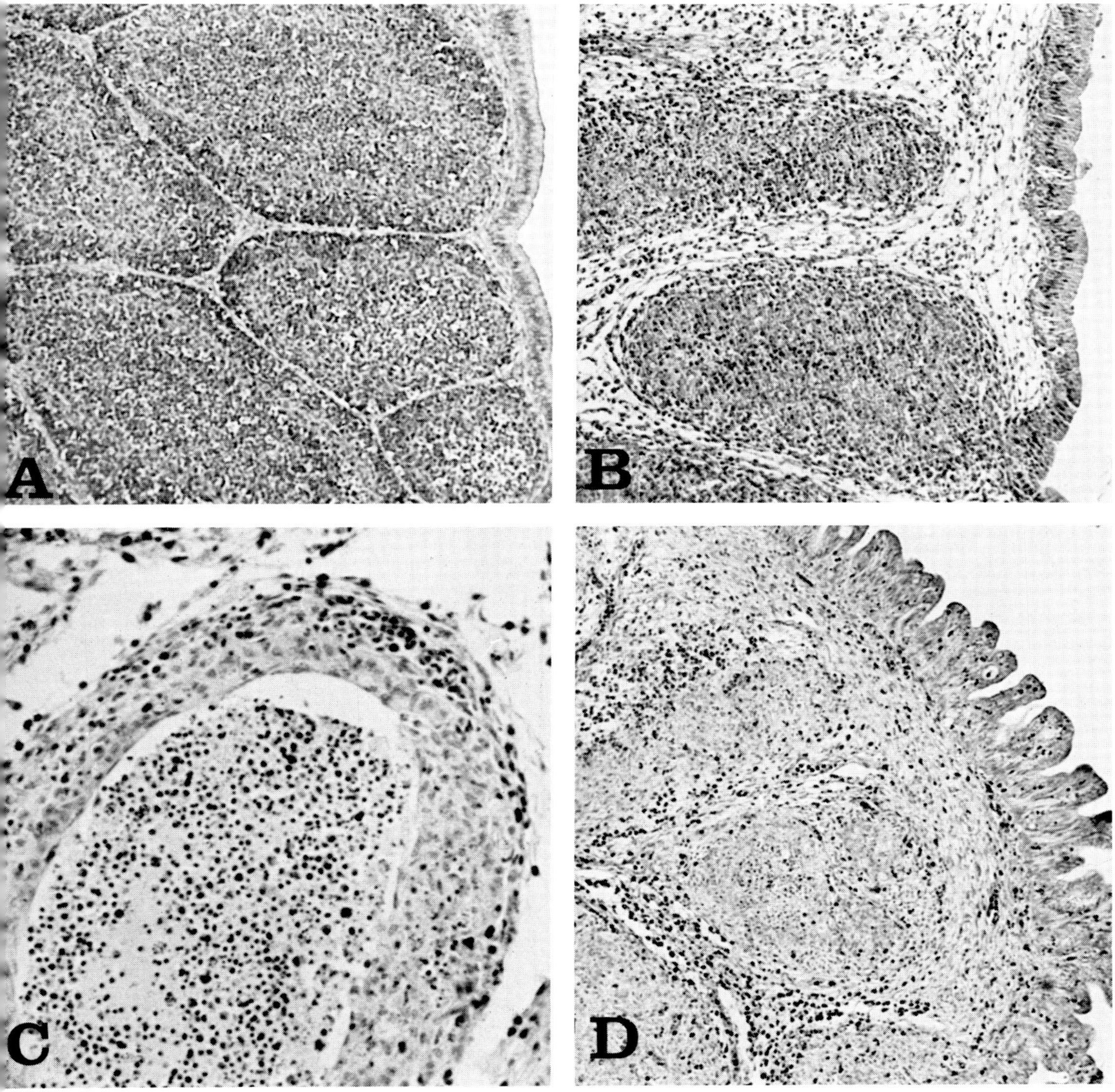

28.4. Photomicrographs of cloacal bursa of 6-wk-old birds affected with IBDV; tissues are fixed in 10% buffered saline and stained with H & E. A. Normal tissue. Large active follicles consist of lymphoid cells that form discrete follicles with little interfollicular tissue. Covering epithelium is simple columnar. ×40. B. Bursa approximately 24 hr postinfection. Note interfollicular edema mixed with phagocytic cells, many of which are heterophils. Follicles are already beginning to degenerate. ×40. C. Single follicle approximately 60 hr postinfection. Medullary portion is now a mass of cellular debris surrounded by cortical remnants. Only reticular cells exist in any number, but scattered among them are a few lymphocytes that will later regenerate. ×250. D. Terminal phase of severe infection. Only ghosts of follicles remain, while heterophils (scattered dark cells) are actively engaged in phagocytosis. ×40. (Helmboldt)

fected by infection of day-old chicks with IBDV. Normally the gland is infiltrated and populated with plasma cells as the chicken ages. Infection with IBDV prevented this infiltration. From 1 to 7 wk of age, glands of infected chickens had populations of plasma cells 5- to 10-fold fewer than uninfected controls (25). In contrast, broilers inoculated with IBDV at 3 wk of age had plasma cell necrosis in the harderian gland from 5–14 days postinoculation and the plasma cells were reduced by 51% at 7 days after inoculation (26). However, reduction in plasma cells was transient and the numbers were normal after 14 days. Follicular necrosis was noticed in the cloacal bursa of infected birds from 1 to 7 days post inoculation.

Histologic lesions of the kidney are nonspecific (103) and probably occur because of severe dehydration of affected chickens. Helmboldt and Garner (35) found kidney lesions in less than 5% of birds examined. Lesions observed were large casts of homogeneous material infiltrated with heterophils.

The liver may have slight perivascular infiltration of monocytes (103).

Naqi and Millar (91) followed the sequential changes in the surface epithelium of the cloacal bursa of IBDV-infected chicks by scanning electron microscopy. They observed a reduction in number and size of microvilli on epithelial cells at 48 hr postinoculation. There was gradual loss of button follicles normally seen at the surface, and by 72 hr most had involuted. By 96 hr there were numerous erosions of the epithelial surface. The surface was intact by the 9th day postinoculation but follicles were involuted, leaving deep pits.

Immunity. Viruses of both serotypes of IBDV share common group antigen(s) that can be detected by the fluorescent antibody test and ELISA (45, 53). Hence, it is not possible to distinguish serotypes or their antibodies by these tests. The common (group) antigens for both serotypes are on VP2 (40 kD) and VP3 (32 kD). VP2 also has serotype-specific group antigens that induce VN antibodies (4, 8). Becht et al. (8) reported that antibodies against VP3 do not have any protective effect. In vivo studies (47, 56) corroborated this observation, since chickens having antibodies to serotype 2 viruses were not protected against serotype 1 viruses. The current thought is that VP2 has the major antigens that induce protection (4, 8).

Traditionally, serotype 1 viruses have been used for studies of the immune response to IBDV. All known isolates of serotype 2 were reported to be nonpathogenic in chickens and turkeys (46, 55, 56) or of very low pathogenicity (17, 93, 101). The discovery of variant strains of serotype 1 has heightened interest in furthering the knowledge of the immune response to IBDV. It was interesting that variants were originally isolated from chickens that had VN antibodies to serotype 1 (107, 112). Inactivated vaccines and a live vaccine made from variant strains protected chickens from disease caused by either variant or standard strains, whereas inactivated vaccines made from standard strains did not protect against challenge with variant strains (47, 111). The molecular basis for the differences in antigenicity, immunogenicity, and pathogenicity between standard and variant strains of serotype 1 currently is not known. In recent studies (45), five different subtypes of serotype 1 IBDV were tested as inactivated vaccines against a variant strain of a different subtype. Vaccines made with 108 but not 10^5 tissue culture infective dose–50% ($TCID_{50}$) were protective against a challenge dose of 102 EID_{50}. Even the higher vaccine dose did not protect against challenge with $10^{3.5}$ EID_{50}. Based on these results it is suggested that all the subtypes of serotype 1 share a minor antigen(s) that elicits protective antibodies.

ACTIVE IMMUNITY. Field exposure to the virus or vaccination with either live or killed vaccines all stimulate active immunity. Antibody response may be measured by several methods – VN, AGP, or ELISA tests. Antibody levels are normally very high after field exposure or vaccination, and VN titers greater than 1:1000 are common. Adult birds are resistant to oral exposure to the virus but produce antibody after intramuscular or subcutaneous inoculation of IBDV (41).

PASSIVE IMMUNITY. Antibody transmitted from the dam via the yolk of the egg can protect chicks against early infections with IBDV, with resultant protection against the immunosuppressive effect of the virus. The half-life of maternal antibodies to IBDV is between 3 and 5 days (125). Therefore, if the antibody titer of the progeny is known, the time that chicks will become susceptible can be predicted. Lucio and Hitchner (68) demonstrated that once antibody titers fell below 1:100, chicks were 100% susceptible to infection, and titers from 1:100 to 1:600 gave approximately 40% protection against challenge. Skeeles et al. (125) reported that titers must fall below 1:64 before chickens can be vaccinated effectively with an attenuated strain of IBDV. Use of killed vaccines in oil emulsions (including variant strains) to stimulate high levels of maternal immunity is extensive in the field. Studies by Lucio and Hitchner (68) and Baxendale and Lutticken (6) indicated that oil emulsion IBD vaccines can stimulate adequate maternal immunity to protect chicks for 4–5 wk, while progeny from breeders vaccinated with live vaccines are protected for only 1–3 wk. As with many diseases, passively acquired immunity to IBDV can interfere with stimulation of an active immune response.

Immunosuppression. Allan et al. (1) and Faragher et al. (30) first reported immunosuppressive effects of IBDV infections. Suppression of the antibody response to Newcastle disease virus was greatest in chicks infected at 1 day of age. There was moderate suppression when chicks were infected at 7 days and negligible effects when infection was at 14 or 21 days (30). Hirai et al. (38) demonstrated decreased humoral antibody response to other vaccines as well. Not only was response to vaccines suppressed but chicks infected early with IBDV were more susceptible to inclusion body hepatitis (27), coccidiosis (2), Marek's disease (15, 115), hemorrhagic-aplastic anemia and gangrenous dermatitis (109), infectious laryngotracheitis, (108), infectious bronchitis (100), chicken anemia agent (145), and salmonellosis and colibacillosis (142).

A paradox associated with IBDV infections of chickens is that while there is immunosuppression against many antigens, the response against IBDV itself is normal, even in day-old susceptible chickens (124). There appears to be a stimulation of the proliferation of B cells committed to anti-IBDV antibody production.

The effect of IBD on cell-mediated immune (CMI) responses is transient and less obvious than on humoral responses. Panigrahy et al. (97) reported that IBDV infections at a young age caused a prolonged skin graft rejection. However, other workers (31, 43) found no effect from early IBDV infections on skin graft rejection or tuberculin-delayed hypersensitivity reaction. Sivanandan and Maheswaran (120) observed suppression of CMI responsiveness, using the lymphoblast transformation assay. They found that maximal depression of cellular immunity occurred 6 wk postinfection. Nusbaum et al. (93) detected a significant suppression of T-cell response to the mitogen concanavalin A in poults from 3 days up to 4 wk postinfection. There was no reduction, however, in tuberculin reactions in IBDV-infected poults. In a sequential study of peripheral blood lymphocytes from chickens inoculated with IBDV, a transient depression of mitogenic stimulation was reported (18). Sharma and Lee (116) reported an inconsistent effect of IBDV infection on natural killer cell toxicity and a transient early depression of the blastogenic response of spleen cells to phytohemagglutinin.

Another component of the immune system is the harderian gland, which is associated with the local immune system of the respiratory tract. Pejkovski et al. (100) and Dohms et al. (25) reported that IBDV infection of 1- to 5-day-old chicks produced a drastic reduction in plasma cell content of the harderian gland that persisted for up to 7 wk. There have been similar observations with IBDV infections of poults (93). In other studies on broilers infected with IBDV at 3 wk of age, extracts from the harderian gland and serum had reduced antibody titers to *Brucella abortus* (a T cell–independent antigen) and sheep red blood cells (SRBC, a T cell–dependent antigen). Compared to SRBC antibody response, diminished antibody responses to *B. abortus* were evident at a later time period. A variant virus of serotype 1 produced a similar effect in chickens (24).

Chickens infected with IBDV at 1 day of age were completely deficient in serum immunoglobulin G (IgG) and produced only a monomeric IgM (48, 49). The number of B cells in peripheral blood was decreased following infection with IBDV but T cells were not appreciably affected (39, 118). The virus appears to replicate primarily in B lymphocytes of chickens (36, 48, 144). Apparently IBDV has a predilection for actively proliferating cells (85), and it was suggested that the virus affected "immature" or precursor B lymphocytes to a greater extent than mature B lymphocytes (119).

In summary, it was shown that infection with IBDV compromises the humoral and local immune systems. The effect of infection on both systems is more pronounced when chickens are infected early in life. The cellular immune system is also affected but that effect is transient and of lower magnitude.

DIAGNOSIS. Acute clinical outbreaks of IBD in fully susceptible flocks are easily recognized and a presumptive diagnosis can be readily made. The rapid onset, high morbidity, spiking mortality curve, and rapid recovery (5–7 days) from clinical signs are characteristic of this disease. Confirmation of the diagnosis can be made at necropsy by examination for characteristic grossly visible changes in the cloacal bursa. It should be remembered that there are distinctive changes in size and color during the course of infection, i.e., enlargement due to inflammatory changes followed by atrophy (see Gross Lesions).

Infections of very young chicks, or chicks with maternal antibody, are usually subclinical and are diagnosed retrospectively at necropsy with observations of macroscopic and histologic bursal atrophy. Infections of chickens of any age with variant strains of IBDV will only be detected by histopathology of the cloacal bursa or by virus isolation.

Isolation and Identification of the Causative Agent. The cloacal bursa and spleen are the tissues of choice for the isolation of IBDV. Other organs contain the virus but at a lower concentration and probably only because of the viremia. Tissues should be macerated in an antibiotic-treated broth or saline and centrifuged to remove the larger tissue particles. The supernatant fluid is then used to inoculate embryonating eggs or cell cultures.

Hitchner (40) demonstrated that the CAM of 9-

to 11-day-old embryos was the most sensitive route for isolation of the virus. The virus could subsequently be adapted to the allantoic sac and yolk sac routes of inoculation. Death of infected embryos usually occurs in 3–5 days. Variant strains of IBD differ from standard viruses in that they induce splenomegaly and liver necrosis of embryos and produce little mortality (110). The embryonating egg may be the most sensitive substrate for isolation of IBDV. McFerran et al. (80) reported that three of seven chicken isolates of IBDV failed to grow in chicken embryo fibroblast (CEF) cells, however, they could be propagated in embryonating eggs.

Isolation and propagation of IBDV in cell culture was discussed previously in this chapter (see Laboratory Host Systems). Since the virus has been shown to replicate in B lymphocytes, either primary cells derived from the cloacal bursa or continuous cell lines of B-cell origin would be the cells of choice for the isolation of the virus. It appears that some strains of virus are very fastidious, and while they may replicate in embryonating eggs or B lymphocytes, they cannot readily be adapted to CEF cells or cells from other organs such as the kidney and liver (67, 80). The use of immunofluorescence and electron microscopy of infected embryos and cell cultures has proven to be of tremendous value for the early detection and identification of IBDV. Cell cultures containing 50% bursal lymphocytes and 50% CEF have been used to successfully isolate and serotype IBD viruses (69). The fibroblasts serve as a matrix for the lymphocytes, and the infected lymphocytes are detected by immunofluorescence. BGM-70 cells may also be used for isolation of IBDV.

Identification of the virus by direct immunofluorescent staining of affected organs or direct examination by electron microscopy have proven to be an adjunct to the isolation and identification of IBDV (80). If antigen or virus is detected by these methods from field cases of disease, then every effort should be made to isolate the virus using both embryonating eggs and cell culture techniques. The broad antigenic diversity of IBDV makes continued isolation and antigenic analysis of field viruses imperative. It would seem that new variants will continue to appear and they should be recognized as soon as possible.

Nucleic acid probes (50) and antigen-capture enzyme immunoassays using monoclonal antibodies (129) to detect and differentiate IBD viruses directly in tissues may prove beneficial for rapid diagnosis and typing of field viruses.

Differential Diagnosis. The sudden onset, morbidity, ruffled feathers, and droopy appearance of the birds in initial disease outbreaks are suggestive of an acute outbreak of coccidiosis. In some cases there is blood in the droppings, which would lead one to suspect coccidiosis. The muscular hemorrhages and enlarged edematous or hemorrhagic cloacal bursae would, however, suggest IBD.

Birds that die from IBD may show an acute nephrosis. Because of many other conditions that may cause nephrosis and the inconsistency of kidney lesions, such lesions should not be sufficient cause for a diagnosis of IBD. Again, involvement of the cloacal bursa will usually distinguish IBD from other nephrosis-causing conditions. Water deprivation will cause kidney changes and possibly gray, atrophied bursae that closely resemble those associated with IBD infection. However, unless this occurs as a flock condition, such changes would be seen in relatively few birds. A history of the flock would be essential in aiding in the differential diagnosis of these cases.

Certain nephrotoxic strains of infectious bronchitis virus cause nephrosis (139). These cases can be differentiated from infectious bursal disease by the fact that there are no changes in the cloacal bursa and deaths are usually preceded by respiratory signs. The possibility that the two diseases may occur simultaneously in a flock should not be overlooked.

The muscular hemorrhages and mucosal hemorrhages seen at the juncture of the proventriculus and gizzard are similar to those reported for hemorrhagic syndrome and could be differentiated on the basis of bursal changes that accompany IBDV infections. It is not unlikely that before IBD was recognized some cases were diagnosed as hemorrhagic syndrome.

Jakowski et al. (58) reported bursal atrophy in experimentally induced infection with four isolates of Marek's disease. The atrophy was observed 12 days postinoculation, but the histologic response was distinctly different from that found in IBD (see Chapter 16).

Grimes and King (33) reported that experimental infections of 1-day-old, specific-pathogen-free (SPF) chickens with a type 8 avian adenovirus produced small bursae and atrophy of bursal follicles at 2 wk postinfection. Several other organs such as the liver, spleen, pancreas, and kidneys were grossly affected and intranuclear inclusion bodies were observed in the liver and pancreas.

Serology. The ELISA procedure is presently the most commonly used serological test for the evaluation of IBDV antibodies in poultry flocks. Marquardt et al. (79) first described an indirect ELISA for measuring antibodies and since that time several workers (11, 77, 128, 131, 135) have reported on the use of ELISA and its comparison to VN test results. The ELISA procedure has the advantage of being a rapid test with the results easily entered into computer software programs. With these programs one can establish an antibody profile on breeder flocks that will indicate the flock immunity level and provide information for developing proper immunization programs for both breeder flocks and their progeny. To perform an antibody profile on a flock for the evaluation of the efficacy of vaccination programs, no less than 30 serum samples should be tested; many producers submit as many as 50–100 samples. The antibody profiles may be performed with serum collected either from the breeders or from day-old progeny. If progeny serums are used, titers will normally be 60–80% lower than those in the breeders. It should be recognized that the ELISA does not differentiate between antibodies to serotypes 1 and 2 (45).

Prior to the use of the ELISA, the most common procedure for antibody detection was the constant virus-diluting serum VN test performed in a microtiter system (123). The VN test is the only serological test that will detect the different serotypes of IBDV and it is still the method of choice to discern antigenic variations between isolates of this virus. The indicator virus used for VN can make a significant difference in test results due to the fact that within a given serotype there are several antigenic subtypes (52). Most chicken serums from the field have high levels of neutralizing antibody to a broad spectrum of antigenically diverse viruses, owing to a combination of field exposure, vaccine exposure, and cross-reactivity from high levels of antibody.

The other method used for the detection of IBDV antibodies is the AGP test. In the UK a quantitative AGP test is routinely used (21); however, as used in the USA, the test is not quantitative. This test does not detect serotypic differences; it measures primarily group-specific soluble antigens.

TREATMENT. No therapeutic or supportive treatment has been found to change the course of IBDV infection (19, 98). Because of the rapid recovery of the affected flock, treatments might appear highly effective if nontreated controls were not maintained for comparison. There are no reports in the literature concerning the use of some of the newer antiviral compounds and interferon inducers for the treatment of IBD.

PREVENTION AND CONTROL. The epizootiology of this infection has not been studied extensively, but it is known that contact with infected birds and contaminated fomites readily causes spread of the infection. The relative stability of this virus to many physical and chemical agents increases the likelihood that it will be carried over from one flock to a succeeding flock. The sanitary precautions that are applied to prevent the spread of most poultry infections must be rigorously used in the case of IBD. The possible involvement of other vectors, e.g., the lesser mealworm, mosquitos, and rats, has already been discussed; they could certainly pose extra problems for the control of this infection.

Management Procedures. At one time, before the development of attenuated vaccine strains, intentional exposure of chicks to infection at an early age was used for controlling IBD. This could be advised on farms that had a history of the disease, and the chicks would normally have maternal antibodies for protection. Also, young chicks less than 2 wk of age did not normally exhibit clinical signs of IBD. When the severe immunosuppressive effect of early IBD infections was discovered, the practice of controlled exposure with virulent strains became less appealing. On many farms the cleanup between broods is not thorough, and due to the stable nature of the virus it easily persists and provides an early exposure by natural means.

Immunization. Immunization is the principal method used for the control of IBD in chickens. Especially important is the immunization of breeder flocks so as to confer parental immunity to their progeny. Such maternal antibodies protect the chick from early immunosuppressive infections. Maternal antibody will normally protect chicks for 1–3 wk, but by boosting the immunity in breeder flocks with oil-adjuvanted vaccines, passive immunity may be extended to 4 or 5 wk (6, 68).

The major problem with active immunization of young maternally immune chicks is determining the proper time of vaccination. Of course, this varies with levels of maternal antibody, route of vaccination, and virulence of the vaccine virus. Environmental stresses and management may be factors to consider when developing a vaccination program that will be effective. Monitoring of antibody levels in a breeder flock or its progeny (antibody profiling) can aid in determining the proper time to vaccinate.

There are many choices of live vaccines available, based on virulence and antigenic diversity. The most virulent vaccine has been discontinued in the marketplace. Presently available in the USA are strains of intermediate virulence and highly attenuated strains. Also available are some cell culture–adapted variant strains. The full impact of the use of variant strain vaccines is still being studied. Highly virulent, intermediate, and avirulent strains break through maternal VN antibody titers of 1:500, 1:250, and less than 1:100, respectively (68, 125). Intermediate strains vary in their virulence and can induce bursal atrophy and immunosuppression in 1-day-old and 3-wk-old SPF chickens (72). If maternal VN antibody titers are less than 1:1000, chicks may be vaccinated by injection with avirulent strains of virus. The vaccine virus replicates in the thymus, spleen, and cloacal bursa where it persists for 2 wk (73). Once the maternal antibody is catabolized there is a primary antibody response to the persisting vaccine virus.

Oil-adjuvant, killed-virus vaccines are used to boost and prolong immunity in breeder flocks, but they are not practical or desirable for inducing a primary response in young chickens. Oil-adjuvant vaccines are most effective in chickens that have been "primed" with live virus, either in the form of vaccine (143) or field exposure to the virus. Oil-adjuvant vaccines presently may contain both standard and variant strains of IBDV. Antibody profiling of breeder flocks is advised to assess effectiveness of vaccination and persistence of antibody.

A universal vaccination program cannot be offered because of the variability in maternal immunity, management, and operational conditions that exist. If very high levels of maternal antibody are achieved and the field challenge is reduced, then vaccination of broilers may not be needed. Vaccination timing with attenuated and intermediate vaccines varies from as early as 7 days to 2 or 3 wk. If broilers are vaccinated at 1 day of age, the IBDV vaccine can be given by injection along with Marek's disease vaccine. Priming of breeder replacement chickens may be necessary and many producers vaccinate with live vaccine at 10–14 wk of age. Killed oil-adjuvant vaccines are commonly administered at 16–18 wk. Revaccination of breeders may be required if antibody profiling should indicate the need.

REFERENCES

1. Allan, W.H., J.T. Faragher, and G.A. Cullen. 1972. Immunosuppression by the infectious bursal agent in chickens immunized against Newcastle disease. Vet Rec 90:511–512
2. Anderson, W.I., W.M. Reid, P.D. Lukert, and O.J. Fletcher. 1977. Influence of infectious bursal disease on the development of immunity to Eimeria tenella. Avian Dis 21:637–641.
3. Azad, A.A., S.A. Barrett, and K.J. Fahey. 1985. The characterization and molecular cloning of the double-stranded RNA genome of an Australian strain of infectious bursal disease virus. Virology 143:35–44.
4. Azad, A.A., M.N. Jagadish, M.A. Brown, and P.J. Hudson. 1987. Deletion mapping and expression in Escherichia coli of the large genomic segment of a birnavirus. Virology 161:145–152.
5. Barnes, H.J., J. Wheeler, and D. Reed. 1982. Serological evidence of infectious bursal disease virus infection in Iowa turkeys. Avian Dis 26:560–565.
6. Baxendale, W., and D. Lutticken. 1981. The results of field trials with an inactivated Gumboro vaccine. Dev Biol Stand 51:211–219.
7. Becht, H. 1980. Infectious bursal disease virus. Curr Top Microbiol Immunol 90:107–121.
8. Becht, H., H. Müller, and H.K. Müller. 1988. Comparative studies on structural and antigenic properties of two serotypes of infectious bursal disease virus. J Gen Virol 69:631–640.
9. Benton, W.J., M.S. Cover, and J.K. Rosenberger. 1967. Studies on the transmission of the infectious bursal agent (IBA) of chickens. Avian Dis 11:430–438.
10. Benton, W.J., M.S. Cover, J.K. Rosenberger, and R.S. Lake. 1967. Physicochemical properties of the infectious bursal agent (IBA). Avian Dis 11:438–445.
11. Briggs, D.J., C.E. Whitfill, J.K. Skeeles, J.D. Story, and K.D. Reed. 1986. Application of the positive/negative ratio method of analysis to quantitate antibody responses to infectious bursal disease virus using a commercially available ELISA. Avian Dis 30:216–218.
12. Brown, F. 1986. The classification and nomenclature of viruses: Summary of results of meetings of the International Committee on Taxonomy of Viruses in Sendai. Intervirology 25:141–143.
13. Cheville, N.F. 1967. Studies on the pathogenesis of Gumboro disease in the bursa of Fabricius, spleen, and thymus of the chicken. Am J Pathol 51:527–551.
14. Chin, R.P., R. Yamamoto, W. Lin, K.M. Lam, and T.B. Farver. 1984. Serological survey of infectious bursal disease virus: Serotypes 1 and 2 in California turkeys. Avian Dis 28:1026–1036.
15. Cho, B.R. 1970. Experimental dual infections of chickens with infectious bursal and Marek's disease agents. I. Preliminary observation on the effect of infectious bursal agent on Marek's disease. Avian Dis 14:665–675.
16. Cho, Y., and S.A. Edgar. 1969. Characterization of the infectious bursal agent. Poult Sci 48:2102–2109.
17. Chui, C.H., and J.J. Thorsen. 1984. Experimental infection of turkeys with infectious bursal disease virus and the effect on the immunocompetence of infected turkeys. Avian Dis 28:197–207.
18. Confer, A.W., W.T. Springer, S.M. Shane, and J.F. Conovan. 1981. Sequential mitogen stimulation of peripheral blood lymphocytes from chickens inoculated with infectious bursal disease virus. Am J Vet Res 42:2109–2113.
19. Cosgrove, A.S. 1962. An apparently new disease of chickens–avian nephrosis. Avian Dis 6:385–389.
20. Cowen, B.S., and M.O. Braune. 1988. The propagation of avian viruses in a continuous cell line (QT35) of Japanese quail origin. Avian Dis 32:282–297.
21. Cullen, G.A., and P.J. Wyeth. 1975. Quantitation of antibodies to infectious bursal disease. Vet Rec 97:315.
22. Dobos, P. 1979. Peptide map comparison of the proteins of infectious bursal disease virus. J Virol 32:1046–1050.
23. Dobos, P., B.J. Hill, R. Hallett, D.T. Kells, H. Becht, and D. Teninges. 1979. Biophysical and biochemical characterization of five animal viruses with bisegmented double-stranded RNA genomes. J Virol 32:593–605.
24. Dohms, J.E. 1988. Personal communication.
25. Dohms, J.E., K.P. Lee, and J.K. Rosenberger. 1981. Plasma cell changes in the gland of Harder following infectious bursal disease virus infection of the chicken. Avian Dis 25:683–695.
26. Dohms, J.E., K.P. Lee, J.K. Rosenberger, and A.L. Metz. 1988. Plasma cell quantitation in the gland of Harder during infectious bursal disease virus infection of 3-week-old broiler chickens. Avian Dis. (In press).
27. Fadley, A.M., R.W. Winterfield, and H.J. Olander. 1976. Role of the bursa of Fabricius in the pathogenicity of inclusion body hepatitis and infectious bursal disease virus. Avian Dis 20:467–477.
28. Fahey, K.J., I.J. O'Donnell, and A.A. Azad. 1985. Characterization by western blotting of the immunogens of infectious bursal disease virus. J Gen Virol 66:1479–1488.
29. Fahey, K.J., I.J. O'Donnell, and T.J. Bagust. 1985. Antibody to the 32K structural protein of infectious bur-

sal disease virus neutralizes viral infectivity in vitro and confers protection on young chickens. J Gen Virol 66:2693-2702.

30. Faragher, J.T., W.H. Allan, and C.J. Wyeth. 1974. Immunosuppressive effect of infectious bursal agent on vaccination against Newcastle disease. Vet Rec 95:385-388.

31. Giambrone, J.J., J.P. Donahoe, D.L. Dawe, and C.S. Eidson. 1977. Specific suppression of the bursa-dependent immune system of chicks with infectious bursal disease virus. Am J Vet Res 38:581-583.

32. Giambrone, J.J., O.J. Fletcher, P.D. Lukert, R.K. Page, and C.E. Eidson. 1978. Experimental infection of turkeys with infectious bursal disease virus. Avian Dis 22:451-458.

33. Grimes, T.M., and D.J. King. 1977. Effect of maternal antibody on experimental infections of chickens with a type-8 avian adenovirus. Avian Dis 21:97-112.

34. Harkness, J.W., D.J. Alexander, M. Pattison, and A.C. Scott. 1975. Infectious bursal disease agent: Morphology by negative stain electron microscopy. Arch Virol 48:63-73.

35. Helmboldt, C.F., and E. Garner. 1964. Experimentally induced Gumboro disease (IBA). Avian Dis 8:561-575.

36. Hirai, K., and B.W. Calnek. 1979. In vitro replication of infectious bursal disease virus in established lymphoid cell lines and chicken B lymphocytes. Infect Immun 25:964-970.

37. Hirai, K., and S. Shimakura. 1974. Structure of infectious bursal disease virus. J Virol 14:957-964.

38. Hirai, K., S. Shimakura, E. Kawamoto, F. Taguchi, S.T. Kim, C.N. Chang, and Y. Iritani. 1974. The immunodepressive effect of infectious bursal disease virus in chickens. Avian Dis 18:50-57.

39. Hirai, K., K. Kunihiro, and S. Shimakura. 1979. Characterization of immunosuppression in chickens by infectious bursal disease virus. Avian Dis 23:950-965.

40. Hitchner, S.B. 1970. Infectivity of infectious bursal disease virus for embryonating eggs. Poult Sci 49:511-516.

41. Hitchner, S.B. 1976. Immunization of adult hens against infectious bursal disease virus. Avian Dis 20:611-613.

42. Howie, R.I., and J. Thorsen. 1981. Identification of a strain of infectious bursal disease virus isolated from mosquitoes. Can J Comp Med 45:315-320.

43. Hudson, L., H. Pattison, and N. Thantrey. 1975. Specific B lymphocyte suppression by infectious bursal agent (Gumboro disease virus) in chickens. Eur J Immunol 5:675-679.

44. Hudson, P.J., N.M. McKern, B.E. Power, and A.A. Azad. 1986. Genomic structure of the large RNA segment of infectious bursal disease virus. Nucl Acids Res 14:5001-5012.

45. Ismail, N., and Y.M. Saif. 1988. Unpublished data.

46. Ismail, N., Y.M. Saif, and P.D. Moorhead. 1988. Lack of pathogenicity of five serotype 2 infectious bursal disease viruses in chickens. Avian Dis 32:757-759.

47. Ismail, N., Y.M. Saif, and P.D. Moorhead. 1988. Unpublished data.

48. Ivanyi, J. 1975. Immunodeficiency in the chicken. II. Production of monomeric IgM following testosterone treatment of infection with Gumboro disease. Immunology 28:1015-1021.

49. Ivanyi, J., and R. Morris. 1976. Immunodeficiency in the chicken. IV. An immunological study of infectious bursal disease. Clin Exp Immunol 23:154-165.

50. Jackwood, D.J. 1988. Detection of infectious bursal disease virus using nucleic acid probes. Proc 125th Annu Meet Am Vet Med Assoc, p. 126. (Abstr).

51. Jackwood, D.J., and Y.M. Saif. 1983. Prevalence of antibodies to infectious bursal disease virus serotypes I and II in 75 Ohio chicken flocks. Avian Dis 27:850-854.

52. Jackwood, D.H., and Y.M. Saif. 1987. Antigenic diversity of infectious bursal disease viruses. Avian Dis 31:766-770.

53. Jackwood, D.J., Y.M. Saif, and J.H. Hughes. 1982. Characteristics and serologic studies of two serotypes of infectious bursal disease virus in turkeys. Avian Dis 26:871-882.

54. Jackwood, D.J., Y.M. Saif, and J.H. Hughes. 1984. Nucleic acid and structural proteins of infectious bursal disease virus isolates belonging to serotypes I and II. Avian Dis 28:990-1006.

55. Jackwood, D.J., Y.M. Saif, P.D. Moorhead, and G. Bishop. 1984. Failure of two serotype II infectious bursal disease viruses to affect the humoral immune response of turkeys. Avian Dis 28:100-116.

56. Jackwood, D.J., Y.M. Saif, and P.D. Moorhead. 1985. Immunogenicity and antigenicity of infectious bursal disease virus serotypes I and II in chickens. Avian Dis 29:1184-1194.

57. Jackwood, D.H., Y.M. Saif, and J.H. Hughes. 1987. Replication of infectious bursal disease virus in continuous cell lines. Avian Dis 31:370-375.

58. Jakowski, R.M., T.N. Fredrickson, R.E. Luginbuhl, and C.F. Helmboldt. 1969. Early changes in bursa of Fabricius from Marek's disease. Avian Dis 13:215-222.

59. Johnson, D.C., P.D. Lukert, and R.K. Page. 1980. Field studies with convalescent serum and infectious bursal disease vaccine to control turkey coryza. Avian Dis 24:386-392.

60. Jones, B.A.H. 1986. Infectious bursal disease serology in New Zealand poultry flocks. NZ Vet J 34:36

61. Kaufer, I., and E. Weiss. 1980. Significance of bursa of Fabricius as target organ in infectious bursal disease of chickens. Infect Immun 27:364-367.

62. Kibenge, F.S.B., A.S. Dhillon, and R.G. Russell. 1988. Biochemistry and immunology of infectious bursal disease virus. J Gen Virol 69:1757-1775.

63. Kibenge, F.S.B., A.S. Dhillon, and R.G. Russell. 1988. Growth of serotypes I and II and variant strains of infectious bursal disease virus in Vero cells. Avian Dis 32:298-303.

64. Kibenge, F.S.B., A.S. Dhillon, and R.G. Russell. 1988. Identification of serotype II infectious bursal disease virus proteins. Avian Pathol 17:679-687.

65. Kosters, J., H. Becht, and R. Rudolph. 1972. Properties of the infectious bursal agent of chicken (IBA). Med Microbiol Immunol 157:291-298.

66. Landgraf, H., E. Vielitz, and R. Kirsch. 1967. Occurrence of an infectious disease affecting the bursa of Fabricius (Gumboro disease). Dtsch Tierärztl Wochenschr 74:6-10.

67. Lee, L.H., and P.D. Lukert. 1986. Adaptation and antigenic variation of infectious bursal disease virus. J Chin Soc Vet Sci 12:297-304.

68. Lucio, B., and S.B. Hitchner. 1979. Infectious bursal disease emulsified vaccine: Effect upon neutralizing-antibody levels in the dam and subsequent protection of the progeny. Avian Dis 23:466-478.

69. Lukert, P.D. 1986. Serotyping recent isolates of infectious bursal disease virus. Proc 21st Nat Meet Poult Health Condemn, pp 71-75.

70. Lukert, P.D. 1988. Unpublished data.

71. Lukert, P.D., and R.B. Davis. 1974. Infectious bursal disease virus: Growth and characterization in cell cultures. Avian Dis 18:243-250.

72. Lukert, P.D., and L.A. Mazariegos. 1985. Viru-

lence and immunosuppressive potential of intermediate vaccine strains of infectious bursal disease virus. J Am Vet Med Assoc 187:306. (Abstr).
73. Lukert, P.D., and D. Rifuliadi. 1982. Replication of virulent and attenuated infectious bursal disease virus in maternally immune day-old chickens. J Am Vet Med Assoc 181:284. (Abstr).
74. Lukert, P.D., J. Leonard, and R.B. Davis. 1975. Infectious bursal disease virus: Antigen production and immunity. Am J Vet Res 36:539-540.
75. Lunger, P.D., and T.C. Maddux. 1972. Fine-structure studies of the avian infectious bursal agent. I. In vivo viral morphogenesis. Avian Dis 16:874-893.
76. MacDonald, R.D. 1980. Immunofluorescent detection of double-stranded RNA in cells infected with reovirus, infectious pancreatic necrosis virus, and infectious bursal disease virus. Can J Microbiol 26:256-261.
77. Mallinson, E.T., D.B. Snyder, W.W. Marquardt, E. Russek-Cohen, P.K. Savage, D.C. Allen, and F.S. Yancey. 1985. Presumptive diagnosis of subclinical infections utilizing computer-assisted analysis of sequential enzyme-linked immunosorbent assays against multiple antigens. Poult Sci 64:1661-1669.
78. Mandelli, G., A. Rinaldi, A. Cerioli, and G. Cervio. 1967. Aspetti ultrastrutturali della borsa di Fabrizio nella malattia di Gumboro de pollo. Atti Soc Ital Sci Vet 21:615-619.
79. Marquardt, W., R.B. Johnson, W.F. Odenwald, and B.A. Schlotthober. 1980. An indirect enzyme-linked immunosorbent assay (ELISA) for measuring antibodies in chickens infected with infectious bursal disease virus. Avian Dis 24:375-385.
80. McFerran, J.B., M.S. McNulty, E.R. McKillop, T.J. Conner, R.M. McCracken, D.S. Collins, and G.M. Allan. 1980. Isolation and serological studies with infectious bursal disease viruses from fowl, turkey, and duck: Demonstration of a second serotype. Avian Pathol 9:395-404.
81. McNulty, M.S., and Y.M. Saif. 1988. Antigenic relationship of non-serotype 1 turkey infectious bursal disease viruses. Avian Dis 32:374-375.
82. McNulty, M.S., G.M. Allan, and J.B. McFerran. 1979. Isolation of infectious bursal disease virus from turkeys. Avian Pathol 8:205-212.
83. Meroz, M. 1966. An epidemiological survey of Gumboro disease. Refu Vet 23:235-37.
84. Morgan, M.M., I.G. Macreadie, V.R. Harley, P.J. Hudson, and A.A. Azad. 1988. Sequence of the small double-stranded RNA genomic segment of infectious bursal disease virus and its deduced 90-kD product. Virology 163:240-242.
85. Müller, H. 1986. Replication of infectious bursal disease virus in lymphoid cell. Arch Virol 87:191-203.
86. Müller, H., and H. Becht. 1982. Biosynthesis of virus-specific proteins in cells infected with infectious bursal disease virus and their significance as structural elements for infectious virus and incomplete particles. J Virol 44:384-392.
87. Müller, H., C. Scholtissek, and H. Becht. 1979. Genome of infectious bursal disease virus consists of two segments of double-stranded RNA. J Virol 31:584-589.
88. Müller, H., H. Lange, and H. Becht. 1986. Formation, characterization and interfering capacity of a small plaque mutant and of incomplete virus particles of infectious bursal disease virus. Virus Res 4:297-309.
89. Nagy, E., R. Duncan, P. Krell, and P. Dobos. 1987. Mapping of the large RNA genome segment of infectious pancreatic necrosis virus by hybrid arrested translation. Virology 158:211-217.
90. Nakai, T., and K. Hirai. 1981. In vitro infection of fractionated chicken lymphocytes by infectious bursal disease virus. Avian Dis 25:831-838.
91. Naqi, S.A., and D.L. Millar. 1979. Morphologic changes in the bursa of Fabricius of chickens after inoculation with infectious bursal disease virus. Am J Vet Res 40:1134-1139.
92. Nick, H., D. Cursiefen, and H. Becht. 1976. Structural and growth characteristics of infectious bursal disease virus. J Virol 18:227-234.
93. Nusbaum, K.E., P.D. Lukert, and O.J. Fletcher. 1988. Experimental infection of one-day-old poults with turkey isolates of infectious bursal disease virus. Avian Pathol 17:51-62
94. Okoye, J.O.A., and U.E. Uche. 1986. Serological evidence of infectious bursal disease virus infection in wild rats. Acta Vet Brno 55:207-209.
95. Ozel, M., and H. Gelderblom. 1985. Capsid symmetry of viruses of the proposed birnavirus group. Arch Virol 84:149-161.
96. Page, R.K., O.J. Fletcher, P.D. Lukert, and R. Rimler. 1978. Rhinotracheitis in turkey poults. Avian Dis 22:529-534.
97. Panigrahy, B., L.K. Misra, S.A. Naqi, and C.F. Hall. 1977. Prolongation of skin allograft survival in chickens with infectious bursal disease. Poult Sci 56:1745.
98. Parkhurst, R.T. 1964. On-the-farm studies of Gumboro disease in broilers. Avian Dis 8:584-596.
99. Pattison, M., D.J. Alexander, and J.W. Harkness. 1975. Purification and preliminary characterization of a pathogenic strain of infectious bursal disease virus. Avian Pathol 4:175-187.
100. Pejkovski, C., F.G. Davelaar, and B. Kouwenhoven. 1979. Immunosuppressive effect of infectious bursal disease virus on vaccination against infectious bronchitis. Avian Pathol 8:95-106.
101. Perelman, B., and E.D. Heller. 1983. The effect of infectious bursal disease virus on the immune system of turkeys. Avian Dis 27:66-76.
102. Petek, M., P.N. D'Aprile, and F. Cancellotti. 1973. Biological and physicochemical properties of the infectious bursal disease virus (IBDV). Avian Pathol 2:135-152.
103. Peters, G. 1967. Histology of Gumboro disease. Berl Muench Tierärztl Wochenschr 80:394-396.
104. Rinaldi, A., G. Cervio, and G. Mandelli. 1965. Aspetti epidemiologici, anatomo-clinici ed istologici di una nuova forma morbosa dei polli verosimilmente identificabile con la considdetta Malattia di Gumboro. Societa Italiana de Patologia Aviare. Atti Conv Patol Aviare, pp. 77-83
105. Rinaldi, A., E. Lodetti, D. Cessi, E. Lodrini, G. Cervio, and L. Nardelli. 1972. Coltura del virus de Gumboro (IBA) su fibroblast de embrioni di pollo. Nuova Vet 48:195-201.
106. Rosenberger, J.K., and S.S. Cloud. 1985. Isolation and characterization of variant infectious bursal disease viruses. J Am Vet Med Assoc 189:357. (Abstr).
107. Rosenberger, J.K., and S.S. Cloud. 1986. Isolation and characterization of variant infectious bursal disease viruses. Proc 123rd Annu Meet Am Vet Med Assoc, Abstr 181.
108. Rosenberger, J.K., and J. Gelb, Jr. 1978. Response to several avian respiratory viruses as affected by infectious bursal disease virus. Avian Dis 22:95-105.
109. Rosenberger, J.K., S. Klopp, R.J. Eckroade, and W.C. Krauss. 1975. The role of the infectious bursal agent and several avian adenoviruses in the hemorrhagic-aplastic-anemia syndrome and gangrenous dermatitis. Avian Dis 19:717-729.
110. Rosenberger, J.K., S.S. Cloud, J. Gelb, Jr., E. Odor, and J.E. Dohms. 1985. Sentinel bird survey of Delmarva broiler flocks. Proc 20th Nat Meet Poult

Health Condemn, pp 94–101.
111. Rosenberger, J.K., S.S. Cloud, and A. Metz. 1987. Use of infectious bursal disease virus variant vaccines in broilers and broiler breeders. Proc 36th West Poultry Dis Conf, pp 105–109.
112. Saif, Y.M. 1984. Infectious bursal disease virus types. Proc 19th Nat Meet Poult Health Condemn, pp. 105–107.
113. Saif, Y.M. 1988. Unpublished data.
114. Schat, K.A., B. Lucio, and J.C. Carlisle. 1981. Pathogenesis of infectious bursal disease in embryonally bursectomized chickens. Avian Dis 25:996–1004.
115. Sharma, J.M. 1984. Effect of infectious bursal disease virus on protection against Marek's disease by turkey herpesvirus vaccine. Avian Dis 28:629–640.
116. Sharma, J.M., and L.F. Lee. 1983. Effect of infectious bursal disease virus on natural killer cell activity and mitogenic response of chicken lymphoid cells: Role of adherent cells in cellular immune suppression. Infect Immun 42:747–754.
117. Sharma, J.M., J.E. Dohms, and A.L. Metz. 1989. Comparative pathogenesis of serotype 1 and variant serotype 1 isolates of infectious bursal disease virus and the effect of those viruses on humoral and cellular immune competence of specific-pathogen-free chickens. Avian Dis 33:112–124.
118. Sivanandan, V., and S.K. Maheswaran. 1980. Immune profile of infectious bursal disease. I. Effect of infectious bursal disease virus on peripheral blood T and B lymphocytes in chickens. Avian Dis 24:715–725.
119. Sivanandan, V., and S.K. Maheswaran. 1980. Immune profile of infectious bursal disease (IBD). II. Effect of IBD virus on pokeweed-mitogen-stimulated peripheral blood lymphocytes of chickens. Avian Dis 24:734–742.
120. Sivanandan, V., and S.K. Maheswaran. 1981. Immune profile of infectious bursal disease. III. Effect of infectious bursal disease virus on the lymphocyte responses to phytomitogens and on mixed lymphocyte reaction of chickens. Avian Dis 25:112–120.
121. Sivanandan, V., J. Sasipreeyajan, D.A. Halvorson, and J.A. Newman. 1986. Histopathologic changes induced by serotype II infectious bursal disease virus in specific-pathogen-free chickens. Avian Dis 30:709–715.
122. Skeeles, J.K., and P.D. Lukert. 1980. Studies with an attenuated cell-culture-adapted infectious bursal disease virus: Replication sites and persistence of the virus in specific-pathogen-free chickens. Avian Dis 24:43–47.
123. Skeeles, J.K., P.D. Lukert, E.V. De Buysscher, O.J. Fletcher, and J. Brown. 1979. Infectious bursal disease virus infections. I. Complement and virus-neutralizing antibody response following infection of susceptible chickens. Avian Dis 23:95–106.
124. Skeeles, J.K., P.D. Lukert, E.V. De Buysscher, O.J. Fletcher, and J. Brown. 1979. Infectious bursal disease virus infections. II. The relationship of age, complement levels, virus-neutralizing antibody, clotting, and lesions. Avian Dis 23:107–117.
125. Skeeles, J.K., P.D. Lukert, O.J. Fletcher, and J.D. Leonard. 1979. Immunization studies with a cell-culture-adapted infectious bursal disease virus. Avian Dis 23:456–465.
126. Skeeles, J.K., M.F. Slavik, J.N. Beasley, A.H. Brown, C.F. Meinecke, S. Maruca, and S. Welch. 1980. An age-related coagulation disorder associated with experimental infection with infectious bursal disease virus. Am J Vet Res 41:1458–1461.
127. Snedeker, C., F.K. Wills, and I.M. Moulthrop. 1967. Some studies on the infectious bursal agent. Avian Dis 11:519–528.
128. Snyder, D.B., W.W. Marquardt, E.T. Mallinson, E. Russek-Cohen, P. K. Savage, and D.C. Allen. 1986. Rapid serological profiling by enzyme-linked immunosorbent assay. IV. Association of infectious bursal disease serology with broiler flock performance. Avian Dis 30:139–148.
129. Snyder, D.B., D.P. Lana, B.R. Cho, and W.W. Marquardt. 1988. Group and strain-specific neutralization sites of infectious bursal disease virus defined with monoclonal antibodies. Avian Dis 32:527–534.
130. Snyder, D.B., D.P. Lana, P.K. Savage, F.S. Yancey, S.A. Mengel, and W.W. Marquardt. 1988. Differentiation of infectious bursal disease viruses directly from infected tissues with neutralizing monoclonal antibodies: Evidence of a major antigenic shift in recent field isolates. Avian Dis 32:535–539.
131. Solano, W., J.J. Giambrone, and V.S. Panangala. 1985. Comparison of a kinetic-based enzyme-linked immunosorbent assay (KELISA) and virus-neutralization test for infectious bursal disease virus. I. Quantitation of antibody in white leghorn hens. Avian Dis 29:662–671.
132. Spies, U., H. Müller, and H. Becht. 1987. Properties of RNA polymerase activity associated with infectious bursal disease virus and characterization of its reaction products. Virus Res 8:127–140.
133. Steger, D., H. Müller, and D. Riesner. 1980. Helix-core transitions in double-stranded viral RNA: Fine resolution melting and ionic strength dependence. Biochem Biophys Acta 606:274–285.
134. Survashe, B.D., I.D. Aitken, and J.R. Powell. 1979. The response of the harderian gland of the fowl to antigen given by the ocular route. I. Histological changes. Avian Pathol 8:77–93.
135. Thayer, S.G., P. Villegas, and O.J. Fletcher. 1987. Comparison of two commercial enzyme-linked immunosorbent assays and conventional methods for avian serology. Avian Dis 31:120–124.
136. Todd, D., and M.S. McNulty. 1979. Biochemical studies with infectious bursal disease virus: Comparison of some of its properties with infectious pancreatic necrosis virus. Arch Virol 60:265–277.
137. Weisman, J., and S.B. Hitchner. 1978. Infectious bursal disease virus infection attempts in turkeys and coturnix quail. Avian Dis 22:604–609.
138. Winterfield, R.W. 1969. Immunity response to the infectious bursal agent. Avian Dis 13:548–557.
139. Winterfield, R.W., and S.B. Hitchner. 1962. Etiology of an infectious nephritis-nephrosis syndrome of chickens. Am J Vet Res 23:1273–1279.
140. Winterfield, R.W., S.B. Hitchner, G.S. Appleton, and A.S. Cosgrove. 1962. Avian nephrosis, nephritis and Gumboro disease. L & M News and Views 3:103.
141. With, L.G. 1985. Infectious bursal disease serology in New Zealand meat chicken flocks. NZ Vet J 33:174.
142. Wyeth, P.J. 1975. Effect of infectious bursal disease on the response of chickens to S. typhimurium and E. coli infections. Vet Rec 96:238–243.
143. Wyeth, P.J., and G.A. Cullen. 1978. Transmission of immunity from inactivated infectious bursal disease oil-emulsion vaccinated parent chickens to their chicks. Vet Rec 102:362–363.
144. Yamaguchi, S., I. Imada, and H. Kawamura. 1981. Growth and infectivity titration of virulent infectious bursal disease virus in established cell lines from lymphoid leucosis. Avian Dis 25:927–935.
145. Yuasa, N., T. Taniguchi, T. Noguchi, and I. Yoshida. 1980. Effect of infectious bursal disease virus infection on incidence of anemia by chicken anemia agent. Avian Dis 24:202–209.

29 MISCELLANEOUS VIRUS INFECTIONS

INTRODUCTION

B.W. Calnek

This chapter includes material on infections that are newly reported, or of limited importance, or simply require only a brief description. Two previously included conditions, reovirus infection and infectious bursal disease, have been moved to Chapters 27 and 28, respectively, and rotavirus infections are now described in Chapter 26, along with other enteric viral infections. Only the subchapter on arbovirus infections remains.

Miscellaneous herpesviruses have been added; of these, the pigeon herpesvirus is the most significant. Pseudorabies (Aujesky's disease) is briefly mentioned only because chickens and pigeons are susceptible to infection with that virus. Herpesviruses that infect wild and exotic birds are not included, in keeping with the scope of this book.

Pneumovirus, chicken anemia agent (CAA) and the picornavirus that causes infectious nephritis are newly described viruses first detected in Europe and/or Japan. Infectious anemia, caused by CAA, appears to be widespread and has probably been seen for many years but without knowledge of the etiology. Very likely it was sometimes confused as one of the consequences of Marek's disease virus or adenovirus infection. Although lesions characteristic of the so-called "hemorrhagic syndrome" are associated with CAA infection, there may be other causes of this condition (see Chapter 34). Pneumovirus infections have been described only in Europe, South Africa, and Israel, and evidence of infectious nephritis has been limited to Japan and Europe. These may be truly emerging diseases about which we may become more concerned worldwide in the future.

There is some confusion over the relationship between CAA and the chicken parvovirus described by Kisary in this chapter. The parvovirus is reported to be antigenically similar or identical to CAA, and many of the lesions described for infections with the two viruses are similar. Yet, the buoyant densities of the two viruses are reportedly different, and only the parvovirus is reported to grow in chicken embryo fibroblasts. CAA, while still unclassified, does not appear to be a parvovirus. Because of these conflicting data, it would seem that either the serologic comparisons or some of the characterization studies may be in error. The risk of possibly offering two subchapters describing the same infection is considered to be an acceptable one until additional studies to resolve the issue are completed. The goose parvovirus, also described in this chapter, does not appear to be involved in this controversy.

A similar dilemma is associated with the so-called "malabsorption syndrome" or "infectious stunting syndrome" attributed to chicken parvovirus infection. Descriptions of this condition(s) also appear elsewhere (Chapter 27, Reovirus Infections; Chapter 34, Developmental, Metabolic and Miscellaneous Disorders), and several other viruses claimed to be involved in the condition are mentioned in the Introduction to Chapter 26, Viral Enteric Infections. Until there is agreement about the etiology(ies) of this complex disorder, some potential overlap is inevitable.

Turkey viral hepatitis was previously included in the chapter on adenovirus infections. However, because the classification of the causative virus is still unknown, the material is more appropriately included here.

Arbovirus infections can be significant in domestic poultry, as illustrated by those causing meningoencephalitis in turkeys or equine encephalitis in pheasants, but additionally they are important as human pathogens originating from avian reservoirs.

MISCELLANEOUS HERPESVIRUS INFECTIONS

H. Vindevogel and J.P. Duchatel

INTRODUCTION. Herpesvirus infections have been described in several species of domestic and wild birds including pigeons (9, 37), psittacine birds (30), falcons (22), owls (4), cormorants (11), cranes (5), storks (16), and bobwhite quail (15).

To date, all herpesvirus strains isolated from pigeons have been found to be antigenically similar and to possess the same cultural characteristics (37, 39). Therefore, only one pigeon herpesvirus type, *pigeon herpesvirus 1* (PHV1), appears to exist. A virus isolated from the brain of pigeons showing signs of encephalomyelitis, called pigeon encephalomyelitis herpesvirus (PEHV) was found to be antigenically related to PHV1 but to differ in its pathogenicity (23, 32, 33). However, Kaleta et al. (17) later found PEHV to be contaminated with a paramyxovirus type 1 (PMV1), which was the likely cause of the encephalitis in the pigeons from which the herpesvirus was isolated.

PHV1 is antigenically different from turkey herpesvirus, Marek's disease virus, infectious laryngotracheitis virus, and duck virus enteritis herpesvirus (24, 37). PHV1 can also be clearly distinguished from the psittacine herpesvirus (Pacheco's disease virus) based on antigenic composition and plaque size in cell cultures (49).

On the contrary PHV1 can not be serologically distinguished from the falcon (FHV) and the owl (OHV) herpesviruses and it remains to be established whether these three herpesviruses are different isolates of the same virus (22, 24). All other herpesviruses isolated from wild birds differ antigenically from each other and from other avian herpesviruses except for the bobwhite quail herpesvirus and the crane herpesvirus, which are serologically related (15).

This subchapter will cover PHV1 infections in pigeons and will briefly mention pseudorabies virus infections, which can be experimentally induced in pigeons and young chickens.

PIGEON HERPESVIRUS INFECTION

HISTORY. The first observation of intranuclear inclusion bodies in the liver of pigeons, probably associated with PHV1 infection, was reported in 1945 (31). Since 1967 PHV1 has been isolated from diseased pigeons in numerous countries (9, 37).

INCIDENCE AND DISTRIBUTION. The suspected geographic distribution of PHV1 is worldwide. The virus has been isolated in the UK (8), Czechoslovakia (19), Australia (3), Belgium (43), Hungary (36), Germany (12), France (20), and Italy (56). Infection has also been observed in the USA (25). In Europe the vast majority of pigeons are infected, since more than 50% of them possess specific antibodies (14, 20, 37, 50). In Belgium the presence of PHV1 was demonstrated in 60% of dovecotes where pigeons were permanently affected with respiratory disease, and PHV1 could be isolated from the pharynx of 82% of pigeons affected with acute coryza (37, 51).

ETIOLOGY. PHV1 belongs to the family of Herpesviridae (most probably alpha) and is called *Columbid herpesvirus 1* in the new nomenclature. It possesses the morphology and has the physicochemical properties of a typical herpesvirus (58).

All avian cell cultures tested to date were susceptible to PHV1 but the cytopathic effects varied (7, 44, 45). In chicken embryo fibroblast (CEF) cultures, the most consistent change is an increase in the size of cells with syncytia containing two to four nuclei. Initial alterations consist of margination of chromatin and the appearance of Cowdry type-A intranuclear inclusion bodies 10 hr after inoculation. Viral antigen is first detected in the nucleus and later throughout the cytoplasm. Virus can be detected by 12 hr, and peak titers are reached by 36 hr after inoculation (44). The baby hamster kidney cell line (BHK) is also susceptible to infection with PHV1, but all the other mammalian cell lines tested so far have been refractory to the virus (45).

Plaques develop in cultures overlaid with carboxymethylcellulose, agarose, or specific antiserum (42, 43). Virus multiplication in cell cultures is inhibited by trisodium phosphonoformate (26, 27, 37) and acycloguanosine (34). Extracellular virus can be protected by the addition of 5% dimethylsulfoxide to the medium before freezing (43).

PATHOGENESIS AND EPIZOOTIOLOGY

Natural and Experimental Hosts. The pigeon seems to be the natural host of PHV1 with virus infection remaining latent (37).

PHV1 has been isolated from budgerigars (*Nymphicus hollandicus*) accidently infected after close contact with pigeons (46). Pigeons are susceptible to experimental infection by pharyngeal painting, which causes a mainly localized disease (42, 48), or by the intraperitoneal route, causing a systemic infection (10). Systemic infections can also be produced in budgerigars (*Melopsittacus undulatus*) by intranasal inoculation of the virus (38). Chickens, ducks, canaries, and hamsters are resistant to infection (10, 37, 40).

Transmission. Susceptible pigeons can be infected through direct contact with infected birds. Egg transmission of PHV1 seems unlikely (41). Mature pigeons in infected flocks are asymptomatic carriers of the virus and some of them may shed virus from time to time (48).

The vast majority of latently infected mature pigeons reexcrete virus in their throat during the breeding season and during squab gorging (60). They are therefore able to directly transmit the infection to the squabs soon after hatching. Although the squabs become infected, they are protected from the disease by maternal antibodies acquired through the egg yolk. Therefore, most of the squabs themselves become asymptomatic carriers after this initial infection (41).

Incubation Period, Shedding, Latency. Virus excretion begins 24 hr after inoculation and persists at a high titer for a minimum of 7–10 days in inoculated squabs. Typical lesions appear 1–3 days after infection when viral excretion reaches its peak. Mild episodes of recurrence, without clinical signs, occur spontaneously. High titers of specific antibodies do not prevent these recurrences and conversely, recurrent episodes are not more frequent when the animals are nearly devoid of specific antibodies. PHV1 reexcretion can also be provoked by cyclophosphamide (Cy)-treatment of pigeons, and this period of reexcretion may be accompanied by lesions (48).

Distribution of PHV1 in the Host. In classical PHV1 infection, virus generally remains localized in the upper respiratory and digestive tracts. However, natural or experimental pharyngeal infection may be followed by viral dissemination throughout the body with viral localization and development of lesions in organs such as trachea, spleen, liver, kidney, and brain (6, 8, 42, 43). Indeed, during the primary infection and during episodes of reexcretion following Cy-treatment, a transient viremia may occur (42). Moreover, PHV1 can be transmitted from cell to cell in the presence of high titers of specific antibodies (42). PHV1 can thus be spread either by tissue contiguity or by viremia, especially when pigeons are immunodepressed (37).

Signs. In the acute form of the disease, pigeons sneeze frequently and show conjunctivitis, and nostrils become obstructed with nasal mucus and moisture. Caruncles, which are normally white, turn yellow-grey.

In the chronic form, sinusitis and intense dyspnea may be observed if the primary viral infection is complicated by *Trichomonas columbae* or secondary mycoplasmal or bacterial invaders (*Mycoplasma columbinum, Mycoplasma columborale, Pasteurella multocida, Pasteurella hemolytica, Escherichia coli, Staphylococcus beta-hemolysin, Streptococcus beta-hemolytic*) (28, 37).

Morbidity and Mortality. Clinical disease is observed principally following primary infection of young pigeons not protected by maternal antibodies and in virus carriers in which the infection is complicated by virtue of debilitating factors (41).

Gross Lesions. The mucous membranes of the mouth, pharynx and larynx are congested and, in severe cases, covered with foci of necrosis and small ulcers. The mucous membrane of the pharynx may be coated with diphtheritic membranes. When the viral infection is generalized (viremia), foci of necrosis can be observed in the liver. If the initial infection becomes complicated by bacterial infections, the trachea may be obstructed by caseous material and some birds may show air-sacculitis and pericarditis (pigeon chronic respiratory disease) (37).

Histopathology. Multiple foci of necrosis are observed in the pharyngeal stratified squamous epithelium and in the salivary glands. Foci contain cells at different stages of degeneration and necrosis, and intranuclear inclusions are present in adjacent epithelial cells. Large foci may extend and form ulcers. Similar foci of necrosis can also be observed in the laryngeal and tracheal epithelium (42).

In generalized infections, pigeons present hepatitis; intranuclear inclusion bodies are found in many hepatic cells widely spread throughout the organ (8, 42, 43). Lesions have also been described in the pancreas and the brain (6, 8,10).

Immunity. Neutralizing antibodies appear in squabs at the end of the 1st week following infection. Importance of these antibodies is difficult to evaluate with regard to re-emergence of active infection (48), but when acquired passively in the form of maternally derived antibodies, they are protective for squabs (41). As a herpesvirus infection, it might be presumed that cell- mediated immunity is important in PHV1 infections.

DIAGNOSIS

Isolation and Identification of Causative Agent. PHV1 can be easily isolated in CEF cultures from pharyngeal swabs of infected pigeons; also, but with more difficulty, from internal organs such as trachea, lungs or liver. Isolates should be characterized by immunological means such as immunofluorescence (37, 47).

Serology. Specific antibodies can be titrated by virus-neutralization tests or by indirect immunofluorescence and can be detected by counter-immuno-electro-osmophoresis (37, 47).

Differential Diagnosis. Clinically acute PHV1 infection disease may be confused with Newcastle disease virus infection (lentogenic pneumotropic paramyxovirus 1 strains) and chronic PHV1 infection disease complicated by secondary bacterial invaders must be distinguished from the diphtheroid form of pox virus infection (57, 59). A diagnosis of PHV1 infection requires virus isolation or serologic evidence. However, both techniques may fail to demonstrate PHV1 infection in individual pigeons, the first because the animal may not be actively excreting virus and the second because of an absence of seroconversion in a latent carrier. For these reasons, several animals from the same dove-cote must be simultaneously examined (37, 47).

TREATMENT, PREVENTION, CONTROL. After primary infection, pigeons become asymptomatic carriers and may reexcrete virus. Chemotherapy trials with trisodium phosphonoformate and acycloguanosine failed to prevent infection (26, 27, 34, 52). Vindevogel et al. (53–55), therefore, compared the ability of inactivated (in oil adjuvant), or attenuated, vaccines to prevent clinical disease, the carrier state, and virus reexcretion. Both types of vaccine were able to reduce primary viral excretion and clinical signs after challenge. Nevertheless, neither attenuated nor inactivated vaccines were able to prevent appearance of carriers, since most of the pigeons reexcreted virus after Cy-treatment. However, vaccination did help to prevent spontaneous viral reexcretion, thereby helping to control viral dissemination.

PSEUDORABIES (AUJESZKY'S DISEASE)

Pseudorabies virus (*Sus herpesvirus 1,* SHV1) produces a generally mild disease in swine, its natural host, but a fatal disease in cattle. Other animals found infected in nature are dogs, cats, sheep, and rats (18, 21). SHV1 multiplies very well in chicken embryo fibroblast cultures (2).

Experimentally, SHV1 can infect chickens, chicken embryos, and pigeons (13, 18, 35). Chicken embryos succumb with encephalitis after inoculation on the chorioallantoic membrane, as do 2-day-old chicks after being inoculated subcutaneously (1). Adult chickens, however, are resistant to subcutaneous inoculation (29).

Toneva (35) attenuated a strain of SHV1 by serial passages in pigeons combining intramuscular and subcutaneous routes of inoculation (pigeon strain 80). Inoculated pigeons developed classical symptoms of encephalitis, i.e., torticollis and disordered balance. The SHV1 pigeon strain 80 is avirulent for rabbits, mice, guinea pigs, and piglets after subcutaneous injection but remains lethal after intracerebral inoculation.

REFERENCES

1. Bang, F.B. 1942. Experimental infection of the chick embryo with the virus of pseudorabies. J Exp Med 76:263–270.

2. Beladi, I. 1962. Study on the plaque formation and some properties of the Aujeszky disease virus on chicken embryo cells. Acta Vet Acad Sci Hung 12:417–422.

3. Boyle, D.B., and J.A. Binnington. 1973. Isolation of a herpesvirus from a pigeon. Aust Vet J 49:54.

4. Burtscher, H. 1965. Die virusbedingte Hepatosplenitis infectiosa strigum. 1. Mitteilung: Morphologische Untersuchungen. Pathol Vet 2:227–255.

5. Burtscher, H., and W. Grünberg. 1979. Herpesvirus-Hepatitis bei Kranichen (Aves Gruidae). I. Pathomorphologische Befunde. Zentralbl Veterinaermed [B] 26:561–569.

6. Callinan, R.B., B. Kefford, R. Borland, and R. Garrett. 1979. An outbreak of disease in pigeons associated with a herpesvirus. Aust Vet J 55:339–341.

7. Cornwell, H.J.C., and A.R. Weir. 1970. Herpesvirus infection of pigeons. IV. Growth of the virus in tissue-culture and comparison of its cytopathogenicity with that of the viruses of laryngotracheitis and pigeon pox. J Comp Pathol 80:517–523.

8. Cornwell, H.J.C., and N.G. Wright. 1970. Herpesvirus infection of pigeons. I. Pathology and virus isolation. J Comp Pathol 80:221–227.

9. Cornwell, H.J.C., A.R. Weir, and E.A.C. Follett. 1967. A herpes infection of pigeons. Vet Rec 81:267–268.

10. Cornwell, H.J.C., N.G. Wright, and H.B. McCusker. 1970. Herpesvirus infection of pigeons. II. Experimental infection of pigeons and chicks. J Comp Pathol 80:229–232.

11. French, E.L., H.G. Purchase, and K. Nazerian. 1973. A new herpesvirus isolated from a nestling cor-

morant (Phalacrocorax melanoleucos). Avian Pathol 2:3-15.
12. Fritzche, K., U. Heffels, and E.F Kaleta. 1981. Ubersichtreferat: Virusbedingte Infektionen der Taube. Dtsch Tierärztl Wochenschr 88:72-76.
13. Glover, R.E. 1939. Cultivation of the virus of Aujeszky's disease on the chorioallantoic membrane of the developing egg. Br J Exp Pathol 20:150-158.
14. Heffels, U., K. Fritzche, E.F. Kaleta, and U. Neumann. 1981. Serologische Untersuchungen zum Nachweis virusbedingter Infektionen bei der Taube in der Bundesrepublik Deutschland. Dtsch Tierärztl Wochenschr 88:97-102.
15. Kaleta, E.F., H. J. Marschall, G. Glünder, and B. Stiburek. 1980. Isolation and serologial differentiation of a herpesvirus from Bobwhite Quail (Colinus virginianus, L. 1758). Arch Virol 66:359-364.
16. Kaleta, E.F., T. Mikami, H.J. Marschall, U. Heffels, M. Heidenreich, and B. Stiburek. 1980. A new herpesvirus isolated from black storks (Ciconia nigra). Avian Pathol 9:301-310.
17. Kaleta, E.F., D.J. Alexander, and P.H. Russell. 1985. The first isolation of the avian PMV1 virus responsible for the current panzootic in pigeons? Avian Pathol 14:553-557.
18. Kaplan, A.S. 1969. Herpes simplex and pseudorabies viruses. In S. Gard, C. Hallauer, and K.F. Meyer (eds.), Virology Monographs, pp. 66-68, 80-82. Springer-Verlag, Vienna/New York.
19. Krupicka, V., B. Smid, L. Valicek, and V. Pleva. 1970. Isolation of a herpesvirus from pigeons on the chorio-allantoic membrane of embryonated eggs. Vet Med (Praha) 15:609-612.
20. Landré, F., H. Vindevogel, P.P. Pastoret, A. Schwers, E. Thiry, and J. Espinasse. 1982. Fréquence de l'infection du pigeon par le Pigeon herpesvirus 1 et le virus de la maladie de Newcastle dans le Nord de la France. Recl Méd Vét 158:523-528.
21. Lautié, R. 1969. Les maladies animales à virus. La maladie d'Aujeszky. Collection de monographies, direction scientifique P. Lépine, P. Goret. L'expansion scientifique française éditeur.
22. Mare, C.J., and D.L. Graham. 1973. Falcon herpesvirus, the etiologic agent of inclusion body disease of falcons. Infect Immun 8:118-126.
23. Mohammed, M.A., S.M. Sokkar, and H.H. Tantawi. 1978. Contagious paralysis of pigeons. Avian Pathol 7:637-643.
24. Purchase, H.G., C.J. Mare, and B.R. Burmester. 1972. Antigenic comparison of avian and mammmalian herpesviruses and protection tests against Marek's disease. Proc 76th Annu Meet US Anim Health Assoc, pp. 484-492.
25. Saik, J.E., E.R. Weintraub, R.W. Diters, and M.A.E. Egy. 1986. Pigeon herpesvirus: Inclusion body hepatitis in a free-ranging pigeon. Avian Dis 30:426-429.
26. Schwers, A., P.P. Pastoret, H. Vindevogel, P. Leroy, A. Aguilar-Setien, and M. Godart. 1980. Comparison of the effect of trisodium phosphonoformate on the mean plaque size of pseudorabies virus, infectious bovine rhinotracheitis virus, and pigeon herpesvirus. J Comp Pathol 90:625-633.
27. Schwers, A., H. Vindevogel, P. Leroy, and P.P. Pastoret. 1981. Susceptibility of different strains of pigeon herpesvirus to trisodium phosphonoformate. Avian Pathol 10:23-29.
28. Shimizu, T., H. Erno, and H. Nagatomo. 1978. Isolation and characterization of Mycoplasma columbinum and Mycoplasma columborale, two new species from pigeons. Int J Syst Bact 28:538-546.
29. Shope, R.E. 1931. An experimental study of mad itch with special reference to its relationship to pseudorabies. J Exp Med 45:233-248.
30. Simpsons, C.F., J.E. Hanley, and J.M. Gaskin. 1975. Psittacine herpesvirus resembling Pacheco's parrot disease. J Infect Dis 131:390-396.
31. Smadel, J.E., E.B. Jackson, and J.W. Harman. 1945. A new virus of pigeons. I. Recovery of the virus. J Exp Med 81:385-398.
32. Tantawi, H.H., M.M. Al Falluji, and F. Al Sheikhly. 1979. Viral encephalomyelitis of pigeons: Identification and characterization of the virus. Avian Dis 23:785-793.
33. Tantawi, H.H., Z.I. Iman, C.J. Mare, R. El-Karamany, M.A. Shalaby, and F. Tayeb. 1983. Antigenic relatedness of pigeon herpes encephalomyelitis virus to other avian herpesviruses. Avian Dis 27:563-568.
34. Thiry, E., H. Vindevogel, P. Leroy, P.P. Pastoret, A. Schwers, B. Brochier, Y. Anciaux, and P. Hoyois. 1983. In vivo and in vitro effect of acyclovir on pseudorabies virus, infectious bovine rhinotracheitis virus and pigeon herpesvirus. Ann Rech Vét 14:239-245.
35. Toneva, V. 1961. Obtention d'une souche nonvirulente du virus de la maladie d'Aujeszky au moyen de passages et de l'adaptation des pigeons. C R Acad Bulg Sci 14:187-190.
36. Vetesy, F., and J. Tanyi. 1975. Occurrence of a pigeon disease in Hungary caused by a herpesvirus. Magyar Allatorv Lapja, 193-197.
37. Vindevogel, H. 1981. Le coryza infectieux du pigeon, thesis of "Agrégation de l'Enseignement Supérieur," Univ Liège, Fac Vét Méd.
38. Vindevogel, H., and J.P. Duchatel. 1977. Réceptivité de la perruche au virus herpès du pigeon. Ann Méd Vét 121:193-195.
39. Vindevogel, H., and J.P. Duchatel. 1978. Contribution á l'étude de l'étiologie du coryza infectieux du pigeon. Ann Méd Vét 122:507-513.
40. Vindevogel, H., and J.P. Duchatel. 1979. 1. Etude de la récéptivité de différentes espèces animales au virus herpès du pigeon. 2. Résistance du pigeon au virus de la laryngotrachéite infectieuse aviaire. Ann Méd Vét 123:63-65.
41. Vindevogel, H., and P.P. Pastoret. 1980 . Pigeon herpes infection: Natural transmission of the disease. J Comp Pathol 90:409-413.
42. Vindevogel, H., and P.P. Pastoret. 1981. Pathogenesis of pigeon herpes infection. J Comp Pathol 91:415-426.
43. Vindevogel, H., P.P. Pastoret, G. Burtonboy, M. Gouffaux, and J.P. Duchatel. 1975. Isolement d'un virus herpès dans un elevage de pigeons de chair. Ann Rech Vét 6:431-436.
44. Vindevogel, H., J.P. Duchatel, and M. Gouffaux. 1977. Pigeon herpesvirus. I. Pathogenesis of pigeon herpesvirus in chicken embryo fibroblasts. J Comp Pathol 87:597-603.
45. Vindevogel, H., J.P. Duchatel, M. Gouffaux, and P.P. Pastoret. 1977. Pigeon herpesvirus. II. Susceptibility of avian and mammalian cell cultures to infection with pigeon herpesvirus. J Comp Pathol 87:605-610.
46. Vindevogel, H., J.P. Duchatel, and G. Burtonboy. 1978. Infection herpétique de psittacidés. Ann Méd Vét 122:167-169.
47. Vindevogel, H., A. Aguilar-Setien, L. Dagenais, and P.P. Pastoret. 1980. Diagnostic de l'infection herpétique du pigeon. Ann Méd Vét 124:407-418.
48. Vindevogel, H., P.P. Pastoret, and G. Burtonboy. 1980. Pigeon herpes infection: Excretion and re-excretion of virus after experimental infection. J Comp Pathol 90:401-408.
49. Vindevogel, H., P.P. Pastoret, P. Leroy, and F.

Coignoul. 1980. Comparaison de trois souches de virus herpétique isolées de psittacidés avec le virus herpès du pigeon. Avian Pathol 9:385–394.

50. Vindevogel, H., L. Dagenais, B. Lansival, and P.P. Pastoret. 1981. Incidence of rotavirus, adenovirus and herpesvirus infection in pigeons. Vet Rec 109:285–286.

51. Vindevogel, H., A. Kaeckenbeeck, and P.P. Pastoret. 1981. Fréquence de l'ornithose-psittacose et de l'infection herpétique chez le pigeon voyageur et les psittacidés en Belgique. Rev Méd de Liège 36:693–696.

52. Vindevogel, H., P.P. Pastoret, and A. Aguilar-Setien. 1982. Assays of phosphonoformate-treatment of pigeon herpesvirus infection in pigeons and budgerigars, and Aujeszky's disease in rabbits. J Comp Pathol 92:177–180.

53. Vindevogel, H., P.P. Pastoret, and P. Leroy. 1982. Vaccination trials against pigeon herpesvirus infection (Pigeon herpesvirus 1). J Comp Pathol 92:484–494.

54. Vindevogel, H., P.P. Pastoret, and P. Leroy. 1982. Essais de vaccination contre l'infection herpétique du pigeon (Pigeon herpesvirus 1). 17th Int Congr Herpesvirus Man Anim: Stand Immunol Proced Dev Biol Stand 52:429–436.

55. Vindevogel, H., P.P. Pastoret, and P. Leroy. 1982. Comportement d'une souche atténuée de Pigeon herpesvirus 1 et de souches pathogènes lors d'infections successives chez le pigeon. Ann Rech Vét 13:143–148.

56. Vindevogel, H., P.P. Pastoret, E. Thiry, and N. Peeters. 1982. Réapparition de formes graves de la maladie de Newcastle chez le pigeon. Ann Méd Vét 126:5–7.

57. Vindevogel, H., E. Thiry, P.P. Pastoret, and G. Meulemans. 1982. Lentogenic strains of Newcastle disease virus in pigeons. Vet Rec 110:497–499.

58. Vindevogel, H., P.P. Pastoret, and E. Thiry. 1983. Pigeon herpesvirus 1. WHO Collaborating Centre for Collection and Evaluation of Data on Comparative Virology. Munich, W Ger.

59. Vindevogel, H., J.P. Duchatel, and P.P. Pastoret. 1984. Les dominantes pathologiques respiratoires chez le pigeon. Recl Méd Vét 160:1031–1036.

60. Vindevogel, H., H. Debruyne, and P.P. Pastoret. 1985. Observation of Pigeon herpesvirus 1 re-excretion during the reproduction period in conventionally reared homing pigeons. J Comp Pathol 95:105–112.

PNEUMOVIRUS INFECTIONS (TURKEY RHINOTRACHEITIS AND SWOLLEN HEAD SYNDROME OF CHICKENS)

D.J. Alexander

INTRODUCTION. A disease of turkeys termed turkey coryza or, more frequently, turkey rhinotracheitis (TRT) has been reported from many countries. The etiology of the disease has not always been clear or has been attributed to different organisms in different countries despite the similarity of clinical signs. These aspects of the disease have been reviewed in detail by Lister and Alexander (17). In some countries a virus, now recognized as a probable member of the *Pneumovirus* genus (7, 16), has been implicated in the disease. TRT, caused by avian pneumovirus, should not be confused with turkey bordetellosis (also called rhinotracheitis), which is covered in Chapter 12.

A disease of chickens, termed swollen head syndrome (SHS) has often been reported from countries experiencing TRT and occasionally from countries where there is no substantial turkey population. There is now strong evidence that this condition involves infection with the same avian pneumovirus as TRT, although it appears that the "swollen head" occurs as a result of infection with secondary, adventitious bacteria, usually *Escherichia coli.*

HISTORY. A clinical disease syndrome indistinguishable from conditions now known to be related to avian pneumovirus infections has been reported from a number of countries since the late 1960s. However, in some of these countries, most notably the USA, it has been established that the causative organism is *Bordetella avium* and this organism and disease are dealt with in Chapter 12. Because of the differing etiologies and the difficulty in isolating the causative virus it is impossible to state categorically when the condition was first recognized. Early reports attributing a viral etiology to both TRT and SHS in chickens came from South Africa where both diseases had appeared during the 1970s (5, 19). But it was not until the isolation of the causative virus and the development of a serological test in 1986 that some estimation of the true prevalence and distribution of the disease could be made.

INCIDENCE AND DISTRIBUTION. Lister and Alexander (17) listed the countries reporting disease signs similar to TRT and the prevalence of the disease in those countries prior to the isolation and identification of avian pneumoviruses. Retrospective assessment of serology or isolation of viruses indicated that the disease seen in many of these countries was related to avian pneumovirus infections. The virus has been isolated from turkeys in France, Great Britain, and Italy, and viruses reported in South Africa (5) and Israel (24) are probably also avian pneumoviruses. Antibodies to the virus have been demonstrated in chickens and/or turkeys in Great Britain, France, Italy, South Africa, Israel, Federal Republic of Germany, the Netherlands, Spain, and Greece. In South Africa, SHS, or "dikkop" as it is termed there, appears to have been prevalent for a number of years.

ETIOLOGY

Classification. The virus family Paramyxoviridae is formed from enveloped RNA viruses that have a nonsegmented, single-stranded genome of negative polarity; have helical capsid symmetry; undergo capsid assembly in the cytoplasm; and are budded from the cell surface. The family is divided into three genera: *Morbillivirus*–measles, distemper, rinderpest; *Paramyxovirus*–Newcastle disease virus, etc; *Pneumovirus*–the respiratory syncytial viruses. Pneumoviruses are distinguished from other paramyxoviruses by the lack of both hemagglutinating and neuraminidase activities, by the characteristic diameter of the nucleocapsid (12–15 nm), and by a larger number of structural and nonstructural polypeptides. The virus associated with TRT and SHS appears to fulfil all these criteria and it has been considered to represent a member of the Pneumovirus genus, along with respiratory syncytial viruses (human and bovine) and mouse pneumonia virus (7, 11, 16).

Morphology. Negative contrast electron microscopy of the virus reveals pleomorphic fringed particles, usually roughly spherical, of 80–200 nm in diameter, although occasionally round particles with diameters of 500 nm or more can be seen (Fig. 29.1). Fringed filamentous forms 80–100 nm in diameter and up to 1000 nm long may be present (Fig. 29.2), particularly in preparations from organ culture propagation. Collins and Gough (7) reported the surface projections to be 13–14 nm in length and the helical nucleocapsid to be 14 nm in diameter with an estimated pitch of 7 nm per turn.

Structure. Characteristically, pneumoviruses have been reported to have about seven structural and three nonstructural virus-specified proteins of which two are glycosylated (22). Collins and Gough (7) described seven structural polypeptides for a TRT virus isolate of which two were glycosylated. In in vitro and in vivo polypeptide synthesis studies, Ling and Pringle (16) reported

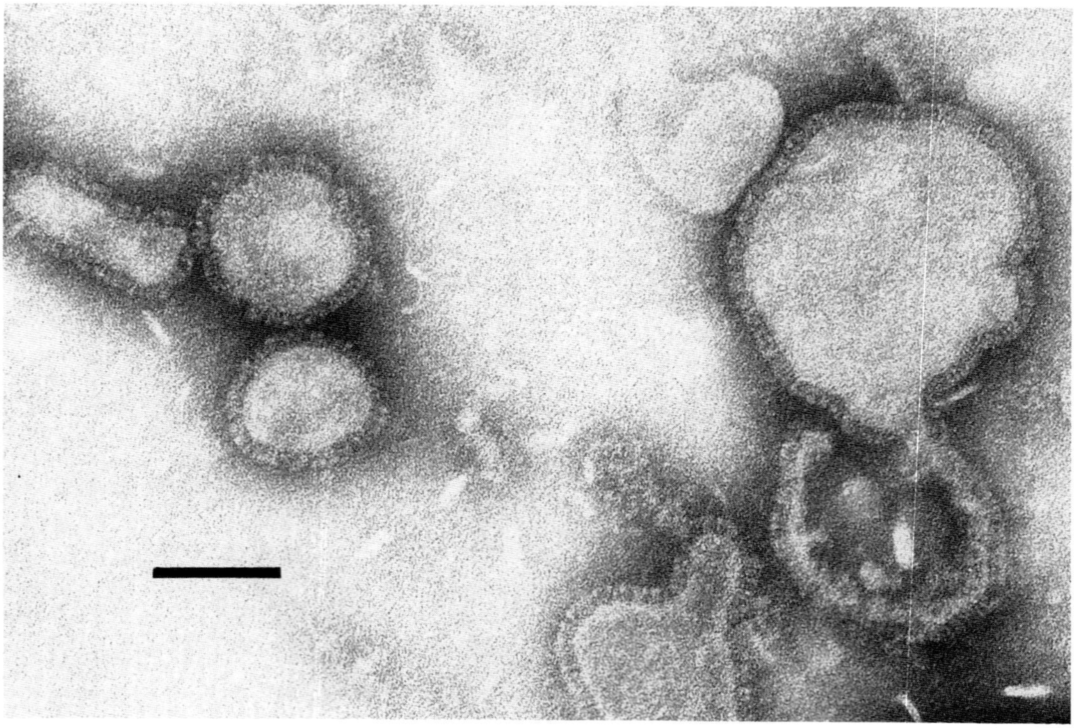

29.1. Negative-contrast electron micrograph of avian pneumovirus particles. ×160,000, bar = 100 nm. (Collins)

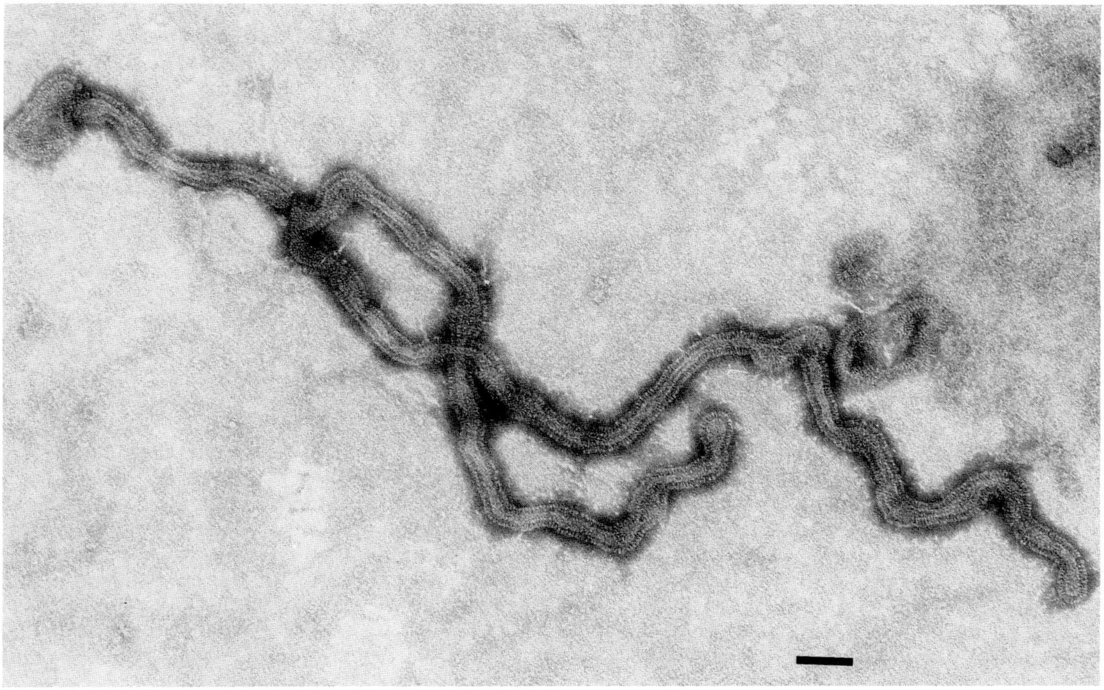

29.2. Negative-contrast electron micrograph of avian pneumovirus filamentous particles. ×100,000, bar = 100 nm. (Collins)

similar structural polypeptides and at least two nonstructural proteins. These authors considered their results to be consistent with classification of the virus as a member of the *Pneumovirus* genus.

Strain Classification. To date there have been relatively few isolations of the virus. Studies using isolates from different laboratories propagated under different conditions have indicated no significant variation detectable by enzyme-linked immunosorbent assay (ELISA), virus-neutralization (VN), microimmunofluorescence, and immunodiffusion cross-antibody tests or polypeptide profiles (4, 12).

Laboratory Host Systems. Initial problems in the laboratory diagnosis and determination of the etiology of TRT were due primarily to a lack of a suitable laboratory propagation system. The infectious nature of the disease could be demonstrated by typical clinical signs appearing in susceptible turkey poults placed in contact with infected birds or inoculated with filtered mucus from affected birds (1).

Inoculation of infective mucus into the yolk sac of turkey or chicken embryos resulted in embryo mortality after four or five passages but virus was demonstrated to be at a very low titer (1). Similarly, inoculation of turkey or chicken tracheal organ cultures resulted in ciliostasis, but again virus only replicated to low titers (9, 18). However, isolates adapted to embryos or tracheal organ cultures were capable of replication in cultures of chick embryo cells, turkey embryo cells, Vero cells and BS-C-1 cells with a characteristic cytopathic effect of syncytium formation and relatively high virus titers.

Pathogenicity. Despite the high morbidity and often high mortality associated with TRT in the field, the pathogenicity of isolates has been difficult to assess in the laboratory. Experimentally infected birds often show recognizable signs of TRT but these are milder than those seen in the field. Chickens show, at most, only mild respiratory disease in laboratory infections. The single isolate of avian pneumovirus from chickens with SHS was able to produce TRT in infected turkey poults (21). Presumably the difference in pathogenicity between laboratory and field infections is related to the conditions under which the birds are kept and the presence or absence of exacerbative organisms.

PATHOGENESIS AND EPIZOOTIOLOGY

Natural and Experimental Hosts. Turkeys and chickens are known natural hosts. Additionally, Picault et al. (21) found avian pneumovirus antibodies in flocks of Guinea fowl (*Numida meleagris*) and were able to produce a rhinotracheitislike disease in this species with virus isolated from TRT-affected turkeys. In experimental infections with a TRT isolate, Gough et al. (13) demonstrated susceptibility with clinical signs in turkeys, chickens, and pheasants, and an immune response to the virus in Guinea fowl. Pigeons, geese, and ducks appeared to be refractory to the virus.

The virus appears to be capable of infecting chickens and turkeys of any age.

Transmission. The infectious nature of the disease has been established by contact transmission from affected to susceptible turkey poults, or by inoculation with filtered or unfiltered mucus, nasal washings, or other materials from the respiratory tract of affected birds (17).

In most countries where TRT has appeared as a new disease it has spread rapidly. For example, in Great Britain the disease had been reported from most of the turkey-producing areas of England and Wales within 9 wk of the first outbreak of the disease (1). The methods by which such spread takes place are unclear and even on a single site, spread is unpredictable. Contaminated water, movement of affected or recovered poults, movement of personnel and equipment, feed trucks etc. have all been implicated in some outbreaks, while airborne spread or vertical transmission have also been put forward as possibilities. At present only contact spread has been confirmed.

Signs, Morbidity, Mortality. Lister and Alexander (17) summarized the various clinical signs reported for TRT. Much of the variation reported may relate to the secondary adventitious organisms that frequently appear as a problem with TRT. Signs in young poults typically include snicking, rales, sneezing, nasal discharge (often frothy), foamy conjunctivitis, swelling of infraorbital sinuses, and submandibular edema. In laying birds there may be a drop in egg production of up to 70% (23), along with slight respiratory distress. In some adult flocks of turkeys serological conversion to the virus has been recorded without any observation of clinical signs. When disease is seen, morbidity is usually described as 100%, or very high, in birds of all ages. There is considerable variation in mortality, ranging from as low as 0.4% to as high as 90% of the flock. It is usually highest in young poults.

The clinical signs of SHS in broiler breeders were described by O'Brien (20) as swelling of the periorbital and infraorbital sinuses, torticollis, cerebral disorientation, and depression. Usually less than 4% of the flock were affected, although on occasions widespread respiratory signs were also present (26). Marked egg production losses have also been associated with SHS. Broiler chickens with confirmed avian pneumovirus infections have had more severe respiratory disease and a greater proportion showing head swelling than has been seen in adult birds (19).

DIAGNOSIS

Isolation and Identification of Virus. Initially, virus isolation proved extremely difficult due to the fastidious nature of the virus, the frequency with which other organisms could be isolated, and the timing of the virus isolation attempts (17). Successful virus isolation was achieved in chicken or turkey embryos or chicken organ cultures and these have been used on a routine basis.

CHOICE AND TIMING OF SAMPLES FOR ISOLATION. Although virus has been isolated from trachea, lung, and viscera of affected turkey poults, by far the most fruitful source of virus has been nasal secretions or tissue scraped from the sinuses of affected birds. It is extremely important to obtain samples as early as possible after infection. Isolation of virus is rarely successful from birds showing severe signs; presumably, the extreme signs are a result of secondary, adventitious bacterial infections in birds predisposed by earlier virus infection. This probably accounts for the lack of success in isolating virus from chickens with SHS, as the characteristic signs appear to be due to secondary *E. coli* infection.

ISOLATION PROCEDURES. Twenty-percent (v/v) suspensions of nasal secretions/exudate and sinus material in phosphate-buffered saline containing antibiotics are held at room temperature for 1–2 hr, clarified by centrifugation at 1000 g's for 10 min, and then passed through a 450 nm porosity membrane filter. Six- to 7-day-old, specific-pathogen-free embryonated chickens eggs should be inoculated via the yolk sac. Tracheal organ cultures from chick embryos or young chicks are susceptible to infection, but those from turkeys are generally more sensitive and should be used if they are from a specific-pathogen-free flock, or at least a flock free of specific antibodies. Blind passages should be made using allantoic-amniotic fluid harvested 10 days after inoculation, or supernatant fluids from tracheal organ cultures 7 days after inoculation. On passage in eggs, the virus first causes stunting of the embryo; after 4–5 passages, it consistently causes death. In organ cultures the virus may cause ciliostasis within 2–3 passages.

Viruses adapted so that they are lethal to embryos or cause rapid ciliostasis generally grow to only very low titers. At this stage they are usually capable of growth in chicken embryo fibroblast (CEF) cell cultures, although production of full cytopathic effects may require further passaging in CEF cells. Viruses adapted to CEF cultures grow to high titers, enabling electron microscopy and VN tests with specific antiserum to confirm the identity of the virus. As an alternative, VN tests for confirmatory diagnosis may be done in tracheal organ cultures, observing inhibition of ciliostasis by specific antiserum.

Serology. Antibodies to avian pneumovirus may be detected in standard VN tests in organ cultures (4) or CEF microcultures (12). Immunofluorescence assays (4) and immunodiffusion tests with N-lauroylsarcosine-disrupted virus (12) can also detect antibodies. However, the most frequently used method to assess antibodies to avian pneumovirus has been the ELISA (4, 6, 9, 14, 25).

PREVENTION AND CONTROL

Management Procedures. TRT is greatly exacerbated by poor management practices such as inadequate ventilation, over stocking, poor litter conditions, poor general hygiene, and mixed age groups (8, 23). Debeaking or vaccination with live Newcastle disease virus, if done at a critical time, might also increase the incidence and severity of clinical signs and mortality. Andral et al. (2) stressed the difficulty in eradicating TRT from multiage sites where complete cleaning and disinfection can not take place.

Chemotherapy. Attempts to treat TRT with antibiotics have met with varied success. Dayon and Pecquerie (8) reported some success in reducing the severity of the disease with an antibiotic regimen, presumably by controlling secondary adventitious bacteria. However, similar attempts at treatment of the disease in Great Britain met with little success (3).

Vaccination. At present no vaccine is commercially available. In a preliminary study by French workers poor results were obtained with a single dose of oil-emulsion, inactivated vaccine but a live attenuated vaccine given at 1 day old resulted in lower mortality and condemnations than were observed in nonvaccinated birds (10, 15).

REFERENCES

1. Alexander, D.J, E.D. Borland, C.D.Bracewell, N.J. Chettle, R.E. Gough, S.A. Lister, and P.J. Wyeth. 1986. A preliminary report of investigations into turkey rhinotracheitis in Great Britain. State Vet J 40:161–169.
2. Andral, B., C. Louzis, D. Trap, J.A. Newman, D. Toquin, and G. Bennejean. 1985. Respiratory disease (rhinotracheitis) in turkeys in Brittany, France, 1981–1982. I. Field observation and serology. Avian Dis 29:35–42.
3. Anonymous. 1985. Turkey rhinotracheitis of unknown etiology in England and Wales. Vet Rec 117:653–654.
4. Baxter-Jones, C., J.K.A. Cook, J.A. Frazier, M. Grant, R.C. Jones, A.P.A. Mockett, and G.P. Wilding. 1987. Close relationship between TRT virus isolates. Vet Rec 120:562.
5. Buys, S.B., and J.H. Du Preez. 1980. A preliminary report on the isolation of a virus causing sinusitis in turkeys in South Africa and attempts to attenuate the virus. Turkeys (June):36, 46.
6. Chettle, N.J., and P.J. Wyeth. 1988. The use of an ELISA test to detect antibodies to turkey rhinotracheitis. Br Vet J 144:282–287.
7. Collins, M.S., and R.E. Gough. 1988. Characterisation of a virus associated with turkey rhinotracheitis. J Gen Virol 69:909–916.
8. Dayon, J.F., and F. Pecquerie. 1982. Rhinotracheite 81 de la dinde: Le constat sur le terrain. L'Aviculteur 423:65–70.
9. Giraud, P., G. Bennejean, M. Guittet, and D. Toquin. 1986. Turkey rhinotracheitis in France: Preliminary investigations on a ciliostatic virus. Vet Rec 118:81.
10. Giraud, P., M. Guittet, D. Toquin, F.X. Le Gros, J.F. Bouquet, and G. Bennejean. 1987. Rhinotracheite infectieuse de la dinde (R.T.I.): Progres recents dans l'etiologie et la prevention. L'Aviculteur 477:47–53.
11. Giraud, P., F.X. Le Gros, D. Toquin, J.F. Bouquet, and G. Bennejean. 1988. Turkey rhinotracheitis: Viral identification of the causal agent. Proc 37th West Poult Dis Conf, pp. 61–62.
12. Gough, R.E., and M.S. Collins. 1989. Antigenic relationships of three turkey rhinotracheitis viruses. Avian Pathol 18:227–238.
13. Gough, R.E., M.S. Collins, W.J. Cox, and N.J. Chettle. 1988. Experimental infection of turkeys, chickens, ducks, geese, Guinea fowl, pheasants, and pigeons with turkey rhinotracheitis virus. Vet Rec 123:58–59.
14. Grant, M., C. Baxter-Jones, and G.P. Wilding. 1987. An enzyme-linked immunosorbent assay for the serodiagnosis of turkey rhinotracheitis infection. Vet Rec 120:279–280.
15. Le Gros, F.X., G. Magand, P. Giraud, J.F. Bouquet, M. Guittet, and G. Bennejean. 1988. Turkey rhinotracheitis: Field results of the vaccination of day-old turkeys with a live attenuated virus. Proc 37th West Poult Dis Conf, pp. 63–66.
16. Ling, R., and C.R. Pringle. 1988. Turkey rhinotracheitis virus: In vivo and in vitro polypeptide synthesis. J Gen Virol 69:917–923.
17. Lister, S.A., and D.J. Alexander. 1986. Turkey rhinotracheitis: A review. Vet Bull 56:637–663.
18. McDougall, J.S., and J.K.A. Cook. 1986. Turkey rhinotracheitis: Preliminary investigations. Vet Rec 118:206–207.
19. Morley, A.J., and D.K. Thomson. 1984. Swollen head syndrome in broiler chickens. Avian Dis 28:238–243.
20. O'Brien, J.D.P. 1985. Swollen head syndrome in broiler breeders. Vet Rec 117:619–620.
21. Picault, J.P., P. Giraud, P. Drouin, M. Guittet, G. Bennejean, I. Lamande, D. Toquin, and C. Gueguen. 1987. Isolation of a TRT-like virus from chickens with swollen head syndrome. Vet Rec 121:135.
22. Pringle, C.R. 1985. Pneumoviruses. In B.W.J. Mahy (ed.), Virology–A Practical Approach, pp. 95–117, IRL Press, Oxford.
23. Stuart, J.C. 1986. Field experience in the UK with turkey rhinotracheitis. Turkeys 34:24–26.
24. Weisman, Y., C. Strengel, R. Blumenkranz, and Y. Segal. 1988. Turkey rhinotracheitis (TRT) in turkey flocks in Israel–virus isolation and serological response. Proc 37th West Poult Dis Conf, pp. 67–69.
25. Wyeth, P.J., R.E. Gough, N.J. Chettle, and R. Eddy. 1986. Preliminary observations on a virus associated with turkey rhinotracheitis. Vet Rec 119:139.
26. Wyeth, P.J., N.J. Chettle, R.E. Gough, and M.S. Collins. 1987. Antibodies to TRT in chickens with swollen head syndrome. Vet Rec 120:286–287.

ARBOVIRUS INFECTIONS

Marius Ianconescu

INTRODUCTION. The arboviruses comprise a large group of viruses clustered together by their ability to replicate in, and to be transmitted to other hosts by, arthropod vectors. The name arboviruses stands for an abbreviation of ARthropod-BOrne-VIRUSES.

The first known arbovirus, that causing bluetongue disease, was isolated at the turn of this century. The list of arboviruses is growing. At the beginning of the 1950s, 35 arboviruses were known. The first *International Catalog of Arboviruses,* published in 1972, listed 204 viruses, and in December 1987, 530 agents were included in this group (33).

INCIDENCE AND DISTRIBUTION. The dependency on an arthropod vector confers to arbovirus-caused diseases some special characteristics such as seasonal incidence and geographical distribution. Arboviruses have been isolated all over the world, even in arid and/or frozen areas, and from a multitude of hosts including humans, domestic animals, birds, and even lower vertebrates such as reptiles and amphibians (23). Some of these represent the habitual hosts, not necessarily because their susceptibility to the arboviruses is especially high, but rather because they live in a natural habitat rich in potential arthropod vectors and so have higher chances of becoming infected. Under certain conditions new "occasional" hosts like humans or domestic animals and birds are also infected, but usually, even in cases of real outbreaks, they represent accidental "spill-over" hosts, outside the normal arthropod-vertebrate-arthropod life cycle of the arbovirus (18, 20). Periodic changes in the weather, such as temperature and rainfall; changes in the local ecology due to irrigation, forestation, or deforestation; changes in the type, methodology, and localization of agriculture (40); and demographic and zoographic movements all can increase either the number of susceptible hosts or the chances of a given host coming in contact with the vector. Thus, they can serve as triggering factors for cases or even outbreaks of arbovirus infections outside their usual geographical and biological habitat (18, 36).

Most arboviruses associated with avian species were isolated from wild birds; only a few have come from domestic and paradomestic birds. Again, this difference is due more to the habitat than to a difference in susceptibility as was proven by placing domestic "sentinel birds" in the natural habitat of wild birds (16, 21, 27, 35, 57, 62).

Thus birds, both wild and domestic, together with rodents and any other potential hosts represent a natural reservoir and possible disseminator of these agents by way of their vector(s). Even viruses that are apathogenic or of low pathogenicity for birds can be important from an epidemiological point of view, considering that 30 of the 116 arboviruses associated with birds are also able to infect humans. For the maintenance and spread of an arbovirus, the level and duration of viremia are more important than its pathogenicity for the respective host.

ETIOLOGY

Virus Classification and Characteristics. The arboviruses, according to their morphologic, biochemical, and antigenic characteristics, belong to 12 families. Each may contain one or more genera, which in turn may be subdivided into groups of agents closely related antigenically but clearly distinguishable. This classification is very complex and is under continuous change and improvement. One hundred sixteen arboviruses, belonging to 6 families, have been isolated from birds or ornitophilic vectors. Due to the heterogeneousness of these viruses the main characteristics of each family for which there are avian isolates are presented (18, 19, 37, 42, 47, 54).

TOGAVIRIDAE AND FLAVIVIRIDAE. These are spheroid viruses, 40–70 nm diameter with a genome of positive-sense infective single-stranded RNA with a molecular weight (MW) of about 4 megadaltons (mD) in a lipid-containing envelope. Multiplication takes place in the cytoplasm; assembly occurs during budding through the cell membrane. Examples of viruses from these families are Eastern and Western equine encephalitis, Sindbis, Israel turkey meningoencephalitis, and St. Louis encephalitis viruses.

BUNYAVIRIDAE AND ARENAVIRIDAE. These viruses are 90–120 nm diameter with a lipid-containing envelope and a genome with circular molecules of negative-sense single-stranded RNA (MW 4.5–7 mD and 3.2–4.8 mD, respectively). Multiplication occurs in the cytoplasm with budding through the membrane of Golgi. Representatives of the Bunyaviridae family that are able to infect birds include Hughes, Avalon, and Uukuniemi viruses. Quaranfil and Johnston Atoll viruses belong to the Arenaviridae.

REOVIRIDAE. Not all the viruses of this family are

transmitted by an arthropod vector. Arboviruses of this family isolated from birds all belong to the genus *Orbivirus.* They are nonenveloped, are spheroidal with a diameter of 70–90 nm, and have a segmented genome with 10 linear fragments of double-stranded RNA (MW 12–20 mD). Kemerovo and Umatilla viruses are representative members of this family.

RHABDOVIRIDAE. These viruses have a characteristic bullet-shaped morphology, 130–380 nm long and 50–90 nm in diameter, and they have a lipid-containing envelope. The genome is one molecule of negative-sense single stranded RNA (MW 3.5–4.6 mD) coiled in a cylindrical structure. Flanders and Hart Park are examples of viruses belonging to this family.

Three arboviruses isolated from birds (Nyamanini, Kammavanpettai, and Sembalam) have not been classified as to family.

Laboratory Host Systems. Arboviruses are pathogenic for newborn and baby mice by intracerebral (IC) and some also by peripheral inoculations. IC inoculation is the method of choice for their isolation. They can be propagated in a variety of vertebrate cell cultures, inducing a cytopathic effect (CPE), and in arthropod cell cultures, where usually no CPE can be detected. Their antigenic structure is rather complex. Some tests detect group-specific antigens; others are able to differentiate various serotypes of the same group. Many arboviruses have hemagglutinating properties although hemagglutination and hemagglutination-inhibition (HI) tests have to be done with erythrocytes from day-old chickens or geese at stringent pH conditions for each virus (22).

ARBOVIRUS DISEASES OF BIRDS

There are three arbovirus-induced diseases of economic importance in domestic poultry and farm-reared game birds: Eastern and Western equine encephalitis (EEE, WEE) and Israel turkey meningoencephalitis (IT). The first two diseases, caused by Togaviridae (alphaviruses) were reported mainly in the Americas (39), but sporadic cases of EEE also have been described in other continents except Africa. The IT virus belongs to Flaviviridae and was reported in Asia and Africa. It can be a major problem for the turkey industry.

EASTERN EQUINE ENCEPHALITIS

EEE is transmitted by an ornitophil mosquito *Culiseta melanura* (11, 40, 41, 52), but the virus has also been isolated from a variety of other mosquitoes such as *Aedes sollicitans* (13), *Culex panocossa, Cx. dunni,* and *Cx. sacchettae* (58) and even from mites, culicoides, etc. (59).

Natural Hosts. Outbreaks of EEE have been reported mainly in pheasants but also in turkeys, ducks, chukars, and pigeons. In an infected pheasant flock, besides vector transmission, horizontal spread of the virus may occur by feather picking; debeaking effectively reduced the spread of the disease (59). Chickens are susceptible to the infection but no disease signs are observed in birds older than 3 wk. EEE has been isolated from numerous wild birds (61), mainly from passerine and columbiform species but they rarely become ill and are important primarily as a virus reservoir (49) and as a source of infection for domestic birds, animals, and humans.

Clinical Features and Pathology. Clinical manifestations differ among birds but are mainly signs of nervous involvement such as somnolence, incoordination, and paresis. Mortality may be as high as 75% or more. Gross lesions are not seen, but histologic changes in the central nervous system (CNS) are those normally associated with viral encephalitis (perivascular lymphocytic infiltration, microgliosis, focal meningitis, and neuronal degeneration).

Isolation and Identification of Causative Agent. Virus can be isolated (12, 22) by inoculation of blood and/or organ homogenate (brain, spleen, liver) into newborn mice (IC), freshly hatched chicks (subcutaneous), or guinea pigs (IC); 9- to 11-day-old chicken embryos (intraamniotic); and cultures of chick or duck embryo fibroblasts, baby hampster kidney (BHK-21), or Vero cells. Inoculated animals die of encephalitis in 2–5 days. Infected embryos die within 18–72 hr, presenting a purplish hemorrhagic appearance. Cell cultures develop CPE in 24–48 hr, and under agar, plaques develop in 36–48 hr. The conditions under which the collected materials are stored, transported, and processed are important, since arboviruses are sensitive to temperature, pH, and many solvents. Although embryo mortality or cell culture CPE can signal that a virus was isolated, its identification requires virus neutralization (VN) or other methods.

The complement-fixation (CF) test is also useful for virus identification or antibody determination (55). New methods such as enzyme-linked immunosorbent assay (ELISA), radio-immunoassay and molecular hybridization were introduced and are able to detect viral antigens and/or their nucleic acids with much more accuracy and in much smaller quantities than the classical methods (5, 6). The highly sensitive ELISA was able to detect EEE virus in experimentally infected birds at 12 hr postinfection and in pools of mosquitoes in which only 1% of the insects were infected (25, 26, 51, 53).

Serology. The presence of EEE antibody (17, 56) is also of diagnostic value. Available methods include VN, CF, HI, radio-immunoassay, and ELISA. The latter two methods offer advantages in sensitivity, specificity, and speed compared to the classical methods (44). Special care must be taken in interpreting results taking into consideration the persistency of antibody and the presence of group-specific reactions that, in some of the serological tests, can interfere with the precise identification or the typing of the virus, especially if various serotypes exist. Even among viruses of the same serotype, minor antigenic differences have been found, and erroneous or confusing results can be obtained by using "standard," or nonlocal strains of virus or commercial antibody (3, 58). Interestingly, Griffiths and McClain (21) found that anti-EEE class IgM antibody persisted longer than class IgG antibody. If this finding is confirmed with other arboviruses, many of the reports of short persistency of antibody, determined by methods detecting IgG, may have to be revised.

PREVENTION AND CONTROL. The best way to prevent EEE is to monitor and control the vector population (15, 60). There are no vaccines specifically prepared for bird immunization and the vaccine used for horses may give unsatisfactory results (14).

WESTERN EQUINE ENCEPHALITIS

WEE has many characteristics in common with EEE and only some will be emphasized here. Its vectors are mosquitoes (*Culiseta tarsalis, C. melanura*) (23, 24) and among the farm-reared birds, it affects pheasants, turkeys, and chukars. Based on the presence of antibody, WEE virus also infects chickens and many free-flying birds but no clinical manifestations have been reported. Laboratory diagnostic procedures are similar to those useful with EEE. Because minor antigenic variations have been found between WEE virus strains isolated in different areas, it is recommended that diagnostic antigens and immune sera should be prepared using locally isolated strains of virus.

ISRAEL TURKEY MENINGOENCEPHALITIS

It was described by Komarov and Kalmar in 1960 (34) as a paralytic disease affecting turkey flocks. Afflicted birds first showed incoordination and an unwillingness to move. When disturbed, they walked with their wings hanging down and stumbled. In more advanced stages they would lie down, unable to move. If such a bird was raised and then put down quickly, the legs generally were extended unequally or not at the same time. Under field conditions only turkeys older than 10 wk were affected (50). A severe drop in egg production sometimes occurred. Mortality was usually 10–30% but in some cases it reached over 80%. The etiologic agent isolated by Komarov and Kalmar was identified by Porterfield (46) as a new virus belonging to Flaviviridae. Experimentally it was shown that the IT virus (ITV) is able to infect mosquitoes (*Ae. aegypti* and *Cx. molestus*) (43), and the virus was isolated from pools of engorged mosquitoes and culicoides captured in or near turkey runs (4).

Natural and Experimental Hosts. Under field conditions, IT has been reported only in turkeys. Experimentally, chickens, ducks, geese, and pigeons were refractory to infection (34), but Japanese quail (*Coturnix coturnix japonica*) (31) and 2- to 3-day-old mice were highly susceptible. In contrast with the field observation that only turkeys older than 10 wk are affected, newly hatched poults are highly susceptible to IT following inoculation of virus by either the intracerebral or intramuscular route (32).

INCIDENCE AND DISTRIBUTION. The disease has a clear seasonal incidence starting toward the end of summer, reaching its peak in late autumn, and then declining at the beginning of winter, a period corresponding to the activity of the arthropod vectors. From 1958, when the disease was first observed, until 1973, all recorded cases were in northern Israel (50). In 1974 numerous flocks located in southern Israel also were affected, and in 1978 outbreaks of IT were recorded in South Africa (2).

PATHOLOGY. Some gross lesions such as splenomegaly or splenoatrophy, catarrhal enteritis, peritonitis, and myocarditis (2, 29, 34) are nonpathognomonic. More helpful are microscopic lesions such as nonpurulent meningoencephalitis (submeningeal and perivascular lymphocytic infiltration), focal myocardial necrosis, and grossly atretic and ruptured follicles in the ovary (2).

DIAGNOSIS

Isolation and Identification of Causative Agent. The ITV could be detected in turkey blood within 24 hr after infection and it persisted for 5–8 days in blood and in various organs such as brain, spleen, and liver (28, 30). Virus can be isolated by inoculating these materials into the yolk sac of 7- to 8-day-old chicken embryos. In positive cases embryo mortality occurs between 3 and 5 days postinoculation and the embryo presents a cherry-red discoloration. Virus identification has to be done by VN assays in cell cultures, chicken embryos, or baby mice. A retrospective diagnosis can be made by HI tests using goose RBCs and an antigen prepared from infected mouse brains (28, 43), or by VN in CEF or BHK cell cultures (2, 29, 30, 45).

Differential Diagnosis. Differential diagnosis with Newcastle disease, EEE, WEE, and avian encephalomyelitis must be considered. Newcastle disease can be excluded by testing the allantoic fluid from inoculated eggs in HI tests with Newcastle disease virus antisera, and EEE and WEE by HI or CF tests. Avian encephalomyelitis in turkeys can be excluded based on the age of birds (over 10 wk) and by the lack of disease in poults hatched from eggs of affected flocks.

CONTROL. IT can be controlled by vaccination. A live attenuated vaccine prepared by serial passage of the virus in chicken embryos was efficient, but it caused severe postvaccinal reactions (29, 32). A new vaccine prepared by passage of ITV in Japanese quail (32) is currently in use. Attenuation of the virus has also been achieved by serial propagation in BHK-21 cells (1) but no field vaccinations with this material have been reported.

ST. LOUIS ENCEPHALITIS

Although no clinical disease in birds has been reported, infection with St. Louis encephalitis virus (SLE) deserves some attention considering the high pathogenicity of this virus for humans and the fact that both domestic and wild birds represent the main source for its spread (27, 38, 39). The vectors are mosquitoes (*Cx. pipiens, Cx. tarsalis, Cx. quinquefasciatus, Cx. nigripalpus*), and the transovarial (vertical) transmission of this virus was demonstrated in a number of these vectors. Outbreaks of SLE in humans can be predicted by an increase of serocoversion in sentinel flocks or free-flying birds and they can be prevented or abated by appropriate control measures.

OTHER AVIAN ARBOVIRUSES

Chastel et al. (8, 9, 10) and Quillien et al. (48) reported a high prevalence of antibody to arboviruses among sea birds. They isolated Avalon, Meaban, Tyuleniy, Soldado, and Zaliv Terpenya viruses from various sea birds and ticks collected in their habitat. Some of these viruses are pathogenic for humans, and one of the main hosts for such viruses is the herring gull (*Larus argentatus*), which is known for its tendency to invade nonmarine biotopes and even urban dumping grounds (7), increasing the danger of virus dissemination in populated areas.

Only a few of the 116 avian arboviruses identified to date are described in this chapter and we must be aware that they represent only the very tip of the iceberg. Changes in climate or ecology, and accidental introduction of exotic arthropods can facilitate the colonization of new potential vectors and arboviruses in different areas of the world. Such an intrusion creates conditions of "virgin territory" where the susceptible host population (humans, animal, birds) is lacking any degree of immunity. Diseases, which in endemic areas are of low pathogenicity, can cause outbreaks of severe diseases.

REFERENCES

1. Barnard, B.J.H., and H.J. Geyer. 1981. Attenuation of turkey meningo-encephalitis virus in BHK21 cells. Onderstepoort J Vet Res 48:105–108.

2. Barnard, B.J.H., S.B. Buys, J.H. Du Preez, S.P. Greyling, and H. J. Venter. 1980. Turkey meningo-encephalitis in South Africa. Onderstepoort J Vet Res 47:89–94.

3. Bowen, G.S., T.P. Monath, G.E. Kemp, J.H. Kerschner, and L.J. Kirk. 1980. Geographic variations among St. Louis encephalitis virus strains in the viremic responses of avian hosts. Am J Trop Med Hyg 29:1411–1419.

4. Braverman, Y., M. Rubina, and K. Frish. 1981. Pathogens of veterinary importance isolated from mosquitoes and biting midges in Israel. Insect Sci Appl 2:157–161.

5. Burrell, C.J. 1985. Use of nucleic acid probes in virus diagnosis. In A.J. Della-Porta (ed.), Veterinary Viral Diseases: Their Significance in South-east Asia and the Western Pacific, pp. 71–81. Academic Press, Sydney, Aust.

6. Calisher, C.H., H.N. Fremount, W.L. Vesely, A.O. El-Kafrawi, and M.I. Al-Deen Mahmud. 1986. Relevance of detection of immunoglobulin M antibody response in birds used for arbovirus surveillance. J Clin Microbiol 24:770–774.

7. Chastel, C., and G. Le Lay-Rogues. 1981. Le virus Soldado, un arbovirus associé a des tiques et a des oiseaux de mer. Lyon Méd 245:29–35.

8. Chastel, C., J.Y. Monnat, G. Le Lay, C. Guiguen, M.C. Quillien, and J.C. Beaucournu. 1981. Studies on Bunyaviridae including Zaliv Terpeniya virus isolated from Ixodes Uriae ticks (Acarina:Ixodidae) in Brittany, France. Arch Virol 70:357–366.

9. Chastel, C., A.J. Main, C. Guiguen, G. Le Lay, M.C. Quillien, J. Y. Monnat, and J.C. Beaucournu. 1985. The isolation of Meaban virus, a new Flavivirus from the seabird tick Ornithodorus (Alectorobius) maritimus in France. Arch Virol 83:129–140.

10. Chastel, C., C. Guiguen, G. Le Lay, J.Y. Monnat, E. Hardy, G. Kerdraon, and J.C. Beaucournu. 1985. Enquete serologique arbovirus chez des oiseaux marins et non marins de Bretagne. Bull Soc Pathol Exot 78:594–605.

11. Coleman, P.H. 1984. Arbovirus infections. In M.S. Hofstad, H.J. Barnes, B.W. Calnek, W.M. Reid, and H.W. Yoder, Jr. (eds.), Diseases of Poultry, 8th Ed., pp. 576–580. Iowa State Univ Press, Ames.

12. Coleman, P.H., and C.H. Calisher. 1980. Arbovirus infections. In S.B. Hitchner, C.H. Domermuth, H.G. Purchase, and J.E. Williams (eds.), Isolation and Identification of Avian Pathogens, pp. 81–82. Am Assoc Avian Pathol, Kennett Square, PA.

13. Crans, W.J., J. McNelly, T.L. Sulze, and A. Main. 1986. Isolation of Eastern equine encephalitis virus from Aedes sollicitans during an epizootic in southern New Jersey. J Am Mosq Control Assoc 2:68–72.

14. Eisner, R.J., and S.R. Nusbaum. 1983. Encephalitis vaccination of pheasants: A question of efficacy. J Am Vet Med Assoc 183:280–281.

15. Eldridge, B.F. 1987. Strategies for surveillance, prevention, and control of arbovirus diseases in western North America. Am J Trop Med Hyg 37:77S-86S.

16. Emmons, R.W., D.V. Dondero, C.S. Chan, M.M. Milby, J.D. Walsh, W. C. Reeves, E.V. Bayer, L.T. Hui, and R.A. Murray. 1987. Surveillance for arthropod-borne viral activity and disease in California during 1986. Calif Mosq and Vector Control Assoc Inc 55:1–11.

17. Emord, D.E., C.D. Morris. 1984. Epizootiology of Eastern equine encephalomyelitis virus in upstate New York, USA. 6. Antibody prevalence in wild birds during an interepizootic period. J Med Entomol 21:395–404.

18. Fenner, F., P.A. Bachmann, E.P.J. Gibbs, F.A. Murphy, M.J. Studdert, and D.O. White. 1987. Epidemiology of viral infections. In Veterinary Virology, pp. 283–303. Academic Press, New York.

19. Fenner, F., P.A. Bachmann, E.P.J. Gibbs, F.A. Murphy, M.J. Studdert, and D.O. White. 1987. Togaviridae and Flaviviridae. In Veterinary Virology, pp. 451–472. Academic Press, New York.

20. Gordon-Smith, C.E. 1987. Factors influencing the transmission of Western equine encephalomyelitis virus between its vertebrate maintenance hosts and from them to humans. Am J Trop Med Hyg 37:33S-39S.

21. Griffiths, B.B., and O. McClain. 1985. Immunological response of chickens to Eastern equine encephalomyelitis virus. Res Vet Sci 38:65–68.

22. Halstead, S.B. 1985. Arboviruses. In E.H. Lennette (ed.), Laboratory Diagnosis of Viral Infections, pp. 147–169. M. Dekker, New York.

23. Hardy, J.L. 1987. The ecology of Western equine encephalomyelitis virus in the central valley of California, 1945–1985. Am J Trop Med Hyg 37:18S-32S.

24. Hayes, C.G., and R.C. Wallis. 1977. Ecology of Western equine encephalomyelitis in the Eastern United States. In M.A. Lauffer, F.B. Bang, K. Marmorosh, and K.M. Smith (eds.), Advances in Virus Research, Vol. 21, pp. 37–83. Academic Press, New York.

25. Hildreth, S.W., and B.J. Beaty. 1984. Detection of Eastern equine encephalomyelitis virus and Highlands J virus antigens within mosquito pools by enzyme immunoassay (EIA). 1. A laboratory study. Am J Trop Med Hyg 33:965–972.

26. Hildreth, S.W., B.J. Beaty, H.K. Maxfield, R.F. Gilfillan, and B. J. Rosenau. 1984. Detection of Eastern equine encephalomyelitis virus and Highlands J virus antigens within mosquito pools by enzyme immunoassay (EIA) 2. Retrospective field teast of the EIA. Am J Trop Med Hyg 33:973–980.

27. Hughes, P.E., and C.P. Ryan. 1985. Birds and the 1984 St.Louis encephalitis epidemic in Southern California. Proc 34th West Poult Conf, pp.69–70.

28. Ianconescu, M. 1980. Turkey meningo-encephalitis. In S.B. Hitchner, C.H. Domermuth, H.G. Purchase, and J.E. Williams (eds.), Isolation and Identification of Avian Pathogens, pp. 83–84. Am Assoc Avian Pathol, Kennett Square, PA.

29. Ianconescu, M., A. Aharonovici, Y. Samberg, M. Merdinger, and K. Hornstein. 1972. An aetiological and immunological study of the 1971 outbreak of Turkey meningo-encephalitis. Refu Vet 29:110–117.

30. Ianconescu, M., A. Aharonovici, Y. Samberg, K.

Hornstein, and M. Merdinger. 1973. turkey meningo-encephalitis: Pathogenic and immunological aspects of the infection. Avian Pathol 2:251-262.
31. Ianconescu, M., A. Aharonovici, and Y. Samberg. 1974. The Japanese quail as an experimental host for turkey meningo-encephalitis virus. Refu Vet 31:100-108.
32. Ianconescu, M., K. Hornstein, Y. Samberg, A. Aharonovici, and M. Merdinger. 1975. Development of a new vaccine against turkey meningo-encephalitis using a virus passaged through the Japanese quail (Coturnix coturnix japonica). Avian Pathol 4:119-131.
33. Karabatsos, N. 1988. Personal communication.
34. Komarov, A., and E. Kalmar. 1960. A hitherto undescribed disease–turkey meningo-encephalitis. Vet Rec 72:257-261.
35. Main, A.J., K.S. Anderson, H.K. Maxfield, B. Rosenau, and C. Oliver. 1988. Duration of Alphavirus neutralizing antibody in naturally infected birds. Am J Trop Med Hyg 38:208-217.
36. Monath, T.P. 1985. Epidemiology and control of vector-borne viral diseases. In A.J. Della-Porta (ed.), Veterinary Viral Diseases: Their Significance in Southeast Asia and the Western Pacific, pp. 85-99. Academic Press, Sydney, Aust.
37. Monath, T.P. 1985. Flaviviruses. In B.N. Fields (ed.), Virology, pp. 955-1004. Raven Press, New York.
38. Monath, T.P., and T.F. Tsai. 1987. St. Louis encephalitis: Lessons from the last decade. Am J Trop Med Hyg 37:40S-59S.
39. Monath, T.P., M.S. Sabattini, R. Pauli, J.F. Daffner, C.J. Mitchell, G.S. Bowen, and C.B. Cropp. 1985. Arbovirus investigations in Argentina 1977-1980. 4. Serological survey and sentinel equine program. Am J Trop Med Hyg 34:966-975.
40. Morris, C.D., M.E. Corey, D.E. Emord, and J.J. Howard. 1980. Epizootiology of Eastern equine encephalomyelitis virus in upstate New York, USA. 1. Introduction, demography, and natural environment of an endemic focus. J Med Entomol 17:442-452.
41. Morris, C.D., R.H. Zimmerman, and J.D. Edman. 1980. Epizootiology of Eastern equine encephalomyelitis virus in upstate New York, USA. 2. Population dynamics and vector potential of adult Culiseta melanura (Diptera:Culicidae) in relation to distance from breeding site. J Med Entomol 17:453-465.
42. Murphy, F.A. 1985. Virus taxonomy. In B.N. Fields (ed.), Virology, pp. 7-27. Raven Press, New York.
43. Nir, Y. 1972. Some characteristics of Israel turkey virus. Arch ges Virusforsch 36:105-114.
44. Oprandy, J.J., J.G. Olson, and T.W. Scott. 1988. A rapid dot immunoassay for the detection of serum antibody to Eastern equine encephalomyelitis and St. Louis encephalitis viruses in sentinel chickens. Am J Trop Med Hyg 38:181-186.
45. Peleg, B.A. 1963. A small-scale serological survey of Israel turkey meningo-encephalitis. Refu Vet 20:253-250.
46. Porterfield, J.S. 1961. Israel turkey meningo-encephalitis virus. Vet Rec 73:392-393.
47. Porterfield, J.S. 1989. Bunyaviridae infecting birds. In J.B. McFerren (ed.), Viral Infections of Vertebrates, Vol. 3. Elsevier, Amsterdam. (In press).
48. Quillien, M.C., J.Y. Monnat, G. Le Lay, F. Le Goff, E. Hardy, and C. Chastel. 1986. Avalon virus, Sakhalin group (Nairovirus, Bunyaviridae) from the seabird tick Ixodes (Ceratixodes) Uriae White 1852 in France. Acta Virol 30:418-427.
49. Rosen, L. 1987. Overwintering mechanisms of mosquito-borne arboviruses in temperate climates. Am J Trop Med Hyg 37:69S-75S.
50. Samberg, Y., M. Ianconescu, and K. Hornstein. 1972. Epizootiological aspects of turkey meningo-encephalitis. Refu Vet 29:103-110.
51. Scott, T.W., and J.G. Olson. 1986. Detection of Eastern equine encephalomyelitis viral antigen in avian blood by enzyme immunoassay: A laboratory study. Am J Trop Med Hyg 35:611-618.
52. Scott, T.W., S.W. Hildreth, and B.J. Beaty. 1984. The distribution and the development of Eastern equine encephalitis virus in its enzootic mosquito vector: Culiseta melanura. Am J Trop Med Hyg 33:300-310.
53. Scott, T.W., J.G. Olson, T.E. Lewis, J.W. Carpenter, L.H. Lorenz, L.A. Lembeck, S.R. Joseph, and B.B. Pagac. 1987. A prospective field evaluation of an enzyme immunoassay: Detection of Eastern equine encephalomyelitis virus antigen in pools of Culiseta melanura. J Am Mosq Control Assoc 3:412-417.
54. Shope, R.E. 1985. Alphaviruses. In B.N. Fields (ed.), Virology, pp. 931-953. Raven Press, New York.
55. Shope, R.E., and G.E. Sather. 1979. Arboviruses. In E.H. Lenette and N.J. Schmidt (eds.), Diagnostic Procedures for Viral, Rickettsial and Chlamydial Infections, pp. 767-814. Am Pub Health Assoc, Washington, DC.
56. Srihongse, S., M.A. Grayson, C.D. Morris, R. Deibel, and C.S. Duncan. 1978. Eastern equine encephalomyelitis in upstate New York: Studies of a 1976 epizootic by a modified serologic technique, hemagglutination reduction, for rapid detection of virus infections. Am J Trop Med Hyg 27:1240-1245.
57. Tidwell, M.A., D.M. Forsythe, M.A. Tidwell, R.L. Parker, and A.J. Main. 1984. Eastern equine encephalomyelitis virus activity in South Carolina. J Agric Entomol 1:43-52.
58. Walder, R., O.M. Suarez, and C.H. Calisher. 1984. Arbovirus studies in the Guajira region of Venezuela: Activities of Eastern equine encephalitis and Venezuelan equine encephalitis viruses during an interepizootic period. Am J Trop Med Hyg 33:699-707.
59. Wallis, R.C., and A.J. Main. 1974. Eastern equine encephalitis in Connecticut, progress and problems. Mem Conn Entomol Soc, pp. 117-144.
60. Wallis, R.C., J.J. Howard, A.J. Main, C. Frazier, and C. Hayes. 1974. With an epizootic of Eastern equine encephalitis in Connecticut. Mosq News 34:63-65.
61. Williams, J.E., O.P. Young, D.M. Watts, and T.J. Reed. 1971. Wild birds as Eastern equine encephalomyelitis and Western equine encephalomyelitis sentinels. J Wildl Dis 7:188-194.
62. Wong, F.C., and J.L. Neufeld. 1982. Sentinel flock monitoring procedure for Western equine encephalomyelitis in Manitoba. In L. Sekla (ed.), Western Equine Encephalomyelitis in Manitoba, pp. 86-97. Manitoba Dep Health, Winnepeg.

INFECTIOUS NEPHRITIS

T. Imada and H. Kawamura

INTRODUCTION. Infectious nephritis, caused by a newly recognized picornavirus (enterovirus), is an acute, highly contagious, typically subclinical disease of young chickens that produces lesions in the kidneys.

The causative agent, avian nephritis virus (ANV), was isolated in chicken kidney cell (CKC) cultures from the rectal contents of apparently normal, 1-wk-old broiler chickens in Japan in 1976 (12). It has been shown to be a picornavirus, which is distinct from avian encephalomyelitis virus and duck hepatitis virus, based on pathological (2, 7) and immunological (1, 8, 12) criteria. The pathogenicity of this virus was established by experimental infection of chickens and chicken embryos (2, 4, 5–7). As there have been few reports on the disease associated with this virus infection in the field, the economic importance is not well known, and public health significance is not known.

INCIDENCE AND DISTRIBUTION. The true incidence and distribution of the disease are not well known owing to the transient, usually subclinical nature of the infection and difficulties with virus isolation. Runting and diarrhea in chickens associated with an enteroviruslike particle serologically identical to ANV, but different biologically, have been reported in Northern Ireland (8–10). ANV has been shown to be widely distributed in chicken flocks in Japan (3), Northern Ireland, and some European specific-pathogen-free (SPF) flocks (1). Antibody to ANV has been also detected in turkeys in Northern Ireland (1).

ETIOLOGY

Classification and Morphology. ANV has been tentatively classified as a picornavirus based on the following properties: 1) the presence of RNA; 2) replication in the cytoplasm (Fig. 29.3); 3) 28 nm in diameter; 4) resistance to ethyl ether, chloroform, trypsin, and acid (pH 3.0); 5) relative heat lability; 6) partial stabilization at 50 C by molar magnesium chloride (12). The density in cesium chloride (CsCl) of the intact particles was not estimated because the virus is very unstable in a strong solution of CsCl. When the density is defined, the virus will probably be classified as an enterovirus belonging to the family Picornaviridae. ANV grew in CKC with round-cell type cytopathic effect (CPE) and maximum virus titers at 24 hr postinoculation (PI) (12). It did not grow in duck embryo fibroblasts, duck embryo kidney cells, or some established mammalian cell lines (HeLa, Vero, MDBK, PK-15, and MDCK).

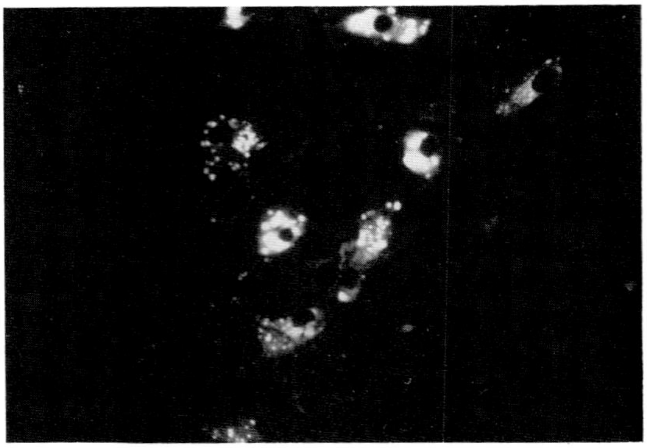

29.3. Fluorescent antigens in chicken kidney cells infected with ANV. Lumpy and granular antigens are seen in the cytoplasm. ×300.

Pathogenicity

CHICKENS. Following intraperitoneal inoculation with ANV, no clinical signs were seen in 1-day-old chicks, but there was growth retardation. Virus was widely distributed, with maximum titers in the kidney and jejunum and lower titers in the bursa of Fabricius, spleen, and liver (2). There were focal lesions in the kidney cortex (7). Imada et al. (4) showed that chickens could be infected by a variety of routes. Oral inoculation was the best, producing gross lesions in the kidney, characterized microscopically as nephritis. Only birds infected at 1 and 14 days of age developed gross lesions; 28-day-old birds developed only microscopic lesions of nephritis. At 58 and 300 days of age, all inoculated birds became infected. The chick infective dose–50% (CID_{50}) of the virus was calculated to be between 100.9 and 101.7 plaque-forming units (4). ANV had no apparent effect on egg production or egg quality in laying hens (6).

CHICKEN EMBRYOS. When inoculated with ANV, 6-day-old embryos died 3–14 days PI. They manifested hemorrhage and edema of the whole body (3–6 days PI) and stunting (7–14 days PI). When inoculated by the chorioallantoic membrane (CAM) route, high virus doses killed all embryos, but low virus doses allowed some infected embryos to hatch normally. In these eggs the CAM showed edematous thickening at the inoculation site, and the embryos were stunted. Embryos inoculated by the allantoic cavity route sometimes became infected, but no virus was detected in allantoic fluids (5).

PATHOGENESIS AND EPIZOOTIOLOGY

Natural and Experimental Hosts. Infection has been recognized in chickens and turkeys. Attempts to establish active infection in other animals have not yet been carried out. Chickens of all ages may be infected, but it has been observed that 1-day-old chicks are the most susceptible. Transmission readily occurs by direct or indirect contact. Egg transmission has been suggested on the basis of field observations (1), and virus can be isolated from chicks hatched from artificially infected embryonating eggs (5). In experimentally infected chicks, the virus was first detected in feces 2 days PI, with maximum virus shedding at 4–5 days PI. Not all infected chicks showed clinical signs but there was variation of growth at 7 days PI, and at necropsy at 7–21 days PI, a mild yellowish discoloration of the kidneys was observed. The virus was consistently isolated from kidney, jejunum, and rectum, but not from brain and trachea during the first 10 days PI. No mortality was observed (2, 4).

Under field conditions, clinical signs associated with this virus infection in broiler chickens have varied from none (subclinical) to outbreaks of the so-called runting syndrome (3, 8, 9, 12). Nothing is known about clinical signs in turkeys.

Histopathology. Histopathological lesions in the kidneys of experimentally infected chickens have been studied (4–7). The primary changes consisted of degeneration of epithelial cells of the proximal convoluted tubules with infiltration of granulocytes. The degenerating epithelial cells had acidophilic granules of various sizes in the cytoplasm (Fig. 29.4). Also, there was interstitial lymphocyte infiltration and moderate fibrosis. In later stages, at 21–28 days PI, lymphoid follicles developed. ANV particles and viral antigens were demonstrated by electron microscopy in the degenerating epithelium (Fig. 29.5) and immunofluorescence (IF) (Fig. 29.6), respectively. Specific viral antigens were recognized by IF also in the jejunum, but distinct microscopic lesions were not observed in the small intestine.

DIAGNOSIS

Isolation and Identification of Causative Agent. For isolation of the virus from infected chickens, suspensions of either the kidneys or the rectal contents made in cell culture medium can be used as inoculum. After freezing and thawing three times, and centrifuging to remove the large tissue particles, the supernatant fluid is inoculated onto monolayers of CKCs or injected by the yolk sac route into 6-day-old embryonating eggs that originated from a SPF flock. In infected CKC cultures, round cell–type CPE, without inclusion bodies or hemagglutinin, develops within 72 hr

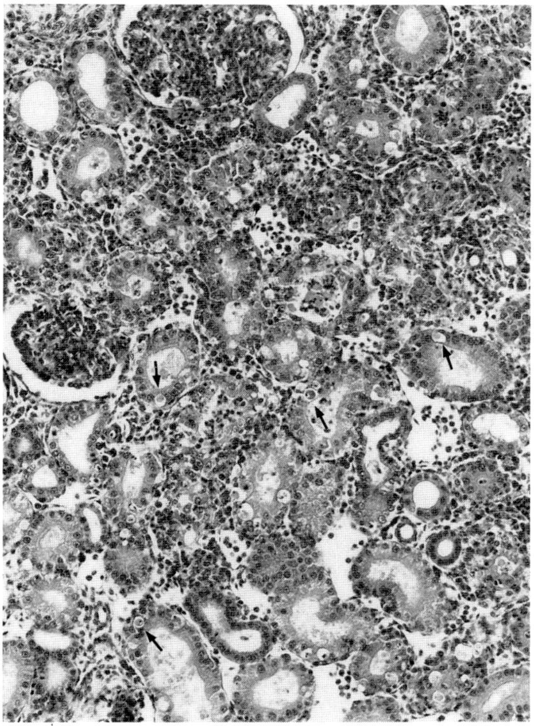

29.4. Degenerated proximal convoluted tubules containing acidophilic granules (*arrows*) in epithelial cell cytoplasm, and lymphocytic infiltration in interstitium, 5 days postinfection. H & E, ×300.

PI. There may be difficulties associated with isolation of enteric viruses in cell cultures (see Chapter 26, ROTOVIRUS INFECTIONS, DIAGNOSIS).

In embryonating eggs, infected embryos display hemorrhage and edema of the whole body, or stunting. Virus isolates may be further characterized by filtration through 50-nm-porosity membrane filters, or by inoculation of 1-day-old chicks with a 50% suspension of tissues harvested from embryos, followed by examination for lesions in the kidneys 3–7 days PI.

The IF technique is a useful diagnostic procedure. Viral antigens can be detected in the early acute phase of the disease by staining infected kidneys with specific anti-ANV fluorescent antibodies. This technique can also be used to detect viral antigens in cell cultures and embryos. In CKC infected with ANV, lumpy and granular antigens are seen in the cytoplasm as early as 12 hr PI.

Serology. Chickens recovered from natural and experimental infections manifest an immunological response that can be measured with a conventional virus-neutralization test or the indirect IF test.

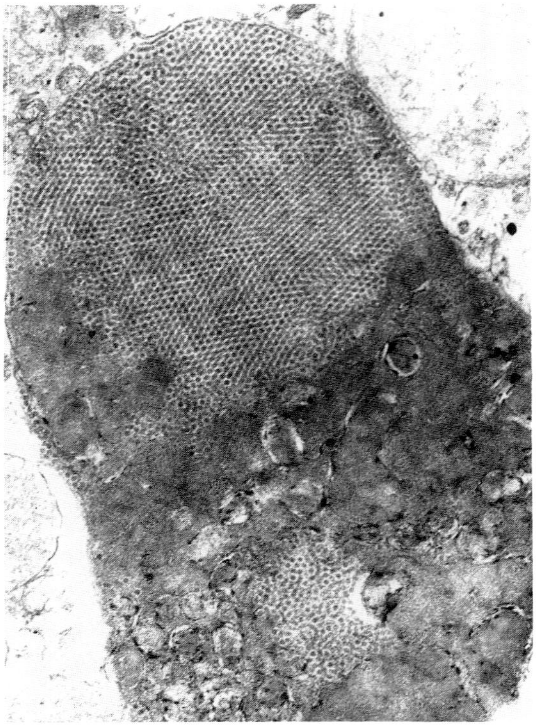

29.5. Crystalline array of virus particles in the cytoplasm of a kidney epithelial cell, 3 days postinfection. ×30,000.

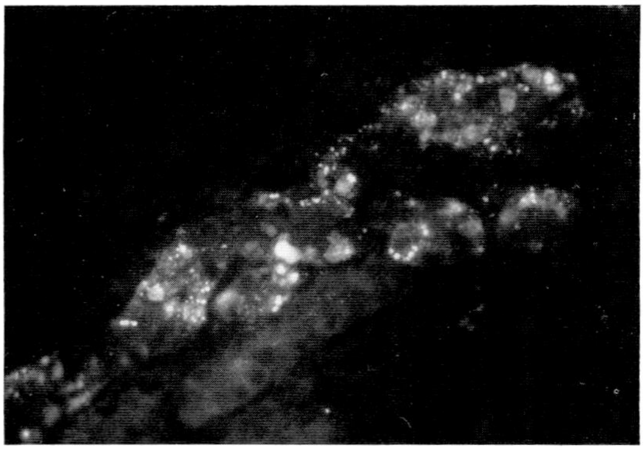

29.6. Immunofluorescent staining of ANV antigens in the epithelium of renal tubules, 3 days postinfection. ×200.

Differential Diagnosis. Certain nephrotoxic strains of infectious bronchitis virus (IBV) cause interstitial nephritis. It would be difficult to separate the two conditions on the basis of the histological lesions (11). These cases may be differentiated from ANV infections by the fact that with infectious bronchitis there are some changes in the trachea, and infections in kidneys are usually preceded by respiratory signs. When a nephritis is noticed in especially young chickens, it is necessary to isolate the causative agent or conduct seriological tests. The possibility that the two diseases may occur simultaneously in a flock should not be overlooked.

TREATMENT, PREVENTION, CONTROL.

There is no specific treatment. Additional knowledge is needed to formulate measures for prophylaxis and control.

REFERENCES

1. Connor, T.J., F. McNeilly, J.B. McFerran, and M.S. McNulty. 1987. A survey of avian sera from Northern Ireland for antibody to avian nephritis virus. Avian Pathol 16:15–20.
2. Imada, T., S. Yamaguchi, and H. Kawamura. 1979. Pathogenicity for baby chicks of the G-4260 strain of the picornavirus "avian nephritis virus." Avian Dis 23:582–588.
3. Imada, T., S. Yamaguchi, and H. Kawamura. 1980. Antibody survey against avian nephritis virus among chickens in Japan. Nat Inst Anim Health Q (Japan) 20:79–80.
4. Imada, T., T. Taniguchi, T. Minetoma, M. Maeda, and H. Kawamura. 1981. Susceptibility of chickens to avian nephritis virus at various inoculation routes and ages. Avian Dis 25:294–302.
5. Imada, T., T. Taniguchi, S. Sato, S. Yamaguchi, and H. Kawamura. 1982. Pathogenicity of avian nephritis virus for embryonating hen's eggs. Nat Inst Anim Health Q (Japan) 22:8–15.
6. Imada, T., M. Maeda, K. Furuta, S. Yamaguchi, and H. Kawamura. 1983. Pathogenicity and distribution of avian nephritis virus (G-4260 strain) in inoculated laying hens. Nat Inst Anim Health Q (Japan) 23:43–48.
7. Maeda, M., T. Imada, T. Taniguchi, and T. Horiuchi. 1979. Pathological changes in chicks inoculated with the picornavirus "avian nephritis virus." Avian Dis 23:589–596.
8. McFerran, J.B., and M.S. McNulty. 1986. Recent advances in enterovirus infections of birds. In J.B. McFerran and M.S. McNulty (eds.), Acute Virus Infections of Poultry, pp. 195–202. Martinus Nijhoff, Dordrecht, Neth.
9. McNulty, M.S., G.M. Allan, T.J. Connor, J.B. McFerran, and R.M. McCracken. 1984. An entero-like virus associated with the runting syndrome in broiler chickens. Avian Pathol 13:429–439.
10. McNulty, M.S., G.M. Allan, and J.B. McFerran. 1987. Isolation of a novel avian entero-like virus. Avian Pathol 16:331–337.
11. Siller, W.G. 1981. Renal pathology of the fowl—a review. Avian Pathol 10:187–262.
12. Yamaguchi, S., T. Imada, and H. Kawamura. 1979. Characterization of a picornavirus isolated from broiler chicks. Avian Dis 23:571–581.

PARVOVIRUS INFECTION OF CHICKENS

Janos Kisary

INTRODUCTION. Although the causative agent of the condition variously known as "stunting-runting syndrome," "helicopter disease," or "chicken anemia" has not been definitively identified, a parvovirus isolated from the intestinal tracts of stunted broilers has induced these manifestations in broiler chickens under experimental conditions.

HISTORY. The first hint of the existence of a self-replicating, autonomous fowl parvovirus was reported in 1977 (9). Small viral particles of 18–22 nm in diameter were seen within intranuclear inclusions in myocardial cells of white leghorn chickens, which died due to a nonsuppurative myocarditis. Later, a condition was observed in Japan (10) that was characterized by a significant decrease in the number of erythrocytes accompanied with low hematocrit values and atrophy of the femoral bone marrow. These changes were attributed to infection by a small virus with several properties typical of parvoviruses. Further studies (1) confirmed the possible role of parvoviruses, but no decisive biochemical characteristics were published that would allow taxonomic classification.

In 1984 Kisary et al. (6) reported the presence of parvoviruslike particles in intestinal homogenates from stunted broiler chickens. Subsequent molecular-biological studies (7) proved that the newly identified virus was, indeed, a parvovirus.

INCIDENCE AND DISTRIBUTION. The fowl parvovirus has been demonstrated in intestinal tracts, and specific virus-neutralizing antibodies have been detected in sera of broiler chickens in Hungary, Belgium, and the Netherlands (5).

ETIOLOGY. The chicken parvovirus belongs to the genus *Parvovirus* (self-replicating parvoviruses) of the family Parvoviridae (7). Viral particles are 19–25 nm in diameter and hexagonal. They band in cesium chloride (CsCl) at a density range of 1.42–1.44 g/ml (6, 7). The sedimentation (S) value of the infectious particles is 110 (5). The genome contains single-stranded DNA of one polarity, consisting of about 5200 bases (7). It has a palindrome at the 3′end to serve as a natural primer for in vitro conversion into a double-stranded form. No hemagglutination was recorded when the erythrocytes of mouse, rabbit, hamster, guinea pig, chicken, pigeon, dog, sheep, or goat were tested in a temperature range between 4 and 37 C. Infectious particles were resistant to treatment with chloroform or to heating at 65 C for 1 hr (5).

In cross-neutralization tests the virus showed a strong antigenic relationship (or identity) with the chicken anemia agent but not with the goose parvovirus (5).

The virus replicates in the chicken embryo cell line CEC32 (2) and in primary or secondary chicken embryo fibroblast tissue cultures provided the cells are actively dividing at the time of infection (5). The cytopathic effect in both types of cells is characterized by swelling and subsequent shrinking of infected cells. In cells stained by hematoxylin-eosin intranuclear Cowdry type-A inclusion bodies can be seen.

PATHOGENICITY AND EPIZOOTIOLOGY. Under experimental conditions the virus induces clinical signs only in fast-growing broiler chickens infected not older than 7 days of age (3, 5). In white leghorn chickens no, or very mild, signs develop due to the experimental infection (3).

The virus apparently spreads from bird to bird by both horizontal and vertical transmission. The first is presumed because viral particles could be demonstrated in intestinal homogenates from broilers (6). Possible vertical transmission is concluded from the demonstration of fowl parvovirus particles in fibroblast cell cultures prepared from uninoculated chicken embryos (8).

The clinical signs presented herein are based on observations in chickens infected experimentally with a CsCl-purified parvovirus suspension (3, 5). When antibody-free, 3-day-old, fast-growing broiler chickens are infected per os or intraperitoneally, the first clinical signs appear within 3–5 days. The droppings become watery or mucoid and they are mustard yellow in color. Despite a normal or voracious appetite, a proportion of the chickens become seriously retarded in growth. In some of the stunted birds, growth of the juvenile feathers is delayed and, due to an abnormal growth of new feathers, the chickens develop the so-called "helicopter" appearance. Between 10 and 20 days of age a variable number of the most seriously stunted chickens succumb. A temporary leg weakness can also be observed during this same period. The most pronounced weight-gain retardation (average of 40–50%) is observed around 4 wk of age. A relatively high proportion of the infected chickens (about 50–70%) have a marked decrease in the number of erythrocytes between 8 and 20 days of age (5). The average number of red blood cells in affected birds is around 2×10^6/mm^3 compared to 3×10^6/mm^3 in normal birds.

Under experimental conditions the morbidity rate is between 50 and 80% and the mortality is about 5–10%, provided the chickens infected are free from maternal antibodies against parvovirus.

At postmortem examination the most obvious finding is the reduced body size compared to that expected, along with abnormal development of feathers. An extremely white color of the small intestines is the most characteristic feature in internal organs. The cecae are often enormously enlarged and filled with gaseous, foul-smelling contents. The pancreas is frequently shrunken, white, and firm, either along its whole length or only at the apex of the duodenal loop. The femoral bone marrow of chickens with anemia is yellowish or whitish. The metatarsal bones are often more flexible than those of uninfected controls.

Day-old chickens hatched with maternal antibodies against parvovirus are protected against experimental challenge with a high dose of the virus (5).

DIAGNOSIS. Uneven growth of broiler chickens at the flock level can be an indication of parvovirus infection. Virus particles can be relatively easily detected by electron microscopic examination of purified intestinal homogenates (6). Another rapid method for diagnosis is the indirect immunofluorescence assay performed on smears prepared from the duodenal mucosa (4). In positive cases fluorescing antigen can be seen in the nucleus of detatched epithelial villus cells. For the isolation of the parvovirus, subconfluent primary or secondary chicken embryo fibroblast, or CEC32 cell cultures, should be inoculated with a purified intestinal homogenate (5, 6). In all cases the parvovirus should be identified either with specific antiparvoviral serum or with further biochemical studies.

As mentioned in the introductory part of this subchapter, the relationship between the etiology of stunting-runting syndrome and parvovirus infection of broilers is not yet clear. Therefore, to definitively determine whether it is a parvovirus infection or some other unknown etiologic agent that is responsible for the sydrome in question, very thorough laboratory and epizootiological investigations are needed.

PREVENTION AND CONTROL. No specific control methods have been published to date. Based on the observation that chicks are protected by yolk-derived antibodies, a vaccination scheme for the dams seems worthy of consideration. In the absence of other control methods, basic veterinary hygienic measures should be followed.

REFERENCES

1. Goryo, M., T. Suwa, S. Matsumoto, T. Umemura, and C. Itakura. 1987. Serial propagation and purification of chicken anaemia agent in MDCC-MSB1 cell line. Avian Pathol 16:149–163.
2. Kaaden, O.R., S. Lange, and B. Stiburek. 1982. Establishment and characterization of chicken embryo fibroblast clone LSCC-H32. In Vitro 18:827–834.
3. Kisary, J. 1985. Experimental infection of chicken embryos and day-old chickens with parvovirus of chicken origin. Avian Pathol 14:1–7.
4. Kisary, J. 1985. Indirect immunofluorescence as a diagnostic tool for parvovirus infection of chickens. Avian Pathol 14:269–273.
5. Kisary, J. 1988. Unpublished data.
6. Kisary, J., B. Nagy, and Z. Bitay. 1984. Presence of parvoviruses in the intestine of chickens showing stunting syndrome. Avian Pathol 13:339–343.
7. Kisary, J., B. Avalosse, A. Miller-Faures, and J. Rommelaere. 1985. The genome structure of a new chicken virus identifies it as a parvovirus. J Gen Virol 66:2259–2263.
8. Kisary, J., A. Miller-Faures, and J. Rommelaere. 1987. Presence of fowl parvovirus in fibroblast cell cultures prepared from uninoculated White Leghorn chicken embryos. Avian Pathol 16:115–121.
9. Parker, G.A., M.A. Stedham, and A. Van Dellen. 1977. Myocarditis of probable viral origin in chickens. Avian Dis 21:123–132.
10. Yuasa, M., T. Taniguchi, and Yoshida. 1979. Isolation and some characteristics of an agent inducing anemia in chicks. Avian Dis 23:366–385.

GOOSE PARVOVIRUS INFECTION

R.E. Gough

INTRODUCTION. Goose parvovirus infection, variously known as Derzsy's disease, so-called goose influenza, goose or gosling plague, goose hepatitis, goose enteritis, infectious myocarditis, and ascitic hepatonephritis, is a highly contagious disease affecting young geese and Muscovy ducks (*Cairina moschata*). The diverse names given to the condition reflect the multiple pathological features of the disease. Depending on the age of affected goslings the disease may be present in either acute, subacute, or chronic forms (6, 48, 53). The acute form of the disease can result in 100% mortality in goslings under 10 days of age. Apart from geese and Muscovy ducks, the disease has not been reported in other avian species or mammals, including humans.

HISTORY. The first detailed description of a serious disease of goslings, which occurred in China in 1956 and was later shown to be caused by a parvovirus, was reported by Fang and Wang in 1981 (16) and later confirmed by Zheng et al. (62). During the 1960s a similar disease was reported from many European countries, including Poland (58), W. Germany (39), Hungary (36), Bulgaria (1), Holland (57), France, USSR, and Czechoslovakia (10). Initially, many authors referred to the disease as "goose influenza," which caused some confusion as this name had originally been used for a disease of geese thought to be caused by a hemophilic bacterium (10). To distinguish the two diseases it was suggested that the "new" disease be known as "so-called goose influenza" (12). During the following years the disease was reported from all the major goose-farming countries of Europe and a variety of names were given to the condition.

Although several viruses had been implicated, it was not until 1971 that Schettler (55) confirmed that the disease was caused by a parvovirus. In 1978 it was recommended that the disease be called goose parvovirus (11).

INCIDENCE AND DISTRIBUTION. Goose parvovirus has been reported from all the major goose-farming countries of Europe, including the USSR and Israel. The disease has also been reported from the Peoples' Republic of China, several of its autonomous regions, Taiwan, and Vietnam. A disease with similar clinical and postmortem features has also been reported from Canada (50), although parvoviruses were not isolated. In countries such as France and W. Germany, where Muscovy ducks are farmed intensively, the disease is a serious problem.

ETIOLOGY. During the past 20 yr several etiological agents have been proposed for the disease. Some early reports attributed the disease to reoviruses (8, 13, 39). It was suggested that adenoviruses were the etiological agents as they were frequently isolated or detected from outbreaks of disease in goslings (7, 26, 49). However, in subsequent, more detailed, studies it has been confirmed that the etiological agent is a parvovirus (6, 9, 21, 34, 37, 55).

Classification. The virus is a member of the family Parvoviridae. No antigenic relationships with other parvoviruses have been demonstrated (32, 45).

Morphology. Intact virions are unenveloped and hexagonal in shape (Fig. 29.7A) with an estimated 32 capsomeres and a diameter of 20–22 nm (9, 21, 34, 55). The density of the virus in cesium chloride is approximately 1.38 g/ml (29).

Chemical Composition. Goose parvovirus, like its mammalian counterparts, has a single-stranded DNA genome (34, 55). No information is available on the structural polypeptide composition of goose parvovirus. Unlike several mammalian parvoviruses, hemagglutination activity, using a variety of red blood cells under different conditions, has not been demonstrated with goose parvovirus (55).

Virus Replication. The replication of goose parvovirus has not been investigated in detail although in vitro studies by Kisary and Derzsy (34) have shown that viral replication takes place in the nucleus; electron microscopy studies by Bergmann (2) have demonstrated the presence of large aggregates of parvovirus in the nuclei of cells from the hearts and bursae of infected goslings. Like other parvoviruses that are able to replicate without the presence of a helper virus, goose parvovirus is dependent on cells actively synthesizing DNA for its replication cycle (31).

Resistance to Chemical and Physical Agents. Goose parvovirus is very resistant to chemical and physical inactivation. Gough et al. (21) reported no loss of titer when the virus was heated at 65 C for 30 min. These authors also found that the virus was stable at pH 3.0 for 1 hr at 37 C. Schettler (55) tested an isolate against a variety of chemicals under different conditions and detected no significant loss of activity.

Strain Classification. The results of early studies using cross-neutralization and gosling-protection tests suggested that several serologically distinct strains of the virus existed (14). However, at the time of these studies the etiology of the disease had not been confirmed; later work showed that several of the virus strains used were contaminated with reoviruses (15). Subsequent studies have shown that all the goose parvoviruses tested are antigenically closely related (18, 22, 28).

Laboratory Host Systems. Goose parvovirus has only been isolated in embryonated goose or Muscovy duck eggs or primary cell cultures prepared from the embryos.

PATHOGENESIS AND EPIZOOTIOLOGY

Natural and Experimental Hosts. Geese and Muscovy ducks are the only species in which natural clinical disease has been observed. All breeds of domestic geese are susceptible and the disease has also been reported to occur in Canada geese

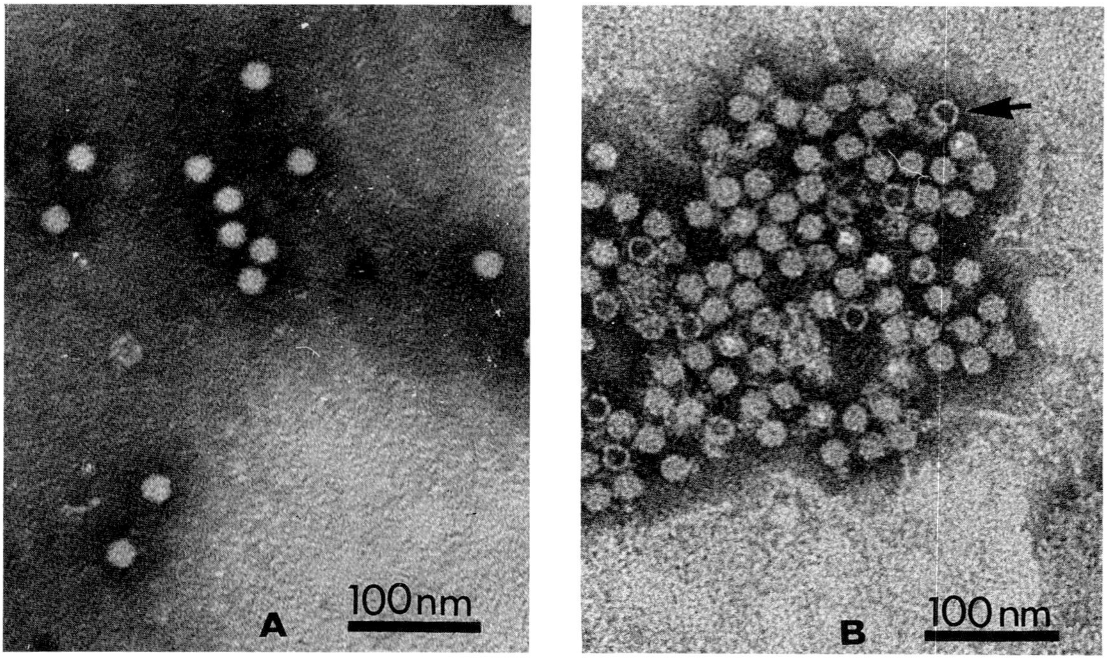

29.7. Electron micrographs of purified goose parvovirus. A. Purified virions. B. Virions in the feces of a naturally infected 10-day-old gosling, showing intact and hollow (*arrow*) particles.

(*Branta canadensis*) and snow geese (*Chen hypoborea atlantica*) following accidental infection (54). Other breeds of domestic poultry and ducks appear refractory to experimental infection (21, 25).

AGE OF HOST COMMONLY AFFECTED. The disease is strictly age dependent; thus, 100% mortality may occur in goslings under 1 wk of age, with negligible losses occurring in 4- to 5-wk-old birds. However, while older geese do not show clinical signs of infection, they respond immunologically (12, 18, 30). Similar findings apply to the clinical disease in Muscovy ducks (25, 38, 64).

Transmission, Carriers, Vectors. Infected birds excrete large amounts of virus in their feces resulting in a rapid spread of infection by direct and indirect contact. The most serious outbreaks occur in susceptible goslings following vertical transmission of the virus. In older geese that become subclinically infected, a latent infection may become established. These birds may then act as carriers of the disease and transmit the virus through their eggs to susceptible goslings in the hatchery (10, 33). No biological vectors have been identified.

Incubation Period, Signs, Morbidity, Mortality. In susceptible goslings the incubation period is age dependent. Experimental infection of day-old goslings results in the appearance of clinical signs 3–5 days later. In 2- to 3-wk-old birds the incubation period may vary between 5 and 10 days (33, 53).

The clinical signs; morbidity, and mortality in susceptible goslings also vary according to the age of the birds. In goslings under 1 wk of age the course of the disease may be very rapid with anorexia, prostration, and death occurring within 2–5 days. In older birds, or those with variable levels of maternally derived antibody, the disease follows a more protracted course with the appearance of characteristic clinical signs. Initially, affected birds exhibit anorexia, polydipsia, and weakness with a reluctance to move. There is a nasal and ocular discharge in many birds with associated headshaking. The uropygial glands and eyelids are often red and swollen, and a profuse white diarrhea is evident in many of the birds. Examination of the birds at this stage may reveal a fibrinous pseudomembrane covering the tongue and oral cavity. Goslings that survive the acute phase may develop a more prolonged disease characterized by profound growth retardation, loss of down around the back and neck, and marked reddening of the exposed skin. There may be an accumulation of ascitic fluid in the abdomen, which causes the goslings to stand in a "penguinlike" posture.

Mortality sometimes reaches 100% in goslings

infected in the hatchers. In 2- to 3-wk-old goslings mortality levels may be below 10% although morbidity levels may be high. Complicating factors such as poor management and secondary bacterial, fungal, or viral infections may influence the final mortality levels (33, 38). Goslings over 4 wk of age rarely show clinical signs although a "late form" of the disease has been described in goslings 1–3 mo of age (6). Geese of all ages respond immunologically to goose parvovirus infection without necessarily showing clinical signs (30).

Gross Lesions. In acute cases with a short clinical course, lesions are commonly found in the heart, which has a pale myocardium characteristically rounded at its apex (Fig. 29.8). The liver, spleen, and pancreas may be swollen and congested (10). A variety of other gross lesions may also be present in cases with a more prolonged clinical course. Typically, a sero-fibrinous perihepatitis and pericarditis is present with large volumes of straw-colored fluid in the abdominal cavity. Pulmonary edema, liver dystrophy, and catarrhal enteritis may also be present. Less frequently, hemorrhages in the thigh and pectoral muscles may be seen. Diphtheritic and ulcerative lesions may be observed in the mouth, pharynx, and esophagus, depending on the presence of secondary invaders.

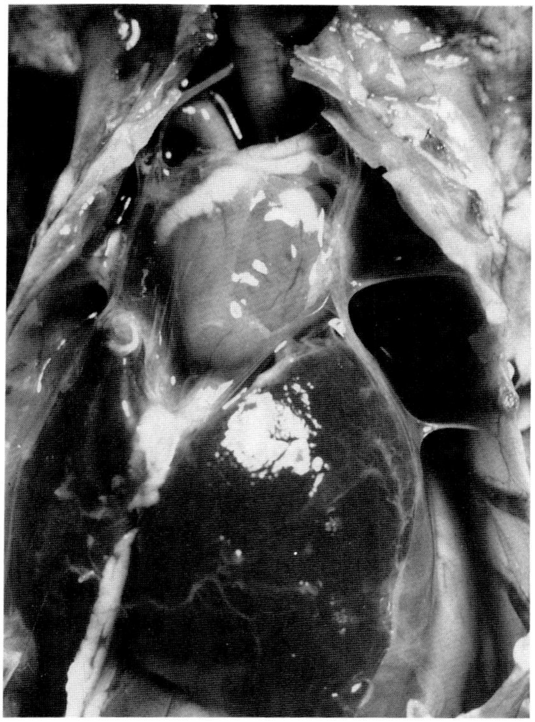

29.8. Postmortem appearance of a 12-day-old gosling infected with goose parvovirus showing hydropericardium and ascites. The liver is coated with a fibrinous membrane.

Histopathology. Detailed histopathology studies of goose parvovirus infection by a number of workers have produced similar findings (5, 44, 46, 47). The main lesions reported were pronounced degenerative changes in myocardial cells with associated loss of striation, fatty infiltration, and the presence of scattered Cowdrey type-A intranuclear inclusions. Similar histological changes were also found in intestinal and smooth muscle cells. In the liver the predominant lesions were degeneration of hepatocytes with vacuolation and fatty infiltration (Fig. 29.9). Small, eosinophilic inclusionlike bodies were sometimes seen in the cytoplasm of the vacuolated hepatocytes. Changes in the pancreas consisted of shrunken, necrotic acinar cells with fatty infiltration. Some lymphoblastic processes were occasionally observed in the spleen, bursa of Fabricius, and thymus, together with marked vacuolation of the kidneys.

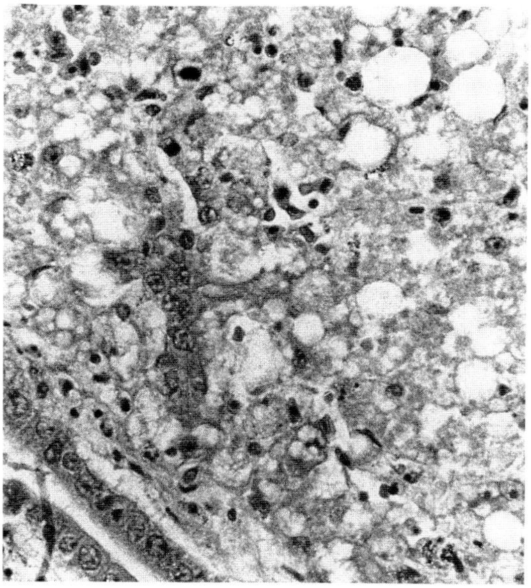

29.9. Liver section from a 10-day-old gosling infected with goose parvovirus showing widespread vacuolation and degeneration of hepatocytes.

Immunity. Adult breeding geese that have been naturally infected with parvovirus, either as goslings or adults, transfer maternal antibody via the egg yolk to their progeny (13, 19, 25). This passively acquired antibody may persist at a relatively high level until about 2 wk of age (30). The primary humoral response of geese to parvovirus infection is characterized by the initial production of IgM- and then IgG-type immunoglobulins (30).

Using virus-neutralization (VN) and agar-gel precipitin tests to measure parvovirus antibodies in the sera of geese that had survived the disease, high and persistent levels of antibody were detected for up to 80 mo after infection. The progeny of these geese were also found to be fully resistant to experimental challenge up to 4 wk of age (19). The results of studies by Kisary (30) suggested that goslings are not fully immunocompetent until 20 days of age.

DIAGNOSIS

Isolation and Identification of the Causative Agent. Goose parvovirus can be isolated from a variety of suitable postmortem specimens following inoculation of 10- to 15-day-old embryonated goose or Muscovy duck eggs via the allantoic cavity. Embryo mortality occurs 5–10 days post inoculation with hemorrhages and ochre-colored livers. The virus can also be isolated in primary cell cultures of goose or Muscovy duck embryos. Isolation of the virus is facilitated by inoculating cultures before they reach confluency (34). The virus produces a well-defined cytopathic effect 3–5 days postinfection. In hemotoxylin-eosin-stained preparations, Cowdrey type-A intranuclear inclusions and syncytium formation are often present (34, 56). The presence of the virus can be confirmed by electron microscopic examination of infected cell cultures or neutralization with specific goose parvovirus antiserum. Immunofluorescence has also been used to detect the presence of antigen in both goose embryos (59) and infected cell cultures (55). Other methods of detecting goose parvovirus have been developed, including the immunoperoxidase technique (51) and reverse indirect hemagglutination test (60).

An agar-gel diffusion technique has been described using hyperimmune rabbit antigoose parvovirus serum to precipitate parvovirus in allantoic fluid from infected goose embryos (3). Aggregates of goose parvovirus virions have also been detected by electron microscopy examination of ultrathin sections of heart and bursa of Fabricius from infected goslings (2), and in concentrated extracts of feces from goslings showing clinical signs of goose parvovirus (Fig. 29.7B) (17).

Serology. Confirmation of goose parvovirus infection can be obtained by serological means. The most commonly used method is the VN test in embryonated goose or Muscovy duck eggs or primary cell cultures to detect the presence of goose parvovirus–neutralizing antibodies. A VN test has also been developed for use in Khaki Campbell or Pekin duck eggs using a duck embryo–adapted goose parvovirus (20). Though less sensitive than the VN test, the agar-gel diffusion test is a useful method of rapidly testing large numbers of sera for the presence of goose parvovirus antibodies (18, 42). Other serological techniques developed include the spermagglutination-inhibition test (43) and enzyme-linked immunosorbent assay tests (24, 40).

Differential Diagnosis. Apart from duck herpesvirus enteritis there are no other known viral infections that cause high mortality in young geese or Muscovy ducklings. However, equivocal results can arise when viruses other than parvovirus are isolated, particularly reoviruses and adenoviruses. In such cases it may be necessary to carry out serological tests in order to confirm the diagnosis.

TREATMENT, PREVENTION, CONTROL. There is no specific treatment for goose parvovirus infection. Antibiotic therapy has been used to reduce losses from secondary bacterial or fungal infections (12).

Because many outbreaks of goose parvovirus are directly attributed to transmission of the disease by congenitally infected goslings during hatching, the practice of incubating and hatching eggs that have originated from different breeding flocks should be discouraged. Only eggs from known parvovirus-free flocks should be incubated together and good hatchery hygiene should be maintained.

On farms where outbreaks of the disease have occurred, the practice of breeding from geese that have survived the disease as goslings should also be discouraged, as these birds are potential carriers of the virus. All contact geese, whether goslings or adults, should be serologically tested in order to identify which birds have been infected horizontally. Positive reactors should be removed from the flock, as these birds may also become carriers of the virus.

Because the disease is confined to young geese or Muscovy ducklings, control measures have been developed to provide adequate immunity during the first 4–5 wk of life. Some of the early outbreaks of goose parvovirus occurring in China in 1962 were controlled by the use of hyperimmune serum in newly hatched goslings (16). Serum therapy was widely used when the disease subsequently appeared in Europe, using serum produced in hyperimmunized geese (10, 23, 25, 52). However, passive immunization was found to be expensive and time consuming, particularly as two doses of serum were often required to produce adequate immunity (35). Active immunization of adult breeding geese and Muscovy ducks with virulent virus has also been reported (25). The results showed that good protection against goose parvovirus was transferred to the progeny via the egg yolk.

One of the first vaccines against the disease

was developed in China, and during the period 1962–79 about four million female geese were vaccinated (16). The virus was attenuated following multiple passage in embryonated goose eggs and good protection to challenge was recorded in the progeny goslings. Other vaccines have been developed by attenuation of the virus in goose or Muscovy duck embryo cell cultures, for use in breeding geese and goslings (27, 35, 41, 61, 63). Duck embryo-adapted goose parvovirus vaccines have also been shown to induce a good immune response in goslings and breeder geese (4, 20).

In flocks of geese where parvovirus has not been diagnosed, inactivated vaccines have been used (33, 48).

REFERENCES

1. Angelacev, A. 1966. Exudative septicaemia of geese (goose influenza). Vet Sb 63:912.

2. Bergmann, V. 1987. Pathology and electron microscopical detection of virus in the tissues of goslings with Derzsy's disease (parvovirus infection). Arch Exp Vet Med 41:212–221.

3. Bondarenko, A.F. 1982. Improved diagnosis of parvoviral enteritis in geese (immunodiffusion test). Vet Moscow 11:68–69.

4. Chen, B.L., B.H. Ye, and J.H. Li. 1985. Duck embryo adapted vaccine for gosling plague. Acta Vet Zootech Sin 16:269–275.

5. Coudert, M., M. Fedida, G. Dannacher, M. Peillon, R. Labatut, and P. Ferlin. 1972. Viral disease of gosling. Recl Med Vet 148:455–471.

6. Coudert, M., M. Fedida, G. Dannacher, and M. Peillon. 1974. Parvovirus disease of goslings. Late form. Recl Med Vet 150:899–906.

7. Csontos, L. 1967. Isolation of an adenovirus from geese. Acta Vet Hung 17:217–219.

8. Dannacher, G., M. Coudert, M. Fedida, M. Peillon, and X. Fouillet. 1972. Etiology of the virus disease of geese. Recl Med Vet 148:1333–1349.

9. Dannacher, G., X. Fouillet, M. Coudert, M. Fedida, and M. Peillon. 1974. Etiology of the virus disease of geese: The beta virus. Recl Med Vet 150:49–58.

10. Derzsy, D. 1967. A viral disease of goslings. Acta Vet Hung 17:443–448.

11. Derzsy, D. 1978. A viral disease of goslings. In H. Rohrer (ed.), Handbuch der Virusinfektionen bei Tieren VI/2, pp. 919–949. VEB Gustav Fischer Verlag, Jena, E Ger.

12. Derzsy, D., and J. Meszaros. 1969. Epidemiological problems of the so-called goose influenza and the possibilities of protection. Magy Allatorv Lapja 10:1–11.

13. Derzsy, D., I. Szep, and F. Szoke. 1966. Investigation on the etiology of the so-called goose influenza. Magy Allatorv Lapja 21:388–389.

14. Derzsy, D., C. Dren, M. Szedo, J. Surjan, B. Toth, and E. Iro. 1970. Viral disease of goslings. III. Isolation, properties and antigenic pattern of the virus strains. Acta Vet Hung 20:419–428.

15. Derzsy, D., J. Kisary, L.M. Kontrimavichus, and G.A. Nadtochey. 1975. Presence of reoviruses in certain goose embryo isolates from outbreaks of viral gosling disease and in chicken embryos. Acta Vet Hung 25:383–391.

16. Fang, D.Y., and Y.K. Wang. 1981. Studies on the etiology and specific control of goose parvovirus infection. Sci Agric Sin 4:1–8.

17. Gough, R.E. 1982. Unpublished data.

18. Gough, R.E. 1984. Application of the agar gel precipitin and virus neutralisation tests to the serological study of goose parvovirus. Avian Pathol 13:501–509.

19. Gough, R.E. 1987. Persistence of parvovirus antibody in geese that have survived Derzsy's disease. Avian Pathol 16:327–330.

20. Gough, R.E., and D. Spackman. 1982. Studies with a duck embryo adapted goose parvovirus vaccine. Avian Pathol 11:503–510.

21. Gough, R.E., D. Spackman, and M.S. Collins. 1981. Isolation and characterisation of a parvovirus from goslings. Vet Rec 108:399–400.

22. Hanh, N.V. 1974. A disease of goslings in Vietnam. Magy Allatorv Lapja 29:262–265.

23. Hansen, H.C. 1980. Derzsy's disease (parvovirus infection in geese). Dansk Vet 63:191–194.

24. Have, P., and H.C. Hansen. 1981. Detection of goose parvovirus antibodies by microneutralisation and enzyme-linked immunosorbent assay. Proc 7th World Vet Poult Assoc, p. 60.

25. Hoekstra, J., T. Smit, and C. van Brakel. 1973. Observations on the host range and control of goose virus hepatitis. Avian Pathol 2:169–178.

26. Kaleta, E.F. 1969. Celo-virus from goslings. Dtsche Tierärztl Wochenschr 76:427–428.

27. Kaleta, E.F. 1985. Immunisation of geese and Muscovy ducks against parvovirus hepatitis (Derzsy's disease). Report of a field trial with the attenuated live vaccine "Palmivax." Dtsche Tierärztl Wochenschr 92:303–305.

28. Kisary, J. 1974. Cross-neutralisation tests on parvoviruses isolated from goslings. Avian Pathol 3:293–296.

29. Kisary, J. 1976. Buoyant density of goose parvovirus strain B. Acta Microbiol Hung 23:205–207.

30. Kisary, J. 1977. Immunological aspects of Derzsy's disease in goslings. Avian Pathol 6:327–334.

31. Kisary, J. 1979. Interaction in replication between the goose parvovirus strain B and duck plague herpesvirus. Arch Virol 59:81–88.

32. Kisary, J. 1985. Indirect immunofluorescence as a diagnostic tool for parvovirus infection of broiler chickens. Avian Pathol 14:269–273.

33. Kisary, J. 1986. Diagnosis and control of parvovirus infection of geese (Derzsy's disease). In J.B. McFerran and M.S. McNulty (eds.), Acute Virus Infections of Poultry, pp. 239–242. Martinus Nijhoff, Dordrecht, Neth.

34. Kisary, J., and D. Derzsy. 1974. Viral disease of goslings. IV. Characterization of the causal agent in tissue culture system. Acta Vet Hung 24:287–292.

35. Kisary, J., D. Derzsy, and J. Meszaros. 1978. Attenuation of the goose parvovirus strain B. Laboratory and field trials of the attenuated mutant for vaccination against Derzsy's disease. Avian Pathol 7:397–406.

36. Kis-Csatari, M. 1965. An outbreak of exudative septicaemia (goose influenza) in goslings. Magy Allatorv Lapja 20:148–151.

37. Kontrimavichus, L.M. 1975. Comparison of strains of virus isolated from goslings with enteritis. Tr Vses Inst Eksp Vet 43:212–224.

38. Kontrimavichus, L.M., V.F. Makogon, and V.V. Navrotskii. 1980. Epidemiological, clinical, and pathological features of goose viral enteritis. Vet Moscow 7:34–35.

39. Krauss, H. 1965. Eine Verlustreiche aufzuchtkrankheit bei gansekuken. Berl Munch Tierärztl Wochenschr 78:372–375.

40. Kwang, M.J., H.J. Tsai, Y.S. Lu, A.C.Y. Fei, Y.L. Lee, D.F. Lin, and C. Lee. 1987. Detection of antibodies against goose parvovirus by an enzyme-linked immunosorbent assay (ELISA). J Chin Soc Vet Sci 13:17–23.

41. Lu, Y.S., Y.L. Lee, D.F. Lin, H.J. Tsai, C. Lee, and T.H. Fuh. 1985. Control of parvoviral enteritis in goslings in Taiwan: The development and field application of immune serum and an attenuated vaccine. Taiwan J Vet Med 46:43-50.
42. Malkinson, M. 1974. Application of the gel diffusion test to the study of the serological response to gosling hepatitis virus. Proc Goose Dis Symp, Doorn, Neth, pp. 47-51.
43. Malkinson, M., B.A. Peleg, N. Ron, and E. Kalmar. 1974. The assay of gosling hepatitis virus and antibody by spermagglutination and spermagglutination-inhibition. II. Spermagglutination-inhibition. Avian Pathol 3:201-209.
44. Mandelli, G., A. Valire, A. Rinaldi, and E. Lodetti. 1971. Histological and ultramicroscopical findings in a viral disease of goslings. Folia Vet Lat 1:121-170.
45. Mengeling, W.L., P.S. Paul, T.O. Bunn, and J.F. Ridpath. 1986. Antigenic relationships among autonomous parvoviruses. J Gen Virol 67:2839-2844.
46. Nadtochei, G.A., and E.V. Petelina. 1985. Ultrastructural changes in the liver and small intestine of geese infected with parvovirus. Tr Vses Inst Eksp Vet 62:103-116.
47. Nagy, Z., and D. Derzsy. 1968. A viral disease of goslings. II Microscopic lesions. Acta Vet Hung 18:3-18.
48. Nougayrede, P. 1980. Virus diseases of Palmipeds or domestic Anatidae. Recl Med Vet 156:471-477.
49. Peter, W. 1985. Parvovirus infection of geese. Monatsh Veterinaermed 40:636-639.
50. Riddell, C. 1984. Viral hepatitis in domestic geese in Saskatchewan. Avian Dis 28:774-782.
51. Roszkowski, J., P. Gazdzinski, W. Kozaczynski, and M. Bartoszcze. 1982. Application of the immunoperoxidase technique for the detection of Derzsy's disease virus antigen in cell culture and goslings. Avian Pathol 11:571-578.
52. Samberg, Y., R. Bock, and Z. Perlstein. 1972. A new infectious disease of goslings in Israel. Refu Vet 29:29-33.
53. Schettler, C.H. 1971. Virus hepatitis of geese. II. Host range of goose hepatitis virus. Avian Dis 15:809-823.
54. Schettler, C.H. 1971. Goose virus hepatitis in the Canada goose and Snow goose. J Wildl Dis 7:147-148.
55. Schettler, C.H. 1973. Virus hepatitis of geese. III. Properties of the causal agent. Avian Pathol 2:179-193.
56. Suvorov, A.V. 1982. Cytopathic changes produced in goose fibroblast cultures by goose parvovirus. Bull Vses Inst Eksp Vet 48:16-18.
57. van Cleef, S.A.M., and J.T. Miltenburg. 1966. A serious virus disease with an acute course and high mortality in goslings. Tijdschr Diergeneesk 91:372-382.
58. Wachnik, Z. and J. Nowaki 1962. Wirusowe zapalenie watroby u gesiat. Med Weter 18:344-347.
59. Winteroll, G. 1974. Fluorescent antibody studies on goose hepatitis. Proc Goose Dis Symp, Doorn Neth, pp. 65-67.
60. Xu, W.Y., and Y.S. Chou. 1981. Preliminary report on the reverse indirect hemagglutination test for goose hepatitis virus. Acta Vet Zootech Sin 12:23-26.
61. Yadin, H., D.J. Roozelaar, and J. Hoekstra. 1977. Vaccines against viral hepatitis in geese. Tijdschr Diergeneesk 102:318-325.
62. Zheng, Y.M., J.B. Li, and Y.S. Zhou. 1985. Determination of the nucleic acid type of goose plague virus. J Jiangsu Agric Coll 6:7-10.
63. Zhou, Y.S., H.F. Tian, J.Y. Guo, and D.Y. Fang. 1984. Safety and potency tests of gosling plague vaccine in newly hatched goslings. Chin J Vet Med 10:2-4.
64. Ziedler, von K., W. Peter, and E. Sobanski. 1984. Studies into the pathogen of entero-hepatitis of Muscovy ducks. Monatsh Veterinaermed 39:374-377.

INFECTIOUS ANEMIA

V. von Bülow

INTRODUCTION. Chicken anemia agent (CAA), an unclassified small virus (14, 18, 36, 39), is the cause of infectious anemia of chickens. The disease is characterized by aplastic anemia and generalized lymphoid atrophy with a concomitant immunosuppression. Consequently, infectious anemia is frequently complicated by secondary viral, bacterial, or fungal infections. CAA appears to play a major role in the etiology of a number of multifactorial diseases associated with hemorrhagic syndrome and aplastic anemia. CAA-induced infectious anemia and closely associated syndromes have commonly been termed hemorrhagic syndrome (45), anemia-dermatitis (32), and blue wing disease (12, 13). Hemorrhagic syndromes that are not clearly CAA-induced (although the possibility does exist) are discussed in Chapter 34.

CAA infection has been confirmed as the cause of disease in several cases where infectious anemia occurred in chicken flocks at 2-4 wk of age (3, 7, 11, 17, 32, 34, 45). Growth is retarded and mortality is generally between 10 and 20%, but occasionally it may reach 60%.

CAA-induced disease, therefore, constitutes a serious economic threat. In chickens 6 or more wk of age, the etiological significance of CAA infection associated with aplastic anemia-hemorrhagic syndromes (16, 25, 42) has not definitely been established.

CAA infection has only been recognized in chickens; it has no known public health significance.

HISTORY. CAA (Gifu-1 strain) was first isolated in 1979 in Japan by Yuasa et al. (39). A major breakthrough was achieved 4 yr later by Yuasa (35) who showed that CAA, which does not replicate in any of the conventional monolayer cell cultures, is cytopathogenic for cultures of certain lymphoblastoid chicken cell lines, e.g., MDCC-MSB1 (MSB1). This enabled virus-neutralization (VN) tests to be performed in vitro (43) rather than in vivo (39), and it facilitated more extensive virological studies. Moreover, the availability of CAA-infected MSB1 cells made it feasible to detect anti-CAA antibody in chicken sera or egg yolk by indirect immunofluorescence tests (5, 44), and to purify the virus from supernatant fluids of CAA-infected cell cultures (14, 18, 36).

Agent identification was followed by studies that unraveled much of the pathogenesis and epizootiology of the infection.

Aplastic anemia syndromes, including inclusion body hepatitis, were described many years before CAA was detected. Their possible etiological association with CAA infection has been reviewed and discussed in several papers dealing with CAA (7, 19, 45).

INCIDENCE AND DISTRIBUTION. CAA appears to be ubiquitous in all major chicken-producing countries of the world. It has frequently been isolated from chickens in Japan (16, 17, 25, 36, 39, 42, 45), Germany (4, 7), Sweden (11), England (10), Canada (21), and the USA (15, 22,28). Serologic evidence of widespread infection has been found with chicken sera from Australia and several European, African, and Asian countries.

ETIOLOGY

Classification and Morphology. Virus particles purified from CAA-infected cell culture fluids appear spherical in negatively stained preparations and are about 19–24 nm in diameter (14, 18, 36). Virions have a buoyant density in cesium chloride density gradients of 1.35–1.36 g/ml (18), which is well below the density of parvoviruses. Chicken anemia virus purified from infected cell cultures apparently shows a type of isometric symmetry (Fig. 29.10), which appears to be unique among animal viruses (14). The virus has been shown to contain single-stranded DNA, and the size of the viral DNA has been estimated to be only 2300 bases (24). The assignment of chicken anemia virus to one of the existing virus groups has not been possible because of these peculiar features.

Virus Replication. Virions probably enter the cell by conventional absorption and penetration. The virus appears to replicate in the nucleus where viral antigens are detectable by indirect immunofluorescence at the peak of infection (5). The multiplication of CAA in MSB1 cells varies with the intensity of cell growth (36).

In chickens, CAA appears to replicate primarily in hematopoietic precursor cells in the bone marrow and in thymic precursor cells in the thymus cortex where it has been shown to cause cytolytic infection (19, 20).

Strain Classification. No antigenic differences have been recognized among various Japanese and European isolates of CAA (1, 5, 11, 36).

Resistance to Chemical and Physical Agents. CAA is resistant to ethyl ether and chloroform and is stable at pH 3 for 3 hr. It is resistant to heating at 56 C or 70 C for 1 hr and at 80 C for 15 min (11, 16, 39), but is only partially resistant to heating at 80 C for 30 min; it is completely inactivated within 15 min at 100 C (16). Infectivity is destroyed by treatment with 50% phenol for 5 min (39). Stability has been tested with crude preparations from liver homogenates and could well be different for virus propagated in cell culture.

CAA passes 25-nm-porosity membrane filters although a considerable proportion of infectivity may be retained by consecutively employed filter membranes with decreasing pore sizes (11, 16, 39).

Laboratory Host Systems. CAA can be propagated and assayed in day-old chicks and in cell cultures. It also can be propagated in chicken embryos but it does not cause any gross lesions.

CHICKENS. Day-old chicks inoculated with CAA develop anemia and gross lesions in lymphoid tissues and bone marrow; they are most pronounced after 12–16 days (39). Mortality occurs between 12 and 28 days postinoculation and usually remains low, rarely exceeding 30%. Response to CAA infection is enhanced by simultaneous inoculation of Marek's disease virus (MDV) or by treatment with betamethasone (6, 7, 9, 26). Chicks with maternal anti-CAA antibody are resistant to CAA infection (40).

CHICKEN EMBRYOS. Propagation of CAA in chicken embryos following yolk sac inoculation has been reported by Bülow and Witt (3). Moderate virus yields were obtained after 14 days from all parts of the embryo, but not from yolk or chorioallantoic membrane.

CELL CULTURES. Cultures of the T-cell lymphoblastoid cell lines MDCC-MSB1 and MDCC-JP2 and the B-cell lymphoblastoid cell line LSCC-1104B1 have been found by Yuasa (35) to be suitable for propagation and assay of CAA. Many other T-cell and B-cell lymphoblastoid cell lines, whether producers or nonproducers of the respective transforming viruses, turned out to be resistant to CAA (7, 35). Also, cell cultures derived from a large variety of tissues of chickens and chicken embryos proved to be resistant to CAA infection (35).

MSB1 cell cultures are presently preferred for in vitro cultivation. Cell-associated infectivity peaks between about 36 and 42 hr after inocula-

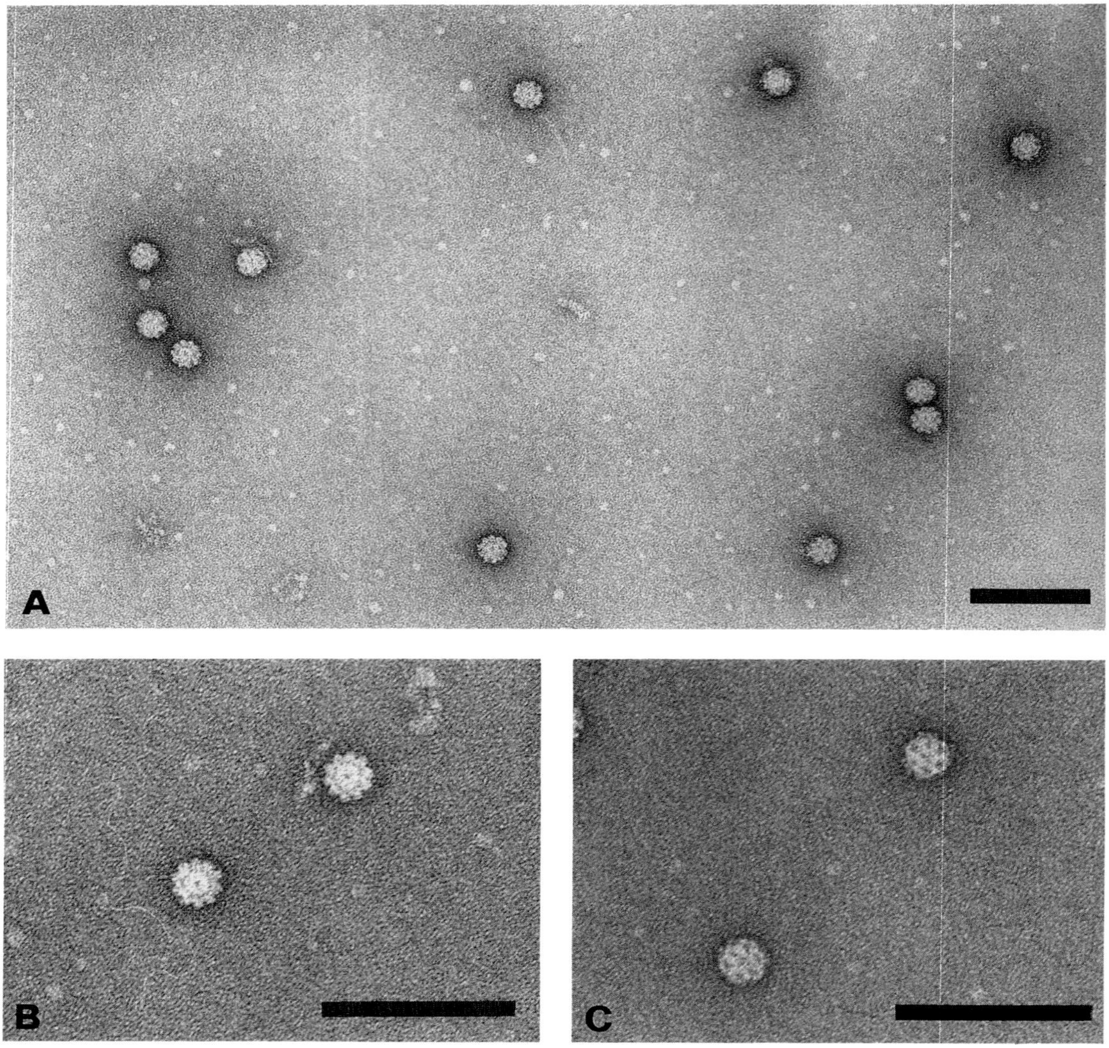

29.10. Chicken anemia virus particles. A. CAA particle preparation taken from a CsCl gradient fraction (density 1.36 g/ml) and negatively stained with 1% uranylacetate. ×150,000, bar = 100 nm. B. At higher magnification, different structural aspects of the CAA capsids become apparent. Two types of particle projections are obvious. Depending on the depth of the stain, the more flattened capsids show 10 peripheral protrusions. ×250,000, bar = 100 nm. C. Other CAA capsids, more deeply stained, exhibit six stain-filled morphological units that surround one central hole. ×250,000, bar = 100 nm. (Gelderblom)

tion, coinciding with the maximum amount of intranuclear antigens detected by immunofluorescence. Cell-free titers peak at 48–72 hr after inoculation, and the rate of multiplication has been reported to range between 10- and 100-fold (5, 35). Virus titrations require subculturing of inoculated cells every 2–4 days until cells inoculated with the endpoint dilution of CAA are destroyed.

Pathogenicity. Virulence of CAA isolates may vary slightly based on the degree of age resistance of chicks to infection (36). Attenuation of CAA by serial passage in cell culture has been reported; however, it is possible that a decrease in infectivity and immunogenicity in vivo was correlated with the attenuation (2).

PATHOGENESIS AND EPIZOOTIOLOGY

Natural and Experimental Hosts. The chicken is the only known host for CAA. All ages are susceptible to infection, but susceptibility to disease rapidly decreases in immunologically intact chicks during the first 2–3 wk of life (16, 36, 39, 41).

Transmission. CAA spreads easily among chickens in a group (41), although vertical transmission through the hatching egg may be the most important means of dissemination (10). Egg transmission only occurred from 8–14 days after experimental infection of hens (38), but field observations indicated that vertical transmission could occur during a period of 3–6 wk (32).

Incubation Period. In experimental infections, anemia and distinct histological lesions can first be detected at 8 days after inoculation. Clinical signs develop after 10–14 days, and mortality occurs beginning at 12–14 days after inoculation (19, 30, 39).

Under field conditions, the incubation period is unknown, but clinical signs and lesions have been noted as early as the 12th day, increasing during 3–4 wk of life.

Signs. The only specific sign of CAA infection is anemia, with a peak at 14–16 days postinoculation as indicated by hematocrit values ranging from 6–27%. Affected birds are depressed and more or less pale. Weight gain is depressed between 10 and 20 days after experimental infection. Usually, no more than 30% of the birds die between 12 and 28 days postinoculation. Surviving chicks completely recover from depression and anemia by 20–28 days after infection (7, 16, 29, 39), although retarded recovery and increased mortality may be associated with secondary bacterial or viral infections. Secondary infections are frequently seen in field cases, but they may inadvertently also occur in experimental chicks (7, 13, 17, 32).

Morbidity and Mortality. The outcome of CAA infection is influenced by a number of viral, host, and environmental factors. Morbidity and mortality may be influenced by the virulence of the CAA strain. The TK-5803 strain described by Goryo et al. (16) appears to be more virulent than either of the isolates studied by Yuasa and Imai (36). Dosage can influence the severity of anemia (39). The route of infection also plays a role in experimental infection, since infection by contact does not cause anemia in immunologically intact chicks.

In immunologically competent chicks, age resistance develops rapidly during the 1st wk of life and becomes complete after 3 wk or even earlier, depending on the virulence of the infecting CAA strain (16, 41). Development of age resistance is delayed by immunosuppression, e.g., by simultaneous infection with infectious bursal disease virus (41) and in bursectomized birds (46).

Morbidity and mortality are considerably enhanced if chicks are dually infected with CAA and MDV, reticuloendotheliosis virus (REV), or infectious bursal disease virus (IBDV), probably due to virus-induced immunosuppression (4, 6, 7, 26, 41). Chemical immunosuppression by betamethasone or cyclosporin A also aggravates signs and lesions (9). In field infections, various environmental and other factors causing a decrease of immunocompetence have therefore been suspected to enhance CAA pathogenicity. The mechanism of the enhancing effect of reovirus infection, resulting in blue wing disease (13), is not completely understood but may also be related to immunosuppression.

Gross Lesions. Thymic atrophy is the most consistent, but bone marrow atrophy the most characteristic, lesion seen in affected chickens. Femoral bone marrow is fatty and yellowish or pink. In some instances, its color appears dark red although distinct lesions can be detected by histologic examination. Thymic atrophy may result in an almost complete regression of the organ, which then has a dark reddish brown color. With increasing age resistance of infected chicks, thymic atrophy may become a much more consistent lesion than grossly visible bone marrow lesions (16). Bursal atrophy is less obvious. In a small proportion of birds, the size of the bursa of Fabricius may be reduced. In many cases, however, the outer bursal wall appears translucent so that plicae become visible. Swelling and a mottled appearance of the liver, hemorrhages in the proventricular mucosa, and subcutaneous and muscular hemorrhages are sometimes associated with severe anemia (7, 16, 29, 30).

Histopathology. Histopathological changes in affected anemic chicks have been characterized as panmyelophthisis and generalized lymphoid atrophy (6, 7, 19, 29, 30).

In the bone marrow, atrophy and aplasia involve all compartments and hematopoietic lineages (Fig. 29.11). Necrosis of residual small cell foci may occasionally be seen. Hematopoietic cells are replaced by adipose tissue or proliferating stroma cells. Regenerative areas consisting of proerythroblasts appear 16–18 days after experimental infection, and there is a hyperplasia of

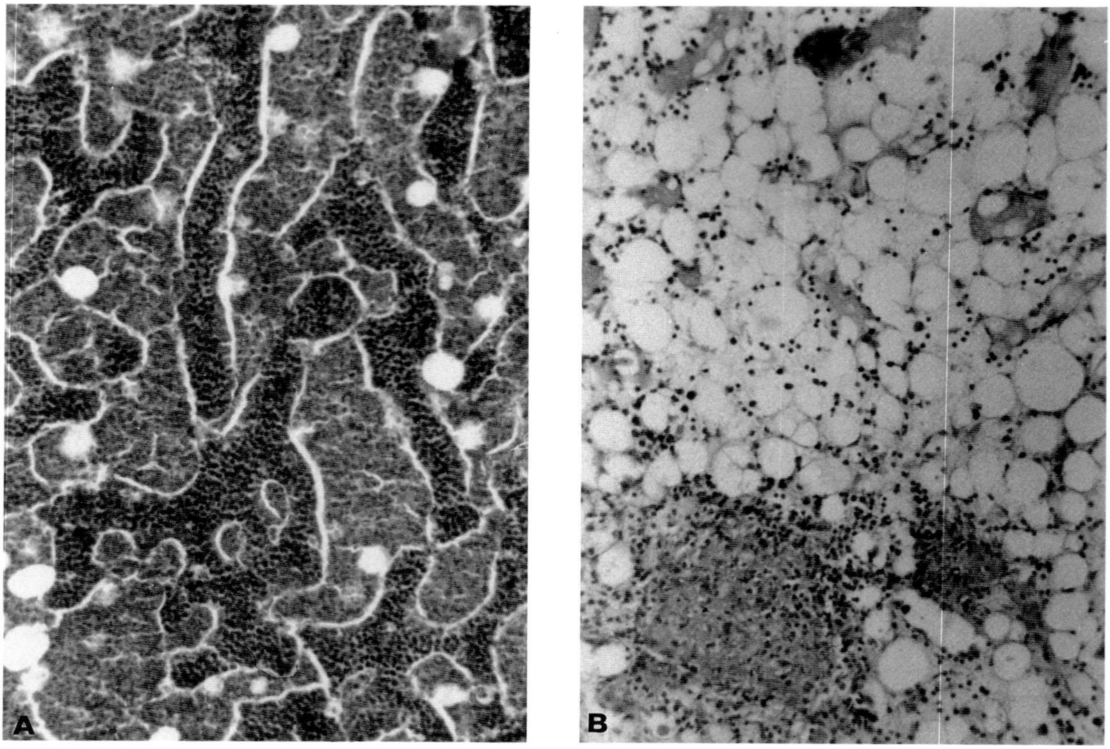

29.11. Femoral bone marrow from 14-day-old chickens. A. Uninfected control. B. CAA-infected, 14 days after inoculation. Atrophy of hematopoietic tissue and a focus with necrotic cells. H & E, ×160. (Rudolph)

bone marrow between 24 and 32 days post inoculation in birds that recover.

Severe lymphoid depletion is seen in the thymus, bursa of Fabricius, spleen, and cecal tonsils, as well as in a wide range of other tissues. The thymic cortex and medulla become equally atrophic, with hydropic degeneration of residual cells and occasional necrotic foci (Fig. 29.12). In chicks that recover, repopulation of the thymus with lymphocytes becomes distinct at 20–24 days, and the morphology returns to normal by 32–36 days after infection.

Lesions in the bursa of Fabricius consist of atrophy of the lymphoid follicles with occasional small necrotic foci, infolded epithelium, hydropic epithelial degeneration, and proliferation of reticular cells (Fig. 29.13). Repopulation of lymphocytes until complete recovery is similar to that in the thymus.

In the spleen, atrophy of lymphoid tissue with hyperplasia of reticular cells is seen in the lymphoid follicles as well as in the Schweiger-Seidel sheaths. Necrotic foci in follicles or sheaths have rarely been observed.

In the liver, kidneys, lungs, proventriculus, duodenum, and cecal tonsils, lymphoid foci are depleted of cells, are smaller, and are less dense than in unaffected birds. Liver cells are swollen, and hepatic sinusoids may be dilated.

Pathogenesis. The pathogenesis of CAA infection has been partially elucidated by chronological studies of affected tissues (19, 30). It may be concluded from the findings of Goryo et al. (19, 20) that hematopoietic precursor cells in the bone marrow and thymic precursor cells in the thymus cortex are primarily involved in early cytolytic infection at 6–8 days postinoculation. Besides enlarged proerythroblasts and degenerating hematopoietic cells, macrophages with ingested degenerated hematopoietic cells have been observed in the bone marrow. Eosinophilic, intranuclear inclusion bodies have been found in altered cells in the bone marrow as well as in the thymus, but the significance of these inclusions is not known (19, 20). In contrast to the thymus, depletion of lymphoid cells and occasional necrosis in the bursa of Fabricius, spleen, and in lymphoid foci of other tissues have not been detected before 12 days postinoculation (19, 30). Repopulation of the bone marrow with proerythroblasts and promyelocytes and recovery of hematopoietic

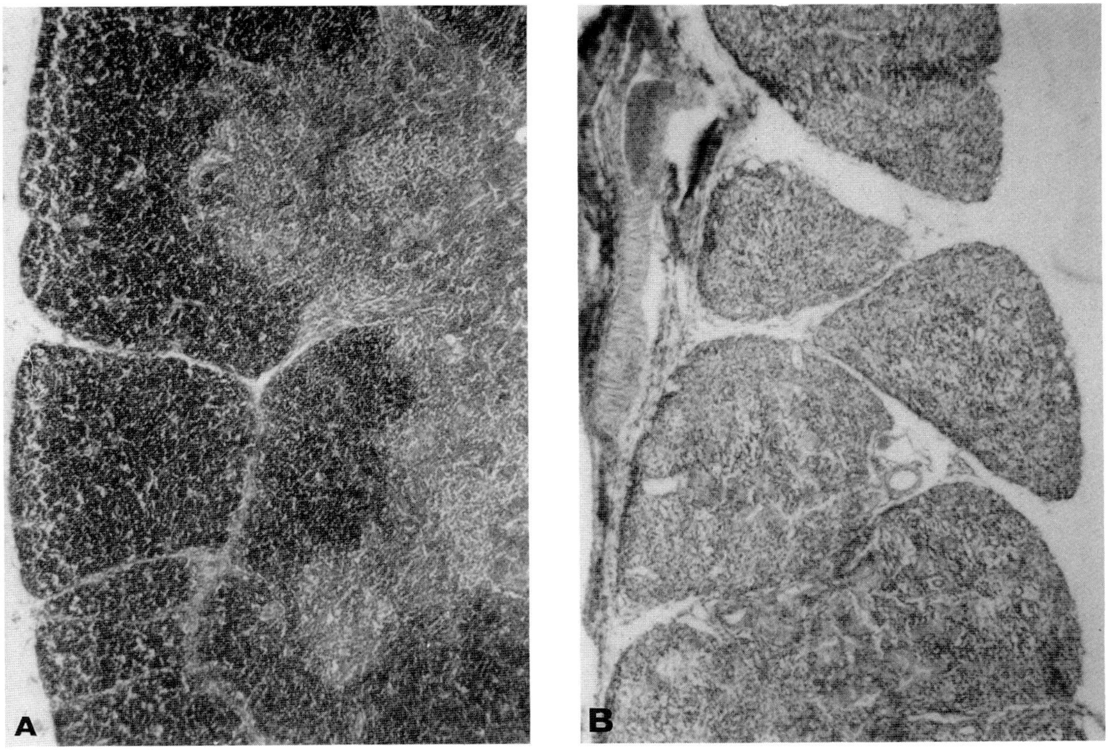

29.12. Chicken thymus. A. Normal, from a 14-day-old uninfected chicken. B. Atrophic, at 14 days after inoculation of CAA. H & E, ×63. (Rudolph)

activity at 16 days after inoculation appear to coincide with the beginning of antibody formation (see Immunity).

Hematology. Blood of severely affected chicks is more or less watery, the clotting time is increased, and the blood plasma is paler than normal. Hematocrit values begin to decrease at 8–10 days after inoculation, are mostly in the range of 10–20% at 14–20 days, and may even drop to 6% in moribund birds. In convalescent chicks, hematocrit values increase after 16–20 days and return to normal by 32 days postinfection (19, 30, 39).

Low hematocrit values are due to a pancytopenia (29, 30, 39) with markedly decreased numbers of erythrocytes, white blood cells, and thrombocytes. Anisocytosis has been noticed as early as 8 days postinfection. Juvenile forms of erythrocytes, granulocytes, and thrombocytes begin to appear in the peripheral blood by 16 days after inoculation, and the incidence of immature erythrocytes may exceed 30% several days later. The blood picture in convalescent chicks returns to normal by 40 days (30).

Immunity

ACTIVE. There is only a poor antibody response in susceptible chickens inoculated with CAA at 1 day of age. Neutralizing antibody cannot be detected until 3 wk after inoculation. Even then, titers are low (1:80) with little increase (1:320) until 4 wk. The antibody response is considerably enhanced in chickens inoculated intramuscularly at 2–6 wk of age, with neutralizing anti-CAA antibody detectable as early as 4–7 days and with maximum titers (1:1280–1:5120) at 12–14 days postinoculation (43, 44). Humoral antibody formation is delayed by about 1 wk if chickens are infected orally rather than intramuscularly. Yuasa et al. (43) reported that increasing antibody production coincides with decreasing virus concentrations in chicken tissues.

PASSIVE. Maternal antibodies provide complete protection of young chicks against CAA-induced infectious anemia (40), provided that the chicks are not immunologically compromised by other factors (6, 7). Outbreaks of infectious anemia in the field have in fact been found to be correlated with the absence of anti-CAA antibody in the respective parent flocks (31, 32, 45).

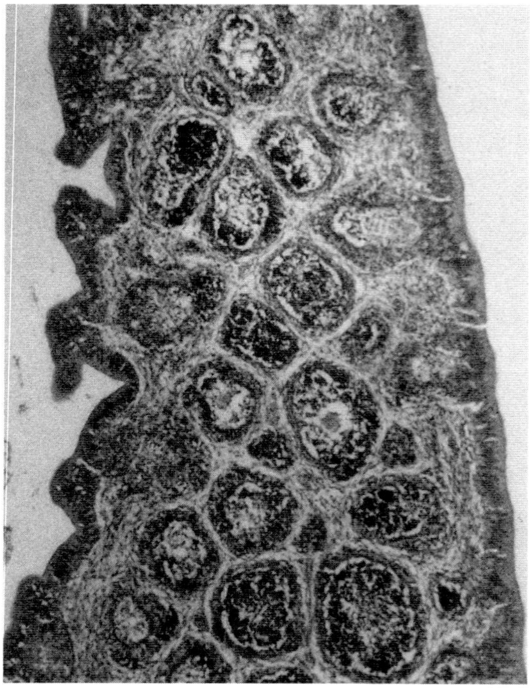

29.13. Bursa of Fabricius from a CAA-infected chicken at 14 days after inoculation, showing lymphoid depletion and atrophy of follicles. H & E, ×63. (Rudolph)

IMMUNOSUPPRESSION. There is strong circumstantial evidence that CAA infection is immunosuppressive, at least in susceptible young chicks during clinical stages of the disease. Immunosuppression in anemic birds is indicated by an increased susceptibility to bacterial and fungal infections (7, 17, 29, 34), and by enhanced pathogenicity of adenovirus (8) and reovirus (13) in dually infected chicks. Under certain conditions, vaccinal immunity, e.g., against Marek's disease, is depressed by CAA infection (26, 27, 37). Impairment of the immune response may result directly from CAA infection, i.e., from damage of hematopoietic and lymphopoietic tissues (see Histology).

DIAGNOSIS

Isolation and Identification of the Causative Agent.

CAA can be isolated from virtually all tissues of infected chickens (43). Maximum virus titers have been detected at 7 days after infection. In chickens inoculated at 1 day of age, the CAA content of tissues and rectal contents remains almost constant until 21 days and rapidly declines thereafter. Serum, however, loses its infectivity after 14 days (43). Bülow (4) found whole blood infectious for least 14 days. In chickens inoculated at 4–6 wk of age, maximum virus titers occurred in a variety of tissues and in rectal contents at 7 days after infection, rapidly decreasing to rather low levels until 14–21 days. However, CAA has never been detected in the brain or serum of such birds (43).

Liver is preferred as a source of CAA because it most consistently contains high concentrations of the agent. Clarified liver homogenate can be heated for 5 min at 70 C (16) or treated with chloroform to eliminate or inactivate possible contaminants before inoculation in cell cultures.

Bioassay by intramuscular or intraperitoneal inoculation of susceptible 1-day-old chicks is the most specific method available for primary isolation of CAA. The infectivity is up to 100-fold lower than in cell culture but can be increased by immunosuppression of experimental chicks (2). At 14–16 days after inoculation, chicks are examined for anemia, as indicated by hematocrit values below 27%, and for typical gross lesions that may also be present in some nonanemic birds. Histopathological examination of suspected tissues may be included but is usually not necessary to confirm the diagnosis.

MDCC-MSB1 cell cultures can be used for in vitro isolation attempts (5, 17, 35, 42). Freshly prepared cultures (2–3 × 10^5 cells/ml in RPMI 1640 culture medium, 105 cells/cm^2) should be inoculated with $^1/_{10}$ volume of 1:20 or greater dilution, or serial 10-fold dilutions, of appropriately prepared tissue homogenate. Cell damage occurring after 1–6 subcultures (7–24 days) is suggestive of CAA infection, but there are no CAA-specific features of cytopathology that could be recognized by light microscopy. Isolation of CAA should be verified by serological procedures.

Serology.

Anti-CAA antibody in chicken sera or egg yolk can be detected by virus-neutralization (VN) tests (5, 43) or by indirect fluorescent antibody (FA) tests (5, 23, 44). In the VN test, serial twofold serum dilutions are mixed with equal parts of a CAA suspension (200–500 $TCID_{50}$/0.1 ml), and the mixture is incubated at 37 C for 60 min or at 4 C overnight before assay in MSB1 cell culture. It may take up to 5 wk, i.e., nine subcultures, before the assay is completed and the antibody titer of the tested serum can be estimated. In a semi-quantitative VN test, a constant serum dilution of 1:20 - 1:80 is mixed with an equal volume of CAA suspension with about 105.5 $TCID_{50}$/0.1 ml. With this procedure, absence of neutralizing anti-CAA antibody in the tested serum can be recognized after only one to two subcultures of inoculated cells, and presence of antibody after three to four subcultures. The relative antibody titer may be estimated by the number of subcultures in which the inoculated cells stay alive. Chicken sera may occasionally exhibit a toxic effect on cultured MSB1 cells, even if diluted 1:50 or 1:80. Therefore, it is necessary to include appropriate serum controls to avoid false negative results.

In the indirect FA test, CAA-infected MSB1 cells collected just before the beginning of cell lysis, usually 36–42 hr after inoculation, are smeared on glass slides and acetone-fixed for use as antigens. Cells are reacted first with test serum and then with a fluorescein-labelled mammalian antiserum against chicken gamma globulin. Fluorescent staining of small, irregularly shaped granules in the nucleus of enlarged cells is considered evidence for antibody in the test serum (Fig. 29.14). Positive control serum should always be included. Negative control sera are of little or no use, since they are usually selected for being nonreactive in the indirect FA test. Noninfected cells as internal controls enable the evaluation of several types of nonspecific nuclear fluorescence. Sometimes there are test sera, particularly from adult specific-pathogen-free chickens, which cause nonspecific intranuclear fluorescence that is virtually indistinguishable from CAA-specific fluorescence. The indirect FA test is less sensitive and less specific than the VN test (1). On the other hand, the VN test is more laborious and it takes much more time to get results.

CAA-infection of inoculated MSB1 cells can be verified by indirect FA tests with positive anti-CAA reference serum, provided that a sufficient proportion of cells is infected and that cells are harvested at an appropriate time after infection.

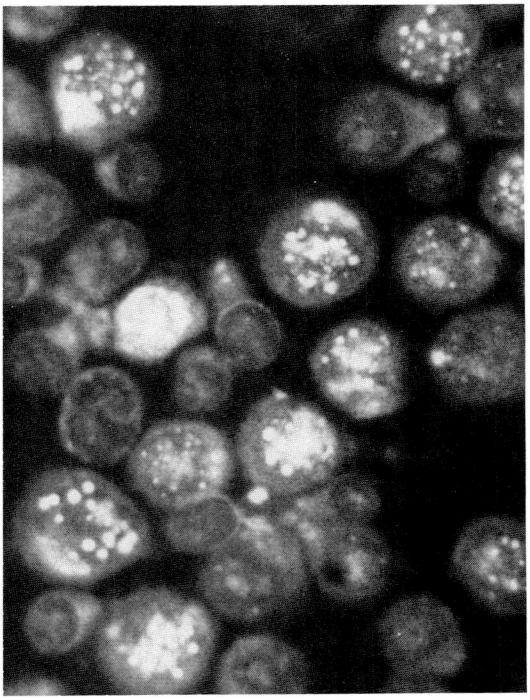

29.14. CAA antigens detected by immunofluorescent staining in MSB1 cells harvested at 40 hr after inoculation. Antigens are seen in enlarged cells with characteristic intranuclear granular fluorescence. ×400.

Differential Diagnosis. Infection criteria have only limited value in diagnosis of CAA-induced disease, because CAA is virtually ubiquitous among chickens. In chickens under 6 wk of age, a typical combination of signs, hematological changes, gross and microscopic lesions, and flock history (see PATHOGENESIS AND EPIZOOTIOLOGY) are suggestive of CAA infection. There are no particular lesions per se, however, that can be considered pathognomonic.

Aplastic anemia, but not a pancytopenia, with a concurrent atrophy of thymus and bursa of Fabricius, and depressed immune response can also be caused by osteopetrosis virus. Anemia induced by erythroblastosis virus can be distinguished from CAA-induced anemia by microscopic examination. Marek's disease virus and infectious bursal disease virus induce atrophy of lymphoid tissues with typical histological lesions, but do not cause anemia in naturally infected chickens.

Intoxication with high doses of sulfonamides, or mycotoxins such as aflatoxin, can result in aplastic anemia and "hemorrhagic syndrome." Aflatoxin may also impair the immune system. In the field, however, chickens are rarely exposed to doses of aflatoxin or sulfonamides that are sufficient to cause acute disease. On the other hand, subclinical intoxication of chickens might add to the pathogenicity of CAA.

TREATMENT. There is no specific treatment for chickens affected by CAA infection. Treatment with broad-spectrum antibiotics to control bacterial infections usually associated with infectious anemia might be indicated, but its efficacy is usually poor.

PREVENTION AND CONTROL. Immunization of parent flocks several weeks before egg production efficiently prevents outbreaks of infectious anemia caused by CAA in their progeny. Artificial exposure by transfer of litter from CAA-infected flocks to young breeder flocks has been shown to be effective but is a dubious and risky procedure with regard to hygiene (32). CAA infection of breeders via the drinking water with tissue homogenates from naturally affected chicks has also been effective (31, 32). This method, however, cannot be recommended as a standard procedure, because it is almost impossible to be sure of a sufficient CAA concentration and the absence of other pathogens in the tissue preparations.

Bülow and Witt (3) had suggested that virulent CAA production in embryos could provide a vaccine with little or no risk of attenuation. Indeed, efficacious and safe vaccines free from extraneous agents have been produced in that manner (33). Cell culture-propagated CAA may also be suitable as a vaccine provided that the titer (chicken ID_{50}) is adequate. Vaccination should be performed at about 16-18 wk of age, but never later than 3-4 wk before the first collection of hatching eggs to avoid the hazard of vaccine virus spread through the egg. CAA does not cause immunosuppression in birds of that age (33). Vaccination can be omitted if humoral anti-CAA antibody has been detected in the growing breeder chickens.

Attention should be paid to management and hygiene procedures to prevent immunosuppression by environmental factors or infectious diseases, and to prevent early exposure to CAA. Monitoring of breeder flocks for the presence of anti-CAA antibody should be done to avoid vertically transmitted CAA infections.

REFERENCES

1. Bülow, V.v. 1988. Unsatisfactory sensitivity and specificity of indirect immunofluorescence tests for the presence or absence of antibodies to chicken anaemia agent (CAA) in sera of SPF and broiler breeder chickens. J Vet Med B 35:594-600.

2. Bülow, V.v., and B. Fuchs. 1986. Attenuierung des Erregers der aviären infektiösen Anämie (CAA) durch Serienpassagen in Zellkulturen. J Vet Med B 33:568-573.

3. Bülow, V.v., and M. Witt. 1986. Vermehrung des Erregers der aviären infektiösen Anämie (CAA) in embryonierten Hühnereiern. J Vet Med B 33:664-669.

4. Bülow, V.v., B. Fuchs, E. Vielitz, und H. Landgraf. 1983. Frühsterblichkeitssyndrom bei Küken nach Infektion mit dem Virus der Marekschen Krankheit (MDV) und einem Anämie-Erreger (CAA). Zentralbl Veterinärmed [B] 30:742-750.

5. Bülow, V.v., B. Fuchs, und M. Bertram. 1985. Untersuchungen über den Erreger der infektiösen Anämie bei Hühnerküken (CAA) in vitro: Vermehrung, Titration, Serumneutralisationstest und indirekter Immunfluoreszenztest. Zentralbl Veterinärmed [B] 32:679-693.

6. Bülow, V.v., B. Fuchs, and R. Rudolph. 1986. Avian infectious anaemia caused by chicken anaemia agent (CAA). In J.B. McFerran and M.S. McNulty (eds.), Acute Virus Infections of Poultry, pp. 203-212. Martinus Nijhoff, Dordrecht, Boston, and Lancaster.

7. Bülow, V.v., R. Rudolph, and B. Fuchs. 1986. Erhöhte Pathogenität des Erregers der aviären infektiösen Anämie bei Hühnerküken (CAA) bei simultaner Infektion mit dem Virus der Marekschen Krankheit (MDV), Bursitisvirus (IBDV), oder Reticuloendotheliosevirus (REV). J Vet Med B 33:93-116.

8. Bülow, V.v., R. Rudolph, and B. Fuchs. 1986. Folgen der Doppelinfektion von Küken mit Adenovirus oder Reovirus und dem Erreger der aviären infektiösen Anämie (CAA). J Vet Med B 33:717-726.

9. Bülow, V.v., M. Witt, and R. Rudolph. 1987. Auswirkungen immunologischer Defekte bei Hühnerküken im Zusammenhang mit der aviären infektiösen Anämie. In Bericht des 17. Kongresses der Deutschen Veterinärmedizinischen Gesellschaft, pp. 384-390. Deutsche Veterinärmedizinische Gesellschaft, Giessaen.

10. Chettle, N.J., R.K. Eddy, P.J. Wyeth, and S.A. Lister. 1989. An outbreak of disease due to chicken anaemia agent in broiler chickens in England. Vet Rec 124:211-215.

11. Engström, B.E. 1988. Blue wing disease of chickens: Isolation of avian reovirus and chicken anaemia agent. Avian Pathol 17:23-32.

12. Engström, B.E., and M. Luthman. 1984. Blue wing disease of chickens: Signs, pathology, and natural transmission. Avian Pathol 13:1-12.

13. Engström, B.E., O. Fossum, and M. Luthman. 1988. Blue wing disease of chickens: Experimental infection with a Swedish isolate of chicken anaemia agent and an avian reovirus. Avian Pathol 17:33-50.

14. Gelderblom, H., S. Kling, R. Lurz, I. Tischer, and V.v. Bülow. 1989. Morphological characterization of chicken anaemia agent (CAA). Arch Virol 109:115-120.

15. Goodwin, M.A., J. Brown, S.L. Miller, M.A. Smeltzer, W.L. Steffens, and W.D. Waltman. 1989. Infectious anemia caused by a parvoviruslike virus in Georgia broilers. Avian Dis 33:438-445.

16. Goryo, M., H. Sugimura, S. Matsumoto, T. Umemura, and C. Itakura. 1985. Isolation of an agent inducing chicken anaemia. Avian Pathol 14:483-496.

17. Goryo, M., Y. Shibata, T. Suwa, T. Umemura, and C. Itakura. 1987. Outbreak of anemia associated with chicken anemia agent in young chicks. Jpn J Vet Sci 49:867-873.

18. Goryo, M., T. Suwa, S. Matsumoto, T. Umemura, and C. Itakura. 1987. Serial propagation and purification of chicken anaemia agent in MDCC-MSB1 cell line. Avian Pathol 16:149-163.

19. Goryo, M., T. Suwa, T. Umemura, C. Itakura, and S. Yamashiro. 1989. Histopathology of chicks inoculated with chicken anaemia agent (MSB1-TK5803 strain). Avian Pathol 18:73-89.

20. Goryo, M., T. Suwa, T. Umemura, C. Itakura, and S. Yamashiro. 1989. Ultrastructure of bone marrow in chicks inoculated with chicken anaemia agent (MSB1-TK5803 strain). Avian Pathol 18:329-343.

21. Goryo, M., R.J. Julian, J. Thorsen, and S. Yamashiro. 1989. Isolation of the chicken anemia agent from field chickens in Ontario. Avian Dis. (In press).

22. Lucio, B., K.A. Schat, and H.L. Shivaprasad. 1989. Identification of the chicken anemia agent, reproduction of the disease, and serological survey in the United States. Proc 38th West Poult Dis Conf, pp. 35-38.

23. McNulty, M.S., T.J. Connor, F. McNeilly, K.S. Kirkpatrick, and J.B. McFerran 1988. A serological survey of domestic poultry in the United Kingdom for antibody to chicken anaemia agent. Avian Pathol 17:315-324.

24. McNulty, M.S., T.J. Connor, F. McNeilly, D. Todd, K.A. Mawhinney, J. Creelan, D.P. Mackie, D. Pollock, J. McNair, W.L. Curran, and M.F. McLoughlin. 1989. Current status of chicken anemia agent. Proc 38th West Poult Dis Conf, pp. 12-13.

25. Otaki, Y., T. Nunoya, M. Tajima, H. Tamada, and Y. Nomura. 1987. Isolation of chicken anaemia agent and Marek's disease virus from chickens vaccinated with turkey herpesvirus and lesions induced in chicks by inoculating both agents. Avian Pathol 16:291-306.

26. Otaki, Y., T. Nunoya, M. Tajima, A. Kato, and Y. Nomura 1988. Depression of vaccinal immunity to Marek's disease by infection with chicken anemia agent. Avian Pathol 17:333-347.

27. Otaki, Y., M. Tajima, K. Saito, and Y. Nomura. 1988. Immune response of chicks inoculated with chicken anemia agent alone or in combination with Marek's disease virus or turkey herpesvirus. Jpn J Vet Sci 50:1040-1047.

28. Rosenberger, J.K., and S.S. Cloud. 1989. The isolation and characterization of chicken anemia agent (CAA) from broilers in the United States. Avian Dis 33:707–713.

29. Taniguchi, T., N. Yuasa, M. Maeda, and T. Horiuchi. 1982. Hematopathological changes in dead and moribund chicks induced by chicken anemia agent. Nat Inst Anim Health Q (Tokyo) 22:61–69.

30. Taniguchi, T., N. Yuasa, M. Maeda, and T. Horiuchi. 1983. Chronological observations on hematopathological changes in chicks inoculated with chicken anemia agent. Nat Inst Anim Health Q (Tokyo) 23:1–12.

31. Vielitz, E., and H. Landgraf. 1986. Zur Epidemiologie und Prophylaxe der infektiösen Anämie (CAA)-Dermatitis des Huhnes. In M. Larbier (ed.), 7th Euro Poult Conf, Vol. 2, pp. 1124–1129. World's Poult Sci Assoc, French Branch, Tours.

32. Vielitz, E., and H. Landgraf. 1988. Anaemia-dermatitis of broilers: Field observations on its occurrence, transmission, and prevention. Avian Pathol 17:113–120.

33. Vielitz, E., V. v. Bülow, H. Landgraf, and C. Conrad. 1987. Anämie des Mastgeflügels–entwicklung eines Impfstoffes für Elterntiere. J Vet Med B 34:553–557.

34. Weikel, J., P. Dorn, H. Spiess, and E. Wessling. 1986. Ein Beitrag zur Diagnostik und Epidemiologie der infektiösen Anämie (CAA) beim Broiler. Berl Münch Tierärztl Wochenschr 99:119–121.

35. Yuasa, N. 1983. Propagation and infectivity titration of the Gifu-1 strain of chicken anemia agent in a cell line (MDCC-MSB1) derived from Marek's disease lymphoma. Nat Inst Anim Health Q (Tokyo) 23:13–20.

36. Yuasa, N., and K. Imai. 1986. Pathogenicity and antigenicity of eleven isolates of chicken anaemia agent (CAA). Avian Pathol 15:639–645.

37. Yuasa, N., and K. Imai. 1988. Efficacy of Marek's disease vaccine, herpesvirus of turkeys, in chickens infected with chicken anemia agent. In S. Kato, T. Horiuchi, T. Mikami, and K. Hirai (eds.), Advances in Marek's Disease Research, pp. 358–363. Japanese Association on Marek's Disease, Osaka.

38. Yuasa, N., and I. Yoshida. 1983. Experimental egg transmission of chicken anemia agent. Nat Inst Anim Health Q (Tokyo) 23:99–100.

39. Yuasa, N., T. Taniguchi, and I. Yoshida. 1979. Isolation and some characteristics of an agent inducing anemia in chicks. Avian Dis 23:366–385.

40. Yuasa, N., T. Noguchi, K. Furata, and I. Yoshida. 1980. Maternal antibody and its effect on the susceptibility of chicks to chicken anemia agent. Avian Dis 24:197–201.

41. Yuasa, N., T. Taniguchi, T. Noguchi, and I. Yoshida. 1980. Effect of infectious bursal disease virus infection on incidence of anemia by chicken anemia agent. Avian Dis 24:202–209.

42. Yuasa, N., T. Taniguchi, M. Goda, M. Shibatani, T. Imada, and H. Hihara. 1983. Isolation of chicken anemia agent with MDCC-MSB1 cells from chickens in the field. Nat Inst Anim Health Q (Tokyo) 23:75–77.

43. Yuasa, N., T. Taniguchi, T. Imada, and H. Hihara. 1983. Distribution of chicken anemia agent (CAA) and detection of neutralizing antibody in chicks experimentally inoculated with CAA. Nat Inst Anim Health Q (Tokyo) 23:78–81.

44. Yuasa, N., K. Imai, and H. Tezuka. 1985. Survey of antibody against chicken anaemia agent (CAA) by an indirect immunofluorescent antibody technique in breeder flocks in Japan. Avian Pathol 14:521–530.

45. Yuasa, N., K. Imai, K. Watanabe, F. Saito, M. Abe, and K. Komi. 1987. Aetiological examination of an outbreak of haemorrhagic syndrome in a broiler flock in Japan. Avian Pathol 16:521–526.

46. Yuasa, N., K. Imai, and K. Nakamura. 1988. Pathogenicity of chicken anaemia agent in bursectomised chickens. Avian Pathol 17:363–369.

TURKEY VIRAL HEPATITIS

G.H. Snoeyenbos

INTRODUCTION. Turkey viral hepatitis (TVH) is an acute, highly contagious, typically subclinical disease of turkeys that produces lesions of the liver and less frequently the pancreas.

The disease was first described simultaneously by Mongeau et al. (4) from Ontario and Snoeyenbos et al. (10) from Massachusetts in 1959. Diagnostic summaries indicate that TVH has been observed in a number of states. Mandelli et al. (3) recognized it in Italy in 1966 and suggested hepatopancreatitis as a more appropriate designation. The true incidence and distribution are unknown owing to the transient, usually subclinical nature of the infection and lack of serologic means to detect previous infection.

ETIOLOGY. The etiologic agent is a virus that passes a 100-nm-porosity membrane filter and is resistant to ether, chloroform, phenol, and creoline but not to formalin. In a yolk menstruum it survived for 6 hr at 60 C, 14 hr at 56 C, and 4 wk at 37 C. It retained viability for 1 hr at pH 2 but not at pH 12 (12).

The virus may be propagated in the yolk sac of chicken and turkey embryos injected not later than 7 and 10 days of age, respectively. Mandelli et al. (3) found 6-day-old chicken embryos much superior to older embryos. Viral replication has been demonstrated 66 hr postinoculation, and virus titers peaked at approximately 90 hr. Rapid embryo passage did not greatly enhance the final titer, which was seldom greater than $10^{3.5}$ embryo-infective dose-50% (11). Other routes of embryo inoculation did not always result in viral replication. A variety of tissue culture systems failed to support viral replication (13). A one-way antigenic relationship has been reported between TVH rabbit antiserum and duck hepatitis virus in an agar-gel diffusion test (13).

Macdonald et al. (2) reported finding picornalike virions in degenerative hepatocytes from lesions in a turkey. Growth patterns of the virus in chicken embryos and lesions produced in exposed turkey poults closely resembled those reported earlier for TVH virus. However, because repeated attempts by Snoeyenbos (8) had failed to reveal virions in affected tissues by electron microscopy, there remains a question of whether more than one virus may produce the syndrome.

PATHOGENESIS AND EPIZOOTIOLOGY.

Infection has been recognized only in the turkey. White Pekin ducks, chickens, pheasants, and Coturnix quail were refractory to experimental exposure. Transmission readily occurs by direct or indirect contact. The possibility of transmission via the egg has been suggested on a basis of field observations and isolation of virus from an ovum of an artificially infected turkey hen. The virus has been consistently isolated from liver and feces of infected birds and less frequently from bile, blood, and kidneys during the first 28 days postinfection. After that time the virus apparently disappears (9, 13).

Based on the time of appearance of lesions, the incubation period in poults injected intraperitoneally with TVH virus was as short as 48 hr and usually no longer than 7 days in either injected or contact-exposed poults.

Signs, Morbidity, Mortality. The disease is usually subclinical and is thought to become apparent only in presence of other stressor agents. Variable degrees of flock depression and sudden death of apparently normal birds are usually noted in clinical cases. There is suggestive evidence that affected breeder flocks may exhibit decreased production, fertility, and hatchability. Morbidity and mortality appear to be largely determined by severity of concurrent stressor agents. Nearly 100% morbidity has been reported by some flock owners. A mortality rate of 25% in one flock was reported, but usually mortality is very low and occurs during a 7- to 10-day period. Mortality in birds over 6 wk of age has not been reported.

Pathology. Distinct gross lesions have been observed only in the liver and pancreas. Mandelli et al. (3) also observed catarrhal enteritis, bronchopneumonia, and peritonitis or airsacculitis in specimens that may have had intercurrent infections. Hepatic lesions consist of focal, gray, sometimes slightly depressed areas up to several millimeters in diameter. Lesion distribution is variable. Birds that die usually exhibit very extensive lesions, often coalescing, which may be partially masked by vascular congestion and focal hemorrhage. Bile staining is not uncommon. Pancreatic lesions, less consistently observed than hepatic lesions, are often prominent and consist of roughly circular gray-pink areas, often extending across a lobe.

Bickford (1) examined tissues from experimentally infected poults and failed to find inclusion bodies. Lesions found were similar to those reported earlier by Mongeau et al. (4), Snoeyenbos et al. (10), and Mandelli et al. (3) and consisted of early vacuolation of hepatocytes, dense infiltration by mononuclear leukocytes and a few heterophils, and some proliferation of bile ductules. Lesions progressed to overt focal necrosis with pooling of blood around the focus. The necrotic area consisted of necrotic cells scattered among infiltrating leukocytes and proliferating reticuloendothelial cells that sometimes formed giant cells. The necrotizing effect of virus infection appeared to continue during the 16-day postinfection period in which tissues were examined. Pancreatic lesions were of the same general character.

Immunity. Some immunity develops following infection. Exposure of recovered birds resulted in less frequent and less extensive lesions than in initially infected controls (9). Progeny of recovered breeders developed extensive lesions following exposure (13). Using direct or indirect complement-fixation, virus-neutralization, or agar-gel diffusion tests, Tzianabos and Snoeyenbos (13) were unable to demonstrate antibodies from recovered birds or rabbits repeatedly injected with antigen. Rahn (7) reported significant virus neutralization with some of the same serums. Prince (6) found no relationship between TVH and human serum hepatitis antigen.

DIAGNOSIS.

Presence of lesions in the liver and pancreas is highly suggestive of TVH. The relationship to the picornalike viral infection reported by Macdonald et al. (2) is not clear. Page and Kleven (5) reported somewhat similar lesions in breeding turkeys from which a serotype 1 avian adenovirus was isolated. Bacterial infections producing hepatic lesions can be identified by appropriate bacteriologic examination. Histomoniasis, particularly if suppressed by medication, may produce confusing gross hepatic lesions without cecal involvement. These cases can be diagnosed by demonstration of the histomonad (see Chapter 33).

Virus may be demonstrated by injecting liver suspension into the yolk sac of 5- to 7-day-old chicken embryos. Most embryos die between 4 and 10 days postinoculation and exhibit marked cutaneous congestion and hemorrhage. Low dosage results in delayed mortality; embryos are stunted and show less cutaneous congestion. Embryonic fluids are nonhemagglutinating. Isolates may be further characterized by yolk sac or intraperitoneal injection of poults with yolk harvested from infected embryos, and examination for lesions 5–10 days postinoculation.

TREATMENT. There is no effective treatment. Secondary bacterial invasion does not appear to be an important problem. Prevention of stress, including treatment of concurrent diseases, is indicated.

REFERENCES

1. Bickford, A. 1973. Personal communication.
2. Macdonald, J.W., C.J. Randall, and M.D. Dagless. 1982. Picorna-like virus causing hepatitis and pancreatitis in turkeys. Vet Rec 111:323.
3. Mandelli, G., A. Rinaldi, and C. Giulio. 1966. Hepato-pancreatitis of a probable viral nature in the turkey. G Pollicoltori 16:101–104.
4. Mongeau, J.D., R.B. Truscott, A. E. Ferguson, and M.C. Connell. 1959. Virus hepatitis in turkeys. Avian Dis 4:388–396.
5. Page, L.A., and S.H. Kleven. 1975. Personal communication.
6. Prince, R.P. 1969. Personal communication.
7. Rahn, D.P. 1962. Susceptibility of turkeys to duck hepatitis virus–serologic comparison of duck hepatitis virus and turkey hepatitis virus. MS thesis, Univ Illinois.
8. Snoeyenbos, G.H., and H.I. Basch. 1960. Further studies of virus hepatitis of turkeys. Avian Dis 4:477–484.
9. Snoeyenbos, G.H., H.I. Basch, and M. Sevoian. 1959. An infectious agent producing hepatitis in turkeys. Avian Dis 4:377–388.
10. Snoeyenbos, G.H. 1965. Unpublished data.
11. Tzianabos, T. 1965. Turkey viral hepatitis: Some clinical, immunological, and physiochemical properties. PhD diss, Univ Massachusetts, Amherst.
12. Tzianabos, T. and G.H. Snoeyenbos. 1965. Some physiochemical properties of turkey hepatitis virus. Avian Dis 9:152–156.
13. Tzianabos, T., and G.H. Snoeyenbos. 1965. Clinical, immunological, and serological observations on turkey virus hepatitis. Avian Dis 9:578–595.

30 EXTERNAL PARASITES AND POULTRY PESTS

James J. Arends

INTRODUCTION. External parasites of poultry are arthropods that live on or in the skin and feathers. A few parasites of internal organs are included. Also important are insects that develop in poultry manure, dead carcasses, and moist organic debris, thereby causing sanitation and public relations problems. There is a large number of parasite species of bird hosts and other arthropods related to poultry production; this chapter emphasizes those of the domesticated chicken, turkey, fowl, duck, goose, and pigeon of North America. Reference texts on these parasites are those by Georgi (23), Soulsby (42) Williams et al. (48), Lancaster and Meisch (34), and Kettle (31).

The external parasite problem has changed completely with evolution of the poultry industry to high-density confinement production units. Pests that were once common in poultry flocks are less frequently seen in modern poultry production facilities, and some of the previously minor pests have become major pest problems. Pests such as lice depend upon bird-to-bird transmission. Lice problems are less common in modern poultry practice than formerly, since fewer ages of birds are maintained on a single farm. However, with the increase in integrated poultry production, the chance of human management practices spreading a pest is increased. For example the northern fowl mite, which can live off the host for long periods of time, may be transported on egg flats, other equipment, and clothing of company service personnel as well as on wild birds and rodents. Thus mites remain major problems. Type of housing can be a deciding factor mitigating against some species of mites and flies. The chicken mite seldom infests caged-layer houses, since there are fewer hiding places, such as manure-coated roosts, in which to complete its life cycle. Instead, the crowding of birds favors the northern fowl mite, which completes its life cycle on the birds and moves freely among them. The house fly can be a problem in all types of poultry housing. If a breeding area is present and the temperature requirements are met, flies can increase to large numbers. While the house fly does not generally cause problems to birds, it is a possible nuisance to the surrounding human dwellings and the frequency of complaints against poultry producers about fly numbers is increasing. Modern broiler facilities seldom have ectoparasite problems; chicks arrive with few or no parasites, and there is not enough time for parasites to increase to damaging numbers before birds are slaughtered.

Integrated pest management, which can capitalize on the advantages of modern poultry systems, should be stressed for the control of pests. External parasite problems will be minimized by thorough cleaning of houses between flocks of birds, whole flock replacement rather than partial culling and replacement, smooth-house construction and mesh to keep out wild birds, a sound rodent management program, and keeping manure dry to discourage fly breeding.

Certain ectoparasites of birds (lice) actually eat the dead cells of the skin and its appendages. However, for many, skin merely serves as a medium through which they draw blood or lymph and from which they obtain warmth and shelter. Ectoparasites may be closely confined to their hosts during the entire life cycle (lice), with transmission taking place by host contact. Others wander freely from bird to bird. Some are highly host-specific, contradicting the viewpoint that chicken lice, e.g., can live on horses or other animals. Also, some species may maintain a rather loose relationship and do not always limit their activities to one particular host species or even to birds (gnats, mosquitoes, bedbugs, fleas). Fowl ticks and chicken mites attack birds only at night, hiding in cracks and nests during the day.

These variations in habit and pest biology are important when control measures are considered. Mites cannot be successfully controlled by any single method of attack because of habit variations among species. This indicates the prime necessity for accurate parasite identification to insure that the proper integrated control approach is chosen. In case of doubt, various state and national diagnostic services may be called on for assistance.

Grateful acknowledgement is given for background materials, figures, references, and copyright permissions taken from earlier editions of this chapter written by E.A. Benbrook and E.C. Loomis.

CLASSIFICATION. Poultry ectoparasites are members of the animal phylum Arthropoda, characterized by possession of externally segmented bodies, jointed appendages, and chitinous exoskeletons. However, adaptation to the parasitic mode of life frequently involves modification in form and reduction in characters so that recognition is difficult.

Lice, flies, bugs, and fleas are members of the Class Insecta, characterized by possession of a body divided into three regions (head, thorax, abdomen), one pair of antennae attached to the head, three pairs of legs attached to the thorax, and tracheae (air tubes) for breathing. Some adult insects have wings.

Insects undergo metamorphosis, whereby immature stages may appear totally different from adults, and do not show the characteristics given for the Class Insecta; for example, some fly maggots possess no legs, antennae, or obvious body divisions. Lice, on the other hand, are easily recognized as insects regardless of stage. For classification of insects see Borror and DeLong (7).

Mites are members of the class Arachnida, order Acarina, characterized by fused body divisions, no antennae, and four pairs of legs (the first motile stage, larva, has three pairs). Ticks are very large mites, contrasting sharply with most mites, which are much smaller than most insects. Acarina never possess wings. For classification of mites see Krantz (33).

Common names and scientific binomials used are those accepted by the Entomological Society of America (46).

DETECTION. Poultry seriously infested with the common parasites exhibit irritation and react by scratching and preening. Incipient infestations may be less obvious. Any unexplained production drop or increase in feed conversion is cause to look for external parasites. Lice and northern fowl mites can be found by examining the skin after parting the feathers. Good light and good eyes are needed to see these small parasites. An adequate light is a battery-pack lamp held on the head by its elastic band, leaving the hands free to ruffle the feathers. To monitor birds in a production facility, 20–50 birds should be checked a minimum of two times a month. Birds should be checked at random and should be chosen from all parts of the house. The vent, head, and legs should be closely examined. If parasites are found and cannot be identified at first glance, specimens should be sent to a laboratory or to an entomologist to have the specific identity determined.

Bloodsucking parasites (bed bugs and chicken mites) that come to the birds only to feed are more difficult to detect. It is necessary to examine bedding, roosts, walls, cracks and crevices, and beneath manure clods. A sharp-pointed probe may be useful in prying under splintered wood to reveal ectoparasites. Nest material, dust, and other material collected in the house can be spread out on a white pan and examined. The arthropods can be seen crawling on the pan. This material can also be placed in a Berlese funnel, which is a funnel with a light over it, and the arthropods are collected in a container placed below the funnel. The collection container should have alcohol in it to preserve arthropods that emerge from the funnel. Nighttime examination of birds may detect parasites that feed on them at night. A necropsy examination in the laboratory is required to locate parasites in internal organs.

GENERAL PESTICIDE CONTROL PROCEDURES. Control techniques and strategies will be discussed under sections describing each parasite. For a full description see *Integrated Pest Management Manual* for North Carolina (2). General recommendations of specific chemicals is difficult due to their ever changing availability. Prior to choosing a particular chemical for use, a specialist should be consulted on the best choice and use of the chemical. General information on insecticides, tolerances and residues, and methods of application are presented here to avoid repetition.

The synthetic and natural pyrethroid insecticides, organophosphorus, and carbamate are the main ectoparasite and fly control chemicals used for direct application to poultry, litter, or buildings. In general chemical insecticides and disinfectants should not be mixed for application together (21). There is little reason to use the relatively ineffective older inorganic insecticides such as sulfur and lime. Application methods for many older insecticides require too much labor to be pertinent to modern poultry production. Among the botanical insecticides, pyrethrum remains very effective against flies and is a main ingredient of mist and aerosol fly sprays, particularly with synergists.

In the USA, insecticides for use on poultry must be accepted by the Environmental Protection Agency (EPA) as causing no hazardous residues in eggs, meat, or other edible poultry products. The EPA has set tolerances for use of a few insecticides on poultry or poultry premises. A few others have been declared safe after absence of food residues hazardous to consumers has been demonstrated. The Pesticides Regulation Division of the EPA issues label approvals after all regulations have been met. Each label should be checked to see sure that poultry or poultry housing is listed on the label. The list of approved insecticides is constantly changing.

The chlorinated hydrocarbon insecticides are banned from use on poultry or in poultry houses because of residues in eggs and meat. Under no circumstances should DDT, benzene hexachloride, toxaphene, chlordane, aldrin, dieldrin, endrin, or heptachlor be used on poultry houses or on poultry feed or feed ingredients.

Insecticides are available as wettable powders (WP), emulsifiable concentrates (EC), and water dispersible liquids (WDL), all of which are intended to be applied as a spray or mist. Insecticides are also available as dusts and as baits. These low-assay products are prepared, premixed, and ready to use. Care should be taken to insure that feed and water are not contaminated and that all label directions are strictly adhered to so that tolerances are not exceeded.

Tolerances and Residues. Listed in Table 30.1 are residue tolerances for common pesticides used for control of poultry pests, and time that must elapse between application and slaughter or sale of eggs to meet legal requirements. This time is often spoken of as "withdrawal time," in days prior to slaughter.

All other insecticides (except sulfur and lime sulfur, which require no tolerances) must be accepted as having no tolerance, thus no allowable residue. Fly spray ingredients (pyrethrin and piperonyl butoxide) may be used on poultry or in poultry houses with no interval required between treatment and slaughter or gathering of eggs.

Insecticides should not be used on poultry or in poultry houses without carefully reading all precautions on the label. Illegal insecticide residues in eggs and meat will result if the wrong insecticides are used, the wrong concentration or volume is used, or the application method is wrong. In all treatment of poultry, contamination of feed and water must be avoided. All eggs should be gathered before starting to treat with insecticides. Off-flavors in eggs can be caused by direct contamination of eggshells. Ventilation should be supplied during dusting, spraying, or misting.

Pesticide residues may occur in eggs or meat from contaminants in feed water, litter, or soil. Persistent chlorinated hydrocarbons (particularly DDT and dieldrin) have occasionally been found in poultry feeds, causing illegal residues. In some cases contaminated carcasses have been seized and destroyed after processing. Residue levels in eggs approximate levels in feed, and contaminated eggs continue to be produced long after pesticide ingestion ceases. Because the EPA and Food and Drug Administration (FDA) are concerned with contamination of foods by pesticides, industrial chemicals (PCBs), and toxins (aflatoxin), regular collections are made of poultry, meat, and eggs from market shelves for laboratory analysis of residues. Thus feed manufacturers should buy only pesticide-free ingredients, and poultry producers should not use contaminated local ingredients or keep birds in a known contaminated environment. Grain fumigants can be hazardous to chickens. Fumigated grain should be thoroughly aerated before feeding to poultry.

Application. Laborious individual bird application methods such as dusting or dipping are inappropriate to modern poultry production. The key to any successful application of an insecticide, and resulting control that meets expectations, is to make sure that the insecticide is applied directly to the site where the pest is located. If birds are being sprayed, the treatment must thoroughly cover the entire bird and the bird should be wet to the skin. If buildings are being treated, the sites where the pests are located must be

Table 30.1. Generic or common and trade names of insecticides with specific regulations regarding use with poultry

Generic or Common Name	Trade Name	Primary US Manufacturer	Tolerance, if Established (ppm)	Required Withdrawal Days before Slaughter
Cyromazine	Larvadex	Ciba-Geigy	0.05, MBY[a]	ND[b]
Carbaryl	Sevin	Union Carbide	5, MF 0, E	7
Chlorpyrifos	Dursban	Dow Chemical	0.05, FMBY; 1, E	ND
Coumaphos	Co-Ral	Bayvet	1, MBY	0
Dichlorvos	Vapona	Fermenta Animal Health	0.05, FMEBY	ND
Dimethoate	Cygon	American Cyanamid	0.02, MFEBY	0
Fenthion	Baytex	Bayvet	0.1, MFBY	ND
Fenvalerate (a pyrthroid)	Ectrin	Fermenta Animal Health	Pending	ND
Malathion	Malathion	American Cyanamid	4, MBY 0.1, E	0
Methomyl	Malrin	E.I. DuPont de Nemours	0[c]	ND
Naled	Dibrom	Chevron Chemical	0.05, FMBYE	0
Permethrin (a pyrethroid)	Ectiban Atroban	Coopers Animal Health	0.05, FMEBY	ND
Propoxyr	Baygon	Bayvet	0[c]	ND
Stirofos	Rabon	Fermenta Animal Health	0.75, F; 0.1, E	ND

[a]M = meat, BY = by-products, F = fat, E = eggs.
[b]ND = No documentation for drug withdrawal listed.
[c]Pesticides are listed as having a zero degree tolerance unless special documentation is approved.

treated if control is to be good. Methods of choice for caged layers include high-pressure sprays (125 pounds per square inch [psi]) from outside the cages. Other types of equipment can be used, but if the birds are not treated to insure the wetting of the skin and feathers, control will not be acceptable.

Dusting. For conventional houses the easiest way to use dust is to apply it to litter; figure floor area, weigh amount of dust necessary for this area, and scatter it with a grain scoop or large can, attempting to cover the area evenly including under roosts, feeders, and nest boxes. Dust boxes may be used for birds kept on conventional litter or in cages. Put dilute insecticides in a shallow (3-in.) dusting box, about 1 × 1.5 ft; use one box for every 30 birds, or put one box in each colony cage. Because of the large number of boxes required, this method is seldom used in modern poultry facilities. The use of electrostatic dusters and other dust application equipment has not been used in commercial poultry production. While these methods work well in small-scale tests, they have not worked well in large commercial houses where the dusts do not penetrate the feathers of the birds and control is poor due to the lack of penetration to the skin.

Spraying. The usual cylindric compressed-air sprayers are satisfactory, although slow, for treating roosts and walls, as are knapsack sprayers (continuously pumped during spraying) that give a continuous spray. Sprayers powered by an electric or gasoline motor that deliver pressures of 125 psi and use a spray gun with a solid-stream nozzle are much more rapid and efficient. When spraying houses, high-pressure and large-volume output are most desirable to drive spray into all cracks and crevices. Be sure the sprayer is equipped with an agitator or pump bypass to ensure constant agitation, particularly if wettable powders are used. Dunning et al. (14) and Arends (2) describe portable spray units that are highly adaptable and versatile for use on poultry farms.

Misting. Electric mist machines (foggers) are efficient, rapid, and often laborsaving. Mist machines are concentrate applicators and do not use the same mixtures as ordinary sprayers. Generally they use 5–10 times the concentration and $1/3$–$1/10$ the volume. In all fog work, the container should be shaken frequently during spraying to keep insecticide from settling. Mist machines can be used efficiently to dispense fly spray.

Recommended Treatments. Annual recommendations and guides for use of insecticides listed in Table 30.1, plus information on limitations of use and new EPA label information, can be obtained from state departments of agriculture, cooperative extension offices, or entomology departments at state universities in major poultry-producing regions of the USA.

INSECTS

LICE. Lice are common external parasites of birds. They belong in the order Mallophaga, the chewing lice, and are characterized by possession of chewing-type mandibles located ventrally on the head, incomplete metamorphosis, no wings, dorsoventrally flattened body, and short antennae with 3–5 segments. More than 40 species have been reported from domesticated fowl. Fortunately, as far as the poultry producer is concerned, all the various species of bird lice are controlled by the same methods. Birds frequently harbor several species at the same time.

The list of lice of North American poultry is from Emerson (17, 18), who also includes keys and illustrations of lice on chickens and turkeys. There are many species of bird lice, however, only a few are commonly seen. Bird lice can be found on hosts that are not commonly produced commercially, that is, you may see lice from guinea fowl on chickens and turkeys if these birds have physical contact. Pigeon lice are frequently found on domestic fowl if the pigeons nest above the fowl. The species of louse on infested birds should be determined if cross-contamination from another bird species is suspected. If the lice are not controlled on both birds at the same time, the control program will fail. The more common louse species are listed below.

Chicken lice:
- *Cuclotogaster heterographa,* chicken head louse (Fig. 30.1)
- *Goniocotes gallinae,* fluff louse (Fig. 30.2)
- *Goniodes dissimilis,* brown chicken louse
- *Lipeurus caponis,* wing louse
- *Menacanthus stramineus,* chicken body louse (also turkey, guinea fowl)
- *Menopon gallinae,* shaft louse (also on guinea fowl) (Fig. 30.3)

Turkey lice:
- *Chelopistes meleagridis,* large turkey louse
- *Oxylipeurus polytrapezius,* slender turkey louse
- *O. corpelentus* (common on wild turkeys)

Guinea fowl lice:
- *Goniodes numidae,* guinea feather louse
- *Lipeurus numidae,* slender guinea louse

Duck and goose lice:
- *Anaticola anseris,* slender goose louse
- *A. crassicormis,* slender duck louse
- *Trinoton anserinum,* goose body louse
- *T. querquedulae,* large duck louse

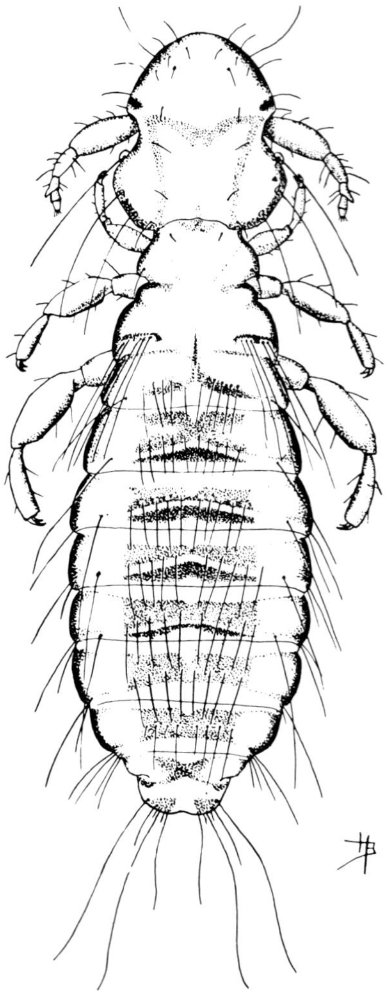

30.1. *Cuclotogaster heterographa,* chicken head louse. (USDA)

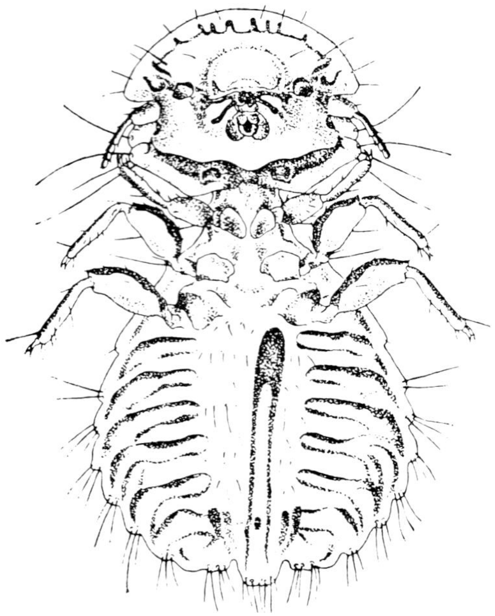

30.2. *Goniocotes,* probably *gallinae,* fluff louse. ×20. (Reis and Nobrega)

Pigeon lice:
- *Campanulotes bidentatus compar,* small pigeon louse
- *Columbicola columbae,* slender pigeon louse (Figs. 30.4, 30.5)

Lice will transfer from one bird species to another if these hosts are in close contact. However, the slender pigeon louse is known to transfer between hosts by transmission with the hippoboscid pigeon fly (*Pseudolynchia canariensis*) (32). Only lice included in the host-parasite list for any one species of bird are likely to become established. Some species of lice occur wherever domestic birds are raised, but they are less frequently found on modern intensive poultry production facilities. Lousiness (pediculosis) of birds is diagnosed by finding the straw-colored lice on

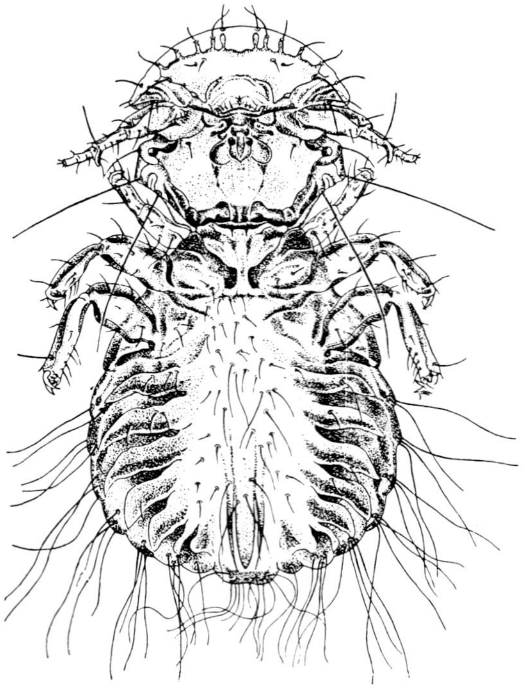

30.3. *Menopon gallinae,* shaft louse. (Kriner)

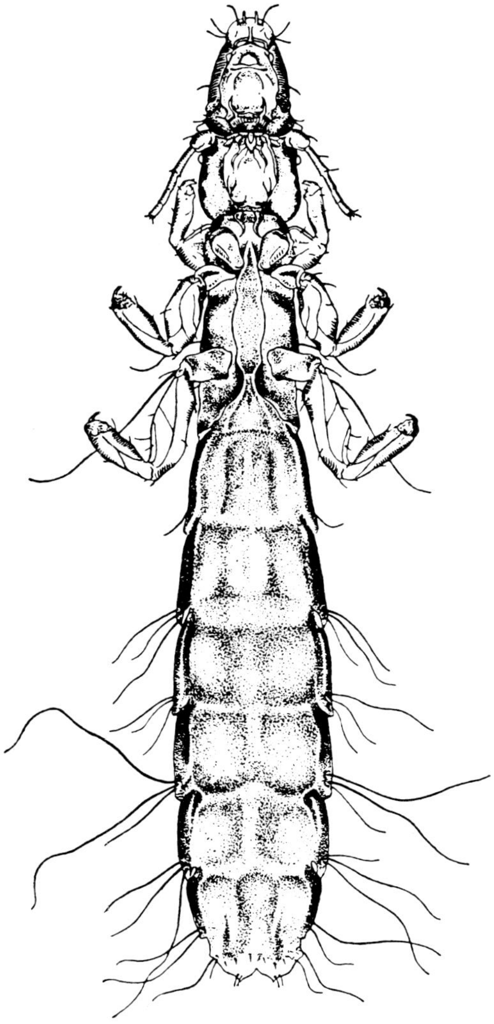

30.4. *Columbicola columbae,* slender pigeon louse. ×42. (Reis and Nobrega)

skin or feathers of birds. Lice of domestic birds vary in size from less than 1 mm to over 6 mm in length. Mallophaga up to 10 mm long occur on wild birds. Lice spend the entire life cycle on the host. Eggs are attached to the feathers, often in clusters, and require 4–7 days to hatch (Fig. 30.5). The entire life cycle takes about 3 wk for completion, including 4–5 days for incubation and three nymphal instars of 3 days each. One pair of lice may produce 120,000 descendants within a few months. Their normal life span is several months, but away from the birds they can remain alive only 5 or 6 days. Although bird lice ordinarily eat feather products, *Menacanthus stramineus* may consume blood by puncturing soft quills near the bases and gnawing through the covering layers of the skin itself.

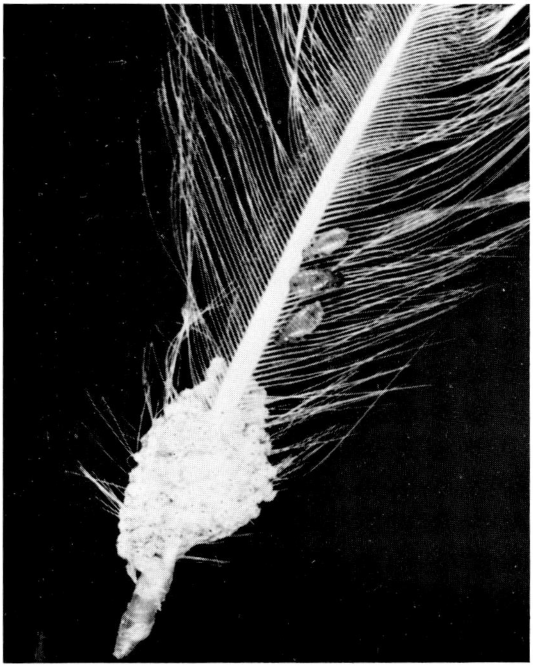

30.5. Eggs of *Columbicola columbae,* slender pigeon louse, at base of feather. ×48. (Reis and Nobrega)

Severe lousiness in poultry originally was thought to follow malnutrition and lead to weight loss as well as low production. There is conflicting evidence on these hypotheses. Warren et al. (45) and Stockdale and Raun (43) found no effect on laying hens, even following rather heavy body louse infestation. Edgar and King (15) concluded that louse-free hens averaged about 11% greater egg production than did those moderately infested. Gless and Raun (24) revealed that an average of 23,000 chicken body lice/hen reduced egg production by 15%. DeVaney (10, 11) showed a decrease in egg production, hen weight, clutch size, and feed consumption when lice-infested birds were compared to uninfested birds, and all decreases correlated with populations of lice. Further research is needed to quantify economic effect and determine differences in effect according to the louse species involved. Breeding lines of chickens also may vary in louse susceptibility. Factors of grooming (related to birds without trimmed beaks) and relative humidity may also be important in determining variations in densities of chicken body lice on birds.

Lice are not highly pathogenic to mature birds, but louse-infected chicks may die. Clinical evidence indicates that lice may irritate nerve endings, thus interfere with the rest and sleep so necessary to immature animals. Lousiness frequently accompanies manifestations of poor health such as internal parasitism, infectious disease, and malnutrition, as well as poor sanitation.

The virus of equine encephalomyelitis has been isolated from *M. stramineus,* as has chlamydia of ornithosis from *Menopon gallinae* and from mites on chickens and turkeys. However, there is little data to support the fact that these lice are actually important in transmission of these agents in the field.

Turkeys may be infested with the common chicken body louse (*M. stramineus*), large turkey louse (*Chelopistes meleagridis*), and slender turkey louse (*Oxylipeurus polytrapezius*), which is occasionally found on wild turkeys. Rearing turkeys in close confinement and unsanitary quarters favors lice more than does range management. It is important that breeding males and females be examined frequently since parasites may contribute to infertility. A common method of introducing lice to an uninfested facility is by the use of infested shipping crates or egg flats or cartons that have been brought on the facility. All equipment used to transfer birds should be cleaned and disinfected before being used on another farm.

Control. Galliform wild or domestic birds should never be allowed to contact poultry flocks. Lice tend to increase during autumn and winter, so flocks should be examined for lice on a regular basis (two times/mo minimum) and treated if needed. If treatment is required, the birds should be treated two times on a 7- to 10-day interval. Only the mature and immature forms will be controlled as none of the available chemicals are ovicidal (eggs are not killed). Retreatment (the second spraying) is necessary to control the lice that will hatch after the initial treatment. In all poultry houses, the egg-laden feathers will continue to be a source of reinfestation and when the house is depopulated, a thorough cleanup should be completed. In many cases, spraying of birds is the best choice for most poultry operations. Spraying when properly done insures that all birds in a house are treated, and with large numbers of birds it is the most practical means currently available. Care should be taken when spraying the birds to insure that the whole bird is treated, as it is common for lice to move to the neck from the vent when populations are large. In caged-layer flocks it is important that the birds are checked on a regular basis. Monitoring is done by randomly checking birds twice a month throughout the house. By following this procedure, infestations can be seen prior to the time that the whole house is infested and control can be implemented on 100–200 birds instead of 60,000. Lice on pigeons can be controlled by using the same methods and materials that are used on commercial poultry.

BUGS. The family Cimicidae in the order Hemiptera includes several bloodsucking parasites of birds. These insects are flattened dorsoventrally, and adults are 2–5 mm long × 1.5–3 mm wide with small padlike wing remnants. Thus they are able to creep into crevices and hide in the daytime. Color varies according to species from brown to yellow or red. The piercing-sucking mouthpart or "beak" is attached far forward on the head and is jointed, folding under the head and part of the thorax when not in use. Stink glands provide the common bedbug and its surroundings with an unpleasant odor. If attacked by large numbers of bugs, young birds may become anemic. Bites are usually followed by swelling and itching caused by injection of saliva into the wound.

Bedbug. The most widespread of these bugs is the common bedbug (*Cimex lectularius*) (Fig. 30.6), which attacks most mammals, including humans, and poultry. It is most prevalent in temperate and subtropical climates. Poultry houses and pigeon lofts may become heavily invaded.

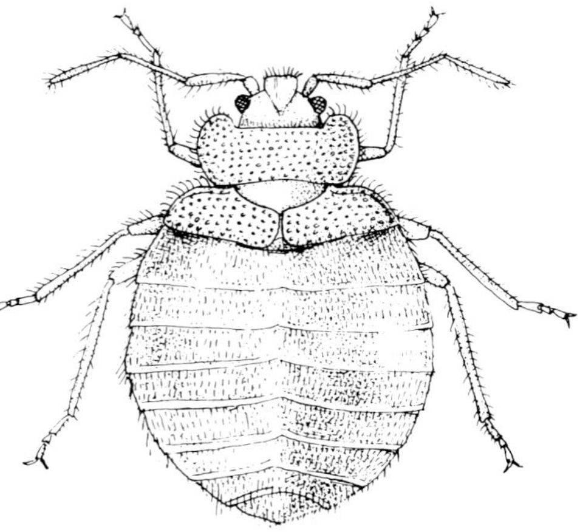

30.6. *Cimex lectularius,* common bedbug. (USDA)

The female bedbug lays several eggs per day in crevices until about 200 have been deposited. Depending on temperature, the eggs hatch in 4–20 days, followed by five nymphal stages that feed at each stage and hide in crevices to digest the blood meal and molt their skins. From egg hatching to adulthood requires 1–3 mo. Nymphs may withstand starvation for about 70 days, while adults live without food for 1–12 mo, depending on temperature. Feeding usually occurs at night, the bugs becoming engorged within 10 min. Large numbers of bed bugs can have a severe impact on production of poultry. Infested breeder houses have shown decreased egg production, increased feed consumption, and lower peak production.

In the tropics and subtropics the closely related

bedbugs *C. hemipterus* and *C. boueti* will also attack poultry. *C. columbarius* attacks pigeons in Europe.

Bird Bug. The most important bird bug is the poultry bug (*Haematosiphon modoru*), also known as the Mexican chicken bug, adobe bug, or "curuco." It occurs in the southern and western USA and Central America and has been found in nests of the California condor, on the great horned owl in Oklahoma, and on the turkey in New Mexico and Arizona. It also attacks humans.

The swallow bug (*Oeciacus vicarius*) is commonly found in nests of swallows (particularly barn swallows) and may spread to poultry and humans.

Other cimicid bugs may be found occasionally on poultry in various countries outside the USA. *Ornithocoris toledoi* is a South American poultry pest known as the Brazilian chicken bug, *O. pallidus,* another South American species, has been found on chicks in Florida and Georgia.

Assassin Bug. The family Reduviidae in the order Hemiptera includes many predacious bugs, but a few known as cone-nose bugs are minor bloodsucking pests of poultry (Fig. 30.7).

The body is cylindrical in shape, and the narrow head bears a stout beak that is curved back into a groove in the prosternum. They are larger than true bedbugs (up to 25 mm in length) and have well-developed wings; otherwise, their morphology, life cycles, and behavior are somewhat similar. Species of reduviid bugs reported as attacking poultry in the USA include the bloodsucking cone-nose (*Triatoma sanguisuga*) (Maryland, Florida, California, Texas) and the western bloodsucking cone-nose (*T. protracta*) (Utah, California). *T. sanguisuga* was found to harbor the virus of equine encephalomyelitis in Kansas, with natural viral infections found in pigeons and pheasants.

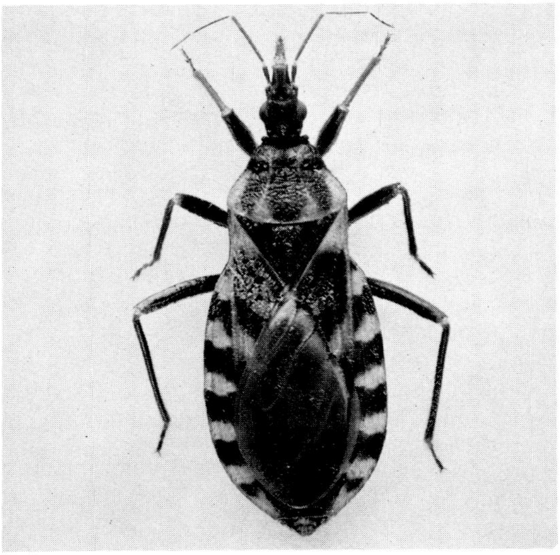

30.7. *Triatoma,* probably *lectularia,* cone-nose assassin bug. (USDA)

Control. Treatment should be directed against daytime hiding places of the bugs–in cracks and crevices of walls and floors and under roosts, nest boxes, and feeders. Spraying the birds will also be helpful if an infestation is large. In a house infested with bedbugs it will be necessary to treat the house and all contents at cleanout. A residual chemical in combination with a fumigant is needed to flush the bugs from their hiding places and give control.

FLEAS. Fleas (order Siphonaptera) are parasites in the adult stage but free-living as larvae. The larvae, which are legless and wormlike and pupate in tiny cocoons, undergo complete metamorphosis. Adults vary in size from 1.5 to 5 mm and possess a tough, laterally compressed body, piercing-sucking mouthparts, short antennae in grooves, and long legs adapted for leaping.

Fleas are brown to black in color and suck blood from various host species. They are cosmopolitan in distribution although more abundant in temperate and warm climates. Females deposit several white spherical eggs per day, which roll off the host into surrounding litter, where they incubate. Dampness and warmth are essential for further development. Within 1–2 wk eggs hatch, liberating tiny maggotlike larvae that feed chiefly on flea feces and on organic matter found in dust and litter. Flea larvae of nesting birds also feed on feather sheaths and epidermal scales of young birds. Fully grown larvae proceed to spin silken cocoons, entangling the threads with various particles of dust and dirt. The inactive pupal stage varies from 1 wk to several months, depending on the temperature. Emerging from the pupal cocoons, young fleas seek a host, suck blood, and are ready to reproduce within a few days. Immature fleas may live for weeks or months without food. Adult fleas may also live for weeks without feeding but live many months to a year when hosts are available. Their life cycle varies greatly, depending on such factors as temperature, humidity, exposure, and host availability. Birds returning to old haunts can become infested with fleas that have remained quiescent for long periods. Many species of fleas have been found on birds, but only three of six species reported from poultry in North America are important for review. To identify fleas and for distributional data, see Fox (19) and Hubbard (30).

Sticktight Flea. The sticktight flea (*Echidnophaga gallinacea*) (Fig. 30.8) occurs more often in the southern USA, although occasionally it is found as far north as New York. Adults usually attach to skin of the head, often in clusters of 100 or more. Mouthparts are deeply embedded in the skin, so they are difficult to dislodge. The sticktight is unique among poultry fleas in that adults become sessile parasites and usually remain attached for days or weeks. Adult females forcibly eject their eggs so that they reach surrounding litter. *E. gallinacea* has been reported from bird hosts (chickens, turkeys, pigeons, blackbirds, bluejays, hawks, owls, pheasants, quail, sparrows) as well as mammals (humans, horses, cattle, swine, dogs, fox, cats, badgers, coyotes, deer, ground squirrel, lynx, mice, opossums, rabbits, racoons, rats, ring-tailed cats, skunks).

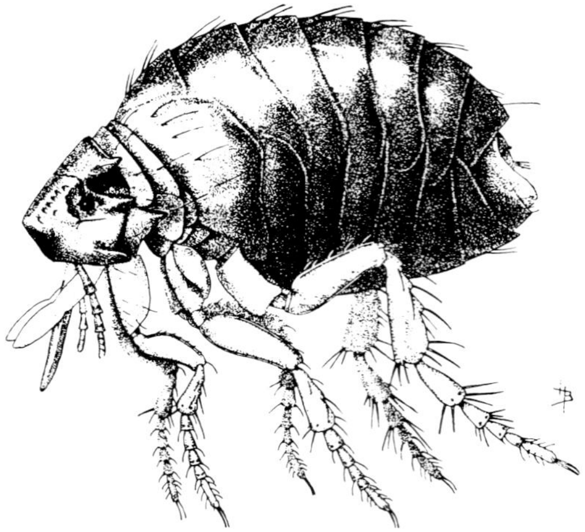

30.8. *Echidnophaga gallinacea,* sticktight flea. (USDA)

This flea does not transmit infectious disease agents to chickens; however, irritation and blood loss may damage poultry seriously, especially young birds in which death may occur. Production is lowered in older birds. The rickettsia that causes human endemic (murine) typhus has been experimentally transmitted from infected rats to guinea pigs through sticktight fleas, thus indicating a possible public health importance of this parasite.

European Chicken Flea. The European chicken flea (*Ceratophyllus gallinae*) (Fig. 30.9) has been reported from Maine, Massachusetts, Connecticut, New York, Delaware, Michigan, and Iowa. Undoubtedly it has a much wider distribution. Hosts include chickens, pigeons, bluebirds, sparrows, and tree swallows as well as humans, dogs, chipmunks, rats, and squirrels. This flea stays on birds only long enough to feed while its immature stages occur in nests and other surroundings.

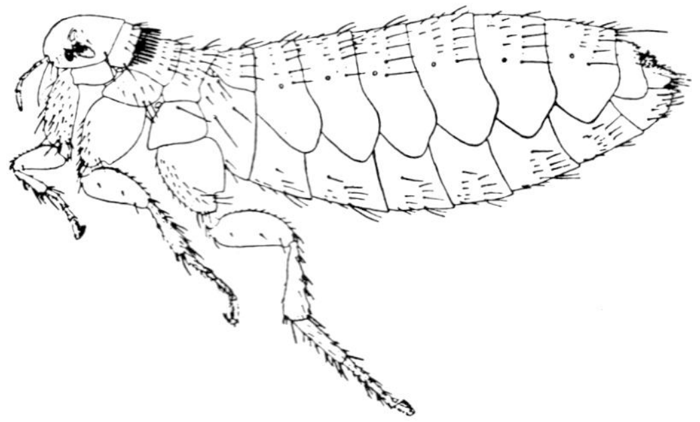

30.9. *Ceratophyllus gallinae,* European chicken flea. (Reis and Nobrega)

Western Chicken Flea. The western chicken flea (*Ceratophyllus niger*) is reported mainly from the Pacific coast and north to Alberta. It may attack various birds and mammals, including chickens, turkeys, cormorants, gulls, magpies, sparrows, and woodpeckers as well as humans, mice, and rats. It resembles *C. gallinae* in appearance and biology.

Others. The cat flea (*Ctenocephalides felis*) has been found in poultry houses at pest levels. Most of these houses are using cats as a rodent control program and it appears as if the cats start the fleas in the house and they then move to the birds. Other pests are accidental, such as is *Orchopeas howardii,* ordinarily found on squirrels. Similarly, the human flea (*Pulex irritans*) occasionally attacks poultry.

Control. The most important control measures are removal of infested litter and thorough house spraying to kill immature fleas. Fresh litter should be put in the house and treated to kill adult fleas on birds and those that drop into litter. In Scotland, tests have shown control of *C. gallinae* by using the pyrethroid permethrin as a 0.125–0.25% spray for nest boxes and litter (44).

Poultry, dogs, cats, and rats should be screened from access under buildings, since they may serve to perpetuate flea invasions. Sunlight, hot dry weather, excessive moisture, and freezing hinder development of fleas.

BEETLES. Beetles (order Coleoptera) possess chewing mouthparts and two pairs of wings, the first pair modified to horny wing covers and the second pair folded under the wing covers except during flight; they experience complete metamorphosis, with a wormlike grub stage followed by the resting pupal stage. No beetles are true parasites of birds, but a few may occasionally feed on living skin. Poultry will feed on beetles found in litter or on the range, thus providing an opportunity for ingestion of parasites or debris associated with the beetles. The following tapeworms can be transmitted by beetles: *Raillietina cesticillus, R. magninumida, Choanotaenia infundibulum, Hymenolepis carioca, H. diminuta,* and *H. cantaniana* (see Chapter 33 for specific host-parasite relationships). Some bacterial and viral infections are probably transmitted by beetles that have fed on infected carcasses. Styrofoam insulation used in enclosed poultry houses may be invaded by various beetle species (lesser or yellow mealworms and dermestids), and severe damage particularly to ceiling areas requires expensive repair (20).

Darkling Beetle or Lesser Mealworm. Darkling beetles are cosmopolitan insects infesting poultry houses around the world. The beetles live in the litter where they feed on spilled poultry feed, manure, and dead or moribund birds. The life cycle of darkling beetles (Fig. 30.10) requires from 1 to 3 mo for the development of the larvae, and the adults can live for 2 yr (20). Darkling beetles are small (0.5 cm), and can be most easily seen under feeders or along the walls of the poultry house. The larvae are wormlike and will avoid light. It should be noted that there will be other species of beetles found in the litter as well as darkling beetles. The other species of beetles are beneficial insects such as histerids and staphylinids and should not be confused with the litter beetle.

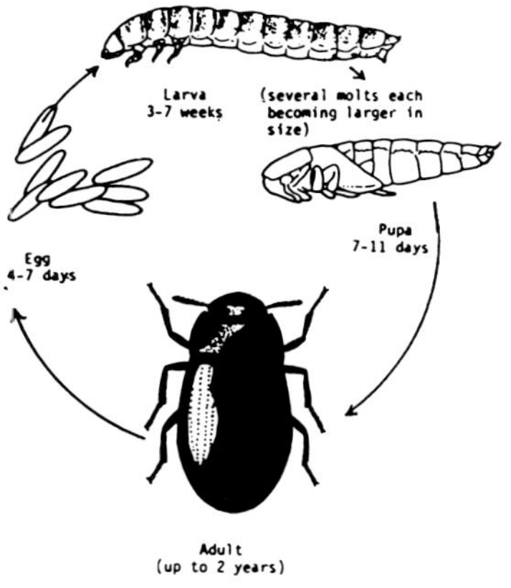

30.10. Life cycle of the darkling beetle.

Beetles within a poultry house can number up to 1000/m^2. They are important to the poultry industry as possible disease vectors, by damage to insulation and as pests. Geden and Axtell (20) reported that only adults and late instar larvae seeking pupation sites were tunnelling in the insulation and that the climbing activity was taking place at night. Beetles can be found throughout the poultry house; eggs, larvae, pupae, and adults are in litter and soil. Due to the beetles' ability to utilize many niches in the poultry house, control is difficult to achieve with any single approach.

Others. The yellow mealworm (*Tenebrio molitor*) is ordinarily found consuming grain products stored in mills, warehouses, bakeries, and groceries. Adult beetles are shiny brown to black in color and about 15 mm long. The yellow larvae or grubs (flour, meal, or branworms) are smooth, cylindrical wormlike creatures up to 30 mm long. They may infest setting hens, mainly attacking the feet, where loss of skin may be followed by severe hemorrhage. These grubs have been found to erode skin of young pigeons; other related mealworm beetle larvae may produce similar damage.

The larder beetle (*Dermestes lardarius*) and related species (*D. maculatus*) ordinarily destroy stored grain products and meats (especially ham and bacon) and feed on hides, skins, furs, museum specimens, or decaying animal matter (notably accumulated droppings in pigeon lofts). The adult is black and about 7 mm long; the basal half of each wing cover is brownish yellow crossed by a band of three black spots. The larvae are up to 12 mm long, dark brown above, gray below, and covered with brown hairs. The larvae may attack skin of nestling pigeons. *D. maculatus* has emerged as a problem in high-rise layer housing where deep-pit manure is used. The beetles feed on dead birds, feathers, and feed in the pits. This beetle will tunnel insulation when seeking pupation sites, and they also tunnel into the structure itself. In some instances the beetles have tunnelled support beams so extensively that the building collapsed.

Silpha thoracica, S. opaca, Necrophorus vestigator, and possibly other species of the beetle family Silphidae (carrion beetles) may also develop in pigeon droppings. Larvae, which are black and up to 15 mm long, are reported to invade the skin of squabs; wounds produced may be secondarily infested by fly maggots.

Control. Generally there is little point in attempting to control beetles on poultry ranges, but control in confined large-scale poultry housing is necessary. Stored grains and feeds should not be allowed to become infested with insects; infested material should be fumigated.

Control of lesser mealworms and hide beetles should be part of an integrated approach that utilizes all possible approaches to manage the population. Any control strategy that is chosen must take into account that there will be a number of eggs, larvae, pupae, and adults in the soil and walls of a building. These life stages will not come into immediate contact with an insecticide and if the insecticide chosen does not have a long residual life, control of the beetles will be shortened. The best control approach is to clean out each house after each flock; however, due to the cost of bedding and labor, this practice is rarely followed. Another approach is to utilize carefully timed insecticide treatments. Houses should be treated with an insecticide immediately after the flock is removed. If treatment is delayed, a number of the beetles will move to inaccessible areas in the house and the insecticide will not come into contact with the beetles. Posts and support poles and braces can be treated as a barrier to the beetles. At the present time there is no one insecticide that would be a best choice for treatment when a flock is removed; any of the currently registered products is acceptable. To monitor the population of beetles in the house, a tube trap can be used (2). By examining the traps weekly, the population trend can be determined.

The darkling beetle is not tolerant of temperatures below 40 F. If the air temperature is less than 40, the house should be opened up at clean-out to allow the temperature of the litter to drop as low as possible. By using cultural controls, low temperature, clean-out schedules, and chemicals, beetle populations can be managed and maintained below damaging levels.

FLIES, MOSQUITOES, MIDGES. The order Diptera includes several families whose members annoy or suck blood from birds as well as mammals. All dipterans have two wings in the adult stage (except degenerate wingless forms) and pass through a complete metamorphosis including a maggotlike larva and a puparium resting stage. Adult mouthparts are of the piercing-sucking or sponging types. The intermittent nature of their feeding and extensive flight range render adult flies ideal vectors of disease. Certain species develop in poultry manure and may become so numerous as to create a health and public relations problem. For identification and information on flies associated with manure, see Axtell, (6).

Mosquitoes. Although mosquitoes are not as important to poultry as to humans and other mammals, many species feed on poultry and transmit disease. Some 140 species have been described from North America; a number of these are known to suck avian blood.

Most mosquito species are about 5 mm in length, and wings are characteristically veined and scaled. Legs and abdomen are long and slender, and the female is provided with elongated mouthparts for piercing the skin (Fig. 30.11). The male does not suck blood but feeds on plant juices, nectar, and other fluids. Mosquitoes deposit eggs on pools of water, moist soil, or surfaces subject to flooding. Larval and pupal stages develop in water, with adults emerging from pupal cases to mate and then seek a host. In warm weather the life cycle is completed in about 7–14 days. Adults are most active on dull, quiet days, especially toward evening and at night.

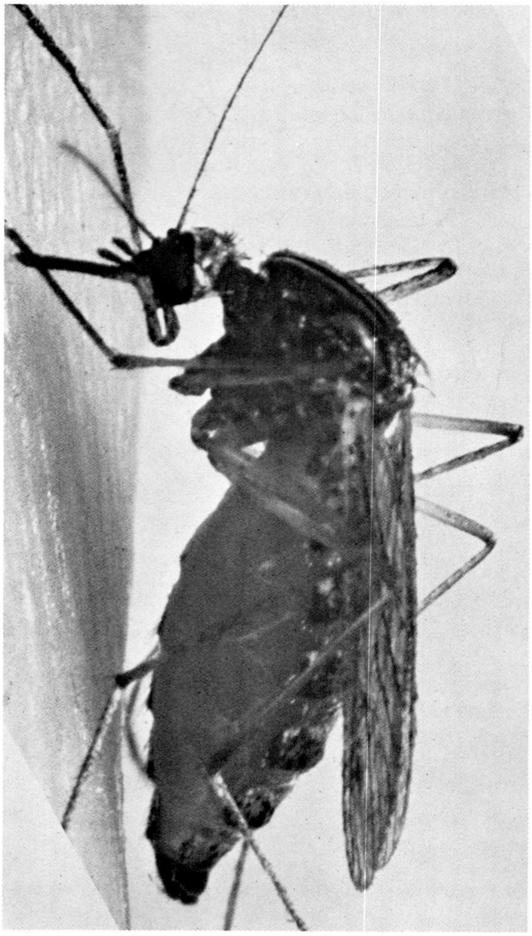

30.11. *Culex tarsalis,* adult female taking a blood meal. (Dunning)

Poultry production facilities that utilize lagoons can have problems with mosquitoes breeding in the lagoon if it is not properly maintained. Lagoons should have steep banks that are free of vegetation along the shoreline and be relatively deep to provide the proper environment for anaerobic decomposition of the waste. If mosquito breeding is a problem and the lagoon requires chemical treatment, Dursban would be the chemical of choice.

Mosquitoes may attack poultry in dense numbers. *Psorophora confinnis* was responsible for the deaths of numerous chickens in Florida. The southern house mosquito (*Culex quinquefasciatus*) was found in dense numbers in chicken houses in Alabama, and their attacks on birds appeared to reduce egg production. The encephalitis mosquito in the western United States (*Culex tarsalis*) shows a host preference for birds, including chickens. Other mosquito species have been found to carry and transmit viral agents of eastern equine encephalomyelitis (EEE), St. Louis encephalitis (SLE), and western equine encephalomyelitis (WEE). Reeves (40) reviewed avian virus reservoirs and mosquito vectors and their relation to human disease. Fowl poxvirus is transmitted by *Aedes stimulans, A. aegypti, A. vexans,* and many species of culicoides biting midges. *A. stimulans* may harbor the virus for 2 days, whereas *A. vexans* may infect birds up to 39 days after contacting the virus of fowl pox and pigeon pox. Vaccination programs for fowl pox are often instituted during seasons when dense mosquito populations are expected.

CONTROL. The best attack is prevention of mosquito development. The farm should be surveyed for all water areas that may produce mosquitoes, including swamps, ponds, stagnant pools, and water-filled containers of all types. Mosquito production can be stopped by removal of such containers, covering cisterns and water barrels, clearing pool and pond edges of emergent vegetation, drainage operations, and filling low areas that collect water.

For housed poultry, mosquitoes landing on surfaces inside or outside the house may be killed by residual insecticide deposits of the type recommended for fly control. Poultry in open houses or on range are most difficult to protect from mosquitoes. Pyrethrum fly sprays can be fogged in houses or on ranges to obtain quick kill of mosquitoes in an outbreak, but control will not last more than a few hours. Residual sprays of carbaryl, malathion, propoxpur, or stirofos can be applied to exterior surfaces of buildings or outdoors to vegetation from which poultry are excluded. If needed, breeding areas can be larvicided using temephos (Abate), or Bti (*Bacillus thuringiensis* var. *israelenis*), a biological control agent that has been shown to be effective.

Area treatment with insecticides is fraught with danger of water contamination and wildlife and fish kills. In many states a permit must be obtained to treat stream and pond drainage basins. Mosquito control and local public health authorities should be consulted for current information prior to outdoor use of pesticides. Promotion of communitywide mosquito control is usually necessary, since water sources may be far from the poultry farm.

Biting Midges. *Culicoides* spp. (family Ceratopoginidae) are biting midges, "punkies," or "no-see-ums"; some 35 species have been reported from North America, and many attack birds and mammals. These are extremely small although easily seen as small blackish specks moving on the skin. In Virginia some 20 species have been taken in chicken coops or found to feed on chickens and turkeys; *C. obsoletus, C. furens, C. sanguisuga,* and *C. crepuscularis* were most abundant. The agent of avian infectious synovitis remains alive in *C. variipennis* for at least 24 hr, but transmission by bites has not been proved for any culicoides species. Some species may serve as intermediate hosts for *Haemoproteus nettionis,* a blood protozoan of domesticated ducks in Canada. Culicodies midges have been incriminated in the transmission of fowl pox.

CONTROL. Controlling biting midges is very difficult. They will pass through ordinary screen mesh, but screens treated with 6% malathion solution have killed midges for more than 3 wk. Fogging with mosquito or fly sprays may alleviate the problem. Residual deposits applied for fly control will also help. Since habitats where these species develop are so variable, it is difficult and often impractical to use measures for source reduction. However, one area that has become a breeding area near poultry housing is improperly managed lagoons. In many cases the midges can be controlled by maintaining the lagoon properly on these facilities.

Blackflies. Blackflies (family Simuliidae) (Fig. 30.12) are also known as turkey or buffalo gnats. They are similar in size to mosquitoes but are dark, short, chunky, and humpbacked, with short legs; wing venation is distinctive. More than 20 species have been reported to attack domestic poultry in North America. Blackflies usually suck blood during the day and may cause serious damage to humans and livestock; in dense numbers on poultry they may cause a severe anemia. They also transmit certain blood protozoans belonging to the genus *Leucocytozoon.*

Blackfly production sources are restricted to running water such as creeks, streams, or irrigation supply and drainage systems. Eggs are laid

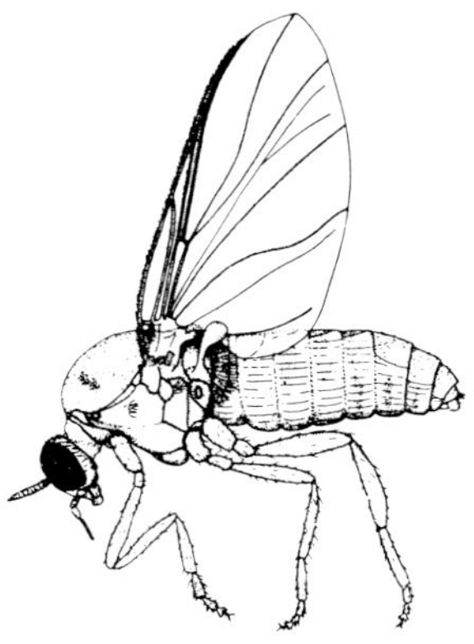

30.12. Blackfly, family Simuliidae. (Travis)

on rocks, sticks, or floating vegetation, or are dropped into streams. They may hatch in a few days, but some remain through summer or even until the following spring. Larvae attach to stones or other objects and reach the pupal stage after 3–10 wk. The pupal stage also occurs under water, lasting from a few days to 1 wk or more. Adults of some species emerge in spring, others during summer or early fall. Overwintering occurs in the egg or larval stage. Most temperate zone species have one generation a year.

Simuliids are most troublesome in the northern part of the temperate zone and the subarctic, but some important species are found in the tropics. Reports in the USA date back to the last century when buffalo gnats were noted to swarm on poultry, forcing setting chickens and turkeys to leave their nests. It is reported that *Simulium bracteatum* fatally attacked goslings and that other *Simulium* species caused losses to chickens and turkeys in Canada. Some species may travel several miles to seek a blood meal; *S. jenningsi* and *S. slossonae* were found to attack turkeys in Virginia as far as 15 mi from their breeding places. In Kansas, egg losses of 50% in 8 days were recorded from chickens attacked by the turkey gnat *S. meridionae*.

Disease transmission by gnats to poultry was initially proved in Nebraska, where *S. occidentale* transmitted *Leucocytozoon smithi,* a blood protozoan of turkeys. Many other blackfly species have been found to transmit *Leucocytozoon* spp. to poultry. *S. venustum* transmits *L. simondi* to tame and wild ducks in Michigan, while in Canada this organism is transmitted to ducks by *S. croxtoni, S. euryadminiculum,* and *S. rugglesi. S. slossonae* and *S. congareenarum* are vectors of *Leucocytozoon* spp. to turkeys in South Carolina. Noblet et al. (39) showed differences in seasonal incidence, levels of transmission, and blackfly vector habits related to *L. smithi* in turkeys in the coastal plains and sandhill areas of South Carolina. This information was overlooked in locating a new turkey industry, and disease outbreaks resulted in great financial losses to a major poultry-producing company. Anderson (1) found that six species of blackflies in Canada transmitted the blood microfilariae of the nematode *Ornithofilaria fallinsensis* to domesticated and wild ducks. Ducks are no longer produced commercially in these localities.

CONTROL. Control is difficult because these pests develop in streams, often some distance from the poultry farm, where insecticide treatment may be harmful to fish. Successful reduction of larval and subsequent adult blackfly populations (and no fish kill) were obtained in infested streams treated monthly by helicopters using 2% temephos granules. Areawide control programs have been developed using biological control agents such as *Bacillus thuringiensis* var. *israelenis* (Bti). These programs involve weekly treatment of all breeding areas in a defined geographical area. Measures recommended for mosquito control as well as cautions on watershed contamination by pesticides are also pertinent to blackfly control.

Housefly and Its Relatives. Nonbiting flies produced on poultry farms are a health and sanitation problem to the poultry producer and neighbors. Public pressure against poultry enterprises can force producers to move or go out of business if flies, odors, or blowing feathers are not controlled. Intensive modern poultry farms produce a tremendous amount of manure, which must be properly managed to insure that it is not attractive to flies for breeding or causing an odor problem.

Location of poultry houses and manure disposal areas needs to be carefully planned to prevent filth fly problems from developing. The entire poultry industry has an important role in community responsibility to control flies in suburban and urban areas. Many poultry producers have met financial disaster as new residential developments have invaded formerly suburban locations where they had built their facilities. In many regions, state and county legislative action has strengthened public health codes, and local ordinances have resulted whereby poultry farms can be closed because of unabated fly sources found on their property. Poultry associations have assisted in drafting legislation and policing the few careless producers who have permitted public health problems to develop.

The common nonbiting flies on poultry farms in the USA include housefly (*Musca domestica*) (Fig. 30.13); *Fannia* spp. (Fig. 30.14) including the little housefly (*Fannia canicularis*), coastal fly (*F. femoralis*), and latrine fly (*F. scalaris*); false stable fly (*Muscina stabulans*); several species of blowflies (Calliphoridae); and flesh flies (Sarcophagidae). So-called filth flies are a worldwide problem on poultry farms, with many other species of *Musca,* other genera, and indigenous Calliphoridae and Sarcophagidae involved. Identification of biting and nonbiting flies and notes on their biology were reported by Loomis et al. (37) and a monograph on fly biology and control by Axtell (6).

Filth flies lay eggs in manure (some sarcophagids deposit living larvae), in moist spilled feed, or on dead-bird carcasses. In hot weather the housefly can complete its life cycle in 8 days, but in colder weather it may require over 6 wk. Larvae (maggots) develop in moist manure and then move to drier areas for pupation. The housefly does not diapause and survives northern winters by slow development in warm indoor locations such as enclosed poultry houses and dairy barns and in towns and cities. Other filth flies survive northern winters by hibernation as diapausing

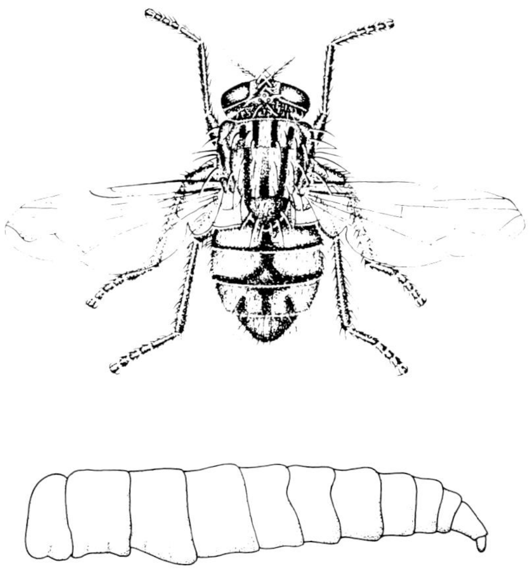

30.13. *Musca domestica,* housefly adult and smooth-tapered larva. (Coop Ext, Univ Calif)

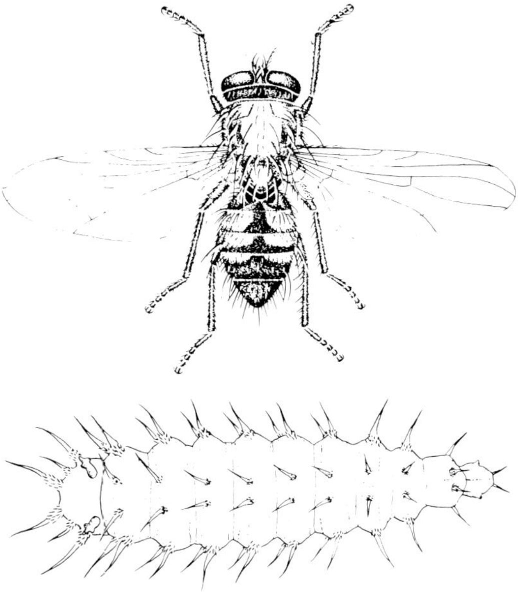

30.14. *Fannia* spp. adult and spinose larva. (Coop Ext Univ Calif)

adults or in immature stages.

Flies have been incriminated as vectors of many mammalian as well as avian gastrointestinal diseases, largely through their habit of feeding on inoculum in excrement and regurgitation onto food or feeds (47). Newcastle disease virus was isolated from adult *F. canicularis, F. femoralis,* and *M. domestica* larvae during an outbreak of this disease in California. Houseflies and maggots are readily eaten by birds, thus affording transmission of helminths for they are intermediate hosts for the tapeworm *Choanotaenia infundibulum* of chickens and turkeys. Common housefly and blowfly species are capable of carrying eggs of the cecal worm *Heterakis gallinae,* which may contain the protozoan agent of histomoniasis of turkeys.

Certain fly larvae feed on decomposing cadavers and may ingest toxins of the bacterium *Clostridium botulinum.* If poultry eat such maggots, botulism ("limberneck") may occur. Larvae of the following species of flies have been incriminated as transmitters of botulinus toxins, types A and C: *Lucilia illustris* and *Phaenicia sericata* (Calliphoridae); sarcophagid larvae; larvae of *Cochliomyia macellaria* (Calliphoridae), the secondary screwworm fly. Prompt burial, burning, or use of disposal pits for animal cadavers will do much to prevent botulism from these sources.

It is known that common houseflies feeding on infected fowl cholera blood can transmit this disease when fed to turkeys. Larvae of fly species that often develop in tuberculous chicken cadavers can also transmit *Mycobacterium tuberculosis* when fed to nontuberculous chickens.

Invasion of birds by fly larvae (maggots) is not as common as in mammals. The black blowfly (*Phormia regina*) can deposit eggs in wounds on chickens, turkeys, and geese, and the ensuing maggots may destroy living tissue. Nests of wild birds may become infested by maggots of other species of flesh flies and blowflies, with disastrous effects on nestlings.

CONTROL. Fly control on poultry farms should be based on integrated pest management (IPM) principles that include judicious use of cultural (manure management), biologic (parasites and predators), and chemical (insecticides) control strategies. By utilizing such an IPM approach, flies can be maintained below threshold levels (5). Manure should be maintained in a moisture range of less than 60%. Manure moisture of 60–90% is ideal for fly development. Sufficient air flow should be provided over the manure to aid in its drying. All tall vegetation that might reduce the flow of air into the house should be cut. All watering devices should be maintained and water leaks repaired. The selection of building site is also very important. The site should be well drained and constructed properly. Roofs should be in good condition in order to keep manure cones dry and the roof overhang should be large enough to insure that rain will be carried away from the building and not pool next to the foundation where it is often found leaking back into the manure. Clean-out should be completed on a schedule, remembering that in hot weather the housefly maggot can develop in less than 1 wk and other pest species in 2–3 wk. On-farm storage can be done by proper composting of manure in short windrows or covering with a black polyethylene tarpaulin to prevent fly production. If manure is stored in a shallow or deep pit under the birds, clean-out should be completed in the winter, which will allow time for a new dry pad of manure to develop prior to fly season. This will act as an absorbent pad as well as a reservoir for parasites and predators.

After all possible physical methods of maintaining dry manure have been completed, attention should be directed to the use and fostering of the natural and introduced biologic control organisms–mites, beetles, and parasitic wasps. Biologic methods include retention of indigenous as well as introduced predators and parasites of eggs, larvae, and pupae of filth flies such as predator mites (*Macrocheles muscaedomesticae, Fuscuropoda vegetans*); predator beetles (*Carcinops pumilo*) and other Histeridae; and parasitic hymenopterous wasps (*Muscidifurax, Spalangia sp.*) and other parasites of the eggs, larvae, and pupae of filth flies (5).

The success of releasing parasites into a poultry house to control a fly population has been mixed (5). In general, due to strain differences and rearing problems, the most successful approach with parasites has been to insure that the environment of the poultry house is conducive to natural reproduction of the parasites.

Predators of filth flies include histerid beetles, macrochelid mites, and the muscid fly *Ophyra aenescens*. Geden et al. (22) reported that the daily destruction of fly larvae and eggs would range from 5 to 30/predator. By maintaining the manure in the poultry house in a dry condition, the effectiveness of predators can be enhanced and in many cases chemicals will not be needed to maintain the fly population below threshold.

It is useful to have a method of evaluating a fly population within the poultry house. Monitoring methods should be simple and give an accurate assessment of the population so that the effectiveness of a control program can be measured. By using a monitoring system, treatment can be timed to give the maximum level of control before the population reaches problem levels. Methods for monitoring flies are grid counts, sticky fly ribbons, baited jug traps, and spot cards. The two simplest methods of monitoring are the baited jug trap and the spot cards. Jug traps consist of a plastic 1-gal milk jug with four 3-in. holes cut in the upper ⅓ of the jug. One ounce of fly bait that contains Muscalure is placed in the bottom (38). Flies enter to feed in the jugs and die, with the number of flies being counted weekly in each trap to determine the level of flies in the house. A minimum of 6 traps should be used in each house and a threshold of an average of 350 flies/trap/week would indicate a need for treatment. This threshold will vary depending upon the location of the poultry house and the nearness of neighbors. A second method of fly monitoring is the use of spot cards. Index cards (3 × 5 in.) should be placed on fly resting sites, rafters, etc. A minimum of 10 cards should be used with a threshold of 50 specs/card indicating a need for treatment (38). Visual monitoring should be done for fly larvae. Areas where manure is wet should be checked and if larvae are seen, these areas should be treated.

The use of insecticides for fly control is an important component in an integrated fly control program. Insecticides that are registered for use in poultry buildings for fly control are the only insecticides that should be used to avoid residues in eggs or meat. Insecticides that are efficacious against flies will also kill predators and parasites, and care must be taken when using insecticides to insure that the predator and parasite population is not decreased due to improper application of an insecticide.

Insecticides can be applied in four basic ways: space sprays/fogs; surface sprays/residuals; baits; larvicides. Each method has merit and can be an aid in reducing the fly population in the poultry facility but must be used properly for the maximum benefit and lowest cost.

Space Sprays, Fogs, Mists. The use of space sprays gives temporary control of adult flies. There is no residual or long-term effect of these applications with all the flies being killed at the time of application. Space sprays and mists should be applied early in the morning or late in the evening when most of the flies will be resting within the building. They can be applied with hand-held or tractor-mounted units. The equipment should break the insecticide into fine droplets, and in general, formulations that have an oil or petroleum product base will be more effective, although the oil may irritate animals. Piped-in systems that are designed to deliver a small amount of insecticide on a regular basis (hourly or six times daily) can also be installed in the facility. One key point that should be remembered when using a mist for fly control is that the mist must hang in the air as long as possible for full effectiveness. If a house is well ventilated and air is being rapidly moved at the time of application, control will be decreased due to the short time that the product and flies can come into contact. It may be necessary to close the curtains or stop the fans until after the treatment is completed.

Surface Sprays/Residuals. Residual surface sprays should be applied as a coarse spray to areas that adult flies rest on. These surfaces include posts, overhead beams/rafters, vertical surfaces, etc. Surface sprays may be applied with any type of sprayer at low pressure (40 psi) with the resting surfaces treated until thoroughly wet but without runoff. Insecticide formulations used are water dispersable liquids, wettable powders (WP), and emulsifiable concentrates. In general the WP formulations will give a longer lasting residue than the other formulations. Dust, type of surface, and amount of sunlight on the surface will all have an effect on how long the product remains active.

Baits. Commercial baits are generally formulated as granules and should be placed in pans or in protected areas. Bait can also be placed in fly traps. To increase effectiveness of dry baits such as methomyl, one part field-grade molasses may be diluted with three parts water in a 5-gal can and covered with a removable window screen lid on which the dry bait is placed. Some commercial baits add a fly attractant such as muscamone, which greatly increases their effectiveness.

Larvicides. Control of fly larvae in the manure is done with a larvicide, which can be applied as a liquid, dry, or in the bird feed. Penetration of the manure with a liquid is difficult, and it is adding water to manure, which will make it more difficult to dry to reduce breeding. Larviciding manure is also devastating to the predators and parasites living in the manure causing a further imbalance of the fly larvae and predators and parasites. Larvaciding should only be done on a spot treatment basis where large numbers of larvae are seen. One exception to this is the larvicide cyromazine, which is toxic to fly larvae but not to the predators and parasites.

Stable Fly. The stable fly (*Stomoxys calcitrans*) attacks most mammals and birds. This fly is similar in size and appearance to the common housefly but possesses a piercing beak. Stable flies develop in manure with high fiber content or in wet crop refuse such as straw left in the field after grain harvest. Near the seacoast they can be very annoying, since they develop in windrows of wet seaweed.

CONTROL. Stable flies can be controlled in poultry houses by the same measures used against houseflies. Prevention requires cleanup of crop and other plant refuse and proper manure management to prevent mixing of moist manure with spilled feed.

Pigeon Fly. The pigeon fly (*Pseudolynchia canariensis*), a member of the parasitic fly family Hippoboscidae, or louse flies, is a rather important parasite of domesticated pigeons in warm or tropical areas (Fig. 30.15). It has been known since 1896 in the southern half of the USA and also occurs in many other countries. The body is dorsoventrally flattened, and the head is provided with a short stout beak. The life cycle is unusual in that the larva matures inside the female and pupates immediately upon being ejected. The pupal stage requires about 30 days; adults live about 45 days and deposit four or five young.

The adult pigeon fly is dark brown, about 6 mm in length, with two transparent wings somewhat longer than the body. These flies move rapidly through the feathers and suck blood, particularly from nestling pigeons 2–3 wk of age. They may

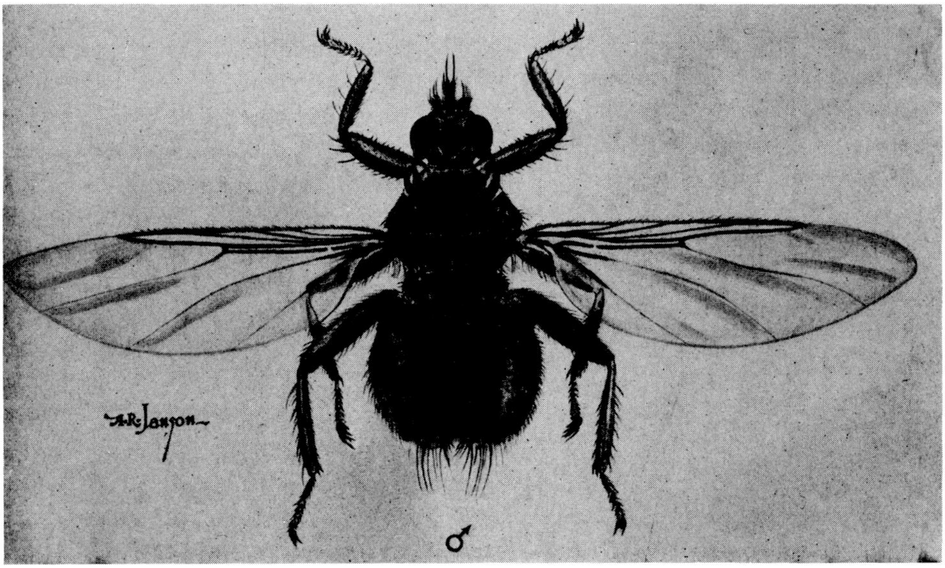

30.15. *Pseudolynchia canariensis,* pigeon fly. (Drake and Jones)

also bite humans, inflicting a painful skin wound that persists for several days. Infested pigeons suffer from blood loss and irritation. The pigeon fly may also transmit a protozoan blood-cell parasite (*Haemoproteus columbae*), the cause of a malarialike disease of pigeons.

CONTROL. See control of mites.

MITES. The common free-living ectoparasitic mites of poultry belong to the family Dermanyssidae and include the chicken mite, northern fowl mite, and tropical fowl mite. These mites possess relatively well-sclerotized, free dorsal and ventral plates; claws and caruncles on the tarsi; one lateroventral stigma near each third coxa; and small chelicerae on long, sheathed bases. They are bloodsuckers and can run rapidly on skin and feathers. Of lesser importance are members of many other mite families that bore into the skin or infect various internal passages and organs.

Chicken Mite. The chicken mite (*Dermanyssus gallinae*), also called red mite, roost mite, or poultry mite, is found worldwide and is particularly serious in warmer parts of the temperate zone in older poultry houses with roosts. The mite is rare in modern large commercial caged-layer operations but is seen frequently in modern broiler breeder farms. It can be identified by the shape of the dorsal plate and by the long whiplike chelicerae that appear to be stylets (Fig. 30.16). The adult female measures about 0.7 × 0.4 mm, varying in color from gray to deep red, depending on its blood content. The life cycle may be completed in as little as 7 days. Adult females lay eggs in surroundings of the hosts 12–24 hr after their first blood meal. Eggs hatch in 48–72 hr when warm. The 6-legged larvae molt in 24–48 hr without feeding, becoming first-stage bloodsucking nymphs; they then molt to second-stage nymphs in another 24–48 hr and soon afterward molt to the adult stage. Chicken mites have lived up to 34 wk without food.

Chickens are the commonest hosts, but these mites may occur on turkeys, pigeons, canaries, and several species of wild birds. Humans may also be attacked, and invasions of human dwellings (apartments, hospitals, doctor's offices) by mites from outdoor pigeon nests are frequently seen. English sparrows may transmit this parasite because of the habit of lining their nests with chicken feathers. These mites may not only produce anemia, thereby seriously lowering production and increasing feed consumption, but actually kill birds, particularly chicks and setting or laying hens. Birds in production may refuse to lay in infested nests.

An increase in feed consumption accompanied by lower production are signs that poultry houses should be examined for mites. These mites often can be found by looking under loose clods of manure, under slats in a breeder house, in nests or in cracks and crevices of posts and roof bracing. They are evident as tiny red to blackish dots, often clustered together. Inspection during the night is usually necessary to find mites on birds. Occasionally these mites may be found on the shanks of both hens and roosters but care must be taken to differentiate them from northern fowl mites that also appear on the legs.

Northern Fowl Mite. The northern fowl mite (NFM) (*Ornithonyssus sylviarum*) is the com-

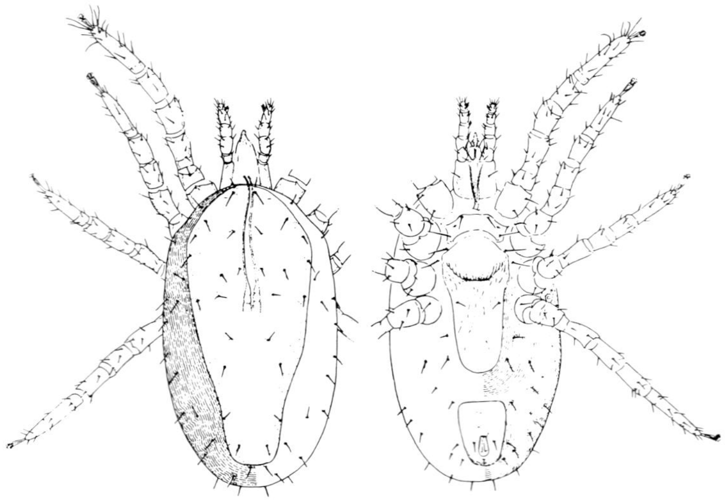

30.16. *Dermanyssus gallinae,* chicken mite. (Baker)

monest and most important permanent parasite of poultry in all major poultry production areas of the USA. It is also recognized as a serious pest throughout the temperate zone of other countries. It is extremely common in almost all types of production facilities. It has been reported from many species of birds, including domesticated poultry, English sparrows, numerous wild birds, and also from rats and humans.

This mite is often confused with the chicken mite but can be distinguished by its possession of easily visible chelicerae and the shape of dorsal and anal plates (Fig. 30.17). Unlike the chicken mite, the northern fowl mite can easily be found on birds in the day as well as night, since it breeds continuously. In heavy infestations feathers are blackened (Fig. 30.18) and skin is scabbed and cracked around the vent; when birds are handled, mites quickly crawl over the examiner's hands and arms. Parting the feathers reveals mites, their eggs, cast-off skins, and excrement on the body surface and feathers. Poultry producers often diagnose NFM infestation by seeing mites crawling on eggs. However, the proper way to monitor for NFM is to check a sample of 20–60 birds in the house. In layer houses birds should be removed from cages at random throughout the house and the vents examined. Turkeys and broiler breeders should be caught and checked, with more males being checked than females. Birds from all sections of a house need to be examined as it is common for NFM to start in one section and then slowly spread throughout the house. If the birds are monitored twice monthly, a NFM infestation can be caught before it causes economic damage and a smaller number of birds can be treated.

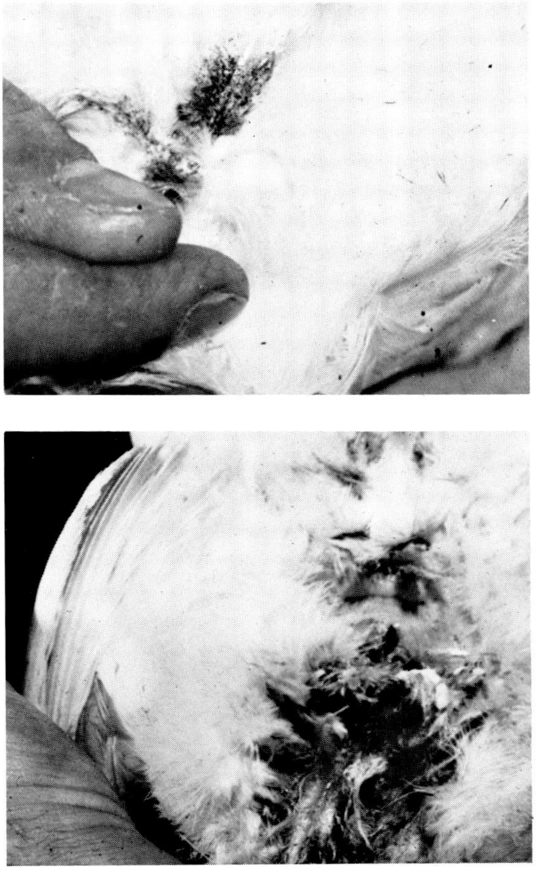

30.18. Two levels of feather blackening and soiling by northern fowl mite. (Matthysse)

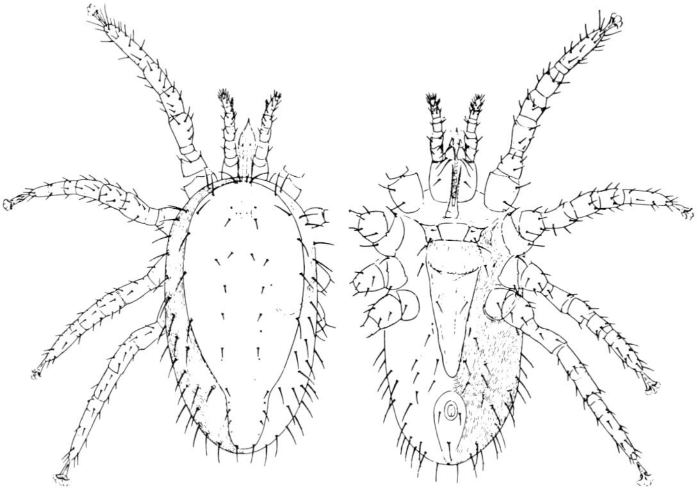

30.17. *Ornithonyssus sylviarum,* northern fowl mite. (Baker)

The life cycle of the northern fowl mite is completed in less than 1 wk on the birds. Eggs are laid on the feathers and hatch in 1 day. The larval instar and two nymphal instars develop in less than 4 days. In the north, mite densities increase in winter and usually drop to low numbers by summer. Occasionally, however, infestations are found in summer. This contrasts with the chicken mite, which is a pest during warm weather in northern areas but inactive in cold houses during winter. Mites may survive 3–4 wk in absence of avian hosts.

The NFM is introduced into laying hen flocks from four main sources: infested hatcheries and contract-started pullet farms; trucks and crates used to carry old birds or infested pullets; personnel, equipment, or egg flats and crates; and wild birds. Sparrows, pigeons, etc. that nest in or near poultry houses are suspected, although tests to infest chicks with northern fowl mites taken from sparrows have not proved successful.

These mites suck blood, and the resulting scabs may injure the appearance of dressed poultry. Of greater concern is the economic importance of this mite to egg production from infested caged layers. Recent investigations indicate the following factors relating to mite densities on hens showing normal or reduced egg production: breed or strain differences (11, 36); plasma corticosterone levels and cage stress (26); estrogen levels (27); and immune responses and genetic heritability (12, 16). Arends et al. (3) showed that in broiler breeder laying hens, NFM-infested birds produced 7.7 eggs/hen less than NFM-free birds and that feed costs were increased from $.01 to $.06/dozen eggs produced. These and other investigators agree that the northern fowl mite is deleterious to male birds, with extremely dense infestations causing lowered semen production, anemia, and even death.

Although WEE and SLE viruses have been recovered from the northern fowl mite obtained from wild birds, it is doubtful that this mite plays any important role in the epidemiology of encephalitides. The northern fowl mite may harbor the viruses of fowl pox and Newcastle disease of poultry after feeding on infected chickens, but proof of transmission is lacking. Chlamydia have been isolated from fowl mites (*Ornithonyssus* sp.) and from nonparasitic mites found in nests of turkeys 2½ mo after their abandonment because of ornithosis in the flock (8).

Tropical Fowl Mite. The tropical fowl mite (*Ornithonyssus bursa*) (Fig. 30.19) is distributed throughout the warmer regions of the world and possibly replaces the northern fowl mite in these regions. It is a much less important pest in the USA. Hosts include poultry, pigeons, sparrows, myna birds, and humans. The tropical fowl mite closely resembles the northern fowl mite but can be distinguished by the shape of the dorsal plate and pattern of setae. This mite can pass its entire life cycle on chickens. Its biology and habits are similar to those of the northern fowl mite, although a greater proportion of its eggs are laid in the nests.

Control. The chicken mite, northern fowl mite, and tropical fowl mite may be controlled by the same insecticides applied to birds, litter, nests, and the walls and roosts of the facility.

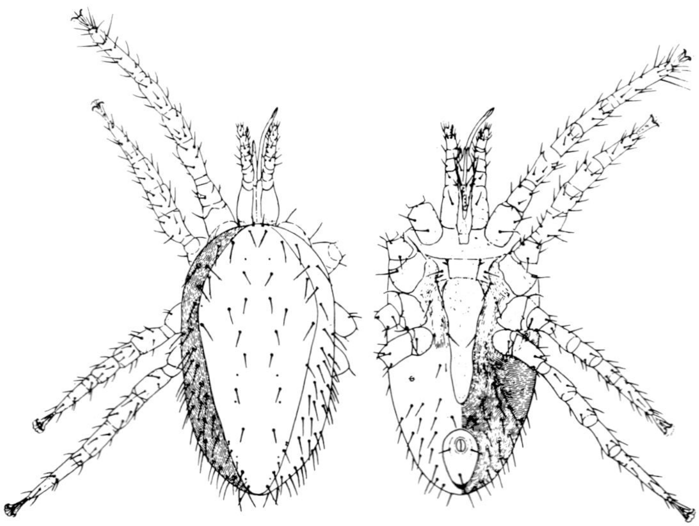

30.19. *Ornithonyssus bursa,* tropical fowl mite. (Baker)

Initial control strategy should be focused on monitoring all birds and the facilities. Proper monitoring will reduce the spread of ectoparasites from farm to farm on service personnel, flats, repair personnel, replacement birds, and live-haul equipment. By following an active monitoring system, infestations can be identified and movement on and off these facilities restricted. By reducing the number of houses that are infested, the cost of control can be drastically reduced. This is especially true for most modern, vertically integrated companies that may have large numbers of houses that are linked by feed trucks, egg trucks, and service personnel.

All egg flats and cases should be checked if they are coming off an infested farm. Operations that use plastic flats on racks should be sure that they are washed with hot water and detergent prior to being redelivered to another farm. Operations that use fiber flats and cardboard cases should inspect them prior to sending them back to a farm. Data from the North Carolina State Integrated Pest Management Program for Poultry has shown that as many as 19 adult NFM/egg case can be transported from an infested farm through the hatchery and back on another farm.

Birds can be treated with any of the registered insecticides. All flocks should be treated twice on a 5- to 7-day interval for NFM and longer with other parasites. With lice and NFM, the birds should be treated to insure that the skin is wet, since this is where the pests reside. The most efficient method to use in most poultry facilities is a solid stream spray at 40–125 psi. Care should be taken to insure that the birds are wet to the skin or control will be less than desired. Arthur and Axtell (4) found permethrin EC spray to be the most effective chemical registered, lasting up to 9 wk after treatment when applied at .05%. Red mites can be controlled by treating both the birds and the facility. If the red mites persist in a house, the house should be retreated at clean-out.

Laelaptidae. Occasionally, mites of the family Laelaptidae will infest chickens, e.g., *Haemolaelaps casalis,* which has also been found on pigeons.

Uropodidae. Heavy infestations of scavenger mites found in the litter have frequently alarmed broiler producers as they prepare for a new batch of chicks. These mites, which are fungus feeders, often multiply in old litter and then climb through to the surface of new pine shavings used as top dressing. If examined with some magnification (×10) and identified as a member of the Uropodidae family, the producer may rest assured that the mite is harmless and that treatment or a last minute clean-out is unnecessary.

Chigger. Chigger infestations are sporadic and localized; a heavily infested site may adjoin a habitat that appears similar to it in all respects but is free of these mites. Chiggers affect poultry mainly in the southern states and only birds that are housed outside on the ground. Larval mites of the family Trombiculidae are called chiggers. Nymphs and adults are free-living, usually in or on soil. Although over 700 species are known, only a few attack poultry. The larval chigger is 6-legged and possesses a single dorsal plate bearing a pair of sensillae and 4–6 setae. The legs are 7-segmented and bear 2 claws and an empodial bristle. Unfed chigger larvae are 0.1–0.45 mm in diameter, hence hardly visible unless engorged, when they appear as minute red dots. Adults occur on the ground, especially along fence rows or in undisturbed wooded or bushy areas. Larvae attach to the skin, often in groups, and inject a highly irritating substance into the wound, thereafter feeding on liquefied host tissue but not blood. Itching vesicles or even abscesses surrounded by a zone of hyperemia and edema may form at the points of attachments. Apparently, a toxemia may occur, as indicated by the mortality that follows infestation of chicks, especially quail.

The most important poultry chigger in the USA is *Neoschongastia americana* (Fig. 30.20), which is a serious pest of turkeys and wild birds and a minor pest of chickens all across the South (particularly Georgia, the Carolinas, Texas, Alabama, Arkansas, Missouri, and Kentucky) as well as Nebraska. This chigger also occurs in Central America and the West Indies. *N. americana* was not important in past years when turkeys were marketed almost exclusively for the Thanksgiving and Christmas holidays in contrast to current

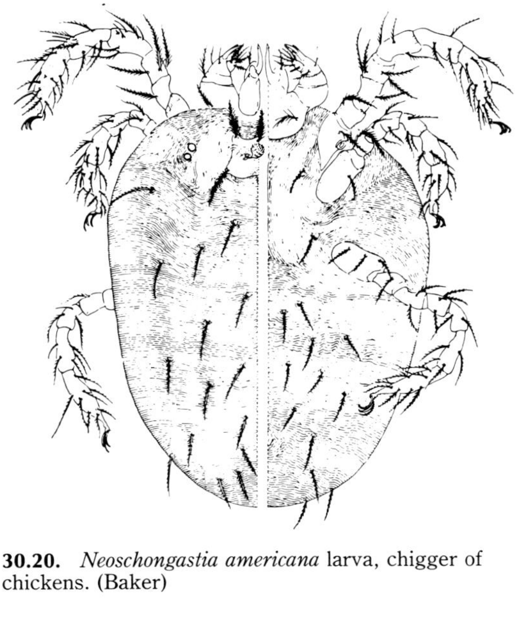

30.20. *Neoschongastia americana* larva, chigger of chickens. (Baker)

marketing throughout the year, including the summer period of chigger activity.

Feather Mites. Most mites in the families Analgesidae, Pterolichidae, and Proctorphyllodidae and a few in Cheyletidae live on the feathers of birds or in the quills. These feather mites are rather host specific, and over 25 species are found on poultry throughout the world. Feather mites are rarely found on modern chicken farms because the cycle is broken by separation of the hatchery from producing flocks. Although reports from Germany cite no pathogenicity caused by feather mites on ducks, Indian workers claim pathogenicity with loss of vigor, poor laying performance, and with clinical signs similar to those of the depluming mite.

Feather mites (except *Syringophilus*) belong to the superfamily Analgesoidae of the suborder Sarcoptiformes.

The quill mite (*Syringophilus hipectinatus*) occurs inside quills of poultry, and wild birds harbor related species: *S. columbae* in pigeons and *S. minor* in house sparrows. These mites are elongate, with long setae on the body. Females measure up to 0.9 mm in length and 0.15 mm in width. The cycle of development from eggs to sexually mature adults takes from 38 to 41 days, and only males develop from eggs deposited by unfertilized females (parthenogenesis).

This species has been found on chickens, turkeys, and golden pheasants in Ohio and on chickens in New Jersey, Maryland, and Pennsylvania. These mites appear to cause partial or complete loss of feathers. The remaining quill stumps contain a powdery material in which mites may be detected under low-power magnification. No specific method for control has yet been described. It would appear advisable to dispose of affected birds, then disinfect and clean their quarters.

Other feather-damaging mites (family Pterolichidae) include *Falculifer rostratus* (Europe, USA) and *F. cornutus,* occurring chiefly between the barbs of the large wing feathers of pigeons; *Freyana chanayi* (USA), in the grooves on the underside of shafts on wing feathers of turkeys; *Dermoglyphus minor* and *D. elongatus* (USA), from inside chicken and turkey quills; and *Pterolichus obtusus* (USA), on flight and tail feathers of chickens. *Megninia cubitalis* (family Analgesidae) occurs on chickens and less so on turkeys in the USA, with *M. gallineulae* (Canada) on the legs and head region of chickens, *M. ginglymura* (depluming mite in India) on chickens and turkeys, and *M. columbae* (USA) on the neck and body areas of pigeons.

Records of economic damage by these mites are rare, although a few reports cite possible reduced egg production in relation to malnutrition, feather loss, and dermatitis in mite-infested body regions where crustlike lesions appear on the lower legs and the skin of combs and wattles. Other skin lesions of poultry can be caused by ectoparasite mites of the families Sarcoptidae and Epidermoptidae, but these parasites are rarely encountered on large poultry production farms.

Scaly-Leg Mites. *Knemidocoptes mutans* (Sarcoptidae) (Fig. 30.21) is one of a dozen related species of scaly-leg mites occurring on various birds. They are most commonly found on older birds that should ordinarily be culled from flocks. The mites are almost spherical in shape and short-legged, with strongly striated epidermis, and the dorsal striations are not interrupted. Adult females are about 0.5 mm in diameter. The mites pass through their entire life cycle in the skin, with transmission to uninfested birds by contact with infested birds and their surroundings. Lesions are produced on unfeathered portions of the host's legs and occasionally on skin of the comb and wattles. Tunnels are bored into the epithelium, causing proliferation and formation of scales and crusts (Fig. 30.22). Affected birds may be crippled if the infestation is severe.

CONTROL. Control of scaly-leg mites should begin by culling or isolating affected birds. Additions to the flock should be covered with an application of warm vegetable oil to loosen scabs, which can then be scraped from the leg, placed in a vial, and sent to a diagnostic laboratory for microscopic examination. If scaly-leg mites are found, it is best

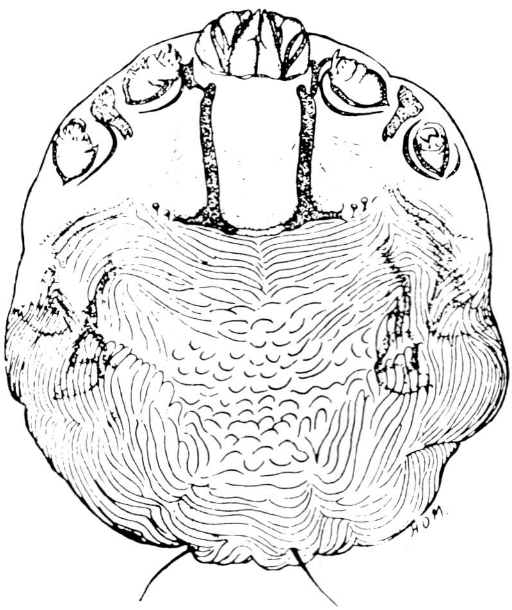

30.21. *Knemidocoptes mutans,* scaly-leg mite. (Soulsby)

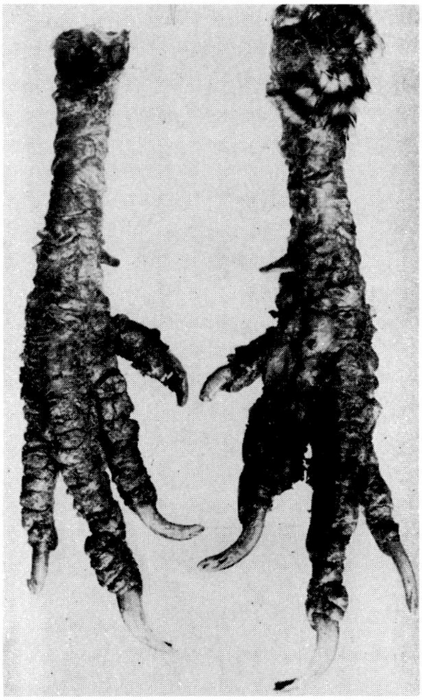

30.22. Lesions caused by scaly-leg mites. (Benbrook and Sloss)

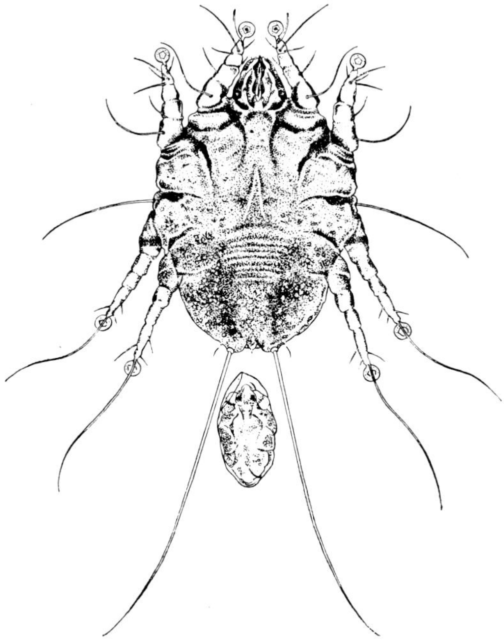

30.23. *Epidermoptes bilobatus,* epidermoptic scabies (or skin) mite. ×200. (Reis and Nobrega)

to dip the legs in a warm acaricidal solution recommended by a veterinarian. Houses should be cleaned frequently, especially the roosts, which should be sprayed as recommended for the chicken mite.

Depluming Mite. The depluming mite (*Knemidocoptes gallineae*) resembles the scaly-leg mite in general structure although it is smaller, the adult female being about 0.3 mm in diameter. Striations are interrupted on the dorsal surface to form raised sculpturing. The mites are more prevalent in spring and summer, at which time infestation may spread rapidly by contact. Mites burrow into basal shafts of feathers on the epidermis of chickens, pigeons, and pheasants. Intense irritation induces the host to pull out body feathers. These mites injure the bird by interfering with control of body heat. Some affected birds will lose weight and show lowered production.

CONTROL. Control of depluming mites is not easily accomplished. Prompt isolation of affected birds and disinfection of houses as recommended for chicken mites should come first.

Skin Mites. *Epidermoptes bilobatus* (Epidermoptidae) (Fig. 30.23) is a skin mite frequently reported from Europe and more rarely from South and North America. The adult female is about 0.17–0.22 mm long. It occurs on chickens and apparently may or may not produce lesions but has been described as a cause of pityriasis. When lesions are produced, they consist first of a fine scaly dermatitis, followed by formation of thick, brownish, sharply edged scabs. The more severe lesions may be due partly to a concomitant fungus infection by *Lophophyton gallinae;* also, birds affected with epidermoptid mites often have depluming mites at the same time. Epidermoptic scabies may at times result in emaciation and even death. Pruritis is a common sign.

CONTROL. Treatment of infested birds is recommended as for depluming mites.

Internal Parasitic Mites. Internal passages of the respiratory system, air sacs, and subcutaneous tissue can be infested with sarcoptiform mites of the families Cytoditidae and Laminosioptidae, the mesostigmatid family Rhinonyssidae, and the prostigmatid family Speleogmatidae. These mites are an odd occurrence on modern poultry farms but may be commoner than reports would indicate, since diagnostic procedures seldom include a search for them.

Cyst Mite. The fowl cyst mite (*Laminosioptes cysticola,* family Laminosioptidae) (Fig. 30.24) has been reported mainly from chickens and also from turkeys, pheasants, geese, and pigeons in many parts of the world. The female mite

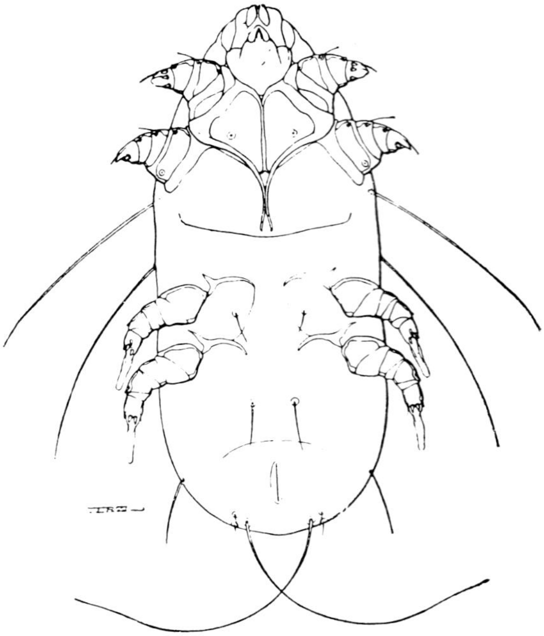

30.24. *Laminosioptes cysticola,* fowl cyst mite. ×376. (Hirst)

measures about 0.25 × 0.11 mm. The gnathosoma is reduced and not visible from above, and the body bears a few long setae. The life cycle is unknown except that the female lays embryonated eggs and mites pass through all stages of their development under the skin or even in the deeper tissues of the host.

Initial infestation is on the skin, with more frequent findings in the loose subcutaneous connective tissue, occurring in the muscles, abdominal viscera, lungs (pigeons), and on the peritoneum. These mites do not appear to influence the health of infested birds, although lesions may make carcasses unpalatable as food for humans. If lesions or mites are detected by the inspection service, the carcass is condemned.

Subcutaneous mites occur inside yellowish nodules up to several millimeters in diameter in the subcutis. These areas are often mistaken for tuberculous lesions. The nodules appear to be caseocalcareous deposits formed by the bird to enclose mites after they die in the tissues. Large numbers of nodules are most often found in aged emaciated birds. *L. cysticola* has been reported in pigeons in which mites were surrounded by nodules in the lungs, causing death.

Careful examination of skin and subcutis of birds under a dissecting microscope might reveal presence of this parasite more frequently. Otherwise, diagnosis will depend on finding characteristic nodular lesions and by seeing mites or their remains in nodules that have been crushed under a coverglass in a drop of acidulated water.

CONTROL. No attempt has been made to control subcutaneous mites except by destruction of affected birds.

Air Sac Mite. Respiratory system mites of poultry include the air sac mite (*Cytodites nudus,* family Cytoditidae) (Fig. 30.25), which is found in bronchi, lungs, air sacs, and bone cavities. Air sac mites have been found in chickens, turkeys, pheasants, pigeons, canaries, and ruffled grouse from many parts of the world. Although not of common occurrence, these mites are often overlooked because of their small size and peculiar habitat.

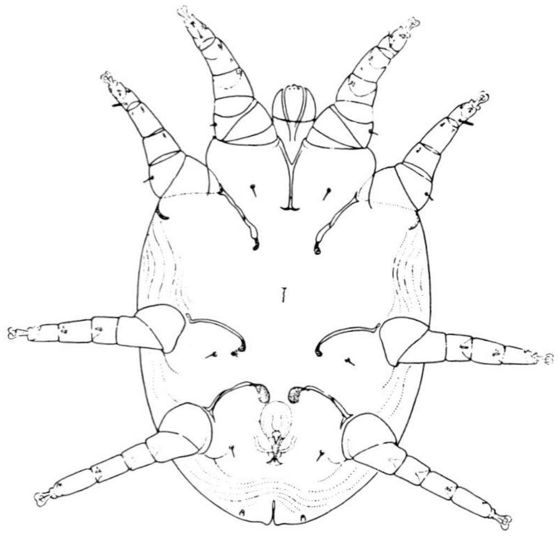

30.25. *Cytodites nudus,* air sac mite. (Baker)

The adult female mites are whitish specks, measuring about 0.6 × 0.4 mm. The mites appear nude because they bear but a few short setae. The gnathosoma is reduced, with minute chelicerae in a tube formed by coalescence of the palpi and gnathosoma. No details are known of the life cycle; speculation is that the mites lay eggs in the lower air passages and these are coughed up and probably swallowed, reaching the ground in droppings. The mode of infection is not known.

There is considerable conflict as to the damage done by air sac mites. Some observers claim they are practically harmless because their presence has been noted in apparently healthy birds. Others state that the mites are responsible for emaciation, peritonitis, pneumonia, and obstruction of air passages and are predisposing factors for tuberculosis. Dense infestations have definitely been associated with weakness and grave loss in weight so that affected birds resemble clinical cases of tuberculosis. Lindt and Kutzer (35) found *C. nudus* to cause granulomatous pneumonia, which can be fatal.

Close inspection of the opened cadaver of an affected bird soon after death will show whitish dots moving slowly over the transparent air sac surfaces. Identification requires examination under ×100 magnification.

CONTROL. Limited publications on control suggest destruction of the cadavers of affected birds, followed by disinfection and cleaning of the poultry house.

Other Respiratory System Mites. Other respiratory system mites of poultry and pigeons include a few members of the genera *Neonyssus, Rhinonyssus,* and *Sternostoma* of the family Rhinonyssidae and *Speleognathus* of the family Speleognathidae. None is an important pest of commercial poultry. *N. columbae, N. melloi,* and *S. striatus* are nasal mites from pigeons and *R. rhinolethrum* is from ducks and geese. These mites are about 0.5 mm long, oval, bear no setae, possess two dorsal plates, and have stigmata without peritremes.

CONTROL. *S. tracheacolum* has been controlled in Gouldian finches with 0.04 g carbaryl on 50 g millet and 1 ml cod liver oil fed three times within 18–24 hr at weekly intervals.

TICKS. Ticks are large mites belonging to the superfamily Ixodoidea of the Acarina, characterized by having a pair of oval or kidney-shaped stigmata posterior or lateral to the coxae; the hypostome is modified as a piercing organ provided with recurved teeth, and there is a pitlike sensory organ on the tarsi of the first pair of legs (Haller's organ). Unengorged adults of most common ticks are 2–4 mm long, but fully engorged females may reach more than 10 mm. However, unengorged tick larvae are similar in size to adult mites. Ticks inhabiting poultry houses belong to the family Argasidae. They have no scutum (dorsal shield) and except for larvae feed intermittently in all stages. The integument is leathery, wrinkled, and granulated in appearance. The capitulum (head) is ventrally placed near the anterior margin of the body (Fig. 30.26). Many hard-bodied ticks in the family Ixodidae will feed on range poultry. These ticks possess a scutum in all stages and feed only once in each stage, remaining on the host for several days. The scutum usually appears shiny, and the capitulum is terminal at the anterior of the tick (Fig. 30.27). Diagnostic keys by Cooley and Kohls (9) and Diamant and Strickland (13) are most useful to determine North American tick species.

Losses caused by ticks are threefold: loss of host blood, which may cause death; reduced production associated with anemia but also possibly due to tick-produced toxic substances; and transmission of disease such as avian spirochetosis, tularemia, piroplasmosis, anaplasmosis, dirofilariasis, certain rickettsial diseases (notably Rocky Mountain spotted fever), and many viruses, including encephalitis.

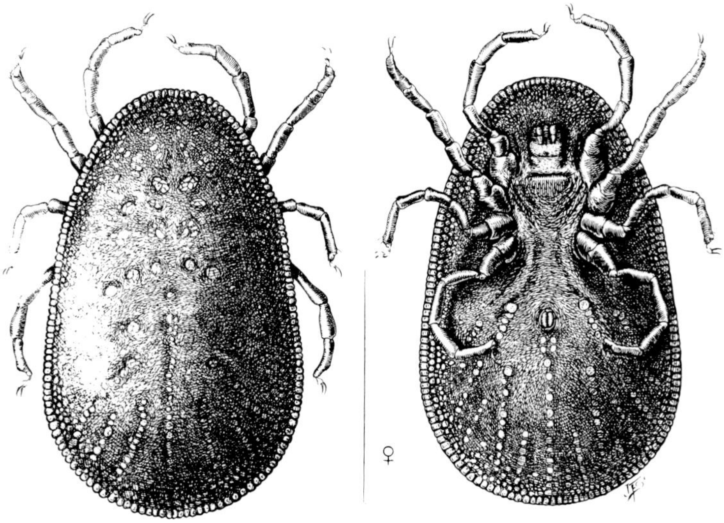

30.26. *Argas persicus* group, fowl tick. Dorsal view (*left*); ventral view (*right*). (USDA)

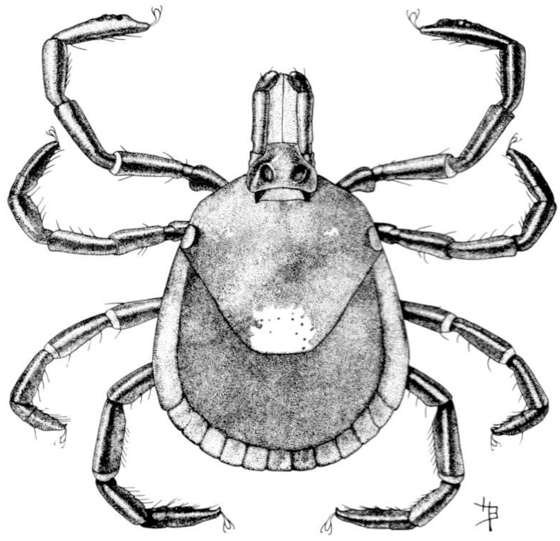

30.27. *Amblyomma americanum,* lone star tick. (USDA)

Fowl Ticks. Soft-bodied ticks (Argasidae) are the most important ticks of poultry. The genus *Argas* (*persicus* group) consists of three species found on poultry, other fowl, and pigeons in the USA: *Argas persicus, A. sanchezi,* and *A. radiatus.* Other species include *A. miniatus* in Central and South America, *A. robertsi* along with *A. persicus* in Australia, and *A. aboreus* on wild birds and chickens in South Africa.

Life cycles are about equal in time for *A. radiatus* and *A. sanchezi,* but temperature sensitivity limits *A. sanchezi* to two or three generations per year in southern Texas. These fowl ticks (chicken ticks, blue bugs, tampans, adobe ticks) are distributed mainly in states along the Gulf of Mexico and the Mexican border. They are also established in many other tropical and temperate areas of the world. Although primarily parasites of birds, they may be found on mammals. In North America they have been reported from the following hosts: chickens, turkeys, ducks, geese, guinea fowl, pigeons, canaries, doves, hawks, magpies, owls, quail, sparrows, thrushes, vultures, ostriches, and wild turkeys; also rarely from cattle, dogs, and humans.

Mature blood-engorged females measure about 10 × 6 mm. Unfed ticks are relatively easily recognized by their flattened ovoid shape and tan to reddish brown color. Females may lay a total of 500–875 eggs in four or five separate batches but require a blood meal before laying each batch of eggs. Eggs are laid in sheltered crevices, including bark of trees. They hatch in from 6–10 days in warm weather to 3 mo during cool periods. Larvae (seed ticks) become hungry in 4–5 days and seek a host, although they may live for several months without feeding. They blood-feed for 4–5 days and then leave the host for a hiding place nearby and molt (shed skins) in 3–9 days to the first nymphal stage. Nymphs are active and feed only at night but can do without food for as long as 15 mo. The first-stage nymphs feed in 10–45 min, leave the host and hide for 5–8 days, and molt to a second nymphal stage that is ready to feed in 5–15 days. Similarly, these second-stage nymphs feed and hide; adult ticks emerge from the nymphal skins ready to engorge with blood and mate about 1 wk later. Oviposition commences 3–5 days after mating. This complete life cycle takes about 7–8 wk during warm weather and longer during cold seasons. Fowl ticks remain inactive in cracks and crevices during cold weather, and adults may live without a blood meal for more than 4 yr.

Birds suffer chiefly from attacks of these ticks during the warm dry season. Loss of blood may reach proportions of a fatal anemia; at least there may be emaciation, weakness, slow growth, and lowered production. Ruffled feathers, poor appetite, and diarrhea are signs suggesting tick infestation.

The fowl tick is the most important poultry ectoparasite in many tropical countries, being a limiting factor in successful rearing of standard breeds of poultry (41). Turkeys usually suffer even more than chickens; recently hatched poults and chicks show the highest mortality. These ticks cause skin blemishes on turkeys, reducing market price.

The fowl tick is capable of transmitting the highly pathogenic spirochete *Borrelia anserina* in many parts of the world. Tick-borne avian spirochetosis has been reported in chickens and turkeys in the USA, with epizootics of avian spirochetosis in Arizona associated with infestations by the fowl tick. Fowl ticks have been reported to transmit *Aegyptianella pullorum* and fowl cholera (*Pasteurella multocida*) in some regions of the world. All postembryonal stages of the common fowl tick have been found infected with *A. pullorum* in some areas. However, in other areas transmission of fowl cholera was not shown even though fowl ticks harbored *P. multocida* for 25 days. Aegyptianellosis has not been reported from the Americas.

Tick paralysis in chickens–a flaccid, afebrile motor paralysis–may result from attacks by *A. persicus* as well as by *A. walkerae* in Africa (25). Etiology of this sporadic disease is not understood, but most probably a specific paralytic toxin is contained and transmitted in the tick salivary secretions. Clinical signs may be confused with botulism, neural signs of Marek's disease, transient paralysis, Newcastle disease, and possibly conditions caused by other bacterial or chemical toxins.

The pigeon tick (*A. reflexus*) is not in the persicus group. The subspecies *A. reflexus* attacks pigeons in Europe and Asia; *A. reflexus hermanni* is the pigeon tick of Africa (28, 29). In most areas these ticks are not pests of chickens, but *A. reflexus hermanni* and *A. persicus* are found together on chickens in West Africa. *A. neghmei* is a pest of both chickens and pigeons in Chile. These argasid ticks (except *A. refexus hermanni*) have been reported as pests of humans, and *A. neghmei* is known to bite children in homes adjacent to adobe wall poultry houses in Chile. Probably both subspecies of *A. reflexus* are important vectors of fowl spirochetosis. *A. reflexus hermanni* in Egypt is suspected of transmitting West Nile and Chenuda virus and the Quaranfil virus group among pigeons and is implicated in transmission of Q fever rickettsia.

CONTROL. Control requires treatment of premises because adult and nymphal ticks are on their hosts only a short time and then hide in the surroundings. The litter, walls, floors, and ceilings must be sprayed thoroughly, forcing spray into cracks and behind nest boxes. Outdoor runs and feed troughs, woodpiles, and tree trunks may be treated using approved insecticides. Other methods for fowl tick control include use of metal construction, elimination of tree roosting, using roosts suspended from ceilings, and converting to cage operation. Frequent inspection is necessary to combat ticks before their number has increased to a harmful extent. Fowl ticks are rarely found in modern, large commercial cage-layer operations.

Hard Ticks. Hard ticks (Ixodidae) of many species will feed on poultry as well as wild ground birds. Birds are preferred hosts of larvae and nymphs of some species of *Hyalomma* (Old World only) and *Amblyomma* ticks that are common in the adult stage on mammals. Ixodid ticks attach to hosts, mate, feed to repletion, and then drop off. Females oviposit several thousand eggs in a single batch on the ground and then die. The eggs hatch in 1–2 mo, and the 6-legged larvae climb up on the vegetation to await a new vertebrate host. There is only one larval and one nymphal stage, and each feeds from 5 to 7 days on the host. Hard ticks are likely to be found only on birds that are on range or have access to range.

In the temperate zone many ixodid ticks have but one generation a year, spending the winter in diapause as eggs or immature or mature ticks. Even in the tropics some ticks require a year to complete their life cycle; others may complete the cycle in 2–4 mo. Ticks that do not find a host will live for a long period (over 2 yr has been recorded), so the cycle may be very prolonged. Premises and ranges will remain infested for long periods even when unoccupied.

RODENTS

Rodents are very common pests in and around poultry facilities, and a facility that does not have at least a few rodents is unusual. Rodents do a tremendous amount of damage if an effective control program is not implemented and maintained; burrowing and gnawing activity can undermine foundations and destroy curtains and insulation. Rodents can eat or contaminate feed, which increases feed costs and affects feed conversions. Additional problems can be produced by the presence of these pests since they are capable of carrying a variety of diseases and ectoparasites.

RATS. The Norway rat (*Rattus norvegicus*) is the most common rat found around poultry houses. Rats have three basic requirements: food, water, and harborage. If one of these items is missing from an area, there will not be a rat problem. Unfortunately, all of these items are usually present in and around poultry production facilities. Rats eat almost any type of food, including eggs and poultry feed; however, rats prefer fresh food. When fresh food is available, rodents will totally ignore spoiled food. An adult rat will eat and drink approximately 0.5–2 oz of food and water each day with 200 adult rats consuming 25 lb of feed daily.

Rat harborage around a poultry house is seen in the form of burrows in the ground and under the foundation, litter under the slats, and in wood piles, old nests, and other debris near the poultry houses. This type of harborage must be removed for any control program to be successful. Most rat activity, including feeding, occurs at night. Rats observed outside their harborage during the day indicate a large population. Rats are very territorial, and when crowded they become increasingly aggressive. The stronger and more aggressive rats drive the weaker rats away from the food, forcing them to feed during the day.

Rats have high reproductive rates, which can lead to large numbers of rodents in a fairly short period of time. A single pair of rats and their offspring could produce as many as 1500 rats in 1 yr if all the offspring survived. Rats will breed at 3–5 mo of age and give birth approximately 3 wk after mating. Four to seven litters are produced in 1 yr with each litter having 6–12 young; the female will breed again 1–2 days after giving birth. Although breeding will occur all year, increased breeding frequently occurs during the spring and fall. Generally, rodent populations decrease during the winter; however, in a poultry house, the opposite is frequently true because of immigration of rats into the building when the weather cools, not because of increased reproduction.

MICE. The house mouse (*Mus musculus*) is the most common mouse found in and around poultry facilities. Mice require food, water, and harborage, and will eat almost any kind of food with about 0.1 oz of food consumed by an adult mouse each day. Mice are frequently active throughout the day, often feeding every hour. However, peak activity usually occurs at dusk and dawn. Mice require much less water than rats and are capable of utilizing water from the food they eat. Mice will burrow in the ground and in insulation or live in rolled-up curtains. Mice are able to reproduce at 6–8 wk of age. They will give birth to five or six young approximately 3 wk after mating; the female can breed again 2–4 days after giving birth. Generally, five to eight litters are produced in a year. Mice breed regularly throughout the year with no seasonal peak.

CONTROL. There are three general aspects to rodent control: rodentproofing, sanitation, and rodent killing. Rodentproofing can be an effective long-term control measure. However, it is impractical, if not impossible, to rodentproof a poultry facility. Access to the poultry building can be restricted by patching or screening holes in the foundation, thus forcing the rodents to burrow into the house, which makes them easier to detect.

Sanitation is a form of cultural control and simply involves cleaning up around the poultry facility. Rodents are secretive creatures, they do not like to move about in open areas; therefore, mowing the grass and weeds on a regular basis creates a less favorable habitat. Removing piles of old wood, nests, or any other debris helps to make the area less attractive to rodents and aids in making early detection possible. When debris or tall grass is present, rodents can burrow into a facility and go unnoticed. Rolling the house curtains up and down a couple of times a week during summer months will disturb any rodents that are in the curtains and discourage them from living and/or nesting in them.

After the cultural control measures have been completed, a rodent-killing program should be implemented. Rodent killing can take the form of baiting, fumigating, trapping, or even shooting. Under most circumstances, a properly conducted baiting program is easiest and most effective.

There are many products on the market that will kill rodents. The first group of safe and commonly used baits are the multiple-dose anticoagulants (Table 30.2). Products that contain warfarin, fumarin, chlorophacinone, or diphacinone as an active ingredient are examples of this type of bait. Multiple-dose anticoagulants must be consumed for several days in a row to be lethal. The effects are cumulative: if a rodent feeds on this type of bait for a day or so, then feeds on something else before returning to the bait for another few feedings, the rodent will not be controlled. Therefore, it is imperative that enough bait be available for the rodents to eat for several days. The specific number of days that a rat or mouse must feed on a multiple-dose anticoagulant poison depends on the bait being used and amount consumed. These chemicals are relatively safe for humans and nontarget animals, because a single dose will not cause death.

Table 30.2. Rodenticides for use in poultry facilities

Active Ingredient	Type of Bait
Warfarin	Multiple-dose anticoagulant
Pival	Multiple-dose anticoagulant
Diphacinone	Multiple-dose anticoagulant
Chlorophacinone	Multiple-dose anticoagulant
Zinc Phosphide[a]	Acute single dose, rapid death
Bromethalin	Single dose, affects central nervous system
Brodifacoum	Single-dose anticoagulant
Bromadiolon	Single-dose anticoagulant
Cholecalciferol	Single dose/multiple dose, affects blood calcium levels

[a]Restricted to use by licensed pest-control operators.

The second type of rodenticide includes the single-dose anticoagulants. Products that contain brodifacoum are examples of this category of baits. A single feeding is sufficient to kill a rodent. They are safe; however, care should be taken to keep them out of reach of pets, livestock, and children. They are potentially lethal if a large dose is consumed.

Currently, there are two other types of single-dose baits that are not anticoagulants. The first contains the active ingredient bromethalin, which affects the central nervous system. Baits containing bromethalin are effective, but they are also fairly toxic so extra care should be taken when using this compound. The second type of bait contains cholecalciferol, which is vitamin D_3. Cholecalciferol causes a calcium imbalance in the blood. Since other mammals can tolerate much larger changes in their blood calcium level, this compound is very safe for humans and nontarget animals.

The last category of baits includes acute single-dose rodenticides such as zinc phosphide. These chemicals are very effective and useful for a quick knockdown of a large rodent population. However, these chemicals are highly toxic, and most of them are restricted to use by licensed pest-control operators. Except under extreme circumstances, the other types of bait are equally effective and they are much safer.

For any baiting program to be effective, rodents must consume a lethal amount of bait. In order to accomplish this, care must be taken in the placement of bait. Random placement of bait around a poultry facility is rarely very effective. Always remember that rodents will not go out of their way to eat poison bait if they have food readily available. Therefore, placing the bait in or closer to their harborage than their regular food source is important. One of the best and safest places to put the bait is in the active rodent burrow. A great deal of bait, time, and money can be saved by determining which burrows are active before the baiting begins. This can be done by filling in all burrows around the facility with soil or newspaper and checking the next day; all burrows that have been reopened should be baited.

When using a multiple-dose rodenticide, be sure to put bait in all active burrows *daily* until the bait is no longer consumed. When bait is no longer taken, remove the uneaten bait and fill in the burrow. If a single-dose anticoagulant is used, the active burrows should be baited for 2 consecutive days and 4 or 5 days later all of the burrows should be filled and any that are active baited for 2 more days. When baiting for mice at ground level, the above procedure should be used. However, mice frequently inhabit the upper areas of a poultry house. When this occurs, baiting at ground level will be ineffective. The bait must be placed within the mouse's territory. To accomplish this, put out a small amount of bait in many places rather than putting out a large quantity in a few places. The bait can be placed on the sill, in the feed rooms, or scattered in the attic area if the facility has a dropped ceiling. There are also baits that are sold in a block form that can be nailed or wired to the rafters, or a bait station can be used.

Acute rodenticides should only be used in extreme cases. The best time to use these compounds is when a very high rodent population is present and after the birds have been removed. Then the bait can be placed in the poultry houses so that no animals, other than rodents, could be accidentally poisoned. Since the rodents' normal food source is absent during this period, the bait placement is not that crucial. The location of all bait placements should be recorded on paper and checked off when they are removed to make sure that no bait station is missed. Always *remove* and carefully *dispose* of any uneaten bait before the building is cleaned out.

Tracking powders and fumigants can also be used to kill rodents. Tracking powders are mixtures of rodent poisons and nontoxic powders that are spread on the floor in active rodent runways. Rats and mice pick up the poisoned powder on their fur, tail, and feet as they run across it and then ingest the poison when grooming.

Until recently, fumigants were frequently used to gas rodents trapped in their burrows or enclosed areas. Methyl bromide gas, chloropicrin fumigant, and other control measures are now being used as fumigants. Fumigants are extremely hazardous to humans and nontarget animals. All humans, pets, and livestock must be removed from the area until the gas is totally dissipated. When using any pesticide, always read and follow label instructions carefully.

Claims that rodents can be driven away or negatively affected by ultrasonic sound or electromagnetic radiation are as yet unproven. In fact, several studies have indicated that ultrasonic sound and electromagnetic radiation do not drive rodents away or affect them adversely. The devices involved are very expensive and should be viewed skeptically until further research proves them worthwhile.

A rodent control program must be a continual effort if it is to be effective and efficient. Too often, control programs are implemented only after a severe problem exists. At that point, control requires a great deal of effort and expense and, when most of the rodents are killed, the control effort stops until the rodents become a serious problem again. This type of program is a waste of time and money. It is much easier and less expensive to control and/or totally eliminate a small rodent population by checking the facility for rodent activity on a regular basis even after the control program has killed most of the rodents. Look for signs both inside and outside at least every 2 wk, and start baiting as soon as any activity is observed. It is especially important to check inside partially slatted broiler breeder facilities. Frequently, rodents will enter this type of facility through a small number of burrows from outside and then live and reproduce in the litter under the slats. If rodents are under slats, the severity of the infestation can be underestimated if just the outside of the building is checked and the area under the slats left uninspected.

REFERENCES

1. Anderson, R.C. 1956. The life cycle and seasonal transmission of Ornithofilaria fallisensis Anderson, a parasite of domestic and wild ducks. Can J Zool 34:485.
2. Arends, J.J. 1982. Integrated Pest Management Manual. North Carolina State Univ Ext Publ, Raleigh, NC.
3. Arends, J.J., S.H. Robertson, and C.S. Payne. 1984. Impact of northern fowl mite on broiler breeder flocks in North Carolina. Poult Sci 63:1457–1461.
4. Arthur, F.H., and R.C. Axtell. 1982. Comparisons of permethrin formulations and application methods for northern fowl mite control on caged laying hens. Poult Sci 61:879–884.
5. Axtell, R.C. 1986. Fly management in poultry production: Cultural, biological, and chemical. Poult Sci 65:657–667.
6. Axtell, R.C. 1987. Fly control in confined livestock and poultry production. Ciba-Geigy Corp, Greensboro, NC.
7. Borror, D.J., and D.M. DeLong. 1976. An Introduction to the Study of Insects. Holt, Rinehart & Winston, New York.
8. Chamberlain, R.W. 1968. In K. Maramorosch (ed.), Curr Top Microbiol Immunol 42:38–58. Springer-Verlag, Berlin.
9. Cooley, R.A., and G.M. Kohls. 1944. The Argasidae of North America, Central America, and Cuba. Notre Dame Univ Press, South Bend, IN.
10. DeVaney, J.A. 1976. Effects of the chicken body

louse, Menacanthus stramineus, on caged layers. Poult Sci 55:430–435.

11. DeVaney, J.A. 1979. The effects of the northern fowl mite, Ornithonyssus sylviarum, on egg production and body weight of caged white leghorn hens. Poult Sci 191–194.

12. DeVaney, J.A., and R.L. Ziprin. 1980. Acquired immune response of white leghorn hens to populations of northern fowl mite, Ornithonyssus sylviarum. Poult Sci 59:1742–1744.

13. Diamant, G., and R.K. Strickland. 1965. Manual on Livestock Ticks, pp. 91–94. US Dep Agric, ARS, Washington, DC.

14. Dunning, L.L., E.C. Loomis, and V.E. Burton. 1971. Portable spray unit serves many farm and ranch purposes. Calif Agric 25:8–10.

15. Edgar, S.A., and D.F. King. 1950. Effect of the body louse, Eomenacanthus stramineus, on mature chickens. Poult Sci 29:214–219.

16. Eklund, J., E. Loomis, and H. Abplanalp. 1980. Genetic resistance of white leghorn chickens to infestation by the northern fowl mite, Ornithonyssus sylviarum. Arch Gefluegelkd 44:195–199.

17. Emerson, K.C. 1956. Mallophaga (chewing lice) occurring on the domestic chicken. J Kans Entomol Soc 29:63–79.

18. Emerson, K.C. 1962. Mallophaga (chewing lice) occurring on the turkey. J Kans Entomol Soc 35:196–201.

19. Fox, I. 1940. Fleas of Eastern United States. Iowa State Coll Press, Ames.

20. Geden, C.J., and R.C. Axtell. 1987. Factors affecting climbing and tunneling behavior of the lesser mealworm (Coleoptoia: Tenebrionidae) J Econ Entomol 80:1197–1204.

21. Geden, C.J., T.D. Edwards, J.J. Arends, and R.C. Axtell. 1987. Efficacies of mixtures of disinfectants and insecticides. Poult Sci 66:659–665.

22. Geden, C.J., R.E. Stinner, and R.C. Axtell. 1988. Predation by predators of the house fly in poultry manure: Effects of predator density, feeding history, interspecific interference, and field conditions. Environ Entomol 17:320–329.

23. Georgi, J.R. 1980. Parasitology for Veterinarians, 3rd Ed. Saunders, Philadelphia.

24. Gless, E.E., and E.S. Raun. 1959. Effects of chicken body louse infestation on egg production. J Econ Entomol 52:358–359.

25. Goethe, R., and K. Kunze. 1973. Neuropharmacological investigations on tick paralysis of chickens induced by larvae of Argas (Persicargas) walkerae. In E.J.L. Soulsby (ed.), Parasitic Zoonosis. Clinical and Experimental Studies, pp. 369–382. Academic Press, New York.

26. Hall, R.D., and W.B. Gross. 1975. Effect of social stress and inherited plasma corticosterone levels in chickens on populations of the northern fowl mite, Ornithonyssus sylviarum. J Parasitol 61:1096–1100.

27. Hall, R.D., W.B. Gross, and E.C. Turner, Jr. 1978. Preliminary observations on northern fowl mite infestations on estrogenized roosters and in relation to initial egg production in hens. Poult Sci 57:1088–1090.

28. Hoogstraal, H., and G.M. Kohls. 1960. Observations on the subgenus Argas (Ixodoidea, Argasidae, Argas). 1. Study of A. reflexus reflexus (Fabricius, 1794), the European bird argasid. Ann Entomol Soc Am 53:611–618.

29. Hoogstraal, H., and G.M. Khols. 1960. Observations on the subgenus Argas (Ixodoidea, Argasidae, Argas). 3. A biological and systematic study of A. reflexus hermanni Audouin, 1827 (revalidated), the African bird argasid. Ann Entomol Soc Am 53:743–755.

30. Hubbard, C.A. 1947. Fleas of Western North America. Iowa State Coll Press, Ames.

31. Kettle, D.S. 1985. Medical and Veterinary Entomology. John Wiley & Sons, New York.

32. Kiernans, J.E. 1975. A review of the phoretic relationship between Mallophaga (Phthiraptera: Insecta) and Hippoboscidae (Diptera: Insecta). J Med Entomol 12:71–76.

33. Krantz, G.W. 1970. A Manual of Acarology. Oregon State Univ Press, Corvallis.

34. Lancaster, J.L., Jr., and M.V. Meisch. 1986. Arthropods in Livestock and Poultry Production. Halsted Press, New York.

35. Lindt, S., and E. Kutzer. 1965. Luftsackmilben (Cytodites nudus) als Ursache einer granulomatosen Pneumonic beim Huhn. Pathol Vet 2:264–276.

36. Loomis, E.C., E.L. Bramhall, J.A. Allen, R.A. Ernst, and L.L. Dunning. 1970. Effects of the northern fowl mite on white leghorn chickens. J Econ Entomol 63:1885–1889.

37. Loomis, E.C., J.P. Anderson, and A.S. Peal. 1980. Coop Ext Univ Calif Leafl 2506.

38. Lysyk, T.J., and R.C. Axtell. 1986. Field evaluation of three methods for monitoring populations of house flies (Musca domestica) (Diptera:Muscidae) and other filth flies in three types of poultry housing systems. J Econ Entomol 79:144–151.

39. Noblet, R., J.B. Kissam, and T.R. Atkins, Jr. 1975. Leucocytozoon smithi: Incidence of transmission by black flies in South Carolina (Diptera: Simuliidae). J Med Entomol 12:111–114.

40. Reeves, W.C. 1965. Ecology of mosquitoes in relation to arboviruses. Annu Rev Entmol 10:25–46.

41. Reid, W.M. 1956. Incidence and economic importance of poultry parasites under different ecological and geographical situations in Egypt. Poult Sci 35:926–933.

42. Soulsby, E.J.L. 1982. Helminths, Arthropods, and Protozoa of Domesticated Animals, 7th Ed. Williams & Wilkins, Baltimore, MD.

43. Stockdale, H.J., and E.S. Raun. 1960. Economic importance of the chicken louse. J Econ Entomol 53:421–422.

44. Titchener, R.N. 1983. The use of permethrin to control an outbreak of hen fleas (Ceratophyllus gallinae). Poult Sci 62:608–611.

45. Warren, D.C., R. Eaton, and H. Smith. 1948. Influence of infestations of body lice on egg production in the hen. Poult Sci 27:641–642.

46. Werner, F.G. 1982. Common names of insects and related organisms. Entomol Soc Am, College Park, MD.

47. West, L.S. 1951. The Housefly: Its Natural History, Medical Importance and Control. Comstock, Ithaca, NY.

48. Williams, R.E., R.D. Hall, A.B. Broce, and P.J. Scholl. 1985. Livestock Entomology. John Wiley & Sons, New York.

31 NEMATODES AND ACANTHOCEPHALANS

M.D. Ruff

INTRODUCTION. Nematodes constitute the most important group of helminth parasites of poultry. In both number of species and amount of damage done, they far exceed the trematodes and cestodes.

This chapter is designed to aid the diagnostician in identifying predominant nematodes of poultry in North America. Those reported in chickens are listed in Table 31.1; those found in other domestic poultry and/or commercially raised game birds are in Table 31.2. Nematodes from areas other than North America are mentioned in the text but not listed in the tables. Avian nematodes often have a broad host range. Accordingly, nematodes found in wild birds may constitute a hazard for commercially raised birds (Table 31.3). Only species commonly found are described in any detail in this chapter. For a more detailed description of individual species, early works, and additional information, the reader should refer to the original references listed in the previous editions of this book (72, 89) or to other reviews (1, 16, 18, 20, 57). A checklist and descriptions are available for parasites reported from the bobwhite quail and waterfowl (53, 63).

The genus and species names used in this chapter are those of Yamaguti (92), except where usage by recognized authorities supersedes his classification. Yamaguti described 25 families of nematodes from 9 orders in avian species; 13 of these families (Strongyloididae, Trichuridae, Syngamidae, Trichostrongylidae, Subuluridae, Heterakidae, Ascarididae, Spiruridae, Thelaziidae, Gnathostomatidae, Physalopteridea, Acuariidae, Dipetalonematidae) contain species that infect poultry. Levine (57) used a similar classification but substituted Onchocercidae for Dipetalonematidae. The classification used for families in this chapter is that given in the CIH keys in a series on the Nematode Parasite of Vertebrates (3), which elevates many of the families (57, 92) to superfamily rank; thus, the number of families containing parasites of poultry is increased to 21. Yorke and Maplestone (93) provided yet another key to orders and families.

GENERAL MORPHOLOGY. Nematodes, or roundworms, are usually spindle shaped with the anterior and posterior ends attenuated. The body covering, or cuticle, is often marked by transverse grooves. Cuticular fins, or alae, may be present at the anterior (cervical alae) or posterior (caudal alae, Fig. 31.14) part of the body. The latter are found on the tail of the male worm and, in the case of certain groups, are modified to form a bursa (Fig. 31.18B). Cuticular ornamentations are occasionally found on the anterior extremities and may take the form of spines, cordons, or shields (Fig. 31.6A).

The mouth opening, located at the anterior end of the body, is usually surrounded by lips bearing sensory organs (Fig. 31.5A). In more generalized types of nematodes the mouth leads directly into a cavity immediately anterior to the esophagus (Fig. 31.24A). The mouth cavity may be considerably reduced or absent in more specialized groups of nematodes. The esophagus may be simple (consisting of one undivided part) or more complex (consisting of a short anterior muscular part and a long posterior glandular part). A bulb may or may not be present at the posterior end (Fig. 31.20C). The intestine follows the esophagus and is connected with the anal or cloacal opening in the posterior end of the body by a short rectum.

The nematodes are, with very few exceptions, sexually distinct. Sexual dimorphism is remarkably demonstrated by some species of nematodes such as *Tetrameres americana* (Fig. 31.7), in which the elongate male worm is much smaller than the globular-shaped female. The male can usually be distinguished from the female by the presence of two (rarely one) chitinous structures known as spicules, located in the posterior end of the body. The spicules (Fig. 31.20) have been considered as intromittent organs for use during copulation, keeping the vulva and vagina open and, to some extent, guiding the sperm into the female. Eggs or larvae are discharged through the vulva, the position of which varies considerably in different groups of nematodes.

DEVELOPMENT. Nematodes of poultry have either a direct or an indirect type of development; about one-half require no invertebrate intermediate hosts, whereas the others depend on such intermediate hosts as insects, snails, and slugs for the early stage of development.

Nematodes normally pass through four devel-

Table 31.1. Nematodes reported from chickens in the USA

Nematode	Location	Intermediate Hosts	Other Definitive Hosts
Baylisascaris procyonis	Brain		Racoons (accidental parasite in chicken, turkey, partridge, quail)
Oxyspirura mansoni	Eye	Cockroach	Turkey, duck, grouse, guinea fowl, peafowl, pigeon, quail
Syngamus trachea	Trachea	None	Turkey, goose, guinea fowl, pheasant, peafowl, quail
Capillaria contorta	Mouth, esophagus, crop	None or earthworm	Turkey, duck, guinea fowl, partridge, pheasant, quail
C. annulata	Esophagus, crop	Earthworm	Turkey, goose, grouse, guinea fowl, partridge, pheasant, quail
Gongylonema ingluvicola	Crop, esophagus, proventriculus	Beetle, cockroach	Turkey, partridge, pheasant, quail
Dispharynx nasuta	Proventriculus	Sowbug	Turkey, grouse, guinea fowl, partridge, pheasant, pigeon, quail
Tetrameres americana	Proventriculus	Grasshopper, cockroach	Turkey, duck, grouse, pigeon, quail
T. fissispina	Proventriculus	Amphipod, grasshopper, cockroach, earthworm	Turkey, duck, goose, guinea fowl, pigeon, quail
Cheilospirura hamulosa	Gizzard	Grasshopper, beetle	Turkey, grouse, guinea fowl, pheasant, quail
Ascaridia galli	Small intestine	None	Turkey, duck, goose, quail
Capillaria anatis	Small intestine, cecum, cloaca	None	Turkey, duck, goose, partridge, pheasant
C. bursata	Small intestine	Earthworm	Turkey, goose, pheasant
C. caudinflata	Small intestine	Earthworm	Turkey, duck, goose, grouse, guinea fowl, partridge, pheasant, pigeon, quail
C. obsignata	Small intestine, cecum	None	Turkey, goose, guinea fowl, pigeon, quail
Heterakis gallinarum	Cecum	None	Turkey, duck, goose, grouse, guinea fowl, partridge, pheasant, quail
Subulura brumpti	Cecum	Earwig, grasshopper, beetle	Turkey, dove, duck, grouse, guinea fowl, partridge, pheasant, quail
S. strongylina	Cecum	Beetle, cockroach, grasshopper	Guinea fowl, quail
Strongyloides avium	Cecum	None	Turkey, goose, grouse, quail
Trichostrongylus tenuis	Cecum	None	Turkey, duck, goose, guinea fowl, pigeon, quail

opmental stages before reaching the fifth or final stage. Successive stages are preceded by shedding of the skin (molting). In some nematodes the loosened skin or cuticle is retained for a short time as a protective covering; in others it is shed at once.

Eggs deposited in the location in which the female worms are found ultimately reach the outside in the droppings. Excorporeal existence is necessary for eggs to become infective for avian or arthropod hosts. The conditions existing within the definitive host are usually inimical to the development of the eggs. Outside the host in the required optimum moisture and temperature, these undergo development. Eggs of some nematodes require only a few days to complete embryonation; others require several weeks. For nematodes with direct life cycles, the final host becomes infected by eating embryonated eggs or free larvae; for those with indirect life cycles, the intermediate host ingests embryonated eggs or free larvae and retains the larvae within the body tissues. The final host becomes infected either by eating the infected intermediate host or by injection of the larvae by a blood-feeding arthropod.

Table 31.2. Nematodes reported from poultry or commercially raised game birds other than chickens

Nematode	Location	Intermediate Hosts	Other Definitive Hosts
Cyathostoma bronchialis	Trachea	None or earthworm	Turkey, duck, goose, (chicken)[a]
Cyrnea colini	Proventriculus	Cockroach	Turkey, grouse, prairie chicken, quail, (chicken)[a]
Tetrameres crami	Proventriculus	Amphipod	Duck
Microtetrameres helix	Proventriculus	Grasshopper	Pigeon
Amidostomum anseris	Gizzard	None	Duck, goose, pigeon
A. skrjabini	Gizzard	None	Duck, pigeon, (chicken)[a]
Ascaridia columbae	Small intestine	None	Pigeon, dove
A. dissimilis	Small intestine	None	Turkey
A. numidae	Small intestine	None	Guinea fowl
Ornithostrongylus quadriradiatus	Small intestine	None	Pigeon, dove
Heterakis dispar	Cecum	None	Duck, goose
H. isolonche	Cecum	None	Duck, grouse, pheasant, prairie chicken, quail
Capillaria columbae	Large intestine	None	Pigeon, dove

[a]Experimental.

Table 31.3. Nematodes reported from wild birds in the USA that pose a potential problem for poultry or commercially raised game birds

Nematode	Location	Intermediate Hosts	Definitive Hosts
Oxyspirura petrowi	Eye	Unknown	Grouse, quail, pheasant, prairie chicken
Splendidofilaria californiensis	Heart	Unknown	Quail
Singhfilaria hayesi	Subcutaneous	Unknown	Turkey, quail
Splendidofilaria pectoralis	Subcutaneous	Unknown	Grouse
Chandlerella chitwoodae	Connective tissues	Unknown	Grouse
Aproctella stoddardi	Body cavity	Unknown	Turkey, dove, quail
Cardiofilaria nilesi	Body cavity	Mosquito	Chicken
Echinura uncinata	Esophagus, gizzard, proventriculus, small intestine	Water flea	Duck, goose
E. parva	Proventriculus, gizzard	Unknown	Duck, goose
Tetrameres pattersoni	Proventriculus	Grasshopper, cockroach	Quail
T. ryjikovi	Proventriculus	Unknown	Duck
Cyrnea neeli	Proventriculus, gizzard	Unknown	Turkey
C. pileata	Proventriculus	Unknown	Quail
Physaloptera acuticauda	Proventriculus	Unknown	Chicken, pheasant
Amidostomum acutum	Gizzard	None	Duck
A. raillieti	Gizzard	None	Duck, dove
Cheilospirura spinosa	Gizzard	Grasshopper	Grouse, partridge, pheasant, quail, turkey
Cyrnea eurycerea	Gizzard	Unknown	Pheasant, quail, turkey
Epomidiostomum uncinatum	Gizzard	None	Chicken, duck, goose, pigeon
Streptocara crassicauda	Gizzard	Amphipod	Chicken, duck
Ascaridia bonasae	Small intestine	None	Grouse
A. compar	Small intestine	None	Grouse, partridge, pheasant, quail
Porrocaecum ensicaudatum	Small intestine	Earthworm	Chicken, duck
Capillaria phasianina	Small intestine, cecum	Unknown	Partridge, pheasant, guinea fowl
C. tridens	Small intestine	Unknown	Turkey
Aulonocephalus lindquisti	Cecum, large intestine	Unknown	Quail
A. pennula	Cecum	Unknown	Turkey
A. quaricensis	Cecum	Unknown	Quail

Note: Some of these have been reported from domestic poultry outside of the USA.

NEMATODES

NEMATODES OF THE DIGESTIVE TRACT

CAPILLARIA ANNULATA MOLIN 1858, CAPILLARIIDAE

Synonyms. *C. oblata* Graham, Thorpe, and Hectorne 1929; *Trichosoma delicatissum* Godoelst 1903 (61, 62).

Hosts. Chickens, turkeys, geese, grouse, guinea fowl, partridges, pheasants, quail.

Location. Mucosa of esophagus and crop.

Morphology. Long, slender worms similar in appearance to *C. contorta* but easily differentiated by a cuticular swelling just back of the head (Fig. 31.1A). *Male:* Usually 1-26 mm long, 52–74 μm wide; tail ends in 2 inconspicuous round lateral flaps, united dorsally by a cuticular flap; spicule sheath beset with fine spines (Fig. 31.1B); spicule 1.12–11.63 mm long. *Female:* Usually 25–60 mm long, 77–120 μm wide; posterior portion of body (posterior to vulva) about seven times as long as anterior portion; vulva circular, located about opposite the termination of the esophagus; eggs operculated (Fig. 31.1C), 55–66 × 26–28 μm.

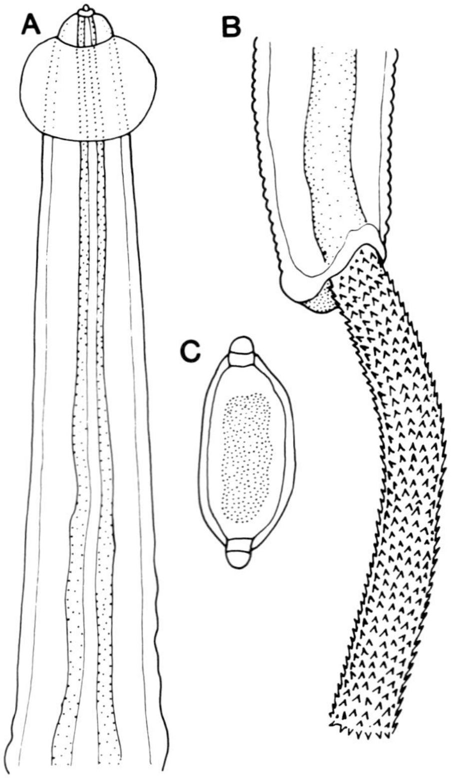

31.1. *Capillaria annulata.* A. Head end. B. Male tail. (After Ciurea). C. Egg.

Life Cycle. Eggs pass out in the droppings of infected birds. They develop to active embryos very slowly (24 days to over 1 mo). Wehr (87) demonstrated that two species of earthworms, *Eisenia foetidus* and *Allolobophora caliginosus,* serve as intermediate hosts of this crop worm.

Pathogenicity. This worm has been associated with deaths of turkeys in Maryland. Burrowing into the crop mucosa causes a thickening of the crop wall and enlargement of the glands. Usually there is inflammation of the crop and esophageal walls. In heavy infections the inner surface of the crop becomes thickened, roughened, and badly macerated, with masses of worms concentrated primarily in the sloughing tissue.

In pheasants, quail, and other gallinaceous game birds, infections often prove fatal. Signs are principally malnutrition and emaciation, associated with severe anemia.

CAPILLARIA CONTORTA CREPLIN 1839, CAPILLARIIDAE

Synonyms. *C. vanelli* Yamaguti 1935.

Hosts. Chickens, turkeys, ducks, guinea fowl, partridges, pheasants, quail.

Location. Mucosa of esophagus, crop, and sometimes the mouth.

Morphology. Body threadlike, attenuated anteriorly and posteriorly; head without a cuticular swelling. *Male:* 8–17 mm long, 60–70 μm wide; 2 terminal laterodorsal prominences on tail end; spicule very slender and transparent, about 800 μm long; spicule sheath covered with fine hairlike processes (Fig. 31.2B). *Female:* 15–60 mm long, 120–150 μm wide; vulva prominent, circular, 140–180 μm posterior to beginning of intestine (Fig. 31.2A).

Life Cycle. Eggs are apparently deposited in tunnels in the crop mucosa and escape into the lumen of crop and esophagus with the sloughed mucosa. They are abundant in droppings from infected birds. Approximately 1 mo or slightly longer is required for embryos to develop. Worms mature in susceptible avian hosts 1–2 mo after embryonated eggs are ingested.

Pathogenicity. When present in large numbers, these worms are extremely pathogenic. In light infections, the wall of the crop and esophagus becomes slightly thickened and inflamed. In heavy infections there is a marked thickening and in-

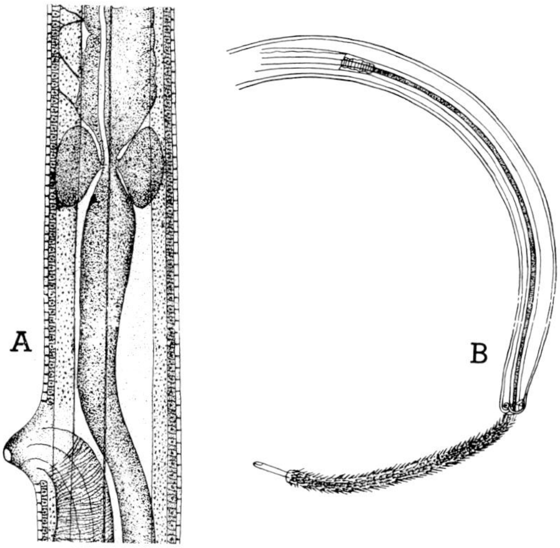

31.2. *Capillaria contorta.* A. Region of vulva. (After Eberth). B. Male tail. (After Travassos)

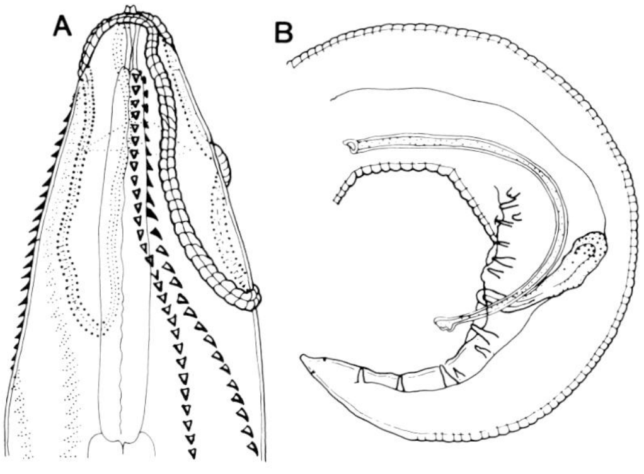

31.3. *Echinura uncinata.* A. Head. B. Male tail. (After Romanova)

flammation with a flocculent exudate covering the mucosa, with more or less sloughing of the mucosa. The crop may become nonfunctional. In extremely heavy infections the worms may invade the mouth and upper esophagus.

Infected birds become droopy, weak, and emaciated. Deaths have been observed among infected wild turkeys, Hungarian partridges, and quail in the USA. The birds are not inclined to move unless forced to; occasionally they assume a penguinlike posture, with the head drawn close to the body.

Echinura uncinata (Rudolphi 1819) Soloviev 1912, Acuariidae

Hosts. Wild and domestic ducks and geese. Reported in wild and domestic birds in Canada.

Location. Mucosa of the esophagus, proventriculus, gizzard, and small intestine. There is one report of this parasite in air sacs.

Morphology. Similar to *Cheilospirura* and *Dispharynx;* however, the cordons are not recurrent and anastomose posteriorly (Fig. 31.3A). *Male:* 8–10 mm long, 300–500 μm wide; left spicule 700–900 μm long, right spicule 350 μm long (Fig. 31.3B). *Female:* 12–18.5 mm long, 515 μm wide; tail 250 μm long; vulva 1.0–1.4 mm from end of tail, eggs 28–37 × 17–23 μm and embryonated when laid.

Life Cycle. Eggs are ingested by water fleas of the genus *Daphnia.* Larvae become infective after 12–14 days. Adults mature 51 days after ingestion.

Pathogenicity. Death is sometimes quite rapid and can occur without any previous signs. Nodules may form in the proventriculus; however, in chronic infections these may contain only inspissated pus, the worms having disappeared. Emaciation and listlessness can occur.

Gongylonema ingluvicola Ransom 1904, Gongylonematidae

Hosts. Chickens, turkeys, partridges, pheasants, quail.

Location. Mucosa of the crop and sometimes esophagus and proventriculus.

Morphology. Anterior end of body with a zone of shieldlike markings, few and scattered near head, numerous and arranged in longitudinal rows farther back (Fig. 31.4A). *Male:* 17–20 mm long, 224–250 μm wide; cervical papillae about 100 μm from head end; tail with 2 narrow bursal asymmetrical membranes; genital papillae variable in number and asymmetrical; preanal papillae up to 7 on left side and up to 5 on right side (Fig. 31.4B); left spicule as long or nearly as long (17–19 mm) as body and 7–9 μm wide, with a barbed point; right spicule 100–120 μm long 15–20 μm wide. *Female:* 32–55 mm long, 320–490 μm wide; vulva 2.5–3.5 mm from tip of tail.

Life Cycle. Larval roundworms collected from the beetle *Copris minutus* and fed to a chicken permitted recovery of a single male specimen of species *Gongylonema,* tentatively identified as *G. ingluvicola* (20). Subsequently cockroaches were infected by feeding embryonated eggs of *G. ingluvicola* derived from a mountain quail (19). Some of the larvae recovered from the cockroaches were fed to a chicken, but no worms were found on necropsy 79 days later.

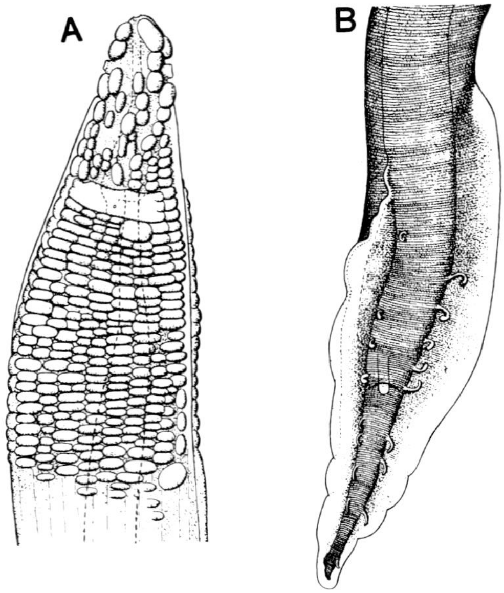

31.4. *Gongylonema ingluvicola.* A. Head. B. Male tail. (After Ransom)

Pathogenicity. The only damage associated with these worms is local lesions in the form of burrows in the crop mucosa. The worms and burrows appear as white convoluted tracks in the crop wall and can be confused with *Capillaria* unless examined microscopically.

CYRNEA COLINI CRAM 1927, HABRONEMATIDAE

Synonym. *Seurocyrena colini* Strand 1929.

Hosts. Turkeys, grouse, prairie chickens, quail (chickens, experimentally). Common in bobwhite quail of southeastern states and occasionally in this or closely related birds in some northeastern states. Also reported from turkeys in Georgia and prairie chickens in Wisconsin and Montana.

Location. Wall of the proventriculus, preferentially at its junction with the gizzard.

Morphology. Slender yellowish white worms, similar in appearance to *Cheilospirura hamulosa* but smaller and lacking the so-called cordons or cuticular ornamentations on anterior part of the body; the tail of the male has winglike expansions or alae (Fig. 31.5B); the head structures are complicated with 4 lips; dorsal and ventral lips prominent and bearing 4 conspicuous projecting papillae and a prominent thumblike projection (Fig. 31.5A); lateral lips very large, each bearing 2 digitiform processes on inner surface and 2 winglike expansions on lateral surface. *Male:* 6 mm long, 250 μm wide; buccal cavity 58 μm deep; esophagus 2 mm long; caudal alae nearly circular, with 10 pairs of pedunculated papillae, the anterior ones larger than posterior; spicules very unequal, the left 2 mm long and the right 365–400 μm. *Female:* 14–18 mm long, 315 μm wide; buccal cavity 75 μm deep; esophagus about 2.8 mm long; vulva 915 μm anterior to anus; eggs 40.5 x 22.5 μm (Fig. 31.5C).

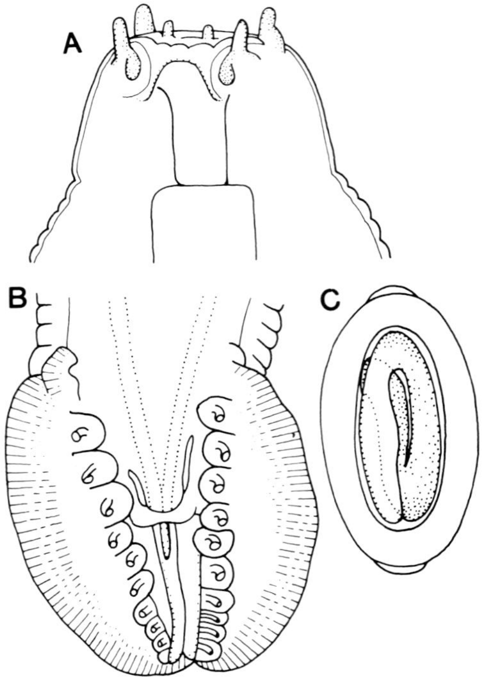

31.5. *Cyrnea colini.* A. Head. B. Male tail. (After Cram). C. Egg.

Life Cycle. The cockroach *Blattella germanica* was infected with *C. colini* by feeding eggs (18). Larvae entered the body cavity, developed into the third stage in the tissues without encysting, and appeared fully developed by 18 days. Larvae were fed to quail 27 days later; mature worms were recovered 41 days subsequently.

Pathogenicity. Little or no pathological change has been observed.

DISPHARYNX NASUTA (RUDOLPHI 1819) STILES AND HASSELL 1920, ACUARIIDAE

Synonyms. All forms of *Dispharynx* recorded from galliform, columbiform, and passiform birds in the Western Hemisphere are nonspecific, and a morphological study indicates their identity as *D. nasuta* (40). *D. nasuta* (Rudolphi 1819) Stiles and

Hassall 1920, has priority over *D. spiralis* (Molin 1858) Skrjabin 1916.

Hosts. Chickens, turkeys, grouse, guinea fowl, partridges, pheasants, pigeons, quail, and a number of passerine birds in the USA.

Location. Wall of the proventriculus, sometimes the esophagus, rarely the small intestine.

Morphology. Four wavy cuticular cordons on anterior end, originating at base of lips, recurrent, the distal extremity of the cordons turning forward and extending anteriorly a short distance (Fig. 31.6A); postcervical papillae small, bicuspid, situated between the recurrent branches of the cordons; body usually rolled in a spiral (Fig. 31.6B). *Male:* 7–8.3 mm long, 230–315 μm wide; 5 pairs of postanal and 4 pairs of preanal papillae (Fig. 31.6C); long spicule 400 μm long, slender and curved; short spicule 150 μm long, navicular. *Female:* 9–10.2 mm long, 360–565 μm wide; vulva in posterior portion of body; eggs embryonated when oviposited.

Life Cycle. The pillbug (*Armadillidium vulgare*) and the sowbug (*Porcellio scaber*) serve as intermediate hosts in experimental infections (18). Within 4 days after ingestion of embryonated eggs, larvae escape from the eggs and are found among the tissues of the body cavity. The larva completes its development to third or infective stage in the isopod within approximately 26 days. Female worms become sexually mature and deposit eggs 27 days after ingestion by a susceptible vertebrate host (18).

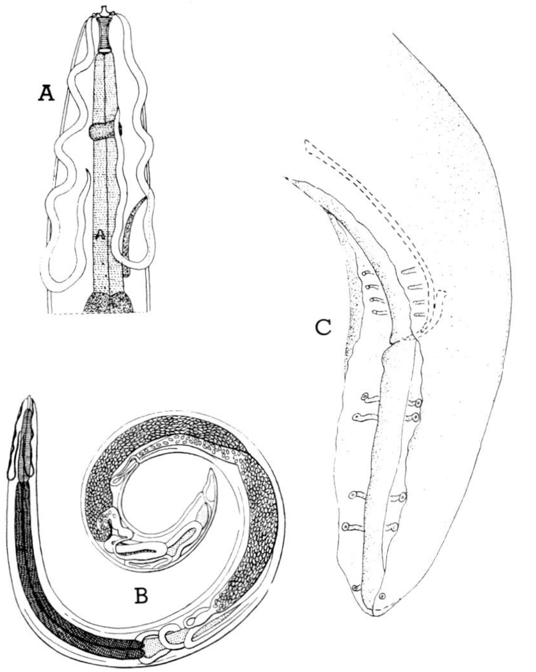

31.6. *Dispharynx nasuta.* A. Head. (After Seurat). B. Female. (After Piana). C. Male tail. (After Cram)

Pathogenicity. These roundworms are usually found with their heads buried deep in the mucosa. Ulcers are often observed in the proventriculus. In a heavy infection, the wall of the proventriculus becomes tremendously thickened and macerated, tissue layers being indistinguishable, and the parasites become almost completely concealed beneath the proliferating tissue.

Dispharynx nasuta has been considered the chief cause of "grouse disease" in northeastern USA. Heavy infections have resulted in the death of many carrier pigeons. Wild pigeons trapped at the Balboa Zoological Park, San Diego, California, were heavily infected with this parasite.

TETRAMERES AMERICANA CRAM 1926, TETRAMERIDAE

Hosts. Chickens, turkeys, ducks, grouse, pigeons, quail.

Location. Proventriculus.

Morphology. Mouth surrounded with 3 small lips; buccal cavity present (Fig. 31.8A). Marked sexual dimorphism. *Male:* 5–5.5 mm long, 116–133 μm wide (Fig. 31.7A); 2 double rows of poste-

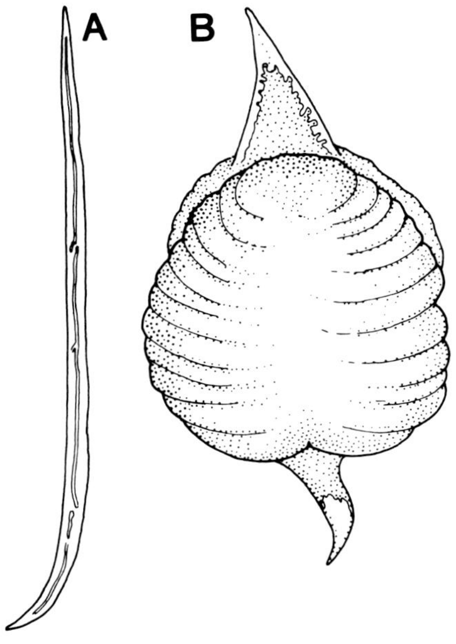

31.7. *Tetrameres americana.* A. Male. B. Female. (After Cram)

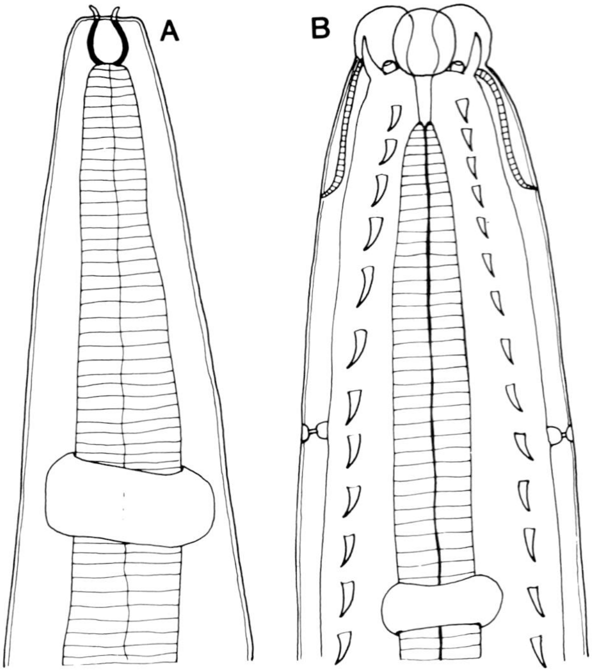

31.8. A. *Tetrameres americana*, head. (Courtesy Graybill). B. *Tetrameres fissispina*, head. (Travassos)

riorly directed spines extend throughout whole body length in the submedian lines; cervical papillae present; tail long and slender; 2 unequal spicules, 100 μm and 290–312 μm long respectively. *Female:* 3.5–4.5 mm long, 3 mm wide; body globular (Fig. 31.7B), blood red in color, with 4 longitudinal furrows; uteri and ovaries very long, their numerous coils filling the body cavity; eggs 42–50 × 24 μm and embryonated when laid.

Life Cycle. At necropsy these bright red worms are often observed through the wall of the unopened proventriculus. The nematode-shaped male of this species is very small, almost microscopic in size, and is seldom observed elsewhere other than on the surface of the mucosa of the proventriculus. The male apparently enters the glands of the proventriculus only long enough to mate with the female. However, the males of some species of *Tetrameres* occurring in wild birds have been found together with the females in the same glands, indicating that the two sexes were permanent residents of the glands in which they were found.

T. americana requires an intermediate host for its complete development (18). Embryonated eggs fed to two species of grasshoppers (*Melanoplus femurrubrum* and *M. differentialis*) and a species of cockroach (*Blatella germanica*) produced infective (third stage) larvae recovered from the body cavities of these insects about 42 days later. After ingestion, the larvae escape and spend at least 14 days in the gastric mucosa, molting to the fourth stage. Females then enter the gastric glands, mate, and contain embryonated eggs by the 45th day.

Pathogenicity. Infected chickens become emaciated and anemic as a result of heavy infections. *T. americana* did not produce any damage in quail (20). In chickens the walls of the proventriculus may be thickened so that the lumen is almost entirely obliterated.

T. americana has been reported both from wild (33) and laboratory-raised pigeons (38). Mild infections produced little evidence of clinical disease; heavy infections resulted in diarrhea, emaciation, and possibly death.

TETRAMERES CRAMI SWALES 1933, TETRAMERIDAE

Hosts. Wild and domestic ducks.

Location. Proventriculus.

Morphology. Smaller than *T. americana*. *Male:* 2.9–4.1 mm long, 70–92 μm wide; a narrow curved right spicule 136–185 μm long, a twisted left spicule 272–350 μm long. *Female:* 1.5–3.3 mm long, 1.2–2.2 mm wide; tail 113–156 μm long; vulva 319–350 μm from posterior end; eggs 41–57 × 26–34 μm and embryonated when laid.

Life Cycle. The intermediate hosts of *T. crami* are the amphipods *Gammarus fasciatus* and *Hyalella knickerbocki* (79). The larvae become infective in 29 days. Adults mature 33 days after infection.

TETRAMERES FISSISPINA (DIESING 1861) TRAVASSOS 1915, TETRAMERIDAE

Hosts. Chickens, turkeys, ducks, guinea fowl, geese, pigeons, quail. Most commonly a parasite of wild or domestic ducks and geese and wild birds, rarely found in the other poultry.

Location. Proventriculus.

Morphology. Similar in appearance to *T. americana*. *Male:* 3–6 mm long, 90–200 μm wide; 4 longitudinal rows of spines along the median and lateral lines (Fig. 31.8B); spicules 280–490 and 82–150 μm long. *Female:* 1.7–6.0 mm long, 1.3–5.0 mm wide; tail 71 μm long; vulva 310 μm from posterior end; eggs 48–56 × 26–30 μm and embryonated when laid.

Life Cycle. Intermediate hosts include amphipods, grasshoppers, earthworms, and cockroaches. Larvae are infective by the 10th day. Worms mature about 18 days after ingestion. Fish are known to serve as a transport host.

Pathogenicity. Considerable tissue reaction occurs together with degeneration of the glandular tissue, edema, and extensive leukocyte infiltration (84).

TETRAMERES PATTERSONI CRAM 1933, TETRAMERIDAE

Host. Quail.

Location. Proventriculus.

Morphology. Bright red female worms found embedded in the glands of the proventriculus, males on surface of mucosa. *Male:* 4.2–4.6 mm long, 140–170 μm wide; body with 2 rows of spines ending just anterior to cloacal aperture; 3 pairs of lateral and 4 pairs of subventral spines posterior to cloacal aperture; only 1 spicule, 1.2–1.5 mm long with conspicuous cross-striations. *Female:* 5 mm long, 2–2.3 mm wide; vulva about 235 μm from tail end, anus 156 μm from tail end; bulbous enlargement between vulva and anus; eggs 42–46 × 25–30 μm.

Life Cycle. Eggs fed to grasshoppers (*Melanoplus femurrubrum* or *Chortophaga viridifasciata*) or cockroaches (*Blattella germanica*) developed into larvae (19). By 24 days third-stage characteristics were fully developed. Larvae were encysted in the muscles and the mesenteries of the body cavity, each cyst containing 1–3 larvae. The tail end of the larva had a small protuberance, thus differing from *T. fissispina* and *T. americana.* Attempts to infect chickens, turkeys, pigeons, or ducks with this species were unsuccessful.

Pathogenicity. The extent of damage in quail is not fully known. Worms can be so numerous that little uninfected stomach wall remains. Hosts from which the original collections were made died shortly after capture, but whether this was from the infection or other causes was not determined.

AMIDOSTOMUM ANSERIS ZEDER 1800, AMIDOSTOMATIDAE

Hosts. Ducks, geese, pigeons. In the USA, parasites have been reported from domestic geese in New York, Delaware, Pennsylvania, and Washington but no doubt there is a wider distribution.

Location. Under the horny lining of the gizzard, less frequently in the proventriculus.

Morphology. Worms slender and reddish; short, wide buccal capsule has 3 pointed teeth at its base (Fig. 31.9A). *Male:* 10–17 mm long, 250–350 μm wide; bursa with 2 large lateral lobes and a small median lobe (Fig. 31.9B); dorsal ray short, bifurcating posteriorly, the bifurcations forked and terminating in 2 tips; spicules 200 μm long, slender, and cleft near their middle; gubernaculum slender and 95 μm long. *Female:* 12–24 mm long, 200–400 μm wide at vulva, thinning toward both extremities; vulva transverse, in posterior part of the body; eggs thin-shelled, 85–110 × 50–82 μm.

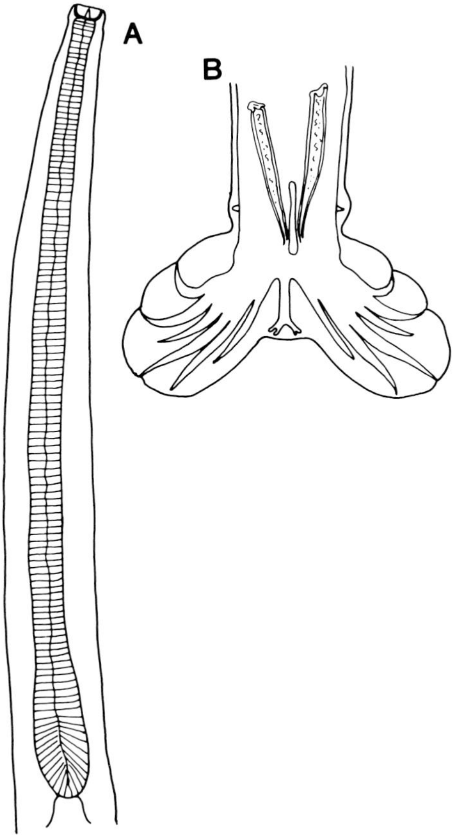

31.9. *Amidostomum anseris.* A. Anterior. (After Boulenger). B. Male bursa. (After Railliet)

Life Cycle. Eggs pass out in the droppings in a partly developed stage; active embryos develop within a few hours, and hatch within a few days. Susceptible birds become infected by swallowing food or drinking water contaminated with infective larvae. This parasite is quite host-specific; attempts to infect a variety of other hosts (whooper swans, coots, avocets, godwits, gulls, blackbirds, crows, doves, quail, chickens, and turkeys) were unsuccessful, even though geese serving as controls all became infected (28).

Third-stage larvae placed directly on the skin of birds are also infective. Larvae remain viable for several weeks if kept in clean aerated water. Enigk and Dey-Hazra (27) showed that larvae migrate via the lungs when given percutaneously but not when given orally. Adult worms are recovered approximately 40 days after the feeding of infective larvae.

Pathogenicity. Heavy losses among geese have been attributed to this nematode. Young birds show loss of appetite, dullness, and emaciation. The lining of the gizzard of a heavily parasitized bird appears necrotic, loosened, often sloughed in places, and dark brown or black in areas adjacent to the site of the worms. Extreme blood loss may contribute to the effects.

AMIDOSTOMUM SKRJABINI BOULENGER 1926, AMIDOSTOMATIDAE

Synonym. *A. fuligulae* Maplestone 1930.

Hosts. Ducks, pigeons, (chickens, experimentally).

Location. Horny lining of gizzard.

Morphology. Smaller than *A. anseris.* Can be distinguished from *A. raillieti* by the latter's posterior bulblike enlargement of esophagus (Fig. 31.10A); each branch of the dorsal ray further divided into 2 equal branches; spicules 115–125 µm long. *Male.* 7.5–8.8 mm long, 100–130 µm wide; bursa resembling that of *A. raillieti* (Fig. 31.10B); each branch of the dorsal ray further divided into 2 equal branches; spicules 115–125 µm long. *Female:* 9–11 mm long, 1001–20 µm wide; vulva 1.7–2.1 mm from posterior end; eggs 70–80 × 40–50 µm, in the morula stage when laid.

Life Cycle. Similar to *A. anseris.*

Pathogenicity. Involved in some outbreaks of amidostomiasis in young ducks.

CHEILOSPIRURA HAMULOSA (DIESING 1851) DIESING 1861, ACUARIIDAE

Synonym. *Acuaria hamulosa* Diesing 1851.

Hosts. Chickens, turkeys, grouse, guinea fowl, pheasants, quail.

Location. Under the horny lining of the gizzard, usually in the cardiac and/or pyloric regions where the lining is soft and pliable.

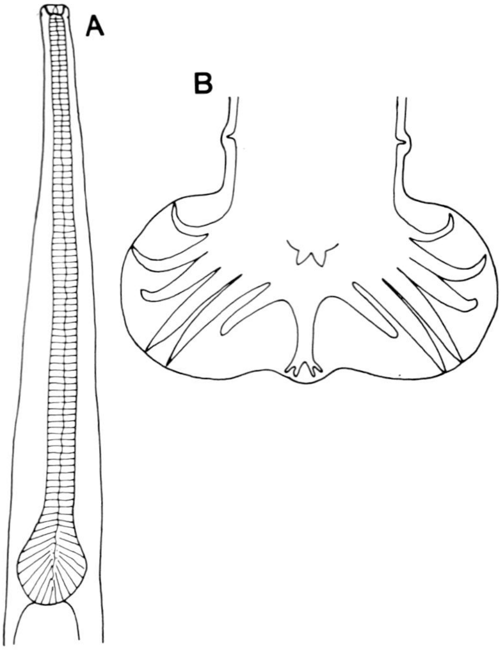

31.10. A. *Amidostomum raillieti,* head. B. *Amidostomum skrjabini,* male bursa. (After Boulenger)

Morphology. Two large triangular lateral lips; the 4 cuticular cordons double, irregularly wavy (Fig. 31.11A), and extending at least 2/3 the length of the body and sometimes almost to posterior extremity, not anastomosing or recurring anteriorly. *Male:* 9–19 mm long; spicules unequal and dissimilar, the left long and slender, 1.6–1.8 mm by 12 µm, the right short and curved, 180–200 × 64 µm; tail tightly coiled; 2 very wide caudal alae present; 10 pairs of caudal papillae (Fig. 31.11B). *Female:* 16–25 mm long; vulva slightly posterior to middle of body; tail pointed; eggs embryonated when deposited, 40 × 27 µm.

Life Cycle. Grasshoppers, beetles, weevils, and sandhoppers serve as intermediate hosts. When eggs are fed to grasshoppers (*Melanoplus femurrubrum* and *M. differentialis*), the *C. hamulosa* larvae hatch and migrate into the body cavity (18). They develop, chiefly in the muscles, to the third stage, which is infective for the bird. This larva is easily recognized by the 2 prominent liplike structures at the anterior end of the body, the dorsal curvature of the posterior portion of the body, and the 4 digitiform processes at the tip of the tail.

Larvae are infective for chickens as early as 22 days and as late as 67 days after ingestion of eggs by the grasshoppers. At 11 days after feeding to chicks, larvae are on the underside of the corneous lining of the gizzard; 16 days after feeding, larvae show characteristics of immature adults.

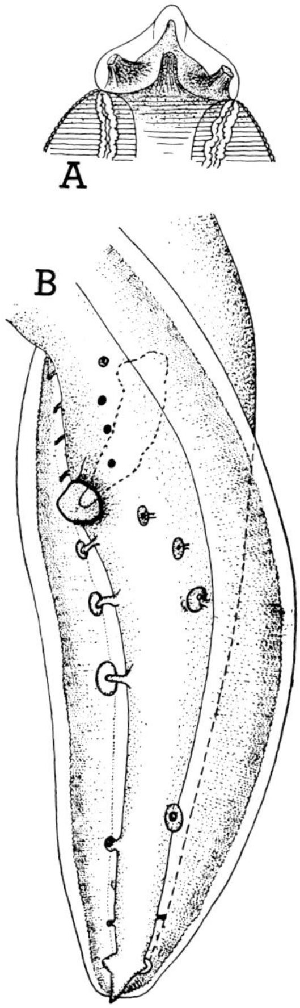

31.11. *Cheilospirura hamulosa.* A. Head. (After Drasche). B. Male tail. (After Cram)

By 25 days, worms begin penetrating the muscular wall. Maturity is reached at about 76 days.

Pathogenicity. When present in small numbers, these worms are relatively nonpathogenic, although the lining of the gizzard may show small local lesions that may also involve the muscular tissue. Soft nodules enclosing parasites may be found in the muscular portion of the gizzard. In heavy infections the wall of the gizzard may be seriously weakened, causing a rupture, with ultimate formation of a sac or pouch. There has been only a single human infection reported (in the Philippines), a tumor in the conjunctiva.

CHEILOSPIRURA SPINOSA CRAM 1927, ACUARIIDAE

Hosts. Grouse, partridges, pheasants, quail, wild turkeys.

Location. In the gizzard underneath the corneous lining.

Morphology. Four spiny cordons originating in pairs between the lips (Fig. 31.12A), not extending beyond the anterior 1/3 of the anterior esophagus. *Male:* 14–20 mm long, 183–232 μm wide; spicules unequal and very dissimilar, one 660–720 μm long, the other 192 μm long; caudal alae broad, similar in appearance to *C. hamulosa* (Fig. 31.12B). *Female:* 34–40 mm long, 315–348 μm wide; vulva anterior to middle of body; anus 250–300 μm from posterior end; eggs 39–42 × 25–27 μm.

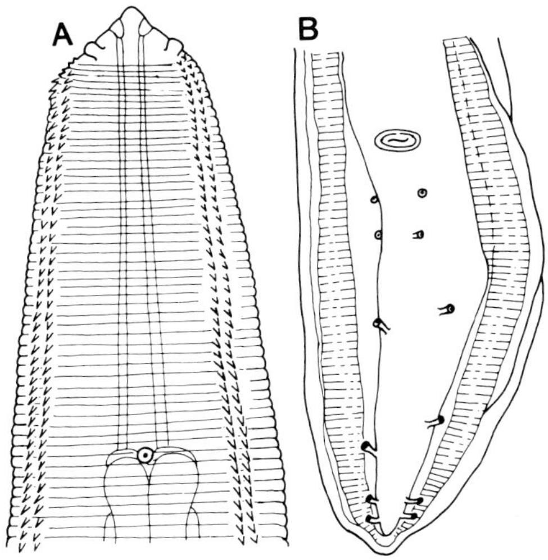

31.12. *Cheilospirura spinosa.* A. Head. B. Male tail. (After Cram)

Life Cycle. This worm, originally a parasite of grouse, probably then spread to quail (18). Grasshoppers serve as the intermediate host, where development is similar to that seen with *C. hamulosa.* The tail structures on the third-stage larvae are similar in *C. spinosa* rather than in *C. hamulosa.* In the bobwhite quail, fourth-stage larvae were found underneath the gizzard lining 14 days after feeding (18). Worms with fully developed sexual characteristics were seen at 32 days.

Pathogenicity. Light infections seem to produce few problems in quail, although tortuous paths are found between the lining and muscular wall of the gizzard. In cases of heavy infection the gizzard lining may become hemorrhagic and necrotic. Marked proliferative changes in the gizzard wall can occur with prolonged heavy infection.

Epomidiostomum uncinatum (Lundahl 1841) Seurat 1918, Amidostomatidae

Synonym. *E. anatinum* Skrjabin 1915.

Hosts. Ducks, geese, pigeons (chickens, experimentally).

Location. Under horny lining of gizzard.

Morphology. Differs from *Amidostomum* in that the buccal capsule contains no teeth and the head has a pair of nodules (Fig. 31.13A). *Male:* 6.5–7.3 mm long, 150 μm wide; spicules 120–130 μm long (Fig. 31.13B), dividing to form 3 terminations. *Female:* 10–11.5 mm long, 230–240 μm wide; tail 140–170 μm long (Fig. 31.13C); vulva 2.2–3.2 mm from posterior end; eggs 74–90 × 45–50 μm.

Life Cycle. In larval development the ensheathed, third-stage larvae are infective 4 days after hatching (55).

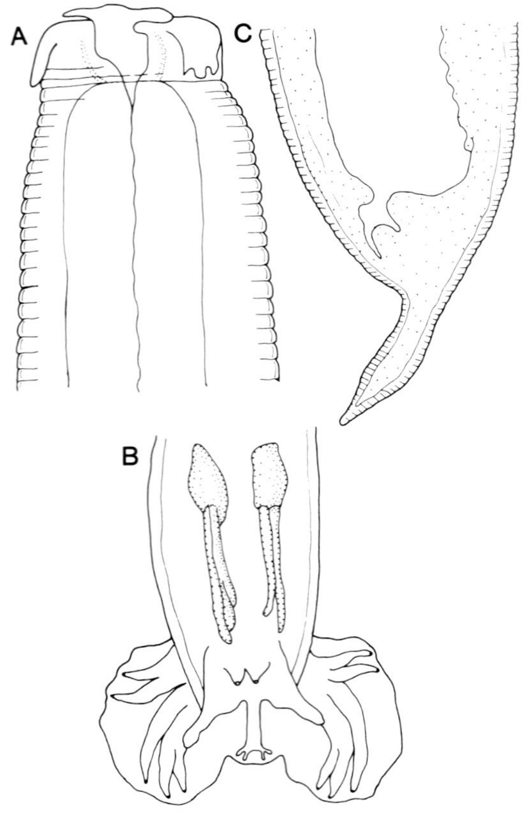

31.13. *Epomidiostomum uncinatum.* A. Head. B. Male tail. C. Female tail. (After Skrjabin)

Ascaridia bonasae Wehr 1940, Ascaridiidae

Host. Grouse.

Location. Lumen of small intestine.

Morphology. Apparently this has been reported as *A. galli,* although *A. bonasae* is small and does not infect chickens. *Male:* 10–35 mm long; spicules 1.8–2.7 mm long and equal. *Female:* 30–50 mm long.

Life Cycle. Similar to *A. galli.*

Ascaridia columbae (Gmelin 1790) Travassos 1913, Ascaridiidae

Hosts. Pigeons, doves.

Location. Usually the lumen of the small intestine but sometimes in the esophagus, proventriculus, gizzard, liver, or body cavity.

Morphology. *Male:* 50–70 mm long; spicules 1.2–1.9 mm long and equal; fourth pair of ventral papillae located adjacent to the anus (Fig. 31.14A). *Female:* 20–95 mm long.

Life Cycle. Similar to *A. galli* but more invasive. Second-stage larvae frequently penetrate the intestinal mucosa and reach the liver and lungs (90) but do not develop further. Worms mature in about 37 days after embryonated eggs are consumed.

Pathogenicity. The invasion of the liver produces little effect until the larvae die, then granulomatous lesions form with leukocyte infiltration.

Ascaridia compar Schrank 1790, Ascaridiidae

Hosts. Grouse, partridges, pheasants, quail.

Morphology. Smaller than *A. galli* but similar in appearance. *Male:* 36–48 mm long; spicules 1.8 mm long; 4 pairs of preanal papillae (2 near the preanal sucker, 2 just anterior to the anus, Fig. 31.14B). *Female:* 84–96 mm long.

Life Cycle. Similar to *A. galli.*

Ascaridia dissimilis Perez Vigueras 1931, Ascaridiidae

Host. Turkeys.

Location. Lumen of the small intestine.

Morphology. Although the literature contains numerous reports of both *A. galli* and *A. dissimilus* in turkeys, probably only *A. dissimilis* is the parasite found (49). Only males can be accurately identified based on caudal papillae and spicule tips. *Male:* 35–65 mm long; spicules 1.3–2.2 mm long, distal ends of the spicules rounded; the first pair of preanal papillae are opposite the preanal sucker, the ventral pair of postanal papillae are only slightly separated and just behind the anus (Fig. 31.14C). *Female:* 50–105 mm long.

Life Cycle. Similar to *A. galli.* Eggs embryonate in 9–10 days. Larvae enter the intestinal mucosa, then mature in the lumen in about 30 days.

ASCARIDIA GALLI SCHRANK 1788, ASCARIDIIDAE

Synonyms. *A. lineata* Schneider 1866 and *Heterakis granulosa* Linstow 1906.

Hosts. Chickens, turkeys, doves, ducks, geese.

Location. Lumen of the intestine, occasionally in the esophagus, crop, gizzard, oviduct, and body cavity.

Morphology. Worms large, thick, yellowish white; head with 3 large lips. *Male:* 50–76 mm long, 490 μm to 1.21 mm wide; preanal sucker oval or circular, with strong chitinous wall with a papilliform interruption on its posterior rim; tail with narrow caudal alae or membranes and 10 pairs of papillae; first pair of ventral caudal papillae are anterior to the preanal sucker, fourth pair are widely separated (Fig. 31.14D, compare with *A. dissimilis*); spicules nearly equal and narrow, end blunt with a slight indentation. *Female:* 60–116 mm long, 900 μm to 1.8 mm wide; vulva in anterior part of body; eggs elliptical, thick-shelled, not embryonated at time of deposition (Fig. 31.15).

Life Cycle. The life history is simple and direct. Infective eggs hatch in either the proventriculus or the duodenum of the susceptible host. The young larvae, after hatching, live free in the lumen of the posterior portion of the duodenum for the first 9 days, then penetrate the mucosa and cause hemorrhages. The young worms enter the lumen of the duodenum by 17 or 18 days and remain there until maturity, at approximately 28–30 days after ingestion of embryonated eggs. Larvae may enter the tissues as early as the 1st day and remain there as long as 26 days after infection. The large majority spend from 8 to 17 days in the intestinal mucosa. A few of the larvae penetrate deep into the tissue while the majority undergo only a brief and shallow association with the intestinal mucosa during the "tissue phase." *A. galli* eggs ingested by grasshoppers or earthworms hatch and are infective to chickens, although no development of the larvae occurs.

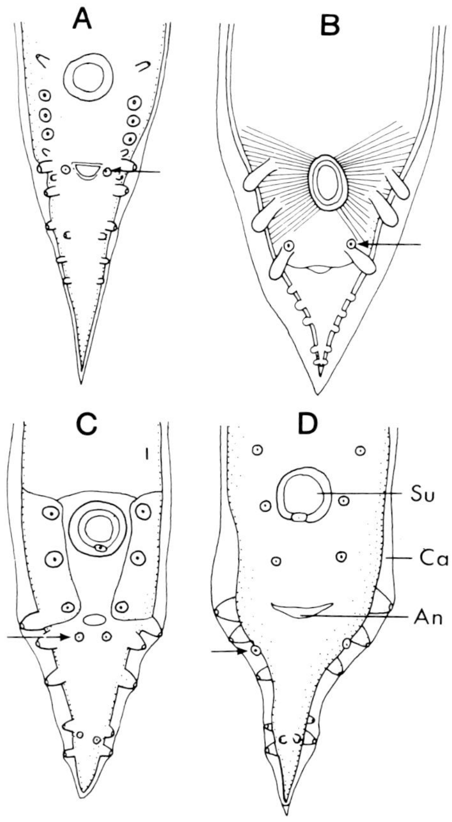

31.14. Male tails showing anal or caudal papillae (*arrows*). A. *Ascaridia columbae.* (After Wehr and Hwang). B. *Ascaridia compar.* (After Linstow). C. *Ascaridia dissimilis.* D. *Ascaridia galli. An* = anus; *Ca* = caudal alae; *Su* = sucker. (After Wehr)

Under optimum temperature and moisture conditions, eggs in the droppings become infective in 10–12 days; under less favorable conditions a longer time is necessary. Eggs are quite resistant to low temperatures. Larvae were recovered from experimental birds fed embryonated eggs that had been exposed continuously to outdoor conditions at Beltsville, MD, for 66 wk (34). A 12-hr exposure to 43 C proved lethal for eggs in all stages of development.

Pathogenicity. *A. galli* infection causes weight depression in the host, which correlates with increasing worm burden (70). In severe infections, intestinal blockage can occur. The nutritional state of the host is also important, since weight depression is greater with high dietary levels of protein (15%) than with low levels (12.5%) (48). Chickens infected with a large number of ascarids suffer from loss of blood, reduced blood sugar

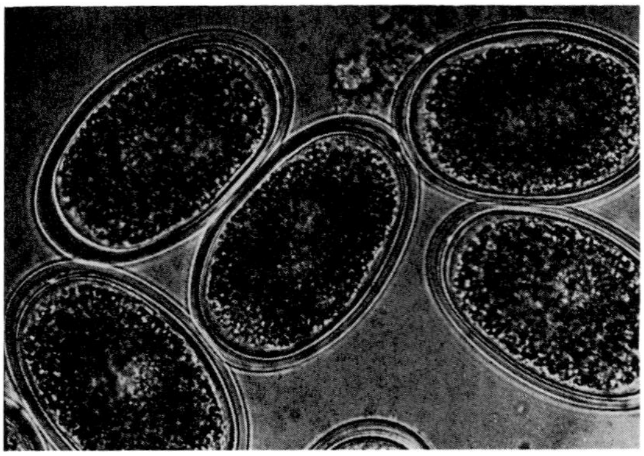

31.15. *Ascaridia galli* eggs freshly voided from a chicken. ×400. (Benbrook)

content, increased urates, shrunken thymus glands, retarded growth, and greatly increased mortality. However, no effects of infection on blood protein level, packed-cell volume, or hemoglobin levels were found (46). *A. galli* can also have detrimental effects through interaction (synergism) with other disease conditions such as coccidiosis and infectious bronchitis. *A. galli* has also been shown to contain and transmit avian reoviruses.

One of the most striking effects of infection, at least from an aesthetic standpoint, is the occasional finding of this parasite in the hen's egg. Numerous reports of this phenomenon have been made in the literature (71). Presumably the worms migrate up the oviduct via the cloaca, with subsequent inclusion in the egg. Infected eggs can be detected by candling, thus eliminating a potential consumer complaint. Some embarrassing law suits against the poultry industries could be avoided if egg candlers were encouraged to remove such eggs in packing plants.

Immunity. Age of the host and severity of exposure play roles in *A. galli* infections. Chickens 3 mo or older manifest considerable resistance to infection with *A. galli*. In older fowl, larvae are recovered that have undergone little or no development since emerging from the egg (83). Larval development is arrested in the third stage at high-dose rates as a result of resistance rather than a density-dependent phenomenon (47). Heavier breeds such as Rhode Island Reds and White and Barred Plymouth Rocks are more resistant to ascarid infections than are the lighter White Leghorns and White Minorcas.

The nutritional state of the bird also influences the development of immunity. Diets consisting chiefly of animal proteins with little or no plant protein aid the chicken in building resistance to infection with ascarids. Birds given a diet consisting principally of animal protein developed fewer worms than those given a diet low in animal protein. Diets high in vitamins A and B (complex) increase the fowl's resistance to *A. galli*, and diets low in these vitamins definitely favor parasitism. Increasing levels of dietary calcium and lysine decreased the length and number of worms recovered (21).

ASCARIDIA NUMIDAE LEIPER 1908, ASCARIDIIDAE

Synonym. *Heterakis numidae* Leiper 1908.

Host. Guinea fowl.

Location. Lumen of small intestine, sometimes cecum.

Morphology. Much smaller than *A. galli*. *Male:* 19–35 mm long; 10 pairs of caudal papillae, 2 of them preanal and 2 adanal; spicules equal, 3 mm long. *Female:* 30–50 mm long.

Life Cycle. The larvae remain in the lumen for 4–14 days before penetrating the intestinal mucosa.

TAXONOMY OF *CAPILLARIA* FROM THE INTESTINE OF BIRDS. Most species of *Capillaria* from birds have been described under a variety of names. Likewise, many species names have been used for several different capillaria. As a result, descriptions, host specificity, location in the intestine, geographic distribution, and even the validity of some species is confused (57, 59, 61, 69). This chapter uses essentially the species accepted by Levine (57) except for *C. dujardini*, which is considered a synonym of *C. obsignata*. The species *C. retusa*, *C. collaris*, and *C. longicallis* commonly used in the literature have been synonymized. The species *C. columbae* Rudolphi 1819 is retained for the capillaria in the large intestine of pigeons that possess a vulva with a projecting appendage (Table 31.4 and Fig. 31.16).

Table 31.4. Characteristics of *Capillaria* from chickens in the USA

Characteristic	*C. anatis*	*C. bursata*	*C. caudinflata*	*C. obsignata*
Male				
Lateral caudalae	–	+	+	–
Spicule sheath	Spines	No spines	Minute spines	No spines
Female				
Vulvar appendage	None	Semicircular	Pronounced	None

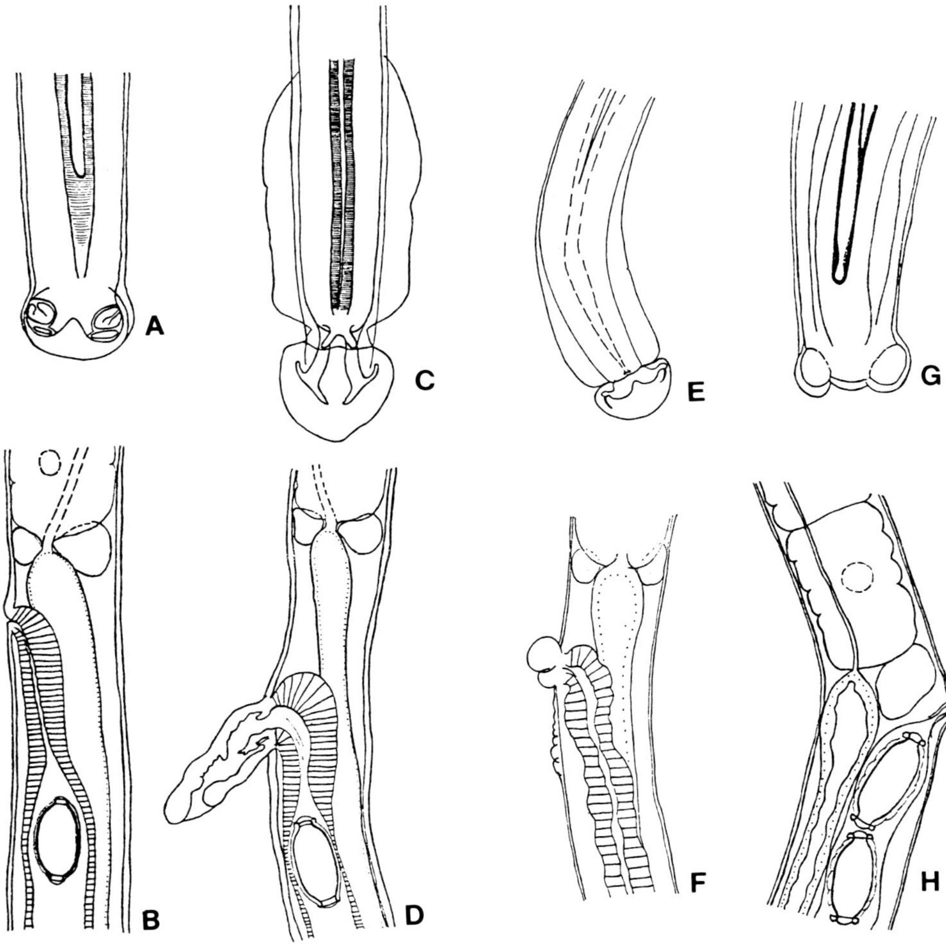

31.16. Male bursa (A, C, E, G) and female vulva (B, D, F, H) of *Capillaria obsignata* (A, B), *Capillaria caudinflata* (C, D), *Capillaria bursata* (E, F), and *Capillaria anatis* (G, H). (After Wakelin)

Capillaria anatis (Schrank 1790) Travassos 1915, Capillariidae

Synonym. *Capillaria brevicollis* Walton 1935.

Hosts. Chickens, turkeys, ducks, geese, partridges, pheasants.

Location. Usually cecum, sometimes small intestine.

Morphology. Threadlike worms. *Male:* 8–15 mm long; spicule 0.7–1.9 mm long with a spiny sheath; tail with 2 lobes but no lateral caudal alae (Fig. 31.16G). *Female:* 11–28 mm long; vulva without appendage (Fig. 31.16H); eggs 46–67 × 22–29 μm with a thick rugous outer shell.

Capillaria bursata Freitas and Almeida 1934, Capillariidae

Hosts. Chickens, turkeys, geese, pheasants.

Location. Mucosa of small intestine.

Morphology. Although some authors consider *C. bursata* a synonym of *C. caudinflata,* others gives reasons for their being recognized as separate species (69, 86). *Male:* 11–20 mm long, 44–51 μm wide; spicule 1.1–1.6 mm long; sheath without spines; bursa round, supported by 2 dorsal and 2 ventral projections (Fig. 31.16E). *Female:* 16–35 mm long, 53–64 μm wide; vulva with 2 semicircular valves (Fig. 31.16F); eggs 51–62 × 22–24 μm, shell with fine longitudinal ridges.

Life Cycle. Eggs are passed in the feces; larval development is complete in 8–15 days, depending on temperature. Eggs hatch after ingestion by earthworm. Larvae are infective after 22–25 days. Worms mature in final host 20–26 days after ingestion.

CAPILLARIA CAUDINFLATA (MOLIN 1858) WAWILOWA 1926, CAPILLARIIDAE

Synonym. *C. longicollis* (Mehlis 1931) of Madsen 1945.

Hosts. Chickens, turkeys, ducks, geese, guinea fowl, grouse, partridges, pheasants, pigeons, quail.

Location. Mucosa of small intestine.

Morphology. *Male:* 9–18 mm long, 33–51 μm wide; spicule 0.7–1.2 mm, tapering to a fine point distally; spicule sheath with fine thornlike spines on proximal portion; bursa present, supported dorsally by 2 T-shaped processes (Fig. 31.16C). *Female:* 12–25 mm long, 38–62 μm wide; vulva with characteristic appendage (Fig. 31.16D); eggs 47–58 × 20–24 μm, shell thick and finely sculptured.

Life Cycle. Turkeys were experimentally infected by feeding earthworms (*Allolobophora caliginosa*) from infected poultry yards (2). This earthworm is an essential intermediate host for the successful transmission of *C. caudinflata* from turkey to turkey. Attempts to transmit this threadworm by using the earthworm *Lumbricus terrestris* were unsuccessful. When earthworms (*Eisenia foetida*) were fed embryonated eggs of *C. caudinflata,* adults were recovered at necropsy from turkeys to which these earthworms had been fed.

CAPILLARIA OBSIGNATA MADSEN 1945, CAPILLARIIDAE

Synonym. *C. collaris* Linstow 1873.

Hosts. Chickens, turkeys, geese, guinea fowl, pigeons, quail.

Location. Small intestine, cecum.

Morphology. Hairlike worms (Fig. 31.17). *Male:* 7–13 mm long, 49–53 μm wide, cloacal aperture almost terminal, with a small bursal lobe on either side, the 2 lobes connected dorsally by a delicate bursal membrane (Fig. 31.16A); spicule 1.1–1.5 mm long; sheath with transverse folds without spines. *Female:* 10–18 mm long, approximately 80 μm wide; vulva on slight prominence slightly posterior to union of esophagus and intestine (Fig. 31.16B); eggs 44–46 × 22–29 μm, shell with reticulate pattern.

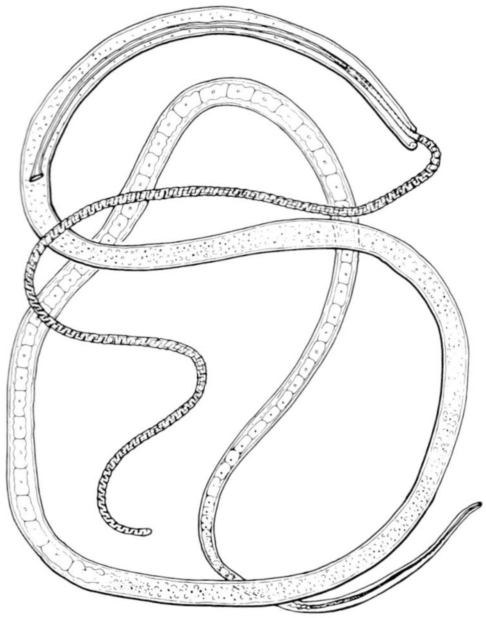

31.17. *Capillaria obsignata.* (After Gagarin)

Life Cycle. *C. obsignata* has a direct development as detailed by Wakelin (86). Embryonation of the eggs was dependent on environmental conditions. No development occurred at 4 C. Development was complete in 13 days at 20 C and in 65–72 hr at 35 C. Temperatures above 37 C were detrimental to embryonation. Storage of embryonated eggs at low (−3.5 C) or high (50 C) temperatures reduced infectivity. No molting was observed in the egg; the larva, which hatched only after ingestion by the host, was considered first stage. Worms reached maturity in about 18 days. The prepatent period was 20–21 days after infection. Pigeons experimentally infected with *C. obsignata* and held under conditions designed to preclude reinfection will remain infected for about 9 mo.

Pathogenicity. Birds heavily infected with *C. obsignata* spend much of their time apart from the rest of the flock huddled on the ground, underneath the roosts, or in some corner of the room. Signs include emaciation, diarrhea, hemorrhagic enteritis, and death. A catarrhal exudate in the upper intestine and some thickening of the wall are the most severe gross pathological changes seen in heavy experimental infections (86). Changes, however, are variable and are not an inevitable consequence of massive infection. Effects on weight gain are also variable, with some weight depression with as few as 14 worms (56); in other cases infections of 100–1000 worms cause no weight change (86). Perhaps the most significant effect of infection from a practical standpoint is the less efficient utilization of feed.

No significant differences in total white blood cells or packed-cell volume between infected and uninfected birds were found (86). A significant increase in B and V globulin, total globulin, and total protein in infected chickens compared with uninfected controls was demonstrated (8). Conversely, in the pigeon, there was a marked decrease in total protein and albumen. A significant reduction in levels of plasma carotenoids and liver vitamin A with heavy infection was shown, although plasma vitamin A levels were only slightly reduced (11).

ORNITHOSTRONGYLUS QUADRIRADIATUS (STEVENSON 1904) TRAVASSOS 1914, HELIGMOSOMIDAE

Hosts. Pigeons, doves.

Location. Lumen of small intestine.

Morphology. Worms delicate, slender, red when freshly collected, apparently from ingested blood in intestine; cuticle about head inflated to form vesicular enlargement (Fig. 31.18A). *Male:* 9–12 mm long; bursa bilobed, with no distinct dorsal lobe; dorsal ray much shorter than other rays, not extending halfway to bursal margin, bifurcating near its tip to form 2 short tips; a stumpy process present on each side near base of ray; spicules equal, 150–160 μm long, somewhat curved, each terminating in 3 pointed processes (Fig. 31.18B); telamon 57–70 μm long, with 2 longitudinal processes extending backward and forward along dorsal wall of cloaca, and 2 lateral processes forming a partial ring through which the spicules protrude. *Female:* 18–24 mm long; vulva near end of tail; vagina short, followed by 2 powerful muscular ovejectors; tail tapers to a narrow blunt end, bearing a short spine; eggs segmenting when deposited.

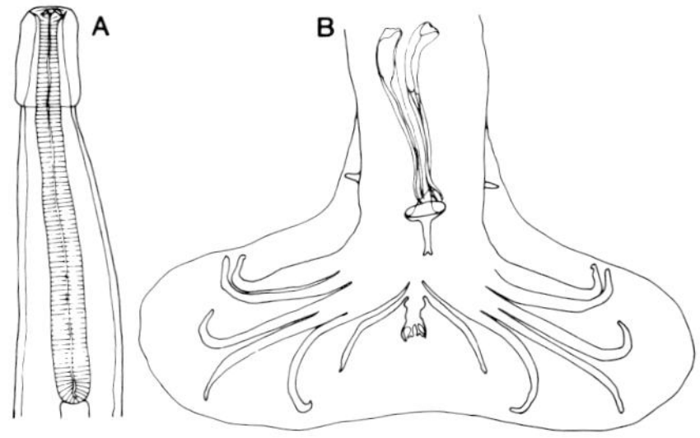

31.18. *Ornithostrongylus quadriradiatus.* A. Head. B. Bursa of male. (After Stevenson)

Life Cycle. This bloodsucking nematode occurs in the small intestine of pigeons and mourning doves in the USA. The oval thin-shelled eggs are voided in the droppings and hatch in approximately 19–25 hr under favorable conditions of moisture and temperature. After hatching the larva molts twice within the next 3 or 4 days to reach the infective stage. The infective larva is swallowed by a pigeon or other susceptible host and grows to maturity in the small intestine. The female worm deposits eggs 5–6 days following ingestion of the larva.

Pathogenicity. This roundworm can cause serious losses in pigeons due to catarrhal enteritis and blood loss during hemorrhage. Birds heavily infected become droopy, remain squatted on the ground or floor, and if disturbed try to move but usually tip forward on the breast and head. Food is eaten sparingly and is frequently regurgitated, along with bile-stained fluid. There is a pronounced greenish diarrhea, and the bird gradually wastes away. Signs of difficult and rapid breathing usually precede death. Intestines of fatally infected birds are markedly hemorrhagic and have a greenish mucoid content with masses of sloughed epithelium.

HETERAKIS DISPAR (SCHRANK 1790) DUJARDIN 1845, HETERAKIDAE

Hosts. Ducks, geese.

Location. Lumen of the cecum.

Morphology. Somewhat larger than *H. gallinarum* but similar in appearance except for spicules. *Male:* 7–18 mm long; preanal sucker 109–256 μm in diameter; spicules short and essentially equal, 390–730 μm long (Fig. 31.19A). *Female:* 16–23 mm long; eggs 59–62 × 39–41 μm.

Life Cycle. Similar to *H. gallinarum.*

Pathogenicity. Considered relatively nonpathogenic.

HETERAKIS GALLINARUM (SCHRANK 1788) MADSEN 1950, HETERAKIDAE

Synonyms. See Madsen (60).

Hosts. Chickens, turkeys, ducks, geese, grouse, guinea fowl, partridges, pheasants, quail.

Location. Lumen of the cecum.

Morphology. Worms small, white; head end bent dorsally; mouth surrounded by 3 small equal-sized lips; 2 narrow lateral membranes extend almost entire length of body; esophagus ending in a

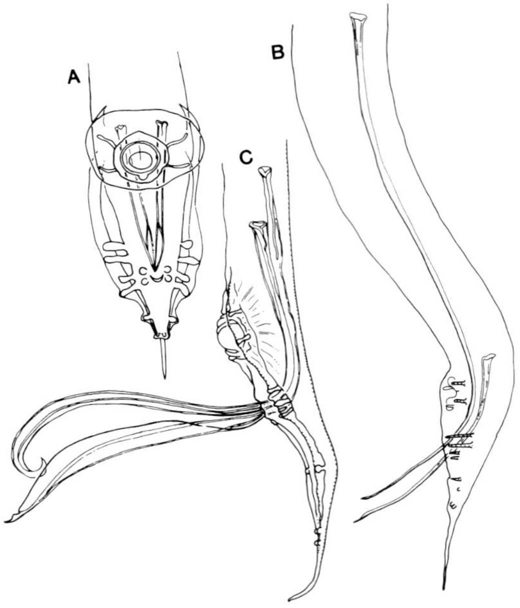

31.19. Male tails. A. *Heterakis dispar.* (After Madsen). B. *Heterakis gallinarum.* (After Lane). C. *Heterakis isolonche.* (After Cram et al.)

well-developed bulb containing a valvular apparatus (Fig. 31.20A). *Male:* 7–13 mm long; tail straight, ending in a subulate point; 2 large lateral bursal wings; well-developed preanal sucker, with strongly chitinized walls and small semicircular incision in posterior margin of the sucker wall; 12 pairs of caudal papillae, the 2 most posterior pairs stout and superimposed; spicules dissimilar, the right one 0.85–2.8 (generally 2) mm long, the left one 0.37–1.1 mm long with a curved tip (Fig. 31.19B). *Female:* 10–15 mm long; tail long, narrow, and pointed; vulva not prominent, slightly posterior to middle of body; eggs thick-shelled, ellipsoidal, unsegmented when deposited, similar in appearance to those of *A. galli,* 63–75 × 36–50 μm.

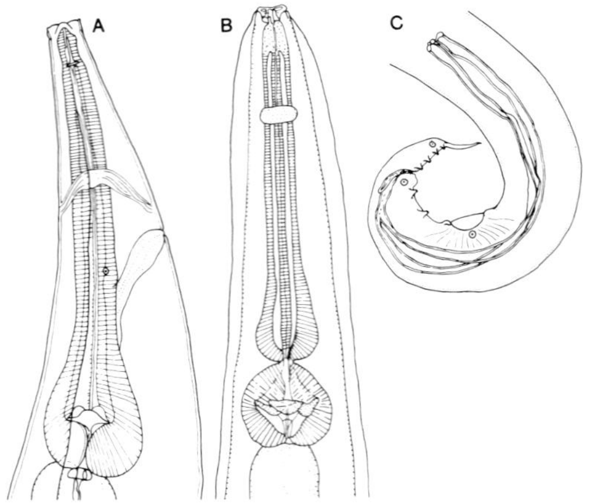

31.20. A. *Heterakis gallinarum,* head. B. *Subulura suctoria,* head. (After Skrjabin and Shikhobalova). C. *Subulura strongylina,* male tail. (After Barreto)

Life Cycle. Lund and Chute (58) found the greatest production of eggs for each egg ingested was with the ring-necked pheasant, followed by the guinea fowl and chicken. Eggs pass out in the feces in an unsegmented state. Oogenesis and eggshell formation have been described by Lee and Lestan (54). In approximately 2 wk or less, under favorable conditions of temperature and moisture, eggs reach the infective stage. When these are swallowed by a susceptible host, the embryos hatch in the upper part of the intestine; at the end of 24 hr most of the young worms have reached the ceca. The larvae are closely associated with or occasionally embedded in the cecal tissue until 12 days postexposure, with peak association at 3 days. Tissue association increases with age of birds; nevertheless, a true tissue phase rarely occurs with *H. gallinarum.* At necropsy most of the adult worms are found in the tips or blind ends of the ceca. Earthworms may also ingest the eggs of the cecal worms and may be the means of causing infection in poultry.

Pathogenicity. The ceca of experimentally infected birds show marked inflammation and thickening of the walls. In heavy infections nodules form in the mucosa and submucosa, as the response of already sensitized ceca to subsequent infection (51).

The chief economic importance of the cecal worm lies in its role as a carrier of the blackhead organism *Histomonas meleagridis.* Blackhead may be produced in susceptible birds by feeding embryonated eggs of *H. gallinarum* taken from blackhead-infected birds. The protozoan parasite was found incorporated in the worm egg (85), and its presence was identified in the gut wall and in the reproductive systems of the male and female and in the developing eggs of this cecal worm (39). Direct transmission of *Histomonas meleagridis* was accomplished using larvae (73) and male worms (77).

HETERAKIS ISOLONCHE LINSTOW 1906, HETERAKIDAE

Synonym. *Heterakis bonasae* Cram 1927.

Hosts. Ducks, grouse, pheasants, prairie chickens, quail.

Location. Adults in lumen of the cecum or mucosa, larvae in mucosa.

Morphology. Similar to *H. gallinarum* but easily differentiated based on the spicules. *Male:* 5.9–15 mm long; preanal sucker 70–15 μm in diameter; spicules long, 0.72–2.33 (generally 1.4–1.9) μm, and essentially equal (Fig. 30.19C). *Female:* 9–12 mm long; eggs 65–75 × 37–46 μm.

Life Cycle. Similar to *H. gallinarum* but with a more extensive tissue phase. The second-stage larvae mature in the cecal mucosa and sometimes the adults are still found there.

Pathogenicity. *H. isolonche* can be quite pathogenic and mortality in pen-reared pheasants can exceed 50%. Diarrhea and weight depression are common. The invasion of the mucosa causes lymphocyte infiltration and granulation that leads to the formation of nodules in the cecal wall. These nodules may coalesce to form a thickened wall. However, in quail and grouse these nodules do not seem to form and there is little pathology, even when worms are present in the large numbers.

SUBULURA BRUMPTI (LOPEZ-NEYRA 1922) CRAM 1926, SUBULARIDAE

Synonyms. Some authors consider *S. brumpti* a synonym of *S. suctoria,* others consider it a separate species.

Hosts. Chickens, turkeys, doves, ducks, grouse, guinea fowl, partridges, pheasants, quail.

Location. Lumen of the cecum.

Morphology. Small nematodes with anterior end curved dorsally; mouth hexagonal, surrounded by 6 weakly developed lips, each with median papillae; 2 pairs of larger papillae located dorsally and ventrally; well-developed amphids laterally; anterior portions of esophageal wall cuticularized, forming 3 toothlike structures; esophagus dilated posteriorly, followed by a bulb (Fig. 31.20B); cephalic alae extending to anterior portion of intestine. *Male:* 6.9–10 mm long, 340–420 μm wide; esophagus 0.98–1.1 mm long; lateral alae extending to middle of esophagus; tail curved ventrally and ending in prolongation; caudal papillae (10 pairs) consist of 3 preanal pairs, 2 adanal pairs, and 5 postanal pairs; caudal alae narrow and not well developed; preanal sucker 170–220 μm long; spicules similar and equal, 1.22–1.5 mm long; gubernaculum 150–210 μm long. *Female:* 9–13.7 mm long, 460–560 μm wide; esophagus 1–1.3 mm long; tail straight and conical, ending in sharp point; vulva anterior to middle of body; eggs almost spherical, thin-shelled, 82–86 × 66–76 μm, fully embryonated when deposited.

Life Cycle. Eggs pass from definitive hosts in cecal droppings. At this time they contain embryos infective to beetles and cockroaches, the reported intermediate hosts (5, 22). Larvae hatch in 4–5 hr, penetrate the intestinal wall, and enter the body cavity where further development occurs (4, 22). The first larval molt occurs on the 4th or 5th day after infection and by the 7th or 8th day the larva encapsulates on the intestinal wall. The molt to the second stage occurs 13–15 days after ingestion; shortly thereafter the larva contracts in length and coils within the capsule, becoming the third or infective stage. When the definitive host swallows an infected intermediate host, the larva migrates to the ceca and develops to the fourth stage within about 2 wk. The final molt takes place about 18 days after infection. The young adults continue to grow and develop, and eggs appear in the feces in about 6 wk after infection.

Pathogenicity. The cecum showed no evidence of larval penetration or any extensive inflammatory reactions, even though infection could persist as long as 8 mo (22). No noticeable lesions were produced by this worm in the ceca of the quail (20).

SUBULURA STRONGYLINA (RUDOLPHI 1819) RAILLIET AND HENRY 1912, SUBULURIDAE

Hosts. Chickens, guinea fowl, quail. This parasite has been reported in chickens in South America and Puerto Rico but not in the USA. It has, however, been found in quail in southeastern USA.

Location. Lumen of cecum.

Morphology. The lateral cephalic alae are well developed and extend from head to the median part of the esophageal bulb. *Male:* 4.4–12 mm long; lateral alae extending to median part of bulb; tail curved into V or O shape; preanal sucker long and slender, 169 μm long; 11 pairs of caudal papillae; spicules equal, 890 μm–1.2 mm long (Fig. 31.20C). *Female:* 5.6–18 mm long; vulva slightly anterior to middle of body; eggs 84 × 67 μm, embryonated when deposited.

Pathogenicity. No noticeable lesions are produced in the ceca of quail.

SUBULURA SUCTORIA (MOLIN 1860) RAILLIET AND HENRY 1912, SUBULURIDAE

Synonym. *Heterakis suctoria* Molin 1860.

Hosts. Chickens, turkeys, guinea fowl, partridges, pheasants, quail.

Location. Lumen or mucosa of the cecum, although sometimes in the small intestine.

Morphology. This worm is larger than *S. brumpti*. Apparently it has not been reported from the USA but has been found in the chicken in Mexico, Africa, South America, Middle East, and Asia. The lateral cephalic alae are small and extend to the middle of the esophagus. *Male:* 11.8–13.8 mm long; 359 μm wide; spicules equal and curved, 1–1.5 mm long. *Female:* 20–33 mm long; eggs 51–70 × 45–64 μm.

Life Cycle. Similar to *S. brumpti*. Beetles serve as intermediate hosts.

Pathogenicity. Barus and Blazek (7) reported little pathology.

STRONGYLOIDES AVIUM CRAM 1929, STRONGYLOIDIDAE

Hosts. Chickens, turkeys, geese, grouse, quail. This extremely small roundworm has been reported from chickens in Puerto Rico (17). The junco *Junco hyemalis* in Virginia and the coot *Fulica americana* in North Carolina harbor natural infections.

Location. Cecum, sometimes in the small intestine.

Morphology. Parasitic generation consisting of only parthenogenic females in intestine of avian host; free-living generation consisting of both males (Fig. 31.21A) and females in soil. *Parasitic adult:* 2.2 mm long, 40–45 μm wide; vulva with projecting lips, located 1.4 mm from head (Fig. 31.21B, C); uteri divergent from vulva; ovaries recurrent with simple "hairpin" bends and course not sinuous; eggs 52–56 × 36–40 μm, very thin-shelled, segmenting when deposited.

Life Cycle. Unlike most species of nematodes, the parasitic cycle of *S. avium* consists of females only. Eggs hatch as soon as 18 hr after being passed in droppings. Young worms develop in the soil to adult males and females. Shortly thereafter the females give rise to young that feed, molt, and develop into other adult free-living males and females, or they transform into another type of larvae known as the infective larvae that develop into parthenogenic females after being swallowed by a susceptible host.

Pathogenicity. During the early or acute stage of infection the walls of the ceca are greatly thickened; typical pasty cecal contents almost disappear, the discharge being thin and bloody. If the fowl survives this acute stage, the ceca gradually become functional again and the thickening of the walls decreases. Young birds suffer most from infections. If infection is light or the birds are adults, little if any clinical effect is noted.

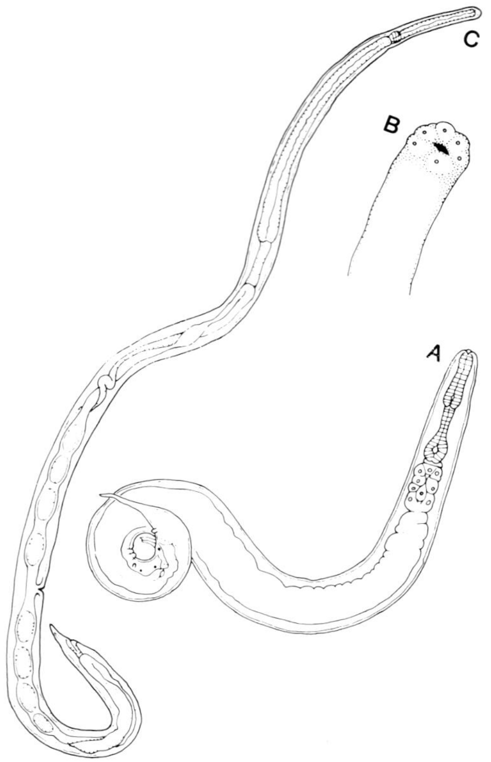

31.21. *Strongyloides avium*. A. Free-living male. (After Cram). B. Parasitic female, head. C. Parasitic (parthenogenic) female. (B and C after Sakamoto and Sarashina)

TRICHOSTRONGYLUS TENUIS MEHLIS 1846, TRICHOSTRONGYLIDAE

Hosts. Chickens, turkeys, ducks, geese, guinea fowl, pigeons, quail.

Location. Cecum, sometimes small intestine.

Morphology. Worms small and slender; body gradually attenuated in front of genital opening; mouth surrounded by 3 small, inconspicuous lips; cuticle anterior end of body lacking conspicuous striations about 200–250 μm from extremity, then with distinct serrated appearance about 1–2 mm more. *Male:* 5.5–9 mm long, 48 μm wide near center of body; cuticle inflated on ventral surface just anterior to bursa; bursa with 1 dorsal and 2 lateral lobes, the dorsal one not distinctly marked off from the lateral; each lateral lobe supported by 6 rays (Fig. 31.22); the dorsal ray bifurcates at its distal third, and each of these divisions again bifurcates and is very finely pointed; spicules dark

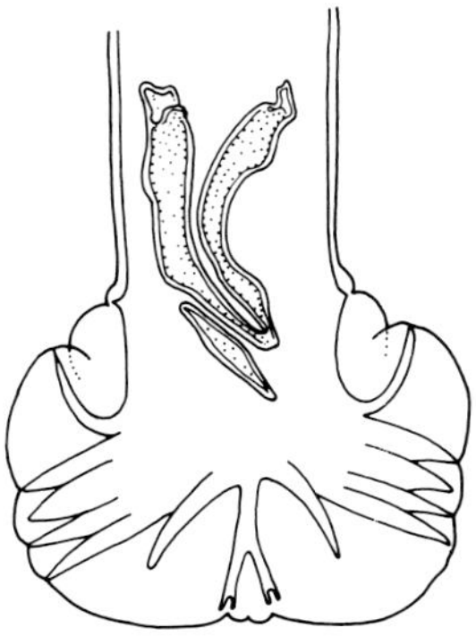

31.22. *Trichostrongylus tenuis,* bursa of male. (After Railliet)

brown, slightly unequal in length (the longer 120–164 μm and the shorter 104–150 μm), both much twisted, especially at distal ends, and provided with an earlike structure on proximal end, both apparently surrounded in distal 2/3 by a thin membrane extending for a short distance beyond distal ends. *Female:* 6.5–11 mm long, 77–100 μm wide at level of vulva; vulva in posterior end of body, with crenelated edges; uteri divergent; eggs thin-shelled.

Life Cycle. This worm has a direct life cycle. *T. tenuis* from pheasants has been successfully transmitted to domestic turkey, guinea fowl, and chicken. Eggs hatch within 36–48 hr after being passed in the droppings, and the larvae become infective within approximately 2 wk. Within this time the larvae have molted twice. When picked up by a susceptible host, the infective larvae molt twice more within the ceca of the bird before finally becoming adults.

Pathogenicity. *T. tenuis* was associated with the disease that decimated the red grouse population in Scotland. A fatal dose can be as low as 500 infective larvae. Ceca become extended, and blood vessels show congestion. The mucosa of the ceca is inflamed, and the ridges are greatly thickened. Severe infection causes loss of weight and anemia. *T. tenuis* can also be fatal to young goslings under certain conditions.

Heavy mortality occurs usually in the fall, mainly in the young birds in that year's hatching, and again in the spring. These two seasons are not isolated epidemics but rather peaks of a disease that continues in a chronic form the entire year.

AULONOCEPHALUS LINDQUISTI CHANDLER 1934, SUBULURIDAE

Host. Bobwhite quail and blue or scaled quail. The distribution seems somewhat restricted, being found mainly in western Texas.

Location. Most common in cecum, although sometimes in large intestine.

Morphology. Bright pink worms; cuticle finely striated; cervical alae present, 45–65 μm broad in female but only 20–25 μm broad in male; head with 6 troughlike grooves about 65–70 μm long radiating from the mouth (Fig. 31.23A); esophagus club-shaped, 1.3–1.8 mm long, bulb slightly longer than broad. *Male:* 8–10.6 mm long, 420–490 μm wide; gubernaculum 170–190 μm long; spicules approximately equal, 1.16–1.3 mm long (Fig. 31.23B). *Female:* 10–14.8 mm long, 530–590 μm wide; vulva inconspicuous, ranging from slightly anterior to slightly posterior to middle of the body; tail terminates in a thin spike; eggs broadly oval, 58 × 42–45 μm.

Pathogenicity. The pathologic effects of this species is unknown, but as many as 300 worms have been recovered from a single host.

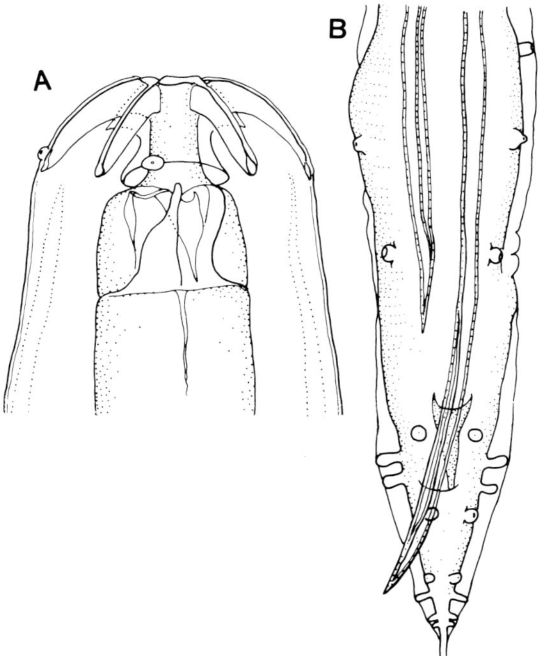

31.23. *Aulonocephalus lindquisti.* A. Head. B. Male tail. (After Chandler)

OTHER NEMATODES OF THE DIGESTIVE TRACT. Numerous species of nematodes have been found in domestic poultry in other parts of the world, but have not yet been reported from North America. The diagnostician should, however, be aware of their existence because the potential always remains for their appearance. Some of these species are as follows.

Esophagus and Crop. These include *Gongylonema crami* Smit 1927 from chickens in Java, *G. congolense* Fain 1944 from chickens and ducks in Africa, and *G. Sumani* Bhalerao 1933 from chickens in India. *Capillaria cairinae* Freitas and Almeida 1935 is found in the esophagus of ducks in Brazil and *C. combologiodes* Erlich and Mikacie 1940, in the crop of turkeys in Europe. Larvae of *Spirocerca lupi* have been found encysted in the crop of chickens in the southern USA.

Proventriculus. *Parhadjelia neglecta* Lent and Freitas 1939 is a Habronematide resembling *Cyrnea* that has been reported in the submucosa of the proventriculus of domestic ducks in Brazil. *Echinuria jugadornata* Soloviev 1912 causes nodules at the junction of the proventriculus and gizzard of domestic ducks in the USSR. *Physaloptera acuticauda* Molin 1860 has been reported from chickens and pheasants in Brazil and falconiform birds in the USA. *Tetrameres* include *T. confusa* Travassos 1919 from chickens, turkeys, and pigeons in South America and Asia; *T. gigas* Travassos 1919 from domestic ducks in South America; *T. mohtedae* Bhalerao and Rao 1944 from chickens in India; and *T. spinosa* Maplestone 1913 from chickens and domestic ducks in India.

Gizzard. Several other nematodes are found under the gizzard lining of domestic poultry. *Histiocephalus laticaudatus* (Rudolphi 1819) Diesing 1851 has been recovered from chickens and ducks, and *Streptocara pectinifera* (Neumann 1900) Skrjabin 1916 from chickens and guinea fowl in Europe. *Epomidiostomum orispinum* (Molin 1861) Seurat 1981 is in domestic ducks and geese in Europe and Africa and *E. skrjabini* Petrov 1926 in domestic geese in Asia.

Small Intestine. *Abbreviata gemina* Linstow 1899, a *Physaloptera*-like worm, occurs in chickens in Egypt. The anisakid *Contracaecum microcephalum* (Rudolphi 1809) Railliet and Henry 1912 infects domestic ducks in Europe, Asia, and Africa, while *Porrocaecum crassum* (Deslongchamps 1824) Railliet and Henry 1912 is in domestic ducks and guinea fowl in Europe. *Capillaria anseris* occurs in domestic geese in Europe. *Hartertia gallinrum* (Theiler 1919) Cram 1927, which uses termites as an intermediate host, causes diarrhea and decreased growth and egg production in chickens in Africa.

Cecum. Numerous other species of *Heterakis* are found in chickens throughout the world. These include *H. beramporia* Lane 1914, Asia; *H. bervispiculum* Gendre 1911, South America and Africa; *H. caudabrevis* Popova 1929, USSR; *H. indica* Maplestone 1931, India; and *H. linganensis* Li 1933, China. Turkeys in China are infected with *H. meleagris* Hsu 1957. *Subulura differens* Sonsino 1890 is widespread in chickens, guinea fowl, and quail in South America, Europe, Africa, and Asia; sometimes it is also found in the small intestine. Several *Capillaria* have been described including *C. monteividensis* Calzada 1937 and *C. uruguayensis* Calzada 1937 from chickens in Uruguay, and *C. spinulosa* (Linstow 1890) Travassos 1915 from ducks in Europe.

NEMATODES OF THE RESPIRATORY TRACT

CYATHOSTOMA BRONCHIALIS (MUEHLIG 1884) CHAPIN 1925, SYNGAMIIDAE

Hosts. Ducks, geese, turkeys, (chickens experimentally).

Location. Larynx, trachea, bronchi, and sometimes in the abdominal air sacs.

Morphology. Very similar to *Syngamus* but larger and less firmly united in copula; buccal capsule somewhat wider than deep, usually 6 but occasionally 7 triangular buccal teeth (Fig. 31.24A). *Male:* 8–12 mm long, 200–600 μm wide; spicules long and slender, 540–870 μm, with tips slightly incurved (Fig. 31.24B). *Female:* 16–30 mm long, 750 μm–1.5 mm wide; vulva with fairly prominent lips, situated in posterior part of anterior third of body; tail acute; eggs 68–90 × 43–60 μm, with slight operculum in mature ones.

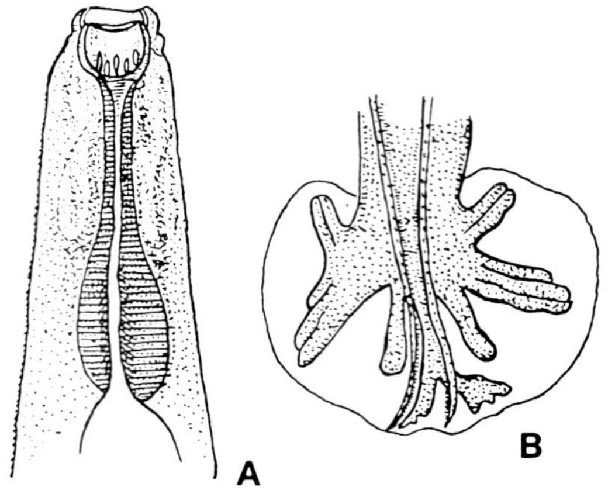

31.24. *Cyathostoma bronchialis.* A. Head. B. Male tail.

Life Cycle. This species of gapeworm can involve direct infections with third-stage larvae, but infections using infected earthworms are more successful. The third-stage larvae migrate to the lungs through the peritoneal cavity and air sacs (36) rather than through the bloodstream as does *S. trachea.* The larvae molt twice in the lung at 1 and 4 days postinfection. They migrate into the trachea at 6 days, copulate at 7 days, and reach maturity by 13 days postinfection. Eggs are first found in the tracheal mucus 13 days postinfection.

Pathogenicity. Morbidity of 80% with a mortality of 20% has been reported in a flock of domestic geese near Duluth, Minnesota (41). The course of the disease extended over 5 mo, during which time the birds showed signs of respiratory distress by throwing back their heads and gasping for air. Severely affected birds died soon after the appearance of respiratory disturbances. The signs were similar to those of laryngotracheitis. Recovered birds showed growth retardation.

Experimentally infected domestic geese developed bronchitis of the primary, secondary, and tertiary bronchi (37). During prepatency, hyperplasia of the epithelium of the primary bronchi was the predominant lesion. During patency, generalized pneumonitis was most prominent in response to the aspirated nematode eggs.

Syngamus trachea (Montagu 1811) Chapin 1925, Syngamidae

Synonyms. *S. gracilis* Chapin 1925 and *S. parvis* Chapin 1925.

Hosts. Chickens, turkeys, geese, guinea fowl, pheasants, peafowl, quail.

Location. Trachea, bronchi, and bronchioles.

Morphology. Sometimes designated as "redworm" because of its color or "forked worm" because the male and female are in permanent copulation so that they appear like the letter Y (Fig. 31.25A). Mouth orbicular, with a hemispheric chitinous capsule, usually with 8 sharp teeth at the base, surrounded by a chitinous plate, the outer margin of which is incised to form 6 festoons opposite each other. *Male:* 2–6 mm long, 200 μm wide; bursa obliquely truncated, provided with rays, sometimes with strikingly asymmetrical dorsal rays; spicules equal, slender, short (57–64 μm). *Female:* 5–20 mm long (longer in the turkey), 350 μm wide; tail end conical, bearing a pointed process; vulva prominent, about 1/4 of body length from anterior end, but the position varies with age; eggs 90 × 49 μm, ellipsoidal, operculated (Fig. 31.25B).

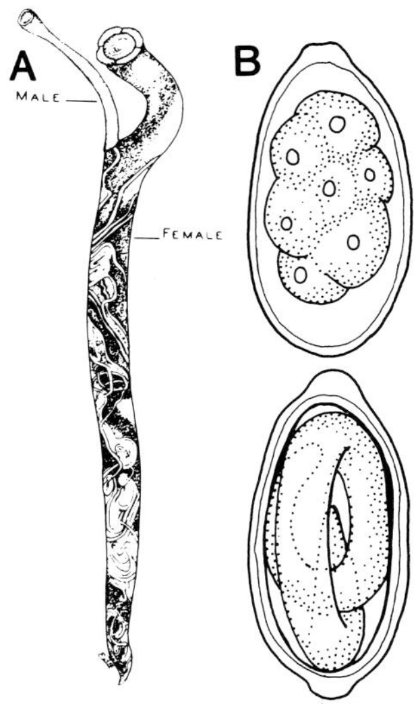

31.25. *Syngamus trachea.* A. Male and female worms. (After Wehr). B. Eggs.

Life Cycle. The life history of this cosmopolitan gapeworm is peculiar in that transmission from bird to bird may be successfully accomplished either directly (by the feeding of embryonated eggs or infective larvae) or indirectly (by ingestion of earthworms containing free or encysted gapeworm larvae they had obtained by feeding on contaminated soil). The female gapeworm deposits eggs through the vulvar opening underneath the bursa of the attached male onto the lumen of the trachea. The eggs reach the mouth, are swallowed, and pass to the outside in the droppings. Following incubation of approximately 8–14 days under optimum moisture and temperature, eggs embryonate, and soon after some may hatch, with the larvae living free in the soil. The earthworms *Eisenia foetidus* and *Allolobophora caliginosus* become infected with gapeworm larvae. Within the earthworm the larvae penetrate the intestinal wall, enter the body cavity, and finally invade the body musculature in which they may encyst for an indefinite period. Gapeworm larvae in the earthworm remain infective to young chickens for as long as 4 1/3 yr. Slugs and snails may also serve as transfer or auxiliary hosts of larvae, and live larvae have been recovered from snails over a year after infection. Snails are not true intermediate hosts in the strict sense, since they are not necessary for the transfer of gapeworms to other bird hosts. *S. trachea* taken from various wild and domestic birds were more readily transferred to young chickens and with a greater degree of success if the earthworm was employed as an intermediary.

Some infective larvae penetrate the wall of the crop and esophagus and then penetrate the lungs directly. However, the majority penetrate the duodenum and are carried to the lungs by the portal bloodstream via the liver and heart (6, 35). Larvae are found in the liver as early as 2 hr postinoculation and in the lungs as early as 4 hr. Larvae probably break out of the capillaries in the lung into the interlobular connective tissue and migrate into the parabronchia and atria via air capillaries. Molting and development to the adult stage can occur as early as 4 days postinfection, with copulation by 5 days in pheasants. Copulation of the worms in chickens is seen 1 day later. Larvae can be recovered in the lungs up to 7 days. Worms are also found in the parabronchi and secondary bronchi up to 9 days. Adults enter the trachea as early as 7 days, and males are firmly attached to the tracheal wall by 11 days postinfection. Approximately 2 wk are required for the infective larvae to reach sexual maturity and for eggs to appear in the droppings. Although the role played by wild birds in the spread of gapeworm disease is still undecided, wild birds probably do not spread the disease in this country.

Pathogenicity. In the USA, *S. trachea* is the causative agent of "gapes" (labored breathing due to parasites) in chickens, turkeys, peacocks, and pheasants (Fig. 31.26); *Cyathostoma bronchialis* is the causative agent of this disease in geese.

In artificial rearing of pheasants, gapes is a serious menace in the USA. Confinement rearing of young birds has reduced the problem in chickens compared to a few years ago. However, this parasite continues to present an occasional problem with turkeys raised on range.

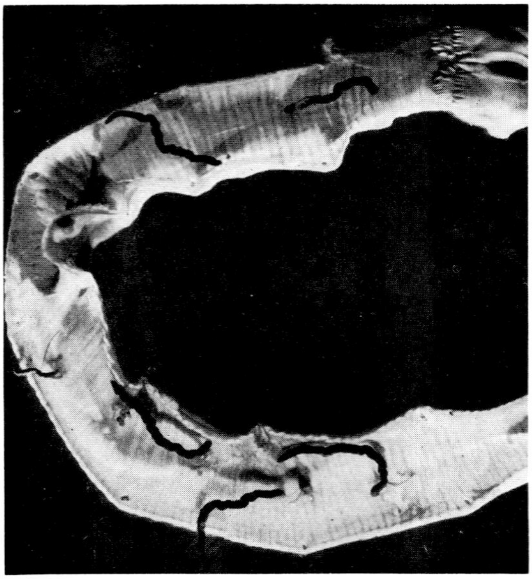

31.26. *Syngamus trachea,* trachea showing attached gapeworms. (After Wehr)

Young birds are most seriously affected with gapeworms. The rapidly growing worms soon obstruct the lumen of the trachea and cause suffocation. Turkey poults, baby chicks, and pheasant chicks are most susceptible to infection. Turkey poults usually develop gapeworm signs earlier and begin to die sooner after infection than young chickens. Experimentally infected guinea fowl, pigeons, and ducks do not exhibit characteristic signs of gapeworm infections. Full-grown birds rarely show characteristic signs unless heavily infected.

Birds infected with gapeworms show signs of weakness and emaciation and usually spend much of their time with eyes closed and head drawn back against the body. From time to time they throw their heads forward and upward and open the mouth wide to draw in air. An infected bird may give its head a convulsive shake in an attempt to remove the obstruction from the trachea so that normal breathing may be resumed. Little or no food is taken by birds in the advanced stages of infection, and death usually ensues.

Examination of the trachea of infected birds shows that the mucous membrane is extensively irritated and inflamed; coughing is apparently the result of this irritation to the mucous lining. Lesions are usually found in the trachea of turkeys and pheasants but seldom if ever in the trachea of young chickens and guinea fowl. These lesions or nodules are produced as a result of an inflammatory reaction at the site of attachment of the male worm, which remains permanently attached to the tracheal wall throughout the duration of its life. The female worms apparently detach and reattach from time to time in order to obtain a more abundant supply of food. Studies with radioactive isotopes have shown that the net blood loss with *S. trachea* is minimal. A marked heterophilia, monocytosis, eosinophilia, lymphocytopenia, and a decreased packed-cell volume in infected turkey poults has been reported (45).

NEMATODES OF THE EYE

OXYSPIRURA MANSONI COBBOLD 1879, THELAZIIDAE

Hosts. Chickens, turkeys, ducks, grouse, guinea fowl, peafowl, pigeons, quail.

Location. Beneath the nictitating membrane, conjunctival sacs, and nasolacrimal ducts.

Morphology. Body attenuated at both ends, anterior rounded, posterior pointed; cuticle smooth; no membranous appendages; mouth circular, surrounded by a 6-lobed chitinous ring with 2 lateral and 4 submedian papillae in relation to the clefts of this ring; 2 pairs of subdorsal and 1 pair of subventral teeth in mouth cavity; buccal cavity with a short wide anterior portion and a long narrow posterior portion (Fig. 31.27A). *Male:* 8.2–16 mm long, 350 μm wide; tail curved ventrally, without alae; 4 pairs of preanal and 2 pairs of postanal papillae; spicules unequal (Fig. 31.27B), one 3–4.55 mm long, the other 180–240 μm long. *Female:* 12–20 mm long, 270–430 μm wide; vulva 0.78–1.55 mm; anus 400–530 μm from tip of tail (Fig. 31.27C); eggs embryonated when deposited, 50–65 × 45 μm (Fig. 31.27D).

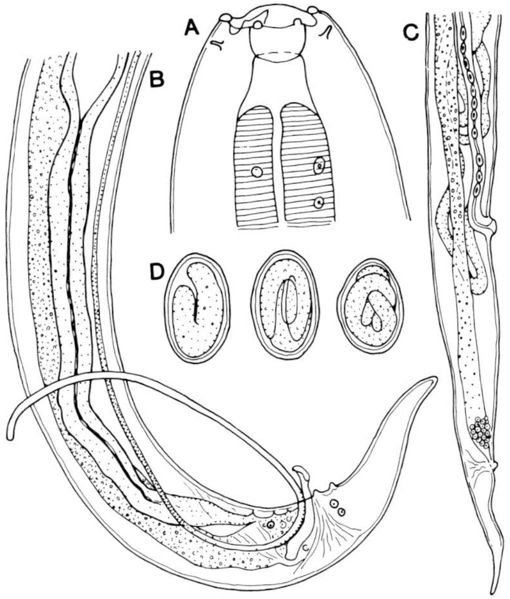

31.27. *Oxyspirura mansoni.* A. Head. B. Male tail. C. Female tail. D. Eggs. (B–D after Ransom)

Life Cycle. Eggs of the mature female eyeworm are deposited in the eyes of the bird host, washed down the tear ducts, swallowed, and passed in the droppings. The cockroach *Pycnoscelus* (*Leucophaea*) *surinamensis,* which is an omnivorous feeder, ingests the eggs in the feces. Within approximately 50 days, the body cavity of the cockroach contains mature larvae, which are capable of infecting a susceptible host. Mature larvae are often contained within cysts deep in the adipose tissue or along the course of the alimentary tract of the insect host. Some larvae release themselves from the capsules and are found free in the body cavity and legs of the cockroach. When an infected cockroach is swallowed by a chicken or other susceptible host, the infective larva is freed in the crop, passes up the esophagus to the mouth and through the nasolacrimal duct to the eye.

Various wild birds become infected with the eyeworm of poultry and may serve as sources of infection for domestic birds. Such birds as the blackbird (*Agelaius phoeniceus*), bobolink (*Dolichonyx oryzivorus*), wild pigeon (*Columbia livia*), loggerhead shrike (*Lanius ludovicianus*), and blue jay (*Aphelocoma cyanea*) have been experimentally infected with the eyeworm of poultry. This worm occurs naturally in English sparrows, mynahs, Chinese doves, Japanese quail, and pheasants (*Phasianus torquatus torquatus* and *P. versicolor versicolor*) in Hawaii. In Hawaii the local wild birds appear to be of little importance in the dissemination of this poultry parasite (75).

Pathogenicity. Infected birds show a peculiar ophthalmia. They appear uneasy and continuously scratch at the eyes, which are usually watery and show severe inflammation. The nictitating membrane becomes swollen, projects slightly beyond the eyelids at the corners of the eyes, and is usually kept in continual motion as if trying to remove some foreign object from the eye. The eyelids sometimes become stuck together, and a white cheesy material collects beneath them. If left untreated, severe ophthalmia may develop; as a result the eyeball may be destroyed. The worms are seldom if ever found in the eyes when severe signs are manifested, presumably due to unfavorable conditions existing there.

OXYSPIRURA PETROWI SKRYJABIN 1929, THELAZIIDAE

Synonym. *O. lumsdeni* Addison and Anderson 1969.

Hosts. Grouse, pheasants, prairie chickens.

Location. Beneath nictitating membrane of eye.

Morphology. Body slender, yellow to cream color, bluntly rounded anteriorly, attenuated posteriorly; cervical alae present; cuticle transversely striated; mouth with 4 submedian pairs and 3 circumoral pairs of cephalic papillae; cuticularized bursal capsule undivided. *Male:* 6.3–8.6 mm long, 185–330 μm wide; right spicule 121–320 μm long and slender with a sharp tip. *Female:* 7.7–12.3 μm long, 200–455 μm wide; vulva 500–700 μm from tip of tail; anus 242–400 μm from posterior extremity; eggs 35–44 μm × 15–31 μm, embryonated.

Life Cycle. Over 70 species of *Oxyspirura* have been described as parasites in the eyes of birds. Of these species only *O. mansoni, O. petrowi,* and *O. pusillae* have been reported from North America north of Mexico. *O. petrowi* is a species of wide geographic range. It shows little host specificity (68) and has been found in 14 species of wild birds in Louisiana and 5 species in Michigan. Although this species has not been reported from chickens, it is found in grouse and prairie chickens.

Pathogenicity. Infection with *O. petrowi* produces a condition similar to that seen with *O. mansoni.*

TISSUE-DWELLING NEMATODES OUTSIDE OF THE ENTERIC TRACT

APROCTELLA STODDARDI CRAM 1931, DIPETALONEMATIDAE

Synonym. *Microfilaria fallisi* Brinkmann 1950.

Hosts. Turkeys, doves, quail, grouse. This species has been recovered from the bobwhite quail in southern USA and from grouse in New England.

Location. Body cavity.

Morphology. Body slender; cuticle divided into 4 fields, 2 medians longitudinally striated, 2 laterals smooth; mouth simple without definite lips (Fig. 31.28A). *Male:* 6–7.6 mm long, 60–140 μm wide; spicules stout and curved, right 50–60 μm, left 73–90 μm (Fig. 31.28B); caudal papillae absent. *Female:* 13–16.5 mm long, 71–260 μm wide; vulva 1.3–1.6 mm from anterior end, not opening on protuberance; anus 140–180 μm from caudal extremity; no eggs, unsheathed larvae in uteri.

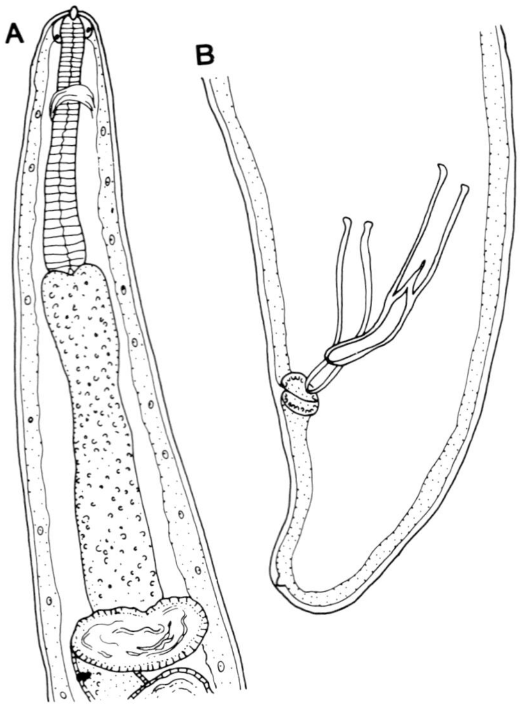

31.28. *Aproctella stoddardi.* A. Head. B. Male tail. (After Anderson)

Life Cycle. The life cycle is unknown, but a biting arthropod is hypothesized as intermediate host.

Pathogenicity. Small numbers are not pathogenic; however, heavy infection may result in mortality in doves. A granulomatous pericarditis has also been reported.

SINGHFILARIA HAYESI ANDERSON AND PRESTWOOD 1969, ONCHOCERCIDAE

Host. Turkeys, quail. Recovered from the wild turkey in southern USA, thus representing a potential problem in domestic turkeys.

Location. Subcutaneous tissues in the region of the esophagus, crop, and trachea.

Morphology. No structures on head (Fig. 31.29A); cuticle with innumerable tiny, transverse thickenings. *Male:* 13.6 mm long, 250 μm wide; spicules markedly dissimilar, right tooth shaped 81 μm long, left 125 μm long divided into broad shaft and blade and short filament (Fig. 31.29B); anus subterminal, 28 μm from caudal extremity; caudal papillae consisting of 1 large pair postanal papillae and 1 large medial papilla anterior to anus. *Female:* 35–40 mm long, 420–500 μm wide; vulva 390–400 μm from cephalic extremity; microfilariae in uteri.

Pathogenicity. Few pathologic lesions are found.

OTHER TISSUE-DWELLING NEMATODES.

The guinea worm *Avioserpens taiwana* (Sugimoto 1919) Chabaud, Campana, and Truong-Tan-Ngoc 1950 causes fibrous tumors in the subcutaneous tissue under the mandible and on the thigh of domestic ducks in Asia.

Fifteen genera of filaroids that infect birds have been recognized (3). Many species are not host-specific. *Cardiofilaria pavlovsky* and *Aproctella stoddardi* have been reported from at least seven families of birds. In general, filaroids cause few problems in domestic poultry. Those species shown in Table 31.3 are from game birds in North America. Other species that infect chickens in India but have not been reported in North America include *Aprocta babamii* Bhalerae and Rao 1944 from the heart, *Cardiofilaria mhowensis* (Jain, Alwar, Adwadhiya, and Pandit 1965) from the body cavity, and experimentally *Chandlerella quiscali* (Linstow 1904) Robinson 1971 (3).

Baylisascaris procynois and *B. columnaris* from raccoons and skunks, respectively, are reported

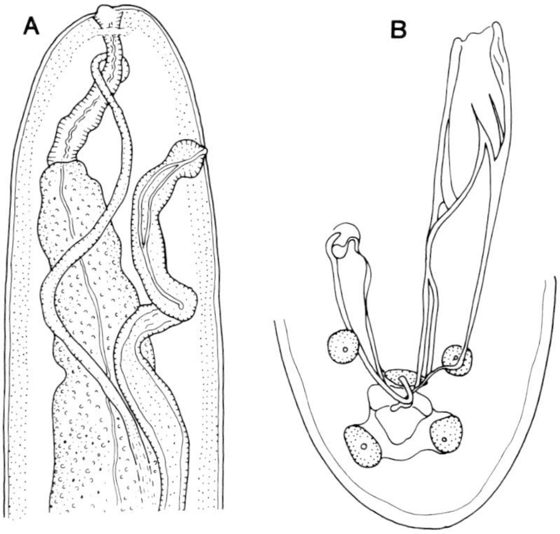

31.29. *Singhfilaria hayesi.* A. Head. B. Male tail. (After Anderson and Prestwood)

to cause avian cerebrospinal nematodiasis in a variety of birds including chickens, bush turkeys, partridges, and quail. This disease has been experimentally produced in chickens (52).

PREVENTION AND CONTROL.

Modern poultry practices, especially confinement-rearing of broilers and pullets and caging of laying hens, have significantly influenced the quantity and variety of nematode infections in poultry. Many that caused extensive problems in "backyard" or "farmyard" flocks are seldom seen in commercial operations. Others such as *Ascaridia* are still found in older birds. In addition, increased pen rearing of game birds has led to increasing nematode problems in these species.

For most nematodes control measures consist of sanitation and breaking the life cycle rather than chemotherapy. Confinement-rearing on litter largely prevents infections with nematodes using outdoor intermediate hosts such as earthworms or grasshoppers. Conversely, nematodes with direct life cycles or those that utilize indoor intermediate hosts such as beetles may prosper. Treatment of the soil or litter to kill intermediate hosts may be beneficial (64). Insecticides suitable for litter treatment include carbaryl, tetrachlorvinphos (stirofos), or Ronnel; however, treatment is usually made only between grow-outs. Extreme care should be taken to insure that feed and water are not contaminated. Treatment of range soil to kill ova is only partially successful. Changing litter can reduce infections, but treating floors with oil is not very effective. After the old litter has been removed, spraying with permethrin or Ravap (a mixture of Rabon and Vapona) has proven effective for beetle control. Edgar (24) feels that changing litter is unnecessary if medication is given on a regular basis.

Raising different species or different ages of birds together or in close proximity is a dangerous procedure as regards parasitism. Adult turkeys, which are carriers of gapeworms, can transmit the disease to young chicks or pheasants, although older chickens are almost entirely resistant to infection.

Chemotherapy.

Because of economics, investigations into the efficacy of chemotherapy have been limited to parasites widespread enough to suggest a potential drug market. The increasing cost of testing to obtain Food and Drug Administration (FDA) approval for new compounds or new uses for approved compounds also makes unlikely future studies on chemical control of rare or infrequently occurring nematodes. Investigations may continue on the ascarids, capillarids, heterakids, and *Syngamus.* The reported types of drugs, effective levels, and means of administering compounds for control of these parasites vary considerably. Only certain compounds have been approved by the FDA. Poultry producers should be aware that the use of unapproved drugs is not legal in birds that will produce eggs or meat for market, and that approvals for drugs and levels are continually changing. Extreme care should be taken to obtain current information from appropriate sources before any medication is used. Label directions and dosages should be followed explicitly.

Ascaridia

APPROVED COMPOUNDS. Drugs currently approved for use in chickens are Hygromycin B or coumaphos (Meldane) in feed, and piperazine in feed or water. Only piperazine is approved for turkeys. Hygromycin B is fed at a level of 0.00088–0.00132%. Coumaphos is only approved for use in replacements (0.004%) or layers (0.003%). It is more commonly used for control of capillarids (see below) than for ascarids.

Piperazine compounds have been widely adopted as a method of treatment for ascaridiasis, since they are practically nontoxic. Piperazine may be administered to chickens in the feed (0.2–0.4%), water (0.1–0.2%), or as a single treatment (50–100 mg/bird). The rate for feed or water medication in turkeys is the same, however, the single-treatment dose is 100 mg/bird (under 12 wk) and 100–400 mg/bird (over 12 wk). A high concentration of piperazine in contact with worms at a given time is very important for maximum elimination. Therefore, to be most effective, piperazine should be consumed by birds in a period of a few hours. Piperazine in drinking water is the most practical method of application for commercial flocks. Since piperazine is available as a wide variety of salts, the level should be calculated on the basis of milligrams of active piperazine (25). Piperazine compounds exert a narcotizing effect, thus enabling worms to be removed and expelled alive by means of natural peristalsis. A combination of piperazine (0.11%) and phenothiazine (0.50–0.56%) as a 1-day treatment only is used for removal of both heterakids and ascarids.

EXPERIMENTAL DATA. Piperazine citrate administered at the rate of 8, 10, and 16 g/gal of drinking water for 1–4 days effectively removed all ascarids but not heterakids (9, 76). Piperazine carbon bisulfide, piperazine adipate, and piperazine citrate, tested against *A. galli* in chickens, completely eliminated all adult worms (44). The compounds were administered as single doses of 100–500 mg/kg body weight. Fenbendazole at 8–10 mg/kg for 3 or 4 days was also effective (78).

Poultry producers sometimes utilize knowledge of the *Ascaridia* life cycle to plan a routine medication program at fixed time periods rather than waiting until worms are present. This is most beneficial when large numbers of *A. galli* eggs are present in built-up litter.

EXPERIMENTAL COMPOUNDS. The three common nematodes of chickens, *Ascaridia galli, Heterakis gallinarum,* and *Capillaria obsignata,* were effectively removed with 40 mg/kg of body weight of dl-tetramisole (10, 81). Levotetramisole (levamisole) given to turkeys naturally infected with *A. dissimilis, H. gallinarum,* and *C. obsignata* at the rate of 30 mg/kg of body weight was also effective (50). Levels of 0.06% or 0.03% levamisole in the drinking water removed 99% of adult *A. dissimilis,* 94–98% of larval *A. dissimilis,* and 99–100% of *H. gallinarum* and *C. obsignata* (67). Clarkson and Beg (13) found 25 mg/kg of body weight to be effective.

Pyrantel tartrate has a high efficacy against *A. galli* and some against *C. obsignata.* A single dose of 15–25 mg/kg body weight gave 99.6–100% removal of all adult *A. galli* from chicks but was relatively ineffective against the larval stages (66).

Capillaria

APPROVED COMPOUNDS. Coumaphos and Hygromycin B are both approved only for use in chickens. Coumaphos is given to replacement pullets in feed (0.004%) for 10–14 days prior to the onset of egg production. It is given to layers (0.003%) for 14 days as needed, but no sooner than 3 wk after the end of the preceding treatment. Coumaphos was reported (26) to be effective against *A. galli, H. gallinarum,* and *C. obsignata.*

EXPERIMENTAL COMPOUNDS. Capillariasis due to *C. obsignata* can be controlled in pigeons and chickens by administration of 1 cc of 10% methyridine solution subcutaneously in the pectoral region or into the leg (pigeons) and dorsal regions between the wings (chickens) (80). These authors stated that this drug must be administered with great care: 1) spilling of the drug on the skin may produce a small lesion; 2) nausea, slight ataxia, and incoordination were observed to some degree even with subeffective doses; and 3) death may sometimes result. The drug has no marked effect on coccidiosis and trichomoniasis and was only slightly effective against *Ascaridia.* Methyridine is an excellent drug for the removal of adults and larvae of *C. obsignata* from chickens (42, 43, 65).

Methyridine injected subcutaneously beneath the wing as a 5% aqueous solution was an effective anthelmintic for the removal of *C. obsignata* from the pigeon (91). Injections of 25–45 mg/bird were 99–100% effective in naturally infected birds, but doses of 23 mg/bird removed only 62% of the worms. The anthelmintic action of the drug was relatively rapid, as indicated by elimination of the majority of the worms within 24 hr after treatment. Maretin (*N*-hydroxynaphthalimide diethyl phosphate) was more effective than Coumaphos against *C. obsignata* in quail (23).

Individual doses of 25 and 50 mg/kg body weight of haloxon against *Capillaria* infections in chickens eliminated practically all the worms (12). Doses of 50–60 mg/kg haloxon were effective against adult worms, but larvae and immature stages were less sensitive (65). Piperazine citrate, phenothiazine, thiabendazole, and bephenium were inactive against *C. obsignata.*

Haloxon was apparently 46–100% effective against *C. contorta* in quail when administered at levels of 0.05–0.5% of the feed for 5–7 days (15). Results were best at the 0.075–0.5% levels. However, the highest concentration was toxic, and one-fourth of the birds died. Single oral doses of the drug were not uniformly effective and produced undesirable side effects, primarily ataxia.

Heterakis

APPROVED COMPOUNDS. Phenothiazine is highly effective in the control of cecal worms in chickens (0.5 g/bird) and turkeys (1 g/bird) when given for 1 day only. Hygromycin B and Coumaphos (see above) are also approved for use in chickens but not in turkeys.

EXPERIMENTAL DATA. Phenothiazine in 1 g doses removed 94% of the heterakids but only 24% of the ascarids (14). Piperazine citrate, given by capsule in single 200-mg doses, removed 66% of the heterakids and was completely effective against the ascarids. However, single 1-g doses of a 7:1 mixture or a 12:1 mixture of phenothiazine and piperazine removed 94% of the heterakids and 91% of the ascarids. It seems, therefore, that the combination of the two drugs is more effective against these roundworms than either alone.

Hygromycin B has been used extensively in controlling combinations of ascaridiasis, heterakidiasis, and capillariasis. It shows greatest efficacy against *H. gallinarum* and may completely eliminate them when fed at the rate of 0.0018–0.0026% for a period of 2 mo or longer. Reductions in worm numbers of *A. galli* and *C. obsignata* are less dramatic, but continuous use in successive flocks grown in the same house may drastically reduce worm numbers and can improve egg production. Economic benefits (including drug costs) have not been fully demonstrated, but the product has been found useful in cases where few other drugs are cleared for use. Hygromycin B has found some acceptance on pen-raised game-bird farms where losses due to intestinal nematodes have been severe.

SYNGAMUS

APPROVED COMPOUNDS. Thiabendazole is currently approved for use only in pheasants at a level of 0.05% for 2 wk.

EXPERIMENTAL COMPOUNDS. Thiabendazole is effective when administered in the feed. Mash containing 0.5% thiabendazole fed to 4-wk-old turkey poults for 9–20 days removed 98% of the gapeworms from 117 birds (88). The drug appeared effective whether treatment was initiated on postinfection-day 30 or started on the day of infection. Continuous medication of pen-reared birds at levels of 0.1–4% has been recommended but is not economical.

Several other compounds have been shown effective against *Syngamus*. Mebendazole (methyl 5-benzoyl-2-benzimidazole carbarmate) was 100% efficacious when fed prophylactically at 0.0064% and curatively at 0.0125% to turkey poults (82). A level of 0.044% for 14 days has also been effective.

Cambendazole [5-isopropoxycarbonylamino-2-(4-thizolyl)-benzimidizole] was found to be more efficacious than thiabendazole or disophenol (2, 6-diiodo-4-nitrophenol) (29). The level of control with three treatments of cambendazole on days 3–4, 6–7, and 16–17 postinfection was 94.9% in chickens (2 × 50 mg/kg) and 99.1% in turkeys (2 × 20 mg/kg).

Levamisole, fed at a level of 0.04% for 2 days or 2 g/gal drinking water for 1 day each month, has proven effective in game birds. Fenbendazole at 20 mg/kg for 3–4 days is also effective (78).

OTHER NEMATODES. *Amidostomum anseris* in geese can be treated with a variety of compounds. Cambendazole (60 mg/kg) was the most effective against both adults and larvae (30). Pyrantel (100 mg/kg) was effective against adults. Some success was also obtained with citarin (40 mg/kg). Mebendazole at 10 mg/kg given for 3 consecutive days completely eliminated *A. anseris* (32). Fenbendazole is also effective.

Tetramisole is not effective against *Dispharynx nasuta* although mebendazole has some efficacy. *Subulura brumpti* can be partially controlled with several different tin compounds or tetramisole. Tetramisole also has some effect against *Strongyloides avium*. Piperazine has been used against *Tetrameres fissispina*.

Trichostrongylus tenuis can be controlled by cambendazole (30 mg/kg), pyrantel tartrate (50 mg/kg), thiabendazole (75 mg/kg), and citarin (40 mg/kg) (31). Mebendazole was completely effective at 10 mg/kg given for 3 consecutive days (32).

ACANTHOCEPHALANS

The Acanthocephala, or thorny-headed worms, are parasites occurring as adults in the intestinal tract of vertebrates.

They are elongate, roughly cylindrical, or spindle shaped. Several distinct body regions are recognizable: retractile proboscis, neck, and body proper. The retractile proboscis always bears a considerable number of recurved hooks arranged in rows. The number, form, and arrangement of the hooks are valuable diagnostic characteristics. The body proper forms the major portion of the worm. It is usually unarmed but may bear small spines of definite form and arrangement on some portion of the external surface. This group of worms has no digestive tract. Nutrition is obtained entirely by absorption through the body wall. The sexes are separate in all cases. The male is smaller and more slender than the female and often distinguished externally by a bell-shaped bursa that surrounds the genital pore.

Apparently, all species of Acanthocephala require one or more intermediate hosts before reaching a stage of development where they are infective for the final host. Various arthropods, snakes, lizards, and amphibians serve as hosts of the larval stages.

Only four species of thorny-headed worms have been reported as parasites of domestic poultry in North America, three of these as immature forms.

***ONCICOLA CANIS* KAUPP 1909.** This worm was found in about 10% of young turkeys around San Angelo, TX (Fig. 31.30). The worms were encysted under the epithelial lining of the esophagus in numbers varying from a few to 100 or more. They were reported as the possible cause of death.

Adults occur in the dog and coyote. The pres-

39. Gibbs, B.J. 1962. The occurrence of the protozoan parasite Histomonas meleagridis in the adults and eggs of the cecal worm Heterakis gallinae. J Protozool 9:288–293.

40. Goble, F.C., and H.L. Kutz. 1945. Notes on the gapeworms (Nematoda: Syngamidae) of galliform and passeriform birds in New York State. J Parasitol 31:323-331.

41. Griffiths, H.J., R.M. Leary, and R. Fenstermacher. 1954. A new record for gapeworm (Cyathostoma bronchialis) infections of domestic geese in North America. Am J Vet Res 15:298-299.

42. Hendriks, J. 1962. The use of Promintic as anthelmintic against experimental infections of Capillaria obsignata Madsen, 1945, in chickens. Tijdschr Diergeneeskd 87:314-322.

43. Hendriks, J. 1963. Methyridine in the drinking water against Capillaria obsignata, Madsen, 1945, in experimentally infected chickens. Tijdschr Diergeneeskd 88:418-424.

44. Horton-Smith, C., and P.L. Long. 1956. The antelmintic effect of three piperazine derivatives on Ascaridia galli (Schrank 1788). Poult Sci 35:606-614.

45. Hwang, J.C. 1964. Hemogram of turkey poults experimentally infected with Syngamus trachea. Avian Dis 8:380-390.

46. Ikeme, M.M. 1971. Observations on the pathogenicity and pathology of Ascaridia galli. Parasitology 63:169-179.

47. Ikeme, M.M. 1971. Effects of different levels of nutrition and continuing dosing of poultry with Ascaridia galli eggs on the subsequent development of parasite populations. Parasitology 63:233-250.

48. Ikeme, M.M. 1971. Weight changes in chickens placed on different levels of nutrition and varying degrees of repeated dosage with Ascaridia galli eggs. Parasitology 63:251-260.

49. Kates, K.C., and M.L. Colglazier. 1970. Differential morphology of adult Ascaridia galli (Schrank 1788) and Ascaridia dissimilis Perez Vigueras, 1931. Proc Helminthol Soc Wash 37:80-84.

50. Kates, K.C., M.L. Colglazier, and F.D. Enzie. 1969. Comparative efficacy of levo-tetramisole, parbendazole, and piperazine citrate against some common helminths of turkeys. Trans Am Microsc Soc 88:142–148.

51. Kaushik, R.K., and V.P.S. Deorani. 1969. Studies on tissue responses in primary and subsequent infections with Heterakis gallinae in chickens and on the process of formation of caecal nodules. J Helminthol 43:69-78.

52. Kazacos, K.R., and W.L. Wirtz. 1983. Experimental cerebrospinal nematodiasis due to Baylisascaris procyonis in chickens. Avian Dis 27:55-65.

53. Kellogg, F.E., and J.P. Calpin. 1971. A checklist of parasites and diseases reported from the Bobwhite Quail. Avian Dis 15:704-715.

54. Lee, D.L., and P. Lestan. 1971. Oogenesis and egg shell formation in Heterakis gallinarum (Nematoda). Proc Zool Soc London 164:189-196.

55. Leiby, P.D., and O.W. Olsen. 1965. Life history studies on Nematodes of the genera Amidostomum (Strongloidea) and Epomidiostomum (Trichostrongyloidea) occurring in the gizzards of waterfowl. Proc Helminthol Soc Wash 32:32-49.

56. Levine, P.P. 1938. Infection of the chicken with Capillaria columbae (RUD). J Parasitol 24:45-52.

57. Levine, N.D. 1980. Nematode Parasites of Domestic Animals and of Man, 2nd Ed. Burgess Publ Co., Minneapolis.

58. Lund, E.E., and A.M. Chute. 1972. Reciprocal responses of eight species of galliform birds and three parasites: Heterakis gallinarum, Histomonas meleagridis, and Parahistomonas wenrichi. J Parasitol 58:940–945.

59. Madsen, H. 1945. The species of (Capillaria, Nematodes, Trichinelloidea) parasite in the digestive tract of Danish gallinaceous and anatine game birds, with a revised list of species of Capillaria in birds. Dan Rev Game Biol 1:1-112.

60. Madsen, H. 1950. Studies on species of Heterakis (nematodes) in birds. Dan Rev Game Biol 1:1-42.

61. Madsen, H. 1951. Notes on the species of Capillaria zeder, 1800 known from gallinaceous birds. J Parasitol 37:257-265.

62. Madsen, H. 1952. A study on the nematodes of Danish gallinaceous gamebirds. Dan Rev Game Biol 2:1-126.

63. McDonald, M.E. 1969. Catalogue of helminths of waterfowl (Anatidae). Spec Sci Rep Wildl (126), Fish Wildl Ser.

64. McGregor, J.K., A.A. Kingscote, and F.W. Remmler. 1961. Field trials in the control of gapeworm infections in pheasants. Avian Dis 5:11-18.

65. Norton, C.C., and L.P. Joyner. 1965. Experimental chemotherapy of infection with Capillaria obsignata. J Comp Pathol 75:137-145.

66. Okon, E.D. 1975. Anthelmintic activity of pyrantel tartrate against Ascaridia galli in fowls. Res Vet Sci 18:331-332.

67. Pankavich, J.A., G.P. Poeschel, A.L. Shor, and A. Gallo. 1973. Evaluation of levamisole against experimental infections of Ascaridia, Heterakis, and Capillaria spp. in chickens. Am J Vet Res 34:501-505.

68. Pence, D.B. 1972. The genus Oxyspirura (Nematoda: Thelaziidae) from birds in Louisiana. Proc Helminthol Soc Wash 39:23-28.

69. Read, C.P. 1949. Studies on North American helminths of the genus Capillaria zedor, 1800 (Nematoda). III. Capillarids from the lower digestive tract of North American birds. J Parasitol 35:240-249.

70. Reid, W.M., and J.L. Carmon. 1958. Effects of numbers of Ascarida galli in depressing weight gains in chicks. J Parasitol 44:183-186.

71. Reid, W.M., J.L. Mabon, and W.C. Harshbarger. 1973. Detection of worm parasites in chicken eggs by candling. Poult Sci 52:2316-2324.

72. Ruff, M.D. 1984. Nematodes and acanthocephalans. In M.S. Hofstad, H.J. Barnes, B.W. Calnek, W.M. Reid, and H.W. Yoder, Jr. (eds.), Diseases of Poultry, 8th Ed., pp. 614-648. Iowa State Univ Press, Ames.

73. Ruff, M.D., L.R. McDougald, and M.F. Hansen. 1970. Isolation of Histomonas meleagridis from embryonated eggs of Heterakis gallinarum. J Protozool 17:10–11.

74. Schmidt, G.D., and O.W. Olsen. 1964. Life cycle and development of Prosthorynchus formosus (Van Cleave, 1918) Travassos, 1926, an acanthocephalan parasite of birds. J Parasitol 50:721-730.

75. Schwabe, C.W. 1951. Studies on Oxyspirura manson: The tropical eyeworm of poultry. II Life history. Pac Sci 5:18-35.

76. Shumard, R.F., and D.F. Eveleth. 1955. A preliminary report on the anthelmintic action of piperazine citrate on Ascardia galli and Heterakis gallinae in hens. Vet Med 50:203-205.

77. Springer, W.T., J. Johnson, and W.M. Reid. 1969. Transmission of histomoniasis with male Heterakis gallinarum (Nematoda). Parasitology 59:401-405.

78. Ssenyonga, G.S.Z. 1982. Efficacy of fenbendazole against helminth parasites of poultry in Uganda. Trop Anim Health Prod 14:163-166.

79. Swales, W.E. 1933. Tetrameres crami sp. nov., a nematode parasitizing the proventriculus of a domestic duck in Canada. Can J Res 8:334-336.

80. Thienpont, D., and J. Mortelmans. 1962. Methyridine in the control of intestinal capillariasis in birds. Vet Rec 74:850-852.

81. Thienpont, D., O.F.J. Vanparijs, A.H.M. Raeymaekers, J. Vanderberk, P.J.A. Demoen, R.P.H. Marsboom, C.J.E. Niemegeers, K.H.L. Schellekens, and P.A.J. Janssen. 1966. Tetramisole (R-8299), a new potent broad spectrum anthelmintic. Nature 209:1084-1086.

82. Thienpont, D.C., O.F.J. Vanparijs, and L.C. Hermans. 1973. Mebendazole, a new potent drug against Syngamus trachea in turkeys. Poult Sci 52:1712-1714.

83. Tongson, M.S., and B.M. McCraw. 1967. Experimental ascaridiasis: Influence of chicken age and infective egg dose on structure of Ascaridia galli populations. Exp Parasitol 21:160-172.

84. Tsvetaeva, N.P. 1960. Pathomorphological changes in the proventriculus of the ducks by experimental tetrameriasis. Helminthologia 2:143-150.

85. Tyzzer, E.E. 1926. Heterakis vesicularis Froelich 1791: A vector of an infectious disease. Proc Soc Exp Med 23:708-709.

86. Wakelin, D. 1965. Experimental studies on the biology of Capillaria obsignata, Madson, 1945, a nematode parasite of the domestic fowl. J Helminthol 39:399-412.

87. Wehr, E.E. 1936. Earthworms as transmitters of Capillaria annulata, the crop-worm of chickens. N Am Vet 17:18-20.

88. Wehr, E.E. 1967. Anthelmintic activity of thiabendazole against the gapeworm (Syngamus trachea) in turkeys. Avian Dis 11:44-48.

89. Wehr, E.E. 1972. Nematodes and acanthocephalans. In M.S. Hofstad, B.W. Calnek, C.F. Helmboldt, W.M. Reid, and H.W. Yoder, Jr. (eds.), Diseases of Poultry, 6th Ed., pp. 844-883. Iowa State Univ Press, Ames.

90. Wehr, E.E., and J.C. Hwang. 1964. The life cycle and morphology of Ascaridia columbae (Gmelin, 1790) Travassos. 1913. (Nematoda: Ascarididae) in the domestic pigeon (Columba livia domestica). J Parasitol 50:131-137.

91. Wehr, E.E., M.I. Colglazier, R.H. Burtner, and L.M. Wiest, Jr. 1967. Methyridine, an effective antihelmintic for intestinal threadworm, Capillaria obsignata in pigeons. Avian Dis 11:322-326.

92. Yamaguti, S. 1961. The nematodes of vertebrates. Parts I and II. Systema Helminthum, Vol 3, Nematodes, pp. 1-679; 681-1261. Interscience, New York.

93. Yorke, W., and P.A. Maplestone, 1962. The Nematode Parasites of Vertebrates. Hafner, New York.

32 CESTODES AND TREMATODES

W. Malcolm Reid

INTRODUCTION. Many species of worm parasites may appear during necropsy examination of the digestive tract or other internal organs of poultry. Some of these are large enough to cause concern for the damage they may be inflicting on the host. Others are so small that a hand lens may be required to distinguish them from other debris. If flattened in shape they are probably "flatworms" belonging to the phylum Platyhelminthes, which contrast with the roundworms or Nemathelminthes discussed in Chapter 31. Before control methods can be considered, accurate identification is essential. Species identification may give direction to control measures aimed at eliminating the intermediate host, thus breaking the life cycle. Marked differences between cestodes (class Cestoda) and trematodes (class Trematoda) require separate sections to describe these two classes in this phylum.

CESTODES

INTRODUCTION. Fifty percent of the intestinal tracts of chickens or turkeys may contain tapeworms if they are reared on range or in backyard flocks. These parasites are found more frequently late in the summer when intermediate hosts are abundant. In contrast, birds confined within poultry houses seldom become infected. Tapeworm infections are now considered rare in intensive poultry-rearing regions. Beetles and houseflies inhabiting poultry houses still act as intermediate hosts for the two large chicken tapeworms known only by the scientific names *Raillietina cesticillus* and *Choantaenia infundibulum.*

Some larger tapeworms may appear to completely block the intestine of infected birds, thus producing concern on the part of the poultry producer. Different species vary considerably in pathogenicity so identification to species is desired.

Unfortunately, diagnosticians have often been satisfied with a diagnosis of "cestodiasis" or "taeniasis" without making further attempts at identification. Prevention, flock prognosis, and treatment suggestions may vary with each species of tapeworm. Only after the species has been determined can an assessment of flock damage and possible control measures be considered (Table 32.1). For identification of the less common specimens, specialized textbooks (9, 12, 16, 17) may be needed to supplement the keys and illustrations included in this text.

Tapeworms or cestodes are flattened, ribbon-shaped, usually segmented worms. The term proglottid is used to describe these individual "segments," since the latter term is reserved by classical zoologists as a characteristic demonstrated in other phyla (Fig. 32.1). One to several gravid proglottids are shed daily from the posterior end of the worm. Millions of eggs may be required to complete the complicated two- or three-host life cycle. Each proglottid contains one or more sets of reproductive organs, which may be crowded with a mass of eggs as the maturing proglottid becomes gravid.

Tapeworms are characterized by complete absence of a digestive tract and obtain their nourishment by absorption from the gut contents of the host. Although the duodenum, jejunum, or ileum is the usual site for attachment of the scolex ("head"), one species (*Hymenolepis megalops*) from ducks is found attached to the cloaca or bursa of Fabricius. Birds become infected by eating an intermediate host, which transmits a larval stage of the tapeworm to the intestine of the definitive host. This larval tapeworm is known as a cysticercoid (Fig. 32.2C). The intermediate host may be an insect, crustacean, earthworm, slug, snail, or leech depending upon the species of tapeworm.

Most cestodes are usually host specific for a single or a few closely related birds. Identification of the genus and species may provide a clue to the probable intermediate host. The diagnostician may then be able to suggest practical control measures. Completion of a two-host life cycle depends upon a unique set of ecologic conditions. Thus minor changes in flock management may cause a break in the life cycle and thus effect a useful control measure.

HISTORY, INCIDENCE, DISTRIBUTION. Over 4000 species of tapeworms have been described from animals (15) with many of the ear-

E.E. Wehr authored the chapter on cestodes in earlier editions of this text while W.W. Price, E.E. Byrd, and Newton Kingston authored a chapter on trematodes. Their contributions to materials included in this edition are gratefully acknowledged.

Table 32.1. Tapeworms and hosts from poultry in the USA

Tapeworm	Definitive Hosts (Occasional Hosts)	Intermediate Hosts	Degree of Pathogenicity
Amoebotaenia cuneata	Chicken (turkey)	Earthworm	Mild
Choanotaenia infundibulum	Chicken (turkey)	Housefly, beetle	Moderate
Davainea proglottina	Chicken	Slug, snail	Severe
Hymenolepis carioca	Chicken (turkey, bobwhite quail)	Stable fly, dung beetle	Unknown
H. cantaniana	Chicken (turkey, peafowl, bobwhite quail)	Beetle	Mild or harmless
Raillietina cesticillus	Chicken (turkey, guinea fowl, bobwhite quail)	Beetle	Mild or harmless
R. tetragona	Chicken (guinea fowl, peafowl, bobwhite quail, turkey?)	Ant	Moderate to severe
R. echinobothrida	Chicken (turkey?)	Ant	Moderate to severe
R. magninumida	Guinea fowl (chicken, turkey)	Beetle	Unknown
Davainea meleagridis	Turkey	Unknown	Unknown
Drepanidotaenia watsoni	Wild turkey	Unknown	Unknown
Imparmargo baileyi	Wild turkey	Unknown	Unknown
Raillietina georgiensis	Wild turkey (domestic turkey)	Ant	Unknown
R. ransomi	Wild turkey	Unknown	Unknown
R. williamsi	Wild turkey	Unknown	Unknown
Metroliasthes lucida	Turkey (guinea fowl, chicken)	Grasshopper	Unknown
Diorchis nyrocae	Wild and domestic duck	Copepod crustacean	Unknown
Fimbriaria fasciolaris	Duck (chicken)	Copepod crustacean	Unknown
Hymenolepis anatina	Wild and domestic duck	Freshwater crustacean	Severe
H. compressa	Duck, goose	Unknown	Unknown
H. collaris	Wild and domestic duck (chicken)	Freshwater crustacean (snail = auxiliary)	Unknown
H. coronula	Duck	Crustacean, snail	Unknown
H. lanceolata	Goose, duck	Crustacean	Severe
H. megalops	Duck	Unknown	Unknown
H. parvula	Wild and domestic duck	Leech	Unknown

lier species bearing the genus name *Taenia*. Since no poultry tapeworms are currently listed in this genus, the term "taeniasis" is no longer appropriate and the term "cestodiasis" would be a better substitute for infection with poultry tapeworms. Slender threadlike forms (*Hymenolepis carioca*) may require some magnification to distinguish individual proglottids, thus indicating that they are tapeworms. Some short forms, e.g., *Davainea proglottina* are so small they have been called "microscopic" tapeworms. To differentiate them from villi, which they superficially resemble, may require examining the mucosal surface with low magnification. However, these tapeworms are still large enough to be recognized unmagnified after they have been removed from the intestine.

CLASSIFICATION. Over 1400 species of tapeworms have been described from wild and domestic birds. Since most of them have no common name, they are best recognized by their genus and species names. Descriptions of species together with keys and more complete classification into higher taxa will be found in separate works.

The 3 families (Davainidae, Dilepididae, Hymenolepidae) and 10 genera (*Amoebotaenia, Choanotaenia, Davainea, Diorchis, Drepanidotaenia, Imparmargo, Metroliasthes, Raillietina, Hymenolepis, Fimbriaria*) recognized here may appear in birds brought to diagnostic laboratories in the USA.

MORPHOLOGY AND LIFE CYCLES

ADULTS. The anatomic features needed to identify poultry tapeworms are illustrated by *Davainea proglottina* (Fig. 32.1). This species differs from most other tapeworms in possessing only one or two each of immature, mature, and gravid proglottids compared to dozens or hundreds in other species. The entire connected chain of proglottids constitutes the strobila. Besides the strobila, the scolex and the neck are recognized. Anchorage is accomplished by the scolex with the assistance of four pairs of suckers or acetabula, which may possess one or two rows of acetabular hooks. If hooks are present, the species is described as armed; if absent, it is unarmed. A plunger-shaped organ known as the rostellum is frequently present at the anterior end. The rostellum may assist in anchorage by means of one or two rows of rostellar hooks and by the suction created by partial withdrawal of the rostellum into the scolex. The host tissue thus becomes firmly embedded in the rim of the scolex. The neck is an elongated undifferentiated area between the scolex and the strobila from which new proglottids proliferate. The neck area in *D. proglottina* is so

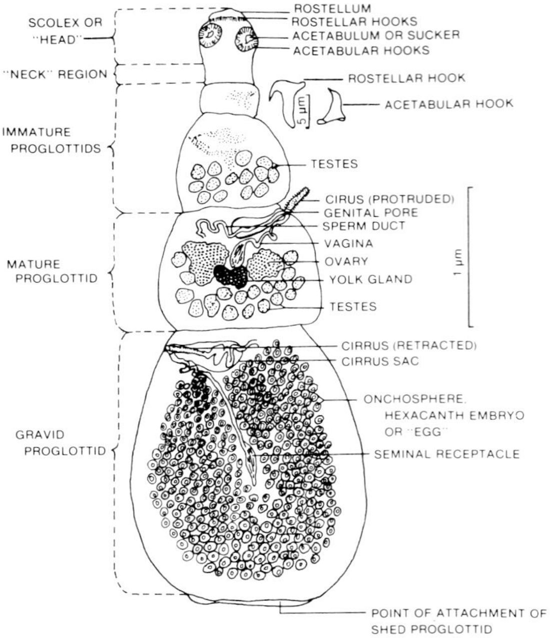

32.1. Adult tapeworm (*Davainea proglottina*). Although readily seen with the naked eye, this species has been called a "microscopic" tapeworm, since it is often overlooked among villi in gross examination of the intestine.

short that it is sometimes listed as missing.

A set of both male and female reproductive organs are found in each proglottid. Morphological differences in size and location of these organs are used in taxonomic descriptions of different species. Older gravid proglottids containing numerous eggs are shed individually or in short chains late in the day after the worm has absorbed and stored glycogen from the gut contents of the host. *D. proglottina* generally sheds 1 gravid proglottid per day while *Raillietina cesticillus* may produce as many as 10–12.

ONCHOSPHERE. Within the uterus the fertilized egg develops into a multicellular embryo; 6 hooks are a prominent feature (Fig. 32.2A, B). The onchosphere (6-hooked or hexacanth embryo) represents a multicellular larva that contains penetration glands and has numerous muscular attachments to activate the hooks. Each proglottid may contain several hundred of these multicellular embryos or "eggs," which may be surrounded by distinctive membranes (Fig 32.2A) and which may be useful in identifying the species of chicken tapeworm.

CYSTICERCOID. Intermediate hosts such as beetles, houseflies, slugs, or snails become infected by swallowing individual eggs from the feces or they devour the entire proglottid after being attracted by odor or movement. The 6-hooked embryo hatches from the egg in the gut of the intermediate host by action of the hooks and penetrates the gut wall. After radical reorganization and a change in polarity, the larva transforms into a cysticercoid (Fig. 32.2C, D). This development requires a minimum of 2 wk depending upon outside temperatures. The cysticercoid remains within the body cavity of the intermediate host until the latter is eaten by the bird host. The cysticercoid is activated by the bile in the definitive host and the scolex becomes attached to the intestine. The first gravid proglottids appear in the feces 2–3 wk after the cysticercoid is swallowed by the definitive host.

DIAGNOSIS AND IDENTIFICATION. Distinctive characteristics of different species of chicken tapeworms may best be demonstrated by examining the scolex (Figs. 32.1, 32.3), the eggs (Figs. 32.2, 32.5), or individual proglottids of recently shed, live specimens (Figs. 32.1, 32.4) (12). Although differential staining to show internal organs of mature proglottids is sometimes recommended, this procedure is too slow for most diagnostic laboratories. Preservation in alcohol or formalin, although required before staining, often obscures useful characteristics needed for rapid identification. The intestine is best opened with scissors under water thus permitting the strobila to float free revealing the area to which the scolex is attached. Recovery of the scolex is worth considerable effort as its characteristics alone may indicate the species. Freeing the scolex, which is frequently lost, may be accomplished by 1) teasing apart the mucosa with two dissecting needles, 2) cutting a deep gouge into the mucosa under the attachment point with a sharp scalpel, or 3) leaving the intestine submerged in saline for a few hours in the refrigerator. Wet-mount preparations of the scolex examined under a cover glass with 100× or higher magnification may reveal sufficient characteristics to make a species identification. Hook characteristics may require measurement with an ocular micrometer under higher magnification. Semipermanent cleared preparations of scolices may be made by using a drop of Hoyer's solution (prepared by adding to 50 ml of distilled water the following ingredients in this order: 30 g gum arabic flakes, 200 g chloral hydrate, 20 g glycerin). If a gravid proglottid is present, distinctive egg characteristics may be demonstrated after teasing it apart or crushing it under a coverglass (Fig. 32.5). Wet preparations of mature or gravid proglottids under low magnification may reveal diagnostic characteristics such as the location, size and shape of the cirrus pouch and location of the genital pore and the gonads. If further details of the internal structure of the proglottid are required for identification, it may be necessary to kill, fix, stain, destain, dehydrate and permanently mount the specimen (1).

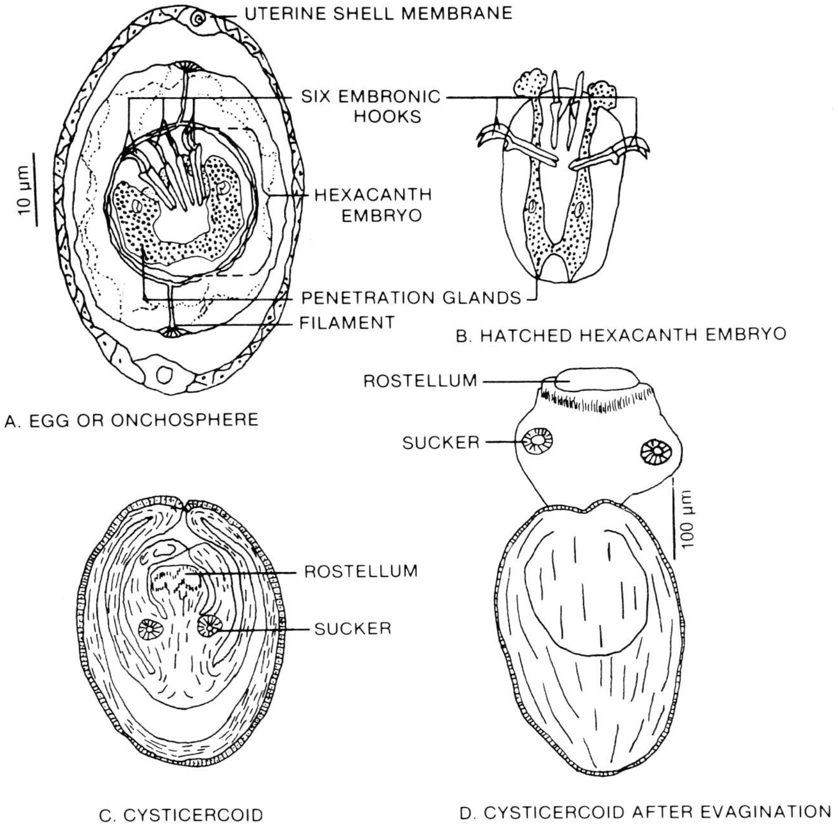

32.2. Larval stages of the chicken tapeworm (*Raillietina cesticillus*). A. The egg is encapsulated by a membrane derived from the uterine wall. Eggs are occasionally found free in feces, but more often several hundred are enclosed in a single gravid proglottid. B. Hexacanth embryos escape from shell membranes. Active hooks and enzymes from secretory glands assist in penetration of gut wall of the beetle intermediate host. C. Cysticercoid that has developed from the hexacanth embryo in the hemocoele of a beetle. D. Scolex in the cysticercoid has evaginated after exposure to bile and enzymes in gut of the fowl.

TAPEWORMS OF CHICKENS. A dichotomous key is given to the eight species of tapeworms commonly found in chickens from the continental USA. In such keys successive selections must be made between 1a and 1b, 2a and 2b, etc. until a species name is designated. After viewing a portion of the worm under the microscope, make a comparison of the appropriate figures organized under scolices (Fig. 32.3), eggs (Fig 32.5), or proglottids (Fig. 32.4). With rare species additional descriptions from other texts may be required (17).

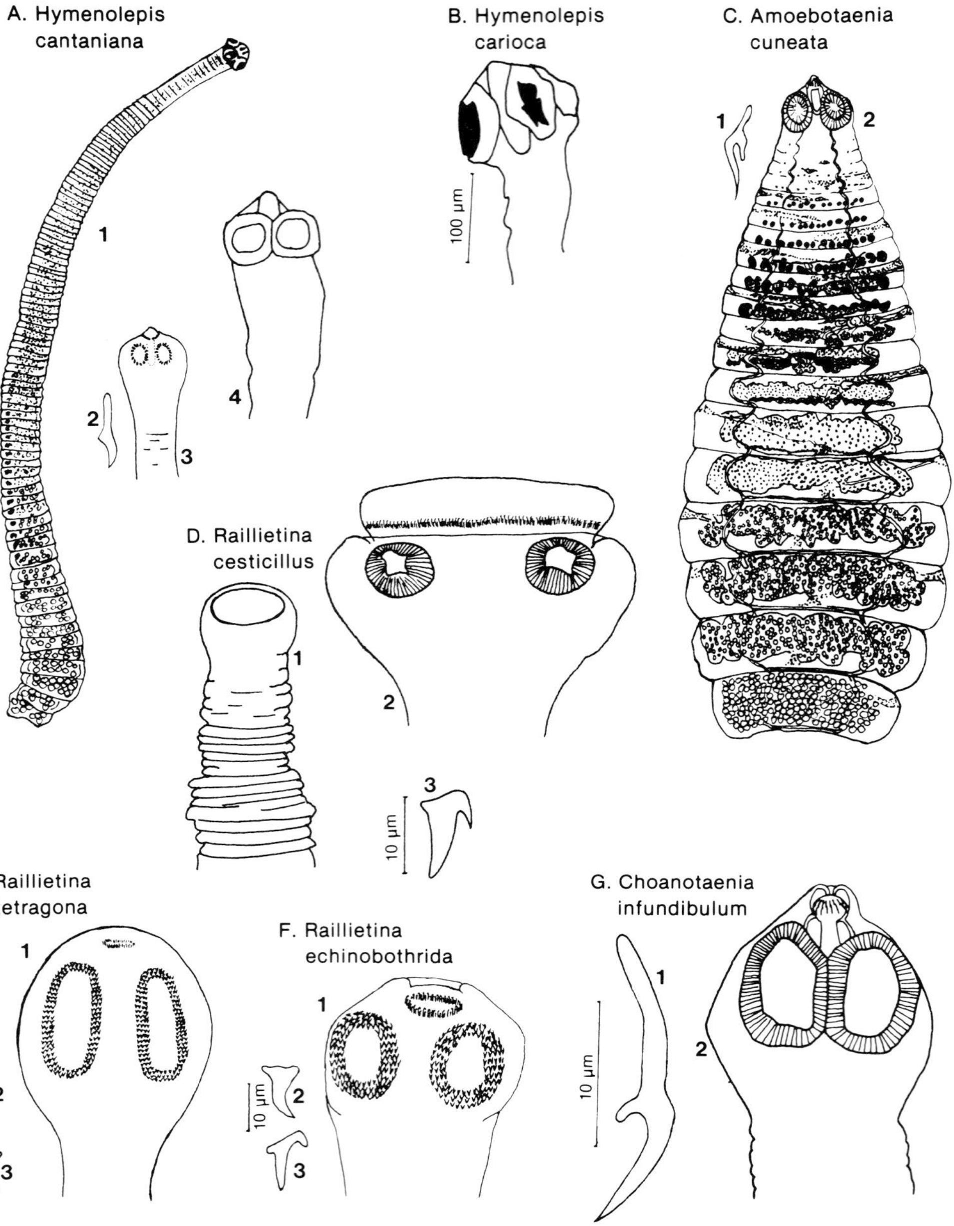

32.3. Scolex characteristics of chicken tapeworms. A. *Hymenolepis cantaniana: 1.* Scolex and strobilia. (Ransom); *2.* Hook. (Yamaguti); *3.* Scolex. (Neveu-Lemaire); *4.* Scolex. (Wehr). B. *H. carioca* scolex. C. *Amoebotaenia cuneata: 1.* Rostellar hook; *2.* Entire worm. (Monnig). D. *Raillietina cesticillus: 1.* Scolex. (Ackert); *2.* Scolex. (Monnig); *3.* Rostellar hook. (Ransom). E. *R. tetragona: 1.* Scolex. (Monnig); *2, 3.* Rostellar and acetabular hooks. (Ransom). F. *R. echinobothrida: 1.* Scolex (Monnig); *2, 3.* Rostellar and acetabular hooks. (Ransom). G. *Choanotaenia infundibulum: 1.* Hook. (Ransom); *2.* Scolex (Monnig)

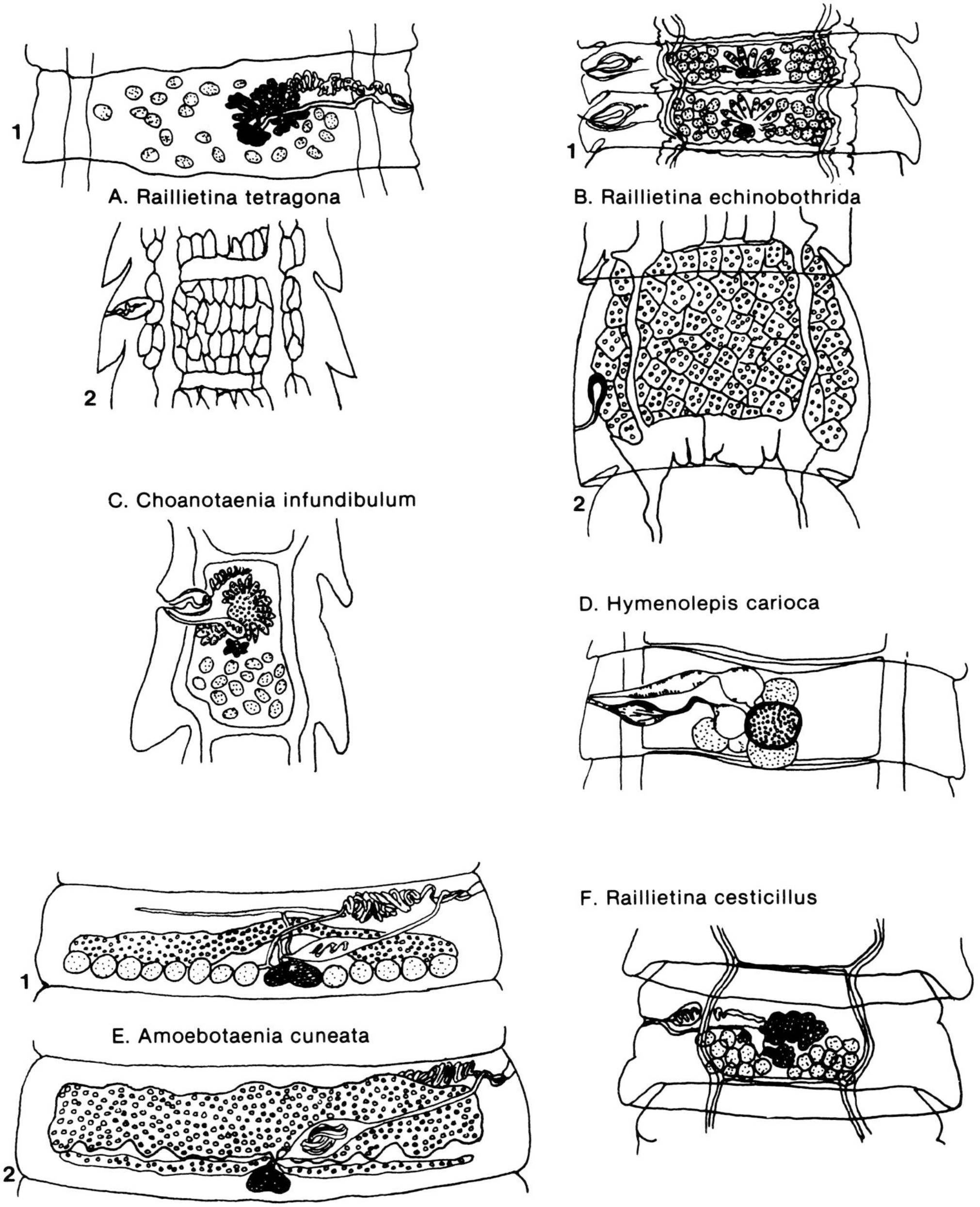

32.4. Mature and gravid proglottids of chicken tapeworms. A. *Raillietina tetragona: 1.* Mature proglottid. (Ransom); *2.* Gravid proglottid showing egg capsules. (Neveu-Lemaire). B. *R. echinobothrida: 1.* Mature proglottid. (Fuhrmann); *2.* Gravid proglottid. (Lang). C. *Choanotaenia infundibulum*. (Fuhrmann). D. *Hymenolepis carioca.* (Sawada). E. *Amoebotaenia cuneata: 1.* Mature proglottid; *2.* Gravid proglottid filled with eggs. (Fuhrmann). F. *Raillietina cesticillus:* Mature proglottid. (Monnig)

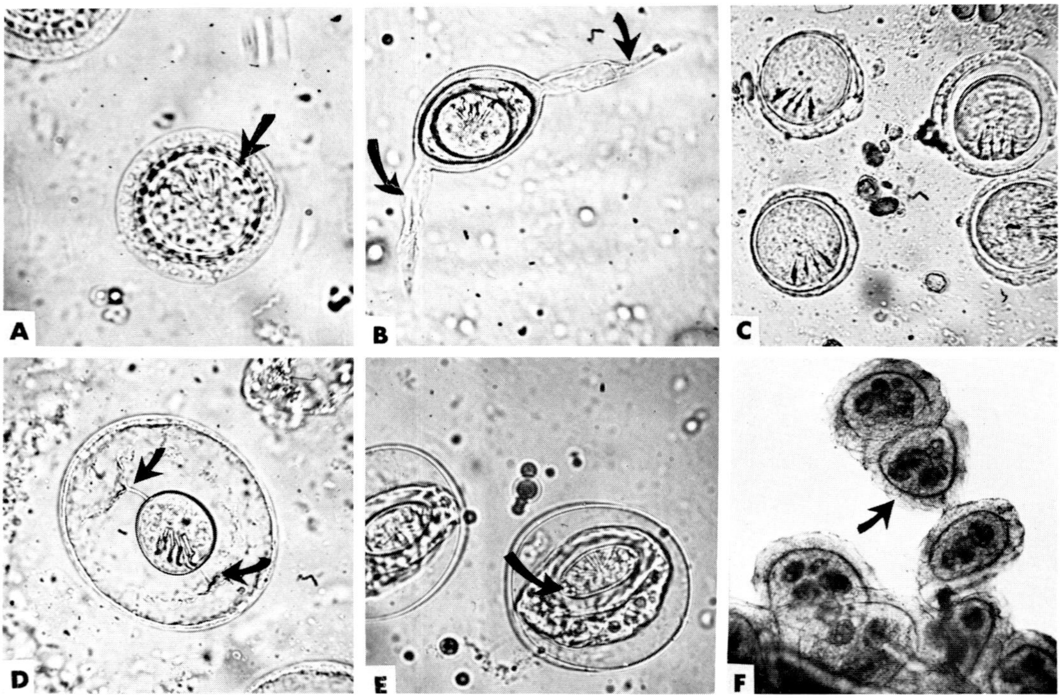

32.5. Eggs of chicken tapeworms (high power). A. *Amoebotaenia sphenoides* showing distinctive granular layer. B. *Choanotaenia infundibulum* with elongated filaments. C. *Davainea proglottina.* D. *Raillietina cesticillus* showing distinctive funnel-shaped structures between membranes found only in fully developed gravid proglottids. E. *Hymenolepis carioca* or *H. cantaniana* showing football-shaped embryophore with granular accumulations at the poles. F. Capsules containing 6–12 eggs; found in the chicken (*Raillietina tetragona, R. echinobothrida*) and two turkey tapeworms (*R. georgiensis, R. williamsi*).

Key to Species

1a. Minute forms, less than 1 cm in length ("microscopic tapeworms"). A very limited number of proglottids with the terminal proglottid being gravid with eggs 2
1b. Longer than 1 cm 3
2a. Wedge-shaped worm. Contains about 20 proglottids. Posterior proglottids wide, short (Figs. 32.3C, 32.4E, 32.5) . . . . . *Amoebotaenia cuneata*
2b. Contains only 2–5 proglottids, rarely 9. Posterior proglottids as long as wide (Fig. 32.1) . . . . . *Davainea proglottina*
3a. Threadlike, never more than 1.5 mm wide; fragile scolex is usually lost; often more than 100 worms in a single bird; proglottids short and wide, genus *Hymenolepis* 4
3b. Robust worms, gravid proglottids wider than 2 mm 5
4a. Mature worms with gravid proglottids present less than 12 mm in length (Fig 32.3A) . . . . . *H. cantaniana*
4b. Mature specimens with a total length including gravid proglottids of more than 12 mm (Figs 32.3B, 32.4D) . . . . . *H. carioca*
5a. 5–12 embryos enclosed in single capsule; verify by opening terminal proglottid; view under a coverglass (Fig. 32.5F) 6
5b. Embryos in single egg capsules enclosed in distinct membranes (examine under high power) . . . 7
6a. Cirrus sac small (75–100 μm in length). Suckers markedly oval in shape (Figs. 32.3E, 32.4A) . . . . . *Raillietina tetragona*
6b. Cirrus sac large (130–180 μm). Suckers round (Figs. 32.3F, 32.4B) . . . . . *R. echinobothrida*
7a. Outer membrane prolonged in 2 elongated filaments (Fig 32.5B) . . . . . *Choanotaenia infundibulum*
7b. Outer membrane smooth and round, 2 elongated filaments (Fig. 32.2A, 32.5D) . . . . . *R. cesticillus*

AMOEBOTAENIA CUNEATA LINSTOW 1872

Diagnostic Characteristics. This short (<4 mm, 25–30 proglottids) tapeworm may be recognized as whitish projections among the villi of the duodenum (Fig. 32.3C); a triangular anterior end with a pointed scolex gives the entire worm a wedge-shaped anterior; suckers unarmed, rostellum armed with a single row of 12–14 distinctive hooks 25–32 μm long; 12–15 testes located transversely in a single row across the posterior end of the proglottid (32.4E); genital pores usually alternate regularly, located at extreme anterior point of proglottid margin; 6-hooked embryos single, surrounded by a distinctive granular layer (Fig. 32.5A); embryonal hooks 6 μm.

Life History. Several species of earthworms belonging to the genera *Allotophora, Pheritima, Ocnerodrilus,* and *Lumbricus* act as intermediate hosts for this tapeworm. Literature descriptions of pathogenicity range from "comparatively slight" to "cause of death." No controlled experiments have been reported.

CHOANOTAENIA INFUNDIBULUM BLOCH 1779

Diagnostic Characteristics. This large robust tapeworm is extremely white and is readily seen attached to the upper half of the intestine. Mature worms up to 23 cm in length; large rostellum armed with a single row of 16–22 large (25–30 μm) hooks, suckers unarmed (Fig. 32.3G); genital pores irregularly alternate; 25–60 testes grouped in posterior portion of proglottid (Fig. 32.4C); eggs with distinctive elongated filaments (Fig. 32.5B); embryonal hooks 18 μm long.

Life History and Pathogenicity. Houseflies and several species of beetles are proven natural hosts. Other insects including nine families of beetles, grasshoppers, and termites are proven experimental hosts. Gravid proglottids are released 13 days after swallowing an infected fly. No controlled experiments testing pathogenicity have been reported.

DAVAINEA PROGLOTTINA DAVAINE 1860

Diagnostic Characteristics. This microscopic tapeworm may be recognized in the duodenal mucosa by protrusion of the gravid proglottids above the villi if the open intestine is floated in water. Eggs without distinctive membranes but embryonal hooks are distinctive, 10–11 μm long (Fig. 32.5C); mature worms up to 4 mm in length; never more than 9 proglottids; suckers armed with 3-6 rows of hooks (Fig. 32.1); rostellum armed; genital pores regularly alternate, located near the anterior margin; cirrus disproportionately large.

Life History. Several species of slugs and snails host larval stages of this tapeworm. Slugs, whose presence may be unsuspected by poultry producers, emerge from hiding at night and travel some distance. More than 1500 cystericercoids have developed along the digestive tract of susceptible slugs where they have remained infective for more than 11 mo. Tapeworms may live as long as 3 yr; over 3000 worms have been recovered from a single bird.

Pathogenicity. This parasite is one of the more harmful species in young birds. In controlled experiments a 12% reduction in growth rate has been reported (6). Uncontrolled reports include emaciation, dull plumage, slow movements, breathing difficulties, thickened mucosal membranes that produce hemorrhage and fetid mucus, leg weakness, paralysis, and death.

HYMENOLEPIS CANTANIANA POLONIO 1860

Diagnostic Characteristics. This short hymenolepid tapeworm (maximum length 2 cm) superficially resembles *H. carioca,* which is much longer. Usually listed as unarmed, but rostellar hooks have been described by European investigators (Fig. 32.3A); fragile rostellum is frequently lost; genital pores unilateral, anterior to middle of proglottid; eggs similar to *H. carioca;* embryonal hooks 13–14 μm.

Life History. Dung beetles (Scarabeidae) are intermediate hosts; each beetle may carry 100 or more cysticercoids. A unique larval development involves budding, which produces many cysticercoids from a single onchosphere. This tapeworm is considered relatively nonpathogenic although no controlled experiments have been reported.

HYMENOLEPIS CARIOCA MAGALHAES 1898

Diagnostic Characteristics. Several thousand specimens of this extremely slender species have been found in the duodenum of a single chicken or turkey. The worm is so slender (about 1 mm in diameter) that the hundreds of inconspicuous proglottids look more like a thread than a worm. Suckers unarmed; rostellar sac present; rostellum rudimentary (Fig. 32.3B); 3 testes, usually in a straight row; genital pores unilateral, located anterior to middle of proglottid margin (Fig. 32.4D); an inner membrane enveloping the onchosphere is elongated into a football shape with granular deposits at poles (Fig. 32.5E); embryonal hooks 10–12 μm.

Life History. Twenty-six species belonging to nine families of beetles and one species of termite are experimental or natural intermediate hosts; dung and ground beetles are the most common source of infection. Reports incriminating the housefly are probably erroneous.

Pathogenicity. Experimental infections establishing several hundred worms per bird produced no retardation in weight gains compared to unparasitized controls of the same age. These results indicate that this species is relatively nonpathogenic.

RAILLIETINA CESTICILLUS MOLIN 1858

Diagnostic Characteristics. Scolex of this large robust tapeworm (15 cm long) embeds deeply in the mucosa of the duodenum or jejunum; distinctive, wide, flat, rostellum bears a double row of 300–500 hammer-shaped hooks; flattened rostellum acts as a retractable piston drawing into an outer sleeve of the scolex thus providing a firm grip on the mucosa (Fig. 32.3D*1, 2*); 4 unarmed weak suckers; genital pores alternate irregularly (Fig. 32.4F); 20–30 testes posteriad in proglottid; single eggs encapsulated in uterine membranes, mature eggs with 2 distinctive funnel-shaped filaments between the middle and inner membranes (Fig. 32.5D).

Life History. Over 100 species of beetles belonging to 10 families are proven natural or experimental intermediate hosts. A minute histerid beetle (*Carcinops pumilio*) is the natural intermediate host in broiler houses. Darkling beetles (*Alphitobius diaperinus*), houseflies, grasshoppers, ants, and lepidopterous larvae have proved negative as experimental hosts. As many as 930 cysticercoids have been found in a single ground beetle.

Pathogenicity. Early reports attribute this parasite with causing emaciation, degeneration and inflammation of villi, reduction of blood sugar and hemoglobin, and reduced growth rate. None of these early reports could be confirmed in extensive controlled experiments with broilers and layers maintained on optimum nutritional diets (3). Experimental infections (135 worms/bird) produced by feeding 300 cysticercoids caused no reduction in weight gain in broilers or reduced egg production in layers when compared to uninfected controls.

RAILLIETINA TETRAGONA MOLIN 1858

Diagnostic Characteristics. These are moderately large tapeworms, up to 25 cm long, 3 mm wide; scolex (Fig. 32.3E*1*) anchors in posterior half of the intestine; rostellum armed with 90–100 hooks 6–8 μm long, arranged in a single or double row (Fig. 32.3E*2*); suckers oval-shaped, armed with 8–12 rows of minute hooks 3–8 μm long (Fig. 32.3E*1*); genital pores usually unilateral (Fig. 32.4A); uterus breaks up into capsules containing 6–12 eggs (Figs. 32.4A*2*, 32.5F), similar to *R. echinobothrida* from chickens, and *R. williamsi* and *R. georgensis* from turkeys; cirrus sac small (75–100 μm long), more anterior in proglottid margin than with *R. echinobothrida.*

Life History. Several species of small ants that nest under rocks or boards act as intermediate hosts. The minimum prepatent period after feeding cysticercoids to chickens is 13 days.

Pathogenicity. Weight loss was demonstrated in controlled experiments (10) with white leghorns and hybrids infected with an average of 12–16 worms/bird. Decreases in egg production in four breeds of hens occurred after administering 50 cysticercoids/bird causing reduced glycogen levels in livers and the intestinal mucosa of infected chickens.

RAILLIETINA ECHINOBOTHRIDA MEGNIN 1881

Diagnostic Characteristics. This species resembles *R. tetragona* but differs in the following characteristics: Strobila larger (34 cm long, 4 mm wide); rostellum containing 200–250 hooks 10–13 μm long (Fig. 32.3F*1*); suckers rounded with 8–15 rows of hooks 5–15 μm long (Fig. 32.3F*2, 3*); genital pores in posterior half of proglottid (Fig. 32.4B*2*); cirrus sac large (130–180 μm long); gravid proglottids frequently loosen from each other in the center making a windowlike arrangement not found in *R. tetragona.*

Life History. As with *R. tetragona,* numerous species of ants have been found naturally infected with cysticercoids. Concurrent infections with both *R. echinobothrida* and *R. tetragona* cysticercoids have been found in ants.

Pathogenicity. *R. echinobothrida* is usually listed as one of the most pathogenic tapeworms, since its presence has often been associated with nodular disease of chickens. Nadakal et al. (11) reported parasitic granulomas approximately 1–6 mm in diameter at the sites of worm attachment 6 mo after experimental infection with 200 cysticercoids. The condition was associated with catarrhal hyperplastic enteritis as well as lymphocytic, polymorphonuclear, and eosinophilic infiltration.

TAPEWORMS OF TURKEYS. Six species of tapeworms from domestic and/or wild turkeys have been reported from the USA (13). Since these tapeworms are readily transferred between wild and domestic turkeys, wild turkeys sometimes present problems for poultry producers. No controlled experiments on pathogenicity have been reported for any species. Descriptions included here are limited to the two species with known life cycles. Scolex (Fig. 32.6) and proglottid characteristics (Fig. 32.7) of different species are organized in separate figures to facilitate comparisons if complete specimens are unavailable.

Raillietina georgiensis Reid and Nugara 1961

Diagnostic Characteristics. Large (15–38 cm long, 3.5 mm wide) robust tapeworm from domestic and wild turkeys; rostellum armed with double row of 230 moderate length (12–23 μm) hooks (Fig. 32.6A*1, 2*); suckers circular with 8–10 rows of hooks 8–13 μm long (Fig. 32.6A*1, 3*); genital pores unilateral, located in middle of proglottid (Fig. 32.7A); eggs in uterine capsules, similar to *R. tetragona* and *R. echinobothrida.*

Life History. A small brownish ant (*Pheidole vinelandica*) that frequents turkey ranges has

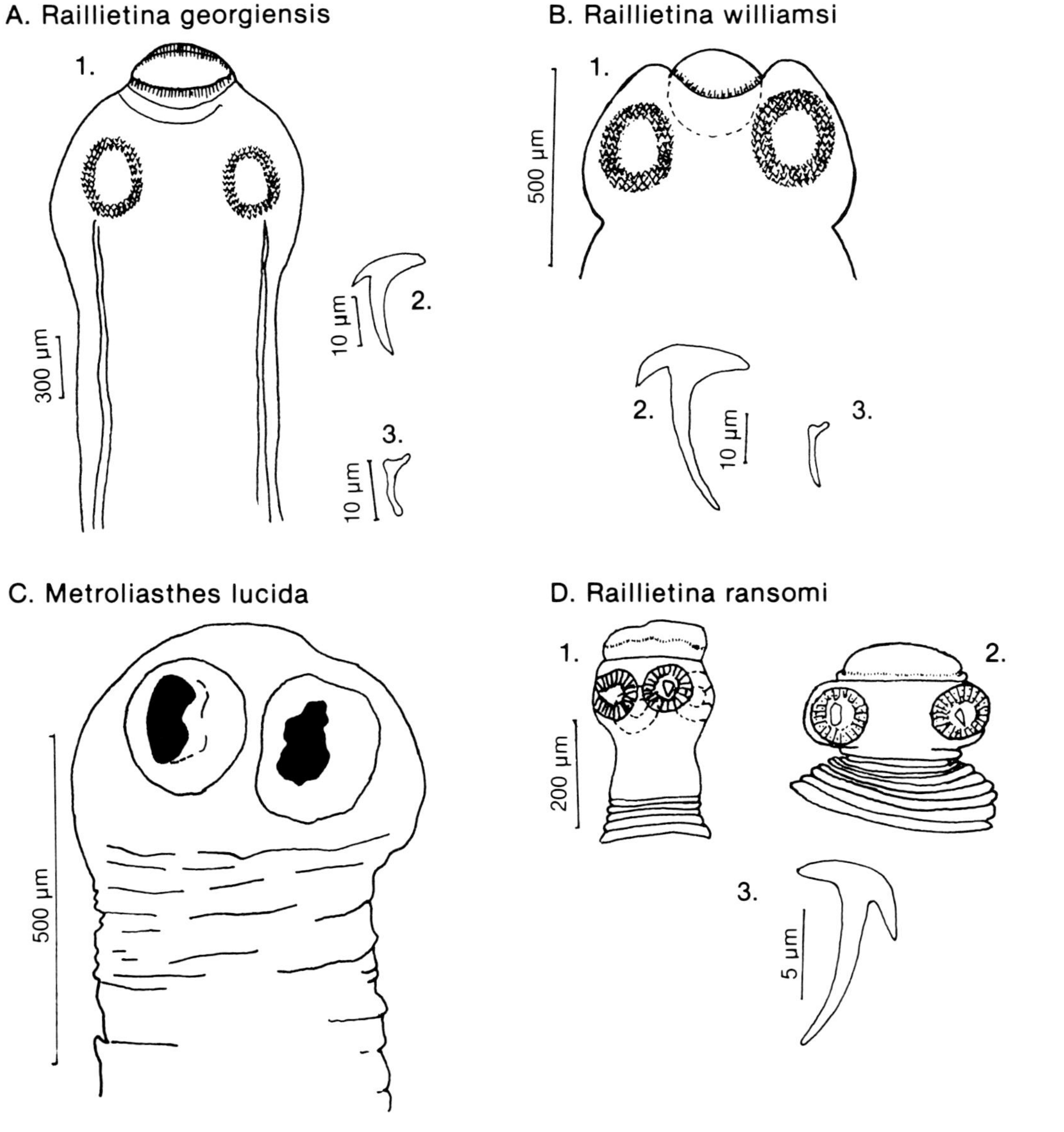

32.6. Scolices of turkey tapeworms. A. *Raillietina georgiensis: 1.* Scolex; *2.* Rostellar hook; *3.* Acetabular hook. (Reid and Nugara). B. *R. williamsi: 1.* Scolex; *2.* Rostellar hook; *3.* Acetabular hook. (Williams). C. *Metroliasthes lucida* scolex. (Ransom). D. *R. ransomi: 1, 2.* Scolex; *3.* Rostellar hook. (Williams)

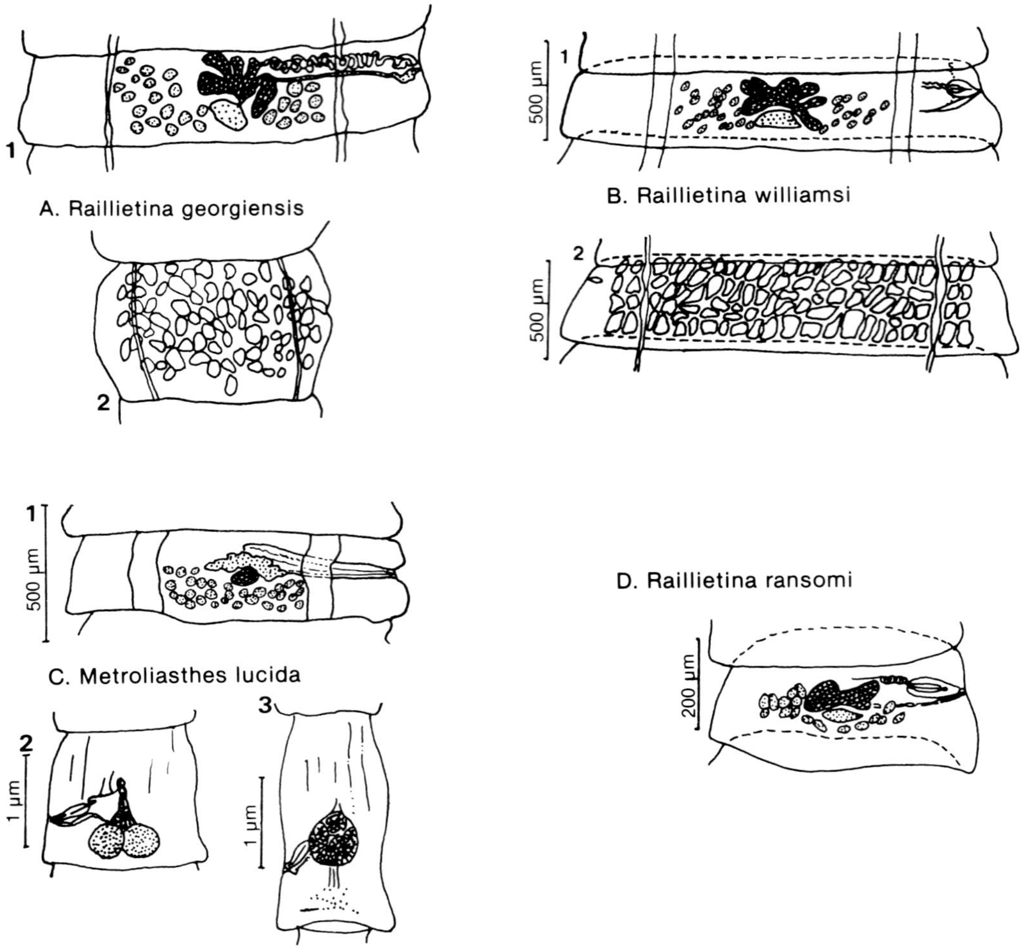

32.7. Mature and gravid proglottids of domestic and wild turkey tapeworms. A. *Raillietina georgiensis.* (Reid and Nugara). B. *R. williamsi: 1.* Mature proglottid; *2.* Gravid proglottid showing position of egg capsules, each containing several eggs. (Williams). C. *Metroliasthes lucida: 1.* Mature proglottid; *2.* Proglottid showing two-part uterus and developing parauterine organ; *3.* Gravid proglottid. (Ransom). D. *R. ransomi* mature proglottid. (Williams)

been found naturally infected; gravid proglottids appear in droppings within 3 wk after turkeys have fed on infected ants. This tapeworm was introduced to a domestic farm by wild turkeys.

Pathogenicity. Enteritis is present if parasites are found in large numbers. Some host damage is assumed on the basis of a close relationship to *R. echinobothrida* from chickens.

METROLIASTHES LUCIDA RANSOM 1900

Diagnostic Characteristics. Long tapeworm (20 cm) from turkeys and guinea fowl, rarely in chickens. Unarmed scolex and suckers, 200–250 µm in diameter (Fig. 32.6C); genital pores irregularly alternate, near middle of margin in mature proglottids but posterior in gravid proglottids; uterus consists of 2 sacs side by side visible to the naked eye in gravid proglottids, is known as the parauterine organ (Fig. 32.7C*2, 3*); eggs with 3 membranes, 75 × 50 µm.

Life History. Several species of grasshoppers serve as intermediate hosts; cysticercoid development requires 15–42 days depending on temperature.

TAPEWORMS OF DUCKS AND GEESE. Domestic ducks and geese frequently become infected with numerous species of tapeworms introduced by wild ducks and geese. Some of these species have occasionally been reported in chickens. Two of the more common species are described below. Life cycles usually involve crustaceans or other aquatic invertebrates. No controlled pathogenicity studies have been made on any of these species.

FIMBRIARIA FASCIOLARIS PALLAS 1781

Diagnostic Characteristics. This large (5–43 cm long, 1–5 mm wide) twisted tapeworm of ducks also occurs in chickens and 31 species of wild birds. The distinctive flaring anterior neck region is known as the pseudoscolex; strobila unsegmented, but cross-striations give the impression of segmentation (Fig. 32.8A*1*); minute scolex (Fig. 32.8A*3, 4*) attached to pseudoscolex 100–130 μm wide; suckers unarmed; retractile rostellum with 10–12 hooks 17–22 μm long (Fig. 32.8A*2*); genital pores unilateral, closely crowded together; onchospheres 35–45 μm, hooks 16 μm long.

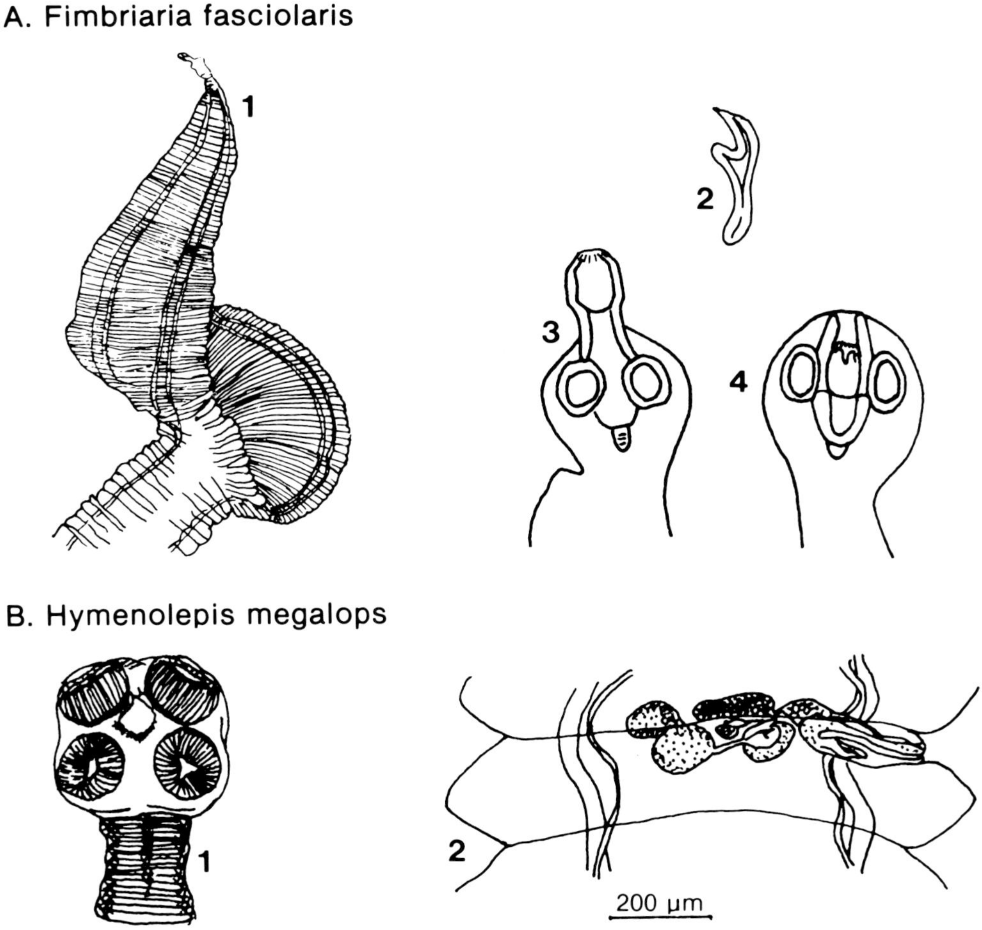

32.8. Tapeworms of ducks and geese. A. *Fimbriaria fasciolaris: 1.* Pseudoscolex showing irregular distension of the anterior end and the minute scolex. (Todd); *2.* Rostellar hook. (Fuhrmann); *3.* Scolex with rostellum extended; *4.* Scolex with rostellum withdrawn. (Neveu-Lemaire). B. *H. megalops: 1.* Scolex; *2.* Mature proglottid. (Yamaguti)

Life History. Cysticercoids develop in copepod crustaceans (*Diaptomus* sp. *Cyclops* sp.); intermediate hosts are ingested with drinking water to infect the definitive host.

HYMENOLEPIS MEGALOPS NITZSCH, IN CREPLIN 1829

Diagnostic Characteristics. This cosmopolitan tapeworm of waterfowl (Fig. 32.8B) is 3–6 mm long and readily recognized by the large scolex (1–2 mm wide) attached to the cloaca or the bursa of Fabricius. Suckers and rostellum unarmed, the latter contains a rudimentary central pit; eggs not in capsules.

Life History. Onchospheres develop into cysticercoids after 18 days in ostracod crustacea. The definitive host is infected by eating ostracods.

Pathogenicity. Reports range from "severe damage" to "mortality if other cestodes (*H. coronula, H. furcigera*) are also present."

PREVENTION AND CONTROL. Establishing a tapeworm infection requires a delicate balance between the habits of the host and of the parasite. During the past 40 yr changes from backyard or range management to confinement rearing in large houses has brought on marked reductions in tapeworm infections in chickens and turkeys. Many flocks no longer have easy access to the required insect or other invertebrate hosts. *Davainea proglottina,* one of the most pathogenic species, was reported from 23% of the chickens submitted to the diagnostic laboratory in New York State in 1932. No cases have been found in recent years after confinement rearing became the common commercial poultry practice. Poultry no longer has easy access to garden slugs.

Preventing the birds from having contact with the intermediate host is the first step to consider in tapeworm control. Eliminating the intermediate hosts may provide additional benefits besides tapeworm control. If *Choanotaenia infundibulum* appears in a cage-layer facility, housefly control will benefit the producer by preventing nuisance and public health complaints (see Chapter 30). If *Raillietina cesticillus* tapeworms appear in broiler houses, beetle control measures for the darkling beetle (*Alphitobius diaperinus*) may also eliminate the true intermediate host *Carcinops pumilio,* which is a minute histerid beetle. After species identification has given an indication of the intermediate host, some specific control measures may be recommended.

TREATMENT. If a tapeworm infection appears during a necropsy examination in a diagnostic laboratory, the client usually asks first for a drug to remove the worms. The diagnostician should warn the client that expulsion of the parasite will be a very short-term remedy if the intermediate host as a source of infection is still present.

Unfortunately little success in flock improvement has come from treatment recommendations. After extensive screening tests, several drugs have been found to have efficacy against tapeworms. In the USA approval of the Food and Drug Administration (FDA) has been obtained for a single drug that is an organic tin compound. The basic ingredient is known by the generic name butynorate (dibutyltin dilaurate). It is approved for treatment against six species of chicken tapeworms (*Raillietina cesticillus, R. tetragona, Choanotaenia infundibulum, D. proglottina, Hymenolepis carioca,* and *Amoebotaenia sphenoides*) (4). Butynorate is available in granular form in a combination with piperazine and phenothiazine as a feed additive or in individual tablets under the trade name Wormal. The latter two drugs are included for control of two common nematodes (*Ascaridia galli* and *Heterakis gallinarum*). Although butynorate (trade name Tinostat) is available as a feed additive for prevention of turkey coccidiosis, requests have yet to be submitted to FDA for use against tapeworms. Recommended dosage indicated on the label should never be exceeded, since higher levels reduce growth rate and egg production.

Other experimental drugs showing efficacy that have not been approved by FDA include hexachlorophene and niclosamide (Yomesan) (2). Increasing costs of demonstrating efficacy without producing toxicity to satisfy standards of FDA make it unlikely that such products will become commercially available in the USA.

TREMATODES

INTRODUCTION. Trematodes (flukes) are flat, leaflike, parasitic organisms belonging to the phylum Platyhelminthes, and they represent a distinct class (Trematoda). They differ from the cestodes (class Cestoda) by having a digestive system, but trematodes do not have separate proglottids. The life cycle of all trematodes parasitizing birds requires a molluscan intermediate host; many species also use a second intermediate host. Since adult trematodes and larval metacercariae invade almost every cavity and tissue of birds, they may show up unexpectedly at necropsy. The diagnostician may need a general knowledge of trematode morphology and life cycles to interpret such findings.

Over 500 species belonging to some 125 genera and 27 families are known to occur in the four orders of birds most likely to be submitted to diagnostic laboratories as domestic or pet birds

(5); 20 of these flukes are considered potentially dangerous to poultry in the Western Hemisphere. These flukes belong to four orders: Anseriformes (ducks and geese), Galliformes (chickens and turkeys), Columbiformes (pigeons and allies), and Passeriformes (perching birds). Flukes are less host-specific than tapeworms, so wild birds often introduce infection in areas where domestic poultry is reared. Since many snails live in ponds and streams, ducks and geese are the most frequently parasitized. The oviduct fluke (*Prosthogonimus* sp.), which is a frequent parasite of many species of wild birds, sometimes causes problems with ducks and chickens (7). This species will be used to illustrate fluke morphology and life history. *P. macrorchis* is the species name recognized in the USA, while this fluke is known as *P. ovatus* or by other specific names in other countries.

MORPHOLOGY AND LIFE HISTORY. The body of the adult fluke (Fig. 32.9) is leaflike and bears two suckers. The digestive system consists of the mouth entering the oral sucker, the pharynx, a short esophagus, and two intestinal ceca. An anus is lacking in the trematodes. Two testes and one ovary are present in the same individual. After fertilization the zygote is enclosed along with yolk cells from the vitellaria by an egg shell. Large numbers of eggs are stored in a prominent convoluted uterus. The excretory system, which originates in a series of flame cells bearing a tuft of cilia, drains with a series of collecting tubules that empty through an excretory pore near the posterior end of the parasite. The arrangement pattern of these collecting tubules is used as a family characteristic in classification of flukes.

LIFE CYCLE. Adult flukes are continually shedding eggs, which pass out with the feces of the host. These eggs contain an embryo that develops into a larval stage known as a miracidium. In this group of trematodes the miracidium hatches after the egg is swallowed by a susceptible snail. Larval development continues within the snail through a succession of stages known as sporocysts and cercariae. The cercariae emerge from the snail and swim about in a lake or pond. Some are drawn into the brachial basket of a dragon fly naiad. The cercaria encysts (metacercaria) and remains in the insect until either the naiad or an infected adult dragonfly is eaten by a bird (Fig 32.10).

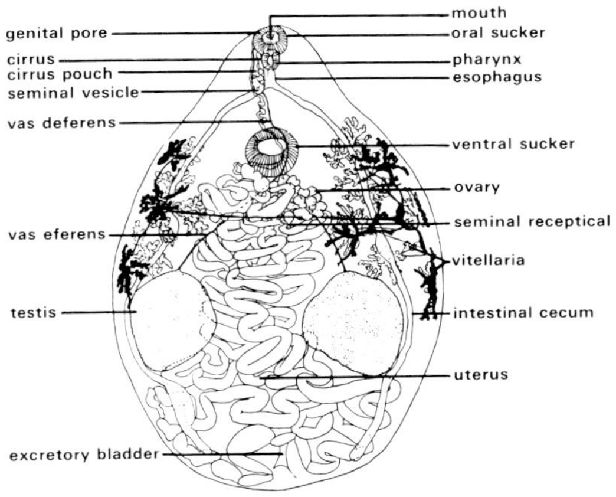

32.9. Morphology of an adult trematode (*Prosthogonimus macrorchis*). (Macy)

IDENTIFICATION. Twenty-four trematodes, which occasionally appear in diagnostic laboratories, have been described with keys by Kingston (5). More extensive listings of species is provided by Yamaguti (18), McDonald (8), and Schell (14). The latter text also describes methods of identifying, collecting, preserving, and staining trematodes with emphasis on North American families and genera.

PATHOGENICITY. *Prosthogonimus* sp., popularly known as the oviduct fluke, has caused economic losses to poultry producers by 1) drastically reducing egg production after a recent infection and 2) occasionally being enveloped within a hen's egg and later discovered by a complaining customer. Other organs of the bird invaded by flukes include 1) metacercarial cysts in the skin of chickens and turkeys (*Collyriclum faba*); 2) small adult flukes in the conjunctival sac of the eye (*Philophthalmus gralli*); 3) adults in the liver, pancreas, and bile duct of ducks and turkeys (*Amphimerus elongatus*); 4) adults in the collecting tubules of the excretory system of chickens, turkeys, and pigeons (*Tanaisia bragai*); 5) adults and eggs in the circulatory system of ducks by three species of blood fluke; and 6) 14 species of flukes that invade various areas of the digestive tract.

Severe pathogenicity may be regarded as relatively rare. Fluke parasites and their hosts have both survived by living together for thousands of years. Only when habitat conditions permit large numbers of parasites to infect, does severe damage occur.

CONTROL. If the life cycle is known and evidence of pathogenicity or economic loss is clear, changes in poultry management may prevent the problem. For example, with oviduct flukes control was effected by fencing in chicken flocks, which prevented access to the lake shores where they were eating dragonfly naiads (7). This prevented troublesome decreases in egg production and customer complaints after finding worms inside market eggs.

With poultry, neither chemical control of snails

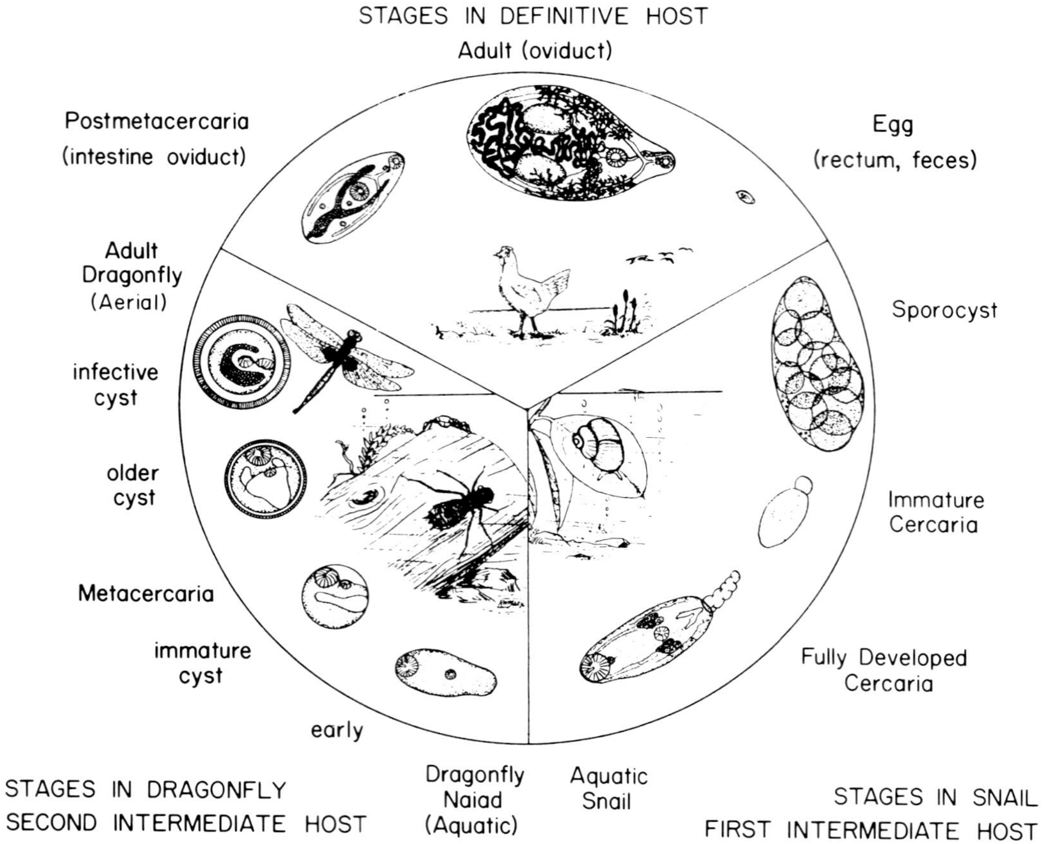

32.10. Life cycle of a typical digenetic trematode (*Prosthogonimus macrorchis*). (Macy)

to prevent trematode infections nor drug treatments for adult flukes appear to be practical solutions to trematode infections.

REFERENCES

1. Ash, L.R., and T.C. Orihel. 1987. Parasites: A Guide to Laboratory Procedures and Identification. Am Soc Clinical Pathol, Chicago.
2. Boisvenue, R.J., and J.C. Hendrix. 1965. Prophylactic treatment of experimental Raillietina cesticillus infections in chickens with Yomesan™. J Parasitol 51:519–522.
3. Botero, H., and W.M. Reid. 1969. The effects of the tapeworm Raillietina cesticillus upon body weight gains of broilers, poults, and on egg production. Poult Sci 48:536–542.
4. Kerr, K.B. 1952. Butynorate, an effective and safe substance for the removal of R. cesticillus from chickens. Poult Sci 31:328–336.
5. Kingston, N. 1984. Trematodes. In M.S. Hofstad, H.J. Barnes, B.W. Calnek, W.M. Reid, and H.W. Yoder, Jr. (eds.), Diseases of Poultry, 8th Ed., pp. 668–690. Iowa State Univ Press, Ames.
6. Levine, P.P. 1938. The effect of infection with Davainea proglottina on the weights of growing chickens. J Parasitol 24:550–551.
7. Macy, R.W. 1934. Studies on the taxonomy, morphology, and biology of Prostogonimus macrorchis Macy, a common oviduct fluke of domestic fowls in North America. Minnesota Agric Exp Tech Bull 98:1–64.
8. McDonald, M.E. 1981. Key to trematodes reported in waterfowl. US Dept Int Fish Wildl Serv Resour Publ 142, Washington, DC.
9. Monnig, H.O. 1934. Veterinary Helminthology and Entomology. Baillerie, Tindall and Cox, London.
10. Nadakal, A.M., and K.V. Nair. 1979. Studies on the metabolic disturbances caused by Raillietina tetragona (Cestoda) infection in domestic fowl. Indian J Exp Biol 17:310–311.
11. Nadakal, A.M., K. Mohandas, K.O. John, and K. Muraleedharan. 1973. Contribution to the biology of the fowl cestode Raillietina echinobothrida with a note on its pathogenicity. Trans Am Microsc Soc 92:273–276.
12. Reid, W.M. 1962. Chicken and turkey tapeworms. Handb Univ Georgia Poult Dep, Athens.
13. Reid, W.M. Cestodes. 1984. In M.S. Hofstad, H.J., Barnes, B.W. Calnek, W.M. Reid, and H.W. Yoder, Jr. (eds.), Diseases of Poultry, 8th Ed., pp. 649–667. Iowa State Univ Press, Ames.
14. Schell, S.C., 1985. Handbook of Trematodes of North America North of Mexico. Univ Press, Moscow, ID.
15. Schmidt, G.D. 1986. Handbook of Tapeworm Identification. CRC Press, Boca Raton, FL.
16. Wardle, R.A., and J.A. McLeod. 1952. The Zoology of Tapeworms. Univ Minnesota Press, Minneapolis.
17. Yamaguti, S. 1959. Systema Helminthum. Vol 2, The Cestodes of Vertebrates. Interscience, New York.
18. Yamaguti, S. 1958. The Digenetic Trematodes of Vertebrates, Vols 1 and 2. Interscience, New York.

33 PROTOZOA

INTRODUCTION

W. Malcolm Reid

Several poultry diseases are caused by parasitic protozoa that produce severe morbidity and mortality. These parasites range in length between 1 and 50 μ.

Parasitic diseases often differ from viral and bacterial diseases by the 1) presence of a complicated life cycle, 2) methods of transmission, 3) absence of serological methods for diagnosis, and 4) usefulness of disinfection and quarantine measures for their control.

Changes in poultry management practices such as confinement-rearing with high-density flocks have increased seriousness of diseases such as coccidiosis. In contrast other parasitic diseases have decreased in importance if an intermediate host has been eliminated by the confinement.

The discovery that anticoccidial drugs could prevent disastrous economic losses from coccidiosis has resulted in their constant use in broiler production. This discovery has resulted in responsibility for the control of this disease being shifted from the farm to the feedmill operator.

Rational control measures for all parasitic diseases depends upon accurate diagnosis of the parasite causing the problem. Since few parasites have a universally acceptable common name, the double latinized scientific name is usually applied.

For many years the protozoa were placed in a single phylum and defined as one-celled organisms. Others recognizing the presence of a unique complex organelle within the cell defined the protozoa as acellular organisms. More recently protozoa have been elevated to a subkingdom status containing seven phyla (1). Two of these phyla contain protozoa parasitic in poultry. The phylum Apicomplexa is characterized by the presence of an apical complex, which can be demonstrated by electron microscopy. Parasitic genera in this phylum described in this chapter include *Eimeria, Isopora, Haemoproteus, Leucocytozoon, Plasmodium, Toxoplasma, Sarcocystis, Wenonella, Tyzzeria,* and *Cryptosporidium.* Due to recent increased interest in the latter genus, a new section has been added entitled *Cryptosporidium.*

Members of the phylum Sarcomastigophora have a single-type nucleus, flagella or pseudopodia, or both types of locomoter organelles. Genera in this phylum discussed in this text include *Histomonas, Trypanosoma, Chilomastix, Entamoeba, Endolimax, Hexamita, Cochlosoma,* and *Haemoproteus.*

REFERENCE

1. Levine, N.D., J.O. Corliss, F.E.G. Cox, G. Deroux, J. Grain, B.M. Honigberg, G.F. Leedale, A.R. Loeblich, III, J. Lom, D. Lynn, E.G. Merinfeld, F.C. Page, G. Poljansky, V. Sprague, J. Varva, and F.G. Wallace. 1980. A newly revised classification of the Protozoa. J Protozool 27:37–58.

Grateful acknowledgement is made to Elery R. Becker, author of this chapter in the first four editions of this book and to Everett E. Lund and Marion M. Farr, authors of the fifth edition.

COCCIDIOSIS

Larry R. McDougald and W. Malcolm Reid

INTRODUCTION. Coccidiosis is a disease of almost universal importance in poultry production. The protozoan parasites of the genus *Eimeria* multiply in the intestinal tract and cause tissue damage with resulting interruption of feeding and digestive processes or nutrient absorption, dehydration, blood loss, and increased susceptibility to other disease agents. Historically, the spectacular onset of coccidiosis with bloody diarrhea and high mortality inspired awe and dread on the part of poultry growers and fanciers. Like many parasitic diseases, coccidiosis is largely a disease of young animals because immunity quickly develops after exposure and gives protection against later disease outbreaks. Unfortunately, there is no cross-immunity between species of *Eimeria* in birds, and later outbreaks may be the result of different species. The short, direct life cycle and high reproductive potential of coccidia in poultry intensifies the potential for severe outbreaks of disease in the modern poultry house, where 15–30,000 chickens may be reared in total confinement.

Coccidiosis may strike any type of poultry in any type of facility. The disease may be mild, resulting from ingestion of a few oocysts, and may escape notice, or may be severe as a result of ingestion of millions of oocysts. Most infections are relatively mild, but because of the potential for the disastrous outbreak and the resulting financial loss, almost all young poultry are given continuous medication with low levels of anticoccidial drugs, which prevent the infection or reduce infections to a low, immunizing level. Immunity is not as important in broiler chickens, which may be kept only for 6–8 wk before market, as in layers, turkeys, and breeder birds, which may be kept much longer. Vaccines against coccidiosis have met with limited success, and have been used mostly in breeder pullets and in turkeys. Vaccination of broilers has rarely been practiced because even light infections with some species of coccidia can affect weight gain, feed conversion, and pigmentation of the skin.

CLASSIFICATION AND TAXONOMIC RELATIONSHIPS. The biology and taxonomy of coccidia were reviewed by Long (18) and Pellerdy (25). Although several genera of coccidia are known to infect some types of birds, those most often encountered in poultry belong to the genus *Eimeria* described in this section or the genus *Cryptosporidium* discussed in another section. Species of *Eimeria* are frequently described from the morphology of the oocyst, a thick-walled zygote shed in fecal matter by the infected host. Oocysts are enclosed in a thick outer shell and consist of a single cell that begins the process of sporulation to yield the infective stage in about 48 hr. Infective oocysts contain four sporocysts, which in turn contain two sporozoites (Fig. 33.1).

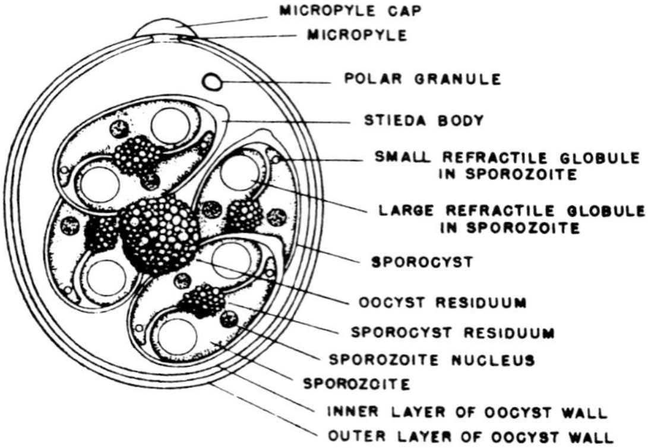

33.1. Diagram of sporulated oocyst of genus *Eimeria*.

When oocysts are ingested, the oocyst wall is crushed in the gizzard, and the sporozoites are released from sporocysts by the action of chymotrypsin and bile salts in the small intestine. Sporozoites enter epithelial cells or are taken into intraepithelial lymphocytes where development may begin. Species of coccidia are identified on the basis of 1) oocyst morphology, 2) host specificity, 3) immune specificity, 4) appearance and location of gross lesions within the natural host, and 5) length of the prepatent period. The host specificity of *Eimeria* in birds and mammals is very strict, so that parasites from different species of birds or animals can be considered different species even though they may have similar-appearing oocysts.

Life Cycle. Coccidiosis differs from bacterial and viral diseases in the self-limiting nature of its development. The life cycle of *E. tenella* (Fig. 33.2) is typical of all *Eimeria,* although some species vary in the number of asexual generations and the time required for each developmental stage. After the oocyst wall is crushed in the gizzard and the sporozoites are released, the sporozoites enter cells in the mucosa of the intestine and begin the cell cycle leading to reproduction. At least two generations of asexual development, called schizogony or merogony, lead to a sexual phase, where small, motile microgametes seek

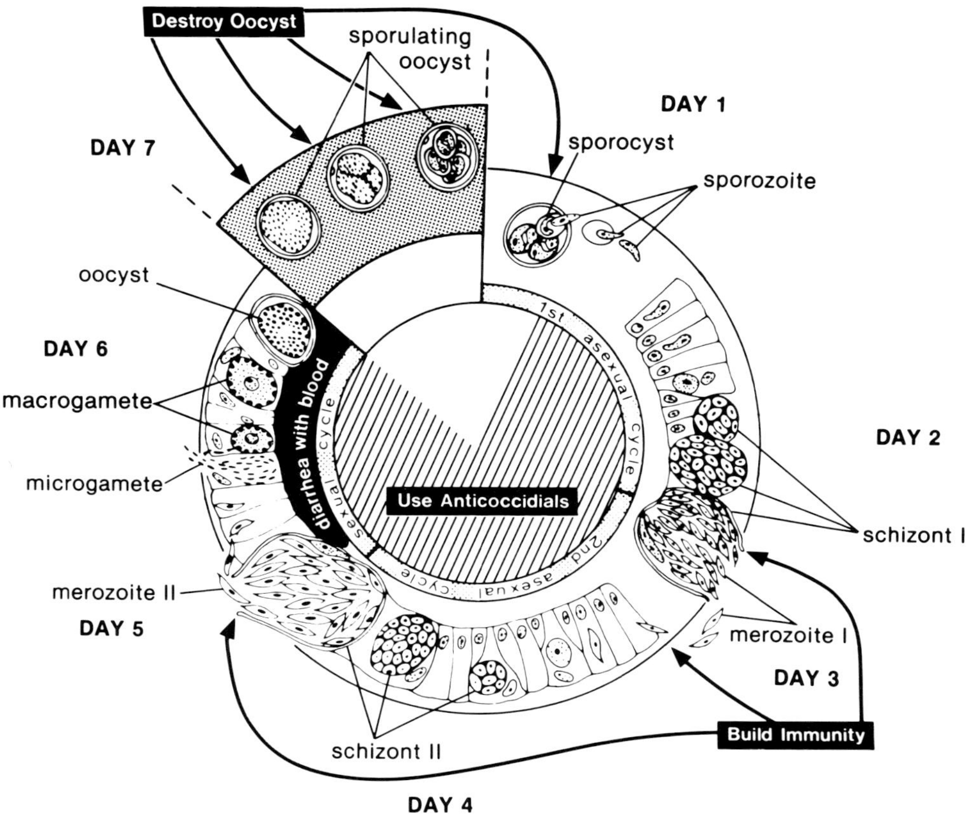

33.2. The 7-day life cycle of *E. tenella* includes two or more asexual and one sexual cycle during the 6 days after an oocyst has been swallowed by the host. The new generation of oocysts must sporulate (day 7) after being passed by the host before becoming infective.

out and unite with macrogametes. The resulting zygote matures into an oocyst, which is released from the intestinal mucosa and is shed in the feces. With each species, the reproductive potential from a single ingested oocyst is fairly constant. The entire process takes 4–6 days, depending on species, although oocysts may be shed for several days after patency is reached. In some species (*E. tenella, E. necatrix*), the maximum tissue damage may occur when second-generation schizonts rupture to release merozoites. Other species may have small schizonts that cause little damage, but the sexual stages may elicit a strong reaction with cellular infiltration and thickened, inflamed tissues.

Relationship between Coccidiosis and Other Poultry Diseases. The tissue damage and changes in intestinal tract function may allow colonization by various harmful bacteria, such as *Clostridium perfringens,* leading to necrotic enteritis (12, 19), or *Salmonella typhimurium* (2, 3).

Immunosuppressive diseases may act in concert with coccidiosis to produce a more severe disease. Marek's disease may interfere with development of immunity to coccidiosis (4), and infectious bursal disease (IBD) may exacerbate coccidiosis, placing a heavier burden on anticoccidial drugs (21).

COCCIDIOSIS IN CHICKENS. Coccidiosis remains one of the most expensive and common diseases of poultry production in spite of advances in chemotherapy, management, nutrition, and genetics. The disease is often diagnosed in birds brought to diagnostic laboratories (1), but the vast majority of cases are diagnosed in the field, and handled by poultry service personnel. The current expense for preventive medication exceeds $90 million in the USA and over $300 million worldwide.

Incidence and Distribution. Coccidia are almost universally found wherever chickens are raised. Their strict host specificity eliminates wild birds as sources of infection. The most common means of spread of coccidia is mechanical, by personnel who move between pens, houses, or farms. Coccidial infections are self-limiting and depend largely on the number of oocysts ingested, and on the immune status of the bird. Surveys in North and South America revealed coccidia present in almost all broiler farms (22, 23). Very high percentages of positive flocks were also reported from Europe (5, 17). Oocysts in the litter or droppings of broiler chickens are usually most numerous at 4–5 wk of age, and generally decline thereafter (Fig. 33.3). Few oocysts are found after birds are removed from a farm, because poultry litter or droppings are poor environments for their survival. The ubiquitous nature of poultry coccidia precludes the possibility of elimination or prevention of coccidia by quarantine, disinfection, and sanitation.

Etiology. Nine species of *Eimeria* have been described from chickens (Table 33.1), but some are questionable. Similarly, several species of *Cryptosporidium* were described, but possibly only one or two names are valid owing to the lack of species specificity. *Cryptosporidium* spp. are often diagnosed, but clinical disease is not often seen (9). Concurrent infection with two or more species of coccidia is common.

Characteristics useful in identification of species are 1) location of the lesions in the intestine; 2) appearance of the gross lesion; 3) oocyst size, shape, and color; 4) size of schizonts and merozoites; 5) location of parasites in tissues (type of cell parasitized); 6) minimum prepatent period in experimental infections; 7) minimum time for sporulation; and 8) immunogenicity against pure strains. In recent years, more emphasis has been placed on biochemical and physiological identification of coccidia. A promising new tool for species identification is electrophoresis of metabolic enzymes (28). For diagnostic purposes, the traditional characteristics are adequate, and a satisfactory diagnosis can usually be made from Table 33.2. Cross-immunity and biochemical studies require pure species isolates propagated from single oocysts. Monoclonal antibodies are useful in serological diagnosis, but have not been suitably specific to distinguish species, probably because of common antigens. The severity of infection is often graded on a scale of 0 to 4+ as described by Johnson and Reid (16), where 0 = normal and 4+ = maximum lesion.

***EIMERIA ACERVULINA* TYZZER 1929.** This species is the most frequently encountered in commercial poultry in North and South America. Oocysts are ovoid and often show thinning of the shell at the small end. The average size of oocysts is 18.3 × 14.6 μm but the range is 17.7–20.2 × 13.7–16.3 μm.

PATHOGENICITY. Severity of infection may vary with the isolate, the number of oocysts ingested, and the immune state of the bird. Ingestion of 1000, 30,000, 100,000, or 1,000,000 oocysts by young White Rock chicks resulted in mild to severe coccidiosis, with lesion scores ranging from 1+ (1000 oocysts) to 4+ (1,000,000 oocysts) (26). Reduction in rate of weight gain was also proportional to the infective dose. Heavy infections often cause lesions to coalesce, and sometimes mortality may result. Light to moderate infections may produce little effect on weight gain and feed conversion, but may cause loss of carotenoid and xanthophyll pigments from the blood and skin because of reduced absorption in the small intestine. The intestinal mucosa may be thickened, resulting in poor feed conversion. Egg production may be reduced in laying birds.

GROSS LESIONS AND HISTOPATHOLOGY. Lesions can often be seen from the serosal surface of the small intestine. The intestinal mucosa may at first be thin and covered with white plaques that tend to arrange in transverse fashion and cause a ladder-like appearance because of the striations. The intestine may be pale and contain watery fluid. The gross lesion in light infections is limited to the duodenal loop, with only a few plaques per centimeter, but in heavy infections lesions may extend some distance through the small intestine and plaques may overlap or coalesce; they are generally smaller in heavy infections due to crowding. The lesions consist of schizonts, gametocytes, and developing oocysts. Microscopy of smears from intestinal lesions usually reveals numerous oocysts.

Histopathology of the small intestine reveals the ovoid gametocytes lining the mucosal cells on the villi. In moderate to heavy infections, the tips of villi are broken off, leading to truncation and fusion of villi and thickening of the mucosa. Some cells may contain more than one parasite. Schiff's reagent will stain the macrogametes and developing oocysts a brilliant red, because of the polysaccharide used in oocyst wall formation.

***EIMERIA BRUNETTI* LEVINE 1942.** About 10–20% of field isolates in recent surveys in the USA and South America contained *E. brunetti* (22). The oocysts of *E. brunetti* average 24.6 × 18.8 μm, and are easily confused with *E. tenella*. This species is found in the lower small intestine, usually from the yolk sac diverticulum to near the cecal juncture. In severe cases the lesion may extend from the gizzard to the cloaca and extend into the ceca (Fig. 33.4 E–H). Most field infections are difficult to recognize based on gross le-

TABLE 33.1 DIFFERENTIAL CHARACTERISTICS FOR 9 SPECIES OF CHICKEN COCCIDIA ◉

DIAGNOSTIC CHARACTERISTICS IN RED

										SPECIES OF DOUBTFUL VALIDITY
	CHARACTERISTICS	E. acervulina	E. brunetti	E. maxima	E. mitis †	E. mivati ‡	E. necatrix	E. praecox	E. tenella	E. hagani
MACROSCOPIC LESIONS	ZONE PARASITIZED	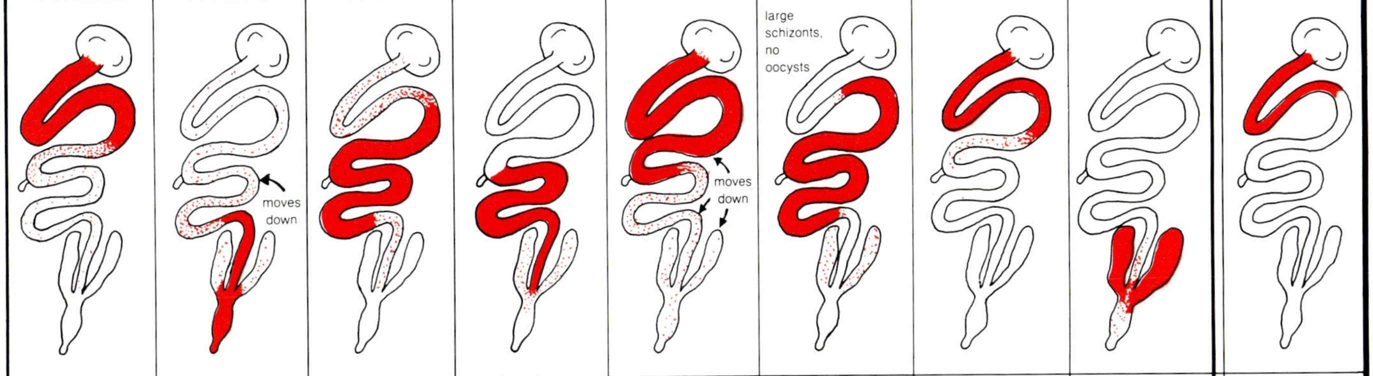	moves down			moves down	large schizonts, no oocysts			
	MACROSCOPIC LESIONS	light infection: whitish round lesions sometimes in ladder-like streaks heavy infection: plaques coalescing, thickened intestinal wall	coagulation necrosis mucoid, bloody enteritis in lower intestine	thickened walls, mucoid, blood - tinged exudate, petechiae	no discrete lesions in intestine, mucoid exudate	light infection: rounded plaques of oocysts heavy infection: thickened walls coalescing plaques	ballooning, white spots (schizonts), petechiae, mucoid blood - filled exudate	no lesions, mucoid exudate	onset: hemorrhage into lumen later: thickening, whitish mucosa, cores clotted blood	pinhead hemorrhages petechiae
MICROSCOPIC CHARACTERISTICS	MILLIMICRONS / OOCYSTS REDRAWN FROM ORIGINALS	10 20 30 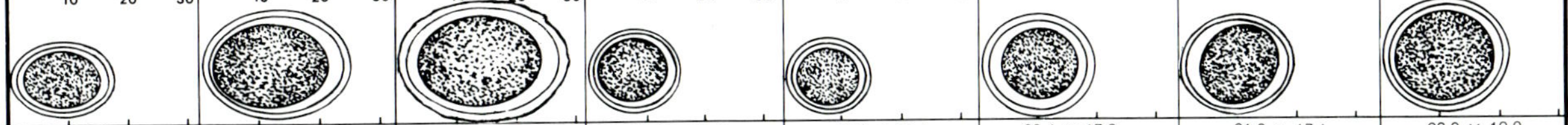	10 20 30	10 20 30	10 20 30	10 20 30	10 20 30	10 20 30	10 20 30	non available
	LENGTH × WIDTH / μ LENGTH = / WIDTH =	AV = 18.3 × 14.6 17.7 - 20.2 13.7 - 16.3	24.6 × 18.8 20.7 - 30.3 18.1 - 24.2	30.5 × 20.7 21.5 - 42.5 16.5 - 29.8	15.6 × 14.2 11.7 - 18.7 11.0 - 18.0	15.6 × 13.4 11.1 - 19.9 10.5 - 16.2	20.4 × 17.2 13.2 - 22.7 11.3 - 18.3	21.3 × 17.1 19.8 - 24.7 15.7 - 19.8	22.0 × 19.0 19.5 - 26.0 16.5 - 22.8	19.1 × 17.6 15.8 - 20.9 14.3 - 19.5
	OOCYST SHAPE AND INDEX-LENGTH/WIDTH	ovoid 1.25	ovoid 1.31	ovoid 1.47	subspherical 1.09	ellipsoid to broadly ovoid 1.16	oblong ovoid 1.19	ovoidal 1.24	ovoid 1.16	broadly ovoid 1.08
	SCHIZONT, MAX IN MICRONS	10.3	30.0	9.4	15.1	17.3	65.9	20	54.0	
	PARASITE LOCATION IN TISSUE SECTIONS	epithelial	2nd generation schizonts subepithelial	gametocytes subepithelial	epithelial	epithelial	2nd generation schizonts subepithelial	epithelial	2nd generation schizonts subepithelial	epithelial
LIFE HISTORY CHARACTERISTICS	MINIMUM PREPATENT PERIOD-HR	97	120	121	93	93	138		115	99
	SPORULATION TIME MINIMUM (HR)	17	18	30	15	12	18	12	18	18

† = From Norton and Joyner (1980)
‡ = As described by Edgar and Siebold (1964)
◉ = Compiled from various sources (1982)

Peter L. Long and W. Malcolm Reid
Department of Poultry Science
The University of Georgia, Athens

Table 33.2. Anticoccidial drugs for treatment of coccidiosis in chickens

Trade or Empirical Name (Manufacturer)	Feed or water	Active Ingredient: Treatment, Duration	First Approval by FDA	Drug Withdrawal (Days before Slaughter)
Sulfamethazine (American Cyanamid)	Water	0.1%: 2 days; 0.05%: 4 days	1947	10
SQ[a], sulfaquinoxaline (Merck); Sulquin[a] (Salsbury)	Feed	0.1%: 2–3 days on, 3 days off followed by 0.05%: 2 days on, 3 days off, 2 days on	1948	10
Amprol[a], amprolium (Merck)	Water	0.012–0.024%: 3–5 days; 0.006%: 1–2 weeks	1960	0
Esb_3[a], sodium sulfachloropyrazine monohydrate (Squibb)	Water	0.03%: 3 days	1967	4
Agribon[a], Albon[a], sulfadimethoxine (Hoffmann-La Roche)	Water	0.05%: 6 days	1968	5

[a]Registered trade name.

sions and can be confirmed only with the aid of microscopy.

PATHOGENICITY. Although less serious than *E. tenella* or *E. necatrix, E. brunetti* is capable of producing moderate mortality, loss of weight gain, poor feed conversion, and other complications. Inoculation with 100–200,000 oocysts will frequently cause 10–30% mortality and reduced weight gain in survivors. Light infections of *E. brunetti* are easily overlooked unless careful attention is paid to the lower small intestine. Such infections can cause reduced weight gain and poor feed conversion even though gross lesions are not clearly apparent.

GROSS LESIONS AND HISTOPATHOLOGY. At early stages of infection, the mucosa of the lower small intestine may be covered with tiny petechiae and have some thickening and loss of color. In heavy infections the mucosa is badly damaged, with coagulation necrosis appearing on days 5–7 postinfection (PI), and with a caseous eroded surface over the entire mucosa. The coagulated blood and mucosa will be apparent in the droppings. Thickening of the mucosa and edematous swelling occurs in severe infections, especially on day 6 PI.

The asexual stages of first- and second-generation schizogony generally occur in the upper small intestine. On day 4 of infection, histopathology reveals schizonts, cellular infiltration, and some damage to the mucosa. By day 5, many of the tips of villi are broken off. Merozoites invade the epithelium and develop into sexual stages in the lower small intestine and ceca. In severe cases the villi may be completely denuded, and in some instances only the basement membranes remain.

***EIMERIA HAGANI* LEVINE 1938.** The taxonomic status of *E. hagani* is in doubt because the original description was incomplete. This species reportedly produced hemorrhagic spots, catarrhal inflammation, and watery intestinal contents and was moderately pathogenic. Unless research is forthcoming to establish the characteristics of this species and existence in field infections, it will likely be declared invalid.

***EIMERIA MAXIMA* TYZZER 1929.** The mid-small intestine is often parasitized with *E. maxima* from below the duodenal loop past the yolk sac diverticulum, but in heavy infections the lesions may extend throughout the small intestine. *E. maxima* is an easy species to recognize because of the characteristic large oocysts, 30.5 × 20.7 μm (21.5–42.5 × 16.5–29.8), which usually have a distinctive yellowish color (Fig. 33.3A, F–J). There is often an abundance of yellow-orange mucus and fluid in the midgut. This species can be differentiated from *E. necatrix* by the lack of large schizonts associated with the lesions, and from *E. brunetti* by the larger oocysts and the appearance of the lesions.

PATHOGENICITY. This species is moderately pathogenic. Infection with 200,000 oocysts is usually sufficient to cause poor weight gain, morbidity, diarrhea, and sometimes mortality. There is often extreme emaciation, pallor, roughening of feathers, and inappetence. Producers interested in maintaining good skin color in chickens must be concerned with subclinical infections because of the effect of this species on absorption of the xanthophyll and carotenoid pigments in the small intestine.

GROSS LESIONS AND HISTOPATHOLOGY. Minimal tissue damage occurs with the first two asexual cycles, which develop superficially in the epithelial cells of the mucosa. When the sexual stages develop in deeper tissues on days 5 and 8 PI, lesions

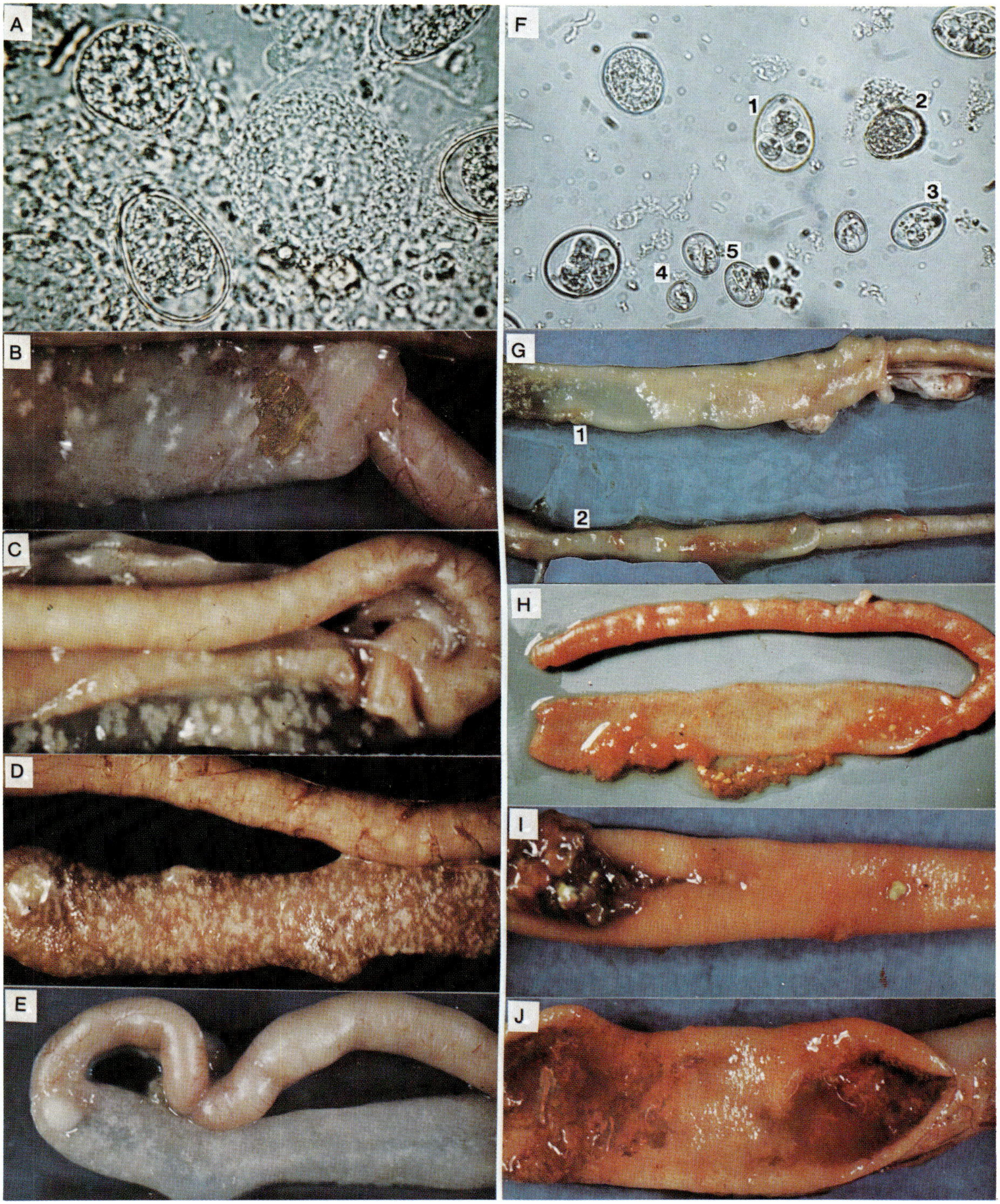

33.3. A. Oocysts and a microgametocyte (*center*) of *E. maxima.* (Long et al., [British] Crown copyright 1976). B. *E. acervulina* (2+). C. *E. acervulina* (2+). D. *E. acervulina* (3+). E. *E. acervulina* (4+). F. *1.* Sporulated *E. maxima* with distinctive brownish walls; *2.* Unsporulated *E. maxima* showing roughened outer wall; *3.* Probably *E. tenella; 4.* End view, probably *E. mitis; 5.* Side view, probably two *E. mitis.* G. *1.* Normal midgut; *2. E. maxima* midgut (1+). H. *E. maxima* midgut (2+ or 3+) (Long et al., [British] Crown copyright 1976). I. *E. maxima* (3+). J. *E. maxima* close-up view (4+).

develop because of congestion and edema, cellular infiltration, and thickening of the mucosa. Infected host cells become enlarged, pushing into the subepithelial zone. Microscopic hemorrhages occur near the tips of the villi, and foci of infection can be seen from the serosal surface. The intestine may be flaccid and filled with fluid, and the lumen often contains yellow or orange mucus and blood. This condition has been described as "ballooning." Microscopic pathology is characterized by edema and cellular infiltration, developing schizonts through day 4 and sexual stages (macrogametes and microgametes) in deeper tissues on days 5–8. In severe infections there is considerable disruption of the mucosa.

Eimeria mitis **Tyzzer 1929.** The lower small intestine is the normal site of this parasite, from the yolk sac diverticulum to the cecal necks. The lesions are normally indistinct with this species, but the potential for pathogenic effects on weight gain and morbidity were recently demonstrated.

PATHOGENICITY. Infection with 1–1.5 million oocysts will reduce weight gain and cause morbidity and loss of pigmentation. The lack of distinct gross lesions causes this species to be overlooked or misdiagnosed in subclinical infections.

GROSS LESIONS AND HISTOPATHOLOGY. Clinically, the gross lesion is very slight and can be easily overlooked. The lower small intestine appears pale and flaccid, and microscopic examination of smears from the mucosal surface may reveal numerous tiny oocysts (15.6 × 14.2 μm). The infection is easily distinguished from *E. brunetti* by the smaller, round oocysts. In light infections the appearance of the gross lesion may be similar with *E. brunetti.* The gross lesion of this species is unremarkable because the developing parasites do not tend to localize in colonies as do other species, and the schizonts and gametocytes are superficial in the mucosa.

Eimeria mivati **Edgar and Siebold 1964.** This parasite was first identified as a small strain of *E. acervulina* (7). The parasitized zone reportedly extends from the duodenal loop to the ceca and cloaca. Early lesions appear in the duodenum, and later in the midgut and lower small intestine. In light infections, isolated lesions resemble those of *E. acervulina* but are more circular in shape. These lesions, representing colonies of gametocytes and developing oocysts, may be seen from the serosal surface of the gut. Infection with 1,000,000 oocysts of *E. mivati* causes reduced weight gain and morbidity. Occasional mortality occurs in experimental infections.

Recent work with isoenzymes has caused some workers to question the validity of *E. mivati.* Examination of laboratory cultures has failed to produce a bona fide culture of *E. mivati,* but there have been no extensive field studies aimed at settling this controversy. While there is no convincing evidence for the existence of this species, not all field observations can be easily explained within the taxonomic limits of other described species. Further work will be needed to settle the taxonomic status of this species.

Eimeria necatrix **Johnson 1930.** Because of the spectacular lesions in the small intestine, this species was one of the best known by early poultry producers. The lesion is found in the small intestine in approximately the same location as *E. maxima* (Fig. 33.4A–D). Probably because of the low reproductive capability of *E. necatrix,* it is not able to compete with other coccidia and is diagnosed mostly in older birds such as brooder pullets or layer pullets 9–14 wk old. The intestine is often dilated to twice its normal size (ballooning) and the lumen may be filled with blood. The oocysts are near in size to those of *E. tenella,* and are found only in the ceca. The sexual stages do not develop in the intestine where the lesions are found, but in the ceca where they compete for space with *E. tenella.* The developing gametocytes are scattered and not found in colonies.

PATHOGENICITY, GROSS LESIONS, HISTOPATHOLOGY. Some gross lesions may be associated with first-generation schizogony at 2–3 days PI. By the 4th day PI, the intestine may be ballooned, the mucosa thickened, and the lumen filled with fluid, blood, and tissue debris. From the serosal surface the foci of infection can be seen as small white plaques or red petechiae. Smears examined microscopically on the 4–5th days may contain numerous clusters of large (66 μm) schizonts, often containing hundreds of merozoites. The clusters of schizonts deep in the mucosa often penetrate the submucosa and damage the layers of smooth muscle and destroy blood vessels. In these instances, the foci are large enough to be seen from the serosal surface. Later, scar tissue may be seen where epithelial regeneration is incomplete. Few pathogenic effects are seen with the invasion of the cecal mucosa by the third-generation parasites and sexual stages because of the scattered, noncolonizing nature of these parasites. The third-generation schizonts produce only 6–16 merozoites, compared with the hundreds of merozoites produced by the second-generation schizonts in the small intestine.

Lesions may extend throughout the small intestine in severe infections, causing dilation (ballooning) and thickening of the mucosa. The lumen may be filled with blood and pieces of mucosal tissue. From the serosal surface, the infection may be seen as white or red foci, or in dead birds the foci will be white and black, giving the appearance of "salt and pepper." Microscopic examination of smears from the mucosal surface reveals numerous clusters of large schizonts that are characteristic for this species and distinguishes it from others that overlap in habitat. Also, oocysts are never associated with lesions of this species.

Infection with 75–100,000 oocysts is sufficient to cause severe weight loss, morbidity, and mortality. Survivors may be emaciated, suffer secondary infections, and lose pigmentation. Droppings of infected birds often contain blood, fluid, and mucus. This species and *E. tenella* are the most pathogenic of the chicken coccidia. Natural infections have caused mortality in excess of 25% in commercial flocks, and in experimental infections 100% mortality is possible.

***EIMERIA PRAECOX* JOHNSON 1930.** This species is named from the short prepatent period (about 83 hr); hence a "precocious" parasite. Even though *E. praecox* is often overlooked because there are no prominent lesions, there may be reduced weight gain, loss of pigmentation, extreme loss of fluids, and poor feed conversion.

PATHOGENICITY, GROSS LESIONS, HISTOPATHOLOGY. The gross lesion consists of watery intestinal contents and sometimes mucus and mucoid casts. Most of the infection is confined to the duodenal loop. Small pinpoint hemorrhages may be seen on the mucosal surface on the 4–5th days of infection. Recent studies suggest that this species may cause morbidity and reduced weight gain (10). Dehydration may result from the extreme fluid loss caused by severe infections. The epithelial cells of the sides of the villi (but not the tips) are most often infected. There may be several parasites in each cell. Three to four asexual generations are followed by the sexual stages. The oocysts are generally larger than those of other species found in the duodenum. At 21.3 × 17.1 μm, they are larger than *E. acervulina, E. mivati,* and *E. mitis,* and smaller than *E. maxima.* Little tissue reaction has been described.

***EIMERIA TENELLA* (RAILLIET AND LUCET 1891) FANTHAM 1909.** Coccidiosis caused by *E. tenella* is the best known of the avian types, partly because of the spectacular disease it causes and partly because of its widespread importance in commercial broilers. This species inhabits the ceca and adjacent intestinal tissues causing a severe disease characterized by bleeding, high morbidity and mortality, lost weight gain, emaciation and other signs attributed to coccidiosis. Diagnosis is dependent upon finding cecal lesions with accompanying clusters of large schizonts or (later) oocysts (Fig. 33.4I-L).

PATHOGENICITY, PATHOGENESIS, EPIZOOTIOLOGY. Experimental inoculation with 100,000 sporulated oocysts can cause morbidity, mortality, and greatly reduced weight gain, making this one of the most pathogenic species in chickens. Inoculation with 1–3000 oocysts is sufficient to cause bloody droppings and other signs of infection. The most pathogenic stage is the second-generation schizont, which matures at 4 days PI. Like *E. necatrix,* this species produces colonies of large schizonts that may contain hundreds of merozoites. The schizonts develop deep in the lamina propria, so that the mucosa is badly disrupted when the schizonts mature and merozoites are released. Onset of mortality in a flock is rapid. Most of the mortality occurs between 5 and 6 days PI, and in acute infections it may follow the first signs of infection by only a few hours. Blood loss may reduce the erythrocyte count and hematocrit value as much as 50%. The maximum effect on weight gain is seen at 7 days PI. Some of the weight lost from dehydration may be regained quickly, but growth will always lag behind that of uninfected birds. The exact cause of death is not known, but toxic factors are suspected. Blood loss alone does not account for mortality. In a few cases death may result from gangrenous or ruptured cecal pouches. Extracts of infected cecal pouches produce acute blood coagulation and death when injected intravenously into other chicks. The possible role of bacterial products in mortality from coccidiosis is suggested by the lack of mortality from *E. tenella* in germ-free chicks.

GROSS LESIONS AND HISTOPATHOLOGY. Even during maturation of the first-generation schizonts, small foci of denuded epithelium may be seen. By the 4th day PI the second-generation schizonts are maturing and hemorrhages are apparent. The cecal pouch may become greatly enlarged and distended with clotted blood and pieces of cecal mucosa in the lumen. On the 6th and 7th days the cecal core becomes hardened and drier; eventually it is passed in the feces. Regeneration of the epithelium is rapid, and may be complete by the 10th day. The infection can usually be seen from the serosal surface of the ceca as dark petechiae and foci that become coalesced in more severe infections. The cecal wall is often greatly thickened because of edema and infiltration, and later scar tissue.

Microscopically, the first-generation schizonts are widely scattered and mature at 2–3 days PI. Small focal areas of hemorrhage and necrosis may appear near blood vessels of the inner circular muscles of the muscularis layer. Heterophil infiltration of the submucosa proceeds rapidly as the large second-generation schizonts develop in the lamina propria. These are found in clusters or

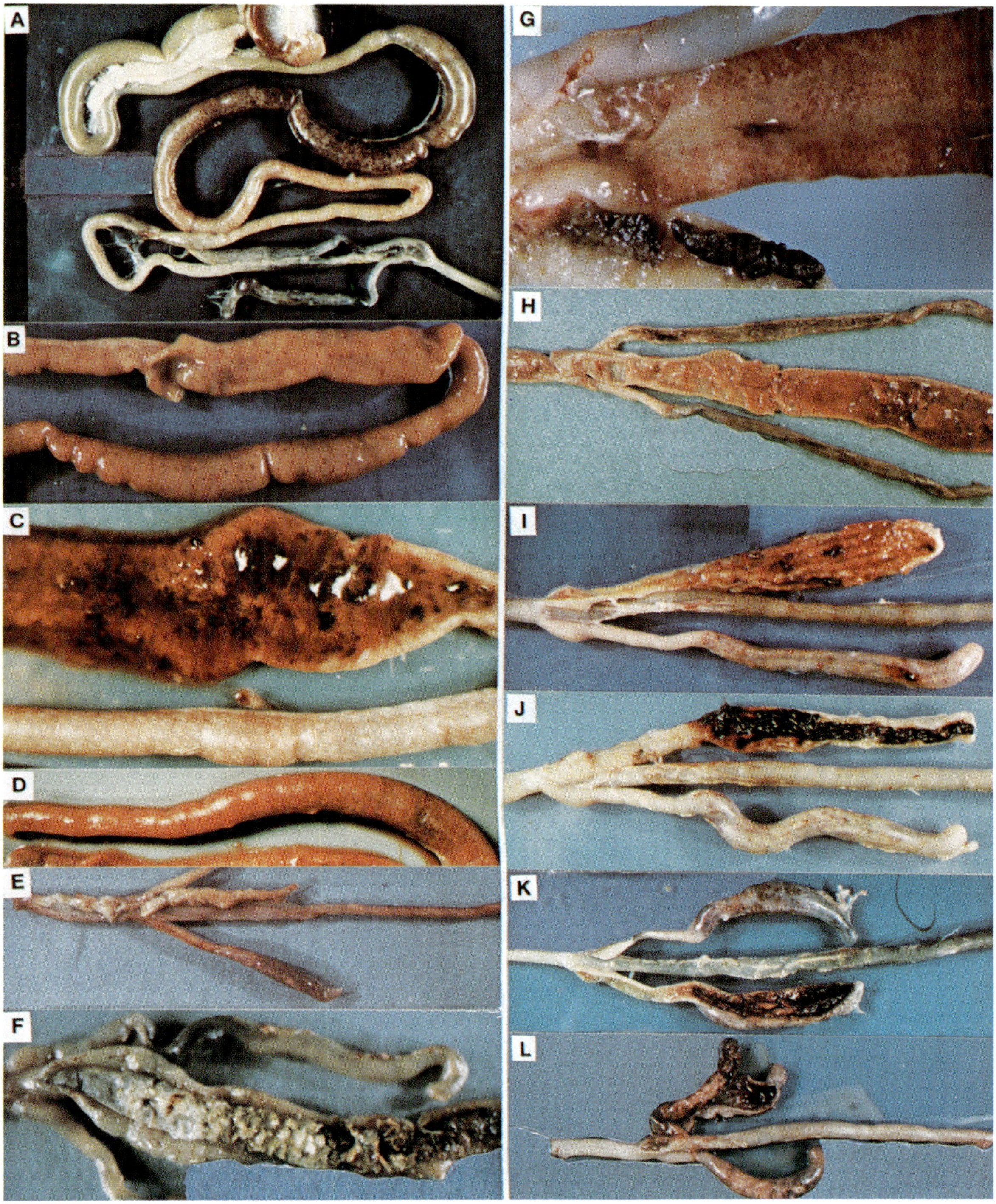

33.4. A. *E. necatrix* showing ballooning in midgut. B. *E. necatrix* (2+). C. *E. necatrix* (3+). D. *E. necatrix* (4+). (Long et al., [British] Crown copyright 1976). E. *E. brunetti* from bacteria-free chick. F. *E. brunetti* (4+). G. *E. brunetti* (3+). H. *E. brunetti* (4+). (Long et al. [British] Crown copyright 1976). I. *E. tenella* (2+). J. *E. tenella* (3+). K. *E. tenella* (4+). L. *E. tenella* (4+) with cecal core.

colonies that generally are progeny of a single first-generation schizont. Maturation of the second-generation parasites is accompanied by excessive tissue damage, bleeding, disruption of the cecal glands, and often complete destruction of the mucosa and muscularis layer. Oocysts are seen on microscopic examination on the 6th and 7th days, when macrogametes and motile microgametes can often be seen. Regeneration of the epithelium and glands may be complete by the 10th day in light infections, but the epithelium may never completely recover in severe infections. Lost muscularis mucosa is not replaced and the submucosa becomes densely fibrosed.

Epizootiology

NATURAL AND EXPERIMENTAL HOSTS. The chicken is the only natural host of the species described above, and reports of these species infecting other birds can be considered spurious. Cross-transmission of *Eimeria* spp. from chickens to other host species has been unsuccessful except for a few instances where immunocompromised birds were used.

Chickens of all ages and breeds are susceptible to infection, but immunity develops quickly, thus limiting further infection. Newly hatched birds are sometimes not fully susceptible to infection because of insufficient chymotrypsin and bile salts in the intestines to cause excystation. Outbreaks are common at 3–6 wk of age, and are rarely seen in poultry flocks at less than 3 wk. Surveys of coccidia in broiler houses in Georgia demonstrated the manner in which oocysts of coccidia build up during growth of a flock, then decline as the birds become immune to further infection (27). This "self-limiting" nature of coccidial infections is widely known in chickens and other poultry. There is no stimulation of cross-immunity between species of coccidia. Thus, several outbreaks of coccidiosis are possible in the same flock, with different species involved in each. Breeder and layer pullets are at greatest risk because they are kept on litter for 20 wk or more. Normally, the infections with *E. acervulina, E. tenella,* and *E. maxima* are seen at 3–6 wk of age, then *E. necatrix* at 8–18 wk of age.

Coccidiosis rarely occurs in layers and breeders because of prior exposure to coccidia and resulting immunity. In a few instances a flock may not be exposed to a particular species, or the immunity may lapse because of other diseases. Outbreaks of any species in layers can reduce or eliminate egg production for several weeks.

TRANSMISSION AND VECTORS. Ingestion of viable sporulated oocysts is the only natural method of transmission. Infected chickens may shed oocysts in the feces for several days or weeks. The oocysts in feces become infective through the process of sporulation within 2 days. Susceptible birds in the same flock may ingest the oocysts through the litter-pecking activities common to chickens.

Although there are no natural intermediate hosts for the *Eimeria* spp., oocysts can be spread mechanically by many different animals, insects, contaminated equipment, wild birds, and dust. Oocysts are generally considered resistant to environmental extremes and to disinfectants, although survival time varies with conditions. Oocysts may survive for many weeks in soil, but survival in poultry litter is limited to a few days because of the ammonia released by composting and the action of molds and bacteria. Viable oocysts have been reported from the dust inside and outside broiler houses, as well as from insects in poultry litter (27). The darkling beetle, common in broiler litter, is a mechanical carrier of oocysts. Transmission from one farm to another is facilitated by movement of personnel and equipment between farms, and by the migration of wild birds, which may mechanically spread the oocysts. New farms may remain free of coccidia for most of the first grow-out of chickens until the introduction of coccidia to a completely susceptible flock. Such outbreaks, which are usually more severe than those experienced on older farms, are often called "the new-house coccidiosis syndrome."

Oocysts may survive for many weeks under optimal conditions, but will be quickly killed by exposure to high or low temperatures or drying. Exposure to 55 C or freezing kills oocysts very quickly. Even 37 C is fatal when continued for 2–3 days. Sporozoites and sporocysts can be frozen in liquid nitrogen with appropriate cryopreservation technique, but oocysts cannot be adequately infiltrated with cryoprotectants to effect survival. Threat of coccidiosis is less during hot dry weather and greater in cooler wetter weather.

HISTOPATHOLOGY. Ordinary methods in histopathology are satisfactory for routine examination of tissues infected with coccidia. Staining of sections with H & E or other common histological stains will demonstrate developing stages. There are specialized techniques which will identify specific stages: Staining with Schiff's reagent gives a brilliant red color with the polysaccharide associated with the refractile body and with wall-forming bodies in the macrogamete. Monoclonal antibodies conjugated with fluorescent markers such as fluorescein are highly useful in research because specific stages of parts of cells can be readily identified.

Diagnosis. Coccidiosis can best be diagnosed from birds killed for immediate necropsy. Attempts to identify characteristic lesions in birds that have been dead for 1 hr or longer are frustrated by the postmortem changes that begin quickly in the intestine. The entire intestinal tract should be examined. A microscope should be available for identifying special diagnostic characteristics such as the large schizonts of *E. necatrix* or the small round oocysts of *E. mitis*. The finding of a few oocysts by microscopic examination of smears from the intestine indicates the presence of infection, but not a diagnosis of clinical coccidiosis. Coccidia are often present in the intestines of birds 3–6 wk old in most flocks. Coccidiosis should be diagnosed if the gross lesions are serious, or if other economic parameters are threatened. Diagnosis should be based on finding of lesions and confirmatory microscopic stages on necropsy of typical birds from the flock, rather than from culls.

Microscopic Examination. Many stages of coccidia can be seen in smears taken from the suspected lesion. A small amount of mucosal scraping should be diluted with saline on a slide, then covered with a coverslip. Oocysts or macrogametes are most easily seen, but in many cases the lesion is caused by maturing schizonts. Presence of clusters of large schizonts in the midgut area is pathognomonic for *E. necatrix,* while a similar finding in the ceca indicates *E. tenella.*

Oocyst size and shape are less useful as diagnostic characteristics in chickens than once thought, because of the extensive overlapping in size of the species. Measurement of 30–50 oocysts of the predominant type of oocyst usually gives a good indication of the size of the unknown species. This information is useful in conjunction with other observations in the identification of species in field cases.

Lesion Scoring. The severity of lesions is generally proportionate to the number of oocysts ingested by the bird, and correlates with other parameters such as weight loss and droppings scores. The most commonly used system was devised by Johnson and Reid (16). By this system a score of 0 to 4+ is assigned to a bird where 0 = normal and 4+ = most severe case. This technique is most useful in experimental infections, where the dose of oocysts and medicaments are controlled, and the species are known. In the field, lesion scoring is generally useful in gauging the severity of infections. Even though there are several species of coccidia that may be present at some time, only four separate sections of the intestine are usually scored. These are 1) the duodenum (upper), 2) the midgut from the duodenum past the yolk sac diverticulum, 3) the lower small intestine from the yolk sac diverticulum to the cecal junctures, and 4) the ceca.

Droppings Score. In laboratory infections the droppings score may be used in the same manner as lesion score for a rapid and fairly reliable rating of the infection (24). The extent of abnormal droppings is rated on a scale of 0 to 4+, where 4+ = maximum diarrhea, with mucus, fluid, and/or blood.

Procedures Used in Species Identification. One of the oldest techniques takes advantage of the lack of cross-immunity when birds are infected with one species of coccidia. If pure cultures of coccidia are used to repeatedly infect groups of birds, they will become immune to that species. If a test culture produces patent infections in immunized birds, it must be of a different species. In this way, by process of elimination, the species can be determined. This technique is time consuming, and requires extensive laboratory isolation facilities and access to pure cultures of known species of coccidia. However, it has proved extremely useful as a research tool. Pure species cultures of coccidia are difficult to maintain because they must be propagated in strict isolation to prevent contamination.

Preservation of Coccidia for Experimental Work. Droppings or litter collected in the field or intestinal contents in the diagnostic lab can be saved for isolation of coccidia in a solution of 2–4% potassium dichromate. Aeration of oocyst suspensions is necessary to allow sporulation. A good-quality aquarium pump is highly effective and can be regulated with valves and tubes to service several bottles at one time. For short-term storage, suspensions of oocysts may be refrigerated.

Prevention and Control

CONTROL OF COCCIDIOSIS BY CHEMOTHERAPY. Early emphasis in chemotherapy was centered on the treatment of outbreaks with sulfonamides or other compounds after signs of infection were apparent. Soon the concept of preventive medication emerged with the realization that most of the damage is done once signs of coccidiosis are widespread in a flock. Today, almost all broiler flocks receive preventive medication, and treatment is used as a last resort (Table 33.3). The historical aspects of chemotherapy were reviewed extensively by McDougald (20).

CHARACTERISTICS OF ANTICOCCIDIAL DRUGS. All types of drugs used for coccidiosis control are unique in the mode of action, the way in which parasites are killed or arrested, and the effects of the drug on the growth and performance of the bird.

Spectrum of Activity. There are several important species of coccidia in chickens, several more in turkeys, and many others in other hosts. A

Table 33.3. Preventive anticoccidials approved by FDA for use in feed formulation

Trade or Empirical Name, Approved Level (Manufacturer)	Trade Name	First Approval by FDA	Drug Withdrawal (Days before Slaughter)
Sulfaquinoxaline, 0.015–0.025% (Merck)	SQ, Sulquin	1948	10
Nitrofurazone, 0.0055% (Hess & Clark; Smith-Kline)	nfz, Amifur	1948	5
Arsanilic acid or sodium arsanilate, 0.04% for 8 days (Abbott)	Pro-Gen	1949	5
Butynorate, 0.0375 for turkeys (Salsbury)	Tinostat	1954	28
Nicarbazin, 0.0125% (Merck)	Nicarb	1955	4
Furazolidone, 0.0055–0.011% (Hess & Clark)	nf-180	1957	5
Nitromide, 0.025% + sulfanitran, 0.03% + roxarasone, 0.005% (Salsbury)	Unistat-3	1958	5
Oxytetracycline, 0.022% (Pfizer)	Terramycin	1959	3
Amprolium, 0.0125–0.025% (MSD-AGVET)	Amprol	1960	0
Chlortetracycline, 0.022% (American Cyanamid)	Aureomycin	1960	(See feeding restrictions)
Zoalene, 0.004–0.0125% (Salsbury)	Zoamix	1960	(Higher levels, 5 days)
Amprolium, 0.0125% + ethopabate, 0.0004/0.004% (Merck)	Amprol Plus Amprol Hi-E	1963	0
Buquinolate, 0.00825% (Norwich-Eaton)	Bonaid	1967	0
Clopidol or meticlorpindol, 0.0125–0.025% (A. L. Laboratories)	Coyden	1968	0 days at 0.0125%; 5 days at 0.025%
Decoquinate 0.003% (Rhone-Poulenc)	Deccox	1970	0
Sulfadimethoxine, 0.0125% + ormetoprin, 0.0075% (Hoffmann-La Roche)	Rofenaid	1970	5
Monensin, 0.01–0.0121% (Elanco)	Coban	1971	0
Robenidine, 0.0033% (American Cyanamid)	Robenz, Cycostat	1972	5
Lasalocid, 0.0075–0.125% (Hoffmann-La Roche)	Avatec	1976	3
Salinomycin, 0.004–0.0066% (Agri-Bio)	Bio-Cox	1983	0
Halofuginone, 3 ppm (Hoechst-Roussell Agri-Vet)	Stenorol	1987	5
Narasin, 54–72 g/T (Elanco)	Monteban	1988	0
Madurimicin, 5–6 ppm (American Cyanamid)	Cygro	1989	5
Narasin + nicarbazin, 54–90 g/T (Elanco)	Maxiban	1989	5

Source: (8).

drug may be efficacious against one or several of these parasites; very few drugs are equally efficacious against all.

Mode of Action. Each class of chemical compound is unique in the type of action exerted on the parasite, and even in the developmental stage of the parasite most affected. The chemical mode of action of some drugs is known to be highly detailed, while the action of other drugs remains a mystery. The sulfonamides and related drugs compete for the incorporation of PABA and metabolism of folic acid. Amprolium competes for absorption of thiamine by the parasite. The quinoline coccidiostats and clopidol inhibit energy metabolism in the cytochrome system of the coccidia. The polyether ionophores upset the osmotic balance of the protozoan cell by altering the permeability of cell membranes for alkaline metal cations.

The coccidia are prone to attack by drugs at various stages of development in the host. Totally unrelated drugs may attack the same stage of parasite. The quinolones and ionophores arrest or kill the sporozoite or early trophozoite. Nicarbazin, robenidine and zoalene destroy the first- or second-generation schizont, and the sulfonamides act on the developing schizonts and also on the sexual stages. Diclazuril acts in early schizogony with *E. tenella,* but is delayed to later schizogony with *E. acervulina* and to the maturing macrogamete with *E. maxima.* The time of action in the life cycle has been construed as having significance in the use of drugs in certain types of programs where immunity is desired, but there is no good evidence that this is true under practical conditions.

Coccidiocidal vs. Coccidiostatic. Some drugs kill the parasite but others only arrest development. When coccidiostatic medication is withdrawn, arrested parasites may continue to develop and contaminate the environment with oocysts. In such cases a relapse of coccidiosis is possible. In general, the coccidiocidal drugs have been more successful than those that are coccidiostatic.

Effects of Drugs on the Chicken. Most compounds used in animal feeds have good "selective toxicity," providing toxicity for the parasite but being nontoxic to vertebrates. Unfortunately, toxicity and side effects of drugs on the host are possible where formulation errors lead to overdose. Sometimes a drug may exhibit side effects at the recommended use level. Some of the toxicity may be the result of management, genetics, nutrition, or other interaction, and in other cases the margin of safety is just too narrow. Environmental interaction is possible with nicarbazin, which interacts with high temperatures to produce excess mortality. Also nicarbazin is highly toxic to layers, first causing a bleaching of brown-shelled eggs, mottling of yolks, reduced hatchability, and reduced production. The ionophores are highly toxic at elevated doses, causing a transient paralysis in mild overdoses, or a permanent paralysis and mortality in more severe cases. Monensin was once thought to interact with methionine to reduce feather growth, but this relationship is not clear. Under some conditions lasalocid will stimulate water consumption and excretion, resulting in wet litter. With slight overdoses, most of the ionophores depress weight gain under laboratory conditions. A withdrawal period of 5–7 days is often practiced to allow "compensatory growth" to make up for the lost gain. The ionophores are known for their toxicity to other animals. Thus, monensin and salinomycin are highly toxic to horses. The LD_{50} for monensin in horses is about 2 mg/kg body weight. Salinomycin is highly toxic to turkeys at levels above 15 g/ton and causes excessive mortality at the level recommended for use in chickens (60 g/ton), while monensin and lasalocid are well tolerated in turkeys at the level used for chickens.

PROGRAMS FOR USE OF ANTICOCCIDIAL DRUGS IN BROILERS. In broilers the objective is usually to produce the maximum growth and feed efficiency with minimum disease, while in layers or breeders the objective may be immunization. (Fig. 33.5).

Continuous Use of a Single Drug. Often a single product will be used from day 1 to slaughter, or with a withdrawal period of 3–7 days. Most products are approved for use until slaughter, but producers withdraw medication for economic or other reasons.

Shuttle or Dual Programs. The use of one product in the starter and another in the grower feed is called a "shuttle" program in the USA and a "dual" program in other countries. The shuttle program is usually intended to improve coccidiosis control. Intensive use of the polyether ionophore drugs for many years produced strains of coccidia in the field that have "reduced sensitivity" to the ionophores. It is a common practice to use another drug such as nicarbazin or halofuginone in either the starter or grower feed to bolster the anticoccidial control and take some pressure off the ionophore. The use of shuttle programs is thought to reduce build-up of drug resistance. In 1988 approximately 80% of the producers used some type of shuttle program.

Rotation of Products. It is considered sound management to make changes in anticoccidial drug use. Most producers consider changes in the spring and in the fall. Rotation of drugs may improve productivity because of the build-up of isolates or species of coccidia that have reduced sensitivity after products have been used for a long time. Producers often notice a boost in productivity for a few months after a change of anticoccidial drugs.

DRUG RESISTANCE. The development of tolerance of drugs by coccidia after exposure to medication is the most serious limitation to the effectiveness of products. Surveys reveal widespread drug resistance in coccidia in the USA, South America, and Europe (11, 14, 15, 17, 20, 23). Even though coccidia develop less resistance to some drugs than to others, long-term exposure to any drug will produce a loss in sensitivity and eventually resistance.

Drug resistance is a genetic phenomenon, and once established in a line of coccidia, it will remain for many years or until selection pressure and genetic drift forces return to sensitivity in the population. Drugs such as the quinolones and clopidol have a well-defined mode of action and resistance develops quickly as coccidia are selected with cytochromes, which do not bind as readily to the drug. The polyether ionophores, in contrast, have a more complicated mode of action involving the mechanisms of active transport of alkaline metal cations across cell membranes, and it has

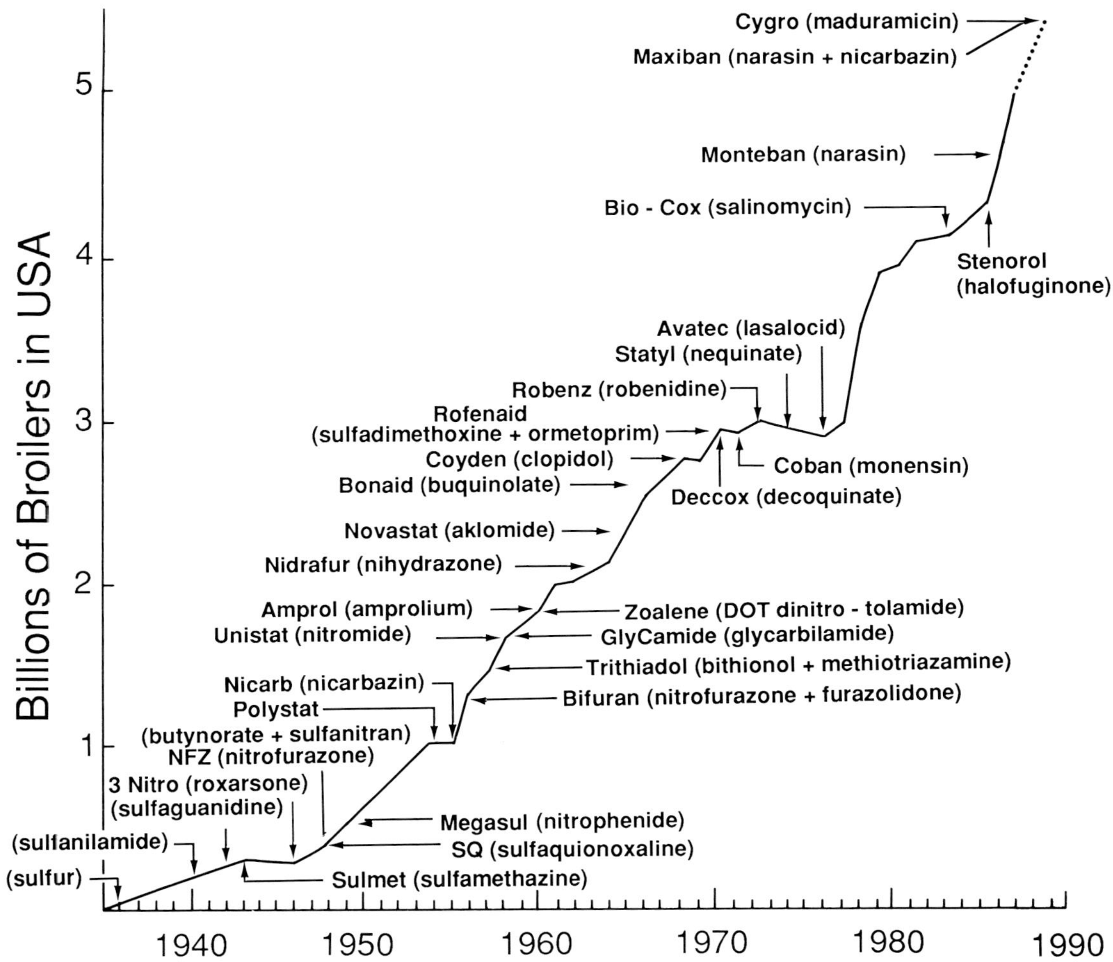

33.5. Broiler production (USDA figures) and year of introduction of new anticoccidial drugs. Generic names begin with lower case letters while trade names begin with a capital letter. (Avian Dis)

taken many years for coccidia to become tolerant, and in some cases completely resistant. Many other drugs appear to be intermediate in selecting resistance in coccidia.

The primary defense against drug resistance is the use of less intensive programs, shuttle programs, and frequent rotation of drugs. Rotation of programs, used alone, will not prevent the development of resistance because the periods of use of drugs between changes is often adequate for resistance development.

DRUGS USED FOR BROILERS IN THE USA. The products currently approved for use in chickens in the USA are listed in Table 33.3. Not all are still available commercially, but the approvals remain. Those used at present include monensin, salinomycin, lasalocid (polyether ionophores), nicarbazin, amprolium + ethopabate, decoquinate, clopidol, sulfadimethoxine + ormetoprim, and sulfaquinoxaline. Other products listed with approvals but lacking in significant activity include chlortetracycline, oxytetracycline, and nitrofurans. These products may prevent mortality from coccidiosis when given at high levels because of antibacterial activity but are not of much value in general use. The polyether ionophores became the drugs of choice for prevention of coccidiosis in 1972, and remain the most extensively used today. Other drugs, such as nicarbazin and halofuginone, are used mostly in shuttle programs as an adjunct to the ionophores.

New drugs pending approval in the USA that are used in Europe, South America, or Asia include diclazuril and toltazuril (synthetic triazines).

DRUGS AND PROGRAMS USED IN BREEDERS AND LAYERS. Pullets started on the floor and later reared as caged layers do not need immunity to coccidiosis. They are often protected with preventive medication as with broilers until they are moved to cages. Breeder pullets that will be kept on the floor during lay should have an immunity to coccidiosis. Natural immunity after mild infection is usually achieved by one of two approaches. Controlled exposure can be given by means of a commercial product (Coccivac). The program calls for a light, harmless initial exposure that must be reinforced by two to three repeated natural life cycles. Careful supervision of management is required to provide adequate immunity. The second approach relies upon a natural exposure assuming the presence of oocysts of important species. A broad-spectrum anticoccidial drug is fed to provide protection for 6–12 wk. Some producers reduce the level of the drug during the final 4 wk in a "step-down" program. Occasionally oocyst numbers may be insufficient to provide adequate exposure to all species. Outbreaks of *E. necatrix* have sometimes occurred at 8–16 wk after all medication has been stopped. Climatic and seasonal conditions may add to the inherent uncertainties of this method. Neither program is fool-proof, and damaging outbreaks may occur.

NEW VACCINES TO PREVENT COCCIDIOSIS. The considerable research on coccidiosis vaccines in recent years has produced interesting results and may eventually lead to a commercial product. Along conventional lines, Coccivac-style vaccines have been prepared from live but attenuated lines of oocysts. The success of these vaccines may depend more on a novel approach to administration rather than attenuation. One product is encapsulated in alginate beads, then mixed into the starter feed for "trickle administration." Another is given by spraying the oocysts directly into feed or water in the poultry house.

Monoclonal antibody technology has led to identification of coccidial proteins that protect against infection when inoculated into young chicks. These proteins can be made in quantity if the gene that encodes the protein is cloned into a bacterial cell. Research is in progress to identify broad-spectrum antigens and appropriate routes of administration.

DISINFECTION AND SANITATION. Older recommendations for coccidiosis control often suggest directions for sanitation and disinfection to prevent outbreaks. Most of these are no longer considered valid since 1) there have been too many failures in such programs, 2) oocysts are extremely resistant to common disinfectants, 3) complete house sterilization is never complete, and 4) an oocyst-sterile environment for floor-maintained birds could prevent early establishment of immunity.

If birds are kept in self-cleaning cages, immunity is not essential, and outbreaks of coccidiosis occur only rarely, usually in single rows of cages in which there has been accidental fecal contamination of feed or water.

COCCIDIOSIS IN TURKEYS.

Coccidiosis in turkeys is common but often unrecognized because the lesions are less spectacular than those in chickens. Several species infect turkeys, but only about four are economically important. Typical signs of coccidiosis in turkeys are watery or mucoid diarrhea, ruffled feathers, anorexia, and general signs of illness. Recovery is quick, so that lesions could go undetected at necropsy. Several species have been found in commercial turkey farms throughout the USA (6). Coccidia infecting domestic turkeys also infect wild turkeys. Range-rearing can add significantly to the exposure of wildlife to coccidiosis and other diseases.

Turkeys of all ages are susceptible to primary infection, but birds older than 6–8 wk are considered more resistant to the disease; they can suffer weight loss and morbidity, but are not killed as easily as are younger birds. Reductions in rate of weight gain are often unrecognized until adequate coccidiosis control measures have been instituted.

Etiology.

Seven species of *Eimeria* have been described turkeys in the USA. Identifying characteristics of each species are listed in Table 33.4. *E. innocua* and *E. subrotunda* have been so rarely recovered that the validity of these species should be listed as doubtful.

Species described from the turkey include *Isospora* spp. and *Cryptosporidium* spp. (see next section) as well as *Eimeria* spp. The strictly intestinal *Eimeria* spp. contrast with *Cryptosporidium* spp., which may cause both respiratory and intestinal infection (13). The pathogenic species of *Eimeria* are *E. adenoeides, E. meleagrimitis, E. gallopavonis,* and *E. dispersa.* Differentiation of oocysts of the pathogenic species from those of milder species is difficult, because some of the species are poorly described.

EIMERIA ADENOEIDES MOORE AND BROWN 1951. Gross lesions appear primarily in the ceca but extend to the lower small intestine and cloaca. Cecal contents are often hardened into a core consisting of mucosal debris. The cecal and/or intestinal wall is often swollen and edematous. Oocysts are ellipsoidal and have a high shape index (length/width = 1.54). The oocysts average 25.6 × 16.6 μm.

Table 33.4. Diagnostic characteristics of *Eimeria* in turkeys

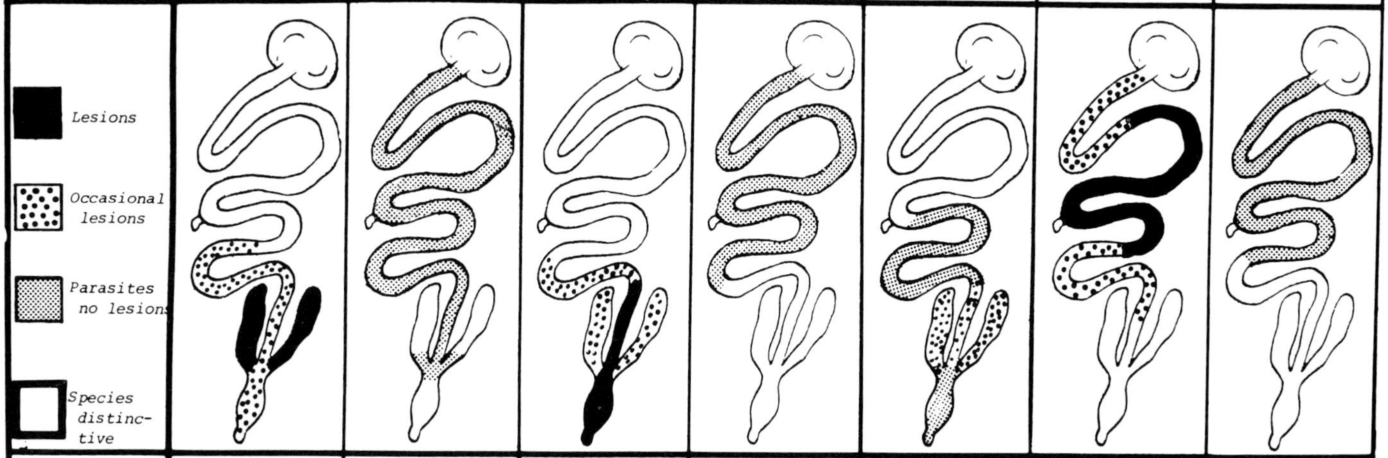

SPECIES → CHARACTERISTICS ↓	*E. adenoeides*	*E. dispersa*	*E. gallopavonis*	*E. innocua*	*E. meleagridis*	*E. meleagrimitis*	*E. subrotunda*
Macroscopic lesions	liquid feces with mucus and flecks of blood, **loose whitish cecal cores**	cream-colored serosal surface, dilation of intestine, yellowish mucoid feces	edema, ulceration of mucosal ileum, yellow exudate, flecks of blood in feces	none	cream-colored ceca, formation of caseous plug, a few petechial hemorrhages	spotty congestion and petechiae from duodenum to ileum, dilation of jejunum, casts	none
Length × Width (in μm)	Av = 25.6 × 16.6	Av = 26.1 × 21.0	Av = 27.1 × 17.2	Av = 22.4 × 20.9	Av = 24.4 × 18.1	**Av = 19.2 × 16.3**	Av = 21.8 × 19.8
Length =	18.9 - 31.3	21.8 - 31.1	22.7 - 32.7	18.57 - 25.86	20.3 - 30.8	**15.8 - 26.9**	16.48 - 26.42
Width =	12.6 - 20.9	17.7 - 23.9	15.2 - 19.4	17.34 - 24.54	15.4 - 20.6	**13.1 - 21.9**	14.21 - 24.44
Oocyst shape and index length/width	ellipsoidal **1.54**	broadly oval **1.24**	ellipsoidal **1.52**	subspherical **1.07**	ellipsoidal **1.34**	ovoid **1.17**	subspherical **1.10**
Minimum sporulation	24 hr	35 hr	**15 hr**	**under 45 hr**	24 hr	**18 hr**	**48 hr**
Prepatent period (minimum)	103 hr	**120 hr**	**105 hr**	**114 hr**	110 hr	103 hr	**95 hr**
Refractile body	yes	no	yes	no	yes	yes	no
Pathogenicity	**+ + + +**	+	**+ + + +**	none	**none**	**+ + + +**	none

NOTE: *Characteristics compiled from original descriptions.*

PATHOGENICITY. *E. adenoeides* is one of the most pathogenic of the turkey coccidia. Experimental infections of 25,000–100,000 oocysts in young poults may produce mortality up to 100% on the 5th or 6th day PI. Turkeys several months old may lose considerable weight after infection. Outward signs of infection are apparent after 4 days PI. Feces are frequently fluid, may be blood-tinged, and may contain mucous casts. White or grey caseous cores may be produced in the ceca. The lesions heal quickly, so that no evidence of infection may be seen soon after the acute phase unless the cecal core remains.

GROSS LESIONS AND HISTOPATHOLOGY. By the 4th day PI the intestine may suffer congestion, edema, petechial hemorrhage, and mucus secretion. Five days PI the ceca contain white caseous material that condenses into a core. The serosal surface of the intestine appears pale and may be edematous and dilated.

Invasion of the submucosa by heterophils occurs throughout the intestine, especially in the lower small intestine and ceca. Epithelial cells at the tips of villi are most often invaded, but deep glands may also be parasitized. Edema is common deep in the muscular layers as the infection progresses. After 5 days regeneration of lost mucosa is rapid.

***EIMERIA DISPERSA* TYZZER 1929.** The small intestine, principally the midgut region, is commonly parasitized, but some infection may occur in the cecal necks. Oocysts are large (averaging 26.1 × 21.0 μm) and broadly ovoid (index = 1.24). Sporozoites lack a refractile body, and the oocyst wall is distinctively contoured and lacks the double wall common to other species. The prepatent period is 120 hr, longer than for other species.

PATHOGENICITY. Compared to some of the other species the pathogenicity is low, but infection with 1–2,000,000 oocysts can cause reduction in rate of weight gain and diarrhea in young poults.

NATURAL AND EXPERIMENTAL HOSTS. The natural host of this species is apparently the bob-white quail, in which the parasite is more pathogenic than in turkeys. This is the only *Eimeria* in chickens or turkeys known to infect more than one species. Experimental inoculation has produced patent infections in domestic and wild turkeys, Hungarian partridge (*Perdix perdix*), ruffed grouse (*Bonasa umbellus*), sharp-tailed grouse (*Pediocetes phasianellus campestris*), Japanese and bob-white quail, and other pheasants. Infection of chickens often requires immunosuppression.

GROSS LESIONS AND HSITOPATHOLOGY. Three days PI the duodenum appears cream colored on the serosal surface. Later the entire intestine may become dilated with thickening of the wall. Dilation continues on the 5th and 6th day along with secretion of a cream-colored mucoid material containing denuded epithelium from the duodenum. Individual villi may become so dilated as to be visible to the naked eye.

The duodenum shows edema and progressively increasing congestion of capillaries. Separation of the epithelium and basement membranes may result in the lamina propria being exposed to a fibrin network or an open fluid-filled space. Necrosis is common on distal tips of villi. Parasites do not invade the glands.

***EIMERIA GALLOPAVONIS* HAWKINS 1952.** Lesions are restricted to the area posterior to the yolk sac diverticulum and tend to be most severe in the lower small intestine and large intestine. Some foci of infection may be seen in the ceca. Oocysts are elongate, averaging 17.1 × 17.2 μm (index = 1.52).

PATHOGENICITY. Experimental infection with 50–100,000 oocysts causes mortality of 10–100% in 2- to 6-wk-old poults. Mortality occurs 5–6 days PI.

GROSS LESIONS AND HISTOPATHOLOGY. Marked inflammatory and edematous changes in 5–6 days are followed by sloughing of soft white caseous necrotic material containing numerous oocysts and flecks of blood in 7–8 days.

***EIMERIA MELEAGRIDIS* TYZZER 1929.** Visible lesions may be seen in the ceca with yellow-white caseous cores, but this species is considered virtually nonpathogenic. Oocysts resemble those of other pathogenic species in the ceca, and differentiation is difficult.

PATHOGENICITY. Most studies have characterized this species as almost nonpathogenic. Two to five million oocysts produce little effect on growth of 4- to 8-wk-old poults. Earlier reports indicating greater pathogenicity may have come from mixed infections with *E. adenoeides*.

GROSS LESIONS AND HISTOPATHOLOGY. Nonadherent cream-colored caseous cecal cores are characteristics of infection in young poults. The core may be passed intact. The mucosa is somewhat thickened and may contain petechial hemorrhages in dilated portions of the ceca. The plugs disappear 5.5–6 days PI, and many oocysts may be found in cecal contents.

Edema and lymphocytic infiltration may be seen histologically, but less extensively than with *E. adenoeides* and *E. gallopavonis*. First-generation schizonts develop in surface epithelium of the small intestine but later stages occur in the cecal epithelium.

***Eimeria meleagrimitis* Tyzzer 1929.** Infection with *E. meleagrimitis* is primarily upper intestinal but may spread throughout the small intestine in heavy infections. This is the most pathogenic of the upper intestinal coccidia in turkeys. The oocysts are small (averaging 19.2 × 16.3 μm) and ovoid.

PATHOGENICITY. Experimental infection of young poults produces morbidity and mortality, lost weight gain, dehydration, and general unthriftiness. Inoculation of 200,000 oocysts produces some mortality and morbidity, but this species is not as pathogenic as *E. adenoeides.*

GROSS LESIONS AND HISTOPATHOLOGY. Infected birds show signs of dehydration. In the duodenum, enlargement and congestion are marked on the 5th and 6th day of infection. Large amounts of mucus and fluid may be found in the lumen. Feces may contain occasional flecks of blood and mucous casts 5–7 days PI.

The tips of villi are most commonly parasitized, and the epithelium may be completely denuded, although hemorrhage is rare. Eosinophilic infiltration may begin as early as 2 hr PI and is extensive at the height of the infection.

Undescribed Species. Several species of coccidia that do not fit descriptions of established species have been isolated from wild or domestic turkeys, but have not been adequately described or named. Thus, some difficulty may be expected in speciating coccidia found in field cases unless the pathology and appearance are distinctive.

Prevention and Control. Drugs effective in chickens are generally effective in turkeys, but the optimal level of application may vary and the toxicity of some drugs is significantly higher in turkeys than in chickens.

TREATMENT. As in chickens, treatment of outbreaks in turkeys is less desirable than prevention by chemotherapy or immunization. When treatment is necessary, application of amprolium (0.012–0.025% in water) or a sulfonamide (dosage depending on drug, often given 2 days on drug, 3 days off, and 2 days on, sometimes repeated a second week). The toxicity of sulfonamides limits their usefulness for turkeys.

CONTROL BY CHEMOTHERAPY. Most producers use anticoccidial drugs continuously in the feed for at least 8 wk. Generally, poults are confined to a brooding facility at that time. Later, the birds may be moved to range or to other facilities. Drugs approved for use in feed include amprolium (0.0125%-0.25%), butynorate (.0275%), sulfaquinoxaline (0.0175%), sulfadimethoxine (0.006–0.25%) + ormetoprim (.00375%), or monensin (54–90 g/ton). Approvals for halofuginone (1.5–3.0 ppm) and lasalocid (75–125 ppm) are pending.

PREVENTION WITH PLANNED IMMUNIZATION. The principle of immunization by exposure to a small number of pathogenic oocysts of the important species of *Eimeria* was developed with chickens and is represented by a single product for turkeys in the USA (Coccivac-T, Sterwin, Millsboro, DE). The inoculum is delivered in the water during the first 7–10 days and causes a mild infection. There are risks inherent in using virulent strains of coccidia, and occasional treatment at 3–4 wk of age is necessary if one of the species multiplies too rapidly, but the program is used with success in most instances.

COCCIDIOSIS IN GEESE.

Numerous species of coccidia have been described from domestic and wild geese. The most prevalent and damaging in commercial flocks is *E. truncata,* which causes renal coccidiosis, and *E. anseris,* which causes intestinal coccidiosis. Renal coccidiosis may produce high mortality from blockage of kidney function in young goslings. Coccidia may be introduced into domestic flocks by migrating and resident wild geese.

***Eimeria truncata* Railliet and Lucet 1891.** Flock losses due to renal coccidiosis have been reported as high as 87% in Iowa. Geese aged 3–12 wk are affected, although the disease is most acute in younger goslings. Signs of infection include depression, weakness, diarrhea with whitish feces, and anorexia. Eyes become dull and sunken and wings are drooped. Survivors may show vertigo and torticollis. Birds quickly develop immunity to reinfection.

Oocysts and endogenous stages of *E. truncata* are found only in the kidneys or cloaca near the junction of the ureters. Diagnosis of *E. truncata* is assured by finding the distinctive oocysts in the kidneys and ureters. Oocysts average 21.3 × 16.7 μm and have truncated ends.

NATURAL AND EXPERIMENTAL HOSTS. Although thorough cross-infection experiments have not been done in most cases, *E. truncata* has been reported from domestic and wild geese, ducks, and swans.

GROSS LESIONS AND HISTOPATHOLOGY. The kidneys may be enlarged and protrude from the sacral bed. The normal reddish brown is altered to light grayish yellow or grayish red. Pinhead-sized grayish white foci or hemorrhagic petechiae may be seen; they contain numerous oocysts and accumulations of urates. Invading and growing parasites may distort the kidney tubules to many times the normal size. Eosinophils and signs of necrosis are present in focal areas.

EIMERIA ANSERIS KOTLAN 1933. The oocysts average 19.2 × 16.6 μm. Differentiation from the 14 species listed by Pellerdy (25) may be difficult.

PATHOGENICITY. *E. anseris* may produce anorexia, tottering gait, debility, diarrhea and morbidity, and sometimes mortality. The small intestine becomes enlarged and filled with thin reddish brown fluid. Catarrhal inflammatory lesions are most intense in middle and lower portions of the small intestine. There may be large whitish nodules or a fibrinous diphtheroid necrotic enteritis. Under dry pseudomembranous flakes the oocysts and endogenous stages of the parasite are found in large numbers. Parasite stages invade epithelial cells of the posterior half of the intestine in closely packed rows. Developing gametocytes penetrate deeply into subepithelial tissues of the villi.

TREATMENT. Various sulfonamide drugs have been used in treatment of renal and intestinal coccidiosis of geese. Some studies indicated a favorable response, but unfortunately there have been no controlled experiments.

COCCIDIOSIS IN DUCKS.

Coccidiosis in ducks is sporadic but of sufficient frequency to warrant more attention from researchers. Cases involving moderate to heavy mortality have been reported on domestic duck farms in New York, New Jersey, Hungary, and Japan. Coccidia were recovered from every farm sampled on Long Island, New York. Clinical and subclinical coccidiosis appears to be quite common, and can produce morbidity and mortality as well as poor performance.

SPECIES OF COCCIDIA AND DESCRIPTIONS. Although 13 species of coccidia have been reported from domestic and wild ducks, the descriptions are often insufficient to use in diagnosis (25). Many species will remain in doubt until further work is completed. Coccidia in ducks may be of *Eimeria, Wenyonella,* or *Tyzzeria.* The genus can readily be determined from the sporulated oocyst. The oocysts of *Eimeria* have 4 sporocysts, each containing 2 sporozoites; *Wenyonella* have 4 sporozoites, each with 4 sporozoites; and *Tyzzeria* have 8 naked sporozoites not contained with sporocysts.

Tyzzeria perniciosa Allen 1936, from domestic ducks in the USA, have thin-walled oocysts measuring 10–12.3 × 9–10.8 μm, and sporulate to produce 8 free sporozoites.

Wenyonella philiplevinei Leibovitz 1968 is the best described of the coccidia from ducks. It is found in the lower intestine from the posterior jejunal annular band to the cloaca. The prepatent period is 93 hr. The oocysts have 3-layered walls, measure 15.5–21 × 12.5–16 μm (averaging 18.7 × 14.4), have a micropyle at one end, 1–2 polar granules and no oocyst residuum. Sporulation of the oocyst yields 4 sporocysts, each containing 4 sporozoites.

PATHOGENICITY. Signs of infection with *T. perniciosa* usually include anorexia, weight loss, weakness, distress, morbidity, and up to 70% mortality. Hemorrhagic areas are common in the anterior portion of the intestine, but may be found throughout. Bloody or cheesy exudate is common. The epithelial lining may be sloughed in long sheets. Parasite invasion may extend through the mucosal and submucosal layers as deep as the muscular layers. Acute hemorrhage as early as the 4th day may be followed by death on the 5th to 6th day.

With *W. philiplevinei* the effects are limited to 72–96 hrs PI. Occasional petechial hemorrhages appear in the posterior ileal mucosa. Diffuse congestion is found in lower intestinal mucosa. In severe infections mortality may occur on the 4th day.

COCCIDIOSIS IN PIGEONS.

Coccidiosis in pigeons is similar to, but less severe than, that caused in chickens by *E. necatrix.* Young pigeons suffer the greatest losses, but mortality may occur in birds as old as 3–4 mo.

The most frequently occurring species of coccidia in pigeons is *E. labbeana* (Labbe 1896) Pinto 1928. Oocysts are spherical or subspherical, averaging 19.1 × 17.4 μm.

PATHOGENICITY. Mortality of 15–70% has been reported in young pigeons in various parts of the world. Subclinical infections may persist in older birds for long periods. Immunity does not appear to be as "self-limiting" as reported for other species. Common signs of infection are anorexia, greenish diarrhea, marked dehydration, and emaciation. Droppings may be blood-tinged, and the entire digestive tract may be inflamed. The common condition of "going light" is frequently attributed to coccidiosis.

TREATMENT. Favorable response has been reported after use of sulfonamides in drinking water at the same or half the level recommended for chickens. A product was introduced in 1987 in France and Belgium for specific use in pigeons. The active ingredient is Clazuril, a close relative of the Diclazuril under development for use in chickens. This product is highly effective in treating coccidiosis in pigeons.

REFERENCES

1. AAAP Committee on Disease Reporting. 1987. Summary of commercial poultry disease reports. Avian Dis 31:926–982.

2. Arakawa, A., E. Baba, and T. Fukata. 1981. Eime-

ria tenella infection enhances Salmonella typhimurium infections in chickens. Poult Sci 60:2203–2209.

3. Baba, E., T. Fukata, and A. Arakawa. 1982. Establishment and persistence of Salmonella typhimurium infection stimulated by Eimeria tenella in chickens. Poult Sci 61:1410.

4. Biggs, P.M., P.L. Long, S.G. Kenzy, and D.G. Rootes. 1969. Investigations into the association between Marek's disease and coccidiosis. Acta Vet 38:65–75.

5. Braunius, W.W. 1986. Incidence of Eimeria species in broilers in relation to the use of anticoccidial drugs. Proc Georgia Coccidiosis Conf, Univ Georgia, Athens, pp. 409–414.

6. Edgar, S.A. 1986. Coccidiosis in turkeys: Biology and incidence. Proc Georgia Coccidiosis Conf, Univ Georgia, Athens, pp. 116–123.

7. Edgar, S.A., and C.T. Siebold. 1964. A new coccidium of chickens, Eimeria mivati sp. n. (Protozoa: Eimeriidae), with details of its life history. J Parasitol 50:193–204.

8. Feed Additive Compendium. 1989. Miller Publ Co., Minneapolis, MN.

9. Fletcher, O.J., J.F. Munnell, and P.K. Page. 1975. Cryptosporidiosis of the bursa of Fabricius in chickens. Avian Dis 19:630–639.

10. Gore, T.C., and P.L. Long. 1982. The biology and pathogenicity of a recent field isolate of Eimeria praecox, Johnson 1930. J Protozool 29:82–85.

11. Hamet, N. 1986. Resistance to anticoccidial drugs in poultry farms in France from 1975 to 1984. Proc Georgia Coccidiosis Conf, Univ Georgia, Athens, pp. 415–421.

12. Helmbolt, C.F., and E.S. Bryant. 1971. The pathology of necrotic enteritis in domestic fowl. Avian Dis 15:775–780.

13. Hoerr, J.F., F.M. Ranck, and T.F. Hastings. 1978. Respiratory cryptosporidiosis in turkeys. J Am Vet Med Assoc 173:1591–1593.

14. Jeffers, T.K. 1974. Eimeria tenella: Incidence, distribution, and anticoccidial drug resistance of isolants in major broiler producing areas. Avian Dis 18:74–84.

15. Jeffers, T.K. 1974. Eimeria acervulina and Eimeria maxima: Incidence and anticoccidial drug resistance of isolants in major broiler producing areas. Avian Dis 18:331–342.

16. Johnson, J., and W.M. Reid. 1970. Anticoccidial drugs: Lesion scoring techniques in battery and floor-pen experiments with chickens. Exp Parasitol 28:30–36.

17. Litjens, J.B. 1986. The relationship between coccidiosis and the use of anticoccidials in broilers in the southern part of the Netherlands. Proc Georgia Coccidiosis Conf, Univ Georgia, Athens, pp. 442–448.

18. Long, P.L. 1982. The Biology of the Coccidia. University Park Press, Baltimore, MD.

19. Maxey, B.W., and R.K. Page. 1977. Efficacy of lincomycin feed medication for the control of necrotic enteritis in broiler-type chickens. Poult Sci 56:1909–1913.

20. McDougald, L.R. 1986. Current drugs and programs. Proc Georgia Coccidiosis Conf, Univ Georgia, Athens, pp. 237–238.

21. McDougald, L.R., T. Karlsson, and W.M. Reid. 1979. Interaction of infectious bursal disease and coccidiosis in layer replacement chickens. Avian Dis 23:999–1005.

22. McDougald, L.R., A.L. Fuller, and J. Solis. 1986. Drug sensitivity of 99 isolates of coccidia from broiler farms. Avian Dis 30:690–694.

23. McDougald, L.R., J.M.L. DaSilva, J. Solis, and M. Braga. 1987. A survey of sensitivity to anticoccidial drugs in 60 isolates of coccidia from broiler chickens in Brazil and Argentina. Avian Dis 31:287–292.

24. Morehouse, N.F., and R.R. Barron. 1970. Coccidiosis: Evaluation of coccidiostats by mortality, weight gains, and fecal scores. Exp Parasitol 28:25–29.

25. Pellerdy, L.P. 1974. Coccidia and Coccidiosis, 2nd Ed. Akademine Kiado, Budapest.

26. Reid, W.M., and J. Johnson. 1970. Pathogenicity of Eimeria acervulina in light and heavy coccidial infections. Avian Dis 14:166–177.

27. Reyna, P.S., G.F. Mathis, and L.R. McDougald. 1982. A survey of sensitizing anticoccidial drugs to 60 isolates from broiler chickens in Brazil and Argentina. Avian Dis 31:287–292.

28. Shirley, M.W. 1986. Studies on the immunogenicity of the seven attenuated lines of Eimeria given as a mixture to chickens. Avian Pathol 15:629–638.

CRYPTOSPORIDIOSIS

William L. Current

INTRODUCTION. Cryptosporidiosis is caused by small coccidian parasites of the genus *Cryptosporidium* that live within the microvillous region of epithelial cells of the respiratory and gastrointestinal tracts of vertebrates. Natural infections have been reported from at least nine different avian hosts. In chickens, turkeys, and quail, these parasites are primary pathogens that can produce respiratory and/or intestinal disease resulting in morbidity and mortality. Recent reviews of the biology of *Cryptosporidium* spp. are now available (5, 11).

HISTORY AND TAXONOMY. Clarke (2) in 1895, observed what may have been a species of *Cryptosporidium* in mice. The type species *C. muris* was described 12 yr later from laboratory mice by Tyzzer (37), who later also described many of the life cycle stages and a second species, *C. parvum* (38, 39). Only a few of the 19 additional named species of *Cryptosporidium* from a variety of vertebrate hosts are now considered valid. At the time of this writing, there appears to be two species (*C. baileyi* and *C. meleagridis*) infecting both chickens and turkeys, and perhaps a third, unnamed species infecting quail. *Cryptosporidium baileyi* is believed to be responsible for both intestinal (cloaca and bursa of Fabricius) and respiratory infections in chickens and turkeys. The species believed to be responsible for intestinal (small intestine) infections associated with diarrheal disease in turkeys is *C. meleagridis*. A species believed to be distinct from *C. baileyi* and *C. meleagridis* is responsible for intestinal (small intestine) cryptosporidiosis associated with high mortality in quail.

LIFE CYCLE AND MORPHOLOGY. Taxonomic distinctions among the genera of coccidia are based mainly on the differences in oocyst structure. In contrast to other coccidia found in poultry, *Cryptosporidium* spp. oocysts do not have sporocysts surrounding the sporozoites, four of which lie naked within the oocyst wall (Fig. 33.6).

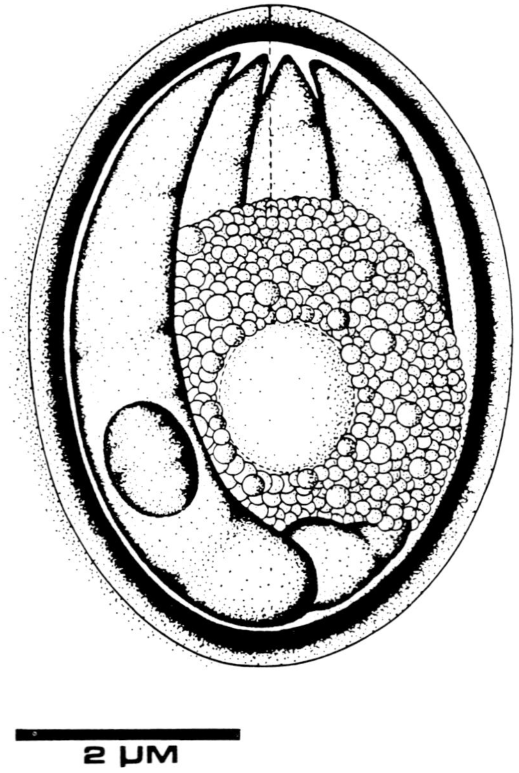

33.6. Composite line drawing of an oocyst of *Cryptosporidium baileyi.* Note the four sporozoites surrounding the oocyst residuum, and the suture in the two-layered oocyst wall. (J Protozool)

The life cycle of *Cryptosporidium,* like other true coccidia belonging to the suborder Eimeriorina, can be divided into six major developmental events (Fig. 33.7): excystation (release of infective sporozoites), merogony (asexual multiplication within epithelial cells), gametogony (formation of male and female gametes), fertilization (union of gametes), oocyst wall formation (to produce an environmentally resistant form), and sporogony (the formation of infective sporozoites within the oocyst wall).

The life cycle (8) differs in several respects from that of *Eimeria* spp. infecting poultry. The intracellular stages of *Cryptosporidium* spp. are confined to the microvillous region of the host cell and the oocysts, which sporulate within the host cell, are infective when released in the feces. Some oocysts do not form environmentally resistant walls; their sporozoites are surrounded by only a single unit membrane. When released from the parasitophorous vacuole of the host cell, the unit membrane ruptures and these invasive forms penetrate adjacent host cells and reinitiate the developmental cycle. However, the majority of oocysts develop a multilayered, environmentally resistant, thick wall and are passed in the feces. It is this thick-walled form that transmits the infection to other susceptible hosts. The thin-walled, autoinfective oocysts and the type I meronts (asexual stages) can recycle, allowing a small number of ingested oocysts to produce a severe infection. In the absence of new exposures, the immune-deficient host may develop a persistent, life-threatening disease. Another feature of *Cryptosporidium* spp., which differs from *Eimeria* spp. in mammalian and avian hosts, is frequent establishment of infections in the mucosal epithelium of a wide variety of organs. For example, *C. baileyi* can infect the cloaca, the bursa of Fabricius, the upper and lower respiratory tracts, and the eye lids.

Oocyst morphology may be useful for species identification (Table 33.5). Only *C. baileyi* can be identified on the basis of morphology alone, since it is larger and more ovoid than *C. meleagridis* or the other species infecting quail. *Cryptosporidium* isolated from quail will not infect chickens or turkeys. Thus, the species infecting quail can be distinguished from *C. meleagridis* on the basis of the host in which it is found. Oocysts of all three species are fully sporulated when passed in feces and contain four crescent-shaped sporozoites that surround a centrally located oocyst residuum. Oocyst walls of all three species are about 0.5 μm thick, colorless, and have no micropyle (Fig. 33.6).

INCIDENCE AND DISTRIBUTION. *Cryptosporidium* spp. appear to be present wherever avian hosts are raised commercially. The reported worldwide distribution in avian hosts corresponds to the regions in which poultry health specialists have used appropriate diagnostic tools, and will continue to expand as awareness of their importance as primary pathogens increases.

CRYPTOSPORIDIOSIS IN CHICKENS. *Cryptosporidium* (probably *C. baileyi*) was diagnosed in 6.8% of 1000 consecutive histology cases of chickens in Georgia (15). In North Carolina, *Cryp-*

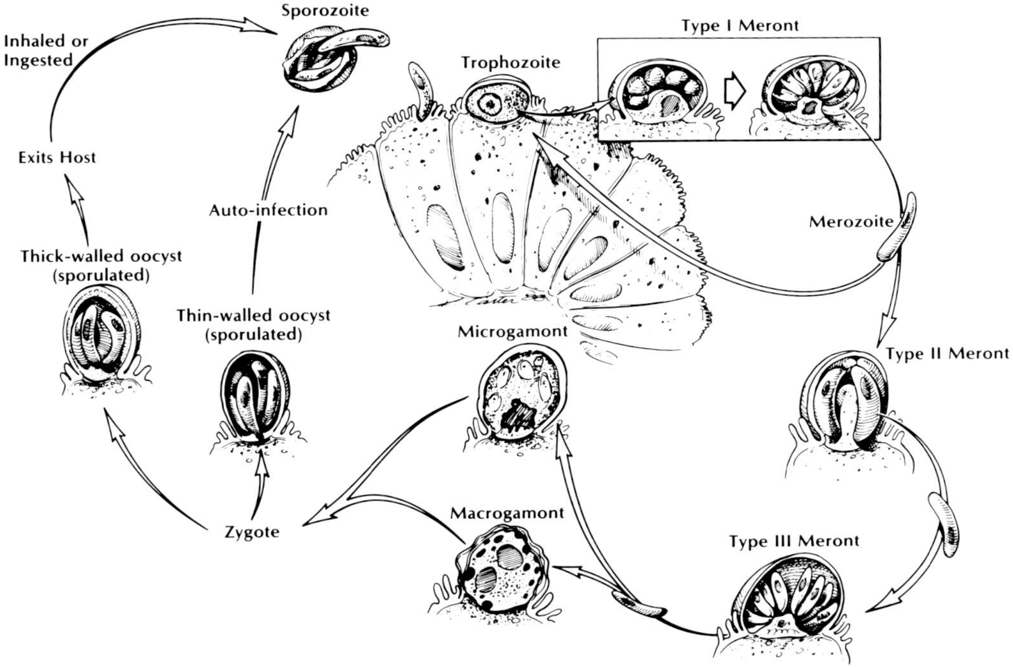

33.7. Proposed life cycle of *Cryptosporidium baileyi* as it occurs in the mucosal epithelium of the intestine (bursa of Fabricius and cloaca) and the respiratory tract of broiler chickens.

Table 33.5. Distinguishing features of *Cryptosporidium* spp. infecting poultry

Species	Host(s)	Site of Infection	Measurements of Oocysts (μm)
C. baileyi	Chicken, turkey, duck	Bursa of Fabricius, cloaca, respiratory epithelium	6.2 × 4.6 (mean), 6.3–5.6 × 4.8–4.5 (range)
C. meleagridis	Turkey, chicken	Small intestine	5.2 × 4.6 (mean), 6.0–5.6 × 4.8–4.5 (range)
Cryptosporidium sp.	Quail	Small intestine	Approximately 5

Source: (4, 21, 24).

tosporidium spp. oocysts were found in the feces of 9 of 33 (27.3%) broilers, 3 of 30 (10%) broiler breeders, and 1 of 17 (5.9%) layers (24). Using an enzyme-linked immunosorbent assay, 22% of 454 broiler flocks in Delmarva region had birds that were seropositive for *Cryptosporidium* spp. at the time they were processed (6, 33). The number of positive flocks among different companies sampled ranged from 2.8 to 40%. Serologic data demonstrated less cryptosporidiosis in the best 10 than in the worst 10 broiler flocks (ranked by overall mortality). Such investigations do not distinguish between intestinal and respiratory infections (4, 6). These and other data indicate that *Cryptosporidium* spp. are common intestinal infections in broiler chickens in the USA and Japan (10, 12, 22, 27, 30).

Although less common, respiratory cryptosporidiosis can be a major cause of morbidity and mortality. The factors responsible for natural outbreaks of respiratory cryptosporidiosis between 4 and 17 wk of age are not understood. *C. baileyi* is believed to be responsible for intestinal (bursa of Fabricius and cloaca) and respiratory cryptosporidiosis in chickens (8). Experimentally induced respiratory and intestinal infections in broiler chickens have established the primary pathogenic potential of this parasite (1, 26).

Pathogenesis and Epizootiology. *C. baileyi* generally invades the epithelium of the cloaca and bursa of Fabricius. Oocysts are picked up from heavy fecal contamination of the litter or cages. Respiratory infections apparently result from inhalation or aspiration of oocysts that are present in the environment. As few as 100 oocysts can result in intestinal infections when given orally or in respiratory infections when inoculated intratracheally. Oocysts of *C. baileyi* are infective at the time they are passed in the feces and no vectors have been identified. Since *C. baileyi* can infect a variety of avian hosts, it is possible that wild birds may serve as carriers. Although *C. baileyi* is not infective for mammals, it is possible that rodents (mice and rats) or perhaps insects could serve as mechanical carriers. Studies of the potential for carrier or transport hosts to spread cryptosporidiosis are needed.

Mild to heavy intestinal and respiratory infections can be demonstrated as early as 3 days after inoculation of oocysts. Intestinal disease is usually mild. No overt signs of gastrointestinal disease occur in chickens receiving oocysts by gavage into the crop.

Signs of respiratory disease may appear within 1 wk after intratracheal (IT) inoculation of *C. bailey* oocysts into 7- or 9-day-old broiler chickens. Severe morbidity and sometimes mortality may result (1, 9). IT inoculation of broilers with 4×10^5 *C. baileyi* oocysts produced severe respiratory disease, while equal numbers of oocysts produced asymptomatic intestinal infections. The experimental disease appeared similar to that reported in several natural outbreaks (10, 22, 27).

Respiratory signs of sneezing and coughing occur in most IT-inoculated chickens by 6 days postinoculation (PI). By 12 days PI, respiratory signs are more severe and many of the birds extend their heads to facilitate breathing. The more severely affected chickens lie on their sterna and are reluctant to move. Severe signs of respiratory disease are present in most IT-inoculated birds for about 3–4 wk PI, after which there may be gradual improvement. Birds with respiratory infection had significantly lower weights than birds with intestinal or no *C. baileyi* infection when they were inoculated at 7 days of age and sampled 14, 21, and 28 days later (9). The total mean weights of surviving birds in each group did not differ significantly at the end of the 50 day experiment, suggesting a compensatory weight gain following recovery from respiratory cryptosporidiosis. However, this apparent compensatory weight gain may have been due in part to death of 14% of the smallest birds in the group of chickens with respiratory cryptosporidiosis. Chickens were more resistant to IT inoculation at 28 days than at 7 or 14 days of age (26).

Airsacculitis and pneumonia can occur as early as 6 days but are more common 12–28 days following IT inoculation of *C. baileyi* oocysts. Early in the disease process, posterior thoracic air sacs are slightly thickened and contain foamy, clear to white or gray fluid. By 12 days, air sacs may become very thick and contain white caseous exudate. The lungs of birds with severe airsacculitis are almost always affected and exhibit focal consolidation (10–80%), particularly in the ventral region. Abdominal air sacs may also be affected.

Histopathology of IT-inoculated chicks shows large numbers of parasites throughout the microvillous region of the epithelium lining the trachea and bronchi. Deciliation by replacement with developing parasites becomes apparent by 4 days PI (Fig. 33.8). By 12 days almost all cilia may be replaced by developing parasites and the mucociliary elevator function ceases in affected trachea and bronchi. Histologic lesions include epithelial cell hyperplasia, thickening of the mucosa by mononuclear cell infiltrates with some heterophils, loss of cilia, and discharge of mucocellular exudate into the airways. There is accumulation of mucus, sloughed epithelial cells, lymphocytes, macrophages, and parasites in the tertiary bronchi and atria of the lungs. Affected lobules are expanded by accumulation of exudate and infiltration of mononuclear cells (Fig. 33.9). Affected air sacs lined with respiratory epithelium also contain large numbers of parasites and suffer similar changes.

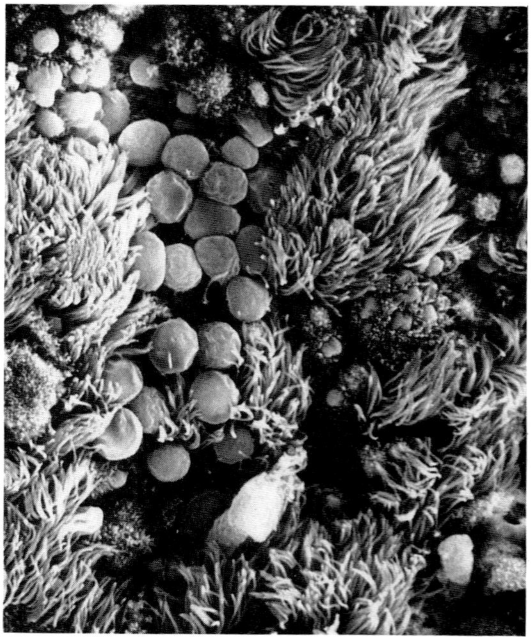

33.8. Scanning electron micrograph of the mucosal surface of the primary bronchi obtained from a broiler chicken 4 days after IT inoculation of *Cryptosporidium baileyi*. Some developmental stages of the parasite can be seen among the cilia of the respiratory surface. At this stage of infection, the mucociliary elevator is probably still functional and the bird would not have overt signs of respiratory distress. On days 10–18 after IT inoculation, developmental stages of the parasite form a virtual monolayer on the respiratory surface. Few or no cilia can be found. (S.L. White, Lilly Research Laboratories)

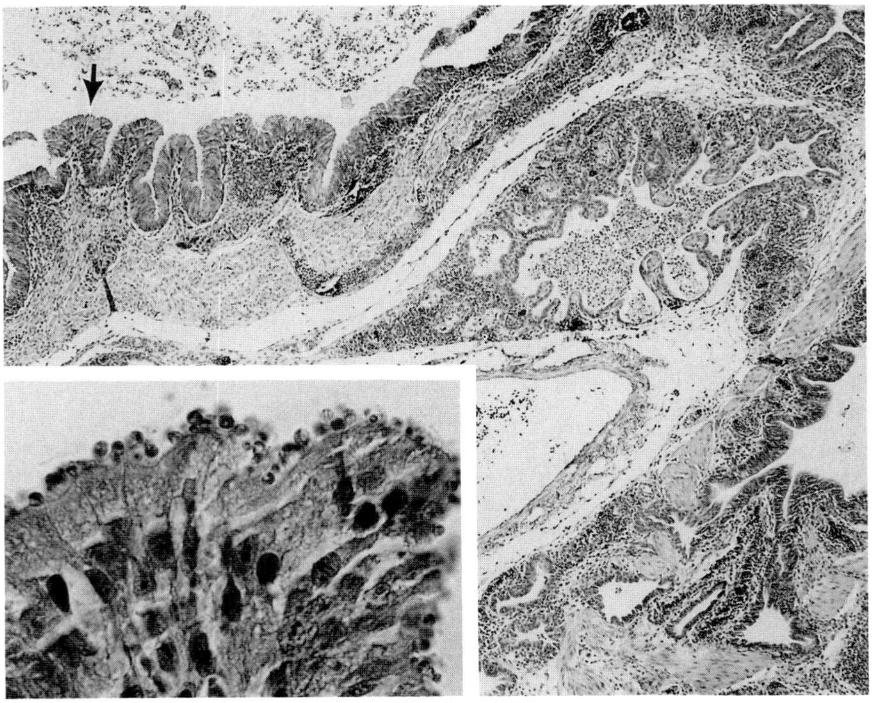

33.9. Histologic section showing accumulation of lymphoid cells around bronchi in the lungs of a broiler chicken 6 days after IT inoculation of *Cryptosporidium baileyi* oocysts. Inset: A higher magnification of the villus (*arrow*), showing the numerous developmental stages of the parasite on the epithelial surface. H & E.

Respiratory cryptosporidiosis caused high mortality and morbidity in a flock of 16,000 7-wk-old broiler chickens (10). In addition to increased mortality, the performance of birds with respiratory infections is also adversely affected by lower weight gains and higher feed:gain ratios.

Intestinal (cloaca and bursa of Fabricius) cryptosporidiosis in chickens (produced by *C. baileyi*) may result in histologic lesions but does not result in gross lesions or in overt signs of disease. However, several reports suggest that performance of broilers can be adversely affected. An unusually high mortality was associated with *C. baileyi* infection in the bursa of Fabricius, and there were lower pigmentation scores when inoculated birds were compared with noninfected controls (1, 17).

Interaction of *C. baileyi* and other respiratory pathogens predisposes birds to secondary invasion by *Escherichia coli* because of disruption of the mucociliary elevator (9). Infectious bronchitis virus and *E. coli* also enhance the severity of *C. baileyi*-induced respiratory disease in chickens.

CRYPTOSPORIDIOSIS IN TURKEYS. Two valid species of *Cryptosporidium* found in turkeys are *C. meleagridis* (32) and *C. baileyi*. The intestinal (bursa of Fabricius and cloaca) and respiratory infections produced by *C. baileyi* are similar to those described above for chickens (8, 9, 25).

Slavin (32) reported small intestinal cryptosporidiosis in 1955 due to *C. meleagridis* in a flock of 10- to 14-day-old turkey poults. Illness was associated with diarrhea, unthriftiness, and moderate mortality. More than 30 yr later, several outbreaks of this disease were reported (16, 40).

Turkey poults infected with *C. meleagridis* may develop severe diarrhea. Numerous parasites are present within the brush border of the intestinal mucosa lining the middle and lower small intestine, which becomes pale and distended with cloudy mucoid fluid and gas bubbles. Villi in the affected regions of the intestine become atrophic, the crypts become hypertrophic, and large numbers of lymphocytes, heterophils, and some macrophages and plasma cells accumulate within the lamina propria (16).

There are several case reports of severe respiratory cryptosporidiosis in commercial turkeys caused by *Cryptosporidium* spp. (14, 20, 29, 35). There appear to be two different manifestations of the disease, an upper respiratory involvement that includes sinusitis and a lower respiratory involvement that includes colonization of the trachea and bronchi with concomitant airsacculitis and pneumonia. The case reports of upper respiratory tract infections described acute signs of bilateral swelling of infraorbital sinuses, similar to that reported for birds infected with *Mycoplasma* spp., and serous conjunctivitis (14, 20). Case reports of lower respiratory tract infections described signs including rattling, coughing, sneezing, and gasping (29, 35). Microscopic lesions of the infected tissues included deciliation of the epithelium and inflammation.

Inoculation of oocysts of *C. baileyi* isolated from the intestinal tract of broiler chickens into the trachea of turkeys produced respiratory signs the same as those observed in natural outbreaks (25).

The importance of *Cryptosporidium* spp. as agents of intestinal and respiratory disease in commercially reared turkeys is not clear. More study is needed.

CRYPTOSPORIDIOSIS IN QUAIL. Both respiratory and intestinal cryptosporidiosis have been reported in commercially grown quail, but the species involved has not been adequately described. A case of respiratory cryptosporidiosis was reported in a flock of 4-wk-old quail (*Coturnix coturnix*) in southern Australia (36). Clinical signs included depression, sneezing, and respiratory distress; mortality was approximately 10%. Histologic examination revealed parasites in the microvillous region of epithelial cells lining the nasal cavity, trachea, bronchi, salivary glands of the roof of the mouth, esophageal glands, and bursa of Fabricius. Pathologic changes in the respiratory mucosa were similar to those described above for chickens infected experimentally with *C. baileyi*. In five successive hatches of 25,000 young quail (*Colinus virginianus*), there was severe, fatal intestinal cryptosporidiosis (21). Diarrhea developed 4–6 days after hatching and mortality soon exceeded 90%. At necropsy, carcass dehydration was marked. The small intestine had clear, watery contents and the cecum was distended by brown, foamy fluid. Histologic examination of the small intestine revealed shortened villi and enterocytes detached from the tips of villi. Numerous developmental stages of the parasite were observed in the microvillous border of the small intestine, being most numerous in the proximal half. No parasites were observed in the cecum, colon, bursa of Fabricius, respiratory tract, or other tissues. Oocysts measuring approximately 5 μm, which were obtained from the intestines of these infected quail, were not orally infective to day-old broilers.

A similar outbreak was reported from young quail due to a combination of *Cryptosporidium* spp. and a reovirus isolated from intestinal contents (31). Subsequent laboratory studies (18) suggested that the *Cryptosporidium* and not the reovirus was responsible for the intestinal disease.

The organism responsible for this disease in quail appears to be a distinct species of *Cryptosporidium,* since its oocysts are smaller than those of *C. baileyi* and they are not infective to chickens or turkeys.

PREVENTION AND CONTROL. There are no effective anticryptosporidial drugs for prevention or treatment, and other approaches to the control are still experimental. Sanitation and immunity may provide some help, but there are no proven programs that can be recommended.

Sanitation. The oocysts of *Cryptosporidium* spp. infecting poultry are remarkably resistant to chemical agents that readily kill most viral, bacterial, and fungal pathogens. This resistance to chemical agents can be exploited by laboratory researchers trying to separate oocysts from other contaminating microbes; however, destruction of oocysts in commercial production facilities is not considered practical. In the laboratory, oocysts remain viable for months when stored at 4 C in solution of 2.5% potassium dichromate. Oocyst viability is also maintained after a 10–15 min incubation in 25% commercial bleach (sodium hypochlorite), a treatment used to remove other contaminating organic matter. Incubation of *C. baileyi* oocysts for 30 min at room temperature in each of nine commonly used disinfectants mixed with water at the highest concentration recommended by the manufacturers had little or no effect on viability (34). Incubation in 50% ammonia resulted in the greatest reduction in excystation and 50% commercial bleach destroyed many of the oocysts. Unless a more effective chemical agent is found, large-scale disinfection for cryptosporidiosis in commercial poultry facilities is impractical. The use of a steam-cleaner may be a more effective and safer means of disinfecting contaminated cages, since exposure to temperatures above 65 C tends to destroy the oocysts.

Immunity. A single intestinal and/or respiratory infection with *C. baileyi* can stimulate an immune response in broiler chickens of sufficient magnitude to clear the parasite from the infected mucosae and to render the host resistant to subsequent intestinal or respiratory challenge with oocysts of the same species (4, 6, 9). Oral or IT inoculation of oocysts into 8- to 14-day-old broilers results in heavy infections of the exposed mucosae for 14–16 days and then a rapid clearance of the parasite. At the time chickens clear primary infections, high titers of circulating antibodies specific to *C. baileyi* can be detected, and the birds exhibit a delayed hypersensitivity reaction to *C. baileyi* oocyst antigens. Data from laboratory studies and from a serologic survey suggest that acquired immunity may protect broilers from cryptosporidiosis during the last several weeks of growout. Studies are needed to identify antigens of *Cryptosporidium* spp. that may be candidates for use as vaccines.

DIAGNOSIS. Active infections in poultry, both respiratory and intestinal, can be diagnosed by identifying oocysts from fluids obtained from the respiratory tract or from the feces. Identification of *Cryptosporidium* oocysts differs somewhat from techniques used for the oocysts of *Eimeria*. Techniques include concentration procedures coupled with standard bright-field or with phase contrast microscopy (7), acid-fast staining (13, 28), negative-staining (3, 19), and staining with auramine-O for examination under a florescence microscope (24). These techniques allow one to readily distinguish *Cryptosporidium* oocysts from yeast cells that are often present in specimens.

Fecal or respiratory specimens can be collected and submitted fresh, in 10% formalin, or in an aqueous solution of 2.5% potassium dichromate. The most effective way of obtaining specimens in the field and in the laboratory is by the use of moist cotton-tipped swabs. Vigorous swabbing of the tracheal or cloacal epithelium will remove oocysts from the microvillous border. The swabs are placed in a tube containing 1 ml of water or fixative for transportation to the laboratory. Cryptosporidiosis infection can also be detected by demonstrating other stages of the life cycle from fresh or stained (23) mucosal scrapings from the microvillous region of the mucosae. These parasites also appear in histologic sections stained with hematoxylin and eosin as 2–6 μm basophilic bodies within the brush border of the epithelial cells. The diagnosis can be confirmed by transmission electron microscopy as this procedure reveals the distinct morphology of developmental stages of *Cryptosporidium* spp. within the mucosal epithelium.

Previous exposure to the parasite can be demonstrated by testing for serum antibodies specific to *Cryptosporidium* sp. (4, 6, 33).

REFERENCES

1. Blagburn, B.L., D.S. Lindsay, J.J. Giambrone, C.A. Sundermann, and F.J. Hoerr. 1987. Experimental cryptosporidiosis in broiler chickens. Poult Sci 66:442–449.
2. Clarke, J.J. 1895. A study of coccidia met with in mice. J Microsc Sci 37:277–302.
3. Current, W.L. 1983. Human cryptosporidiosis. N Engl J Med 309:1326–1327.
4. Current, W.L. 1986. Cryptosporidium sp. in chickens: Parasite life cycle and aspects of acquired immunity. In L.R. McDougald, P.L. Long, and L.P. Joyner (eds.), Proc Georgia Coccidiosis Conf, pp. 124–133. Univ Georgia, Athens.
5. Current, W.L. 1989. Cryptosporidium spp. In P.D. Walzer and R.M. Genta (eds.), Parasitic Infections in the Compromised Host, pp.281–341. Marcel Dekker, Inc., New York.
6. Current, W.L., and D.B. Snyder. 1988. Development of and serologic evaluation of acquired immunity to Cryptosporidium baileyi by broiler chickens. Poult Sci 67:720–729.
7. Current, W.L., N.C. Reese, J.V. Ernst, W.S. Bailey, M.B. Heyman, and W.M. Weinstein. 1983. Human cryptosporidiosis in immunocompetent and immunodeficient persons. Studies of an outbreak and experimental transmission. N Engl J Med 308:1252–1257.
8. Current, W.L., S.J. Upton, and T.B. Haynes. 1986. The life cycle of Cryptosporidium baileyi n. sp. (Apicomplexa, Cryptosporidiidae) infecting chickens. J Protozool 33:289–296.
9. Current, W.L., M.N. Novilla, and D.B. Snyder. 1987. Cryptosporidiosis in poultry: An update (Are Cryptosporidium spp. primary pathogens?). Proc 22nd Nat Meet Poultry Health Condemn, pp. 17–29. Delmarva Poultry Industry, Inc.
10. Dhillon, A.S., H.L. Thacker, A.V. Dietzel, and R.W. Winterfield. 1981. Respiratory cryptosporidiosis in broiler chickens. Avian Dis 25:747–751.
11. Fayer, R., and B.L.P. Ungar. 1986. Cryptosporidium spp. and cryptosporidiosis. Microbiol Rev 50:458–483.
12. Fletcher, O.J., J.F. Munell, and R.K. Page. 1975. Cryptosporidiosis of the bursa of Fabricius of chickens. Avian Dis 19:630–639.
13. Garcia, L.S., D.A. Bruckner, T.C. Brewer, and R.Y. Shimizu. 1983. Techniques for the recovery and identification of Cryptosporidium oocysts from stool specimens. J Clin Microbiol 18:185–190.
14. Glisson, J.R., T.P. Brown, M. Brugh, R.K. Page, S.H. Kleven, and R.B. Davis. 1984. Sinusitis in turkeys associated with respiratory cryptosporidiosis. Avian Dis 28:783–790.
15. Goodwin M.A., and J. Brown. 1987. Histologic incidence and distribution of Cryptosporidium sp. infection in chickens. J Am Vet Med Assoc 190:1623.
16. Goodwin, M.A., W.L. Steffens, I.D. Russell, and J. Brown. 1988. Diarrhea associated with intestinal cryptosporidiosis in turkeys. Avian Dis 32:63–67.
17. Gorham, S.L., E.T. Mallinson, D.B. Snyder, and E.M. Odor. 1987. Cryptosporidiosis in the bursa of Fabricius–a correlation with mortality rates in broiler chickens. Avian Pathol 16:205–211.
18. Guy, J.S., M.G. Levy, D.H. Ley, H.J. Barnes, and T.M. Craig. 1987. Experimental reproduction of enteritis in bobwhite quail (Colinus virginianus) with Cryptosporidium and Reovirus. Avian Dis 31:713–722.
19. Heine, J. 1982. Ein einfache Nachweismethode fur Kryptosporidien im Kot. Zentralbl Veterinaermed [B] 29:324–327.
20. Hoerr, F.J., F.M. Ranck, Jr., and T.F. Hastings. 1978. Respiratory cryptosporidiosis in turkeys. J Am Vet Med Assoc 173:1591–1593.
21. Hoerr, F.J., W.L. Current, and T.B. Haynes. 1986. Fatal cryptosporidiosis in quail. Avian Dis 30:421–425.
22. Itakura, C., M. Goryo, and T. Unemura. 1984. Cryptosporidial infection in chickens. Avian Pathol 13:487–499.
23. Latimer, K.S., M.A. Goodwin, and M.K. Davis. 1988. Rapid cytologic diagnosis of respiratory cryptosporidiosis in chickens. Avian Dis 32:826–830.
24. Ley, D.H., M.G. Levy, L. Hunter, W. Corbett, and H.J. Barnes. 1988. Cryptosporidia-positive rates of avian necropsy accessions determined by examination of auramine O-stained fecal smears. Avian Dis 32:108–113.
25. Lindsay, D.S., B.L. Blagburn, and F.J. Hoerr.

1987. Experimentally induced infection in turkeys with Cryptosporidium baileyi isolated from chickens. Am J Vet Res 48:104-108.
26. Lindsay, D.S., B.L. Blagburn, C.A. Sundermann, and J.J. Giambrone. 1988. Effect of broiler chicken age on susceptibility to experimentally induced Cryptosporidium baileyi infection. Am J Vet Res 49:1412-1414.
27. Nakamura, K., and F. Abe. 1988. Respiratory (especially pulmonary) and urinary infections of Cryptosporidium in layer chickens. Avian Pathol 17:703-711.
28. Payne, P., L.A. Lancaster, M. Heinzman, and J.A. McCutchan. 1983. Identification of Cryptosporidium in patients with the acquired immunologic syndrome. N Engl J Med 309:613-614.
29. Ranck, F.M., Jr., and F.J. Hoerr. 1986. Cryptosporidia in the respiratory tract of turkeys. Avian Dis 31:389-391.
30. Randall, C.J. 1982. Cryptosporidiosis of the bursa of Fabricius and trachea of broilers. Avian Pathol 11:95-102.
31. Ritter, G.D., D.H. Ley, M. Levy, J. Guy, and H.J. Barnes. 1986. Intestinal cryptosporidiosis and reovirus isolated from Bobwhite quail (Colinus virginianus) with enteritis. Avian Dis 30:603-608.
32. Slavin, D. 1955. Cryptosporidium meleagridis (sp. nov.). J Comp Pathol 65:262-266.
33. Snyder, D.B., W.L. Current, E. Russek-Cohen, S. Gorham, E.T. Mallison, W.W. Marquardt, and P.K. Savage. 1988. Serologic incidence of Cryptosporidium in Delmarva broiler flocks. Poult Sci 67:730-735.
34. Sundermann, C.A., D.S. Lindsay, and B.L. Blagburn. 1987. Evaluation of disinfectants for ability to kill avian Cryptosporidium oocysts. Compan Anim Pract 2:36-39.
35. Tarwid, J.N., R.J. Cawthorn, and C. Riddell. 1985. Cryptosporidiosis in the respiratory tract of turkeys in Saskatchewan. Avian Dis 29:528-532.
36. Tham, V.L., S. Kniesberg, and B.R. Dixon. 1982. Cryptosporidiosis in quails. Avian Pathol 11:619-626.
37. Tyzzer, E.E. 1907. A sporozoan found in the peptic glands of the common mouse. Proc Soc Exp Biol Med 5:12-13.
38. Tyzzer, E.E. 1910. An extracellular coccidium, Cryptosporidium muris (gen et sp. nov.) of the gastric glands of the common mouse. J Med Res 23:487-509.
39. Tyzzer, E.E. 1912. Cryptosporidium parvum (sp. nov.), a coccidium found in the small intestine of the common mouse. Arch Protistenkd 26:394-412.
40. Wages, D.P. 1987. Cryptosporidiosis and turkey viral hepatitis in turkey poult. J Am Vet Med Assoc 190:1623.

OTHER PROTOZOAN DISEASES OF THE INTESTINAL TRACT

Larry R. McDougald

HISTOMONIASIS. Histomoniasis is a parasitic disorder of the ceca and liver of many gallinaceous birds. The disease (caused by the protozoan *Histomonas meleagridis*) is characterized by necrotic foci in the liver and ulceration of the ceca and has also been called infectious enterohepatitis or blackhead. The signs leading to the use of the term blackhead are neither pathognomonic nor distinctive, since many other diseases may produce a similar appearance (Fig. 33.10A). The roles of the cecal worm *Heterakis gallinarum* and earthworms as accessory hosts of *Histomonas* comprise one of the most intriguing relationships in parasitology.

Although the economic significance of the disease is difficult to ascertain, annual losses from mortality in turkeys has been estimated to exceed $2 million. Decreased production from morbidity and chemotherapy expense increase cost of the disease. Although histomoniasis is less severe in chickens, losses from morbidity and mortality are estimated to be greater than in turkeys because of the frequency of occurrence and the numbers of birds involved (1). Outbreaks of histomoniasis in leghorn pullets in Georgia caused up to 20% mortality and high morbidity. Chicken houses may become badly contaminated by *Heterakis* worm eggs, causing outbreaks in flock after flock.

History. The disease complex has been reviewed in depth (16, 17, 22, 27). Histomoniasis in turkeys was first described in 1895. Discovery that a milder form of the disease occurs in chickens that often remained carriers resulted in the first useful recommendation for control. Every poultry producer has learned that turkeys should not be reared with chickens or on range where chickens have been produced during the previous several years. The role of the cecal worm (*Heterakis*) and its eggs and of the earthworm as carriers of the parasite explain this long period of infectivity on uninhabited range.

Although Smith recognized the primary etiologic agent as a protozoan in 1895, Tyzzer was the first to observe that the parasite had flagella as well as pseudopodia (30, 31). The pathogenesis of histomoniasis was elucidated further between 1964 and 1974 by studies showing that certain bacteria are necessary in addition to the histomonads to produce disease. This interesting *His-*

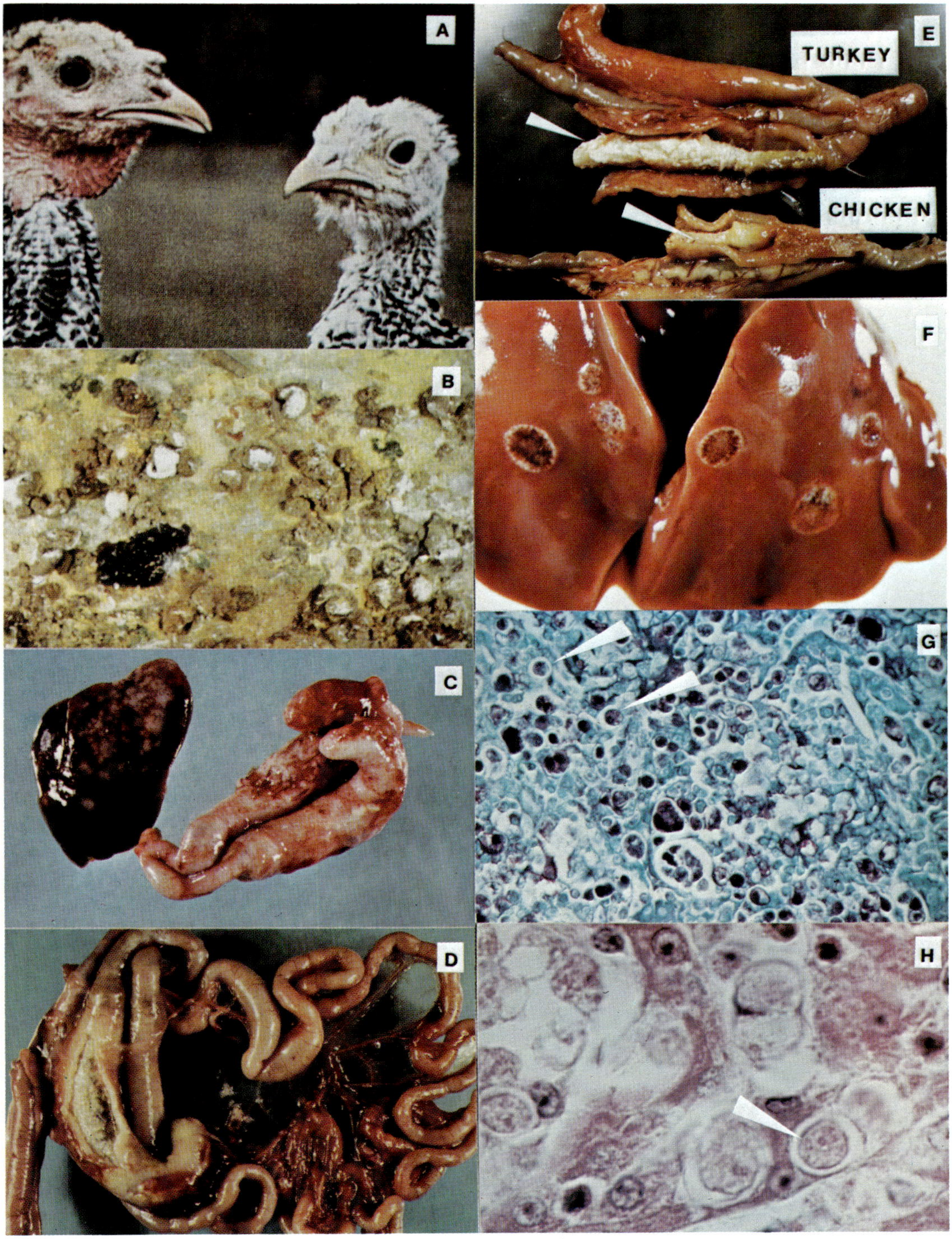

33.10. Histomoniasis infections. A. Normal uninfected poult (*left*); histomonas-infected poult of the same age (*right*). Sickly appearance occurs later in course of infection and is not distinctive to histomoniasis. (Hilbrich). B. Sulfur-colored feces often constitute the first sign of histomoniasis outbreaks in turkeys. C. Liver and cecum from poult 14 days after feeding on *Heterakis gallinarum* ova. Note engorgement of ceca and diffuse nature of liver lesions. (McDougald). D. Intestinal tract from experimentally infected turkey showing engorged cecum, core, and inflamed mesenteries. E. Chicken and turkey ceca 10 days PI with *Histomonas meleagridis.* Note cecal cores (*arrows*). F. Discrete pathognomonic lesions with raised surface in liver from a turkey infected with histomoniasis. G. Liver section showing histomonad PAS stain (*arrows*). H. Liver sections showing histomonads (*arrows*). H & E., ×1000. (Page)

tomonas-bacteria connection was discovered using germ-free techniques at the Universities of Georgia and Notre Dame.

Incidence and Distribution. Histomoniasis occurs wherever suitable avian hosts exist. In general, it is more prevalent in areas favoring coexistence of the cecal worm *Heterakis gallinarum* and various earthworm species, but it is regularly reported by diagnostic laboratories in the USA, Canada, and Mexico (1).

Despite improved management and availability of antihistomonal drugs, histomoniasis remains an important, if occasional, disease in chickens, turkeys, and other fowl.

Etiology and Classification. The causative agent, *Histomonas meleagridis,* was first described under the name *Amoeba meleagridis,* but discovery of flagellate characteristics led Tyzzer to rename the protozoan *H. meleagridis.* A larger (17 μm), nonpathogenic, 4-flagellated histomonad found in the cecum was named as a separate species, *H. wenrichi.*

Other agents such as trichomonads and fungi (*Candida albicans*) have been advanced as etiologic agents of blackhead (27). The term "pseudoblackhead" has been popularly applied to cases that did not respond to antihistomonals. Differential diagnosis including demonstration of the organism may be required in such cases.

MORPHOLOGY. *H. meleagridis* in its nonamoeboid state is nearly spherical (3–16 μm in diameter). The amoeboid phase is highly pleomorphic. Pseudopodia may be observed if the slide is warmed during microscopy (Fig. 33.11). There is a single stout flagellum 6–11 μm long. There is a large pelta and an axostyle wholly contained within the body of the organism. The parabasal body is V-shaped and anterior to the nucleus, which is spheroid to ellipsoid or ovoid and averages 2.2 × 1.7 μm.

The tissue forms lack flagella and exist in several different stages: 1) parasites in the "invasive" stage at the peripheral areas of the lesions (2) 8–17 μm in size, amoeboid, and appear to form pseudopods; 2) larger (12–21 μm), more numerous "vegetative" stage clustered in vacuoles in degenerating tissue; 3) a third stage present in older lesions is eosinophilic and smaller, may represent a degenerating form.

LIFE CYCLE. The existence of this organism is intimately associated with the cecal nematode *Heterakis gallinarum* and several species of earthworms common to poultry-yard soil. Early attempts to find histomonads in cecal worm eggs were inconclusive until Gibbs (10) demonstrated small bodies seen with the light microscope. Lee (14) observed a small form (3 μm) by electron microscopy and histomonads have been cultured from heterakid eggs in vitro (28).

Histomonads are found in intestinal epithelial cells of very young juveniles or newly hatched worms. The mechanism of egg infection by histomonads has not been determined. Springer et al. (29) found that triturated male worms recently removed from chickens carry viable histomonads. Female worms are less likely to transmit viable histomonads until the heterakid eggs mature. The female worms probably become infected with the histomonads during copulation and incorporate the protozoan into eggs before shell formation.

Earthworms can serve as transport hosts in which heterakid eggs hatch, and the juvenile worms survive in tissues in an infective state. The earthworm thus serves as a means for collection and concentration of heterakid eggs from the poultry-yard environment. On range, where climate and soil types favor survival of heterakids and earthworms, the latter must be considered in attempts to control a recurrent histomoniasis problem.

Earthworm transmission of *H. meleagridis* to the ring-necked pheasant (*Phasianus colchicus torquatus*) has been of documented importance in a partridge-pheasant histomoniasis outbreak at a game-rearing station in central Iowa.

Although direct infection of turkeys by oral ingestion of viable histomonads in fresh droppings is possible, their extremely delicate nature makes this route rather unlikely. Histomonads cannot survive outside the host for more than a few minutes unless protected by the heterakid egg or earthworm.

PATHOGENICITY. Characteristics of the definitive host influence clinical manifestations of infection by *Histomonas meleagridis* more than variations of pathogenicity of the parasite. These characteristics include species, breed, age, and intestinal flora.

Although natural infections occur in several species, the turkey is considered the most susceptible host because most infected turkeys die. Chickens are easily infected, but often have a milder form of the disease. Some variation in susceptibility has been found among different breeds of chickens. Chickens 4–6 wk old and turkeys 3–12 wk old are highly susceptible to infection.

Bacterial flora also plays a role with *H. meleagridis* in development of disease. Lesions of histomoniasis were more severe in turkeys when *Clostridium perfringens* was present as a monospecific contaminant than when *Escherichia coli* was present.

Isolates of *H. meleagridis* grown in vitro frequently lose pathogenicity in successive passages. Defined strains of *H. meleagridis* with varying pathogenicity have not been characterized, with the exception of *H. wenrichi,* now listed as a separate species.

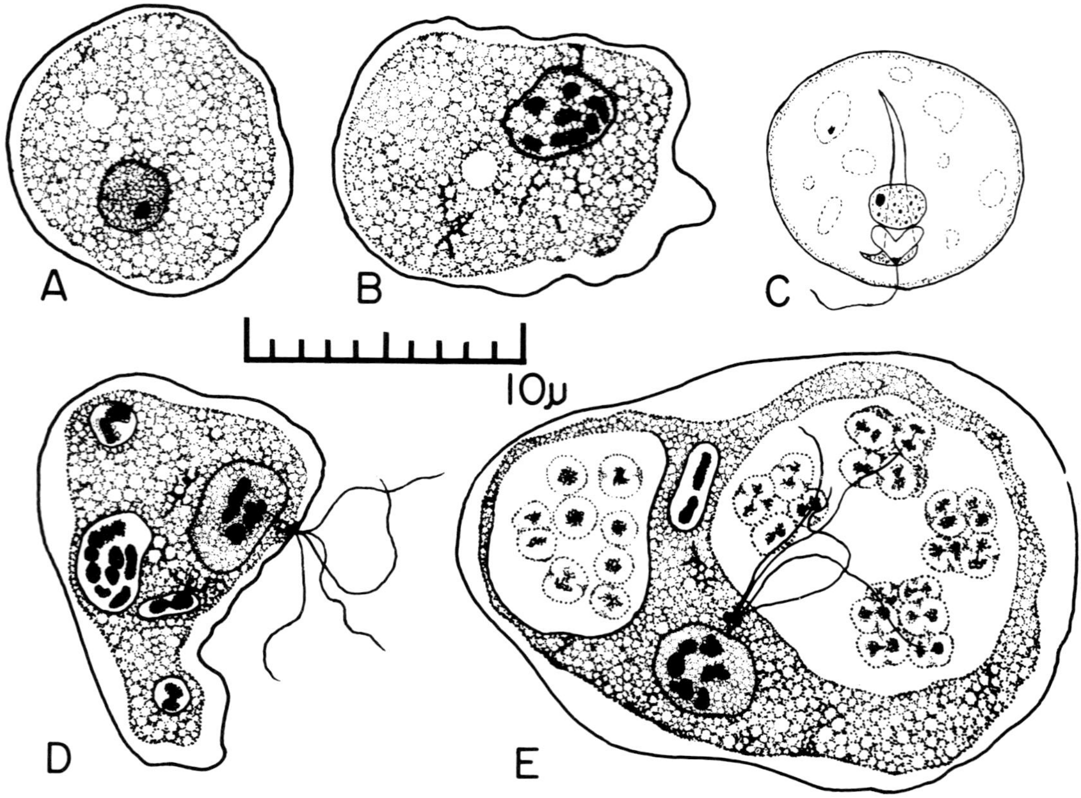

33.11. Examples of *H. meleagridis* (A, B, C) compared with *H. wenrichi* (D, E) showing variations for each species associated with environmental conditions. A. Tissue type *H. meleagridis* in fresh preparation from liver lesion, viewed with phase-contrast. B. *H. meleagridis* in transitional stage in lumen of the cecum. Pseudopodia have been formed; distribution of chromatin suggests that binary fission is approaching. However, the flagellum has not yet appeared. C. An organism from culture, with free flagellum typical of lumen-dwelling forms. (Honigberg and Bennett). D. Small *H. wenrichi,* structurally distinguishable from *H. meleagridis* by presence of 4 flagella. E. *H. wenrichi* as viewed in stained smear from cecum in which packets of *Sarcina* were abundant. Figures A, B, D, E from camera lucida tracings. Organisms B and D from portions of ceca fixed in Zenker's fluid, sectioned at 6 or 8 µm, and stained with Heidenhain's (B) or Wiegert's (D) iron hematoxylin. Specimen pictured in E was fixed in Schaudinn's fluid with 10% glacial acetic acid.

Pathogenesis and Epizootiology

NATURAL AND EXPERIMENTAL HOSTS. Numerous gallinaceous birds are reported as hosts for *H. meleagridis.* Turkeys, chukar partridges, and ruffed grouse may be severely affected by histomoniasis; chickens, peafowl, guinea fowl, bobwhite quail, and pheasants have a milder form of the disease. Experimentally, the coturnix quail can be infected but it is a poor host for the parasite.

VECTORS. The role of heterakids as vectors for histomonads is extremely important because they too are parasites of gallinaceous birds and protect the histomonad within their egg during transmission from bird to bird. The chicken, by serving as an inapparent host for both heterakids and histomonads, can be an important vector; however, with onset of confinement-rearing of chickens and other changes in management of poultry and game-bird production, their importance in disseminating *H. meleagridis* was diminished. Wild populations of game fowl, pheasants, and bobwhite quail may serve as vectors. Besides the earthworm, arthropods including flies, grasshoppers, sowbugs, and crickets may serve as mechanical vectors.

INCUBATION PERIOD. Disease is caused by histomonads penetrating the cecal wall, multiplying, entering the bloodstream, and eventually parasitizing the liver. Overt signs of histomoniasis are apparent from 7 to 12 days and occur most commonly 11 days postinfection (PI). The incubation period is similar following all natural methods of infection, i.e., histomonad-containing heterakid egg, earthworm, and arthropod transmission. Experimentally, lesions develop about 3 days earlier after cloacal inoculation of turkeys with cultured histomonads compared with infection via heterakid eggs.

CLINICAL SIGNS. Early signs of histomoniasis in turkeys include sulfur-colored feces (Fig. 33.10B), drowsiness, dropping of the wings, walking with a stilted gait, closed eyes, head down close to the body or tucked under a wing, and anorexia. The head may or may not be cyanotic, a sign observed by those who gave the disease the name blackhead. About 12 days PI, turkeys become emaciated. Infections in chickens may be mild and go unnoticed, or may be severe and cause high mortality. Sulfur-colored droppings associated with histomoniasis in turkeys are seldom found in chickens, but bloody cecal discharges have been observed. Sometimes gross pathology in chickens may resemble cecal coccidiosis.

CLINICAL PATHOLOGY. Total leukocytes are increased to a maximum count of 70,000/mm^3 after 10 days PI and return to normal levels after 21 days PI. The increase in leukocytes is composed mainly of heterophils; lymphocyte, basophil, and erythrocyte counts are unchanged.

There is a decline in serum nitrogen, uric acid, and hemoglobin levels during the incubation period but these return to normal prior to death. Blood sugar levels rise during the cecal phase, decrease during liver lesion development, and drop below normal prior to death. Serum albumin falls very low, but the alpha and beta globulins increase slightly, and the gamma globulins increase greatly during the acute infection in turkeys (20).

Plasma levels of glutamic oxaloacetic transaminase (GOT) and lactic dehydrogenase (LDH) increase as liver lesions develop in turkeys (21), but glutamic pyruvic transaminase (GPT) remains essentially unchanged. There is very little GPT activity in avian liver or other tissues, suggesting that it is not an important enzyme in birds. Appearance of a brilliant yellow urine pigment coincides with depressed liver function and elevated enzyme resulting from tissue damage. In chickens with cecal lesions but without liver lesions, there is an actual decline in plasma levels of GOT, LDH, malic dehydrogenase, and other enzymes, suggesting impaired liver function. Cholinesterase is also depressed, further suggesting depressed liver function, even though gross liver lesions are not apparent. In acutely ill turkeys the proportion of hemoglobins in the methemoglobin state in the blood is greatly elevated, possibly contributing to cyanosis and the purported blackhead appearance.

MORBIDITY AND MORTALITY. Host response to the infective agent may be variable and is influenced by method and amount of exposure. In natural infections mortality usually reaches a peak at about 17 days and then subsides by the end of 4 wk. Farmer and Stephenson (8) reported that turkeys confined to areas contaminated by chickens have had 89% morbidity and 70% mortality. Experimentally, mortality has reached 100% in turkeys. Although mortality from histomoniasis in chickens is generally low, mortality has exceeded 30% in some natural infections. Occasionally, a strain of *Histomonas* with high virulence for chickens is found.

GROSS LESIONS. The primary lesions of histomoniasis develop in the ceca and liver (Fig. 33.10). Lesions are observed initially in ceca about the 8th day. After tissue invasion by histomonads, cecal walls become thickened and hyperemic. Serous and hemorrhagic exudate from the mucosa fills the lumen of ceca, distends the walls with a caseous or cheesy core, and ulceration of the cecal wall may lead to perforation of the organ and cause generalized peritonitis.

Liver lesions in turkeys are often apparent on the 10th day of infection and are highly variable in appearance. Often the lesion is described as a circular depressed area of necrosis up to 1 cm in diameter and is circumscribed by a raised ring. While these lesions are seen often (Fig. 33.10C, F), they may take on other appearances. In heavy infections lesions may be small, numerous, and mostly subsurface, and they may involve a large part of the liver. In rare cases of recovery, lesions leave purulent scars on the surface of the liver. The liver may be enlarged and discolored green or tan. Lesions in lung, kidney, spleen, and mesenteries are sometimes recognized as white rounded areas of necrosis.

HISTOPATHOLOGY. Initial invasion of the cecal wall results in hyperemia and heterophil leukocyte infiltration, probably a combined response to bacteria, histomonads, and heterakid juveniles (2). Within 5–6 days, numerous histomonads are visible as pale, lightly stained, ovoid bodies within lacunae in the lamina propria and muscularis mucosa. Large numbers of lymphocytes and macrophages have infiltrated tissues by this time, and the heterophil population has also increased. There is a core in the cecal lumen composed of sloughed epithelium, fibrin, erythrocytes, and leukocytes along with trapped cecal ingesta. The core may initially be amorphous and red-tinged, but by about 12 days it appears laminated, dry, and yellowish from buildup of successive layers of exudate. By 12–16 days giant cells appear in cecal tissues. Coagulation necrosis and histomonad invasion extend well into the muscular tunic, extending nearly to the serosa. At about 17–21 days histomonads are scarce within the tissues, mostly concentrated near the serosal layers. Large numbers of giant cells form and may appear grossly as granulomata bulging upon the serosal aspect of the cecum. Old lesions, after recovery, are characterized by lymphoid centers scattered throughout the cecal tissue. Expulsion of cores and regeneration of epithelium may occur, but the cecum is often abnormally thin and crypts are shallow.

The earliest microscopic lesions are visible in the liver by about 6–7 days PI and consist of small clusters of heterophils, lymphocytes, and monocytes near portal vessels. Histomonads are difficult to locate in these areas. After about 10–14 days the lesions are enlarged, becoming confluent in some areas. There is extensive lymphocytic and macrophage infiltration, and heterophils are present in moderate numbers. Hepatocytes in centers of the lesions necrose and disintegrate. Many individual or clustered histomonads are visible in lacunae near the periphery of lesions. From 14 to 21 days PI necrosis becomes increasingly severe, resulting in large areas consisting of little more than reticulum and cellular debris. Histomonads at this stage are present mostly as small bodies in macrophages. If recovery occurs, foci of lymphoid cells remain, along with areas of fibrosis and regenerating hepatocytes.

IMMUNITY

Active. Immunity arising in turkeys naturally or experimentally infected with histomonads is not sufficient to give complete protection against reinfection. Most work with immunity in turkeys has relied on drug-limiting infections, since turkeys usually die from the disease.

Attempts to immunize chickens and turkeys with in vitro attenuated or nonpathogenic histomonads have been only partially successful. Some protection has been demonstrated against cloacal inoculation of pathogenic or attenuated strains of histomonads but very little against histomonad-containing heterakid eggs (18). Although reports are not in agreement, some protective immunity may be obtained while drug therapy is being administered.

Precipitating antibodies against antigens prepared from infected livers and ceca have been demonstrated in serum of chickens and turkeys 10–12 days PI. Antibodies in turkeys and fowl apparently did not confer resistance to reinfection, but were connected with infection of cecal mucosa and persisted in turkeys and fowl for a considerable time (3). Birds recovering from histomoniasis may harbor parasites in the ceca without signs or lesions of the disease (5).

Passive. Attempts to transfer immunity from resistant to susceptible chickens and turkeys by repeated intraperitoneal injections of serum from immune birds have been unsuccessful. When birds receiving immune serum were challenged by cloacal inoculation of infected liver homogenates, turkeys died from histomoniasis and all chickens developed typical cecal lesions (4, 5).

Diagnosis.

Most experienced poultry workers make a diagnosis on the basis of gross appearance of lesions, but laboratory confirmation by poultry disease specialists should be sought to rule out concurrent infections with other agents that affect the ceca or liver (coccidiosis, salmonellosis, aspergillosis, upper digestive tract trichomoniasis).

Presence of characteristic lesions is sufficient for presumptive diagnosis. Identification of histomonads requires careful microscopy, preferably with phase-contrast using fresh specimens from birds recently killed in the laboratory and maintained with reasonable warmth during preparation. Histomonads remain active and are more easily identified if the microscope stage is warmed, either with a special stage incubator or small incandescent light bulb.

Histomonads found in the cecal lumen are easily seen and identified, but histomonads found in tissue lesions are nonflagellated and can be differentiated from macrophages and yeast cells only with difficulty.

For routine diagnostic histopathology any of several stains, including hematoxylin and eosin or periodic acid–Schiff, may be used (13). Excellent cytologic preparations have been made from fresh cultures using Hollande's cupric picroformol and a protein-silver stain.

Where freshly killed birds are available, it is a simple matter to cultivate histomonads in vitro as a diagnostic aid (19), using a modification of Dwyer's (6) medium. If samples are taken from freshly killed birds (before body heat has been lost), the test is over 75% accurate. The medium consists of 85% Medium 199 in Hank's balanced salt solution, 5% chicken embryo extract (CEE50, Gibco), and 10% horse or sheep serum adjusted to pH 7.2. A small amount (10–20 mg) of rice powder (Difco) is added, then tubes are sealed, incubated at 40 C overnight, and observed with an inverted microscope. Cultures obtained in this way can be maintained by subculturing every 2–3 days, but they will become nonpathogenic within 6–8 wk.

Prevention and Control. Since primary means of transmission of histomoniasis occurs through the vehicle of heterakid eggs, successful control measures are directed in large part toward reduction or exclusion of the eggs.

Exclusion of domestic chickens from turkey-raising operations is essential, since chickens may often harbor large numbers of egg-laying cecal worms. Turkey ranges can become severely contaminated with long-lived heterakid eggs, thus creating a situation in which histomoniasis recurs in turkey flocks for many years. Because of the longevity of infectious eggs, range rotation is not practical as a solution. Survival of heterakid eggs may be diminished by providing sunny, well-drained ranges so that lethal effects of solar radiation and dryness can have maximum effect.

Rearing turkeys indoors seems to reduce incidence of blackhead, possibly by eliminating access to earthworms, but this has not helped with chickens. Leghorn pullets often become infected in problem houses where worm eggs have built up in number for several years. In Australia, histomoniasis has been a problem in broilers for many years. In some instances disinfection may have value in killing worm eggs, but there is little published data.

Management practices alone are rarely adequate to keep the disease at a low level in commercial turkey flocks; therefore, preventive chemotherapy is usually practiced during the high-risk part of the grow-out. Preventive chemotherapy is not ordinarily practiced with chickens except on problem farms or in localities where there is high incidence of outbreaks.

Five drugs were at one time registered for use in the USA (9), including two arsenicals, two nitroimidazoles, and one nitrofuran (Table 33.6), but recent regulatory action has removed the most useful drugs (nitroimidazoles) from the market. Other drugs are available outside the USA. For preventive use nitarsone may be effective, but the arsenicals are generally not strong enough for treatment of established infections. The nitroimidazoles (dimetridazole, ipronidazole, or ronidazole) were highly effective for prevention or treatment in chickens or turkeys. These important drugs are still available in many countries. Furazolidone has also been used for treatment of blackhead disease. There is no reported sign of drug resistance in histomonads. For a historical review of older literature on these drugs, see Joyner et al. (12) and Joyner (11).

TRICHOMONIASIS. Trichomoniasis in birds, affecting the upper digestive tract, is caused by the flagellated protozoan *Trichomonas gallinae* (Fig. 33.12). In pigeons, it causes a condition known as "canker." Turkeys, chickens, and a wide variety of wild birds are parasitized with varying degrees of pathogenicity (15).

Description. These intestinal flagellates are rapidly moving, pear-shaped protozoa that range in size from 5–9 μm in length and 2–9 μm in width (Fig. 33.13). There are typically 4 free flagella arising from a basal granule at the anterior pole of the organism. A slender axostyle usually extends well beyond the posterior end of the body. An undulating membrane originates at the anterior pole of the body and ends short of the posterior pole, with the enclosed flagellum not trailing free at the posterior end. The flagella and internal structures can only be seen with the aid of phase-contrast microscopy or special stains.

Incidence and Distribution. Squabs usually become infected with their first taste of "pigeon milk" from the crop of adults and usually remain carriers throughout life. With virulent strains, mortality may be as high as 50% before sufficient

Table 33.6. Feed additives used in the USA for prevention or treatment of blackhead disease in turkeys. Some products are also available for water treatment

Drug	Trade Name	Supplier	Conditions of Use: Use Level	Conditions of Use: Withdrawal	Approval for Chickens
Carbarsone[a]	Carb-O-Sep	Whitmoyer	0.025–0.037%	5	No
Dimetridazole[a]	Emtrymix	Salsbury	0.015–0.02%[b] or 0.16–0.08%[c]	5	No
Furazolidone	nf-180	Rhodia/Hess & Clark	0.011%[b]	5	Yes
	Furox	Smith-Kline	0.022%[c]	5	Yes
Ipronidazole[a]	Ipropan	Hoffmann-La Roche	0.00625%[b]	4	No
			0.0625%[c]	4	No
Nitarsone	Histostat-50	Salsbury	0.01875%	5	Yes

[a]No longer available.
[b]Preventive level.
[c]Treatment level.

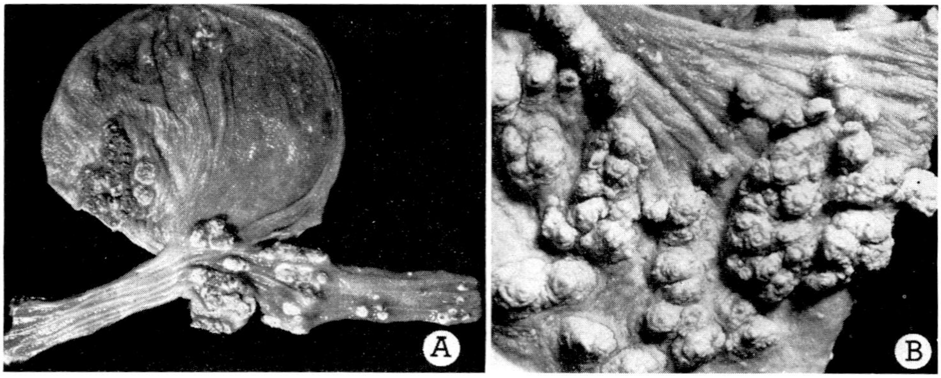

33.12. Trichomoniasis. A. Necrotic ulceration of esophagus and crop. B. Close-up of typical pyramidlike necrotic ulcers characteristic of trichomoniasis of upper digestive tract. (Hinshaw and Rosenwald)

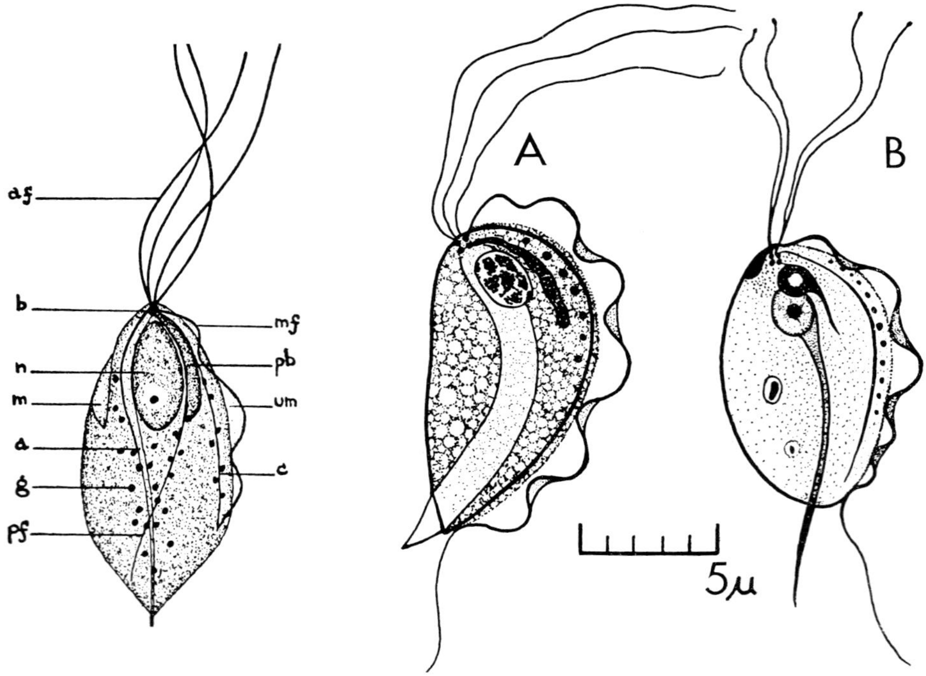

33.13. *Trichomonas gallinae,* semidiagrammatic (*left*): (*a*) axostyle, (*af*) anterior flagellum, (*b*) blepharoplast, (*c*) costa, (*g*) cytoplasmic granules, (*m*) mouth, (*mf*) marginal filament, (*n*) nucleus, (*pb*) parabasal body, (*pf*) parabasal fibril, (*um*) undulating membrane. (Stabler). Diagrammatic representations of two common trichomonads of lower digestive tract of domestic birds (*right*), as favorable specimens fixed in Schaudinn's fluid and stained with Heidenhain's hematoxylin may appear. A. *Tritrichomonas eberthi.* B. *Trichomonas gallinarum.* (Lund)

protective immunity develops. Pigeons are often blamed for transmission of trichomoniasis to turkeys and chickens. The economic impact of the disease in turkeys and chickens is difficult to assess, although infections are occasionally reported. When captive birds of prey such as falcons are allowed to feed on pigeons, infection may result in a condition known as "frounce" among falconers.

Life Cycle. *T. gallinae* reproduces by longitudinal binary fission. Cysts, sexual stages, or vectors are not known. The organism is transferred to squabs by infection of "pigeon milk" from adults. In chicken and turkey flocks, infection is spread by contamination of drinking water and perhaps feed.

Pathogenesis and Pathology. Nearly all pigeons are carriers of this organism. Affected birds may cease to feed and become listless, ruffled in appearance, and emaciated before death. A greenish to yellowish fluid may be seen in the oral cavity and may drip from the beaks of infected birds.

GROSS LESIONS. *T. gallinae* invade the mucosal surface of the buccal cavity, sinuses, pharynx, esophagus, crop, and occasionally the conjunctiva and proventriculus. The liver is frequently invaded, and occasionally other organs, but not the digestive tract below the proventriculus.

Lesions appear initially as small, circumscribed caseous areas on the surface of the oral mucosa, which may be surrounded by a thin zone of hyperemia. These may enlarge and become confluent. The buildup of caseous material may be sufficient to partially or completely occlude the lumen of the esophagus. These lesions may eventually penetrate tissue and extensively involve other regions of the head and neck, including the nasopharynx, orbits, and cervical soft tissues. In the liver, lesions appear on the surface and extend into the parenchyma as solid, white to yellow circular or spherical masses.

HISTOPATHOLOGY. Pigeons infected with a virulent strain of *T. gallinae* had purulent inflammation with caseation necrosis as the predominant lesion (26). Trichomonads multiplied locally in secretions and on the mucosal surface of the oropharynx. Ulceration of the mucosa with a massive inflammatory response, primarily heterophils, was well established by the 4th day of infection. In the liver, focal necrotic abscesses occurred in all zones of lobules, with an inflammatory reaction characterized by mononuclear cells and heterophils. As liver lesions progressed, no intact hepatocytes remained in the center of foci; trichomonads were most numerous at the periphery.

IMMUNITY. Relatively high incidence of infections in otherwise normal pigeons can be attributed to strain variations, acquired immunity, or both. Pigeons are immune to disease from virulent strains of trichomonads after recovery from sublethal trichomoniasis. Plasma from pigeons harboring any of three strains of *T. gallinae* was capable of protecting other pigeons against disease but not infection from a virulent strain.

Antigens of *T. gallinae* have been studied in regard to taxonomy with the conclusion that virulence and antigenic composition were related (7).

Diagnosis. Clinical signs and gross lesions are highly suggestive and may be confirmed by microscopic observation of organisms in direct wet smears from the mouth or crop. Histopathologic examination or cultivation of organisms in artificial media may help in cases where the parasites are absent in fresh smears. Trichomoniasis must be differentiated from candidiasis and hypovitaminosis-A, which can produce somewhat similar lesions. History, cultivation for fungi, and histopathologic examination may prove useful in resolving problem diagnoses.

Several other species of flagellates that inhabit the avian gastrointestinal tract are frequently misidentified as *T. gallinae.* These other species of trichomonads and more distantly related flagellates have never been unequivocally demonstrated to be pathogenic for the avian host. Their recognition as harmless commensals will prevent unnecessary expenditures for therapeutic measures.

One trichomonad, *Tetratrichomonas gallinarum* (*Trichomonas gallinarum*), is a common inhabitant of the cecum of chickens and other gallinaceous birds. This trichomonad or a closely related species has occasionally been isolated from liver and blood. Although lesions have been ascribed to this organism, no confirmation of pathogenicity has come from experimental infection.

Other lower intestinal protozoa such as *Chilomastix gallinarum* (Fig. 33.14), a cyst-forming flagellate with a large cytostomal cleft but no undulating membrane, and *Cochlosoma anatis,* with a ventral sucker covering half the surface of the body, are apparently nonpathogenic. Although additional controlled experiments with flagellates found in the lower intestine are needed, for the present they should not be considered important.

Prevention and Control. Since *T. gallinae* is transmitted from parent to squab in pigeons, and by contamination of feed and water by oral fluids in the case of domestic fowl, every effort should be made to remove infected birds from a flock. Experimentally, several drugs are active against trichomoniasis in pigeons or turkeys. McLoughlin (24) found dimetridazole useful at a level of 0.05%

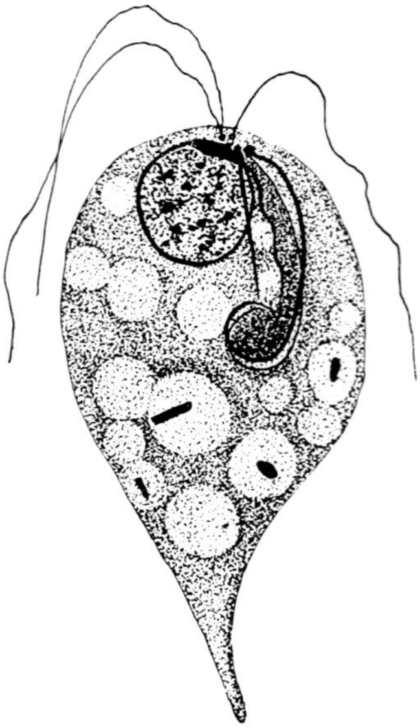

33.14. *Chilomastix gallinarum,* semidiagrammatic, illustrating details of morphology. ×5000. (Boeck and Tanabe)

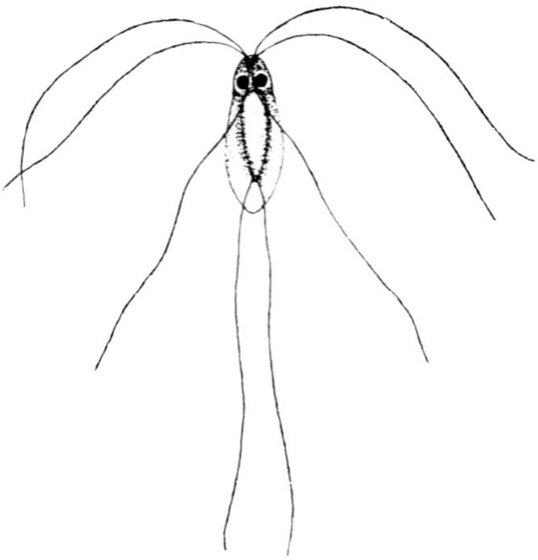

33.15. *Hexamita meleagridis* from intestine of turkey. ×1875. (25)

in drinking water for pigeons. This drug is no longer available in the USA.

HEXAMITIASIS

Etiology and Distribution. Hexamitiasis, or infectious catarrhal enteritis, of poults is caused by the protozoan *Hexamita meleagridis.* The USDA (32) estimated that an annual loss of $667,000 occurred from hexamitiasis in turkeys from 1942 to 1951. However, only 10 cases were reported in the USA in 1986 (1). The disease has been reported from several areas of the USA, Canada, Scotland, England, and Germany. The organism has also been found in pheasants, quail, chukar partridges, and peafowl, which may be a source of infection for turkey poults. The 8 prominent flagella include 4 anterior, 2 anterolateral, and 2 posterior. The 4 anterior flagella are recurved along the body (Fig. 33.15). McNeil et al. (25), who named the species, described it as being 6–12.4 × 2–5 μm in size with binucleate large endosomes.

Pathology. Affected poults do not show specific signs, but a watery diarrhea occurs that may become yellowish later in the course of the disease. The poults at first are nervous and active but later tend to become listless and huddled. Convulsions and coma may occur as the terminal stage is approached.

Lesions include catarrhal inflammation and atony resulting in distention, especially in the upper small intestine. Intestinal contents are watery, and large numbers of hexamitae may be seen in the crypts upon microscopic examination. A yellowish discoloration of the liver surface was described in an outbreak in Germany.

Diagnosis. Presence of watery diarrhea and demonstration of hexamitae in fresh smears of duodenal contents are sufficient to establish the diagnosis. Since carrier birds may occur among survivors, presence of *H. meleagridis* without signs may occur. Hexamitae move very rapidly, with a darting motion, and are quite small compared to other flagellates that may be encountered in the avian digestive tract.

Control and Treatment. Removal of carrier birds, separation of older stock from poults, and exclusion of other avian host species from the area of the poult flock, along with cleanliness around feeders and waterers should minimize transmission. Approved drugs (9) for feed medication include butynorate (0.0375%), chlortetracycline (0.0055%), and furazolidone (0.022%) alone or in combination with oxytetracycline (0.044%).

MISCELLANEOUS PROTOZOA IN THE DIGESTIVE TRACT. Several species of the genera *Entamoeba* and *Endolimax* occur naturally in ceca or feces of various domestic fowl or are capable of being established experimentally. Apparently none of these are pathogenic; they exist by feeding on intestinal contents.

The amoebas have irregularly shaped trophozoites and a single nucleus with a more or less prominent endosome and produce cysts that when mature contain 1, 4, or 8 nuclei. These organisms may be difficult to see without using warm smears and phase-contrast microscopy or stained preparations. Accounts of a number of species have been reported by McDowell (23), Lund (17), or Levine (15).

REFERENCES

1. AAAP Committee on Disease Reporting. 1986. Summary of commercial poultry disease reports. Avian Dis 31:926–987.

2. Clarkson, M.J. 1962. Studies on the immunity to Histomonas meleagridis in the turkey and the fowl. Res Vet Sci 3:443–448.

3. Clarkson, M.J. 1963. Immunity to Histomoniasis (blackhead). Immunology 6:156–168.

4. Clarkson, M.J. 1966. Progressive serum protein changes in turkeys infected with Histomonas meleagridis. J Comp Pathol 76:387–397.

5. Cuckler, A.C. 1970. Coccidiosis and histomoniasis in avian hosts. In G.J. Jackson, R. Herman, and I. Singer (eds.), Immunity to Parasitic Animals, pp. 371–397. Appleton-Century-Crofts, New York.

6. Dwyer, D.M. 1970. An improved method for cultivating Histomonas meleagridis. J Parasitol 56:191–192.

7. Dwyer, D.M. 1974. Analysis of the antigenic relationships among Trichomonas, Histomonas, Dientamoeba, and Entamoeba. J Protozool 21:139–145.

8. Farmer, R.K., and J. Stephenson. 1949. Infectious enterohepatitis (blackhead) in turkeys: A comparative study of methods of infection. J Comp Pathol 59:119–126.

9. Feed Additive Compendium. 1988. Miller Publishing Co., Minneapolis, MN.

10. Gibbs, B.J. 1962. The occurrence of the protozoan parasite Histomonas meleagridis in the adult and eggs of the cecal worm Heterakis gallinae. J Protozool 59:877–884.

11. Joyner, L.P. 1966. Chemotherapy of histomoniasis. In R.J. Schnitzer and F. Hawking (eds.), Experimental Chemotherapy, Vol 4, pp. 425–428. Academic Press, New York.

12. Joyner, L.P., S.F.M. Davies, and S.D. Kendall. 1963. Chemotherapy of histomoniasis. In R.J. Schnitzer and F. Hawking (eds.), Experimental Chemotherapy, Vol 1, pp. 333–349. Academic Press, New York.

13. Kemp, R.L., and W.M. Reid. 1966. Staining techniques for differential diagnosis of histomoniasis and mycosis in domestic poultry. Avian Dis 10:357–363.

14. Lee, D.L. 1969. The structure and development of Histomonas meleagridis (Masticamoebidae: Protozoa) in the female reproductive tract of its host, Heterakis gallinae (Nematoda). Parasitology 59:877–884.

15. Levine, N.D. 1973. Protozoan Parasites of Domestic Animals and of Man, 2nd Ed. Burgess, Minneapolis, MN.

16. Lund, E.E. 1969. Histomoniasis. Adv Vet Sci Comp Med 13:355–390.

17. Lund, E.E. 1972. Other protozoan diseases. In M.S. Hofstad, B.W. Calnek, C.F. Hembold, W.M. Reid, and H.W. Yoder Jr. (eds.), Diseases of Poultry, 6th Ed., pp 990–1046. Iowa Sate Univ Press, Ames.

18. Lund, E.E., P.C. Augustine, and D.J. Ellis. 1966. Earthworm transmission of Heterakis and Histomonas to turkeys and chickens. Exp Parasitol 18:403–407.

19. McDougald, L., and R.B. Galloway. 1973. Blackhead disease in vitro isolation of Histomonas meleagridis as a potentially useful diagnostic aid. Avian Dis 17:847–450.

20. McDougald, L.R., and M.F. Hansen. 1969. Serum protein changes in chickens subsequent to infection with Histomonas meleagridis. Avian Dis 13:673–677.

21. McDougald, L.R., and M.F. Hansen. 1970. Histomonas meleagridis: Effect on plasma enzymes in chickens and turkeys. Exp Parasitol 27:229–235.

22. McDougald, L.R., and W.M. Reid. 1976. Protozoa of Medical and Veterinary Interest, Vol. 1, pp. 140–161. Academic Press, New York.

23. McDowell, S., Jr. 1953. A morphological and taxonomic study of the caecal protozoa of the common fowl, Gallus gallus L. J Morphol 92:337–399.

24. McLoughlin, D.K. 1966. Observations on the treatment of Trichomonas gallinae in pigeons. Avian Dis 10:288–290.

25. McNeil, E., W.R. Hinshaw, and C.A. Kofoid. 1941. Hexamita meleagridis sp. nov. from the turkey. Am J Hyg 34:71–82.

26. Perez Mesa, C., R.M. Stabler, and M. Berthrong. 1961. Histopathological changes in the domestic pigeon infected with Trichomonas gallinae (Jones' Barn Strain). Avian Dis 5:48–60.

27. Reid, W.M. 1967. Etiology and dissemination of the blackhead disease syndrome in turkeys and chickens. Exp Parasitol 21:249–275.

28. Ruff, M.D., L.R. McDougald, and M.F. Hansen. 1970. Isolation of Histomonas meleagridis from embryonated eggs of the Heterakis gallinarum. J Protozool 17:10–11.

29. Springer, W.T., J. Johnson, and W.M. Reid. 1969. Transmission of Histomoniasis with male Heterakis gallinarum (Nematoda). Parasitology 59:401–405.

30. Tyzzer, E.E. 1920. The flagellate character of the parasite producing "blackhead" in turkeys, Histomonas meleagridis. J Parasitol 6:124–130.

31. Tyzzer, E.E. 1934. Studies on histomoniasis, or "blackhead" infection, in the chicken and turkey. Proc Am Acad Arts Sci 69:189–264.

32. USDA. 1954. Losses in Agriculture. US Dept Agric, ARS, Washington, DC.

OTHER BLOOD AND TISSUE PROTOZOA

Wilfred T. Springer

LEUCOCYTOZOONOSIS. This parasitic disease of birds affects blood and tissue cells of internal organs. The disease has been named after the parasites belonging to the protozoan genus *Leucocytozoon*. Reviews of this and other parasitic diseases were summarized from: Lund (54), Levine (49), and Fallis et al. (21).

Leucocytozoon was assigned to the suborder Haemospororina of the phylum Apicomplexa by a committee of the Society of Protozoologists (52). Levine (49) suggested that similarities in life cycle and ultrastructure of some life stages of *Leucocytozoon, Haematroteus,* and *Plasmodium* warrant inclusion of all three genera in a single family, Plasmodiidae.

Criteria for species designation include host range and gametocyte characteristics, such as staining characteristics, size, nature, and extent of distortion of the host cell and altered shape and position of the host cell nucleus (21). Approximately 67 valid species and 34 synonyms have been described. With the exception of a species observed in the teiid lizard in Brazil, all species of *Leucocytozoon* are found in birds (34).

The life cycle includes reproduction by sporogony in insects with schizogony (merogony) in tissue cells, and gametogony in erythrocytes or leukocytes. The disease is prevalent in areas with a suitable ecology and ethology for dipterous invertebrate hosts, simuliid flies and culicoid midges. At least 3 species of *Leucocytozoon* reported in domestic fowl are known to have caused outbreaks in North America resulting in economic losses in ducks, geese, turkeys and chickens.

LEUCOCYTOZOON SIMONDI **MATHIS AND LEGER 1910.** Infection with *L. simondi* has been reported from 27 species of ducks and geese in USA, Canada, Europe, and Vietnam by Hsu et al. (34). They consider *L. anatis* from ducks and *L. anseris* from geese as synonyms of *L. simondi.* Approximately 20% of ducks and geese along the northeastern seaboard of North America each year carry *Leucocytozoon* infections (6). Eighty percent of geese at Seney Wildlife Refuge had some parasitemia in 1963 just prior to the egg-laying season, and each year all goslings become infected (33).

ETIOLOGY. Sporogony occurs in the insect vector and may be completed in 3–4 days. Ookinetes develop following fertilization of the macrogametocyte and may be found in the stomach of the insect within 12 hr after a blood meal. Oocysts form from the ookinetes within the stomach of the invertebrate host and produce sporozoites that migrate to the salivary glands after emerging from the oocyst. Viable sporozoites have been found in vectors up to 18 days after the last blood meal.

Schizogony takes place in such internal organs of the vertebrate host as liver, brain, spleen, and lungs. "Hepatic schizonts" in liver cells measure up to 45 μm when mature. Merozoites and syncytia are released from hepatic schizonts (syncytium refers to cytoplasm bounded by a plasma membrane and containing two or more nuclei). There is some indication that some merozoites may enter parenchymal cells of the liver and initiate another schizogonic cycle while others enter erythrocytes or erythroblasts to develop into gametocytes. Apparently, syncytia are phagocytized by macrophages or reticuloendothelial cells throughout the body, where they develop into megaloschizonts up to 400 μm in size. Merozoites released from the megaloschizont enter lymphocytes and other leukocytes to form gametocytes.

The gametocytes of *L. simondi* found in the blood average 14.5 × 5.5 μm, and usually inhabit elongate spindle-shaped host cells averaging about 48 μm in length. The parasite lies beside the nucleus of the host cell, which is about 30 μm in length. Round gametocytes have been reported also. Elongate gametocytes probably develop exclusively in leukocytes, predominantly lymphocytes and monocytes, while mature round gametocytes are found in erythrocytes. According to Allan and Mahrt (2), each *Leucocytozoon* species has gametogony in only one type of host cell; therefore, the presence of two morphological types in the same bird indicates a concurrent host infection with two species. Desser et al. (16) observed infections in some areas of northern Michigan that were characterized by presence of both hepatic schizonts and round gametocytes, which he attributed to different strains of *L. simondi.*

Gamonts may be differentiated with a Romanowsky stain based on the dark blue–staining cytoplasm of the macrogamete with its red nucleus and the very pale blue–staining cytoplasm of the microgamont with its pale pink nucleus. The microgamonts are more delicate and subject to distortion (49).

PATHOGENESIS AND EPIZOOTIOLOGY. Ducks and geese are suitable hosts for *L. simondi* but chickens, turkeys, pheasants, and ruffed grouse are not.

Simulium venustum, a blood-sucking fly, was first demonstrated to be the vector among ducks. Others species of this insect shown to be transmitters of *Leucocytozoon* are *S. croxtoni, S. euradminiculum,* and *S. rugglesi.*

The pathogenicity of *L. simondi* in ducks and geese is well documented. An outbreak of *L. simondi* among ducks in Michigan resulted in 35% mortality. Extensive losses of young goslings attributed to infections of *L. simondi* are observed annually at Seney Wildlife Refuge, with mortality greater than 70% occurring every 4 yr (33).

Clinical signs vary with age and condition of the host. Young ducklings manifest inappetence, weakness, listlessness, dyspnea, and sometimes death within 24 hr. Signs in adults appear less abruptly and consist of listlessness and low mortality. About 60% of fatalities occur 11–19 days postexposure. Some pathologic effects of the disease are anemia, leukocytosis, splenomegaly, and liver degeneration and hypertrophy. Extensive tissue damage was noted in the spleen and heart of ducks carrying megaloschizonts.

Kocan (48) described an antierythrocyte factor in sera from acutely infected ducks, which agglutinated and hemolyzed normal untreated duck erythrocytes as well as infected cells. This factor was believed to be a product of the parasite, and its action was intravascular; it may account for the osmotic fragility of erythrocytes and anemia associated with *L. simondi* infections (55).

The greatest number of infections in northern Michigan occur mostly in July, the hottest part of the summer. Gametocytes decrease in number in the blood until midwinter, when they disappear or become scarce and then reappear in the spring.

***LEUCOCYTOZOON SMITHI* LAVERAN AND LUCET 1905.** *L. smithi* was first seen in turkeys in the eastern USA by T. Smith, after whom it is named, and since reported in turkeys in North Dakota, Minnesota, Nebraska, California, Texas, Missouri, France, Germany, the Crimea, and Canada.

In the USA it is widespread in adult turkeys (75); 289 of 357 turkeys were found infected in Georgia, 60 of 67 in Florida, 4 of 12 in Alabama, and 7 of 9 in South Carolina. The incidence of infection in pen-raised and free-ranging mature wild turkeys in the Cumberland State Forest in Virginia was 100%.

ETIOLOGY. *L. smithi* may be observed in the blood as rounded gametocytes that later become elongate, averaging 20–22 μm in length. They inhabit elongate cells averaging 45 × 14 μm, with pale cytoplasmic "horns" extending out beyond the enclosed parasite. The host cell forms a long, thin dark band along each side of the parasite; often it is split, forming a band on each side. Gamonts are found only in leukocytes. The staining characteristics of the gamonts with a Romanowsky stain are similar to those of *L. simondi* (49) (Fig. 33.16A).

Intracellular schizogonous forms are found in the liver. Both schizonts and megaloschizonts were observed and illustrated by Siccardi et al. (67).

Several aspects of the life cycle were described in detail by Newberne and Wehr (see 54); the ultrastructure of gametocytes was defined by Milhous and Solis (59).

PATHOGENESIS AND EPIZOOTIOLOGY. *L. smithi* generally resembles *L. simondi* of Anseriformes, but turkeys are probably not susceptible to the latter. *L. smithi* is not transmissible experimentally to chickens or ducks.

Simulium occidentale, S. aureum, S. meridionale, S. nigroparvum, and *S. slossonae* have been listed as vectors for *L. smithi* (21, 47).

The progress of leucocytozoonosis in susceptible young turkeys may be rapid and fatal. Clinical signs include anorexia, excessive thirst, depression, somnolence, and sometimes muscular incoordination. Death may occur suddenly during the acute stage of the disease.

Heavy infections of *L. smithi,* comparable to those reported for *L. simondi* in ducks, do not seem to occur in mature wild turkeys. Few signs of infection are observed in wild turkeys possibly because of local factors such as time at which suitable vectors are prevalent and age of birds at first exposure.

Domestic hens infected with *Leucocytozoon* spp. had decreased egg production, egg weight, and hatchability, and higher mortality than uninfected hens (42).

Recovered birds may harbor the parasite in their blood for more than 1 yr (17). There is often loss of vigor, and birds may suffer moist tracheal rales and coughing. Some birds die when subjected to stress. Males showed reduced mating activity (49).

Johnson et al. (40) reported that death results from obstruction of the circulatory system by large numbers of parasites. Congestion of the lungs, small intestine, liver, and spleen, and enlargement of the liver and spleen are frequently observed in affected turkeys. Lund (54) cites descriptive reports of the pathogenesis of the disease.

***LEUCOCYTOZOON CAULLERYI* MATHIS AND LEGER 1909.** *L. caulleryi* is frequently found in chickens in southern and eastern Asia. Infections occur frequently in Japan (61). Reports of leucocytozoonosis in South Carolina, probably caused by *L. caulleryi,* are the only known cases of the disease in chickens in North America. In one survey 13.6% of domestic yard chickens in South Carolina were infected (64).

ETIOLOGY. *L. andrewsi* and *L. schueffneri* are considered by some protozoologists to be synonymous with *L. caulleryi* (49).

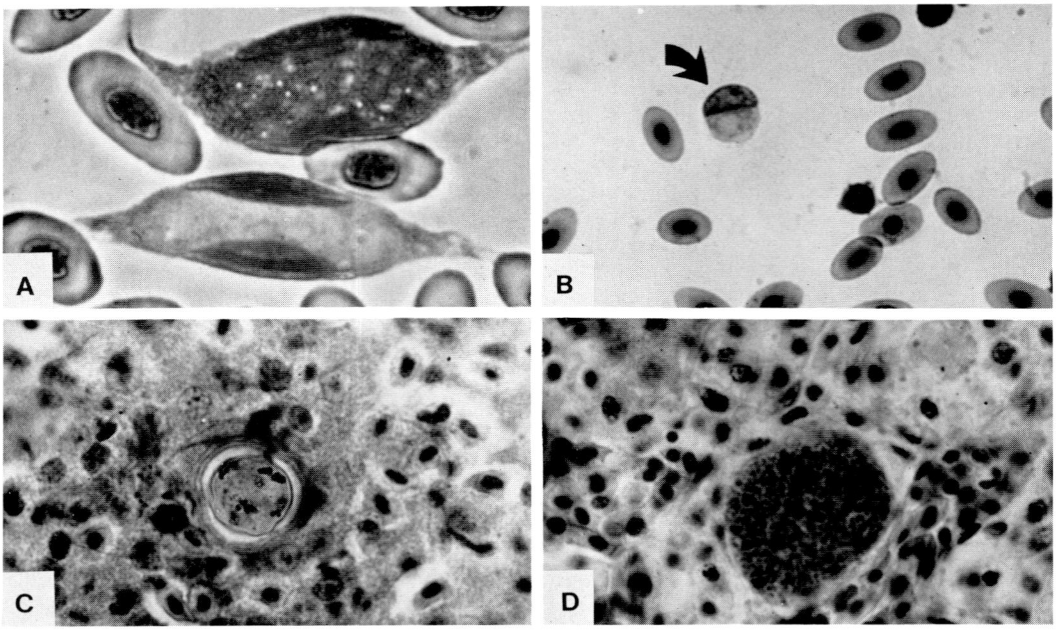

33.16. Photomicrographs of turkey blood containing various stages of *Leucocytozoon smithi*. A. Darkly stained macrogametocyte (*upper*) and lightly stained microgametocyte (*lower*). Giemsa stain, ×1250. B. "Round form" often found early in infection (day 16), ×140. C. Megaloschizont in turkey liver, day 9. H & E. ×1000. D. Megaloschizont turkey kidney, day 10. (Dick)

Mature gamonts are round and occupy round host cells, erythrocytes, and leukocytes about 20 μm in diameter. The nucleus of the host cell reportedly disappears after infection, a characteristic that differs from other species with round gametocytes. Others observed that the nucleus was always present in infected cells leading them to designate the parasite as a new species, *L. andrewsi* (54). Macrogametes (12–15 μm) stain more darkly with Romanowsky stain than microgamonts (10–15 μm) according to Levine (49).

Schizogony occurs in many organs, but more often in lungs, liver, and kidneys. Megaloschizonts and their location in tissues are similar to those of *L. simondi* (21).

PATHOGENESIS AND EPIZOOTIOLOGY. The domestic chicken is the only reported host for this parasite. Insect vectors are *Culicoides arakawa, C. circumscriptus,* and *C. odibilis*. Akiba's discovery that the vector was a species of *Culicoides* and not *Simulium* prompted some to place *L. caulleryi* in a new genus called *Akiba* (21). Leucocytozoonosis epizootics, widespread during summer months in Japan, are serious enough to cause deaths in growing chicks and reduced egg production in hens (61). Serious outbreaks of *L. caulleryi* in chickens are characterized by hemoptysis and severe renal lesions. Apparently, extensive hemorrhage results in the kidneys when merozoites are released from megaloschizonts. Clopidol has been successfully used in preventive medication, while combinations of pyrimethamine and a sulfonamide have been used in treatment.

***LEUCOCYTOZOON SABREZI* MATHIS AND LEGER 1910.** *L. sabrezi* (*L. schueffneri,* probably a synonym) has been found in domestic chickens in Southeast Asia, causing anemia, thickened oral discharge, and paralysis of the legs. Megaloschizont formation has not been reported for this parasite. Merozoites enter both erythroblasts and leukocytes to form elongate gametocytes within spindle-shaped host cells (6–7 × 4–6 μm), whose nuclei appear as thin bands beside the parasite (21). Macrogametes (22 × 6.5 μm) have a more compact nucleus and stain more darkly with a Romanowsky stain than the microgamonts (20 × 6 μm) (49). The insect vector is unknown.

***LEUCOCYTOZOON SCHOUTEDENI* RODHAM, PONS, VANDENBRANDEN, AND BEQUAERT 1913.** *L. schoutedeni,* which was found in 50% of chickens in East Africa (21), is unknown elsewhere. Gametocytes are round (11–13 μm) and found in round host cells (18 μm), whose nuclei surround the parasite about 1/2 its length. Staining characteristics of the gametocytes have not been reported. The *Simulium* fly serves as the invertebrate host for *L. schoutedeni.*

Diagnosis. *Leucocytozoon* infections are diagnosed by direct microscopic observation and identification of gametocytes in stained blood or schizonts in tissue sections. Solis (71) described the high staining contrast of *Leucocytozoon* in peripheral blood films stained with brilliant cresyl blue.

Treatment and Control. Drug treatment of leucocytozoonosis has had limited success. No effective treatment has been found for *L. simondi.* Pyrimethamine (1 ppm) and sulfadimethoxine (10 ppm) administered simultaneously reportedly will prevent, but not cure, infections of *L. caulleryi.* Clopidol in feed effectively controlled *L. smithi* according to Siccardi et al. (67). This drug (0.0125–0.0250% in feed) has been approved by the FDA for medication of turkeys.

Control requires eliminating the insect vector from the environment of the vertebrate host. A large-scale aerial treatment program using 2% Abate Celatom granules for control of larval *Simulium* substantially reduced adult and larval blackfly populations and reduced the level of *L. smithi* blood parasitemia in turkeys in one study (46).

Repellents sprayed within houses to discourage entrance of the insect vector lowered mortality and incidence of disease but did not completely prevent infection in the flock (21). Had proper control measures been implemented, an economic disaster might have been avoided when a new turkey enterprise was established in the coastal plain area of South Carolina. It is advisable to grow susceptible birds in areas free of blackflies and midges.

AVIAN MALARIA. Avian malarial infections are caused by parasites of the genus *Plasmodium* and are characterized by the presence of pigment in erythrocytes. Schizogony occurs in blood and gametocytes are found in mature erythrocytes. Transmission is by mosquitoes. These characteristics distinguish them from other members of the family Plasmodiidae and *Haemoproteus* and *Leucocytozoon* species.

About 65 species of *Plasmodium* from over 1000 different birds have been described, but some 35 or less are considered to be valid (44). The species pathogenic for domestic fowl are found mostly in Asia, Africa, and South America. Malaria outbreaks in birds on the North American continent are sometimes found in species of the orders Anseriformes, Passeriformes, and Columbiformes.

Etiology. Although many species of *Plasmodium* can be introduced into various domestic fowl, only a few appear to be natural parasites of these birds. *P. gallinaceum* occurs in jungle fowl and domestic hens; *P. juxtanucleare* parasitizes domestic hens and turkeys; *P. durae* and *P. griffithsi* occur in turkeys; *P. lophurae* of the fire-backed pheasant can also parasitize chickens and has been host-adapted to other domestic fowl and ducks; *P. fallax* of guinea fowl has been adapted to various domestic fowl; *P. hermani* will infect domestic and wild turkeys and bobwhite quail (27).

A number of other species that occur primarily in passerine birds can infect domestic fowl or have been experimentally transmitted to them. These include *P. relictum, P. elongatum, P. cathemerium,* and *P. circumflexum* (44).

Life Cycle. Only a general outline of the malarian life cycle can be given here. Garnham (30) detailed the life cycles extensively and should be consulted for specific information on various species. Greiner et al. (32) presented color plates of 24 species.

Avian plasmodia characteristically develop in culicine mosquitoes of the genera *Culex* and *Aedes,* and rarely in *Anopheles.* Gametocytes from an avian blood meal are taken up by the mosquito, after which gamete formation, oocysts development, and sporogony occur. Infective sporozoites entering the avian host from the bite of a mosquito invade cells of the reticuloendothelial system and typically progress through two generations of primary exoerythrocytic schizonts: cryptozoites and metacryptozoites. Merozoites produced by the second generation are released into the bloodstream and invade erythrocytes. An interchange of parasites between blood and reticuloendothelial tissues may occur, resulting in secondary exoerythrocytic schizonts (phanerozoites) in many tissues, especially spleen, kidney, and liver endothelial cells. These may be responsible for subsequent heavy parasitemias.

The initial stage of the merozoite after invasion of the erythrocyte, the trophozoite, is known as the ring form because of its appearance. A vacuole is formed within the parasite surrounded by a band of blue cytoplasm containing a peripheral red-stained nucleus after Romanowsky staining. A characteristic malarial pigment is formed as the parasite consumes and metabolizes the host cell hemoglobin and this is visible in stained smears. Subsequently, nuclear division leads to formation of a mature schizont containing a variable number of nuclei. Merozoites differentiate from the schizont, and the host cell ruptures to release merozoites for infection of other erythrocytes. After several asexual cycles, some merozoites differentiate into gametocytes and await ingestion by a suitable mosquito. The species of avian plasmodia vary in numbers of merozoites formed in exoerythrocytic and erythrocytic stages, in timing of the life cycle, and in morphology of different stages.

Pathology and Pathogenesis. The pathologic effects in avian hosts range from no apparent signs to severe anemia and death. *P. gallinaceum, P. juxtanucleare,* and *P. durae* are the most pathogenic for domestic fowl, and may cause 90% mortality. Intense and severe anemia and generalized hypoxia may occur in acute *P. gallinaceum* malaria (44). A similar situation occurs in ducks affected with *P. lophurae.* Severe anemia may also occur in *P. juxtanucleare* infections.

Other pathologic manifestations occur in avian malaria. The exoerythrocytic stages of *P. gallinaceum* may block capillaries in the brain resulting in death due to central nervous system dysfunction. *P. durae,* which can cause high mortality in turkeys, causes extensive fibrosis in many tissues.

Immunity. Immunologic factors such as antigen-antibody complex and hemagglutinins, and such conditions as splenomegaly, anemia, and nephritis have been studied extensively in *P. gallinaceum* infections (57, 73).

Treatment and Control. The life cycle of the malaria parasite must be broken by eradication of mosquitoes or by isolation of the flock from the vector by suitable housing. Quarantine and import controls diminish the chances of importing malarious fowl into areas such as the USA, which are free from the pathogenic species. Although avian models have been used extensively in chemotherapeutic studies, there are no commercially available medications for treatment of avian malaria. Steck (76) reviewed the literature on malaria chemotherapy.

HAEMOPROTEUS INFECTIONS. *Haemoproteus* infections are characterized by schizogony (merogony) in visceral endothelial cells, gametocyte development in circulating erythrocytes, and presence of pigment in granules in infected erythrocytes. Transmission is by various biting dipterans of the families Hippoboscidae and Ceratopogonidae. Characteristics of *Haemoproteus* are similar enough to *Plasmodium* and *Leucocytozoon* that the genera are placed in the same family, Plasmodiidae. Infections occur throughout tropical and temperate areas of the New and Old World wherever vector species and avian hosts coexist.

Over 120 species of *Haemoproteus* have been reported from birds, mostly in wild waterfowl, raptors, passerines, and some other families of birds (51). Synonymization of many of these species may result as life cycles are defined and cross-transmission studies are conducted. Many of the species designations for avian haemoproteids were evaluated by Bennett and coworkers (5, 79).

Species sometimes found in domestic poultry and pet birds include *Haemoproteus meleagridis,* which has been diagnosed in domestic and wild turkeys (31); *H. columbae* and *H. saccharovi* in pigeons and doves; and *H. nettionis* in waterfowl (54).

Etiology. *H. columbae* of pigeons and doves is the most extensively studied of these parasites. The process of sporogony occurs in two families of flies where development time differs. Sporogony is completed in 6–7 days in the ceratopogonids or in 7–14 days in the hippoboscids. Schizonts (meronts) of various sizes and numbers of merozoites occur in the pulmonary vascular endothelium in alveolar septa of pigeons. These merozoites invade erythrocytes and mature into gametocytes (1). Further development requires that erythrocytic forms be ingested by a suitable vector in a blood meal.

Vectors include the hippoboscid *Pseudolynchia canariensis* for *H. columbae* and the ceratopogonid *Culicoides* for *H. nettionis* according to Lund (54). Vectors for *H. meleagridis* include *C. edeni, C. hinmani, C. arboricoli, C. knowltoni,* and *C. haemoproteus* (3).

Atkinson (3) studied experimental infections of *H. meleagridis* in turkeys and partially defined the life cycle. He observed developmental stages of ookinetes, oocysts, sporozoites, and megaloschizonts. At least two generations of schizogony occurred. Maturation of the first generation schizonts occurred 5 and 8 days postinfection (PI), and produced elongate merozoites. Second generation megaloschizonts developed after 8 and 17 days in cardiac and skeletal muscles and yielded spherical merozoites that developed into erythrocytic gametocytes (Fig. 33.17).

Pathology and Pathogenesis. Apparently most haemoproteid species are well adapted to their host, since few clinical signs have been reported. Signs include severe lameness, diarrhea, severe depression, emaciation, and anorexia in turkeys experimentally infected with *H. meleagridis* (3). There are occasional reports of anemia and enlarged livers attributed to infections. At necropsy, myopathy associated with megaloschizonts was found in wild turkeys infected with *H. meleagridis.* Skeletal muscles contained numerous fusiform cysts oriented in parallel order with muscle fibers (4), and eight pigeons with *H. saccharovi* had enlarged gizzards. *H. nettionis* caused lameness, dyspnea, and sudden death with hemorrhage on the heart as well as edematous lungs and swollen firm livers, spleens, and kidneys in mus-

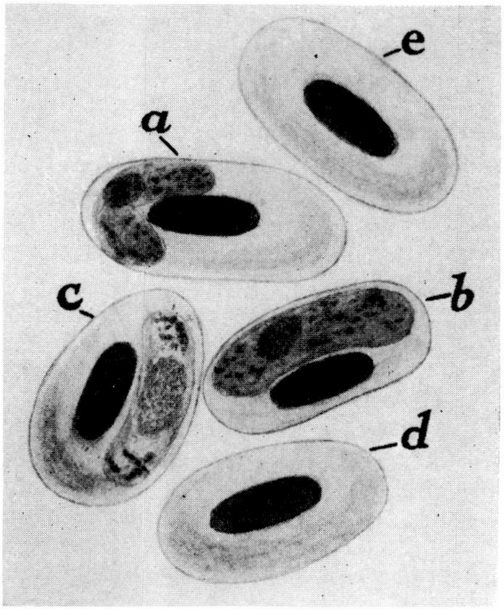

33.17. *Haemoproteus columbae,* pigeon blood: Macrogametocyte in erythrocyte (*a, b*); microgametocyte (*c*); normal erythrocyte (*d, e*). (Drake and Jones)

covy ducks (*Carina moschata*); it was nonpathogenic for other species of ducks (43).

Treatment and Control. Since life cycles are incompletely known for most species, specific control measures are difficult to recommend. The control of hippoboscids or ceratopogonids may be of use in local situations (44). Atebrin and plasmochin may have marginal effects against *H. columbae,* but these drugs are not approved for commercial use.

TRYPANOSOMIASIS. Although trypanosomes have been reported from many species of wild birds, and some species of domestic birds, their pathologic significance appears to be minimal or nil. Even the taxonomic grouping of these organisms is unclear.

Several species have been named, including *Trypanosoma avium, T. numidae, T. calmetti,* and *T. gallinarum.* The possibility that the latter three are synonyms of *T. avium* cannot be ruled out in absence of a rigorous taxonomic study (20).

Observations on *T. avium* and its life cycle were given by Molyneaux (62), who summarized vector relationships for all avian trypanosomes and listed culicine mosquitoes and simuliids as known vectors.

SARCOSPORIDIOSIS. Sarcosporidiosis is a parasitic infection caused by protozoa of the genus *Sarcocystis* Lankester 1882. The disease is recognized by presence of elongated cysts (sarcocysts) located in muscles of mammals, birds, and reptiles. The nature of the causative organism was unclear until discovery that coccidian oocysts appeared when flesh containing sarcocysts was eaten by a suitable final host.

Sarcosporidiosis is not economically important to the poultry industry, but its extensive occurrence in wild ducks must be considered significant because many infected game birds are discarded annually by hunters for aesthetic reasons. Sarcosporidiosis does not appear to be a public health hazard; the parasite is killed by cooking and storage at subfreezing temperatures. Mild signs were reported, however, by infected human volunteers (56).

The true biologic nature of *Sarcocystis,* a controversial subject for the past century, and the historic aspects of sarcosporidiosis were reported by Spindler (74), Levine (49), Long (53), and Melhorn and Heydorn (58).

Incidence and Distribution. Avian sarcosporidiosis is found throughout the world in individual birds, but the disease has been reported only six times in domestic chickens. The incidence is as high as 40% in ducks and 93% in grackles (23), and is influenced by species, age, and geographic location of the host. *Sarcocystis* occurs more often in puddling than diving ducks.

Etiology. *Sarcocystis horwathi* (*S. gallinarum, S. horwathi*) is regarded as the etiologic agent for sarcosporidiosis in chickens (50), and *S. rileyi* (*Balbiani rileyi, S. anatina*) the cause of sarcosporidiosis in ducks. Based on microscopic differences in the wall substance of microcysts, however, at least five different species of *Sarcocystis* are present in birds (18). Duszynski and Box (19) successfully infected the opossum with tissue cysts from only one of three species of ducks, suggesting that different definitive hosts are required to complete the life cycle.

Sarcocystis is classified in the phylum Apicomplexa (50) and the family Sarcocystidae, characterized as having endodyogeny, cysts, or pseudocysts containing zoites in parenteral cells of the host, and is a monoxenous parasite of vertebrates (49). The protozoan classification of *Sarcocystis* is based on discovery of its coccidial nature with a disporocystid (a tetrazoic isosporanlike oocyst), an obligatory two-host life cycle, and characteristic ultrastructure (56, 69). These findings and the lack of evidence of endodyogeny in its life cycle place the genus *Sarcocystis* within the suborder Eimeriorina.

MORPHOLOGY. Sarcocysts (third-generation meronts) of *S. rileyi,* also called Miescher's tubules, are elongate, with their long axis parallel to the muscle fibers (Fig. 33.18). They are whitish and smooth-walled and appear cylindroid or spindle-shaped when removed from the musculature. They are 1.0–6.5 × 0.48–1.0 μm (74). They have

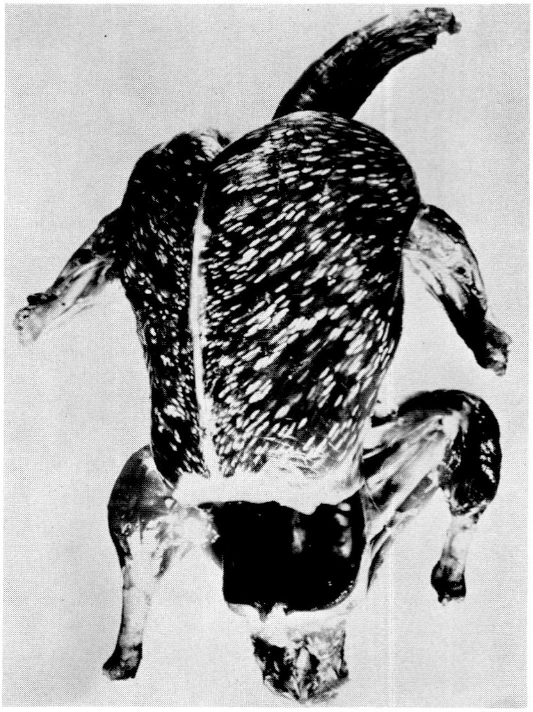

33.18. Severe sarcosporidiosis in wild mallard, natural infection. (US Dep Int)

double-layered walls, an inner spongy fibrous layer, and an outer dense limiting membrane (49). Sarcocysts are divided into compartments, each of which contains numerous banana-shaped cystozoites (bradyzoites), also called Rainey's corpuscles. Cystozoites are 8–15 μm long and 2–3 μm wide. Other developmental stages of *S. rileyi* are less well defined. The ultrastructure of *Sarcocystis* was described by Mehlhorn and Heydorn (58).

LIFE CYCLE. Obligatory two-host life cycles have been described from many species of *Sarcocystis* (56). Two vertebrate hosts are required in the life cycle of all these species, usually a carnivorous predator or scavenger and the prey or food animal. Sexual reproduction occurs in the predator (definitive host) and asexual reproduction in the prey (intermediate host). The intermediate host becomes infected by fecal contamination from an infected definitive host.

Studies on transmission of *Sarcocystis* from shoveler ducks (*Anas dypeata*) to the striped skunk (*Mephitis mephitis*) demonstrated an obligatory two-host life cycle (15, 80). When muscle containing sarcocysts was eaten by skunks, sporocysts (1.4 × 12.4 μm) were shed sporadically from 19 to 63 days PI. Shoveler ducks orally administered sporocysts developed microcysts (80 × 16 μm) in skeletal muscle 85 days later and macrocysts (1–3 × <1 mm) 154 days PI (15). In another study (70) the transmission of *S. falcatula* was demonstrated with the opossum (*Didelphis virginiana*) serving as the definitive host. Although asexual parasites were not found in ducks (*Anas platyrhynchos*) given fecal sporocysts from opossums, the intermediate host spectrum of some avian species of *Sarcocystis* is apparently quite broad (12). Sarcocysts from grackles and cowbirds are also infective to the opossum.

Levine (50) lists the chicken as the intermediate host and the dog as the definitive host for *S. horvathi.* The life cycle for *S. horvathi* is not completely defined.

All species of *Sarcocystis* apparently have similar developmental stages in their life cycle. Sarcocysts in cardiac, smooth, or skeletal muscle tissues are eaten by a definitive host, releasing cystozoites, which penetrate the intestinal wall and develop into macrogametocytes and microgametocytes in subepithelial tissues. Oocysts (containing two sporocysts, each with four sporozoites) are produced, and are shed in feces as fully sporulated sporocysts. Sporozoites are released when sporocysts are ingested by the intermediate host, and invade the mucosa of the intestine. Schizogony (merogony) occurs in endothelial cells of various organs. After several asexual generations the merozoites develop into young cyst stages, containing metrocytes and later cystozoites, and mature into the third-generation meronts (sarcocysts) in myocardial, skeletal, and smooth muscle tissues (56, 70).

The life cycles of *Sarcocystis* spp. that infect most species of birds remain incompletely known. More recent findings make earlier postulations of a simple one-host life cycle for any species of *Sarcocystis* less tenable (12, 15).

PATHOGENICITY. The pathogenicity of sarcosporidiosis in most birds is unknown. Box and Duszynski (10) attributed death of 4 of 12 sparrows and morbidity of 3 of 6 canaries to an experimental sarcosporidial infection but observed no adverse effect from infection in the definitive host (opossum).

Sarcocystin, an endotoxin found in sarcocysts, is toxic for rabbits, mice, and sparrows and may slightly affect other animals. Acting on the central nervous, cardiovascular, and digestive systems, it may cause diarrhea, collapse, and death. There was petechiation of the musculature, anemia, and nephrosis appearing in chickens within 24 hr after subcutaneous (SC) and oral administration of *S. tenella* sarcocysts (72).

Pathogenesis and Epizootiology. Natural and experimental sarcosporidial infections have been observed in 58 species and 11 orders of birds, including the domestic duck and chicken but not the turkey (9, 74).

TRANSMISSION, CARRIERS, VECTORS. Unsuccessful attempts to transmit *S. rileyi* to young ducks by oral, intramuscular (IM), and intravenous (IV) administration of cystozoites and cohabitation with infected ducks indicate that direct transmission through a one-host cycle does not occur (75).

Sporocyst-contaminated food is the common source of infection for the intermediate host; infection in the carnivorous definitive host results from ingestion of sarcocyst-infected tissues of the intermediate hosts. Cystozoites from sarcocysts in confined migratory ducks were found to be viable at the end of a 3-yr observation period. Thus, intermediate hosts may serve as an available source of infection for prolonged periods over a widespread area. Sarcosporidiosis appears to be most prevalent in hosts that frequently drink from shallow or stagnant water (puddling ducks, cattle, sheep, or swine) (74).

INCUBATION PERIOD. Infections are seldom found in juvenile grackles (23) or in juvenile ducks, which may indicate that the incubation period is long. Cawthorn et al. (15) stated that microcysts and macrocysts were found in ducks 85 and 154 days PI respectively. Macrocysts were observed in sparrows and canaries 70 days PI (11).

CLINICAL SIGNS. Sarcosporidiosis is usually found in birds that appear normal. Spindler (74) reported that very heavy infections may cause signs of disease and ducks may fly low and slowly. Adverse signs were not observed in experimentally infected ducks (15); however, Box and Duszynski (10) noted labored breathing and morbidity in canaries and sudden death in sparrows given oocysts.

GROSS LESIONS. Sarcocysts running lengthwise in the musculature of the breast, thigh, neck, or esophagus are the usual lesions associated with avian sarcosporidiosis. Lung consolidation and splenomegaly were observed in infected canaries (10). Lesions have not been seen in definitive hosts with experimental infections.

HISTOPATHOLOGY. Fatty degeneration of muscles, enlargement and rupture of parasitized muscle fibers, and inflammatory responses around sarcocysts in muscles resulting from avian sarcosporidiosis were reported (74).

IMMUNITY. Active and passive immunity have not been demonstrated. Animals have been immunized against sarcocystin by repeated injections of untreated or formalin-treated toxin, and serum from immunized animals gives protection to other animals against the toxin (74).

Diagnosis.

Diagnosis is based on identification of sarcocysts or cystozoites in tissues. Large sarcocysts are easily seen in gross specimens; smaller ones and cystozoites can be identified by histologic examination of muscle tissue.

Infections by species of *Sarcocystis* whose life cycles have been defined may be diagnosed in the definitive host by identification of sporocysts in feces and in the intermediate host on the basis of gross lesions or by detecting schizonts in or near endothelial cells of blood vessels in nearly all organs.

SEROLOGY. *Sarcocystis* reacts with cytoplasm-modifying antibody in the Sabin-Feldman dye test but cross-reacts with *Toxoplasma* (74). An indirect fluorescent antibody test in which cystozoites were used as the antigen was successful (77). Munday and Corbould (63) devised a complement-fixation test using an antigen prepared from sarcocysts and found that a titer of 1:10 was indicative of sarcosporidial infections.

Serologic reactions have not been applied in diagnosis of sarcosporidial infections in birds.

Treatment.

Administration of potassium iodide was reported to be beneficial in treating sarcosporidial infections (74). Sulfamethoxine successfully arrested sarcosporidian sporocyst shedding in cats (65); an anticoccidial compound (amprolium) reduced severity of sarcosporidial infections in calves (22). However, chemotherapy of avian sarcosporidiosis has no practical application at this time.

Prevention and Control.

The lack of chemotherapeutic or biologic control agents places the burden of control on prevention by breaking the infection cycle. Better knowledge of the parasite life cycles will be necessary for any progress in elimination of these parasites.

TOXOPLASMOSIS.

Toxoplasmosis is a parasitic disorder of mammals, birds, and reptiles affecting primarily the central nervous system but sometimes also the reproductive system, skeletal muscles, and visceral organs. The majority of infections are inapparent or latent, with overt toxoplasmosis resulting under favorable ecologic conditions.

Only sporadic outbreaks of toxoplasmosis in chickens have been reported (68). Studies of avian tissues using the mouse inoculation test and histologic examination indicate that a somewhat higher incidence of infection may exist than is apparent. Nevertheless, the disorder is uncommon in chickens and is of little significance to the poultry industry.

Toxoplasmosis is a zoonotic disorder and a human health problem of great concern. The total annual cost of neonatal toxoplasmosis in the USA in 1973 was estimated at $31–$40 million (41). Serologic surveys of human populations have shown evidence of 68% infection in some geographic areas, with an average of 14% throughout the USA (25).

The literature presents extensive overviews of history and current knowledge of toxoplasmosis (25, 28, 37, 41, 49).

Etiology. A single species, *Toxoplasma gondii,* is the cause of toxoplasmosis in all hosts. Synonyms for the agent in avian hosts are *T. avium* and *T. paddae.*

T. gondii is a coccidian with sexual stages similar to *Isospora bigemina* (28, 35). However, endodyogeny, which is not known to occur in *I. bigemina,* is a characteristic of *T. gondii.* Thus current knowledge supports classification close to the family Eimeriidae, which contains the coccidia. Levine (49) classifies *Toxoplasma* in the family Sarcocystidae along with *Sarcocystis.*

Numerous *Toxoplasma* isolates have been designated strains based on varying pathogenicity in different hosts rather than on immunologic variation, although the latter may occur with some strains.

In the free stage, *T. gondii* is crescent-shaped (4–6 × 2–3 μm), with one extremity more rounded than the other and a nucleus near the rounded end. No pseudopods, cilia, or flagella are present. Ultrastructure of developmental stages was reviewed by Levine (49) and Ferguson et al. (26).

LIFE CYCLE. Both schizogonic and gametogenic developmental cycles are known to occur in the intestinal epithelium of some members of the family Felidae. Both an "enteroepithelial" cycle and an "extraintestinal" cycle have been described.

The enteroepithelial cycle occurs only in Felidae, resulting from infection by encysted organisms (bradyzoites), free or intracellular individual organisms (tachyzoites), or oocysts (24). The prepatent period is 24 days or longer if oocysts are ingested, 5–10 days after ingestion of tachyzoites, and only 3–5 days if bradyzoites are the source of infection. Five multiplicative stages (type A-E), resulting only from infection by bradyzoites, have been identified on the basis of type of cellular division; sequence of development; number of merozoites; presence or absence of a rosette pattern or residual body; and shape, size, location, duration, and effect on the host cell (28). The type of cellular division for each type is type A, endodyogeny (division into two by internal budding); type B, endodyogeny and endopolygeny (division following formation of four or more nuclei); type C, schizogony; type D, schizogony, endopolygeny, and splitting; and type E, schizogony. Asexual development may start as early as 12 hr after ingestion, with schizogony occurring in the intestinal epithelium. These stages have not been clarified in cats following infection with tachyzoites and oocysts. From 4 to 24 merozoites form by endopolygeny deep within the schizont, not near the surface as in *Eimeria* and *Isospora.* The number of generations of merozoites that may occur prior to gametogony is undetermined.

The sexual phase of the enteroepithelial cycle occurs also only in intestinal epithelial cells of Felidae. Gametocytes develop throughout the small intestine, but more commonly in the ileum. Microgametocytes (7–10 × 5–8 μm) give rise to 12–32 microgametes (2–5 μm). Following fertilization of the macrogamete (13 μm), oocysts develop and detach unsporulated from the intestinal epithelium. Oocysts are shed for 7–20 days. Sporulation (mode of division unknown) then occurs in 1–5 days, depending on environmental temperature and oxygen, and results in development of two sporocysts (6–8 × 5–7 μm), each containing four sporozoites.

The extraintestinal (tissue) cycle apparently constitutes the entire cycle of *T. gondii* in nonfelines but occurs simultaneously with the enteroepithelial cycle in Felidae. After oral infection, rapidly multiplying *T. gondii* forms (tachyzoites), reproducing by endodyogeny, develop within vacuoles of many cell types. Tachyzoites in the free form spread from cell to cell and may be found in brain, eye, heart, liver, lungs, and nucleated red blood cells of birds. About eight or more organisms tend to accumulate in a host cell, forming pseudocysts (terminal colonies, aggregated), before it disintegrates.

Tachyzoites usually develop into bradyzoites (cells resting or slowly reproducing by endodyogeny with cysts) as chronic toxoplasmosis ensues. Encysted bradyzoites begin to develop intracellularly in the brain, heart, eyes, and skeletal muscles within 1–2 wk as immunity develops. Cysts may persist for the life of the host or, if immunity wanes, bradyzoites may be released and a proliferation of tachyzoites renewed. The tissue cycle may reverse again and cysts form from tachyzoites (28, 38, 41).

Pathogenesis and Epizootiology. Only members of the Felidae (domestic cats, ocelots, pumas, jaguarundi, bobcats, Asian leopards) are known natural and experimental definitive hosts for *T. gondii* (41). Intermediate or incomplete hosts include reptiles and more than 63 species of birds and 27 species of mammals (68). Natural infections have been diagnosed in the chickens, turkeys, ducks and many wild birds (13, 54). Ruiz and Frenkel (66) isolated *T. gondii* from 54% of chickens and 16% of sparrows examined in Costa Rica. *T. gondii* has been reisolated from Japanese quail, bluejays, crows, and chickens after experimental infections (60).

TRANSMISSION, CARRIERS, VECTORS. The known modes of transmission for the parasite are carnivorism, fecal contamination, and transplacental infection. Tachyzoites and bradyzoites may be spread by carnivorous ingestion; sporozoites in sporulated oocysts are spread by fecal contamination; and tachyzoites from ingestion of encysted bradyzoites or sporulated oocysts from the mother may be spread by transplacental infection.

The question of congenital infection occurring in chicks from naturally infected parents remains unresolved. Jacobs and Melton (39) found that 12 of 62 pools of reproductive tract tissues from chickens were infected with *T. gondii,* but the parasite could not be isolated from any of 108 eggs from these hens. In another study, 1 of 327 eggs from hens with chronic toxoplasmosis was positive. Iannuzzi and Renieri (36) concluded that toxoplasmas did not survive in unembryonated eggs and was not a factor in transmission. Caballero-Servin (14) reported successful transovarian transmission of the parasite by experimentally infecting hens, which resulted in embryonic mortality and congenital malformation of 18% of the surviving chicks.

Coprophagous arthropods such as flies and cockroaches can serve as transport hosts for the parasite (78). Earthworms ingest toxoplasma oocysts and are a source of infection for chickens (66).

COURSE OF THE DISEASE. The chicken is quite resistant to *T. gondii,* but disease has been observed from both natural and experimental infections. Variations in the clinical syndrome are attributed to age of host, strain of infective agent, and methods of infection. Clinical signs become apparent in chicks when they are inoculated by the intracerebral (IC) route before 3 wk of age (8) and in chicks inoculated by the intraperitoneal (IP) route before 1 day of age (45). Parasitemia and chronic toxoplasma infections occur in older birds via IV, IP, IM, and SC inoculations.

Clinical signs in chickens include anorexia, emaciation, paleness and shrinking of the comb, drop in egg production, whitish feces, diarrhea, incoordination, ataxia, trembling, opisthotonos, torticollis, and blindness. Clinical signs are apparent 3–12 days after IC inoculation and all chicks die within 24 hr after onset of clinical signs (7, 8, 45, 54). A rapidly developing outbreak was reported in which most of a flock of chickens were affected and total mortality reached 50% (54). Death occurred in 2/3 of the chicks fed toxoplasma oocysts from cats. Siim et al. (68) noted that infections in turkeys and ducks were mild and suggested that many may be undetected.

GROSS LESIONS. Gross lesions include enlargement of liver and spleen, necrotic hepatitis, pericarditis, myocarditis, ulcerative enteritis, lung congestion, and encephalitis (8, 54).

HISTOPATHOLOGY. In chickens inoculated by IC and IM routes, encysted toxoplasmas were found in the cerebrum, brain stem, optic chiasma, and, most frequently, around ventricles and in molecular and Purkinje layers of the cerebellum. Free toxoplasmas were seldom found, and then only in the brain. Toxoplasma cysts were found in the myocardium, pancreas, and testes of chickens infected intramuscularly (8).

Coagulation necrosis and diffuse sinusoidal congestion were observed in the liver. The myocardium, pancreas, and testes were diffusely infiltrated with lymphocytes, plasma cells, and heterophils. In the brain, infection caused lymphocytic lesions and plasma cell–cuffing of blood vessels; lymphocytic infiltration of choroid villi; ependymal proliferation of the lateral ventricle; thickening of leptomeninges; and gliosis of the lateral ventricle and around vessels of the cerebrum, brain stem, and cerebellum.

Diagnosis.

T. gondii may be isolated and identified by injecting suspensions of infected tissues into various species of laboratory animals, chicken embryos, or cell cultures. IP or IC inoculation of mice with suspensions of brain, liver, lung, or spleen are preferred methods of isolation (29). Mice inoculated with virulent strains die within a few days. When less virulent isolates are suspected, brains should be examined for cyst forms 8–10 wk after mouse inoculation. The isolated organisms should be identified serologically.

Impression smears of peritoneal fluids or tissues stained with Giemsa, or tissue sections of brain, liver, spleen, lung, lymph nodes, and eye often suffice for direct microscopic observation of toxoplasmas.

Toxoplasmas can be grown in the chorioallantoic cavity of 6- to 12-day-old embryonated chicken eggs. Embryos succumb 7–10 days PI with hemorrhage and nodular lesions in skin and viscera. Numerous yellow-white plaques 0.5–3.0 mm in diameter develop on the chorioallantoic and amniotic membranes. Smears of the chorioallantoic membrane and yolk sac stained with Wright's stain reveal numerous free and intracellular toxoplasmas.

SEROLOGY. The complement-fixation (CF), enzyme-linked immunosorbent assay (ELISA), indirect fluorescent antibody (FA), and Sabin-Feldman dye tests are currently used to diagnose toxoplasma infections with the agglutination and agar-gel diffusion tests having less practical applications. The dye, ELISA, and indirect FA tests detect early antibodies that persist indefinitely, whereas the CF test detects antibodies that appear about 14 days PI and disappear within 1–2 yr (41).

Present serologic tests for *T. gondii* are not adequate for detecting the presence of the carrier state in most birds. Chickens, Japanese quail, bluejays, and crows did not develop appreciable levels of antibody detectable by the dye test, although *T. gondii* could be isolated from all birds and up to 14 mo PI in chickens (60, 66, 78). With the dye test, low antibody titers (1:16 or less) were measurable in only 3 of 34 infected chickens (45); doves and pigeons, however, develop high antibody levels.

TREATMENT, PREVENTION, CONTROL. Chemotherapy is generally used to suppress proliferation of the parasite until some immunity has developed. Treatment of choice for humans and laboratory animals is a combination of sulfadiazine and pyrimethamine, which act synergistically (49). Sulfamerazine and triple sulfonamides are also efficacious; spiramycin, tetracycline, and clindamycin inhibit the parasite less effectively (37). Neither prophylactic nor therapeutic treatment has been used to control avian toxoplasmosis. There are no reports of therapeutic control of the enteroepithelial cycle in cats.

Prevention of avian toxoplasmosis requires management practices that eliminate the source of infective tachyzoites and oocysts, by preventing exposure to rodents, coprophagous arthropods, and cats. Oocysts disseminated throughout the premises are resistant to common laboratory detergents, acids, and alkalis and are therefore difficult to destroy. However, they may be destroyed by ammonia, drying, and a temperature of 55 C (49).

REFERENCES

1. Ahmed, F.E., and A.H.H. Mohammed. 1978. Studies of growth and development of gametocytes in Haemoproteus columbae Kruse. J Protozool 25:174-177.
2. Allan, R.A., and J.L. Mahrt. 1987. Populations of Leucocytozoon gametocytes in blue grouse (Dendragapus obscurus) from Hardwicke Island, British Columbia. J Protozool 34:363-366.
3. Atkinson, C.T. 1985. Epizootiology and pathogenicity of Haemoproteus meleagridis Levine 1961 from Florida turkeys. PhD diss, Univ Florida.
4. Atkinson, C.T., and D.J. Forrester. 1987. Myopathy associated with megaloschizonts of Haemoproteus meleagridis in a wild turkey from Florida. J Wildl Dis 23:495-498.
5. Bennett, G.F., and M. Cameron. 1974. Seasonal prevalance of avian hematozoa in passerine birds of Atlantic Canada. Can J Zool 52:1259-1284.
6. Bennett, G.F., and M. Laird. 1973. Collaborative investigation into avian malaria: An international research programme. J Wildl Dis 9:26-28.
7. Biancifiori, F., C. Rondini, V. Grelloni, and T. Frescura. 1986. Avian toxoplasmosis: Experimental infection of chicken and pigeon. Comp Immunol Microbiol Infect Dis 9:337-346.
8. Bickford, A.A., and J.R. Saunders. 1966. Experimental toxoplasmosis in chickens. Am J Vet Res 116:308-318.
9. Borst, G.H., and P. Zwort. 1973. Sarcosporidiosis in Psittaciformes. Z Parasitenkd 42:293-298.
10. Box, E.D., and D.W. Duszynski. 1978. Experimental transmission of Sarcocystis from icterid birds to sparrows and canaries by sporocysts from the opossum. J Parasitol 64:682-688.
11. Box, E.D., and D.W. Duszynski. 1980. Sarcocystis of passerine birds: Sexual stages in the opossum (Didelphis virginiana). J Wildl Dis 16:209-215.
12. Box, E.D., and J.H. Smith. 1982. The intermediate host spectrum in a sarcocystis species of birds. J Parasitol 68:668-673.
13. Burridge, M.J., W.J. Bigler, D.J. Forrester, and J.M. Henneman. 1979. Serologic survey for Toxoplasma gondii in wild animals in Florida. J Am Vet Med Assoc 175:964-967.
14. Caballero-Servin, A. 1974. Congenital malformations in Gallus gallus induced by Toxoplasma gondii. Rev Invest Salud Publica (Mexico) 34:87-94.
15. Cawthorn, R.J., D. Rainnie, and G. Wobeser. 1981. Experimental transmission of Sarcocystis sp. (protozoa: Sarcocystidae) between the Shoveler (Anas clypeata) duck and the striped skunk (Mephitis mephitis). J Wildl Dis 17:389-394.
16. Desser, S.S., J. Stuht, and A.M. Fallis. 1978. Leucocytozoonosis in Canada geese in upper Michigan. 1. Strain differences among geese from different localities. J Wildl Dis 14:124-131.
17. Dick, J. 1978. Leucocytozoon smithi: Persistence of gametocytes in peripheral turkey blood. Avian Dis 22:82-85.
18. Drouin, T.E., and J.L. Mahrt. 1980. The morphology of cysts of Sarcocystis infecting birds in western Canada. Can J Zool 58:1477-1482.
19. Duszynski, D.W., and E.D. Box. 1978. The opossum (Didelphis virginiana) as a host for Sarcocystis debonei from cowbirds (Molothrus ater) and grackles (Cassidiz mexicanus, Quiscalus quiscula). J Parasitol 64:326-329.
20. Fallis, A.M., R.L. Jacobson, and J.N. Raybould. 1973. Haematoza in domestic chickens and guinea fowl in Tanzania and transmission of Leucocytozoon neavet and Leucocytozoon schoutedent. J Protozool 20:436-437.
21. Fallis, A.M., S.S. Desser, and R.A. Khan. 1974. On species of Leucocytozoon. Adv Parasitol 12:1-67.
22. Fayer, R., and A.J. Johnson. 1975. Effect of amprolium on acute Sarcocystis in experimentally infected calves. J Parasitol 61:932-936.
23. Fayer, R., and R.M. Kocan. 1971. Prevalence of Sarcocystis in grackles in Maryland. J Protozool 18:547-548.
24. Fayer, R., A.J. Johnson, and P.K. Hildebrandt. 1976. Oral infection of mammals with Sarcocystis fusiformis bradyzoites from cattle and sporocysts from dogs and coyotes. J Parasitol 62:10-14.
25. Feldman, H.A. 1974. Toxoplasmosis: An overview. Bull NY Acad Med 50:110-127.
26. Ferguson, D.S., W.M. Hutchinson, J.F. Dunachie, and J.C. Siim. 1974. Ultrastructural study of early stages of asexual multiplication and microgametogony of Toxoplasma gondii in the small intestine of the cat. Acta Pathol Microbiol Scand 82:167-181.
27. Forrester, D.J., J.K. Nayar, and M.D. Young. 1987. Natural infection of Plasmodium hermani in the Northern Bobwhite, Colinus virginianus, in Florida. J Parasitol 73:865-866.
28. Frenkel, J.K. 1973. Toxoplasmosis: Parasite life cycle, pathology, and immunology. In D.M. Hammond and P.L. Long (eds), The Coccidia. Eimeria, Isopora, Toxoplasma, and Related Genera, pp. 343-410. Univ Park Press, Baltimore, MD.
29. Frenkel, J.K. 1981. False-negative serologic tests

for Toxoplasma in birds. J Parasitol 67:952-953.

30. Garnham, P.C.C. 1966. Malaria Parasites and Other Haemosporidia. Blackwell, Oxford, Engl.

31. Greiner, E.C., and D.J. Forrester. 1980. Haemoproteus meleagridis Levine 1961: Redescription and developmental morphology of the gametocytes in turkeys. J Parasitol 66:652-688.

32. Greiner, E.D., G.F. Bennett, M. Laird, and C.M. Herman. 1975. Avian Hematozoa. I. A color pictorial guide to some species of Haemoproteus, Leucocytozoon, and Trypanosoma. Wildl Dis 68 (WD75-3). (Color fiche).

33. Herman C.M., J.H. Barrows, Jr., and I.B. Tarshis. 1975. Leucocytozoonosis in Canada geese at the Seney National Wildlife Refuge. J Wildl Dis 11:404-411.

34. Hsu, C.-K., G.R. Campbell, and N.D. Levine. 1973. A checklist of the species of the genus Leucocytozoon. J Protozool 20:195-203.

35. Hutchinson, W.M., J.F. Dunachie, K. Work, and J.C. Siim. 1971. The life cycle of the coccidian parasite, Toxoplasma gondii, in the domestic cat. Trans R Soc Trop Med Hyg 65:380-399.

36. Iannuzzi, L., and G. Renieri. 1971. The egg in the epidemiology of Toxoplasmosis. Tests of expermimental infections by injection through the shell. Acta Med Vet 17:311-317.

37. Jacobs, L. 1973. New knowledge of Toxoplasma and toxoplasmosis. Adv Parasitol 11:631-669.

38. Jacobs, L. 1974. Toxoplasma gondii: Parasitology and transmission. Bull NY Acad Med 50:128-145.

39. Jacobs, L., and M.L. Melton. 1966. Toxoplasmosis in chickens. J Parasitol 52:1158-1162.

40. Johnson, E.P., G.W. Underhill, J.A. Cox, and W.L. Threlkeld. 1968. A blood protozoan of turkeys transmitted by Simulium nigroparvum (Twinn). Am J Hyg 27:649-665.

41. Jones, S.R. 1973. Toxoplasmosis: A review. J Am Vet Med Assoc 163:1038-1042.

42. Jones, J.E., B.D. Barnett, and J. Solis. 1972. The effect of Leucocytozoon smithi infection on production, fertility, and hatchability of broad breasted white turkey hens. Poult Sci 51:543-545.

43. Julian, R.J., and D.E. Galt. 1980. Mortality in Muscovy ducks (Cairina moschata) caused by Haemoproteus infection. J Wildl Dis 16:39-44.

44. Kemp, R.L. 1978. Haemoproteus. In M.S. Hofstad, B.W. Calnek, C.F. Helmbodt, W.M. Reid, and H.W. Yoder, Jr. (eds.), Diseases of Poultry, 7th Ed., pp. 824-825. Iowa State Univ Press, Ames.

45. Kinjo, T. 1972. Experimental toxoplasmosis in fowls. III. Reactions of chicks at 30-40 days old and one day old. IV. Susceptibility of chick embryos. Sci Bull Coll Agric (Okinawa) 19:407-420.

46. Kissam, J.B., R. Noblet, and G.I. Garris. 1975. Large scale aerial treatment of an endemic area with abate granular larvicide to control black flies (Diptera simuliidae) and suppress Leucocytozoon smithi of turkeys. J Med Entomol 12:359-362.

47. Kiszewski, A.E., and E.W. Cupp. 1986. Transmission of Leucocytozoon smithi (Sporozoa: Leucocytozoidae) by black flies (Diptera simulidae) in New York, USA. J Med Entomol 23:256-262.

48. Kocan, R.M. 1968. Anemia and mechanism of erythrocyte destruction in ducks with acute Leucocytozoon infections. J Protozool 15:455-462.

49. Levine, N.D. 1973. Protozoan Parasites of Domestic Animals and of Man. 2nd Ed. Burgess, Minneapolis.

50. Levine, N.D. 1986. The taxonomy of Sarcocystis (Protozoa: Apicomplexa) species. J Parasitol 72:372-382.

51. Levine, N.D., and G.R. Campbell. 1971. A checklist of the species of the genus Haemoproteus (Apicomplexa, Plasmodiidae). J Protozool 18:475-484.

52. Levine, N.D., J.O. Corliss, F.E.G. Cox, G. Deroux, J. Grain, B.M. Honigberg, G.F. Leedale, A.R. Loeblich III, J. Lom, D. Lynn, E.G. Merinfeld, F.C. Page, G. Poljansky, V. Sprague, J. Vavra, and F.G. Wallace. 1980. A newly revised classification of the protozoa. J Parasitol 27:37-58.

53. Long, P.L. 1982. The Biology of the Coccidia. Univ Park Press, Baltimore, MD.

54. Lund, E.E. 1972. Other protozoan diseases. In M.S. Hofstad, B.W. Calnek, C.F. Helmboldt, W.M. Reid, and H.W. Yoder, Jr. (eds.), Diseases of Poultry, 6th Ed., pp. 990-1046. Iowa State Univ Press, Ames.

55. Maley, G.J.M., and S.S. Desser. 1977. Anemia in Leucocytozoon simondi infections. I. Quantification of anemia, gametocytemia, and osmotic fragility of erythrocytes in naturally infected Pekin ducklings. Can J Zool 55:255-258.

56. Markus, M.B., R. Killick-Kendrick, and P.C.C. Garnham. 1974. The coccidial nature and life-cycle of Sarcocystis. J Trop Med Hyg 77:248-259.

57. McGhee, R.B. 1970. Avian malaria. In D.J. Jackson, R. Herman, and I. Singer (eds.), Immunity to Parasitic Animals, Vol. 2, pp. 295-329. Appleton-Century-Crofts, New York.

58. Melhorn, H., and A.O. Heydorn. 1978. The Sarcosporidia (Protozoa, Sporozoa): Life cycle and fine structure. Adv Parasitol 16:43-91.

59. Milhous, W., and J. Solis. 1973. Turkey leucocytozoon infection. 3. Ultrastructure of Leucocytozoon smithi: Gametocytes. Poult Sci 52:2138-2146.

60. Miller, N.L., J.K. Frenkel, and J.P. Dubey. 1972. Oral infections with Toxoplasma cysts and oocysts in felines, other mammals, and in birds. J Parasitol 58:928-937.

61. Miura, S., K. Ohshima, C. Itakura, and S. Yamogiwa. 1973. A histopathological study on Leucocytozoonosis in young hens. Japan J Vet Sci 35:175-181.

62. Molyneux, D.H. 1977. Vector relationships in the trypanosomatidae. Adv Parasitol 15:1-82.

63. Munday, B.L., and A. Corbould. 1974. The possible role of the dog in the epidemiology of ovine sarcosporidiosis. Br Vet J 130:9-11.

64. Noblet, R., H.S. Moore IV, and G.P. Noblet. 1976. Survey of Leucocytozoon in South Carolina. Poult Sci 55:447-449.

65. Powell, E.C., and J.B. McCarley. 1975. A murine Sarcocystis that causes isospora-like infection in cats. J Parasitol 61:928-931.

66. Ruiz, A., and J.K. Frenkel. 1980. Intermediate and transport hosts of Toxoplasma gondii in Costa Rica. Am J Trop Med Hyg 29:1161-1166.

67. Siccardi, F.J., H.O. Rutherford, and W.T. Derieux. 1974. Pathology and prevention of Leucocytozoon smithi infection in turkeys. Avian Dis 18:21-32.

68. Siim, J.C., U. Biering-Sorenson, and T. Moller. 1963. Toxoplasmosis in domestic animals. Adv Vet Sci 8:335-429.

69. Simpson, C.R., and D.J. Forrester. 1973. Electron microscopy of Sarcosystis sp: Cyst wall, micropore, rhoptries, and an unidentified body. Int J Parasitol 3:467-470.

70. Smith, J.H., J.L. Meier, P.J.G. Neill, and E.D. Box. 1987. Pathogenesis of Sarcocystis falcatula in the budgerigar. II. Pulmonary pathology. Lab Invest 56:72-84.

71. Solis, J. 1973. Nonsusceptibility of some avian species to turkey Leucocytozoon infection. Poult Sci 52:498-500.

72. Sominski, Z.F., D.I. Panasiuk, and R.P. Vilkova.

1971. Pathological-morphological changes during experimental sarcocystis in chickens. Veterinariia 6:68–69.

73. Soni, J.L., and H.W. Cox. 1975. Pathogenesis of acute avian malaria. II. Anemia mediated by a cold-active autohemagglutinin from the blood of chickens with acute Plasmodium gallinaceum infection. Am J Trop Med Hyg 24:206–213.

74. Spindler, L.A. 1972. Sarcosporidiosis. In M.S. Hofstad, B.W. Calnek, C.F. Helmboldt, W.M. Reid, and H.W. Yoder, Jr. (eds.), Diseases of Poultry, 6th Ed., pp. 1046–1054. Iowa State Univ Press, Ames.

75. Springer, W.T. 1984. Other blood and tissue protozoa. In M.S. Hofstad, H. John Barnes, B.W. Calnek, W.M. Reid, and H.W. Yoder, Jr. (eds.), Diseases of Poultry, 8th Ed., pp. 727–740. Iowa State Univ Press, Ames.

76. Steck, E.A. 1971. Chemotherapy of Protozoan Disease, Vol. 3, Sect. 4A, pp. 1–376. Walter Reed Arm Res Inst (Unnumbered monogr).

77. Wallace, G.D. 1973. Sarcocystis in mice inoculated with Toxoplasma-like oocysts from cat feces. Science 180:1375–1377.

78. Wallace G.D. 1973. Intermediate and transport hosts in the natural history of Toxoplasma gondii. Am J Trop Med Hyg 22:456–464.

79. White, E.M., and G.F. Bennett. 1979. Avian Haemoproteidae. 12. The hemoproteids of the grouse family Tetraonidae. Can J Zool 57:1465–1472.

80. Wicht, R.J. 1981. Transmission of Sarcocystis rileyi to the striped skunk (Mephitis mephitisy). J Wildl Dis 17:387–388.

34 DEVELOPMENTAL, METABOLIC, AND MISCELLANEOUS DISORDERS

C. Riddell

INTRODUCTION. The diseases and conditions discussed in this chapter represent a heterogeneous group; in some cases the etiology is quite clear, whereas in others it is questionable or unknown. They vary in economic importance and frequency of occurrence. Emphasis has been placed on metabolic diseases of economic importance to the modern poultry industry. Diseases have been classified by body system primarily affected except for the conditions that are discussed under cannibalism or environmental diseases.

CANNIBALISM. Many forms of cannibalism occur in domestic fowl and game birds reared in captivity. Weaver and Bird (254) indicated that light breeds of the Mediterranean class are much more prone to these vices than heavier breeds of the American and Asiatic classes.

Vent Picking. Picking of the vent or region of the abdomen several inches below the vent is the most severe form of cannibalism. This is generally seen in high-production pullet flocks. Predisposing factors are prolapse or tearing of the tissues by passage of an abnormally large egg. Vent picking can cause high mortality in turkeys as young as 1 wk of age. Dead poults are anemic and there is generally blood on the tail feathers around the injured vent and on the back of the legs.

Feather Pulling. Feather pulling is most frequently seen in flocks kept in close confinement resulting in lack of sufficient exercise. Nutritional and mineral deficiencies may be contributing factors. Feather picking causes "blueback" in bronze turkeys. Injury to the feather quills allows pigment to escape and tattoo the surrounding area.

Toe Picking. Toe picking is most commonly seen in domestic chicks or young game birds and is often initiated by hunger. Chicks may not find feed because hoppers are too high or too far from the heat source. Feeder space may be inadequate, and the smaller or more timid chicks may be kept from eating by aggressive birds. If the chick cannot find feed, it may pick at its own or a neighbor's toes. It is good practice to put feed on chick box covers or trays and place them under the hover the first few days of brooding.

Head Picking. Head picking usually follows injuries to the comb or wattles caused by freezing or fighting among males. A different form of cannibalism is now being observed in beak-trimmed birds kept in cages. The area about the eyes is black and blue due to subcutaneous hemorrhage, wattles are dark and swollen with extravasated blood, and ear lobes are black and necrotic. Even though birds have trimmed beaks and are kept in separate cages, they will reach through the wire and peck at a neighbor or grasp its ear lobes or wattles and shake their heads in much the same fashion as a terrier shaking a rat.

Nose Picking in Quail. Bass (5) reported an unusual form of cannibalism in quail. It is termed "nose picking," since the birds peck at the top of the nose where the fleshy portion merges with the beak. The condition is generally seen in birds 2–7 wk of age kept under crowded conditions. The bird may die as the result of blood loss. If the bird survives, the beak will be permanently deformed and males will be unsatisfactory for breeding stock. This vice occurs only when birds are brooded under artificial conditions. It seldom develops in large pens on the ground in which there is opportunity to pick and scratch. Bass also observed that addition of raw meat to the ration was very effective in preventing and controlling outbreaks.

Etiology. Many causes of cannibalism have been suggested, but often outbreaks of cannibalism occur in one pen, while similar environmental conditions or feeding practices in other pens on the same farm do not cause difficulty. Conditions reported as predisposing to cannibalism are feed-

Grateful acknowledgement is made to Dr. M.C. Peckham, previous author of this chapter, for much of the material on cannibalism and environmental disease, reviews of several conditions, and many figures.

ing only pellets or compressed feed, cafeteria system of feeding, excess corn in the ration, insufficient feeder or drinker space, being without feed too long, insufficient nests, nests too light, excessively light pens, high-density rearing systems, too much heat, nutritional and mineral deficiencies, and irritation from external parasites (105, 180). After birds have started picking they will continue their cannibalistic habits without provocation.

Prevention. Cannibalism can best be prevented by providing adequate feed and water space and not permitting birds to go without feed for extended periods. Overcrowding should be avoided; in cages where high-density rearing is practiced it may be necessary to trim beaks before housing. Careful attention to ventilation and light intensity may preclude an outbreak of cannibalism. In many large scale commercial operations beak trimming is necessary to prevent cannibalism. Peckham (187) reviewed old remedies for controlling cannibalism and methods of beak trimming.

ENVIRONMENTAL DISEASE

Heat Prostration. Birds in production are particularly susceptible to high temperatures accompanied by high humidity. Lacking sweat glands, birds' only method of cooling is rapid respiration with mouths open and wings relaxed and hanging loosely at their sides. If body temperatures rise birds become weak and die due to respiratory, circulatory, or electrolyte imbalances. An attempt to cool the birds can be made by dipping them in or spraying them with water. Every effort should be made to increase circulation of air by running ventilation equipment at full capacity. Cooling the air can be accomplished by hosing down the floor, walls, ceiling, and outside roof. Adequate drinking water should be available. Preventive measures consist of installation of fans, proper construction of ventilating ducts, insulation of the building, and use of white or aluminum paint on the outside to reflect heat. In southern climates where low production and mortality from heat are constant problems, installation of foggers and sprinklers or evaporative coolers is essential.

Smothering. Smothering is generally caused by birds crowding or piling in a corner. It may occur when birds are moved to new quarters, when they are frightened, or in young birds when they are chilled. The history of the case often indicates that mortality occurs only at night and the flock in general looks healthy. Smothering of baby chicks can occur in chick boxes that are piled too high without an air space between each box, in boxes that do not have sufficient ventilation holes, or in boxes placed in a closed compartment such as the trunk of a car. Necropsy of chicks that have smothered usually does not reveal enough gross pathology to make a positive diagnosis but a thorough examination will eliminate other possible causes of death. In broilers and older birds that have smothered there is congestion of the trachea and lungs, and feathers will be worn off where birds have been trampled.

Smothering of chicks in the brooder house can be controlled by putting a circle of corrugated cardboard around the hover for the 1st wk and gradually widening the diameter as chicks get older. This will prevent piling in a corner during the night. When birds are moved to new quarters, the use of a dim light or lantern the first few nights will decrease the possibility of smothering. Birds transferred to new quarters should be checked late in the evening for signs of piling. Frequent observation of the flock is very important the first few days after acquiring a group of new chicks or grown birds.

Dehydration. Dehydration is generally caused by failure of birds to find water, an inability to reach the water, or in some cases by a deterring factor in the water, such as an electrical charge caused by faulty heating devices that prevent freezing. Chicks can survive several days without water but will start to die in 4–5 days. Mortality peaks in 5–6 days and terminates abruptly if water is provided. Chicks that are not drinking will have succumbed by this period, and survivors are those that have found the water and are drinking. Dehydration can be detected by the chick's inability to "peep" during the later stages, insufficient weight for size and age, and dehydrated and wrinkled skin on the shanks. Other changes are blue discoloration of the beak, dry and dark breast musculature, dark kidneys, accumulation of urates in the ureters, and darkening of the blood. Signs and lesions in older birds are similar to those in chicks, and weight loss is much more noticeable.

To prevent dehydration in chicks, water fountains should be placed at the edge of the hover directly on the litter without any platform. When a small drinker is replaced by a large type or automatic drinkers, the old type should be kept for a few days and gradually moved toward the new water supply to accustom birds to the change.

SKELETON DISEASES

Crooked Neck. Moorhead and Mohamed (163) reported a crooked-neck syndrome in a flock of 18-wk-old turkeys, with approximately 10% of 8000 birds affected. The principal lesion was an osteodystrophy of the cervical vertebrae. The clinical signs were similar to those of a crooked-neck syndrome attributed to a single recessive gene in brown leghorns. It appears unlikely that the syndrome in turkeys was a genetic defect.

The syndrome was common in many turkey flocks in North America circa 1970 and was associated with airsacculitis due to *Mycoplasma meleagridis.* The incidence was reduced by dipping hatching eggs in tylosin tartrate to control *M. meleagridis* infection (202).

Spondylolisthesis. It is postulated that spondylolisthesis is a development disorder influenced by conformation and growth rate, resulting in a deformity of the 6th thoracic vertebra, which causes spinal cord compression and posterior paralysis in broiler chickens. It is commonly called "kinky back." Wise (266) and Riddell (206) have written reviews on the condition. Most broiler flocks have a few birds affected with spondylolisthesis. In some flocks the incidence of affected birds has reached 2%. The peak incidence occurs at 3–6 wk of age. Affected birds are alert, remain sitting on their hocks with their feet slightly raised off the ground (Fig. 34.1), and use their wings in an attempt to escape when approached. Severely affected birds often become laterally recumbent. Affected birds often die from dehydration if not culled.

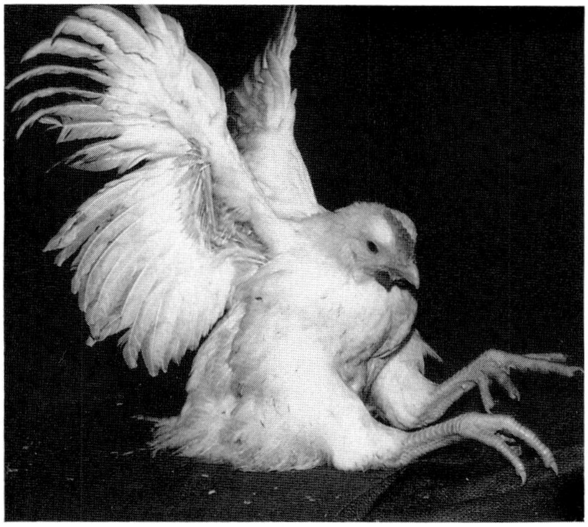

34.1. Broiler chicken with spondylolisthesis. (Avian Dis)

The posterior paralysis results from rotation of the body of the 6th vertebra along the axis of the spine with the posterior part of the body moving dorsal and anterior, relative to the anterior part. This rotation causes a kyphotic angulation of the floor of the spinal canal between the 6th and 7th thoracic vertebrae, and spinal cord compression (Fig. 34.2). The deformation of the spinal column can be readily recognized by palpating the ventral surface of the spinal column during necropsy. A diagnosis of spondylolisthesis is best confirmed by removing, decalcifying, and splitting the spinal column along a midline longitudinal plane to allow visualization of the spinal cord compression.

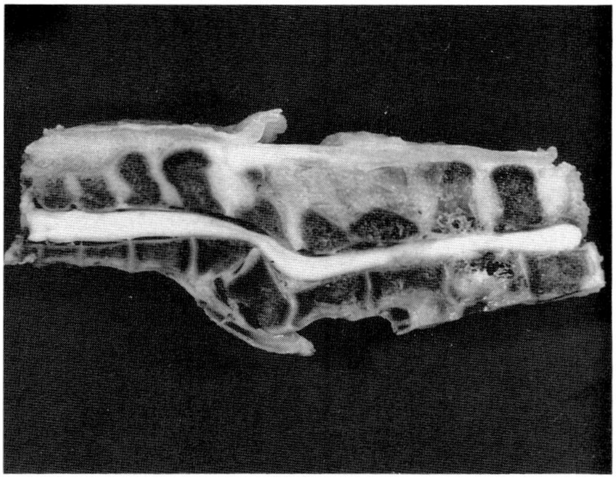

34.2. Midline longitudinal section through thoracic-lumbar region of the spinal column of a broiler chicken with spondylolisthesis, cervical end to the right. Rotation of the body of vertebra T6, deformation of T7, and spinal cord compression. (Avian Dis)

Lordosis and subclinical spondylolisthesis are common in broiler chickens. The lordosis develops after hatching. It can be decreased by slowing the growth rate of the broiler chicken. The incidence of spondylolisthesis can be increased by genetic selection.

Other Abnormalities of the Spine. Several other spinal deformities occur sporadically at a low incidence in commercial poultry. These deformities include scoliosis and rumplessness and have been reviewed by Riddell (202).

Valgus and Varus Deformation of the Intertarsal Joint. Deformation of the long bones of broiler chickens and turkeys is a significant cause of economic loss due to culling and death of affected birds. Such deformation includes many different types of twisting or bending of the bones and has been described as long-bone distortion, twisted legs, or crooked legs. The general topic of deformation of the long bones in domestic poultry was reviewed by Riddell (206). The most common type of long-bone deformation in broiler chickens is valgus or varus deformation (VVD) of the intertarsal joint (118, 196, 214). Similar deformation of the intertarsal joint is also common in turkeys but is often associated with varus deformation of the femoral-tibial joint (205). The incidence of broiler chickens affected with VVD varies from 0.5–2.0% in normal broiler flocks but occasionally affects 5–25% of male broilers in problem flocks (118).

SIGNS AND PATHOLOGY. Broilers may be affected with VVD before 1 wk of age, and the incidence increases with birds becoming affected throughout the life of a flock (214). Approximately 70% of affected birds are males (214). The defect may affect both legs but is often unilateral with the right leg more commonly affected than the left leg (59, 214). Most birds have either valgus or varus deformation but occasionally birds will have valgus deformation of one leg and varus deformation of the other leg. These birds have been described as "windswept" (47). The major deformity is outward or inward angulation of the distal tibia with similar but less severe angulation in the proximal metatarsus (Fig. 34.3, 34.4). In some birds there is an associated outward or internal rotation of the distal tibia. Abnormal rotation of the femur may also be present (59). The degree of angulation varies from mild to very severe. As the severity of the angulation increases, the gastrocnemius tendon becomes displaced and the distal tibial condyles become flattened. In some cases the angulation progresses to displacement and separation of the tarsal bones from the shaft of the tibia. With severe angulation birds are forced to walk on the posterior surface of the hock, which becomes bruised and swollen. In some instances the distal shaft of the tibia will penetrate the skin. Detailed descriptions of the deformity are provided by Randall and Mills (196), Julian (118), and Riddell (207).

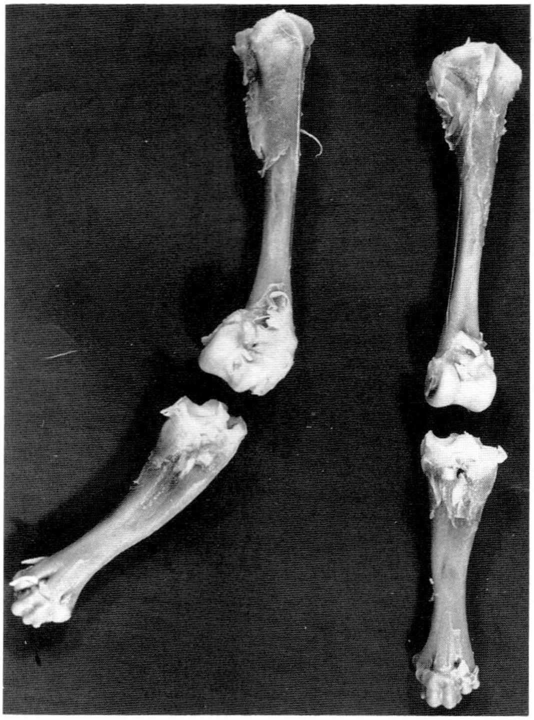

34.4. Tibiotarsal and tarsometatarsal bones from a broiler chicken with unilateral valgus deformation. (Avian Dis)

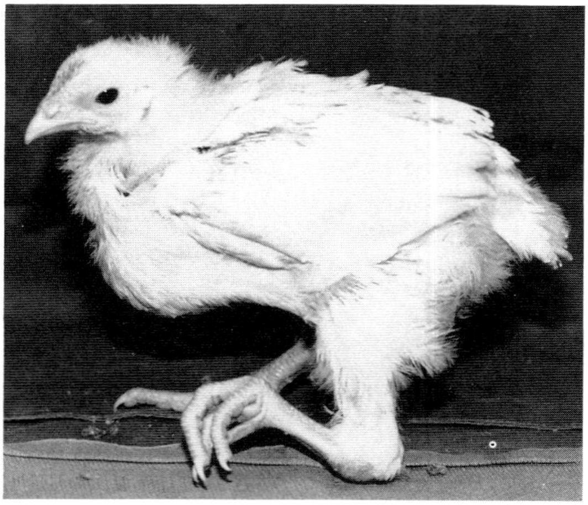

34.3. Broiler chicken with unilateral valgus deformation of the intertarsal joint. (Avian Dis)

PATHOGENESIS AND ETIOLOGY. The pathogenesis of the deformation has not been defined. Similar gross deformation has been reproduced experimentally with several nutritional deficiencies in which there was a generalized disorder of the growth plates of the long bones (206). The classical example of such a deficiency is manganese deficiency and the syndrome produced was called perosis. Wise (266) proposed the term chondrodystrophy to replace perosis and this terminology is now widely accepted. No evidence of the microscopic growth plate lesions found in chondrodystrophy has been recognized in VVD (211, 196). The possibility that submicroscopic lesions of the growth plate due to marginal nutritional deficiencies may result in VVD should not be ignored. Some workers (32, 108, 109) have noted a delay in cortical bone differentiation, which precedes the angulation. Young normal broiler chickens have slight valgus deformation. The angulation is greater in the right leg (58). This small inclination of the growth plate in a rapidly growing chicken may promote deviant growth (196, 215). An association between VVD and dyschondroplasia has been noted (191, 196, 207). Although dyschondroplasia may weaken bones and predispose to deformation it may be secondary to the deformation (268). In a breeding study it was observed that VVD was unrelated to dyschondroplasia (203).

The incidence of VVD is influenced by genotype (32) and can be reduced by slowing growth rate (90, 102, 207). A higher incidence of VVD occurs in broiler chickens raised in cages compared with broiler chickens raised in floor pens (90, 199, 207). This may be explained by a lack of exercise in cages (90). Stronger cortical bone in chickens occurs with exercise (217). Different photoperiods will affect the incidence of VVD (24). It is unknown whether this is due to a change in growth rate, amount of exercise, or a hormonal factor.

Rotated Tibia. Rotated tibia was reported initially as a significant cause of lameness in turkeys and guinea fowl (206). More recently it has been reported in broilers (214). Affected birds often have the affected leg extended laterally. Either or both legs may be affected. The defect is restricted to the shaft of the tibia, which is rotated externally, often to 90° or greater. There is no angulation of bones and the hock joint is normal with no displacement of the gastrocnemius tendon. In some extreme cases the rotation reaches 180°. In such cases if both legs are extended ventrally the two foot pads face in opposite directions (Fig. 34.5). Rotation or torsion of the femur, tibiotarsus, and tarsometatarsus is normal during early development of the chicken. Femurs and tibiotarsi rotate externally while the tarsometatarsi rotate medially when the axis of the distal articular surface is compared with that of the proximal articular surface (58). Rotated tibia represents excessive and abnormal rotation during development. The cause is unknown though early rickets has been suggested as a predisposing factor in guinea fowl (6). Rotated tibia differs from VVD in that no angulation of bones is present and that in broiler flocks the peak incidence occurs at 3 wk of age, no sex predisposition is apparent, and the number of birds with either the right leg or left leg affected is approximately equal (214).

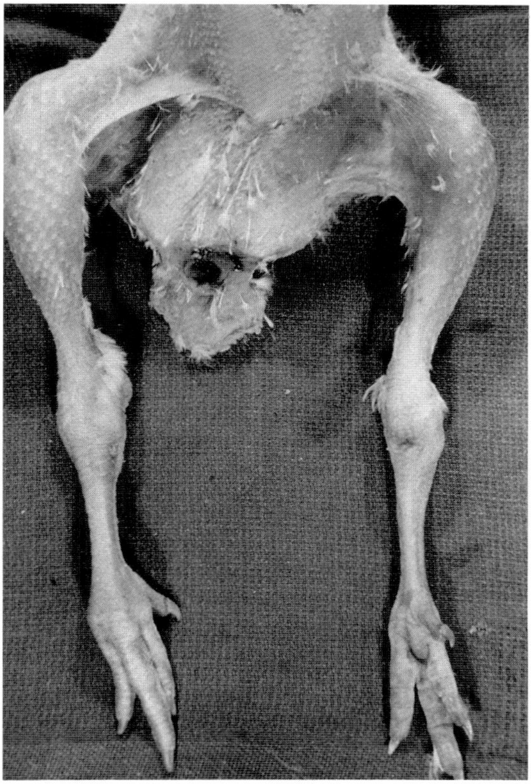

34.5. Turkey with rotated tibia of left leg. Rotation is nearly 180°, and the foot pads face in opposite directions.

Crooked Toes. Crooked toes are a common finding in meat-type chickens and turkeys. The syndrome was reviewed by Riddell (202). An incidence of 4.8–7.7% was reported in broiler chickens in Europe (191) while incidences exceeding 50% were reported in broiler chickens in Australia (164). The deformity unless very severe has limited clinical significance. It may interfere with the reproductive performance of breeding cockerels (164). Most digits or a single digit may be bent laterally or medially. Rotation of the phalanges often is present.

The pathogenesis is not understood though it has been proposed that shortening of flexor tendons may cause the deformation. A negative correlation between the presence of twisted legs and slipped tendons and the presence of crooked toes has been reported. The tension in flexor tendons is probably decreased when legs are twisted (191). An increased incidence of crooked toes has been associated with certain types of flooring, infrared brooding, pyridoxine deficiency, and some toxins (202). The syndrome should be differentiated from curly-toe paralysis due to riboflavin deficiency.

Dyschondroplasia. Dyschondroplasia is a very common defect associated with the growth plates of meat-type chickens, ducks, and turkeys. It is most commonly recognized in the proximal tibiotarsus and hence the condition is often described as tibial dyschondroplasia. The condition has also been called osteochondrosis by some authors. Osteochondrosis has been used in mammalian pathology to describe a wide range of lesions of growing cartilage, including degenerative and developmental changes in both physeal and articular cartilage. The defect that has been called dyschondroplasia in poultry is primarily an abnormal development of physeal cartilage and in the author's opinion dyschondroplasia is the most appropriate name. Reviews on the condition have been written by Wise (267) and Riddell (206).

SIGNS AND PATHOLOGY. In many broiler chicken and turkey flocks up to 30% of birds may have lesions of dyschondroplasia characterized by abnormal masses of cartilage below the growth plate, primarily in the proximal tibiotarsus (Fig. 34.6) but also at many other sites. Most birds show no clinical signs. If masses of cartilage are

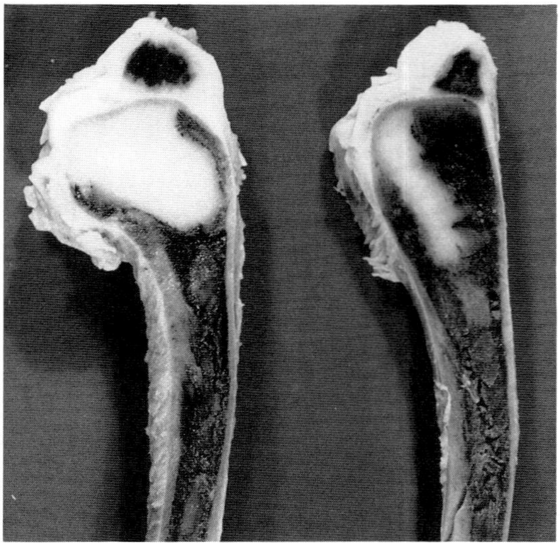

34.6. Medial view of sagittal sections of two proximal tibiotarsal bones from broiler chickens with tibial dyschondroplasia. Abnormal cartilage is only present in the posterior part of the metaphysis (*right*); abnormal cartilage fills the whole metaphysis and the proximal end of the bone is enlarged (*left*).

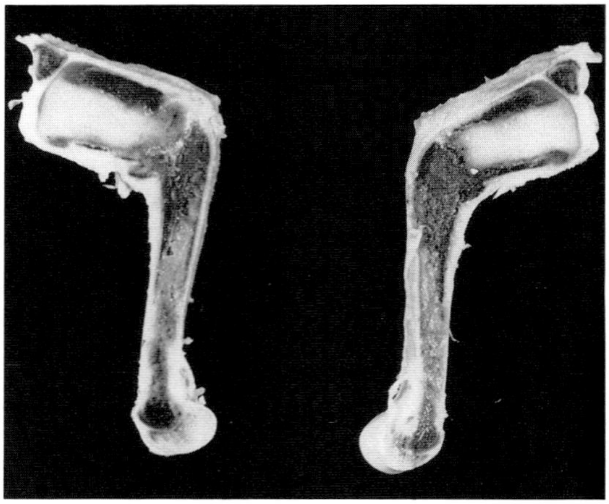

34.7. Sagittal sections of tibiotarsal bones from a roaster chicken with tibial dyschondroplasia. Severe angulation of the bones is due to fractures below the abnormal cartilage.

very large, signs will include a reluctance to move, a stilted gait, and bilateral swelling of the femoral-tibial joints often associated with bowing of the legs. In a recent survey of leg weakness in broiler chicken flocks processed at 7 wk of age or earlier, few birds were culled because of dyschondroplasia (214). Downgrading of carcasses and trimming of deformed legs at processing have been attributed to dyschondroplasia (19, 214). If broiler chickens are kept to roaster weights, lesions due to dyschondroplasia may be much more severe. In such birds fractures below the abnormal cartilage in the tibia may cause severe crippling (Fig. 34.7). A high association between leg deformities and tibial dyschondroplasia has been described in turkeys (252).

The abnormal masses of cartilage in the proximal tibia tend to be cone shaped. In mild cases these cones of abnormal cartilage mainly develop below the posterior medial part of the growth plate, but in severe cases they develop from the whole growth plate and fill the whole metaphysis. Anterior lateral bowing of the tibia is often associated with larger masses of cartilage. The concave surfaces of such bones have hypertrophied cortices. This is considered an adaptive change (59). Resolution of the abnormal cartilage may start as early as 48 days of age but sequestra of abnormal cartilage separated from the growth plate and bowing of the tibia may persist to as late as 30 wk of age even though the proximal growth plate of the tibiotarsus in a chicken closes at 16–17 wk of age. Fractured fibulae have been associated with tibial dyschondroplasia and bowing of the tibia (191). These fractures occur at the *Tuberculum M. iliofibularus* but are not always associated with abnormal tibiotarsal curvature (45). Dyschondroplasia also occurs but is less severe in the proximal and distal femur, the distal tibia, the proximal tarsometatarsus, and the proximal humerus (191). Dyschondroplasia in the femoral head in broiler chickens has been associated with a widened and shortened femoral neck and in some cases with fractures of the femoral head (39–41).

Microscopically, dyschondroplasia is characterized by persistence and accumulation of prehypertrophic cartilage. The separation of the prehypertrophic cartilage from the proliferating cartilage is not sharply demarcated and few vessels penetrate the abnormal cartilage from the metaphysis. Chondrocytes in the abnormal cartilage are small and shrunken and the matrix is more abundant than in normal hypertrophic cartilage. The matrix is not mineralized. Ultrastructural studies have demonstrated that the lesion begins in the prehypertrophic zone and that the chondrocytes in the abnormal cartilage undergo necrosis (80, 91).

PATHOGENESIS AND ETIOLOGY. The pathogenesis of dyschondroplasia is not well understood. At least three different mechanisms have been suggested. A failure in chondrocyte hypertrophy may result in abnormal cartilage that cannot be invaded by metaphyseal vessels (191). This failure may be a result of rapid bone growth. The presence of the most severe lesions of dyschondroplasia in the proximal tibiotarsus may be due to the growth plate at that site having the most rapid growth. The incidence of tibial dyschondroplasia has been decreased by reducing the growth rate of experimental birds, but there was no direct correlation between growth of individual birds and the development of tibial dyschondroplasia (206). Occlusion of vascular canals from the epiphysis has been described in the physes of femoral heads with dyschondroplasia. It has been proposed that patent vascular canals from the epiphysis may be necessary for normal chondrocyte hypertrophy (39). Such occlusion of vascular canals is not seen in dyschondroplasia in the proximal tibiotarsus and may in the opinion of the present author be an unrelated lesion. A second possible mechanism is that vascular invasion of the cartilage from the metaphysis may be inadequate. Such inadequacy may be genetically determined or due to trauma in a rapidly growing immature skeleton. Increased weight bearing may increase the incidence of dyschondroplasia (51). A third possible mechanism is defective chondrolysis. In *Fusarium*-induced tibial dyschondroplasia a paucity of chondroclasts has been described (92, 253). The possibility that dyschondroplasia may be the common endpoint of several different mechanisms cannot be ignored (92).

The incidence and severity of tibial dyschondroplasia can be influenced by genetic selection and cation-anion ratio in the ration (206). Though in original reports calcium and phosphorus levels in the ration were considered to have no effect, it has recently been shown that the incidence and severity of tibial dyschondroplasia in broiler chickens can be increased by feeding high levels of phosphorus relative to the level of calcium (61, 63, 213). Dyschondroplasia in broiler chickens was not eliminated by feeding a ration containing 1.5% calcium and 0.5% available phosphorus (213). The incidence of tibial dyschondroplasia in broiler chickens was reduced by daily fasting (62). A high incidence of tibial dyschondroplasia in broiler chickens has been produced with rations containing grain contaminated with a fungus, *Fusarium roseum* (253), and with rations containing a fungicide, tetramethylthiuram disulfide (246). Tetramethylthiuram disulfide has also been used recently to produce tibial dyschondroplasia in white leghorn chickens. This is the first time dyschondroplasia has been reported in egg-type chickens (247).

Osteochondrosis. A variety of microscopic degenerate lesions, including eosinophilic streaks or scars, occlusion and thrombosis of vascular canals, and necrosis in the growth plate and epiphysis, have been described in growing meat-type birds. Though these lesions may be associated with dyschondroplasia and in some cases may cause dyschondroplasia (39), in most cases they appear histologically, morphologically, and etiologically dissimilar to dyschondroplasia (152, 215). In this discussion the term osteochondrosis will be used for these degenerate lesions. Osteochondrosis has primarily been described in cervical and thoracic vertebrae of broiler chickens (152, 215), and in the femoral head (39, 40, 57, 119, 215) and the antitrochanter (42) of broiler chickens and turkeys.

SIGNS AND PATHOLOGY. Fifty percent of broiler chickens may have osteochondrosis, often without any clinical signs (152, 215). In many studies osteochondrosis has been described in birds with other skeletal lesions causing lameness, but in two studies osteochondrosis of the femoral head was the only abnormality detected that could have caused lameness (41, 119).

In affected vertebrae there is often focal thickening of growth plates associated with eosinophilic streaks following the zone of proliferation or transversing obliquely the growth plate (Fig. 34.8). Many of the streaks enlarge into clefts containing red blood cells and the adjacent cartilage is necrotic (152, 215). The eosinophilic streaks probably represent microscopic tears and the focal thickening of the growth plates appears to be

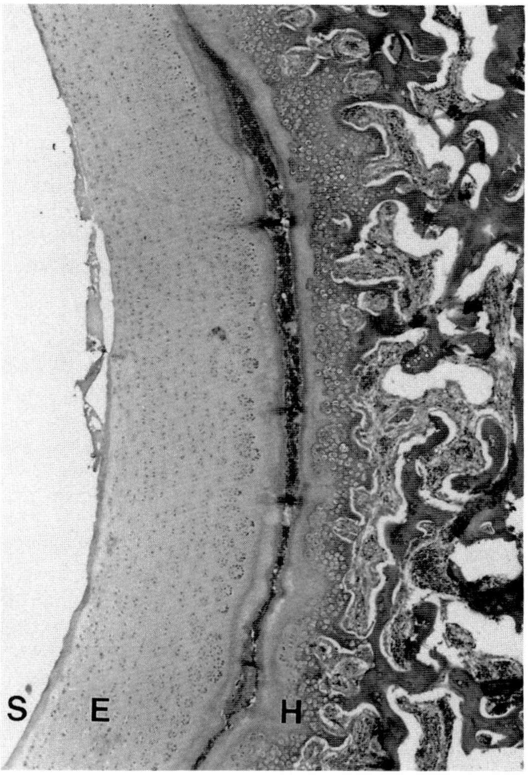

34.8. Osteochondrosis. Midline section of the end of a 6th thoracic vertebral body adjacent to a synovial joint from a broiler chicken. Synovial space (*S*), epiphysis (*E*), and top of zone of hypertrophy (*H*). An eosinophilic streak containing red blood cells follows the zone of proliferation. (Avian Dis)

secondary to the tears interfering with endochondral ossification (215).

In affected femoral heads similar eosinophilic streaks are seen in growth plates. Lakes of amorphous eosinophilic material may also be present. In addition vascular canals in the epiphysis and penetrating the zone of proliferation from the epiphysis are occluded with fibrinoid material and contain intact and hemolyzed red blood cells and thrombosed vessels. The growth plate is often thickened and disorganized. Lesions mainly occur on the medial side of the growth plate but also occur laterally. A widened or shortened femoral neck can be associated with these microscopic changes (39). Partial or total femoral head infarction may be associated with the vascular canal occlusion (40). In turkeys, lame because of osteochondrosis, there is often complete separation of the epiphysis and growth plate from the metaphysis. In such birds the joint capsule may contain brown fluid and necrotic debris (119). In mature chickens the lesions in the femoral head appear to result in abnormal persistence of growth plate cartilage, often with granulation tissue between the cartilage and adjacent trabeculae in the metaphysis. The retained cartilage is disorganized and often necrotic in part, with cystic spaces and fracture lines close to the trabeculae in the metaphysis (41). Such degenerative changes may result in detachment of the femoral head (55). Similar changes have been reported in the antitrochanter of broiler chickens and turkeys (42) and in the femoral trochanter of broiler chickens (43). Detachment of the proximal femoral epiphysis was observed in broilers that were being downgraded at slaughter as a result of hemorrhage into the thigh musculature. The detachment was probably caused by trauma and it was suggested that the detachment be described as fracture separation or traumatic epiphysiolysis. It is possible that osteochondrosis may have predisposed to the detachment (57).

Osteochondrosis has been described as a cause of femoral head necrosis in turkeys (119). In the opinion of the author the term femoral head necrosis is nonspecific and has been misused. The use of the term should be discontinued. Necrosis of the femoral head can result from osteochondrosis, dyschondroplasia, or osteomyelitis (119). The term has been applied to the shattering of the femoral head when the femur is osteoporotic and to the common separation of the proximal femoral epiphysis from the shaft of the femur, which occurs as an artifact when the coxofemoral joint is disarticulated at postmortem. In an experimental study no evidence was found to support the theory that osteochondrosis might predispose the separation induced at postmortem (215).

PATHOGENESIS AND ETIOLOGY. The lesions of osteochondrosis may be due to mechanical forces acting on rapidly growing cartilage (57, 152). The predominance of lesions in the growth plates of vertebrae and the femoral head may be explained by the greater exposure to shear forces of these growth plates than other growth plates (215).

Degenerative Joint Disease. Degenerative changes in joints have been recognized primarily in coxofemoral joints of mature male turkeys (37, 42) and mature meat-type chickens (42, 52), and in the spine of laying hens (271). They have also been reported in the femoral-tibial and intertarsal joint of turkeys (38, 60) and male broiler breeding fowl (52, 55). Duff (37) reviewed early reports of degenerative hip disease in poultry.

SIGNS AND PATHOLOGY. Turkeys with degenerative hip disease assume a stance with abducted pelvic limbs, constantly shift weight from one leg to another, and are reluctant to move. The primary gross lesions are found in the articular surface of the antitrochanter. Lesions include areas of surface irregularity, fissures along the dorsocaudal border, and formation of a flap of cartilage that breaks free to give fragments of cartilage within the joint. Erosions and thinning of the articular cartilage of the trochanter, marginal osteophytes, and periarticular fibrosis accompany severe lesions (37). Microscopic changes in the cartilage of the antitrochanter include loss of normal structure, areas of necrosis, fissures, and massive chondrocyte clusters. Surface fibrillation occurs in the articular cartilage (36).

In the femoral-tibial and intertarsal joints focal erosions occur in the articular cartilage with or without free cartilage bodies in the joint. Flaps of articular cartilage and osteophytes around the joint have also been found. Microscopic changes similar to those described above for lesions in the femoral head were found associated with evidence of disturbed endochondral ossification in some cases. It was proposed that the lesion in such cases could be described as osteochondrosis dissecans (38).

PATHOGENESIS AND ETIOLOGY. The pathogenesis of many of the joint lesions described above is not clear. Many may result from primary damage to the articular cartilage while others may be sequelae to osteochondrosis (42, 52).

Ligament Failure and Avulsion. Lesions of ligaments of the intertarsal joint were first described as a significant cause of lameness in meat-type poultry by Craig (27). Lesions have since been reported in the capital femoral ligament in young adult broiler chickens (44), in the posterior cruciate and other ligaments of the femoral-tibial joint in young adult broiler chickens (46, 49, 50, 55) and turkeys (37, 60), and in the intercondylar and collateral ligaments of the intertarsal joint of turkeys (60, 117) and broiler chickens (48, 55).

SIGNS AND PATHOLOGY. Lameness has been attributed to lesions in the capital femoral ligament. Lesions found include stretching, partial or total rupture, and avulsion, sometimes with a piece of cartilage or bone, from the femoral head insertion. Stretched ligaments sometimes contain hematomas or are infiltrated with fat. Microscopic lesions include fraying of collagen bundles, acellularity, and hyalinization of the collagen in the tendon along with necrosis, fissures, and hemorrhage in cartilage adjacent to the site of insertion (44). Lameness has also been associated with lesions in ligaments of the femoral-tibial joint. The posterior cruciate ligament has been the most commonly affected but the cranial cruciate, collateral, and caudal meniscofemoral ligaments have also been affected. In the cruciate ligament total or partial rupture near the tibial insertion or avulsion from the tibial insertion occurs. Microscopic lesions are similar to those described for affected capital femoral ligaments. In addition multicellular clusters and mucoid degeneration in the tendons and disorganization of subchondral bone with cysts and granulation at the avulsion site are found (46). Some abnormalities of the menisci of the knee joint have been associated with ligament disruption (53). Lameness has also been associated with partial or total rupture of the intercondylar ligament and with rupture or avulsion of the collateral ligaments. Most microscopic changes in affected ligaments have been similar to those described for other affected ligaments (48, 117).

PATHOGENESIS AND ETIOLOGY. Ligament rupture is probably due to trauma. Microscopic lesions similar to these described in ruptured ligaments have been described in intact ligaments of broiler-type chickens indicating that these changes precede the rupture (49). In individual male broiler breeding chickens tendon or ligament failure is often found at more than one site, suggesting a predisposition to ligament and tendon failure in these birds (50). Ligament failure may in part be age related as the incidence appears to increase with age (55). Ligament lesions were less severe in turkeys fed a restricted amount of feed when compared to turkeys fed ad libitum (60). Rupture of ligaments may be secondary to stress induced by limb angulation (48). In converse, it has been suggested that ligament rupture may result in limb angulation (117, 206).

Cage Layer Osteoporosis (Fatigue).

Cage layer osteoporosis (fatigue) is the most significant disease of the skeleton in modern chickens used for egg production. As the name implies the major feature of the condition is poor bone structure in laying chickens kept in cages. In the past, loss of birds in excess of 3% per month would occur in severely affected flocks. Recent losses have been much smaller but poor bone structure in caged laying hens still causes considerable economic loss due to bone breakage when birds are processed. The literature relative to the condition was reviewed by Riddell (206).

SIGNS AND PATHOLOGY. Birds initially are found paralyzed in their cages. They often are alert but later become depressed and die from dehydration. Some birds die acutely. The paralysis gave rise to the term fatigue. Paralyzed birds, if removed from their cages and given ready access to feed and water, will often recover in 4–7 days. On postmortem examination paralyzed or dead birds have bones that are easily broken. Fractures may be found in leg and wing bones and in the thoracic spine. Sterna are often deformed and there is characteristic infolding of the ribs at the junction of the sternal and vertebral components. Parathyroid glands are enlarged. Many birds have regressive ovaries and are dehydrated, while some dead birds have an egg in the oviduct and have died acutely.

Histologically the cortices of bones are thin with enlarged absorption spaces. Medullary bone is reduced in amount and largely consists of osteoid. The deformation of the ribs is due to small fractures and often damage to the spinal cord is associated with the fractures in the thoracic spine.

PATHOGENESIS AND ETIOLOGY. The paralysis in some birds may be explained by the spinal cord fractures but these cannot always be found. It is possible that paralysis in some birds and acute death in others may be due to hypocalcemia but this has not been proved. Similar skeletal changes and clinical syndromes have been produced experimentally with low-phosphorus, low-calcium, and vitamin D–deficient diets. Low-calcium and vitamin D–deficient diets produced a severe decrease in egg production while the low-phosphorus diet only produced a slight decrease. The modern laying hen has a very active calcium metabolism and high egg production may result in a physiological osteoporosis. Marginal nutritional deficiencies may result in severe osteoporosis and clinical signs. The formation of strong cortical bone and adequate medullary bone prior to egg production may be helpful in reducing cage layer fatigue. Increased calcium in the ration prior to egg production may be necessary, but it has been suggested that if increased calcium is fed for too long before egg production the parathyroid gland may be suppressed. Strain of bird and type of housing have been shown to affect the incidence of cage layer osteoporosis. The condition has been restricted to birds kept in cages. This can be due to less exercise causing poorer skeletal development but also in part due to birds not in cages obtaining some nutritional benefits from litter.

DISEASES OF MUSCLES AND TENDONS

Deep Pectoral Myopathy. Deep pectoral myopathy has also been called green muscle disease. Ischemia following exercise in heavily muscled meat-type turkeys and chickens causes the condition. Condemnation of affected muscles has resulted in economic loss in breeder turkeys. The condition was first described in Oregon in breeder turkey hens older than 10 mo of age with up to 9% of some flocks being affected (34). Several strains of bronze, as well as large, medium, and small white turkeys are affected. Both sexes have the defect (85). The lesion has been recognized in turkeys elsewhere in North America (77) and in the UK (113). The lesion has also been described in meat-type breeding chickens (86, 114) and in 7-wk-old broiler chickens (201).

SIGNS AND PATHOLOGY. The lesion can be unilateral or bilateral and does not affect the general health of birds. It is generally only found at processing. Chronic lesions result in dimpling or flattening of the breast muscles. These lesions can be detected by palpation (87). Comprehensive descriptions of the pathology of the lesion in turkeys have been provided by Siller and Wight (227) and in broiler breeder chickens by Wight and Siller (262). Lesions in both types of birds are similar. In early lesions the whole deep pectoral muscle is swollen, pale, and edematous with necrosis in the middle 1/3–3/5 of the muscle. The overlying fascia is often opaque with edema between the deep and superficial muscles. In older lesions the edema disappears and the necrotic muscle becomes more prominent and drier with greenish areas. In chronic lesions (Fig.34.9) the necrotic muscle has shrunk and is uniformly green, dry and friable, and enclosed by a fibrous capsule. It may shrink to a fibrous scar. The muscle posterior to the necrotic muscle becomes atrophied, pale, and sometimes fibrosed. The sternum adjacent to the necrotic muscle is roughened and irregular.

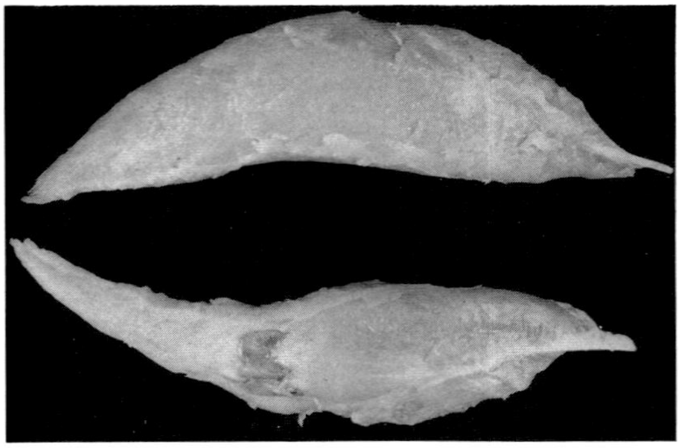

34.9. Deep pectoral myopathy in a turkey. Normal deep pectoral muscle (*upper*); shrunken deep pectoral muscle with a colored central core of necrotic muscle and a pale fibrotic posterior portion on the left (*lower*).

When examined microscopically the fibers in the green necrotic muscle are swollen and uniformly eosinophilic with discoid necrosis. Nuclei are absent or faint. Blood vessels within the necrotic tissue often contain only nuclei of lysed red blood cells. Surrounding the necrotic tissue there is an inflammatory reaction with heterophils, macrophages, and giant cells, and a fibrous capsule in chronic cases. Viable, degenerate, and regenerating muscle fibers are often enveloped by the capsule. Brown pigment and cystlike structures containing yellow material are also found within the capsule. In the muscle posterior to the necrotic tissue fibers may be atrophied and replaced by fat and in some instances fibrosis is present. Vascular lesions consisting of thromboses, intimal proliferation, and aneurysm formation are found in and around the necrotic tissue. Ultrastructural studies on affected muscles have been conducted (113, 262).

PATHOGENESIS AND ETIOLOGY. In an elegant series of experiments Wight, Siller, and Martindale (142, 229, 230, 263) have demonstrated that deep pectoral myopathy is the result of ischemia, secondary to the swelling in a tight fascia of a vigorously exercised muscle. In prior studies surgical occlusion of arteries to the pectoral muscles in both turkeys and chickens resulted in infarcts similar in appearance to the lesions of deep pectoral myopathy (178, 228). In subsequent studies temporary occlusion of the subclavian artery combined with electrically induced contractions of the deep pectoral muscle induced necrosis of the muscle in both light-weight and broiler strains of chickens. Similar electrically induced contractions alone produced necrosis of the muscle in the broiler strains but not in the light-weight chickens (263). Subsequently it was demonstrated that the necrosis could be produced by voluntary wing movements (229). However, surgical incision of the fascia around the deep pectoral muscle prior to exercise would prevent development of the lesion (230). Angiography demonstrated a complete ischemia in the deep pectoral muscle associated with an increase in subfascial pressure following electrical stimulation of the muscle. After 24 hr the ischemia only persisted in the middle of the muscle (142).

It is possible that the high incidence of deep pectoral myopathy in turkey breeder hens is in part the result of the extensive handling these birds receive during artificial insemination. Modification of handling procedures may reduce the incidence (264). Some evidence has been produced for a hereditary predisposition (87). This predisposition may be related to inadequate vasculature in muscles of meat-type birds (263). No specific nutritional factors are known to influence the condition (77, 84) but food restriction may reduce the incidence (262).

Rupture of the Gastrocnemius Tendon. For many years lameness due to rupture of the gastrocnemius tendon has been recognized commonly in meat-type chickens and rarely in turkeys. It can cause considerable economic loss in broiler breeder flocks and in broiler chickens raised to roaster weights. The early literature on the condition was reviewed by Peckham (187).

SIGNS AND PATHOLOGY. Up to 20% of a flock may be affected. Most outbreaks have been in broiler breeder chickens older than 12 wk of age but the condition has been recognized in broiler chickens as early as 7 wk of age. The rupture can be unilateral or bilateral. Onset of lameness is acute. Birds with bilateral rupture have a characteristic posture in which the bird sits on its hocks with its toes flexed (Fig. 34.10). In affected birds a swelling can be palpated on the posterior surface of the leg just above the hock. With acute lesions hemorrhage can be seen through the skin. With older lesions there is green discoloration while with chronic lesions no discoloration may be apparent but a very firm mass of abnormal subcutaneous tissue can be palpated. Dissection of acute lesions reveals a blood-filled swelling under the skin on the posterior surface of the leg. Within the hematoma the free end of the ruptured tendon can be found. The rupture generally occurs as an irregular transverse break just above the hock joint. In older and chronic lesions the blood is partially or completely reabsorbed and fibrous tissue encloses the end of the ruptured tendon and surrounding tissue. Microscopic lesions are variable. In many acute lesions there is hemorrhage only. In older lesions there is fibrous tissue surrounding resolving hematomas and the ruptured tendon. Synovial hyperplasia and infiltration of heterophils and macrophages vary from very little to massive. The infiltration of inflammatory cells occurs within the tendon and in the synovial membranes and cavities and may be associated with masses of heterophil debris and some bacterial colonies.

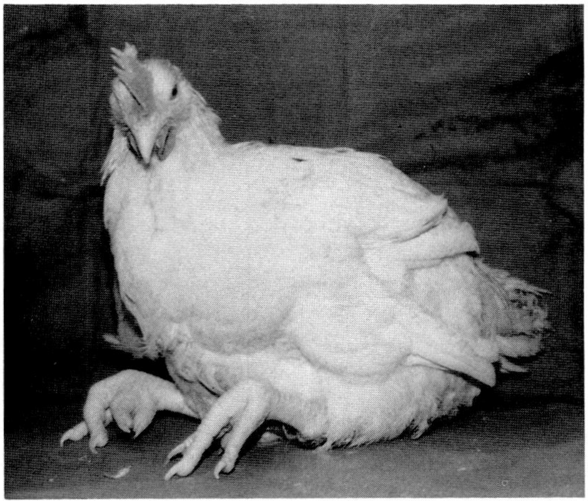

34.10. Roaster chicken with bilateral rupture of the gastrocnemius tendon. Hock-sitting posture with toes directed ventrally is characteristic.

PATHOGENESIS AND ETIOLOGY. Duff and Randall (56) reviewed the literature on the causes of rupture of the gastrocnemius tendon. They concluded that tenosynovitis, in particular that due to reoviruses, may be implicated in some cases. In other cases the rupture appears to be spontaneous. In such cases a frequent concurrent finding is rupture of other pelvic limb tendons or ligaments. In cases associated with tenosynovitis there was a marked inflammatory response while in spontaneous rupture there was a minimal inflammatory response.

The tensile strength of the flexor digitus perforatus and perforans tendon to the third digit is less in meat-type chickens than in egg-type chickens. It has been suggested that this could predispose meat-type birds to tenosynovitis (243). This could also predispose to spontaneous rupture of tendons. Tissue of the gastrocnemius tendon in meat-type birds has a less organized appearance than that in egg-type birds (244). In addition many meat-type birds have a hypovascular area in the gastrocnemius tendon just above the hock joint. This hypovascular area is associated with thickened chondrocyte plaques, chondrocyte death, and excessive lipid accumulation in the tendon. These changes may predispose to noninfectious tendon rupture (54). Little research has been conducted on the effect of nutrition on tendon strength. In one study administration of glycine, vitamin C or E, or copper had no effect on tensile strength of tendons (245). In another study restricted feeding had no effect on tensile strength of tendons but the ratio of tensile strength to body weight was less in chickens fed ad libitum than in those fed a restricted amount of feed (215).

DISEASES OF THE CIRCULATORY SYSTEM

Round Heart Disease in Chickens. Round heart disease is an acute cardiac failure due to myocardial degeneration in chickens commonly between 4 and 8 mo of age. It used to have a worldwide distribution but has not been reported in commercial poultry flocks for 20 yr. In the past 20 yr the author has diagnosed a few cases a year in backyard flocks in Saskatchewan but has never diagnosed the condition in large commercial flocks. The literature on the condition was extensively reviewed by Peckham (187). The reader is referred to the review for specific citations. In that review some papers on round heart disease in turkeys were also discussed. Round heart disease of turkeys in the opinion of the author is a different syndrome and will be discussed under spontaneous cardiomyopathy in turkeys in this book.

SIGNS AND PATHOLOGY. Morbidity in affected flocks is very low or absent while mortality may reach 50%. Birds are generally not diagnosed as sick prior to death. The most striking and consistent lesion found at necropsy is an enlarged and yellowish heart. The apex of the heart is blunt and may be dimpled. Both ventricles are hypertrophied (Fig. 34.11). In some birds there may be excess gelatinous fluid in the pericardial sac and in a few birds excess fluid is present in the abdominal cavity. Lungs are often edematous and the liver, kidneys, and spleen may be congested. Microscopic lesions consist of vacuolated myocardial fibers with very prominent cell membranes (Fig. 34.12). The vacuolation is due to distension of fibers with fat. Interstitial and perivascular lymphocyte and interstitial heterophil infiltration have been described in some reports and intranuclear inclusion bodies in other reports.

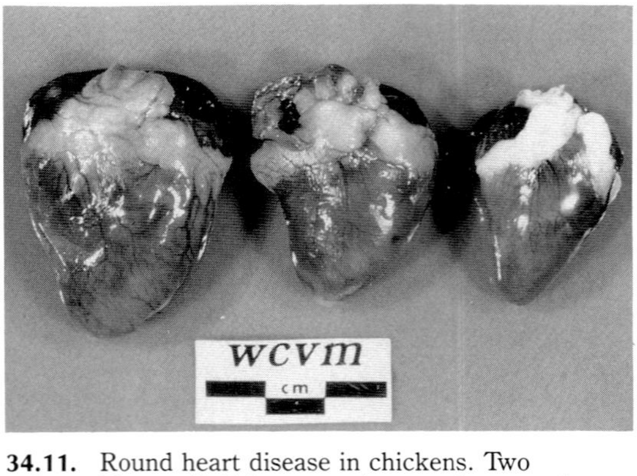

34.11. Round heart disease in chickens. Two enlarged hearts (*left*) in comparison to the normal heart (*right*).

PATHOGENESIS AND ETIOLOGY. The etiology is unknown. Numerous attempts to transmit the disease have been unsuccessful. Unspecified toxins, particularly those associated with built up litter, have been suggested as causes. Successful treatment of the syndrome with sodium selenite was reported once but has not been confirmed. In the author's opinion the restriction of the syndrome in Saskatchewan to backyard flocks fed marginal rations supports the concept that round heart disease in chickens may be due to a nutritional deficiency. Microscopic lesions of round heart disease differ from those reported in experimental vitamin E/selenium deficiency in chickens (209).

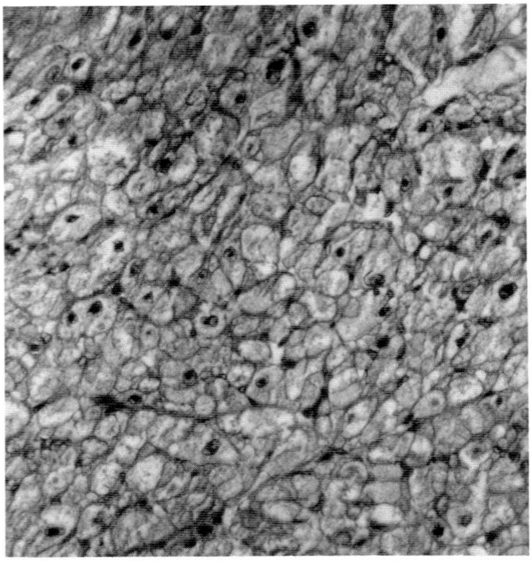

34.12. Histologic section of myocardium from a chicken with round heart disease. The fibers are dilated and vacuolated with prominent membranes. H & E, ×330.

Spontaneous Cardiomyopathy in Turkeys. Spontaneous cardiomyopathy causes mortality in turkey poults between 1 and 4 wk of age. The condition has more commonly been called round heart disease and less commonly the cardiohepatic syndrome. It is desirable that the term round heart disease be discontinued as the syndrome in turkeys is different in many respects from round heart disease in chickens (139). The literature on the syndrome has been reviewed by Czarnecki (31) and the reader is referred to this review for more detail and specific citations.

SIGNS AND PATHOLOGY. The highest rate of mortality due to spontaneous cardiomyopathy occurs in young poults peaking at 2 wk of age and disappearing at 3 wk of age. Losses have totalled as high as 22% in some flocks. The lesions of spontaneous cardiomyopathy persist after 3 wk of age but mortality is then sporadic. Affected young turkeys may die suddenly or may have ruffled feathers, drooping wings, and labored gasping prior to death. On postmortem examination affected young turkeys have greatly enlarged hearts due to dilation of both ventricles. Often the right ventricle is more dilated. Hydropericardium and ascites may or may not be present. Lungs are generally congested and edematous. Livers may be slightly swollen with rounded edges. In older turkeys from affected flocks enlarged hearts can still be found but in these hearts the prominent lesion is an enlargement and hypertrophy of the left ventricle.

Microscopic changes in abnormal hearts are nonspecific and include congestion, minor possible degeneration of myofibers, focal infiltration of lymphocytes, and in older turkeys increased fibroelastic tissue under the endocardium of the left ventricle. Vacuolization of hepatic cells, focal necrosis, bile duct hyperplasia, and intracytoplasmic periodic acid–Schiff (PAS)-positive globules in hepatocytes have been described in the swollen livers.

PATHOGENESIS AND ETIOLOGY. The etiology of spontaneous cardiomyopathy is unknown. A genetic influence was demonstrated by breeding trials. Birds with spontaneous cardiomyopathy were selected using electrocardiography and, by mating affected males to affected females, the incidence of the condition was increased in the progeny. Management stresses such as chilling, fumes, and poor nutrition have been implicated in spontaneous cardiomyopathy without any scientific proof. A suggestion that spontaneous cardiomyopathy might be due to an inherited serum trypsin inhibition has not been confirmed. Further work is needed to determine any relationship between the viral particles seen with the electron microscope in affected hearts and spontaneous cardiomyopathy. Furazolidone is toxic for turkey poults in concentrations as low as 300 ppm in the feed and produces a syndrome that is indistinguishable from spontaneous cardiomyopathy. Furazolidone may have a toxic effect on the myocardium but the exact mechanism is unknown. Sodium toxicity should be considered as a differential diagnosis but mortality generally occurs at an earlier age.

Ascites and Right Ventricular Failure in Broiler Chickens and Ducks. Ascites secondary to right ventricular failure (ARVF) occurs worldwide in growing broiler chickens and is a significant cause of mortality in many flocks. The incidence appears to be increasing. A similar syndrome has been reported in meat-type ducklings (122). The disease was first reported in flocks reared at high altitudes in Bolivia (78). It has since been described in flocks at high altitudes in Peru (28), Mexico (138), and South Africa (21, 99). Losses of up to 30% of the birds in some flocks may occur (138). More recently it has been reported in flocks at low altitude in the UK (2, 240), Canada (125, 208), and South Africa (99). A low incidence of the syndrome has been found in most broiler flocks at processing (208) and mortality may be above 1% in many broiler flocks and occasionally 15–20% in some roaster flocks (126) in Canada.

SIGNS AND PATHOLOGY. The condition may manifest itself as sudden death (125, 240), but often affected birds are smaller than normal and listless with ruffled feathers. Severely affected birds have abdominal distension (Fig. 34.13), may be reluctant to move, and are dyspneic and cyanotic (149). Gross lesions include ascites, right-side cardiac enlargement, and variable liver changes. More than 300 ml of straw-colored ascitic fluid with or without fibrin clots explains the abdominal distension (78, 149, 265). The right-side cardiac enlargement is due to both dilation and hypertrophy (Fig. 34.14). The hypertrophy involves both the right ventricle and right muscular atrioventricular valve. Measurement of the ratio of the weight of the right ventricle to the weight of the total ventricles (18) shows a greatly increased ratio in affected birds (99). Nodular thickenings of the endocardium particularly in the region of the right atrioventricular valve have been described (78). The livers in affected birds vary from congested or mottled to shrunken with a grayish capsule and irregular surface (78, 149, 265). Blood from affected birds has an increased packed-cell volume, hemoglobin, and red and white blood cell counts. Heterophils and monocytes are increased at the expense of lymphocytes (149).

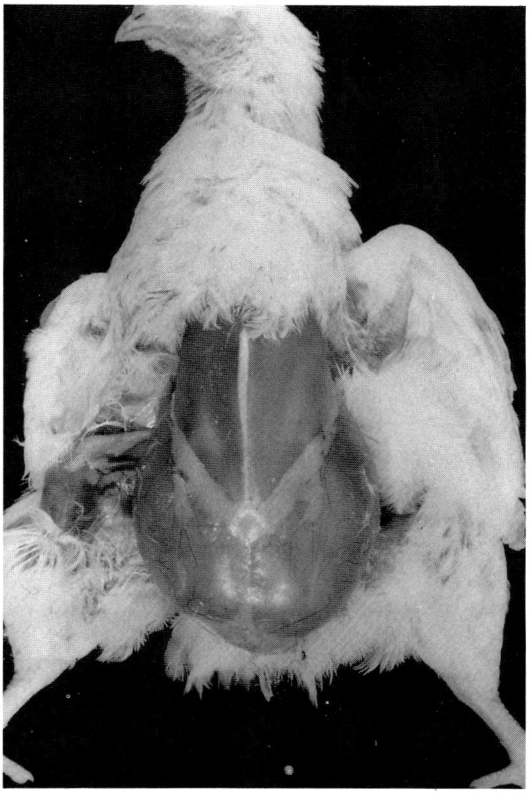

34.13. Broiler chicken with abdomen distended with fluid, secondary to right ventricular heart failure.

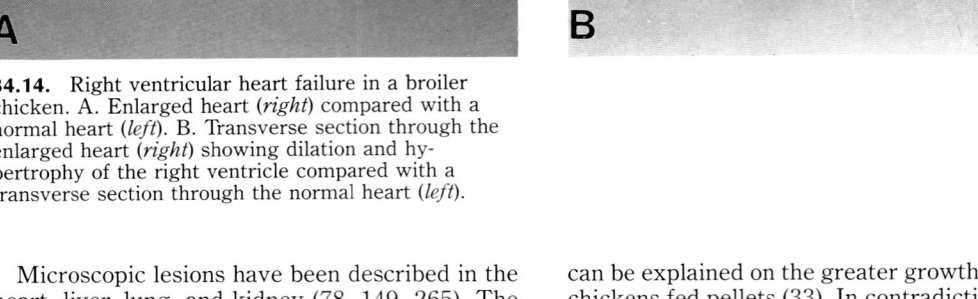

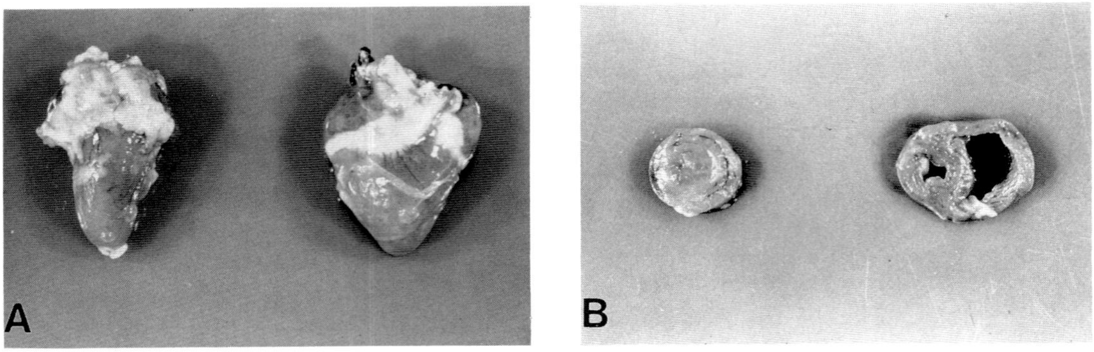

34.14. Right ventricular heart failure in a broiler chicken. A. Enlarged heart (*right*) compared with a normal heart (*left*). B. Transverse section through the enlarged heart (*right*) showing dilation and hypertrophy of the right ventricle compared with a transverse section through the normal heart (*left*).

Microscopic lesions have been described in the heart, liver, lung, and kidney (78, 149, 265). The myocardial fibers are mildly disorganized, with edema and some proliferation of loose connective tissue between fibers, focal hemorrhages, and infiltrations of heterophils. The liver sinusoids may be distended and often the capsule is greatly thickened. Foci of lymphocytes and heterophils in the liver are common. The lungs are often hyperemic with visible evidence of hemorrhage, edema, and hypertrophy of smooth muscle around the parabronchi, and collapse of the atria and air capillaries. Increased numbers of cartilaginous and osseous nodules have been found in the lungs of birds affected with ascites (148). Kidneys may have congested glomeruli with thickened basement membranes and scattered foci of lymphocytes (149).

PATHOGENESIS AND ETIOLOGY. The pathogenesis and possible causes of ARVF have been discussed by Julian (121) and Julian and Wilson (124). Broiler chickens raised at high altitudes and exposed to hypoxia develop increased pulmonary arterial pressure and right ventricle dilation and hypertrophy. There is a high correlation between pulmonary arterial pressure and the ratio of right ventricular weight to total ventricular weight. Severely affected birds develop ascites (28). In studies with white leghorn chickens kept at high altitudes, similar cardiac and liver changes to those in broiler chickens were described but excessive ascitic fluid was not reported (175). The broiler chicken is probably more susceptible to ARVF because of its greater metabolic rate producing a greater demand for oxygen. Rapidly growing broilers appear to be more susceptible to ARVF than slower-growing broilers (126). An increased incidence of ARVF in broiler chickens fed pellets compared to broiler chickens fed mash can be explained on the greater growth rate of the chickens fed pellets (33). In contradiction to these two studies in a comparison of the incidence of ARVF between two strains of broilers, the strain with the lowest incidence of ARVF had the greatest body weight at 51 days (101). The increased incidence of ascites in cold weather (21, 99, 138, 250) may be explained by an increased metabolic rate due to the cold weather. Increased right ventricular mass has been reported in chickens infected with *Aegyptianella pullorum* (100) and in turkeys infected with *Plasmodium durae* (98). It is postulated that hypoxia secondary to anemia caused by the parasites results in right ventricular hypertrophy.

Interference with respiration may produce an alveolar hypoxia. ARVF has been described in broilers with phosphorus-deficient rickets. It is postulated that such birds may experience respiratory difficulty because of rib softening and deformation (125). Lung pathology may interfere with oxygen diffusion across membranes or pulmonary capillary blood flow with resulting increased pulmonary arterial pressure. Amiodarone, an antiarrhythmic drug with serious side effects, has been shown to produce interstitial fibrosis in the lung of chickens with associated ascites and right ventricular failure (123). A high incidence of cartilaginous and osseous nodules has been found in the lungs of birds with ARVF (148, 265). Though it has been suggested that they may be secondary to hypoxia (148), it is possible that they may interfere with pulmonary blood flow.

Sodium toxicosis may cause ARVF as a result of hypervolemia (121). Cardiomyopathy is another possible cause of ARVF. ARVF has been produced experimentally in ducklings by feeding high levels of furazolidone. The pathogenesis has not been clearly defined but it was proposed that furazolidone induced biochemical changes in the myocardium (242). ARVF has been reported in broiler chickens fed excessive levels of furazolidone in their feed (66, 179). ARVF has also been produced experimentally in ducks and chickens fed high levels of rapeseed oil containing 40% erucic acid. The erucic acid caused degenerative changes in the myocardium and this was presumed to be the cause of the ARVF (198). Enveloped viruslike particles with an external diameter of between 77 and 128 nm were seen between myocardial fibers in an ultrastructural study of chickens affected with ARVF. Similar viruslike particles were also seen in the livers, lungs, and kidneys of affected birds but not in the tissues of unaffected control birds. A relationship of the viruslike particles to ARVF was not established (150).

In many reported cases of ascites in poultry the pathology and pathogenesis have not been clearly defined. In differential diagnosis of ascites in poultry consideration must be given to ascites occurring secondary to liver or vascular damage rather than to right heart failure. Ascites in meat-type ducklings is commonly secondary to hepatic amyloidosis, while hepatic fibrosis is the second most common cause of ascites in broiler chickens (122). Ascites following intravenous injection of carbon particles in chickens has been attributed to overloading of Kupffer cells with carbon (174). Ascites in poultry has also been associated with poisoning due to cresol, chlorinated biphenyls, coal tar, and toxic fat. In some of these poisonings damage to blood vessels has been described (188).

Acute Death Syndrome. Acute death syndrome (ADS) describes a condition in which healthy broiler chickens die suddenly for no discernible cause. The syndrome has also been described as sudden death syndrome, heart attack, and flip-over. The latter term has been used because birds dead from the syndrome are commonly found on their backs. The condition was first described as "edema of lungs" in England (94) and subsequently as "died in good condition" in Australia (110). Later it was reported in Eastern Europe (251), Canada (13, 22), and the USA (17). Birds dead from ADS are found in most broiler flocks. The incidence varies from 0.5 to 4.0% (13, 22, 110, 214, 234).

SIGNS AND PATHOLOGY. ADS has been reported to occur from 1 to 8 wk of age with the greatest losses occurring from 2 to 3 wk of age in most flocks (13, 214, 234). In some broiler flocks the weekly incidence appears to increase throughout the growing period suggesting an error in diagnosis or a different syndrome (214). Groups of dead birds may be found adjacent to feeder motors or heaters or within feed pans suggesting the birds may have been startled prior to death (234). In contradiction, no evidence was found in a behavioral study that ADS was precipitated by any environmental event occurring immediately prior to death (171).

Affected chickens show no clinical signs or unusual behavior until less than a minute before death. Birds may squawk during a sudden attack characterized by loss of balance, convulsions, and violent flapping (171). Most birds die on their backs with one or both legs extended or raised, but some may die on their sterna or sides (212, 234). Comparison of blood from birds just after death from ADS with blood from killed healthy birds revealed no consistent differences in serum levels of sodium, potassium, chloride, calcium, phosphorus, magnesium, or glucose. Total lipids were raised in some birds dying from ADS (212).

At necropsy birds dying from ADS are well fleshed with a full gastrointestinal tract. Livers are enlarged, pale, and friable and generally the gall bladder is empty. Kidneys may be pale and the lungs are often congested and edematous (176, 234). The congestion and edema of the lungs may be a postmortem artifact as it is not found in freshly dead birds (212). The ventricles of the heart are generally contracted and the thyroid, thymus, and spleen may be congested; there may be hemorrhages in the kidney (176). Microscopic lesions reported are nonspecific and consist of congestion, edema, and lymphoid cell infiltration in the lungs; hemorrhages in the kidneys; mild bile duct hyperplasia and periportal lymphoid infiltration in the liver; and mild degeneration and infiltration of lymphoid cells and heterophils in the heart (176). The cellular infiltrations described in the heart of birds dying from ADS have been considered to be normal lymphoid foci and foci of ectopic hemopoiesis (212). Use of an allochrome stain and a hematoxylin-basic fuchsin-picric acid stain did not demonstrate any degenerative changes in hearts of birds dying from ADS (212). In a study of organ weights, relative liver weights of broilers dead from ADS were significantly greater than the liver weights of control birds but no significant differences were noted between ADS and control birds in relative weights of lungs, hearts, and intestines (10).

PATHOGENESIS AND ETIOLOGY. The etiology of ADS is unknown. It has been suggested that it is a metabolic disease and that genetic, nutritional, and environmental factors may affect the incidence (212). ADS has primarily been described in broiler-type chickens. White Rock strains are more susceptible than the Light Sussex and New Hampshire crosses used in the early days of intensive broiler chicken production (94). Most modern broiler chicken strains are susceptible (13, 214) but the heritability is low (23). ADS was associated with rapid growth in a trial comparing crumble-pellet feeding with all-mash feeding

(193). In other experimental studies the incidence of ADS has not been affected by growth rate (104). Under field conditions no correlation was found between growth rate and incidence of ADS (214). A higher incidence of ADS in birds fed a pelleted feed compared with birds fed a mash feed may be due to a factor in the pelleting process rather than due to the more rapid growth in birds fed the pelleted feed (195).

Several nutritional factors have been studied with regard to the incidence of ADS. In a field survey a higher incidence of ADS was noted in flocks fed wheat-based rations low in corn (214), but no difference was found in incidence of ADS between experimental broilers fed wheat-soy diets and those fed corn-soy diets (104). It has been suggested that the addition of biotin to broiler rations will reduce the incidence of ADS (103) but this has not been confirmed (104, 235, 255). The content of biotin in liver samples from birds dead from ADS was not significantly different from that in normal flock-mates in one study (234) but was lower than that of flock-mates dying from other causes in another study (17). Biotin will prevent fatty liver and kidney syndrome (256). A syndrome has been described in which postmortem signs of both fatty liver and kidney syndrome and ADS have been found in dead birds. In particular, affected birds have fatty infiltration in liver, kidney, and heart. It was suggested that an abnormality occurring as a result of fatty liver and kidney syndrome may contribute to the initiation of ADS (255). The total lipid content of livers from birds dead from ADS is increased in a similar amount to that which occurs in livers of birds deficient in biotin, but the alterations in fatty-acid composition that occur in livers of biotin-deficient birds are not found in livers of birds dying from ADS (17). A number of other dietary studies also suggest that an alteration in lipid metabolism may be involved (162, 220, 236). Increased amounts of calcium, phosphorus, and magnesium (120) or potassium (104) in rations had no effect on the incidence of ADS.

In an epizootiological study of ADS, multiple regression analysis demonstrated negative correlations between incidence of ADS and flocks with more growing space, larger flocks, flocks raised on hammer-milled straw, and flocks raised in barns with hot-water heating. The authors commented that the correlations did not necessarily indicate causes but suggested areas for future study. No correlations were found with many other management factors including light intensity (214). In an experimental study it was also shown that light intensity did not affect the incidence of ADS (170), but a field trial suggested that intermittent light may decrease the incidence of ADS (177). Increased light intensity alternating from side to side within pens when superimposed on a background of low light intensity had no effect on the incidence of ADS (168, 169). Both acetylsalicylic acid (194) and reserpine (68) have been added to the diet with no effect on the incidence of ADS.

Hemorrhagic Anemia Syndrome. Severe mortality in chicken flocks associated with hemorrhages in muscles and internal organs and aplasia of the bone marrow has been recognized for many years. Early reports of the syndrome from England, USA, Israel, and Europe were reviewed by Peckham (187). Considerable confusion as to the cause of the hemorrhagic anemia syndrome (HAS) in many poultry flocks was apparent until the early 1970s when some studies indicated the syndrome might be due to a viral infection (64, 218). As a result of these studies the term "infectious anemia" was used by some workers to describe the syndrome (237). In this book that term is used to refer to the specific disease caused by the chicken anemia agent (CAA) (see Chapter 29). CAA may, in fact, be involved in all cases that have collectively been called HAS based on clinical and pathological features of the syndrome. However, the matter of etiology is still somewhat confused and the condition will be described in this chapter at the possible expense of overlap with the description of CAA-induced infectious anemia in Chapter 29.

SIGNS AND PATHOLOGY. The disease occurs in young growing birds between 3 and 14 wk of age and the mortality may vary from 1 to 40%. Gross and microscopic lesions have been described by Gray et al. (73), Cover et al. (25), and Marthedal and Velling (141). Affected birds show a paleness or icteric discoloration of tissues about the head. Hemorrhage may be present in the anterior chamber of the eye. Feathers are ruffled and birds are droopy and have a tendency to huddle. Diarrhea has been noted in some cases.

At necropsy, hemorrhages may be found in skin, musculature, and viscera. Blood may be cherry red and have a watery consistency. An occasional bird may have hydropericardium. The most consistent lesion, a great aid in diagnosis if extensive hemorrhagic changes have not occurred, is pale and fatty bone marrow (Fig. 34.15E). This change in appearance of bone marrow is due to a decrease in hematopoietic elements that are replaced by fatty tissue. Irregular scattered hemorrhages may be present in breast and thigh muscles (Fig. 34.15B, C). Punctate hemorrhages may be present in the proventriculus at its junction with the gizzard (Fig. 34.15F), and hemorrhage may occur beneath the gizzard lining, causing blackening and sloughing. Focal hemorrhages may be found on the external surface of the crop, and "paintbrush" splotches may occur in the myocardium. The intestine may have punctate hemorrhages in mucosal and serosal surfaces (Fig. 34.15D), and occasionally a bloody core is present in the cecum. Subcutaneous hemorrhage of shanks and feet may result in formation of ulcers. Hemorrhages may be present in liver, spleen, and kidney. The liver may be ocher-colored and studded with small hemorrhages (Fig. 34.15A), or it may present a reticulated network, particularly along the edges. Kidneys may show evidence of nephritis.

Marthedal and Velling (141) noted hemorrhages and fungal granulomas in the lungs that they regarded as a manifestation of reduced resistance. This observation has been confirmed by others, and the diagnostician should make a differentiation between primary and secondary fungal granulomas. Gray et al. (73) described liver necrosis and intestinal ulcers in HAS occurring during the terminal course of the disease. These liver and intestinal lesions are the hallmark of ulcerative enteritis, which may follow in the wake of debilitating diseases.

Leukopenia and anemia in HAS are associated with depressed bone marrow activity. The anemia is the normocytic, normochromic type. Abnormal thrombocytes are observed in blood smears. These cells are enlarged, more circular than normal, and highly vacuolated (73). The prothrombin time is not prolonged (25). Chickens with HAS have packed-cell volumes in the range of 8–19 in contrast to 22–26 in normal-appearing birds (130).

When examined microscopically the bone marrow of affected birds is devoid of hematopoietic elements, which are replaced by fatty tissue. Most of the sinusoids are collapsed. Hypoplastic bone marrow has a conspicuous reduction of myelocytic elements (73). Microscopic lesions described in other tissues include hemorrhage and necrosis in the liver, irregular areas of hemorrhage in the red pulp, hyalinized material in the adenoid sheaths and lymphoid nodules of the spleen, and evidence of coagulation necrosis in the tubular epithelium of the kidney (25).

In early reports of HAS (25, 73) there was no mention of inclusion body hepatitis. More recently inclusion body hepatitis has been described as a common finding in outbreaks of HAS (64, 130). Aplastic anemia and hemorrhage have been reported as variable features in outbreaks of inclusion body hepatitis (93, 96, 154, 190). In one report of inclusion body hepatitis no anemia was reported (97). More study is needed to clarify the nature of the relationship between HAS and inclusion body hepatitis. In field outbreaks gangrenous dermatitis has also been associated with HAS (35, 96, 141, 219).

PATHOGENESIS AND ETIOLOGY. Peckham (187) reviewed early studies on the etiology of HAS. Many of these early studies were directed at toxins including trichloroethylene, mycotoxins and sulfonamides, and vitamin K deficiency. None were conclusively proven to be a cause of HAS and more recent studies have been directed toward viral agents. Circumstantial evidence has suggested that adenoviruses may cause HAS (64, 218, 219, 237). Immunosuppression of young chickens by infectious bursal disease may predispose to HAS and gangrenous dermatitis (219). Significant anemia has also been reported in birds infected with Marek's disease virus (MDV), some of the leukosis/sarcoma viruses, and reticuloendotheliosis viruses (see Chapter 16). Of the infectious agents, however, CAA must be considered the most likely candidate; it could also be involved in the anemia attributed to MDV, adenoviruses, and other agents discussed previously.

Aortic Rupture in Turkeys. Aortic rupture or dissecting aneurysm of turkeys is characterized by sudden death in growing turkeys due to internal hemorrhage. The condition has been recognized throughout North America, in Europe, and in Israel. Mortality in the past has been reported to reach 50% but losses in affected flocks at present usually only reach 1–2%. References to early reports and studies of the syndrome may be found in a review by Peckham (187).

SIGNS AND PATHOLOGY. The condition occurs in birds between 7 and 24 wk of age with a peak mortality between 12 and 16 wk of age. The incidence is higher in male turkeys. Affected birds die suddenly. Gross and microscopic lesions have been described by McSherry et al. (158) and Pritchard et al. (192). At necropsy the head, skin, and musculature are anemic. Occasionally blood will run out of the mouth or the oral cavity will be bloodstained. Upon internal examination, large clots of blood will be found in the abdominal cavity and beneath the capsule of the kidney. Clotted blood may be present in the pericardial sac, lungs, and leg muscle. Invariably a longitudinal slit will be present in the aorta between the external iliac and sciatic arteries. In this region the aorta is dilated; the wall is thin and has lost its elasticity. The tunica intima and media may be thrown into deep folds and partially separated from the tunica adventitia. Fibers of the tunica media may show mild to severe degenerative changes and may be infiltrated with heterophils and macrophages. The media may be thickened due to an increase in ground substance and fibroblastic proliferation. Dissolution or disappearance of the elastic laminae of the media occurs at the site of rupture. Degenerative changes, areas of erosion, and cellular infiltration may be present in the adventitia. A marked intimal thickening or a large fibrous intimal plaque often occurs in the region of rupture. Sudan II stains reveal lipid accumulations in the affected intima.

PATHOGENESIS AND ETIOLOGY. Several reports have emphasized the possible role of intimal plaques in the pathogenesis of aortic rupture in turkeys. It has been suggested that these plaques and the absence of an intramural vasa vasorum around the abdominal aorta result in impaired nutrition to and degeneration of the media (165). High blood pressure in young male turkeys may also be a precipitating factor, but paradoxically the administration of diethylstilbestrol decreased blood pressure and increased the incidence of aortic aneurysm (134, 135). Diets containing high levels of protein and fat may increase the incidence of aortic rupture (192). Copper is important in collagen synthesis and it has been suggested that copper deficiency may play a role in aortic rupture. It has been shown that liver levels of copper are low in turkeys dying from aortic aneurysm (72). This was a limited study and further investigation of the possible role of copper in aortic rupture is needed. Beta-aminoproprionitrile, a toxic product that occurs in the sweet pea (*Lathyrus odoratus*), will produce aortic rupture in the turkey but has not been incriminated in the field syndrome (187). Uncontrolled field studies suggest favorable results in treatment of ruptured aorta with reserpine. This has not been confirmed experimentally and such treatment may depress growth rate (187).

Sporadic Renal Hemorrhage in Turkeys. Sporadic renal hemorrhage is an unexplained syndrome that also is associated with sudden death in growing male turkeys. Its etiology is obscure. It should be differentiated from aortic aneurysm. Extravasated blood surrounds the kidneys and is confined underneath the renal capsule. The birds are not anemic and the source of the hemorrhage may be rupture of small renal veins (166).

Endocarditis. Vegetative endocarditis is rarely reported as a flock problem but a low incidence of affected birds may be found if hearts of all birds necropsied are examined carefully. Peckham (187) reviewed some of the literature on endocarditis. Lesions generally consist of yellow irregular masses on any of the heart valves (Fig. 34.16). Infarcts in the liver, spleen, myocardium, and brain are associated with lesions on the left side of the heart. Cultures of affected heart valves generally yield staphylococci or streptococci but *Pasteurella* spp. and *Erysipelothrix insidiosa* have also been found, the latter particularly in turkeys. In experimental reproduction of the condition bacteremia preceded the valvular vegetation.

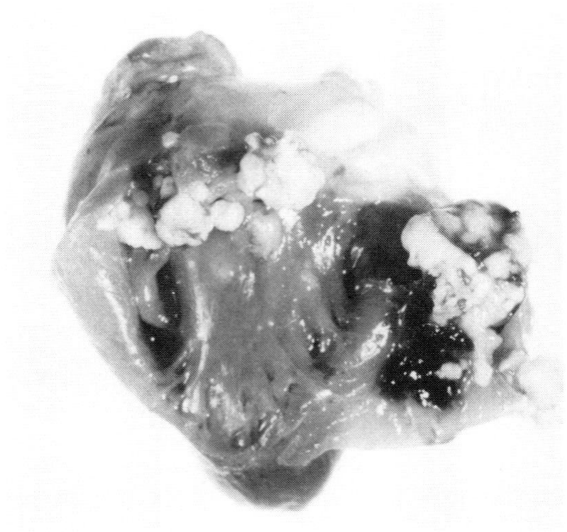

34.16. Vegetative endocarditis. Nodular vegetations on heart valve caused by *Streptococcus zooepidemicus*. (Peckham)

DISEASES OF THE RESPIRATORY SYSTEM

Emphysema. Subcutaneous emphysema is caused by an injury or defect in the respiratory tract that permits accumulation of air beneath the skin. This condition has been observed following rough handling and caponizing. After the caponizing operation the skin incision may heal before the opening in the body wall, with a subsequent accumulation of air beneath the skin. This condition, commonly called a "windpuff," can be alleviated by puncturing the skin with a sharp instrument. In aquatic or flying birds some of the pneumatic bones such as the humerus, coracoid, and sternum may fracture, allowing air to accumulate beneath the skin. Minor emphysematous bullae are common under the skin ventral to the proximal end of humerus in both turkeys and chickens. It is possible that they may be related to invasion of the humerus by the air sac during the first few weeks of life.

Cartilaginous and Osseous Lung Nodules in Broiler Chickens. A low incidence of cartilaginous and osseous nodules have been reported in the lungs of birds for several years. Early reports were listed by Maxwell (148). More recent reports from Canada (116, 223) and the UK (260) indicate that a high incidence of such nodules is common in the modern broiler chicken. The nodules are much less common in egg-type chickens, turkeys, ducks, and geese (223, 260). The incidence of broiler chickens with nodules has been reported to be circa 60% or greater (148, 223, 260). The incidence is probably 100% as the nodules can only be seen under the microscope and in surveys conducted to date only a limited number of sections of the lungs have been examined. The nodules have been recognized in meat-type chickens from 1 day to 52 wk of age (260). They may be more numerous at 3 wk of age (223), in the left

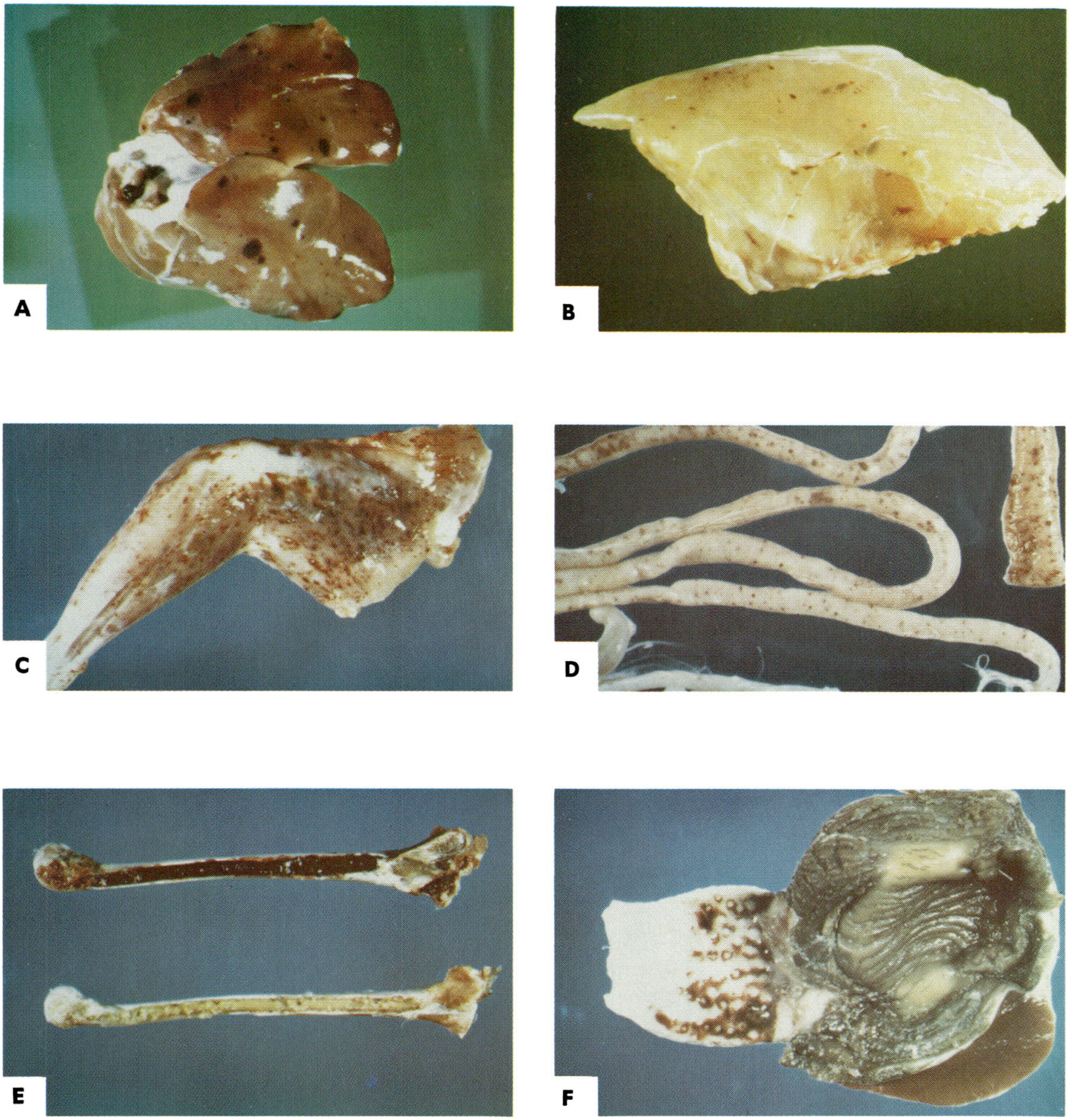

34.15. Lesions of hemorrhagic anemia disease. A. Punctate hemorrhages in pale liver. B. Hemorrhages in breast muscle of chicken. C. Hemorrhage in thigh and leg muscles of chicken. D. Punctate hemorrhages in mucosal surface of duodenum. E. Pale aplastic marrow in tibia from chicken with hemorrhagic anemia disease (*bottom*) contrasted with the dark red marrow in tibia from normal bird (*top*). F. Hemorrhages in proventriculus. (Peckham)

as compared to the right lung (151), and in males (260).

PATHOLOGY. The nodules, though only visible under the microscope, may be as large as 240 μm in diameter (148) and have been classified into hyaline cartilaginous, fibrous cartilaginous, mineralized cartilaginous, and osseous (Fig. 34.17) (148, 223). Hyaline cartilaginous nodules consist of a circular mass of bluish to pink cartilage containing numerous chondrocytes in lacunae. The matrix of fibrous cartilaginous nodules is pink and has a fibrous appearance, lacunae are not apparent, and the chondrocytes are pyknotic. Mineralized cartilaginous nodules are similar to fibrous nodules but are in part stained dark blue due to mineralization. The osseous nodules have a variable shape and stain red to purple and contain small cells resembling osteocytes. The nodules are found in the parenchyma of lung lobules. All are located some distance from large airways and blood vessels. No reaction is visible around hyaline cartilaginous nodules but the other types of nodules may be surrounded by a thin layer of fibrous cells, heterophils, and macrophages. The nodules appear to change with age from hyaline to fibrous to mineralized cartilaginous types and finally to an osseous type.

PATHOGENESIS AND ETIOLOGY. The cause and significance of these nodules are unknown. It has been suggested that the nodules may be derived from embolic chondrocytes arising from embryonic cartilage in developing bones (116) or from abnormal growth plates (223). No correlation could be found between incidence of nodules and skeletal deformities (116, 223). It is more probable that the nodules may be derived from chondrocytes displaced from nearby bronchi during early development (260). Recently an increased incidence of nodules has been described in birds suffering from ascites and right heart failure (148, 151, 265). An increase in fibrous tissue in the lungs of such birds may lead to an increase in the number of nodules (148). An increased number of nodules has also been reported in broilers dying from other diseases but the data could be questioned as the control birds were kept in separate accommodations (151). The number of nodules is greater in broiler chickens fed ad libitum than in broiler chickens fed a restricted amount of food (223). A theory that the nodules may arise from inhaled dietary bonemeal has been disproven by the finding of the nodules in broiler chickens fed rations free of bonemeal and animal protein (260).

DISEASES OF THE DIGESTIVE SYSTEM

Miscellaneous Conditions of the Upper Digestive System. Peckham (187) reviewed four minor conditions of the upper digestive system. These conditions are rarely recognized today and are of limited importance. A stomatitis characterized by diphtheritic patches in the oral cavity of chickens was attributed to *Spirillum pulli*. Beak necrosis, in which the mandible sloughs in chickens, and curled tongue in turkeys were associated with impaction of fine mash feeds in the mouths of affected birds. Crop impaction occurred when large amounts of fibrous material were ingested and formed a ball in the crop.

Pendulous Crop. Pendulous crop occurs at a low incidence in many chicken and turkey flocks. In some flocks the incidence may reach 5%. In severely affected birds the crop is greatly distended and full of feed, particles of bedding, and fluid that is often foul smelling (Fig. 34.18). The lining of the crop may be ulcerated. Birds continue to eat but digestion is impaired and birds become emaciated. Death may result and carcasses of affected birds are generally condemned at processing. The possible etiologies of pendulous crop were discussed by Peckham (187). A hereditary predisposition has been suggested in turkeys. An increased incidence has been noted in turkeys after increased liquid intake in hot weather. Neither of these factors appear to be important when a high incidence is encountered in modern poultry flocks. The possibility that diet may influence the incidence of pendulous crop is supported by the experimental production of pendulous crops with rations containing cerelose as a substitute for starch. Further research is needed on the etiology of pendulous crop.

Dilation of the Proventriculus in Chickens. In 4-wk-old chicks fed a purified diet, dilation of the proventriculus was first reported as proventricular hypertrophy by Newberne et al. (167). The abnormality is commonly observed as an incidental finding in broiler chickens. Occasionally a high incidence in a broiler chicken flock may cause significant carcass contamination when enlarged proventriculi rupture at processing. The enlarged proventriculi have greatly dilated, thin walls and are full of feed. The gizzards in affected birds are poorly developed and there is no sharp demarcation between the gizzard and proventriculus (Fig. 34.19). The poor development of the gizzard is generally the result of a finely ground diet lacking in fiber and the dilation of the proventriculus is secondary (204).

Gizzard Impaction. Gizzard impaction can cause high mortality during the first 3 wk of life in turkey flocks. The condition is rare in chickens. Affected poults are emaciated with empty intestinal tracts but gizzards are full of a solid mass of interwoven fibrous material. This fibrous mass often extends into the first part of the duodenum and in some birds masses of fibrous material are

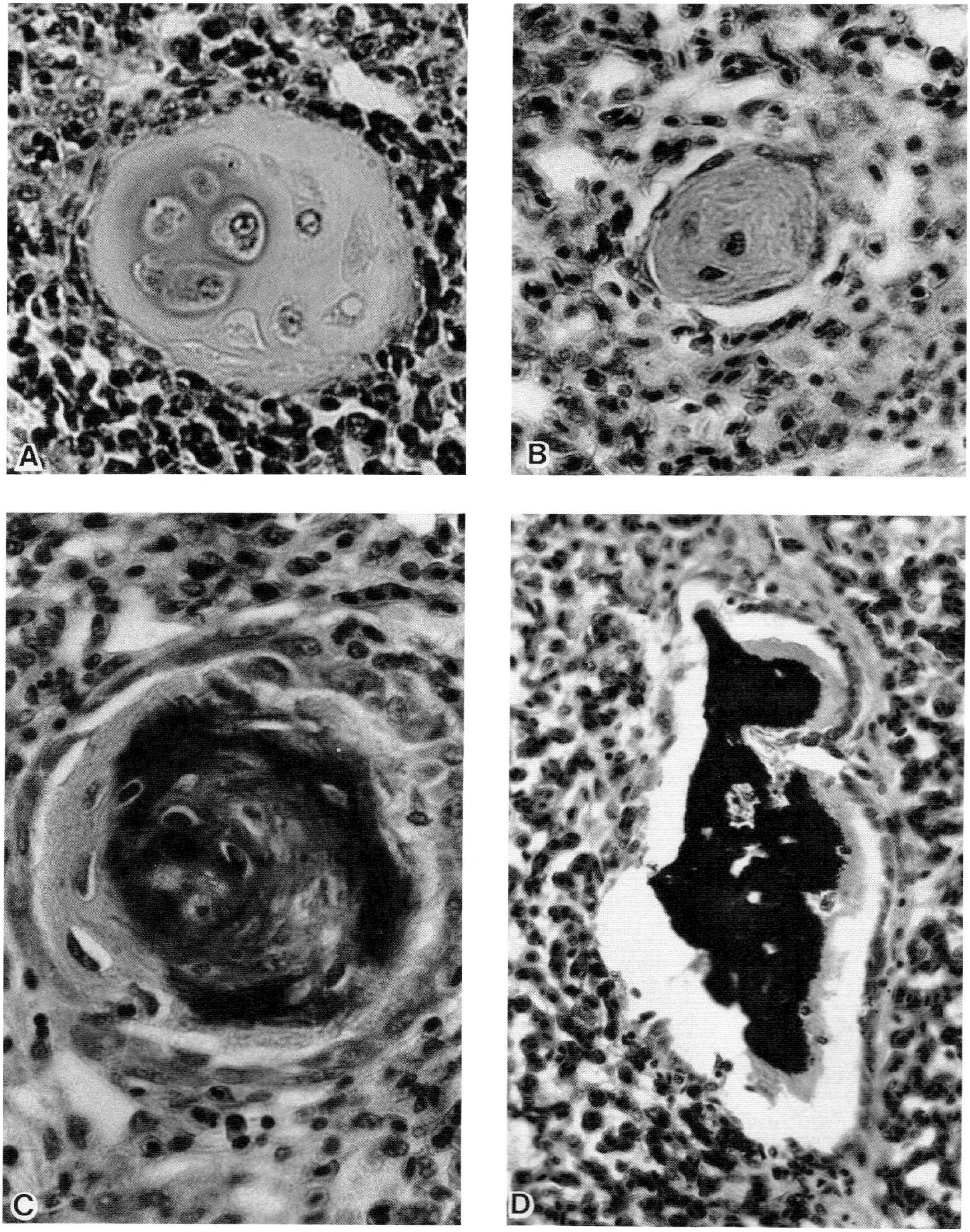

34.17. Cartilaginous and osseous nodules in microscopic sections from the lungs of broiler chickens. A. Hyaline cartilaginous nodule. H & E, ×528. B. Fibrous cartilaginous nodule. H & E, ×528. C. Mineralized cartilaginous nodule. H & E, ×528. D. Osseous nodule. Van Kossa stain, ×528. (Avian Dis.)

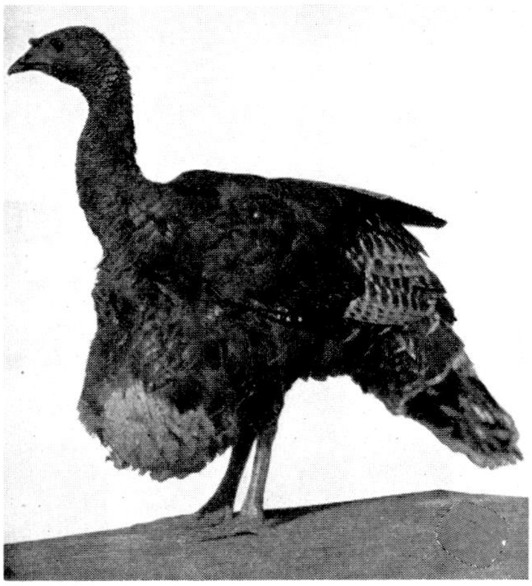

34.18. An 8-mo-old female turkey with pendulous crop of about 5 mo duration. (Peckham)

found lower in the intestine. The impaction results from the birds eating litter, which the gizzard is unable to handle. Prevention is aimed at discouraging the eating of litter by young poults.

Infectious Stunting Syndrome. Infectious stunting syndrome (ISS) was first reported in the Netherlands in 1978 (131, 132), in the UK in 1981 (12), in Australia in 1982 (183), and in Canada in 1985 (210). ISS is characterized by severe growth depression. At the time ISS was first recognized in Europe other syndromes in which severe growth depression occurred were described as malabsorption syndrome (182), pale bird syndrome (173), and brittle bone disease (241) in the USA. Though it is possible that all these syndromes were variations of a new disease affecting the broiler industry worldwide this has not been proven. Striking differences have been noted in clinical signs and postmortem findings between different countries and even between different parts of the same country (11). ISS continues to cause significant economic loss for the broiler industry. Although ISS has been reported primarily in broiler chickens, a similar syndrome has been reported in replacement pullets (239) and in turkeys (29, 156).

SIGNS AND PATHOLOGY. Bracewell and Randall (11) reviewed early reports of ISS and described its common and variable features. Later descriptions (133, 200, 210) do not differ markedly. ISS is characterized by uneven growth, which is obvious by 1 wk of age or earlier. From 5 to 20% of birds in a flock may be affected and these birds will be half the size or less of their penmates by 4 wk of age. Between 6 and 14 days of age a small rise in mortality may occur and there may be excessive drinking and diarrhea. Affected flocks have poor feed conversions. The small chicks are active. They retain chick down and development of primary feathers is delayed and irregular. Many have abdominal distension. Their intestines are pale and dilated and may contain undigested feed.

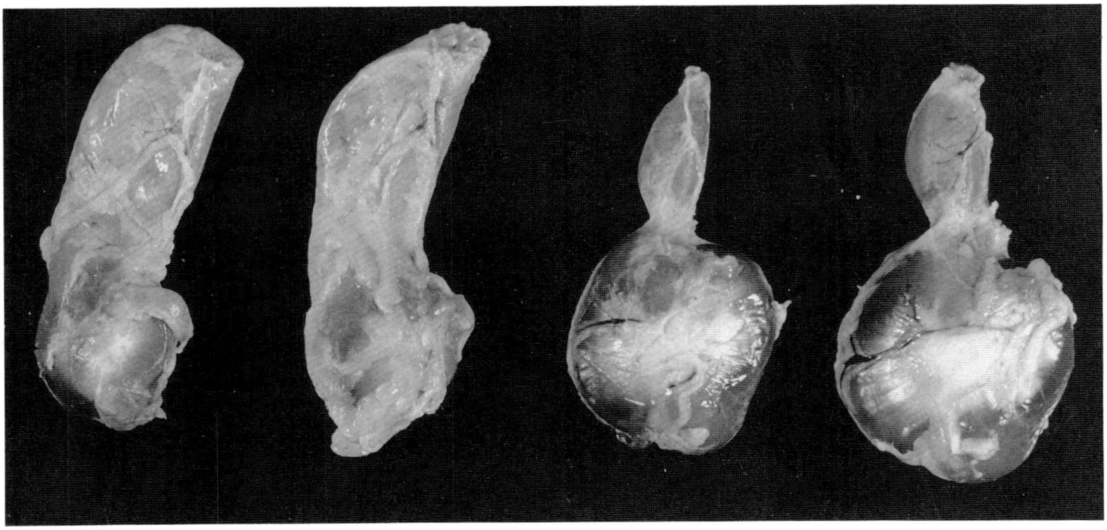

34.19. Gizzards and dilated proventriculi from broiler chickens fed only a commercial broiler starter (*left*) compared with those from broiler chickens fed a broiler starter containing oat hulls (*right*). The former gizzards are small and the proventriculi enlarged. (Avian Dis)

The proventriculus may be enlarged. The bursa of Fabricius is often small and the thymus atrophied. A striking but variable lesion affects the pancreas. Affected pancreases are thin, white, and firm particularly in the distal third (Fig. 34.20). Long bones may be soft with associated thickening of the growth plates. The femoral head may disintegrate on disarticulation of the coxofemoral joint.

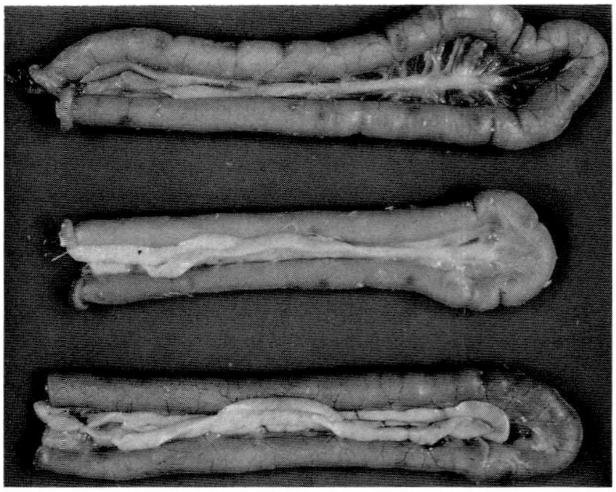

34.20. Abnormal pancreases (*top*) from broiler chickens with infectious stunting syndrome compared with a normal pancreas (*bottom*). The upper pancreas is most severely affected and thin and fibrotic for ⅔ of its length while only the distal ⅓ of the middle pancreas is affected.

Microscopic lesions reported have been confined to organs in which gross lesions have been recognized. Some blunted villi and dilation of the crypts of Lieberkuhn have been seen in intestines. In some cases infiltration of the interglandular tissue in the proventriculus with mononuclear cells has been observed. This lesion, which has been described as proventriculitis, may be a separate cause of growth retardation (133). The bursae exhibit some atrophy of follicles while in the thymus the cortex is thinner and it may be difficult to differentiate the cortex and medulla. Early lesions in affected pancreases consist of vacuolation and shrinkage of exocrine cells leading to atrophy of acini. Later much of the exocrine tissue is obliterated by fibroplasia. Scattered foci of lymphoid cells occur and remnants of exocrine tissue persist, ringing the islets of Langerhans. Abnormal growth plates have a thickened zone of proliferation with no sharp demarcation from the zone of hypertrophy, which is poorly eroded by vessels from the metaphysis. These lesions suggest a vitamin D or calcium deficiency.

Low plasma carotenoid and an increased alkaline phosphatase activity have been found in the blood of affected experimental birds in Holland (248, 249), while increased plasma protein and a decreased plasma pigment in the blood and sometimes an increased glycogen level in the liver were found in affected birds in the USA (221). Increased plasma amylase and reduced glutathione peroxidase, vitamin E concentration, and alkaline phosphatase activity were found in the blood of affected birds in outbreaks of ISS in Australia (231).

PATHOGENESIS AND ETIOLOGY. The pathogenesis and etiology of ISS are poorly understood. Impaired nutrient utilization has been described in stunted birds (70, 137, 221). Prolonged gastrointestinal times have been reported in experimental birds (71). Impaired nutrient utilization may be due to malabsorption but it may also be due to maldigestion (76). Maldigestion could result from the pancreatic lesions but it is probable that the pancreatic lesions are secondary. Similar pancreatic lesions have been caused by selenium deficiency (75) or pancreatic duct obstruction (145). A togaviruslike agent has recently been seen in the pancreatic duct of chickens with ISS and it has been suggested that it may cause pancreatic duct obstruction (67, 146). In many field outbreaks the infectious nature of ISS has been based on field observations and laboratory reproduction of the syndrome with intestinal contents from affected birds. Reoviruses (11, 95, 182, 241, 248), caliciviruses (270), enterolike viruses (157, 159), parvoviruses (128, 129), coronaviruslike particles (70), and togalike viruses (67) have been demonstrated in intestinal contents or enterocytes or isolated from birds with ISS. The possible association of reoviruses with a malabsorption syndrome is further discussed in Chapter 27. However, it should be noted that ISS has not been completely reproduced with any of these viruses after they have been purified. Kouwenhoven et al. (133) have suggested that bacteria as well as viruses may be involved in the etiology.

Similar field syndromes have been attributed to mycotoxins (238) and the possibility of mycotoxins or other toxins being the cause of some field outbreaks should not be ignored. Thorough cleaning and disinfection between flocks and good husbandry, in particular reducing stocking density, has been reported to ameliorate the condition (11, 65, 161). A stunted chick disease occurred between 1943 and 1953 in North America (216). Typical signs reported were rough feathering with brittle and broken primary and secondary wing feathers, encrustations at the commissures of the mouth, and granulations on the eyelids. Growth was severely depressed. Mortality ranged from 25 to 75% by the 4th wk. Survivors at 5–6 wk of age recovered and grew normally. The cause was not determined. Stunted chick disease has not been reported recently and is different in several aspects from ISS.

DISEASES OF THE LIVER

Fatty Liver–Hemorrhagic Syndrome (FLHS).

This syndrome has been recognized in laying hens in many countries of the world. It occurs primarily in egg-type birds kept in cages but has also been recognized as a less significant problem in birds kept on litter; outbreaks occur sporadically. A review by Butler (20) formed the basis of the following description.

SIGNS AND PATHOLOGY. In outbreaks of FLHS there is often a sudden drop in egg production. Hens may be overweight with large pale combs and wattles covered with dandruff. The first sign of disease is often an increase in mortality with birds in full production being found dead with pale heads. Mortality usually does not reach 5%. Dead birds have large blood clots in the abdomen often partially enveloping the liver and arising from the liver (Fig. 34.21). The liver is generally enlarged, pale, and friable. It may have smaller hematomas within the parenchyma. These hematomas may be recent and dark red or older and green to brown. Similar hematomas may be seen in clinically healthy birds in the same flock if such are examined during or after an outbreak. Large amounts of fat are present in the abdominal cavity and around the viscera. Dead birds are in full production and often have a developing egg in the oviduct.

Microscopic examination of the liver shows hepatocytes distended with fat vacuoles, varying sized hemorrhages and organizing hematomas, and often small irregular masses of uniform eosinophilic material. These masses, which are amyloidlike in appearance, have been identified as a possible derivative of plasma protein and similar to fibrin (261). The fat content of livers generally exceeds 40% dry weight and may reach 70%. The proportion of oleic acid in the lipids is increased. No changes have been found in concentrations of major plasma proteins; the glucose level; or the activities of glutamate-oxalactate transaminase, β-glucuronidase, and lactate dehydrogenase.

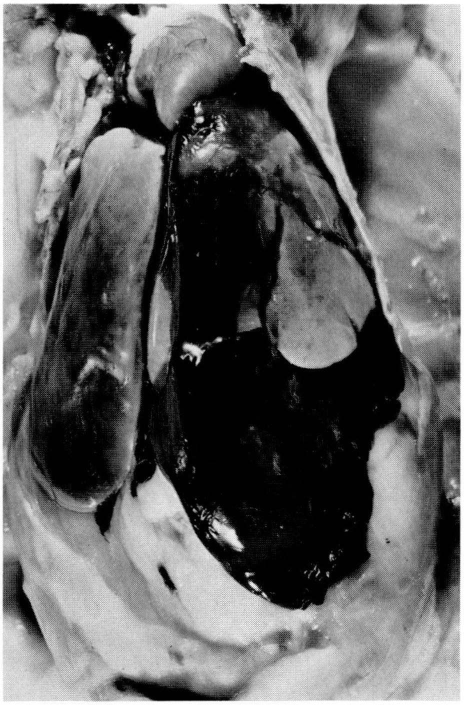

34.21. Fatty liver–hemorrhagic syndrome. A large blood clot is molded over one lobe of the liver. Note excess abdominal fat. (Peckham)

PATHOGENESIS AND ETIOLOGY. Excessive consumption of high-energy diets in birds whose exercise is restricted in cages is considered to result in a positive energy balance and excessive fat deposition. This may be compounded by hot weather. However, laying hens can have high levels of fat in their livers without hemorrhage. The pathogenesis and cause of the hemorrhage has not been defined. Excessive fat may disrupt architecture of the liver and result in weakening of the reticular framework and blood vessels in the liver. A pathogenic relationship between hepatic steatosis and hemorrhage has been suggested (184). Lysis of the reticulin framework of the liver has been reported in FLHS. A strong association of reticulolysis with severity of liver hemorrhage has been described in experimental birds. Rupture of intrahepatic portal veins associated with degenerative changes in the veins was described in the same birds (147). Focal necrosis of hepatocytes leading to vascular injury has been described as another mechanism to explain the hemorrhage (107, 272). The observation of greatly elevated serum calcium and cholesterol in chickens from flocks with FLHS suggests that the syndrome may be due to a hormone imbalance (82, 160). Injection of immature chickens with oestradiol has been shown to result in hepatic steatosis and hemorrhage (185). Similar injection of laying hens caused liver enlargement, death from liver hemorrhage, and neurologic disorders (233).

Dietary factors other than excess caloric intake have been considered as causes of FLHS. Many papers describing the field treatment of FLHS with specific nutrients and experiments testing the effect of specific nutrients added to the diet of laying hens on the level of hepatic fat were reviewed by Butler (20). He concluded that the results were inconsistent and provided no useful conclusions as to the etiology or treatment of FLHS. Stake et al. (233) listed some more recent papers in which the incidence and severity of FLHS were reported to have been reduced by unidentified nutritional factors in alfalfa, dried brewer's grains, soybean mill feed, wheat bran, vitamin E, dried brewer's yeast and torula yeast, fish meal, and fermentation by-products.

In several reports mortality in laying hens due to liver hemorrhage has been associated with the use of rapeseed meal in the diet (186). In addition rapeseed meal has been shown experimentally to increase the extent and severity of liver hemorrhage, but in these experiments liver hemorrhage has also occurred in birds not fed rapeseed meal (147, 186). The possibility of toxins causing FLHS should not be ignored. Aflatoxin has been considered as a possible cause but produces different liver lesions.

DISEASES OF THE URINARY SYSTEM. An excellent review of renal pathology of the fowl by Siller (226) formed the basis for the following descriptions. The present descriptions are brief and only cover conditions of major importance commonly seen in commercial poultry and the reader is referred to the above review for more detailed information and descriptions of miscellaneous conditions such as congenital malformations and baby chick nephropathy.

Gout. Gout is a common finding during necropsy of poultry. It is the result of abnormal accumulation of urates and occurs as two distinct syndromes. Articular gout is characterized by tophi, deposits of urates, around joints particularly those of the feet. The joints are enlarged and the feet appear deformed (Fig. 34.22). When these joints are opened the periarticular tissue is white due to urate deposition, and white semifluid deposits of urates may be found within the joints. Articular gout is a sporadic individual bird problem of little economic importance in poultry. As it has been reproduced by feeding high-protein diets, it is tempting to infer that it results from excess production of uric acid. However, studies in a line of chickens bred for susceptibility to articular gout indicate that they may have a defect in tubular secretion of uric acid.

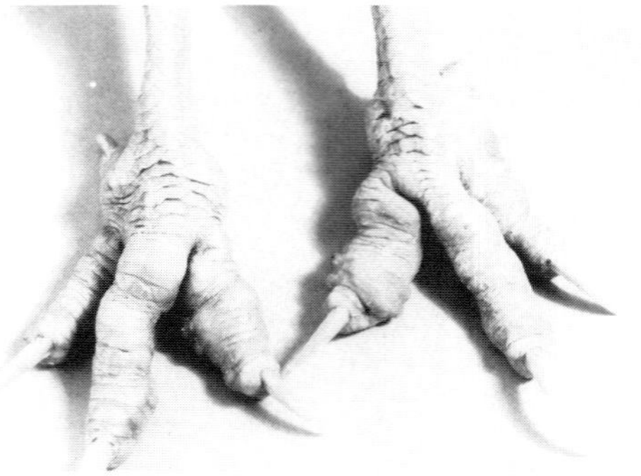

34.22. Gout in a mature chicken, causing enlargement and deformity of toes and feet. (Peckham)

Visceral gout, which has also been called visceral urate deposition, is characterized by precipitation of urates in the kidneys and on serous surfaces of the heart, liver, mesenteries, air sacs, and peritoneum. In severe cases, surfaces of muscles and synovial sheaths of tendons and joints may be involved, and precipitation may occur within the liver and spleen. The deposits on serosal surfaces appear grossly as a white chalky coating while those within viscera may only be recognized microscopically. Much urate is lost when tissues are processed for histology but evidence of its presence is often seen as blue or pink amorphous material under the microscope. Feathery crystals or basophilic spherical masses may be seen within tissues under the microscope in some cases.

Visceral urate deposition is generally due to a failure of urinary excretion. This may be due to obstruction of ureters, renal damage, or dehydration. Raised levels of uric acid in the blood have been reported in both renal disease and articular gout in the absence of visceral urate deposition. A change in concentration of some constituent of the intercellular fluid due to renal disease is probably needed to cause precipitation of the urates. Dehydration due to water deprivation is a common cause of visceral gout in domestic poultry. Outbreaks in poultry have also been attributed to vitamin A deficiency, excess dietary calcium, treatment with sodium bicarbonate, and a mycotoxin, oosporein (189). Kidney damage can cause death of birds without visceral gout occurring. Outbreaks of renal gout in which kidneys are enlarged and often distended with urates results when flocks of young chickens are infected with nephrotropic strains of infectious bronchitis virus.

Avian Monocytosis. The term avian monocytosis has been used to describe a variable condition in young laying hens. Prominent features of the condition include cyanosis of the head, diarrhea, monocytosis, hepatic necrosis, and renal gout. The condition was widely reported throughout the world from 1929 to circa 1960. Published reports decreased after 1960 but it was still reported in the American Association of Avian Pathologists summary of disease reports until 1982 (232). A review of the condition was written by Jungherr and Pomeroy (127). Avian monocytosis is rarely recognized today.

SIGNS AND PATHOLOGY. In an affected flock many birds develop inappetence, depression, and diarrhea. Combs and wattles become shrunken and cyanotic. Egg production decreases and up to

50% mortality may occur. Dead birds are often dehydrated and pectoral muscles may have white streaks. The ovaries exhibit regressive changes and free yolk may be present in the abdominal cavity. Catarrhal enteritis and a chalky pancreas have been reported. Livers are often dark and may have scattered pinpoint foci of necrosis. The kidneys are generally swollen and contain prominent urate deposits. Microscopic lesions include Zenker's degeneration of breast muscle, focal necrosis in the liver, thickening of basement membranes and dilation of Bowman's space in glomeruli, and degeneration of tubules with casts and urate crystals associated with heterophils and giant cells in the kidneys. A relative and absolute monocytosis has been reported in the blood of affected birds.

PATHOGENESIS AND ETIOLOGY. Cumming (30) reviewed the possible etiology of avian monocytosis. He stated that avian monocytosis has never been clearly defined and that the great number of synonyms used exemplifies the confusion regarding the condition. The condition was often called bluecomb. Many different entities may have been included in the bluecomb complex. He noted that a decrease in outbreaks of avian monocytosis in North America in the 1940s coincided with deliberate exposure of young pullets to infectious bronchitis virus. In flocks that were range-reared many pullets may have reached sexual maturity without exposure to infectious bronchitis. At the same time soybean meal replaced meat meal in poultry rations. Nephrotropic infectious bronchitis viruses will cause higher mortalities in susceptible chickens if they are fed diets containing meat meal. Other causes of avian monocytosis that have been postulated include water deprivation, nephrotoxic substances in new wheat, overheating, a sodium-potassium imbalance, and other infectious agents (127).

Urolithiasis.

In recent years outbreaks of mortality in laying flocks have been attributed to urolithiasis in both the UK (9, 197) and the USA (16, 26, 140). Urolithiasis is characterized by severe atrophy of one or both kidneys, distended ureters often containing uroliths, and varying degrees of renal and visceral gout.

SIGNS AND PATHOLOGY. Mortality from all causes in affected flocks may exceed 2% for several months and in excess of 50% of this mortality may be due to urolithiasis (9, 140). Renal lesions have been recognized in clinically normal birds in flocks undergoing an outbreak and 3.2–6.3% of hens in some affected flocks had renal lesions at processing (140). Laying chickens die suddenly and may be in good condition and in full lay (9) or they may have a reduced muscle mass, small pale combs, and white pasting on pericloacal feathers (16). Diffuse visceral urate deposits, atrophied kidneys, and dilated ureters are found in affected birds (9, 16, 140) (Fig. 34.23). The kidney atrophy is often more severe in anterior lobes and unilateral but it may be bilateral. The surviving ipsilateral or contralateral lobes may be enlarged. The ureters arising from the atrophied lobes are dilated and full of clear mucus and often contain white irregular concretions consisting of 100% calcium urate (16). Microscopic lesions in affected kidneys consist of dilation of ureter branches and tubules, tubular degeneration and loss of tubules, cellular casts and urate crystals, and varying degrees of fibrosis (9, 16). Urolithiasis has been primarily recognized as a disease of laying birds but recent reports indicate that lesions and mortality may start during the rearing period (16, 26). In a sequential study of one outbreak minor focal cortical tubular necrosis was found by microscopic study in grossly normal kidneys of 4-wk-old pullets. In 7-wk-old pullets the kidneys were grossly swollen with tubular necrosis and casts, eosinophilic globules in glomeruli, and interstitial infiltration of heterophils and lymphocytes. Typical lesions of urolithiasis were found in 14-wk-old birds (16).

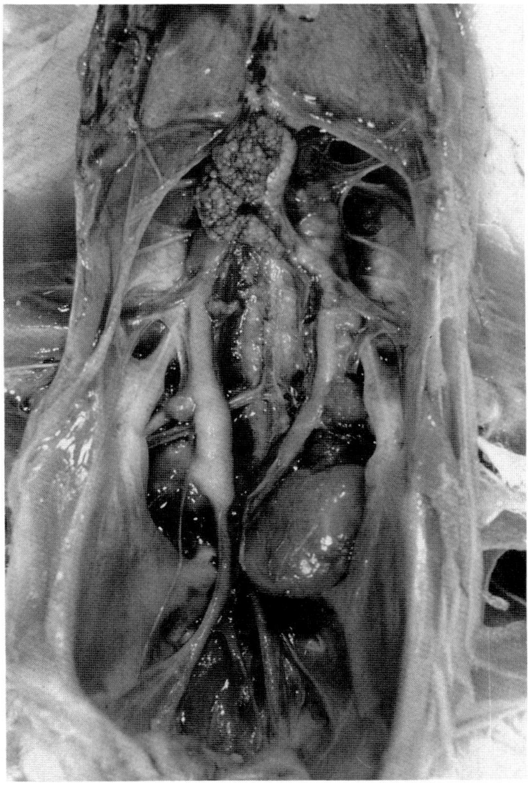

34.23. Urolithiasis in a chicken. Severe atrophy of the right kidney and anterior lobes of the left kidney. The right ureter is distended with white material.

PATHOGENESIS AND ETIOLOGY. Wideman et al. (257) conducted renal function studies on chickens during outbreaks of urolithiasis and concluded that the physiological impact of the kidney damage was the result of reduced renal mass rather than from inappropriate renal handling of minerals or electrolytes. A significant reduction in number of glomeruli has also been reported in birds affected by urolithiasis (172). The uroliths may cause sudden death by plugging ureters but probably occur secondary to kidney damage (140). The lesions described in outbreaks of urolithiasis are similar to those described in a long-term study of the pathogenesis of infection of chickens with infectious bronchitis virus (1). In many outbreaks of urolithiasis it has been difficult to isolate infectious bronchitis virus from affected laying birds (9, 16, 140). This would not be unexpected as recovery of infectious bronchitis virus was erratic in the long-term study mentioned above. Infectious bronchitis viruses, which have been shown to cause renal damage in experimental chickens, have been isolated in recent outbreaks of urolithiasis (16, 26). In several outbreaks potential problems in vaccination programs against infectious bronchitis have been identified (9, 26, 140). Excess dietary calcium, in particular if combined with low available dietary phosphorus, fed to growing pullets has been considered as a possible cause of urolithiasis. Such diets have produced lesions similar to those of urolithiasis in experimental trials (225, 258). Water deprivation has been suggested as a cause of urolithiasis on the basis of field observations (115). The fact that some mycotoxins are nephrotoxic led to the suggestion that they should be considered as a potential cause of urolithiasis (140).

DISEASES OF THE EYE

Ammonia Burn. Ammonia burn describes a keratoconjunctivitis in poultry caused by exposure to ammonia fumes resulting from unsanitary conditions. Peckham (187) reviewed the condition. Affected birds keep their eyelids closed and are reluctant to move. They may rub their head and eyelids against their wings. The cornea has a grey cloudy appearance and may be ulcerated. Edema and hyperemia may be present in the conjunctiva but often may not be very obvious. The condition is generally bilateral and affected birds do not eat and become emaciated. Many birds recover if exposure to ammonia fumes is eliminated. Time of recovery depends on the severity of damage to the cornea and may take 1 mo or longer if lesions are severe. Prevention of the condition is based on proper ventilation and litter management. The ammonia fumes are formed in wet litter.

Blepharoconjunctivitis in Turkeys. Bierer (7, 8) and Sanger et al. (222) described a disease of breeder turkeys characterized by inflammation of the eyelids, excess lacrimation, and in severe cases destruction of the eyeball. Mortality was low but morbidity reached 15–40% and resulted in economic loss from poor production performance. White frothy foam at the anterior canthus of the eye was followed by accumulation of caseous exudate and swelling of eyelids, which became encrusted and closed. Ulceration of the cornea resulted in panophthalmitis and destruction of the eyeball. The cause was not determined. Treatment with antibiotics, supplemental vitamin A, and a change to clean warm quarters caused improvement.

Eye-Notch Syndrome. Eye-notch syndrome refers to a widespread lesion in the eyelid of caged layers (187). The condition appears to start as a small scab or erosion on the lower lid that develops into a fissure with a tag of flesh attached to one side. The significance and cause of the condition is unknown.

Chorioretinitis and Buphthalmos. A turkey blindness syndrome due to chorioretinitis and buphthalmos was described in turkeys by Barnett et al. (4). Similar eye abnormalities were previously described in turkeys (224) and in chickens (259).

SIGNS AND PATHOLOGY. The turkey blindness syndrome occurred in turkey breeder flocks (4). The incidence of eye lesions ranged from 2–30% and egg production was reduced. Blind poults could be recognized by a wandering movement, a tendency to peer at objects in a short sighted manner, and occasionally by holding their heads to one side. Blind poults grew normally and were able to locate feed and water. Eyeballs were enlarged by 5–7 wk of age and the corneas flattened. The palpebral fissures became oval. By 16–20 wk of age many birds had cataracts. Ophthalmoscopic examination of affected eyes revealed pale areas in the retina. On section severely affected eyes contained an abnormal fluid and some were hard to cut due to bone formation within the eye. Microscopic changes in affected eyes included choroid thickening, degeneration and detachment of the retina, and in severe cases fibroplasia and islands of ossifying cartilage in the posterior chamber.

PATHOGENESIS AND ETIOLOGY. Similar lesions to the above have been induced in experimental turkeys by rearing them on continual artificial light (3, 4). Rearing experimental chickens under continuous light has caused enlargement of eyeballs, decreased corneal curvature, thinning of the retina, and an accumulation of fluid in the vitreous body (136). Birds reared on low-intensity but diurnal light also develop enlarged eyes but in such eyes the corneas protrude rather than become flattened (89). Eye enlargement in chickens may also be induced by darkness (111).

DISEASES OF THE REPRODUCTIVE SYSTEM

Cystic Right Oviduct. In the female chicken embryo two Muellerian ducts start to develop into oviducts. The left duct develops into a functional oviduct while the right duct regresses. If this regression is not complete partial development will result in a cystic right oviduct. Cystic right oviducts are common incidental findings in postmortem examination of chickens. They vary in size from small 2-cm elongated cysts to large fluid filled sacs up to 10 cm or more in diameter (Fig. 34.24). Small cysts are of little consequence but large cysts compress the abdominal viscera. The large sacs can result in a bird with a pendulous abdomen and should be differentiated from ascites.

False Layer. The term "false layer" has been used to describe a bird that has the characteristics of a bird in production, visiting the nest regularly but not laying eggs (106). This bird has a normal-appearing ovary and oviduct, but the infundibulum fails to engulf the ovum after it has been ovulated. At necropsy these birds show excessive amounts of orange-colored fat and have liquid yolk or coagulated yolk in the body cavity. This defect may result as a sequel to infectious bronchitis at an early age (14, 15).

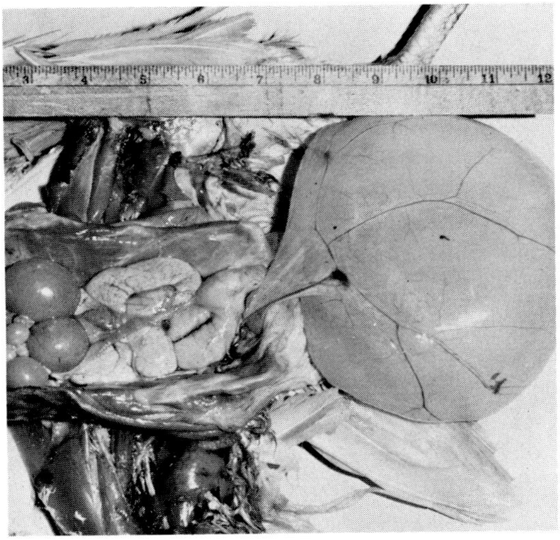

34.24. Cystic right oviduct in a chicken. (Peckham)

Internal Layer. In some birds, soft-shelled eggs or fully formed eggs may be found in the peritoneal cavity. This indicates that the yolk progressed normally through the oviduct to a certain point and then reverse peristalsis discharged the egg into the body cavity. A bird with a large accumulation of eggs in the peritoneal cavity may assume a penguinlike posture.

Impacted Oviduct. Occasionally an oviduct is occluded by masses of yolk, coagulated albumen, shell membranes, and in some instances fully formed eggs. Large masses of yolklike material may also be found in the oviduct, and upon transection these masses have the appearance of concentric rings.

Egg Bound. This term is used to describe a condition in which an egg is lodged in the cloaca but cannot be laid. It may result from inflammation of the oviduct, partial paralysis of the muscles of the oviduct, or production of an egg so large that it is physically impossible for it to be laid. Young pullets laying an unusually large egg are more prone to the problem.

Abnormal Eggs and Depressed Production. Poor egg quality and depressed egg production are common problems that cause great economic loss to the poultry industry. They can be due to a multitude of factors involving nutrition, management, environment, and disease. Reviews related to the topic have been written by Hanson (79), Overfield (181), Wolford and Tanaka (269) and Peckham (187).

DISEASES OF THE INTEGUMENT

Contact Dermatitis and Pododermatitis. Erosive lesions affecting the skin on the plantar surface of the feet, the posterior surface of the hocks, or overlying the sternum have been recognized as a significant problem in turkeys in the UK (143, 267) and in North America (69, 164) and in broiler chickens in the UK (74, 155), North America (81), and Australia (164). Ulcers and erosions of the skin covering the thigh of broiler chickens have been described as scabby hip syndrome in North America (88). A common feature of all these skin lesions is that they appear to be due to contact irritation and are associated with poor litter conditions.

SIGNS AND PATHOLOGY. The lesions have been described by Martland (143) and Greene et al.

(74). Pododermatitis appears as dark black scabs filling ulcers on the ventral metatarsal and digital foot pads. Early changes include enlargement of foot scales, cracks, abrasions, and a superficial scab. These changes proceed to a deep ulcer. Histological lesions include defective keratin in the *stratum intermedium,* particularly adjacent to the ulcer, and infiltration of heterophils in adjacent epidermis. The center of the lesion is occupied by a necrotic mass of cellular debris that may enclose plant material and bacteria. The base of the mass is underlain by heterophils and often macrophages and a line of giant cells. Many birds, in addition to the foot lesions, have similar ulcers filled with black scabs on the posterior of the hock and on the breast. In some focal ulcers on the breasts of turkeys a granulomatous response with giant cells was not noted, but connective tissue proliferation occurred below the ulcers (69). Scabby hip syndrome in broiler chickens in North America is characterized by ulcers and erosions covered by scabs on the skin of the thigh of broilers. It differs from other syndromes in that foot and breast lesions were not reported (88). Contact dermatitis has resulted in downgrading of broiler carcasses (155) and experimental studies have demonstrated that severe foot lesions may result in lameness and a depression of body weight (143, 144).

PATHOGENESIS AND ETIOLOGY. Field outbreaks of contact dermatitis have been associated with poor litter conditions (74). In an epidemiological study lesions were more frequent with increased stocking density, increased age, particular feeds, and in male birds in winter (155). In experimental studies the incidence of dermatitis has been increased by deliberate wetting of litter (83, 143, 144). In an early report of pododermatitis in experimental birds it was suggested that soybean-based diets may contribute to the condition (112). This has not been confirmed (164). In other early experimental studies it was also suggested that marginal deficiencies of biotin may cause the condition (81, 83). This appears to be an unlikely cause under modern conditions. Breast blisters involving the formation of a subcutaneous cyst between the skin and the sternum (153) should be distinguished from the ulcerative lesions of contact dermatitis in the skin overlying the sternum. Both may be found in the same flock (144) but the breast blisters are more probably due to prolonged pressure from sitting (153) rather than contact irritation.

Vesicular Dermatitis and Photosensitization. Vesicular dermatitis characterized by vesicle and scab formation on feet and toes and occasionally on unfeathered portions of the head has been described in chickens, turkeys, ducks, and geese. Peckham (187) reviewed the condition and the reader is referred to his review for specific citations. In outbreaks, up to 20% mortality and severe drops in egg production have occurred. Erythema may precede vesicle and scab formation. Beak deformation (Fig. 34.25) and scarring of foot webs with upturning of toes (Fig. 34.26) may be sequelae in ducks. The condition in some outbreaks has been shown to be due to photosensitization following ingestion of *Ammi visnaga* and *A. majus* seeds and *Cymopterus watsonii* and *C. longipes* plants and seeds. In some outbreaks of vesicular dermatitis the photodynamic agent has not been identified. Vesicular dermatitis has been reproduced with *Lolium temulentum* contaminated with *Cladosporium herbarum* without exposure to sunlight.

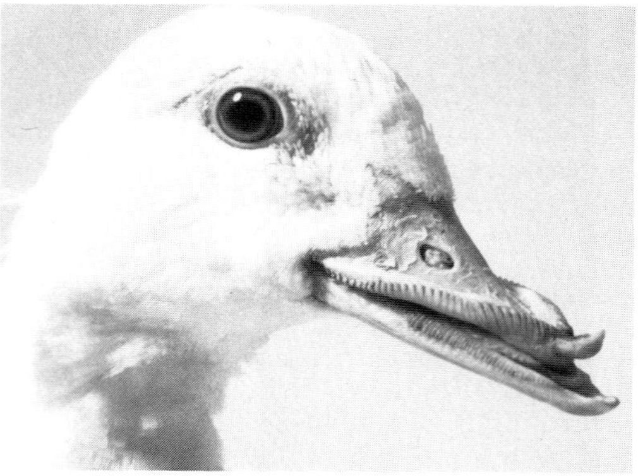

34.25. Chronic lesion of photosensitization in Muscovy duck. Loss of normal epithelium on surface of beak, upturning of edges of beak, and foreshortening of upper beak. (Peckham)

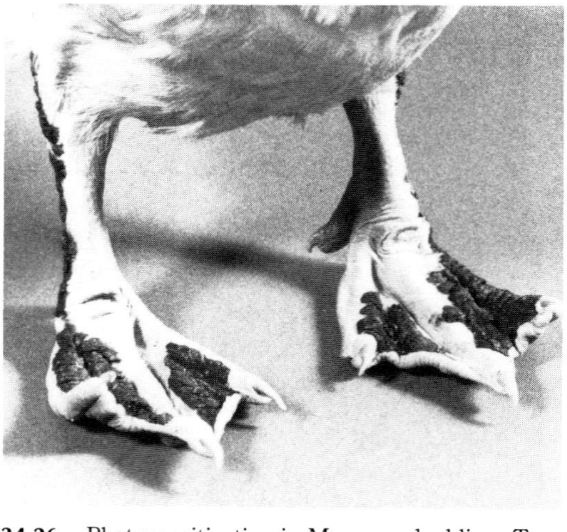

34.26. Photosensitization in Muscovy duckling. Toes upturned and thick brown scabs on footwebs and lateral aspect of legs. (Peckham)

Xanthomatosis. This unusual condition characterized by an accumulation of semifluid yellowish material under the skin of chickens was reported as a significant flock problem around 1960. Peckham (187) reviewed case reports and studies of the condition. White leghorn hens were primarily affected and the incidence of affected birds in flocks reached 60%. Birds with lesions were bright, active, and in production. Wattles were often swollen. Swellings also occurred on the breast, abdomen, and feathered portions of the legs. The swellings often became nodular and pendulous (Fig. 34.27). Initially the lesions were soft and fluctuating and contained a honey-colored fluid. Later they became firm with chalky white areas of cholesterol interspersed through the abnormal, thickened subcutaneous tissue. Histopathologic changes included massive infiltration of foamy macrophages (Fig. 34.28), cholesterol clefts (Fig. 34.29), and giant cells. The cause is unknown but as the xanthomatous tissue contained high levels of hydrocarbons, it was postulated that a hydrocarbon in animal feed may have caused the condition.

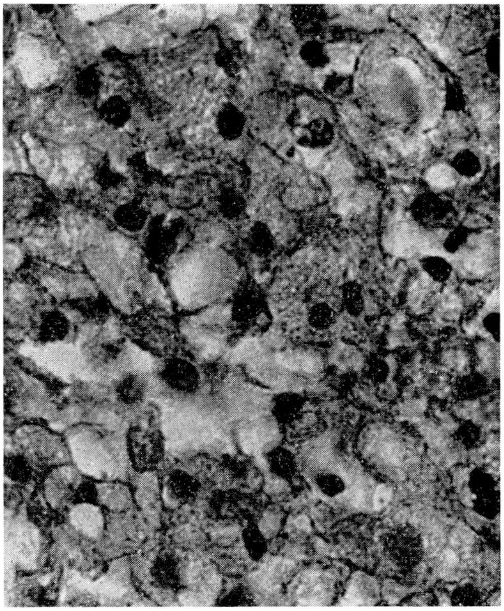

34.28. Histologic section of xanthomatous lesion illustrating vacuolated cytoplasm in foam cells. ×470. (AFIP 54-7256)

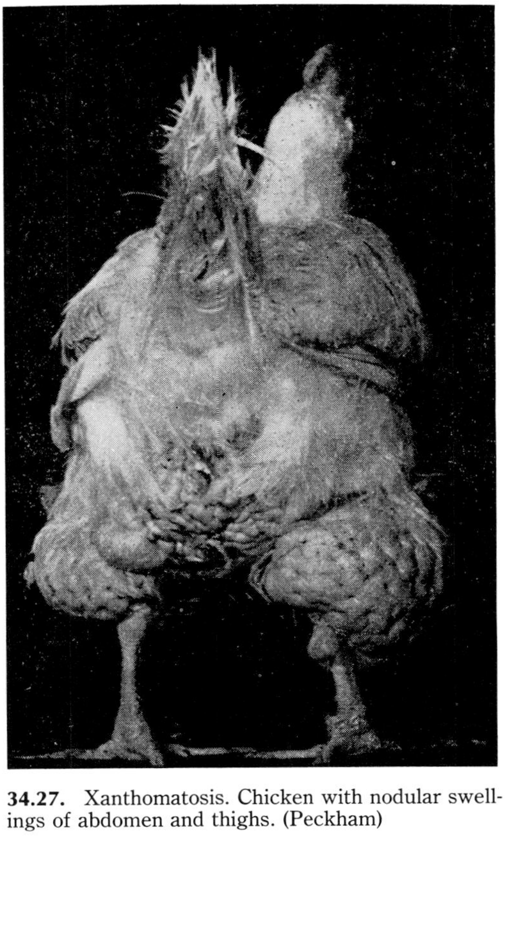

34.27. Xanthomatosis. Chicken with nodular swellings of abdomen and thighs. (Peckham)

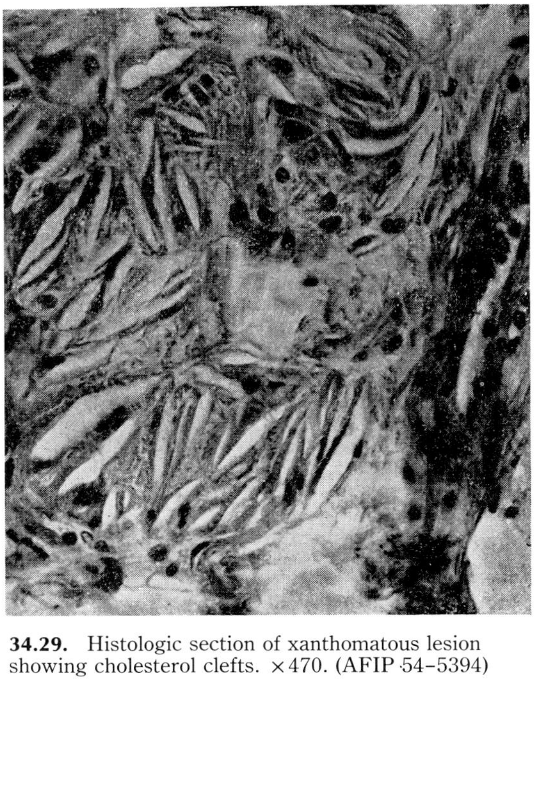

34.29. Histologic section of xanthomatous lesion showing cholesterol clefts. ×470. (AFIP 54–5394)

REFERENCES

1. Alexander, D.J., R.E. Gough, and M. Pattison. 1978. A long-term study of the pathogenesis of infection of fowls with three strains of avian infectious bronchitis virus. Res Vet Sci 24:228–233.

2. Anonymous. 1985. Upsurge of ascites in broilers. Vet Rec 116:559.

3. Ashton, W.L.G., M. Pattison, and K.C. Barnett. 1973. Light-induced eye abnormalities in turkeys and the turkey blindness syndrome. Res Vet Sci 14:42–46.

4. Barnett, K.C., W.L.G. Ashton, G. Holford, I. MacPherson, and P.D. Simm. 1971. Chorioretinitis and buphthalmos in turkeys. Vet Rec 88:620–627.

5. Bass, C.C. 1939. Control of "nose-picking" form of cannibalism in young closely confined quail fed raw meat. Proc Soc Exp Biol Med 40:488–489.

6. Bergmann, V., and M. Pietsch. 1976. Beiträge zur diffentialdiagnose der bewegungsstörungen beim junghuhn. 4. Mitt.: Tibiatorsion beim perlhuhn-eine perosisähnliche erkrankung in einem perlhuhnmastbetrieb. Monatsh Veterinaermed 31:581–585.

7. Bierer, B.W. 1956. Keratoconjunctivitis in turkeys: A preliminary report. Vet Med 51:363–366.

8. Bierer, B.W. 1958. Keratoconjunctivitis in turkeys. II. The relationship of vitamin A, infectious agents and environmental factors to the disease. Vet Med 53:477–483.

9. Blaxland, J.D., E.D. Borland, W.G. Siller, and L. Martindale. 1980. An investigation of urolithiasis in two flocks of laying fowls. Avian Pathol 9:5–19.

10. Bowes, V.A., and R.J. Julian. 1988. Organ weights of normal broiler chickens and those dying of sudden death syndrome. Can Vet J 29:153–156.

11. Bracewell, C.D., and C.J. Randall. 1984. The infectious stunting syndrome. World's Poult Sci J 40:31–37.

12. Bracewell, C.D., and P. Wyeth. 1981. Infectious stunting of chickens. Vet Rec 109:64.

13. Brigden, J.L., and C. Riddell. 1975. A survey of mortality in four broiler flocks in western Canada. Can Vet J 16:194–200.

14. Broadfoot, D.I., B.S. Pomeroy, and W.M. Smith, Jr. 1954. Effects of infectious bronchitis on egg production. J Am Vet Med Assoc 124:128–130.

15. Broadfoot, D.I., B.S. Pomeroy, and W.M. Smith Jr. 1956. Effects of infectious bronchitis in baby chicks. Poult Sci 35:757–762.

16. Brown, T.P., J.R. Glisson, G. Rosales, P. Villegas, and R.B. Davis. 1987. Studies of avian urolithiasis associated with an infectious bronchitis virus. Avian Dis 31:629–636.

17. Buenrostro, J.L., and F.H. Kratzer. 1982. A nutritional approach to the "flip-over" syndrome. Proc 31st West Poult Dis Conf, pp. 76–79.

18. Burton, R.R., and A.H. Smith. 1967. Effect of polycythemia and chronic hypoxia on heart mass in the chicken. J Appl Physiol 22:782–785.

19. Burton, R.W., A.K. Sheridan, and C.R. Howlett. 1981. The incidence and importance of tibial dyschondroplasia to the commercial broiler industry in Australia. Br Poult Sci 22:153–160.

20. Butler, E.J. 1976. Fatty liver diseases in the domestic fowl: A review. Avian Pathol 5:1–14.

21. Buys, S.B., and P. Barnes. 1981. Ascites in broilers. Vet Rec 108:266.

22. Cassidy, D.M., M.A. Gibson, and F.G. Proudfoot. 1975. The histology of cardiac blood clots in chicks exhibiting the "flip-over" syndrome. Poult Sci 54:1882–1886.

23. Chambers, J.R. 1986. Heritability of crippling and acute death syndrome in sire and dam strains of broiler chickens. Poult Sci 65 (Suppl 1):23.

24. Classen, H.L., and C. Riddell. 1989. Photoperiodic effects on performance and leg abnormalities in broiler chickens. Poult Sci 68:873–879.

25. Cover, M.S., W.J. Mellen, and E. Gill. 1955. Studies of hemorrhagic syndromes in chickens. Cornell Vet 45:366–386.

26. Cowen, B.S., R.F. Wideman, H. Rothenbacher, and M.O. Braune. 1987. An outbreak of avian urolithiasis on a large commercial egg farm. Avian Dis 31:392–397.

27. Craig, F. 1967. Traumatic hock disorder in poultry. Proc 16th West Poult Dis Conf, pp. 11–12.

28. Cueva, S., H. Sillau, A. Valenzuela, and H. Ploog. 1974. High altitude induced pulmonary hypertension and right heart failure in broiler chickens. Res Vet Sci 16:370–374.

29. Cullen, G.A. 1988. Runting and stunting syndrome in turkeys. Vet Rec 122:48.

30. Cumming, R.B. 1969. What has happened to avian monocytosis? World's Poult Sci J 25:218–222.

31. Czarnecki, C.M. 1984. Cardiomyopathy in turkeys. Comp Biochem Physiol 77A:591–598.

32. Dämmrich, K., and G. Rodenhoff. 1970. Skeletveränderungen bei mastküken. Zentralbl Veterinaermed [B] 17:131–146.

33. Da Silva, J.M.L., N. Dale, and J.B. Luchesi. 1988. Effect of pelleted feed on the incidence of ascites in broilers reared at low altitudes. Avian Dis 32:376–378.

34. Dickinson, E.M., J.O. Stevens, and D.H. Helfer. 1968. A degenerative myopathy in turkeys. Proc 17th West Poult Dis Conf, p.7.

35. Dorn, P., J. Weikel, and E. Wessling. 1981. Anemia, involution of lymphatic tissues and dermatitis–observations on a new picture of disease in poultry fattening. Tierärztl Wochenschr 88:313–315.

36. Duff, S.R.I. 1984. The histopathology of degenerative hip disease in male breeding turkeys. J Comp Pathol 94:115–125.

37. Duff, S.R.I. 1984. The morphology of degenerative hip disease in male breeding turkeys. J Comp Pathol 94:127–139.

38. Duff, S.R.I. 1984. Osteochondrosis dissecans in turkeys. J Comp Pathol 94:467–476.

39. Duff, S.R.I. 1984. Dyschondroplasia of the caput femoris in skeletally immature broilers. Res Vet Sci 37:293–302.

40. Duff, S.R.I. 1984. Capital femoral epiphyseal infarction in skeletally immature broilers. Res Vet Sci 37:303–309.

41. Duff, S.R.I. 1984. Consequences of capital femoral dyschondroplasia in young adult and skeletally mature broilers. Res Vet Sci 37:310–319.

42. Duff, S.R.I. 1985. Further studies of degenerative hip disease; antitrochanteric degeneration in turkeys and broiler type chickens. J Comp Pathol 95:113–122.

43. Duff, S.R.I. 1985. Dyschondroplasia/osteochondrosis of the femoral trochanter in the fowl. J Comp Pathol 95:363–371.

44. Duff, S.R.I. 1985. Hip instability in young adult broiler fowls. J Comp Pathol 95:373–382.

45. Duff, S.R.I. 1985. Fractured fibulae in broiler fowls. J Comp Pathol 95:525–536.

46. Duff, S.R.I. 1985. Cruciate ligament rupture in young adult broiler knee joints. J Comp Pathol 95:537–548.

47. Duff, S.R.I. 1986. Windswept deformities in poultry. J Comp Pathol 96:147–158.

48. Duff, S.R.I. 1986. Rupture of the intercondylar ligament in intertarsal joints of broiler fowls. J Comp

Pathol 96:159–169.
49. Duff, S.R.I. 1986. Further studies on cruciate and collateral knee ligaments in adult broiler fowls. Avian Pathol 15:407–420.
50. Duff, S.R.I. 1986. Further studies on knee ligament failure in broiler breeding fowls. J Comp Pathol 96:485–495.
51. Duff, S.R.I. 1986. Effect of unilateral weight-bearing on pelvic limb development in broiler fowls: Morphological and radiological findings. Res Vet Sci 40:393–399.
52. Duff, S.R.I. 1987. Destructive cartilage loss in the joints of adult male broiler breeding fowls. J Comp Pathol 97:237–246.
53. Duff, S.R.I. 1987. Meniscal lesions in the knee joints of broiler fowls. J Comp Pathol 97:451–462.
54. Duff, S.R.I., and I.A. Anderson. 1986. The gastrocnemius tendon of domestic fowl: Histological findings in different strains. Res Vet Sci 41:402–409.
55. Duff, S.R.I., and P.M. Hocking. 1986. Chronic orthopaedic disease in adult male broiler breeding fowls. Res Vet Sci 41:340–348.
56. Duff, S.R.I., and C.J. Randall. 1986. Tendon lesions in broiler fowls. Res Vet Sci 40:333–338.
57. Duff, S.R.I., and C. J. Randall. 1987. Observations on femoral head abnormalities in broilers. Res Vet Sci 42:17–23.
58. Duff, S.R.I., and B.H. Thorp. 1985. Patterns of physiological bone torsion in the pelvic appendicular skeletons of domestic fowl. Res Vet Sci 39:307–312.
59. Duff, S.R.I., and B.H. Thorp. 1985. Abnormal angulation/torsion of the pelvic appendicular skeleton in broiler fowl: Morphological and radiological findings. Res Vet Sci 39:313–319.
60. Duff, S.R.I., P.M. Hocking, and R.K. Field. 1987. The gross morphology of skeletal disease in adult male breeding turkeys. Avian Pathol 16:635–651.
61. Edwards, H.M., Jr. 1984. Studies on the etiology of tibial dyschondroplasia in chickens. J Nutr 114:1001–1013.
62. Edwards, H.M., Jr., and P. Sorensen. 1987. Effect of short fasts on the development of tibial dyschondroplasia in chickens. J Nutr 117:194–200.
63. Edwards, H.M., Jr., and J.R. Veltmann, Jr. 1983. The role of calcium and phosphorus in the etiology of tibial dyschondroplasia in young chicks. J Nutr 113:1568–1575.
64. Fadly, A.M., and R.W. Winterfield. 1973. Isolation and some characteristics of an agent associated with inclusion body hepatitis, hemorrhages, and aplastic anemia in chickens. Avian Dis 17:182–193.
65. Farmer, H. 1985. Stunting syndrome of broilers. Vet Rec 117:154.
66. Feron, V.J., and P.G.C. Van Stratum. 1966. The effect of furazolidone on broiler chickens fed rations containing amprolium or zoalene. II. Intoxication after continuous administration during six weeks. Tijdschr Diergeneesk 91:571–579.
67. Frazier, J.A., H. Farmer, and M.F. Martland. 1986. A togavirus-like agent in the pancreatic duct of chickens with infectious stunting syndrome. Vet Rec 119:209–210.
68. Gardiner, E.E., and J.R. Hunt. 1984. Effect of dietary reserpine on the incidence of sudden death syndrome in chickens. Can J Anim Sci 64:1015–1018.
69. Gonder, E., and H.J. Barnes. 1987. Focal ulcerative dermatitis ("breast buttons") in marketed turkeys. Avian Dis 31:52–58.
70. Goodwin, M.A., M.A. Dekich, K.S. Latimer, and O.J. Fletcher. 1985. Quantitation of intestinal D-xylose absorption in normal broilers and in broilers with pale-bird syndrome. Avian Dis 29:630–639.
71. Goodwin, M.A., B.N. Nersessian, J. Brown, and O.J. Fletcher. 1985. Gastrointestinal transit times in normal and reovirus-inoculated turkeys. Avian Dis 29:920–928.
72. Graham, C.L.G. 1977. Copper levels in livers of turkeys with naturally occurring aortic rupture. Avian Dis 21:113–116.
73. Gray, J.E., G.H. Snoeyenbos, and I.M. Reynolds. 1954. Hemorrhagic syndrome of chickens. J Am Vet Med Assoc 125:144–151.
74. Greene, J.A., R.M. McCracken, and R.T. Evans. 1985. A contact dermatitis of broilers–clinical and pathological findings. Avian Pathol 14:23–38.
75. Gries, C.L., and M.L. Scott. 1972. Pathology of selenium deficiency in the chick. J Nutr 102:1287–1296.
76. Griffiths, G.L., and W. Williams. 1985. Runting in broilers associated with temporary maldigestion. Vet Rec 116:160–161.
77. Grunder, A.A., K.G. Hollands, and J.S. Gavora. 1979. Incidence of degenerative myopathy among turkeys fed corn or wheat based rations. Poult Sci 58:1321–1324.
78. Hall, S.A., and N. Machicao. 1968. Myocarditis in broiler chickens reared at high altitude. Avian Dis 12:75–84.
79. Hanson, B.S. 1968. Disease and egg quality. In T.C. Carter (ed.), Egg Quality. A Study of the Hen's Egg. Br Egg Marketing Board Symp #4, pp. 171–180. Oliver and Boyd, Edinburgh.
80. Hargest, T.E., R.M. Leach, and C.V. Gay. 1985. Avian dyschondroplasia. I. Ultrastructure. Am J Pathol 119:175–190.
81. Harms, R.H., and C.F. Simpson. 1975. Biotin deficiency as a possible cause of swelling and ulceration of foot pads. Poult Sci 54:1711–1713.
82. Harms, R.H., and C.F. Simpson. 1979. Serum and body characteristics of laying hens with fatty liver syndrome. Poult Sci 58:1644–1646.
83. Harms, R.H., B.L. Damron, and C.F. Simpson. 1977. Effect of wet litter and supplemental biotin and/or whey on the production of foot pad dermatitis in broilers. Poult Sci 56:291–296.
84. Harper, J.A., and D.H. Helfer. 1972. The effect of vitamin E, methionine and selenium on degenerative myopathy in turkeys. Poult Sci 51:1757–1759.
85. Harper, J.A., P.E. Bernier, J.O. Stevens, and E.M. Dickinson. 1969. Degenerative myopathy in the domestic turkey. Poult Sci 48:1816.
86. Harper, J.A., D.H. Helfer, and E.M. Dickinson. 1971. Hereditary myopathy in turkeys. Proc 20th West Poult Dis Conf, p. 76.
87. Harper, J.A., P.A. Bernier, D.H. Helfer, and J.A. Schmitz. 1975. Degenerative myopathy of the deep pectoral muscle in the turkey. J Hered 66:362–366.
88. Harris, G.C., M. Musbah, J.N. Beasley, and G.S. Nelson. 1978. The development of dermatitis (scabby hip) on the hip and thigh of broiler chickens. Avian Dis 22:122–130.
89. Harrison, P.C., and J. McGinnis. 1967. Light induced exophthalmos in the domestic fowl. Proc Soc Exp Biol Med 126:308–312.
90. Haye, U., and P.C.M. Simons. 1978. Twisted legs in broilers. Br Poult Sci 19:549–557.
91. Haynes, J.S., and M.M. Walser. 1986. Ultrastructure of Fusarium-induced tibial dyschondroplasia in chickens: A sequential study. Vet Pathol 23:499–505.
92. Haynes, J.S., M.M. Walser, and E.M. Lawler. 1985. Morphogenesis of Fusarium sp.-induced tibial dyschondroplasia in chickens. Vet Pathol 22:629–636.
93. Helmboldt, C.F., and M.N. Frazier. 1963. Avian

hepatic inclusion bodies of unknown significance. Avian Dis 7 446-450.

94. Hemsley, L.A. 1965. The causes of mortality in fourteen flocks of broiler chickens. Vet Rec 77:467-472.

95. Hieronymus, D.R.K., P. Villegas, and S.H. Kleven. 1983. Identification and serological differentiation of several reovirus strains isolated from chickens with suspected malabsorption syndrome. Avian Dis 27:246-254.

96. Hoffmann, R., E. Wessling, P. Dorn, and H. Dangschat. 1975. Lesions in chickens with spontaneous or experimental infectious hepato-myelopoietic disease (inclusion body hepatitis) in Germany. Avian Dis 19:224-236.

97. Howell, J., D.W. Macdonald, and R.G. Christian. 1970. Inclusion body hepatitis in chickens. Can Vet J 11:99-101.

98. Huchzermeyer, F.W. 1988. Avian pulmonary hypertension syndrome. IV. Increased right ventricular mass in turkeys experimentally infected with Plasmodium durae. Onderstepoort J Vet Res 55:107-108.

99. Huchzermeyer, F.W., and A.M.C. De Ruyck. 1986. Pulmonary hypertension syndrome associated with ascites in broilers. Vet Rec 119:94.

100. Huchzermeyer, F.W., J.A. Cilliers, C.D.D. Lavigne, and R.A. Bartkowiak. 1987. Broiler pulmonary hypertension syndrome. 1. Increased right ventricular mass in broilers experimentally infected with Aegyptianella pullorum. Onderstepoort J Vet Res 54:113-114.

101. Huchzermeyer, F.W., A.M.C. De Ruyck, and H. Van Ark. 1988. Broiler pulmonary hypertension syndrome. III. Commercial broiler strains differ in their susceptibility. Onderstepoort J Vet Res 55:5-9.

102. Hulan, H.W., F.G. Proudfoot, D. Ramey, and K.B. McRae. 1980. Influence of genotype and diet on general performance and incidence of leg abnormalities of commercial broilers reared to roaster weight. Poult Sci 59:748-757.

103. Hulan, H.W., F.G. Proudfoot, and K.B. McRae. 1980. Effect of vitamins on the incidence of mortality and acute death syndrome ("flip-over") in broiler chickens. Poult Sci 59:927-931.

104. Hunt, J.R., and E.E. Gardiner. 1982. Effect of various diets on the incidence of acute death syndrome ("flip-over") of chickens. Poult Sci 61:1481.

105. Huston, T.M., H.L. Fuller, and C.K. Laurent. 1956. A comparison of various methods of debeaking broilers. Poult Sci 35:806-810.

106. Hutt, F.B., K. Goodwin, and W.D. Urban. 1956. Investigations of nonlaying hens. Cornell Vet 46:257-273.

107. Ibrahim, I.K., R.D. Hodges, and R. Hill. 1980. Haemorrhagic liver syndrome in laying fowl fed diets containing rapeseed meal. Res Vet Sci 29:68-76.

108. Itakura, C., and S. Yamagiwa. 1970. Histopathological studies on bone dysplasia of chickens. I. Histopathology of the bone. Jpn J Vet Sci 32:105-117.

109. Itakura, C., and S. Yamagiwa. 1971. Histopathological studies on bone dysplasia of chickens. III. A collective occurence of bowleg (genu varum) among broiler chicks. Jpn J Vet Sci 33:11-16.

110. Jackson, C.A.W., D.J. Kingston, and L.A. Hemsley. 1972. A total mortality survey of nine batches of broiler chickens. Aust Vet J 48:481-487.

111. Jenkins, R.L., W.D. Ivey, G.R. McDaniel, and R.A. Albert. 1979. A darkness induced eye abnormality in the domestic chicken. Poult Sci 58:55-59.

112. Jensen, L.S., R. Martinson, and G. Schumaier. 1970. A foot pad dermatitis in turkey poults associated with soybean meal. Poult Sci 49:76-82.

113. Jones, J.M., N.R. King, and M.M. Mulliner. 1974. Degenerative myopathy in turkey breeder hens: A comparative study of normal and affected muscle. Br Poult Sci 15:191-196.

114. Jones, H.G.R., C.J. Randall, and C.P.J. Mills. 1978. A survey of mortality in three adult broiler breeder flocks. Avian Pathol 7:619-628.

115. Julian, R. 1982. Water deprivation as a cause of renal disease in chickens. Avian Pathol 11:615-617.

116. Julian, R. 1983. Foci of cartilage in the lung of broiler chickens. Avian Dis 27:292-295.

117. Julian, R.J. 1984. Tendon avulsion as a cause of lameness in turkeys. Avian Dis 28:244-249.

118. Julian, R.J. 1984. Valgus-varus deformity of the intertarsal joint in broiler chickens. Can Vet J 25:254-258.

119. Julian, R.J. 1985. Osteochondrosis, dyschondroplasia and osteomyelitis causing femoral head necrosis in turkeys. Avian Dis 29:854-866.

120. Julian, R.J. 1986. The effect of increased mineral levels in the feed on leg weakness and sudden death syndrome in broiler chickens. Can Vet J 27:157-160.

121. Julian, R.J. 1987. The effect of increased sodium in the drinking water on right ventricular hypertrophy, right ventricular failure, and ascites in broiler chickens. Avian Pathol 16:61-71.

122. Julian, R.J. 1988. Ascites in meat-type ducklings. Avian Pathol 17:11-21.

123. Julian, R.J., and J.A. Frazier. 1987. Right ventricular hypertrophy, right ventricular failure, and ascites in broiler chickens caused by amiodarone-induced lung fibrosis. Proc 23rd World Vet Congr, pp 314-315.

124. Julian, R.J., and J.B. Wilson. 1986. Right ventricular failure as a cause of ascites in broiler and roaster chickens. Proc 4th Int Symp Vet Lab Diagnost, pp. 608-611.

125. Julian, R.J., J. Summers, and J.B. Wilson. 1986. Right ventricular failure, and ascites in broiler chickens caused by phosphorus-deficient diets. Avian Dis 30:453-459.

126. Julian, R.J., G.W. Friars, H. French, and M. Quinton. 1987. The relationship of right ventricular hypertrophy, right ventricular failure, and ascites to weight gain in broiler and roaster chickens. Avian Dis 31:130-135.

127. Jungherr, E., and B.S. Pomeroy. 1965. Avian monocytosis (so-called pullet disease), infectious nephrosis, and bluecomb diseases of turkeys. In H.E. Biester, and L.H. Schwarte (eds.), Diseases of Poultry, 5th Ed., pp. 844-862. Iowa State Univ Press, Ames.

128. Kisary, J. 1985. Indirect immunofluorescence as a diagnostic tool for parvovirus infection of broiler chickens. Avian Pathol 14:269-273.

129. Kisary, J., B. Nagy, and Z. Bitay. 1984. Presence of parvoviruses in the intestine of chickens showing stunting syndrome. Avian Pathol 13:339-343.

130. Klopp, S., J.K. Rosenberger, and W.C. Krauss. 1975. Diagnosis of inclusion body hepatitis and hemorrhagic anemia syndrome in Delmarva broiler chickens. Avian Dis 19:608-611.

131. Kouwenhoven, B., F.G. Davelaar, and J. Van Walsum. 1978. Infectious proventriculitis causing runting in broilers. Avian Pathol 7:183-187.

132. Kouwenhoven, B., M. Vertommen, and J.H.H. Van Eck. 1978. Runting and leg weakness in broilers; involvement of infectious factors. Vet Sci Commun 2:253-259.

133. Kouwenhoven, B., M.H. Vertommen, and E. Goren. 1986. Runting in broilers. In J.B. McFerren and M.S. McNulty (eds.), Acute Virus Infections of Poultry, pp. 165-178. Martinus Nijhoff, Dordrecht, Neth.

134. Krista, L.M., P.E. Waibel, and R.E. Burger.

1965. The influence of dietary alterations, hormones, and blood pressure on the incidence of dissecting aneurysms in the turkey. Poult Sci 44:15–22.

135. Krista, L.M., P.E. Waibel, R.N. Shoffner, and J.A. Sautter. 1967. Natural dissecting aneurysm (aortic rupture) and blood pressure in the turkey. Nature 214:1162–1163.

136. Lauber, J.K., J.V. Shutze, and J. McGinnis. 1961. Effects of exposure to continuous light on the eye of the growing chick. Proc Soc Exp Biol Med 106:871–872.

137. Lilburn, M.S., H.M. Edwards, Jr., and L.S. Jensen. 1982. Impaired nutrient utilization associated with pale bird syndrome in broiler chicks. Poult Sci 61:608–609.

138. Lopez Coello, C., L. Paasch, R. Rosiles, and C. Casas. 1982. Ascites in broilers due to undetermined causes. Proc 31st West Poult Dis Conf, pp. 13–15.

139. Magwood, S.E., and D.F. Bray. 1962. Disease condition of turkey poults characterized by enlarged and rounded hearts. Can J Comp Med 26:268–272.

140. Mallinson, E.T., H. Rothenbacher, R.F. Wideman, D.B. Snyder, E. Russek, A.I. Zuckerman, and J.P. Davidson. 1984. Epizootiology, pathology, and microbiology of an outbreak of urolithiasis in chickens. Avian Dis 28:25–43.

141. Marthedal, H.E., and G. Velling. 1961. Haemorrhagic syndrome in poultry. Br Vet J 117:357–365.

142. Martindale, L., W.G. Siller, and P.A.L Wight. 1979. Effects of subfascial pressure in experimental deep pectoral myopathy of the fowl: An angiographic study. Avian Pathol 8:425–436.

143. Martland, M.F. 1984. Wet litter as a cause of plantar pododermatitis leading to foot ulceration and lameness in fattening turkeys. Avian Pathol 13:241–252.

144. Martland, M.F. 1985. Ulcerative dermatitis in broiler chickens: The effects of wet litter. Avian Pathol 14:353–364.

145. Martland, M.F. 1986. Histopathology of the chick pancreas following pancreatic duct ligation. Vet Rec 118:526–530.

146. Martland, M.F., and H. Farmer. 1986. Pancreatic duct obstruction in a stunting syndrome of broiler chickens. Vet Rec 118:531–534.

147. Martland, M.F., E.J. Butler, and G.R. Fenwick. 1984. Rapeseed induced liver haemorrhage, reticulolysis and biochemical changes in laying hens: The effects of feeding high and low glucosinolate meals. Res Vet Sci 36:298–309.

148. Maxwell, M.H. 1988. The histology and ultrastructure of ectopic cartilaginous and osseous nodules in the lungs of young broilers with an ascitic syndrome. Avian Pathol 17:201–219.

149. Maxwell, M.H., G.W. Robertson, and S. Spence. 1986. Studies on an ascitic syndrome in young broilers. 1. Haematology and pathology. Avian Pathol 15:511–524.

150. Maxwell, M.H., G.W. Robertson, and S. Spence. 1986. Studies on an ascitic syndrome in young broilers. 2. Ultrastructure. Avian Pathol 15:525–538.

151. Maxwell, M.H., I.A. Anderson, and L.A. Dick. 1988. The incidence of ectopic cartilaginous and osseous lung nodules in young broiler fowls with ascites and various other diseases. Avian Pathol 17:487–493.

152. McCaskey, P.C., G.N. Rowland, R.K. Page, and L.R. Minear. 1982. Focal failures of endochondral ossification in the broiler. Avian Dis 26:701–717.

153. McCune, E.L. and H.-D. Dellmann. 1968. Developmental origin and structural characters of "breast blisters" in chickens. Poult Sci 47:852–858.

154. McFerran, J.B., R.M. McCracken, T.J. Connor, and R.T. Evans. 1976. The isolation of viruses from clinical outbreaks of inclusion body hepatitis. Avian Pathol 5:315–324.

155. McIlroy, S.G., E.A. Goodall, and C.H. McMurray. 1987. A contact dermatitis of broilers–epidemiological findings. Avian Pathol 16:93–105.

156. McLoughlin, M.F., D.A. McLoone, and T.J. Connor. 1987. Runting and stunting syndrome in turkeys. Vet Rec 121:583–586.

157. McNulty, M.S., G.M. Allan, T.J. Connor, J.B. McFerran, and R.M. McCracken. 1984. An entero-like virus associated with the runting syndrome in broiler chickens. Avian Pathol 13:429–439.

158. McSherry, B.J., A.E. Ferguson, and J. Ballantyne. 1954. A dissecting aneurism in internal hemorrhage in turkeys. J Am Vet Med Assoc 124:279–283.

159. Meulemans, G., M. Decaesstecker, and G. Charlier. 1986. Runting syndrome in broiler chickens. Experimental reproduction studies. In J.B. McFerren and M.S. McNulty (eds.), Acute Virus Infections of Poultry, pp. 179–189. Martinus Nijhoff, Dordrecht, Neth.

160. Miles, R.D., and R.H. Harms. 1981. An observation of abnormally high calcium and phosphorus levels in laying hens with fatty liver syndrome. Poult Sci 60:485–486.

161. Miltenburg, J.T., B. Kouwenhoven, and M. Vertommen. 1981. Infectious stunting of chickens. Vet Rec 109:477.

162. Mollison, B., W. Guenter, and B.R. Boycott. 1984. Abdominal fat deposition and sudden death syndrome in broilers: The effects of restricted intake, early life caloric (fat) restriction, and calorie:protein ratio. Poult Sci 63:1190–1200.

163. Moorhead, P.D., and Y.S. Mohamed. 1968. Case report: Pathologic and microbiologic studies of crookedneck in a turkey flock. Avian Dis 12:476–482.

164. Nairn, M.E., and A.R.A. Watson. 1972. Leg weakness of poultry–a clinical and pathological characterisation. Aust Vet J 48:645–656.

165. Neumann, F., and H. Ungar. 1973. Spontaneous aortic rupture in turkeys and the vascularization of the aortic wall. Can Vet J 14:136–138.

166. Neumann, F., M.S. Dison, U. Klopfer, and T.A. Nobel. 1973. Sporadic renal haemorrhage in turkeys. Refu Vet 30:59–61.

167. Newberne, P.M., M.E. Muhrer, R. Craghead, and B.L. O'Dell. 1956. An abnormality of the proventriculus of the chick. J Am Vet Med Assoc 128:553–555.

168. Newberry, R.C., J.R. Hunt, and E.E. Gardiner. 1985. Effect of alternating lights and strain on roaster chicken performance and mortality due to sudden death syndrome. Can J Anim Sci 65:993–996.

169. Newberry, R.C., J.R. Hunt, and E.E. Gardiner. 1985. Effect of alternating lights and strain on behavior and leg disorders of roaster chickens. Poult Sci 64:1863–1868.

170. Newberry, R.C., J.R. Hunt, and E.E. Gardiner. 1986. Light intensity effects on performance, activity, leg disorders, and sudden death syndrome of roaster chickens. Poult Sci 65:2232–2238.

171. Newberry, R.C., E.E. Gardiner, and J.R. Hunt. 1987. Behavior of chickens prior to death from sudden death syndrome. Poult Sci 66:1446–1450.

172. Niznik, R.A., R.F. Wideman, B.S. Cowen, and R.E. Kissell. 1985. Induction of urolithiasis in single comb white leghorn pullets: Effect on glomerular number. Poult Sci 64:1430–1437.

173. Odor, E.M., R.K. Page, O.J. Fletcher, and P. Villegas. 1981. Pale bird syndrome–clinical picture and etiology. J Am Vet Med Assoc 179:273.

174. Olah, I., R.L. Taylor, Jr., and B. Glick. 1983.

Ascites formation in the chicken. Poult Sci 62:2095-2098.
175. Olander, H.J., R.R. Burton, and H.E. Adler. 1967. The pathophysiology of chronic hypoxia in chickens. Avian Dis 11:609-620.
176. Ononiwu, J.C., R.G. Thomson, H.C. Carlson, and R.J. Julian. 1979. Pathological studies of "sudden death syndrome" in broiler chickens. Can Vet J 20:70-73.
177. Ononiwu, J.C., R.G. Thomson, H.C. Carlson, and R.J. Julian. 1979. Studies on effect of lighting on "sudden death syndrome" in broiler chickens. Can Vet J 20:74-77.
178. Orr, J.P., and C. Riddell. 1977. Investigation of the vascular supply of the pectoral muscles of the domestic turkey and comparison of experimentally produced infarcts with naturally occurring deep pectoral myopathy. Am J Vet Res 38:1237-1242.
179. Orr, J.P., K.S. Little, M. Schoonderwoerd, and A.J. Rehmtulla. 1986. Ascites in broiler chickens. Can Vet J 27:99-100.
180. Ostrander, C.E. 1957. Control cannabilism in your poultry flock. Cornell Ext Bull 992.
181. Overfield, N.D. 1970. Factors affecting egg quality– field observations. In B.M. Freeman and R.F. Gordon, (eds.), Factors Affecting Egg Grading. Br Egg Marketing Board Symp #6, pp. 29-52. Oliver and Boyd, Edinburgh.
182. Page, R.K., O.J. Fletcher, G.N. Rowland, D. Gaudry, and P. Villegas. 1982. Malabsorption syndrome in broiler chickens. Avian Dis 26:618-624.
183. Pass, D.A., M.D. Robertson, and G.E. Wilcox. 1982. Runting syndrome in broiler chickens in Australia. Vet Rec 110:386-387.
184. Pearson, A.W., and E.J. Butler. 1978. Pathological and biochemical observations on subclinical cases of fatty liver– haemorrhagic syndrome in the fowl. Res Vet Sci 24:65-71.
185. Pearson, A.W., and E.J. Butler. 1978. The oestrogenised chick as an experimental model for fatty liver-haemorrhagic syndrome in the fowl. Res Vet Sci 24:82-86.
186. Pearson, A.W., E.J. Butler, R.F. Curtis, G.R. Fenwick, A. Hobson-Frohock, D.G. Land, and S.A. Hall. 1978. Effects of rapeseed meal on laying hens (Gallus domesticus) in relation to fatty liver-haemorrhagic syndrome and egg taint. Res Vet Sci 25:307-313.
187. Peckham, M.C. 1984. Vices and miscellaneous diseases and conditions. In M.S. Hofstad, H.J. Barnes, B.W. Calnek, W.M. Reid, and H.W. Yoder, Jr. (eds.), Diseases of Poultry, 8th Ed., pp. 741-782. Iowa State Univ Press, Ames.
188. Peckham, M.C. 1984. Poisons and toxins. In M.S. Hofstad, H.J. Barnes, B.W. Calnek, W.M. Reid, and H.W. Yoder, Jr. (eds.), Diseases of Poultry, 8th Ed., pp. 783-818. Iowa State Univ Press, Ames.
189. Pegram, R.A., and R.D. Wyatt. 1981. Avian gout caused by oosporein, a mycotoxin produced by Chaetomium trilaterale. Poult Sci 60:2429-2440.
190. Pettit, J.R., and H.C. Carlson. 1972. Inclusion-body hepatitis in broiler chickens. Avian Dis 16:858-863.
191. Poulos, P.W., Jr., S. Reiland, K. Elwinger, and S.E. Olsson. 1978. Skeletal lesions in the broiler with special reference to dyschondroplasia (osteochondrosis). Acta Radiol Suppl 358:229-275.
192. Pritchard, W.R., W. Henderson, and C.W. Beall. 1958. Experimental production of dissecting aneurysms in turkeys. Am J Vet Res 19:696-705.
193. Proudfoot, F.G., and H.W. Hulan. 1982. Effect of reduced feeding time using all mash or crumble-pellet dietary regimens on chicken broiler performance, including the incidence of acute death syndrome. Poult Sci 61:750-754.
194. Proudfoot, F.G., and H.W. Hulan. 1983. Effects of dietary aspirin (acetylsalicylic acid) on the incidence of sudden death syndrome and the general performance of broiler chickens. Can J Anim Sci 63:469-471.
195. Proudfoot, F.G., H.W. Hulan, and K.B. McRae. 1982. The effect of crumbled and pelleted feed on the incidence of sudden death syndrome among male chicken broilers. Poult Sci 61:1766-1768.
196. Randall, C.J., and C.P.J. Mills. 1981. Observations on leg deformity in broilers with particular reference to the intertarsal joint. Avian Pathol 10:407-431.
197. Randall, C.J., T.B. Blandford, E.D. Borland, N.H. Brooksbank, and S.A. Hall. 1977. A survey of mortality in 51 caged laying flocks. Avian Pathol 6:149-170.
198. Ratanasethkul, C., C. Riddell, R.E. Salmon, and J.B. O'Neil. 1976. Pathological changes in chickens, ducks, and turkeys fed high levels of rapeseed oil. Can J Comp Med 40:360-369.
199. Reece, F.N., J.W. Deaton, J.D. May, and K.N. May. 1971. Cage versus floor rearing of broiler chickens. Poult Sci 50:1786-1790.
200. Reece, R.L., P.T. Hooper, S.H. Tate, V.D. Beddome, W.M. Forsyth, P.C. Scott, and D.A. Barr. 1984. Field, clinical, and pathological observations of a runting and stunting syndrome in broilers. Vet Rec 115:483-485.
201. Richardson, J.A., J. Burgener, R.W. Winterfield, and A.S. Dhillon. 1980. Deep pectoral myopathy in seven-week-old broiler chickens. Avian Dis 24:1054-1059.
202. Riddell, C. 1975. Pathology of developmental and metabolic disorders of the skeleton of domestic chickens and turkeys. I. Abnormalities of genetic or unknown aetiology. Vet Bull 45:629-640.
203. Riddell, C. 1976. Selection of broiler chickens for a high and low incidence of tibial dyschondroplasia with observation on spondylolisthesis and twisted legs (perosis). Poult Sci 55:145-151.
204. Riddell, C. 1976. The influence of fiber in the diet on dilation (hypertrophy) of the proventriculus in chickens. Avian Dis 20:442-445.
205. Riddell, C. 1980. A survey of skeletal disorders in five turkey flocks in Saskatchewan. Can J Comp Med 44:275-279.
206. Riddell, C. 1981. Skeletal deformities in poultry. Adv Vet Sci Comp Med 25:277-310.
207. Riddell, C. 1983. Pathology of the skeleton and tendons of broiler chickens reared to roaster weights. I. Crippled chickens. Avian Dis 27:950-962.
208. Riddell, C. 1985. Cardiomyopathy and ascites in broiler chickens. Proc 34th West Poult Dis Conf, p. 36.
209. Riddell, C. 1987. Avian Histopathology, pp. 32-33. Am Assoc Avian Pathol. Kennett Square, PA.
210. Riddell, C., and D. Derow. 1985. Infectious stunting and pancreatic fibrosis in broiler chickens in Saskatchewan. Avian Dis 29:107-115.
211. Riddell, C., and J. Howell. 1972. Spondylolisthesis ("kinky back") in broiler chickens in western Canada. Avian Dis 16:444-452.
212. Riddell, C., and J.P. Orr. 1980. Chemical studies of the blood, and histological studies of the heart of broiler chickens dying from acute death syndrome. Avian Dis 24:751-757.
213. Riddell, C., and D.A. Pass. 1987. The influence of dietary calcium and phosphorus on tibial dyschondroplasia in broiler chickens. Avian Dis 31:771-775.
214. Riddell, C., and R. Springer. 1985. An epizootiological study of acute death syndrome and leg

weakness in broiler chickens in western Canada. Avian Dis 29:90-102.

215. Riddell, C., M.W. King, and K.R. Gunasekera. 1983. Pathology of the skeleton and tendons of broiler chickens reared to roaster weights. II. Normal chickens. Avian Dis 27:980-991.

216. Robertson, E.I., C.I. Angstrom, H.C. Clark, and M. Shimm. 1949. Field research on "stunted chick" disease. Poult Sci 28:14-18.

217. Rodenhoff, G., and K. Dämmrich. 1973. Untersuchungen zur beeinflussung der röhrenknochenstruktur durch verschiedene haltungssysteme bei masthähnchen. Berl Muench Tierärztl Wochenschr 86:230-233, 241-244.

218. Rosenberger, J.K., R.J. Eckroade, S. Klopp, and W.C. Krauss. 1974. Characterization of several viruses isolated from chickens with inclusion body hepatitis and aplastic anemia. Avian Dis 18:399-409.

219. Rosenberger, J.K., S. Klopp, R.J. Eckroade, and W.C. Krauss. 1975. The role of the infectious bursal agent and several avian adenoviruses in the hemorrhagic-aplastic-anemia syndrome and gangrenous dermatitis. Avian Dis 19:717-729.

220. Rotter, B., W. Guenter, and B.R. Boycott. 1985. Sudden death syndrome in broilers: Dietary fat supplementation and its effect on tissue composition. Poult Sci 64:1128-1136.

221. Ruff, M.D. 1982. Nutrient absorption and changes in blood plasma of stunted broilers. Avian Dis 26:852-859.

222. Sanger, V.L., E.N. Moore, and N.A. Frank. 1960. Blepharoconjunctivitis in turkeys. Poult Sci 39:482-487.

223. Sarango, J.A., and C. Riddell. 1985. A study of cartilaginous nodules in the lungs of domestic poultry. Avian Dis 29:116-127.

224. Saunders, L.Z., and E.N. Moore. 1957. Blindness in turkeys due to granulomatous chorioretinitis. Avian Dis 1:27-36.

225. Shane, S.M., R.J. Young, and L. Krook. 1969. Renal and parathyroid changes produced by high calcium intake in growing pullets. Avian Dis 13:558-567.

226. Siller, W.G. 1981. Renal pathology of the fowl – a review. Avian Pathol 10:187-262.

227. Siller, W.G., and P.A.L. Wight. 1978. The pathology of deep pectoral myopathy of turkeys. Avian Pathol 7:583-617.

228. Siller, W.G., P.A.L. Wight, L. Martindale, and D.W. Bannister. 1978. Deep pectoral myopathy: An experimental simulation in the fowl. Res Vet Sci 24:267-268.

229. Siller, W.G., P.A.L. Wight, and L. Martindale. 1979. Exercise-induced deep pectoral myopathy in broiler fowls and turkeys. Vet Sci Commun 2:331-336.

230. Siller, W.G., L. Martindale, and P.A.L. Wight. 1979. The prevention of experimental deep pectoral myopathy of the fowl by fasciotomy. Avian Pathol 8:301-307.

231. Sinclair, A.J., D.H. Embury, I.J. Smart, D.A. Barr, R.L. Reece, P.T. Hooper, and J.A. Gould. 1984. Pancreatic degeneration in broilers with runting and stunting syndrome. Vet Rec 115:485-488.

232. Springer, W.T. 1984. AAAP 1982 summary of disease reports. Avian Dis 28:816-843.

233. Stake, P.E., T.N. Fredrickson, and C.A. Bourdeau. 1981. Induction of fatty liver-hemorrhagic syndrome in laying hens by exogenous β-estradiol. Avian Dis 25:410-422.

234. Steele, P., and J. Edgar. 1982. Importance of acute death syndrome in mortalities in broiler chicken flocks. Aust Vet J 58:63-66.

235. Steele, P., J. Edgar, and G. Doncon. 1982. Effect of biotin supplementation on incidence of acute death syndrome in broiler chickens. Poult Sci 61:909-913.

236. Steele, P., P. O'Malley, and M.C. McGrath. 1983. Personal communication.

237. Stein, G., and C.R. Wills. 1974. Isolation and identification of infectious anemia virus. J Am Vet Med Assoc 165:742.

238. Stuart, B.P., R.J. Cole, E.F. Waller, and R.F. Vesonder. 1981. Proventricular hyperplasia (Malabsorption syndrome) in broilers: Involvement of mycotoxins and other dietary factors. J Am Vet Med Assoc 179:273.

239. Swarbrick, O. 1986. Probable infectious stunting syndrome in replacement pullets. Vet Rec 119 352-355.

240. Swire, P.W. 1980. Ascites in broilers. Vet Rec 107:541.

241. Van der Heide, L., D. Lütticken, and M. Horzinek. 1981. Isolation of avian reovirus as a possible etiologic agent of osteoporosis ("brittle bone disease"; "femoral head necrosis") in broiler chickens. Avian Dis 25:847-856.

242. Van Vleet, J.F., and V.J. Ferrans. 1983. Congestive cardiomyopathy induced in ducklings fed graded amounts of furazolidone. Am J Vet Res 44:76-85.

243. Van Walsum, J. 1975. Contribution to the aetiology of synovitis in chickens, with special reference to noninfective factors. II. Tijdschr Diergeneeskd 100:76-83.

244. Van Walsum, J. 1977. Contribution to the aetiology of synovitis in chickens, with special reference to noninfective factors. III. Tijdschr Diergeneeskd 102:793-800.

245. Van Walsum, J. 1979. Contribution to the aetiology of synovitis in chickens, with special reference to noninfective factors. IV. Vet Q 1:90-96.

246. Vargas, M.I., J.M. Lamas, and V. Alvarenga. 1983. Tibial dyschondroplasia in growing chickens experimentally intoxicated with tetramethylthiuram disulfide. Poult Sci 62:1195-1200.

247. Veltmann, J.R., Jr., G.N. Rowland, and S.S. Linton. 1985. Tibial dyschondroplasia in single-comb white leghorn chicks fed tetramethylthiuram disulfide (a fungicide). Avian Dis 29:1269-1272.

248. Vertommen, M., J.H.H. Van Eck, B. Kouwenhoven, and Nel Van Kol. 1980. Infectious stunting and leg weakness in broilers. I. Pathology and biochemical changes in blood plasma. Avian Pathol 9:133-142.

249. Vertommen, M., A. Van der Laan and H.M. Veenendaal-Hesselman. 1980. Infectious stunting and leg weakness in broilers. II. Studies on alkaline phosphatase isoenzymes in blood plasma. Avian Pathol 9:143-152.

250. Villasenor, J., and E. Rivera-Cruz. 1980. What happened to ascites? Proc 29th West Poult Dis Conf, pp. 89-92.

251. Volk, M., M. Herceg, B. Marzan, M. Kralj, S. Meknic, and V. Tadic. 1974. Investigations of fatal syncope of fowl in broilers. I. Incidence, clinical symptoms, pathomorphological findings and pathogenesis. Vet Arh 44:14-23.

252. Walser, M.M., F.L. Cherms, and H.E. Dziuk. 1982. Osseous development and tibial dyschondroplasia in five lines of turkeys. Avian Dis 26:265-271.

253. Walser, M.M., N.K. Allen, C.J. Mirocha, G.F. Hanlon, and J.A. Newman. 1982. Fusarium-induced osteochondrosis (tibial dyschondroplasia) in chickens. Vet Pathol 19:544-550.

254. Weaver, C.H., and S. Bird. 1934. The nature of cannibalism occurring among adult domestic fowls. J Am Vet Med Assoc 85:623-637.

255. Whitehead, C.C., and C.J. Randall. 1982. Interrelationships between biotin, choline, and other B-vitamins and the occurrence of fatty liver and kidney syndrome and sudden death syndrome in broiler chickens. Br J Nutr 48:177–184.

256. Whitehead, C.C., R. Blair, D.W. Bannister, A.J. Evans, and R. Morley Jones. 1976. The involvement of biotin in preventing the fatty liver and kidney syndrome in chicks. Res Vet Sci 20:180–184.

257. Wideman, R.F., E.T. Mallinson, and H. Rothenbacher. 1983. Kidney function of pullets and laying hens during outbreaks of urolithiasis. Poult Sci 62:1954–1970.

258. Wideman, R.F., J.A. Closser, W.B. Roush, and B.S. Cowen. 1985. Urolithiasis in pullets and laying hens: Role of dietary calcium and phosphorus. Poult Sci 64:2300–2307.

259. Wight, P.A.L. 1965. Histopathology of a chronic endophthalmitis of the domestic fowl. J Comp Pathol 75:353–361.

260. Wight, P.A.L., and S.R.I. Duff. 1985. Ectopic pulmonary cartilage and bone in domestic fowl. Res Vet Sci 39:188–195.

261. Wight, P.A.L., and D.W.F. Shannon. 1977. Plasma protein derivative (amyloid-like substance) in livers of rapeseed-fed fowls. Avian Pathol 6:293–305.

262. Wight, P.A.L., and W.G. Siller. 1980. Pathology of deep pectoral myopathy of broilers. Vet Pathol 17:29–39.

263. Wight, P.A.L., W.G. Siller, L. Martindale, and J.H. Filshie. 1979. The induction by muscle stimulation of a deep pectoral myopathy in the fowl. Avian Pathol 8:115–121.

264. Wight, P.A.L., L. Martindale, and W.G. Siller. 1979. Oregon disease and husbandry. Vet Rec 105:470–471.

265. Wilson, J.B., R.J. Julian, and I.K. Barker. 1988. Lesions of right heart failure and ascites in broiler chickens. Avian Dis 32:246–261.

266. Wise, D.R. 1975. Skeletal abnormalities in table poultry–a review. Avian Pathol 4:1–10.

267. Wise, D.R. 1979. Nutrition-disease interactions of leg weakness in poultry. In W. Haresign and D. Lewis (eds.), Recent Advances in Animal Nutrition–1978, pp. 41–57. Butterworths, London.

268. Wise, D.R., and A.R. Jennings. 1972. Dyschondroplasia in domestic poultry. Vet Rec 91:285–286.

269. Wolford, J.H., and K. Tanaka. 1970. Factors influencing egg shell quality–a review. World's Poult Sci J 26:763–780.

270. Wyeth, P.J., N.J. Chettle, and J. Labram. 1981. Avian calicivirus. Vet Rec 109:477.

271. Yamasaki, K., and C. Itakura. 1983. Pathology of degenerative osteoarthritis in laying hens. Jpn J Vet Sci 45:1–8.

272. Yamashiro, S., M.K. Bhatnagar, J.R. Scott, and S.J. Slinger. 1975. Fatty haemorrhagic liver syndrome in laying hens on diets supplemented with rapeseed products. Res Vet Sci 19:312–321.

35 POISONS AND TOXINS

Richard J. Julian

INTRODUCTION. Paracelsus recognized 400 yr ago it is "the dose that makes the poison." Although that may be obvious with known toxic material, it is also true for products such as growth promotants and chemotherapeutic agents usually considered safe. Deliberate overdose may cause illness, and a misplaced decimal in water or feed medication frequently results in toxicity. Sulfaquinoxaline poisoning occurs in meat-type chickens even at recommended doses because of high water intake in warm buildings, particularly in hot weather, or because of poor feed mixing. Disease may also be caused by toxic levels of some nutrients, e.g., excess dietary sodium causes significant losses in chickens and turkeys around the world. High levels of vitamins A and D will result in toxicity. There may be a species or age susceptibility as occurs with the ionophore anticoccidials. Waterfowl are sensitive to some drugs at a dose safe for chickens and turkeys. The immune system seems to be affected by many toxic agents. In addition to disease caused by poisons, the problem of residues in eggs and meat must also be considered. For information on withdrawal times and drug and chemical residues see Booth (29). It must be remembered, material starts to be deposited in an egg yolk 10 days before that egg is laid.

Poisonous substances are widely distributed in nature. Mycotoxins, covered in a separate subsection of this chapter, are important to the poultry industry, but toxic agents are also produced by bacteria (botulinus toxin, methylmercury, toxic amines) or occur naturally (selenium, phytotoxins). Pesticides, herbicides and other manufactured chemicals, metals such as lead, and industrial contaminants add to the list of toxic materials. Many chemicals and human drugs have been given to birds in feed and water to study their toxic effects. These experimental toxicities have not been included in this chapter.

Poisons and toxins are not major causes of production loss or disease in poultry in most countries, although some, such as lead, pesticides, and botulism, are significant in wild birds. However, in 1985, Terzic and Curcic (250) reported 40% of 2065 poisoning cases seen at the Belgrade Veterinary Facility over a 17-yr period were in poultry. Poisoning occurs more frequently in free-range and backyard flocks and in village poultry where birds forage in neighboring gardens and fields or receive household waste and weeds cut from roadsides and fields. Some of these poisonings are malicious. Contaminated litter on the floor and in nest boxes is an added source of toxins in chickens. Since suspected toxicity cases are more likely than other sick birds to be submitted to a diagnostic laboratory, statistics collected from that source may not be an accurate indication of the incidence of poisoning compared to other disease.

Toxicants covered in this chapter are grouped for presentation by primary use.

ANTIBACTERIALS, ANTICOCCIDIALS, AND GROWTH PROMOTANTS. Most reports of poisoning with chemotherapeutic agents involve inappropriate use or overdose of anticoccidials or growth promotants. Toxicity of a variety of chemotherapeutic agents in poultry and pigeons has recently been reviewed (203).

Sulfonamides. Sulfonamides were used as the primary form of prevention and treatment for coccidiosis in poultry between the early 1940s and late 1950s. Sulfaquinoxaline and sulfamethazine were most widely used. The toxic level of sulfonamides is close to the therapeutic level in poultry, and even the therapeutic level has a detrimental effect on hemopoietic and immune systems. Previous low-level or continuous preventive medication has a protective effect against subsequent higher doses (79).

Sulfonamides are difficult to mix evenly in feed, which may cause some chickens to receive a toxic dose even when a treatment level is used. This is less likely at preventive levels. Both feed and water medication require accurate estimates of feed and water consumption if each chicken is to receive the correct daily dose. Sulfa poisoning has occurred when no allowance was made for increased water and feed consumption of the modern broiler that eats to its physical capacity rather than to its metabolic need, or, more frequently, for the effect of increased water consumption at high environmental temperature or in hot broiler houses. For broilers, the author recommends 1/2 of the therapeutic dose, and at temperatures over 27 C, 1/3 of the therapeutic dose for water medication. Repeat treatment is hazardous and should not be recommended without a postmortem diagnosis to make sure there is no evidence of sulfa toxicity. Even the newer "safe" sulfas need to be used with care (60, 203).

Hemorrhagic syndrome, which occurred frequently when sulfas were in widespread use, is a manifestation of sulfa toxicity and occurs even at therapeutic doses (275). In addition to blood dyscrasia, bone marrow depression, and thrombocytopenia, sulfonamides depress the lymphoid system and immune function in birds. Focal bacterial granulomas are found in tissues and organs of chickens dying from sulfa poisoning. Epithelial degeneration in liver, kidney, and other organs may be caused by the direct effect of the drug, but is more likely due to hypoxia secondary to anemia. When considering withdrawal times in layers, the fact that yolk is laid down over a period of 10 days must be considered (26).

Signs. Chickens and turkeys with sulfa toxicity are depressed, pale, and frequently underweight. In adults there is a marked decrease in egg production and shell quality. Brown eggs may be depigmented (10, 64, 81, 126, 140, 185, 219). Secondary bacterial infections including septicemia and gangrenous dermatitis may follow sulfonamide toxicity (60).

Pathology. For descriptions of gross and microscopic pathology see (64, 79).

Hemorrhage in skin, muscles, and internal organs is the most consistent and extensive gross lesion of sulfonamide intoxication. Hemorrhage may be present in comb, eyelids, face, wattles, anterior chamber of the eye, and musculature of breast and thighs. Normal dark red bone marrow in growing birds changes to pink in mild cases and yellow in severe cases. The entire length of the intestinal tract may be spotted with petechial and ecchymotic hemorrhages, and cecal lumen may contain blood. Hemorrhage may be present in the proventriculus and beneath the gizzard lining. There may be ulcers at the proventricular-gizzard junction. The liver is swollen, pale red or icteric, and may be studded with petechiae or focal necrosis. The spleen is commonly enlarged, has hemorrhagic infarcts, and contains gray nodular areas (82). "Paintbrush" hemorrhages occur in the myocardium. Thymus and bursa of Fabricius are small.

Microscopically, areas of caseation necrosis surrounded by a mantle of giant cells occur in liver, spleen, lungs, and kidneys. Lymphocytic and heterophilic infiltration is present at the periphery of necrotic foci. Lymphoid hypoplasia around splenic adenoid sheaths, edema and fibroplasia of the capsule, and macrophages containing hemosiderin are common. Early changes in the liver are periportal mononuclear infiltration associated with bile duct hyperplasia. Hemosiderin deposits are present in necrotic areas, and thrombosis of portal vessels is present. An early change in kidneys is interstitial lymphocytic infiltration. Degeneration and necrosis of tubular epithelium are associated with albuminous casts. Glomeruli are hyperplastic and Bowman's capsule is dilated with albuminous casts. Lungs are congested with interlobular and interstitial edema. Interstitial tissues contain mononuclear foci. There is degeneration and necrosis of lymphocytes and depletion of bursal follicles.

In femoral bone marrow there is decreased intrasinusoidal erythropoiesis, focal increase in extrasinusoidal lymphopoiesis, and, in some instances, myelopoiesis. There are also focal areas of hyalinization, necrosis, and fibroplasia. Hemosiderin deposits and extrasinusoidal edema are present.

Nitrofurans. Prominent signs of nitrofurazone (NFZ) toxicity in chicks include depression, ruffled feathers, and growth retardation (94, 116, 127, 185). Poor growth may be partially related to feed aversion since feed consumption drops as the level of NFZ increases. Ducklings on toxic levels of NFZ die suddenly without clinical signs (145). Nervous signs and hyperexcitability have been described in acute toxicity in chicks and poults (115, 138, 168). Loud vocalization, opisthotonos, aimless running and flying, and convulsions may be seen.

Furazolidone (FZ) toxicity mainly affects the heart in turkeys, ducks, and chickens (28, 54–56, 101, 178, 204, 240). Marked individual susceptibility to FZ occurs. Some poults, chicks, and ducklings grow well without cardiac damage when fed 400–700 mg FZ/kg feed, whereas others fail to grow, develop ascites, and signs associated with heart failure. Frequency and severity of clinical signs are dose related. There is field evidence FZ may also cause nervous signs in chicks and poults.

FZ causes dose-related biventricular cardiomyopathy with prominent dilation of ventricles and thinning of either the right or left ventricular wall. Secondary heart failure results in passive congestion with lung edema, or marked congestion of liver and other organs, and ascites depending on whether heart failure is mainly left- or right-sided. Right-sided heart failure with marked cardiac enlargement is usually more common up to 3 wk of age.

In turkeys, FZ-induced cardiomyopathy cannot be distinguished from spontaneous turkey cardiomyopathy (STC). The cause of STC is not known, but clinically it is associated with rapid growth, low serum protein, and stressors such as low incubator oxygen, poor ventilation, fumes from brooders, etc., which might induce ischemic cardiomyopathy. Why high doses of FZ cause dilatory cardiomyopathy is not known. FZ is a free-radical inducer and primary free-radical damage may be involved; alternatively, FZ may be inhibiting glutathione peroxidase activity or producing primary ischemic cardiomyopathy making the heart muscle more susceptible to free-radical injury.

Most microscopic lesions result from heart failure. Cardiac lesions include edema, thinning of myocardial muscle fibers, and multifocal myocytolysis with increased connective tissue. Epicardial fibrosis and endocardial fibroelastosis may also occur. Ultrastructural changes include myofibrillar lysis, clumps of Z-band material (204), and increased glycogen in myocardial fibers. Changes in heart muscle enzyme levels accompany tissue alterations.

Ionophores. Ionophores (ion carriers) move some alkali metallic cations, such as sodium (Na^+), across cell membranes. They have both anticoccidial and antibacterial activity, and the group is extensively used in broiler and ruminant feed. Ionophores are coccidiocidal because of their ability to move Na^+ into cells.

Toxic levels of ionophores cause potassium to leave and calcium to enter cells, particularly myocytes, resulting in cell death. Signs of toxicity are related to high extracellular potassium and high intracellular (intramitochondrial) calcium. For more specific information on metabolism and toxicity of monensin see (29, 179). Ionophore toxicity varies with species and age; equidae are very susceptible and adult poultry, particularly turkeys, are more susceptible than broilers (107). There is a synergistic effect with antibiotics in the same family of drugs (253), and increased toxicity with nonrelated antibiotics, other drugs (31, 35, 70, 188, 189, 196), and low-protein rations (203). Monensin, lasalocid, salinomycin, and narasin have been associated with toxicity in poultry, guinea fowl, and other species (17, 61, 108, 144, 193, 246).

Signs. Signs vary from anorexia with depression, weakness, and reluctance to move to complete paralysis in which birds lie in sternal recumbency with neck and legs extended. Less severely affected birds may show posterior paralysis with legs extended laterally. Dyspnea has occurred in affected adult turkeys. Signs are associated with muscle damage. Death may follow respiratory failure or be secondary to dehydration. Mortality is variable but may exceed 70% (85). Stunting is prominent in chronic cases.

Pathology. Subchronic monensin toxicity (258) resulted in opaque fibrin plaques on the epicardium, hemorrhage in coronary fat, and decreased liver weight. In acutely affected turkeys, pallor and atrophy of mainly type I fibers of legs and back has been observed associated with monensin use (257). Gross lesions are often absent in breeders ingesting high levels of monensin (85).

Microscopic changes are seen in heart and skeletal muscle. There are scattered areas of hyalinization with muscle necrosis and myofiber degeneration and necrosis. Type I fibers appear to be selectively affected (108). Heterophils, macrophages, and occasionally lymphocytes may be present. Frequently, when exposed to low doses or interaction with other drugs occurs, affected areas are very cellular with large numbers of sarcolemmal nuclei, indicating regeneration is occurring. Ultrastructural changes have been described (253).

Differential Diagnosis. Since there is a marked age and species variation in susceptibility, and the toxic effect may be potentiated by other drugs, normal levels of ionophores should not be dismissed if clinical signs and histologic changes suggest ionophore toxicity. Ionophore toxicity must be distinguished from selenium deficiency and *Cassia* ingestion, which may produce similar signs and lesions.

Organic Arsenical Feed Additives. Phenylarsonic acids such as arsanilic acid (*p*-amino-benzene arsanilate), sodium arsanate, roxarsone (3-nitro-4-hydroxyphenylarsonic acid), and 4-nitrophenylarsonic acid are used to improve feed efficiency in livestock. Para-ureidobenzenearsonic acid (Carb-o-sep, Carbarsone) and dimetridazole (1,2-dimethyl-5-nitroimidazole (Nitrazol, Emtryl) are used for prevention and control of histomoniasis. Toxicity occurs with accidental or deliberate overdose or in dehydrated animals or birds (179). Peripheral neuropathy causing lameness in turkeys developed after they were given twice the recommended level of 3-nitro-4-hydroxyphenylarsonic acid (272). Toxicity, with liver lesions suggestive of inorganic trivalent arsenite, occurred in broilers receiving 10 times the recommended dose of this same growth promotant. Lesions may have resulted from degradation and reduction of the organic product to the trivalent state, or more likely, from biliary excretion of inorganic arsenic present as a contaminant (224). Cysteine exacerbates toxicity, perhaps by reducing arsenical to the more toxic trivalent state (59).

Signs. Ataxia and incoordination are usually reported, but stunting and depression may be the most prominent signs. Lameness may be evident in turkey poults.

Pathology. Gross changes are absent although affected birds are usually small and the digestive tract is empty. Microscopically, peripheral nerves may show loss of myelin, fragmentation of axons, and proliferation of neurilemmal cells (203, 208).

Others

ANTIBIOTICS. After subcutaneous injection, gentamicin causes depression in turkey poults with edema and hemorrhage at the injection site, and large pale and degenerated kidneys (21, 208). Streptomycin and dihydrostreptomycin sulfate injected intramuscularly for sinusitis in turkey poults causes respiratory distress, paresis, and mild convulsions (131, 203). Aminoglycosides and various other antibiotics, when used for egg inoculation, have caused embryo mortality (95, 96, 163).

ANTICOCCIDIALS. 3,5-dinitro-o-toluamide (dinitrotolumide, dinitolmide, DNOT, Zoalene, Zoamix) can cause ataxia, torticollis, incoordination, and reduced growth (38, 139, 185). Nicarbizine (Nicarb) can make broiler chicks listless, dull, and ataxic; in older birds there can be reduced egg production, shell depigmentation, yolk mottling and reduced hatchability. No gross lesions have been reported but there may be hepatic and renal epithelial degeneration (185, 203). Nitrophenide (Megasul) has caused nervous signs but with rapid recovery (27, 185). Ducks and geese may have depressed growth from halofuginone (Sternorol) (18), and *t*-butylaminoethanol may reduce growth due to a choline deficiency (165).

ANTIPROTOZOALS. Organic arsenicals such as dimetridazole (Nitrazol, Emtryl), used for histomoniasis, have caused growth depression, drop in egg production, nervous signs (ataxia, incoordination, tremors), convulsions, and death in various geese, ducks, pigeons, or turkeys (203, 207). Waterfowl may be poisoned by doses safe for other poultry. Quinacrine hydorchloride or atabrine, used for hemoproteus in pigeons, was fatal at a dose of approximately 50 mg/kg (251).

NUTRIENTS AND OTHER FEED- AND WATER-RELATED TOXICANTS

Amino Acids. Interaction among some amino acids relate to growth, but only methionine is toxic in poultry. Methionine toxicity affects chicks and quail (143, 223), and has caused depressed growth and cervical paralysis in turkey poults (105). Ethinone (a methionine antagonist) toxicity in chicks can be relieved by methionine (276).

Minerals. For information on trace mineral deficiency and toxicity (tissue levels, signs, etc.) see (198). Information on poultry is included for the following minerals: aluminum, arsenic, cadmium, calcium, chloride, chromium, cobalt, copper, fluoride, iodine, iron, lead, magnesium, manganese, mercury, molybdenum, nickel, phosphorus, potassium, selenium, sodium, tungsten, vanadium, and zinc.

CALCIUM. Excess absorbed calcium is excreted through kidneys; high levels cause ureter and kidney impaction resulting in nephrosis. Very young birds are most susceptible. High mortality from hyperuricemia with visceral urate deposits may result from kidney damage because of high dietary calcium. Lung pathology with damage to parenchyma from calcium deposits may also occur in young chicks. It is possible that nephrosis and visceral urate deposits in young and dead-in-shell chicks may result from kidney obstruction by calcium. Excess unabsorbed calcium remaining in the intestine increases fecal water content of pullets and hens on high calcium rations. If the source of calcium is dicalcium phosphate, the alkaline solution formed in the upper digestive tract may result in epithelial necrosis (183, 185, 262), particularly if the mineral has been "top-dressed" on feed and birds eat undiluted material.

Urolithiasis in pullet and adult layer flocks may be caused by high calcium and low phosphorus in pullet rations (267).

COPPER. Copper sulfate is added to water for treatment of enteritis or yeast infection, or to clean algae or scum from water lines and drinkers. Addition to feed is another method for treating enteritis and candidiasis. It may also be sprayed on litter to control aspergillus or used as an antifungal preparation on wood. Birds are occasionally poisoned by eating copper sulfate crystals. Mortality in turkeys offered water containing copper sulphate may have resulted from dehydration caused by water refusal rather than copper poisoning. Toxicity signs are depression and weakness with convulsions and coma terminally (185) or anemia (117, 179, 208). Gross lesions include necrosis of proventriculus and gizzard epithelium and koilin sloughing (122).

FLUORINE. Growth, production, and egg quality were reduced by 700 and 1000 mg NaF/kg feed (104). Leg deformity has also been described (206).

MAGNESIUM. Excess magnesium causes bone abnormalities by replacing calcium and affecting phosphorus utilization (151, 206).

PHOSPHORUS. Excess phosphorus affects growth plate development of bones and increases tibial dyschondroplasia and leg deformities (209).

POTASSIUM. Potassium in the form of fertilizer or potassium permanganate is toxic. $KMnO_4$ causes epithelial necrosis of the digestive tract (185).

SODIUM (SODIUM CHLORIDE, SODIUM BICARBONATE). Excess ionic sodium, usually from sodium chloride in feed or water, causes significant economic losses in poultry in many countries. Most toxicity results from consuming saline water, not water deprivation. Sodium in feed can be toxic for young chicks and poults with (202) or without water deprivation. In some cases of toxicity at apparently low salt levels, analysis may have been for chloride, with salt level calculated from chloride level. When Na^+ toxicity is suspected, both feed and water should be analyzed for Na^+, not estimated from chloride content. There may be sources of Na^+ in feed or water other than sodium chloride. Levels of Na^+ in feed and water are additive.

Chicks and poults are much more sensitive to Na^+ toxicity than adults and mammals, probably because their kidney is not fully developed. Water with Na^+ above 0.4% (4000 parts per million [ppm]) is quite toxic and will cause high mortality within a few days. Lower levels may be toxic as well, depending on amount of Na^+ in feed. Levels of Na^+ above 0.12% (1200 ppm) are toxic for some chicks and poults and produce heart failure with edema and ascites (141). Feed with Na^+ above 0.85% is toxic for some chicks and poults. Much lower levels will cause heart failure and ascites even when water is available free choice. Since steroids increase Na^+ and water retention (222), resulting in hypervolemia, hypertension, right ventricular failure, and ascites, stress may also contribute to Na^+ susceptibility. Birds have poor renal concentrating ability and difficulty reducing plasma osmolality by excretion of salt in excess of water (30). Some waterfowl have nasal salt glands that allow them to excrete Na^+ if an excess is ingested.

Two forms of disease result from Na^+ toxicity in young birds. At high Na^+ levels birds develop acute, severe diarrhea and dehydration, lose weight, and die. There is often acute kidney damage, particularly with sodium bicarbonate (185), which may be caused by urate nephrosis resulting from dehydration. Potassium may have a protective effect (234). At lower Na^+ levels loose droppings also occur, but birds gain weight, at least for 1–2 days, because of associated water retention. Depending on Na^+ level, they may subsequently eat less and grow poorly, or continue to eat and grow well. Water retention, with hypervolemia and hypertension, can lead to functional cardiac overload causing marked right ventricular hypertrophy and dilation, valvular insufficiency, edema, and ascites in chicks (141).

At intermediate levels of excess sodium, a variety of clinical signs and pathologic changes are seen, depending partly on how long birds survive with hypertension before heart failure occurs and how long they survive afterwards. Many lesions described for Na^+ can be attributed to heart failure.

Signs. At low levels of excess Na^+ only watery droppings are seen until ascites occurs. At this stage chicks and poults are dyspneic, depressed, and have a swollen abdomen. At high Na^+ levels birds are obviously depressed and sick with thirst and diarrhea within a few hours. They may have rough, dirty, wet feathers or down. Nervous signs may be present and some birds may be prostrate. At intermediate levels stunting of some birds may be prominent.

Pathology. Chicks with ascites and edema frequently have excess fluid in lungs and hydropericardium. Young males may have cystic dilation of seminiferous tubules (208). There is cardiac hypertrophy, which in chickens is mainly right-sided. Poults have biventricular hypertrophy with dilatory cardiomyopathy. At levels of Na^+ that cause dehydration, cyanosis, myocardial hemorrhage, nephrosis, and enteritis may also be seen.

Microscopic lesions are frequently secondary to heart failure or dehydration. For a detailed description of histologic lesions see (167). Glomerulosclerosis (222, 234) may be hypertensive in origin. Ultrastructural changes in heart muscle (177) include glycogen accumulation, myofibrillar disarray, Z-band streaming, and disruption of intercalated discs.

SELENIUM. Decreased growth and feed intake was seen at 4 and 8 mg/liter drinking water (40). Selenium can accumulate in the food chain of aquatic birds causing emaciation, hepatitis, and ascites. Embryo deformity has also been reported (175, 190).

Protein Supplements. Uncooked soybean (antitrypsin) and rapeseed toxicity (erucic acid, glucosinolate, tannins, and goiterogenic effect) are presented under Phytotoxins.

FISH MEAL. Gizzerosine, histamine, histidine, and other amines cause digestive disturbances, stunting, and osteoporosis. These and other toxic amines result from bacterial spoilage of fish. Toxic products get into poultry feed through fish meal. Excess acid secretion in the proventriculus is stimulated causing gizzard erosion and hemorrhage (125, 218). Broiler chickens may die from hypovolemic shock. Black ingesta and blood may run from the mouth (vomito negro) and contents of the digestive tract are melanic.

Vitamins

VITAMIN A. Excess vitamin A reduces growth rate and causes osteodystrophy and osteoporosis (206, 247, 255).

VITAMIN B_6 (PYRIDOXINE). Pyridoxine is toxic for pigeons at levels safe for poultry (90–100 mg/bird, i.e., approximately 200 mg/kg body weight given by injection) (186).

VITAMIN D_3. Toxicity occurred when feed was top-dressed with vitamin D_3 powder, and 4% of the chicks died from kidney failure. Nephrosis with focal mineralization was present throughout the kidneys. Excess vitamin D_3 has also been shown to increase leg abnormalities in broilers (53, 206). Experimentally induced toxicity indicated 25-hydroxycholecalciferol was 100 times as toxic as cholecalciferol. A variety of lesions were seen but renal damage was most significant (169).

Miscellaneous

LIGNOSOL. Calcium lignosulfonate, a pellet binder, may produce black, sticky cecal contents that adhere to the skin of processed broilers causing increased condemnation from contamination. It has no effect on body weight or feed conversion (197).

NITRATE AND NITRITE. Nitrate is converted to nitrite by bacteria in the digestive tract and is much less toxic than nitrite. High levels of nitrate cause diarrhea, dyspnea, and death. Lower levels affect growth and egg production (103). Blood hemoglobin is changed to methemoglobin. Most reports of toxicity are experimental (4), although there are some reports of toxic nitrate levels in leaves and stems of plants (269).

PEN- AND LITTER-RELATED TOXICANTS.

Pen- and litter-related toxicants include products accidentally or intentionally incorporated into litter or applied to the pen that result in illness. Some are disinfectants and fumigants discussed below. Insecticides that might be mixed in the litter, such as fire ant control products, and insecticides applied to walls, floor, or ceiling are covered later in the chapter. Copper sulfate, often used as a fungicide in litter, has been discussed with food- and water-related toxicants above. Toxic mixtures such as copper-chrome-arsenic formulations are used as preservatives in the timber industry (173). Occasionally, part of the building structure is toxic; geese have been poisoned from eating urea-formaldehyde foam insulation picked from the wall.

IRON. Ferrous sulfate hepatahydrate added to litter to reduce ammonia formation was toxic to broilers (261). Affected chicks were depressed and lethargic. Those that died had severe gizzard ulceration and liver degeneration.

PENTACHLOROPHENOL. Pentachlorophenol has been used as a pesticide in industry and agriculture, but its primary use is as a wood preservative. Logs may be treated before they leave the forest, or wood may be treated after cutting. Sawdust and shavings from treated wood have frequently been used as poultry litter, and chickens can become contaminated from the shavings. Because the product is used for many other purposes, pentachlorophenol may also contaminate broilers or table egg poultry in other ways.

Illness associated with pentachlorophenol has been caused by toxic impurities such as dioxins (see below). Pure pentachlorophenol can reduce growth, cause kidney hypertrophy, and decrease humoral immune responses (194, 241). It has also been associated with musty taint in eggs and broiler meat. Chlorophenols in litter are metabolized by bacteria and fungi to chloroanisoles. Anisoles have a musty or earthy odor even at a very low concentration, and are responsible for the taint in eggs and meat from chickens in contact with contaminated litter (90). Reduced hatchability has also been associated with pentachlorophenol contamination (93).

DISINFECTANTS AND FUMIGANTS.

Fumigants are products producing toxic gases used to control rodents, insects, fungi, and bacteria. They can cause toxicity when inhaled or ingested. Phenolic disinfectant can be toxic when inhaled or absorbed through skin.

Phenolic Compounds and Coal Tar Derivatives. Phenol, cresol, creolin, carbolineum, and creosote products cause damage to vascular endothelium, epithelia of respiratory and digestive tracts, and parenchymal organs such as liver and kidney (185). Thymus and bursa of Fabricius are small, but this may result from stunting rather than being a direct effect on the immune system. Hydropericardium is prominent, but ascites and subcutaneous edema are also frequently present if contact is severe. Mortality may be high. Diagnosis is based on a history of contact and elimination of other causes of ascites and edema. Odor may also provide a useful clue. Cases of creolin toxicity still appear in the literature (154). Coal tar poisoning has been induced in ducks by feeding clay pigeons (43).

Quaternary Ammonium (Cationic) Detergents. Use of sanitizers to clean poultry drinkers or treat water has resulted in reduced growth or production, and occasionally, severe lesions and death in young chicks. High levels of quaternary ammonia cause epithelial irritation of mouth, pharynx, and upper respiratory tract resulting in oral, ocular, and nasal discharges. Necrosis of epithelium leads to pseudomembranes in the mouth and epithelial thickening in esophagus, crop, and proventriculus, with ulcers at the gizzard-proventricular junction (68, 185). Similar lesions have been reported in poults (48, 162).

Chlorine. Low levels (37.5–150 mg/kg) may have a beneficial effect, but high levels (300–1200 mg/kg) result in reduced growth and increased mortality (132).

Formaldehyde. Formaldehyde gas and formalin (a 37% solution of the gas in water, which is then 100% formalin) have been widely used for many years as antibacterial and antiviral agents in the poultry industry. Photophobia and respiratory signs in newly hatched or recently delivered baby chicks and poults from contact with high levels of formaldehyde are seen occasionally. Prolonged exposure to high levels of formaldehyde (which dissolves in liquids on mucous membranes to produce formalin) in the hatcher or delivery truck causes epithelial degeneration and necrosis of eyes, mouth, and trachea. Necrotic pseudomembranous plaques may be found in the mouth and trachea. Edematous swellings under the lower beak (98), subcutaneous edema (20) during the acute phase, and ascites or edema later (220) have been reported in poults.

Other Fumigants. It must be assumed most or all chemicals used as fumigants are toxic to poultry (179). A few reports of deliberate or accidental poisoning of poultry by other fumigants appear in the literature (229, 265).

ANTHELMINTICS. All anthelmintics are probably toxic if a sufficient overdose is given, but in general, birds are more resistant to anthelmintics than mammals.

Benzimidazoles. Cambendazole, mebendazole, and fenbendazole are well tolerated by birds (211).

Imidazathiazoles. Levamisole and tetramisole are not quite as safe. The lethal dose–50% (LD_{50}) of tetramisole for chickens is 2.75 g/kg. Geese and captive birds are more susceptible (211); 300 mg/kg is toxic for geese and as little as 66 mg/kg of levamisole is toxic for some wild birds. The anthelmintic activity of dl-tetramisole resides in the l-isomer (levamisole), so the effective dose of levamisole is ½ that of tetramisole. This doubles the safety margin. Tetramisole is no longer available in most countries. Levamisole poisoning has been reported in geese being treated for *Amidostomum* infection (279). Levamisole was toxic for ducks parenterally at 40 and 80 mg/kg (106).

Organophosphates. Organophosphorus compounds have caused poisoning in birds eating treated feed intended for horses (134, 157). The resin pellet form of dichlorvos (DDVP) is toxic because it is retained in the gizzard. Colored breeds of chickens are more susceptible to coumaphos than white breeds, and naphthaphos has a narrow safety range for chickens with 50 mg/kg being fatal (211).

Ivermectin. Ivermectin has a wide safety margin in birds. An oral or injectable dose of 0.1 mg/kg has been suggested (211). Ivermectin is effective against a wide range of parasites. Zeman (280) tried 1.8 mg/kg for *Dermanyssus gallinae*. This dose was more effective in chickens weighing over 450 g. The toxic dose for chickens is 5.4 mg/kg, which causes 4-hr somnolence; 16.2 mg/kg, which causes 24-hr listlessness and ataxia; 48.6 mg/kg, which resulted in death 5 hr postinjection. Canaries given 20–60 fg/bird intramuscularly showed temporary immobility (33).

Other Anthelmintics. Phenothiazine is relatively nontoxic for birds and hygromycin B is safe at 8 g /900 kg feed (211).

FUNGICIDES. Fungicides are used as seed dressings (protectants), wood preservatives, in paint and plastic, and on cereal crops, fruits, vegetables, and flowers. Previously, poisoning in poultry has usually been from incorporation of treated seed in poultry feed.

Organic Mercurials. Mercurial fungicides, frequently ethyl or methyl mercuric chloride, that cause poisoning with central and peripheral nervous lesions in poultry, wild birds, animals, and humans consuming treated seed, are no longer in use (100, 120, 121, 129, 208, 238). Signs of organic mercury poisoning may be nonspecific or affected birds may show progressive paralysis or other neurologic signs. Specific gross lesions may be lacking, but microscopically, Wallerian degeneration in peripheral nerves and spinal cord and neuronal damage in the brain may be present. Vasculitis may also be obvious in some vessels, particularly in the brain.

Arasan. Arasan (active ingredient thiram, a dithiocarbamate) has caused poisoning in poultry, producing lameness and leg deformity in chicks and poults, and soft-shelled eggs in layers (185). It is also teratogenic (181). Thiram increases the incidence and severity of tibial dyschondroplasia (75).

Captan. Captan is an organic seed protectant. It is less toxic than Arasan. It depresses feed consumption, slows growth, and reduces egg production (185, 245).

For descriptions of other organic synthetic fungicides see (179); pentachlorophenol, a widely used wood preservative, and copper sulfate, a litter treatment, are covered elsewhere in the chapter.

HERBICIDES

Chlorates. Sodium and potassium chlorates used as herbicides and defoliants are moderately toxic for poultry. They act by converting hemoglobin to methemoglobin. The lethal dose for chickens is 5 g/kg (179).

Organic Synthetic Herbicides. Amitrate (3-amino-1,2,4-triazole) causes hypothyroidism and reduces weight gain in chickens (273). Phenoxy-herbicides such as 2-4-D cause kidney enlargement. Some herbicides are toxic for embryos (72). See (179) for additional information.

Dipyridyl Herbicides (Diquat and Paraquat). Paraquat toxicity results from free-radical-induced membrane damage caused by inhibition of the glutathione peroxidase system. Selenium is protective (166). Experimental oral paraquat poisoning in turkeys produced diarrhea, listlessness, and anorexia with terminal convulsions. Gastroenteritis was present at necropsy (237). Turkeys are more resistant than mammals (117, 179).

INSECTICIDES. Insecticides may be referred to by either their common or registered name. The common name is not capitalized, e.g., carbaryl, while the trade name is, e.g., Sevin (179). Organic insecticides, organophosphates, organochlorides, and carbamates have been widely used; some on animals and birds as systemic larvicides and anthelmintics, as well as on buildings and pens. Many are quite toxic for animals as well as insects, arthropods, and helminths. Some more toxic products are used on crops, wood, trees, as soil insecticides, and as seed dressings.

Tables of insecticides by trade name, common name and basic manufacturer; insecticides by common name, class (1. organochlorines or chlorinated hydrocarbons, 2. organophosphates, 3. carbamates, 4. botanicals, bacterials and derivatives and growth regulators, 5. fumigants, 6. sulfonates, sulfides, sulfonis, 7. miscellaneous), and rat LD_{50}; common organochlorine insecticides with specific information on the product and species toxicity (including poultry, waterfowl, and other birds in some cases); common organophosphorus and carbamate insecticides with specific identification of the product and species toxicity, including a variety of birds can be found in (179).

Organochloride Insecticides. Organochloride insecticides tend to persist in the environment. Some more persistent products have been taken off the market or have restricted use. Because they are fat soluble, organochlorides tend to build up in the food chain and be present in yolk of eggs.

Signs. Nervous signs varying from excitement with vocalization to tremors, ataxia, and convulsions are prominent. Prostration and death may occur without other signs. Salivation, vomition, diarrhea, and depression have also been reported (221). There may be decreased egg production, a drop in hatchability, embryo mortality, loss of pigment on pigmented eggs, a change in shell texture (chalky), and eggshell thinning. Lameness and leg deformity have also been described (206).

Pathology. Specific lesions do not occur in organochloride toxicity. Nonspecific changes such as congestion and hemorrhage may be present.

Organophosphorus and Carbamate Insecticides. These products inhibit acetylcholinesterase causing acetylcholine to accumulate, which results in overstimulation of parasympathetic nerves and muscles. Some organophosphates have delayed neurotoxic effects. Chickens and other birds are highly susceptible to this type of toxicity.

Signs. Chicks and poults may die quickly showing few signs except dyspnea and paralysis, or they may exhibit lacrimation, salivation, diarrhea, tremors, depression, dullness, lethargy, cyanosis, ataxia, incoordination, and convulsions prior to death. Because of respiratory signs and salivation in early stages, respiratory infection may be suspected initially (202).

Pathology. Few gross lesions occur. There may be congestion with dark blood and hemorrhages may be present in heart muscle, on serosal surfaces, and on mucosa of intestines. No specific microscopic changes have been identified.

Delayed Organophosphorus Neurotoxicity. Delayed neurotoxicity may result from ingestion or absorption of a variety of phenylphosphothioate insecticides such as leptophos (Phasvel), cyanopenphas, and their analogues. Malathion and dimethoate may also cause delayed neurotoxicity. Chickens, and presumably other birds, are very susceptible to the neurotoxic effect of fire retardants, tri-aryl-cresyl-phosphate chemicals, and phenylphosphothioate insecticides and are used as models. These cause axon and myelin degeneration in peripheral nerves and spinal cord with die-back of axons in long tracts of the cord. There are many reports of delayed neurotoxicity in chickens from these products. Most describe experimentally induced lesions (1, 2, 73, 149). Chicks hatched after in ovo exposure also show clinical signs (80). The author has seen turkeys in Ontario, Canada, with typical clinical signs of ataxia and paralysis and histological lesions of delayed organophosphorus neurotoxicity in spinal cord and peripheral nerves. Clinical cases have also been reported from Europe where chickens ate scraps of synthetic leather containing tri-ortho-cresyl-phosphate (185).

Signs. Ataxia, falling sideways, inability to rise, lack of leg reflexes, and prostration may be evident. Birds appear bright and eat and drink if given access to food and water for several days.

Pathology. There are no gross lesions. Degeneration of axons and myelin in peripheral nerves and long tracts of the spinal cord are diagnostic. Axons may be swollen, and spheroids may be present in axon spaces. Digestion chambers containing macrophages and debris may be present in subacute cases.

Pyrethrum and Synthetic Pyrethroids. These products are not very toxic to animals or birds, and there are no reports of illness.

Rotenone. Rotenone (derris powder) is prepared from roots of the derris plant. Chickens are resistant (lethal dose is 1000–3000 mg/kg) (179). Fish are very susceptible to rotenone.

Nicotine. Nicotine sulfate (Black Leaf 40) has been used to paint chicken roosts to control insects and arthropods, particularly northern fowl mites (44). It has also been used for internal parasites (24, 25).

Signs. Sudden death, occasionally preceded by depression and coma, is seen in affected birds.

Pathology. Since death is from respiratory failure, cyanosis and congestion may be marked. Hemorrhages may be present on the heart and in other tissues.

Organochlorine

CHLORDANE. Chicks develop ataxia and hyperexcitability; hens have reduced body weight, decreased egg production, atrophy and cyanosis of the comb and wattles, and hydropericardium (185).

DDT AND DDE. Hens develop tremors, production drop, and weight loss, and there is eggshell thinning (32, 88, 185, 233).

DIELDRIN. Pigeons, gulls, and other birds may show nervous signs (8, 185, 233).

HEPTACHLOR. This may cause ataxia, salivation, prostration, and death (184, 259).

LINDANE. Diarrhea, vomition, anorexia, depression, convulsions, and sudden death have been associated with lindane poisoning (23, 185).

MIREX (DECHLORANE). This has caused embryo mortality (3).

TOXAPHENE. Lameness, thin shells and osteomalacia may occur (182, 185).

Organophosphates

DIAZANON. This can cause incoordination, paralysis, and respiratory signs (71, 97, 202).

DICHLORVOS (VAPONA, DDVPR). Dichlorvos has been reported to induce staggering, frothing from the mouth, paralysis, and convulsions (76, 202).

DIMETHOATE (CYGONE). Toxic effects include reduced growth and egg production (226, 227).

MALATHION (CYTHION). Malathion causes dullness, salivation, loose droppings, cyanosis, paralysis, and death; lesions include injected subcutaneous vessels and a dark congested heart (34, 92, 185, 202). In geese, there may be flaccid paralysis.

MONOCROTOPHOS (AZODRIN). Monocrotophos toxicity has been associated with salivation, mortality in quail, and weight loss and embryo abnormalities in chickens (216, 231).

PARATHION (NIRAN). Parathion induces lacrimation, salivation, dyspnea, tremors, and convulsions (185).

FAMPHUR (FAMIX, WARBIX, FAMPHOS). Mortality in raptors has resulted from famphur toxicity (123).

Carbamates. Various carbamates such as carbaryl (Sevin), carbofuran (Furadan), and others have been reported to be toxic for pheasants, pigeons, turkey poults, chickens, and ducks (11, 36, 200, 239). Signs include reduced growth, retarded testicular development, lameness, weakness, ataxia, and death. There may be tibial dyschondroplasia, degeneration of seminiferous epithelium, nerve fiber degeneration, and congestion of organs and tissues.

RODENTICIDES, AVICIDES, AND MOLLUSCACIDES

Rodenticides

ALPHA-NAPHTHYL THIOUREA (ANTU). ANTU causes depression, anorexia, weakness, prostration, and death. Lesions include pulmonary edema, hydropericardium, fatty change in liver, and myocardial degeneration (9).

ARSENIC. See METALS AND METALOIDS.

SODIUM MONOFLUOROACETATE (COMPOUND 1080). Signs are reluctance to move, edema of wattles, dyspnea, cyanosis, and nervous signs. Lesions include dark unclotted blood, pulmonary hemorrhage and edema, clotted blood in the trachea and air sacs, petechiation, enteritis, and hydropericardium (52, 117, 179, 217).

STRYCHNINE. Toxic effects are tonic spasms and respiratory failure (119, 179, 185).

WARFARIN AND BRODIFACOUM. These anticoagulant rodenticides cause fluttering and gasping, and hemorrhages in eyes and mouth. The onset is sudden. Anemia occurs (12, 117, 179, 202).

PHOSPHORUS. Elemental yellow, red, and white phosphorus can induce depression, anorexia, diarrhea, ataxia, gastroenteritis, and death (179, 185).

ZINC PHOSPHIDE. Weakness, diarrhea, opisthotonos, and convulsions occur. There is enteritis, ascites, and hydorpericardium (111).

For birds, the toxic doses of several rodenticides (alpha-chloralase, crimidine, pyriminil, phosphorus, alpha-chlorohydrim) are given in *Clinical and Diagnostic Veterinary Toxicology* (179).

Avicides

AVITROL (4-AMINOPYRIDINE or 4-AP). This is reported to cause disorientation and vocalization (distress calls). Affected pigeons may be molested by normal pigeons. Lesions include congestion (89, 171).

2-CHLORO-4-ACETOTOLUIDINE (CAT) AND 3-CHLORO-*P*-TOLUIDINE (CPT). No clinical signs are reported, but kidney necrosis (from CAT) and liver and kidney necrosis (from CPT) occur (99).

Molluscacides

METALDEHYDE. Toxicity of this agent was reported by Osweiler et al. (179) and Hatch (117).

TOXIC GASES

AMMONIA. Ammonia level should be less than 25 cm^3/m^3 (ppm), but in poorly ventilated litter-type houses, ammonia may exceed 100 ppm (142). High levels of ammonia (50–75 ppm) reduce food consumption and growth rate (63). Egg production is also reduced. Ammonia dissolves in the liquid on mucous membranes and eyes to produce ammonium hydroxide, an irritating alkali causing keratoconjunctivitis. If levels above 100 ppm persist, corneal ulceration and blindness can occur. The condition is painful and photophobia and stunting are marked. At levels of 75–100 ppm changes in respiratory epithelium include loss of cilia (180) and increased numbers of mucus-secreting cells (7). Heart rate and breathing may be affected and there may be hemorrhages in trachea and bronchi. For a recent literature review see (42).

CARBON MONOXIDE. Carbon monoxide (CO) poisoning may occur in buildings where defective or unventilated gas catalytic or open flame brooders or furnaces are in use, or where poultry are exposed to internal-combustion engine exhaust fumes. Affected chicks or poults show drowsiness, labored breathing, and incoordination. Spasms and convulsions may occur prior to death. At postmortem, blood is bright red. Sublethal levels cause stunting (185, 242). In suspected cases CO should be measured at several locations in the pen with the ventilation system shut off. Carboxyhemoglobin can be measured in blood of affected birds. The author found levels of 70 ppm CO in pens where a repeated high incidence of ascites due to pulmonary hypertension and right ventricular failure occurred. Toxic levels of CO for chickens are 600 ppm for 30 min, which causes distress, and 2000–3600 ppm, which is lethal in 1.5–2 hr (179).

Other Toxic Gases. Levels of methane, carbon dioxide, hydrogen sulfide, methyl mercaptan, dimethyl sulfide, and dimethyl disulfide were found to be low in poultry and other livestock buildings in Finland (142), but toxic fumes from liquid manure pits in pig barns have killed humans and pigs in North America, and nitrogen dioxide formed in freshly filled silos has also killed humans and animals in Canada and the USA. Toxic gases associated with livestock production, including poultry, have been reviewed (179). The effect of sulfur dioxide in chickens has been described (83).

HOUSEHOLD AND COMMERCIAL PRODUCTS

ANTIFREEZE (ETHYLENE GLYCOL). Ethylene glycol is toxic when ingested because it breaks down to oxalic acid, which combines with calcium to form calcium oxalate. Calcium oxalate crystals block renal tubules and cause tubular epithelial necrosis leading to hyperuricemia and urate nephrosis with visceral urate deposits. Diagnosis is usually based on finding typical crystals and tubular changes on microscopic examination of kidney (208, 210, 244). Liver necrosis has been reported in pigeons (158). Other forms of toxicity may occur in other species (179). Coccidia oocysts treated with ethylene oxide were toxic to chicks and caused kidney lesions similar to ethylene glycol (264).

CARBON TETRACHLORIDE. Carbon tetrachloride has been used previously as a household solvent and cleaner. It has also been used to treat tapeworms in chickens (212). It is toxic to animals and birds, interfering with fat metabolism and causing liver and kidney damage. Chicks are more resistant than rats, but low levels cause decreased growth (91).

FERTILIZER. Lawn, garden, and farm fertilizers contain nitrogen, phosphorus, and potassium. These elements have been discussed above (see NUTRIENTS AND OTHER FEED- AND WATER-RELATED TOXICANTS). Fertilizer may be attractive to birds because it is frequently in the form of small hard pellets. Some phosphate fertilizers contain very low levels of radioactive material.

NAPHTHALENE. Moth balls are frequently recommended to keep pets and other animals away from gardens or out of attics. They have also been used in chicken nests for ectoparasite control. Moth balls are toxic and poisoning has been reported in poultry (130).

UREA. Urea is relatively nontoxic for birds. Because it is used in feed preparations for ruminants, the pellets are occasionally found in poultry feed.

METALS AND METALOIDS

ARSENIC. Most reports of arsenic toxicity in birds are experimental except those associated with grasshopper bait (185). Organic arsenicals are discussed above with other growth promotants and feed additives.

Inorganic, aliphatic, and trivalent organic arsenic are used as pesticides, weed and brush killers, and defoliants. Toxic effects include diarrhea, nervous signs, and cyanosis. There is inflammation of crop, proventriculus, and gizzard, and hepatosis and nephrosis occur (13, 133, 179, 224, 263).

CADMIUM. Experimental cadmium toxicity in chicks, poults, and ducklings and induction of free-radical-induced lesions by cadmium, silver, and other minerals have been reported (58, 137, 254).

Toxic levels of cadmium, found in industrial waste and sewage sludge, cause decreased feed intake and decreased growth (133, 195, 198).

CHROMIUM AND POTASSIUM DICHROMATE. Chromium from industrial waste or coated metal objects may cause depression, anorexia, and paralysis (133, 198).

COBALT, COPPER, IRON. See FEED- AND WATER-RELATED TOXICANTS.

LEAD. All species of birds are susceptible to lead poisoning. Lead is the only metallic poison causing significant disease in birds, and most toxicity occurs in wild species, especially waterfowl. Chickens are more resistant than waterfowl (198). Birds as a group are at risk from metallic lead because the material is retained in the gizzard, ground down, and absorbed slowly. Experimental poisoning trials with chickens show an interaction with some nutrients (74, 150) and inhibition of avian bone healing (155).

Lead is widespread in the environment, and there are many possible sources for ingested lead when toxicity occurs. Wild water birds are at greatest risk from ingesting lead shot, which is the main hazard in North America (215, 266), or lead weights from fishing lines, which are the most important source in England. Pigeons may also ingest lead shot (66). Birds that eat carrion may be poisoned by lead shot ingested with tissues. Backyard and free-range poultry may pick up lead from paint chips, lead batteries, or other lead objects. Caged birds may be poisoned from the same environmental sources as children and dogs—mainly paint chips, leaded windows, toys, and lead objects (274). Chicks have been poisoned by eating contaminated grit (185).

Signs. Most lead poisoning in birds is chronic. Clinical disease is usually noted as wasting, ataxia, lameness or paralysis, and anemia. In acute cases anorexia, weakness, prostration, and anemia may be prominent. Green diarrhea may result from anorexia, or it may be a direct effect of lead on digestive and nervous systems.

Hematology. Basophilic stippling and abnormal erythrocytes occur in lead poisoning in birds but are of doubtful diagnostic value (185). Anemia with large numbers of immature cells may be more significant. Mitosis of erythrocytes has also been reported (235).

Pathology. Most lesions probably result from anorexia and debility. Impaction of proventriculus is frequently seen and likely secondary to vagus nerve damage (see Fig. 35.1). Emaciation may be prominent, but many ducks and geese that die from lead poisoning are in good body condition. The carcass may be pale with watery blood.

Microscopically, the most diagnostic lesions are demyelination of peripheral nerves and focal areas of vascular damage in the cerebellum (135), and acid-fast intranuclear inclusion bodies in kidney (Fig. 35.2), liver, and spleen (156, 185, 208). Inclusions are composed of protein-bound lead and can be demonstrated by special staining or electron microscopy (65). Nephrosis with degeneration and necrosis of tubular epithelial cells and brown pigment in epithelial cells has been described (50, 235). Hemosiderosis is prominent in spleen and other organs. Scattered myocardial necrosis associated with hyaline or fibrinoid necrosis of blood vessels (50) and arrested mitotic activity in proventriculus epithelial cells have also been identified (49).

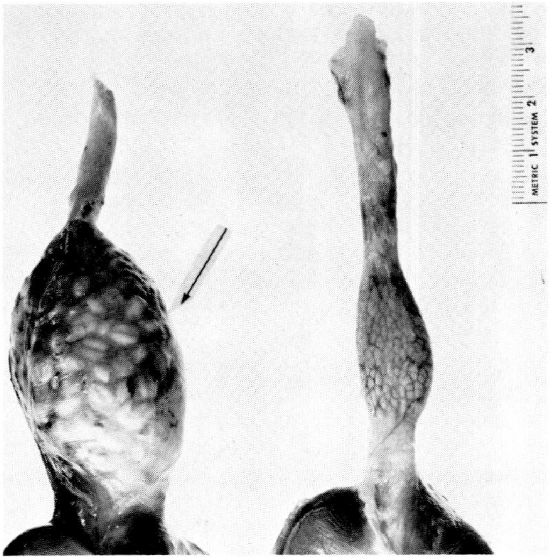

35.1. Lead poisoning, showing distended proventriculus (*arrow*); there were 15 lead shot in gizzard.

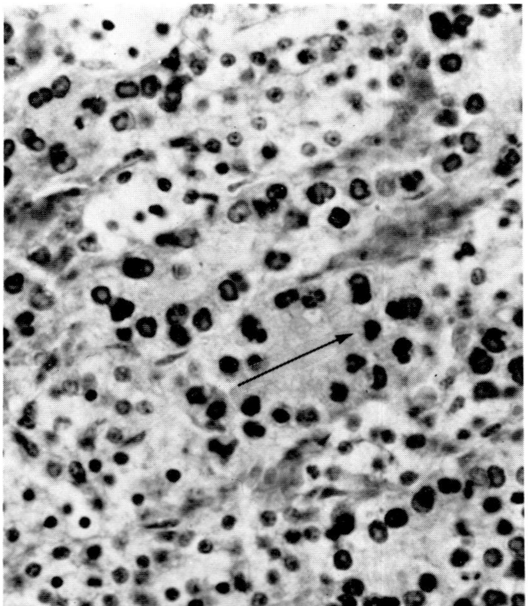

35.2. Lead poisoning. Acid-fast intranuclear inclusion bodies (*arrow*) in kidney of mallard duck. ×480. (Locke)

Diagnosis. The final diagnosis of lead poisoning is based on blood and tissue levels. In chickens a blood lead level above 4 ppm, liver lead level above 18 ppm wet weight, and 20 ppm wet weight in kidney would be considered diagnostic (198). Lead levels in bone can also be determined. Acid-fast inclusions in kidney epithelial cells suggest lead poisoning but may be found in birds that ingested lead and died from some other cause. Peripheral nerve lesions, in conjunction with fibrinoid necrosis of blood vessels that may be found throughout the body, not just in brain and heart, are useful in diagnosis, but similar changes are seen in methylmercury poisoning (208). However, in lead poisoning, lesions in the central nervous system are related only to vascular damage.

MERCURY. Organic mercury, used previously as a seed protectant, is discussed above with fungicides. Most organic mercury in the environment today results from methylation by aquatic organisms and action of methogenic bacterial enzymes on elemental mercury from nature (decaying trees) or industry. Tons of mercury as bivalent inorganic mercury, elemental mercury, and phenyl mercury have been discharged into waterways around the world.

Methylmercury, a direct product of biotransformation, gets into small water organisms and enters the food chain when fish eat contaminated plants, insects, or animals (bioconcentration). Fish-eating birds, particularly ducks, may become poisoned from mercury in the food they eat (179).

Inorganic mercury of medicinal or industrial waste origin may induce anorexia, enteritis and nephrosis (179, 198).

TIN. Tin from medicinal sources can cause depression, hunching up, and yellow diarrhea (230).

URANIUM (URANYL NITRATE). Industrial uranium causes depression, anorexia, hyperuricemia, nephrosis, and visceral urate deposits (114).

VANADIUM. Reduced egg quality, growth, and hatchability all have been attributed to vanadium toxicity (148, 198). Also, there are many reports of experimental vanadium toxicity in the literature.

INDUSTRY-RELATED TOXICANTS

Toxic Fat Syndrome, Chick Edema Disease, Dioxin Toxicity. Over 30 yr ago the most toxic dioxin, 2,3,7,8-tetrachlorodibenzodioxin (TCDD), and other dioxins in the same polychlorinated dibenzodioxin group were found as contaminants in industrial fat (tallow from cattle hides) added to feed. This material, which could be distilled from fat, was called "chick edema factor" until it was identified. It caused widespread disease in the broiler industry and in other poultry for several years. Occasional cases of dioxin toxicity (chick edema disease) occurred until about 1970. More recently TCDD toxicity followed environmental contamination in Italy, where adult fowl died with lesions of chick edema disease (191).

Chickens are more susceptible than some mammals to the toxic effect of TCDD (179). In chickens dioxin damages vascular endothelium causing vascular leakage and extensive movement of fluid into body cavities and subcutaneous tissue. The epithelium of some parenchymal organs is damaged and there is degeneration of heart and skeletal muscle.

Since right ventricular hypertrophy and dilation has been described (5) and many lesions in dioxin toxicity are similar to right-sided heart failure from other causes, the possibility that dioxin may be contributing to the pathogenesis of right ventricular failure should be considered.

Depending on the level of TCDD in feed, many broilers in a flock will show severe signs of stunting, respiratory distress, weakness, ataxia, and edema. Mortality can occasionally be very high. For a description and review of the syndrome see (185).

TCDD may be present as a contaminant in herbicides. It and other dioxins are produced by incineration (179) and by industry (77).

Polybrominated Biphenyl (PBB) and Polychlorinated Biphenyl (PCB). PBBs or PCBs may be accidentally added to feed, get into feed as contaminants (as in oil or grease from equipment), or be present in the environment from industrial contamination and deliberate dumping. Both PBBs and PCBs are toxic to birds. At low levels they affect production, reproduction, hatchability, and offspring viability (192, 221). Hepatocyte damage and bursal depletion also occur with low-level PBB toxicity (67). Residues may be found in eggs and meat from birds without clinical signs. It has been reported (179) that PBBs are concentrated in eggs at 1.5 times the dietary level.

At high levels, lesions of PCB toxicity are similar to dioxin toxicity (232). It is likely in some cases PCBs were contaminated with TCDD. Dioxin was probably the material causing lesions in toxicity caused by paint containing chlorinated hydrocarbon (164).

Crude Petroleum and Oils. Most information on toxicity of oil to birds deals with environmental contamination and the effect of oil spills on waterfowl. Ingested oil causes anorexia, weight loss, incoordination, and tremors. Anemia has also been reported (153). Lesions included lipid pneumonia, enteritis, hepatosis with fatty infiltration, nephrosis and degeneration of pancreas, spleen, and bursa (113, 174). Impaired immune response has been reported (213). In herring gulls and puffins, lesions suggested a primary toxic hemolytic disease (152) with lymphoid depletion being secondary and stress related.

Oils and oil products on the feathers and skin can be removed with detergents.

Alcohol. Ethyl alcohol may be used to dissolve experimental chemicals or drugs given to poultry in feed or water. Clinical signs of intoxication include ataxia and reduced feed consumption. Fatty change in the liver and heart lesions may occur (6, 57, 91).

BIOTOXINS. Biotoxins are poisonous substances produced by living organisms including bacterial toxins such as botulinum, which in birds is frequently associated with toxin-contaminated maggots; bacterial food poisoning; and diseases such as necrotic and ulcerative enteritis, gangrenous dermatitis, and mycotoxins. Perhaps even methylmercury produced by bacteria should be classed as a biotoxin. Insect and snake venoms are also biotoxins. Most of these conditions are of little importance or discussed in other parts of the text. Only algae poisoning and rose chafer toxicity will be mentioned here.

Algae. Several species of blue-green algae produce a toxin that, when concentrated by rapid algal growth (bloom) in warm bodies of fresh water and a constant light wind blowing the toxic material to the side of the lake, may poison animals and birds consuming it. Toxicity varies directly with concentration. Affected chickens may show nervous signs and paralysis before death. Ducks and turkeys have also been poisoned (133). Cyanosis, congestion, and dilated, distended heart may be seen at necropsy (185). Liver is swollen with necrosis of hepatocytes (146). Diagnosis is based on identifying toxin in the water (179).

Rose Chafers. Rose chafers (*Macrodactylus subspinosus*) are insects appearing in spring and early summer in eastern and central North America. Young chicks may be poisoned by 15–30 insects (185). Clinical signs include drowsiness, weakness, prostration, and convulsions (185).

PHYTOTOXINS. Phytotoxins that are reported to affect poultry are briefly discussed in this section.

BEANS (SEVERAL SPP.—TRYPSIN INHIBITION)

Part of Plant. Raw bean.

Signs and Lesions. Reduced growth, pancreatic hypertrophy, acinar cell hypertrophy and hyperplasia (147, 159, 260, 278).

BLACK LOCUST (*ROBINIA PSEUDOACACIA*)

Part of Plant. Leaf.

Signs and Lesions. Depression and paralysis; hemorrhagic enteritis (15).

CACAO (*THEOBROMA CACAO*—THEOBROMINE TOXICITY)

Part of Plant. Bean waste.

Signs and Lesions. Acute cases—nervous signs followed by convulsions and death; cyanosis, cloacal prolapse, mottled kidneys. Chronic cases—anorexia, diarrhea (22, 62, 185).

CASTOR BEAN (*RICINUS COMMUNIS*)

Part of Plant. Bean.

Signs and Lesions. Progressive paralysis with prostration (like botulism); diarrhea, emaciation, swollen pale mottled liver, hemmorhagic catarrhal enteritis, petechiae, degeneration of lymphoid tissue and parenchymal cells of liver and kidney, bile duct proliferation (136, 176, 185).

COFFEE BEAN (*CASSIA OCCIDENTALIS, C. OBTUSIFOLIA*)

Part of Plant. Seed.

Signs and Lesions. Weakness, ataxia, paralysis, decreased egg production, diarrhea; toxic myopathy, pectoralis and semitendonosis muscles pale and edematous, muscle degeneration and necrosis (45, 185, 236, 256).

CORN COCKLE (*AGROSTEMMA GITHAGO*—GITHAGENIN TOXICITY)

Part of Plant. Seed.

Signs and Lesions. Depression, rough feathers, decreased respiratory and heart rate, diarrhea, depressed growth; hydropericardium; caseous necrosis of crop, pharyngeal mucosa, and mouth (124, 185).

COTTON SEED MEAL (GOSSYPOL TOXICITY)

Signs and Lesions. Cyanosis, inappetence, emaciation, reduced egg production and quality; enteritis, degeneration of liver and kidney (185).

COYOTILLO (*KARWINSKIA HUMBOLDTIANA*)

Part of Plant. Fruit and seed.

Signs and Lesions. Depressed growth, cyanosis, paralysis (161).

CROTALARIA SPP. (MONOCROTALINE OR SPECTABILINE TOXICITY)

Part of Plant. Seed, leaf, stem.

Signs and Lesions. Dull, inactive, reduced feed consumption, stunting, and bright yellow-green urates; subcutaneous edema, ascites, hydropericardium, lung edema, hepatitis, bile duct hyperplasia (37, 46, 69, 185, 270).

DAUBENTONIA (*DAUBENTONIA LONGIFOLIA, SESBANIA DRUMMONDII*)

Part of Plant. Seed.

Signs and Lesions. Weakness, depression, stunting, diarrhea, emaciation; proventriculitis with ulceration and enteritis; liver and kidney degeneration (86, 225).

DEATH CAMAS (*ZYGADENUS* SPP.)

Part of Plant. Leaf, stem, root.

Signs and Lesions. Weakness, salivation, diarrhea, prostration (160, 172).

EUCALYPTUS CLADOCALYX (CYANIDE OR PRUSSIC ACID)

Part of Plant. Leaf.

Signs and Lesions. Specimens found dead (41, 202).

GLOTTIDIUM (*GLOTTIDIUM VESICARIUM*)

Part of Plant. Seed.

Signs and Lesions. Diarrhea, cyanosis, prostration; necrotic enteritis, gizzard ulceration (78).

HEMLOCK (*CONIUM MACULATUM*—CONIINE TOXICITY)

Part of Plant. Seed.

Signs and Lesions. Salivation, weakness, diarrhea, reduced growth; hepatic congestion, enteritis (87).

JIMSONWEED (*DATURA STRAMONIUM*)

Part of Plant. Seed.

Signs and Lesions. Reduced growth (62).

LATHYRUS SPP. (LATHYRISM)

Part of Plant. Seed (pea).

Signs and Lesions. Skeletal deformity, osteolathyrism (*L. odoratus*); or neurologic disease, neurolathyrism (*L. sativus*) (47, 170, 199, 243).

LEUCAENA LEUCOCEPHALA (*Mimosine? Toxicity*)

Part of Plant. Leaf.

Signs and Lesions. Depressed growth (118).

LILY OF THE VALLEY (*CONVALLARIA MAJALIS*) (14)

MILKWEED (*ASCLEPIAS* SPP.—ASCLEPIDIN TOXICITY)

Signs and Lesions. Weakness and incoordination, convulsions; recovery; prostration and death (185)

NIGHTSHADE (*SOLANUM NIGRUM*—BELLADONNA TOXICITY)

Part of Plant. Immature fruit.

Signs and Lesions. Dilated pupils, incoordination, prostration (109, 110).

NITRATE (See NUTRIENTS AND OTHER FEED- AND WATER-RELATED TOXICANTS)

OLEANDER (*NERIUM OLEANDER*)

Part of Plant. All parts.

Signs and Lesions. Depression, weakness, diarrhea; gastroenteritis, liver degeneration (14, 185).

OXALATE (OXALIC ACID)

Part of Plant. Leaf and stem.

Signs and Lesions. See ethylene glycol (HOUSEHOLD AND COMMERCIAL PRODUCTS) for signs; oxalate nephrosis (269).

PARSLEY, *AMMI MAJUS,* OTHERS (PHOTOSENSITIZATION)

Part of Plant. All parts.

Signs and Lesions. Dermatitis (unfeathered areas); hepatitis (187, 228).

POKEBERRY (*PHYTOLACCA AMERICANA*)

Part of Plant. Fruit.

Signs and Lesions. Ataxia, leg deformity, ascites (16, 221).

POTATO (*SOLANUM TUBEROSUM*—SOLANINE TOXICITY)

Part of Plant. Green or spoiled tubers, peelings, sprouts.

Signs and Lesions. Incoordination, prostration (teratogenic) (110, 249).

RAGWORT (*SENECIO JACOBEA*—PYRROLIZIDINE ALKALOID)

Part of Plant. All parts.

Signs and Lesions. Focal hepatic necrosis and portal fibrosis (46, 221).

RAPESEED MEAL (ERUCIC ACID/GLUCOSINOLATE/TANNIN TOXICITY—ANTITHRYOID ACTIVITY)

Part of Plant. Seed.

Signs and Lesions. Egg taint, depressed growth, anemia, sudden death, ruptured liver, hepatitis, ascites, hydropericardium; periacinar hepatic necrosis, fatty change in skeletal and heart muscle (19, 39, 51, 84, 102, 201, 268, 277).

RYE (GRAIN)

Part of Plant. Seed.

Signs and Lesions. Poor growth, pasting, lameness, soft bones (147, 214).

SAPONIN (Alfalfa [Lucerne]—MEDICAGENIC ACID)

Part of Plant. Leaf and stem.

Signs and Lesions. Reduced growth (252)

SORGHUM (GRAIN—TANNIN TOXICITY)

Part of Plant. Seed.

Signs and Lesions. Depressed growth, leg deformity (147, 248).

TOBACCO (*NICOTIANA TABACUM*—NICOTINE SULFATE TOXICITY)

Part of Plant. Leaf and stem.

Signs and Lesions. Stunting, reduced production (teratogenic) (185).

VETCH (*VICIA* SPP.—B-CYANO-*L*-ALANINE TOXICITY—SEE LATHYRISM, ABOVE)

Part of Plant. Seed (pea).

Signs and Lesions. Excitability, respiratory distress, convulsions (112, 128, 205).

YELLOW JESSAMINE (*GELSEMIUM SEMPERVIRENS*)

Part of Plant. Whole plant.

Signs and Lesions. Depressed growth (185, 271).

YEW (*TAXUS* SPP.—TAXINE TOXICITY)

Part of Plant. All parts.

Signs and Lesions. Labored breathing, incoordination, collapse; cyanosis.

REFERENCES

1. Abou-Donia, M.B., and A.A. Komeil. 1979. Delayed neurotoxicity of o-ethyl o-4-cyanophenyl phenylphosphonothioate (cyanofenphos) in hens. Toxicol Lett 4:455–459.
2. Abou-Donia, M.B., D.G. Graham, M.A. Ashry, and P.R. Timmons. 1980. Delayed neurotoxicity of leptophos and related compounds: Differential effects of subchronic oral administration of pure technical grade and degradation products on the hen. Toxicol Appl Pharmacol 53:150–163.
3. Abuelgasim, A., R. Ringer, and V. Sanger. 1982. Toxicosis of mirex for chick embryos and chickens hatched from eggs inoculated with mirex. Avian Dis 26:34–39.
4. Adams, A.W. 1974. Effects of nitrate in drinking water on Japanese quail. Poult Sci 53:832–834.
5. Allen, J.R. 1964. The role of "toxic fat" in the production of hydropericardium and ascites in chickens. Am J Vet Res 25:1210–1219.
6. Allen, N.K., S.R. Aakhus-Allen, and M.M. Walser. 1981. Toxic effects of repeated ethanol intubations to chicks. Poult Sci 60:941–943.
7. Al-Mashhadani, E.H., and M.M. Beck. 1985. Effect of atmospheric ammonia on the surface ultrastructure of the lung and trachea of broiler chicks. Poult Sci 64:2056–2061.
8. Amure, J., and J.C. Stuart. 1978. Dieldrin toxicity in poultry associated with wood shavings. Vet Rec 102:387.
9. Anderson, W.A., and C.P. Richter. 1946. Toxicity of alpha naphthyl thiourea for chickens and pigs. Vet Med 41:302–303.
10. Asplin, F.D., and E. Boyland. 1947. The effects of pyrimidine sulfonamide derivatives upon the blood-clotting system and testes of chicks and the breeding capacity of adult fowls. Br J Pharmacol 2:79–82.
11. Bahl, A.K., and B.S. Pomeroy. 1978. Acute toxicity in poults associated with carbaryl insecticide. Avian Dis 22:526–528.
12. Bai, K.M., and M.K. Krishnakumari. 1986. Acute oral toxicity of Warfarin to poultry, Gallus domesticus: A nontarget species. Bull Environ Contam Toxicol 37:544–549.
13. Barber, P.G. 1933. Arsenic poisoning in poultry. Vet Med 28:500–502.
14. Bardosi, Z. 1939. [Toxicity of lily of the valley and oleander leaves for fowls.] Thesis, Budapest. Vet Bull 10:624. (Abstr).
15. Barnes, M.F. 1921. Black locust poisoning of chickens. J Am Vet Med Assoc 59:370–372.
16. Barnett, B.D. 1975. Toxicity of pokeberries (fruit of Phytolacca americana, large) for turkey poults. Poult Sci 54:1215–1217.
17. Beck, B.E., and W.N. Harries. 1979. The diagnosis of monensin toxicosis: A report on outbreaks in horses, cattle, and chickens. Proc 22nd Annu Meet Am Assoc Vet Lab Diag, pp. 269–282.
18. Behr, K.-P., H. Lüders, and C. Plate. 1986. Safety of halofuginone (Sternorol[R]) in geese, muskovy ducks and peking ducks. Tierärztl Wochenschr 93:4–8.
19. Bhatnagar, M.K., S. Yamashiro, and L.L. David. 1980. Ultrastructural study of liver fibrosis in turkeys fed diets containing rapeseed meal. Res Vet Sci 29:260–265.
20. Bierer, B.W. 1958. The ill effects of excessive formaldehyde fumigation on turkey poults. J Am Vet Med Assoc 132:174–176.
21. Bird, J.E., M.M. Walser, and G.E. Duke. 1983. Toxicity of gentamicin in red-tailed hawks. Am J Vet Res 44:1289–1293.
22. Black, D.J.G., and N.S. Barron. 1943. Observations on the feeding of a cacao waste product to poultry. Vet Rec 55:166–167.
23. Blakley, B.R. 1982. Lindane toxicity in pigeons. Can Vet J 23:267–268.
24. Bleecker, W.L., and R.M. Smith. 1933. Further studies on the relative efficiency of vermifuges for poultry. J Am Vet Med Assoc 83:76–81.
25. Bleecker, W.L., and R.M. Smith. 1933. Nicotine sulfate as a vermifuge for the removal of ascardis from poultry. J Am Vet Med Assoc 83:645–655.
26. Blom, L. 1975. Residues of drugs in eggs after medication of laying hens for eight days. Acta Vet Scand 16:396–404.
27. Blount, W.P. 1955. Recent advances in poultry therapeutics. Vet Rec 67:1087–1097.
28. Bogin, E., D. Ratner, and Y. Avidar. 1983. Biochemical changes in blood and tissue associated with round heart disease in turkey poults. Avian Pathol 12:437–442.
29. Booth, N.H. 1988. Drugs and chemical residues in the edible tissue of animals. In N.H. Booth and L.E. McDonald (eds.), Veterinary Pharmacology and Therapeutics, 6th Ed., pp 1149–1205. Iowa State Univ Press, Ames.
30. Braun, E.J., and W.H. Dantzler. 1972. Function of mammalian-type and reptilian-type nephrons in kidney of desert quail. Am J Physiol 222:617–629.
31. Braunius, W.W. 1986. Monensin/sulfachlorpyrazine intoxicatie bij kalkoenen. Tijdschr Diergeneeskd 111:676–678.
32. Britton, W.M. 1975. Toxicity of high dietary levels of DDT in laying hens. Bull Environ Contam Toxicol 13:703–706.
33. Brownell, J.R. 1984. Sternostoma tracheacolum. Continuing studies. Proc 33rd West Poult Dis Conf, pp. 91–93.
34. Brown, C., W.B. Gross, and M. Ehrich. 1986. Effects of social stress on the toxicity of malathion in young chickens. Avian Dis 30:679–682.
35. Broz, J., and M. Frigg. 1987. Incompatability between lasalocid and chloramphenicol in broiler chicks after a long-term simultaneous administration. Vet Res Commun 11:159–172.
36. Bunyan, P.J., and D.M. Jennings. 1976. Carbamate poisoning. Effect of certain carbamate pesticides on esterase levels in the pheasant (Phasianius colchicus) and pigeons (Columba livia): J Agric Food Chem 24:136–143.
37. Burguera, J.A., G.T. Edds, and O. Osuna. 1983. Influences of selenium on aflatoxin B, or crotalaria toxicity in turkey poults. Am J Vet Res 44:1714–1717.
38. Cameron, I.R.D., and D. Spackman. 1982. Coccidiostat toxicity. Vet Rec 111:307.
39. Campbell, L.D. 1987. Effect of different intact glucosinolates on liver hemorrhage in laying hens and the influence on vitamin K. Nutr Rep Int 35:1221–1227.
40. Cantor, A.H., D.M. Nash, and T.H. Johnson. 1984. Toxicity of selenium in drinking water of poultry. Nutr Rep Int 29:683–688.
41. Carew, S.N., R.H. Davis, and A.H. Sykes. 1986. Methionine, sulphate, and thiosulphate as sources of dietary sulphur for chicks chronically intoxicated with

cyanide. Nutr Rep Int 34:655-665.
42. Carlile, F.S. 1984. Ammonia in poultry houses: A literature review. World's Poult Sci J 40:99-113.
43. Carlton, W.W. 1966. Experimental coal tar poisoning in the White Pekin duck. Avian Dis 10:484-502.
44. Carpenter, C.D. 1931. The use of nicotine and its compounds for the control of poultry parasites. J Am Vet Med Assoc 78:651-657.
45. Charles, O.W. 1976. Coffee weed toxicity in animals. Proc Georgia Nutr Conf Feed Ind, pp. 67-76.
46. Cheeke, P.R. 1988. Toxicity and metabolism of pyrrolizidine alkaloids. J Anim Sci 66:2343-2350.
47. Chowdhury, S.D. 1988. Lathyrism in poultry: A review. World's Poult Sci J 44:7-16.
48. Christensen, N. 1980. QAC poisoning from drinking apparatus. Vet Rec 107:363.
49. Clemens, E.T., L. Krook, A.L. Aronson, and C.E. Stevens. 1975. Pathogenesis of lead shot poisoning in the mallard duck. Cornell Vet 65:248-285.
50. Cook, R.S., and D.O. Trainer. 1966. Experimental lead poisoning of Canada geese. J Wildl Manage 30:1-8.
51. Corner, A.H., H.W. Hulan, D.M. Nash, and F.G. Proudfoot. 1985. Pathological changes associated with the feeding of soybean oil or oil extracted from different rapeseed cultivars to single comb white leghorn cockerels. Poult Sci 64:1438-1450.
52. Cottral, G.E., G.D. Dibble, and B. Winton. 1947. The effect of sodium fluoroacetate ("1080" rodenticide) on White Leghorn chickens. Poult Sci 26:610-613.
53. Cruickshank, J.J., and J.S. Sim. 1987. Effects of excess vitamin D_3 and cage density on the incidence of leg abnormalities in broiler chickens. Avian Dis 31:332-338.
54. Czarnecki, C.M. 1980. Furazolidone-induced cardiomyopathy biomedical model for the study of cardiac hypertrophy and congestive heart failure. Avian Dis 24:120-138.
55. Czarnecki, C.M. 1984. Cardiomyopathy in turkeys (a review). Comp Biochem Physiol 77A:591-598.
56. Czarnecki, C.M. 1986. Quantitative morphological alterations during the development of furazolidone-induced cardiomyopathy in turkeys. J Comp Pathol 96:64-75.
57. Czarnecki, C.M., and H.A. Badreldin. 1987. Graded ethanol consumption in young turkey poults: Effect on body weight, feed intake and development of cardiomegaly. Res Commun Subst Abuse 8:93-96.
58. Czarnecki, G.L., and D.H. Baker. 1982. Tolerence of the chick to excess dietary cadmium as influenced by dietary cysteine and by experimental infection with Eimeria acervulina. J Anim Sci 54:983-988.
59. Czarnecki, G.L., D.H. Baker, and J.E. Gorst. 1984. Arsenic-sulfur amino acid interactions in the chick. J Anim Sci 59:1573-1581.
60. Daft, B.M., A.A. Bickford, and M.A. Hammarlund. 1989. Experimental and field sulfaquinoxaline toxicosis in leghorn chickens. Avian Dis 33:30-34.
61. Davis, C. 1983. Narasin toxicity in turkeys. Vet Rec 113:627.
62. Day, E.J., and B.C. Dilworth. 1984. Toxicity of Jimson weed seed and cocoa shell meal to broilers. Poult Sci 63:466-468.
63. Deaton, J.W., F.N. Reece, and F.D. Thornberry. 1986. Atmospheric ammonia and incidence of blood spots in eggs. Poult Sci 65:1427-1428.
64. Delaplane, J.P., and J.H. Milliff. 1948. The gross and micropathology of sulfaquinoxaline poisoning in chickens. Am J Vet Res 9:92-96.
65. Del Bono, G., and G. Braca. 1973. Lead poisoning in domestic and wild ducks. Avian Pathol 2:195-209.
66. De Ment, S.H., J.J. Chisolm, M.A. Eckhaus, and J.D. Strandberg. 1987. Toxic lead exposure in the urban rock dove. J Wildl Dis 23:273-278.
67. Dharma, D.N., S.D. Sleight, R.K. Ringer, and S.D. Aust. 1982. Pathologic effect of 2,2′,4,4′,5,5′- and 2,3′,4,4′,5′,5-hexabromobiphenyl in White Leghorn cockerels. Avian Dis 26:542-552.
68. Dhillon, A.S., R.W. Winterfield, and H.L. Thacker. 1982. Quaternary ammonium compound toxicity in chickens. Avian Dis 26:928-931.
69. Dickinson, J.O., and R.C. Braun. 1987. Effect of 2(3)-tertbutyl-4-hydroxyanisole (BHA) and 2-chloroethanol against payrole production and chronic toxicity of monocrotaline in chickens. Vet Hum Toxicol 29:11-15.
70. Dorn, P., R. Weber, J. Weikel, and E. Wessling. 1983. Intoxikation durch gleichzeitige verabreichung von chloramphenicol und monensin bei puten. Prakt Tierärztl 64:240-243.
71. Dougherty, E., III. 1957. Thiophosphate poisoning in White Pekin ducks. Avian Dis 1:127-130.
72. Dunachie, J.F., and W.W. Fletcher. 1970. The toxicity of certain herbicides to hens' eggs assessed by the egg injection technique. Ann Appl Biol 66:515-520.
73. Durham, H.D., and D.J. Ecobichon. 1986. An assessment of the neurotoxic potential of fenitrothion in the hen. Toxicology 41:319-332.
74. Edelstein, S., C.S Fullmer, and R.H. Wasserman. 1984. Gastrointestinal absorption of lead in chicks: Involvement of the cholecalciferol endocrine system. J Nutr 114:692-700.
75. Edwards, H.M., Jr. 1987. Effects of thiuram disulfiram and a trace element mixture on the incidence of tibial dyschondroplasia in chickens. J Nutr 117:964-969.
76. Egyed, M.N., and U. Bendheim. 1977. Mass poisoning in chickens caused by consumption of organophosphorus (dichlorvos) contaminated drinking water. Refu Vet 34:107-110.
77. Elliott, J.E., R.W. Butler, R.J. Norstrom, and P.E. Whitehead. 1988. Levels of polychlorinated dibenzodioxins and polychlorinated dibenzofurans in eggs of Great Blue Herons (Ardea herodias) in British Columbia, 1983-87: Possible impacts on reproductive success. Progress Notes No. 176. Can Wildl Serv.
78. Emmel, M.W. 1935. The toxicity of Glottidium vesicarium (Jacq) Harper seeds for the fowl. J Am Vet Med Assoc 87:13-21.
79. Faddoul, G.P., S.V. Amato, M. Sevoian, and G.W. Fellows. 1967. Studies on intolerance to sulfaquinoxaline in chickens. Avian Dis 11:226-240.
80. Farage-Elawar, M., and B.M. Francis. 1988. Effects of fenthion, fenitrothion and desbromoleptophos on gait, acetylcholinesterase, and neurotoxic esterase in young chicks after in ovo exposure. Toxicology 49:253-261.
81. Farr, M.M., and D.S. Jaquette. 1947. The toxicity of sulfamerazine to chickens. Am J Vet Res 8:216-220.
82. Farr, M.M., and E.E. Wehr. 1945. Sulfamerazine therapy in experimental cecal coccidiosis of chickens. J Parasitol 31:353-358.
83. Fedde, M.R., and W.D. Kuhlmann. 1979. Cardiopulmonary responses to inhaled sulfur dioxide in the chicken. Poult Sci 58:1584-1591.
84. Fenwick, G.R., C.L. Curl, E.J. Butler, N.M. Greenwood, and A.W. Pearson. 1984. Rapeseed meal and egg taint. J Sci Food Agri 35:749-756.
85. Ficken, M.D., D.P. Wages, and E. Gonder. 1989. Monensin toxicity in turkey breeder hens. Avian Dis 33:186-190.
86. Flory, W., and C.D. Hebert. 1984. Determination of the oral toxicity of Sesbania drummondii seeds in

chickens. Am J Vet Res 45:955–958.
87. Frank, A.A., and W.M. Reed. 1987. Conium maculatum (poison hemlock) toxicosis in a flock of range turkeys. Avian Dis 31:386–388.
88. Frank, R., M. van H. Holdrinet, and W.A. Rapley. 1975. Residue of organochlorine compounds and mercury in birds' eggs from the Niagara Peninsula, Ontario. Arch Environ Contam Toxicol 3:205–218.
89. Frank, R., G.J. Sirons, and D. Wilson. 1981. Residues of 4-aminopyridine in poisoned birds. Bull Environ Contam Toxicol 26:389–392.
90. Frank, R., N. Fish, G.J. Sirons, J. Walker, H.L. Orr, and S. Leeson. 1983. Residues of polychlorinated phenols and anisoles in broilers raised on contaminated wood shaving litter. Poult Sci 62:1559–1565.
91. Friedman, L., J. Sage, and E.M. Blendermann. 1970. Growth and liver response of chicks and rats to carbon tetrachloride and ethanol. Poult Sci 49:298–309.
92. Gaafar, S.M., and R.D. Turk. 1957. The toxicity of malathion in chickens. Am J Vet Res 18:180–182.
93. Galt, D.E. 1988. Reduced hatchability of eggs associated with pentachlorophenol-contaminated shavings. Can Vet J 29:65–67.
94. Gardiner, J.L., and M.M. Farr. 1954. Nitrofurazone for the prevention of experimentally induced Eimeria tenella infections in chickens. J Parasitol 40:42–49.
95. Gentry, R.F. 1958. The toxicity of certain antibiotics and furazalidone for chicken embryos. Avian Dis 2:76–82.
96. Ghazikhanian, G.Y., R. Yamamoto, R.H. McCapes, W.M. Dungan, and H.B. Ortmayer. 1980. Combination dip and injection of turkey eggs with antibiotics to eliminate Mycoplasma meleagridis infection from a primary breeding stock. Avian Dis 24:57–70.
97. Gifford, D.H., R.K. Page, and O.J. Fletcher. 1988. Diazinon toxicity in broilers. Proc 37th West Poult Dis Conf, Davis, CA. p. 105–116.
98. Gilead, M., and U. Bendheim. 1986. Formalin poisoning in turkeys. Isr J Vet Med 42:193–194.
99. Giri, S.N., A.A. Bickford, and A.E. Barger. 1979. Effects of 2-chloro-4-acetotoluidine (CAT) toxicity on biochemical and morphological alterations in quail. Avian Dis 23:794–811.
100. Glover, J.S. 1932. Mercurial poisoning in fowl. Rep Ont Vet Coll 1931, p. 56.
101. Good, A.L., and C.M. Czarnecki. 1980. The production of cardiomyopathy in turkey poults by the oral administration of furazolidone. Avian Dis 24:980–988.
102. Gough, A.W., and L.J. Weber. 1978. Massive liver hemorrhage in Ontario broiler chickens. Avian Dis 22:205–210.
103. Guberlet, J.E. 1922. Potassium nitrate poisoning in chickens with a note on its toxicity. J Am Vet Med Assoc 62:362–365.
104. Guenter, W., and P.H.B. Hahn. 1986. Flourine toxicity and laying hen performance. Poult Sci 65:769–778.
105. Hafez, Y.S.M., E. Chavez, P. Vohra, and F.H. Kratzer. 1978. Methionine toxicity in chicks and poults. Poult Sci 57:699–703.
106. Haigh, J.C. 1979. Levamisole in waterfowl: Trials on effect and toxicity. J Zoo Anim Med 10:103–105.
107. Halvorson, D.A., C. Van Dijk, and P. Brown. 1982. Ionaphore toxicity in turkey breeders. Avian Dis 26:634–639.
108. Hanrahan, L.A., D.E. Corrier, and S.A. Naqi. 1981. Monensin toxicosis in broiler chickens. Vet Pathol 18:665–671.
109. Hansen, A.A. 1925. Nightshade poisoning in chickens and ducks. J Am Vet Med Assoc 66:502–503.
110. Hansen, A.A. 1927. Stock poisoning by plants in the nightshade family. J Am Vet Med Assoc 71:221–227.
111. Hare, T., and A.B. Orr. 1945. Poultry poisoned by zinc phosphide. Vet Rec 57:17.
112. Harper, J.A., and G.H. Arscott. 1962. Toxicity of common and hairy vetch seed for poults and chicks. Poult Sci 41:1968–1974.
113. Hartung, R., and G.S. Hunt. 1966. Toxicity of some oils to waterfowl. J Wildl Manage 30:564–570.
114. Harvey, R.B., L.F. Kubena, S.L. Lovering, H.H. Mollenhauer, and T.D. Phillips. 1986. Acute toxicity of uranyl nitrate to growing chicks: A pathophysiologic study. Bull Environ Contam Toxicol 37:907–915.
115. Harwood, P.D., and D. Stunz. 1949. Nitrofurazone in the medication of avian coccidiosis. J Parasitol 35:175–182.
116. Harwood, P.D., and D. Stunz. 1949. Nitrofurazone and coccidiosis. Ann NY Acad Sci 52:538–542.
117. Hatch, R.C. 1988. Veterinary Toxicology. In N.H. Booth and L.E. McDonald (eds.), Veterinary Pharmacology and Therapeutics, 6th Ed., pp. 1001–1148. Iowa State Univ Press, Ames.
118. Hathcock, J.N., M.M. Labadan, and J.P. Mateo. 1975. Effects of dietary protein level on toxicity of Leucaena leucocephala to chicks. Nutr Rep Int 11:55–62.
119. Heinekamp, W.J.R. 1925. The resistance of fowl to strychnine. J Lab Clin Med 11:209–214.
120. Heinz, G.H. 1979. Methylmercury: Reproductive and behavioral effects on three generations of mallard ducks. J Wildl Manage 43:394–401.
121. Heinz, G.H., and L.N. Locke. 1976. Brain lesions in mallard ducklings from parents fed methylmercury. Avian Dis 20:9–17.
122. Henderson, B.M., and R.W. Winterfield. 1975. Acute copper toxicosis in the Canada goose. Avian Dis 19:385–387.
123. Henny, C.J., E.J. Kolbe, E.F. Hill, and L.J. Blus. 1987. Case histories of bald eagles and other raptors killed by organophosphorus insecticides topically applied to livestock. J Wildl Dis 23:292–295.
124. Heuser, G.F., and A.E. Schumacher. 1942. The feeding of corn cockle to chickens. Poult Sci 21:86–93.
125. Hino, T., T. Noguchi, and H. Naito. 1987. Effect of gizzerosine on acid secretion by isolated mucosal cells of chicken proventriculus. Poult Sci 66:548–551.
126. Hinshaw, W.R., and E. McNeil. 1943. Experiments with sulfanilamide for turkeys. Poult Sci 22:291–294.
127. Horton-Smith, C., and P.L. Long. 1952. Nitrofurazone in the treatment of cecal coccidiosis in chickens. Br Vet J 108:47–57.
128. Horvath, A.A. 1945. Toxicity of vetch seed for chickens. Poult Sci 24:291–295.
129. Howell, J. 1969. Mercury residues in chicken eggs and tissues from a flock exposed to methylmercury dicyandiamide. Can Vet J 10:212–213.
130. Hudson, C.B. 1936. Naphthalene poisoning in poultry. J Am Vet Med Assoc 89:219.
131. Huebner, R.A., J.M. Glassman, G.M. Hudyma, and J. Seifter. 1956. The toxic dose of dihydrostreptomycin in fowl. Cornell Vet 46:219–222.
132. Hulan, H.W., and F.G. Proudfoot. 1982. Effect of sodium hypochlorite (Javex) on the performance of broiler chickens. Am J Vet Res 43:1804–1806.
133. Humphreys, D.J. 1979. Poisoning in poultry. World's Poult Sci J 35:161–176.
134. Humphreys, D.J., J.B.J. Stoduliski, R.R. Fysh, and N.M. Howie. 1980. Haloxon poisoning in geese. Vet Rec 107:541.
135. Hunter, B., and G. Wobeser. 1980. Encephalopathy and peripheral neuropathy in lead-poisoned mallard ducks. Avian Dis 24:169–178.

136. Jensen, W.I., and J.P. Allen. 1981. Naturally occurring and experimentally induced castor bean (Ricinus communis) poisoning in ducks. Avian Dis 25:184-194.

137. Jensen, L.S., R.P. Peterson, and L. Falen. 1974. Inducement of enlarged hearts and muscular dystrophy in turkey poults with dietary silver. Poult Sci 53:57-64.

138. Jordan, F.T.W. 1955. Accidental nitrofurazone poisoning in baby chicks. Vet Rec 67:514-516.

139. Jordan, F.T.W., J.M. Howell, J. Howorth, and J.K. Rayton. 1976. Clinical and pathological observations on field and experimental zoalene poisoning in broiler chicks and the effect of the drug on laying hens. Avian Pathol 5:175-186.

140. Joyner, L.P., and S.F.M. Davies. 1956. Sulfaquinoxaline poisoning in chickens. J Comp Pathol Therap 66:39-48.

141. Julian, R.J. 1987. The effect of increased sodium in the drinking water on right ventricular hypertrophy, right ventricular failure and ascites in broiler chickens. Avian Pathol 16:61-71.

142. Kangas, J., K. Louhelainen, and K. Husman. 1987. Gaseous health hazards in livestock confinement buildings. J Agr Sci (Fin) 59:57-62.

143. Katz, R.S., and D.H. Baker. 1975. Methionine toxicity in the chick: Nutritional and metabolic implications. J Nutr 105:1168-1175.

144. Kemp, J. 1978. Monensin poisoning in turkeys (toxicity for guinea fowl). Vet Rec 102:467.

145. Klimes, B., and B. Kruza. 1962. Toxicity of nitrofurazone for young ducklings. Vet Rec 74:167-168.

146. Konst, K., P.D. McKercher, P.R. Gorham, A. Robertson, and J. Howell. 1968. Symptoms and pathology produced by toxic Microcystic aeruginosa NRC-1 in laboratory and domestic animals. Can J Comp Med 29:221-227.

147. Kratzer, F.H. 1979. Poultry Nutrition Research 1978. Proc Pfizer 27th Annu Res Conf, pp. 7-52.

148. Kubena, L.F., and T.D. Phillips. 1983. Toxicity of vanadium in female leghorn chickens. Poult Sci 62:47-50.

149. Larsen, C., B.S. Jortner, and M. Ehrich. 1986. Effect of neurotoxic organophosphorus compounds in turkeys. J Toxicol Environ Health 17:365-374.

150. Latta, D.M., and W.E. Donaldson. 1986. Lead toxicity in chicks: Interactions with dietary methionine and choline. J Nutr 116:1561-1568.

151. Lee, S.R., W.M. Britton, and G.N. Rowland. 1980. Magnesium toxicity: Bone lesions. Poult Sci 59:2403-2411.

152. Leighton, F.A. 1986. Clinical, gross and histological findings in herring gulls and Atlantic puffins that ingested Prudhoe Bay crude oil. Vet Pathol 23:254-263.

153. Leighton, F.A., D.B. Peakall, and R.G. Butler. 1983. Heinz-body hemolytic anemia from the ingestion of crude oil: A primary toxic effect in marine birds. Science 220:871-873.

154. Lekkas, S., P. Iordanidis, and E. Artopios. 1986. Intoxication by creolin in broilers. Isr J Vet Med 42:114-119.

155. Lessler, M.A., and D.A. Ray. 1986. Dietary lead inhibits avian bone fracture healing. J Physiol 371:223.

156. Locke, L.N., G.E. Bagley, and H.D. Irby. 1966. Acid-fast intranuclear inclusion bodies in the kidneys of mallards fed lead shot. Bull Wildl Dis Assoc 2:127-131.

157. Ludke, J.L., and L.N. Locke. 1976. Duck deaths from accidental ingestion of anthelmintic. Avian Dis 20:607-608.

158. Lumeij, J.T., M. Meidam, J. Wolfswinkel, M.H. Van Der Hage, and G.M. Dorrestein. 1988. Changes in plasma chemistry after drug-induced liver disease or muscle necrosis in racing pigeons (Columba livia domestica). Avian Pathol 17:865-874.

159. Madar, Z., and M. Klein. 1979. Composition and histological observations of enlarged pancreases of chicks adapted to raw soybean meal diets. Nutr Methods 23:117-126.

160. Marsh, C.D., A.B. Clawson, and H. Harsh. 1915. Zygadenus or death camas. US Dep AgricTech Bull 125.

161. Marsh, C.D., A.B. Clawson, and G.C. Roe. 1928. Coyotillo (Karwinskia humboldtiana) as a poisonous plant. US Dep Agric Tech Bull 29.

162. Mayeda, B. 1968. Toxic effect in turkey poults of a quaternary ammonia compound in drinking water at 150 and 200 ppm. Avian Dis 12:67-74.

163. McCapes, R.H., R. Yamamoto, H.B. Ortmayer, and W.F. Scott. 1975. Injecting antibiotics into turkey hatching eggs to eliminate Mycoplasma meleagridis infection. Avian Dis 19:506-514.

164. McCune, E.L., J.E. Savage, and B.L. O'Dell. 1962. Hydropericardium and ascites in chicks fed a chlorinated hydrocarbon. Poult Sci 41:295-299.

165. McManus, E.C., E.F. Rogers, B.M. Miller, F.R. Judith, K.D. Schleim, and G. Olson. 1979. Eimeria tenella: Specific reversal of t-butylaminoethanol toxicity for parasite and host by choline and dimethylaminoethanol. Exp Parasitol 47:13-23.

166. Mercurio, S.D., and G.F. Combs Jr. 1986. Selenium-dependent glutathione peroxidase inhibitors increase toxicity of prooxidant compounds in chicks. J Nutr 116:1726-1734.

167. Mohanty, G.C., and J.L. West. 1969. Pathologic features of experimental sodium chloride poisoning in chicks. Avian Dis 13:762-773.

168. Moore, E.N., and J.A. Brown. 1950. The effect of nitrofurazone on normal and coccidiosis infected turkeys. J Parasitol 36:43. (Suppl).

169. Morrissey, R.L., R.M. Cohn, R.N. Empson, H.L. Greene, O.D. Taunton, and Z.Z. Ziporin. 1977. Relative toxicity and metabolic effects of cholecalciferol and 25-hydroxycholecalciferol in chicks. J Nutr 107:1027-1034.

170. Moslehuddin, A.B.M., Y.D. Hang, and G.S. Stoewsand. 1987. Evaluation of the toxicity of processed Lathyrus sativus seeds in chicks. Nutr Rep Int 36:851-855.

171. Nelson, H.A., R.A. Decker, and D.L. Osheim. 1976. Poisoning in zoo animals with 4-aminopyridine. Vet Toxicol 18:125-126.

172. Niemann, K.W. 1928. Report of an outbreak of poisoning in the domesticated fowl, due to death camas. J Am Vet Med Assoc 73:627-630.

173. Norton, J., M. Evans, and J. Connor. 1987. Timber treatment and poultry litter. Queensl Agric J 113:105-107.

174. Nwokolo, E., and L.O.C. Ohale. 1986. Growth and anatomical characteristics of pullet chicks fed diets contaminated with crude petroleum. Bull Environ Cont Toxicol 37:441-447.

175. Ohlendorf, H.M., A.W. Kilness, J.L. Simmons, R.K. Stroud, D.J. Hoffman, and J.F. Moore. 1988. Selenium toxicosis in wild aquatic birds. J Toxicol Environ Health 24:67-92.

176. Okoye, J.O.A., C.A. Enunwaonye, A.U. Okorie, and F.O.I. Anugwa. 1987. Pathological effects of feeding roasted castor bean meal (Ricinus communis) to chicks. Avian Pathol 16:283-290.

177. Onderka, D.K., and R. Bhatnagar. 1982. Ultrastructural changes of sodium chloride-induced cardiomyopathy in turkey poults. Avian Dis 26:835-841.

178. Orr, J.P., K.S. Little, M. Schoonderwoerd, and A.J. Rehmtulla. 1986. Ascites in broiler chickens. Can Vet J 27:99-100.

179. Osweiler, G.D., T.L. Carson, W.B. Buck, and G.A. Van Gelder. 1985. Clinical and Diagnostic Veteri-

nary Toxicology. Kendall/Hunt Publ Co, Dubuque, Iowa.
180. Oyetunde, O.O.F., R.G. Thomson, and H.C. Carlson. 1978. Aerosol exposure of ammonia, dust, and Escherichia coli in broiler chickens. Can Vet J 19:187–193.
181. Page, R.K. 1975. Teratogenic activity of arasan fed to broiler breeder hens. Avian Dis 19:463–472.
182. Page, R.K., O.J. Fletcher, S. Vezey, P. Bush, and N. Booth. 1978. Effects of continuous feeding of toxaphene to white leghorn layers. Avian Pathol 7:289–294.
183. Page, R.K., O.J. Fletcher, and P. Bush. 1979. Calcium toxicosis in broiler chicks. Avian Dis 34:1055–1059.
184. Panigraphy, B., L.C. Grumbles, and C.F. Hall. 1979. Insecticide poisoning in peafowls and lead poisoning in a cockatoo. Avian Dis 23:760–762.
185. Peckham, M.C. 1982. Poisons and Toxins. In M.S. Hofstad, H.J. Barnes, B.W. Calnek, W.M. Reid, H.W. Yoder, Jr. (eds.), Diseases of Poultry, 8th Ed., pp. 783–818. Iowa State Univ Press, Ames.
186. Peeters, N., N. Viaene, and L. Devriese. 1978. Poisoning in pigeons after administration of vitamin B_6 (pyridoxine). Poult Abstr 4:108. (Abstr).
187. Perelman, B., and E.S. Kuttin. 1988. Parsley-induced photosensitivity in ostriches and ducks. Avian Pathol 17:183–192.
188. Perelman, B., J.M. Abarbanel, A. Gur-Lavie, Y. Meller, and T. Elad. 1986. Clinical and pathological changes caused by the interaction of lasalocid and chloramphenicol in broiler chickens. Avian Pathol 15:279–288.
189. Pietsch, W., and E. Ruffle. 1986. Zur toxizität des monensins und zu problemen seines einsatzes im broilerfutter. Monatsh Veterinaermed 41:851–854.
190. Poley, W.E., A.L. Moxon, and K.W. Franke. 1937. Further studies of the effects of selenium poisoning on hatchability. Poult Sci 16:219–225.
191. Poli, A., and G. Renzoni. 1983. Chick oedema disease in fowls naturally contaminated with 2,3,7,8-tetrachlorodibenzyl-p-dioxin (TCDD). Poult Abstr 10:273. (Abstr).
192. Potter, L.M. 1976. Poultry Nutrition Research 1975. Proc Pfizer 24th Annu Res Conf, pp. 113–149.
193. Potter, L.M., J.P. Blake, M.E. Blair, B.A. Bliss, and D.M. Denbow. 1986. Salinomycin toxicity in turkeys. Poult Sci 65:1955–1959.
194. Prescott, C.A., B.N. Wilkie, B. Hunter, and R.J. Julian. 1982. Influence of a purified grade of pentachlorophenol on the immune response of chickens. Am J Vet Res 43:481–487.
195. Pritzl, M.C., Y.H. Lie, E.W. Kienholz, and C.E. Whiteman. 1974. The effect of dietary cadmium on development of young chicks. Poult Sci 53:2026–2029.
196. Prohaszka, L., E. Hajdu, E. Dworschak, and T. Rozsnyai. 1987. Growth depression in broiler chicks caused by incompatability of feed ingredients. Acta Vet Hung 35:349–358.
197. Proudfoot, F.G., and W.F. DeWitt. 1976. The effect of the pellet binder "Lignosol FG" on the chicken's digestive system and general performance. Poult Sci 55:629–631.
198. Puls, R. 1988. Mineral Levels in Animal Health. Diagnostic Data. Sherpa International, Clearbrook, BC, Canada.
199. Raharjo, Y.C., P.R. Cheeke, and G.H. Arscott. 1988. Effects of dietary butylated hydroxyanisole and cysteine on toxicity of Lathyrus odoratus to broiler and Japanese quail chicks. Poult Sci 67:153–155.
200. Rasul, A.R., and J.McC. Howell. 1974. The toxicity of some dithiocarbamate compounds in young and adult domestic fowl. Toxicol Appl Pharmicol 30:63–78.
201. Ratanasethkul, C., C. Riddell, R.E. Salmon, and J.B. O'Niel. 1976. Pathological changes in chickens, ducks, and turkeys fed high levels of rapeseed oil. Can J Comp Med 40:360–369.
202. Reece, R.L., and P. Handson. 1982. Observations on the accidental poisoning of birds by organophosphate insecticides and other toxic substances. Vet Rec 111:453–455.
203. Reece, R.L., D.A. Barr, W.M. Forsyth, and P.C. Scott. 1985. Investigations of toxicity episodes involving chemotherapeutic agents in Victorian poultry and pigeons. Avian Dis 29:1239–1251.
204. Reed, W.M., J.F. Van Vleet, W.L. Wigle, and R.M. Fulton. 1987. Furazolidone-associated cardiomyopathy in two Indiana flocks of ducklings. Avian Dis 31:666–672.
205. Ressler, C. 1962. Isolation and identification from common vetch of the neurotoxin B-cyano-L-alanine, a possible factor in neurolathyrism. J Biol Chem 237:733–735.
206. Riddell, C. 1975. Pathology of developmental and metabolic disorders of the skeleton of domestic chickens and turkeys. 2. Abnormalities due to nutritional or toxic factors. Vet Bull 45:705–718.
207. Riddell, C. 1984. Toxicity of dimetridazole in waterfowl. Avian Dis 28:974–977.
208. Riddell, C. 1987. Avian Histopathology. Am Assoc Avian Pathol, Kennett Square, PA.
209. Riddell, C., and D.A. Pass. 1987. The influence of dietary calcium and phosphorus on tibial dyschondroplasia in broiler chickens. Avian Dis 31:771–775.
210. Riddell, C., S.W. Nielsen, and E.J. Kersting. 1967. Ethylene glycol poisoning in poultry. J Am Vet Med Assoc 150:1531–1535.
211. Roberson, E.L. 1988. Antinematodal Drugs. In N.H. Booth and L.E. McDonald (eds.), Veterinary Pharmacology and Therapeutics, 6th Ed., pp. 882–927. Iowa State Univ Press, Ames.
212. Roberson, E.L. 1988. Anticestodal and Antitrematodal Drugs. In N.H. Booth and L.E. McDonald (eds.), Veterinary Pharmacology and Therapeutics, 6th Ed., pp. 928–949. Iowa State Univ Press, Ames.
213. Rocke, T.E., T.M. Yuill, and R.D. Hinsdill. 1984. Oil related toxicant effects on mallard immune defences. Environ Res 33:343–352.
214. Roland, D.A., Sr. 1984. Poultry nutrition research 1983. Proc Pfizer 32nd Annu Res Conf, pp. 74–108.
215. Sanderson, G.C., and F.C. Bellrose. 1986. A review of the problem of lead poisoning in waterfowl. Illinois Natural History Survey, 2nd Ed., Champaign, IL.
216. Schom, C.B., U.K. Abbott, and N.E. Walker. 1979. Adult and embryo responses to organophosphate pesticide: Azodrin. Poult Sci 58:60–66.
217. Schwarte, L.H. 1947. The toxicity of sodium monofluoroacetate (1080) for swine and chickens. J Am Vet Med Assoc 111:301–303.
218. Scott, M.L. 1985. Gizzard erosion. Anim Health Nutr Large Anim Vet, Sept 1985: 22–29.
219. Scott, H.M., E. Jungherr, and L.D. Matterson. 1944. The effect of feeding sulfanilamide to the laying fowl. Poult Sci 23:446–453.
220. Scrivner, L.H. 1946. Experimental edema and ascites in poults. J Am Vet Med Assoc 108:27–32.
221. Sell, J.L. 1978. Poultry nutrition research 1977. Proc Pfizer 26th Annu Res Conf, pp. 27–70.
222. Selye, H., and H. Stone. 1943. Role of sodium chloride in production of nephrosclerosis by steroids. Proc Soc Exp Biol Med 52:190–193.
223. Serafin, J.A. 1981. Factors influencing methionine toxicity in young bobwhite quail. Poult Sci 60:204–214.

224. Shapiro, J.L., R.J. Julian, R.J. Hampson, R.G. Trenton, and I.H. Yo. 1988. An unusual necrotizing cholangiohepatitis in broiler chickens. Can Vet J 29:636-639.

225. Shealy, A.L., and E.F. Thomas. 1928. Daubentonia seed poisoning of poultry. Univ Florida Agric Exp Stn Bull 196.

226. Sherman, M., E. Ross, F.F. Sanchez, and M.T.Y. Chang. 1963. Chronic toxicity of dimethoate to hens. J Econ Entomol 56:10-15.

227. Sherman, M., E. Ross, and M.T.Y. Chang. 1964. Acute and subacute toxicity of several organophosphorus insecticides to chicks. Toxicol Appl Pharmacol 6:147-153.

228. Shlosberg, A., M.N. Egyed, and A. Eilat. 1974. The comparative photosensitizing properties of Ammi majus and Ammi visnaga in goslings. Avian Dis 18:544-550.

229. Shlosberg, A., D. Hadash, S. Tromperl, and M. Meroz. 1976. Poisoning in a flock of chickens after exposure to vapours of methyl bromide and chloropicrin. Refu Vet 33:135-137.

230. Shlosberg, A., S. Held, and R. Bircz. 1978. Poisoning of palm doves with dibutyltin dilurate. J Am Vet Med Assoc 173:1183-1184.

231. Shlosberg, A., M.N. Egyed, and V. Hanji. 1980. Monocrotophos poisoning in geese caused by drift from crop spraying. Refu Vet 37:42-44.

232. Shoya, S., T. Horiuchi, and M. Kohanawa. 1979. Pathological changes of experimental polychlorinated biphenyl poisoning in chickens. Nat Inst Anim Health Q (Tokyo) 19:53-64.

233. Sileo, L., L. Karstad, R. Frank, M.V.H. Holdrinet, E. Addison, and H.E. Braun. 1977. Organochlorine poisoning of ring-billed gulls in Southern Ontario. J Wildl Dis 13:313-322.

234. Siller, W.G. 1981. Renal pathology of the fowl: A review. Avian Pathol 10:187-262.

235. Simpson, C.F., B.L. Damron, and R.H. Harms. 1970. Abnormalities of erythrocytes and renal tubules of chicks poisoned with lead. Am J Vet Res 31:515-523.

236. Simpson, C.F., B.L. Damron, and R.H. Harms. 1971. Toxic myopathy of chicks fed Cassia occidentalis seeds. Avian Dis 15:284-290.

237. Smalley, H.E. 1973. Toxicity and hazard of the herbicide paraquat in turkeys. Poult Sci 52:1625-1628.

238. Snelgrove-Hobson, S.M., P.V.V.P. Rao, and M.K. Bhatnagar. 1988. Ultrastructural alterations in the kidneys of Pekin ducks fed methylmercury. Can J Vet Res 52:89-98.

239. Soenardi. 1987. Personal communication.

240. Staley, N.A., G.R. Noren, C.M. Bandt, and H.L. Sharp. 1978. Furazolidone-induced cardiomyopathy in turkeys. Am J Pathol 91:531-544.

241. Stedman, T.M., N.H. Booth, P.B. Bush, R.K. Page, and D.D. Goetsch. 1980. Toxicity and bioaccumulation of pentachlorophenol in broiler chickens. Poult Sci 59:1018-1026.

242. Stiles, G.W. 1940. Carbon monoxide poisoning of chicks and poults in poorly ventilated brooders. Poult Sci 19:111-115.

243. Stockman, R. 1931. Poisonous principle of Lathyrus and some other leguminous seeds. J Hyg 31:550-562.

244. Stowe, C.M., D.M. Barnes, and T.D. Arendt. 1981. Ethylene glycol intoxication in ducks. Avian Dis 25:538-541.

245. Stromborg, K.L. 1975. Sublethal effects of seed treatment pesticides on breeding hen pheasants. Dis Abst Int 36B:2547-2548.

246. Stuart, J.C. 1978. An outbreak of monensin poisoning in adult turkeys. Vet Rec 102:303-304.

247. Tang, K.N., G.N. Rowland, and J.R. Veltmann. 1985. Vitamin A toxicity: Comparative changes in bone of the broiler and leghorn chicks. Avian Dis 29:416-429.

248. Teeter, R.G., S. Sarani, M.O. Smith, and C.A. Hibberd. 1986. Detoxification of high tannin sorghum grains. Poult Sci 65:67-71.

249. Temperton, H. 1944. Effect of green and sprouted potatoes on laying pullets. Vet Med 39:13-14.

250. Terzic, L., and M. Curcic. 1985. Toxic chemicals and poisoning of farm animals: Survey of cases examined toxicologically and chemically. Vet Glas 39:965-973.

251. Tudor, D.C. 1988. Personal communication.

252. Ueda, H., and M. Ohshima. 1987. Effects of alfalfa saponin on chick performance and plasma cholesterol level. Jpn J Zootech Sci 58:583-590.

253. Umemura, T., H. Nakamura, M. Goryo, and C. Itakura. 1984. Ultrastructural changes of monensin-oleandomycin myopathy in broiler chickens. Avian Pathol 13:743-751.

254. Van Vleet, J.F., G.D. Boon, and V.J. Ferrans. 1981. Induction of lesions of selenium-vitamin E deficiency in ducklings fed silver, copper, cobalt, tellurium, cadmium or zinc: Protection by selenium or vitamin E supplements. Am J Vet Res 42:1206-1217.

255. Veltmann, J.R., Jr., and L.S. Jensen. 1986. Vitamin A toxicosis in the chick and turkey poults. Poult Sci 65:538-545.

256. Venugopalan, C.S., W. Flory, C.D. Hebert, and T. Tucker. 1984. Assessment of smooth muscle toxicity in Cassia occidentalis toxicosis. Vet Hum Toxicol 26:300-302.

257. Wages, D.P., and M.D. Ficken. 1988. Skeletal muscle lesions in turkeys associated with the feeding of monensin. Avian Dis 32:583-586.

258. Wagner, D.D., R.D. Furrow, and B.D. Bradley. 1983. Subchronic toxicity of monensin in broiler chickens. Vet Pathol 20:353-359.

259. Wagstaff, D.J., J.R. McDowell, and H.J. Paulin. 1980. Heptachlor residue accumulation and depletion in broiler chickens. Am J Vet Res 41:765-768.

260. Waibel, P.E. 1974. Poultry nutrition research 1973. Proc Pfizer 22nd Annu Res Conf, pp. 40-75.

261. Wallner-Pendleton, E., D.P. Froman, and O. Hedstrom. 1986. Identification of ferrous sulfate toxicity in a commercial broiler flock. Avian Dis 30:430-432.

262. Wallner-Pendleton, E.A., O. Hedstrom, T. Savage, and H. Nakaue. 1987. Dicalcium phosphate toxicity in a flock of turkey poults. Proc 36th West Poult Dis Conf, pp. 97-98.

263. Weber, A.L., F.R. Beaudette, and C.B. Hudson. 1932. Arsenic poisoning in poultry. North Am Vet 13(12):46-47.

264. Wescott, R.B., and H.C. McDougle. 1967. Ethylene oxide toxicosis in chickens. J Am Vet Med Assoc 151:935-938.

265. Westlake, G.E., P.J. Bunyan, P.I. Stanley, and C.H. Walker. 1981. A study on the toxicity and the biochemical effects of ethylene dibromide in the Japanese quail. Br Poult Sci 22:355-364.

266. Wickware, A.B. 1940. Lead poisoning in ducks following ingestion of shot. Can J Comp Med Vet Sci 4:201-203.

267. Wideman, R.F., and B.S. Cowen. 1987. Effect of dietary acidifcation on kidney damage induced in immature chickens by excess calcium and infectious bronchitis virus. Poult Sci 66:626-633.

268. Wight, P.A.L., R.K. Scougall, D.W.F. Shannon, J.W. Wells, and R. Mawson. 1987. Role of glucosinolates in the causation of liver haemorrhages in laying hens fed water-extracted or heat-treated rapeseed cakes. Res Vet Sci 43:313-319.

269. Williams, M.C. 1979. Toxicological investigations on Galenia pubescens. Weed Sci 27:506–508.

270. Williams, M.C., and R.J. Molyneux. 1987. Occurrence, concentration, and toxicity of pyrrolizidine alkaloids in Crotalaria seeds. Weed Sci 36:476–481.

271. Williamson, J.H., F.R. Craig, C.W. Barber, and F.W. Cook. 1964. Some effects of feeding Gelsemium sempervirens (yellow jessamine) to young chickens and turkeys. Avian Dis 8:183–190.

272. Wise, D.R., W.J. Hartley, and N.G. Fowler. 1974. Pathology of 3-nitro-4-hydroxy-phenylarsonic acid toxicity in turkeys. Res Vet Sci 16:336–340.

273. Wishe, H.I. 1976. The effect of aminotriazole on the thyroid gland and development of the white leghorn chick. Dis Abst Int 37B:1066–1067.

274. Woerpel, R.W., and W.J. Rosskopf. 1982. Heavy-metal intoxication in caged birds. Compend Cont Ed 4: Pt 1, pp. 729–738; Pt 2, pp. 801–806.

275. Yacowitz, H., E. Ross, V.L. Sanger, E.N. Moore, and R.D. Carter. 1955. Hemorrhagic syndrome in chicks fed normal rations supplemented with sulfaquinoxaline. Proc Soc Exp Biol Med 89:1–7.

276. Yamada, M., and J. Takahashi. 1977. Reversal of ethionine toxicity in the domestic fowl with methionine and adenine sulphate. Br Poult Sci 18:567–571.

277. Yamashiro, S., and T. Bast. 1978. Ultrastructure of livers of broiler chickens fed diets containing rapeseed meal. Res Vet Sci 25:21–24.

278. Young, R.J. 1973. Poultry nutrition 1972. Proc Pfizer 21st Annu Res Conf, pp. 9–39.

279. Zajicek, J., O. Kypetova, and P. Matejka. 1985. Levamizole toxicity in breeding geese. Poult Abstr 12:35. (Abstr).

280. Zeman, P. 1987. Systematic efficacy of ivermectin against Dermanyssus gallinae (De Geer, 1778) in fowls. Vet Parasitol 23:141–146.

MYCOTOXICOSES

Frederic J. Hoerr

INTRODUCTION. A mycotoxicosis is a disease caused by a toxic fungal metabolite affecting either humans or animals. Poultry mycotoxicoses are usually caused by fungi colonizing and invading grains and feeds, but other environmental aspects may be involved.

The economic significance of mycotoxicoses to the poultry industry is probably considerable, but yet insidious. The public health significance of mycotoxin residues in poultry meat and eggs is another concern.

Mycotoxins received worldwide attention in the early 1960s when aflatoxicosis caused overt disease and mortality in food animals. The significance of aflatoxins was accentuated by discovery of their carcinogenicity. Diseases in humans and animals caused by consumption of moldy food have been recognized, however, far before the chemistry and conditions of aflatoxin formation were discovered. Ergotism, moldy corn poisoning of horses, stachybotryotoxicosis, alimentary toxic aleukia, various hemorrhagic syndromes, yellow rice poisoning, and other acute food poisonings are just some of the historically significant mycotoxicoses. From this early knowledge, fungal metabolites have been defined toxicologically. Some metabolites are used for the betterment of humankind as pharmacological agents, while some are used detrimentally as agents of chemical warfare (yellow rain) (382).

The significance of aflatoxin is so well impressed upon those in the modern poultry industry, it is nearly synonymous with the term mycotoxin. Actually, hundreds of mycotoxins have been identified as members of defined biochemical pathways (see review 372). The toxicity, frequency of occurrence, and target organs of this large group of natural toxins vary considerably.

One area of mycotoxicology, yet unresolved, is the apparent discrepancy in establishing defined concentrations at which specific production problems will occur. Variations occur according to the experimental approach chosen by investigators. This review defines conditions under which spontaneous disease and changes in experimental parameters occur.

The complexity of mycotoxicology invites two extremes in diagnosis. Mycotoxin problems may be disregarded, possibly because of the cost and difficulty in confirming the diagnosis, or mycotoxicosis can be used as a diagnosis for any problem; for much the same reason, it's difficult to disprove. The impact of mycotoxins on poultry production may be measured best indirectly and by improvements in weight gain, feed efficiency, pigmentation, egg production, and reproductive performance that accompany mycotoxin control programs. Overt intoxication is uncommon and diagnostic confirmation even less so, but capabilities are improving and the number of confirmed reports is steadily increasing.

This section presents the biologic effects of mycotoxins now recognized, or potentially able, to influence poultry production.

ERGOTISM

HISTORY AND ETIOLOGY. Ergotism (reviewed in 228) is an important mycotoxicosis that literally influenced the course of history. Epidemics killed thousands of people in Europe during the Middle Ages. Descriptions of ergot date back to the Roman Empire, and even earlier, to China 5000 yr ago.

Ergotism is caused by species of *Claviceps*, fungi attacking cereal grains. Rye is especially affected, but also wheat and other leading cereal grains, with regional differences throughout the world. *Claviceps purpurea* is a frequent cause of ergotism because of its wide host range among cereals.

Mycotoxins form in the sclerotium, a visible, hard, dark mass of mycelium displacing grain tissue. In the normal cycle, the sclerotium falls to the ground, germinates, and produces spores that infect the flower of the new crop, and the cycle repeats. Harvest channels the sclerotium into the food chain.

Within the sclerotium are ergot alkaloids, first described in 1864, which cause ergotism. Lysergic acid is the chemical building block. The 40 or more alkaloids produced by *Claviceps* spp. comprise four chemical groups. With individual variation, alkaloids affect the nervous system, causing convulsive and sensory neurological disorders; the vascular system, causing vasoconstriction and gangrene of extremities; and the endocrine system, influencing neuroendocrine control of the anterior pituitary (255). Characteristics responsible for toxicity also have important pharmacological uses.

Tolerances for ergot in international trade vary, but the USA, Canada, and EEC countries classify various grains as "ergoty" with sclerotium concentrations of 0.1–0.33%.

Ergotism due to *Claviceps* spp. has serious implications for food-producing animals. Poultry experience reductions in feed intake and growth; necrosis of the beak, comb, and toes; and also enteritis.

NATURAL DISEASE. Ergotism in leghorns (vesicular dermatitis, sod disease) reflects vasoconstrictive injury and occurs as coalescing fluid-distended vesicles on the comb and wattles, face, and eyelids (285), which eventually rupture to form crusts. Combs and wattles become permanently atrophied and disfigured. Vesicles also develop on leg shanks and tops and sides of toes, rupture, and form ulcers. Leg lesions are more severe in leghorn pullets, heavy breeds, and breeds with a small comb. In one episode, ergotism spared young chickens, while development of those over 6 wk of age was severely retarded, with high morbidity and mortality of 25%. Ergotism in laying hens adversely affects feed consumption and egg production. At necropsy, chickens with ergotism may show no consistent lesions other than those on the skin.

Cladiosporium hebarum colonization of *Lolium temulentum,* a weed seed contaminant of wheat used in poultry feed formulation, was incriminated in an outbreak of ergotism in poultry in Israel (285).

Muscovy ducks fed wheat dockage contaminated with 1.17% ergot became listless and lethargic, stopped eating and drinking, and developed diarrhea (354). In contrast to the earlier report for chickens, most ducklings aged 12 wk or younger died, but older birds were resistant. At necropsy, lesions were confined to marked congestion of the liver and kidney.

EXPERIMENTAL DISEASE. Wheat ergot has appetite- and growth-depressant effects on broiler and leghorn chicks, but the detrimental effects, including mortality, are quite variable (322–324). Broilers are more sensitive than leghorns. Although toxicity is mostly in the alkaloid fraction of the ergot extract, the predictive value of total alkaloid content is not highly accurate.

Ergotamine tartrate is one of the most common alkaloids and induces toe necrosis and skin necrosis in leghorn chicks at levels of 243 and 739 mg/kg diet, respectively (407). Cardiac enlargement is also seen, which is thought to reflect increased cardiac work load due to hypertension caused by vasoconstriction.

Triticale ergot ($>0.8\%$ of diet as contaminated grain) in broiler chicks causes depression of growth, poor feathering, nervousness, loss of coordination, and inability to stand (24). Intoxication can be fatal. A wheat-based diet containing triticale ergot is more detrimental than a triticale-based diet, suggesting triticale contains factors antagonistic to ergotism. Pelleting increases toxicity of ergot diets, perhaps through increased liberation of toxins.

Ergot is common in rye, but rye as a feedstuff for poultry has other inherent problems. These include an appetite-suppressing factor in bran, and a growth-depressing factor found in bran, flour and millings. Rye ergot at concentrations that might be encountered naturally (0.33%) has no interaction with these detrimental factors in poultry (247, 248).

METABOLISM AND RESIDUES. Only trace amounts of ergotamine tartrate accumulate in broiler chicken tissues when fed at relatively high concentrations (800 mg/kg diet). About 5% of the alkaloid is excreted unchanged and 15–20% is excreted as a complex mixture containing as many as 16 possible metabolites (407).

FUSARIUM MYCOTOXINS. The genus *Fusarium* produces numerous mycotoxins injurious to poultry. Trichothecenes, the largest group, produce caustic and radiomimetic patterns of disease exemplified by T-2 toxin and diacetoxyscirpenol (DAS). Deoxynivalenol (DON, vomitoxin), a prevalent trichothecene of lesser toxicity in poultry, causes feed refusal and emesis in pigs. Water-soluble extracts of certain fusarial species affect bone growth (fusarochromanone) and can affect hatchability. Metabolites of *Fusarium moniliforme* (moniliformin) cause severe disease in equine species and may impact on poultry production.

Zearalenone, an environmental estrogen of potential concern to poultry, is often formed coincidental with DON, and causes significant disease in swine.

Trichothecenes

ETIOLOGY AND TOXICOLOGY. Trichothecene mycotoxins are produced by *Fusarium* and its perithecial stages *Calonectria* and *Gibberella,* and the genera *Myrothecium, Stachybotrys, Cephalosporium, Trichoderma,* and *Trichothecium* (244, 370). These common soil and plant saprophytes are found worldwide. In one study, about 20% of investigated isolates were capable of trichothecene production. Of the more than 50 trichothecenes, about half are produced by *Fusarium* (371). Toxin production is greatest with high humidity and temperatures of 6–24 C.

Trichothecene mycotoxins have a tetracyclic sesquiterpene nucleus with a characteristic epoxide ring at carbon positions 12 and 13. They are stable toxins that resist deterioration during prolonged storage. Toxicity resides in the epoxide ring, which is shielded from backside nucleophilic attack by the nucleus configuration (244, 370). Normal cooking temperatures will not destroy trichothecenes (16). As a group, but with individual variation, trichothecenes are potent inhibitors of protein synthesis (236), some inhibit DNA synthesis (370), and some inhibit synthesis of structural lipids (63).

NATURAL DISEASE. T-2 toxin, DAS, DON, and nivalenol have been identified throughout the world in numerous feedstuffs, including corn, sorghum, barley, safflower seed, oats, mixed feed, and brewer's grains (see 166). Many trichothecenes are caustic irritants, a feature used in bioassay detection screens. Positive bioassays are more common than unequivocal analytical confirmations, due, in part, to the numerous toxins and complexity of confirmation procedures.

Both historical and recent accounts of trichothecene mycotoxicosis reflect their caustic and radiomimetic effects, expressed as feed refusal, extensive necrosis of oral mucosa and skin in contact with the mold, acute digestive tract disease, and altered bone marrow and immune system function.

Avian fusariotoxicosis occurred in Russia in the same regions where alimentary toxic aleukia was endemic in humans at certain times during the first half of this century. *Fusarium poae* and *F. sporotrichioides* isolated from grain and green vegetation feedstuffs were likely sources of toxins. In the Russian literature (see 219) it was reported that chickens with fusariotoxicosis (probable trichothecene mycotoxicosis) had reduced growth, severe depression, and bloody diarrhea. At necropsy, necrosis of oral mucosa, reddening of the remainder of the gastrointestinal mucosa, mottling of the liver, gallbladder distention, atrophy of the spleen, and visceral hemorrhages were observed.

Presumed trichothecene mycotoxicosis caused by *Stachybotrys* fungi was recognized in poultry during the 1940s as necrosis of oral and crop mucosa, digestive and neurological disturbances, blood dyscrasias, and hemorrhagic disease (see 164).

Broiler Chickens. T-2 toxin, produced in culture by isolated *Fusarium tricinctum,* was considered the etiology of trichothecene mycotoxicosis in the USA. Contamination of feed and litter caused reduced growth and vesicular lesions on the feet and legs (396). Oral mucosa was ulcerated and covered by caseous exudate.

T-2 toxin, neosolaniol, verrucarol, fusarenon-X, and crotocol were trichothecenes identified in feed produced from crib-stored corn that caused digestive disturbance, reduced growth, rickets, nervous disorders, abnormal feathering, pigmentation defects, and hemorrhages in broiler chickens in France (310). Mycotoxin concentrations of 1–4 mg/kg were identified. The problems resolved when unadulterated corn was fed. Infectious bursal disease was a concurrent problem.

Laying Hens. In Israel 5 days after a delivery of feed to a flock of 2800 hens, egg production decreased from normal production of 2423 to 150 (336). This production decrease, which began the day after the feed was delivered, was accompanied by depression, recumbency, feed refusal, and cyanotic comb and wattles. At necropsy, atrophy of the ovary and oviduct was observed. T-2 toxin and HT-2 toxin were identified in the feed. Clinical disease and egg production improved when uncontaminated feed was provided.

In the USA, a decrease in egg production in 60, 000 leghorn hens was accompanied by reductions in feed intake and thin-shelled eggs (157). Some hens had yellow crusts on the oral mucosa, with underlying ulcers, to the degree that closing the mouth was difficult. Feathers of these hens were uneven and poorly formed. Oral and feather lesions were neither uniform throughout the facility (cage operation), nor were lesions uniform within a cage. At necropsy birds with oral lesions had yellow-tan, friable livers; swollen kidneys with urates in the ureters; yellow exudate and focal ulceration of crop mucosa; and thickened, rough lining in the gizzard. Analysis of feed collected from the trough revealed 3 mg T-2 toxin/kg feed. Oral lesions and abnormal feathering occurred in broilers fed the toxic feed.

Geese and Ducks. Barley contaminated with T-2 toxin (25 mg/kg) caused reduced spontaneous activity, feed refusal, and increased water consumption in geese and ducks in Canada (141, 299). Geese that ate toxic grain died within 2 days and, at necropsy, had necrosis and pseudomembranes in the esophagus, proventriculus, and gizzard. Microscopic lesions included mucosal necrosis of the upper enteric tract and degeneration of intestinal epithelium. Interstitial edema and necrosis of tubular epithelium occurred in the kidney.

EXPERIMENTAL DISEASE. Experimental trichothecene mycotoxicosis in poultry has required three approaches to fully reproduce the disease spectrum observed naturally: purified toxin administered either in solution or in the diet, and toxigenic fungal cultures (see 197). The single oral lethal dose-50% (LD_{50}) have been reported as 140 mg/kg body weight (bw) for DON (187), 3.82–5.0 mg/kg bw for DAS (58, 168), 7.22 mg/kg bw for HT-2 toxin (58), 24.87 mg/kg bw for neosolaniol (58), and 4.0–6.27 mg/kg bw for T-2 toxin (55, 56, 58, 168). Other dose effect studies on trichothenes have been reported (7, 8, 33, 34, 170–172, 212, 251, 252, 348). These toxins cause feed refusal, impaired growth and reproductive capability, and whole-body pathologic events including caustic injury to skin and alimentary mucosa; radiomimetic injury to bone marrow, lymphoid tissues, gastrointestinal tract, and feathers; hepatosis; and thyroid alterations.

Pathology. Most trichothecenes are caustic toxins and induce erosive and exudative injury to the oral mucosa of poultry fed toxin-appended diets (54, 69, 396, 397). Broiler chickens develop focal, yellow oral plaques that progress to yellow-gray raised accumulations of exudate with underlying ulcers located near major salivary duct openings on the palate, tongue, and buccal floor. Thick crusts of exudate accumulate along the interior margin of the beak. Oral lesions are illustrated in Figure 35.3A, B. Histopathology confirms mucosal necrosis and ulceration, submucosal granulation tissue and inflammatory cells, and crusts composed of exudate, bacterial colonies, and feed components.

T-2 toxin and DAS, structurally similar, naturally occurring trichothecenes, have been given separately and in combinations to broiler chickens (168, 169). Acute lethal intoxication by either toxin causes necrosis of lymphoid and hematopoietic tissues within 1 hr, then rapid cellular depletion, followed by repletion after 72 hr. Necrosis of hepatocytes is accompanied by hemorrhage, mild proliferation of bile ductular epithelium, and necrosis and inflammation of the gallbladder mucosa. Necrosis of intestinal epithelium is followed by transient shortening of villi and reduced numbers of mitotic figures in crypt epithelium. Necrosis also occurs in the mucosa of the proventriculus and gizzard, and in feather epithelium.

Multiple oral doses of either T-2 toxin or DAS in broiler chickens cause dehydration, emaciation, and death (171, 398, 403); changes were also observed in some dietary studies using pure toxins and fungal cultures. Survivors have reduced body weight and pigmentation, anemia, and malformed feathers (Fig. 35.4) (402). At necropsy, lymphoid tissues are atrophic, bone marrow is

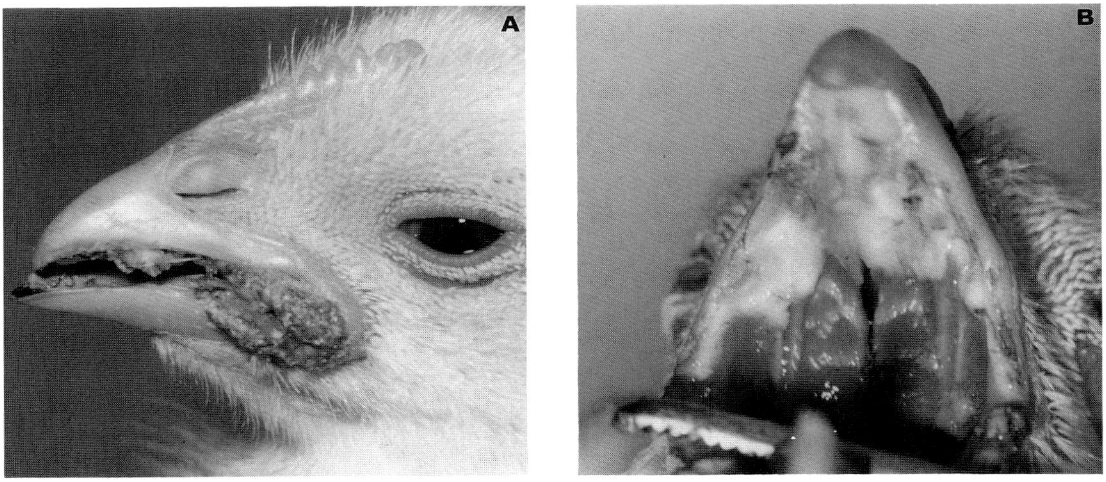

35.3. Fusariotoxicosis. Trichothecene mycotoxins cause chemical irritation of the upper digestive tract mucosa. A. Crusts at the beak commissure of a broiler chicken fed diacetoxyscirpenol for 8 days. B. Beak and palate ulceration and crusting in a broiler chicken following 14 days of consuming diacetoxyscirpenol (4 mg/kg diet).

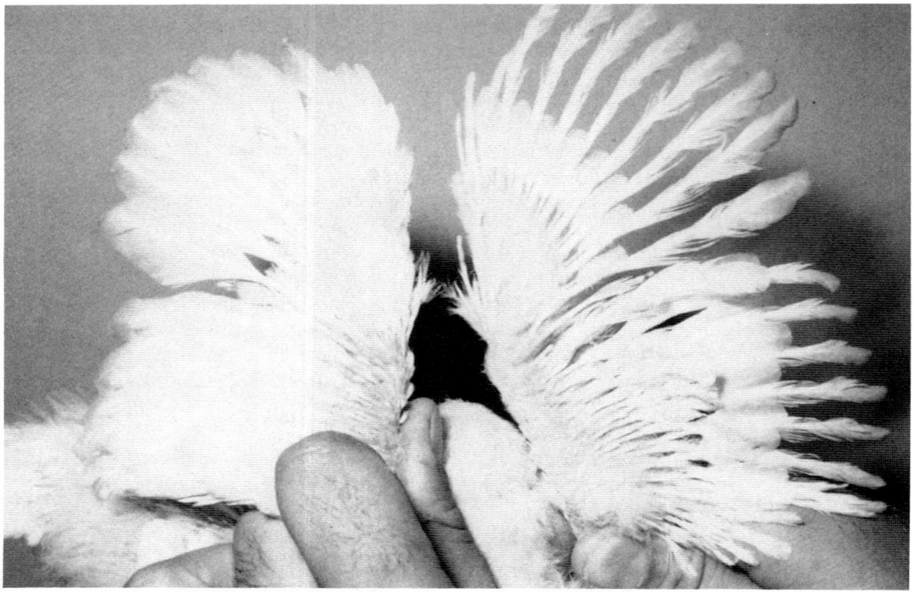

35.4. Feathers from a chicken fed T-2 toxin for 24 days (*right*) are narrow because of radiomimetic injury to the developing barbs; control (*left*).

pale red or yellow, and the liver is yellow and sometimes hemorrhagic (Figs. 35.5A, B). Histopathologic changes include necrosis with cell depletion of lymphoid and hematopoietic tissues and necrosis of hepatocytes, bile ducts, enteric mucosa, and germinal epithelium of feather barbs. Hepatocytes have vacuolar change due to lipid accumulation, accompanied by hyperplasia of bile ducts. Thyroid gland follicles are small, contain pale colloid, and have tall epithelial cells.

Broiler chickens fed trichothecene-producing cultures of *Fusarium* develop clinical disease and postmortem lesions as described collectively for models using purified toxin, either as dissolved oral doses or as appended diets (172, 198). Toxigenic cultures of *Stachybotrys atra* produce identical, severe lesions in the upper gastrointestinal tract (331). Trichothecenes in fungal cultures (a model closer to natural intoxication) appear more toxic than purified compounds. This suggests certain trichothecenes, even in low concentrations, may be significant in naturally contaminated feedstuffs.

In mallard ducks, T-2 toxin causes caseonecrotic plaques throughout the upper alimentary tract, especially in the oropharynx and proventriculus (159). Severely affected ducks develop ulcerative, proliferative esophagitis and proventriculitis. The gizzard lining is thickened, fissured, and ulcerated. Lymphoid tissues are severely atrophied. Muscovy ducks are particularly sensitive to trichothecene injury of oral mucosa, and have been recommended as a bioassay (337).

Reproduction and Egg Production. Trichothecenes T-2 toxin, DAS, and monoacetoxyscirpenol cause reductions in feed intake, body weight, and egg production in leghorn chickens and Nicholas large white turkey hens (7, 55, 348, 403). Decreases in egg production may be abrupt. Hatchability is impaired, although toxins other than trichothecenes may also be involved in this aspect. Leghorn hens recover from impaired egg production, but over consume feed in the process (404).

Immunosuppression. Despite the profound effects of many trichothecenes on lymphoid organs and bone marrow (357), no measurable evidence of immunosuppression is apparent in chickens and turkeys (22, 311). This may result from using purified toxin–appended diets rather than feeding fungal cultures or oral dosing, which allow greater expression of toxicity by trichothecenes (172).

Neurotoxicity. T-2 toxin–induced neurotoxic behavior in broiler chickens is characterized by abnormal wing positioning, hysteroid seizures, and loss of righting response (400). Toxigenic cultures of *Fusarium* inconsistently affect the righting reflex (172). These findings are unconfirmed by similar experiments using purified toxins (56, 170, 171). Brain dopamine concentration is in-

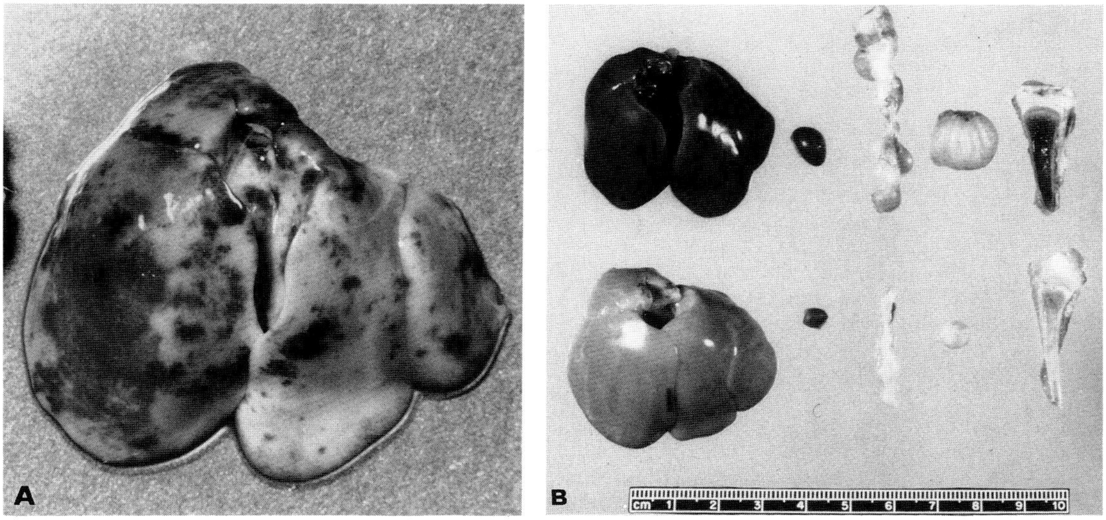

35.5. Experimental trichothecene mycotoxicosis in broiler chickens. A. Hemorrhage in the liver occurring 20 hr after consumption of feed mixed with a culture of *Fusarium sporotrichiella* that produced T-2 toxin and neosolaniol. (Avian Pathology). B. Fourteen daily oral doses of T-2 toxin cause yellow discoloration of the liver; radiomimetic effects are evidenced by atrophy of the spleen, thymus, and bursa of Fabricius, and yellow discoloration (aplasia) of the bone marrow (*bottom row*). Control (*top row*). (Avian Pathology)

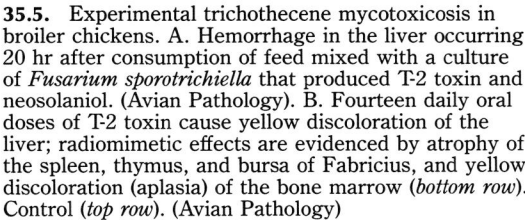

creased while norepinephrine is decreased in broiler chickens with acute T-2 mycotoxicosis (62). T-2 toxin has no effect on electroretinograms of broiler chickens (80).

Nutrition. T-2 toxin reduces plasma vitamin E concentrations in broiler chickens (74). The sparing effect of micelle-promoting compounds suggests T-2 toxin impairs lipid metabolism in the intestine.

Hematology. Purified T-2 toxin and DAS given as daily oral doses, or trichothecene-producing cultures of *Fusarium,* cause anemia in conjunction with marked hematopoietic depletion in the bone marrow of broiler chickens (171, 172). However, purified T-2 toxin- and DAS-appended diets are much less toxic, suggesting the manner of toxin presentation is important in toxicity (171). T-2 toxin causes leukopenia in leghorn hens (403).

Coagulation. Broiler chickens fed growth inhibitory levels of T-2 toxin develop prolonged prothrombin times and have suppressed activity of factor VIII and fibrinogen (95, 98).

Serum Chemistry. Chickens given intramuscular doses of T-2 toxin have transient changes (decrease, then increase) in plasma triglyceride and total cholesterol; increases in activity of plasma aspartate transaminase, alanine transaminase, and lactate dehydrogenase; and decreases of plasma acid and alkaline phosphatases. These changes reflect toxicity to the liver, intestine, and muscle (278), and correlate with gross and microscopic findings. In broiler chickens with subacute dietary T-2 mycotoxicosis, uric acid is increased and alkaline phosphatase, lactate dehydrogenase, and cholesterol are decreased (57). Serum parameters are unchanged after 10 days following sublethal T-2 intoxication (55).

T-2 toxin in leghorn hens increases serum concentrations of alkaline phosphatase, lactate dehydrogenase, and uric acid (56). Plasma protein and lipids are reduced (403).

METABOLISM AND RESIDUES. Liver is the major organ for T-2 toxin metabolism and excretion in the chicken. In broiler chickens, oral T-2 toxin reaches highest concentration in liver at 4 hr, and bile and intestine at 12 hr (59). Eighty-two percent of T-2 toxin and its metabolites are excreted from the body within 48 hr.

Metabolites recovered from chickens given oral T-2 toxin indicate hydroxylation occurs at major substitution points on the parent compound (321). T-2 toxin is the only trichothecene found in liver, but T-2 toxin, HT-2 toxin, neosolaniol, T-2 tetraol, and eight unidentified metabolites, quantitatively in higher concentrations than the preceding four, appear in feces (406). One of these eight metabolites is 4-deacetylneosolaniol.

Relatively small amounts of T-2 toxin are excreted into the egg. For hens given a single oral dose of T-2 toxin, the first egg receives 0.17% of the dose (59). Hens given T-2 toxin for 8 days as oral doses excrete progressively greater amounts of metabolites into yolk, whereas concentrations in egg white peak after the third dose and remain constant thereafter. The average amount of T-2 toxin excreted into an egg is about 0.9 μg.

Deoxynivalenol (DON, Vomitoxin)

ETIOLOGY AND TOXICOLOGY. In addition to hyperestrogenism in swine (see zearalenone), many feeds contaminated with *Fusarium roseum* (*Gibberella zeae, F. roseum* "Graminearum") also caused feed refusal and emesis in pigs. The idea was advanced in 1966 that the feed refusal factor was separate from the one causing estrogenic syndrome (82). In 1973, a trichothecene, deoxynivalenol (DON, vomitoxin), was identified as the emetic factor (374) and was later determined to cause both feed refusal and emesis (375). Trichothecenes less common than DON also induce refusal and emesis, and *Fusarium* spp. produce uncharacterized metabolites that cause feed refusal (376). DON is the most prevalent trichothecene, occurring on corn, wheat, and other grains, often with zearalenone, aflatoxin, and other mycotoxins (140, 146, 375).

Like zearalenone, grains contaminated with DON may be fed to poultry because of their relative insensitivity to this mycotoxin. For this reason, experimental DON mycotoxicosis in poultry has received considerable study.

NATURAL DISEASE. No reports were found of natural, overt poultry intoxication by DON. Feed taken from a commercial turkey farm where poults refused to eat and high mortality occurred contained 0.81 mg DON and 2.2 mg salinomycin/kg diet (232). Poults fed the commercial diet in a feeding trial had lower feed consumption and higher mortality. Poults test fed diets containing much higher concentrations of DON and salinomycin, alone and in combination, were not adversely affected.

EXPERIMENTAL DISEASE. DON is substantially less toxic to chickens than aflatoxin, T-2 toxin, or ochratoxin A. DON mycotoxicosis has been studied experimentally in broiler and leghorn chickens, and in turkeys.

Pathology. In acute lethal intoxication in broiler chickens, birds gasp, have reduced spontaneous activity, assume a squatting postural change, loose balance, repeatedly swallow, develop diarrhea, and die (187). At necropsy, diffuse subcutaneous hemorrhage, visceral gout, and ecchymotic hemorrhages in viscera are seen.

Broiler and leghorn chicks and turkey poults can tolerate up to 5 mg DON/kg diet formulated with contaminated winter or spring wheat. No adverse effects occur in feed intake, weight gain, feed efficiency, mortality, or dressing percentage (154, 194, 212). Broiler chickens consuming highly contaminated diets develop oral plaques and gizzard erosions proportional to the level of DON (251). Toxin concentrations required to produce these lesions are much higher than other trichothecenes, and in excess of levels causing feed refusal and emesis in swine.

The only lesion from numerous experiments with leghorn hens is mild erosions in the gizzard lining (230). DON induces either mild or no oral lesions in chickens, in contrast to other trichothecenes.

Reproduction. DON mycotoxicosis in hens essentially does not occur at concentrations likely to be encountered in naturally contaminated grain (154, 155, 214, 215, 230, 252). Adverse effects are limited to minor changes in percentages of yolk and white, shell quality, and embryo mortality. Mild changes in dietary intake are likely due to palatability or olfactory responses, and not direct anorexic effects.

Hematology. Male leghorn chicks experience decreased hemoglobin and hematocrit when fed relatively high concentrations of DON for 35 days (212). Broiler chicks develop leukopenia, also at relatively high concentrations (60).

METABOLISM AND RESIDUES. DON has low absorption from the intestine of leghorn hens, as plasma concentration reaches only 1% of an oral dose (292). Maximum tissue concentrations are achieved in 3 hr, with kidney, liver, and spleen having the highest levels. The tissue half-life is 16.8 hr, and 98% of the dose is eliminated in excreta within 72 hr. With repeated low doses of deoxynivalenol, tissue levels are not achieved.

Only low concentrations occur in eggs; these do not continue once the contaminated diet is withdrawn (293). Only about 10% of egg metabolites are the parent DON compound. DON is undetectable in skeletal muscle of broilers fed diets contaminated to field levels (115). Gizzard may contain low concentrations (230).

Zearalenone

ETIOLOGY AND TOXICOLOGY. Grains infected with the fungus *Gibberella zeae* (*Fusarium graminearum, F. roseum* "Graminearum") are sources of zearalenone (F-2), a mycotoxin with estrogenic activity. Vulvovaginitis in swine was associated with moldy grain in 1927 (see 68), and in 1962 *Fusarium*-invaded grain was unequivocally established as the cause (352).

Zearalenone, a resorcyclic acid lactone, has at least seven derivatives produced in fungal culture, but only zearalenone and zearalenol occur naturally. While zearalenone occurs more commonly and has been closely examined for effects in poultry, zearalenol is three to four times more active estrogenically (245). In the USA, zearalenone prevalence is higher in corn belt states, but toxin formation also occurs on grain sorghum in the south (90). Adverse effects in food animals are seen chiefly in swine as reproductive failure. In prepuberal gilts, the vulva becomes swollen, sometimes accompanied by vaginal or rectal prolapse. The uterus is enlarged, edematous, and tortuous, and ovaries are atrophied. Young males experience feminization, atrophy of testes, and mammary development.

Broiler and leghorn chickens are more tolerant of zearalenone than either turkeys or swine, and provide an outlet for grains unfit for swine (3, 118). Although most data show zearalenone as safe for chickens, recent information suggests it may adversely affect poultry.

NATURAL DISEASE. Zearalenone was considered detrimental to broiler breeders in Israel (21). High mortality occurred in 24,000 broiler breeders kept in four houses. Peak egg production was reduced, but not fertility, hatchability, or progeny performance. Affected hens had ascites in conjunction with many oviduct cysts and distention of the oviduct with fibrinous material. Histopathologic findings in the oviduct and peritoneum were caseous cysts accompanied by a chronic inflammatory response. Serum progesterone was lowered but estradiol was unaffected. Zearalenone was identified at concentrations of >0.5–5.0 mg/kg in feed from three houses, and was considered a factor in the disease and production problems.

EXPERIMENTAL DISEASE. Experimental zearalenone mycotoxicosis has been studied in broiler and leghorn chickens, turkeys, quail, and geese. In general, poultry are tolerant of this mycotoxin, turkeys being the least tolerant, with the reproductive tract and sex hormone–sensitive tissues being targeted. Dose-effect studies on zearalenone have been reported by several workers as varying from as low as 100 to >800 mg/kg in the diet, or 5 mg/kg body weight, or 10 mg/bird (6, 8, 60, 86, 246).

Pathology. In leghorn chicks, the weight of the bursa of Fabricius increases (347), possibly related to hormone-induced regional swelling in birds. Cysts develop on the peritoneal surface, and apparently within the immature oviduct as thin-walled, fluid-filled sacs (347). The incidence of ovarian cysts is also increased in leghorn hens.

Broiler chickens are highly tolerant of zearalenone. Lesions are limited to decreased comb and testes weight (4) and oviduct enlargement (61).

Male turkey poults fed starter feed appended with zearalenone develop strutting behavior, increased size and coloration of the caruncles and dewlaps, and soft-tissue swelling of the vent (4). No adverse effects are seen in Japanese quail (14).

Reproduction. Egg specific gravity, eggshell thickness, and interior egg quality are reduced in leghorns given corn diets contaminated with *F. roseum.* (347). A water-soluble component of *F. roseum* cultures, containing neither zearalenone nor trichothecenes, is responsible for reduced hatchability of fertile eggs produced by leghorns fed the cultures (227). Other studies show leghorns highly tolerant of zearalenone (61) and of corn contaminated with *F. roseum* (3, 235).

Eggs produced by Nicholas large white turkey hens fed *F. roseum* cultures have reduced hatchability, but neither zearalenone nor trichothecenes are responsible (7), indicating other metabolites contribute to the toxicity.

Spermatogenesis inhibition by *Fusarium* spp. in geese (275) affects fertility (274). Egg production is unaffected (273).

Hematology and Serum Chemistry. In broiler chickens, total leukocytes are decreased by zearalenone due to a decrease in lymphocytes (60). No effect is observed with other parameters of the hemogram, total protein, calcium, phosphorus, alkaline phosphatase, and cholesterol. In leghorn hens, serum calcium is decreased and phosphorus is increased (61).

METABOLISM AND RESIDUES. The public health danger of zearalenone residues in broiler chicken edible tissues is low. Zearalenone distributes chiefly to liver and gallbladder (246), and is excreted mainly in feces. Muscle, abdominal fat, skin, and heart have transient, low residues. Zearalenone and alpha- and beta-zearalenol are metabolites in liver and feces. Muscle contains only zearalenone.

Dietary zearalenone metabolizes to alpha-zearalenol and only traces of beta-zearalenol in turkeys (264). Zearalenone and alpha-zearalenol both occur in plasma, fecal droppings, lung, heart, liver, and kidney, and the percentage of alpha-zearalenol increases with time. Most plasma zearalenone and alpha-zearalenol is conjugated with glucuronides and sulfates.

In leghorn hens, about 94% of zearalenone is excreted in feces within 72 hr of oral dosing (86). One-third of identified metabolites is zearalenone, and another third is a polar metabolite. Yolk residues occur 72 hr after a single oral dose. Muscle has no residues at 72 hr.

Fusarochromanone

ETIOLOGY AND TOXICOLOGY. Tibial dyschondroplasia is a defect in endochondral ossification. A cone of cartilage forms most commonly in the tibiotarsus, but also in the long bones of growing, heavy breeds of chickens, turkeys, and ducks. Lack of cartilage penetration by metaphyseal vascular sprouts leads to failure of normal ossification. Rapid growth, genetic predisposition, and various nutritional and management factors influence the lesion.

In 1972 cultures of *Aspergillus niger, A. flavus, Fusarium moniliforme,* and *F. roseum* caused varus and valgus deformities in broiler chicken legs (332). In 1982 *F. roseum*–contaminated grain induced a high incidence of tibial dyschondroplasia in broiler chickens (378). Defective chondroclasis was suggested as a possible pathogenesis. Chondroclastic activity was found in the water-soluble extract, which had six components (227). One of three fluorescent components (UV light), TDP-1 (fusarochromanone), was lethal to chick embryos and induced a 100% incidence of tibial dyschondroplasia when fed to broiler chickens at 75 mg/kg diet. The fungal strain, originally isolated from overwintered barley in Alaska, also produced trichothecenes, but they were not considered involved in the pathogenesis. Aflatoxin has also been excluded as a primary etiology of tibial dyschondroplasia in broilers (177).

EXPERIMENTAL DISEASE. Chicks fed fusarochromanone-producing cultures of *Fusarium* develop lesions in the tibial physis within 4 days (162). It becomes thickened and has histopathologic alterations of a thickened transitional zone, especially prominent in the center of the growth plate. The zone is unmineralized, avascular, and contains chondrocytes, which are crenated and densely eosinophilic. Cartilage matrix is pale and contains eosinophilic foci. Compared to normal chicks, affected broilers have increased distance between the proliferative/transitional junction and metaphyseal sprout tips. The lesion resembles spontaneous and chloride-induced tibial dyschondroplasia, and is probably a common endpoint arrived at by several pathogenetic mechanisms.

The primary site of fusarochromanone action at the cellular and biochemical level has proven elusive. Sections of hypertrophic cartilage have a lower density of chondroclasts, a secondary factor in the pathogenesis (225). The ultrastructural lesion in hypertrophic chondrocytes from the cartilage core is intracellular lipid accumulation, autophagic vacuole formation, and necrosis. This lesion too is considered secondary, due to the increased distance of chondrocytes from their vascular source of nutrients (161). Fusarochromanone is only moderately toxic to chondrocytes in vitro (390), and much less than T-2 toxin, a trichothecene mycotoxin. The following have also been excluded as primary events: defective or deficient metaphyseal vascular front, biochemical abnormalities in cartilage composition, and excessive protease inhibitor (160).

Another water-soluble toxin of *Fusarium roseum* "Graminearum" that is not a trichothecene or zearalenone causes marked decreases in hatchability of fertile chicken embryos (227). Embryo mortality occurs during the first 5 days of incubation.

Fusarium moniliforme

ETIOLOGY AND TOXICOLOGY. *Fusarium moniliforme* causes ear rot, kernel rot, and stalk rot of unharvested corn, and may be involved in advanced decay of stored high-moisture shelled corn (37). The fungus also occurs on oats, soybeans, sorghum, barley, and wheat, and corn that may appear perfectly sound.

Moniliformin, a toxin produced by *F. moniliforme* and other *Fusarium* spp. (303), is considered a causative agent of equine leukoencephalomalacia (147), a highly fatal disease of horses and other equidae (386). The chick is used as a bioassay for presence of moniliformin in cultures. Although moniliformin is quite toxic to poultry as defined by the LD_{50}, purified moniliformin–appended diets are much less toxic than toxigenic fungal cultures. *F. moniliforme* also produces zearalenone, fusariocin A (37), and other toxic fractions (81).

NATURAL DISEASE. Research and laboratory verification of *F. moniliforme* mycotoxicosis is relatively lacking, although industry reports indicate it is a problem for poultry. Broiler breeders and leghorns eating corn contaminated with *F. moniliforme* have reduced rate of lay and delayed peaks in production (81). Intermittent over- and underconsumption of feed occurs in conjunction with diarrhea, dark fecal droppings with undigested feed, fecal-stained eggshells, and blood smears on eggshells. Contaminated corn is high in moisture, low in protein, and high in crushing strength. The latter causes large particle sizes in corn meal leading to digestive disturbance.

EXPERIMENTAL DISEASE. *F. moniliforme* causes reductions in feed consumption and weight gain, and can be fatal to broiler chicks while producing no overt lesions (5). Lethal intoxication by purified moniliformin (single oral LD_{50}, 4 mg/kg bw) produces gross lesions of mesenteric edema, ascites, and hemorrhages in the digestive tract and skin

(76). Purified moniliformin–appended diets with the same concentrations however, have no adverse effects.

Although *F. moniliforme* is thought to have a necrotizing vascular effect in the pathogenesis of equine leukoencephalomalacia, no vascular necrosis has been found in chicks other than the initial toxicity studies (76) described above. In one study, chicks fed *F. moniliforme* diets developed signs of thiamine deficiency and responded to thiamine therapy (121). Diet analysis indicated that either the thiamine had been destroyed or the mold was competing with the chicks for thiamine in the feed.

Fusarium moniliforme var. *subglutinans*, which produced moniliformin, caused rapid, fatal intoxication when fed to ducklings (207). Ducks were not examined at necropsy, but rats fed the same cultures developed lesions in heart, liver, and kidney.

Aflatoxins

ETIOLOGY AND TOXICOLOGY. Aflatoxins are highly toxic and carcinogenic fungal metabolites produced by *Aspergillus flavus, A. parasiticus,* and *Penicillium puberulum* (112). Almost any feed or grain for poultry and livestock will support fungal growth and aflatoxin formation. Aflatoxins are relatively stable compounds in normal food and feed products, but are reactive to ultraviolet light at pH extremes and are sensitive to oxidizing agents such as hypochlorite (commercial bleach).

Aflatoxins are chemically a fusion of two dihydrofuran rings with various moieties, and comprise a group with members designated B1, B2, G1, and G2, after their blue and green color reaction to fluorescent light (365-nm wavelength) and their chromatographic Rf values. Aflatoxin B1 is the most toxic, and hepatotoxicity is the primary effect in nearly all animals.

Chronic aflatoxicosis results in neoplasia in rats, mice, trout, ducks, monkeys, and possibly humans (272). The primary tumor is usually in liver, but gallbladder, pancreas, urinary tract, and bone may also be primarily involved. Although several aflatoxin metabolites are carcinogenic, aflatoxin B1 is most potent. Like other carcinogens, it binds to nuclear and mitochondrial DNA in a selective, nonrandom manner (176). Aflatoxin B1 is a model hepatocarcinogen used to elucidate mechanisms of initiation in the liver. It may also be active in promotion through oncogene activation, hormonal alteration, and dietary interaction.

NATURAL DISEASE. Detailed descriptions of the first cases of aflatoxicosis, reviewed in the previous edition (280), will be briefly described to serve as a reference point. Lethal aflatoxicosis in ducklings began with inappetence and reduced growth about 2 wk after initial consumption of toxic feed (13). Abnormal crying vocalizations were heard, ducks picked at their feathers, legs and feet became discolored purple, and lameness developed. Ataxia, convulsions, and opisthotonos preceded death. At necropsy, liver and kidneys were enlarged and pale. With chronicity, livers became shrunken, firm, and nodular, and gallbladder was distended. Hemorrhages occurred on kidneys and pancreas and in the subcutis of the legs. Hydropericardium and ascites frequently developed.

The principal microscopic lesions in ducks occurred in liver. Hepatocytes were swollen with vacuolated cytoplasm and enlarged, often degenerated nuclei. Bile ductule proliferation and fibrosis became extensive, leaving only islands of hepatocytes. Phlebitis was sometimes severe. Acinar cell swelling and karyorrhexis occurred in the pancreas. Hemorrhage was present in the kidneys.

Turkeys developed a similar disease: inappetence, reduced spontaneous activity, unsteady gait, recumbency, and death (340). Hematologic alterations were decreased erythrocyte count, an increased leukocyte count with increased heterophils and monocytes, and decreased lymphocytes (379). Lethal aflatoxicosis can cause either dark red or yellow discoloration of the liver due to congestion or fat accumulation, respectively (Fig. 35.6).

At necropsy, body condition was good but there was generalized congestion and mild edema. Livers were congested, enlarged, and firm, and the gallbladders were distended. Kidneys were swollen and congested. The duodenum was distended with catarrhal content. Microscopic lesions in turkey livers consisted of swollen hepatocytes with homogenous, sometimes vacuolated, cytoplasm. Nuclei were large with marginated chromatin and prominent spherical nuclei. Irregular zones of hepatocyte necrosis occurred in centrilobular areas. With toxicity of longer duration, regenerating hepatocytes with basophilic, vacuolated cytoplasm and occasional multiple nuclei were seen. Reticuloendothelial cells were hyperplastic and moderate increases in collagen and reticulum fibers occurred. There was moderate bile duct proliferation. Kidneys had glomerular changes of pronounced thickening of the capillary basement membrane. Proximal tubular and collecting duct epithelium contained hyalin droplets. Other lesions included catarrhal enteritis and granular degeneration of myocardial fibers.

Gross and microscopic lesions in chickens were similar to ducks and turkeys (11, 13), but the early report from Australia described, in addition, white discoloration and necrosis of skeletal muscle, unique to the chicken (130). The interaction of selenium and aflatoxicosis may have been involved (see **EXPERIMENTAL DISEASE**).

Aflatoxin-producing fungi and aflatoxin-contaminated animal feedstuffs are now identified

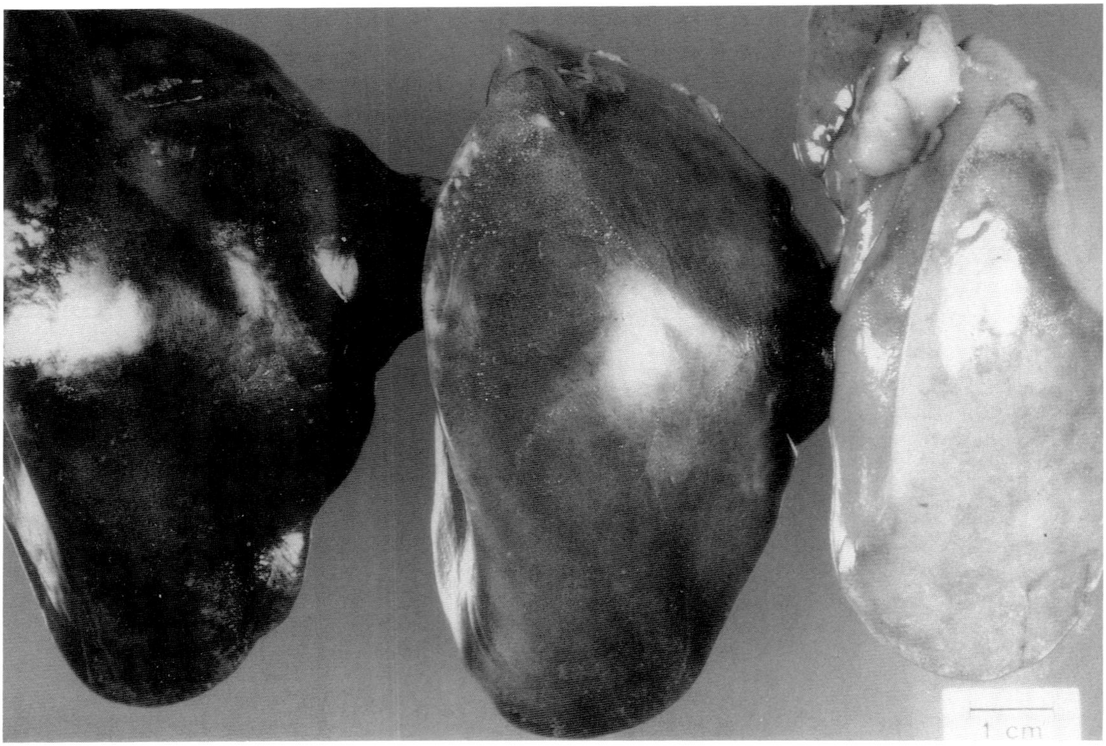

35.6. Lethal aflatoxicosis in turkeys causes liver discoloration ranging from dark red (*left*) due to congestion and necrosis, to yellow (*right*) owing to fat accumulation in hepatocytes. Aflatoxin B1 (200 ppb) was detected in the feed that killed these turkeys.

and reported throughout the world (91, 167, 261, 335), usually with adverse implications for poultry production (199, 202, 231, 253).

Worldwide recognition of aflatoxin in feedstuffs has also resulted in identification of aflatoxicosis. Overt intoxication occurred recently in ducks in India (306), Malaysia (1), and Indonesia (163); chickens in Sudan (84), Nigeria (263, 339), UK (220), Australia (32), USA (148, 342), and India (65, 291, 305); and quail in the USA (387).

Concurrent with aflatoxin hepatosis are increased mortality from heat stress in broiler breeders (84); loss of egg production in egg-type chickens (32); anemia, hemorrhages, liver condemnations (220), paralysis and lameness (263), and impaired performance (202) in broilers; nervous symptoms (1), impaired performance, and mortality in ducks (32); impaired ambulation and paralysis in quail (387); and increased susceptibility to infectious disease in multiple avian species (32, 291).

Cases of both mycosis (aspergillosis) and mycotoxicosis (aflatoxicosis) are increasingly common and confirm that *Aspergillus* spp. are a threat to poultry production in the feed, litter, and environment (306, 339).

EXPERIMENTAL DISEASE. Aflatoxicosis impairs all important production parameters, including weight gain, feed intake, feed-conversion efficiency, pigmentation, processing yield, egg production, and both male and female reproductive performance. Some influences are direct effects of intoxication, while others are indirect to factors such as reduced feed intake.

Susceptibility of poultry to aflatoxins varies among species, breeds, and genetic lines. In general, ducklings, turkeys, and pheasants are susceptible, while chickens, Japanese quail, and guinea fowl are relatively resistant (10, 144). Wide variation exists among breeds, with age and sex being important, depending on the parameter (31, 78, 383). Dose-effect studies on aflatoxin in broilers, ducklings, geese, leghorns, quail, and turkeys have been reported (10, 40, 48, 52, 96, 100, 133, 134, 175, 191, 195, 223, 243, 267, 270, 300, 308, 312, 326, 333, 361, 368, 389).

Pathology. Acute and subacute experimental aflatoxicosis reflects natural disease. Acute lethal intoxication in ducks is characterized by gross hepatic lesions of pale yellow-green discoloration and atrophy, with the left hepatic lobe being more affected (260). Microscopic lesions chiefly involve hepatocytes as cytoplasmic vacuolation and massive necrosis, often accompanied by hemorrhage. Necrosis of tubular epithelium in kidneys may be seen. Bile duct proliferation is evident in 2 days and progresses rapidly. Subacute lethal intoxication of ducks, especially those fed cultures of *Aspergillus flavus,* causes extensive necrosis and loss of hepatocytes, and explosive bile duct proliferation. In nonlethal aflatoxicosis, prominent hepatic lesions are clear vacuolation of swollen hepatocytes, karyomegaly, and numerous mitotic figures (173). Bile duct proliferation occurs in the portal areas. Histologic changes in liver and kidney are illustrated in Figures 35.7A, B, C.

Subacute, nonlethal aflatoxicosis in chickens is characterized by hepatic lesions of pale yellow-ocher discoloration, multifocal hemorrhage, and a reticulated pattern on the capsular surface (43). In time, chicken livers develop white foci, and hepatic lipid content increases. Histologic lesions are progressively severe fatty vacuolation of hepatocyte cytoplasm, karyomegaly and prominent nucleoli in hepatocytes, bile duct proliferation, and fibrosis. Basophilic, vacuolated, regenerative hepatocytes and cellular inflammation comprising heterophil and mononuclear cells occur in portal zones (43, 173).

In turkeys with subacute aflatoxicosis, ductular proliferation in the trabecular and, less commonly, tubular form is prevalent in portal areas but extends to all of the lobule (173, 259). Turkey livers develop nodules of regenerative, densely eosinophilic hepatocytes that compress adjacent parenchyma. Vacuolar change and fibrosis are mild, even in turkeys that die following prolonged toxin ingestion.

For the studies above, no aflatoxin-related lesions occurred in either the kidney or major lymphoid tissues. Membranous glomerular lesions and interstitial fibrosis occurred in ducks and goslings of another study (254).

Reproduction and Egg Production. Mature white leghorn males experience lowered semen volume, testis weight, spermatocrits, and testosterone values caused indirectly by reduced feed intake during aflatoxicosis (333, 334). Lower testosterone plasma concentration and responsiveness in younger, maturing leghorn males are direct effects (73). Aflatoxin causes reduction in body weight and mild anemia in broiler breeder males, but semen characteristics are not altered (25. 401).

Hatchability declines before egg production

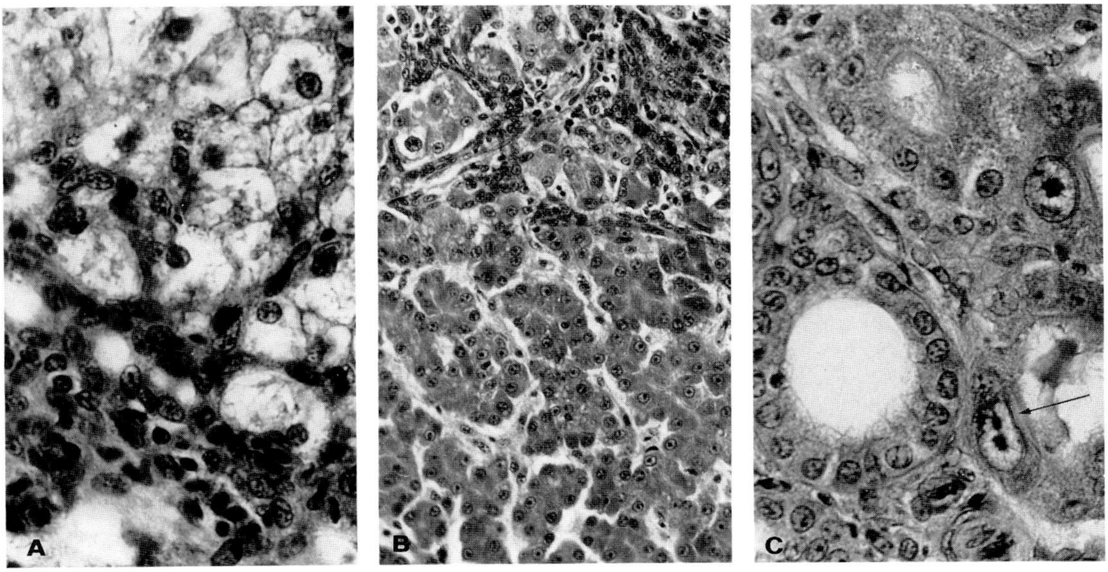

35.7. Aflatoxicosis in ducks fed toxic peanut meal. A. Early liver lesion showing degenerative changes in parenchyma and bile duct hyperplasia. H & E, ×1000. B. Nodular hyperplasia of liver parenchyma and bile duct hyperplasia. H & E, ×398. C. Proximal tubules of kidney are dilated, epithelium is undergoing necrosis, and some nuclei have enlarged bizarre forms with prominent nucleoli (*arrow*). H & E, ×1000.

and is the most sensitive parameter of aflatoxicosis in broiler breeder hens (175). Loss of hatchability is due to embryonic death during the first 6 days of incubation (79). Fertility and performance of hatched progeny are less affected.

In leghorns, aflatoxin blocks ova maturation and reduces feed efficiency and egg production (195). Like broiler breeders, hatchability is more sensitive than egg production (206). Egg production may be spared despite lesions of hepatotoxicity, although the production decline can be delayed and require several weeks or more to return to normal (117, 131). Aflatoxin impairs egg production by reducing synthesis and transport of yolk precursors in the liver. Egg size, yolk weight, and yolk as percent of total egg size are decreased (181). Aflatoxin metabolites are transferred to the egg (see **METABOLISM AND RESIDUES**), although many studies have shown no transfer.

In Japanese quail, impairment of feed conversion, egg production, egg weight, hatchability, and exterior and interior egg quality occur with hepatosis (325). Maturation of both males and females is delayed (97, 270).

Immunosuppression. The association of spontaneous aflatoxicosis and increased susceptibility to infectious disease is strong (113, 287, 307). Experimental definition of susceptibility through anticipated immunosuppression is less conclusive, but the difficulties lend perspective to the complexity of defining the mechanisms of natural toxins. Among many experimental approaches are a single purified toxin, combinations of purified toxins, crude cultures or culture extracts of cloned fungal species, and naturally contaminated feeds or grains. Potentially numerous metabolite interactions (not to exclude the nutritional interaction) influence both the spectrum of results and accuracy of defining an effect at a given concentration.

In chickens, aflatoxin reportedly increases susceptibility to cecal coccidiosis, Marek's disease (114), and congenitally acquired salmonellosis (394). Higher mortality occurs in chickens fed aflatoxin and then infected with either *Salmonella gallinarum* (343) or infectious bursal disease virus (47). Turkeys experience vaccination failure to *Pasteurella multocida* challenge (288), and increased susceptibility to coccidiosis caused by *Eimeria adenoeides* (389).

Aflatoxin-induced immunosuppression is explained, in part, by atrophy of the bursa of Fabricius, thymus, and spleen (47, 289) regardless of the immune response genetics of the bird (367–369). In ducks, changes in the lymphatic system are accompanied by morphologic changes in the nucleolus of circulating lymphocytes, suggesting functional disablement (341). There is impaired clearance function of blood phagocytes and the reticuloendothelial system in chickens (44, 45, 242, 249). Serum complement activity is reduced in broilers (351). Cell-mediated immune responses are decreased in both turkeys and chickens (133–135).

Despite the above aflatoxin-induced immunosuppression, considerable data show no measurable effect on either the histopathology of lymphoid organs or functional immune responses. This has been tested with aflatoxin concentrations far higher than commonly encountered in spontaneously contaminated feedstuffs (111, 133–135, 173).

Nutrition and Digestion. Broiler chicken skin pigmentation is a desirable characteristic in some markets, and carotenoid pigments are provided in the diet to produce this effect. Aflatoxin causes impaired pigmentation in broiler chickens (366) by inhibiting metabolism and deposition of pigment from the pathway involving the intestinal mucosa, serum, liver, and integument (328), rather than by enhancing pigment depletion from skin (329).

The effect of aflatoxin in poultry is greater with a low-fat diet, (151, 315), a low-protein diet (267, 316), a high–tannic acid diet (88), or a diet deficient in riboflavin or vitamin D_3 (150, 152). Conclusions regarding the need for supplemental vitamin D_3 are equivocal (20, 27). These variables make it difficult to establish minimum-effect or no-effect concentrations for aflatoxin in poultry feeds.

During aflatoxicosis in broiler chickens, the balance of pancreatic enzymes is altered causing a deficiency of amylase and lipase (266), which results in steatorrhea. Egg-type chickens escape this effect (314).

Hematology. Aflatoxin causes hematopoietic suppression and anemia observed as decreases in packed-cell volume, total erythrocytes, and hemoglobin (190, 249). The mean corpuscular volume is decreased, but mean corpuscular hemoglobin concentration is unaffected (223). Iron absorption and retention are initially decreased, but then compensate (222). In broiler chickens, young birds are more susceptible to anemia (223). Total leukocytes are increased, and although differential leukocyte counts vary among studies, there is concurrent lymphopenia (223, 364).

Coagulation. Bruising is a problem during transport and slaughter of poultry. Aflatoxin increases susceptibility to bruising by increasing capillary fragility and reducing shear strength of skeletal muscle (363). It also impairs coagulation in chickens and turkeys by interfering with several coagulation components, notably prothrombin, to affect the extrinsic and common pathways (96, 99,

388). Aflatoxin alters coagulation more than either ochratoxin A and T-2 toxin, but ochratoxin A effects last longer (98, 188).

Serum Chemistry. Aflatoxin decreases total serum protein. In broilers, albumin is the most sensitive component, but decreases are also seen in alpha, beta, and gamma globulins, with IgG being more sensitive than IgM (365). Serum lipoprotein, carotenoid pigment, cholesterol, triglycerides, uric acid, calcium, and lactate dehydrogenase are also decreased (100, 190, 308). Serum sorbital dehydrogenase, glutamic dehydrogenase, and potassium are increased (85). Duckling serum protein changes resemble the broiler chicken (258).

In selected lines of Japanese quail, the degree of total protein and albumin reduction, and increase in beta-glucuronidase, are correlated with resistance to aflatoxin when measured during the stress of intoxication (284). Blood-clotting time and the ratio of aspartate aminotransferase to alanine aminotransferase are resistance indicators in ducks (268).

PHARMACOLOGY. Aflatoxicosis may influence drug effectiveness in poultry through alteration of plasma half-life. In broiler chickens, chlortetracycline plasma concentrations are lowered due to decreased drug binding to plasma protein (243). Conclusions differ on aflatoxicosis being either enhanced by the addition of chlortetracycline to feed (224) or diminished (344).

METABOLISM AND RESIDUES. Poultry reared on diets contaminated with aflatoxin constitute a minimal aflatoxin source in the human food chain. Aflatoxins distribute through the animal body in low concentrations and rapidly clear if unadulterated diets are provided.

In broilers, metabolites of dietary aflatoxins B1 and B2 reach highest concentrations in gizzard, liver, and kidney (51). Aflatoxin-free diets result in no detectable tissue residues within 4 days. In chickens, aflatoxin B1 is metabolized into conjugated aflatoxins B2a and M1 in the liver (64). Also, nicotinamide adenine dinucleotide phosphate (NADP)-linked cytoplasmic enzymes in duck and chicken livers can reduce aflatoxins B1 and B2 to the cyclopentenol and aflatoxicol (277). Aflatoxin B1 is excreted by chickens via bile, urine, and intestinal content at a ratio of 70:15:15 as six major metabolites including B1, B2, B2a, and M1 (156).

Aflatoxins B1 and M1 are the major metabolites in turkeys, with highest concentrations occurring in liver, kidney, gizzard, and feces (143, 312). Aflatoxicol is a minor metabolite. The majority of aflatoxin metabolites are conjugated and tend to clear rapidly from the tissues when the dietary source is removed. Selenium supplementation of turkey diets is protective against aflatoxicosis because it increases the percentage of aflatoxin in the conjugated state (36, 142).

The half-life of a single oral dose of aflatoxin B1 in hens is about 67 hr (326). Most of the toxin, or its metabolites, is excreted via bile and intestine, but metabolites can be identified in eggs for at least 7 days.

In the hen, aflatoxin tissue distribution is widespread, and metabolite studies have confirmed transfer to the ova and eggs (196, 361). Both aflatoxin B1 and aflatoxicol accumulate in eggs, the latter remaining after 7 days on a toxin-free diet. Aflatoxicol is also the major metabolite in hen muscle and blood, B1 in liver, and M1 in kidney. Aflatoxin B1 accumulates in reproductive organs with transfer to eggs (both yolk and albumen) and hatched progeny (yolk sac and liver) in chickens, turkeys, and ducks (346, 408).

Ochratoxins

ETIOLOGY AND TOXICOLOGY. Ochratoxins are among the most toxic mycotoxins to poultry, and several cases have been identified. These nephrotoxic metabolites are produced chiefly by *Penicillium viridicatum* and *Aspergillus ochraceous,* which commonly occur on numerous grains and feedstuffs throughout North America, Europe, and Asia (see review 109).

Ochratoxins are isocoumarin compounds linked to *L*-beta-phenylalanine, and are designated A, B, C, D, and their methyl and ethyl esters. Ochratoxin A is the most common and most toxic, and is relatively stable. Some ochratoxin-producing fungi produce other mycotoxins toxic to poultry, including citrinin.

Ochratoxin is the major determinant in porcine endemic nephropathy in Denmark and Ireland (see review 208). Reports in Denmark date from 1928 and describe chronic wasting disease and failure to thrive in bacon pigs. The condition is caused by chronic renal disease to which mycotoxins have been closely linked as causal factors.

NATURAL DISEASE. Ochratoxin A was first identified in the feed chain in 1969 as a contaminant of corn (338). Since then, ochratoxin A has been found in a variety of grains, including corn, wheat, and barley, and in animal feeds at concentrations ranging from 5–27,000 μg/kg (see review 42). The potential for poultry exposure to ochratoxin from grain sorghum also exists (158). Ochratoxin A readily forms in poultry feed under conditions of high temperature and high moisture (15). The toxin has been identified in North America, in both Canada and the USA; in Europe, including France, Denmark, Yugoslavia, Poland, Italy, and Sweden; and in Asia, including the USSR and

Taiwan. Concentrations of ochratoxins A and B associated with poultry mycotoxicoses varied from 0.3–4.0 mg/kg in feed for chickens (2, 153, 380), 9.6–80 mg/kg in dried bread fed to chickens (377), and 0.09–16.0 mg/kg in turkey feed (153).

A spontaneous toxic nephropathy in poultry associated with ochratoxin A was described in 1975 (116). At a poultry slaughter house in Denmark, 5 of 14 chickens with enlarged pale kidneys had ochratoxin A residues in the kidneys. Four of these five had renal changes of atrophy and degeneration of proximal and distal tubules, and interstitial fibrosis.

Ochratoxin A mycotoxicosis in Canada involved 8,800 broilers and pelleted feed colonized with *Aspergillus ochraceous* and *Penicillium* spp. (2). Mortality was increased threefold and there was failure to gain weight. At necropsy, pale discoloration of liver and kidney and enteritis were seen. In the USA, two episodes of ochratoxicosis involving 12 million broilers were caused by either contaminated corn or corn gluten meal (153). Growth rate, feed conversion efficiency, and pigmentation were affected. Airsacculitis accompanied toxin-induced renal disease. A processing plant problem of fragile intestines that tore and contaminated carcasses with intestinal content was linked to feed contaminated with ochratoxin and aflatoxin (380).

Ochratoxicosis involving ochratoxins A and B formation on moldy bread caused enteritis in chickens (377). Only a few animals were involved. Ochratoxin A occurs in moldy bread and flour (265) as components of bakery by-products used as a poultry feed ingredient.

Ochratoxicosis involving 970,000 turkeys in five independent episodes in the USA was characterized by feed refusal and mortality due to nephrotoxicity and airsacculitis (153). Histopathology confirmed nephrosis as renal edema and necrosis of proximal tubular epithelium. Corn was the ingredient responsible for the toxic feed.

Laying hens experienced reductions in egg production and shell quality, and developed nephropathy during two separate episodes of ochratoxicosis in the USA, again involving contaminated corn (153). Leghorn hens in flocks totaling 600,000 developed chronic renal disease and diarrhea that caused yellow stains on egg shells resulting in decreased market value. Experimental feeding of ochratoxin A caused a diarrhea with high urate content and the eggshells had yellow stains (271).

In the above cases of ochratoxicosis described by Hamilton et al. (153), ochratoxins A, B, and C were identified in seven naturally contaminated feed samples at a ratio of 90:8:2, respectively. Ochratoxins B and C were found only in samples with high concentrations of ochratoxin A.

EXPERIMENTAL DISEASE. Experimental mycotoxicosis caused by ochratoxin A in poultry causes primarily renal disease but also influences hepatic, immunologic, and hematopoietic functions, and has significant interactions with disease agents like bursal disease or coccidia (47, 389), other toxins (168, 178, 188, 191, 192, 216), and nutrients (210, 211). Severe intoxication causes clinical signs of reduced spontaneous activity, huddling, hypothermia, diarrhea, rapid reductions in body weight, and death (128, 295). Dietary ochratoxicosis induces hypotension and bradycardia in broiler chickens (313). Sublethal intoxication can seriously impair performance parameters including weight gain, feed conversion, pigmentation, carcass yield (189), egg production, fertility, and hatchability. Dose-effect studies of ochratoxins for poultry have been reported (49, 50, 66, 67, 70, 102, 108, 128, 180, 184, 188, 210, 294–296, 279, 301, 359, 362).

Pathology. Acute lethal ochratoxin A mycotoxicosis in chickens causes gross lesions of liver, pancreas and kidney pallor, kidney swelling, and white urate deposits in the ureter, on the kidney, heart, pericardium, liver, and spleen (visceral gout) (103, 128, 182, 279). The main histopathologic alteration is acute tubular nephrosis characterized by proteinaceous and urate casts, heterophil inflammation, and focal necrosis of tubular epithelium (279). Some chicks develop cytoplasmic vacuolation and focal necrosis of hepatocytes, followed by foci of fibrosis. Hematopoiesis is suppressed in the bone marrow and lymphocyte depletion occurs in spleen and bursa of Fabricius.

Subacute ochratoxin A mycotoxicosis in turkeys, ducklings, and chickens is characterized by increased weight of liver and kidney and decreased weight of lymphoid organs. The kidney is pale (106). Bile may be pale and less viscous and the intestine has catarrhal content. Intestinal fragility is associated with apparent decreases in collagen (380), although inflammation may play a role (see below).

Broilers provided dietary ochratoxin A develop soft bones (106), manifested as increased diameter of the tibia relative to the body weight (183). The force required to break the tibia is decreased and displacement at the failure is increased. The histologic changes are characterized by generalized skeletal osteopenia with disturbed endochondral and intramembranous bone formation (105). Osteoid formation is defective and osteoporosis develops. Changes in the diaphyseal cortices account for the reduced breaking strength of bones.

In the kidney, histologic alterations including tubular casts, tubular dilation, and hyperplasia of tubular epithelium account for the enlargement seen grossly (182, 234). Interstitial inflammatory cells are found in duck and chicken kidneys (39,

106). Thickening of glomerular basement membranes is dose related.

Ochratoxin A causes vacuolar change in hepatocytes, associated with reversible increases in glycogen content of liver and skeletal muscle in chickens (110, 185, 381). In ducks, hepatocyte vacuolation is due to lipid accumulation (39), and in Japanese quail, is accompanied by bile duct proliferation and enlarged hepatocyte nuclei (102).

Severe lymphoid depletion occurs in the bursa of Fabricius, thymus, spleen, harderian gland, and intestinal lymphoid organs. The intestinal lamina propria is expanded by heterophil infiltration, and there is heterophil inflammation of the muscular zones of the intestine, glands, and crypts (106).

Chronic (341 days) ochratoxicosis in hens (209, 353) reduces renal function, but no lesions are seen at necropsy. Mild histologic lesions occur in proximal and distal tubules as ballooning of epithelial cells, karyomegalic cells, reduction of the brush border, and necrosis. Mitotic figures are increased in number and appear abnormal.

The ultrastructural pathology of ochratoxin A has been studied in broiler and leghorn chickens, and in ducklings. Ochratoxin A nephrotoxicity in broiler chickens originates from sensitivity of mitochondria in the proximal tubules (110). Mitochondria develop ring forms and have increased size and number of dense granules. Increased cytoplasmic peroxisomes, intranuclear and cytoplasmic lipid droplets, and electron-dense round bodies in dilated smooth endoplasmic reticulum are also seen in tubular epithelium. Lesions in duckling and leghorn chicken kidneys closely resemble those in broilers (30, 39). Abnormal mitochondrial forms and swollen endoplasmic reticulum also occur in duck hepatocytes (358). In broiler chicken glomeruli, the basement membrane is thickened and degenerated. This lesion in ducklings is related to the glomerular IgG deposition.

Citrinin-induced ultrastructural lesions are similar to those caused by ochratoxin A, but milder, and chicks fed both compounds in combination develop ultrastructural lesions attributable to both mycotoxins (30). Ultrastructural lesion severity is dose related and is diminished when toxic feed is withdrawn.

Reproduction and Egg Production. Ochratoxicosis in Leghorn pullets delays sexual maturity and may block it entirely (67). For hens in production at the onset of low-level intoxication, egg weight and production begin to decrease within 2 wk (294). Body weight also declines as feed intake is reduced. Leghorn hens have marked reluctance to eat feed contaminated with ochratoxin A (298).

Ochratoxin A reduces egg size, interior quality, and shell specific gravity (a measure of shell quality) at concentrations that have no significant effect on hen-day production (359). Increases in water consumption, paleness of combs, and mortality also occur. At necropsy, hens may have increased weight of the liver and kidneys without overt histopathologic changes.

Japanese quail breeding stock experiencing ochratoxicosis have reduced hatchability due to early embryonic death. Fertility is unaffected. Early deaths are caused by mycotoxin rather than alteration of gametes (296). Hatchability is also reduced for leghorns (66) and progeny have reduced growth. Ochratoxin A is teratogenic for chicken embryos (136).

Immunosuppression. Immunosuppressive effects of ochratoxin A in poultry (see review 38) stem chiefly from thymic atrophy (106, 107), although all lymphoid organs appear subject to atrophy in poultry species. Cell-mediated immunity is impaired in both broiler chickens and turkeys (108).

Humoral immunity is also influenced by ochratoxin A. Lymphoid organ atrophy is attributable, in part, to fewer immunoglobulin-containing cells (107). Serum immunoglobulin concentrations are reduced, but immunoglobulins, especially IgG, are prevalent in the glomerular basement membrane and in the renal parenchyma of hens.

Phagocytic activity of chicken heterophils is impaired by ochratoxin A (46).

Ochratoxin A, like aflatoxin, interacts with coccidiosis (*Eimeria* spp.) to influence body weight, feed efficiency, and pigmentation, greater than either disease alone (179).

Nutrition and Digestion. Addition of ochratoxin A to experimental diets confirmed field observations of feed refusal by turkeys but not broiler chickens (34, 35). Feed refusal is also seen in leghorn hens (298).

Ochratoxin A impairs the ability of broiler chickens to utilize dietary carotenoids for carcass pigmentation by affecting metabolism at five separate loci. Carotenoids are diluted in intestinal contents, uptake is depressed in intestinal mucosa, transport is depressed in the serum, hepatic accumulation is impaired, and acetylation steps are altered in the integument (327).

Vanadium and ochratoxin A, given in dietary combinations at concentrations as occur naturally, have enhanced toxicity in broiler and leghorn chicks. Body weight and serum albumen, calcium, and phosphorus are decreased; serum uric acid is increased; and histologic lesions in the kidneys are more severe as a result of the interaction (211, 213).

Combined ochratoxin A and tannic acid intoxication causes pronounced impairment of body weight and feed efficiency in broiler chickens (210).

Hematology. Ochratoxin A induces iron-deficiency anemia in broiler chickens (184). Reductions in packed-cell volume occur without reduction in circulating erythrocytes, but the mean corpuscular volume and mean corpuscular hemoglobin concentration are reduced. This is accompanied by reduction in the serum iron concentration and transferrin saturation; total iron-binding capacity is unaffected.

Broiler chickens and turkeys develop a reduction in total circulating leukocytes, due to decreases in lymphocytes and monocytes (49, 50).

Coagulation. Ochratoxicosis in broiler chickens has no effect on whole-blood clotting time, but increases recalcification and prothrombin times (98). Ochratoxin severely depresses factor VII and fibrinogen (98). Ochratoxicosis in leghorn hens also causes reduced prothrombin times (294).

Serum Chemistry. Ochratoxin A mycotoxicosis serum chemical alterations reflect nephrotoxicity and hepatotoxicity. Increased serum uric acid is a consistent indicator of toxin-induced renal disease in poultry (50, 210). Creatine, alkaline phosphatase, cholinesterase, and gamma glutamyltransferase are increased (193, 213). Reductions occur in concentrations of serum total protein, albumen, immunoglobulins (107), cholesterol, triglyceride, blood urea nitrogen, carotenoids (327), calcium, phosphorus, potassium, and glucose (193, 211). Indicators of renal function (inulin clearance, para-aminohippuric acid clearance, phenol red clearance, urine concentration) reflect reduced function in both hens and broiler chickens (182, 209, 353).

METABOLISM AND RESIDUES. Dietary ochratoxin A distributes widely in the chicken (129) chiefly to the kidney, with lesser concentrations in liver and muscle (124). The biological half-life in chickens is about 4 hr, and elimination from chicken tissues is almost total within 48 hr.

Ochratoxin A distributes to eggs in yolk and albumin (124), which accounts for its effects on hatchability. Concentrations of ochratoxin A in eggs have low correlation to dose, and several studies found no ochratoxin A in eggs (209, 294).

Intravenous doses of ochratoxin A in Japanese quail rapidly distribute to liver, kidney, and to a lesser extent, proventriculus and ovary. Toxin is excreted in bile and in urine (125). Intestine thus accumulates relatively high concentrations of metabolites from the biliary pathway, and from the proventriculus and gizzard.

Liver and kidney are tissues of choice to monitor for ochratoxin A residues in poultry (241). Residues in skeletal muscle occur in higher concentrations in red (thigh) muscle than in white (breast) muscle. Residues persist for only a short time, 4 days or less, when toxic diets are replaced with feed clear of ochratoxin A (138, 297). Residues may occur in edible tissues without gross or microscopic lesions in kidneys (209).

Citrinin

ETIOLOGY AND TOXICOLOGY. Citrinin (see review 309) is a natural contaminant of corn, rice, and other cereal grains, and is produced by numerous species of *Penicillium* (72) and *Aspergillus*. First purified as a yellow crystalline compound from *P. citrinum* in 1931, it received considerable attention because of antibiotic properties against staphylococci and other gram-positive and gram-negative bacteria before the nephrotoxic properties were discovered. It is a cause of "yellow rice" mycotoxicosis in Japan, and has been implicated in porcine endemic nephropathy, which also involves ochratoxin A.

P. citrinum also produces other, undefined mycotoxins toxic to chickens (see **OTHER MYCOTOXICOSES**).

NATURAL DISEASE. Spontaneous citrinin mycotoxicosis has not been fully documented, but probably occurs. The natural occurrence of citrinin has been reported mainly from Canada and Denmark, suggesting toxigenic *Penicillium* may have a competitive advantage in cooler climates.

P. lanosum was isolated from broiler chicken feed from a house in which the litter was wet and chickens were substantially smaller than expected at slaughter (19). The isolate produced citrinin in culture (256). Corn-based fungal cultures fed to broiler chicks caused watery fecal droppings and reduced weight gain. At necropsy, kidneys were swollen and the gizzard lining was discolored and fissured. Histopathologic changes in kidney were limited to swelling of tubular epithelial cells and occasional pyknosis. Mycotic ventriculitis was confirmed, with fungus invasion of gizzard lining and attendant inflammation. *P. lanosum* was isolated from the gizzard.

EXPERIMENTAL DISEASE. Citrinin is moderately toxic to poultry (72, 234, 237–239, 257, 318, 373). Experimental mycotoxicosis confirms nephrotoxicity, first expressed as diuresis (145, 234). The diuretic effect is destroyed by heating the toxin to 105 C for 16 min (205).

Citrinin acts directly on kidney to transiently alter several tubular transport processes. Increases in urine flow rates and free-water clearance are accompanied by increases in fractional sodium, potassium, and inorganic phosphate excretion (165). Subsequent studies have not confirmed the phosphaturic effect (137). Increased solute excretion does not compensate for increased free-water clearance, and is reflected by a significant decrease in urine osmolality.

Pathology. At the single oral LD_{50}, citrinin is nephrotoxic to chickens, turkey poults, and Pekin ducklings, with turkeys being the most sensitive. Watery fecal droppings and increased water consumption occur with renal lesions of degeneration and necrosis of both proximal and distal tubular epithelium (237, 238). Turkey and chicken livers develop multifocal necrosis of hepatocytes accompanied by hemorrhage. Bile ductule proliferation follows hepatocyte necrosis in turkeys. Lymphocyte necrosis and depletion occur in major lymphoid tissues of each species; this is the most prominent lesion of acute citrinin mycotoxicosis in ducklings (239, 240).

Experimental subacute to chronic dietary toxicity of citrinin in Pekin ducklings results in reduced weight gain, and dose-related nephropathy characterized by degeneration, necrosis, mineralization, and regeneration of tubular epithelial cells in cortical and medullary regions (240). Severely affected kidneys have interstitial inflammation and fibrosis.

Ultrastructural renal pathology of citrinin in leghorn chicks involves proximal tubular epithelium and comprises intranuclear membrane-bound inclusions, elongated tortuous and ring-shaped mitochondria, and an increase in size and number of peroxisomes and secondary lysosomes. Some proximal tubular cells have cytoplasmic aggregates of smooth endoplasmic reticulum (30).

Egg Production. Citrinin-appended diets (250 mg/kg diet) fed to mature laying hens have no effect on egg production or body weight. This dose is capable of producing wet droppings, which resolve when a nontoxic diet is fed (9).

Immunity. Citrinin has no effect on either humoral or cell-mediated immunity in broiler chickens at doses causing nephrotoxicity and diuresis (40).

Hematology. Penicillium citrinum–contaminated corn containing citrinin causes anemia and leukopenia in leghorn chicks (319).

Serum Chemistry. Hyperkalemia and metabolic acidosis characterized by reduced blood pH and base excess occur during intoxication (240).

METABOLISM AND RESIDUES. Citrinin is found only in blood and liver of broiler chicks fed citrinin-appended diets (257).

Oosporein

ETIOLOGY AND TOXICOLOGY. Oosporein is a red, toxic, dibenzoquinone metabolite of *Chaetomium* spp. capable of causing gout and high mortality in poultry (77, 282). Oosporein (282) was originally isolated from *Oospora colorans* in 1944. *Chaetomium* spp. have been isolated from numerous feeds and grains, including peanuts, rice, and corn. Cultures are highly toxic in both plant and animal bioassays. *C. trilaterale* is of particular interest because it produces high concentrations of oosporein on a variety of substrates. *Chaetomium* spp. have been implicated in a growth-inhibition problem in sheep in Nova Scotia.

NATURAL DISEASE. Spontaneous oosporein mycotoxicosis occurs in poultry in both North and South America and is characterized by nephrotoxicity, gout, and mortality (392). In the USA, oosporein forms in milo and corn at concentrations of 1–2 mg/kg (29).

EXPERIMENTAL DISEASE. Experimental oosporein mycotoxicosis in young chickens and turkeys is characterized by visceral and articular gout related to impaired renal function and elevated plasma concentrations of uric acid (233, 281, 282). Chickens are more sensitive to oosporein than turkeys. Water consumption increases during intoxication and fecal droppings may be fluid.

Corn cultures of *Chaetomium*-producing oosporein are more toxic to chickens than the purified organic acid of oosporein. Sodium and potassium salts of oosporein are more toxic than the organic acid. Their existence in cultures and naturally contaminated grains explains apparent enhanced toxicity (233).

Pathology. Acute lethal oosporein toxicosis in chickens and turkeys causes dehydration, swollen pale kidneys, and extensive visceral gout (282, 283, 405). The liver is mottled and has focal necrosis and the gallbladder is distended with translucent green to yellow bile. The proventriculus has enlarged circumference at the isthmus, and the mucosa is covered with pseudomembranous exudate (necrosis may occur at the isthmus). Gizzard lining and intestinal contents are discolored green.

Subacute nonlethal intoxication in chickens and turkeys resembles the above description except visceral gout is either less pronounced or absent, and articular gout is more common. Histopathologic alterations of oosporein mycotoxicosis involve the kidney as proximal tubular nephrosis with periodic acid–Schiff (PAS)-positive granules in the macula densa, during the first 3 days (28). Interstitial granulomas around urate deposits are common. Chicks that survive to 21 days have marked interstitial fibrosis, hyperplasia of remaining proximal tubular epithelial cells, and dilation of centrilobular distal tubules. Glomeruli are atrophic in fibrotic areas, and enlarged in normal areas.

Egg Production. Oosporein reduces both feed consumption and egg production at doses capable of inducing nephrotoxicity and gout (405).

Hematology. Oosporein intoxication of broiler chickens has no effect on the packed cell volume or hemoglobin concentration (282).

Serum Chemistry. Plasma uric acid concentrations are elevated in chickens and turkeys. In turkeys, serum glutamic-oxalacetic transaminase and lactic dehydrogenase are elevated, and albumin, potassium, phosphorus, and calcium are decreased (282, 283). Leghorn hens experience decreases in serum calcium and phosphorus with transient increases in serum sodium (405).

OTHER MYCOTOXICOSES

Cyclopiazonic Acid. Cyclopiazonic acid (CPA) is a frequent metabolite of *Aspergillus flavus,* the predominant producer of aflatoxin in feeds and grains. Some of the features of turkey "X" disease in the UK in 1959 were not fully accountable to aflatoxin and may have been due to CPA (75). The toxin is also produced by *Penicillium* spp. It is a contaminant of meats, outer portions of cheeses (226), peanuts (221), corn, and millet (262).

In chickens, CPA causes impaired feed conversions, decreased weight gain, and mortality. Lesions occur in proventriculus, gizzard, liver and spleen (101). The proventriculus is dilated and the mucosa is thickened by hyperplasia and ulceration. Mucosal necrosis occurs in the gizzard. Liver and spleen contain numerous yellow foci of necrosis and inflammation.

CPA residues in chicken muscle can be detected at a concentration of 14% of a single oral dose, 48 hr after administration (262).

Sterigmatocystin. Sterigmatocystin is a biogenic precursor to aflatoxin B1 and is hepatotoxic and hepatocarcinogenic. It occurs less commonly than aflatoxin and is associated with visibly moldy products (290). Produced on cereal grains, coffee beans, and cheese by *Aspergillus versicolor* and other *Aspergillus* spp., *Chaetomium* spp., and other cereal fungi, sterigmatocystin is less toxic than aflatoxin, but is produced in higher concentrations (330).

Sterigmatocystin mycotoxicosis occurred when commercial crumbled mixed feed colonized with *Aspergillus glaucus* and containing sterigmatocystin (2.3 mg/kg diet) was consumed by 1600 laying hens (2). There was decreased feed intake, a 15–25% reduction in egg production, and pallor of brown-shelled eggs. At necropsy, livers were pale, fatty, and contained hemorrhages.

Experimental sterigmatocystin mycotoxicosis in leghorn chicks affects liver, pancreas, lymphoid organs, and kidney (349, 350). Liver is congested, and has multifocal hemorrhage and necrosis of periacinar hepatocytes, sometimes accompanied by heterophil infiltration. The pancreas has exocrine cell changes of zymogen granule loading and cytoplasmic vacuolation. Lymphocyte necrosis and depletion occur in the bursa of Fabricius and other lymphoid organs. Kidney has mild degenerative changes in tubular epithelium and necrosis of occasional tubular epithelial cells. Accompanying these morphological events are increases in serum aspartate aminotransferase, alanine aminotransferase, lactate dehydrogenase, conjugated bilirubin, amylase, and lipase, and decreases in gamma glutamyltransferase, total proteins, albumen, potassium, magnesium, phosphorus, and triglycerides. Total blood leukocytes are decreased, with mononuclear leukocytes decreased and granulocytic leukocytes increased.

Sterigmatocystin causes reduced embryonic weight, malformations, and mortality in chicken embryos (330).

Rubratoxin. Rubratoxins A and B are hepatotoxic mycotoxins produced by *Penicillium rubrum* and *P. purpurogenum* (384). The significance of these fungi and their effect on poultry was evident even before aflatoxicosis was defined as a distinct mycotoxicosis. In 1958, an investigation of the poultry hemorrhagic syndrome yielded these fungi from the feed and litter of affected chickens (119). It is noteworthy that *Aspergillus flavus* and *Penicillium citrinum,* producers of aflatoxins and citrinin respectively, were also studied (120). Chicks fed cultures of *P. rubrum* and *P. purpurogenum* developed bloody diarrhea. At necropsy, hemorrhages were in muscles and viscera, and erosions and free blood were in the proventriculus and gizzard. *P. rubrum* was more toxic than *P. purpurogenum.*

Despite the above implications, purified rubratoxin (20% A, 80% B) has relatively low toxicity for broiler chickens (393). Acute lethal intoxication produces gross lesions of red mottling and congestion of liver and kidneys, and minor hemorrhages on other viscera. Dietary rubratoxin causes impaired growth, liver enlargement, and atrophy of the bursa of Fabricius. Hemoglobin, serum protein, and serum cholesterol are reduced. Capillary fragility is increased.

Penicillic Acid. Penicillic acid, discovered in 1913, is a metabolite of numerous species of *Penicillium* and *Aspergillus* (186) and is potentially important to poultry because of high concentrations in corn and poultry feed.

Penicillic acid has low toxicity for broiler chickens. Purified toxin has minimal effect when fed at concentrations likely to occur naturally (186).

Tremorgens. Tremorgenic mycotoxins induce tremor, ataxia, and tonic clonic convulsions when administered to animals (83). Clinical disease and losses have occurred in cattle, sheep, and dogs

(12). These toxins are produced by several species of *Penicillium* and *Aspergillus* and include verruculogen, fumitremorgin B, and tremortin (penitrem) A, B, and C (71, 127, 385).

Experimental tremortin A mycotoxicosis in broiler chickens is characterized by acute onset and rapid recovery of dose-dependent tremors and other disorders of the nervous system (395). No impairment occurs in growth, and no lesions are observed at necropsy.

Tenuazonic Acid. Tenuazonic acid is a metabolite of *Alternaria* spp. with a spectrum of toxicologic and pharmacologic effects (132). Investigations of poultry hemorrhagic syndrome revealed marked toxicity of an isolate of *Alternaria* (120). *Alternaria* spp. are common to corn and agricultural commodities.

Tenuazonic acid has moderate toxicity for broiler and leghorn chickens (132). Acute lethal intoxication induces hemorrhages in thigh and breast muscles, on the heart, and in subcutaneous tissues. Subacute nonfatal intoxication has a similar distribution of hemorrhages. Erosions occur in the gizzard lining, and the spleen is pale and mottled.

Cultures of *Alternaria longipes* from tobacco are highly toxic to chicks and produce hemorrhages in the proventriculus and erosion of the gizzard lining (104, 345).

Slaframine. Slaframine toxicosis is a syndrome characterized by excessive salivation in cattle and other farm animals following ingestion of a fungal alkaloid produced by *Rhizoctonia leguminicola,* primarily on red clover forage (41). It causes cholinergic stimulation of exocrine glands, with salivation the most obvious effect.

Slaframine may ultimately benefit poultry. It has been evaluated as a tool to study hydrolytic enzyme activity in the chicken (122). Relatively small amounts affect digestive function of broiler chicks. Slaframine has been used to study cholinergic mechanisms for growth hormone release and effects on plasma glucose (123).

Patulin. Patulin is a mycotoxin produced by several species of *Aspergillus, Penicillium,* and *Byssochlamys.* Patulin-producing *Penicillium* spp. have been isolated from chick starter feed (72, 229). Patulin has relatively low toxicity for chicks. Toxin given by crop intubation produces watery crop content, followed by acute ascites and lumenal hemorrhage in the proventriculus, gizzard, and intestine.

Toxigenic Fungi Significant to Poultry. *Diplodia maydis,* a pathogen of worldwide economic importance in corn production (302), causes a mycotoxicosis in cattle and sheep in South Africa. Diplodiatoxin is the only toxic metabolite characterized for *D. maydis,* and heart is the target organ. Cultures of *D. maydis* from commercial corn are toxic to ducklings (302, 304), broiler chickens, and leghorn hens although apparently no pathology studies have been reported.

Phomopsis leptostromiformis is a fungus that grows on lupine plants and is the etiology of lupinosis, a hepatogenous photosensitizing disease of sheep. *Phomopsis* spp. and *Diaporthe phaseolorum* have been implicated as plant pathogens in the etiology of soybean seed decay. Cultures of each have been examined for toxicity to chickens. All are hepatotoxic in chicks and *P. leptostromiformis* is markedly so (217, 218). Acute intoxication results in focal necrosis and hemorrhage in liver. Subacute intoxication by *Phomopsis* spp. causes fat accumulation in hepatocytes, cholangitis, bile duct proliferation, Kupffer cell hypertrophy, fibrosis, and hepatocyte regeneration.

Helminthosporium maydis Race T, the cause of southern corn blight, is nontoxic to broiler and leghorn chickens (26, 399).

Penicillium citrinum produces, in addition to citrinin, uncharacterized metabolites toxic to poultry (320). Toxigenic cultures fed to leghorn chicks decrease feed intake and growth, and cause mortality. Hepatosis and nephrosis are the principal pathologic changes, but lymphoid tissues, pancreas, bone marrow, intestine, and skeletal and cardiac muscle also have degenerative changes.

DIAGNOSIS.

A definitive diagnosis of mycotoxicosis involves isolation, identification, and quantification of specific toxin(s). This is usually difficult in the modern poultry industry because of the rapid and voluminous use of feed and ingredients. The analytical capability of diagnostic laboratories is also a factor (269). Analyses for aflatoxin and zearalenone are readily available, but analyses for ochratoxins, zearalenol, deoxynivalenol, T-2 toxin, diacetoxyscirpenol, ergot alkaloids, and citrinin are less available. Confirmation of a mycotoxicosis involving other trichothecenes, cyclopiazonic acid, sterigmatocystin, rubratoxin, and other lesser metabolites of potential detriment to poultry, is possible in only a few laboratories.

Analytical techniques for mycotoxins are beyond the scope of this review but include chromatography (thin-layer, gas, liquid), mass spectrometry, and monoclonal antibody–based technology. The black-light evaluation of grains for *Aspergillus flavus* growth is an acceptable presumptive test for aflatoxin, but does not confirm actual toxin (23). Numerous bioassays are defined for mycotoxin screening tests, but positive test results are presumptive. Consult with a laboratory before sending samples, as they differ in their capabilities to conduct screening and confirmation tests for mycotoxins.

A complete diagnostic evaluation including necropsy, histopathology, bacterial and viral cultures, and serology are necessary adjuncts to feed analysis if mycotoxicosis is suspected. Other diseases may be occurring in concert with mycotoxins to adversely affect production. A flock rarely has a single disease stress. Sometimes a mycotoxicosis is suspected but not confirmed by feed analysis. In these situations, a complete laboratory evaluation can exclude other significant diseases (174). Birds that have died recently and those obviously sick should be selected for submission.

Moldy feeds may be unpalatable (33), appear unwholesome, and have diminished nutritive value, especially energy level (18), fats, vitamins, and amino acids (17, 250, 317). Fungal activity in feed may reduce performance, but reduced performance is not definitive evidence of a mycotoxicosis. Many things influence performance. Fungi in feed indicate mycotoxin formation could occur. *Aspergillus, Penicillium,* and *Fusarium,* all mycotoxin-producing fungal genera, are found in most poultry feeds, so the potential is clearly evident (253).

Feed and ingredient samples should be properly collected and promptly submitted to a feed testing laboratory for analysis. Mycotoxin formation is often not uniform in a batch of feed or grain. Multiple samples from different sites increase the likelihood of confirming a mycotoxin formation zone ("hot spot").

Samples should be collected at all possible sites in the chain of ingredient storage, feed manufacture and transport, feed bins, and feeders within poultry houses. Fungal activity increases as feed is moved from the feed mill to feeder pans (200), associated with an increase in fines and higher zinc concentrations. Samples of 500 g (1 lb) should be collected and submitted in separate containers. Clean paper bags, properly labeled, are adequate. Sealed plastic or glass containers are appropriate only for short-term storage and transport because grain rapidly deteriorates in air-tight containers.

TREATMENT. Removal of toxic feed and replacement with unadulterated feed is an important first step. Poultry recover from most mycotoxicoses soon after an uncontaminated diet is available. Treatment of concurrent diseases (parasitic, bacterial) will alleviate additive or synergistic interactions on production parameters. Substandard management practices are especially detrimental to poultry stressed by mycotoxins and should be corrected.

Vitamins, trace minerals (especially selenium), protein, and lipid requirements are increased by some mycotoxins and can be compensated by feed formulation and water-administered treatment.

Nonspecific toxicologic therapies using activated charcoal (digestive tract adsorption) in feed and phenobarbital (enhanced metabolism) in drinking water have been shown to have a sparing effect on aflatoxicosis in poultry (89). These treatments are experimental only but indicate possible additional strategies.

PREVENTION. Prevention of mycotoxicoses requires acquisition of mycotoxin-free feedstuffs, and application of feed manufacturing and management practices that prevent mold growth and mycotoxin formation. This ideally requires access to sufficient laboratory capability to confirm the purchase of ingredients free of mycotoxins, proper storage of ingredients, and feed processing, shipping, and handling procedures to minimize formation. A quality-control program can monitor success of these practices (355).

Rapid, on-site screening tests for several mycotoxins (aflatoxin, T-2 toxin, ochratoxin, zearalenone) are available in monoclonal antibody–based detection kits. Many poultry companies already routinely test grain for aflatoxin contamination by screening grains for green fluorescence under a black light to estimate the degree of *Aspergillus flavus* contamination, and aflatoxin confirmation by a chromatographic procedure (minicolumn technique).

Mycotoxins form in decayed, crusted, built-up feed in feeders, feed mills, and storage bins (149). Regular inspection of feed bins identifies flow problems like feed separation, central-feed-down, and feed bridging (360), which enhance fungal activity and mycotoxin formation. Temperature extremes cause condensation and migration in bins and create high-risk situations for mycotoxin formation (391). Bin inspection and cleaning between flocks to certify absence of feed residue is important. Tandem feed bins allow cleaning between successive feed deliveries. Minimum feed residence time is important, even under cool, dry conditions (139). Poultry house ventilation to reduce relative humidity affects moisture available for fungal growth and toxin formation in feeders (202). Selection of feeder equipment that minimizes surface-area contact with feed diminishes mycotoxin formation (201).

Antifungal agents added to feeds to prevent fungal growth have no effect on toxin already formed, but may be cost-effective management in conjunction with other feed management practices. Organic acids are effective (92, 203), but their effectiveness may be reduced by particle size of feed (93) and buffering by certain ingredients (94). Organic acids are corrosive and irritating to skin, but some have been modified to counteract this characteristic (276). Gentian violet (53, 204) and thiabendazole (126) have shown effectiveness. Copper sulfate is a poor mold inhibitor for poultry feeds (87).

Pelleting feed has among its numerous benefits

destruction of fungal spores (356), and a decrease in the fungal burden. The combination of pelleting and an antifungal agent has additional effectiveness. Pelleting, however, may increase the severity of ergotism (see **ERGOTISM**).

Zeolytes, silica-containing compounds used as anticaking agents and as a shell-quality aid, show promise as practical and economical feed additives to reduce the effects of certain mycotoxins. Hydrated sodium calcium aluminosilicate binds aflatoxin B1 in the digestive tract, possibly by sequestration, and reduces toxicity to chickens (286).

REFERENCES

1. Abdullah, A.S., and O.B. Lee. 1981. Aflatoxicosis in ducks. Kajian Vet 13:33–36.

2. Abramson, D., J.T. Mills, and B.R. Boycott. 1983. Mycotoxins and mycoflora in animal feedstuffs in western Canada. Can J Comp Med 47:23–26.

3. Adams, R.L., and J. Tuite. 1976. Feeding Gibberella zeae damaged corn to laying hens. Poult Sci 55:1991–1993.

4. Allen, N.K., C.J. Mirocha, S.A. Allen, J.J. Bitgood, G. Weaver, and F. Bates. 1981. Effect of dietary zearalenone on reproduction of chickens. Poult Sci 60:1165–1174.

5. Allen, N.K., H.R. Burmeister, G.A. Weaver, and C.J. Mirocha. 1981. Toxicity of dietary and intravenously administered moniliformin to broiler chickens. Poult Sci 60:1415–1417.

6. Allen, N.K., C.J. Mirocha, G. Weaver, S. Aakhus-Allen, and F. Bates. 1981. Effects of dietary zearalenone on finishing broiler chickens and young turkey poults. Poult Sci 60:124–131.

7. Allen, N.K., R.L. Jevne, C.J. Mirocha, and Y.W. Lee. 1982. The effect of a Fusarium roseum culture and diacetoxyscirpenol on reproduction of white leghorn females. Poult Sci 61:2172–2175.

8. Allen, N.K., A. Peguri, C.J. Mirocha, and J.A. Newman. 1983. Effects of Fusarium cultures, T-2 toxin, and zearalenone on reproduction of turkey females. Poult Sci 62:282–289.

9. Ames, D.D., R.D. Wyatt, H.L. Marks, and K.W. Washburn. 1976. Effect of citrinin, a mycotoxin produced by Penicillium citrinum, on laying hens and young broiler chicks. Poult Sci 55:1294–1301.

10. Arafa, A.S., R.J. Bloomer, H.R. Wilson, C.F. Simpson, and R.H. Harms. 1981. Susceptibility of various poultry species to dietary aflatoxin. Br Poult Sci 22:431–436.

11. Archibald, R.M., H.J. Smith, and J.D. Smith. 1962. Brazilian groundnut toxicosis in Canadian broiler chickens. Can Vet J 3:322–325.

12. Arp, L.H., and J.L. Richard. 1979. Intoxication of dogs with the mycotoxin penitrem A. J Am Vet Med Assoc 175:565–566.

13. Asplin, F.D., and R.B.A. Carnaghan. 1961. The toxicity of certain groundnut meals for poultry with special reference to their effect on ducklings and chickens. Vet Rec 73:1215–1219.

14. Bacon, C.W., and H.L. Marks. 1976. Growth of broilers and quail fed Fusarium (Gibberella zeae)-infected corn and zearalenone (F-2). Poult Sci 55:1531–1435.

15. Bacon, C.W., J.G. Sweeney, J.D. Robbins, and D. Burdick. 1973. Production of penicillic acid and ochratoxin A on poultry feed by Aspergillus ochraceus: Temperature and moisture requirements. Appl Environ Microbiol 26:155–160.

16. Bamburg, J.R., and F.M. Strong. 1971. 12,13-epoxytrichothecenes. In S. Kadis, A. Ciegler, and S.J. Ajl (eds.), Microbial Toxins, pp.207–289. Academic Press, New York.

17. Bartov, I., and N. Paster. 1986. Effect of early stages of fungal development on the nutritional value of diets for broiler chicks. Br Poult Sci 27:415–420.

18. Bartov, I., N. Paster, and N. Lisker. 1982. The nutritional value of moldy grains for broiler chicks. Poult Sci 61:2247–2254.

19. Beasley, J.N., L.D. Blalock, T.S. Nelson, and G.E. Templeton. 1980. The effect of feeding corn molded with Penicillium lanosum to broiler chicks. Poult Sci 59:708–713.

20. Bird, F.H. 1978. The effect of aflatoxin B1 on the utilization of cholecalciferol by chicks. Poult Sci 57:1293–1296.

21. Bock, R.R., L.S. Shore, Y. Samberg, and S. Perl. 1986. Death in broiler breeders due to salpingitis: Possible role of zearalenone. Avian Pathol 15:495–502.

22. Boonchuvit, B., P.B. Hamilton, and H.R. Burmeister. 1975. Interaction of T-2 toxin with Salmonella infections of chickens. Poult Sci 54:1693–1696.

23. Bothast, R.J., and C.W. Hesseltine. 1975. Bright greenish-yellow fluorescence and aflatoxin in agricultural commodities. Appl Microbiol 30:337–338.

24. Bragg, D.B., H.A. Salem, and T.J. Devlin. 1970. Effect of dietary triticale ergot on the performance and survival of broiler chicks. Can J Anim Sci 50:259–264.

25. Briggs, D.M., R.D. Wyatt, and P.B. Hamilton. 1974. The effect of dietary aflatoxin on semen characteristics of mature broiler breeder males. Poult Sci 53:2115–2119.

26. Britton, W.M. 1971. The influence of a diet containing Helminthosporium maydis blighted corn on laying hen performance. Poult Sci 50:1209–1212.

27. Britton W.M., and R.D. Wyatt. 1978. Effect of dietary aflatoxin on vitamin D_3 metabolism in chicks. Poult Sci 57:163–165.

28. Brown, T.P. 1986. Comparison of renal changes in chickens due to postmortem interval, estrogen, oosporein, citrinin, or ochratoxin A. Diss Abstr B Sci Eng 47:1445–1446.

29. Brown, T.P. 1988. Personal communication.

30. Brown, T.P., R.O. Manning, O.J. Fletcher, and R.D. Wyatt. 1986. The individual and combined effects of citrinin and ochratoxin A on renal ultrastructure in layer chicks. Avian Dis 30:191–198.

31. Bryden, W.L., R.B. Cumming, and A.B. Lloyd. 1980. Sex and strain responses to aflatoxin B1 in the chicken. Avian Pathol 9:539–550.

32. Bryden, W.L., A.B. Lloyd, and R.B. Cumming. 1980. Aflatoxin contamination of Australian animal feeds and suspected cases of mycotoxicosis. Aust Vet J 56:176–180.

33. Burditt, S.J., W.M. Hagler, Jr., and P.B. Hamilton. 1983. Survey of moulds and mycotoxins for their ability to cause feed refusal in chickens. Poult Sci 62:2187–2191.

34. Burditt, S.J., W.M. Hagler, Jr., J.E. Hutchins, and P.B. Hamilton. 1983. Models of feed refusal syndrome in poultry. Poult Sci 62:2158–2163.

35. Burditt, S.J., W.M. Hagler, Jr., and P.B. Hamilton. 1984. Feed refusal during ochratoxicosis in turkeys. Poult Sci 63:2172–2174.

36. Burguera, J.A., G.T. Edds, and O. Osuna. 1983. Influence of selenium on aflatoxin B1 or crotalaria toxicity in turkey poults. Am J Vet Res 44:1714–1717.

37. Burmeister, H.R., A. Ciegler, and R.F. Vesonder. 1979. Moniliformin, a metabolite of Fusarium monili-

forme NRRL 6322: Purification and toxicity. Appl Environ Microbiol 37:11–13.

38. Burns, R.B., and P. Dwivedi. 1986. The natural occurrence of ochratoxin A and its effects in poultry. A review. II. Pathology and immunology. World Poult Sci J 42:48–55.

39. Burns, R.B., and M.H. Maxwell. 1987. Ochratoxicosis A in young khaki campbell ducklings. Res Vet Sci 42:395–403.

40. Campbell, M.L., Jr., J.A Doerr, and R.D. Wyatt. 1981. Immune status in broiler chickens during citrinin toxicosis. Poult Sci 60:1634. (Abstr).

41. Carlton, W.W. 1976. Mycotoxicoses in animals and humans. Proc Am Phytopathol Soc 3:140–155.

42. Carlton, W.W., and P. Krogh. 1979. Ochratoxins. In W. Shimoda (ed.), Conf Mycotoxins Anim Feeds Grains Related Anim Health, pp. 165–287. US Food and Drug Admin Rep No FDA/BVM-79/139.

43. Carnaghan, R.B.A., G. Lewis, D.S.P. Patterson, and R. Allcroft. 1966. Biochemical and pathological aspects of groundnut poisoning in chickens. Pathol Vet 3:601–615.

44. Chang, C.F., and P.B. Hamilton. 1979. Impairment of phagocytosis in chicken monocytes during aflatoxicosis. Poult Sci 58:562–566.

45. Chang, C.F., and P.B. Hamilton. 1979. Refractory phagocytosis by chicken thrombocytes during aflatoxicosis. Poult Sci 58:559–561.

46. Chang, C.F., and P.B. Hamilton. 1980. Impairment of phagocytosis by heterophils from chickens during ochratoxicosis. Appl Environ Microbiol 39:572–575.

47. Chang, C.F., and P.B. Hamilton. 1982. Increased severity and new symptoms of infectious bursal disease during aflatoxicosis in broiler chickens. Poult Sci 61:1061–1068.

48. Chang, C.F., and P.B. Hamilton. 1982. Experimental aflatoxicosis in young Japanese quail. Poult Sci 61:869–874.

49. Chang, C.F., W.E. Huff, and P.B. Hamilton. 1979. A leukocytopenia induced in chickens by dietary ochratoxin A. Poult Sci 58:555–558.

50. Chang, C.F., J.A. Doerr, and P.B. Hamilton. 1981. Experimental ochratoxicosis in turkey poults. Poult Sci 60:114–119.

51. Chen, C., A.M. Pearson, T.H. Coleman, J.I. Gray, J.J. Peska, and S. K. Aust. 1984. Metabolite deposition and clearance of aflatoxins from broiler chickens fed a contaminated diet. Food Chem Toxicol 22:447–451.

52. Chen, C., A.M. Pearson, T.H. Coleman, J.I. Gray, and A.M. Wolzak. 1985. Br Poult Sci 26:65–71.

53. Chen, T.C., and E.J. Day. 1974. Gentian violet as a possible fungal inhibitor in poultry feed: Plate assays on its antifungal activity. Poult Sci 53:1791–1795.

54. Chi, M.S., C.J. Mirocha. 1978. Necrotic oral lesions in chickens fed diacetoxyscirpenol, T-2 toxin, and crotocin. Poult Sci 57:807–808.

55. Chi, M.S., C.J. Mirocha, H.J. Kurtz, G. Weaver, F. Bates, and W. Shimoda. 1977. Effects of T-2 toxin on reproductive performance and health of laying hens. Poult Sci 56:628–637.

56. Chi, M.S., C.J. Mirocha, H.J. Kurtz, G. Weaver, F. Bates, W. Shimoda, and H.R. Burmeister. 1977. Acute toxicity of T-2 toxin in broiler chicks and laying hens. Poult Sci 56:103–116.

57. Chi, M.S., C.J. Mirocha, H.J. Kurtz, G. Weaver, F. Bates, and W. Shimoda. 1977. Subacute toxicity of T-2 toxin in broiler chicks. Poult Sci 56:306–313.

58. Chi, M.S., T.S. Robison, C.J. Mirocha, and K.R. Reddy. 1978. Acute toxicity of 12,13-epoxytrichothecenes in one-day-old broiler chicks. Appl Environ Microbiol 35:636–640.

59. Chi, M.S., T.S. Robison, C.J. Mirocha, S.P. Swanson, and W. Shimoda. 1978. Excretion and tissue distribution of radioactivity from tritium-labeled T-2 toxin in chicks. Toxicol Appl Pharmacol 45:391–402.

60. Chi, M.S., C.J. Mirocha, H.J. Kurtz, G.A. Weaver, F. Bates, T. Robison, and W. Shimoda. 1980. Effect of dietary zearalenone on growing broiler chicks. Poult Sci 59:531–536.

61. Chi, M.S., C.J. Mirocha, G.A. Weaver, and H.J. Kurtz. 1980. Effect of zearalenone on female white leghorn chickens. Appl Environ Microbiol 39:1026–1030.

62. Chi, M.S., M.E. El-Halawani, P.E. Waibel, and C.J. Mirocha. 1981. Effects of T-2 toxin on brain catecholamines and selected blood components in growing chickens. Poult Sci 60:137–141.

63. Chiba, J., N. Nakano, N. Morooka, S. Nakazawa, and Y. Wanatabe. 1972. Inhibitory effects of fusarenon X, a sesquiterpene mycotoxin, on lipid synthesis and phosphate uptake in Tetrahymena pyriformis. Jpn J Med Sci Biol 25:291–296.

64. Chipley, J.R., M.S. Mabee, K.L. Applegate, and M.S. Dreyfuss. 1974. Further characterization of tissue distribution and metabolism of [14C] aflatoxin B1 in chickens. Appl Microbiol 28:1027–1029.

65. Choudary, C., and M.R. Rao. 1982. An outbreak of aflatoxicosis in commercial poultry farms. Poult Advis 16:75–76.

66. Choudhury, H., and C.W. Carlson. 1973. The lethal dose of ochratoxin for chick embryos. Poult Sci 52:1202–1203.

67. Choudhury, H., C.W. Carlson, and G. Semeniuk. 1971. A study of ochratoxin toxicity in hens. Poult Sci 50:1855–1859.

68. Christensen, C.M. 1979. Zearalenone. In W. Shimoda (ed.), Conf Mycotoxins Anim Feeds Grains Related Anim Health, pp. 1–79. US Food and Drug Admin Rep No FDA/BVM-79/139.

69. Christensen, C.M., R.A. Meronuck, G.H. Nelson, and J.C. Behrens. 1972. Effects on turkey poults of rations containing corn invaded by Fusarium tricinctum (cda.) Sny. & Hans. Appl Microbiol 23:177–179.

70. Chu, F.S., C.C. Chang. 1971. Sensitivity of chicks to ochratoxins. J Assoc Off Anal Chem 54:1032–1034.

71. Ciegler, A. 1969. Tremorgenic toxin from Penicillium palitans. Appl Microbiol 18:128–129.

72. Ciegler, A., R.F. Vesonder, and L.K. Jackson. 1977. Production and biological activity of patulin and citrinin from Penicillium expansum. Appl Environ Microbiol 33:1004–1006.

73. Clarke, R.N., J.A. Doerr, and M.A. Ottinger. 1986. Relative importance of dietary aflatoxin and feed restriction of reproductive changes associated with aflatoxicosis in the maturing white leghorn male. Poult Sci 65:2239–2245.

74. Coffin, J.L., G.F. Combs, Jr. 1981. Impaired vitamin E status of chicks fed T-2 toxin. Poult Sci 60:385–392.

75. Cole, R.J. 1986. Etiology of turkey "X" disease in retrospect: A case for the involvement of cyclopiazonic acid. Mycotoxin Res 2:3–7.

76. Cole, R.J., J.W. Kirksey, H.G. Cutler, B.L. Doupnik, and J.C. Peckham. 1973. Toxin from Fusarium moniliforme: Effects on plants and animal. Science 179:1324–1326.

77. Cole, R.J., J.W. Kirksey, H.G. Cutler, and E.E. Davis. 1974. Toxic effects of oosporein from Chaetomium trilaterale. J Agric Food Chem 22:517–520.

78. Colwell, W.M., R.C. Ashley, D.G. Simmons, and P.B. Hamilton. 1973. The relative in vitro sensitivity to aflatoxin B1 of tracheal organ cultures prepared from

day-old chickens, ducks, Japanese quail, and turkeys. Avian Dis 17:166–172.

79. Cottier, G.J., C.H. Moore, U.L. Diener, and N.D. Davis. 1969. The effect of feeding four levels of aflatoxin on hatchability and subsequent performance of broilers. Poult Sci 48:1797. (Abstr).

80. Coulter, D.B., R.D. Wyatt, and R.G. Stewart. 1977. Electroretinograms from broilers fed aflatoxin and T-2 toxin. Poult Sci 56:1435–1439.

81. Cunningham, P. 1987. Mycotoxin problems appear to be growing worse. Poult Times 34(24):19.

82. Curtin, T.M., and J. Tuite. 1966. Emesis and refusal of feed in swine associated with Gibberella zeae-infected corn. Life Sci 5:1937–1944.

83. Cysewski, S.J. 1973. Paspalum staggers and tremorgen intoxication in animals. J Am Vet Med Assoc 163:1291–1292.

84. Dafalla, R., Y.M. Hassan, and S.E.I. Adam. 1987. Fatty and hemorrhagic liver and kidney syndrome in breeding hens caused by aflatoxin B1 and heat stress in the Sudan. Vet Human Toxicol 29:252–254.

85. Dafalla, R., A.I. Yagi, and S.E.I. Adam. 1987. Experimental aflatoxicosis in Hybro-type chicks: Sequential changes in growth and serum constituents and histopathological changes. Vet Human Toxicol 29:222–225.

86. Dailey, R.E., R.E. Reese, and E.A. Brouwer. 1980. Metabolism of [14C] zearalenone in laying hens. J Agric Food Chem 28:286–291.

87. Dale, N. 1987. Copper sulfate as mold inhibitor. Poult Digest 46:311.

88. Dale, N.M., R.D. Wyatt, and H.L. Fuller. 1980. Additive toxicity of aflatoxin and dietary tannins in broiler chicks. Poult Sci 59:2417–2420.

89. Dalvi, R.R., and C. McGowan. 1984. Experimental induction of chronic aflatoxicosis in chickens by purified aflatoxin B1 and its reversal by activated charcoal, phenobarbital, and reduced glutathione. Poult Sci 63:485–491.

90. D'Andrea, G.H., D.M. Dent, L. Nunley-Bearden, and S.M. Ho. 1987. Zearalenone incidence and toxicosis in Alabama. Auburn Vet 42:4–8

91. D'Andrea, G.H., L. Nunley-Bearden, D.M. Dent, and S.M. Ho. 1987. Aflatoxin incidence and toxicosis in Alabama. Auburn Vet 42:17–23.

92. Dixon, R.C., and P.B. Hamilton. 1981. Evaluation of some organic acids as mold inhibitors by measuring CO_2 production from feed and ingredients. Poult Sci 60:2182–2188.

93. Dixon, R.C., and P.B. Hamilton. 1981. Effect of feed ingredients on the antifungal activity of propionic acid. Poult Sci 60:2407–2411.

94. Dixon, R.C., and P.B. Hamilton. 1981. Effect of particle sizes of corn meal and a mold inhibitor on mold inhibition. Poult Sci 60:2412–2415.

95. Doerr, J.A. 1979. Mycotoxicosis and avian hemostasis. Diss Abstr B Sci Eng:4127.

96. Doerr, J.A., and P.B. Hamilton. 1981. Aflatoxicosis and intrinsic coagulation function in broiler chickens. Poult Sci 60:1406–1411.

97. Doerr, J.A., and M.A. Ottinger. 1980. Delayed reproductive development resulting from aflatoxicosis in juvenile Japanese quail. Poult Sci 59:1995–2001.

98. Doerr, J.A., W.E. Huff, H.T. Tung, R.D. Wyatt, and P.B. Hamilton. 1974. A survey of T-2 toxin, ochratoxin, and aflatoxin for their effects on the coagulation of blood in young broiler chickens. Poult Sci 53:1728–1734.

99. Doerr, J.A., R.D. Wyatt, and P.B. Hamilton. 1976. Impairment of coagulation function during aflatoxicosis in young chickens. Toxicol Appl Pharmacol 35:437–446.

100. Doerr, J.A., W.E. Huff, C.J. Wabeck, G.W. Chaloupka, J.D. May, and J.W. Merkley. 1983. Effects of low level chronic aflatoxicosis in broiler chickens. Poult Sci 62:1971–1977.

101. Dorner, J.W., R.J. Cole, L.G. Lomax, H.S. Gossar, and U.L. Diener. 1983. Cyclopiazonic acid production by Aspergillus flavus and its effects on broiler chickens. Appl Environ Microbiol 46:698–703.

102. Doster, R.C., G.H. Arscott, and R.O. Sinnhuber. 1973. Comparative toxicity of ochratoxin A and crude Aspergillus ochraceus culture extract in Japanese quail (Coturnix coturnix japonica). Poult Sci 52:2351–2353.

103. Doupnik, B., Jr., and J.C. Peckman. 1970. Mycotoxicity of Aspergillus ochraceus to chicks. Appl Microbiol 19:594–597.

104. Doupnik, B. Jr., and E.K. Sobers. 1968. Mycotoxicosis: Toxicity to chicks of Alternaria longipes isolated from tobacco. Appl Microbiol 16:1596–1597.

105. Duff, S.R.I., R.B. Burns, and P. Dwivedi. 1987. Skeletal changes in broiler chicks and turkey poults fed diets containing ochratoxin A. Res Vet Sci 43:301–307.

106. Dwivedi, P., and R.B. Burns. 1984. Pathology of ochratoxicosis A in young broiler chicks. Res Vet Sci 36:92–103.

107. Dwivedi, P., and R.B. Burns. 1984. Effect of ochratoxin A on immunoglobulins in broiler chicks. Res Vet Sci 36:117–121.

108. Dwivedi, P., and R.B. Burns. 1985. Immunosuppressive effects of ochratoxin A in young turkeys. Avian Pathol 14:213–225.

109. Dwivedi, P., and R.B. Burns. 1986. The natural occurrence of ochratoxin A and its effects in poultry. A review. Part I. Epidemiology and toxicity. World Poult Sci J 42:32–47.

110. Dwivedi, P., R.B. Burns, and M.H. Maxwell. 1984. Ultrastructural study of the liver and kidney in ochratoxicosis A in young broiler chicks. Res Vet Sci 36:104–116.

111. Dzuik, H.E., G.H. Nelson, G.E. Duke, S.K. Maheswaran, and M.S. Chi. 1978. Acquired resistance in poults to Pasteurella multocida (P-1059 strain) during aflatoxin consumption. Poult Sci 57:1251–1254.

112. Edds, G.R. 1979. Aflatoxins. In W. Shimoda (ed.), Conf Mycotoxins Anim Feeds Grains Related Anim Health, pp. 80–164. Rep No. FDA/BVM-79/139.

113. Edds, G.T., and O. Osuna. 1976. Aflatoxin B1 increases infectious disease losses in food animals. Proc US Anim Health Assoc 80:434–441.

114. Edds, G.T., K.P.C. Nair, and C.F. Simpson. 1973. Effect of aflatoxin B1 on resistance in poultry against cecal coccidiosis and Marek's disease. Am J Vet Res 34:819–826.

115. El-Banna, A.A., R.M.G. Hamilton, P.M. Scott, and H.L. Trenholm. 1983. Nontransmission of deoxynivalenol (vomitoxin) to eggs and meat in chickens fed deoxynivalenol-contaminated diets. J Agric Food Chem 31:1381–1384.

116. Elling, F., B. Hald, C. Jacobsen, and P. Krogh. 1975. Spontaneous toxic nephropathy in poultry associated with ochratoxin A. Acta Pathol Microbiol Scand [A] 83:739–741.

117. Exarchos, C.C., and R.F. Gentry. 1982. Effect of aflatoxin B1 on egg production. Avian Dis 26:191–195.

118. Featherston, W.R. 1973. Utilization of Gibberella-infected corn by chicks and rats. Poult Sci 52:2334–2335.

119. Forgacs, J., H. Koch, W.T. Carll, and R.H. White-Stevens. 1958. Additional studies on the relationship of mycotoxicoses to the poultry hemorrhagic syndrome. Am J Vet Res 19:744–753.

120. Forgacs, J., H. Koch, W.T. Carll, and R.H. White-Stevens. 1962. Mycotoxicoses I. Relationship of

toxic fungi to moldy-feed toxicosis in poultry. Avian Dis 6:363-381.

121. Fritz, J.C., P.B. Mislivec, G.W. Pla, B.N. Harrison, C.E. Weeks, and J.G. Dantzman. 1973. Toxicogenicity of moldy feed for young chicks. Poult Sci 52:1523-1530.

122. Froetschel, M.A., W.M. Hagler, Jr., W.J. Croom, Jr., J. Ort, and H.P. Broquist. 1987. Effects of chronic administration of slaframine on production and digestive function in broiler chicks. Poult Sci 66:357-362.

123. Froetschel, M.A., W.M. Hagler, Jr., W.J. Croom, Jr., J. Ort, T. J. Lauterio, J.M. Fernandez, D.L. Mann, H.P. Broquist, and C.G. Scanes. 1987. Research note: Effects of slaframine on circulating concentrations of growth hormone and glucose. Poult Sci 66:904-906.

124. Frye, C.E., and F.S. Chu. 1977. Distribution of ochratoxin A in chicken tissues and eggs. J Food Safety 1:147-159.

125. Fuchs, R., L.E. Applegren, S. Hagelberg, and K. Hult. 1988. Carbon-14-ochratoxin A distribution in the Japanese quail (Coturnix coturnix japonica) monitored by whole body autoradiography. Poult Sci 67:707-714.

126. Gabal, M.A. 1987. Preliminary study on the use of thiabendazole in the control of common toxigenic fungi in grain feed. Vet Human Toxicol 29:217-221.

127. Gallagher, R.T., and G.C.M. Latch. 1977. Production of the tremorgenic mycotoxins verruculogen and fumitremorgin B by Penicillium piscarium Westling. Appl Environ Microbiol 33:730-731.

128. Galtier, P., J. More, and M. Alvinerie. 1976. Acute and short-term toxicity of ochratoxin A in 10-day-old chicks. Food Cosmetol Toxicol 14:129-131.

129. Galtier, P., M. Alvinerie, and J.L. Charpenteau. 1981. The pharmacokinetic profiles of ochratoxin A in pigs, rabbits, and chickens. Food Cosmetol Toxicol 19:735-738.

130. Gardiner, M.R., B. Oldroyd. 1965. Avian aflatoxicosis. Aust Vet J 41:272-276.

131. Garlich, J.D., H.T. Tung, and R.B. Hamilton. 1973. The effects of short term feeding of aflatoxin on egg production and some plasma constituents of the laying hen. Poult Sci 52:2206-2211.

132. Giambrone, J.J., N.D. Davis, and U.L. Diener. 1978. Effect of tenuazonic acid on young chickens. Poult Sci 57:1554-1558.

133. Giambrone, J.J., U.L. Diener, N.D. Davis, V.S. Panangala, and F.J. Hoerr. 1985. Effects of aflatoxin on young turkeys and broiler chickens. Poult Sci 64:1678-1684.

134. Giambrone, J.J., U.L. Diener, N.D. Davis, V.S. Panangala, and F.J. Hoerr. 1985. Effects of purified aflatoxin on broiler chickens. Poult Sci 64:852-858.

135. Giambrone, J.J., U.L. Diener, N.D. Davis, V.S. Panangala, and F.J. Hoerr. 1985. Effect of purified aflatoxin on turkeys. Poult Sci 64:859-865.

136. Gilani, S.H., J. Bancroft, and M. O'Rahily. 1975. The teratogenic effects of ochratoxin A in the chick embryo. Teratology 11:18A.

137. Glahn, R.P., and R.F. Wideman, Jr. 1987. Avian diuretic response to renal portal infusions of the mycotoxin citrinin. Poult Sci 66:1316-1325.

138. Golinnski, P., J. Chelkowski, A. Konarkowski, and K. Szebiotko. 1982. Mycotoxins in cereal grain. Part IV. The effect of ochratoxin A on growth and tissue residues of the mycotoxin in broiler chickens. Nahrung 27:251-256.

139. Good, R.E., and P.B. Hamilton. 1981. Beneficial effect of reducing the feed residence time in a field problem of suspected moldy feed. Poult Sci 60:1403-1405.

140. Greenhalgh, R., G.A. Neish, and J.D. Miller. 1983. Deoxynivalenol, acetyl deoxynivalenol, and zearalenone formation by Canadian isolates of Fusarium graminearum on solid substrates. Appl Environ Microbiol 46:625-629.

141. Greenway, J.A., and R. Puls. 1976. Fusariotoxicosis from barley in British Columbia. I. Natural occurrence and diagnosis. Can J Comp Med 40:12-15.

142. Gregory, J.F., III, and G.T. Edds. 1984. Effect of dietary selenium on the metabolism of aflatoxin B1 in turkeys. Food Chem Toxicol 22:637-642.

143. Gregory, J.F., III, S.L. Goldstein, and G.T. Edds. 1983. Metabolite distribution and rate of residue clearance in turkeys fed a diet containing aflatoxin B1. Food Chem Toxicol 21:463-467.

144. Gumbmann, M.R., S.N. Williams, A.N. Booth, P. Vohra, R.A. Earnst, and M. Bethard. 1970. Aflatoxin susceptibility in various breeds of poultry. Proc Soc Exp Biol Med 134:683-688.

145. Gustavson, S.A., J.M. Cockrill, J.N. Beasley, and T.S. Nelson. 1981. Effect of dietary citrinin on urine excretion in broiler chickens. Avian Dis 25:827-830.

146. Hagler, W.M., Jr., K. Tyczkowska, and P.B. Hamilton. 1984. Simultaneous occurence of deoxynivalenol, zearalenone, and aflatoxin in 1982 scabby wheat from the midwestern United States. Appl Environ Microbiol 47:151-154.

147. Haliburton, J.C., R.F. Vesonder, T.F. Lock, and W.B. Buck. 1979. Equine leucoencephalomalacia (ELEM): A study of Fusarium moniliforme as an etiologic agent. Vet Human Toxicol 21:348-351.

148. Hamilton, P.B. 1971. A natural and extremely severe occurrence of alfatoxicosis in laying hens. Poult Sci 50:1880-1882.

149. Hamilton, P.B. 1975. Proof of mycotoxicoses being a field problem and a simple method for their control. Poult Sci 54:1706-1708.

150. Hamilton, P.B., and J.D. Garlich. 1972. Failure of vitamin supplementation to alter the fatty liver syndrome caused by aflatoxin. Poult Sci 51:688-692.

151. Hamilton, P.B., H.T. Tung, J.R. Harris, J.H. Gainer, and W.E. Donaldson. 1972. The effect of dietary fat on aflatoxicosis in turkeys. Poult Sci 51:165-170.

152. Hamilton, P.B., H.T. Tung, R.D. Wyatt, and W.E. Donaldson. 1974. Interaction of dietary aflatoxin with some vitamin deficiencies. Poult Sci 53:871-877.

153. Hamilton, P.B, W.E. Huff, J.R. Harris, and R.D. Wyatt. 1982. Natural occurrences of ochratoxicosis in poultry. Poult Sci 61:1832-1841.

154. Hamilton, R.M.G., B.K. Thompson, H.L. Trenholm, P.S. Fiser, and R. Greenhalgh. 1985. Effects of feeding white leghorn hens diets that contain deoxynivalenol (vomitoxin)-contaminated wheat. Poult Sci 64:1840-1851.

155. Hamilton, R.M.G., B.K. Thompson, and H.L. Trenholm. 1986. The effects of deoxynivalenol (vomitoxin) on dietary preference of white leghorn hens. Poult Sci 65:288-293.

156. Harland, E.C., and P.T. Cardeilhac. 1975. Excretion of carbon-14-labeled aflatoxin B1 via bile, urine, and intestinal contents of the chicken. Am J Vet Res 36:909-912.

157. Harris, J.R. 1984. Case report on T-2 mycotoxicosis in chickens. In Keeping Current (CEVA Laboratories, Inc.) Jan-Feb, 1984, pp. 2-3.

158. Harvey, R.B., L.F. Kubena, B. Lawhorn, O.J. Fletcher, T.D. Phillips. 1987. Feed refusal in swine fed ochratoxin-contaminated grain sorghum: Evaluation of toxicity in chicks. J Am Vet Med Assoc 190:673-675.

159. Hayes, M.A., and G.A. Wobeser. 1983. Subacute toxic effects of dietary T-2 toxin in young mallard ducks. Can J Comp Med 47:180-187.

160. Haynes, J.S. 1986. Studies on the pathogenesis

of Fusarium-induced tibial dyschondroplasia. Diss Abstr B Sci Eng 47:868.

161. Haynes, J.S., and M.M. Walser. 1986. Ultrastructure of Fusarium-induced tibial dyschondroplasia in chickens: A sequential study. Vet Pathol 23:499–505.

162. Haynes, J.S., M.M. Walser, and E.M. Lawler. 1985. Morphogenesis of Fusarium sp.-induced tibial dyschondroplasia in chickens. Vet Pathol 22:629–636.

163. Hetzel, D.J.S., D. Hoffman, J. van de Ven, and S. Soeripto. 1984. Mortality rate and liver histopathology in four breeds of ducks following long term exposure to low levels of aflatoxins. Singapore Vet J 8:6–14.

164. Hintikka, E.L. 1978. Stachybotryotoxicosis in poultry. In T.A. Wyllie and L.G. Morehouse (eds.), Mycotoxic Fungi, Mycotoxins, and Mycotoxicoses: An encyclopaedic Handbook II, pp. 203–208. Marcel Dekker, New York.

165. Hnatow, L.L., and R.F. Wideman, Jr. 1985. Kidney function of single comb white leghorn pullets following acute renal portal infusion of the mycotoxin citrinin. Poult Sci 64:1553–1561.

166. Hoerr, F.J. 1981. Trichothecene mycotoxicosis in chickens. PhD diss, pp. 1–78. Purdue Univ.

167. Hoerr, F.J., and G.H. D'Andrea. 1983. Biological effects of aflatoxin in swine. In U.L. Diener, R.L. Asquith, and J.W. Dickens (eds.), Aflatoxin and Aspergillus flavus in Corn, pp. 51–55. Southern Coop Series Bull 279.

168. Hoerr, F.J., W.W. Carlton, and B. Yagen. 1981. The toxicity of T-2 toxin and diacetoxyscirpenol in combination for broiler chickens. Food Cosmetol Toxicol 19:185–188.

169. Hoerr, F.J., W.W. Carlton, and B. Yagen. 1981. Mycotoxicosis caused by a single dose of T-2 toxin or diacetoxyscirpenol in broiler chickens. Vet Pathol 18:652–664.

170. Hoerr, F.J., W.W. Carlton, B. Yagen, and A.Z. Joffe. 1982. Mycotoxicosis caused by either T-2 toxin or diacetoxyscirpenol in the diet of broiler chickens. Fundament Appl Toxicol 2:121–124.

171. Hoerr, F.J., W.W. Carlton, B. Yagen, and A.Z. Joffe. 1982. Mycotoxicosis produced in broiler chickens by multiple doses of either T-2 toxin or diacetoxyscirpenol. Avian Pathol 11:369–383.

172. Hoerr, F.J., W.W. Carlton, J. Tuite, R.F. Vesonder, W.K. Rohwedder, and G. Szigeti. 1982. Experimental trichothecene mycotoxicosis produced in broiler chickens by Fusarium sporotrichiella var. sporotrichioides. Avian Pathol 11:385–405.

173. Hoerr, F.J., G.H. D'Andrea, J.J. Giambrone, and V.S. Panangala. 1986. Comparative histopathologic changes in aflatoxicosis. In J.L. Richard and J.R. Thruston (eds.), Diagnosis of Mycotoxicoses, pp. 179–189. Martinus Nijhoff, Dordrecht, Neth.

174. Hofacre, C.L., R.K. Page, and O.J. Fletcher. 1985. Suspected mycotoxicosis in laying hens. Avian Dis 29:846–849.

175. Howarth, B., Jr., and R.D. Wyatt. 1976. Effect of dietary aflatoxin on fertility, hatchability, and progeny performance of broiler breeder hens. Appl Environ Microbiol 31:680–684.

176. Hsieh, D.P.H. 1987. Mode of action of mycotoxins. In P. Krogh (ed.), Mycotoxins in Food, pp. 149–176. Academic Press, San Diego.

177. Huff, W.E. 1980. Evaluation of tibial dyschondroplasia during aflatoxicosis and feed restriction in young broiler chickens. Poult Sci 59:991–995.

178. Huff, W.E., and J.A. Doerr. 1981. Synergism between aflatoxin and ochratoxin A in broiler chickens. Poult Sci 60:550–555.

179. Huff, W.E., and M.D. Ruff. 1982. Eimeria acervulina and Eimeria tenella infections in ochratoxin A-compromised broiler chickens. Poult Sci 61:685–692.

180. Huff, W.E., R.D. Wyatt, T.L. Tucker, and P.B. Hamilton. 1974. Ochratoxicosis in the broiler chicken. Poult Sci 53:1585–1591.

181. Huff, W.E., R.D. Wyatt, and P.B. Hamilton. 1975. Effects of dietary aflatoxin on certain egg yolk parameters. Poult Sci 54:2014–2018.

182. Huff, W.E., R.D. Wyatt, and P.B. Hamilton. 1975. Nephrotoxicity of dietary ochratoxin A in broiler chickens. Appl Microbiol 30:48–51.

183. Huff, W.E., J.A. Doerr, and P.B. Hamilton. 1977. Decreased bone strength during ochratoxicosis and aflatoxicosis. Poult Sci 56:1724.

184. Huff, W.E., C.F. Chang, M.F. Warren, and P.B. Hamilton. 1979. Ochratoxin A-induced iron deficiency anemia. Appl Environ Microbiol 37:601–604.

185. Huff, W.E., J.A. Doerr, and P.B. Hamilton. 1979. Decreased glycogen mobilization during ochratoxicosis in broiler chickens. Appl Environ Microbiol 37:122–126.

186. Huff, W.E., P.B. Hamilton, and A. Ciegler. 1980. Evaluation of penicillic acid for toxicity in broiler chickens. Poult Sci 59:1203–1207.

187. Huff, W.E., J.A. Doerr, P.B. Hamilton, and R.F. Vesonder. 1981. Acute toxicity of vomitoxin (deoxynivalenol) in broiler chickens. Poult Sci 60:1412–1414.

188. Huff, W.E., J.A. Doerr, C.J. Wabeck, G.W. Chaloupka, J.D. May, and J.W. Merkley. 1983. Individual and combined effects of aflatoxin and ochratoxin A on bruising in broiler chickens. Poult Sci 62:1764–1771.

189. Huff, W.E., J.A. Doerr, C.J. Wabeck, G.W. Chaloupka, J.D. May, and J.W. Merkley. 1984. The individual and combined effects of aflatoxin and ochratoxin A on various processing parameters of broiler chickens. Poult Sci 63:2153–2161.

190. Huff, W.E., L.F. Kubena, R.B. Harvey, D.E. Corrier, and H.H. Mollenhauer. 1986. Progression of aflatoxicosis in broiler chickens. Poult Sci 65:1891–1899.

191. Huff, W.E., L.F. Kubena, R.B. Harvey, W.M. Hagler, Jr., S.P. Swanson, T.D. Phillips, and C.R. Creger. 1986. Individual and combined effects of aflatoxin and deoxynivalenol (DON, vomitoxin) in broiler chickens. Poult Sci 65:1291–1298.

192. Huff W.E., R.B. Harvey, L.F. Kubena, and G.E. Rottinghaus. 1988. Toxic synergism between aflatoxin and T-2 toxin in broiler chickens. Poult Sci 67:1418–1423.

193. Huff, W.E., L.F. Kubena, and R.B. Harvey. 1988. Progression of ochratoxicosis in broiler chickens. Poult Sci 67:1139–1146.

194. Hulan, H.W., and F.G. Proudfoot. 1982. Effects of feeding vomitoxin contaminated wheat on the performance of broiler chickens. Poult Sci 61:1653–1659.

195. Iqbal, Q.K., P.V. Rao, and S.J. Reddy. 1983. Dose-response relationship of experimentally induced aflatoxicosis in commercial layers. Indian J Anim Sci 53:1277–1280.

196. Jacobson, W.C., and H.G. Wiseman. 1974. The transmission of aflatoxin B1 into eggs. Poult Sci 53:1743–1745.

197. Joffe, A.Z. 1986. Fusarium Species: Their Biology and Toxicology, pp. 345–384. John Wiley and Sons, New York.

198. Joffe, A.Z., and B. Yagen. 1978. Intoxication produced by toxic fungi Fusarium poae and F. sporotrichioides in chicks. Toxicology 16:263–273.

199. Johri, T.S., R. Agarwal, and V.R. Sadagopan. 1986. Surveillance of aflatoxin B1 content of poultry feed stuffs in and around Bareilly district of Uttar Pradesh. Indian J Poult Sci 21:227–230.

200. Jones, F.T., and P.B. Hamilton. 1986. Factors influencing fungal activity in low moisture poultry feeds. Poult Sci 65:1522-1525.

201. Jones, F.T., and P.B. Hamilton. 1987. Research notes: Relationship of feed surface area to fungal activity in poultry feeds. Poult Sci 66:1545-1547.

202. Jones, F.T., W.H. Hagler, and P.B. Hamilton. 1982. Association of low levels of aflatoxin in feed with productivity losses in commercial broiler operations. Poult Sci 61:861-868.

203. Jones, G.M., D.N. Mowat, J.I. Elliot, and E.T. Moran, Jr. 1974. Organic acid preservation of high moisture corn and other grains and the nutritional value: A review. Can J Anim Sci 54:499-517.

204. Kingsland, G.C., and J. Anderson. 1976. A study of the feasibility of the use of gentian violet as a fungistat for poultry feed. Poult Sci 55:852-857.

205. Kirby, L.K., T.S. Nelson, J.T. Halley, and J.N. Beasley. 1987. Citrinin toxicity in young chicks. Poult Sci 66:966-968.

206. Kratzer, F.H., D. Bandy, M. Wiley, and A.N. Booth. 1969. Aflatoxin effects in poultry. Proc Soc Exp Biol Med 131:1281-1284.

207. Kriek, N.P.J., W.F.O. Marasas, P.S. Steyn, S.J. van Rensburg, and M. Steyn. 1977. Toxicity of a moniliformin-producing strain of Fusarium moniliforme var. subglutinans isolated from maize. Food Cosmetol Toxicol 15:579-587.

208. Krogh, P., and F. Elling. 1977. Mycotoxic nephropathy. Vet Sci Commun 1:51-63.

209. Krogh, P., F. Elling, B. Hald, B. Jylling, V.E. Petersen, E. Skadhauge, and C.K. Svensen. 1976. Changes of renal function and structure induced by ochratoxin A-contaminated feed. Acta Pathol Microbiol Scand 84:215-221.

210. Kubena, L.F., T.D. Phillips, C.R. Creger, D.A. Witzel, and N.D. Heidelbaugh. 1983. Toxicity of ochratoxin A and tannic acid to growing chicks. Poult Sci 62:1786-1792.

211. Kubena, L.F., R.B. Harvey, O.J. Fletcher, T.D. Phillips, H.H. Mollenhauer, D.A. Witzel, and N.D. Heidelbaugh. 1985. Toxicity of ochratoxin A and vanadium to growing chicks. Poult Sci 64:620-628.

212. Kubena, L.F., S.P. Swanson, R.B. Harvey, O.J. Fletcher, L.D. Rowe, and T.D. Phillips. 1985. Effects of feeding deoxynivalenol (vomitoxin)-contaminated wheat to growing chicks. Poult Sci 64:1649-1655.

213. Kubena, L.F., R.B. Harvey, T.D. Phillips, and O.J. Fletcher. 1986. Influence of ochratoxin A and vanadium on various parameters in growing chicks. Poult Sci 65:1671-1678.

214. Kubena, L.F., R.B. Harvey, D.E. Corrier, W.E. Huff, and T.D. Phillips. 1987. Effects of feeding deoxynivalenol (DON, vomitoxin)-contaminated wheat to female white leghorn chickens from day old through egg production. Poult Sci 66:1612-1618.

215. Kubena, L.F., R.B. Harvey, T.D. Phillips, G.M. Holman, and C.R. Creger. 1987. Effects of feeding mature white leghorn hens diets that contain deoxynivalenol (vomitoxin). Poult Sci 66:55-58.

216. Kubena, L.F., W.E. Huff, R.B. Harvey, D.E. Corrier, T.D. Phillips, and C.R. Creger. 1988. Influence of ochratoxin A and deoxynivalenol on growing broiler chicks. Poult Sci 67:253-260.

217. Kung, H.C., J.R. Chipley, J.D. Latshaw, and K.M. Kerr. 1976. Mycotoxicosis in chicks produced by toxins from Phomopsis sp. or Diaporthe phaseolorum var. sojae. Avian Dis 20:504-518.

218. Kung, H.C., J.R. Chipley, J.D. Latshaw, K.M. Kerr, and R.F. Wilson. 1977. Chronic mycotoxicosis in chicks caused by toxins from Phomopsis grown on soybeans. J Comp Pathol 87:325-333.

219. Kurmanov, I.A., and A. Novacky. 1978. Fusariotoxicosis in chickens in the USSR. In T.A. Wyllie, and L.G. Morehouse (eds.), Mycotoxic Fungi, Mycotoxins, and Mycotoxicoses: An Encyclopaedic Handbook, II, pp. 322-326. Marcel Dekker, New York.

220. Lamont, M.H. 1979. Cases of suspected mycotoxicoses as reported by veterinary investigation centres. Proc Mycotoxins Anim Dis 3:38-39.

221. Lansden J.A., and J.I. Davidson. 1983. Occurrence of cyclopiazonic acid in peanuts. Appl Environ Microbiol 45:766-769.

222. Lanza, G.M., K.W. Washburn, R.D. Wyatt, and H.M. Edwards, Jr. 1979. Depressed 59Fe absorption due to dietary aflatoxin. Poult Sci 58:1439-1444.

223. Lanza, G.M., K.W. Washburn, and R.D. Wyatt. 1980. Strain variation in hematological response of broilers to dietary aflatoxin. Poult Sci 59:2686-2691.

224. Larsen, C., M. Acha, and M. Ehrich. 1988. Research note: Chlortetracycline and aflatoxin interaction in two lines of chicks. Poult Sci 67:1229-1232.

225. Lawler, E.M., T.F. Fletcher, and M.M. Walser. 1985. Chondroclasts in Fusarium-induced tibial dyschondroplasia. Am J Pathol 120:276-281.

226. Le Bars, J. 1979. Cyclopiazonic acid production by Penicillium camemberti Thom and natural occurrence of this mycotoxin in cheese. Appl Environ Microbiol 38:1052-1055.

227. Lee, Y.W., C.J. Mirocha, D.J. Shroeder, and M.M. Walser. 1985. TDP-1, a toxic component causing tibial dyschondroplasia in broiler chickens, and trichothecenes from Fusarium roseum "graminearum." Appl Environ Microbiol 50:102-107.

228. Lorenz, K. 1979. Ergot on cereal grains. Crit Rev Food Sci Nutr 11:311-354.

229. Lovett, J. 1972. Patulin toxicosis in poultry. Poult Sci 51:2097-2098.

230. Lun, A.K., L.G. Young, E.T. Moran, Jr., D.B. Hunter, and J.P. Rodriguez. 1986. Effects of feeding hens a high level of vomitoxin-contaminated corn on performance and tissue residues. Poult Sci 65:1095-1099.

231. Mahipal, S.K., and R.K. Kaushik. 1983. A note on the prevalence of aflatoxicosis in poultry birds in Haryana. Haryana Vet 22:51-52.

232. Manley, R.W., R.M. Hulet, J.B. Meldrum, and C.T. Larsen. 1988. Research note: Turkey poult tolerance to diets containing deoxynivalenol (vomitoxin) and salinomycin. Poult Sci 67:149-152.

233. Manning, R.O., and R.D. Wyatt. 1984. Comparative toxicity of Chaetomium contaminated corn and various chemical forms of oosporein in broiler chicks. Poult Sci 63:251-259.

234. Manning, R.O., T.P. Brown, R.D. Wyatt, and O.J. Fletcher. 1985. The individual and combined effects of citrinin and ochratoxin A in broiler chicks. Avian Dis 29:986-997.

235. Marks, H.L., and C.W. Bacon. 1976. Influence of Fusarium-infected corn and F-2 on laying hens. Poult Sci 55:1864-1870.

236. McLaughlin, C.S., M.H. Vaughan, I.M. Campbell, C.M. Wei, M.E. Stafford, and B.S. Hansen. 1977. Inhibition of protein synthesis by trichothecenes. In J.V. Rodricks, C.W. Hesseltine, and M.A. Mehleman (eds.), Mycotoxins in Human and Animal Health, pp. 263-273. Pathotox Publ, Park Forest South, IL.

237. Mehdi, N.A.Q., W.W. Carlton, and J. Tuite. 1981. Citrinin mycotoxicosis in broiler chickens. Food Cosmetol Toxicol 19:723-733.

238. Mehdi, N.A.Q., W.W. Carlton, and J. Tuite. 1983. Acute toxicity of citrinin in turkeys and ducklings. Avian Pathol 12:221-233.

239. Mehdi, N.A.Q., W.W. Carlton, and J. Tuite. 1984.

Mycotoxicoses produced in ducklings and turkeys by dietary and multiple doses of citrinin. Avian Pathol 13:37–50.

240. Mehdi, N.A.Q., W.W. Carlton, G.D. Boon, and J. Tuite. 1984. Studies on the sequential development and pathogenesis of citrinin mycotoxicosis in turkeys and ducklings. Vet Pathol 21:216–223.

241. Micco, C., M. Miraglia, R. Onori, A. Ioppolo, and A. Mantovani. 1987. Long-term administration of low doses of mycotoxins in poultry. I. Residues of ochratoxin A in broilers and laying hens. Poult Sci 66:47–50.

242. Michael, G.Y., P. Thaxton, and P.B. Hamilton. 1973. Impairment of the reticuloendothelial system of chickens during aflatoxicosis. Poult Sci 52:1206–1207.

243. Miller, B.L., and R.D. Wyatt. 1985. Effect of dietary aflatoxin on the uptake and elimination of chlortetracycline in broiler chicks. Poult Sci 64:1637–1643.

244. Mirocha, C.J. 1979. Trichothecene toxins produced by Fusarium. In W. Shimoda (ed.), Conf Mycotoxins Animal Feeds Grains Related Anim Health, pp. 289–273. US Food and Drug Admin Rep No FDA/BVM-79/139.

245. Mirocha, C.J., B. Schauerhamer, C.M. Christensen, M.L. Niku-Paavola, and M. Nummi. 1979. Incidence of zearalenol (Fusarium mycotoxin) in animal feed. Appl Environ Microbiol 38:749–750.

246. Mirocha, C.J., T.S. Robison, R.J. Pawlosky, and N.K. Allen. 1982. Distribution and residue determination of [3H] zearalenone in broilers. Toxicol Appl Pharmacol 66:77–87.

247. Misir, R., and R.R. Marquardt. 1978. Factors affecting rye (Secale cereale L.) utilization in growing chicks. I. The influence of rye level, ergot, and penicillin supplementation. Can J Anim Sci 58:691–701.

248. Misir, R., and R.R. Marquardt. 1978. Factors affecting rye (Secale cereale l) utilization in growing chicks. III. The influence of milling fractions. Can J Anim Sci 58:717–730.

249. Mohiuddin, S.M., M.V. Reddy, M.M. Reddy, and K. Ramakrishna. 1986. Studies on phagocytic activity and hematological changes in aflatoxicosis in poultry. Indian Vet J 63:442–445.

250. Moran, E.T., Jr., H.C. Carlson, and J.R. Pettit. 1974. Vitamin E–selenium deficiency in the duck aggravated by the use of high-moisture corn and molding prior to preservation. Avian Dis 18:536–543.

251. Moran, E.T., Jr., B. Hunter, P. Ferket, L.G. Young, and L.G. McGirr. 1982. High tolerance of broilers to vomitoxin from corn infected with Fusarium graminearum. Poult Sci 61:1828–1831.

252. Moran, E.T. Jr., P.R. Ferket, and A.K. Lun. 1987. Impact of high dietary vomitoxin on yolk yield and embryonic mortality. Poult Sci 66:977–982.

253. Moreno-Romo, M.A., and G. Suarez-Fernandez. 1986. Aflatoxin-producing potential of Aspergillus flavus strains isolated from Spanish poultry feeds. Mycopathologia 95:129–132.

254. Muller, R.D., C.W. Carlson, G. Semeniuk, and G.S. Harshfield. 1970. The response of chicks, ducklings, goslings, pheasants, and poults to graded levels of aflatoxins. Poult Sci 49:1346–1350.

255. Muller, E.E., A.E. Panerai, D. Cocchi, and P. Mantegazza. 1977. Endocrine profile of ergot alkaloids. Life Sci 21:1545–1558.

256. Nelson, T.S., J.N. Beasley, L.K. Kirby, Z.B. Johnson, and G.C. Ballam. 1980. Isolation and identification of citrinin produced by Penicillium lanosum. Poult Sci 59:2055–2059.

257. Nelson, T.S., J.N. Beasley, L.K. Kriby, Z.B. Johnson, G.C. Ballam, and M.M. Campbell. 1981. Citrinin toxicity in growing chicks. Poult Sci 60:2165–2166.

258. Nemeth, I., and S. Juhasz. 1968. Effect of aflatoxin in serum protein fractions of day-old ducklings. Acta Vet Acad Sci Hung 18:95–105.

259. Newberne, P.M. 1973. Chronic aflatoxicosis. J Am Vet Med Assoc 163:1262–1267.

260. Newberne, P.M., G.N. Wogan, W.W. Carlton, and M.M.A. Kader. 1964. Histopathologic lesions in ducklings caused by Aspergillus flavus cultures, culture extracts, and crystalline aflatoxins. Toxicol Appl Pharmacol 6:542–556.

261. Nichols, T.E. 1983. Economic effects of aflatoxin in corn. In U.L. Diener (ed.), Aflatoxin and Aspergillus Flavus in Corn, pp. 67–71. South Coop Ser Bull 279.

262. Norred, W.P., R.J. Cole, J.W. Dorner, and J.A. Lansden. 1987. Liquid chromatographic determination of cyclopiazonic acid in poultry meat. J Assoc Off Anal Chem 70:121–123.

263. Okoye, J.O.A., I.U. Asuzu, and J.C. Gugnani. 1988. Paralysis and lameness associated with aflatoxicosis in broilers. Avian Pathol 17:731–734.

264. Olsen, M., C.J. Mirocha, H.K. Abbas, and B. Johansson. 1986. Metabolism of high concentrations of dietary zearalenone by young male turkey poults. Poult Sci 65:1905–1910.

265. Osborne, B.G. 1980. The occurrence of ochratoxin A in mouldy bread and flour. Food Cosmetol Toxicol 18:615–617.

266. Osborne, D.J., and P.B. Hamilton. 1981. Decreased pancreatic digestive enzymes during aflatoxicosis. Poult Sci 60:1818–1821.

267. Ostrowski-Meissner, H.T. 1983. Effect of contamination of diets with aflatoxin on growing ducks and chickens. Trop Anim Health Prod 15:161–168.

268. Ostrowski-Meissner, H.T., D.F. Sinclair, I. Komang, and W. Supratman. 1984. Blood analyses in the clinical diagnosis of aflatoxicosis in ducks and chickens. Proc 17th World's Poult Congr, pp. 563–565.

269. Osweiler, G.D. 1986. Mycotoxin diagnosis: A perspective. Proc Am Assoc Vet Lab Diagn 29:221–229.

270. Ottinger, M.A., and J.A. Doerr. 1980. The early influence of aflatoxin upon sexual maturation in the Japanese quail. Poult Sci 59:1750–1754.

271. Page, R.K., G. Stewart, R. Wyatt, P. Bush, O.J. Fletcher, and J. Brown. 1980. Influence of low levels of ochratoxin A on egg production, egg-shell stains, and serum uric-acid levels in leghorn-type hens. Avian Dis 24:777–780.

272. Palmgren, M.S., and A.W. Hayes. 1987. Aflatoxins in food. In P. Krogh (ed.), Mycotoxins in Food, pp. 56–96. Academic Press, San Diego.

273. Palyusik, M., and E.K. Kovacs. 1975. Effect on laying geese of feeds containing the fusariotoxins T-2 and F-2. Acta Vet Acad Sci Hung 25:363–368.

274. Palyusik, M., K.E. Kovacs, and E. Guzsal. 1971. Effect of Fusarium graminearum on the semen production of geese and turkeys. Magy Allatorv Lapja 26:300–303

275. Palyusik, M., G. Nagy, and L. Zoldag. 1974. Effect of different Fusarium species on spermatogenesis in ganders. Magy Allatorv Lapja 29:551–553.

276. Paster, N., E. Pinthus, and D. Reichman. 1987. A comparative study of the efficacy of calcium propionate, agrosil, and adofeed as mold inhibitors in poultry feed. Poult Sci 66:858–860.

277. Patterson, D.S.P., and B.A. Roberts. 1972. Aflatoxin metabolism in duck-liver homogenates: The relative importance of reversible cyclopentenone reduction and hemiacetal formation. Food Cosmetol Toxiçol 10:501–512.

278. Pearson, A.W. 1978. Biochemical changes produced by fusarium T-2 toxin in the chicken. Res Vet Sci 24:92–97.

279. Peckham, J.C., B. Doupnik, Jr., and O.H. Jones,

Jr. 1971. Acute toxicity of ochratoxins A and B in chicks. Appl Microbiol 21:492–494.

280. Peckham, M.C. 1984. Poisons and toxins. In M.S. Hofstad, H.J. Barnes, B.W. Calnek, W.M. Reid, and H.W. Yoder, Jr. (eds.), Diseases of Poultry, 8th Ed., pp. 799–804. Iowa State Univ Press, Ames.

281. Pegram, R.A., and R.D. Wyatt. 1979. Effect of dietary oosporein on broiler chickens. Poult Sci 58:1092. (Abstr).

282. Pegram, R.A., and R.D. Wyatt. 1981. Avian gout caused by oosporein, a mycotoxin produced by Chaetomium trilaterale. Poult Sci 60:2429–2440.

283. Pegram, R.A., Wyatt, R.D., and T.L. Smith. 1982. Oosporein-toxicosis in the turkey poult. Avian Dis 26:47–59.

284. Pegram, R.A., Wyatt, R.D., and H.L. Marks. 1986. The relationship of certain blood parameters to aflatoxin resistance in Japanese quail. Poult Sci 65:1652–1658.

285. Perek, M. 1958. Ergot and ergot-like fungi as the cause of vesicular dermatitis (sod disease) in chickens. J Am Vet Med Assoc 132:529–533.

286. Phillips, T.D., L.F. Kubena, R.B. Harvey, D.R. Taylor, and N.D. Heidelbaugh. 1988. Hydrated sodium calcium aluminosilicate: A high affinity sorbent for aflatoxin. Poult Sci 67:243–247.

287. Pier, A.C. 1973. Effects of aflatoxin on immunity. J Am Vet Med Assoc 163:1268–1269.

288. Pier A.C., and K.L. Heddleston. 1970. The effect of aflatoxin on immunity in turkeys. I. Impairment of actively acquired resistance to bacterial challenge. Avian Dis 14:797–809.

289. Pier, A.C., K.L. Heddleston, S.J. Cysewski, and J.M. Patterson. 1972. Effect of aflatoxin on immunity in turkeys. II. Reversal of impaired resistance to bacterial infection by passive transfer of plasma. Avian Dis 16:381–387.

290. Pohland, A.E., and G.E. Wood. 1987. Occurrence of Mycotoxins in foods. In P. Krogh (ed.), Mycotoxins in Food, pp. 35–64. Academic Press, San Diego.

291. Pramanik, A.K., and H.M. Bhattacharya. 1987. Diseases of poultry in three districts of West Bengal affecting the rural economy. Indian J Vet Med 7:63–65.

292. Prelusky, D.B., R.M.G. Hamilton, H.L. Trenholm, and J.D. Miller. 1986. Tissue distribution and excretion of radioactivity following administration of 14C-labeled deoxynivalenol to white leghorn hens. Fundam Appl Toxicol 7:635–645.

293. Prelusky, D.B., H.L. Trenholm, R.M.G. Hamilton, and J.D. Miller. 1987. Transmission of [14C] deoxynivalenol to eggs following oral administration to laying hens. J Agric Food Chem 35:182–186.

294. Prior, M.G., and C.S. Sisodia. 1978. Ochratoxicosis in white leghorn hens. Poult Sci 57:619–623.

295. Prior, M.G., C.S. Sisodia, and J.B. O'Neil. 1976. Acute oral ochratoxicosis in day-old white leghorns, turkeys and Japanese quail. Poult Sci 55:786–790.

296. Prior, M.G., C.S. Sisodia, J.B. O'Neil, and F. Hrudka. 1979. Effect of ochratoxin A on fertility and embryo viability of Japanese quail (Coturnix coturnix japonica). Can J Comp Med 59:605–609.

297. Prior, M.G., J.B. O'Neil, and C.S. Sisodia. 1980. Effects of ochratoxin A on growth response and residues in broilers. Poult Sci 59:1254–1257.

298. Prior, M.G., C.S. Sisodia, and J.B. O'Neil. 1981. Effects of ochratoxin A on egg production, body weight, and feed intake in white leghorn hens. Poult Sci 60:1145–1148.

299. Puls, R., and J.A. Greenway. 1976. Fusariotoxicosis from barley in British Columbia. II. Analysis and toxicity of suspected barley. Can J Comp Med 40:16–19.

300. Purchase, I.F.H. 1967. Acute toxicity of aflatoxins M1 and M2 in 1-day-old ducklings. Food Cosmetol Toxicol 5:339–342.

301. Purchase, L., and J. Nel. 1967. Recent advances in research on ochratoxin. Pt 1. Toxicological aspects. In R.I. Mateles and G.N. Wogan (eds.), Biochemistry of Some Foodborne Microbial Toxins, pp. 153–156. MIT Press, Cambridge, MA.

302. Rabie, C.J., S.J. van Rensburg, N.P.J. Kriek, and A. Lubben. 1977. Toxicity of Diplodia maydis to laboratory animals. Appl Environ Microbiol 34:111–114.

303. Rabie, C.J., W.F.O. Marasas, P.G. Thiel, A. Lubben, and R. Vleggaar. 1982. Moniliformin production and toxicity of different Fusarium species from southern Africa. Appl Environ Microbiol 43:517–521.

304. Rabie, C.J., J.J. Du Preez, and J.P. Hayes. 1987. Toxicity of Diplodia maydis to broilers, ducklings, and laying chicken hens. Poult Sci 66:1123–1128.

305. Rao, A.G., P.K. Dehuri, S.K. Chand, S.C. Mishra, P.K. Mishra, and B.C. Das. 1985. Aflatoxicosis in broiler chickens. Indian J Poult Sci 20:240–244.

306. Rao, D.G., N.R.G. Naidu, and R.R. Rao. 1985. Observations on the concomitant incidence of aflatoxicosis and aspergillosis (brooder pneumonia) in khaki campbell ducklings. Indian Vet J 62:461–464.

307. Rao, V.S. 1987. Persistent Ranikhet disease in a commercial broiler farm—a report. Poult Advis 20:61–65.

308. Reddy, D.N., P.V. Rao, V.R. Reddy, and B. Yadgiri. 1984. Effect of selected levels of dietary aflatoxin on the performance of broiler chickens. Indian J Anim Sci 54:68–73.

309. Reiss, J. 1977. Mycotoxins in foodstuffs. X. Production of citrinin by Penicillium chrysogenum in bread. Food Cosmetol Toxicol 15:303–307.

310. Renault, L., M. Goujet, A. Monin, G. Boutin, M. Palisse, and A. Alamagny. 1979. Suspected mycotoxicosis due to trichothecenes in broiler fowl. Bull Acad Vet Fr 52:181–188.

311. Richard, J.L., S.J. Cysewski, A.C. Pier, and G.D. Booth. 1978. Comparison of effects of dietary T-2 toxin on growth, immunogenic organs, antibody formation, and pathologic changes in turkeys and chickens. Am J Vet Res 39:1674–1679.

312. Richard, J.L., R.D. Stubblefield, R.L. Lyon, W.M. Peden, J.R. Thurston, and R.B. Rimler. 1986. Distribution and clearance of aflatoxins B1 and M1 in turkeys fed diets containing 50 or 150 ppb aflatoxin from naturally contaminated corn. Avian Dis 30:788–793.

313. Richardi, J.C., and W.E. Huff. 1983. Effects of acute ochratoxicosis on blood pressure and heart rate of broiler chickens. Poult Sci 62:2164–2168.

314. Richardson, K.E., and P.B. Hamilton. 1987. Enhanced production of pancreatic digestive enzymes during aflatoxicosis in egg-type chickens. Poult Sci 66:640–644.

315. Richardson, K.E., L.A. Nelson, and P.B. Hamilton. 1987. Effect of dietary fat level on dose response relationships during aflatoxicosis in young chickens. Poult Sci 66:1470–1478.

316. Richardson, K.E., L.A. Nelson, and P.B. Hamilton. 1987. Interaction of dietary protein level on dose response relationships during aflatoxicosis in young chickens. Poult Sci 66:969–976.

317. Richardson, L.R., S. Wilkes, J. Godwin, and K.R. Pierce. 1962. Effect of moldy diet and moldy soybean meal on the growth of chicks and poults. J Nutr 78:301–306.

318. Roberts, W.T., and E.C. Mora. 1978. Toxicity of Penicillium citrinum AUA-532 contaminated corn and

citrinin in broiler chicks. Poult Sci 57:1221–1226.

319. Roberts, W.T., and E.C. Mora. 1979. Hemorrhagic syndrome of chicks produced by Penicillium citrinum AUA-532 contaminated corn. Poult Sci 58:810–814.

320. Roberts, W.T., and E.C. Mora. 1982. Noncitrinin toxicity of Penicillium citrinum contaminated corn. Poult Sci 61:1637–1645.

321. Robison, T.S., K.R. Reddy, S.B. Swanson, and M.S. Chi. 1977. Metabolism of T-2 toxin in poultry. University of Minnesota Effort in Mycotoxicology. Annu Rep to NC 129.

322. Rotter, R.G., R.R. Marquardt, and J.C. Young. 1985. Effect of ergot from different sources and of fractionated ergot on the performance of growing chicks. Can J Anim Sci 65:953–961.

323. Rotter, R.G., R.R. Marquardt, and G.H. Crow. 1985. A comparison of the effect of increasing dietary concentrations of wheat ergot on the performance of leghorn and broiler chicks. Can J Anim Sci 65:963–974.

324. Rotter, R.G., R.R. Marquardt, and J.C. Young. 1985. The ability of growing chicks to recover from short-term exposure to dietary wheat ergot and the effect of chemical and physical treatment on ergot toxicity. Can J Anim Sci 65:975–983.

325. Sawhney, D.S., D.V. Vadehra, and R.C. Baker. 1973. Aflatoxicosis in the laying Japanese quail. Poult Sci 52:465–473.

326. Sawhney, D.S., D.V. Vadehra, and R.C. Baker. 1973. The metabolism of [14C] aflatoxins in laying hens. Poult Sci 52:1302–1309.

327. Schaeffer, J.L., J.K. Tyczkowski, and P.B. Hamilton. 1987. Alterations in carotenoid metabolism during ochratoxicosis in young broiler chickens. Poult Sci 66:318–324.

328. Schaeffer, J.L., J.K. Tyczkowski, J.E. Riviere, and P.B. Hamilton. 1988. Aflatoxin-impaired ability to accumulate oxycarotenoid pigments during restoration in young chickens. Poult Sci 67:619–625.

329. Schaeffer, J.L., J.K. Tyczkowski, and P.B. Hamilton. 1988. Depletion of oxycarotenoid pigments in chickens and the failure of aflatoxin to alter it. Poult Sci 67:1080–1088.

330. Schroeder, H.W., and W.H. Kelton. 1975. Production of sterigmatocystin by some species of the genus Aspergillus and its toxicity to chicken embryos. Appl Microbiol 30:589–591.

331. Schumaier, G., H.M. DeVolt, N.C. Laffer, R.D. Creek. 1963. Stachybotryotoxicosis of chicks. Poult Sci 42:70–74.

332. Sharby, T.F., G.E. Templeton, J.N. Beasley, and E.L. Stephenson. 1972. Toxicity resulting from feeding experimentally molded corn to broiler chicks. Poult Sci 52:1007–1014.

333. Sharlin, J.S., B. Howarth, Jr., and R.D. Wyatt. 1980. Effect of dietary aflatoxin on reproductive performance of mature white leghorn males. Poult Sci 59:1311–1315.

334. Sharlin, J.S., B. Howarth, Jr., F.N. Thompson, and R.D. Wyatt. 1981. Decreased reproductive potential and reduced feed consumption in mature white leghorn males fed aflatoxin. Poult Sci 60:2701–2708.

335. Sheridan J.J. 1980. Some observations on selected mycoses and mycotoxicoses affecting animals in Ireland. Ir Vet J 34:148–154.

336. Shlosberg, A.S., Y. Weisman, V. Handji, B. Yagen, and L. Shore. 1984. A severe reduction in egg laying in a flock of hens associated with trichothecene mycotoxins in the feed. Vet Human Toxicol 26:384–386.

337. Shlosberg, A.S., Y. Klinger, and M.H. Malkinson. 1986. Muscovy ducklings, a particularly sensitive avian bioassay for T-2 toxin and diacetoxyscirpenol. Avian Dis 30:820–824.

338. Shotwell, O.L., C.W. Hesseltine, and M.L. Goulden. 1969. Ochratoxin A: Occurrence as natural contaminant of a corn sample. Appl Microbiol 17:765–766.

339. Shoyinka, S.V.O., and E.O. Onyekweodiri. 1987. Clinico-pathology of interaction between aflatoxin and aspergillosis in chickens. Bull Anim Health Prod Afr 35:47–51.

340. Siller, W.G., and D.C. Ostler. 1961. The histopathology of an entero-hepatic syndrome of turkey poults. Vet Rec 73:134–138.

341. Slowik, J., S. Graczyk, and J.A. Madej. 1985. The effect of a single dose of aflatoxin B1 on the value of nucleolar index of blood lymphocytes and on the histological changes in the liver, bursa of Fabricius, suprarenal glands, and spleen in ducklings. Folia Histochem Cytobiol 3:71–80.

342. Smith, J.W., and P.B. Hamilton. 1970. Aflatoxicosis in the broiler chicken. Poult Sci 49:207–215.

343. Smith, J.W., W.R. Prince, and P.B. Hamilton. 1969. Relationship of aflatoxicosis to Salmonella gallinarum infections of chickens. Appl Microbiol 18:946–947.

344. Smith, J.W., C.H. Hill, and P.B. Hamilton. 1971. The effect of dietary modifications on aflatoxicosis in the broiler chicken. Poult Sci 50:768–774.

345. Sobers, E.K., and B. Doupnik, Jr. 1972. Relationship of pathogenicity to tobacco leaves and toxicity to chicks of isolates of Alternaria longipes. Appl Microbiol 23:313–315.

346. Sova, Z., L. Fukal, D. Trefny, J. Prosek, and A. Slamova. 1986. B1 aflatoxin (AFB1) transfer from reproductive organs of farm birds into their eggs and hatched young. Conf Eur Avic 7:602–603.

347. Speers, G.M., R.A. Meronuck, D.M. Barnes, and C.J. Mirocha. 1971. Effect of feeding Fusarium roseum f. sp. graminearum contaminated corn and the mycotoxin F-2 on the growing chick and laying hen. Poult Sci 50:627–633.

348. Speers, G.M., C.J. Mirocha, C.M. Christensen, and J.C. Behrens. 1977. Effects on laying hens of feeding corn invaded by two species of Fusarium and pure T-2 mycotoxin. Poult Sci 56:98–102.

349. Sreemannarayana, O., R.R. Marquardt, A.A. Frohlich, and F.A. Juck. 1986. Some acute biochemical and pathological changes in chicks after oral administration of sterigmatocystin. J Am Coll Toxicol 5:275–287.

350. Sreemannarayana, O., A.A. Frohlich, and R.R. Marquardt. 1988. Effects of repeated intra-abdominal injections of sterigmatocystin on relative organ weights, concentration of serum and liver constituents, and histopathology of certain organs of the chick. Poult Sci 67:502–509.

351. Stewart, R.G., J.K. Skeeles, R.D. Wyatt, J. Brown, R.K. Page, I.D. Russell, and P.D. Lukert. 1985. The effect of aflatoxin on complement activity in broiler chickens. Poult Sci 64:616–619.

352. Stob, M., R.S. Baldwin, J. Tuite, F.N. Andrews, and K.G. Gillette. 1962. Isolation of an anabolic, uterotrophic compound from corn infected with Gibberella zeae. Nature 196:1318.

353. Svendsen, C., and E. Skadhauge. 1976. Renal functions in hens fed graded dietary levels of ochratoxin A. Acta Pharmacol Toxicol 38:186–194.

354. Swarbrick, O., and J.T. Swarbrick. 1968. Suspected ergotism in ducks. Vet Rec 82:76–77.

355. Tabib, Z., F.T. Jones, and P.B. Hamilton. 1981. Microbiological quality of poultry feed and ingredients. Poult Sci 60:1392–1397.

356. Tabib, Z., F.T. Jones, and P.B. Hamilton. 1984. Effect of pelleting of poultry feed on the activity of molds and mold inhibitors. Poult Sci 63:70–75.

357. Terao, K., K. Kera, and T. Yazina. 1978. The effects of trichothecene toxins on the bursa of Fabricius in day-old chicks. Virchows Arch 27B:359–370.

358. Theron, J.J., K.J. van der Merwe, N. Liebenberg, H.J.B. Joubert. and W. Nel. 1966. Acute liver injury in ducklings and rats as a result of ochratoxin poisoning. J Pathol Bacteriol 91:521–529.

359. Tohala, S.H. 1983. A study of ochratoxin toxicity in laying hens. Diss Abstr B Sci Eng 44:655.

360. Toleman, W.J. 1981. Overcoming problems with bulk feed bins. Poult Dig 40:406–408.

361. Trucksess, M.W., L. Stoloff, K. Young, R.D. Wyatt, and B.L. Miller. 1983. Aflatoxicol and aflatoxins B1 and M1 in eggs and tissues of laying hens consuming aflatoxin-contaminated feed. Poult Sci 62:2176–2182.

362. Tucker, T.L., and P.B. Hamilton. 1971. The effect of ochratoxin in broilers. Poult Sci 50:1637. (Abstr).

363. Tung, H.T., J.W. Smith, and P.B. Hamilton. 1971. Aflatoxicosis and bruising in the chicken. Poult Sci 50:795–800.

364. Tung, H.T., F.W. Cook, R.K. Wyatt, and P.B. Hamilton. 1975. The anemia caused by aflatoxin. Poult Sci 54:1962–1969.

365. Tung, H.T., R.D. Wyatt, P. Thaxton, and P.B. Hamilton. 1975. Concentrations of serum proteins during aflatoxicosis. Toxicol Appl Pharmacol 34:320–326.

366. Tyczkowski, J.K., and P.B. Hamilton. 1987. Altered metabolism of carotenoids during aflatoxicosis in young chickens. Poult Sci 66:1184–1188.

367. Ubosi, C.O. 1985. The ontogeny of the immune response to sheep erythroctyes and resistance to aflatoxins in chickens. Diss Abstr B Sci Eng 7:45.

368. Ubosi, C.O., P.B. Hamilton, E.A. Dunnington, and P.B. Siegel. 1985. Aflatoxin effects in white leghorn chickens selected for response to sheep erythrocyte antigen. I. Body weight, feed conversion, and temperature responses. Poult Sci 64:1065–1070.

369. Ubosi, C.O., W.B. Gross, P.B. Hamilton, M. Ehrich, and P.B. Siegel. 1985. Aflatoxin effects in white leghorn chickens selected for response to sheep erythrocyte antigen. II. Serological and organ characteristics. Poult Sci 64:1071–1076.

370. Ueno, Y. 1977. Mode of action of trichothecenes. Pure Appl Chem 49:1737–1745.

371. Ueno, Y., K. Ishii, M. Sawano, K. Ohtsubo, Y. Matsuda, T. Tanaka, H. Kurata, and M. Ichinoe. 1977. Toxicological approaches to the metabolites of Fusaria. XI. Trichothecenes and zearalenone from river sediments. Jpn J Exp Med 47:117–184.

372. Uraguchi, K., and M. Yamazaki. 1978. Toxicology Biochemistry and Pathology of Mycotoxins, pp. 1–106. Halstead Press, John Wiley & Sons, New York.

373. Vesela, D., D. Vesely, and R. Jelinek. 1983. Toxic effects of ochratoxin A and citrinin, alone and in combination, on chicken embryos. Appl Environ Microbiol 45:91–93.

374. Vesonder, R.F., A. Ciegler, and A.H. Jensen. 1973. Isolation of the emetic principle from Fusarium-infected corn. Appl Microbiol 26:1008–1010.

375. Vesonder, R.F., A. Ciegler, A.H. Jensen, W.K. Rohwedder, and D. Weisleder. 1976. Co-identity of the refusal and emetic principle from Fusarium-infected corn. Appl Environ Microbiol 31:280–285.

376. Vesonder, R.F., A. Ciegler, and A.H. Jensen. 1977. Production of refusal factors by Fusarium strains on grains. Appl Environ Microbiol 34:105–106.

377. Visconti, A., and A. Bottalico. 1983. High levels of ochratoxins A and B in moldy bread responsible for mycotoxicosis in farm animals. J Agric Food Chem 31:1122–1123.

378. Walser, M.M., N.K. Allen, C.J. Mirocha, G.F. Hanlon, and J.A. Newman. 1982. Fusarium-induced osteochondrosis (tibial dyschondroplasia) in chickens. Vet Pathol 19:544–550.

379. Wannop, C.C. 1961. The histopathology of turkey "X " disease in Great Britain. Avian Dis 5:371–381.

380. Warren, M.F., and P.B. Hamilton. 1980. Intestinal fragility during ochratoxicosis and aflatoxicosis in broiler chickens. Appl Environ Microbiol 40:641–645.

381. Warren, M.F., and P.B. Hamilton. 1981. Glycogen storage disease type X caused by ochratoxin A in broiler chickens. Poult Sci 60:120–123.

382. Watson, S.A., C.J. Mirocha, and A.W. Hayes. 1984. Analysis for trichothecenes in samples from southeast Asia associated with "yellow rain." Fundam Appl Toxicol 4:700–717.

383. Williams, C.M., W.M. Colwell, and L.P. Rose. 1980. Genetic resistance of chickens to aflatoxin assessed with organ-culture techniques. Avian Dis 24:415–422.

384. Wilson, B.J., and R.D. Harbison. 1973. Rubratoxins. J Am Vet Med Assoc 163:1274–1276.

385. Wilson, B.J., and C.H. Wilson. 1964. Toxin from Aspergillus flavus: Production on food materials of a substance causing tremors in mice. Science 144:177–178.

386. Wilson, B.J., R.R. Maronpot, and P.K. Hildebrandt. 1973. Equine leukoencephalomalacia. J Am Vet Med Assoc 163:1293–1294.

387. Wilson, H.R., C.R. Douglas, R.H. Harms, and G.T. Edds. 1975. Reduction of aflatoxin effects on quail. Poult Sci 54:923–925.

388. Witlock, D.R., and R.D. Wyatt. 1981. Effect of dietary aflatoxin on hemostasis of young turkey poults. Poult Sci 60:528–531.

389. Witlock, D.R., R.D. Wyatt, and W.I. Anderson. 1982. Relationship between Eimeria adenoeides infection and aflatoxicosis in turkey poults. Poult Sci 61:1293–1297.

390. Wright, G.C., Jr., W.F.O. Marasas, L. Sokoloff. 1987. Effect of fusarochromanone and T-2 toxin on articular chondrocytes in monolayer culture. Fundam Appl Toxicol 9:595–597.

391. Wyatt, R.D. 1986. Mycotoxicosis of poultry-successful prevention and control. Proc Coban Tech Semin, pp. 1–10. Elanco, Indianapolis, IN.

392. Wyatt, R.D. 1988. Personal communication.

393. Wyatt, R.D., and P.B. Hamilton. 1972. The effect of rubratoxin in broiler chickens. Poult Sci 51:1383–1387.

394. Wyatt, R.D., and P.B. Hamilton. 1975. Interaction between aflatoxicosis and a natural infection of chickens with Salmonella. Appl Microbiol 30:870–872.

395. Wyatt, R.D., P.B. Hamilton, W.M. Colwell, and A. Ciegler. 1972. The effect of tremortin A on chickens. Avian Dis 16:461–464.

396. Wyatt, R.D., J.R. Harris, P.B. Hamilton, and H.R. Burmeister. 1972. Possible outbreaks of fusaritoxicosis in avians. Avian Dis 16:1123–1130.

397. Wyatt, R.D., B.A. Weeks, P.B. Hamilton, and H.R. Burmeister. 1972. Severe oral lesions in chickens caused by ingestion of dietary fusariotoxin T-2. Appl Microbiol 24:251–257.

398. Wyatt, R.D., P.B. Hamilton, and H.R. Burmeister. 1973. The effects of T-2 toxin in broiler chickens. Poult Sci 52:1853–1859.

399. Wyatt, R.D., P.B. Hamilton, and R.E. Welty.

1973. Nontoxigenicity to broiler chickens of corn invaded by a pure culture of Helminthosporium maydis race T. Poult Sci 52:341–344.

400. Wyatt, R.D., W.M. Colwell, P.B. Hamilton, and H.R. Burmeister. 1973. Neural disturbances in chickens caused by dietary T-2 toxin. Appl Microbiol 26:757–761.

401. Wyatt, R.D., D.M. Briggs, and P.B. Hamilton. 1973. The effect of dietary aflatoxin on mature broiler breeder males. Poult Sci 52:1119–1123.

402. Wyatt, R.D., P.B. Hamilton, and H.R. Burmeister. 1975. Altered feathering of chicks caused by T-2 toxin. Poult Sci 54:1042–1045.

403. Wyatt, R.D., J.A. Doerr, P.B. Hamilton, and H.R. Burmeister. 1975. Egg production, shell thickness, and other physiological parameters of laying hens affected by T-2 toxin. Appl Microbiol 29:641–645.

404. Wyatt, R.D., H.L. Marks, and R.O. Manning. 1978. Recovery of laying hens from T-2 toxicosis. Poult Sci 57:1172.

405. Wyatt, R.D., R.O. Manning, R.A. Pegram, and H.L. Marks. 1984. Characterization of oosporein toxicosis in mature laying hens. Poult Sci 63:210. (Abstr).

406. Yoshizawa, T., S.P. Swanson, and C.J. Mirocha. 1980. T-2 metabolites in the excreta of broiler chickens administered H-labeled T-2 toxin. Appl Environ Microbiol 39:1172–1177.

407. Young, J.C., and R.R. Marquardt. 1982. Effects of ergotamine tartrate on growing chickens. Can J Anim Sci 62:1181–1191.

408. Zdenek, Z., Z. Fukal, J. Prosek, A. Slamova, J. Vopalka. 1986. B1 aflatoxin (AFB1) transfer from reproductive organs of farm birds into their eggs and hatched young. Conf Eur Avic 7:618.

INDEX